CURRENT VETERINARY THERAPY

IX

SMALL ANIMAL PRACTICE

W. B. SAUNDERS COMPANY
PHILADELPHIA LONDON TORONTO MEXICO CITY RIO DE JANEIRO SYDNEY TOKYO HONG KONG

W. B. SAUNDERS COMPANY
Harcourt Brace Jovanovich, Inc.

The Curtis Center
Independence Square West
Philadelphia, PA 19106

Library of Congress Cataloging in Publication Data

Current veterinary therapy. 1964/65-

Philadelphia, W. B. Saunders.

v. 26 cm.

"Small animal practice."

Editor: 1964/65- R. W. Kirk.

Key title: Current veterinary therapy, ISSN 0070-2218.

1. Veterinary medicine—Periodicals. 2. Pets—Diseases—Periodicals. I. Kirk, Robert Warren, 1922- ed. [DNLM: W1 CU823]

SF745.C8 636.0896 64-10489
MARC-S

Library of Congress [8308]

Editor: Darlene Pedersen
Designer: Karen O'Keefe
Production Managers: Laura Tarves and Frank Polizzano
Manuscript Editor: Linda Mills
Illustrators: Karen McGarry and Glenn Edelmayer
Illustration Coordinator: Peg Shaw

Current Veterinary Therapy IX ISBN 0–7216–1500–7

Last digit is the print number: 9 8 7

CONTRIBUTORS

SHEHU U. ABDULLAHI, D.V.M., PH.D.; Senior Lecturer, Faculty of Veterinary Medicine, Ahmadu Bello University, Zaria, Nigeria; Internal Medicine Consultant, Veterinary Teaching Hospital, Ahmadu Bello University, Zaria, Nigeria

TERENCE C. AMIS, B.V.SC., M.R.C.V.S., PH.D.; Assistant Professor, Department of Medicine, School of Veterinary Medicine, University of California, Davis, California; Small Animal Internal Medicine Service, Veterinary Medical Teaching Hospital, School of Veterinary Medicine, University of California, Davis, California

ARTHUR L. ARONSON, D.V.M., PH.D.; Professor and Department Head, Department of Anatomy, Physiological Sciences and Radiology, School of Veterinary Medicine, North Carolina State University, Raleigh, North Carolina; Clinical Pharmacology Unit, Teaching Hospital, School of Veterinary Medicine, North Carolina State University, Raleigh, North Carolina

CLARKE E. ATKINS, D.V.M.; Diplomate, American College of Veterinary Internal Medicine; Assistant Professor, University of Wisconsin-Madison, School of Veterinary Medicine, Madison, Wisconsin

LAURIE A. AUER, B.V.SC., PH.D.; Research Scientist, Pathology Branch, Animal Research Institute, Brisbane, Queensland, Australia

E. MURL BAILEY, JR., D.V.M., PH.D.; Professor of Toxicology, Department of Veterinary Physiology and Pharmacology, College of Veterinary Medicine, Texas A & M University, College Station, Texas

JEFFERY E. BARLOUGH, D.V.M., PH.D.; Diplomate, American College of Veterinary Microbiologists; Clinical Instructor, Department of Pathobiological Sciences and Veterinary Medical Teaching Hospital, School of Veterinary Medicine, University of Wisconsin-Madison, Madison, Wisconsin

KATHLEEN P. BARRIE, D.V.M., M.S.; Diplomate, American College of Veterinary Ophthalmologists; Adjunct Assistant Professor, Department of Comparative Ophthalmology, University of Florida, Gainesville, Florida; Ophthalmologist, Animal Eye Clinic, Tampa, Florida

JEANNE A. BARSANTI, D.V.M., M.S.; Diplomate, American College of Veterinary Internal Medicine; Associate Professor, Department of Small Animal Medicine, College of Veterinary Medicine, University of Georgia, Athens, Georgia; Internist, Small Animal Medicine, Veterinary Medical Teaching Hospital, College of Veterinary Medicine, University of Georgia, Athens, Georgia

ROGER M. BATT, B.V.SC., PH.D., M.SC., M.R.C.V.S.; Reader in Veterinary Pathology, University of Liverpool, Liverpool, England

TIMOTHY BAUER, D.V.M.; Lecturer, Department of Medicine, School of Veterinary Medicine, University of California, Davis, California; Private Practitioner, Seattle, Washington

VAL RICHARD BEASLEY, D.V.M.; Assistant Professor of Toxicology, Associate Director, National Animal Poison Control Center, College of Veterinary Medicine, University of Illinois, Urbana, Illinois

FORD WATSON BELL, D.V.M.; Resident, Internal Medicine, Department of Small Animal Clinical Sciences, College of Veterinary Medicine, University of Minnesota, St. Paul, Minnesota

KEVIN BELL, B.V.Sc., Ph.D.; Reader, Department of Physiology and Pharmacology, University of Queensland, St. Lucia, Brisbane, Queenland, Australia

JOHN BENTINCK-SMITH, D.V.M.; Professor of Clinical Pathology, College of Veterinary Medicine, Mississippi State University, Mississippi State, Mississippi

JOHN D. BONAGURA, D.V.M., M.S.; Diplomate, American College of Veterinary Internal Medicine (Cardiology, Internal Medicine); Associate Professor, The Ohio State University, Department of Veterinary Clinical Sciences, Columbus, Ohio; Staff Cardiologist, Veterinary Teaching Hospital, The Ohio State University, College of Veterinary Medicine, Columbus, Ohio

BETSY R. BOND, D.V.M.; Staff Cardiologist, The Animal Medical Center, New York, New York

RICHARD A. BOWEN, D.V.M., Ph.D.; Assistant Professor, Animal Reproduction Laboratory, Colorado State University, Fort Collins, Colorado

EDWARD B. BREITSCHWERDT, D.V.M.; Diplomate, American College of Veterinary Internal Medicine; Associate Professor of Medicine, School of Veterinary Medicine, North Carolina State University, Raleigh, North Carolina; Internist, Veterinary Teaching Hospital, North Carolina State University, Raleigh, North Carolina

DENNIS E. BROOKS, D.V.M.; Diplomate, American College of Veterinary Ophthalmologists; Assistant Professor of Ophthalmology, Department of Urban Practice, College of Veterinary Medicine, University of Tennessee, Knoxville, Tennessee

SCOTT A. BROWN, V.M.D.; Resident in Internal Medicine, University of Georgia, College of Veterinary Medicine, Athens, Georgia

C. A. BUFFINGTON, D.V.M., Ph.D.; Adjunct Instructor, Department of Physiological Sciences, School of Veterinary Medicine, University of California, Davis, California

SUSAN E. BUNCH, D.V.M., Ph.D.; Diplomate, American College of Veterinary Internal Medicine; Assistant Professor of Internal Medicine, School of Veterinary Medicine, North Carolina State University, Raleigh, North Carolina; Small Animal Internist, Veterinary Teaching Hospital, School of Veterinary Medicine, North Carolina State University, Raleigh, North Carolina

THOMAS J. BURKE, D.V.M., M.S.; Associate Professor, College of Veterinary Medicine, University of Illinois, Urbana, Illinois; Consultant, Capitol Illini Veterinary Hospital, Springfield, Illinois

COLIN F. BURROWS, B.vet.med., Ph.D., M.R.C.V.S.; Associate Professor of Medicine, University of Florida, College of Veterinary Medicine, Gainesville, Florida

CLAY A. CALVERT, D.V.M.; Associate Professor, College of Veterinary Medicine, University of Georgia, Athens, Georgia

TERRY W. CAMPBELL, M.S., D.V.M.; Instructor, Kansas State University, Department of Laboratory Medicine, College of Veterinary Medicine, Kansas State University, Manhattan, Kansas

THOMAS L. CARSON, D.V.M., M.S., Ph.D.; Professor of Veterinary Pathology, College of Veterinary Medicine, Iowa State University, Ames, Iowa; Veterinary Toxicologist, Veterinary Diagnostic Laboratory, College of Veterinary Medicine, Iowa State University, Ames, Iowa

SHARON A. CENTER, D.V.M.; Diplomate, American College of Veterinary Internal Medicine; Assistant Professor, New York State College of Veterinary Medicine, Cornell University, Ithaca, New York

DENNIS J. CHEW, D.V.M.; Diplomate, American College of Veterinary Internal Medicine; Associate Professor, Department of Veterinary Clinical Science, College of Veterinary Medicine, The Ohio State University, Columbus, Ohio; Small Animal Clinician, Internal Medicine, Veterinary Teaching Hospital, College of Veterinary Medicine, The Ohio State University, Columbus, Ohio

ANNE CHIAPELLA, D.V.M.; Diplomate, American College of Veterinary Internal Medicine; Private Practitioner, Beltway Internal Medicine Referral, Glenn Dale, Maryland

CHERYL L. CHRISMAN, D.V.M., M.S.; Diplomate, American College of Veterinary Internal Medicine (Neurology); Professor, Assistant Dean for Instruction, College of Veterinary Medicine, University of Florida, Gainesville, Florida; Chief of Neurology Service, Veterinary Medical Teaching Hospital, University of Florida, Gainesville, Florida

DONALD H. CLIFFORD, D.V.M., M.P.H., Ph.D.; Diplomate, American College of Veterinary Surgeons, American College of Laboratory

Animal Medicine; Professor, Division of Laboratory Animal Medicine, Medical College of Ohio at Toledo, Toledo, Ohio

SUSAN L. CLUBB, D.V.M.; Private Practitioner, Pet Farm, Inc., Miami, Florida

GARY L. COCKERELL, D.V.M., PH.D.; Associate Professor of Pathology, College of Veterinary Medicine and Biomedical Sciences, Colorado State University, Fort Collins, Colorado

P. W. CONCANNON, PH.D.; Senior Research Associate, Department of Physiology, New York State College of Veterinary Medicine, Cornell University, Ithaca, New York

ROBERT W. COPPOCK, D.V.M., M.S., PH.D., Diplomate, American Board of Veterinary Toxicology; Head, Clinical Investigation Group, Alberta Environmental Centre, Vegreville, Alberta, Canada

LARRY M. CORNELIUS, D.V.M., PH.D.; Diplomate, American College of Veterinary Internal Medicine; Professor of Small Animal Medicine, The University of Georgia, College of Veterinary Medicine, Athens, Georgia; Small Animal Internist, University of Georgia Veterinary Teaching Hospital, Athens, Georgia

C. GUILLERMO COUTO, D.V.M.; Assistant Professor, Department of Veterinary Clinical Sciences, College of Veterinary Medicine, The Ohio State University, Columbus, Ohio; Assistant Professor, Internal Medicine/Oncology, Veterinary Teaching Hospital, The Ohio State University, Columbus, Ohio

LARRY D. COWGILL, D.V.M., PH.D.; Diplomate, American College of Veterinary Internal Medicine; Associate Professor, Department of Medicine, School of Veterinary Medicine, University of California, Davis, California; Small Animal Internist, Veterinary Medical Teaching Hospital, University of California, Davis, California

STEPHEN W. CRANE, D.V.M.; Professor of Surgery, Department of Companion Animal and Special Species Medicine, School of Veterinary Medicine, North Carolina State University, Raleigh, North Carolina

WAYNE A. CROWELL, D.V.M., PH.D.; Diplomate, American College of Veterinary Pathologists; Professor, Department of Veterinary Pathology, College of Veterinary Medicine, University of Georgia, Athens, Georgia

LLOYD E. DAVIS, D.V.M., PH.D.; Professor of Pharmacology and Veterinary Clinical Medicine, College of Veterinary Medicine, University of Illinois, Urbana, Illinois; Clinical Pharmacology Studies Unit, Veterinary Medicine Teaching Hospital, University of Illinois, Urbana, Illinois

F. JOSHUA DEIN, V.M.D., M.S.; Veterinary Consultant, Tri-State Bird Rescue and Research, Wilmington, Delaware; Veterinary Medical Officer, Endangered Species Research Branch, Patuxent Wildlife Research Center, Laurel, Maryland

ALEXANDER DE LAHUNTA, D.V.M., PH.D.; Diplomate, American College of Veterinary Internal Medicine (Neurology); Professor of Anatomy, Chairman, Department of Clinical Sciences, New York State College of Veterinary Medicine, Cornell University, Ithaca, New York

ROBERT C. DENOVO, JR., D.V.M., M.S.; Diplomate, American College of Veterinary Internal Medicine; Assistant Professor of Medicine, Department of Urban Practice, College of Veterinary Medicine, University of Tennessee, Knoxville, Tennessee

JAMES V. DESIDERIO, M.S., PH.D.; Research Scientist, Department of Microbiological Research, Bristol-Myers Co., Syracuse, New York

STEPHEN P. DIBARTOLA, D.V.M.; Diplomate, American College of Veterinary Internal Medicine; Associate Professor of Medicine, Department of Veterinary Clinical Sciences, College of Veterinary Medicine, The Ohio State University, Columbus, Ohio; Small Animal Clinician, Veterinary Teaching Hospital, The Ohio State University, Columbus, Ohio

AMY DIETZE, D.V.M.; Diplomate, American College of Veterinary Radiology; Assistant Professor, Department of Clinical Sciences, New York State College of Veterinary Medicine, Cornell University, Ithaca, New York

RAY DILLON, D.V.M., M.S.; Diplomate, American College of Veterinary Internal Medicine; Associate Professor, Head, Section of Medicine, Department of Small Animal Surgery and Medicine, Scott-Ritchey Research Program, College of Veterinary Medicine, Auburn University, Auburn, Alabama

GARY M. DUNNY, PH.D.; Associate of Bacteriology, New York State College of Veterinary Medicine, Cornell University, Ithaca, New York

J. E. EIGENMANN, D.V.M., Ph.D.; Assistant Professor, Department of Clinical Studies, School of Veterinary Medicine, University of Pennsylvania, Philadelphia, Pennsylvania

PAMELA H. EISELE, D.V.M.; Associate Veterinarian, Laboratory Animal Medicine, Animal Resources Service, School of Veterinary Medicine, University of California, Davis, California

RICHARD H. EVANS, D.V.M., M.S.; Medical Director, Treehouse Wildlife Center, RR 1 Box 125E, Brighton, Illinois; Project Consultant, Specialty Products, Purina Mills, Inc., St. Louis, Missouri

VALERIE A. FADOK, D.V.M.; Assistant Professor of Dermatology, College of Veterinary Medicine, University of Florida, Gainesville, Florida; Veterinary Medical Teaching Hospital, College of Veterinary Medicine, University of Florida, Gainesville, Florida

BRIAN R. H. FARROW, B.V.Sc., Ph.D., F.A.C.V.Sc., M.R.C.V.S.; Associate Professor of Veterinary Anatomy, University of Sydney, N.S.W., Australia

DANIEL A. FEENEY, D.V.M., M.S.; Associate Professor of Radiology, University of Minnesota, College of Veterinary Medicine, St. Paul, Minnesota; Staff Radiologist, University of Minnesota Veterinary Teaching Hospital, St. Paul, Minnesota

BERNARD F. FELDMAN, D.V.M., Ph.D.; Associate Professor of Clinical Hematology and Biochemistry, Department of Clinical Pathology, School of Veterinary Medicine, University of California, Davis, California; Section Chief, Hemostasis Laboratory and Bone Marrow Cytology Service, Veterinary Medical Teaching Hospital, School of Veterinary Medicine, University of California, Davis, California

EDWARD C. FELDMAN, D.V.M.; Diplomate, American College of Veterinary Internal Medicine; Associate Professor, School of Veterinary Medicine, University of California, Davis, California; Clinician, Small Animal Clinic, Veterinary Medical Teaching Hospital, University of California, Davis, California

PETER J. FELSBURG, V.M.D., Ph.D.; Associate Professor of Clinical Immunology, College of Veterinary Medicine, University of Illinois, Urbana, Illinois

WILLIAM R. FENNER, D.V.M.; Diplomate, American College of Veterinary Internal Medicine (Neurology); Associate Professor, Department of Veterinary Clinical Sciences, College of Veterinary Medicine, The Ohio State University, Columbus, Ohio; Staff Neurologist, Veterinary Teaching Hospital, The Ohio State University, Columbus, Ohio

DUNCAN C. FERGUSON, V.M.D., Ph.D.; Assistant Professor, Department of Pharmacology, New York State College of Veterinary Medicine, Cornell University, Ithaca, New York

DELMAR R. FINCO, D.V.M., Ph.D.; Diplomate, American College of Veterinary Internal Medicine; Professor, Department of Physiology, University of Georgia, Athens, Georgia

KEVEN FLAMMER, D.V.M.; Assistant Professor, Exotic and Wild Bird Medicine, School of Veterinary Medicine, North Carolina State University, Raleigh, North Carolina; Staff Member, Veterinary Medical Teaching Hospital, School of Veterinary Medicine, North Carolina State University, Raleigh, North Carolina

CAROL S. FOIL, M.S., D.V.M.; Assistant Professor of Medicine and Dermatology, Department of Clinical Sciences, School of Veterinary Medicine, Louisiana State University, Baton Rouge, Louisiana; Staff Member, Veterinary Clinics and Teaching Hospital, Louisiana State University, Baton Rouge, Louisiana

MURRAY E. FOWLER, D.V.M.; Diplomate, American College of Zoological Medicine, American College of Veterinary Internal Medicine; Professor of Veterinary Medicine, Department of Medicine, School of Veterinary Medicine, University of California, Davis, California; Chief, Zoological Medicine Service, Veterinary Medical Teaching Hospital, School of Veterinary Medicine, University of California, Davis, California

JAMES G. FOX, D.V.M.; Professor and Director, Division of Comparative Medicine, Massachusetts Institute of Technology, Cambridge, Massachusetts; Adjunct Professor, Department of Comparative Medicine, Tufts University School of Veterinary Medicine, Grafton, Massachusetts

PHILIP R. FOX, D.V.M., M.S.; Diplomate, American College of Veterinary Internal Medicine (Cardiology); Director of Clinics, Staff Cardiologist, The Animal Medical Center, New York, New York

LYNNE S. FRINK, M.A.; Director, Tri-State Bird Rescue and Research, Inc., Wilmington, Delaware

URS GIGER, DR.MED.VET., F.V.H.; Assistant Professor in Medicine, Department of Clinical Studies, School of Veterinary Medicine, University of Pennsylvania, Philadelphia, Pennsylvania; Clinician in Medicine, Veterinary Hospital, University of Pennsylvania, Philadelphia, Pennsylvania

DON GILLESPIE, D.V.M.; Staff Veterinarian, Santa Barbara Zoological Gardens, Santa Barbara, California

N. T. GORMAN, B.V.SC., PH.D., F.R.C.V.S.; Lecturer in Medicine, Department of Clinical Veterinary Medicine, Cambridge University, Cambridge, England; Adjunct Professor, Department of Medical Sciences, College of Veterinary Medicine, University of Florida, Gainesville, Florida

GREGORY F. GRAUER, D.V.M., M.S.; Diplomate, American College of Veterinary Internal Medicine; Assistant Professor, Department of Medical Sciences, School of Veterinary Medicine, University of Wisconsin-Madison, Madison, Wisconsin; Small Animal Internist, Veterinary Medical Teaching Hospital, School of Veterinary Medicine, University of Wisconsin-Madison, Madison, Wisconsin

CRAIG E. GREENE, D.V.M., M.S.; Professor, Department of Small Animal Medicine, College of Veterinary Medicine, University of Georgia, Athens, Georgia

JAMES E. GRIMES, PH.D.; Associate Professor of Veterinary Microbiology and Parasitology, Texas A&M University, College Station, Texas

ROBERT L. HAMLIN, D.V.M., PH.D.; Professor, Department of Veterinary Physiology and Pharmacology, College of Veterinary Medicine, The Ohio State University, Columbus, Ohio; Senior Attending Clinician, Ohio State University Veterinary Hospital, Columbus, Ohio

PREM HANDAGAMA, B.V.SC.; Postdoctoral Research Cell Biologist, Department of Pathology, School of Medicine, University of California, San Francisco, California

ROBERT M. HARDY, D.V.M., M.S.; Associate Professor, Department of Small Animal Clinical Sciences, College of Veterinary Medicine, University of Minnesota, St. Paul, Minnesota

NEIL K. HARPSTER, V.M.D.; Diplomate, American College of Veterinary Internal Medicine (Cardiology); Clinical Professor, Tufts University School of Veterinary Medicine, Grafton, Massachusetts; Director of Cardiology, Angell Memorial Animal Hospital, Jamaica Plain, Massachusetts

COLIN E. HARVEY, B.V.SC., M.R.C.V.S.; Diplomate, American College of Veterinary Surgeons; Professor of Surgery, School of Veterinary Medicine, University of Pennsylvania, Philadelphia, Pennsylvania

WANDA M. HASCHEK, B.V.SC., PH.D.; Associate Professor of Veterinary Pathology, College of Veterinary Medicine, University of Illinois, Urbana, Illinois

DAVID W. HAYDEN, D.V.M., PH.D.; Diplomate, American College of Veterinary Pathologists; Professor of Veterinary Pathology, Department of Veterinary Pathobiology, College of Veterinary Medicine, University of Minnesota, St. Paul, Minnesota

DWIGHT C. HIRSH, D.V.M., PH.D.; Professor of Microbiology, School of Veterinary Medicine, University of California, Davis, California; Chief, Microbiology Diagnostic Service, Veterinary Medical Teaching Hospital, School of Veterinary Medicine, University of California, Davis, California,

MARGARETHE HOENIG, DR.MED.VET., PH.D., Senior Research Associate, Department of Pharmacology, New York State College of Veterinary Medicine, Cornell University, Ithaca, New York

WALTER E. HOFFMANN, D.V.M., PH.D.; Associate Professor, Department of Veterinary Pathobiology and Veterinary Clinical Medicine, College of Veterinary Medicine, University of Illinois, Urbana, Illinois

STEPHEN B. HOOSER, D.V.M.; Research Associate, Veterinary Biosciences, College of Veterinary Medicine, University of Illinois, Urbana, Illinois

WILLIAM E. HORNBUCKLE, D.V.M.; Diplomate, American College of Veterinary Internal Medicine; Associate Professor of Medicine, New York State College of Veterinary Medicine, Cornell University, Ithaca, New York

WILLIAM J. HORNOF, D.V.M., M.S.; Assistant Professor, Department of Radiological Sciences, School of Veterinary Medicine, University of California, Davis, California; Faculty, Veterinary Medical Teaching Hospital, University of California, Davis, California

DENNIS R. HOWARD, M.S., PH.D.; Associate Professor, College of Veterinary Medicine, Kansas State University, Manhattan, Kansas; Veterinary Diagnostic Laboratory, College of Veterinary Medicine, Manhattan, Kansas

PAUL W. HUSTED, V.M.D., M.S.; Assistant Professor, Department of Clinical Sciences, Colorado State University, Fort Collins, Colorado

PETER J. IHRKE, V.M.D.; Diplomate, American College of Veterinary Dermatology; Associate Professor of Dermatology, School of Veterinary Medicine, University of California, Davis, California; Staff Member, Dermatology Service, Small and Large Animal Clinic, Veterinary Medical Teaching Hospital, School of Veterinary Medicine, University of California, Davis, California

NITA L. IRBY, D.V.M.; Lecturer in Ophthalmology, University of Pennsylvania, School of Veterinary Medicine, New Bolton Center, Kennett Square, Pennsylvania; Private Veterinary Ophthalmology Consultation Service, Unionville, Pennsylvania

ELLIOTT R. JACOBSON, D.V.M., PH.D.; Associate Professor, Department of Special Clinical Sciences, University of Florida, Gainesville, Florida; Zoological and Wildlife Medicine Clinician, Veterinary Medical Teaching Hospital, University of Florida, Gainesville, Florida

KENNETH H. JOHNSON, D.V.M., PH.D.; Professor of Veterinary Pathology, Department of Veterinary Pathobiology, College of Veterinary Medicine, University of Minnesota, St. Paul, Minnesota

SUSAN E. JOHNSON, D.V.M., M.S.; Diplomate, American College of Veterinary Internal Medicine; Assistant Professor of Veterinary Medicine, College of Veterinary Medicine, The Ohio State University, Columbus, Ohio; Internist, Veterinary Teaching Hospital, The Ohio State University, Columbus, Ohio

GARY R. JOHNSTON, D.V.M.; Associate Professor of Comparative Radiology, Department of Small Animal Clinical Sciences, College of Veterinary Medicine, University of Minnesota, St. Paul, Minnesota

SHIRLEY D. JOHNSTON, D.V.M., PH.D.; Diplomate, American College of Theriogenologists; Associate Professor of Medicine, Department of Small Animal Clinical Sciences, College of Veterinary Medicine, University of Minnesota, St. Paul, Minnesota

ROBERT L. JONES, D.V.M., PH.D.; Diplomate, American College of Veterinary Microbiologists; Assistant Professor, Department of Microbiology, College of Veterinary Medicine and Biomedical Sciences, Colorado State University, Fort Collins, Colorado; Head, Bacteriology Section, Diagnostic Laboratory, Colorado State University, Fort Collins, Colorado

ANDREW J. KALLET, D.V.M.; Diplomate, American College of Veterinary Internal Medicine; Staff Internist, Madera Pet Hospital, Corte Madera, California

LORRAINE G. KARPINSKI, V.M.D.; Diplomate, American College of Veterinary Ophthalmologists; Adjunct Instructor, Department of Ophthalmology, University of Miami School of Medicine, Miami, Florida; Veterinary Ophthalmologist, South Dade Animal Hospital, and Bascom Palmer Eye Institute, Miami, Florida

BRUCE W. KEENE, D.V.M., M.SC.; Assistant Professor, Department of Medical Sciences, School of Veterinary Medicine, University of Wisconsin-Madison, Madison, Wisconsin; Attending Cardiologist, Veterinary Medical Teaching Hospital, University of Wisconsin-Madison, Madison, Wisconsin

ROBERT J. KEMPPAINEN, D.V.M., PH.D.; Assistant Professor, Department of Physiology and Pharmacology, College of Veterinary Medicine, Auburn University, Auburn, Alabama

THOMAS J. KERN, D.V.M.; Diplomate, American College of Veterinary Ophthalmologists; Assistant Professor of Medicine, Section of Comparative Ophthalmology, Department of Clinical Sciences, New York State College of Veterinary Medicine, Cornell University, Ithaca, New York

ROBERT W. KIRK, D.V.M.; Diplomate, American College of Veterinary Internal Medicine, American College of Veterinary Dermatology; Professor of Medicine Emeritus, New York State College of Veterinary Medicine, Cornell University, Ithaca, New York

MARK D. KITTLESON, D.V.M., PH.D.; Diplomate, American College of Veterinary Internal Medicine (Cardiology); Assistant Professor, Department of Medicine, School of Veterinary Medicine, University of California, Davis, California;

Staff Cardiologist, Veterinary Medical Teaching Hospital, University of California, Davis, California

JEFFREY S. KLAUSNER, D.V.M., M.S.; Diplomate, American College of Veterinary Internal Medicine; Associate Professor, Veterinary Internal Medicine, College of Veterinary Medicine, University of Minnesota, St. Paul, Minnesota

S. K. KNELLER, D.V.M., M.S.; Diplomate, American College of Veterinary Radiology; Associate Professor, Department of Clinical Veterinary Medicine, College of Veterinary Medicine, University of Illinois, Urbana, Illinois; Chief of Radiology Section, Veterinary Medicine Teaching Hospital, University of Illinois, Urbana, Illinois

GRANT G. KNOWLEN, D.V.M., PH.D.; Diplomate, American College of Veterinary Internal Medicine (Cardiology); Visiting Assistant Professor, Department of Veterinary Microbiology and Pathology and Department of Veterinary Comparative Anatomy, Physiology and Pharmacology, Washington State University, Pullman, Washington

GARY J. KOCIBA, D.V.M., PH.D.; Professor, Department of Veterinary Pathobiology, College of Veterinary Medicine, The Ohio State University, Columbus, Ohio

MICHAEL KOCK, B.VET.MED., M.R.C.V.S.; Member, International Wildlife Veterinary Services, Orangevale, California; Graduate Fellow, Department of Epidemiology, School of Veterinary Medicine, University of California, Davis, California

NANCY KOCK, D.V.M., M.S.; Member, International Wildlife Veterinary Services, Orangevale, California; Resident, Department of Veterinary Pathology, School of Veterinary Medicine, Veterinary Medical Teaching Hospital, University of California, Davis, California

JOE N. KORNEGAY, D.V.M., PH.D.; Diplomate, American College of Veterinary Internal Medicine (Neurology); Associate Professor, Neurology, Department of Companion Animal and Special Species Medicine, School of Veterinary Medicine, North Carolina State University, Raleigh, North Carolina; Clinical Neurologist, Veterinary Medical Teaching Hospital, School of Veterinary Medicine, North Carolina State University, Raleigh, North Carolina

DAVID F. KOWALCZYK, V.M.D, PH.D.; Regulatory Affairs Manager, Monsanto Corp., St. Louis, Missouri

JANET M. SCARLETT KRANZ, D.V.M., M.P.H., PH.D.; Assistant Professor, Department of Preventive Medicine, New York State College of Veterinary Medicine, Cornell University, Ithaca, New York

JOHN M. KRUGER, D.V.M.; Veterinary Medical Associate, Department of Small Animal Clinical Sciences, College of Veterinary Medicine, University of Minnesota, St. Paul, Minnesota; Resident, Small Animal Medicine, University of Minnesota Veterinary Teaching Hospital, St. Paul, Minnesota

GAIL A. KUNKLE, D.V.M.; Diplomate, American College of Veterinary Dermatology; Associate Professor, College of Veterinary Medicine, University of Florida, Gainesville, Florida; Chief of Dermatology Service, Veterinary Medical Teaching Hospital, Gainesville, Florida

KENNETH W. KWOCHKA, D.V.M.; Diplomate, American College of Veterinary Dermatology; Assistant Professor of Medicine/Dermatology, School of Veterinary Medicine, University of Wisconsin-Madison, Madison, Wisconsin; Staff Member, Veterinary Medical Teaching Hospital, School of Veterinary Medicine, University of Wisconsin-Madison, Madison, Wisconsin

LOUIS J. LARATTA, D.V.M.; Diplomate, American College of Veterinary Ophthalmologists; Assistant Professor of Ophthalmology, College of Veterinary Medicine, University of Tennessee, Knoxville, Tennessee

RICHARD A. LECOUTEUR, B.V.SC.; Diplomate, American College of Veterinary Internal Medicine (Neurology); Assistant Professor, Neurology, Department of Clinical Sciences, College of Veterinary Medicine and Biomedical Sciences, Colorado State University, Fort Collins, Colorado; Staff Member, Veterinary Teaching Hospital, Colorado State University, Fort Collins, Colorado

GEORGE E. LEES, D.V.M., M.S.; Diplomate, American College of Veterinary Internal Medicine; Associate Professor, Department of Small Animal Medicine and Surgery, Texas A&M University, College Station, Texas; Chief of Medicine Services, Small Animal Clinic, Veterinary Teaching Hospital, Texas A&M University, College Station, Texas

MICHAEL S. LEIB, D.V.M., M.S.; Diplomate, American College of Veterinary Internal Medicine; Assistant Professor, Virginia-Maryland Regional College of Veterinary Medicine, Virginia Polytechnic Institute and State University,

Blacksburg, Virginia; Coordinator, Medical Services, Veterinary Teaching Hospital, Virginia Polytechnic Institute and State University, Blacksburg, Virginia

CONNIE E. LEIFER, D.V.M.; Staff Oncologist, Donaldson-Atwood Cancer Clinic, The Animal Medical Center, New York, New York; Deceased 1985

DONALD H. LEIN, D.V.M., PH.D.; Diplomate, American College of Veterinary Pathologists; Associate Professor of Pathology and Theriogenology, New York State College of Veterinary Medicine, Cornell University, Ithaca, New York; Consultant in Theriogenology, Small Animal Clinic, New York State College of Veterinary Medicine, Cornell University, Ithaca, New York; Assistant Director, Diagnostic Laboratory, New York State College of Veterinary Medicine, Cornell University, Ithaca, New York

HARMON C. LEONARD, D.V.M.; Private Practitioner, Salida, Colorado

GERALD V. LING, D.V.M.; Professor, Department of Medicine, School of Veterinary Medicine, University of California, Davis, California; Chief, Small Animal Medicine, Veterinary Medical Teaching Hospital, University of California, Davis, California

BARRY A. LISSMAN, D.V.M.; Co-Director, Sachem Animal Hospital and Long Island Mobile Veterinary Clinic, Holbrook, New York

ANDREW S. LOAR, D.V.M.; Diplomate, American College of Veterinary Internal Medicine; Staff Oncologist/Internist, Animal Oncology Consultation Service, Coast Pet Clinic, Hermosa Beach, California

MICHAEL R. LOOMIS, D.V.M., A.M.; Adjunct Assistant Professor of Companion Animals and Special Species Medicine, School of Veterinary Medicine, North Carolina State University, Raleigh, North Carolina; Veterinarian, North Carolina Zoological Park, Asheboro, North Carolina

MICHAEL D. LORENZ, D.V.M., B.S.; Professor of Small Animal Medicine, Associate Dean for Academic Affairs, College of Veterinary Medicine, University of Georgia, Athens, Georgia

DONALD G. LOW, D.V.M., PH.D.; Diplomate, American College of Veterinary Internal Medicine; Professor of Medicine, School of Veterinary Medicine, University of California, Davis, California; Staff Member, Veterinary Medical Teaching Hospital, University of California, Davis, California

LINDA J. LOWENSTINE, D.V.M., PH.D.; Diplomate, American College of Veterinary Pathologists; Assistant Professor of Veterinary Pathology, School of Veterinary Medicine, University of California, Davis, California; Pathologist, Veterinary Medical Teaching Hospital, University of California, Davis, California; Collaborative Researcher and Pathology Consultant, California Primate Research Center, Davis, California

HANS LUTZ, DR.MED.VET., PH.D.; Privatdozent, School of Veterinary Medicine, University of Zürich, Zürich, Switzerland

J. M. MACDONALD, D.V.M.; Associate Professor, Department of Small Animal Surgery and Medicine, School of Veterinary Medicine, Auburn University, Auburn, Alabama; Dermatologist, Small Animal Clinic, Auburn University, Auburn, Alabama

ALAN D. MACMILLAN, D.V.M., PH.D.; Diplomate, American College of Veterinary Ophthalmologists; Staff Member, Eye Clinic for Animals, San Diego, California

DENNIS W. MACY, D.V.M., M.S.; Diplomate, American College of Veterinary Internal Medicine; Associate Professor, College of Veterinary Medicine and Biomedical Sciences, Colorado State University, Fort Collins, Colorado

BRUCE R. MADEWELL, V.M.D.; Professor, Department of Veterinary Surgery, School of Veterinary Medicine, University of California, Davis, California; Oncology Service, Veterinary Medical Teaching Hospital, University of California, Davis, California.

MICHAEL L. MAGNE, D.V.M., M.S.; Diplomate, American College of Veterinary Internal Medicine; Staff Internist and Gastroenterologist, Santa Cruz Veterinary Hospital, Santa Cruz, California

EDWARD A. MAHAFFEY, D.V.M., PH.D.; Diplomate, American College of Veterinary Pathologists; Associate Professor, Department of Veterinary Pathology, College of Veterinary Medicine, University of Georgia, Athens, Georgia

MARY B. MAHAFFEY, D.V.M., M.S.; Diplomate, American College of Veterinary Radiology; Assistant Professor of Radiology, Department of

Anatomy and Radiology, College of Veterinary Medicine, University of Georgia, Athens, Georgia; Staff Member, University of Georgia Veterinary Medical Teaching Hospital, Athens, Georgia

LAWRENCE E. MATHES, PH.D.; Assistant Professor, Department of Veterinary Pathobiology, The Ohio State University, Columbus, Ohio

ROBERT E. MATUS, D.V.M., M.S.; Diplomate, American College of Veterinary Internal Medicine; Head, Donaldson-Atwood Cancer Clinic, The Animal Medical Center, New York, New York

SCOTT E. MCDONALD, D.V.M.; Private Practitioner, Midwest Bird and Exotic Animal Hospital, Westchester, Illinois

PATRICK J. MCKEEVER, D.V.M., M.S.; Associate Professor of Veterinary Comparative Dermatology, College of Veterinary Medicine, University of Minnesota, St. Paul, Minnesota; Staff Member, University of Minnesota Veterinary Teaching Hospital, St. Paul, Minnesota

BRENDAN C. MCKIERNAN, D.V.M.; Diplomate, American College of Veterinary Internal Medicine; Associate Professor of Medicine, Department of Veterinary Clinical Medicine, College of Veterinary Medicine, University of Illinois, Urbana, Illinois

MICHAEL F. MCMENOMY, D.V.M.; Director, Kitty Klinic, Minneapolis, Minnesota

MICHAEL S. MILLER, V.M.D., M.S.; Diplomate, American Board of Veterinary Practitioners; Vice President of Clinical Affairs, Cardiopet, a division of Animed Inc., Staff Consultant in Electrocardiography, Roslyn, New York; Staff Clinician, A & A Veterinary Hospital, Franklin Square, New York

T. A. MILLER, D.V.M., PH.D., B.SC. (Agri.), B.V.M.S., M.R.C.V.S.; Director of Research and Development, TechAmerica Group, Inc., Elwood, Kansas

WILLIAM H. MILLER, JR., V.M.D.; Diplomate, American College of Veterinary Dermatology; Assistant Professor of Dermatology, School of Veterinary Medicine, University of Pennsylvania, Philadelphia, Pennsylvania; Faculty Dermatologist, Small Animal Clinic, University of Pennsylvania, Philadelphia, Pennsylvania

NICHOLAS J. MILLICHAMP, B. VET. MED., PH.D, M.R.C.V.S.; Diplomate, American College of Veterinary Ophthalmologists; Visiting Assistant Professor, Department of Small Animal Medicine and Surgery, College of Veterinary Medicine, Texas A & M University, College Station, Texas; Staff Ophthalmologist, Veterinary Teaching Hospital, College of Veterinary Medicine, Texas A & M University, College Station, Texas

MICHELLE S. MOSTROM, D.V.M.; Toxicology Resident, Department of Veterinary Biosciences, College of Veterinary Medicine, University of Illinois, Urbana, Illinois

MICHAEL E. MOUNT, D.V.M., PH.D.; Diplomate, American Board of Veterinary Toxicology; Assistant Professor, Department of Clinical Pathology, School of Veterinary Medicine, University of California, Davis, California; Clinical Pathologist, Veterinary Medical Teaching Hospital, University of California, Davis, California

WILLIAM MUIR, D.V.M., PH.D.; Professor, Department of Veterinary Clinical Sciences, College of Veterinary Medicine, The Ohio State University, Columbus, Ohio; Chairman of Veterinary Clinical Sciences, The Ohio State University, Columbus, Ohio

MICHAEL J. MURPHY, D.V.M.; Research Associate, Texas Veterinary Medical Diagnostic Laboratory, College Station, Texas

A. S. NASH, B.V.M.S., PH.D.; Senior Lecturer, Department of Veterinary Medicine, University of Glasgow Veterinary School, Glasgow, Scotland

MARK P. NASISSE, D.V.M.; Diplomate, American College of Veterinary Ophthalmologists; Assistant Professor, Ophthalmology, Department of Companion Animal and Special Species Medicine, School of Veterinary Medicine, North Carolina State University, Raleigh, North Carolina

DARIEN L. NELSON, D.V.M.; Diplomate, American College of Veterinary Ophthalmologists; Staff Member, Eye Clinic for Animals, Garden Grove, California

RICHARD W. NELSON, D.V.M.; Diplomate, American College of Veterinary Internal Medicine; Assistant Professor, Department of Small Animal Clinics, School of Veterinary Medicine, Purdue University, West Lafayette, Indiana; Internist, Small Animal Clinic, Purdue University, West Lafayette, Indiana

TERRY M. NETT, PH.D.; Associate Professor, Department of Physiology and Biophysics, Colorado State University, Fort Collins, Colorado

STEVEN S. NICHOLSON, D.V.M.; Diplomate, American Board of Veterinary Toxicology; Associate Professor, Department of Physiology, Pharmacology, and Toxicology, School of Veterinary Medicine, Louisiana State University, Baton Rouge, Louisiana

DREW M. NODEN, PH.D.; Associate Professor of Anatomy, Department of Anatomy, New York State College of Veterinary Medicine, Cornell University, Ithaca, New York

KATHLEEN E. NOONE, V.M.D.; Diplomate, American College of Veterinary Internal Medicine; Staff, Department of Medicine, The Animal Medical Center, New York, New York

RICHARD R. NYE, D.V.M.; Chief of Staff, Bird and Small Animal Practice, Des Plaines, Illinois

JOAN A. O'BRIEN, V.M.D.; Diplomate, American College of Veterinary Internal Medicine; Professor of Medicine, School of Veterinary Medicine, University of Pennsylvania, Philadelphia, Pennsylvania; Visiting Professor of Otorhinolaryngology, Hahnemann Hospital and Hospital of the University of Pennsylvania, Philadelphia, Pennsylvania

FREDERICK W. OEHME, D.V.M., PH.D.; Professor of Toxicology, Medicine, and Physiology, College of Veterinary Medicine, Kansas State University, Manhattan, Kansas; Director, Comparative Toxicology Laboratories, Veterinary Medical Hospital, Kansas State University, Manhattan, Kansas

PATRICIA N. OLSON, D.V.M., PH.D.; Diplomate, American College of Theriogenologists; Associate Professor, Department of Clinical Sciences, Colorado State University, Fort Collins, Colorado

E. CHRISTOPHER ORTON, D.V.M., M.S.; Diplomate, American College of Veterinary Surgeons; Assistant Professor, College of Veterinary Medicine and Biomedical Sciences, Colorado State University, Fort Collins, Colorado; Small Animal General Surgeon, Veterinary Teaching Hospital, Colorado State University, Fort Collins, Colorado

CARL A. OSBORNE, D.V.M., PH.D.; Diplomate, American College of Veterinary Internal Medicine; Professor, Department of Small Animal Clinical Sciences, College of Veterinary Medicine, University of Minnesota, St. Paul, Minnesota

GARY D. OSWEILER, D.V.M., M.S., PH.D.; Diplomate, American Board of Veterinary Toxicology; Professor, Veterinary Pathology, Veterinary Diagnostic Laboratory, College of Veterinary Medicine, Iowa State University, Ames, Iowa

MARK G. PAPICH, D.V.M., M.S.; Assistant Professor of Clinical Pharmacology, Western College of Veterinary Medicine, University of Saskatchewan, Saskatoon, Saskatchewan, Canada

JOHN PARROTT, D.V.M.; Clinician/Owner, Pembroke Park Animal Hospital, Pembroke Park, Florida

THERESA PARROTT, D.V.M.; Clinician/Owner, Pembroke Park Animal Hospital, Pembroke Park, Florida

PETER J. PASCOE, B.V.SC., D.V.A., M.R.C.V.S.; Diplomate, American College of Veterinary Anesthesiologists; Assistant Professor, Department of Clinical Studies, Ontario Veterinary College, University of Guelph, Guelph, Ontario, Canada; Service Chief for Anesthesia, Medical Teaching Hospital, Ontario Veterinary College, University of Guelph, Guelph, Ontario, Canada

ROBERT D. PECHMAN, JR., D.V.M.; Diplomate, American College of Veterinary Radiology; Associate Professor of Veterinary Radiology, School of Veterinary Medicine, Louisiana State University, Baton Rouge, Louisiana; Veterinary Radiologist, Veterinary Teaching Hospital and Clinics, Louisiana State University, Baton Rouge, Louisiana

NIELS C. PEDERSEN, D.V.M., PH.D.; Professor, Department of Veterinary Medicine, School of Veterinary Medicine, University of California, Davis, California; Staff Member, Veterinary Medicine Teaching Hospital, University of California, Davis, California

MARK E. PETERSON, D.V.M.; Diplomate, American College of Veterinary Internal Medicine; Staff Endocrinologist, Department of Medicine, The Animal Medical Center, New York, New York; Director of Clinical Medicine, Research Animal Resource Center, Cornell University Medical College, New York, New York

ELLEN M. POFFENBARGER, D.V.M.; Resident in Small Animal Internal Medicine, College of

Veterinary Medicine and Veterinary Teaching Hospital, University of Minnesota, St. Paul, Minnesota

DAVID J. POLZIN, D.V.M., PH.D.; Diplomate, American College of Veterinary Internal Medicine; Assistant Professor, Department of Small Animal Clinical Sciences, College of Veterinary Medicine, University of Minnesota, St. Paul, Minnesota; Staff Internist, Lewis Hospital for Companion Animals, St. Paul, Minnesota

ANNIE K. PRESTWOOD, D.V.M., PH.D.; Professor of Parasitology, College of Veterinary Medicine, University of Georgia, Athens, Georgia

R. WAYNE RANDOLPH, V.M.D.; Diplomate, American Board of Veterinary Practitioners; Owner and Director, Countryside Veterinary Hospital, Flemington, New Jersey

BRUCE M. RANKIN, B.A.; Graduate Research Assistant, New York State College of Veterinary Medicine, Cornell University, Ithaca, New York

CLARENCE A. RAWLINGS, D.V.M., PH.D., Professor, Department of Small Animal Medicine and Department of Physiology and Pharmacology, College of Veterinary Medicine, University of Georgia, Athens, Georgia; Chief of Staff, Small Animal Surgery, Veterinary Teaching Hospital, University of Georgia, Athens, Georgia

JOHN R. REED, D.V.M., M.S.; Diplomate, American College of Veterinary Internal Medicine (Cardiology); Staff Cardiologist, Sacramento Animal Medical Group, Inc., Sacramento, California

RONALD C. RIIS, D.V.M., M.S.; Diplomate, American College of Veterinary Ophthalmologists; Associate Professor of Veterinary Medicine, New York State College of Veterinary Medicine, Cornell University, Ithaca, New York; Comparative Ophthalmologist, New York State College of Veterinary Medicine, Cornell University, Ithaca, New York

J. EDMOND RIVIERE, D.V.M., PH.D.; Associate Professor, Department of Anatomy, Physiological Sciences and Radiology, School of Veterinary Medicine, North Carolina State University, Raleigh, North Carolina; Staff Member, Clinical Pharmacology Unit, Teaching Hospital, School of Veterinary Medicine, North Carolina State University, Raleigh, North Carolina

EDWARD L. ROBERSON, D.V.M., PH.D.; Professor of Parasitology, College of Veterinary Medicine, University of Georgia, Athens, Georgia

ELAINE P. ROBINSON, B.VET.MED.; Assistant Professor, Department of Small Animal Clinical Sciences, College of Veterinary Medicine, University of Minnesota, St. Paul, Minnesota

KAREN E. ROERTGEN, D.V.M.; Staff Member, Mueller Animal Hospital, Sacramento, California

KENITA S. ROGERS, D.V.M.; Veterinary Clinical Associate, Internal Medicine Resident, Department of Small Animal Medicine and Surgery, College of Veterinary Medicine, Texas A&M University, College Station, Texas

JENNIFER L. ROJKO, D.V.M.; Associate Professor, Departments of Veterinary Pathobiology and Comprehensive Cancer Center, The Ohio State University, Columbus, Ohio

ROBERT C. ROSENTHAL, D.V.M., M.S., PH.D.; Diplomate, American College of Veterinary Internal Medicine; Assistant Professor of Medicine/Oncology, Department of Medical Sciences, School of Veterinary Medicine, University of Wisconsin-Madison, Madison, Wisconsin

LINDA A. ROSS, D.V.M., M.S.; Diplomate, American College of Veterinary Internal Medicine; Assistant Professor, Department of Medicine, School of Veterinary Medicine, Tufts University, North Grafton, Massachusetts; Clinician, Foster Hosptial for Small Animals, Tufts New England Veterinary Medical Center, North Grafton, Massachusetts

WALTER J. ROSSKOPF, JR., D.V.M.; Research Associate, California State University, Dominguez Hills, California; Private Practitioner, Animal Medical Centre of Lawndale, Hawthorne, California; Avian and Exotic Animal Hospital of Orange County, Fountain Valley, California

STANLEY I. RUBIN, D.V.M., M.S.; Assistant Professor, Department of Veterinary Internal Medicine, Western College of Veterinary Medicine, University of Saskatchewan, Saskatoon, Saskatchewan, Canada; Attending Clinician, Small Animal Clinic, Veterinary Teaching Hospital, Western College of Veterinary Medicine, University of Saskatchewan, Saskatoon, Saskatchewan, Canada

LAWRENCE P. RUHR, D.V.M., PH.D.; Diplomate, American Board of Veterinary Toxicology; Associate Professor of Veterinary Toxicology, Department of Veterinary Physiology, Pharmacology and Toxicology, School of Veterinary Medicine, Louisana State University, Baton Rouge, Louisiana

ELIZABETH A. RUSSO, D.V.M., M.S.; Diplomate, American College of Veterinary Internal Medicine; Assistant Professor, Department of Small Animal Medicine and Surgery, Texas A&M University, College Station, Texas

ABDULRAHIM SANNUSI, D.V.M., M.Sc.; Senior Lecturer, Faculty of Veterinary Medicine, Ahmadu Bello University, Zaria, Nigeria; Protozoologist (Consultant), Veterinary Teaching Hospital, Ahmadu Bello University, Zaria, Nigeria

THOMAS D. SCAVELLI, D.V.M.; Resident in Surgery, The Animal Medical Center, New York, New York

MICHAEL SCHAER, D.V.M.; Diplomate, American College of Veterinary Internal Medicine; Associate Professor, College of Veterinary Medicine, University of Florida, Gainesville, Florida; Chief, Small Animal Medicine Service, and Head, Small Animal Hospital, College of Veterinary Medicine, University of Florida, Gainesville, Florida

LEE ANN SCHRADER, D.V.M.; Diplomate, American College of Veterinary Internal Medicine; Staff Member, Department of Medicine, The Animal Medical Center, New York, New York

KENNETH L. SCHUNK, D.V.M.; Diplomate, American College of Veterinary Internal Medicine; Assistant Professor of Medicine, School of Veterinary Medicine, Tufts University, North Grafton, Massachusetts; Neurologist, Foster Hospital for Small Animals, North Grafton, Massachusetts

DANNY W. SCOTT, D.V.M.; Diplomate, American College of Veterinary Dermatology; Associate Professor of Medicine, New York State College of Veterinary Medicine, Cornell University, Ithaca, New York

FREDRIC W. SCOTT, D.V.M., Ph.D.; Director, Cornell Feline Health Center, Cornell University, Ithaca, New York; Professor of Virology, Department of Microbiology, New York State College of Veterinary Medicine, Cornell University, Ithaca, New York

HOWARD B. SEIM III, D.V.M.; Diplomate, American College of Veterinary Surgeons; Associate Professor of Veterinary Surgery, Department of Clinical Sciences, Colorado State University, Fort Collins, Colorado; Staff Member, Department of Surgery, Veterinary Medical Teaching Hospital, Colorado State University, Fort Collins, Colorado

N. J. H. SHARP, B.Vet.Med., M.V.M., M.R.C.V.S.; Lecturer, The Veterinary Hospital, University of Liverpool, Liverpool, England

ROBERT G. SHERDING, D.V.M.; Diplomate, American College of Veterinary Internal Medicine; Associate Professor and Head of Small Animal Medicine, Department of Veterinary Clinical Sciences, The Ohio State University, Columbus, Ohio

VICTOR M. SHILLE, D.V.M., Ph.D.; Diplomate, American College of Theriogenologists; Associate Professor of Theriogenology, College of Veterinary Medicine, University of Florida, Gainesville, Florida

JAMES G. SIKARSKIE, D.V.M., M.S.; Zoo and Wildlife Veterinarian, Veterinary Clinical Center, Michigan State University, East Lansing, Michigan

DAVID SISSON, D.V.M.; Diplomate, American College of Veterinary Internal Medicine (Cardiology); Assistant Professor of Medicine, Department of Veterinary Clinical Medicine and Surgery, College of Veterinary Medicine, Washington State University, Pullman, Washington; Staff Cardiologist, Small Animal Clinic, Washington State University, Pullman, Washington

ROBBERT J. SLAPPENDEL, D.V.M., Ph.D., Veterinary Faculty, State University of Utrecht, Utrecht, The Netherlands; Small Animal Clinic, State University of Utrecht, Utrecht, The Netherlands

DAVID L. SMETZER, D.V.M., Ph.D.; Diplomate, American College of Veterinary Internal Medicine; Professor of Cardiology, Department of Veterinary Biosciences, College of Veterinary Medicine, University of Illinois, Urbana, Illinois

FRANCES O. SMITH, D.V.M., Ph.D.; Assistant Clinical Professor, Department of Small Animal Clinical Sciences, University of Minnesota, St. Paul, Minnesota; Private Practitioner, Crossroads Animal Hospital, Burnsville, Minnesota

FRANS C. STADES, D.V.M., Ph.D.; Lecturer, Ophthalmology, Faculty of Veterinary Medicine, State University of Utrecht, Utrecht, The Netherlands; Staff Ophthalmologist, Small Animal Clinic, State University of Utrecht, Utrecht, The Netherlands

ELIZABETH A. STONE, D.V.M., M.S.; Diplomate, American College of Veterinary Surgeons; Associate Professor, School of Veterinary Medicine, North Carolina State University, Raleigh, North Carolina; Small Animal Surgeon, Veterinary Teaching Hospital, School of Veterinary Medicine, North Carolina State University, Raleigh, North Carolina

DONALD R. STROMBECK, D.V.M., PH.D.; Professor, Department of Medicine, School of Veterinary Medicine, University of California, Davis, California; Staff Member, Veterinary Medical Teaching Hospital, University of California, Davis, California

TODD R. TAMS, D.V.M.; Diplomate, American College of Veterinary Internal Medicine; Staff Internist, West Los Angeles Veterinary Medical Group, West Los Angeles, California

ERIK TESKE, D.V.M.; Staff Member, Small Animal Clinic, State University of Utrecht, Utrecht, The Netherlands

KEITH L. THODAY, B.VET.MED., M.R.C.V.S.; Lecturer in Veterinary Medicine, University of Edinburgh, Royal (Dick) School of Veterinary Studies, Edinburgh, Scotland

WILLIAM P. THOMAS, D.V.M.; Diplomate, American College of Veterinary Internal Medicine (Cardiology); Associate Professor, School of Veterinary Medicine, University of California, Davis, California; Chief, Cardiology Service, Veterinary Medical Teaching Hospital, University of California, Davis, California

L. R. THOMSETT, V.V.SC., F.R.C.V.S.; Senior Lecturer, Department of Medicine, Royal Veterinary College, University of London, Hatfield, Hertfordshire, England

MARY ANNA HULL THRALL, D.V.M., M.S.; Diplomate, American College of Veterinary Pathologists; Associate Professor, Department of Pathology, College of Veterinary Medicine, Colorado State University, Fort Collins, Colorado; Clinical Pathologist, Veterinary Teaching Hospital, College of Veterinary Medicine, Colorado State University, Fort Collins, Colorado

LARRY PATRICK TILLEY, D.V.M.; Diplomate, American College of Veterinary Internal Medicine; Staff (Consultant), Department of Medicine, Cardiology, The Animal Medical Center, New York, New York; Vice-Chairman, Animed Inc.; President, Cardiopet, a division of Animed Inc., Roslyn, New York

ERIC J. TROTTER, D.V.M., M.S.; Diplomate, American College of Veterinary Surgeons; Associate Professor of Surgery, New York State College of Veterinary Medicine, Cornell University, Ithaca, New York

JANE M. TURREL, D.V.M., M.S.; Diplomate, American College of Veterinary Radiology; Assistant Professor, Department of Radiological Sciences, School of Veterinary Medicine, University of California, Davis, California; Radiation Oncologist, Veterinary Medical Teaching Hospital, University of California, Davis, California

DAVID C. TWEDT, D.V.M.; Diplomate, American College of Veterinary Internal Medicine; Associate Professor, Department of Clinical Sciences, College of Veterinary Medicine and Biomedical Sciences, Colorado State University, Fort Collins, Colorado; Staff Member, Veterinary Teaching Hospital, Colorado State University, Fort Collins, Colorado

A. J. VENKER-VAN HAAGEN, D.V.M., PH.D.; Lecturer, Small Animal Clinic, State University of Utrecht, Utrecht, The Netherlands

PATRICIA A. WALTER, D.V.M., M.S.; Assistant Professor of Comparative Radiology, Department of Small Animal Clinical Sciences, College of Veterinary Medicine, University of Minnesota, St. Paul, Minnesota; Staff Radiologist, Veterinary Teaching Hospital, University of Minnesota, St. Paul, Minnesota

DONNA K. WALTON, D.V.M.; Diplomate, American College of Veterinary Dermatology; Assistant Professor of Medicine, Dermatology, New York State College of Veterinary Medicine, Cornell University, Ithaca, New York

WENDY A. WARE, D.V.M.; Graduate Research Associate, Department of Veterinary Clinical Sciences, College of Veterinary Medicine, The Ohio State University, Columbus, Ohio; Clinical Instructor of Cardiology and Small Animal Medicine, The Ohio State University Veterinary Teaching Hospital, Columbus, Ohio

ROBERT J. WASHABAU, V.M.D.; Department of Clinical Studies, School of Veterinary Medicine, University of Pennsylvania, Philadelphia, Pennsylvania

M. G. WEISER, D.V.M.; Diplomate, American College of Veterinary Pathologists; Associate Professor of Clinical Pathology, Department of Pathology, College of Veterinary Medicine and Biomedical Sciences, Colorado State University,

Fort Collins, Colorado; Clinical Pathologist, Veterinary Teaching Hospital, Colorado State University, Fort Collins, Colorado

DOUGLAS J. WEISS, D.V.M., PH.D.; Diplomate, American College of Veterinary Pathologists; Assistant Professor, College of Veterinary Medicine, University of Minnesota, St. Paul, Minnesota; Section Chief of Clinical Labs, Veterinary Teaching Hospital, University of Minnesota, St. Paul, Minnesota

MAXEY L. WELLMAN, D.V.M., M.S.; Instructor, Department of Veterinary Pathobiology, College of Veterinary Medicine, The Ohio State University, Columbus, Ohio

L. L. WERNER, D.V.M.; Diplomate, American College of Veterinary Internal Medicine; Adjunct Instructor in Clinical Pathology, Department of Clincial Pathology, College of Veterinary Medicine, University of California, Davis, California

C. SUE WEST, D.V.M.; Diplomate, American College of Veterinary Ophthalmologists; Veterinary Ophthalmologist, Animal Eye Clinic, Tampa, Florida

STEVEN L. WHEELER, D.V.M.; Resident in Small Animal Medicine, Veterinary Teaching Hospital, Colorado State University, Fort Collins, Colorado

STEPHEN D. WHITE, D.V.M.; Diplomate, American College of Veterinary Dermatology; Assistant Professor, Department of Medicine, Tufts University School of Veterinary Medicine, North Grafton, Massachusetts

JEFF R. WILCKE, D.V.M., M.S.; Assistant Professor of Clinical Pharmacology, Virginia-Maryland Regional College of Veterinary Medicine, Virginia Polytechnic and State University, Blacksburg, Virginia; Clinical Pharmacologist, Veterinary Medical Teaching Hospital, Virginia-Maryland Regional College of Veterinary Medicine, Virginia Polytechnic and State University, Blacksburg, Virginia

MICHAEL DUWAYNE WILLARD, D.V.M., M.S.; Diplomate, American College of Veterinary Internal Medicine; Associate Professor of Veterinary Medicine, College of Veterinary Medicine, Michigan State University, East Lansing, Michigan; Internist, Veterinary Clinical Center, East Lansing, Michigan

BENNY J. WOODY, D.V.M.; Assistant Professor, College of Veterinary Medicine, Mississippi State University, Mississippi State, Mississippi; Internist, Animal Health Center, College of Veterinary Medicine, Mississippi State University, Mississippi State, Mississippi

MILTON WYMAN, D.V.M., M.S.; Diplomate, American College of Veterinary Ophthalmologists; Professor of Veterinary Clinical Science, Professor of Veterinary Medicine, College of Veterinary Medicine, The Ohio State University, Columbus, Ohio; Professor of Ophthalmology, Assistant Dean of Student Affairs, College of Medicine, The Ohio State University, Columbus, Ohio

ROGER A. YEARY, D.V.M., PH.D.; Diplomate, American Board of Veterinary Toxicology; Adjunct Professor, College of Veterinary Medicine, The Ohio State University, Columbus, Ohio; Corporate Toxicologist, Chemlawn Services Corporation, Columbus, Ohio

DENNIS A. ZAWIE, D.V.M.; Diplomate, American College of Veterinary Internal Medicine; Staff Gastroenterologist, The Animal Medical Center, New York, New York

ROBERT D. ZENOBLE, D.V.M., M.S.; Diplomate, American College of Veterinary Internal Medicine; Associate Professor, College of Veterinary Medicine, Auburn University, Auburn, Alabama; Staff Member, Small Animal Clinic, Department of Small Animal Surgery and Medicine, College of Veterinary Medicine, Auburn University, Auburn, Alabama

CAROLE A. ZERBE, D.V.M.; Instructor, Department of Small Animal Clinical Sciences, College of Veterinary Medicine, Michigan State University, East Lansing, Michigan; Resident, Small Animal Internal Medicine, Veterinary Clinical Center, Michigan State University, East Lansing, Michigan

JAMES F. ZIMMER, D.V.M., PH.D.; Assistant Professor of Small Animal Medicine, Department of Clinical Sciences, New York State College of Veterinary Medicine, Cornell University, Ithaca, New York

PREFACE

Each edition of *Current Veterinary Therapy* has unique features that document the increasing sophistication and scientific advances in small animal practice. This ninth edition is no exception. The greatest advances in medicine are taking place in areas associated with immunology, so it is no surprise that important changes in this field are noted throughout the text. These are most obvious in the greatly expanded section on immunology, oncology, and hematology. There are also notable changes in the sections on special therapy, chemical and physical disorders, cardiovascular diseases, and gastrointestinal, endocrine, and urinary disorders.

This volume is completely new. There continue to be references to topics in the previous editions, and many appendix tables, charts, and dosage formularies are updated but otherwise repeated for your reference. Some of the new articles may seem exotic to old-timers. They are intended to stretch our thoughts to new principles and new findings that will become foundations for future therapeutic regimens. Some of these ideas are "state of the art" to recent graduates—and only esoteric to us old-timers.

A special thank you is due each of the consulting editors, many of them new, for countless hours of writing, editing, and rushing to meet relentless deadlines.

We are grateful again to a host of regular authors and also to the many first-timers who have joined the team to keep you current with number nine. As always, the people at W. B. Saunders Company have been most efficient and cooperative in bringing this book to fruition. We especially thank Darlene Pedersen and Linda Mills for their unflagging devotion to the project. To one and all, a big thank you for a job well done.

ROBERT W. KIRK, D.V.M.
Ithaca, NY

NOTICE

Extraordinary efforts have been made by the authors, the editors, and the publisher of this book to insure that dosage recommendations are precise and in agreement with standards officially accepted at the time of publication.

It does happen, however, that dosage schedules are changed from time to time in the light of accumulating clinical experience and continuing laboratory studies. This is most likely to occur in the case of recently introduced products.

It is urged, therefore, that you check the manufacturer's recommendations for dosage, especially if the drug to be administered or prescribed is one that you use only infrequently or have not used for some time.

In addition, some drugs mentioned have been used by the authors as experimental drugs. Others have been used after official clearance for use in one species but not in others described here. This is particularly true for rare and exotic species. In these cases the authors have reported on their own considerable experience, but readers are urged to view the recommendations with discretion and precaution.

THE EDITORS

CONTENTS

SECTION

1

SPECIAL THERAPY

Carl A. Osborne
Consulting Editor

SECTION

2

CHEMICAL AND PHYSICAL DISORDERS

Gary D. Osweiler
Consulting Editor

SECTION

3

RESPIRATORY DISEASES

Brendan C. McKiernan
Consulting Editor

SECTION

4

CARDIOVASCULAR DISEASES

John D. Bonagura
Consulting Editor

SECTION

5

IMMUNOLOGY, ONCOLOGY, AND HEMATOLOGY

Bruce R. Madewell
Consulting Editor

Immunology

SECTION

7

OPHTHALMOLOGIC DISEASES

Thomas J. Kern
Ronald E. Riis
Consulting Editors

SECTION

8

DISEASES OF CAGED BIRDS AND EXOTIC PETS

Murray E. Fowler
Consulting Editor

SECTION

9

NEUROLOGIC AND NEUROMUSCULAR DISORDERS

A. de Lahunta
Consulting Editor

SECTION 10
GASTROINTESTINAL DISORDERS

David C. Twedt
Consulting Editor

SECTION 11
ENDOCRINE AND METABOLIC DISORDERS

Mark E. Peterson
Consulting Editor

SECTION 12
INFECTIOUS DISEASES
Fredric W. Scott
Consulting Editor

SECTION 13
URINARY DISORDERS
Jeanne A. Barsanti
Consulting Editor

Diagnosis of Urinary Tract Disorders

Disorders of the Urinary Tract

Management of Urinary Tract Disorders

SECTION 14
REPRODUCTIVE DISORDERS

Donald H. Lein
Consulting Editor

APPENDICES

Robert W. Kirk
Consulting Editor

Section 1

SPECIAL THERAPY

CARL A. OSBORNE, D.V.M.
Consulting Editor

Additional Pertinent Information Found in Current Veterinary Therapy VIII:

Barton, C. L., D.V.M., and Beaver, B. V., D.V.M.: Coping with the Death of a Pet, p. 72.
Beaver, B. V., D.V.M.: Therapy of Behavior Problems, p. 58.
Haskins, S. C., D.V.M.: Shock (The Pathophysiology and Management of the Circulatory Collapse States), p. 2.
Ling, G. V., D.V.M., and Hirsh, D. C., D.V.M.: Principles of Antimicrobial Therapy, p. 41.
Muir, W. W., D.V.M., and DiBartola, S. P., D.V.M.: Fluid Therapy, p. 28.
Pemberton, P. L., B.V.Sc.: Canine and Feline Behavior Control: Progestin Therapy, p. 62.
Venker-van Haagen, A. J., D.V.M.: Managing Diseases of the Ear, p. 47.
Wolski, T. R., D.V.M.: Preventing Canine Behavior Problems, p. 52.

Additional Pertinent Information Found in Current Veterinary Therapy VII:

Glickman, L. T., V.M.D.: Preventive Medicine in Kennel Management, p. 67.
Hoffer, R. E., D.V.M.: Cryotherapy, p. 65.
Rebar, A. H., D.V.M.: Diagnostic Cytology in Veterinary Practice: Current Status and Interpretative Principles, p. 16.
Small, E., D.V.M.: Pediatrics, p. 77.
Staaden, R., B.V.Sc.: Physical Fitness and Training for Dogs, p. 53.

DIAGNOSTIC PERITONEAL LAVAGE

STEPHEN W. CRANE, D.V.M.
Raleigh, North Carolina

Diagnostic peritoneal lavage (DPL) is an effective and practical diagnostic method for detecting intraperitoneal injuries and diseases. It is of no use in the detection of retroperitoneal injuries unless they extend into the peritoneal cavity. Fortunately, radiographic imaging of the sublinear region is a sensitive indicator of extravasations of blood, urine, or both into the retroperitoneal space.

Simple in both concept and practice, DPL consists of lavage of the serosal and parietal peritoneal surfaces and analysis of some portion of the lavage fluid. Cell counts, smears, and other tests of the lavage fluid provide objective data regarding cell populations, biochemical composition, and contamination with gastrointestinal contents. Such information augments the history and physical examination in assessment of the patient. In contrast, indirect observations such as laboratory examination of the peripheral circulation and abdominal radiographic studies often yield delayed or inconclusive information until the injurious process is well advanced.

HISTORY

Generalized, fibrinopurulent peritonitis or massive intraperitoneal hemorrhage is easily detected by recognition of physical findings typical of hypovolemic and endotoxic shock. However, physical examination is not consistently reliable in detection of early hemorrhage or early consequences of viscus rupture caused by blunt or penetrating abdominal trauma. Studies in humans and animals designed to correlate physical examination findings with abdominal injury revealed that recognition of systemic signs and results of abdominal palpation were associated with false-positive and false-negative conclusions.

To reduce mortality and morbidity from abdominal hemorrhage and peritonitis, needle abdominocentesis has been used to facilitate early detection of characteristic fluids. Abdominocentesis techniques vary from a four-quadrant "open" method (no aspiration through needles) to a "closed" method. In the "closed" technique, a syringe and needle combination is used to attempt aspiration of suspected accumulations of fluid within the abdomen.

Unfortunately, abdominocentesis has been associated with a high percentage (up to 50 per cent) of false-negative results (no fluid returns in the presence of significant injury). A false-negative result may be caused by obstruction of the hypodermic needle with omentum or because intraperitoneal fluid becomes loculated within tissues. False-positive results associated with abdominocentesis have been significantly fewer than false-negative results.

To overcome this problem, the rationale, indications, techniques, and results of DPL were established in human trauma management centers between 1965 and 1975. In a large number of cases, the ability of lavage to reveal abdominal injury was excellent. In the mid-1970s, veterinarians also found DPL to be very sensitive in detecting small quantities of intraperitoneal blood and inflammatory cell populations. Subsequent experimental and clinical studies have documented DPL's superiority to physical examination and open or closed abdominocentesis in detection of early illness or injury. Accuracy of DPL has been 95 to 100 per cent; false-negative findings have almost been eliminated, and false-positive results have only occurred as a consequence of iatrogenic injury during catheter placement.

INDICATIONS

DPL should not be performed if the cause of injury is obvious (e.g., the animal has gunshot or major puncture wounds). Exploratory celiotomy is the diagnostic and therapeutic procedure of choice in these cases. Because it is an invasive technique, DPL should follow open-quadrant abdominocentesis. If results of abdominocentesis are inconclusive and a high index of suspicion of abdominal disease or injury remains, DPL should be considered. Cytologic and biochemical evaluation of lavage fluid often permits detection or confirmation of hemorrhage, escape of gastric or intestinal contents into the peritoneal cavity, and chemical peritonitis from bile, urine, or pancreatic enzymes. DPL may also be of value in detection of acute, nonseptic, peritoneal inflammatory or neoplastic reactions in which cells have exfoliated into lavage fluid.

CONTRAINDICATIONS AND PRECAUTIONS

The urinary bladder should be emptied before DPL is performed to minimize laceration or puncture. Gastrointestinal distension or ileus, a gravid uterus, or a torn diaphragm mandates extra caution and care. If a celiotomy scar is present, the catheter should be directed away from this site in order to avoid damage to abdominal structures that may have become adhered to the incision.

TECHNIQUE

The patient's general condition should be assessed prior to DPL. The procedure usually requires local anesthesia; light tranquilization is also suggested for apprehensive or aggressive animals. An area between the umbilicus and pubis should be prepared as for surgery and a four-quadrant open abdominocentesis performed. If positive results are obtained (e.g., appearance of blood or abdominal fluid), DPL may not be required. If no abnormalities are detected, DPL should be performed.

Coexisting injuries and the potential for iatrogenic trauma should be taken into account, and the patient should be restrained in lateral or dorsal recumbency and prepped as for surgery again. The site of needle puncture should be draped with towels to maintain local asepsis. A midline area 2 to 4 cm caudal to the umbilicus and 1 cm long should be infiltrated to the level of the linea alba with 2 per cent xylocaine and epinephrine.

Next, a 1 cm stab wound should be created with a No. 11 or 12 Bard-Parker blade. Subcutaneous fat should be bluntly separated to expose the linea alba. Hemorrhage from the subcutis and fat may be rapidly controlled with pressure. A polyfenestrated plastic peritoneal dialysis catheter (TROCATH, American McGaw Laboratories, Catalogue No. V4901) should then be advanced through the linea alba. The trocar-tipped metal stylet supplied with the dialysis unit is extended beyond the tip of the catheter into the "puncture" position. The catheter should be held in the palm of the hand close to its tip so that when perforation of the linea alba occurs, a sudden and uncontrolled excursion of the catheter into or against the abdominal viscera will not occur. Pressure applied to the end of the stylet will cause the catheter to move through the linea alba. The catheter should be advanced in a dorsocaudal direction. Next, the stylet should be withdrawn until it is just within the catheter tip. The catheter should then be advanced to the paralumbar gutter. Once the catheter is properly positioned within the abdomen, the stylet should be removed.

Aspiration may yield fluid that was previously unobtainable by needle abdominocentesis. If fluid cannot be aspirated, 20 ml/kg of warmed sterile electrolyte solution should be infused into the peritoneal cavity. The procedure should be terminated if excess ventilatory dysfunction suddenly occurs. After infusion of the solution, the abdomen should be gently massaged. The patient may be carefully rolled from the side to side to enhance distribution of fluid within the peritoneal cavity. Next, the mixture of lavage solution and peritoneal fluid should be siphoned into the infusion container, which is placed below the patient. Five-ml aliquots of siphoned fluid should be collected during drainage. One sample should be collected in an aseptic container for microbiologic tests. Another aliquot should be collected in EDTA for determination of PCV, RBC, and WBC counts. The remaining fluid in the same tube may be centrifuged to obtain the sediment. Sediment smeared onto slides may be stained with new methylene blue for leukocytes and Gram's stain for bacteria. Another aliquot of fluid should also be centrifuged; the supernatant may be used for various tests.

After sample collection, as much fluid as possible should be drained from the abdomen. If a slow, continuing hemorrhage is suspected, the catheter may be bandaged in place for further monitoring. When the catheter is removed, a deep skin suture may be used to close the incised tissue.

A "minilaparotomy" technique may be used to reduce the risk of catheter-induced trauma associated with the direct puncture method. To perform this technique, the stab wound in the abdominal wall should be extended for a few centimeters. Then sutures should be placed in the linea alba 1.5 cm apart. After a stab wound is made directly on the midline, the catheter may be threaded to the paralumbar gutter without the metal stylet.

INTERPRETATION

If 20 ml/kg of peritoneal lavage fluid is used, significant intraperitoneal hemorrhage is indicated if the siphoned lavage fluid is bloody and opaque, has a PCV of over 2 per cent, or an RBC count of 200,000/mm^3. In this situation, celiotomy is recommended to identify, isolate, débride, and surgically correct the bleeding areas.

"Pinkish" lavage fluid that is translucent corresponds to a PCV of 1 to 2 per cent and an RBC count of 100,000 to 200,000/mm^3. In this situation, the likelihood of injury is equivocal. Results of other clinical procedures should be considered. It may be advantageous to leave the catheter in place and to repeat the procedure after an appropriate interval. A PCV of less than 1 per cent or a crystal-clear lavage fluid indicates that no significant injury has occurred.

Lavage fluid that is highly turbid and contains feces is indicative of peritonitis. Smears of such fluid are usually populated with high numbers of degenerated leukocytes, bacteria, and particulate debris. Vegetable material is pathognomonic of rupture of the gastrointestinal tract.

If lavage fluid is not yet septic and is grossly turbid, qualitative and quantitative cytological tests of leukocytes should be evaluated. Normal-appearing neutrophils and macrophages beyond 2000/mm^3 indicate the probability of nonseptic peritonitis.

The following points may facilitate proper interpretation of WBC counts. Normally, mature neutrophils are present in lavage fluid in numbers of less than 500/mm^3. Even after uncomplicated abdominal surgery, the neutrophil count will not rise above 750 to 1500/mm^3, but peritoneal leukocystosis can occur if peripheral leukocystosis is present. Leukocyte response to sepsis, chemical contamination, or irritants requires 2 to 4 hours before accumulation in diagnostic numbers occurs. Therefore, detection of bacteria in lavage fluid collected soon after injury is indicative of a serious problem, regardless of the magnitude of peritoneal leukocytosis.

Biochemical examinations are also useful in evaluating the integrity of the peritoneal cavity. When fluid is obtained, it may be tested with Azostix (Ames Laboratories) reagent strips for urea concentration. Creatinine concentrations may also be evaluated. Abnormal concentrations of urea and creatinine in peritoneal fluid are indicative of extravasation of urine into the peritoneal cavity.

Lavage fluid that is green is indicative of the presence of bile, which may be confirmed with the Ictotest (Ames Laboratories) reagent system. Bile may escape into the peritoneal cavity as a result of avulsion or tearing of the extrahepatic biliary tree, liver laceration, or gastrointestinal rupture. Because bile provokes an intense clinical peritonitis, it is typically associated with an intense peritoneal leukocytosis.

COMPLICATIONS

Perforation of abdominal viscera with the catheter stylet is the most common complication of DPL. If enlargement of the spleen causes it to be displaced into caudal portions of the abdomen, it may be lacerated. Perforations of the intestines, mesentery, or bladder may also occur. However, in our experience iatrogenic injury has been uncommon.

References and Suggested Readings

Bjorling, D. E., Latimer, K. S., Rawlings, C. A., et al.: Diagnostic peritoneal lavage before and after abdominal surgery in dogs. Am. J. Vet. Res. 44:816, 1983.

Crowe, D. T., and Crane, S. W.: Diagnostic abdominal paracentesis and lavage in the evaluation of abdominal injuries in dogs and cats: Clinical and experimental investigations. J.A.V.M.A. 168:700, 1976.

Hunt, C. A.: Diagnostic peritoneal paracentesis and lavage. Comp. Cont. Educa. 2:449, 1980.

Powell, D. C., Bivens, B. A., and Bell, R. M.: Diagnostic peritoneal lavage. Surg. Gynecol. Obstet. 155:257, 1982.

DIAGNOSTIC ULTRASONOGRAPHY: PRINCIPLES, APPLICATIONS, AND AVAILABILITY

DANIEL A. FEENEY, D.V.M.,
GARY R. JOHNSTON, D.V.M.,
and PATRICIA A. WALTER, D.V.M.
St. Paul, Minnesota

PRINCIPLES OF ULTRASONIC IMAGING

Diagnostic medical ultrasound (ultrasonography) is a nonionizing imaging technique utilizing high frequency (1–10 MHz), low intensity (< 100 mW/cm^2, spatial peak, temporal average) sound. The concept of ultrasonography consists of a chronologic sequence of sound production, sound transmission into appropriate body tissues, sound reflection within body tissues, detection of reflected sound (usually by the same instrument that produced the sound), and finally reconstruction of returning echoes into a display appropriate to the study. Since each part of this imaging sequence is dependent upon those preceding it, each item will be described in the order that it occurs during imaging.

The production of high frequency sound occurs as a result of electrical stimulation of a piezoelectric crystal of appropriate dimensions that generates sound at the desired frequency. The piezoelectric crystal is housed within a clinically applicable instrument; the portion that touches the patient is termed the transducer. Sound is transmitted from the transducer into the tissues by means of a coupling medium (usually commercially available ultrasonic gel; mineral oil has also been used). The coupling medium is necessary to displace air from the interface between the transducer and the patient's skin or other body surface used as a portal of entry for the sound. Since large quantities of hair interfere with this interface, it is usually necessary to remove it by clipping.

After adequate coupling between the transducer and skin surface, the sound must be of appropriate energy to penetrate to the desired depth of study. In general, penetration is inversely proportional to the frequency of sound. Therefore, care must be used to choose the proper transducer for the study. In general, the smaller the diameter of the crystal producing the sound and the higher the frequency of sound produced, the greater will be the resolving capabilities of the instrument. However, there is a "trade-off" between penetration and resolution. Since sound is progressively attenuated as it is transmitted through tissue, it must be electronically enhanced (so-called time gain compensation) to obtain a uniform display. As ultrasound passes through different types of tissue in its path, varying degrees of reflection versus transmission occur. The relative amounts of reflected energy versus transmitted energy occurring at a given tissue interface is proportional to differences in acoustic impedance (product of the density and the speed of sound transmission through that tissue) of different tissues. Since the frequency range and instrument calibration are designed for use in soft tissues, substances such as air, bone, or metal (which have significantly different sound transmission characteristics than soft tissue) result in complete or very nearly complete sound reflection at the interface between soft tissue and these materials. To permit visualization of tissues deep to a given tissue interface, a portion of the sound must be transmitted through the tissue so that sound is available for reflection at deeper levels of the region to be examined.

Once a portion of the sound beam is reflected (assuming that refraction or scattering has not occurred), it will return to the transducer. At this time, the sound will stimulate the piezoelectric crystal in the transducer to produce an electronic signal. This electronic signal is then reconstructed into an appropriate display for evaluation.

Depending on the type of information desired from the ultrasound study, there are several formats of display. One, called A-mode, is a graphic representation of depth from the position of the transducer (displayed on the abscissa) and the amplitude of the returning echoes (displayed on the ordinate) (Fig. 1). This form of elementary graphic display is

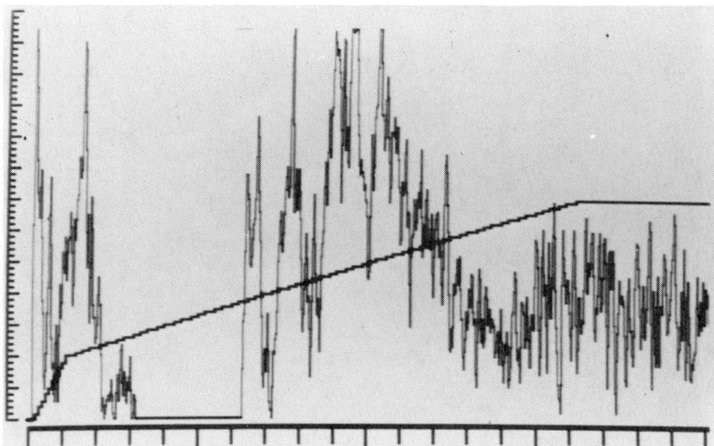

Figure 1. Amplitude (A-mode) scan in which returning echoes (spikes) can be identified at varying distances from point of sound origin (left abscissa is surface). Between 3 and 6 cm from the surface, no returning echoes are identified, indicating that the tissue (probably fluid) lacked sufficient interfaces to create reflection. This proved to be a fluid-filled cyst.

only of limited clinical value. However, the concept of amplitude and distance is the basis for all ultrasonographic display formats. Another display format is called M-mode (also called T-M mode). In this format the distance (depth) from the transducer is measured on the vertical axis, whereas elapsed time is depicted on the horizontal axis (Fig. 2). The amplitudes of returning echoes are displayed visually as varying intensities (or brightness). Because the location of echoes on the display are influenced by the depth of body structures that reflect them, precise measurements of the position and size of an organ (especially the heart) or tissue can be made. This format is somewhat analogous to the display of cardiac electrical activity in time sequence by the electrocardiogram. The M-mode format is most commonly applied to echocardiography (with simultaneous electrocardiography) to assess chamber dimensions, cardiac contractility, and valve motion. Another major mode of display is called two-dimensional B-mode. Currently, most equipment displays two-dimensional anatomic images. Echogenicity (discussed in the next section) is proportional (so-called gray-scale) to the amplitude of returning sound waves. These sound waves (or echoes) are reconstructed into anatomic sections (Fig. 3).

Within the B-mode display, there are basically two types of gray-scale display formats. The first is the "static" scan, which is a display of two-dimensional anatomy without the perception of motion (Figs. 3*A* and 3*B*). It is generated by using an articulated scan arm and offers flexible display capabilities, but the technique is somewhat cumbersome. The other type of B-mode display is so-called real-time ultrasonography. In this format a given area of anatomy is "imaged" and the scan is continuously updated by sequential scans at the rate of approximately 5 to 60 times per second. Displays for the real-time scans are of two basic types. One consists of a pie- or triangular-shaped image with the narrow portion of the display originating at the transducer and diverging with distance away from the transducer (Fig. 3*C*). This type of display is typical of scans generated by mechanical sector scanners, phased-array sector scanners, and annular-array scanners. The other type of display consists of a block (rectangular) image generated by linear array instruments. A linear-array transducer consists of approximately 60 piezoelectric crystals aligned in a single row (thus the rectangular shape of the transducer). Here the transverse dimensions of the image are proportional to the contact surface (cou-

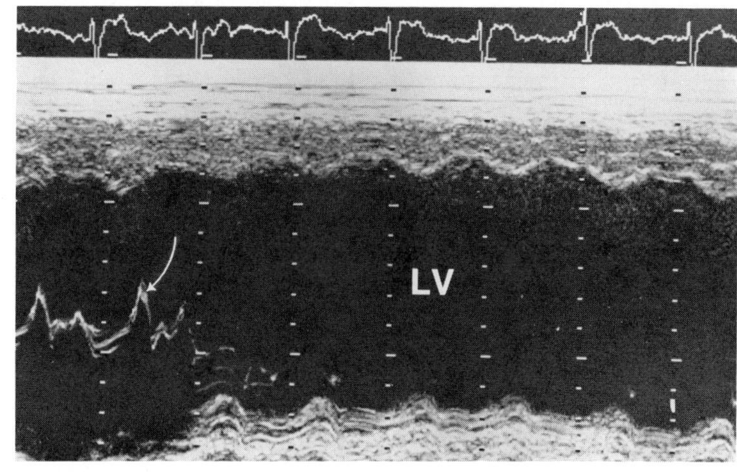

Figure 2. M-mode echocardiogram of the left ventricle (LV) of an adult Doberman pinscher with congestive cardiomyopathy. Left ventricle contractility is poor and the left ventricle chamber is dilated. Anterior mitral valve leaflet is indicated by a white arrow.

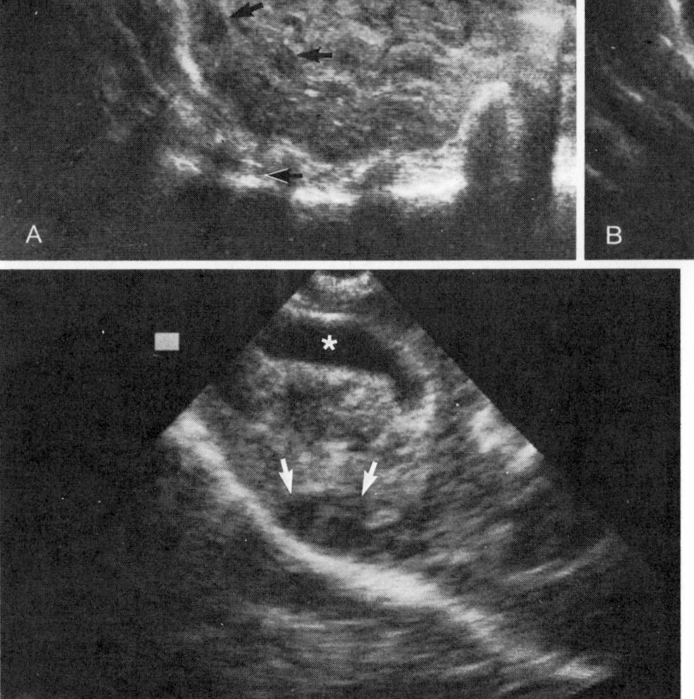

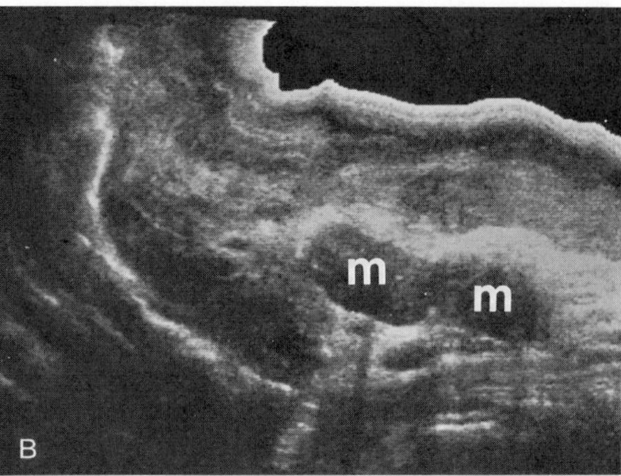

Figure 3. *A*, Supine, sagittal static B-scan of the liver of a young adult German shepherd dog with lymphosarcoma. Note the 1- to 4-cm diameter hypoechoic foci (arrows) in the liver. *B*, Scan similar to that in *A* but in a different sagittal plane. Two well defined, hypoechoic masses (m) in the area of the porta hepatis are illustrated. These proved to be hepatic lymph nodes infiltrated with lymphosarcoma. *C*, Supine, sagittal sector real-time scan of the same patient in which the gallbladder (*) can be identified as well as the hypoechoic foci (arrows) described in *A*. Note: displays are positioned with the patient's head to the left and the ventral body wall at the top.

pling interface) of the transducer. Sound waves penetrate in a rectangular format from the surface to depth. The advantages of a pie-shaped sector scan format is that small surface windows (coupling interfaces) can be used to display structures at various depths of dimensions exceeding those of the coupling interface because of the diverging format. However, resolution decreases with depth because of wider spacing between the scan vectors. The block-format linear-array display has the advantage of wide "near field" image display. It is associated with less image degradation with penetration because it does not consist of a diverging arrangement of scan information. However, any interference at the coupling surface (e.g., surface irregularity or poor coupling) will seriously degrade the image for the entire depth of the scan. All of the modes can be utilized at various frequencies, depending on the degree of resolution and the degree of penetration desired.

GENERAL INTERPRETATIVE PRINCIPLES

Echogenicity is basically a qualitative assessment of the amount of energy reflected within a given tissue or at a given interface. Echogenicity is displayed as brightness (difference between the displayed echo and the scan background). "Gray-scale" imaging, which is generally two-dimensional, is a display format with brightness proportional to the amplitude of the returning echoes. At the organ or tissue level, this intensity of reflected sound is basically determined by collagen and fat content. However, echogenicity without further penetration can also be detected at interfaces of materials that are drastically different from soft tissue, such as bone, air, and metal. Under these circumstances, only the echo at the interface on the transducer side of these materials will be identified, since nearly complete reflection of sound waves occurs. Therefore, greater depth of image cannot be achieved. At the other end of the spectrum are fluids and some solid masses (composed of highly uniform, densely packed internal components), which have few tissue interfaces to reflect echoes. These structures appear the same as the background and are differentiated by a phenomenon (distant enhancement) described in the following paragraph. Degree of echogenicity may be subjectively classified as increased (hyperechoic), normal (isoechoic), decreased (hypoechoic), or absent (anechoic), when compared with normal echo amplitudes expected for a given organ or tissue. Varied combinations of echo amplitudes encountered in pathologic processes such as tumors are described as unstructured (mixed) or as "target" lesions if they have some structural organization (i.e., a core and a rind).

Two artifactual phenomena occur in diagnostic ultrasonography that are of interpretive relevance. On is called distant (far) enhancement. This occurs when sound calibrated for routine soft tissues passes through fluid. The result is increased echogenicity or amplitude of returning echoes from structures deep (as viewed by the transducer) to the fluid-filled structure. This artifact does not occur for tissues located deep to hypo- or anechoic solid masses. The other phenomenon is called shadowing. Here complete or nearly complete reflection occurs at an interface between two vastly different tissues; only the side of the structure toward the transducer can be identified. Beyond this interface either no echoes or diffuse, unstructured echoes are visualized. This phenomenon is commonly associated with intestinal gas or bone encountered within a diagnostic ultrasound beam.

In addition to distant enhancement and shadowing, two other commonly encountered artifacts must be identified. Reverberation artifacts usually appear as evenly spaced bands of sound intensity within an image. These are most likely to be encountered distal (relative to the transducer) to a highly reflective structure such as bone, gas, or metal. However, they may also appear as low-level "dustlike" echoes in the near field (transducer side) of a fluid collection. "Slice thickness" artifacts may also occur. Since the ultrasound beam (even in its focal zone) has a finite diameter, echoes of different amplitudes from the same sample volume at a given depth are averaged when incorporated into the two-dimensional image. This may result in addition of echoes to the edge of an anechoic or hypoechoic structure or deletion of echoes from a hyperechoic interface at the edge of a hypoechoic or anechoic region. Knowledge of this phenomenon is particularly relevant in identification and classification of small fluid collections within parenchymal organs.

APPLICATIONS

Two-dimensional ultrasonography may be used as a primary means of assessing organs and body cavities, or it may be used to complement survey radiography. Our experience with use of this imaging technique has revealed that it provides information of intermediate quality compared with survey radiography and exploratory laparotomy when used to assess abdominal parenchymal organ disease. It will commonly reveal more specific information than will survey radiography, and it is considerably less invasive than pneumoperitonography or organ-specific selective angiography. Two-dimensional ultrasonography is of great value in the differential diagnosis of focal or multifocal disease (e.g., abscesses, cysts, neoplasms, and hematomas), particularly if serial ultrasonographic procedures are used in combination with other data (e.g., history and laboratory findings). Because it does not require use of iodinated contrast media to reveal specific parenchymal organs, it is not associated with risks and complications characteristic of excretory urography, angiocardiography, and parenchymal organ arteriography.

Two-dimensional ultrasonography provides a means by which the internal architecture of a mass or an organ can be identified. This becomes invaluable when it is necessary to determine whether a solid or cystic lesion originates within, invades, or is merely adjacent to a structure. It is also helpful in determining the extent of disease within and adjacent to specific organs, and it can be used to identify focal pathological areas within parenchymal organs. In the abdomen and thorax, ultrasound is not hindered (and in fact may be enhanced) by effusions.

Real-time ultrasonography may also be used to facilitate aspiration or needle biopsy of various organs and tissues. It adds a dimension of safety and accuracy to percutaneous biopsy techniques and has minimized need for exploratory laparotomy.

In small domestic animals, structures such as the liver, gallbladder, kidney, prostate, and spleen have a characteristic ultrasonographic appearance. Alteration of this normal pattern can usually be detected with ultrasonic imaging techniques. However, ultrasound is not a consistently reliable method of distinguishing between lesions caused by neoplasia, infections (usually abscess or granuloma), hematomas, and hyperplasia, Aspiration biopsy, punch biopsy, or surgical biopsy techniques are required to differentiate these abnormalities. Masses involving ovaries, adrenals, intra-abdominal testicles, and various abnormalities of the uterus (excluding pregnancy) must be assessed both by ultrasonographic architecture (which is not usually specific for that organ) and the topographical disruption induced by the change in this organ.

M-mode or two-dimensional echocardiography provides a noninvasive means of assessing cardiac size, internal cardiac structure, great vessels, and cardiac contractility. Echocardiography is particularly useful in detection of pericardial effusions (M-mode or two-dimensional format) and intra- or peri-

Table 1. *Availability of Diagnostic Ultrasonography Among North American Veterinary Institutions*

Institution	Location	M-mode Echocardi-ography	Mechanical Sector Echocardi-ography	Phased-array Sector Echocardiog-raphy	Sector Real-time General Imaging	Linear-array Real-time General Imaging	Static (B-scan) Imaging	High Resolution "Small Parts" Real-time Imaging†	Not Available
Animal Medical Center	New York, NY	x		‡	‡				
Angell Memorial Hosp.	Boston, MA	x							
Auburn University School of Vet. Med.	Auburn, AL	x	x		x	x		x	
University of Calif.-Davis School of Vet. Med.	Davis, CA	x	x		x	x		x	
Colorado State University School of Vet. Med.	Fort Collins, CO	x		x			x	x	
Cornell University New York State College of Vet Med.	Ithaca, NY	x	x		x				
Echo Affiliates, Inc.	Lexington, KY		x		x			x	
University of Florida College of Vet. Med.	Gainesville, FL	x	x		x	x		x	
University of Georgia Ontario Vet. College	Athens, GA	x	x		x		x		
University of Guelph Ontario Vet. College	Guelph, ON, Canada	x		x	x	x			
University of Illinois College of Vet. Med.	Urbana, IL	x	x		x	x	x	x	
Iowa State University College of Vet. Med.	Ames, IA	*			*	x			
Kansas State University College of Vet. Med.	Manhattan, KS	x	x		x	x			
Louisiana State University School of Vet. Med.	Baton Rouge, LA	x		x	x			x	
Michigan State University College of Vet. Med.	East Lansing, MI	x	*		*				
University of Minnesota College of Vet. Med.	St. Paul, MN	x	x		x	x	x		
Mississippi State University College of Vet. Med.	Starkeville, MS	x	x		x			x	
University of Missouri College of Vet. Med.	Columbia, MO								x
University of Montreal Faculty of Vet. Med.	St. Hyacinthe, PQ, Canada								x
North Carolina State Univ. School of Vet. Med.	Raleigh, NC	x	x		x				
Ohio State University College of Vet. Med.	Columbus, OH	x	x	x	x	x		x	
Oklahoma State University College of Vet. Med.	Stillwater, OK	x	x		x				
Oregon State University College of Vet. Med.	Corvallis, OR	Not applicable, Large Animal Clients *only*				x			
University of Pennsylvania School of Vet. Med.	Philadelphia, PA	x			x	x	x		
Purdue University School of Vet. Med.	West Lafayette, IN	x	x		x	x		x	
University of Saskatchewan Western College Vet. Med.	Saskatoon, SK, Canada		x		x			x	
University of Tennessee College of Vet. Med.	Knoxville, TN	x	x		x	x		x	
Texas A & M University College of Vet. Med.	College Station, TX		x		x				
Tufts University School of Vet. Med.	Boston, MA	x		‡	‡	x			
Tuskegee Institute School of Vet. Med.	Tuskegee, AL								x
Virginia-Maryland Regional College of Vet. Med.	Blacksburg, VA								x
Washington State University College of Vet. Med.	Pullman, WA	x		x	x	x		x	
University of Wisconsin School of Vet. Med.	Madison, WI	x	x		x				
Yale University School of Med.—Section of Comparative Medicine	New Haven, CT								x

*Soon to be available.
†Greater than 7.5 MHz for any type of real-time equipment. Need not be a *designated* "small parts" scanner.
‡Mechanical annular phased-array sector.

cardiac masses (best by two-dimensional format). Use of conventional radiography to obtain similar information mandates the use of iodinated contrast media, sedatives, and anesthetics, all of which may have undesirable effects in compromised patients.

To date, ultrasonography appears to be the safest "imaging" modality available to veterinarians. Safety applies to the patient as well as the ultrasonographer. As knowledge about the *in vivo* effects of ultrasound increases, undesirable biologic effects may be identified. However, these are likely to be applicable only to patients directly exposed to the ultrasound beam and not the examiner, since the frequency and intensity of ultrasound produced is not readily transmitted in air.

AVAILABILITY

Diagnostic ultrasonography has achieved widespread acceptance at veterinary referral centers (Table 1). Because of its cost, it is unlikely that "state-of-the-art" equipment will be routinely available in private practice for several years. A plausible alternative, however, is use of mobile ultrasound technical services provided for human patients. Affordable portable ultrasound equipment is becoming available to veterinarians in private practice. However, portable machines have specific limitations. These should be investigated before purchase is considered. If necessary, ultrasonic images can be evaluated by a veterinary specialist.

Although ultrasonography provides much assistance in defining and assessing the extent of disease processes, considerable expertise is required to interpret the images. The clinical specialists most often involved with ultrasonography are either radiologists or cardiologists. In addition to radiologists, internists and theriogenologists are also potential resources for abdominal sonographic investigations.

References and Supplemental Reading

Bonagura, J. D.: M-mode echocardiography: Basic principles. Vet. Clin. North Am. 13:299, 1983.

Cartee, R. E., and Rowles, T.: Transabdominal sonographic evaluation of the canine prostate. Vet. Radiol. 24:156, 1983.

Cartee, R. E., and Rowles, T.: Preliminary study of the ultrasonographic diagnosis of pregnancy and fetal development in the dog. Am. J. Vet. Res. 45:1254, 1984.

Feeney, D. A., Johnston, G. R., and Hardy, R. M.: Two-dimensional gray scale ultrasonography for assessment of hepatic and splenic neoplasia in the dog and cat. J.A.V.M.A. 184:68, 1984.

Feeney, D. A., Johnston, G. R., and Walter, P. A.: Two-dimensional gray scale abdominal ultrasonography: General interpretation and abdominal masses. Vet. Clin. North Am., 15:1225, 1975.

Konde, L. J., Wrigley, R. H., Park, R. D., et al.: Ultrasonographic anatomy of the normal canine kidney. Vet. Radiol. 25:173, 1984.

Leo, F. P.: Real-time ultrasound technology. *In* Saunders, R. C., and Hill, M. (eds): *Ultrasound Annual.* New York: Raven Press, 1983, pp. 47–68.

Nyland, T. G., and Park, R. D.: Hepatic ultrasonography in the dog. Vet. Radiol. 24:74, 1983.

Rantanen, N. W., and Ewing, R. L.: Principles of ultrasound application in animals. Vet. Radiol. 22:196, 1981.

Thomas, W. P.: Two-dimensional real-time echocardiography in the dog: Technique and anatomic validation. Vet. Radiol. 25:50, 1984.

NUCLEAR IMAGING: APPLICATIONS AND AVAILABILITY

GARY R. JOHNSTON, D.V.M.,
DANIEL A. FEENEY, D.V.M.,
and PATRICIA A. WALTER, D.V.M.
St. Paul, Minnesota

NUCLEAR IMAGING

Radioactive isotopes play an important role in clinical medicine in that they are used routinely for *in vitro* and *in vivo* diagnostic procedures and therapy. Diagnostic nuclear imaging consists of parenteral administration of radiolabeled pharmaceuticals for assessment of an organ's structure and function. Diagnostic nuclear imaging provides information about functional capabilities of an organ that cannot be assessed with conventional radiography, ultrasonography, or computed tomography. The purpose of this chapter is to review applications of nuclear imaging for diagnosis of various diseases in companion animals and to provide information about North American veterinary referral centers with nuclear imaging capabilities.

RADIOACTIVE ISOTOPES

All matter is composed of a limited number of elements, which are made up of atoms. An atom is composed of a nucleus and an encircling electron shell that balances the electrical charge of the nucleus. The configuration of electrons in the atom determines the chemical properties (e.g., chemical bonding and valence) of the element, whereas the nuclear composition (e.g., number of protons and neutrons) characterizes the stability and radioactive decay of the nucleus. The nucleus is composed of protons and neutrons, collectively called nucleons. Protons are positively charged; neutrons have no charge. The number of protons in the nucleus is referred to as the atomic number. Mass number consists of the number of protons and neutrons within the nucleus. A nuclide designates any species of atom characterized by the constituents of its nucleus; it may be stable or unstable. If the nuclide is unstable, it is referred to as a radionuclide. Unstable radionuclides decay by spontaneous disintegration from an unstable nuclear configuration to a stable one. During the process of nuclear decay, nuclear disintegration or transformation occurs by spontaneous fission with emission of particles (alpha or beta) or electromagnetic radiation (gamma rays). In this fashion the radionuclide is transformed into a stable nuclide. Nuclides of the same atomic number (i.e., same number of protons) are called isotopes and have the same properties.

Electromagnetic radiation (gamma rays) emitted during nuclear decay provides the major source of energy used in diagnostic nuclear imaging. The decay of radionuclides is a random process. In a population of a specific radionuclide, decay will occur in a predictable manner characteristic of that isotope. Every radionuclide is characterized by its physical half-life ($T\frac{1}{2}$), which is defined as the time required to reduce the initial number of atoms by 50 per cent. Consequently, a radionuclide can be characterized by its physical half-life, particle or gamma ray emission (or both), and gamma ray constant.

The radioactivity of a radionuclide is the number of disintegrations per unit time. A unit of radioactivity is called a curie and is defined as the radioactivity of a sample that is decaying at a rate of 3.7×10^{10} disintegrations per second. The curie is a relatively large unit. A smaller unit more frequently utilized to define the activity of radionuclides used in diagnostic nuclear imaging is the millicurie.

Most radionuclides in human medicine are used for diagnostic nuclear imaging. However, they are also utilized for *in vitro* evaluation of hormones, enzymes, and other biologically active substances. Radionuclides are also used for therapy. For example, radioactive iodine (^{131}I) is routinely used to treat thyroid neoplasia and feline hyperthyroidism. Radioactive phosphorous (^{32}P) is utilized for treatment of polycythemia vera. Other radioisotopes with long half-lives and high-energy gamma emissions are routinely used for interstitial brachytherapy and external beam teletherapy (Feeney and Johnston, 1983).

RADIOPHARMACEUTICALS

Radionuclides may be used separately, or they may be incorporated into a variety of chemical compounds. Chemical compounds are selected because of biochemical, physiologic, or metabolic properties that allow their localization within a specific organ or body system. A chemical compound tagged with a radionuclide and prepared for *in vivo* use is referred to as a radiopharmaceutical. In nuclear medicine, nearly 95 per cent of the radiopharmaceuticals are used for diagnostic purposes; the rest are used for therapeutic applications.

In diagnostic nuclear imaging, the most commonly used radionuclide is technetium-99m (^{99m}Tc). Technetium-99m is a suitable radionuclide because of its short physical half-life (6 hours). In addition, it emits a gamma ray of 140 keV, which is appropriate for most diagnostic nuclear imaging procedures. A technetium-99m generator is used to produce this radionuclide, which is the daughter compound of an unstable parent radionuclide of a longer half-life.

The long physical half-life (8 days) and medium energy (364 keV) of radioactive iodine (^{131}I) makes it less suitable than technetium-99m for diagnostic nuclear imaging. Other radionuclides utilized in diagnostic nuclear imaging include indium-111 (^{111}In), xenon-133 (^{133}Xe), and gallium-67 (^{67}Ga).

The pharmaceutical is selected on the basis of pharmacologic and physiologic properties that allow it to be localized within a desired organ. Mechanisms of localization of various radiopharmaceuticals are variable. For example, an active transport mechanism concentrates radioactive iodine in the thyroid gland. Also, radiolabeled red blood cells are used to determine volume of red blood cells. Bone imaging with technetium-99m–labeled phosphorous compounds is dependent on simple exchange or diffusion mechanisms. Phagocytosis of radiolabeled sulfacolloids by cells in the spleen, liver, and bone marrow allow imaging of these organs. Radiolabeled macroaggregates that cause capillary blockage are utilized in pulmonary perfusion imaging.

DETECTION

Radiopharmaceuticals are administered in millicurie quantities for diagnostic procedures. To determine the quantity and location of a radionuclide within a patient, one must measure the disintegration rate, which is a direct indication of nuclear decay and, therefore, the amount of radioactive material present. A variety of radiation detectors are currently utilized for *in vivo* and *in vitro* detection of radiation. Scintillation detectors convert the energy of the incident gamma ray photon into an electrical impulse. Each incident gamma ray photon produces an electrical impulse whose magnitude is proportional to the energy of the incident photon. Conversion of energy of the gamma ray photon into an electrical impulse is a two-step process. The first step takes place in the scintillation crystal, composed of sodium iodide with a trace amount of thallium. The thickness and dimension of the scintillation crystal is variable and depends upon its intended use. The thallium, used as an activator within the sodium iodide crystal, creates imperfections in the crystal lattice so that atoms within it may readily assume elevated energy states. When a gamma ray photon strikes such a crystal, energy from the gamma ray photon is absorbed. The absorbed energy causes electrons to move to a higher energy level in a number of atoms within the crystal. This higher state of orbital energy is unstable and immediately reverts to its initial stable energy level with subsequent dissipation of light photons. Consequently, the scintillation crystal is an energy-converting device utilized to change the energy of the gamma ray photon into a flash of visible light. The intensity of the light produced is proportional to the energy of the gamma ray photon that excited the crystal.

The second step in the conversion of gamma ray energy into an electrical impulse results when light falls upon the cathode of a photomultiplier tube and causes emission of electrons. The electrons that are ejected from the cathode sequentially strike a series of charged electrodes in such a manner that they cause additional electrons to be ejected from the electrodes. The amplitude of the electrical impulse produced from the photomultiplier tube is proportional to the energy of the gamma ray photon that excited the crystal. Electrical impulses produced within the photomultiplier tube may be further amplified by a linear electronic amplifier to produce either a numerical determination within a well counter or a point source that can form an organ image detected by a stationary or moving scintillation detector.

Gamma ray radiation coming from the patient travels in a straight line, but is emitted in all directions. Therefore, it must be focused onto the detector crystal. It is important to exclude all gamma rays originating outside the area of interest from reaching the detector crystal. This is achieved by use of a lead collimator, a device that limits the field of view of a radiation detector. The collimator will allow incident gamma ray photons to enter only through the holes within it. The design of a collimator for use in nuclear imaging depends on its application. Parallel-hole, converging/diverging, and pinhole collimators are routinely used in diagnostic nuclear imaging equipment.

Two basic types of detectors utilized routinely in diagnostic nuclear imaging include the rectilinear scanner and a scintillation gamma camera. The rectilinear scanner utilizes a moving detector as the basis for image formation. A rigid bar with a scintillation detector and collimator is positioned so that radiation emitted from a point source within the patient passes through the collimator and onto the face of the detector. The electronic impulses arising within the detector are subsequently amplified and passed onto an image-recording device at the end of the bar. The image bar travels in a transverse plane across the area of interest. At the end of the transverse motion, a longitudinal shift is made and the detector moves in a direction opposite to the original motion. This cycle of back-and-forth motion is repeated until the desired area to be scanned by the detector in completed. The terminology of nuclear "scans" was coined from the scanning motion of the moving detector system. Information regarding the intensity of radiation from any given point source is transferred by an electrical impulse from the detector to the recording printer. The printer constructs an image from radiation that strikes the detector as it traverses back and forth across the patient. Because the collimator of a rectilinear scanner will accept radiation from points at a given distance in front of it, it is called a focusing collimator. Focusing collimators of rectilinear scanners exclude information outside the focal zone of the collimator. This is a distinct disadvantage in imaging large organs, because a hot spot may be missed if the lesion is outside the focal plane of the collimator. Another disadvantage of using rectilinear scanners in companion animals is the length of time (30 minutes or longer) required to complete a scan of an organ. This would require heavy sedation or general anesthesia to prevent the patient's motion from interfering with image acquisition during the scanning procedure.

Stationary imaging devices, such as the gamma camera, are most commonly used in veterinary and human diagnostic nuclear imaging. When these devices are used, neither the patient nor the detector moves during image formation. The gamma camera utilizes a scintillation detector that is approximately one-half (½) inch thick and 10 to 12 inches or more in diameter. A collimator plate with holes of varying diameter, number, and configuration covers the surface of the detector crystal. With detector crystals of 10 to 15 inches in diameter, most large organs can be adequately covered without repositioning the patient. An array of 19 to 37 or more photomultiplier tubes is positioned above the crystal to detect light flashes within it. The photomultiplier tube directly above the light flash receives the most light and produces the largest electrical impulse. Adjacent photomultiplier tubes receive less light and accordingly produce weaker electrical impulses. Electrical impulses from all photomultiplier tubes are passed through an electrical network in such a manner that four electrical impulses are obtained. These four electrical impulses carry transverse and longitudinal information about the location of a particular radiation event, and the geometric information obtained for the longitudinal and transverse coordinates is displayed on a cathode ray tube. The process of acquisition of individual light flashes on the photomultiplier tube is repeated thousands of times each second. As a result, an image of the organ builds up on the film of a camera focused on the oscilloscope or on some other recording device.

Gamma cameras are currently utilized in many veterinary institutions and are superior to rectilinear scanners because they are more efficient radiation detectors. Because of the larger field of view of the gamma camera, an organ can be imaged within a few seconds to a few minutes. Image formation by a gamma camera is fast enough to permit dynamic functional studies. In contrast, rectilinear scanners produce stationary views of a static organ. Because of the rapid image formation of a gamma camera, general anesthesia is not required. The spatial resolution of a gamma camera is greatest at the surface of the collimator and diminishes with increased distance from its face. This differs from the rectilinear scanner, in which the best resolution is in the focal plane of the collimator. The use of multiple "scanning" views is consequently employed to obtain the maximum amount of information in the organ scan. Variations in collimator design influence sensitivity and therefore spatial resolution. Collimators vary in thickness of the septum between the collimator holes, in the number of holes, and in their diameter. By using a computer interface with a gamma camera, dynamic functional studies can be performed in which time-activity curves can be constructed to evaluate organ function.

Nuclear imaging equipment available within North American veterinary institutions is listed in Table 1.

APPLICATIONS OF NUCLEAR MEDICINE TO SPONTANEOUS ANIMAL DISEASES

Diagnostic applications of nuclear imaging to spontaneous diseases of companion animals are summarized in Table 2. Although the capacity to perform specific imaging procedures exists at many referral centers, their practicality, risks, and benefits should be carefully assessed before organ scanning begins. The referring clinician should consult with those performing the nuclear imaging procedures to determine if nuclear imaging (compared with other diagnostic procedures) can further characterize the patient's disease.

Thyroid Imaging

Radionuclides are used for *in vivo* and *in vitro* thyroid function tests, anatomic thyroid imaging, and treatment of thyroid disorders. Physiologic processes that facilitate thyroid imaging are related to trapping (uptake from the blood) and organification (such as the iodination of tyrosine to produce diiodotyrosine) of various iodine radionuclides or iodine analogues. In humans, various isotopes of iodine have been used for *in vivo* and *in vitro* imaging. Technetium-99m (^{99m}Tc) and iodine-131 (^{131}I) are the two common radioisotopes utilized for imaging, functional assessment, and treatment of the thyroid gland. Technetium-99m, an iodine analogue, is trapped within the thyroid gland but is not organified. Technetium-99m also localizes within the gastric mucosa, salivary glands, and choroid plexus. The maximum uptake of technetium-99m within the thyroid gland occurs approximately 20 to 30 minutes after intravenous injection. Technetium-99m is currently utilized in thyroid imaging because of its short half-life (6 hours) compared with that for iodine-131 (8 days). The higher energy of iodine-131 increases the risk of radiation exposure and therefore requires more restrictions than does the use of technetium-99m. Technetium-99m has been used as a thyroid imaging agent in cats with feline hyperthyroidism and in dogs with thyroid neoplasms (Fig. 1). Iodine-131 has also been used to treat feline hyperthyroidism and thyroid neoplasia.

Bone Imaging

Bone scans are commonly performed in man and animals. They are much more sensitive than conventional radiography for detecting osseous lesions. Approximately 50 per cent of the bone mineral must be removed before it can be detected by conventional radiographic techniques. Bone scans utilizing technetium-99m–labeled phosphorous compounds can detect lesions within days of the initial insult, whereas the lesion may not be detected by radiography until 10 to 14 days after the insult. Localization of the radiopharmaceutical in bones is dependent upon the skeletal blood supply and mineral exchange at the interface of bone and extracellular

Table 1. *Nuclear Imaging Veterinary Referral Centers in North America*

		Nuclear Imaging Availability			Nuclear Imaging Equipment		
Institution	**Location**	*Not Available*	*Available Through Local Hospital, Medical School, or Allied Hospital*	*Available Within Veterinary Institution*	*Rectilinear Scanner*	*Gamma Camera Without Computer Assistance*	*Gamma Camera With Computer Assistance*
Animal Medical Center	New York, NY			x			x
Angell Memorial Hosp.	Boston, MA		x				x
Auburn Univ. School of Vet. Med.	Auburn, AL			x	x	x	
Univ. of Calif.-Davis, School of Vet. Med.	Davis, CA			x			x
Colorado State Univ., Coll. of Vet. Med.	Fort Collins, CO	x					
Cornell Univ., N.Y. State, Coll. of Vet. Med.	Ithaca, NY			x	x	x	x
Univ. of Florida, Coll. of Vet. Med.	Gainesville, FL	x					
Univ. of Georgia, Coll. of Vet. Med.	Athens, GA			x		x	
Univ. of Illinois, Coll. of Vet. Med.	Urbana, IL			x		x	x
Iowa State Univ., Coll. of Vet. Med.	Ames, IA	x					
Kansas State Univ., Coll. of Vet. Med.	Manhattan, KS			x			x
Louisiana State Univ., School of Vet. Med.	Baton Rouge, LA			x		x	
Michigan State Univ., Coll. of Vet. Med.	East Lansing, MI	x					
Univ. of Minnesota, Coll. of Vet. Med.	St. Paul, MN			x		x	x
Mississippi State Univ. Coll. of Vet. Med.	Starkeville, MS		x				x
Univ. of Missouri-Columbia, Coll. of Vet. Med.	Columbia, MO			x			x
Univ. of Montreal, Faculty of Vet. Med.	St. Hyacinthe PQ, Canada	x					
North Carolina State Univ., Coll. of Vet. Med.	Raleigh, NC						x
Ohio State Univ., Coll. of Vet. Med.	Columbus, OH			x		x	
Oklahoma State Univ., Coll. of Vet. Med.	Stillwater, OK	x					
Ontario Vet. College Univ. of Guelph	Guelph, ON, Canada	x					
Oregon State Univ., Coll. of Vet. Med.	Corvallis, OR	x					
Univ. of Pennsylvania, School of Vet. Med.	Philadelphia, PA		x		x	x	x
Purdue Univ., School of Vet. Med.	West Lafayette, IN			x		x	
Univ. of Saskatchewan, Western Coll. of Vet. Med.	Saskatoon, SK, Canada	x					
Univ. of Tennessee, Coll. of Vet. Med.	Knoxville, TN			x		x	
Texas A & M Univ., Coll. of Vet. Med.	College Station, TX			x	x	x	x
Tufts Univ., School of Vet. Med.	Boston, MA			x			x
Tuskegee Inst., School of Vet. Med.	Tuskegee, AL	x					
Virginia-Maryland Regional Coll. of Vet. Med.	Blacksburg, VA	x					
Washington State Univ., Coll. of Vet. Med.	Pullman, WA			x			x
Yale Univ., School of Med., Section of Comparative Med.	New Haven, CT	x					

***Table 2.** Availability and Types of Nuclear Imaging Procedures Among Veterinary Referral Centers*

Institution	Location	Thyroid Glands		Bone	CNS	Lungs	Hepato-biliary System	Kidneys
		Imaging	*Ablation*					
Animal Medical Center	New York, NY	x	x	x	x	x	x	x
Angell Memorial Hosp.	Boston, MA	x		x		x	x	x
Auburn University, School of Vet. Med.	Auburn, AL	x		x	x	x	x	x
University of Calif.-Davis, School of Vet. Med.	Davis, CA	x	x	x	x	x	x	x
Cornell University, New York State College of Vet. Med.	Ithaca, NY	x	x	x	x	x	x	x
University of Georgia, College of Vet. Med.	Athens, GA	x		x	x	x	x	x
University of Illinois, College of Vet. Med.	Urbana, IL	x	x	x	x	x	x	x
Kansas State University, College of Vet. Med.	Manhattan, KS	x		x	x	x	x	x
Louisiana State University, School of Vet. Med.	Baton Rouge, LA	x		x	x	x		x
University of Minnesota, College of Vet. Med.	St. Paul, MN	x	x	x	x	x		x
Mississippi State University, College of Vet. Med.	Starkeville, MS	x			x	x		
University of Missouri-Col., College of Vet. Med.	Columbia, MO	x		x		x		
North Carolina State Univ., School of Vet. Med.	Raleigh, NC	x		x	x	x	x	x
Ohio State University, College of Vet. Med.	Columbus, OH	x		x	x	x	x	x
University of Pennsylvania, School of Vet. Med.	Philadelphia, PA	x	x	x	x	x	x	x
Purdue University, School of Vet. Med.	West Lafayette, IN	x		x	x	x		
University of Tennessee, College of Vet. Med.	Knoxville, TN	x	x	x	x	x	x	x
Texas A & M University, College of Vet. Med.	College Station, TX	x	x	x	x	x	x	x
Tufts University, School of Vet. Med.	Boston, MA	x		x	x	x	x	x
Washington State University, College of Vet. Med.	Pullman, WA	x		x	x	x	x	x

fluid. It is believed that radiolabeled phosphate compounds bind to the surface of hydroxyapatite crystals by absorption. However, the exact mechanisms are incompletely understood.

Because reactive bone changes are present in most cases of focal bone disease, accumulation of the radiopharmaceutical is not pathognomonic for a specific disease. Localization of the "hot spot" allows localization of a disease process that may then be further evaluated by biopsy techniques. Bone scans have been utilized in veterinary medicine for evaluation of metastatic disease, osteomyelitis, fracture healing, degenerative joint disease, osteonecrosis, and unexplained bone pain and for identification of sites of occult disease. Serial bone scans may also be utilized for monitoring response to therapy, planning of fields for radiation therapy, and finding suitable biopsy sites.

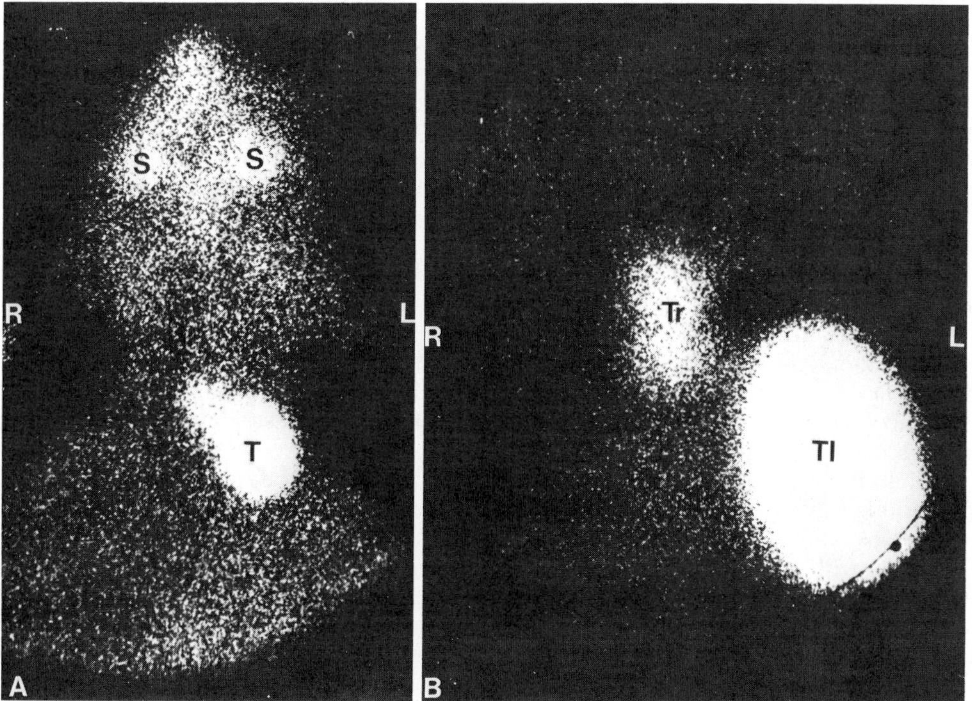

Figure 1. *A*, Ventrodorsal view of a nuclear scan of the thyroid glands of a 12-year-old male castrated domestic longhair cat with hyperthyroidism. Note uptake of the radionuclide pertechnetate (^{99m}Tc) in the region of the thyroid glands *(T)* and salivary glands *(S)*. *B*, A close-up view of the thyroid glands obtained with the aid of a pinhole collimator revealed uptake of ^{99m}Tc in the left *(Tl)* and right *(Tr)* thyroid glands. These findings are indicative of thyroid adenomas.

Imaging of the Central Nervous System

Nuclear imaging provides the clinician with a noninvasive diagnostic modality that can be used for evaluation of lesions within the central nervous system. In the normal healthy patient, an anatomic and physiologic barrier (blood brain barrier) allows entrance of some molecular substances and exclusion of others. In the presence of disease, alteration of this barrier permits radiopharmaceuticals to pass through it and localize within a site of disease. The nuclear scan will show an area of increased radioactivity at a site of uptake within the parenchymal tissue one to two hours after intravenous injection of the radiopharmaceutical.

Nuclear scans have been utilized for evaluation of neoplasias, infarctions, subdural hematomas, and abscesses. However, increased activity within the cortical parenchyma is not pathognomonic for any disease entity. Lesions of neoplastic, inflammatory, or traumatic origin may result in a similar appearance viewed by nuclear imaging. Serial nuclear scans in patients with CNS lesions may be utilized as a prognostic indicator.

Imaging of Lungs

The nuclear imaging of lungs involves perfusion and ventilation studies. Pulmonary perfusion studies utilize radiolabeled macroaggregated albumin or microspheres, which are larger than the pulmonary capillaries and result in obstruction of the lumens of these vessels. After intravenous injection, radiopharmaceuticals pass through the right heart directly into pulmonary capillaries and arterioles, where they become lodged. Distribution of the radiopharmaceutical is dependent upon arterial perfusion of the lungs. Consequently, lung perfusion scans are utilized for evaluation of perfusion defects caused by pulmonary thrombi or emboli. Normal lung perfusion scans are characterized by uniform distribution of radioactivity throughout the lungs. If vascular obstruction has occurred, an area of decreased perfusion ("cold spot") can be detected.

Pulmonary perfusion studies have been performed concurrently with pulmonary ventilation studies for evaluation of human respiratory function. Xenon-133 (^{133}Xe) in either a gaseous state or dissolved in liquid is utilized for ventilation studies, which are infrequently performed in veterinary medicine because the radioactive gas exhaled by the patient must be collected.

Technetium-99m–labeled aerosols delivered by an ultrasonic nebulizer are currently being evaluated for pulmonary ventilation studies. This technique has the advantage of reducing contamination of the environment with a radioactive agent such as xenon-133.

Hepatobiliary Imaging

Hepatic parenchymal and biliary scintigraphy provides information about hepatic architecture, vascular perfusion, and biliary excretion. Radiolabeled sulfacolloids are used for evaluation of hepatic parenchymal disease. Reticuloendothelial cells within the liver (and also spleen and bone marrow) phagocytize the sulfacolloid particles, resulting in a diffuse uptake of the radioisotope. The major limitation of hepatic scintigraphy is its inability to detect lesions beyond a critical distance from the collimator. Lesions 6 to 8 mm in diameter can be identified at the collimator face, but resolution decreases with increased distance. Lesions 10 cm from the collimator must be 2 cm in diameter to be detected.

Hepatic scintigraphy with sulfacolloid can be utilized for evaluation of primary or secondary hepatic neoplasia, abscesses, and traumatic injuries. Space-occupying lesions within the liver displace and disrupt the reticuloendothelial system and result in cold spots. If there is a generalized decrease in reticuloendothelial cell function within the liver, the isotope may become localized in reticuloendothelial cells of the spleen, bone marrow, and lung. The uptake of radiolabeled sulfacolloid by the reticulendothelial cells is proportional to hepatic arterial and portal blood flow. Quantitative estimations of hepatic blood flow have been used for evaluation of dogs with portal vascular anomalies.

Radioisotopes utilized for biliary scintigraphy (cholescintigraphy) are removed from the blood vascular system and excreted into the biliary system. In this technique, radiolabeled isotopes are actively transported through a carrier-mediated process at the cell membrane of the hepatocytes. Excretion of the isotope into biliary canaliculi and subsequent passage into the gallbladder or duodenum provide a functional assessment of bile production and patency of the cystic and common bile ducts. Injection of exogenous cholecystokinin will provide additional information about the functional capabilities of the gallbladder. Biliary scintigraphy is utilized for evaluation of acute cholecystitis in human patients and for differentiating obstructive from nonobstructive jaundice.

The use of ultrasonography for evaluation of hepatic and biliary anatomy has reduced the use of hepatic scintigraphy for evaluation of hepatic architecture.

Renal Imaging

A variety of radiopharmaceuticals have been developed for evaluation of structural and functional abnormalities of the kidneys. However, ultrasonography and computed tomography are superior to nuclear imaging procedures for assessing anatomic detail of renal structure. Noninvasive radionephrology studies are utilized routinely for serial evaluation of renal function in human patients with renal dysfunction and in renal transplant recipients. Quantitative assessments of total or individual renal blood flow, effective renal plasma flow, glomerular filtration rate, and functional renal mass can be achieved with computer-assisted nuclear imaging. The physiologic basis of radiopharmaceuticals utilized for evaluation of renal morphology and function involve glomerular filtration, tubular reabsorption, and tubular secretion.

Miscellaneous Nuclear Imaging Procedures

Gastrointestinal scintigraphy can be used for evaluation of esophageal transit and clearance, gastroesophageal reflux, gastric emptying, and intestinal bleeding. Gastrointestinal hemorrhage may be detected by use of radiolabeled red blood cells injected intravenously and followed by imaging of the abdomen for foci of activity. Application of this technique to companion animals should provide additional information about possible sites of involvement of gastrointestinal bleeding. Radiolabeled amino acids, proteins, immunoglobulins, and fatty acids have been used for evaluation of protein catabolism, anabolism, and protein-losing enteropathies in humans and companion animals.

Lymphoscintigraphy consists of interstitial injection of radiolabeled colloids, which are then cleared from the injection site by the lymphatic system. The radiolabeled colloids are subsequently trapped in lymphatic vessels and sinusoids of the reticuloendothelium system of the draining lymph nodes. Lymphoscintigraphy has been utilized in dogs for evaluation of metastatic spread of mammary neoplasms. Radiolabeled leukocytes have also been utilized for evaluation of the lymph nodes in humans for staging neoplastic disease and for planning surgery or radiation therapy.

Radiolabeled iodocholesterol is used in patients with adrenal disorders, and adrenal imaging is most useful in cases of hypersecretion of adrenal hormones. Use of ^{131}I-labeled cholesterol requires the use of imaging techniques on the patient several days after the intravenous injection of the isotope. Radiolabeled iodocholesterol has been utilized for evaluation of dogs with bilateral adrenal cortical hyperplasia and adrenal tumors.

Radioimmunodiagnosis and radioimmunotherapy are two fields in human medicine that have developed rapidly after recent advances in development of radiopharmaceuticals, production of monoclonal antibodies, and isolation of other immunoglobulins with sufficient specificity for tumor diagnosis. Before the development of monoclonal antibodies, autologous and heterologous antibodies for cancer diagnosis were limited because of insufficient quantities of purified tumor-specific antibodies. Radiolabeled monoclonal antibodies have been used extensively for detecting tumors and tumor byproducts in man.

Gallium citrate (^{67}Ga) has been utilized in imaging the effects of occult inflammatory disease. Gallium citrate will localize within polymorphonuclear leukocytes in areas of inflammatory disease. More recently, leukocytes labeled with indium-111 (^{111}In) have been utilized for localization within occult sepsis.

Nuclear cardiology encompasses computer-assisted nuclear imaging for estimating left and right ventricular function, myocardial perfusion, blood volume, chamber volume, cardiac output, and regurgitant flow.

RADIATION SAFETY

Use of radionuclides in diagnostic and therapeutic nuclear medicine present a potential radiation safety hazard to the client, clinician, and individuals providing supportive care for patients, and consequently, radiation safety requirements must be applied. Isolation facilities with access limited to personnel trained in the safe handling of radioactive wastes may be required by the institution. Patients receiving technetium-99m may require 48 to 72 hours of hospitalization in an isolation facility until surface exposure is reduced to background levels of radiation. Radionuclides with longer half-lives (e.g., iodine-131, T½ = 8 days) may require longer periods of confinement before the level of radiation is reduced to an acceptable level. Hospitalization in an isolation facility to reduce radiation exposure to people working with a patient will result in increased cost for nuclear imaging procedures. The referring clinician should consult with the individual in charge of nuclear imaging at the veterinary institution to determine the cost and duration of hospitalization required for each procedure.

References and Supplemental Reading

Allhonds, R. V., Kallfetz, F. A., and Lust, G.: Radionuclide joint imaging: An ancillary technique in the diagnosis of canine hip dysplasia. Am. J. Vet. Res. 41:230, 1980.

Barber, D. L., and Roberts, R. E.: Imaging nuclear. Vet. Radiol. 24:60, 1983.

Baum, S., and Bromlet, R.: *Basic Nuclear Medicine*. New York: Appleton-Century-Crofts, 1975.

Dijkshovra, N. A., and Rijraberk, A.: Detection of brain tumors in dogs by scintigraphy. J. Am. Vet. Radiol. Soc. 18:147, 1977.

Feeney, D. A., and Johnston, G. R.: Radiation therapy: Applications and availability. *In* Kirk, R. W. (ed.): *Current Veterinary Therapy VIII*. Philadelphia: W. B. Saunders, 1983, pp. 428–434.

Hightower, D., Feldman, R. G., Chester, D. K. et al.: Thyroid scanning in the diagnosis of thyroid neoplasia in two dogs. J.A.M.A. 158:734, 1970.

Hood, D. M., Hightower, D., and Tatum, M. E.: Lung perfusion imaging in the dog. J. Am. Vet. Radiol. Soc. 18:124, 1977.

Hornof, W. J., Koblick, P. D., and Breznock, E. M.: Radiocolloid scintigraphy as an aid to the diagnosis of congenital portocaval anomalies in the dog. J.A.V.M.A. 182:44, 1983.

Kallfetz, F. A., de Lahunta, A., and Allhonds, R. V.: Scintigraphic diagnosis of brain lesions in the dog and cat. J.A.V.M.A. 172:589, 1970.

Koblick, P. D., Hornof, W. J., and Breznock, E. M.: Quantitative hepatic scintigraphy in the dog. Vet. Radiol. 24:226, 1983.

Peterson, M. E., and Becker, D. V.: Radionuclide thyroid imaging in 135 cats with hyperthyroidism. Vet. Radiol. 25:23, 1984.

Powers, T. E., Power, J. D., and Garg, R. C.: Study of the double isotope single-injection method for estimating renal function in purebred beagle dogs. Am. J. Vet. Res. 38:1933, 1977.

Thrall, D. E., and Gillette, E. L.: Canine lung scanning. J. Am. Vet. Radiol. Soc. 12:88, 1971.

Turrel, J. M., Feldman, E. C., Marquerite, H., et al.: Radioactive iodine therapy in cats with hyperthyroidism. J.A.V.M.A. 184:554, 1984.

Ueltschi, G.: Bone and joint imaging with ^{99m} Tc labelled phosphates as a new diagnostic aid in veterinary orthopedics. J. Am. Vet. Radiol. Soc. 18:80, 1977.

CONTROL OF NOSOCOMIAL INFECTIONS

ROBERT L. JONES, D.V.M.

Fort Collins, Colorado

CLINICAL IMPORTANCE

Nosocomial (hospital-acquired) infections are those that occur during hospitalization but were not present or incubating at the time of admission. Such infections may become clinically apparent during hospitalization or after discharge from the hospital. As a general rule, new infections occurring after 48 hours of hospitalization can be considered to be nosocomial. A frequent misconception is that nosocomial infections occur as epidemics caused by an organism from the hospital environment or another patient. Nosocomial infections are frequently caused by endogenous microorganisms inhabiting the patient's flora. Bacteria are the most frequent agents involved in nosocomial infections, but viruses, chlamydia, mycoplasma, fungi, and protozoa can also be involved.

The incidence of nosocomial infections in veterinary hospitals has not been investigated. However, it is probably similar to that found in human hospitals, in which the rate is approximately 5 per cent of hospitalized patients. Although the highest incidence rates are observed in large referral or teaching hospitals, nosocomial infections can occur in any veterinary practice. Urinary tract, respiratory tract, and surgical and wound infections and bacteremia associated with IV catheters are common nosocomial infections.

PREDISPOSING FACTORS

Overview

For a nosocomial infection to develop, a potential pathogen must be transmitted to a susceptible patient. Hospitalized patients are continuously exposed to microorganisms from their own flora and environmental sources that can cause infections. The likelihood that the patient will become infected depends upon the complex interactions of four major factors: (1) the virulence of the agent, (2) the patient's susceptibility to infection by the agent, (3) the nature of exposure to the agent, and (4) the effect of antimicrobial therapy.

Potential Pathogens

The classic contagious diseases of veterinary medicine are usually controlled by immunization, isolation, or hygiene. Occasional transmission of virulent pathogens may occur in the hospital. However, most nosocomial infections are caused by opportunistic bacteria that infrequently cause infections in healthy, nonhospitalized animals. Nosocomial infections are not limited to failures to control infection, but often result from acquisition of bacteria that cause infection as a result of invasive medical procedures. These bacteria commonly acquire resistance to antimicrobials and disinfectants. The modern era of antimicrobial therapy has led to the selection of multiple-drug-resistant (MDR) strains of microbes. Important nosocomial pathogens include gram-negative *Klebsiella, Pseudomonas, Enterobacter, Escherichia coli, Serratia,* and *Salmonella.*

The sources of these opportunistic pathogens include people, animals, inanimate objects, air currents, and occasionally insects or rodents. Once bacteria gain entrance into the hospital, they become a part of the "normal flora" of animals. Therefore, the patient becomes its own major reservoir for endogenous infection. Common sites of colonization include the upper respiratory and the digestive tracts. Antimicrobial therapy plays an important predisposing role in colonization with these microbes.

Patient Susceptibility

Numerous interacting risk factors increase the likelihood of nosocomial infections in hospitalized patients. The most important factors include extremes of age (neonate or geriatric), critical illness, chronic debilitating disease, pre-existing infections, and antimicrobial therapy. Host defenses may be impaired by steroid or immunosuppressive therapy and by altering normal anatomic barriers with invasive instruments such as catheters and endoscopes. Prolonged hospitalization (especially preoperative), the duration of surgery, the site of the operation, and surgical implants are also risk factors for nosocomial infection. Other factors, such as illness and antimicrobial therapy, may alter the normal flora and allow colonization by opportunistic pathogens; others operate by allowing noninvasive bacteria to infect tissues. Finally, some factors compromise the host's immunological and inflammatory reactions.

Antimicrobial Therapy

Widespread use of antimicrobial therapy has prolonged the survival of critically ill patients. As a result, high-risk patients have extended periods of hospitalization that result in more opportunity for nosocomial infections. Use of antimicrobial agents may suppress the normal enteric flora and increase the risk of colonization of the patient with antimicrobial-resistant opportunistic pathogens.

Normally, the host and the anaerobic bacterial flora of the digestive tract act cooperatively and synergistically to limit colonization by potentially pathogenic bacteria. This mechanism is known as "colonization resistance." Oral therapy with partially absorbed antimicrobials, or parenteral therapy with antimicrobials excreted into the intestine in active form, may lead to a decrease in colonization resistance if the anaerobic flora is susceptible to the drug. Antimicrobials have been classified according to the effect they have on colonization resistance (Table 1). In order to minimize nosocomial infections, one must consider the effect of antimicrobials on colonization resistance.

In addition to suppressing normal flora, antimicrobial therapy selects for antimicrobial-resistant bacteria. Resistance to more than one agent frequently occurs and is usually plasmid-mediated.

Table 1. *Effect of Antimicrobial Drugs on Host Resistance to Microbial Colonization*

Antimicrobials that suppress colonization resistance with resulting increase in Enterobacteriaceae colonization:
- Ampicillin
- Cloxacillin
- Metronidazole
- Furazolidone

Antimicrobials with a moderate effect on colonization resistance:
- Amoxicillin
- Tetracycline
- Chloramphenicol

Antimicrobials with no adverse effect on colonization resistance:
- Cephalosporins
- Aminoglycosides
- Trimethoprim
- Sulfonamides
- Doxycycline
- Erythromycin
- Penicillins (parenteral)

Therefore, use of one antimicrobial may select for bacteria with resistance to unrelated agents.

A common example of inappropriate use of antimicrobials in veterinary medicine is the use of oral ampicillin as a prophylactic agent against urinary tract infections (UTIs). Orally administered ampicillin is poorly absorbed. Approximately half the oral dose remains in the lumen of the digestive tract to inhibit anaerobes and suppress colonization resistance. At the time of suppressed colonization resistance, ampicillin-resistant enteric bacteria may multiply. Because species of *Klebsiella* are resistant to ampicillin, they are the most favored organism. If other enterics such as *E. coli* or species of *Enterobacter* or *Proteus* are selected, they will probably become resistant to ampicillin by means of a plasmid-carried resistance factor. Accumulation of large numbers of these organisms in feces increases the risk of UTI. Therefore, the resulting therapy-associated UTI will be ampicillin-resistant. Often these MDR bacterial pathogens are resistant to tetracycline and some aminoglycosides. Recently, resistances to chloramphenicol, cephalothin, and trimethoprim have been observed in MDR nosocomial pathogens isolated from veterinary hospitals.

The therapeutic problem of dealing with MDR bacteria can result from spread of a single strain of bacteria in a hospital. However, several different bacteria with the same resistance pattern are frequently seen in outbreaks of nosocomial infections. This occurs because the plasmid-mediated resistance is readily transferred between gram-negative bacteria. The specific genetic determinant for resistance to an antimicrobial can also readily move between plasmids and the bacterial chromosome. Therefore, antimicrobial therapy may result in selection for an endemic plasmid or resistance factor rather than an endemic strain of bacteria.

In summary, use and misuse of antimicrobials are important risk factors for nosocomial infections. Antimicrobial therapy increases the risk of colonization by MDR bacteria that are difficult to treat once infection becomes established.

EPIDEMIOLOGIC PATTERNS

When the incidence of nosocomial infections is low, they tend to occur sporadically and are caused by a variety of opportunistic organisms. They may not be recognized as nosocomial infections but rather are interpreted as "complications." Serious nosocomial infections are usually first recognized when they occur in epidemic form. Epidemics are usually caused by the same organism and often have a unique pattern of resistance to antimicrobials. However, nosocomial infections caused by a single organism are often associated with outbreaks caused by several strains of gram-negative MDR bacteria. These MDR bacterial strains can occur in either epidemic or endemic patterns.

Epidemic occurrence of MDR bacterial nosocomial infection may result from poor aseptic technique, poor housekeeping associated with crowding of patients, and excessive use of antimicrobials. Attempts to control these discrete episodes usually encompass a search for contaminated objects and efforts to improve asepsis (especially handwashing by hospital personnel). These procedures often control rather than eliminate nosocomial infections. Failure to eradicate the problem occurs because other MDR bacteria or plasmids occur endemically.

This endemic occurrence of MDR bacteria in a hospital environment may result from several factors. Animals admitted or readmitted after antimicrobial therapy are a common source. These animals may not have infection at the time of admission but are colonized with MDR bacteria. During the course of hospitalization, the animal may become infected from its own flora, or MDR bacteria may spread to other patients. Spread from patient to patient is facilitated primarily by the hands of hospital personnel. Less frequently, spread may occur by contact between patients or by environmental contamination. Antimicrobial therapy increases the population of MDR bacteria in patients, facilitating an endemic reservoir.

STRATEGIES FOR CONTROL

General Principles

ENVIRONMENTAL SANITATION. Control of nosocomial infections involves development of standards

Table 2. *Priorities for Control of Nosocomial Infection*

Handwashing
Antiseptics, aseptic techniques
Gloves, gowns
Cleaning, disinfection of facilities and equipment
Sterilization of critical items
Controlled use of antimicrobial drugs
Isolation procedures
Microbiological surveillance

of patient care that prevent spread of microorganisms to patients and introduction of microorganisms into normally sterile body sites (Table 2). The required levels of antisepsis can be classified as critical, semicritical, and noncritical, according to the type of contact an object has with a patient. Critical antisepsis applies to any item introduced directly into sterile areas of the body. In this situation, destruction of all contaminating microorganisms by sterilization is essential. Semicritical antisepsis applies to devices that contact mucous membranes, since they can readily transmit colonizing bacteria from one patient to another. Noncritical antisepsis applies to hospital facilities and surfaces that offer little risk of transmitting infectious agents. Cleaning these surfaces with a detergent is usually adequate; disinfection may also be considered.

Handwashing by all hospital personnel before and after handling each patient is vital for control of nosocomial infections. Abrasive scrubbing and irritating antiseptics should be avoided, because they tend to hinder the desire of hospital personnel to wash their hands frequently. Vigorous washing under running water for 10 seconds will usually remove bacterial contaminants. In some situations, the risk of contamination is so great (e.g., a known infected wound or catheterization procedure) that gloves should be worn.

Environmental monitoring programs are recommended to ensure proper hygiene. The functioning of autoclaves and other methods of sterilization must be checked periodically. Instructions for use of antiseptics and disinfectants should be followed so that proper concentrations and contact times are observed. Microbiological surveillance of the environment by culturing should be restricted to investigation of epidemics caused by a single organism that might be originating from a contaminated object. Usually, visual and white-glove inspections provide adequate evaluations of cleaning procedures when combined with an analysis of possible sources of contamination.

CONTROL OF NOSOCOMIAL EPIDEMICS. Control of epidemics of nosocomial infection requires identification of reservoirs of infectious agents. Colonized and infected patients are the most common sources, although environmental contamination may be important. Transmission from these reservoirs to susceptible, noncolonized patients must be decreased (Table 2). Emphasis should be placed on handwashing, aseptic techniques, and separation of susceptible patients from colonized or infected patients. An important factor in long-term control of nosocomial infections is the restricted use of antimicrobials. It may be necessary to restrict or rotate these agents in high-density areas such as ICUs. Restriction of antimicrobial agents often results in a decrease of outbreaks with MDR bacteria. It is also important to avoid prescribing subinhibitory doses of antimicrobials. Sometimes it is necessary to suspend use of specific antimicrobial agents.

CONTROL OF NOSOCOMIAL ENDEMICS. Control of endemic MDR nosocomial infections requires extension of epidemic control measures to all patients in the hospital. Barrier-type precautions, including segregation, isolation, gloves, and gowns, are recommended. These precautions should be applied to all patients, even before culture results are obtained. Careful surveillance of patients and results from the microbiology laboratory must be maintained to detect miniepidemics of two or more similar MDR isolates. Control of the use of antimicrobials is important but may have limitations in long-term prevention. Because one antimicrobial may select for cross-resistance to other plasmid-carried MDR factors, limiting use of a specific antimicrobial may not eliminate development of resistance to other antimicrobials. Sequential acquisition of MDR characteristics may occur when antimicrobials are rotated.

If control procedures become lax, low numbers of colonizing MDR bacteria may emerge. Therefore, all hospital personnel should be encouraged to maintain ongoing control procedures.

Detection of certain resistance patterns, such as gentamicin resistance or MDR, may indicate nosocomial infection. If a miniepidemic is recognized, aggressive corrective measures must be instituted. Special barrier-type containment procedures should be routine in hospital areas (such as ICUs) that serve as centers for high-risk patients and intensive (and often invasive) therapy. Colonized or infected patients that may be shedding MDR bacteria should be identified with signs on their cages so that all personnel will comply with control procedures.

ISOLATION. Isolation is an important method of prevention and control of nosocomial infections. Infectious diseases should be grouped by their mode of transmission; the patient can then be managed according to the appropriate method of isolation (Table 3). Frequently there is reluctance to initiate isolation procedures because of inadequate physical facilities or because of expected inconveniences. However, practical isolation procedures need not be overly stringent to be effective. When isolation protocols are designed, the objective should be to

Table 3. *Types of Isolation*

Strict isolation
Respiratory isolation
Wound and skin precautions
Enteric precautions
Protective isolation

isolate the disease rather than the patient. Therefore, routes of microbial exit and entry, environmental survival of microbes, and fomite transmission should be considered. In recent years, there has been excessive reliance on disinfectants and antimicrobial drugs. Handwashing and other patient management factors are also important, especially in the face of increasing bacterial resistance.

Special Control Measures

URINARY SYSTEM. Urinary tract infections are the most common type of human nosocomial infection, and although data are lacking, they are probably the most frequent group of nosocomial infections in small animals. An intact urethra is the best safeguard against nosocomial urinary tract infection. Cystocentesis should routinely be performed for collecting diagnostic urine specimens from dogs and cats. When catheterization becomes necessary for proper care of the patient (rather than for the convenience of hospital personnel), aseptic technique must be utilized. The perineal area should be washed and covered with an antiseptic agent. Hands must be washed and sterile gloves worn for insertion of a sterile catheter.

Since the animal's lower urinary tract is usually colonized with potential pathogens before catheterization, nosocomial infection results from endogenous bacteria. Indwelling urinary catheters should be secured to prevent movement and attached to a closed drainage system to prevent reflux of contaminated urine. Special effort must be taken to prevent contamination of the drainage system whenever it is disconnected and reconnected or when urine is removed. Prophylactic antimicrobials should not be used to prevent nosocomial urinary tract infections, since they promote emergence of resistant organisms. When urinalysis or urine culture indicates infection, an appropriate antimicrobial should be prescribed.

RESPIRATORY SYSTEM. Bacteria may enter the lower respiratory system by the hematogenous route, by aspiration, or by inhalation. Prevention of hematogenous pneumonia requires consideration of other sources and sites of infections, such as IV and urinary catheters. Hospitalized and critically ill patients are predisposed to pharyngeal colonization by gram-negative bacilli. Aspiration of these bacteria or introduction of them through endotracheal tubes and endoscopes may lead to serious nosocomial pneumonia. Therefore, gloved hands, sterile equipment, and aseptic techniques should be used for tracheal intubation, bronchial aspiration, and tracheostomy. Equipment placed into the respiratory tract must be cleansed and sterilized or disinfected to prevent inhalation of bacteria. Prophylactic antimicrobials have limited value in prevention of nosocomial pneumonia.

INFECTIONS OF SURGICAL SITES AND WOUNDS. Prevention of surgical infection requires excellent preoperative care. Although wounds frequently are contaminated or infected before treatment, care must be used to prevent superinfections while the animal is hospitalized. Surgical procedures performed on contaminated tissues are associated with increased risk of infection. Other factors that increase the risk of infection include duration of preoperative hospitalization, duration of the operation, magnitude of tissue devitalization, location of the incision or wound, foreign bodies or surgical implants, and remote infections.

Aseptic principles of surgery should be used consistently. Perioperative antimicrobial prophylaxis is often indicated. It must be initiated one to two hours before surgery to attain therapeutic levels of antimicrobials in tissues at the time of surgery. Continued administration of antimicrobials after completion of the operation is seldom indicated, except for wounds already contaminated or infected.

IMMUNOCOMPROMISED PATIENTS. Alteration of normal host defense mechanisms is an important predisposing cause of nosocomial infection. Compromised defenses are frequently associated with malignant disease because of such factors as immunosuppression, physical interference by the neoplastic mass, older age, immunosuppressive therapy, and surgery. Control of nosocomial infections in these patients is best approached by protective isolation rather than by use of prophylactic antimicrobials.

GASTROINTESTINAL INFECTIONS. Epidemic enteric infections are enhanced in hospitals with a high population density of patients. Transmission of most pathogens occurs by oral ingestion of the feces of infected animals. Transmission of enteric pathogens may be prevented by intense cleaning and disinfection of hospital facilities. Hospital wards should be constructed from nonporous surfaces that can be disinfected readily. Personnel must be careful not to spread enteric pathogens with their hands and feet.

Pathogens such as species of *Salmonella* and *Campylobacter* are potential zoonotic agents. Therefore, hospital personnel should follow practices of good hygiene for their own safety. The use of prophylactic antimicrobials is usually contraindicated because they may reduce colonization resistance of the digestive tract and thereby increase the risk of enteritis.

BLOOD-BORNE INFECTIONS. Proper management

of IV infusions is important in prevention of nosocomial bacteremic infections. Contamination of IV catheters and fluids results in delivery of bacteria into the blood stream, bypassing all primary defense barriers. To prevent contamination, catheterization should be performed by using aseptic surgical techniques. The skin must be adequately prepared by shaving, washing, and application of antiseptics. Hands must be washed and covered with sterile gloves.

Movement of catheters should be minimized by firmly securing them in place. Catheters should not be used longer than 48 hours; connecting tubes and bottles should be changed at least every 24 hours. Many IV solutions will support rapid growth of contaminating bacteria at room temperature. Therefore, care must be taken to prevent contamination by reflux into the system or by airborne agents. Prophylactic antimicrobials have limited efficacy while intravenous catheters are in place.

CONCLUSIONS

The ideal approach to preventing nosocomial infections is to preserve and enhance host defenses. However, many patients are in the hospital with primarily or secondarily compromised defenses. Therefore, they are at high risk for developing infections associated with the therapy they receive. The single most important practice that will decrease the incidence of nosocomial infections is handwashing, since disinfectants and antimicrobial drugs have become less effective with emergence of resistant pathogens.

Judicious use of antimicrobials is one factor that veterinarians can control. Overuse of prophylactic antimicrobial therapy must be avoided. Misuse of antimicrobials promotes the selection for resistant opportunistic pathogens and increases the likelihood of nosocomial infections. Clinicians must be knowledgeable of the pharmacodynamics of antimicrobials so that the risk of nosocomial infections can be reduced.

References and Supplemental Reading

Bennett, J. V., and Brachman, P. S. (eds.): *Hospital Infections.* Boston: Little, Brown, 1979.

Finegold, S. M., Mathisen, G. E., and George, W. L.: Changes in human intestinal flora related to the administration of antimicrobial agents. *In* Hentges, D. J. (ed.): *Human Intestinal Microflora in Health and Disease.* New York: Academic Press, 1983, pp. 355–446.

Guidelines for the Prevention and Control of Nosocomial Infections. U.S. Department of Health and Human Services (not dated).

Harris, A. A., Levin, S., and Trenholme, G. M.: Selected aspects of nosocomial infections in the 1980s. Am. J. Med. 77:3, 1984.

Hirsh, D. C., and Enos, L. R.: The use of antimicrobial drugs in the treatment of diseases of the gastrointestinal tract. *In* Kirk, R. W. (ed.): *Current Veterinary Therapy VIII.* Philadelphia: W. B. Saunders, 1983, pp. 794–75

Manual on Control of Infection in Surgical Patients. Philadelphia: J. B. Lippincott, 1976.

Nosocomial Infection Surveillance, 1980–1982. Morbidity and Mortality Weekly Report, CDC Surveillance Summaries. 32:1SS, 1984.

van der Waaji, D.: *Antibiotic Choice: The Importance of Colonization Resistance.* Chichester, UK: Research Studies Press, 1983.

PROPHYLACTIC USE OF ANTIMICROBIAL AGENTS IN SURGICAL PATIENTS

ROBERT W. KIRK, D.V.M.
Ithaca, New York

Prophylaxis refers to the administration of antimicrobials to uninfected patients who are in jeopardy of acquiring a bacterial infection. Factors influencing the risk of infection include age, obesity, diabetes, infection elsewhere in the body, compromised defense due to immunosuppression (either natural or by drugs), time in the hospital, duration of surgery, skill of the surgeon, size of incision, size of inoculum, and incorporation of foreign body.

The prophylactic use of antimicrobial agents remains a controversial subject. Most trials in man or animals have been designed in such a way that conflicting data can be quoted. In essence, one would like to know if the use of antimicrobials prophylactically is effective in preventing infection, and if so, do the benefits clearly outweigh the hazards and costs.

The potential advantages are decreased mortality,

morbidity, hospital stay, and cost. The potential hazards and costs include adverse drug reactions, alteration of the host's normal bacterial flora, and development of resistant organisms. Although impeccable surgical skills and procedures are major deterrents to potential infection, meticulous technique might be relaxed if the surgeon relies too much on antimicrobials to prevent infection. Prophylaxis might also merely delay the onset of infection, and total costs could be increased. Evaluation of a prophylactic protocol involves many variables. One must consider the age and condition of the patient, the underlying diagnosis, the surgical procedure and time, the surgeon's skill, the drug or drugs used, and the dose, route, and duration of treatment.

In man, no study has shown that prophylaxis significantly reduces mortality, and although some trials have demonstrated a decreased morbidity, they failed to delineate the clinical significance of the differences (seriousness of fever and infection, and the impact it had on the clinical course). One should keep in mind that an optimal physiologic status (nutrition, fluid, electrolyte, and acid-base balance) before surgery is just as important as, if not more important than, prophylactic antibiotics in enhancing the patient's resistance to infection. In human trials, allergic and toxic reactions were remarkably uncommon and the incidence of infections caused by resistant bacteria was low. When prophylaxis was effective, the greatest reduction in total antimicrobial use and costs occurred when inexpensive drugs were given for brief periods. Undue duration of drug administration increases the expense and enhances the potential for untoward reactions and development of resistant organisms. In surgical cases, *the presence of adequate tissue levels of an appropriate drug during the operation is the critical determinant of effective prophylaxis.* This can usually be attained by a single parenteral preoperative dose. However, this can be achieved in several ways. Intramuscular therapy initiated 2 to 3 hours before surgery will have a continued effect during the surgical procedure. An alternative and perhaps more desirable procedure is intravenous administration of a bolus of the selected drug during anesthetic induction, with maintenance by intravenous drip throughout the surgical procedure. In most cases, therapy would cease with anesthetic recovery.

Routine use of antibacterial drugs in simple surgical procedures is considered to be a misuse of the drugs. Prophylactic antibiotic therapy is generally considered appropriate for high-risk surgical patients. This group includes:

1. Those whose natural defense mechanisms may be impaired by pre-existing disease or therapeutic regimens (liver cirrhosis, anemia, diabetes mellitus, extensive tissue damage, and corticosteroid or immunosuppressive chemotherapy).

2. Those in which bacterial contamination or bacteremia could result from surgery on an infected site (e.g., to excise an abscess, débride a contaminated wound, or extract infected teeth).

3. Those in which surgery will be extensive and involve prosthetic devices or a high risk of infection, such as major orthopedic or neurosurgical procedures. It is also indicated in those operations that invade the esophagus, lower bowel, bile ducts, or liver parenchyma and in patients with diseases with high mortality or a high morbidity of infection.

Effective prophylaxis requires high tissue levels of an appropriate antibiotic at the time of contamination. The effects of the drug need only be brief. For surgical cases it usually can be given parenterally prior to anesthesia and discontinued when the patient is in the recovery room. Except for surgery of the lower bowel or in cases of obvious contamination, it is almost never necessary or desirable to continue antibiotics for more than 24 hours after surgery. The latent period for most bacterial pathogens is 20 hours or less. The selection of the drug, the dosage form, and time of administration depends on anticipated contaminants, concomitant diseases, and time estimates for surgery.

A combination of oxacillin or ampicillin and gentamicin or kanamycin covers many problem cases. One of the cephalosporins may be useful in orthopedic cases, and erythromycin (in high doses) or metronidazole (alone or in combination) is effective for patients undergoing lower bowel surgery. The latter two drugs should be continued for one week to control anaerobes, which commonly infect tissues contaminated by bowel contents. In man, ampicillin applied topically was effective in preventing infection at the site of lower bowel surgery. Recent evidence suggests that with oral use, nonabsorbable antibiotics (such as the aminoglycosides) are *not* effective.

Ling and Hirsh (1983) have provided current statistical data on bacterial organisms found in several types of small animal infections and on organisms that commonly affect specific body systems. They also documented the antimicrobial agents with the best *in vitro* sensitivities in their series. Davis (1980) provided similar data from a different time period and from different geographic areas. It is emphasized that these results are helpful but should not be considered conclusive. They are useful guidelines. However, actual organisms and sensitivities for individual cases may be influenced by geographic location, environment, nosocomial infection, the individual's bacterial flora, presence of resistant pathogens, age, breed, and sex. In the course of daily practice one should accumulate data on bacterial cultures and antimicrobial susceptibilities from problem cases to build a file of information pertinent to *one's own situation.*

References and Supplemental Reading

Bartlett, S. P., and Burton, R. C.: Effects of prophylactic antibiotics on wound infections after elective colon and rectal surgery. Am. J. Surg. 145:300, 1983.

Burke, J. F.: The effective period of preventive antibiotic action in experimental incisions and dermal lesions. Surgery 50:161, 1961.

Davis, L. E.: Antimicrobial therapy. *In* Kirk, R. W. (ed.): *Current Veterinary Therapy VII.* Philadelphia: W. B. Saunders, 1980, pp. 2–16.

Guglielmo, B. J., Hohn, D. C., Koo, P. J., et al.: Antibiotic prophylaxis in surgical procedures—Critical analysis of the literature. Arch. Surg. 118:943, 1983.

Hirschman, J. V., and Inui, T. S.: Antimicrobial prophylaxis—A critique of recent trials. Rev. Infect. Dis. 2:1, 1980.

Ling, G. V., and Hirsh, D. C.: Principles of antibiotic therapy. *In* Kirk, R. W. (ed.): *Current Veterinary Therapy VIII.* Philadelphia: W. B. Saunders, 1983, pp. 41–47.

Van Scoy, R. E., and Wilkowske, C. J.: Prophylactic use of antimicrobial agents. Mayo Clin. Proc. 58:241, 1983.

Wilkowske, C. J., and Hermans, P. E.: General principles of antimicrobial therapy. Mayo Clin. Proc. 58:6, 1983.

CLINICAL ALGORITHMS: TOOLS THAT FOSTER QUALITY PATIENT CARE

CARL A. OSBORNE, D.V.M.
St. Paul, Minnesota

"No decision can be properly made without obtaining the relevant information"

DEFINITION

Algorithms are defined by Webster's dictionary as special methods of solving specific problems. The name *algorithm* was apparently derived from a ninth-century mathematician named Alkarismi. The change from *Alkarismi* to *algorithm* appears to have been influenced by the word *arithmetic.* Algorithms are reported to have first been used by computer scientists to represent the computer's stepwise solution to a problem (Margolis, 1983).

Clinical algorithms are organized sets of rules of procedures for solving diagnostic or therapeutic problems. Clinical algorithms are often represented graphically by a detailed, step-by-step decision tree for solving problems (Figs. 1 to 9). Each algorithm is a branching network of decision points. Each point branches into at least two paths, each path leading to successive decision points that in turn branch into at least two more points until a defined endpoint is reached. The endpoint is unique to the pathway leading from the point of origin. Properly constructed algorithms concisely, clearly, and consistently inform their users about which procedures to perform and the sequence in which various procedures are to be performed. They represent a "given this, do that" scheme of action.

ADVANTAGES

One reason for adopting use of clinical algorithms is that, like all predetermined rules or orders, they save time by eliminating the need for paramedical personnel to ask questions. Algorithms can be constructed to connect specific decisions to scientific literature that documents the decisions' validity or explains the rationale for the decisions. In this way they facilitate teaching. Algorithms also provide a format that facilitates thought and recall about clinical problems. In the setting of a busy hospital, they minimize the time required by medical personnel to reconstruct diagnostic or therapeutic plans. In addition, algorithms developed by systems or discipline specialists enable primary care veterinarians to manage problems that are otherwise beyond their level of competency. Algorithms can be constructed to emphasize preconceived priorities or probabilities. The use of algorithms facilitates consistency of clinical evaluation and therapy.

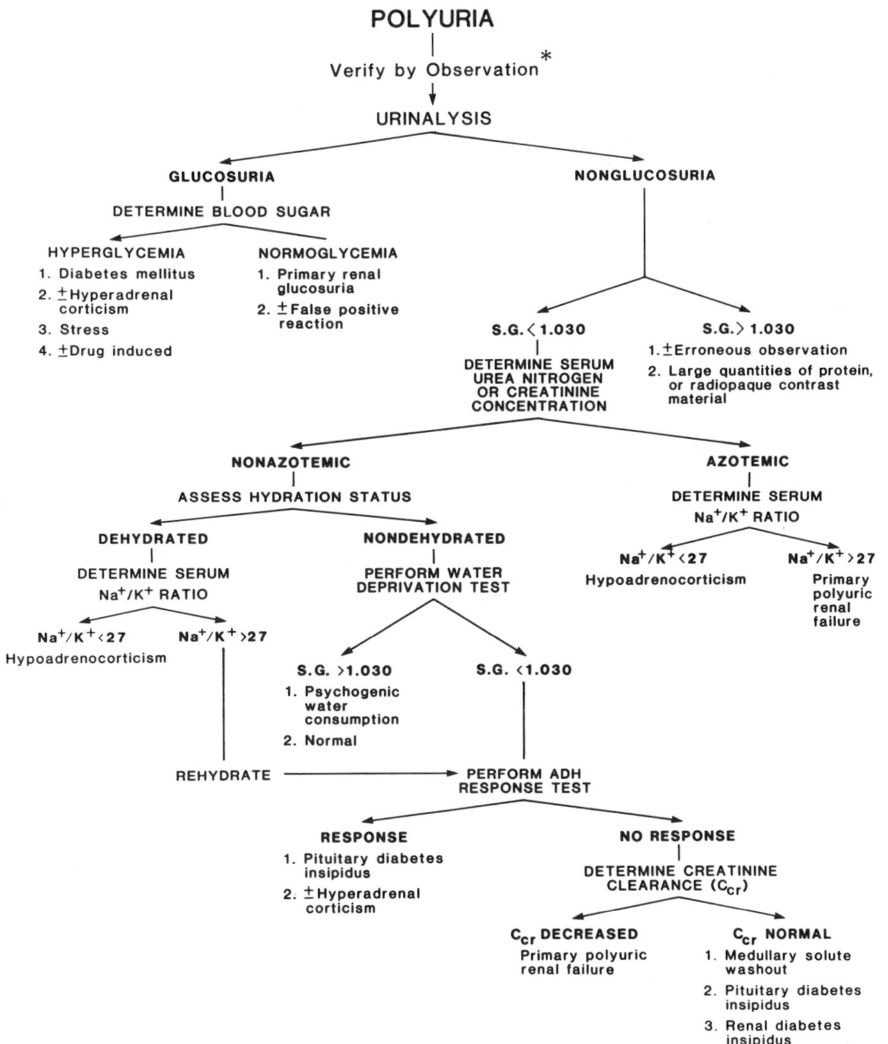

Figure 1. Diagnostic algorithm for canine chronic polyuric renal failure. The algorithm is based on probabilities. Exceptions to these generalities may occur.

*Measurement of 24-hour urine volume is recommended.

(From Polzin and Osborne *in* Kirk: *Current Veterinary Therapy VIII*. Philadelphia: W.B. Saunders, 1983.)

DISADVANTAGES

Despite their advantages, clinical algorithms are not the ultimate answer for consistent delivery of quality patient care. They cannot ensure accuracy of observations, and they have no judgment. Unlike decision analysis (which specifies the probability that a particular clinical state exists and quantitates the value of the outcome of the decision), the innate structure of an algorithm does not specify probability of outcome. If terms and directions are not carefully chosen and explained by their designer, different meanings may be conveyed to different users. Because exceptions to rules are frequent in biological systems, algorithms must be interpreted in the context of relevant probabilities. They rarely encompass all possibilities. However, it is important to recall that the minor exception does not negate the general rule.

DEVELOPMENT

It is beyond the scope of this discussion to provide an in-depth analysis of development of clinical algorithms. However, detailed information is available elsewhere (see list of references and supplemental reading). The following steps summarize the fundamentals involved in construction of a clinical algorithm.

1. Identify the topic that requires problem definition and solution by decision making (i.e., urinary tract disorders in companion animals).

2. Define the problem to be solved (i.e., the starting point). For example, it could be diagnostic evaluation of polyuria (Fig. 1) or therapeutic management of urinary tract infection (Fig. 9).

3. Specify who will solve the problem (such as paramedical staff, primary care veterinarians, or

Text continued on page 33

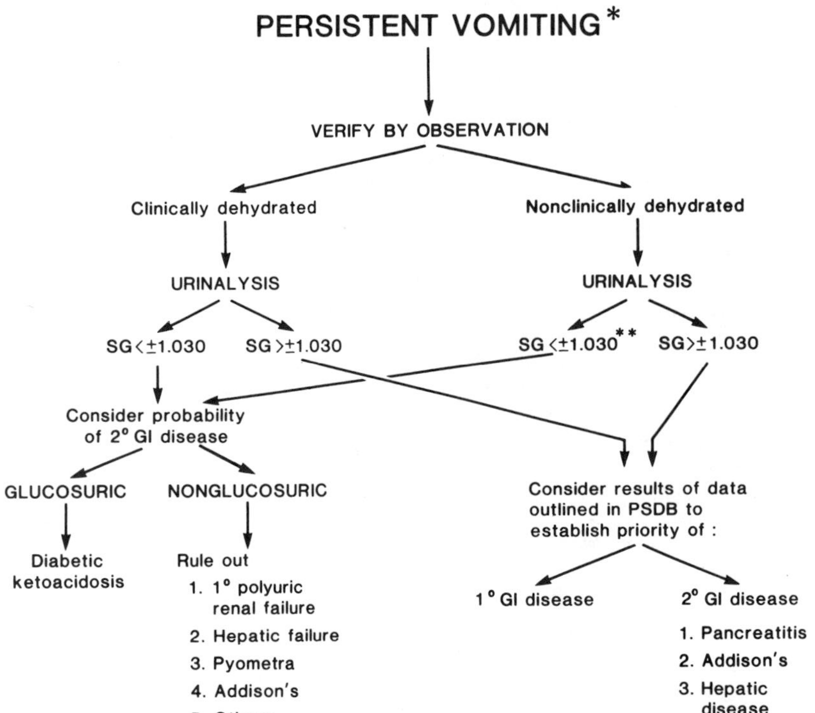

Figure 2. Diagnostic algorithm for persistent vomiting.

PSDB = Problem-specific data base.

*Urinalysis specific gravity calculated for dogs; to adapt for cats, substitute SG of 1.035 for SG of 1.030.

**Assuming patient subclinically dehydrated.

(From Klausner and Osborne: Vet. Clin. North Am. 11:523, 1981.)

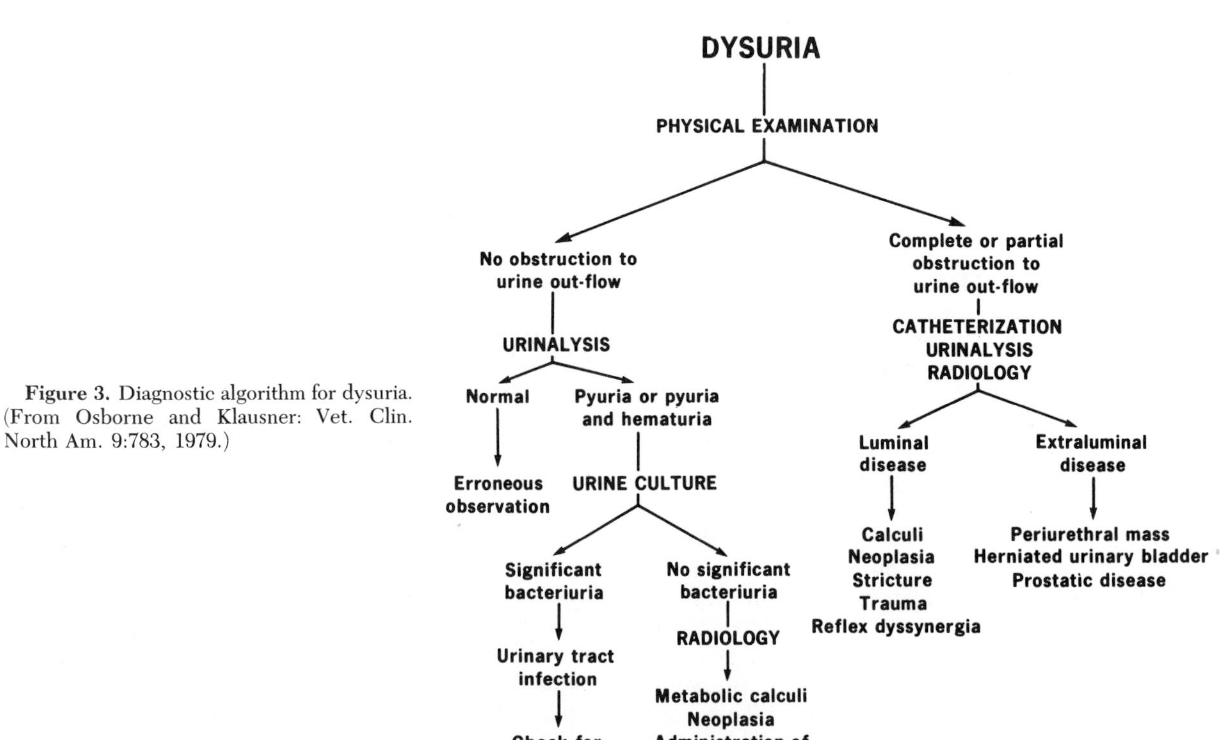

Figure 3. Diagnostic algorithm for dysuria. (From Osborne and Klausner: Vet. Clin. North Am. 9:783, 1979.)

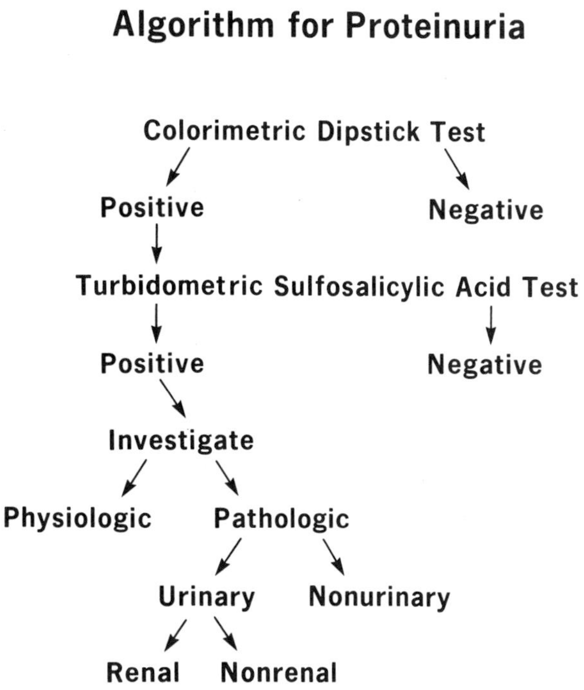

Algorithm for Proteinuria

Colorimetric Dipstick Test

Positive → Turbidometric Sulfosalicylic Acid Test

Negative

Turbidometric Sulfosalicylic Acid Test → Positive / Negative

Positive → Investigate

Investigate → Physiologic / Pathologic

Pathologic → Urinary / Nonurinary

Urinary → Renal / Nonrenal

Figure 4. Diagnostic algorithm for proteinuria. Consult Osborne and Stevens: *Handbook of Canine and Feline Urinalysis.* St. Louis, MO: Ralston Purina Co., 1981, for explanation.

URINARY INCONTINENCE

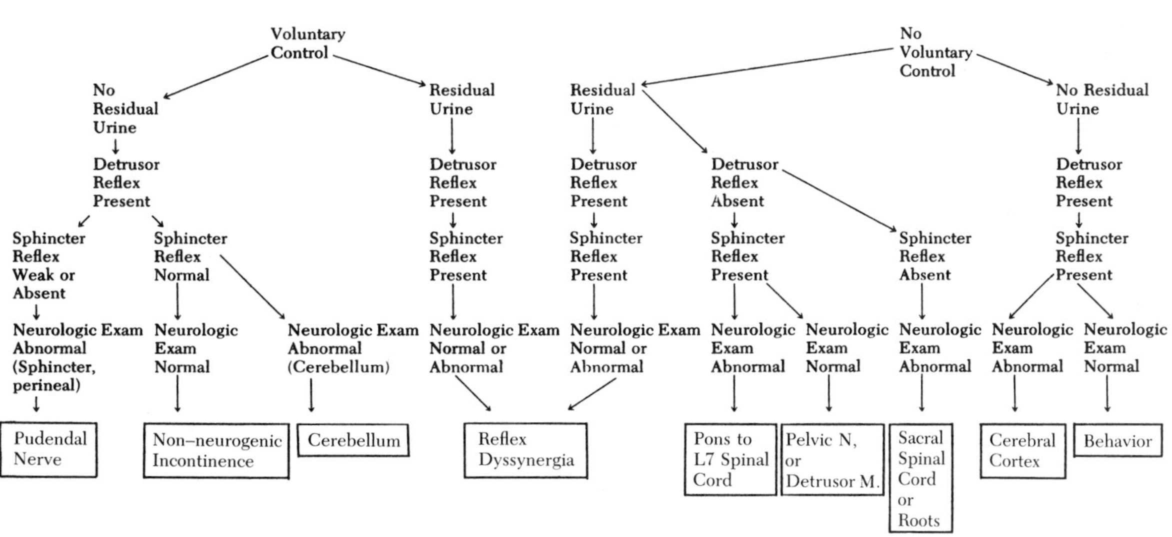

Figure 5. Clinical algorithm for localization of the cause of urinary incontinence. (From Oliver and Osborne *in* Kirk: *Current Veterinary Therapy VII.* Philadelphia: W. B. Saunders, 1980.)

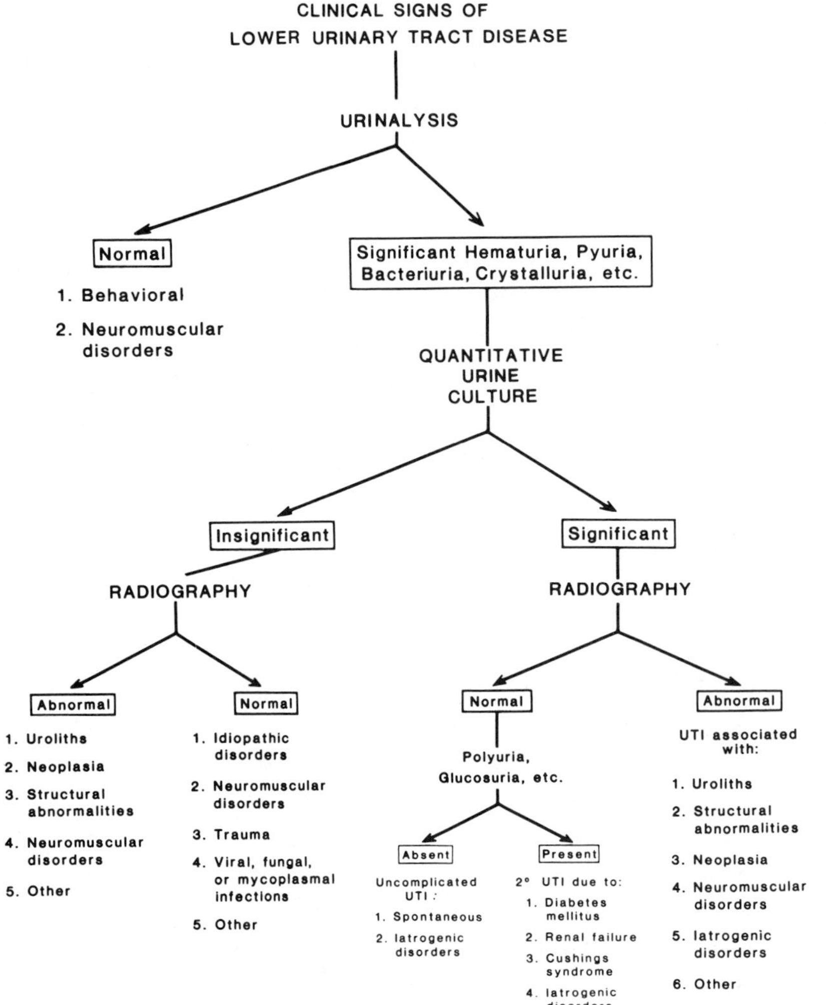

Figure 6. Diagnostic algorithm for feline lower urinary tract disorders. Urine samples for bacterial culture should be obtained by cystocentesis when possible. Recommended radiographic procedures include survey abdominal radiography (including the entire urinary tract from the penile urethra to the kidneys) and positive contrast urethrocystograms. Double contrast cystograms may be required to detect uroliths less than 3 mm in diameter. (From Polzin and Osborne *in* Slatter: *Textbook of Veterinary Surgery.* Philadelphia: W. B. Saunders, 1984.)

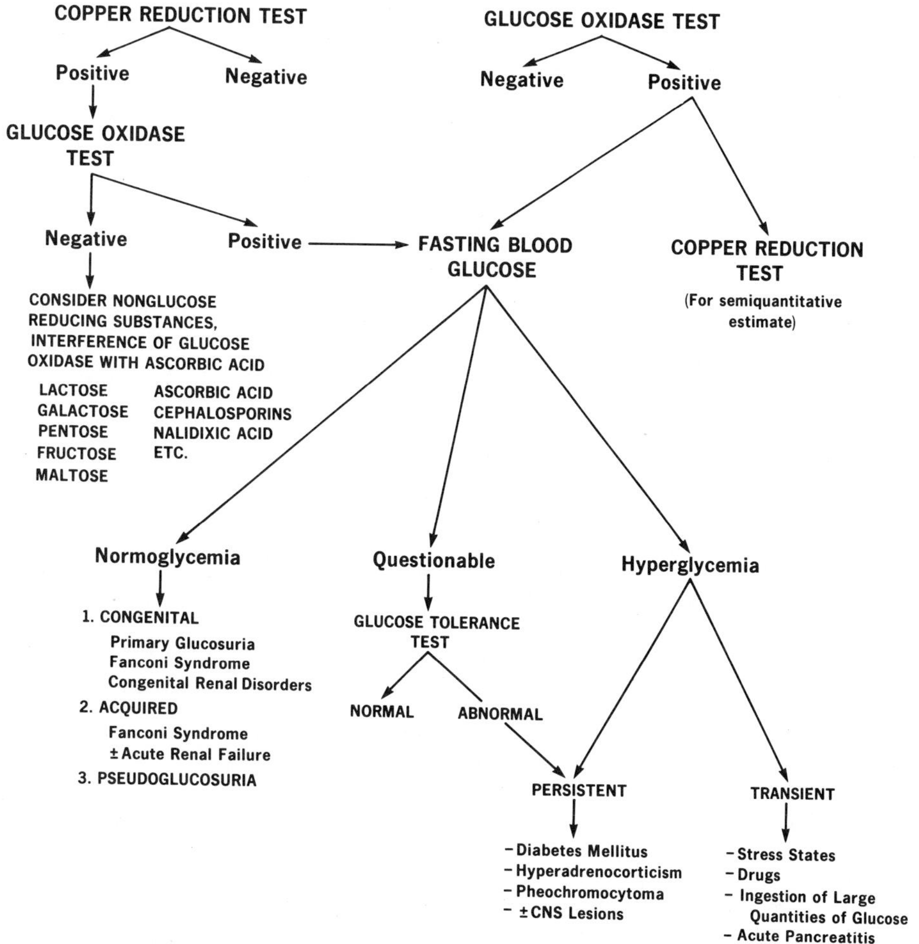

Figure 7. Diagnostic algorithm for glucosuria. Consult Osborne and Stevens: *Handbook of Canine and Feline Urinalysis.* St. Louis, MO: Ralston Purina Co., 1981, for explanation.

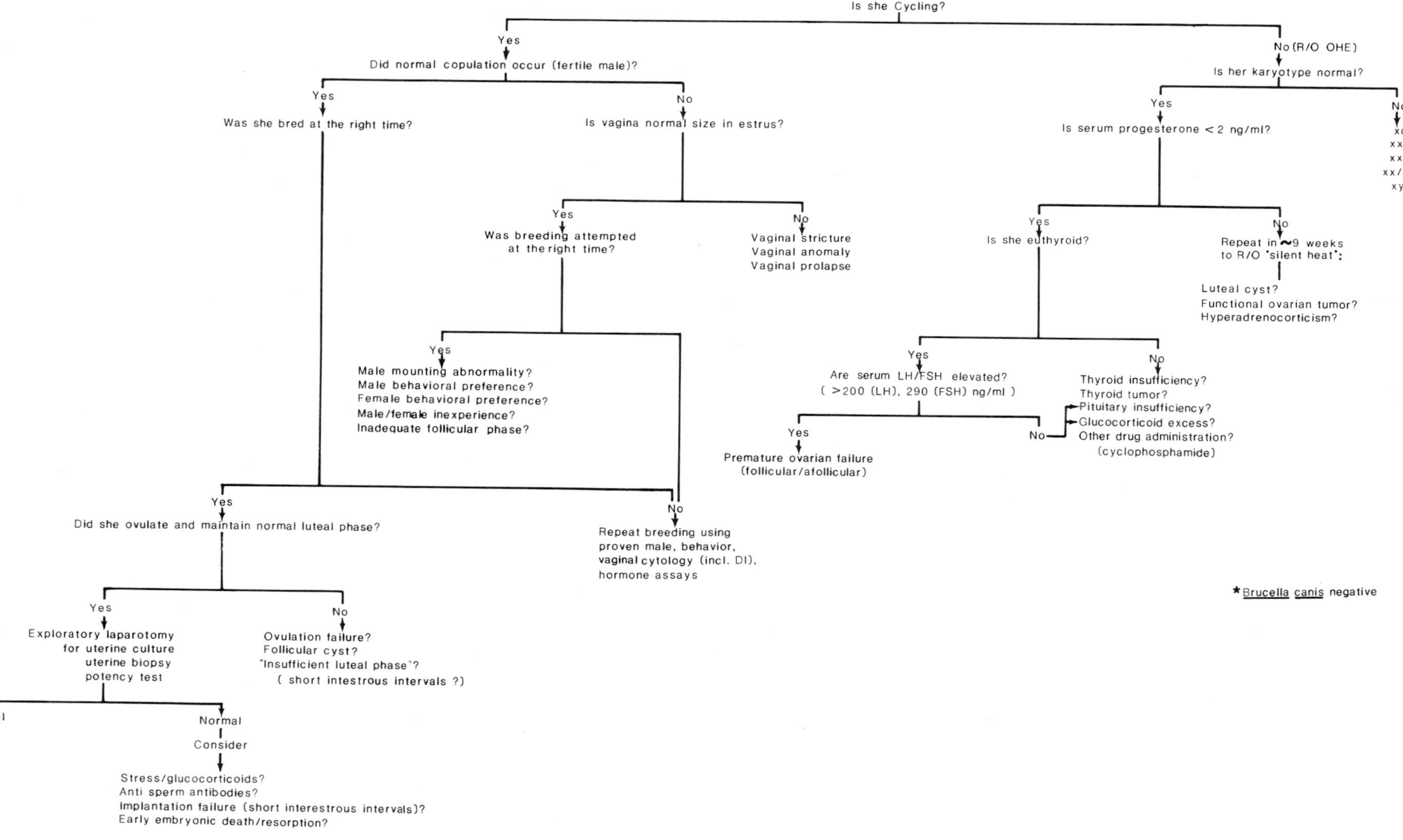

Figure 8. Diagnostic algorithm for canine female infertility (From Johnston: Proc. Soc. Theriogenology Annual Meeting. Denver, CO: 1984, pp. 25–32.)

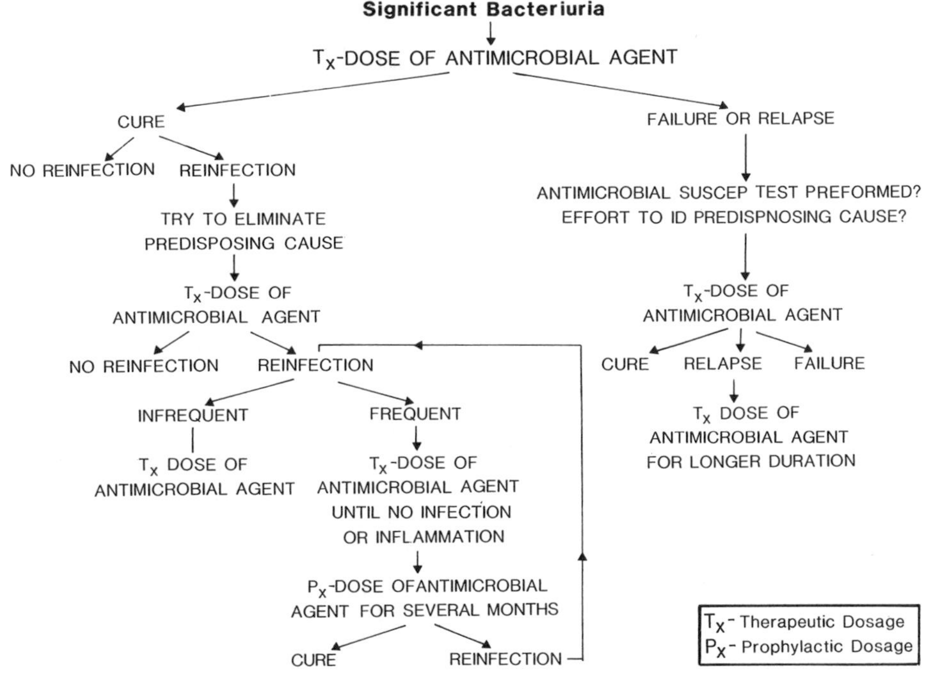

Figure 9. Therapeutic algorithm for urinary tract infections (U.T.I.). Reinfection is defined as UTI caused by a different pathogen. Relapse is defined as UTI caused by the same pathogen. A preventative dose is defined as 1/3 to 1/4 of the therapeutic dosage of trimethoprim-sulfate, nitrofurantoin, or ampicillin, given once per day at night prior to confinement. Consult Osborne in *Bristol Veterinary Handbook of Antimicrobial Therapy,* Princeton Junction, NJ: Veterinary Learning Systems, 1982, for details.

owner). This will influence the terminology used and the degree of complexity of the algorithm.

4. Develop a first draft of decisions that connect the starting point (e.g., polyuria) with the outcome (e.g., recognition of specific causes). At this phase, one must define specific methods that facilitate solution of the problem (e.g., urinalysis, water deprivation test, or contrast radiography). Use of case examples may be very helpful at this phase of development.

5. Evaluate and, if necessary, revise the algorithm until graphic reliability is attained.

6. Test and, if necessary, revise the algorithm until performance effectiveness is attained. It may be useful to consult with a systems, discipline, or species specialist when validating the reliability of the algorithm. It is emphasized that once algorithms are designed, they must be evaluated for reliability and safety before adopted for routine use.

EPILOGUE

Algorithmic pathways frequently must be supplemented with additional information. Rarely can they be designed to be consistently reliable in those circumstances in which two or more different disorders interact in the same patient. *Clinical algorithms typically require judgment in the absence of certainty.* If pertinent new clinical data become available after an algorithmic decision has been made, the algorithm may be reapplied to the entire collection of clinical data.

References and Supplemental Reading

Gorry, G. A.: New perspectives on the art of clinical decision making. Am. J. Clin. Pathol. 75:483, 1981.

Green, G., and Defoe, E. C.: What is a clinical algorithm? Clin. Pediatr. 17:457, 1978.

Margolis, C. Z.: Uses of clinical algorithms. J.A.M.A. 249:627, 1983.

McConell, T. H., Ashworth, C. T., Ashworth, R. D., et al.: Algorithm derived, computer generated interpretative comments in the reporting of laboratory tests. Am. J. Clin. Pathol. 72:32, 1979.

Osborne, C. A.: The problem oriented medical system. Improved knowledge, wisdom, and understanding of patient care. Vet. Clin. North Am., 13:745, 1983.

Osborne, C. A.: Treatment of urinary tract infections in the dog and cat. *In Bristol Veterinary Handbook of Antimicrobial Therapy.* Princeton Junction, NJ: Veterinary Learning Systems, 1982.

Osborne, C. A., and Stevens, J. B.: *Handbook of Canine and Feline Urinalysis.* St. Louis, MO: Ralston Purina, 1981.

Sox, H. G., Sox, C. H., and Tompkins, R. K.: The training of physician's assistants. Use of clinical algorithm system for patient care, audit of performance, and education. N. Engl. J. Med. 288:818, 1973.

THERAPY BY REFERRAL

DONALD G. LOW, D.V.M.
Davis, California

AVAILABILITY OF REFERRAL SERVICES

Better referral services in veterinary medicine are becoming more available each year. Prior to the early 1950s there was relatively little specialization in the practicing segment of the profession. Referral services were infrequently used, except for necropsies at state diagnostic laboratories. In academic institutions, surgery, medicine, radiology, theriogenology, clinical pathology, and pathology were among the first specialties that offered both the sound basis for referrals and a skeleton for later development of many subspecialties of medicine and surgery.

During subsequent years, veterinary specialists have been available only at academic institutions and at a few large nonacademic institutions. However, during the past 15 years, training of clinical specialists has gained substantial momentum. More board-certified veterinarians are being trained. Until recently, clinical specialists trained at one institution would often join another institution; fewer than 20 per cent entered private practice. Now, the clinical faculties at veterinary schools are rapidly filling. Substantially more board-certified specialists will enter private practice. This change will accelerate rapidly during the remaining years of this century and will have two important effects on private practice. First, referral services will become more readily available. Second, there will be a higher standard of practice in the community. This may increase the risk of malpractice suits for those veterinarians who do not inform their clients of availability of specialized services when there is need. The increase in malpractice suits could accelerate even more if awards are made that exceed the monetary value of the animal and include recognition of pain and suffering as well as loss of companionship. With the rapid development of the recognition given in recent years to the human-animal bond and all of its ramifications, this trend is more than a possibility.

UTILIZATION OF REFERRAL SERVICES

There is little reason to believe that the utilization of referral services is developing as fast as their availability and quality. Some veterinarians still tend to guard their clientele and often do not refer to other colleagues out of fear of losing clients. There also remains an attitude among some that they should and can provide a complete veterinary service; to refer is an admission of inadequacy. In fact, a totally different situation exists.

Veterinarians trained in specialties, regardless of whether they are practicing their specialty in an academic institution or in private practice, recognize that referred clients come to them under one of two different conditions. The need for referral may have been initially suggested to a client by their veterinarian, or the referral may have been demanded by the client. The receiving veterinarian usually has an easy public relations task when the referral was initiated by the veterinarian. There is a friendly, coooperative relationship between the client and the referring veterinarian in a high percentage of cases, and it is easy for the client and the patient to return to the referring veterinarian for aftercare as well as for future problems and routine services. The referring veterinarian has clearly demonstrated concern by seeing that the patient receives the best available care. Because the client knows from first-hand experience that the veterinarian has put patient care above monetary gain, the client responds with an increased measure of faith and trust.

By contrast, when the client demands the referral, there is often a total breakdown of relations between the veterinarian and the client. The client has become dissatisfied with the service offered and often loses respect for the veterinarian if there has been failure to discuss openly the pet's problems including the desirability of services of a specialist. When the receiving veterinarian encounters this situation, the client may openly express a feeling of hostility toward the referring veterinarian. It is not unusual under such circumstances for the client to state that he or she has no interest in returning to the referring veterinarian. In fact, the client may ask the receiving veterinarian to recommend a new veterinarian. This may lead to the incorrect assumption that receiving veterinarians are "stealing" clients.

GUIDELINES FOR REFERRAL

Veterinarians in general small animal practice can easily avoid such disagreeable situations by following a few guidelines. First, it is essential to recognize that all pet owners do not demand the same level of veterinary care. The interest of pet owners, in fact, ranges in a continuum. On one hand, some have little or no interest in their pets and will abandon them on a freeway, in a strange part of town, or out in the country. At the other extreme, the pet is an equal member of the family in all respects. In the pet-owning population, there is probably a large bulge between the two extremes of a typical bell-shaped curve that represents pet owners who will request some, but not unlimited, veterinary service for their pets. One of the practitioner's most important tasks is to decide where each client fits into the continuum of pet owners. A reasonable approach to providing an appropriate level of veterinary care is encompassed by the following two important questions.

The veterinarian must first openly and nondefensively determine the nature of the pet's problem and then decide if appropriate resources for handling the diagnostic workup, hospitalization, therapy, and aftercare are immediately available. If the answer is yes, as it most frequently is, the client's veterinary needs can be met. If the answer is no, then the second question arises: does the client want or need more veterinary service given? The practitioner should discuss this with the client rather than make assumptions or decisions for the client without outlining available alternatives. If, for whatever reason, the client's level of interest in the pet is low, and if euthanasia is an easy and an acceptable answer, there may be little need for referral. However, if the client wants to actively pursue additional care, then a referral is in order. By following these recommendations, the veterinarian will establish the need for referral in a timely fashion, will maintain the client's confidence, and will arrange for the referral while the client has some financial resources available and while the patient is in the best possible condition.

A veterinarian should give thought to the possible benefits of referral every time euthanasia is considered. Referral may not be needed or desired at such times, but it should be considered presented as an option to the client.

There is need for the general practitioner to be thoroughly familiar with referral services available locally or regionally. Current listings of board-certified specialists are published in the yellow pages of the AVMA Directory and revised annually. Much information can usually be obtained by regular attendance of local veterinary meetings and by reading publications of the state veterinary medical association.

Practitioners should make an effort to know firsthand what the facilities are like in referral practices, what equipment is available, what nursing care is provided in terms of hours of service and training of personnel, what distances, routes of travel, special skills of receiving veterinarians, and costs are involved, and, in the case of teaching hospitals, what research studies may hold new hope for special patients.

When referring cases, the practitioner should have a staff member arrange the appointment for the client. If possible, the referring veterinarian should talk to the receiving veterinarian. This conversation should be followed by a written summary of the case; it should contain pertinent points from the owner's history, observations and physical findings made by the referring veterinarian, results of tests performed, radiographs, and description of therapy given, including a list of drugs, dosages, routes of administration, and the times the last doses were administered. The best policy to follow is to avoid treatment of referred animals unless a life-threatening situation exists or if the patient has fractures that need stabilization. Rather than facilitate recovery, drugs often interfere with diagnostic tests and their interpretation and can influence observations made by the receiving veterinarian, which may delay and confuse appropriate diagnostic and therapeutic procedures.

When the veterinarian discusses a referred patient with the receiving veterinarian, an opportunity for consultation exists. If a referral is not necessary, a decision can be made at that time and the benefits of a consultation will have already been gained. There is substantial reason to charge the client for this consultation. The best way to handle this situation is to obtain the client's authorization for the consultation and to have the receiving veterinarian bill the client directly for the service at a previously determined rate.

Communication among the referring veterinarian, the receiving veterinarian, and the client is essential. The receiving veterinarian needs to convey diagnosis, prognosis, therapy, needs for follow-up care, schedule of necessary re-examinations, and other pertinent information to both the referring veterinarian and the client. The referring veterinarian should not hesitate to call in order to remain fully informed about the patient's problems. Interaction with the receiving veterinarian can make each referral a valuable learning experience, thus increasing the opportunities for high-quality continuing education.

Decisions about use of referral services need to be periodically re-evaluated. Careful follow-up with the client and the receiving veterinarian provides an opportunity for an ongoing evaluation of the degree of satisfaction provided to all parties involved. Problems need to be identified, discussed, and resolved. Much can be gained by having a personal acquaintance with specialty-trained veterinarians in a community or region. Personal visits and making extra effort to communicate at veterinary association meetings can do much to improve relationships. The exchange of ideas, comments, and suggestions is fostered when a friendly atmosphere prevails.

BENEFITS OF TIMELY REFERRAL

Veterinarians should consider frequent use of referrals:

1. To provide the best available service for their patients.
2. For protection against malpractice suits.
3. For their own continuing education. One can learn a great deal when it can be determined that decisions and actions are right or wrong. The mechanism of referral often provides this information; muddling through difficult clinical problems rarely does.
4. To avoid excessive financial commitment associated with attempts to provide a complete veterinary service. It is not economically feasible to attempt to become equipped, stocked, and staffed to handle all varieties of cases. It is far more reasonable to handle common problems and to refer difficult cases or those requiring specialized diagnosis or treatment to a specialist.
5. To gain a client's confidence and esteem by showing selfless dedication and concern for their pets.
6. For the personal satisfaction of having done the best possible job for the patient.
7. For recognizing the client's greater satisfaction because everything possible was done for the pet, and for the greater confidence the client may have in a decision that was made as a result of a second, highly informed opinion.
8. To support studies of naturally occurring diseases of companion animals when possible.

Referrals may not be beneficial when a patient is moribund or when the client cannot afford extra expense. In situations of economic difficulty, there may be an answer at a teaching hospital. Sometimes research funds or teaching allowances can be used to pay for care, especially when the patient has a disease of research or teaching interest to a receiving specialist. This possibility should always be determined before a referral is made.

ACUPUNCTURE IN VETERINARY MEDICINE

DONALD H. CLIFFORD, D.V.M.
Toledo, Ohio

INTRODUCTION

The place of acupuncture in veterinary as well as human medicine in North America has not been determined; it has been accepted in the Orient and Europe. Since the discovery of beta-endorphin, the scientific community in the United States appears to be altering its position from rejection to limited acceptance of acupuncture. In the broad sense, the palpation or stimulation of peripheral nerves has many uses in the diagnosis and treatment of disease. Pain at an acupuncture locus or acupoint may signify involvement of an associated internal organ. Stimulation of peripheral nerves or acupoints by a needle, vacuum, pressure, superficial electrode, heat, implant, injection, laser, or other means may have immediate or long-term beneficial effects or both. The perception of Teh Chi (a warm, numb, or uncomfortable feeling at the acupuncture site), an important indicator of proper stimulation in humans, may or may not be demonstrated by animals and perceived by the veterinary acupuncturist. Although complications from needle acupuncture have been observed, they are exceedingly rare. Most complications associated with needles are avoided with acupressure, electrical stimulation, transcutaneous electrical neurostimulation (TENS), use of lasers, and other noninvasive techniques. Use of lasers (e.g., 632 nm for 30 seconds) is equivalent to 5 to 8 minutes of electroacupuncture, which usually produces a strong response. A unique aspect of acupuncture or stimulation of peripheral nerves is that these methods have been used successfully in several chronic conditions that respond poorly to conventional treatment.

Animals and humans have over 300 dermal sites of low electrical resistance where superficial nerves may be located anatomically and verified by a galvanometer or acupoint finder. The use of an acupoint finder is stressed by some human acupuncturists, whereas others feel that an experienced person can rely on the response from the patient to verify proper placement. Only about 50 of these points or areas have clinical importance. Acupoints for humans and for various species of animals are similar but often not identical. Comparisons have been complicated by different types of nomenclature to designate the acupoints. The effects of stimulation of these peripheral nerves fall into two major categories: (1) control of pain as mediated through the release of morphinomimetic or other substances in the brain, and (2) stimulation of the autonomic nervous system.

Alleviation of pain, autonomic (physiological) effects, or both in clinical conditions may be interrelated and difficult to evaluate. Lack of understanding of the mechanism of action may account for lack of use of this modality of treatment. Other factors that have deterred use of acupuncture are (1) unreasonable claims by some acupuncturists; (2) variability in treatment, (3) lack of uniformly controlled or well-documented reports of its effectiveness; (4) absence of a strong academic program with a recognized and reliable board to examine, assess, and certify the skills of competent acupuncturists; (5) use of ancient Oriental (Taoist) philosophy to explain the effects of acupuncture rather than the actions of neurohormones (neurotransmitters) and the autonomic nervous system; (6) additional time required to use acupuncture; (7) lack of standardized nomenclature, point locations, and techniques; (8) political and cultural background that surrounded the initial reports of use of acupuncture; and (9) early use of acupuncture by individuals who did not have an adequate background in medicine or who were poorly trained in the techniques of acupuncture.

In animals as in humans, certain conditions or states such as overexertion, previous hysterectomy, prior administration of certain drugs such as atropine, and estrus, among others, will decrease the response to the stimulation of one or many acupoints.

ACUPUNCTURE FOR CONTROL OF PAIN

Acupoints associated with specific organs or areas of the body may become painful when the underlying organ or region is involved with disease. This has been documented in ruminants, horses, and, to a limited extent, dogs and other animals. The treatment of painful conditions of such areas as the osseous structures, digestive tract, and uterus seems more dramatic or apparent in large animals. The pain threshold in horses appears lower than for other animals, which favors this animal as a subject for study and use of acupuncture.

A deterrent to research on acupuncture has been a lack of reliable means of sampling and measuring beta-endorphins and other neurohormones or neurotransmitters such as acetylcholine, dopamine, norepinephrine, epinephrine, histamine, GABA, enkephalins, and serotonin. A radioimmunoassay of beta-endorphin is now available and is specific for this substance in animals and humans. It has been proposed that levels of beta-endorphins in animals are elevated after acupuncture. Increased levels of serotonin have also been associated with reduction of pain following stimulation of peripheral nerves.

The effectiveness of acupuncture in certain types of pain and whether or not the opiate antagonists, naloxone and haltrexone, are capable of blocking or reversing the analgesic effect of acupuncture have not been resolved.

A practical use of acupuncture in animals is the extension of analgesia after surgery. Although acupuncture has been used successfully as the sole "anesthetic" agent in large animals, it has not been frequently used as a local or general anesthetic in small animals. Bilateral electroacupuncture at San Yin Chiao (Sp-6), a traditional acupuncture point for the caudal region, significantly reduced the amount of halothane required to produce anesthesia in dogs.

The administration of naltrexone, IV or intrathecally, did not alter the effect of acupuncture; this suggests that the anesthetic sparing effect was not mediated by endorphins. The administration of beta-endorphin alone depressed the cardiovascular system, but this could be reversed by electroacupuncture at Jen Chung (Go-26), which also suggests that the autonomic effects of acupuncture are mediated through a nonopiate pathway.

ACUPUNCTURE AND THE AUTONOMIC NERVOUS SYSTEM

The beneficial effects of acupuncture in most functional disorders in which pain is not the primary complaint can be directly attributed to the autonomic nervous system. Increased circulation and ventilation, more active peristalsis, enhancement of excretory function, elevations in blood glucose or insulin concentration, and changes in the concentrations of catecholamines are influenced by the autonomic nervous system. There is conflicting information relative to some of the autonomic effects of acupuncture. Most investigators concur that stimulation of Tsu San Li (St-36) on the anterior lateral surface of the hind leg below the knee is associated with a parasympathomimetic effect on the heart and gastrointestinal tract. However, one investigator reported an increase in epinephrine and norepinephrine (presumably a sympathomimetic effect) after stimulation of this acupoint. Further studies are required to resolve these apparent discrepancies. Many other functions, such as increased phagocytosis, antibody production, antipyretic effect, and anti-inflammatory activity, can be related to autonomic mediation.

Major acupoints in the dog are illustrated in Figures 1 and 2. The position of these acupoints is similar for animals and humans. The acupoint Tsu San Li (St-36) is blocked by administration of atropine. The resuscitation acupoint, Jen Chung (Go-26), which is located near the upper lip and base of the nose, causes a sympathomimetic effect that can be blocked by propranolol. The stimulatory effect of acupuncture at Jen Chung (Go-26) on the cardiopulmonary function has been observed in zoo animals as well as domestic animals and humans. The sympathomimetic effect of acupuncture at Jen Chung (Go-26) on the cardiovascular system was not blocked by naloxone, which also leads to the conclusion that the morphinomimetic substances do not mediate the autonomic effects. Clinically, the sympathomimetic effect of acupuncture at Jen Chung (Go-26) in dogs may be enhanced by stimulating the first acupoint on the kidney meridian, which is located under the metatarsal foot pads of both hind feet and approached from the proximal border of the pad. This also may be supplemented by stimulating the ends of the toes distal to each digital pad in members of the family Canidae.

CLINICAL USES OF ACUPUNCTURE

Selected examples of the use of acupuncture in animals are listed below. Although the firing of horses belongs to the past, it is interesting to speculate how the alleged benefits of applying cautery to the legs of horses may have been due to stimulation of peripheral nerves. Acupoints in the horses, cow, hog, chicken, duck, cat, and dog are listed by H. Grady Young, D. Gilchrist, and others. In animals the acupoints should be verified by an acupoint finder or cutaneous impedance equipment to facilitate proper placement of needles, electrodes, or other stimulators.

Cats

Stimulation at Jen Chung (Go-26) in cats is useful in treating shock. The use of acupuncture to treat chronic and unresponsive conditions in cats appears more difficult than in dogs.

Dogs

Chronic painful conditions such as spinal disc syndrome, hip dysplasia arthritis, and osteochondritis have been benefited by acupuncture. Other conditions such as skin disorders (eczema), chronic diarrhea, kennel cough, cardiac disease, incontinence, sterility in males or females, and idiopathic vomiting may respond to acupuncture. Use of acupuncture to treat conditions of the musculoskeletal,

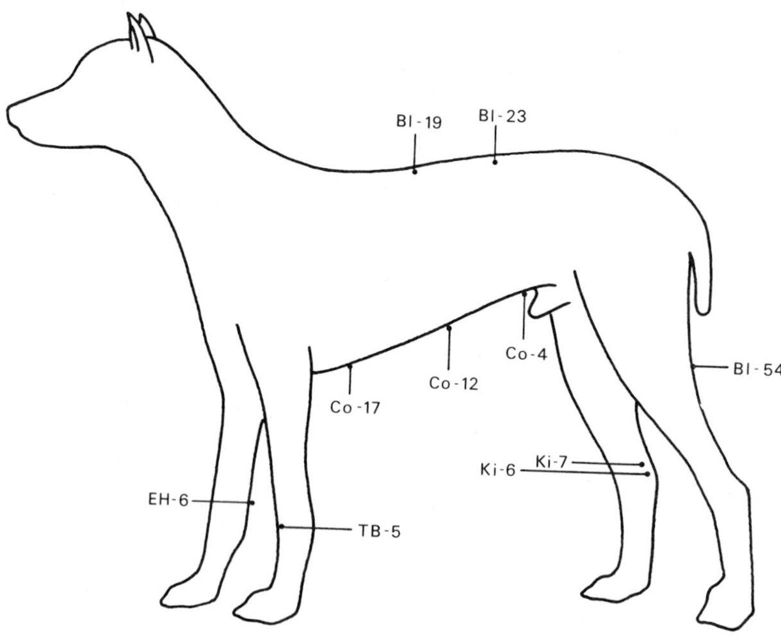

Figure 1. Important acupoints on the bladder (Bl), conception vessel (Co), envelope of the heart (EH), kidney (Ki), and triburner (TB) meridians. Other designations and abbreviations may be used for these same points (e.g., bladder, B; conception vessel, CV; pericardium, P; kidney, K; and triple burner or triple warmer, TW). (Courtesy of Clifford and Lee: V.M./S.A.C. 74:35, 1979.)

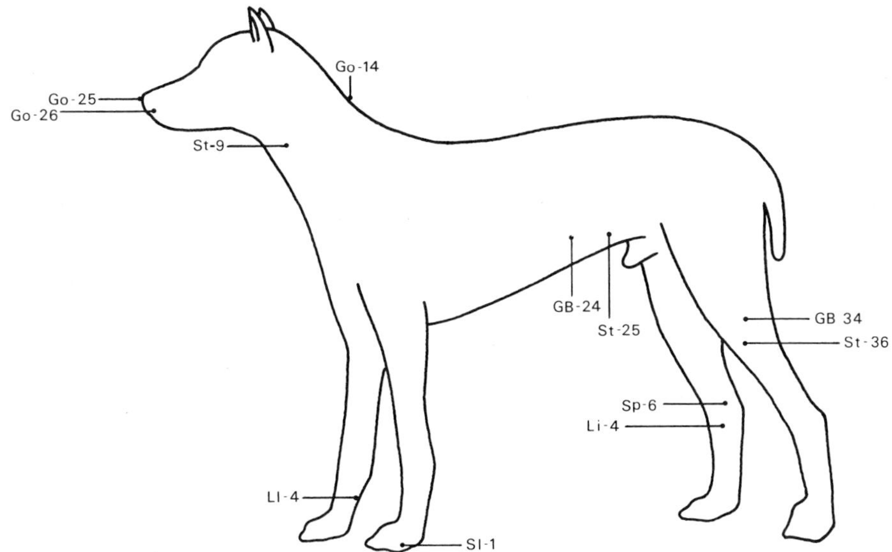

Figure 2. Important acupoints on the gallbladder (GB), governing vessel (Go), large intestine (LI), small intestine (SI), spleen (Sp), liver (Li), and stomach (St) meridians. Other designations and abbreviations may be used for these same points (e.g., governing vessel, GV; liver, LIV; spleen, SP; and stomach, ST). (Courtesy of Clifford and Lee: V.M./S.A.C. 74:35, 1979.)

reproductive, respiratory, and nervous systems, the integument, and organs of special sense in small animals is described by David Gilchrist.

Horses

In horses, acupuncture is useful in controlling painful conditions, in producing local anesthesia, and in treating disease in which the autonomic nervous system appears involved. Examples of disease processes in which acupuncture has been reported are aerophagia, intestinal impaction, colic, lameness, laminitis, sore back, and tendinitis (bowed tendons).

Ruminants

Kothbauer and others have investigated acupoints associated with bladder meridians along the spine in cattle. They have identified and treated a variety of bovine disease processes of underlying thoracic and abdominal cavities, including ovarian dysfunction, placental retention, ketosis, metritis, vaginitis, and ruminal dysfunction. Stimulation of these bladder meridans has also been useful in facilitating teat surgery and in treating mastitis and musculoskeletal conditions. Cesarean section and repair of abdominal herniation have been performed under local anesthesia produced by acupuncture in ruminants.

SUMMARY

Pressure and galvanic recording at cutaneous acupoints can be a useful means of detecting dysfunction of underlying organs. Stimulation of these acupoints can be helpful in the control of certain types of pain. The neurotransmitters appear involved in the alleviation of pain, but their function is not clearly understood. Several systemic dysfunctions can be ameliorated or cured by stimulation of cutaneous acupoints. Strong stimulation (i.e., electrical stimulation of one or more needles) appears more effective than simple pressure (acupressure). The automatic nervous system appears involved in mediating the physiologic effects. The stimulation of superficial acupoints can be very useful in studying pain and providing insight into and relief of many painful conditions. More research is needed to elucidate the mechanism of action and application of this interesting modality of treatment.

INTERNATIONAL VETERINARY ACUPUNCTURE SOCIETY

The stimulation of acupoints as an aid in the diagnosis and treatment of pain and systemic dysfunction is an emerging and complex subject. A person with a serious interest in this form of treatment should contact the International Veterinary Acupuncture Society, c/o Department of Laboratory Animal Medicine, Room R-351, College of Medicine, Mail Location 571, University of Cincinnati, Cincinnati, Ohio 45267.

A list of primary human diseases of the musculoskeletal, respiratory, digestive, and nervous systems and organs of special sense that may be benefited by acupuncture has been prepared and published for the World Health Organization by R. H. Bannerman in *The American Journal of Acupuncture*. This publication is dedicated to dissemination of information on acupuncture in man and animals.

References and Supplemental Reading

Altman, S.: Clinical use of veterinary acupuncture. Vet. Med. Small Anim. Clin. 76:1307, 1981.

Bannerman, R. H.: The World Health Organization viewpoint on acupuncture. Am. J. Acup. 8:231, 1980.

Cheng, R. S., and Pomeranz, B.: Electroacupuncture analgesia could be mediated by at least two pain-relieving mechanisms: endorphin and nonendorphin systems. Life Sci. 25:1957, 1979.

Clifford, D. H., and Lee, M. O.: Trends in acupuncture research—1. Acupuncture in the control of pain. Vet. Med. Small Anim. Clin. 73:1513, 1978.

Clifford, D. H., and Lee, M. O.: Trends in acupuncture research—2. Acupuncture and the autonomic nervous system. Vet. Med. Small Anim. Clin. 74:35, 1979.

Gideon, L.: Acupuncture: Clinical trials in the horse. J.A.V.M.A. 170:220, 1977.

Gilchrist, D.: *Manual of Acupuncture for Small Animals*. Sydney, Australia: Business and Commercial Mailing Service Ltd., 1981.

Grieff, W. K.: Neural therapy based on Kothbauer's points. Its relationship to veterinary acupuncture. Am. J. Acup. 12:61, 1984.

Hymes, A. C., Raab, D. E., Yonehiro, E. G., et al.: Electrical surface stimulation for control of acute postoperative pain and prevention of ileus. Surg. Forum 24:447, 1973.

Janssens, L.: An overview: Veterinary acupuncture in Europe. Am. J. Acup. 9:151, 1981.

Kothbauer, O.: The bladder meridian of the cow. Am. J. Acup. 2:300, 1974.

Lee, D. C., Lee, M. O., Clifford, D. H., et al.: Inhibition of the cardiovascular effects of acupuncture (moxibustion) by propanolol in dogs during halothane anesthesia. Can. Anaesth. Soc. J. 23:307, 1976.

Lee, M. O., Lee, D. C., Clifford, D. H., et al.: Acupuncture in patients unresponsive to conventional treatment. Part 3. Additional examples of treatment involving various systems of the body. Am. J. Acup. 9:311, 1981.

Rogers, P. A. M.: Non-specific immunostimulation by acupuncture in man and animals. Acup. Res. Q. 7:119, 1983.

Westermayer, E.: Acupuncture meridians and ancient points especially in cattle. Am. J. Acup. 11:259, 1983.

Wright, M., and McGrath, C. J.: Physiologic and analgesic effects of acupuncture in the dog. J.A.V.M.A. 178:502, 1981.

Young, H. G.: *Atlas of Veterinary Acupuncture Charts*. 2nd ed. Thomasville, GA: Oriental Veterinary Acupuncture Specialties, 1978.

THERAPEUTIC USE OF VITAMINS IN COMPANION ANIMALS

C. A. BUFFINGTON, D.V.M.
Davis, California

INTRODUCTION

Vitamins are organic compounds essential to life and required in very small quantities for normal metabolism. They are natural components of foodstuffs and are generally present in sufficient amounts in a varied diet. Therapeutic administration of fat- and water-soluble vitamins to companion animals usually occurs in two sets of circumstances. First, they are administered for treatment of signs associated with vitamin deficiency. Second, vitamins are given for various conditions in the absence of classical deficiency signs. Vitamins required by domestic species include fat-soluble vitamins A, D, E, and K, and water-soluble (or B-complex) vitamins, including thiamin, riboflavin, niacin, pyridoxine, pantothenic acid, biotin, folic acid, and B_{12}. Choline is also required; vitamin C may be required in certain conditions.

Many but not all vitamins are required in the diet. Endogenous vitamin D synthesis is generally sufficient if adequate exposure to sunlight occurs, especially in adults. Intestinal microfloral synthesis of vitamin K, folic acid, and biotin may also provide adequate amounts of these vitamins under normal conditions. Adequate vitamin C is normally synthesized in the liver of the common domestic species.

Discovery of the vitamins occurred primarily by isolation of factors in foods that cured signs of such diseases as scurvy (vitamin C), beri-beri (thiamin), and human pellagra or canine black tongue (niacin). The classic deficiency signs of individual vitamin deficiencies are not difficult to identify (Table 1). The clinical problem of identifying most vitamins is

***Table 1.** Summary of Vitamin Requirements, Sources, and Relationships to Clinical Disorders*

Requirement (per kg body weight/day)	Sources (amount/100 gm food)	Signs of Deficiency	Circumstances in Which Deficiency Should Be Suspected	Methods of Diagnosis of Deficiency*	Signs of Toxicity	Clinical Uses
Vitamin A						
Dog: 75–200 IU Cat: 200 IU/kg body weight/day (cats cannot convert carotenes to vitamin A and thus require preformed vitamin A in the diet)	High (>10,000 IU): liver, liver oils, carrots, spinach, pumpkin Low (<1000 IU): milk, most fish, fruits, nuts, and legumes, corn	Decreased growth, night blindness, epithelial hyperkeratinization, uroliths, degeneration of ocular epithelium	Fat malabsorption, liver disease, chronic diarrhea, low-fat diets	Clinical signs, liver vitamin A levels, plasma vitamin A levels	Dog: decreased growth, hyperesthesia, decreased bone density, exophthalmos Cat: deforming cervical spondylosis, osteoporosis	Human: dermatoses, cancer Animal: hypertension (?), vitamin A–responsive dermatoses (dog)
Vitamin D						
Dog: 8–22 IU Cat: 20 IU	High (>1000 IU): liver oils Low (<100 IU): vegetable oils, dairy products, fruits, nuts	Rickets, osteomalacia	See vitamin A; lack of access to ultraviolet light, kidney dysfunction, hypoparathyroidism	Chromatographic determination of blood levels, elevated serum alkaline phosphatase (indirect)	Anorexia, nausea, hypercalcemia, metastatic calcification	Hypoparathyroidism, chronic renal failure
Vitamin E†						
Dog: 0.5–1.2 IU Cat: 1.6 IU	High (>50 mg): vegetable oils, mayonnaise, margarine Low (<5 mg): most vegetables, meat, and dairy products, yeast	Muscle weakness and degeneration, reproductive failure, steatitis (cats)	See vitamin A; high dietary levels of unsaturated fats	Plasma levels of α-tocopherol	No clinical reports (experimental toxicity causes high blood pressure, nausea, and diarrhea, anemia, and prolonged clotting time)	Humans: intermittent claudication, cancer (?), others Animals: none reported
Vitamin K						
Dog: none listed (a dietary requirement has not been demonstrated) Cat: none listed	High (>100 μg): cabbage, soybeans, spinach, beef kidney and liver Low (<10 μg): milk, corn, peas, carrots	Hemorrhage, prolonged clotting times	See vitamin A, ingestion of vitamin K antagonists, use of unabsorbed antibiotics, mineral oil, or cholestyramine	Increased prothrombin time	Humans: hemolysis, hyperbilirubinemia, kernicterus in neonates given vitamin K_3 parenterally Dog: urticaria, flatulence, lacrimation, salivation (case report)	Control of bleeding tendencies
Thiamin						
Dog: 20–54 μg Cat: 100 μg	High (>1000 μg): wheat germ, yeast, ham, soybeans Low (<100 μg): most fruits, fish, and vegetables	Anorexia, growth depression, mydriasis, ataxia, convulsions	Ingestion of raw fish, overcooked foods, severe gastrointestinal disease, prolonged starvation (?)	More than 20% improvement of erythrocyte transketolase activity after addition of thiamin pyrophosphate, absence of increase in urinary thiamin excretion after oral loading test	Decreased blood pressure and death due to respiratory depression have been reported (lethal dose is approximately 350 mg/kg)	No verified uses
Riboflavin						
Dog: 50–100 μg Cat: 100 μg	High (>1000 μg): organ meats, yeast, dairy products Low (<100 μg): most fruits	Anorexia, dermatitis, ocular lesions	Gastrointestinal disease, overcooked foods, diuresis	Humans: erythrocyte glutathione reductase assay (?)	None reported	None reported

Table continued on following page

***Table 1.** Summary of Vitamin Requirements, Sources, and Relationships to Clinical Disorders*
Continued

Requirement (per kg body weight/day)	Sources (amount/100 gm food)	Signs of Deficiency	Circumstances in Which Deficiency Should Be Suspected	Methods of Diagnosis of Deficiency*	Signs of Toxicity	Clinical Uses
Pantothenic Acid						
Dog: 200–400 μg Cat: 200 μg	High (>2 mg): organ meats, eggs, wheat germ, bran, yeast Low (<5 mg): most fruits, milk, honey	Depressed appetite and growth, depressed immune function (dogs), fatty liver, gastrointestinal mucosal damage (cats); neurologic signs are seen in the terminal stages	Pantothenic acid is so widely distributed in nature that the likelihood of a naturally occurring deficiency is extremely low	Humans: estimation of CoA levels by citrate cleavage enzyme assay	None reported	Humans: may reduce symptoms associated with rheumatoid arthritis Animals: none reported
Niacin						
Dog: 225–450 μg Cat: 900 μg	High (>1000 μg): organ meats, yeast, peanuts, tuna Low (<1000 μg): most fruits and vegetables, eggs, milk	Anorexia; growth failure; inflammation and necrosis of gastrointestinal mucosa; fatty infiltration of the liver; ropy, bloody saliva	See riboflavin	Decreased urinary excretion of *N*-methylnicotinamide	Nicotinic acid causes a transient cutaneous flush in dogs when administered in high doses and can lower blood cholesterol levels, depending on the initial level of cholesterol and the dose of nicotinic acid	Humans: none reported, hypocholesterolemic effect is apparently ineffective in avoiding recurrence of atherosclerotic heart disease. Adverse side effects (flushing) limit use of therapeutic doses Animals: none reported
Pyridoxine						
Dog: 22–60 μg Cat: 80 μg (cats cannot convert tryptophan to niacin)	High (>1000 μg): liver, salmon, wheat germ, yeast, blackstrap molasses Low (<100 μg): fruit, cheese, milk	Growth depression, microcytic hypochromic anemia, convulsions, sudden death	See riboflavin; isoniazid administration	Increased urinary excretion of kynurenine, especially after tryptophan loading	None reported	Humans: prolongs clotting time and inhibits platelet aggregation; many other reported therapeutic effects, but confirmation in controlled trials is lacking Animals: none reported
Folic Acid						
Dog: 4–8 μg Cat: 20 μg	High (>90 μg): organ meats, yeast, spinach, dry beans Low (<30 μg): muscle meats, fruit, dairy products, many vegetables	Depressed growth, hypochromic anemia (microcytic in the dog, macrocytic in the cat), leukopenia	See riboflavin; sulfonamide administration	Increased excretion of formiminoglutamic acid after oral histidine load	None reported	None reported
Biotin						
Dog: see vitamin K Cat: see vitamin K	High (>100 μg): yeast, liver Low (<1 μg): fruit, dairy products, many fruits and vegetables	Hyperkeratosis of the skin (dog); oral, nasal and ocular exudata with associated scale dermatitis; generalized alopecia; hypersalivation; bloody diarrhea; anorexia; and emaciation (cat)	Ingestion of large amounts of raw egg white, use of antibiotics and sulfa drugs	Serum biotin concentration	None reported	Clinical reports of biotin-responsive dermatoses are unsubstantiated by controlled trials

Table continued on opposite page

Table 1. *Summary of Vitamin Requirements, Sources, and Relationships to Clinical Disorders* Continued

Requirement (per kg body weight/day)	Sources (amount/100 gm food)	Signs of Deficiency	Circumstances in Which Deficiency Should Be Suspected	Methods of Diagnosis of Deficiency*	Signs of Toxicity	Clinical Uses
Vitamin B$_{12}$						
Dog: 0.5–1 μg Cat: 0.4 μg	High (>50 μg): organ meats, egg yolk Low (<5 μg): fish, fruits, vegetables	Uncomplicated deficiency has not been described (dogs); decreased growth occurred without hematologic changes in kittens	See riboflavin; vegetarian diet	Urinary methylmalonic acid excretion, especially after valine loading	None reported	None reported
Vitamin C						
Dog: supplied by hepatic synthesis Cat: supplied by hepatic synthesis	High (>50 mg): green peppers, citrus fruit, strawberries, liver, fresh meat Low (<25 mg): many fruits and vegetables	None reported	Liver disease, overnutrition of rapidly growing dogs (?)	Leukocyte ascorbate levels	None confirmed in controlled trials	Humans: decreased severity of common cold symptoms (?), increased healing of pressure sores Animals: clinical reports of benefit in bone diseases affecting growing animals and in feline leukemia; no controlled trials
Choline						
Dog: 50 mg‡ Cat: 40 mg‡	High (>400 mg lecithin): liver, egg, soybeans, peanuts Low (<40 mg): most vegetables	Fatty infiltration of the liver, hypoalbuminemia (cats)	Low-protein diets	Serum choline concentration	None reported	Humans: tardive dyskinesia: Animals: resolution of fatty liver caused by dietary choline-lipotropin deficiency

*Diet history, clinical signs, and high index of suspicion are often the only methods available.
†Dietary needs are affected by the polyunsaturated fat content of the diet.
‡Endogenous synthesis also occurs.

that most deficiencies do not occur as the result of a specific dietary deficiency. Vitamin deficiencies more commonly occur because of consumption of inadequate or imbalanced diets prepared by owners with limited nutritional knowledge. Inclusion of a careful diet history in the anamnesis is the only sure method of identification of this problem. Knowledge of dietary sources of nutrients (Table 1) is essential for (1) evaluation of the likelihood of a deficiency, (2) detection of a food with poor vitamin availability, or (3) detection of a vitamin antagonist. Classic signs of vitamin deficiency represent late changes in the course of the disorder. By the time they appear, diagnosis and treatment are near emergencies, and many anatomic lesions are irreversible. A variable period of dietary inadequacy, depletion of body stores of the vitamin, and associated biochemical abnormalities exist before these changes occur. For example, when vitamin A deficiency occurs, liver stores are first depleted. Plasma levels of vitamin A and retinol binding protein then become depressed before night blindness becomes apparent.

FAT-SOLUBLE VERSUS WATER-SOLUBLE VITAMINS

Vitamins are grouped as fat-soluble or water-soluble to distinguish between their biochemical structure and biological function. Provitamins of at least two of the fat-soluble vitamins (A and D) occur in plants; there are no water-soluble provitamins. Fat solubility necessitates adequate dietary fat and bile for absorption of vitamins A, D, E, and K. Diseases of fat malabsorption may inhibit their uptake. Absorption of the water-soluble vitamins is rarely a limiting process.

Once absorbed, fat-soluble vitamins are generally stored in greater quantities in adipose tissue than are the water-soluble vitamins. Thus, deficiencies of fat-soluble vitamins generally take longer to occur. Fat-soluble vitamins are excreted mainly in feces, whereas water-soluble vitamins are excreted in urine. Enhanced excretion by either route may affect vitamin requirements. Because water-soluble vitamins are cofactors in energy transfer and intermediary metabolic reactions, their requirement is proportional to energy needs. Fat-soluble vitamins are involved in a wide variety of reactions that regulate metabolism of structural elements of the body. Owing to limited storage and rapid excretion, water-soluble vitamins generally have very low toxicity. In contrast, chronic ingestion of vitamin A or D at 10 to 100 times the normal requirement may result in signs of toxicity. Signs of B-vitamin deficiencies are frequently nonspecific (e.g., loss of appetite and degenerative changes in the gastrointestinal, integumentary, and nervous systems). Fat-soluble vitamin deficiencies tend to be associated with specific signs (e.g., night blindness in vitamin A deficiency or hemorrhage in vitamin K deficiency).

REQUIREMENTS AND DIETARY NEEDS

NORMAL REQUIREMENTS. To establish the requirement for any nutrient, including vitamins, accurately, one must first define the physiologic state of the animal. Growth, pregnancy, lactation, heavy work, environmental extremes, and disease all affect the animal's metabolic needs for vitamins. The quantity of vitamin required to cure obvious signs of deficiency may be less than that required for maximal filling of body stores (if that is desirable). Recommended intakes, signs of deficiency, and signs of excess, summarized in Table 1, are based on current recommendations of the National Academy of Sciences National Research Council's *Nutrient Requirements of Dogs* (1985) and *Nutrient Requirements of Cats* (1978). These publications are a comprehensive source of vitamin nutritional information in dogs and cats.*

The allowances they describe consist of recommended levels of intake presumed to be adequate for maintenance and growth. They are based on research data obtained from studies of dogs, cats, and other species and on evaluation of satisfactory practical diets.

Although most dogs and cats eat commercially prepared diets, it has previously been difficult to evaluate manufactured foods for nutrient adequacy based on label information. Fortunately, recent regulatory changes now allow the determination of the dietary adequacy of processed foods that have been properly stored. Foods identified as "complete and balanced as determined by AAFCO† protocol testing" have been demonstrated to be nutritionally adequate by sequential feeding trials of pregnant and lactating females, followed by successful completion of a growth trial in their offspring. These tests are currently the best insurance available against a dietary vitamin (nutrient) deficiency, especially of foods fed to animals with this type of increased physiologic need.

AVAILABILITY. A variety of factors that influence dietary vitamin availability may determine whether a vitamin imbalance or deficiency will occur. There is wide variability of vitamins in foods, and all dietary vitamins may not be available for absorption (Table 1). For example, niacin in cereals is almost completely unavailable owing to protein binding and is not included in calculation of the niacin content of these foods. Levels of vitamins in different batches of the same food can also vary. Even when vitamins are present in adequate quantities, their availability may be affected by vitamin antagonists also present in the food. In fact, naturally occurring or synthetic antagonists have been identified for all the vitamins except A and D. One of the most common vitamin antagonists is thiaminase, present in raw flesh of certain species of fish. Because thiamin deficiency may result from the ingestion of these fish, uncooked fish should never be fed to animals. Avidin, a potent biotin-binding protein present in egg white, is a vitamin antagonist. Avidin can completely eliminate the biotin availability of raw whole egg. Although it is possible to produce biotin deficiency by feeding animals large quantities of raw egg white, offering an occasional raw egg is of no consequence. Lanatine, a component of linseed meal, binds pyridoxal phosphate (B_6) and can induce B_6 deficiency in animals fed diets containing large quantities of linseed meal.

EFFECTS OF PROCESSING. Significant vitamin losses can occur during processing. For example, thiamin may be added to cat foods at 1000 times the requirement to ensure that adequate levels survive processing. Significant percentages of many other vitamins may also be lost during preparation of diets, depending on the processing technique. Vitamin K losses during processing of cat food may be 25 per cent in semimoist foods, 50 per cent in canned foods, and up to 75 per cent in extruded diets. Significant vitamin losses can also occur during storage. For example, vitamin A losses may exceed 50 per cent after 6 months of food storage.

PHYSIOLOGIC IMBALANCES. Situations that may result in vitamin imbalances or deficiencies do not occur with equal probability during all stages of life. The maintenance requirements of adult, nonpregnant animals are quite low. They can be fed diets with wide variation in vitamin content and will show few adverse effects. Normal physiologic states that increase vitamin (and all nutrient) requirements

*They may be purchased from the Printing and Publishing Office, National Academy of Sciences, 2101 Constitution Avenue NW, Washington, DC 20418.

†Association of American Feed Control Officials

include growth (especially the early rapid phase), late pregnancy and lactation, and heavy work. Increased requirements are the result of a number of factors, including new tissue synthesis, limited reserves (especially in young), and increased activity.

PATHOLOGIC IMBALANCES. Disease is also often associated with increased nutrient requirements. Diseases that result in rapid catabolism of body stores and protein-calorie malnutrition may result in death if nutrient requirements are not met from exogenous sources. This is one reason for administration of B-vitamin supplements to sick animals. Although it is true that these B vitamins may be lost more rapidly than expected, deficits of protein and energy must also be replaced for nutritional support to be maximally effective. Any disease that results in nutrient malabsorption may decrease body stores of vitamins, especially fat-soluble vitamins. Prolonged diarrhea may lead to increased vitamin losses necessitating parenteral supplementation. However, malabsorption of vitamin B_{12} caused by ileitis in humans is apparently not a problem in cats and dogs. Liver disease may result in deficiencies of the fat-soluble vitamins because the liver is the major organ of vitamin storage and is the site of their conversion to metabolically active forms (e.g., vitamin D). Biliary disease can also lead to decreased absorption of fat-soluble vitamins. Plasma levels of vitamin C were reportedly reduced in dogs with liver disease, although physical signs of vitamin C deficiency were not apparent (Strombeck, 1983).

Renal dysfunction may also affect vitamin requirements because of increased excretion of water-soluble vitamins. Renal failure also results in increased serum levels of retinol-binding protein and vitamin A. Therefore, vitamin A supplements should not be given to patients with renal failure. Vitamin D therapy in patients with renal failure warrants special consideration. Activation of 7-dehydrocholecalciferol occurs in a two-stage process involving the liver (25-hydroxylation) and kidney (1-hydroxylation). Vitamin D deficiency is associated with renal failure because of inadequate kidney hydroxylation of 25-hydroxycholecalciferol (OHCC) to 1,25-dihydroxycholecalciferol (DHCC). DHCC is the most metabolically active form of vitamin D. DHCC has recently become available for use in patients with chronic renal failure. Although this compound may be valuable in the therapy of veterinary patients with chronic renal failure, it should be used only after hyperphosphatemia has been controlled and calcium supplementation has been instituted. If hyperphosphatemia is present, increasing calcium availability may result in metastatic calcification of the kidneys and exacerbation of the problem (Walser, 1984). Variable response to vitamin D therapy has been observed in humans with renal dysfunction (Machlin, 1984).

Another disease that may require the therapeutic use of active vitamin D analogues is hypoparathyroidism (Peterson, 1982). Parathyroid hormone (PTH) enhances conversion of OHCC to DHCC; absence of PTH can result in a deficiency of the active form. Recommended doses of DHCC range from 30 to 60 ng/kg/day. Great care must be taken to avoid overdosage and vitamin D toxicity (consult Treatment of Hypocalcemia).

Erythroleukemia in cats causes megaloblastic changes in red blood cells similar to those seen in folic acid deficiency. Whether or not these changes are due to vitamin deficiency or the disease itself is not clear.

Toxin ingestion also may influence vitamin needs. The most significant clinical entity requiring vitamin K administration is treatment of ingestion of rodenticides that are vitamin K antagonists (the warfarin-related compounds and indanediones) (Mount, 1982).

VITAMIN TOXICITY

Vitamin toxicity, especially of vitamins A and D, is of clinical concern. Vitamin A toxicity has resulted from (1) oversupplementation of the diet, or (2) long-term ingestion of liver as a primary constituent of the diet. Toxicity from vitamin A has been recorded in humans receiving 20 to 30 times the recommended daily allowance (RDA) of vitamin A. Chronic hypervitaminosis A in man leads to fatigue, malaise, and lethargy accompanied by abdominal discomfort, bone and joint pain, severe throbbing headaches, insomnia, restlessness, loss of body hair, dry and scaly rough skin, peripheral edema, and mouth fissures. Exophthalmos also occurs in most individuals. Experimentally induced hypervitaminosis A has produced some of these changes in animals. Naturally occurring hypervitaminosis A in cats has been reported in several countries, including Australia and the United Kingdom, where it is common practice to feed cats beef liver for prolonged periods. The main clinical findings are related to skeletal abnormalities because excess vitamin A intake causes exostoses of cervical vertebrae and tendinous tuberosities of the long bones. Affected cats develop skeletal immobility (e.g., they have difficulty bending their necks to groom themselves) and abnormal gait. In advanced stages, they lose their incisor teeth and appear unkempt. Large doses of vitamin A have been reported to induce congenital harelip.

Most commercial cat and dog foods are well fortified with vitamin A, as it is quite inexpensive. Because it is stable during storage if adequate levels of vitamin E and lipid antioxidants (e.g., BHA, BHT, and ethoxyquin) are present, supplementation is rarely advisable.

Vitamin D is probably the most potentially toxic

of all the vitamins. Toxicity is believed to result from high circulating levels of 25-OHCC, which substitute for 1,25-DHCC on receptors when present in excessive concentrations. Human infants and pregnant women have a low tolerance to excess vitamin D (the RDA for infants is 400 IU/day, whereas levels of 3000 to 4000 IU/day are toxic). The same sensitivity may occur in animals. Hypervitaminosis D is associated with elevation of serum calcium concentration and calcification of soft tissues (especially the kidney, aorta, and heart). Osteopenia occurs in D_3 toxicosis, primarily as a result of decreased formation of bone due to destruction of osteocytes and osteoblasts. Although most living plants have low vitamin D activity, some plants contain compounds with 1,25-DHCC activity. *Cestrum diurnum* (wild jasmine) and *Solanum malocoxylon* have caused hypercalcemia, lameness, osteoporosis, and calcification of soft tissues in cattle, horses, and pigs. Both of these solanaceous plants grow in tropical and subtropical regions. Most cat and dog foods are also well fortified with vitamin D. Since this vitamin is quite resistant to inactivation by heat and oxidation, recovery in the finished product is high. Vitamin D is also synthesized endogenously, so routine dietary supplementation should be avoided.

DRUG-NUTRIENT INTERACTIONS

A variety of drug-vitamin interactions occur in humans and possibly animals. Drugs such as mineral oil or cholestyramine, which affect absorption from the gastrointestinal tract, can depress absorption of fat-soluble vitamins. Nonabsorbed antibiotics such as neomycin and sulfa drugs may depress synthesis of vitamin K, biotin, and folate. Methotrexate and anticonvulsant drugs interfere with folate and vitamin D (25-hydroxylation) metabolism. Enhanced renal excretion of niacin, vitamin C, and pyridoxine has been reported with use of salicylates, indomethacin, and penicillamine. Many other examples of drug-vitamin interactions are known (Hathcock and Coon, 1978); more will undoubtedly be described as new drugs become available. If long-term drug therapy is required, nutritional status should be periodically monitored. If deficits are anticipated, appropriate supplements should be provided.

USE OF VITAMINS IN ABSENCE OF SIGNS OF DEFICIENCY

In addition to use of vitamins for treatment of obvious or subclinical deficiencies, vitamins have been suggested for treatment of a number of disease entities with signs similar to those of vitamin deficiency. Claims for the benefits of administration of supernormal amounts of vitamins are based largely on uncontrolled clinical observations of beneficial responses after vitamin administration. Empirical observations are extremely important to the progress of veterinary medicine and therefore should not be ignored. Uncontrolled clinical observations often suggest possibilities of a particular treatment benefit and the potential for adverse reactions to the therapy. At the same time, it is important to recognize that the next step in the progression of acceptance of an observation as valid is the controlled clinical trial. Reasons for this need include the possibility that (1) adverse consequences may be delayed or unrecognized; (2) use of the therapy may unnecessarily delay development of better methods of treatment; (3) the observed response may have been a placebo effect; and (4) the disease for which vitamins were given may have been self-limiting. Placebo effects are seen in animals as conditioned responses to the therapeutic setting, presence and actions of the therapist, and the nature of the drug or procedure (Presut, 1983). The prospective, double-blind controlled trial is the best safeguard against these hazards.

Therapeutic benefits of vitamins A, E, C, and the B complex in patients without vitamin deficiencies have been proposed (Oveson, 1984). Vitamin A and its derivatives have been used to treat a variety of skin conditions in humans (Ward, 1983). Vitamin A at a dosage of 10,000 IU/day has been recommended for treating dogs with seborrheic disease histologically similar to phrynoderma in man. Because of its regulatory effects on cellular differentiation, beta-carotene and vitamin A have been suggested to have a role in cancer prevention and treatment. Since vitamin A may be toxic, synthetic analogues are generally used (e.g., 13-*cis*-retinoic acid). The value of these compounds in veterinary cancer treatment is largely untested, although much of the research with these compounds has been performed in experimental animals.

High doses of vitamin E have been recommended primarily on the basis of personal experience for a wide variety of human conditions, including immune-mediated diseases, arthritis, and polymyositis. Vitamin E has also been suggested to reduce the risk of cancer by inhibition of nitrosamine formation. No definite conclusions about any of these roles can be made at present; all are the subject of current investigation.

The efficacy of large doses of vitamin C may be as controversial in veterinary as it is in human medicine. Although it is agreed that hepatic synthesis of ascorbate occurs in the dog and cat, a variety of bone disorders in rapidly growing dogs and leukemia in cats have been claimed to respond to "megadose" vitamin C therapy. Use of vitamin C for treatment of such conditions as hip dysplasia and hypertrophic osteodystrophy seems irrational even if it is effective. The most common causes of these diseases are inferior genetics and overnutrition, which should be treated by culling of genetically affected animals and proper feeding of others to limit growth rates to submaximal levels. Excessive intakes of vitamin C may only mask the defects, allowing their persistence in the gene pool. The value of vitamin C in the treatment of feline leukemia has not been carefully tested. The benefit of vitamin C in the treatment of cancer in humans has recently been severely challenged, and the relevance of these findings to veterinary medicine is not yet clear. Although clinical reports of toxicity of vitamin C have appeared from time to time, no controlled studies support the many purported dangers of its administration in large quantities. The primary adverse consequence of excessive intake of vitamin C is diarrhea.

Injections of B-complex vitamins are often given to veterinary patients as a general "tonic" or to stimulate food intake. Although no controlled studies have ever shown the B vitamins to have specific orexigenic effects, administration of reasonable quantities of B vitamins is harmless and may be beneficial. Vitamin administration should always be accompanied by measures to re-establish food intake since deficits of all nutrients occur with anorexia.

For most dogs and cats, commercial diets contain more than adequate levels of vitamins. Vitamin supplementation only enhances the value of the animal's urine. The veterinarian must recognize circumstances such as feeding of home-formulated diets or altered physiologic needs that may increase the possibility of a vitamin deficiency or toxicity. Although some vitamins appear to have beneficial systemic effects on some diseases when given at pharmacologic rather than nutritional levels of intake, controlled trials are required to substantiate their value.

References and Supplemental Reading

Barker, B. M., and Bender, D. A. (eds.): *Vitamins in Medicine* (2 vols.). London: Wm. Heinemann Medical Books, 1980 (vol. 1), 1982 (vol. 2).

Buffington, C. A.: Anorexia. *In* Lewis, L. D., and Morris, M. L. (eds.): *Small Animal Clinical Nutrition*, 2nd ed. Topeka: Mark Morris Associates, 1984, pp. 5-1–5-52.

Hathcock, J. N., and Coon, J. (eds.): *Nutrition and Drug Interrelations*. New York: Academic Press, 1978.

Machlin, L. J. (ed.): *Handbook of Vitamins: Nutritional, Biochemical, and Clinical Aspects*. New York: Marcel Dekker, 1984.

Mount, M. E., Feldman, B. F., and Buffington, T.: Vitamin K and its therapeutic importance. J.A.V.M.A. 180:1354, 1982.

Ovesen, L.: Vitamin therapy in the absence of obvious deficiency. Drugs 27:148, 1984.

Peterson, M. E.: Treatment of canine and feline hypoparathyroidism. J.A.V.M.A. 180:1354, 1982.

Pesut, N., and Kowalczyk, D. F.: Considerations on the use of placebos in veterinary medicine. J.A.V.M.A. 182:675, 1983.

Strombeck, D. R., Harrold, D., Rogers, Q. R., et al.: Plasma amino acid, glucagon, and insulin concentrations in dogs with nitrosamine-induced hepatic disease. Am. J. Vet. Res. 44:2028, 1983.

Taylor, K. B., and Anthony, L. E.: *Clinical Nutrition*. New York: McGraw-Hill, 1983.

DIAGNOSIS AND TREATMENT OF ADVERSE REACTIONS TO RADIOPAQUE CONTRAST AGENTS

PATRICIA A. WALTER, D.V.M.,
DANIEL A. FEENEY, D.V.M.,
and GARY R. JOHNSTON, D.V.M.
St. Paul, Minnesota

Systemic reactions after intravenous injection or regional infusion of diagnostic iodinated radiographic contrast media have been infrequently reported in animals. In part, this may be due to the relatively small numbers of contrast procedures performed in veterinary, as compared with human, medical practice. However, it may also be a reflection of lack of awareness about subtle reactions or failure to associate clinical signs with use of contrast media. Information presented in this article is based on a combination of a review of studies performed in man, collation of experimental data obtained from study of animal models, and retrospective analysis of our personal experiences.

CHEMICAL STRUCTURE AND ACTIVITY OF RADIOGRAPHIC CONTRAST AGENTS

Currently used angiographic and urographic contrast media contain sterile aqueous tri-iodinated benzoic acid derivatives. Common anions include diatrizoate, metrizoate, and iothalamate, which are combined with cations such as methylglucamine or sodium. Calcium, magnesium, or both elements may also be combined with the metrizoate anion. Adverse systemic reactions appear to be caused by the anion components of the contrast media rather than by the free iodine. The anionic components also determine the lipid solubility of the molecule, a factor that influences systemic toxicity, particularly neurotoxic reactions.

The degree of iodine and acetylamino group substitution for the hydrogen ion on the benzoic acid ring influences the degree of protein binding (primarily albumin) and, therefore, the route of excretion of the contrast agent. Fully substituted contrast agents with a low affinity for protein (e.g., diatrizoate) are excreted through glomerular filtration, although the liver and the mucosa of the small intestine are alternate routes of excretion. Protein-bound compounds lack an acetylamino group substitution at position 5 on the benzene ring. These are excreted in bile and therefore are suitable for contrast studies of the gallbladder.

Urographic and angiographic media have a greater osmolarity than that of plasma and therefore function as osmotic diuretics. The anions are not resorbed by the renal tubules. Of the cations, only sodium is resorbed. Plasma hyperosmolality may result in hemodynamic alterations characterized by transiently decreased vascular resistance, hematocrit, and hemoglobin and by erythrocyte shrinkage and clumping.

Metrizamide is a nonionic isotonic contrast medium that is commonly used for myelography. As a myelographic contrast agent, it has an iodine concentration of 166 mg/ml when dissolved in a bicarbonate buffer solution with a pH of 7.4. Nonionic metrizamide is eliminated from the subarachnoid space by cerebrospinal fluid (CSF) circulating into the cranial cisterns or by absorption across the arachnoid into the epidural veins. This latter is probably accomplished by the arachnoid villi.

FREQUENCY OF OCCURRENCE

The incidence of adverse systemic reactions to aqueous iodinated contrast agents in humans is about 5 per cent, with approximately two thirds of these classified as mild and requiring no treatment. During excretory urography, approximately 1 in 2000 humans have had a moderate adverse reaction and 1 in 14,000 had a severe adverse reaction. The incidence of contrast-induced renal failure has been estimated to be 0.1 to 12 per cent. Approximately one death occurred per 40,000 excretory urograms. The frequency appears to be approximately three times greater in atopic patients and is increased in patients who have had previous reactions to contrast media.

In our clinical experience with dogs and cats at the Veterinary Teaching Hospital at the University of Minnesota, approximately 1 in 80 intravenous contrast injection procedures resulted in a fatality. The incidence of mild reactions is unknown but is probably higher.

Underlying cardiovascular or renal disease as well as increasing age affects the frequency of adverse reactions to contrast media. Five per cent of human patients with no history of cardiac disease have developed dysrhythmias. Adverse reactions may be potentiated by dehydration and concurrent use of cardiac glycosides. Pentobarbital enhances adverse reactions to contrast agents with a high affinity for protein-binding (cholegraphic agents).

Iothalamate appears to be the least toxic ionic aqueous contrast agent. Its low toxicity may be related to its low lipid solubility.

CLINICAL SIGNS

Table 1 outlines the clinical signs of adverse reactions to contrast media. Systemic reactions to aqueous iodinated contrast agents may occur acutely or they may be delayed. Most severe acute reactions occur within the first 5 to 10 minutes and have an unpredictable outcome. They range in severity from mild (no treatment required) to fatal. Most severe reactions in humans involve cardiac or respiratory arrest. Cardiovascular toxicity manifested by vascular hypotension and compensatory tachycardia with resultant ischemia has been reported as the initial sign of a severe reaction. The most commonly reported ECG findings after a bolus injection of contrast media are depressed ST segments, increased heart rate, and prolonged Q-T interval. The most frequently observed acute clinical signs in dogs and cats have been vomiting, defecation, urination, and hypotension with or without collapse. Delayed reactions become evident hours or days after the procedure. Contrast media–induced renal failure, disseminated intravascular coagulopathy, and pulmonary edema have been documented as late reactions to contrast media in humans but have not been reported in dogs and cats.

The toxic effects of contrast media on the kidneys

Table 1. Therapeutic Recommendations for Adverse Reactions to Contrast Media

Reaction	Clinical Signs	Therapeutic Options
Early Reactions (<60 minutes after injection)		
MILD		
Neurogenic	Agitation, anxiety	Observe; no treatment*
	Vomiting	Sternal recumbency
	Urination, defecation	No treatment*
Allergic	Erythema, urticaria	Observe; no treatment*; diphenhydramine (Benadryl, Parke-Davis), 5–50 mg IV, and prednisolone (Solu-Delta-Cortef, Upjohn, 10 mg/ml), 10 mg/kg IV
Respiratory	Cough, sneeze	Observe; no treatment
MODERATE		
Cardiovascular	Mild hypotension (pallor, CRT increased)	Often transient (no treatment)*; IV fluids (lactated Ringer's)
	Cardiac arrhythmia	Often transient (no treatment)*; if signs persist, IV fluids, sodium bicarbonate (1 mEq/ml), 0.5 mEq/kg IV. (see Antiarrhythmic Drugs and Management of Cardiac Arrhythmias, p. 346)
	Bradycardia	Atropine (0.5 mg/ml, 0.05–0.2 mg/kg IV; isoproterenol (0.2 mg/ml), 1 mg/250 ml D5W IV drip to effect; epinephrine (1:1000 soln.), 0.1–0.5 ml IV, IC
	Tachycardia (without hypotension)	Lidocaine (2% without epinephrine); canine, 2–6 mg/kg IV (slowly); feline, 0.5 mg/kg IV (slowly)
		Propranolol (1 mg/ml): 0.04–0.06 mg/kg IV slowly (see Antiarrhythmic Drugs and Management of Cardiac Arrhythmias, p. 346)
SEVERE		
Cardiovascular	Refractory hypotension (CRT increased, weak pulse)	IV fluids, prednisolone (Solu-Delta-Cortef 10 mg/ml), 10 mg/kg IV; intubate and ventilate; sodium bicarbonate (1 mEq/ml), 0.5 mEq/kg IV
		Dopamine (40 mg/ml), 5 mg/250 ml D5W IV drip to effect; or dobutamine, 50 mg/250 ml D5W IV drip to effect
	Cardiac arrest (asystole)	Intubate and ventilate, external cardiac massage, IV fluids, sodium bicarbonate (1 mEq/ml), 0.5 mEq/kg IV
		Epinephrine (1:1000 soln.), 0.1–0.5 ml IV, intratracheal, IC; prednisolone (Solu-Delta-Cortef 10 mg/ml), 10 mg/kg IV
		Calcium gluconate (10% soln.), 0.05–0.2 ml/kg IV or IC (slowly); if no effect, isoproterenol (0.2 mg/ml), 1 mg/250 ml D5W IV drip to effect
	Ventricular fibrillation	Lidocaine (2% without epinephrine): canine, 2–6 mg/kg IV (slowly); feline, 1–3 mg/kg IV (slowly)
		Electrical defibrillation, calcium gluconate (10% soln.), 0.05–0.2 mg/kg IV or IC (slowly), or pharmacologic defibrillation; potassium chloride, 1 mEq/kg, and acetylcholine, 6 mg/kg
		Epinephrine (1:1000 soln.), 0.1–0.5 ml IV, IC; prednisolone (Solu-Delta-Cortef 10 mg/ml), 10 mg/kg IV
Respiratory	Respiratory arrest (cyanosis, dyspnea)	Intubate and ventilate with oxygen
		Doxapram (20 mg/ml), 1–4 mg/kg IV
		Prednisolone (Solu-Delta-Cortef 10 mg/ml), 10 mg/kg IV
Late Reactions (>60 minutes after injection)		
	Renal failure (increased creatinine and serum urea nitrogen)	IV fluids (lactated Ringer's) to correct dehydration
		Test dose (2–4 mg/kg IV bolus) of furosemide to initiate diuresis
	Oliguria, anuria	Vasodilators (dopamine, 40 mg/ml), 50 mg/500 ml lactated Ringer's slow IV drip to effect
		Peritoneal dialysis
	Disseminated intravascular coagulopathy	Heparin: canine, 150–250 U/kg SC; feline, 50–100 U/kg SC
	Postmyelographic seizure	Diazepam (5 mg/ml): 0.4 mg/kg IV (slowly); if no effect, phenobarbital, 2 mg/kg at 6–12 hours IV; or pentobarbital, 2–4 mg/kg IV (to effect)
	Pulmonary edema	Furosemide (50 mg/ml), 2–4 mg/kg IV, IM, SC
		Dopamine (40 mg/ml), 5 mg/250 ml D5W IV drip to effect; or dobutamine 50 mg/250 ml D5W IV drip to effect
		Oxygen therapy; IPPV–PEEP

*No treatment required if signs subside within minutes; otherwise, supportive therapy.

Key: CRT = capillary refill time; IC = intracardiac; D5W = 5% dextrose in water; IPPV = intermittent positive pressure ventilation; PEEP = Positive end-expiratory pressure.

may have an acute or delayed onset. Concentration of contrast media in the proximal convoluted tubule after sodium cation resorption may result in damage to epithelial cells. This may result in transitory or irreversible contrast media–induced renal failure characterized by proteinuria, enzymuria, increased serum creatinine and urea nitrogen concentrations, clinical signs of oliguria or anuria, and radiographic findings of a persistent nephrographic opacification.

Nonionic metrizamide has been reported to induce confusion, transient memory loss, nausea, headache, and seizures following myelography in humans. Seizures in dogs usually occur while they are regaining consciousness after myelography but may be observed up to 4 hours thereafter. Death resulting from seizures is uncommon. Mild suppurative meningitis has been described in horses; hemorrhagic leptomeningitis has been reported in dogs. These late complications appear to be directly correlated with increasing concentration of the contrast medium.

PATHOPHYSIOLOGY OF ADVERSE REACTIONS

The pathophysiologic effects of systemic reactions to contrast media have been investigated with both *in vitro* and *in vivo* techniques. Several underlying mechanisms have been implicated in the initiation and perpetuation of adverse reactions.

Contrast media induce histamine release from basophils and mast cells. This may occur through direct interaction between the contrast media and a basophil–mast cell membrane receptor, by the chemical property of hypertonicity (which may induce degranulation), or by activation of the complement cascade.

The complement cascade is probably triggered by plasminogen. Complement activation may alter the coagulation, fibrinolytic, and kinin systems. Release of histamine and anaphylactic substances causes increased vascular permeability, cell membrane disruption, and thrombin activation. The result of release of these pharmacologically active agents is urticaria, laryngeal edema, bronchospasm, hypotension, and other anaphylactoid symptoms.

An immune-mediated response characterized by formation of immunoglobulins directed against contrast agents has been documented. Atopic human patients are more likely to develop this type of adverse reaction. It has been speculated that constant environmental exposure to halogenated benzene derivatives with a similar composition to contrast agents may result in prior antigenic sensitization and possible antibody cross-reaction.

It has also been shown that hyperosmotic contrast agents induce direct injury to vascular endothelium and underlying structures. This chemotoxic effect is a function of time in contact with and concentration of the contrast medium.

The central nervous system has been suggested to be an initiator of reactions to contrast media. Impressions generated within the limbic area of the brain and subsequently transmitted to the hypothalamus may explain the peculiar sensation of chills and flushing described by humans during contrast procedures. It has been hypothesized that anxiety may be involved in the initiation of the central nervous system mechanism. If this were true, mild sedation may prove beneficial in immobilizing animals for procedures and in alleviating their anxieties.

Stimulation of respiratory and vasomotor centers through hypothalamic pathways may result in respiratory arrest and shock. Other brain centers influenced by the reticular formation may result in nausea and vomiting as well as neurogenic pulmonary edema. Stimulation of sympathetic and parasympathetic pathways could explain a variety of symptoms, including cardiac arrhythmias, and disseminated intravascular coagulation due to release of factor VIII during splenic contraction. Bronchospasms are not normally observed in dogs or cats but are common in humans. In man, tachycardia is more often noted than bradycardia, although the latter has been described.

PREDICTABILITY AND RISK OF ADVERSE REACTIONS

The predictability of adverse reactions to contrast media in veterinary medicine is dependent upon the clinician's knowledge of underlying disease processes and recognition of clinical manifestations of contrast reactions. Conditions that appear to increase the risk of an adverse reaction include diabetes mellitus, combined liver and kidney failure, heart failure, and dehydration. Human patients are often asked about known allergies or previous adverse reactions to iodinated media.

In an attempt to screen patients for potential adverse reactions to contrast media, several *in vitro* tests have been proposed. However, they have been unreliable for prediction of adverse reactions. Small test injections of contrast agents have been used as *in vivo* tests for adverse reactions. Because they have failed to predict adverse reactions consistently, they are not recommended.

PREVENTION AND TREATMENT OF ADVERSE REACTIONS

Several measures have been suggested to prevent adverse reactions to contrast media, although none are completely reliable. Since most reactions occur

Table 2. *Protocol for Emergency Treatment of Adverse Reactions to Radiopaque Contrast Media*

Clinical Signs of Contrast Media Reaction	Treatment Plan	Definition of Treatment Plan
Cardiopulmonary arrest	1, 2, 3, 5, 6, 7, 10	1. Establish airway and ventilate 2. External cardiac massage 3. Respiratory center and cardiac stimulant
Cardiac arrhythmia	1, 4, 5, 6, 7, 10	4. Antiarrhythmics
Severe hypotension	1 (if necessary), 5, 6, 7, 10	5. Sodium bicarbonate 6. IV fluids
Mild hypotension	6, 10	7. Steroids
Urticaria	7, 8, 10	8. Antihistamines
Vomiting	9, 10	9. Sternal recumbency
Agitation, urination, defecation, coughing and sneezing	10	10. Observe

within minutes, preparations for emergency care should be made before the injection. The animal's disease state should be assessed. Dehydration must be corrected. An emergency resuscitation kit containing endotracheal tubes, Ambu bag, emergency drugs, and IV fluids should be available prior to injection of contrast agents. We recommend that an IV catheter be utilized instead of a hypodermic needle for injection of contrast media to afford an IV route for administration of medication should an adverse reaction occur. Simultaneous monitoring by electrocardiography may be considered for debilitated patients and those with cardiac dysfunction or previous adverse reactions to aqueous iodinated agents and during selective angiographic studies.

In cooperative patients, sedation may not be necessary for IV contrast procedures. In the dog and cat, premedication with atropine followed by a light dose of morphine, ketamine, or 1 to 2 per cent thiamylal sodium is suggested. Phenothiazines are not recommended because of their vasodilator effects and potentially hypotensive complications. In humans, premedication with steroids and antihistamines has apparently been effective in reducing the number of mild reactions.

Suggested treatment regimens for various clinical manifestations of adverse contrast media reactions are outlined in Table 1. An emergency treatment protocol for adverse reactions is illustrated in Table 2. The most effective therapy of a moderate to severe reaction is IV fluids and ventilation. Steroid therapy is recommended for early adverse reactions, although its efficacy has not been established by controlled studies. It is not known whether tranquilizers administered to dogs and cats after onset of an adverse reaction have any beneficial effect.

ADVERSE EFFECTS ON LABORATORY RESULTS

Changes in clinical laboratory tests are often induced by hypertonic aqueous iodinated contrast agents. Alterations in urinalysis have been reported (consult the article entitled "The Effect of Contrast Media on the Urinalysis"). Potential alterations of other laboratory values after intravenous urography or angiography are summarized in Table 3. Intravenous cholegraphic contrast media have been shown to cause a decrease in serum T_4 (thyroxin) (Jaffiol et al., 1982), and an increase in serum

Table 3. *Potential Alterations in Laboratory Values after Intravenous Urography or Angiography*

Test	Laboratory Value	Reference
Chemistry Profile		
Serum urea nitrogen	↑ (CMIRF)	Alexander et al., 1978
Serum creatinine	↑ (CMIRF)	Alexander et al., 1978
Endogenous creatinine clearance	↓	Feeney et al., 1980
Serum osmolality	↑	Morisette et al., 1980
Serum calcium	↓	Berger et al., 1982; Kutt et al., 1963
Serum magnesium	↓	Kutt et al., 1963
Serum AST (SGOT), ALT (SGPT)	No effect	Måre et al., 1980
Serum total protein	↓	Wisneski et al., 1982
Serum T_4 (thyroxin)	↓	Jaffiol et al., 1982
Serum protein–bound iodine	↑	Caraway and Kammeyer, 1972
Serum parathormone	↑	Berger et al., 1982
Blood pH	↓	Lichtman and Murphy, 1976
Serum Electrophoresis		
γ-globulin	↑	Caraway and Kammeyer, 1972
α,β-globulin	↓	Caraway and Kammeyer, 1972
Albumin	↓	Caraway and Kammeyer, 1972
CBC		
Hematocrit	↓	Morisette et al., 1980; Wisneski et al., 1982
Erythrocyte morphology		
Erythrocyte morphology	Rouleaux formation, crenation	Stäubli et al., 1982
Coagulation Profile		
Prothrombin time (PT)	↑	Parvez et al., 1982
Partial thromboplastin time (PTT)	↑	Parvez et al., 1982
Activated partial thromboplastin time (APTT)	↑	Parvez et al., 1982
Thrombin time (TT)	↑	Parvez et al., 1982
Fibrin degradation products	↑	Simon et al., 1978

Key: CMIRF = Contrast media–induced renal failure.

protein–bound iodine (Caraway and Kammeyer, 1972). Isotonic nonionic myelographic contrast media (metrizamide) result in an increase in leukocytes and protein in CSF samples obtained after myelography (Carakostas et al., 1983).

The duration of most contrast media–induced effects on laboratory findings is unknown. In order to avoid spurious laboratory data, laboratory samples should be obtained before injection of iodinated contrast media.

References and Supplemental Reading

Adams, W. M., and Stowater, J. L.: Complications of metrizamide myelography in the dog: A summary of 107 clinical case histories. Vet. Radiol. 22:27, 1981.

Alexander, P. D., Berkes, S. L., and Abuelo, J. G.: Contrast media-induced renal failure. Arch. Intern. Med. 138:381, 1978.

Ansell, G., Tweedie, M. C. K., West, C. R., et al.: The current status of reactions to intravenous contrast media. Invest. Radiol. *15*:532, 1980.

Berger, R. E., Gomez, I. S., and Mallette, L. E.: Acute hypocalcemic effect of clinical contrast media injections. Am. J. Rad. 138:283, 1982.

Carakostas, M. C., Gossett, K. A., Watters, J. W., et al.: Effects of metrizamide myelography on cerebrospinal fluid analysis in the dog. Vet. Radiol. 24:267, 1983.

Caraway, W. T., and Kammeyer, C. W.: Chemical interference by drugs and other substances with clinical laboratory test procedures. Clin. Chem. Acta. 41:395, 1972.

Feeney, D. A., Osborne, C. A., and Jessen, C. R.: Effect of multiple excretory urograms on glomerular filtration of normal dogs: A preliminary report. Am. J. Vet. Res. 41:960, 1980.

Goldberg, M.: Systemic reactions to intravascular contrast media. Anesthesiology 60:46, 1984.

Harnish, P. P., Morris, T. W., Fischer, H. W., et al.: Drugs providing protection from severe contrast media reactions. Invest. Radiol. 15:248, 1980.

Jaffiol, C., Baldet, L., Bada, M., et al.: The influence on thyroid function of two iodine-containing radiologic contrast media. Br. J. Radiol. 55:263, 1982.

Katzberg, R. W., Morris, T. W., Schulman, G., et al.: Reactions to intravenous contrast media. Radiology 147:331, 1983.

Kutt, H., Milhorat, T. H., and McDowell, F.: The effect of iodinized contrast media upon blood proteins, electrolytes, and red cells. Neurology 13:492, 1963.

Lalli, A. F.: Contrast media reactions: Data analysis and hypothesis. Radiology 134:1, 1980.

Lichtman, M. A., and Murphy, M. S.: Reduced red cell membrane potential and acidification of the plasma in response to contrast materials. Invest. Radiol. 11:588, 1976.

Morisette, M., Gagnon, R. M., Lamoreaux, J., et al.: Effects of angiographic contrast media on colloid oncotic pressure. Am. Heart J. 100:319, 1980.

Måre, K., Almén, T., and Lindell, B.: Liver toxicity of ionic (Diztrizoate) and nonionic (C-29) contrast materials: Effects on serum enzymes after hepatic artery injection in the rat. Invest. Radiol. 11:502, 1980.

Nyland, T., Blythe, L., Pool, R., et al.: Metrizamide myelography in the horse: Clinical, radiographic and pathologic changes. Am. J. Vet. Res. 41:204, 1980.

Parvez, Z., Moncada, R., Messmore, H. L., et al.: Ionic and nonionic contrast media interaction with anticoagulant drugs. Acta Radiol. Diag. 23:401, 1982.

Pfister, R. C., and Hutter, A. M.: Cardiac alterations during intravenous urography. Invest. Radiol. 15:S239, 1980.

Shehadi, W. H.: Contrast media adverse reactions: Occurrence, recurrence and distribution patterns. Radiology 143:11, 1982.

Simon, R. A., Schatz, M., Stevenson, D. D., et al.: Radiograpic contrast media (RCM) infusions: Measurements of mediators and correlation with clinical parameters. Presented at the American Academy of Allergy, Phoenix, Arizona, Abstract 56, 1978.

Spencer, C. P., Chrisman, C. L., Mayhew, I. G., et al.: Neurotoxicologic effects of the monionic agent iopamidol on the leptomeninges of the dog. Am. J. Vet. Res. 43:1958, 1982.

Stäubli, M., Braunschweig, J., and Tillmann, U.: Changes in the rheologic properties of blood as induced by sodium/meglumine ioxaglate compared with sodium/meglumine diatrizoate and metrizamide. Acta Radiol. Diag. 23:71, 1982.

Wise, M.: Non-selective angiography in the normal dog and cat. Vet. Radiol. 23:144, 1982.

Wisneski, J. A., Gertz, E. W., Nesse, R., et al. Myocardial metabolic alterations after contrast angiography. Am. J. Cardiol. 50:239, 1982.

ANION GAP—DIAGNOSTIC AND THERAPEUTIC APPLICATIONS

DAVID J. POLZIN, D.V.M.,
and CARL A. OSBORNE, D.V.M.
St. Paul, Minnesota

CLINICAL IMPORTANCE

The anion gap (AG) is useful in localizing the cause of metabolic acidosis (see Table 1 for definition) and may prompt consideration of disorders that might otherwise be overlooked, including intoxications, lactic acidosis, and renal tubular acidosis. In addition, the AG may be useful in identifying mixed metabolic acid-base disorders. In some cases, it may be the only chemical evidence of metabolic acidosis (e.g., mixed high AG metabolic acidosis and metabolic alkalosis). Serial evaluations of the AG may permit early detection of developing high AG metabolic acidosis, particularly in patients with mixed acid-base disorders. The following generalities are based on experiences with humans and dogs. Although it is logical to assume that these principles do apply for other species such as cats, this assumption must be validated.

Table 1. Definitions and Concepts

Acidemia—A decrease in blood pH below normal. In dogs, acidemia is defined as a blood pH of less than the minimum normal value for blood pH (7.31*).

Acidosis—A process that causes acid to accumulate. Although blood pH tends to decrease when acidosis occurs, the term *acidosis* does not imply that any abnormality in blood pH has occurred.

Alkalemia—An increase in blood pH above normal. In dogs, alkalemia is defined as a blood pH of greater than the maximum normal value for blood pH (7.42*).

Alkalosis—A process that causes alkali (base) to accumulate. Although blood pH tends to increase when alkalosis occurs, the term *alkalosis* does not imply that any abnormality in blood pH has occurred.

Anion—A negatively charged ion (e.g., Cl^-, HCO_3^-, $H_2PO_4^-$).

Buffer—A substance that, when present in a solution, reduces the change of hydrogen ion concentration when acid or alkali is added to the solution.

Cation—A positively charged ion (e.g., Na^+, K^+, Mg^{++}, Ca^{++}).

Metabolic acidosis—A process that causes nonvolatile acid to accumulate in the body. It is characterized by reduced concentration of bicarbonate in the extracellular fluid.

Metabolic alkalosis—A process that causes alkali (usually bicarbonate) to accumulate in the body. It is characterized by increased concentration of bicarbonate in the extracellular fluid.

Nonvolatile acids—Those acids that cannot be eliminated through the lungs and must be excreted by the kidneys.

Organic acids—Nonvolatile acids that contain carbon (e.g., lactic acid, acetoacetic acid, beta-hydroxybutyric acid).

Respiratory acidosis—A process that causes carbon dioxide to accumulate within the body and is detected by an increased concentration of carbon dioxide in the blood (P_{CO_2}).

Respiratory alkalosis—A process that causes increased elimination of carbon dioxide from the body and is detected by a decreased blood P_{CO_2}.

Volatile acids—Those acids that can be eliminated from the body through the lungs (i.e., carbonic acid, H_2CO_3, via the dehydrated form, carbon dioxide, CO_2).

*This value will vary depending on the laboratory being used.

DEFINITION AND CALCULATION

The anion gap (AG) is defined as the difference between measured concentrations of serum cations (sodium and potassium) and measured concentrations of serum anions (chloride and bicarbonate). The AG may be expressed by the following simple equation:

$$AG = (Na^+ + K^+) - (Cl^- + HCO_3^-)$$

The AG is not a true gap between serum anion and cation concentrations but represents the difference between measured cations (which account for approximately 95 per cent of the total serum cations) and measured anions (which account for approximately 85 per cent of the total serum anions). The sum of concentrations of all positively charged particles (cations) in extracellular fluid is equal to the sum of concentrations of all negatively charged particles (anions) in extracellular fluid. The overall relationship between concentrations of total serum anions and total serum cations is expressed in the following equation, where UC represents unmeasured cations and UA represents unmeasured anions:

$$Na^+ + K^+ + UC = Cl^- + HCO_3^- + UA$$

Algebraic rearrangement of this equation reveals that the AG is determined by the difference between undetermined cation concentrations and undetermined anion concentrations:

$$AG = (Na^+ + K^+) - (Cl^- + HCO_3^-) = UA - UC$$

Unmeasured cations include calcium, magnesium, and gamma globulins. Unmeasured anions include phosphate, sulfate, organic anions (e.g., lactate, pyruvate, alpha and beta globulins), and albumin. Increases in unmeasured anion concentrations or decreases in unmeasured cation concentrations increase the AG. Decreases in unmeasured anion concentrations or increases in unmeasured cation concentrations decrease the AG. Changes in unmeasured anion concentrations are the principal determinants of changes in the AG, primarily because alterations in unmeasured cation concentrations large enough to substantially alter the AG are often incompatible with life.

Calculation of the AG requires that concentrations of all anions and cations be expressed as milliequivalents per liter (mEq/L). Because of the low and relatively stable serum concentration of potassium, it is sometimes excluded from calculation of the AG. However, since the concentration of potassium is typically included in serum chemistry profiles obtained with autoanalyzers, we recommend that it be included in the calculation. Another minor modification frequently employed in calculation of the AG is substitution of total serum carbon

Table 2. *Causes of Increased Anion Gap*

1. Metabolic acidosis
2. Therapy with sodium salts of strong acids
   a. Sodium acetate
   b. Sodium lactate (lactated Ringer's solution)
   c. Sodium citrate
3. High doses of certain antibiotics
   a. Carbenicillin
   b. Penicillin
4. Dehydration-induced concentration of normal anions
5. Alkalemia
6. Decreased cation concentrations (calcium, magnesium)
7. Increased serum albumin concentration

dioxide concentration (total CO_2) for serum bicarbonate concentration. Although total CO_2 concentration includes serum CO_2, carbonic acid (H_2CO_2), and bicarbonate (HCO_3^-), it is composed primarily of HCO_3^- (approximately 89 to 90 per cent of CO_2 in plasma is in the form of HCO_3^-). Therefore, total CO_2 concentration provides a close estimate of the concentration of serum HCO_3^-.

The normal range for the AG may vary from laboratory to laboratory. It should therefore be determined for the laboratory utilized by each clinician. When potassium is included in the calculation, the normal range for AG is approximately 15 to 25 mEq/L. The normal range in our laboratory is 12 to 24 mEq/L. When serum potassium concentration is excluded from the calculation, the AG is approximately 4 mEq/L lower (i.e., 8 to 20 mEq/L for our laboratory).

LOCALIZATION OF ACIDOSIS BY USING THE ANION GAP

With a few notable exceptions (Table 2), an elevated AG is highly suggestive of metabolic acidosis. Metabolic acidosis is characterized by increased quantities of organic or inorganic acids in extracellular fluid. Acids (H^+X^-) are buffered by bicarbonate (HCO_3^-), causing loss of HCO_3^- (as carbon dioxide) from extracellular fluid while the acid anion (X^-) remains. Loss of the measured anion (HCO_3^-) is associated with an increase in unmeasured anion (X^-) from the acid, resulting in an increase in AG (unless X^- is chloride). The acid anion (X^-) and how it is metabolized or excreted may influence the AG, acid-base, and electrolyte patterns in several ways:

1. If the unmeasured anion is retained in the extracellular fluid, the magnitude of reduction in serum HCO_3^- concentration will equal the increase in measured anion concentration, which is equal to the increase in AG.

2. If the retained anion (e.g., lactate or ketones) is metabolized, HCO_3^- will be produced in a quantity equal to the quantity of anion metabolized, and acid-base balance and AG will tend to return toward normal.

3. If the anion is excreted, it will be lost in urine with sodium. The obligatory fluid loss associated with urinary sodium loss will induce extracellular fluid volume contraction. Contraction of the extracellular fluid will enhance renal conservation of sodium and chloride. Because the excreted anions are replaced by chloride in the extracellular fluid, the acidosis tends to become hyperchloremic, and the AG becomes normal.

4. Hyperchloremic metabolic acidosis with a normal AG may also occur when the anion derived from acid is chloride. In this case a net change in AG does not occur because as serum HCO_3^- is reduced, serum chloride concentration is increased.

Thus, metabolic acidosis may be associated with normochloremic metabolic acidosis (high AG acidosis) or hyperchloremic metabolic acidosis (normal AG acidosis). Classification of metabolic acidosis as normochloremic or hyperchloremic is useful in localizing the cause of the disturbance (Table 3). The cause of hyperchloremic acidosis may be further localized on the basis of the serum potassium concentration (Table 3). Although these generalities should not be rigidly interpreted, trends toward hypokalemia or hyperkalemia may be helpful in further localizing the cause of hyperchloremic acidosis.

Normochloremic (High AG) Metabolic Acidosis

The hallmark of metabolic acidosis is accumulation of organic or inorganic acids in the extracellular fluid. Accumulated acids may be endogenous or

Table 3. *Causes of Metabolic Acidosis*

High Anion Gap Acidosis	Hyperchloremic Acidosis
Uremia	Diarrhea*
Ketoacidosis	Renal causes
Hyperglycemic nonketotic coma	Early renal failure
Lactic acidosis	Renal tubular acidosis
Toxicity	Distal*
Ethylene glycol	Proximal*
Methanol	Drugs
Salicylate	Carbonic anhydrase inhibitors*
Paraldehyde	Acidifying agents
	NH_4Cl
	Oral $CaCl_2$
	Methionine sulfate
	Hyperalimentation
	Ureteral diversion to the colon*
	Rapid IV hydration
	Sulfur toxicity
	Ketoacidosis with ketone loss in urine

*Often characterized by hypokalemia in addition to hyperchloremic acidosis.

exogenous. Recall that acids (H^+X^-) are buffered by bicarbonate (HCO_3^-), causing loss of HCO_3^- (as CO_2) from extracellular fluid, whereas the acid anion (X^-) remains. The ability of the kidneys to excrete the anion of the accumulated acid determines, in part, whether normochloremic acidosis or hyperchloremic acidosis will occur. If the anion is poorly filtered or is filtered and reabsorbed by the renal tubules, no change in serum chloride concentration will occur. The HCO_3^- lost by titration of the acid will be replaced by the retained anion, resulting in an elevated AG and normochloremic metabolic acidosis.

Detection of an increased AG is not absolute proof of metabolic acidosis. However, other causes of increased AG (Table 2) can usually be ruled out by carefully determining whether drugs were administered or by performing appropriate laboratory tests (e.g., serum protein concentration, blood pH). Dehydration, decreased concentration of calcium or magnesium, and therapy with antibiotics have rarely been associated with detectable increases in AG. Therapy with sodium salts of strong acids may result in elevation of the AG if metabolism of the anion (e.g., acetate, lactate) is impaired or inhibited.

An algorithm may be used as a guide to localization of metabolic acidosis (Fig. 1). Test results depicted in this algorithm *suggest only tentative diagnoses*. Confirmation of the diagnosis is dependent upon careful consideration of the clinical setting and use of confirmatory tests.

UREMIA. Uremic acidosis is a common form of normochloremic acidosis in dogs. However, in early renal failure, hyperchloremic acidosis may occur. In advanced renal failure, decreased glomerular filtration rate causes retention of certain organic and inorganic acids and thus an elevated AG. Diagnosis of uremic acidosis is usually based on detection of acidemia, azotemia, and reduced renal concentrating ability (urine specific gravity < 1.030 in dogs).

DIABETIC KETOACIDOSIS. Metabolic acidosis associated with diabetic ketoacidosis (DKA) may be normochloremic or hyperchloremic, depending upon the balance between production, metabolism, and excretion of ketone anions. Normochloremic acidosis associated with DKA is due to increased hepatic production of ketones. Ketones are strong acids that are rapidly buffered by HCO_3^-. The result is an increase in unmeasured anions in the form of ketones. Diagnosis of diabetic ketoacidosis is based on detection of hyperglycemia, acidemia, ketonemia, and ketonuria.

INTOXICATIONS. Ingestion of large quantities of ethylene glycol, methanol, salicylates, or paraldehyde may be associated with development of normochloremic metabolic acidosis. Large increases in AG often accompany these intoxications. Of these intoxications, only ethylene glycol ingestion is common. The increase in AG associated with ethylene glycol intoxication is caused by ethylene glycol metabolites, including a variety of organic acids. Toxic depression of the citric acid cycle and an altered intracellular oxidation-reduction state result in increased production of lactic acid, which also contributes to the increased AG. Development of acute renal failure may enhance retention of these anions. Diagnosis of ethylene glycol intoxication is based on a history of exposure, characteristic clinical signs, and detection of ethylene glycol or its metabolites in blood or urine.

LACTIC ACIDOSIS. Lactic acidosis results when *in vivo* production of lactic acid exceeds utilization of lactate. Disorders that cause lactic acidosis generally do so by inhibiting oxidative metabolism, either by limiting tissue oxygen delivery or by toxic inhibition of key oxidative enzymes. Conditions that may be associated with lactic acidosis include hypovolemic shock, severe anemia, malignancies, alkalemia, exercise, uremia, diabetic ketoacidosis, and certain intoxications (including ethylene glycol).

When results of the history and routine laboratory evaluation have eliminated renal failure, ketoacidosis, and intoxications from consideration, high AG acidosis has often been assumed to be due to lactic acidosis. A recent study designed to evaluate the accuracy of this generality in humans revealed that elevated concentrations of blood lactate could be demonstrated in only 43 per cent of the patients with the clinical diagnosis of lactic acidosis. Without knowledge of blood lactate concentration, clinical diagnosis of lactic acidosis based solely on AG was frequently inaccurate. In instances in which specific documentation of lactic acidosis is of therapeutic importance, blood lactate concentration should be determined. Blood lactate concentrations in excess of 4.0 mmol/L are indicative of lactic acidosis in humans.

Reliability of Increased AG as an Index of Metabolic Acidosis

The clinical value of the AG has been critically examined in 51 human patients with increased AGs not associated with uremia. It was found that although an increased AG generally indicated organic acidosis, this relationship was not absolute. When the AG exceeded the sum of one half of the patient's serum HCO_3^- concentration plus the upper limit of normal for the AG, an identifiable organic acidosis was readily detected. However, in over 25 per cent of the cases in which the AG did not exceed this calculated quantity, an organic anion could not be identified to explain the observed change in the gap. The size of the AG was a positive indicator of the presence of an identifiable organic acidosis and the accuracy of clinical diagnosis predicted from the

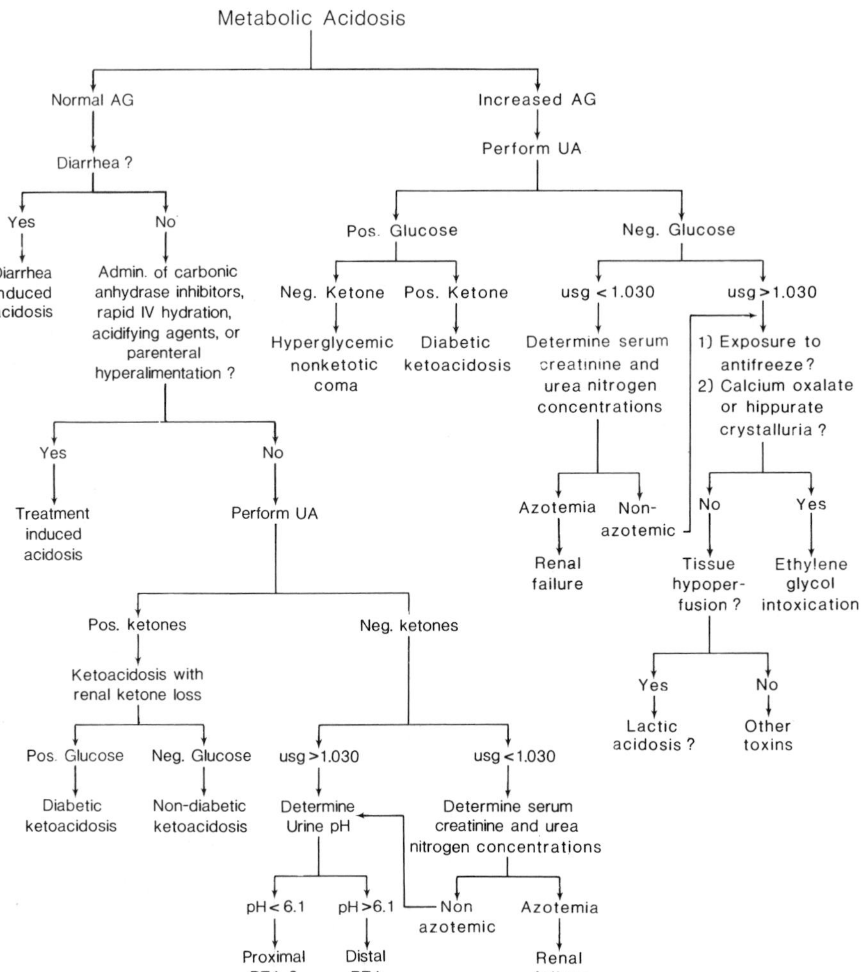

Figure 1. Diagnostic algorithm for localization of the cause of metabolic acidosis using the anion gap (AG). This algorithm provides *a guide* to tentative diagnosis of metabolic acidosis. Refer to the text for further details about confirming these diagnoses. UA = urinalysis; USG = urine specific gravity; RTA = renal tubular acidosis.

elevated AG. Similar clinical evaluations have not been performed in dogs.

Hyperchloremic (Normal AG) Acidosis

Metabolic acidosis unassociated with an increased AG is usually associated with hyperchloremia relative to serum sodium concentration. Hyperchloremia can result from one of three events: hemoconcentration, hyperchloremic metabolic acidosis, or chronic respiratory alkalosis. Hyperchloremia resulting from hemoconcentration (dehydration) can usually be determined by comparison of serum chloride concentration to serum sodium concentration.

Hyperchloremic metabolic acidosis and chronic respiratory alkalosis are characterized by hyperchloremia and reduced serum HCO_3^- concentration. Differentiation of these two forms of acid-base disorders in absence of blood gas determinations should be based on history, clinical signs, and examination of the AG. Patients with clinical and historical evidence of pulmonary or hepatic insufficiency (hepatic coma) and a slightly increased AG may be presumed to have chronic respiratory alkalosis. Patients with clinical and historical evidence of any of the recognized causes of hyperchloremic metabolic acidosis (Table 3) and a slightly reduced AG are presumed to have hyperchloremic metabolic acidosis. However, definitive diagnosis of these conditions requires determination of blood pH and P_{CO_2}.

Hyperchloremic metabolic acidosis results from replacement of bicarbonate by chloride in the extracellular fluid space by one of the following mechanisms: (1) addition of hydrochloric acid (or equivalent); (2) addition of acid other than hydrochloric acid with subsequent buffering by bicarbonate and rapid renal excretion of the acid anion, which is replaced by chloride; (3) gastrointestinal or renal loss of bicarbonate from the body and subsequent chloride retention, (4) defective renal acidification with failure to excrete normal quantities of metabolically produced acid (the conjugate base is excreted as the sodium salt, and sodium chloride is secondarily retained); and (5) rapid dilution of plasma bicarbonate by saline. Except in the cases of dilutional acidosis or addition of hydrochloric acid to extracellular fluid, hyperchloremic metabolic acidosis is almost invariably associated with contraction of effective vascular volume, resulting from loss of sodium bicarbonate or acid anion from the extracellular fluid. Volume contraction results in hyperchloremia through enhanced resorption of sodium chloride in the renal tubules.

Diagnosis of hyperchloremic metabolic acidosis should be based on clinical and laboratory evaluation. Identification of a disease known to result in hyperchloremic metabolic acidosis accompanied by characteristic laboratory values (hyperchloremia, hypobicarbonatemia) confirms the diagnosis. In most cases, an appropriate history, physical examination, and blood chemistry profile (including serum Na^+, K^+, Cl^-, and HCO_3^- or total CO_2 concentrations) permit identification of the condition. Renal tubular acidosis is an exception to this rule; further diagnostic testing is required to detect this disorder.

Renal tubular acidosis (RTA) has been recognized in two forms in dogs: proximal RTA (type II) and distal RTA (type I). Diagnosis of proximal RTA should be confirmed by bicarbonate titration studies. Proximal RTA results from defective proximal tubular reabsorption of filtered bicarbonate ion and loss of HCO_3^- in urine. Loss of sodium bicarbonate leads to volume contraction, subsequent retention of chloride, and hyperchloremic metabolic acidosis.

Distal RTA results from functional impairment of the ability of distal tubules and collecting ducts to secrete hydrogen ions into their lumens against a pH gradient (i.e., inability to acidify urine adequately). Metabolic acidosis occurs as a result of inability to excrete hydrogen ions. The metabolic acidosis is hyperchloremic because the acid anion of the metabolic acid is excreted as a sodium salt, resulting in extracellular volume contraction and consequent retention of sodium and chloride. Distal renal tubular acidosis may be suspected when the urine pH is inappropriately elevated relative to blood pH. Confirmation of this diagnosis should be based on ammonium chloride loading tests or other tests designed to evaluate the ability of the kidney to excrete acids.

Significance of Decreased AG

Although the principal benefits of AG determination have been evaluation of acid-base disorders, recognition of a reduced AG may be useful in evaluation of other types of disorders. The AG may be reduced by increases in unmeasured cations or decreases in unmeasured anions. Causes of decreased AG that have been recognized in humans are summarized in Table 4.

Table 4. *Causes of Reduced Anion Gap*

- Reduced concentration of unmeasured anions
  - Dilution
  - Hypoalbuminemia
- Laboratory error
  - Underestimation of serum sodium
    - Severe hypernatremia
    - Hyperviscosity
  - Overestimation of sodium chloride
    - Bromide intoxication
    - Other causes
  - Overestimation of serum bicarbonate
- Retained nonsodium cations
  - Cationic paraproteins in IgG multiple myeloma
  - Hypercalcemia, hypermagnesemia, or lithium toxicity

Detection of Mixed Acid-Base Disturbances

Principles. Increases in AG may be the only chemical evidence of metabolic acidosis in patients with certain mixed acid-base disturbances (Table 4). In simple high AG metabolic acidosis, the magnitude of increase in AG (ΔAG) should approximate the magnitude of decrease in plasma bicarbonate concentration (ΔHCO_3^-). When ΔAG does not approximate ΔHCO_3^- in a patient with high AG acidosis, the possibility that some other metabolic acid-base disorder may be influencing plasma HCO_3^- concentration or the AG should be considered.

When metabolic alkalosis and high AG metabolic acidosis occur together (e.g., uremic patients that have been vomiting), plasma $HCO^-{}_3$ concentration and blood pH may be modified independently of the high AG (Table 5). This phenomenon occurs because plasma HCO_3^- concentration and blood pH are the net result of the opposing effects of metabolic acidosis (due to decreased plasma HCO_3^- concentration and blood pH) and metabolic alkalosis (due to increased plasma HCO_3^- concentration and blood pH). In contrast, high AG is the result of retained acid anions associated with high AG metabolic acidosis and is only minimally influenced by metabolic alkalosis unless the patient becomes al-

Table 5. *Mixed High Anion Gap Acidosis and Metabolic Alkalosis*

Clinical Data	Normal	High AG Metabolic Acidosis	High AG Metabolic Acidosis Plus Metabolic Alkalosis
Na^+ (mEq/L)	145	145	145
K^+ (mEq/L)	4	4	4
Cl^- (mEq/L)	105	105	95
HCO_3^- (mEq/L)	24	14	24
AG (mEq/L)	20	30	30
P_{CO_2} (torr)	40	35	40
pH	7.40	7.20	7.40
ΔAG (mEq/L)	0	10	10
ΔHCO_3^- (mEq/L)	0	10	0

Key: Δ = change or difference.

kalemic. While metabolic alkalosis increases plasma HCO_3^- concentrations and blood pH values in dogs with high AG metabolic acidosis, acid anions in the blood are not altered by metabolic alkalosis. Therefore, dogs with combined metabolic alkalosis and high AG metabolic acidosis may have decreased, normal, or even increased plasma HCO_3^- concentrations and blood pH values. In some cases only the high AG may remain as a marker of high AG metabolic acidosis.

Combined normochloremic and hyperchloremic metabolic acidosis may also occur in dogs (e.g., advanced uremia with diarrhea). In this case, the magnitude of the decrease in plasma HCO_3^- concentration may exceed the increase in AG because of the combined effects of the two causes of metabolic acidosis on the concentration of plasma HCO_3^- (Table 5).

The relationship between AG and plasma HCO_3^- concentration has been portrayed as a milliequivalent-for-milliequivalent exchange of acid anion (X^-) for HCO_3^-. However, buffers other than HCO_3^- also participate in this reaction; they include plasma proteins, hemoglobin, and intracellular buffers. Also, changes in blood pH may be modified by altered endogenous production of acids (e.g., lactic acid). Because of the influence of these other buffers, the relationship between ΔAG and ΔHCO_3^- may be influenced by many factors, including changes in net plasma protein anion charge, plasma protein concentration, and plasma organic anion concentrations (Emmett and Narins, 1977).

Plasma protein (and other proteins, including hemoglobin) contain large numbers of anionic and cationic groups that may participate in the buffering process. Blood pH influences net ionic charge of proteins. Alkalemia is associated with a decreased cationic or an increased anionic contribution (or a combination of both) to the net charge of the protein. Because plasma proteins contribute to the AG as unmeasured anions or cations, alkalemia may be associated with an increased AG. Similarly, acidemia is associated with increased cationic or decreased anionic contribution (or both) to the protein's net charge. Therefore, acidemia may be associated with a decreased AG. Changes in blood pH may also alter AG by influencing endogenous production of organic acids.

Because albumin is an unmeasured anion, changes in concentration of serum albumin may substantially alter the AG. Overhydration and decreased serum albumin concentration may be associated with decreased AG. Dehydration or blood volume contraction may result in increased serum albumin concentration and increased AG.

APPLICATION. As previously described, some otherwise inapparent acid-base disorders may be detected by comparing ΔHCO_3^- with ΔAG. Methods for calculating and applying this technique are summarized in Table 5. The basic assumption in interpreting results of this comparison is that ΔHCO_3^- and ΔAG will be equal in simple high AG metabolic acidosis and that other concurrent acid-base disturbances may disrupt this equivalency. However, it is emphasized that ΔHCO_3^- and ΔAG are unlikely to be precisely equal, because: (1) the relationship between ΔHCO_3^- and ΔAG is not one of simple equivalency, and (2) precise determinations of ΔHCO_3^- and ΔAG may not be possible because

Table 6. Detection of Mixed Acid-Base Disorders by Using the Anion Gap

Calculations

1. Calculate ΔAG by subtracting the normal AG* from the calculated AG:

   $\Delta AG = AG_{calculated} - AG_{normal}$

2. Calculate ΔHCO_3^- by subtracting the observed plasma HCO_3^- concentration from normal plasma HCO_3^- concentration*†:

   $\Delta HCO_3^- = (HCO_3^-)_{normal} - (HCO_3^-)_{observed}$

Applications

1. When ΔAG is inappropriately large relative to ΔHCO_3^-, mixed metabolic alkalosis and high AG metabolic acidosis should be suspected.
2. When ΔHCO_3^- is inappropriately large relative to ΔAG, mixed hyperchloremic and high AG metabolic acidosis should be suspected.

Precautions

1. The following factors may increase ΔAG relative to ΔHCO_3^- without necessarily indicating mixed metabolic alkalosis and high AG metabolic acidosis:
   a. Alkalemia
   b. Administration of sodium-containing drugs (see Table 2, items 2 and 3)
   c. Dehydration
   d. Increased serum albumin concentration
   e. Hypocalcemia
   f. Hypomagnesemia
2. The following factors may decrease ΔAG relative to ΔHCO_3^- without necessarily indicating mixed hyperchloremic and high AG metabolic acidosis:
   a. Overhydration (dilution)
   b. Hypoalbuminemia
   c. Hypercalcemia, hypermagnesemia
   d. Multiple myeloma (cationic paraproteins)
3. Always consider clinical findings when interpreting the significance of laboratory findings
   a. Evidence for a disease process associated with high AG metabolic acidosis (see Table 3)
   b. Evidence for a disease process associated with hyperchloremic metabolic acidosis (see Table 3)
   c. Evidence for a disease process associated with metabolic alkalosis (e.g., vomiting, administration of diuretics or sodium bicarbonate)

*Normal AG values and HCO_3^- concentrations should be based on normal values for the laboratory being used.

†Use of base excess rather than ΔHCO_3^- will provide a more reliable estimate of the appropriateness of change in the AG. However, if base excess value is unavailable, ΔHCO_3^- is a satisfactory substitute.

actual baseline concentrations of AG and plasma HCO_3^- for each patient are rarely known. Therefore, the clinician must decide whether the relationship between the magnitudes of change in HCO_3^- concentration and AG are appropriate in each case. When ΔHCO_3^- and ΔAG appear to be inappropriate relative to one another, mixed acid-base disorders or factors known to influence the AG independently of plasma HCO_3^- concentration should be considered (Table 6). Comparison of ΔHCO_3^- and ΔAG may be useful in detection of mixed acid-base disorders, but this observation must be interpreted in light of other clinical and laboratory information.

References and Suggested Reading

Emmett, M., and Narins, R. G.: Clinical use of the anion gap. Medicine 56:38, 1977.

Gabow, P. A., and Kaehny, W. D.: The anion gap: Its meaning and clinical utility. The Kidney 12:5, 1979.

Gabow, P. A., Kaehny, W. D., Fennessey, P. V., et al.: Diagnostic importance of an increased anion gap. N. Engl. J. Med. 303:854, 1980.

Narins, R. G., and Emmett, M.: Simple and mixed acid-base disorders: A practical approach. Medicine 59:161, 1980.

Polzin, D. J., Stevens, J. B., and Osborne, C. A.: Clinical application of the anion gap in evaluation of acid-base disorders in dogs. Compend. Cont. Ed. Pract. Vet. 12:1021, 1982.

Shull, R. M.: The value of anion gap and osmolal gap determination in veterinary medicine. Vet. Clin. Pathol. 7:12, 1978.

Thornhill, J. A.: Renal tubular acidosis. *In* Kirk, R. W. (ed.): *Current Veterinary Therapy VI.* Philadelphia: W. B. Saunders, 1977, pp. 1087–1097.

THE DIAGNOSIS AND TREATMENT OF METABOLIC AND RESPIRATORY ACIDOSIS

MICHAEL SCHAER, D.V.M.
Gainesville, Florida

The importance of a basic knowledge of acid-base and blood gas disorders has become very apparent in veterinary medicine over the past ten years. Severely ill patients are commonly encountered that have concomitant severe metabolic or respiratory acidosis. Recognition and appropriate treatment of these complications are essential for recovery. Although a precise diagnosis depends on quantitative laboratory determinations of arterial pH, P_{CO_2} and plasma or serum bicarbonate levels, the clinician should always interpret test results within the clinical context of the patient. This diagnostic approach will facilitate recognition of mixed acid-base disorders as well as possible laboratory errors.

Normal arterial blood gas and acid-base measurements are summarized in Table 1. The methodology of blood sample collection, storage, and measurement has been reviewed elsewhere (Haskins, 1977).

Table 1. *Normal Arterial Blood Gas and pH Levels for the Dog and Cat*

Measurement	Normal Values
pH (units)	7.35–7.45
P_{O_2} (mm Hg)	90–100
P_{CO_2} (mm Hg)	35–45
HCO_3^- or total CO_2 (mEq/L)	24±3

METABOLIC ACIDOSIS

Basic Pathophysiology

The term *metabolic acidosis* describes a fall in pH following a decrease in plasma bicarbonate concentration, $[HCO_3^-]$. This phenomenon can result from three basic mechanisms: (1) addition to body fluids of a strong acid that is buffered by HCO_3^-, (2) loss of HCO_3^- through the kidneys or gastrointestinal tract, and (3) rapid dilution of extracellular fluid (ECF) with a solution that does not contain bicarbonate. The body attempts to offset this reduction of pH by three main processes: (1) chemical buffering, (2) respiratory elimination of carbon dioxide, and (3) renal acid excretion and bicarbonate generation. Various chemical buffers include HCO_3^-, PO_4^{3-}, cell proteins, hemoglobin, and bone. These buffers provide an immediate compensatory response to reduction of pH, but their effect is short-lived and may be incomplete.

The second defense mechanism involves respiratory compensation characterized by an increase in ventilation. As plasma and cerebrospinal fluid (CSF) pH fall, chemoreceptors in the medulla are stimulated to cause an increase in ventilation. This hypocapneic response minimizes the fall in blood pH, but compensation is seldom complete. The appropriate degree of anticipated respiratory compensation in a simple metabolic acidosis can be calculated from the following equation (DuBose, 1983):

$$Pa_{CO_2} = (1.5 \times [HCO_3^-]) + 8 \pm 2$$

If the measured Pa_{CO_2} is greater than the predicted value, the patient probably has a coexisting respiratory acidosis; if it is less, the patient probably has coexisting respiratory alkalosis.

The third and most efficient compensatory mechanism to correct metabolic acidosis involves renal tubular excretion of excess acid and regeneration of HCO_3^-. The kidney eliminates most of the acid through ammonium ion excretion, whereas a lesser amount is excreted as mono- and dibasic phosphates. Substantial renal compensation does not take place for the first 12 to 24 hours after the onset of acidosis and frequently requires several days to reach maximal efficiency. The kidneys generally do not normalize plasma bicarbonate concentration until one or more of the processes maintaining metabolic acidosis have totally abated.

Clinical Signs and Effects

Clinical signs of metabolic acidosis can complicate those caused by the underlying disease. Mild or chronic types may be asymptomatic. However, severe (arterial pH < 7.2) or acute acidemia may be associated with general malaise, nausea, vomiting, and abdominal pain. Characteristic deep respirations (Kussmaul-Kien respiration) may be present. The respiratory rate may be rapid, but it may become depressed if blood pH falls to 7.0 or below. Severe metabolic acidosis can also cause depressed myocardial contractility and a fall in peripheral vascular resistance. These effects may lead to hypotension, tissue hypoxia, pulmonary edema, and ventricular fibrillation.

Laboratory Findings

Accurate assessment of the patient's acid-base status can be made only by measuring arterial pH, P_{CO_2} and plasma HCO_3^- levels. If only two of these values are available, the third can be calculated by using the Henderson-Hasselbalch equation, in which

$$pH = 6.1 + \log \frac{[HCO_3^-]}{Pa_{CO_2} \times 0.03}.$$

Characteristic laboratory findings in simple metabolic acidosis include low arterial pH, P_{CO_2}, and plasma bicarbonate (total CO_2) levels. The serum sodium level is usually normal, and the potassium concentration can range from low to high. Hyperkalemia is usually associated with acute oliguric or anuric renal failure and acute adrenocortical insufficiency. When a lack of complete laboratory facilities prevents in-house blood gas and pH determinations, the clinician might cautiously infer the existence of metabolic acidosis by utilizing the history, physical examination findings, and other laboratory measurements (Table 2).

***Table 2.** Examples of Historical, Physical, and Laboratory Findings Indicative of Metabolic Acidosis*

History
Toxin ingestion (e.g., ethylene glycol, methanol, salicylates)
Polydipsia and polyuria
Previously established diagnosis (e.g., diabetes mellitus, chronic renal insufficiency, shock)

Physical Examination
Dehydration
Hypovolemia
"Fruity" ketone odor of breath
Deep or rapid respirations
Depressed level of consciousness

Laboratory Tests
Isosthenuria (urinary specific gravity of 1.010 to 1.012) in a dehydrated patient
Ketonemia or ketonuria
Azotemia
Oxylate or hippurate crystalluria
Plasma total $CO_2 < 15$ mEq/L
Hyperkalemia

Differential Diagnosis

The differential diagnosis is made after determining whether or not the acidosis is associated with an anion gap (Tables 3 and 4). (Consult the article entitled Anion Gap—Diagnostic and Therapeutic Applications for additional information.) An algorithm may be used to aid in diagnosis of acidosis (Fig. 1).

Treatment

The main therapeutic goal is to eliminate the underlying cause. In general, parenteral alkali therapy should be reserved for patients with organic acidosis only if the causative disorder is not readily reversible or if the degree of acidemia is severe enough to compromise cardiovascular function (arterial pH < 7.2). If respiratory compensation is not appropriate, procedures that improve ventilation will markedly reduce acidemia. The approximate amount of bicarbonate needed to correct an acute metabolic acidosis is determined by the following formula, which accounts for the distribution of bicarbonate ion in the fluid space of the body:

Table 3. *Some Common Causes of Elevated Anion Gap Acidosis in the Dog and Cat*

Cause	Anions Replacing Bicarbonate	Diagnostic Clues
Renal failure	SO_4^{2-}, PO_4^{2-}, various anions	Elevated concentrations of serum urea nitrogen, serum creatinine, and serum phosphorus. Abnormal urine sediment and failure to concentrate urine appropriately.
Lactic acidosis	Lactate	Usually associated with severe hypoxia, hypotension, or various poisons. Marked acidosis in absence of other easily detectable causes (e.g., renal failure, ketoacidosis).
Ketoacidosis	β-hydroxybutyrate; acetoacetate	Detection of hyperglycemia and glycosuria. Positive nitroprusside reaction for urine or serum acetoacetate. The addition of H_2O_2 to urine converts nonreactive β-hydroxybutyrate to reactive acetoacetate.
Ethylene glycol (antifreeze)	Glycolate	History of ingestion followed by acute onset of depressed level of consciousness. Azotemia and hippurate and calcium oxalate crystalluria are usually present.

Modified from Narins et al.: Am. J. Med. 72:496, 1982.

$$\text{mEq } HCO_3^- \text{ needed} = 0.5 \times (\text{kg body weight}) \times (\text{desired total } CO_2 \text{ mEq/L} - \text{measured total } CO_2 \text{ mEq/L})$$

Only half the calculated amount of bicarbonate should be infused over the first 3 to 4 hours; the need for subsequent administration and dosage depends on re-evaluation of blood pH. If acidosis occurs peracutely (e.g., in cardiac arrest), 1 to 2 mEq/kg body weight of $NaHCO_3$ may be injected intravenously as a bolus (so-called IV push dosage).

If offending anions (lactate, acetoacetate, beta-hydroxybutyrate) can be metabolized, correction of the underlying problem will result in conversion of acid organic anions back to bicarbonate by consumption of the hydrogen ion. Thus the amount of anion gap that is above normal (12 to 15 mEq/L) can be used as an approximate amount of plasma bicarbonate that is potentially available to the patient. This consideration is important in order to avoid the iatrogenic development of an "overshoot" alkalosis associated with parenteral administration of sodium bicarbonate.

Specific therapy of metabolic acidosis is influenced by the underlying disease process. Indications for bicarbonate treatment of diabetic ketoacidosis are a blood pH less than 7.1 or a plasma bicarbonate less than 10 mEq/L (Felts, 1983). No attempt should be made to correct the acidosis with sodium bicarbonate when the pH is equal to or greater than 7.2 as long as regular insulin is used to deter further ketone formation and the intravascular fluid volume and serum electrolyte concentrations (especially potassium) are restored to normal. This guideline will help avoid "overshoot" alkalosis.

Table 4. *Causes of Normal Anion Gap Metabolic Acidosis*

General Mechanism	Clinical Examples
Gastrointestinal HCO_3^- loss	Diarrhea; anion exchange resins; ingestion of $CaCl_2$, $MgCl_2$
Renal HCO_3^- loss	Carbonic anhydrase inhibitors (acetazolamide); renal tubular acidosis
Exogenous addition of H^+	Parenteral hyperalimentation solutions; NH_4Cl ingestion; infusion of HCl or its congeners

Therapeutic principles for lactic acidosis include correction of the underlying cause, increasing blood pH through bicarbonate administration, and improving tissue perfusion with intravenous fluids. Vasodilating drugs may also be indicated to reduce peripheral vascular resistance and improve tissue perfusion. Treatment has usually called for large doses of intravenous sodium bicarbonate; however, this method has caused certain iatrogenic complications (Table 5.) One study involving the treatment of lactic acidosis in humans showed that peritoneal dialysis with a bicarbonate-buffered dialysate had fewer alkali-associated side effects (Viziri et al., 1979).

Acute and chronic renal insufficiency commonly cause acidosis due to H^+ retention. In acute renal failure, intravenous alkali therapy is indicated when the concentration of plasma bicarbonate falls below 20 mEq/L. The extrarenal buffering that takes place in chronic renal failure may contribute substantially to maintenance of a nearly normal acid-base status in patients with marked reduction in glomerular filtration rate. However, when moderate metabolic acidosis (pH = 7.2 to 7.3) develops in patients with stable polyuric renal insufficiency, sodium bicarbonate should be given orally at a dose of 25 to 35 mg/kg body weight/day. The dose should be titrated in order to maintain the serum bicarbonate concen-

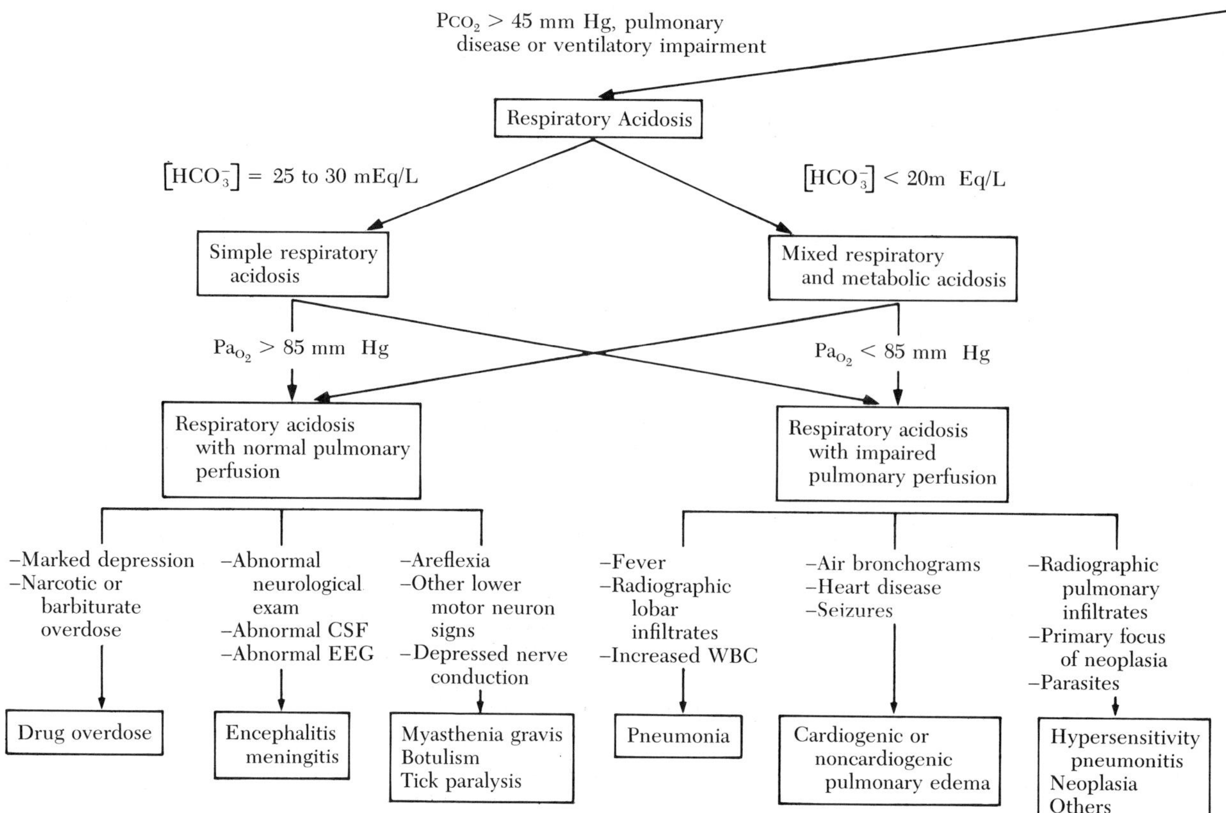

Figure 1. Diagnosis of metabolic and respiratory acidosis. This algorithm illustrates the application of blood gas, acid-base, and other laboratory measurements used to diagnose metabolic and respiratory acidosis.

Table 5. Complications of Sodium Bicarbonate Therapy

Problem	Mechanism and Clinical Setting
Hypernatremia and intravascular volume overload	This problem is a direct complication of the use of large volumes of alkali, which contribute substantial amounts of osmotically active sodium ions to the extracellular fluid space. Patients with acute renal failure, cardiac disease, or both are particularly at risk.
Hypokalemia	Hypokalemia results from cellular influx of potassium ions when plasma pH shifts toward alkalinity. Severe hypokalemia can occur when alkali is given to an acidotic patient that initially is normo- or hypokalemic. The diabetic ketoacidotic patient is particularly at risk if levels of serum potassium ions are not closely monitored and ample amounts of potassium chloride supplementation are not provided.
Hypocalcemia	Enhanced protein binding of calcium induced by alkaline pH may decrease its ionized fraction sufficiently to induce tetany. Patients with renal failure and those that initially have low normal levels of serum calcium are especially prone to this complication.
"Overshoot" alkalosis	Retained organic anions are metabolically converted to HCO_3^- whereas the final serum HCO_3^- concentration is the sum of resynthesized alkali plus that previously given parenterally. Patients with resolving keto- or lactic acidosis are susceptible to "overshoot" alkalosis.
Tissue hypoxia	Tissue hypoxia is a theoretical complication whereby rapid reversal of acidemia increases hemoglobin's binding affinity for oxygen, thereby interfering with oxygen delivery to the tissues.
Paradoxical cerebrospinal fluid acidosis	This phenomenon is a rare complication associated with increased CO_2 diffusion into CSF and brain interstitium, resulting in reduced CSF pH and brain function. It may follow intravenous administration of bicarbonate.

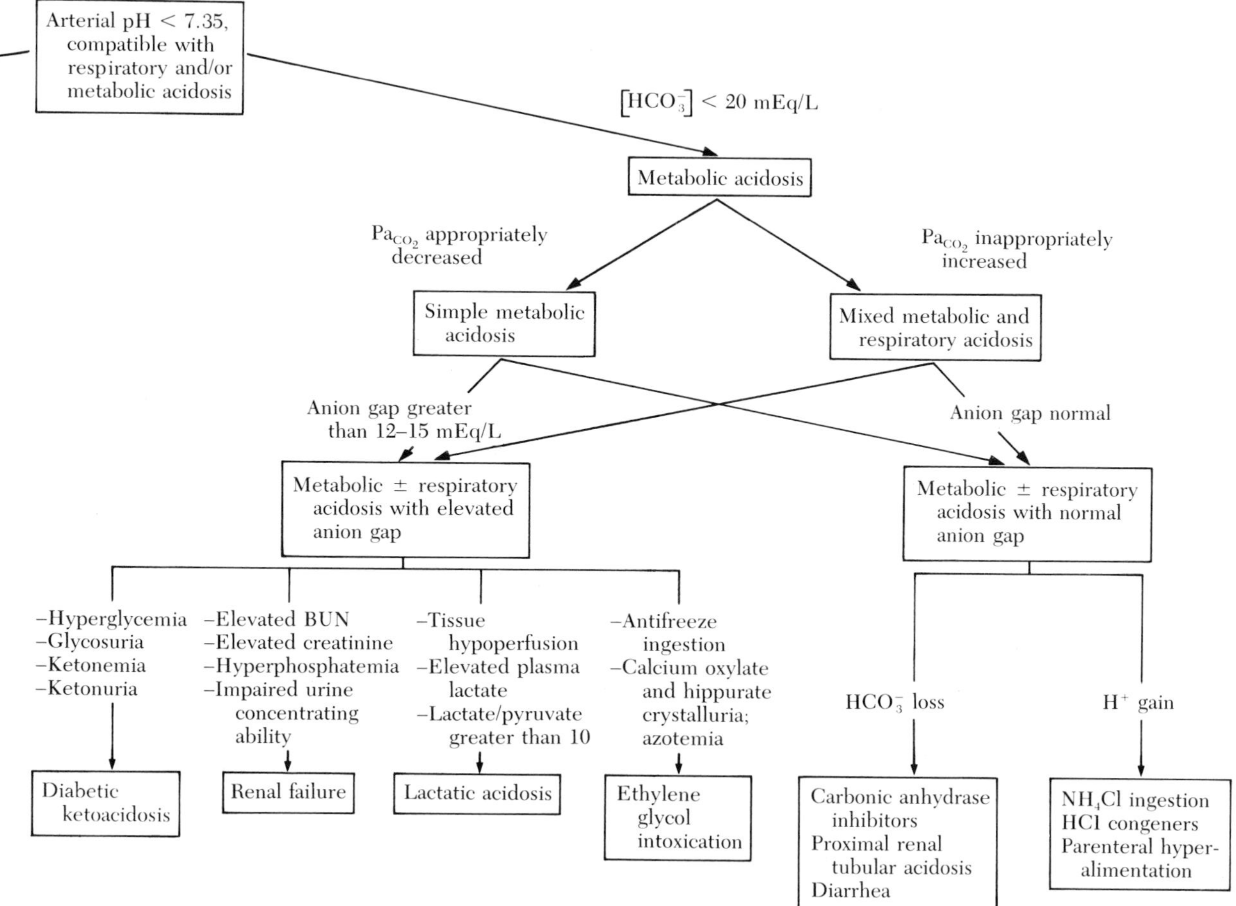

Figure 1. *Continued.*

tration between 18 and 25 mEq/L. This recommendation is restricted to those patients that are neither hypertensive nor edematous (Cowgill and Low, 1980). An algorithm may be used to help formulate treatment of acidosis (Fig. 2).

Other Forms of Alkali Treatment

Sodium bicarbonate has been the most commonly used drug for neutralizing severe acidemia since it has proven efficacy and is readily available. However, other drugs can also be used in appropriate clinical settings in which acidosis is not extreme. Sodium lactate is the buffer present in lactated Ringer's solution. The lactate anion is a bicarbonate precursor that can induce alkalinization after it is metabolized by the liver. Limitations of its use for raising plasma pH include (1) a slow rise toward alkalinity and (2) inability of the liver to convert it to bicarbonate in the clinical conditions of shock, congestive heart failure, and severe liver dysfunction (Hartsfield et al., 1981).

Acetated Ringer's solution contains acetate, which, like lactate, is a bicarbonate precursor. Acetate oxidation occurs in muscle and other tissues rather than in the liver. Therefore, impaired liver function does not restrict its use. An acetate-containing solution should not be used to treat ketoacidosis because it can enhance further ketoacid (acetoacetate) formation.

RESPIRATORY ACIDOSIS

General Pathophysiology

The body must maintain a respiratory, excretory mechanism that collects carbon dioxide produced by cells and transports it to the external environment. In addition, there must be a control center that monitors carbon dioxide levels in the blood and

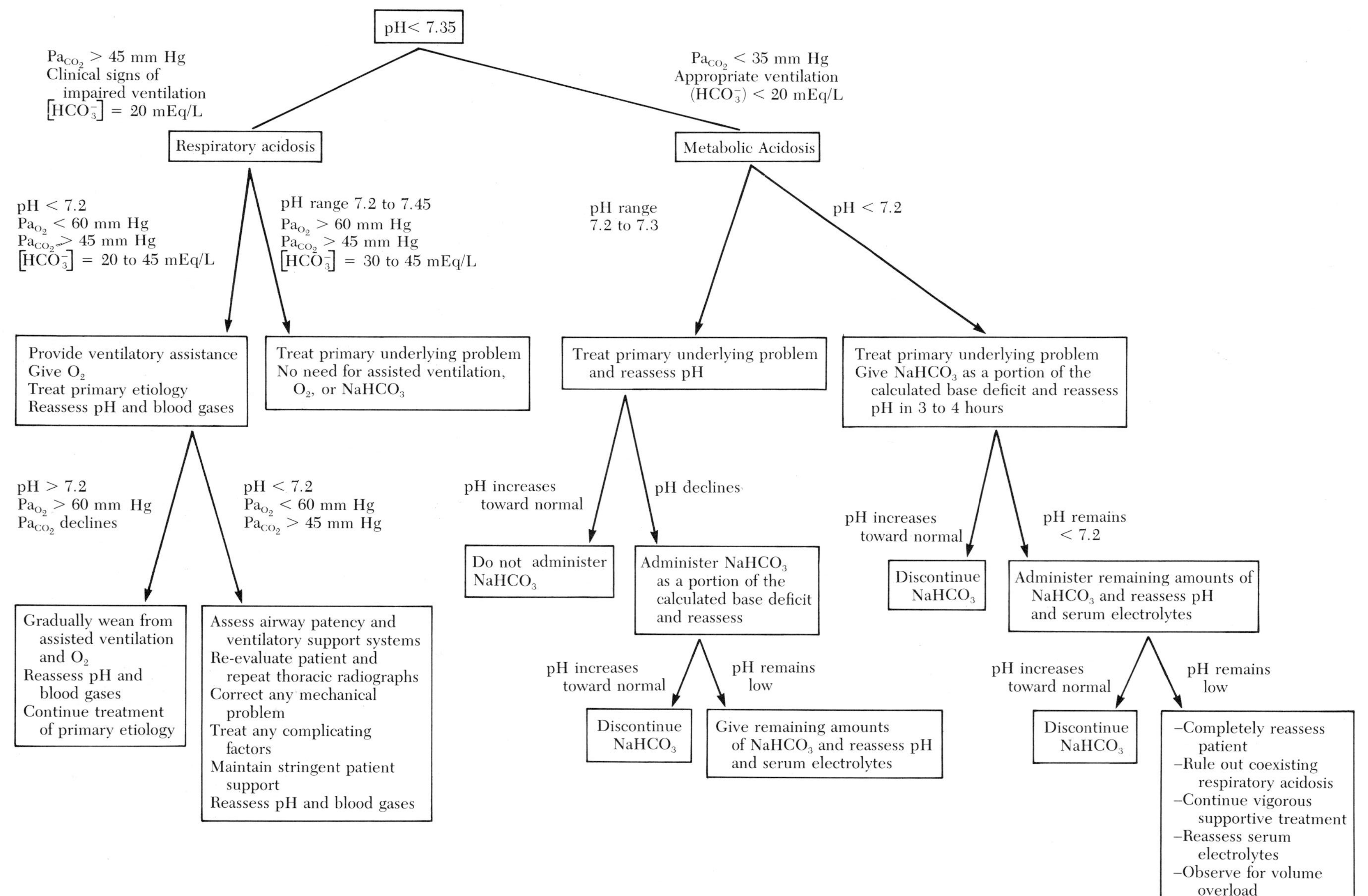

Figure 2. Treatment of simple respiratory and metabolic acidosis. This algorithmic approach provides the general therapeutic guidelines for treating these two causes of acidosis.

regulates activity of the respiratory system. This monitoring system is composed of Pa_{CO_2} chemoreceptors located in the carotid and aortic bodies and the medulla oblongata. There are also chemoreceptors for oxygen and pH in the carotid body, receptors for pH in the central nervous system, and receptors for stretch stimuli in the lungs, upper airways, and thorax. Through this finely integrated network, which feeds into the respiratory control centers located in the medulla and spinal cord, the healthy animal is able to maintain normal Pa_{O_2} and Pa_{CO_2} levels.

Respiratory acidosis results from a primary alteration of pulmonary perfusion, diffusion, or ventilation that allows retention of carbon dioxide (CO_2). The increased dissolved CO_2 is subsequently converted to carbonic acid, which causes a decline of pH.

The H^+ levels that accumulate from acute hypercapnia ($Pa_{CO_2} > 45$ mm Hg) are rapidly buffered by intracellular and extracellular anions. However, this compensatory mechanism is usually incomplete, and respiratory acidosis will persist as long as the primary cause remains uncorrected.

When respiratory acidosis persists for several days, compensation is further attempted through increased renal acid excretion and bicarbonate generation. Hypercapnia associated with high concentrations of serum HCO_3^- and mildly acidemic pH suggests chronic respiratory acidosis, which is associated with a predicted compensatory serum HCO_3^- elevation amounting to 0.4 mEq/L for each mm Hg increase in Pa_{CO_2}. A severely acidemic pH accompanied by minimal elevation of serum HCO_3^- suggests acute disease when the predicted increase in serum HCO_3^- concentration totals 3 to 4 mEq/L (Bia and Thier, 1981).

Clinical Signs and Effects

Signs of the causative disease and hypoxemia usually dominate the clinical picture, but there are specific signs that result directly from respiratory acidosis. Many central nervous system abnormalities, such as anxiety, mental depression, and tremors, are attributed to increased cerebral blood flow produced by the vasodilating property of carbon dioxide (Kaehny, 1983).

Hypercapnia also affects the cardiovascular system by causing tachycardia and vasodilatation. Any accompanying hypoxemia and acidemia can cause ventricular tachyarrhythmias. The acidemia associated with hypercapnia can also cause venoconstriction, which consequently predisposes the patient to overload of intravascular volume and pulmonary edema during the administration of intravenous fluids (Kaehny, 1983).

Laboratory Findings

Acute simple respiratory acidosis characteristically causes hypercapnia, acidemia, and a serum HCO_3^- concentration that measures 25 to 30 mEq/L. The coexistence of metabolic alkalosis or chronic respiratory acidosis should be considered when the serum HCO_3^- concentration exceeds 30 mEq/L. The serum concentrations of sodium, potassium, and chloride are usually normal.

After approximately 5 days, respiratory acidosis usually enters a chronic stage, which is influenced by renal compensation (Kaehny, 1980). Characteristic laboratory findings include acidemia, hypercapnia, hyperbicarbonatemia (serum $[HCO_3^-] > 30$ mEq/L), and hypochloremia. Serum sodium and potassium concentrations are usually normal. Hypoxemia often accompanies hypercapnia in acute and chronic respiratory acidosis.

Differential Diagnosis

Causes of respiratory acidosis can be broadly divided into those associated with the central depression of respiration and those directly involving the thoracic wall and the respiratory apparatus (Table 6). Consideration of the patient's history and physical examination findings will assist identification of the underlying disease process. Further diagnostic tests, such as thoracic radiography, tissue biopsy, cytology, and electromyography, may be required (Fig. 1).

Table 6. *Some Common Causes of Respiratory Acidosis*

Disorder	Usual Type of Acidosis
Central Depression of Respiration	
Sedative and anesthetic drug overdose	Acute
Central nervous system trauma	Acute
Brain tumor, granuloma, or abscess	Chronic
Primary Airway and Thoracic Cavity Disease	
Cardiac arrest	Acute
Pneumothorax and pleural effusions	Acute or chronic
Pulmonary edema	Acute
Pneumonia and other infiltrative lung diseases	Acute or chronic
Bronchial, tracheal, or laryngeal occlusion	Acute
Polyneuropathies	Acute or chronic
Polymyopathies	Acute or chronic

Treatment

The primary therapeutic aims include specific treatment of the underlying cause and supportive therapy consisting of adequate oxygenation and ventilation (Fig. 2). Endotracheal intubation with assisted ventilation may be all that is required when the condition is acute. The duration of this form of treatment depends on the nature and the reversibility of the primary illness. Intensive care monitoring should encompass the patient's level of consciousness, respiratory pattern, and cardiac status. Repeated arterial pH, P_{CO_2}, and P_{O_2} determinations should be done whenever feasible in order to provide an objective assessment of pulmonary ventilation and perfusion. Oxygen supplementation should continue until the Pa_{O_2} is at least 60 mm Hg. Ventilatory support should be gradually discontinued as the patient regains its ability to maintain breathing without assistance. Alkali treatment is usually restricted to those patients with cardiopulmonary arrest or concomitant metabolic acidosis. Inappropriate sodium bicarbonate treatment can be dangerous because the resulting rise in the level of serum HCO_3^- may reduce alveolar ventilation by decreasing stimulation of the central pH chemoreceptors, thereby potentially worsening the hypoxemia and hypercapnia.

Management of chronic respiratory acidosis calls for a more conservative approach consisting of administration of bronchodilators, antibiotics, or other measures needed to treat the underlying disease. Hypercapnia is usually well tolerated, and the acidemia is not severe. Oxygen therapy is provided as needed. However, care should be taken to avoid over-oxygenation ($Pa_{O_2} > 60$ mm Hg) because excessive oxygen might suppress central hypoxic respiratory stimulation. Careful attention is needed to avoid rapid normalization of the Pa_{CO_2} in patients with chronic respiratory acidosis that develop acute respiratory failure ($Pa_{O_2} < 50$ mm Hg, $Pa_{CO_2} > 50$ mm Hg, pH < 7.3), because sudden decreases in chronically elevated levels of Pa_{CO_2} can cause cardiac arrhythmias and seizures (Kaehny, 1983). Furthermore, excess reductions of Pa_{CO_2} levels in chronic hypercapnic patients can cause a posthypercapnic metabolic alkalosis. An adequate intake of chloride and potassium is required to reverse any hyperbicarbonatemia and hypokalemia that might occur. Alkali treatment is not indicated in chronic respiratory acidosis.

References and Supplemental Reading

Bia, M., and Thier, S. O.: Mixed acid base disturbances: A clinical approach. Med. Clin. North Am. 65:347, 1981.

Cowgill, L. D., and Low, D. G.: The medical management of polyuric renal failure: Salt and sodium bicarbonate. *In* Kirk, R. W. (ed.): *Current Veterinary Therapy VII.* Philadelphia: W. B. Saunders, 1980, pp. 1094–1096.

DuBose, T. D., Jr.: Clinical approach to patients with acid-base disorders. Med. Clin. North Am. 67:799, 1983.

Felts, P. W.: Ketoacidosis. Med. Clin. North Am. 67:831, 1983.

Hartsfield, S. M., Thurmon, J. C., and Benson, G. J.: Sodium bicarbonate and bicarbonate precursors for treatment of metabolic acidosis. J.A.V.M.A. 179:914, 1981.

Haskins, S. C.: Sampling and storage of blood for pH and blood gas analysis. J.A.V.M.A. 170:429, 1977.

Kaehny, W. D.: Pathogenesis and management of respiratory and mixed acid-base disorders. *In* Schrier, R. W. (ed.): *Renal and Electrolyte Disorders*, 2nd ed. Boston: Little, Brown, 1980, pp. 159–182.

Kaehny, W. D.: Respiratory acid-base disorders. Med. Clin. North Am. 67:915, 1983.

Kaehny, W. D., and Gabow, P. A.: Pathogenesis and management of metabolic acidosis and alkalosis. *In* Schrier, R. W.: *Renal and Electrolyte Disorders*, 2nd ed. Boston: Little, Brown, 1980, pp. 115–158.

Kreisberg, R. A.: Diabetic ketoacidosis: New concepts and trends in pathogenesis and treatment. Ann. Intern. Med. 88:681, 1978.

Lever, E., and Jaspan, J. B.: Sodium bicarbonate therapy in severe diabetic ketoacidosis. Am. J. Med. 75:263, 1983.

Narins, R. G., and Gardner, L. B.: Simple acid-base disturbances. Med. Clin. North Am. 65:321, 1981.

Narins, R. G., Jones, E. R., Stom, M. C., et al.: Diagnostic strategies in disorders of fluid, electrolyte, and acid-base homeostasis. Am. J. Med. 72:496, 1982.

Sabatini, S.: The acidosis of chronic renal failure. Med. Clin. North Am. 67:845, 1983.

Viziri, N. D., Ness, R., Wellikson, L., et al.: Bicarbonate buffered peritoneal dialysis—an effective adjunct in the treatment of lactic acidosis. Am. J. Med. 67:392, 1979.

TREATMENT OF ALKALOSIS

ROBERT M. HARDY, D.V.M.,
and ELAINE P. ROBINSON, B. VET. MED.
St. Paul, Minnesota

Disease processes that tend to *decrease* acidity or *increase* alkalinity of body fluids induce alkalosis (Haskins, 1977). States of alkalosis are usually characterized by the type of acid-base disorder that led to their development. The most common types are uncomplicated metabolic or respiratory alkaloses, although mixed abnormalities also develop (Tables 1 and 2). Alkalosis occurs much less frequently than acidosis. A recent survey of blood-gas analyses from 220 diseased dogs indicated that alkalemia (pH > 7.51) accounted for 18 per cent of the abnormal blood gas results (Cornelius and Rawlings, 1981). The bulk of these alkalemic dogs had metabolic alkalosis, usually associated with gastrointestinal disorders. Respiratory alkalosis was an uncommon finding in this study.

***Table 1.** Types of Clinical Acid-Base Disturbances**

Simple Acid-Base Disorders
Respiratory
Acidosis
Alkalosis
Metabolic
Acidosis
Alkalosis
Mixed Acid-Base Disorders
Mixed Respiratory and Metabolic Disorders
Respiratory acidosis and metabolic acidosis
Respiratory acidosis and metabolic alkalosis
Respiratory alkalosis and metabolic acidosis
Respiratory alkalosis and metabolic alkalosis
Mixed Metabolic Disorders
Metabolic acidosis and metabolic alkalosis
Anion gap acidosis and hyperchloremic acidosis
Mixed anion-gap acidosis
Mixed hyperchloremic acidosis
"Triple" Disorders
Metabolic acidosis and metabolic alkalosis and respiratory acidosis
Metabolic acidosis and metabolic alkalosis and respiratory alkalosis

*Any of these disorders can be subcategorized as (I) uncompensated (acute), (II) partially compensated (subacute), or (III) compensated (chronic).

From Clark et al.: J. Small Anim. Pract. 18:535, 1977.

METABOLIC ALKALOSIS

Metabolic alkalosis is an acid-base disorder characterized by an increase in the concentration of plasma bicarbonate (HCO_3^-), a reciprocal decrease in plasma chloride (Cl^-) concentration, an increase in blood pH, and, usually, a compensatory increase in the partial pressure of carbon dioxide (P_{CO_2}) in the plasma (i.e., hypercapnia; Tables 2 and 3) (Cogan et al., 1983). Alkalosis develops because of a net gain of HCO_3^-, a loss of hydrogen ions (H^+), or both conditions (Schaer, 1982).

Etiology

There are multiple causes of metabolic alkalosis in humans (Table 4), but the list of *recognized* causes for metabolic alkalosis in dogs is much smaller (Table 4). Clinically important causes include those secondary to (1) loss of hydrochloric acid (HCl) from the stomach after severe vomiting, gastric suction, or gastric outlet obstruction; (2) excessive use of diuretics, which leads to extracellular volume contraction and hypokalemia; and (3) overzealous administration of alkali during therapy of metabolic acidosis.

Pure gastric vomiting is the most important cause of metabolic alkalosis in dogs (Cornelius and Rawlings, 1981). Most vomiting dogs lose both gastric juice (high in HCl) and upper small intestinal secretions (high in HCO_3^-). The net effect usually favors acidosis (Cornelius and Rawlings, 1981). In animals that primarily lose gastric juice without concomitant loss of small bowel fluid, metabolic alkalosis may develop. Conditions such as gastric foreign bodies, gastric neoplasms, or inflammatory lesions that impair pyloric outflow consistently lead to alkalosis if vomiting is severe.

Pathophysiology

Compared with extracellular fluid, gastric juice contains large quantities of hydrogen, chloride, and potassium ions and moderate quantities of sodium ions (Table 5) (Spector, 1956). Gastric parietal cells

Table 2. *Arterial Blood-Gas and Serum Electrolyte Trends Typical of Normal and Alkalotic Dogs and Cats*

	pH (units)	O_2 (mm Hg)	Pco_2 (mm Hg)	HCO_3^- (mEq/L)	Base Excess (mEq/L)	Na^+ (mEq/L)	K^+ (mEq/L)	Cl^- (mEq/L)
Metabolic Alkalosis								
1. Uncompensated	↑	Var	N	↑	↑	N, ↓	N, ↓	N, ↓
2. Partially compensated	↑	Var	↑	↑	↑	N, ↓	N, ↓	N, ↓
Associated with vomiting	↑	Var	N, ↑	↑	↑	↓	↓	↓
Respiratory Alkalosis								
1. Uncompensated	↑	Var	↓	N	N	Var	Var	Var
2. Partially compensated	↑	Var	↓	↓	↓	Var	Var	Var
Associated with hypoxemia	↑	↓	↓	N, ↓	N, ↓	Var	Var	Var
Mixed Metabolic and Respiratory Alkalosis	↑	Var	↑	↓	↑	Var	Var	Var
Normal Dogs*	7.35–7.46	90–110	26–42	18–24	+1–3	140–154	3.8–5.8	99–110
Normal Cats*	7.30–7.45	95–110	26–40	16.5–21	+1–5	150–156	4.1–5.3	115–130

Key: ↑ = increased; ↓ = decreased; N = normal; Var = variable.

*Normal range of values are composite values for arterial blood (Clark et al., 1977; Cornelius and Rawlings, 1981; Haskins, 1983; Middleton et al., 1981; Tan and Simmons, 1981). Venous values would be expected to have lower pH, lower Po_2, higher Pco_2, and higher HCO_3^-, depending on the site of collection.

form carbonic acid (H_2CO_3) from the reaction of H_2O and CO_2, by utilizing the enzyme carbonic anhydrase (CA). Carbonic acid readily dissociates into H^+ and HCO_3^-:

$$H_2O + CO_2 \overset{CA}{\rightleftharpoons} H_2CO_3 \leftrightharpoons H^+ + HCO_3^-$$

Hydrogen ions are secreted from parietal cells into the gastric lumen along with chloride ions, and HCO_3^- is reabsorbed into the blood stream. This process is responsible for a physiologic postprandial alkaline tide (Goldberger, 1980). Normally, excess bicarbonate has only a transient effect on blood pH. Sodium bicarbonate is secreted by the pancreas when gastric acid enters the upper small bowel. The acid-base balance of the blood is thus returned to normal.

When large quantities of gastric acid are lost in vomitus, excess bicarbonate is added to extracellular fluid and leads to metabolic alkalosis. The body has three means of compensating for this increased alkali load: (1) redistribution and cellular buffers, (2) respiratory defense mechanisms, and (3) renal defense mechanisms (DuBoise, 1983).

The first defense against added alkali is redistribution and cellular buffering of the base. As alkali is added to extracellular fluid (ECF), rapid distribution throughout this large tissue space dilutes its effect on ECF pH. Ninety-five per cent of the load of HCO_3^- is redistributed in ECF within 25 min (Cogan et al., 1981). Simultaneously, cellular buffers blunt the ability of added alkali to raise the body's pH (Cogan et al., 1981). Hydrogen ions leave cells to react with the added alkali in exchange for potassium ions. In dogs, the maximal physiologic effects of cellular buffers require about 2 hours. These electrolyte shifts may be expected to produce a decrease in serum potassium concentration of 0.2 to 0.5 mEq/L for each 0.1 unit increase in pH (i.e., if blood pH increases from 7.4 to 7.5, serum potassium decreases by 0.2 to 0.5 mEq/L) (Simmons and Avedon, 1959). Cellular buffering events are unable to normalize blood pH, however. Respiratory and

Table 3. *Blood-Gas Values Indicative of Alkalosis in Alkalemic Dogs and Cats*

	Metabolic Alkalosis (Partially Compensated)	Respiratory Alkalosis (Uncompensated)	Respiratory Alkalosis (Partially compensated)	Mixed Metabolic and Respiratory Alkalosis
pH	> 7.5	> 7.5	> 7.5	> 7.5
Pco_2 (mm Hg)	> 35	< 35	< 35	< 35
HCO_3^- (mEq/L)	> 24	18–24	< 18	> 24
Base excess (mEq/L)	Positive	Normal range	Negative	Positive

*Table 4. Causes of Metabolic Alkalosis in Humans and Dogs**

	Humans	Dogs
Exogenous Sources of Bicarbonate		
Acute alkali administration	Yes	Yes
Milk-alkali syndrome	Yes	Possible
Extracellular Volume Contraction:		
Normotensive Secondary Hyperreninemic Hyperaldosteronism		
Gastrointestinal Origin		
Vomiting	Yes	Yes
Gastric suction	Yes	Possible
Congenital chloridorrhea	Yes	?
Renal Origin		
Diuretics (thiazides, Lasix, ethacrynic acid)	Yes	Yes
Edematous states	Yes	?
Posthypercapneic states	Yes	?
Hypercalcemia or Hypoparathyroidism	Yes	?
Recovery from lactic or ketoacidosis	Yes	Yes
Nonreabsorbable anion excretion	Yes	?
Magnesium deficiency	Yes	?
Bartter's syndrome	Yes	?
Carbohydrate Refeeding After Starvation	Yes	?
Extracellular Volume Expansion:		
Hypertension and Hypermineralocorticoidism		
Associated with Increased Renin Activity		
Renal artery stenotic diseases	Yes	?
Accelerated hypertension	Yes	?
Renin-secreting tumor	Yes	?
Estrogen therapy	Yes	?
Associated with Decreased Renin Activity		
Primary aldosteronism	Yes	?
Adrenal enzymatic defects		
11-Hydroxylase deficiency	Yes	?
17-Hydroxylase deficiency	Yes	?
Cushing's disease or syndrome	Yes	?
Other mineralocorticoids		
Licorice ingestion	Yes	?
Carbenoxolone	Yes	?
Little's disease	Yes	?

*From Cogan et al. *in* Brenner and Rector: *The Kidney*, 2nd ed. Philadelphia: W. B. Saunders, 1981, pp. 841–907.

renal compensatory mechanisms perform this regulatory function (Haskins, 1977).

Hypoventilation, the typical respiratory response to metabolic alkalosis, elevates plasma CO_2 concentrations. The magnitude of change in P_{CO_2} that occurs in response to pure metabolic alkalosis is highly predictable. For each mEq/L increase in HCO_3^- concentration above normal, a 0.55 to 0.7 mmHg increase in P_{CO_2} can be expected (DuBoise, 1983; Harrington, 1984). Retention of CO_2 increases the carbonic acid concentration of blood which, in turn, lowers blood pH toward normal (Cogan et al., 1981). This hypercapneic response requires 8 to 12 hours for maximal effect and is most obvious when plasma HCO_3^- concentrations are 35 to 40 mEq/L or greater (Haskins, 1977; Schwartz, 1979). Arterial P_{CO_2} concentrations rarely exceed 50 mm Hg (normal value = 36.8 ± 3.0 mmHg; Haskins, 1983) in response to metabolic alkalosis, because greater degrees of hypercapnia are associated with hypoxemia (Schwartz, 1979). Hypoxemia stimulates respiratory centers to increase the respiratory rate and eliminate excess CO_2 (Schaer, 1982). Thus, in alert awake patients, it is rare for metabolic alkalosis to cause a significant decrease in alveolar ventilation, and there is a tendency for the alkalemia to remain uncompensated. This "cerebral escape" mechanism may not function in unconscious, semiconscious, or severely debilitated animals. In such animals, metabolic alkalosis may precipitate severe alveolar hypoventilation and result in significant hypoxemia.

Table 5. Comparison of Electrolyte Composition (mEq/L) in Canine Gastric Juice and Extracellular Fluid

Electrolyte	Gastric Juice	Extracellular Fluid
Sodium	46–79	137–149
Potassium	10–22	3.7–5.5
Chloride	98–143	100–112
Free hydrogen	150	1×10^{-7}
Calcium	0.95–3.3	4.5–5.5

Pulmonary compensatory mechanisms are generally not as effective as renal responses in decreasing the severity of metabolic alkalosis. However, they respond faster and attain maximal physiologic effects earlier.

The kidneys are ultimately responsible for elimination of the excess alkali associated with metabolic alkalosis and for returning extracellular pH to normal. Under normal circumstances, when excess alkali from any source accumulates in the body, the renal tubular maximum for HCO_3^- reabsorption is exceeded and bicarbonaturia results (Cogan et al., 1981, 1983; Schwartz, 1980). The kidney is so efficient in this process that it is difficult to induce even mild alkalosis by administering exogenous sodium bicarbonate (Cogan et al., 1981). Unfortunately, this expected renal response to excess alkali is frequently altered during endogenously generated states of metabolic alkalosis (e.g., vomiting, gastrointestinal obstruction, and diuretic excess). In fact, the kidney often fails to excrete the excess HCO_3^- and thus is responsible for *maintaining* the alkalotic state, regardless of its cause.

When metabolic alkalosis occurs secondary to gastric vomiting, alkalosis is caused primarily by loss of acid (H^+), its accompanying anion (Cl^-), and retention of endogenously generated HCO_3^-. Continued loss of fluid (H_2O), acid (H^+), and anions (Cl^-) prevents the kidneys from eliminating excess HCO_3^-.

The most important factors in maintaining metabolic alkalosis associated with vomiting are (1) decreased extracellular volume (ECV), (2) hypochloremia, (3) hypokalemia, and (4) compensatory hypercapnia (Cogan et al., 1981, 1983; Cohen and

Kassirer, 1980; Harrington, 1984). During initial stages of vomiting, the kidneys sense an increased HCO_3^- load and eliminate it in urine. However, if continued fluid and electrolyte losses (Na^+, Cl^-, H^+) result in ECV contraction, decreased glomerular filtration and hypochloremia will develop. The renal response to decreased ECV results in avid HCO_3^- reabsorption by both proximal and distal sites along nephrons. This occurs in spite of elevated concentrations of HCO_3^- in the blood and perpetuates alkalosis. Decreased ECV also enhances sodium reabsorption by proximal tubules. Sodium is reabsorbed with accompanying anions, either chloride or HCO_3^-. Chloride reabsorption is maximal because of vomiting-induced hypochloremia. However, insufficient chloride is present for the sodium, necessitating reabsorption. The only anion availablê in excess is bicarbonate. Thus, sodium will be absorbed primarily as sodium bicarbonate, even though alkalosis exists.

Enhanced mineralocorticoid activity further serves to maintain alkalosis. Reduction in ECV stimulates the renin-angiotensin-aldosterone mechanism. Aldosterone augments sodium reabsorption and potassium excretion by distal nephrons. If chloride anions were readily available, they would accompany sodium cations during reabsorption. However, since vomiting has induced severe chloride deficits, the HCO_3^- again becomes the only available anion to accompany sodium in its reabsorption.

New bicarbonate will also be generated by distal tubular cells through the action of carbonic anhydrase on CO_2 and H_2O:

$$H_2O + CO_2 \overset{CA}{\leftrightharpoons} H_2CO_3 \leftrightharpoons H^+ + HCO_3^-$$

The generated (new) bicarbonate accompanies sodium as it is reabsorbed, perpetuating alkalosis. The reabsorbed Na^+ is exchanged for both H^+ and K^+ ions, both of which are excreted in urine. These processes also maintain the alkalotic state.

Hypokalemia is frequently associated with chronic vomiting-induced metabolic alkalosis, and it aggravates the condition. Loss of potassium in vomitus and mineralocorticoid-augmented renal excretion of potassium are primarily responsible for hypokalemia. Hypokalemia alone serves as a stimulus for HCO_3^- reabsorption by the proximal renal tubules (Kurtzman et al., 1973). Further, if severe hypokalemia exists ($K^+ < 2.0$ mEq/L), Na^+ will be exchanged for H^+ rather than K^+ in the distal nephron. This process leads to additional loss of acid in urine, preventing retention of H^+ to modify systemic alkalosis (Dumler, 1981).

Augmented HCO_3^- reabsorption and exchange of Na^+ for H^+ and K^+ for H^+ in the kidneys can lead to production of acid urine in states of metabolic alkalosis. This phenomenon is called paradoxical aciduria (Dumler, 1981; Van Slyke and Evans, 1947). In dogs with severe metabolic alkalosis experimentally induced with gastric fistulas, urine pH values ranged from 5.0 to 6.4 (Van Slyke and Evans, 1947). Thus, urine pH is not a reliable index of systemic blood-gas disturbances in patients with metabolic alkalosis.

Respiratory compensation (hypercapnia) for metabolic alkalosis may also perpetuate renal "maladaptive" responses to metabolic alkalosis. When the kidney senses an increase in P_{CO_2}, it normally increases HCO_3^- reabsorption and H^+ secretion. These processes enhance the severity of the alkalosis (Harrington, 1984). Although hypercapnia lowers systemic pH in cases of metabolic alkalosis, this renal "maladaptive" response limits the effectiveness of respiratory compensatory mechanisms.

Alkalemia associated with metabolic and respiratory alkalosis increases oxygen affinity of hemoglobin by causing a shift of the oxyhemoglobin curve to the left. As a result there is less transfer of oxygen to tissues (Shapiro et al., 1977).

Diagnosis

An accurate history, determination of blood gases, and an electrolyte profile will confirm the diagnosis of metabolic alkalosis. Clinical signs of alkalosis are similar to those associated with hypocalcemia. Mental confusion, dullness, paresthesia, muscle cramps, and tetany occur in man (Cogan et al., 1981). Preexisting tendencies for seizures and cardiac arrhythmias will also be aggravated. Signs of volume contraction (dehydration, slow capillary refill time, and weak pulse) may also be evident.

Since the body's compensatory mechanisms do not overcompensate in regulating acid-base balance, blood pH is a reliable index of the major abnormality present (i.e., alkalosis or acidosis). Blood pH values greater than 7.50 indicate alkalemia. Evaluation of the HCO_3^- concentration, P_{CO_2}, and base excess will indicate whether the cause is primarily metabolic or respiratory in origin (Tables 2 and 3). In metabolic alkalosis, plasma HCO_3^- concentrations exceed 25 mEq/L and arterial P_{CO_2} values are normal to increased (normal value for dogs is 36.8 ± 3.0 mm Hg) (Haskins, 1983). The calculated base excess will be greater than 2 mEq/L. If the cause for the metabolic alkalosis is vomiting or excessive use of diuretics, hypochloremia and hypokalemia may also be present.

Therapy

Prior to therapy of metabolic alkalosis, it is necessary to establish (1) what factors are responsible for producing alkalosis and (2) what factors are maintaining it (i.e., impairing renal elimination of excess HCO_3^-). Initial therapeutic efforts should be directed at eliminating the cause of alkalosis (e.g., stop vomiting or stop diuretic administration). This action will help to prevent the problem from worsening; however, alkalosis will often persist unless renal mechanisms responsible for avid HCO_3^- retention and H^+ elimination are reversed.

All common types of metabolic alkalosis in dogs are responsive to saline. Adequate quantities of sodium chloride will restore ECV to normal, inhibit further mineralocorticoid secretion, and provide Cl^-. By providing adequate chloride anion, HCO_3^- anion no longer needs to accompany sodium cations during renal reabsorption. Providing Cl^- allows elimination of HCO_3^- in urine and inhibits acid formation of distal tubules (Cohen and Kassirer, 1980).

Chloride concentrations in urine are a good index of the body's need for chloride. In humans with saline-responsive hypochloremic alkalosis, chloride concentrations in the urine are usually lower than 10 mEq/L (Goldberger, 1980). Once chloride stores are replenished, urine pH starts to rise (owing to bicarbonaturia) and urine chloride concentrations will exceed 10 mEq/L.

The quantity of chloride required for replacement therapy may be estimated with the following formula (Dumler, 1981):

$$\text{Extracellular } Cl^- \text{ deficits (mEq/L)} = 0.3\ (\text{L/kg}) \times \text{body weight (kg)} \times (\text{normal } [Cl^-] - \text{measured } [Cl^-])$$

Either physiologic (0.9 per cent) saline or Ringer's solution may be used for both volume and electrolyte replacement. Fifty per cent of the calculated chloride deficit usually should be replaced during the first 24 hours. Because of continuing losses and the approximate nature of these calculations, evaluation of serum electrolyte concentrations and recalculation of deficits should be repeated daily. Once sodium, chloride, and potassium concentrations are normalized, maintenance fluids such as Multisol-M (Abbott) or Plasmalyte-56 (Travenol) should be used for therapy.

Although potassium supplementation is not necessary for correction of alkalosis unless deficits are severe (K^+ <2.0 mEq/L), potassium supplementation may be warranted if surgery is contemplated because cardiac arrhythmias and myocardial depression associated with hypokalemia are of concern during anesthesia. Potassium may be added to replacement fluids to attain final concentrations of 20 to 40 mEq/L. Intravenous flow rates should not exceed 0.5 mEq/kg/hour for potassium. Daily assessment of serum potassium concentrations should be utilized to determine whether or not further supplementation is needed.

Generally, the pH range compatible with life is 6.8 to 7.8 (DuBoise, 1983). Blood pH values between 7.2 and 7.6 are not serious threats to survival (Haskins, 1983). However, pH values greater than 7.6 warrant aggressive therapy (Haskins, 1977). Mortality figures for humans with severe alkalemia are 65 per cent at pH 7.60 to 7.64 and 85 per cent at pH greater than 7.65 (DuBoise, 1983).

Aggressive measures for reversing metabolic alkalosis include use of the following, alone or in combination: cimetidine (Tagamet, Smith Kline & French) (Cogan et al., 1981), carbonic anhydrase inhibitors (Nascimente, 1981), and intravenous acidifying solutions such as hydrochloric acid, ammonium chloride, and arginine monohydrochloride (Kassirer, 1974; Kopple and Blumenkrantz, 1980). For patients that continue to lose large quantities of gastric acid in vomitus, cimetidine (a hydrogen receptor antagonist) may be given to decrease gastric acid hypersecretion (dose = 5 to 10 mg/kg, three to four times daily). Acetazolamide (Diamox, Lederle), a carbonic anhydrase inhibitor, causes bicarbonaturia by inhibiting renal HCO_3^- reabsorption. Owing to its diuretic action, however, this drug may aggravate volume contraction and hypokalemia (Cogan et al., 1983). Dosage recommended for dogs is 10 mg/kg given four times daily. Ammonium chloride is an acidifying agent that can be used to correct metabolic alkalosis rapidly. However, because of the potential for ammonia intoxication after intravenous use of ammonium chloride, it is rarely used. Dilute hydrochloric acid solutions can be given intravenously for rapid correction of life-threatening metabolic alkalosis (Dumler, 1981; Kopple and Blumenkrantz, 1980; Kwun et al., 1983). Hydrochloric acid at a concentration of 1 mEq/ml (1.0 N) may be given intravenously by deep vein catheter. The rate of administration is 1 mEq/min. The quantity required to neutralize the base excess may be calculated as follows (Kurtzman et al., 1973):

$$\text{HCl (mEq) given} = 0.3\ (\text{L/kg}) \times \text{body weight (kg)} \times \text{base excess (mEq/L)}$$

The solution can be sterilized by passing it through a 0.22 μm filter. No more than two thirds of the calculated amount should be given without repeating blood gas determinations. L-Arginine monohydrochloride is considered to be safer than dilute HCl for intravenous neutralization of excess HCO_3^- (Kassirer, 1974). It is available commercially as a 10 per cent intravenous solution (R-Gene, Cutter). During its metabolism approximately 50 mEq HCl

Table 6. *Causes of Respiratory Alkalosis**

Direct Stimulation of Respiratory Center
Anxiety, fear, pain (functional hyperventilation)
Primary CNS lesions
Encephalitis
Neoplasia
Stroke
Decreased blood supply
Hypoxemia
High altitude
Pulmonary shunts
Pulmonary diffusion defects
Hypotension
Anemia
Congestive heart failure
Pneumonia
Interstitial pulmonary edema
Physical stimuli within thorax
Irritation of bronchi
Stiff lungs
Reduced movement of chest wall or diaphragm
Hypermetabolic states
Fever
Heat stroke
Hyperthyroidism
Alcohol intoxication
Salicylate toxicity
Xanthine toxicity
Mechanically assisted ventilation
Specific conditions
Hepatic cirrhosis
Gram-negative sepsis
Progesterone excess

*Compiled from Cohen and Kassirer *in* Maxwell and Kleeman: *Clinical Disorders of Fluid and Electrolyte Metabolism*, 3rd ed. New York: McGraw-Hill, 1980, pp. 197–224; and Goldberger: *A Primer of Water, Electrolyte, and Acid-Base Syndromes*, 5th ed. Philadelphia: Lea & Febiger, 1980.

are liberated for each 100 ml given. Dosage is calculated as described for dilute HCl; the compound should be given slowly over 12 to 24 hours. Because of its nitrogen content, arginine monohydrochloride may be poorly tolerated by patients in renal failure.

RESPIRATORY ALKALOSIS

Primary respiratory alkalosis is synonymous with hyperventilation, since increased alveolar ventilation is the only mechanism that can cause a decrease in P_{CO_2} (hypocapnia) (Cohen and Kassirer, 1980). It is characterized by decreased P_{CO_2}, decreased or normal HCO_3^-, and elevated pH (Tables 2 and 3). Arterial P_{O_2} may or may not be decreased, depending on whether arterial hypoxemia is associated with the respiratory alkalosis.

Etiology

There are multiple causes of respiratory alkalosis (Table 6), which can be divided into three main categories: (1) chemoreceptor response to arterial hypoxemia, (2) central nervous system stimulation, and (3) excessive use of mechanically assisted ventilation. In dogs and cats, the most common causes are arterial hypoxemia from pneumonia or airway obstruction; cortical stimulation by pain, fear, or fever; and incorrect, excessive mechanical ventilation during surgery.

Blood gas analysis is most helpful in delineating the cause of primary respiratory alkalosis because P_{CO_2} can change in minutes. If the animal responds appropriately, serial sampling after therapy may indicate the cause of alkalosis.

Pathophysiology

During hyperventilation, elimination of carbon dioxide exceeds formation, P_{CO_2} falls, and pH rises. Cellular buffers promote a shift of H^+ from cells into the ECF and K^+ from ECF into cells. Hydrogen ions react with HCO_3^-, causing HCO_3^- concentrations to fall. Renal compensation results in decreased renal acid excretion and decreased HCO_3^- reabsorption.

Detection of *alkalemia* is important, since hypocapnia and decreased HCO_3^- concentrations are also typical of compensated metabolic acidosis (Cohen and Kassirer, 1980; Shapiro et al., 1977). During compensation of metabolic acidosis, hyperventilation will continue until pH is normal. Overcompensation characterized by alkalemia will not occur.

Detection of *hypoxemia* associated with respiratory alkalosis is of value in determining the underlying cause and in formulating the therapy. Thus, *arterial* blood samples should be collected from patients suspected of having respiratory alkalosis.

Electrolyte changes associated with respiratory alkalosis are variable, but hyperchloremia is typical. An increase in Cl^- concentration coincides with a decrease in HCO_3^- concentration. Sodium and potassium concentrations may be slightly decreased.

Alkalemia due to respiratory alkalosis gives rise to increased hemoglobin affinity for oxygen, as described in the previous section on metabolic alkalosis.

Hypocapnia may itself produce another detrimental effect if severe ($P_{CO_2} < 25$ mm Hg). Cerebral vasoconstriction during hypocapnia may lead to acute cerebral hypoxia which, in turn, may cause central nervous system depression.

Diagnosis and Therapy

The underlying cause should be identified and corrected. Respiratory alkalosis is the least common blood-gas abnormality; usually it is mild and not life-threatening.

During alveolar hyperventilation, breathing effort and myocardial work are increased. Supportive oxygen therapy (oxygen by mask, oxygen cage) should be initiated while rapid efforts are being made to identify the underlying cause.

If alveolar hyperventilation occurs secondary to hypoxemia, oxygen therapy will (1) decrease alveolar ventilation (i.e., arterial P_{CO_2} will increase toward normal and work of breathing will decrease), (2) decrease heart rate if tachycardia is present, and (3) decrease blood pressure if hypertension is present (Shapiro et al., 1977).

If the cause of respiratory alkalosis is cortical stimulation without pulmonic disease, the Pa_{O_2} will rise dramatically after oxygen therapy with little change in ventilatory status. If pain or fear is the cause, analgesics or sedatives may correct the alkalosis.

Respiratory alkalosis induced by excessive mechanical ventilation may be corrected within minutes by decreasing tidal volume or ventilatory rate or both.

CASE EXAMPLES OF ALKALOSIS

Twenty dogs and one cat with alkalemia (pH > 7.5) were encountered in patients evaluated at the University of Minnesota Veterinary Teaching Hospital between January 1982 and December 1984. Four representative cases are described to illustrate how laboratory data and clinical signs may be used to determine the type of alkalosis present and to formulate therapy (Tables 3 and 7).

Case Example 1

A 4-year-old male standard poodle was admitted with a history of anorexia, lethargy, and vomiting of four weeks' duration. The dog was thin, depressed, and 5 per cent dehydrated. Laboratory data revealed hypochloremic, hypokalemic metabolic alkalosis. Preoperative therapy included intravenous normal saline and normal saline supplemented with potassium chloride. Response to therapy was minimized because of continued vomiting. At surgery an inoperable gastric scirrhous carcinoma affecting the pylorus was found.

Case Example 2

A 12-year-old spayed female boxer was presented to the hospital with a previous history of vomiting and diarrhea after eating garbage. For the past 16 hours she had been anorexic, vomiting (including garbage and plastic), and weak. Examination revealed that she was depressed and dehydrated, and had a distended, painful abdomen. Radiographs revealed a mass of bony material and fluid in the stomach. An arterial blood gas sample (Table 7) taken at the time of admission revealed partially compensated metabolic alkalosis with profound ar-

Table 7. *Case Examples of Alkalosis in Alkalemic Dogs*

Clinical Data	Case 1	Case 2	Case 3	Case 4
pH	7.51	7.55	7.51	7.56
P_{O_2} (mm Hg)	48 (venous)	61.8 (arterial)	77 (arterial)	409 (arterial)
P_{CO_2} (mm Hg)	47 (venous)	63.4 (arterial)	17 (arterial)	17.8 (arterial)
HCO_3^- (mEq/L)	37	54.8	13	18.4
Base excess (mEq/L)	+13	+28.4	−10	0.1
Na^+ (mEq/L)	147	155	145	156
K^+ (mEq/L)	2.2	3.1	4.6	4.1
Cl^- (mEq/L)	94	60	113	115
AG	18	43	24	22
ΔAG	−2	+23	+4	+2
ΔHCO_3^-	−16	−4	+4	0
Clinical diagnosis	Gastric carcinoma	Gastric foreign body	Laryngeal obstruction, pleuritis, lung collapse	Gastric dilatation-volvulus (intraoperative)
Type of alkalosis	Metabolic (partially compensated)	Metabolic (partially compensated)	Respiratory (partially compensated)	Respiratory (partially compensated)

Key: AG (Anion gap) = $(Na^+ + K^+) - (Cl_3^- + HCO_3^-)$; ΔAG = AG calculated − 20 mEq/L (see Polzin et al., 1982); ΔHCO_3^- = (HCO_3^- normal − (HCO_3^- measured) = 21 mEq/L − (HCO_3^- measured).

terial hypoxemia. Hypokalemia and severe hypochloremia were also present.

Muscle weakness due to hypokalemia and central nervous system depression appeared to be responsible for marked secondary alveolar hypoventilation with resultant arterial hypoxemia. The anion gap was inappropriately increased ($\Delta AG = +23.2$ mEq/L) compared with the change in serum bicarbonate concentration ($\Delta HCO_3^- = -33.8$ mEq/L). The high AG may have been due to the alkalemia or a high AG metabolic acidosis (the latter is the more usual reason for a high AG in dogs) (Polzin et al., 1982).

Other significant laboratory data obtained at admission include serum glutamate-pyruvate transaminase, 202 mU/ml; serum alkaline phosphatase, 178 mU/ml; serum urea nitrogen, 61 mg/dl; hematocrit, 55 per cent; and total plasma protein, 9.8 gm/dl.

Intravenous infusion of normal sodium chloride solution with potassium chloride (40 mEq KCl per liter NaCl) was started. After 5 mg diazepam (Valium, Roche) was given IV for restraint and sedation, a stomach tube was passed to relieve gastric distention. Ten hours later electrolyte and arterial blood gas values were improving. Response to saline administration and replacement of the chloride deficit indicated the high AG was due to alkalemia. Intravenous fluids were changed to lactated Ringer's solution with added potassium chloride. Thirty-six hours after admission many bony masses were removed by gastrotomy. Recovery was uneventful.

Case Example 3

A 4-year-old female St. Bernard was presented with a lifelong history of intermittent cough and sudden onset of severe inspiratory dyspnea. The dog was cyanotic, tachypneic (78 breaths/min), tachycardic (150 beats/min), and hyperthermic (T = 107.7°F) with gross edematous swelling and purulent material in the laryngeal area. Evaluation of arterial blood gases at this time (Table 7) revealed respiratory alkalosis with arterial hypoxemia (the fraction of inspired oxygen [F_IO_2] in room air was 0.2; expected Pa_{O_2} was in the range of 95 to 110 mm Hg). Emergency treatment included pentobarbital anesthesia, endotracheal intubation, and administration of oxygen with the aid of an anesthetic machine ($F_IO_2 \approx 1.0$). Dexamethasone sodium phosphate was administered, and the dog was packed with ice and alcohol. Subsequently, a tracheostomy tube was inserted. The dog's agitation was controlled with incremental doses of oxymorphone (Numorphan, DuPont). Other significant data included a total white blood cell count of 28,800/μl (77 per cent segmented neutrophils) and a low T_3 value of 0.43 μg/dl. The owners opted for euthanasia rather than prolonged intensive care, with or without surgery.

At necropsy three days after admission, severe, diffuse suppurative laryngotracheitis, pleuritis, and collapse of one lung were identified.

Case Example 4

An arterial blood-gas sample was measured in a 7-year-old male German Shepherd cross (body weight 92 lb) during surgery for correction of a gastric dilatation-volvulus. Preoperatively, electrolyte values were normal but blood-gas values revealed metabolic acidosis (pH 7.30; Pv_{CO_2}, 33.8; HCO_3^- 16.6; base excess, −7.3). The dog was given 1 L of lactated Ringer's solution and 50 mEq sodium bicarbonate preoperatively. Emergency surgery was performed during which times the dog was mechanically ventilated. Initially the ventilator was set to deliver a tidal volume of 1.6 L 8 times per minute (minute volume of 12.8 L), achieving a peak inspiratory pressure of 20 cm H_2O on the airway pressure gauge. The arterial blood gas values were measured 45 min after the start of mechanical ventilation (Table 7); the inspired oxygen was close to 100 per cent ($F_IO_2 \approx 1.0$). The values indicated respiratory alkalosis without hypoxemia. The ventilator was adjusted to deliver a tidal volume of 1.1 L 8 times per minute (minute volume of 8.8 L), achieving a peak inspiratory pressure of 15 cm. H_2O. An underlying metabolic acidosis was still suspected as the HCO_3^- value remained low. After adjustment of the ventilator, lactated Ringer's solution supplemented with sodium bicarbonate was continued intravenously. Arterial blood gases analyzed one hour later were normal.

References and Supplemental Reading

Clark, W. T., Jones, B. R., and Clark, J.: Blood oxygen and carbon dioxide tensions in normal dogs and in dogs with respiratory failure. J. Small Anim. Pract. 18:535, 1977.

Cogan, M. G., Liu, F. Y., Berger, B. E., et al.: Metabolic alkalosis. Med. Clin. North Am. 67:903, 1983.

Cogan, M. G., Rector, F. C., Jr., and Seldin, D. W.: Acid-base disorders. *In* Brenner, B. M., and Rector, F. C., Jr. (eds.): *The Kidney*, 2nd ed. Philadelphia: W. B. Saunders, 1981, pp. 841–907.

Cohen, J. J., and Kassirer, J. P.: Acid-base metabolism. *In* Maxwell, M. H., and Kleeman, C. R. (eds.): *Clinical Disorders of Fluid and Electrolyte Metabolism*, 3rd ed. New York: McGraw-Hill, 1980, pp. 197–224.

Cornelius, L. M., and Rawlings, C. A.: Arterial blood gas and acid-base values in dogs with various diseases and signs of disease. J.A.V.M.A. 178:992, 1981.

DuBoise, J. D., Jr.: Clinical approach to patients with acid-base disorders. Med. Clin. North Am. 67:799, 1983.

Dumler, F.: Primary metabolic alkalosis. Am. Fam. Physician 23:193, 1981.

Goldberger, E.: *A Primer of Water, Electrolyte, and Acid-Base Syndromes*, 5th ed. Philadelphia: Lea & Febiger, 1980.

Harrington, J. T.: Metabolic alkalosis. Kidney Int. 26:88, 1984.

Haskins, A. C.: Blood gases and acid-base balance: Clinical interpretation and therapeutic implications. *In* Kirk, R. W. (ed.): *Current Veterinary Therapy VIII*. Philadelphia: W. B. Saunders, 1983, pp. 201–215.

Haskins, A. C.: An overview of acid-base physiology. J.A.V.M.A. 170:423, 1977.
Kassirer, J. P.: Serious acid-base disorders. New Engl. J. Med. 291:273, 1974.
Kopple, J. D., and Blumenkrantz, M. J.: Total parenteral nutrition and parenteral fluid therapy. *In* Maxwell, M. H., and Kleeman, C. R. (eds.): *Clinical Disorders of Fluid and Electrolyte Metabolism*, 3rd ed. New York: McGraw-Hill, 1980.
Kurtzman, N. A., White, M. G., and Rogers, P. W.: Pathophysiology of metabolic alkalosis. Arch. Intern. Med. 131:702, 1973.
Kwun, K. B., Boucherit, T., Wong, J., et al.: Treatment of metabolic alkalosis with intravenous infusion of concentrated hydrochloric acid. Am. J. Surg. 146:328, 1983.
Middleton, D. J., Ilkiw, J. E., and Watson, A. D. J.: Arterial and venous blood gas tensions in clinical healthy cats. Am. J. Vet. Res. 42:1609, 1981.
Nascimente, L.: Metabolic alkalosis: Role of the kidney. Contrib. Nephrol. 27:54, 1981.
Polzin, D. J., Stevens, J. B., and Osborne, C. A.: Clinical application of the anion gap in evaluation of acid-base disorders in dogs. Compend. Cont. Ed. Pract. Vet. 4:1021, 1982.
Schaer, M.: A practical review of simple acid-base disorders. Vet. Clin. North Am. (Small Anim. Pract.) 12:434, 1982.
Schwartz, W. B.: Disorders of fluid, electrolyte and acid-base balance. *In* Beeson, P. B., and McDermott, W., and Wyngaarden, J. B. (eds.): *Cecil Textbook of Medicine*, 15th ed. Philadelphia: W. B. Saunders, 1979, pp. 1950–1969.
Shapiro, B. A., Harrison, R. A., and Walton, J. R.: *Clinical Application of Blood Gases*, 2nd ed. Chicago: Year Book Medical Publishers, 1977.
Simmons, D. H., and Avedon, M.: Acid-base alterations and plasma potassium concentrations. Am. J. Physiol. 197:319, 1959.
Spector, W. S. (ed.): *Handbook of Biological Data*. Philadelphia: W. B. Saunders, 1956.
Tan, C. S. H., and Simmons, D. H.: Effect of assisted ventilation on respiratory drive of normal anesthetized dogs. Respir. Physiol. 43:287, 1981.
Van Slyke, K. K., and Evans, E. I.: The paradox of aciduria in presence of alkalosis caused by hypochloremia. Ann. Surg. 126:545, 1947.

TREATMENT OF HYPERCALCEMIA

JOHN M. KRUGER, D.V.M.,
CARL A. OSBORNE, D.V.M.,
and DAVID J. POLZIN, D.V.M.
St. Paul, Minnesota

CLINICAL IMPORTANCE

Hypercalcemia is recognized as a frequent disorder of calcium metabolism in dogs and cats, comprising approximately 2 to 3 per cent of total abnormal serum biochemical determinations (Chew and Meuten, 1982). Calcium plays a central role in a multitude of cellular events, organ functions, and system processes. Aberrations of calcium metabolism producing hypercalcemia may profoundly affect cellular function and result in severe gastrointestinal, cardiovascular, neurological, and renal dysfunction. Over the past decade, remarkable advances in understanding the pathobiology of hypercalcemia and the ability to recognize and evaluate abnormalities of calcium metabolism have resulted in characterization of a diverse number of etiopathogenic mechanisms responsible for hypercalcemia. Increased understanding of abnormal calcium homeostasis has led to an increase in number, specificity, and efficacy of therapeutic agents or modalities used for specific and symptomatic treatment of hypercalcemia. As new products become available, identification of specific applications and evaluation of their therapeutic efficacy in the context of veterinary medicine will minimize their misuse and ultimately simplify and improve management of hypercalcemia.

ETIOPATHOGENESIS

Although a wide variety of disorders have been associated with hypercalcemia in humans, their occurrence in hypercalcemic dogs and cats remain to be critically evaluated (Tables 1 to 3). Nonparathyroid neoplasms, especially lymphomas, are by far the most common cause of hypercalcemia in dogs and cats (Tables 1 and 4) (Meuten, 1984; Meuten et al., 1983). *In vitro* and *in vivo* studies in several species indicate that increased bone resorption is the basic pathogenic mechanism involved in hypercalcemia associated with malignancy (Meuten, 1984; Meuten et al., 1983; Mundy et al., 1984). A variety of humoral and local factors have been identified that may act singly or in combination to stimulate osteoclastic bone resorption or act directly on bone to produce hypercalcemia (Table 1). However, in most patients with malignancy-associated hypercalcemia, the one or more exact mechanisms

Table 1. Etiopathogenic Mechanisms of Hypercalcemia Due to Nonparathyroid Neoplasia

	Species			General Mechanisms				
Cause	*Human*	*Canine*	*Feline*	*Increased Bone Resorption*	*Increased Intestinal Absorption*	*Increased Renal Tubular Resorption*	*Decreased Renal Excretion*	Comments
Hematologic Malignancies								
Lymphoid								Proposed mechanisms for nonpara-
Lymphoma	Yes	Yes	Yes	+	—	—	—	thyroid neoplasia–
Multiple myeloma	Yes	Yes	Unknown	+	—	—	—	induced hypercalcemia
								include:
Myeloid								A. Humoral Factors: Increased
Myeloproliferative disease	Yes	Unknown	Yes	+	—	—	—	general osteoclastic bone
								resorption due to:
Nonhematologic Malignancies								1. PTH
Nonskeletal neoplasms,								2. PTH-like polypeptides
especially of:								3. Prostaglandin E_2
Lung	Yes	Yes	Unknown	+	—	—	—	4. Lymphokines (osteoclast-
Kidney	Yes	Unknown	Unknown	+	—	—	—	activating factor)
Mammary gland	Yes	Yes	Unknown	+	—	—	—	5. Polypeptide growth factors
Integument and adnexa*	Yes	Yes	Unknown	+	—	—	—	a. Epidermal growth factor
Thyroid gland	Yes	Yes	Unknown	+	—	—	—	b. Transforming growth fac-
Pancreas	Yes	Yes	Unknown	+	—	—	—	tor
Liver	Yes	Unknown	Unknown	+	—	—	—	6. Colony-stimulating factor
Colon	Yes	Unknown	Unknown	+	—	—	—	B. Local Factors
Bladder	Yes	Unknown	Unknown	+	—	—	—	1. Increased local osteoclas-
Prostate	Yes	Unknown	Unknown	+	—	—	—	tic bone resorption due
Testicle	Yes	Yes	Unknown	+	—	—	—	to:
Skeletal neoplasms						—		a. Prostaglandin E_2
Metastatic from:						—		b. Lymphokines
Mammary gland	Yes	Yes	Unknown	+	—	—	—	c. Polypeptide growth
Lung	Yes	Unknown	Unknown	+	—	—	—	factors
Kidney	Yes	Unknown	Unknown	+	—	—	—	2. Pressure necrosis
Integument and adnexa*	Yes	Yes	Unknown	+	—	—	—	3. Director resorption by
Thyroid gland	Yes	Yes	Unknown	+	—	—	—	cancer cells
Colon	Yes	Unknown	Unknown	+	—	—	—	4. Direct resorption by
Bladder	Yes	Unknown	Unknown	+	—	—	—	macrophages
Prostate	Yes	Yes	Unknown	+	—	—	—	
Ovary	Yes	Unknown	Unknown	+	—		—	
Primary bone neoplasms	Yes	Unknown	Unknown	+	—		—	

*Neoplasms of skin and associated glandular structures.
Key: PTH = parathyroid hormone.

of increased bone resorption remain undefined. Excellent review articles that discuss specific etiopathogenic mechanisms are available (Meuten, 1984; Mundy et al., 1984).

Hypercalcemia in dogs and cats has been less commonly associated with endocrine, metabolic, and non-neoplastic bone disorders, and with iatrogenic and toxicologic causes (Tables 2 to 4) (Chew and Meuten, 1982, 1983; Finco and Rowland, 1978; Meuten, 1984; Peterson and Feinman, 1982; Spangler et al., 1979). These causes of hypercalcemia represent a diverse group of pathogenic mechanisms involving one or more of the following conditions: increased resorption of bone, increased intestinal absorption of calcium, increased renal tubular resorption of calcium, and decreased renal excretion of calcium (Tables 2 and 3).

CLINICAL MANIFESTATIONS

If one underlying disease is assumed to occur in an untreated patient, hypercalcemia may be associated with a wide variety of clinical signs that are dependent on interaction of one or more of the following: (1) local and systemic effects of the primary disorder, (2) pathophysiologic effects of hypercalcemia, and (3) compensatory responses to alterations in normal homeostasis. Clinical manifestations also reflect the magnitude, duration, and progression of hypercalcemia. The most clinically evident signs are typically referable to the gastrointestinal, cardiovascular, nervous, and urinary systems (Table 5) (Chew and Meuten, 1982).

DIAGNOSTIC CONSIDERATIONS

Overview

Identification of the cause or causes of hypercalcemia in dogs and cats and subsequent formulation of specific therapeutic plans are dependent on careful assessment of historical information, physical examination findings, and results of biochemical, radiographic, and histocytologic evaluations. In addition to biochemical determinations routinely employed in evaluating hypercalcemic patients (e.g., serum concentrations of calcium, inorganic phosphorus, urea nitrogen, creatinine, sodium, potas-

Table 2. Etiopathogenic Mechanisms of Hypercalcemia Due to Endocrinopathies

Cause	Species			General Mechanisms				Comments
	Human	*Canine*	*Feline*	*Increased Bone Resorption*	*Increased Intestinal Absorption*	*Increased Renal Tubular Resorption*	*Decreased Renal Excretion*	
Hyperparathyroidism								
Primary								
Hyperplasia								
Familial	Yes	Yes	Unknown	+	+	+	—	Due to PTH
Multiple endocrine neoplasia	Yes	Yes	Unknown	+	+	+	—	Due to PTH
—Type IIa (MEN II)	Yes	Yes	Unknown	+	+	+	—	Due to PTH
Adenoma								
Multiple endocrine neoplasia —Type I (MEN I)	Yes	Unknown	Unknown	+	+	+	—	
Adenocarcinoma	Yes	Yes	Unknown	+	+	+	—	
Secondary								
Chronic renal failure	Yes	Yes	Unknown	+	+	—	+	Exact mechanism unknown: may involve decreased parathyroid feedback inhibition, increased vitamin D responsiveness, increased anion complexing
Adrenocortical Insufficiency	Yes	Yes	Unknown	—	—	+	—	Exact mechanism unknown: may involve decreased GFR, dehydration, increased plasma protein affinity for calcium, increased anion complexing
Hyperthyroidism	Yes	Unknown	Unknown	+	—	—	+	Increased bone resorption assumed due to direct effect of thyroxin on osteoclast precursor proliferation
Hypothyroidism	Yes	Unknown	Unknown	—	+	—	+	Exact mechanism unknown
Acromegaly	Yes	Unknown	Unknown	+				May also involve increased anion complexing
Pheochromocytoma	Yes	Unknown	Unknown	+	+	+	—	Catecholamines may stimulate PTH secretion or act directly on bone

Key: GFR = glomerular filtration rate; PTH = parathyroid hormone.

sium, and chloride), other biochemical tests allow noninvasive direct and indirect evaluation of calcium homeostasis and parathyroid activity (Table 6) (Blonde et al., 1974; Mallette and Tuma, 1984). Unfortunately, not all determinations useful in distinguishing the causes of hypercalcemia (e.g., immunoreactive PTH, urinary cAMP, or ionized calcium) are available at all laboratories. However, immunoreactive PTH determinations are commercially available to veterinarians and provide the most direct, useful, and cost-effective information concerning circulating plasma PTH concentrations (Table 6). Before samples are collected, laboratories should be asked for specific instructions regarding sample collection and handling and for information about normal values. Laboratory data should be interpreted in light of evaluation of the status of organs and systems that influence laboratory results (Tables 6 and 7). Most causes of hypercalcemia in dogs and cats can readily be differentiated by combining findings from historical and physical examinations with appropriate biochemical determinations (see problem-specific data base and Tables 6 and 7).

Problem-Specific Data Base (Fig. 1)

I. Confirm hypercalcemia by collecting a venous blood sample and repeating serum calcium determinations. When interpreting results, consider age, albumin concentration, presence of lipemia, and the possibility of laboratory error.

II. Obtain an appropriate history and perform a physical examination, including thorough examination of the rectum and perianal tissues for neoplasms.

III. Evaluate serum concentration of inorganic phosphorus, total protein, albumin, urea nitrogen, creatinine, electrolytes (Na, K, Cl), and total bilirubin; determine SGPT (SALT) and alkaline phosphatase activities. Freeze an aliquot of serum and EDTA plasma at −20°C for possible future determinations of immunoreactive parathyroid hormone (iPTH) or other metabolites.

IV. Perform a complete blood count.

V. Perform a complete urinalysis. Freeze an aliquot of urine at −20°C for possible future determination of urine calcium concentration,

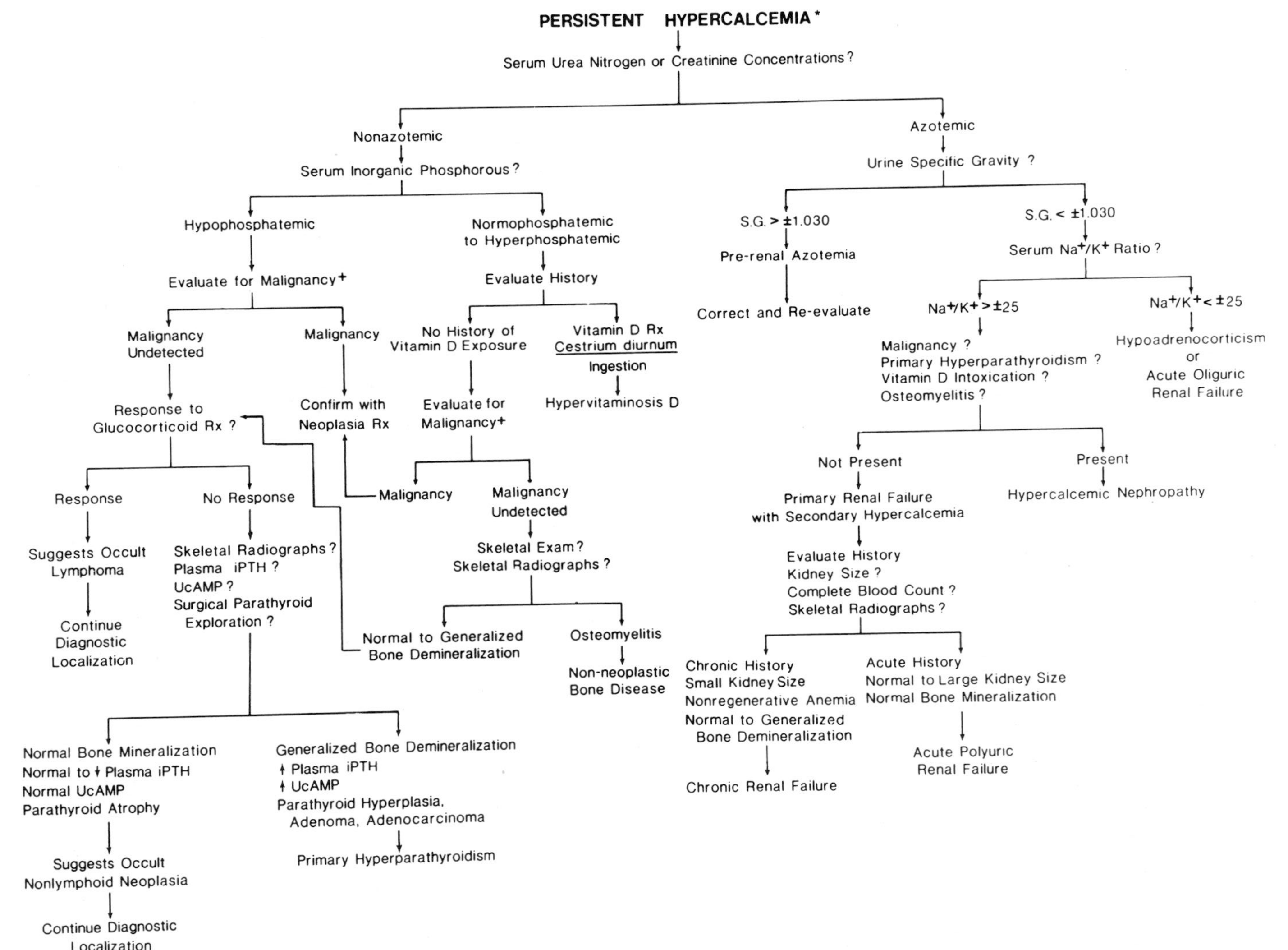

Figure 1. Diagnostic algorithm for persistent hypercalcemia. The algorithm is based on probabilities. Exceptions to these generalities may occur. *Key:* iPTH = immunoreactive parathyroid hormone; UcAMP = urinary cAMP; Rx = therapy.

*See Table 6 for normal values.

†See problem-specific data base.

Table 3. Etiopathogenic Mechanisms of Miscellaneous Causes of Hypercalcemia

	Species			General Mechanisms				
Cause	*Human*	*Canine*	*Feline*	*Increased Bone Resorption*	*Increased Intestinal Absorption*	*Increased Renal Tubular Resorption*	*Decreased Renal Excretion*	Comments
Non-neoplastic Disorders of Bone								
Septic osteomyelitis	Yes	Yes	Unknown	+	—	—	—	Local osteolysis
Disuse osteoporosis	Yes	Unknown	Unknown	+	—	+	—	Associated with variable iPTH levels
Osteitis deformans (Paget's disease of bone)	Yes	Unknown	Unknown	+	—	—	—	Exact mechanism unknown
Idiopathic periostitis	Yes	Unknown	Unknown	+	—	—	—	Exact mechanism unknown
Granulomatous Disorders								
Coccidioidomycosis	Yes	Unknown	Unknown	+	+	—	—	Exact mechanism unknown; may involve production of vitamin D, increased sensitivity to vitamin D, local osteolysis
Histoplasmosis	Yes	Unknown	Unknown	+	+	—	—	
Sarcoidosis	Yes	Unknown	Unknown	+	+	—	—	
Tuberculosis	Yes	Unknown	Unknown	+	+	—	—	
Iatrogenic and Toxicologic Disorders								
Vitamin D intoxication	Yes	Yes	Yes	+	+	—	—	
Cestrum diurnum (day-blooming jasmine)	Unknown	Unknown	Yes	+	+	—	—	Contains a glucuronide of vitamin D
Vitamin A intoxication	Yes	Unknown	Unknown	+	—	—	—	Exact mechanism unknown
Thiazide diuretics	Yes	Unknown	Unknown	—	—	+	+	Increased distal tubular resorption
Total parenteral nutrition	Yes	Unknown	Unknown	—	—	—	+	Regulatory function of the intestine bypassed
Calcium	Yes	Yes	Yes	—	+	—	—	
Lithium	Yes	Unknown	Unknown	+	+	+	—	Exact mechanism unknown; may induce hyperparathyroidism
Unclassified Disorders								
Diuretic phase of acute renal failure	Yes	Yes	Unknown	—	—	—	—	Remobilization of calcium deposited in soft tissue after oliguric phase
Familial hypocalciuric hypercalcemia	Yes	Unknown	Unknown	—	—	+	—	Exact mechanism unknown; may involve incomplete suppression of PTH at higher plasma calcium levels
Idiopathic infantile hypercalcemia	Yes	Unknown	Unknown	—	+	—	—	Exact mechanism unknown; may involve a disorder of vitamin D metabolism
Hyperproteinemia	Yes	Unknown	Unknown	—	—	—	—	Increased plasma protein complexing
Hypothermia	Yes	Yes	Yes	—	—	—	—	Exact mechanism unknown
Laboratory error	Yes	Yes	Yes	—	—	—	—	Lipemia; detergents

Key: iPTH = immunoreactive parathyroid hormone; PTH = parathyroid hormone.

fractional urinary excretion of calcium, urine concentration of cAMP, and other metabolites.

VI. Evaluate serum urea nitrogen and serum creatinine concentration for azotemia.
   A. If nonazotemic, evaluate serum inorganic phosphorus concentration.
      1. If hypophosphatemic:
         a. Evaluate for malignancy.
            1. Thoroughly palpate lymph nodes, rectum, perirectal tissues, and abdomen for evidence of lymphadenopathy, hepatosplenomegaly, or space-occupying mass lesions.
            2. Radiographically evaluate the thorax, abdomen, and skeleton for evidence of lymphadenopathy, hepatosplenomegaly, space-occupying lesions, or disseminated osteolysis.
            3. Evaluate ancillary diagnostic information (CBC, serum chemistries, and urinalysis) to aid further localization, characterization, or identification of neoplastic processes.
            4. Establish or confirm a definitive diagnosis by appropriate microscopic examination of biopsy material obtained from lymph nodes, neoplasms, bone, bone marrow, or any combination of these tissues.
            5. If unable to detect evidence of neoplasia, consider occult malignancy. Perform a therapeutic trial with glucocorticoids. A positive response to glucocorticoid therapy suggests occult lymphoma or other steroid-responsive malignancy. Continue diagnostic efforts di-

Table 4. *Common Causes of Hypercalcemia in Dogs**

Hypercalcemia of Malignancy
Lymphoma
Anal sac apocrine gland adenocarcinoma
Other nonskeletal neoplasms
Other skeletal neoplasms
Errors of Interpretation (young growing dogs)
Adrenocortical Insufficiency
Chronic Renal Failure
Familial renal dysplasia
Other causes
Primary Hyperparathyroidism
Vitamin D Intoxication
Iatrogenic
Toxicity
Non-neoplastic Disorders of Bone
Septic osteomyelitis
Other disorders

*Arranged in approximate order of decreasing likelihood of occurrence.

rected toward localization of neoplastic process.

b. Evaluate for primary hyperparathyroidism.
   1. Evaluate skeletal radiographs for generalized bone demineralization (especially of lamina dura dentes), or increased urinary cAMP.
   2. Confirm diagnosis of primary hyperparathyroidism with iPTH assay or exploratory parathyroid surgery.
   3. If unable to confirm a diagnosis of primary hyperparathyroidism, consider occult nonlymphoid neoplasia. Continue diagnostic efforts directed toward definition and localization of cause.

2. If normophosphatemic or hyperphosphatemic:
   a. Evaluate for hypervitaminosis D. Supporting evidence includes a history of vitamin D therapy or ingestion of plants containing vitamin D sterols and radiographic evidence of soft tissue mineralization.
   b. If there is no historical evidence of vitamin D intoxication, evaluate for malignancy (see VI.A.1.a.).
   c. If malignancy cannot be confirmed, evaluate for non-neoplastic disease of bone.
      1. Perform a thorough skeletal examination. Radiographically evaluate long bones, vertebrae, and skull for evidence of osteolysis, osteomyelitis, or periosteitis.
      2. Establish or confirm a definitive diagnosis with appropriate microscopic examination of biopsy material and appropriate culture for microbial agents.
   d. If findings are inconsistent with non-neoplastic disease of bone, reconsider occult neoplasia or primary hyperparathyroidism (see VI.A.1.a.5. and VI.A.1.b.).

B. If azotemic, evaluate urine specific gravity.
   1. If urine specific gravity is greater than $\approx$ 1.030 (in dogs), azotemia is probably associated with prerenal causes. Correct prerenal factors and re-evaluate for causes of hypercalcemia.
   2. If urine specific gravity is less than $\approx$ 1.030 (in dogs), evaluate serum sodium and potassium concentrations and determine the Na^+/K^+ ratio.
      a. Hyponatremia, hyperkalemia, and a Na^+/K^+ ratio less than $\approx$ 25 are indicative of hypoadrenocorticism or acute anuric or oliguric renal failure.
      b. If serum sodium and potassium concentrations are within normal limits and the Na^+/K^+ ratio is greater than $\approx$ 25, evaluate for malignancy, primary hyperparathyroidism, or non-neoplastic disease of bone.
         1. If malignancy, primary hyperparathyroidism, or non-neoplastic disease of bone is detected, azotemia has probably been caused by hypercalcemia (hypercalcemic nephropathy).
         2. If malignancy, primary hyperparathyroidism, or non-neoplastic disease of bone cannot be detected, consider primary renal failure with secondary hypercalcemia. Evaluate history, kidney size, complete blood count, and bone mineralization.

Table 5. *Clinical Manifestations of Hypercalcemia*

Gastrointestinal	Neurologic
Anorexia	Skeletal muscle weakness
Vomiting	Depression
Constipation	Stupor
Cardiovascular	Coma
Bradycardia	Seizures
Prolonged P-R interval	**Renal**
Shortened Q-T interval	Concentrating defect; polyuria
Ventricular fibrillation	Polydipsia
Vasoconstriction	Decreased GFR
Hypertension	Decreased renal blood flow
Endocardial calcification	Nephrocalcinosis
	Primary renal failure

Table 6. ***Biochemical Measurements Used in Determining Causes of Hypercalcemia in Dogs***

			Normal Range*				
			Dog		*Cat*		
Laboratory Test	**Sample Required**	**Units**	***Adult***	***< 6 Mo***	***Adult***	***< 6 Mo***	**Comments**
Serum calcium	Serum	mg/dl	9.0–11.6	7.0–11.6	7.6–11.0	7.0–11.0	Measures total serum calcium (ionized, complexed, and protein-bound)
Ionized calcium	Heparinized plasma	mg/dl at pH = 7.4	4.83–5.67† (n = 5)	ND	5.05–5.58† (n = 38)	ND	Closely regulated by PTH; influenced by acid-base status; may be useful in cases of "symptomatic hypercalcemia" with episodic or borderline hypercalcemia; little additional diagnostic benefit in cases of persistent hypercalcemia; has not been extensively evaluated in dogs; availability limited to major research centers
Serum inorganic phosphorus	Serum	mg/dl	3.9–6.3	3.9–9.0	3.2–6.3	3.9–8.1	Influenced by PTH and GFR; interpretation complicated by azotemia
Serum urea nitrogen	Serum	mg/dl	7–27	ND‡	18–32	ND‡	Evaluation of renal functional status is absolutely necessary for interpretation of other laboratory data
Serum creatinine	Serum	mg/dl	0.4–1.5	ND‡	0.4–1.85	ND‡	
Serum electrolytes							
Sodium	Serum	mmol/L	144–154	ND‡	147–161	ND‡	
Potassium	Serum	mmol/L	3.8–5.8	ND‡	3.7–4.9	ND‡	
Sodium/potassium ratio			> ≈25	ND‡	> ≈25	ND‡	
Chloride	Serum	mmol/L	105–120	ND‡	115–130	ND‡	
Serum chloride/phosphorus ratio			ND	ND	ND	ND	Value often less than 33 in humans with hyperparathyroidism; PTH reported to produce mild hyperchloremic renal tubular acidosis; significant overlap reported between values for hyperparathyroidism, normal and other causes of hypercalcemia; appears to be of limited diagnostic value in man; invalid if azotemic; has not been evaluated in dogs
Urinary calcium excretion							
Fractional clearance	Serum and urine	Percent	0.05–0.55†	ND	ND	ND	Fractional clearance requires simultaneous serum and urine samples; determine urine calcium and creatinine concentrations, calculated as follows: $\frac{UCa \times SCr}{UCr \times SCa} \times 100\%$
Total urinary excretion	24-hr urine	mg/kg/24 hr	1–3†	ND	0.2–0.45†	ND	
Urinary cAMP	Urine, freeze at −20°C	mmol/dl GF	1.62–2.26§ (n = 15)	ND	ND	ND	Indirect means of assessing levels of PTH or certain polypeptides associated with hypercalcemia of malignancy; glomerular filtration of plasma cAMP responsible for majority of cAMP in urine of dogs; nephrogenous cAMP quantitatively insignificant in the dog; markedly decreased with renal insufficiency; availability limited to major research centers

Table continued on following page

Table 6. Biochemical Measurements Used in Determining Causes of Hypercalcemia in Dogs Continued

			Normal Range*				
			Dog		*Cat*		
Laboratory Test	Sample Required	Units	*Adult*	*< 6 Mo*	*Adult*	*< 6 Mo*	Comments
Immunoreactive PTH‖	EDTA plasma, freeze at −20°C	ng/ml	85–220†	ND	ND	ND	Direct means of assessing levels of certain immunoreactive PTH peptide fragments; midregion assays available, which detect small midmolecular fragments in addition to carboxyterminal fragments; midregion assays appear to have greater sensitivity and allow better discrimination between normal and pathologic states; invalid if azotemic; sample requirements and normal ranges vary considerably with laboratory and methodology employed

Key: ND = not determined; n = number; GF = glomerular filtrate; GFR = glomerular filtration rate; PTH = parathyroid hormone; UCa = urine calcium concentration; UCr = urine creatinine concentration; SCa = serum calcium; SCr = serum creatinine.

*Normal range expressed as mean ±2 standard deviations; ranges vary markedly with laboratory and methodology used; all values adapted from Bentinck-Smith, 1983, unless otherwise indicated.

†Data from University of Minnesota Veterinary Teaching Hospital.

‡Pending further studies, value assumed to be similar to adult value.

§Data from Meuten, 1983.

‖Sample requirements and normal range listed are for midregion PTH assay available through the Minnesota Veterinary Diagnostic Laboratories, University of Minnesota, College of Veterinary Medicine, 1943 Carter Avenue, St. Paul, MN 55108; Phone (612) 373-0774.

a. Consider acute polyuric renal failure, especially if associated with acute onset, extensive soft tissue trauma, normal to large kidneys, normal hemogram, and normal bone mineralization.
b. A history of chronic dysfunction, reduced kidney size, nonregenerative anemia, and normal to generalized bone demineralization are consistent with chronic renal failure and secondary hypercalcemia.

STRATEGIES FOR MANAGEMENT

Specific Treatment

Initiation of specific therapy is the only consistently effective means of long-term management of hypercalcemia. Therefore, every effort should be made to identify the exact cause underlying persistent hypercalcemia before therapy is begun.

Treatment of hypercalcemia-associated neoplasms utilizing surgical excision, chemotherapy, radiotherapy, immunotherapy, or other therapeutic modalities eliminates the direct effects of neoplasia and the source of local or humoral factors (or both) responsible for hypercalcemia mediated by bone resorption. Successful treatment of neoplasms associated with hypercalcemia is usually accompanied by reduction of serum calcium concentration to normal within several days (Weller et al., 1982).

Correction of underlying metabolic, endocrine, inflammatory, iatrogenic, or toxicologic disorders also results in rapid correction of hypercalcemia. Proper treatment of adrenocortical insufficiency with replacement mineralocorticoids, glucocorticoids, and fluids is often the only action required to correct associated hypercalcemia (Peterson and Feinman, 1982). Primary hyperparathyroidism should be corrected by surgical resection of the affected parathyroid glands (Chew and Meuten, 1983). Hypercalcemia due to iatrogenic or toxicologic causes, especially vitamin D intoxication, is readily reversed by eliminating exogenous sources of hypercalcemic agents. Treatment of septic osteomyelitis usually requires a combination of surgical debridement and antimicrobial therapy.

Symptomatic Treatment

OVERVIEW. Although specific therapy is the most effective means of successful long-term management of hypercalcemia, symptomatic therapy may assume an extremely important role in the overall management of hypercalcemic patients. Symptomatic therapy often results in amelioration of cardiac, neurologic, and renal toxicity by temporarily reducing elevated serum calcium concentrations. Short-term control of hypercalcemia allows formulation and initiation of specific diagnostic and therapeutic plans (Osborne and Stevens, 1977). However, premature, overzealous, or inappropriate symptomatic therapy may interfere with identification of specific causes and identification of concurrent but unrelated dis-

Table 7. *Abnormalities* Characteristic of Different Causes of Hypercalcemia in Dogs*

Cause	SCa	ICa	SPO$_4$†	SUN or Creatinine	Serum Electrolytes *Na*$^+$	*K*$^+$	*Na*$^+$/*K*$^+$	*Cl*$^-$	Cl$^-$/SPO$_4$†	UCaE/24h† or FCaE†	UcAMP†	iPTH†	Skeletal Radiographs	Parathyroid
Hypercalcemia of malignancy	↑	Ukn (N, ↑ ?)‡	N, ↓	N	N	N	> ≈25	N	Ukn (< 33?)	↑↑	N, ↑	N, ↓	Variable degrees of bone demineralization or osteolysis	Atrophy
Adrenocortical insufficiency	↑	N	N, ↑	↑	N, ↓	N, ↑	< ≈25	N, ↓	Ukn (< 33?)	↓	Ukn (↓ ?)	Ukn (N, ↑ ?)	N	N
Chronic renal failure	↑	Ukn (N?)	↑↑	↑↑	N, ↓	N	> ≈25	N, ↓	Ukn (< 33?)	Ukn (Variable?)	Ukn (↓ ?)	↑↑	Variable degrees of bone demineralization	Hyperplasia
Primary hyperparathyroidism	↑	Ukn (↑ ?)	N, ↓	N	N	N	> ≈25	Ukn (N, ↑ ?)	Ukn (> 33?)	N, ↑	↑↑	↑	Variable degrees of bone demineralization	Hyperplasia; adenoma; adenocarcinoma
Vitamin D intoxication	↑	Ukn (N?)	N, ↑	N	N	N	> ≈25	N	Ukn (< 33?)	Ukn (↑ ?)	Ukn (↓ ?)	Ukn (N, ↓ ?)	Variable degrees of soft tissue mineralization	Atrophy
Non-neoplastic disorders of bone	↑	Ukn (N, ↑ ?)	N, ↑	N	N	N	> ≈25	N	Ukn (< 33?)	Ukn (↑ ?)	Ukn (↓ ?)	Ukn (N, ↓ ?)	Osteolysis	Ukn (Atrophy?)

Key: SCa = serum calcium; ICa = plasma ionized calcium; SPO$_4$ = serum inorganic phosphorus; SUN = serum urea nitrogen; Na$^+$ = serum sodium; K$^+$ = serum potassium; Cl$^-$ = serum chloride; UCaE = urinary calcium excretion; FCaE = fractional calcium excretion; UcAMP = urinary cAMP; iPTH = immunoreactive parathyroid hormone; N = normal; ↑ = increased; ↑ = decreased; Ukn = unknown.

*See Table 6 for normal values.

†Tests that may be affected by reductions in GFR.

‡Values in parentheses represent predictions based on logic and studies in other species.

orders. It may also expose patients to needless therapy and result in potentially life-threatening complications.

GOALS. Effective symptomatic therapy of hypercalcemia is primarily directed toward reducing serum calcium by one or a combination of the following methods: (1) increasing renal excretion of calcium, (2) inhibiting bone resorption, (3) promoting calcium deposition in soft tissues, (4) altering the intravascular ionic distribution of calcium, and (5) promoting extrarenal loss of calcium. There are many therapeutic agents available for symptomatic treatment of hypercalcemia, each with specific mechanisms of action, indications, limitations, and potential side effects (Tables 8 to 10). Unfortunately, there is no single pharmacologic agent that is uniformly effective and safe, nor are there any absolute guidelines indicating which therapeutic agents are most effective in patients with hypercalcemia. The speed with which symptomatic therapy is initiated and the therapeutic agents employed is dependent upon (1) etiopathogenesis, (2) duration and magnitude of hypercalcemia, (3) severity of associated clinical signs, and (4) other concomitant metabolic, endocrine, hematologic, cardiovascular, or renal abnormalities. A combination of therapeutic manipulations is usually most effective, especially if the agents used are complementary or synergistic in their mechanisms of action. If dehydration is associated with hypercalcemia, it should be immediately corrected by vigorous replacement with 0.9 per cent sodium chloride solution or other types of fluid and electrolyte solutions better suited to patient needs (Tables 8 to 11). Restoration of extracellular fluid volume with isotonic fluids containing large amounts of sodium corrects fluid and electrolyte deficits, increases glomerular filtration rate, and enhances renal excretion of calcium (Chew and Meuten, 1982; Henry et al., 1984; Osborne and Stevens, 1977; Partitt and Kleerekoper, 1980).

SYMPTOMATIC TREATMENT PROTOCOLS. Patients with moderate to severe or rapidly progressing hypercalcemia commonly require a combination of therapeutic agents to promote renal excretion of calcium further and, if appropriate, to inhibit resorption of bone (Table 11). Intravenous administration of furosemide has been effective in promoting renal excretion of calcium in dogs, provided hydration is maintained with concurrent fluid therapy during diuresis (Table 8) (Chew and Meuten, 1982; Henry et al., 1984; Osborne and Stevens, 1977; Partitt and Kleerekoper, 1980). Agents that inhibit bone resorption are indicated if increased bone resorption is a significant cause of hypercalcemia (Tables 1 to 3). Glucocorticoids are often highly effective in treatment of hypercalcemia associated with lymphoma or vitamin D intoxication (Table 9). (Chew and Meuten, 1982; Henry et al., 1984; Partitt and Kleerekoper, 1980). Calcitonin is a popular therapeutic alternative in human patients because of its rapid onset of action, high degree of efficacy, and few known contraindications or adverse effects (Table 9) (Avioli, 1982; Henry et al., 1984; Partitt and Kleerekoper, 1980). Unfortunately, its effectiveness in veterinary medicine has not yet been evaluated. Mithramycin is a potent antihypercalcemic agent successfully used on occasion to treat hypercalcemic dogs (Table 9) (Chew and Meuten, 1983). However, because of its potential serious side effects, difficulty in administration, and unpredictable duration of effect, its use is recommended only in hypercalcemic patients resistant to other conventional forms of therapy (Henry et al., 1984; Kiang et al., 1979; Partitt and Kleerekoper, 1980). Diphosphonates (synthetic analogues of bone pyrophosphates) are a new class of potentially useful therapeutic agents that have been used for symptomatic treatment of hypercalcemia in humans. These agents are potent inhibitors of osteoclastic bone resorption. Because of ease and flexibility of their administration and because they are associated with few adverse effects, they have been used to manage a variety of hypercalcemic disorders in humans (Table 9) (Henry et al., 1984; Jung, 1982). Unfortunately, availability and use of diphosphonates to treat hypercalcemia of dogs, cats, and other animals have been too limited to permit formulation of therapeutic recommendations.

Other therapeutic agents and modalities are available for symptomatic treatment of hypercalcemia in dogs (Tables 8 to 10). Peritoneal dialysis is potentially useful for symptomatic therapy of hypercalcemia, especially if concomitant renal failure has severely limited other therapeutic options (Table 10) (Chew and Meuten, 1982; 1983). Sodium sulfate, a calciuretic agent, has potential for being a safe and effective means of reducing serum calcium (Chew and Meuten, 1982; Osborne and Stevens, 1977; Partitt and Kleerekoper, 1980). However, minimal clinical experience and relative unavailability have limited its use in veterinary medicine (Table 8). Although prostaglandin synthetase inhibitors (such as aspirin) inhibit prostaglandin E_2–mediated bone resorption, their clinical usefulness has been disappointing in humans (Table 9) (Henry et al., 1984). Gallium nitrate, a new antihypercalcemic agent, is currently being evaluated by *in vitro* investigations and *in vivo* studies in human patients. It must be thoroughly evaluated for efficacy and clinical applicability in human and veterinary medicine before specific uses can be recommended (Table 9) (Warrell et al., 1984).

Text continued on page 90

Table 8. Therapeutic Agents That Enhance Urinary Calcium Excretion

		Predicted Therapeutic Response							
Therapeutic Agent	Approximate Dosage and Route of Administration	*Onset of Action**	*Duration of Response*	*Relative Efficacy†*	Indications	Contraindications	Possible Adverse Effects	Relative Safety‡	Comments
0.9% sodium chloride or other fluid that best suits patient needs	Hydration deficit plus 40 to 60 ml/kg IV infusion over 24 hours	Rapid	1 to 3 days	+ + +	Mild to severe hypercalcemia	Congestive heart failure; generalized edema; hypertension	Volume overload; hypokalemia; hypomagnesemia; hypernatremia	+ + + +	Restores and expands ECF volume; increases GFR; decreases renal tubular calcium resorption; enhances calcium and sodium excretion
Furosemide (Lasix, Hoechst-Roussel)	2 to 4 mg/kg IV every 12 hours	Immediate	4 to 6 hours	+ + +	Moderate to severe hypercalcemia	Dehydration; hypovolemia	Volume depletion; hypokalemia; hypomagnesemia; hypochloremic alkalosis	+ + +	Inhibits calcium resorption in ascending loop of Henle; rehydration prior to use essential
Isotonic sodium sulfate	ND (40 to 60 ml/kg IV infusion over 9 hours)§	Rapid	1 to 14 days	+ + +	Mild to severe hypercalcemia	Congestive heart failure; renal failure; generalized edema; hypertension	Vomiting; hypokalemia; hypomagnesemia; hypernatremia	+ + + +	Increases GFR; decreases renal tubular calcium resorption; calcium bound in nonreabsorbable complex; limited experience in dogs

Key: ECF = extracellular fluid; GFR = glomerular filtration rate; ND = not determined.
*Approximate time to beneficial therapeutic effect; maximum effect may occur later; immediate = < 2 hours; rapid = 3 to 12 hours; delayed = > 2 days.
†Percentage of patients expected to show significant decline in serum calcium; + + + = 51–75%.
‡Relative potential of producing adverse effects; + + + + = minimal risk; + + + = generally considered safe.
§Values in parentheses indicate approximate human dosages.

Table 9. Therapeutic Agents That Inhibit Bone Resorption

Therapeutic Agent	Approximate Dosage and Route of Administration	Predicted Therapeutic Response: *Onset of Action*†	*Duration of Response*	*Relative Efficacy*‡	Indications	Contraindications	Possible Adverse Effects	Relative Safety§	Comments
Prednisolone	1 to 1.5 mg/kg PO every 12 hours	Delayed	4 to 8 days	+ to + + +	Moderate to severe hypercalcemia due to steroid-responsive malignancy or vitamin D intoxication	Infectious disease; pancreatitis; hepatic insufficiency; renal failure; ulcerative colitis	Generalized catabolism, immunosuppression; pancreatitis; gastrointestinal ulceration; hepatopathy; myopathy; osteoporois; others	+ + +	Inhibits OAF, PGE_2, and vitamin D; decreases intestinal calcium absorption; promotes renal calcium excretion with chronic administration; direct neoplasm cytoxicity
Calcitonin (Calcimar, USV Laboratories)	ND (4 MRC units/kg IV, then 4 to 8 MRC units/kg SC every 12 to 24 hours)*	Rapid	12 to 24 hours	+ + +	Mild to severe hypercalcemia when other therapy is ineffective or contraindicated	Few	Vomiting	+ + + +	Inhibits osteoclastic bone resorption; direct calciuric effect; transient response; no reported experience in dogs
Diphosphonates EHDP (Didronel, Norwich Eaton)	ND (5 mg/kg every 24 hours PO, 7 to 14 mg/kg every 24 hours IV)*	Delayed	PO:ND IV:ND	PO:ND IV: + + + +	Moderate to severe hypercalcemia when other therapy is ineffective or contraindicated; long-term management of chronic hypercalcemia	Few	Osteomalacia (EDHP); pyrexia (APD); diarrhea; hypocalcemia	+ + + +	Synthetic pyrophosphate analogues resistant to hydrolysis by bone phosphatases; EHDP ineffective orally; intravenous APD associated with toxicity in experimental animals; Cl_2MDP very effective orally and intravenously; CL_2MDP and APD potentially useful for chronic therapy; only oral EHDP currently available; limited experience in dogs
APD	ND (5 mg/kg PO every 8 hours for 5 days, then 4 mg/kg PO every 24 hours maint.)*	Delayed	PO:ND IV:ND	PO: + + + + IV:ND					
Cl_2MDP (Clodronate, Procter and Gamble)	ND (23 mg/kg PO every 12 hours, 5 to 14 mg/kg IV every 24 hours)*	Delayed	PO:ND IV:1 to 8 days	PO: + + + + IV: + + + + + + + +					
Mithramycin (Mithracin, Miles Laboratories)	ND (25 μg/kg IV in D5W slow infusion every 3 to 4 days for 3 to 4 weeks)*	Rapid	2 to 21 days		Moderate to severe hypercalcemia due to glucocorticoid-resistant neoplasia that is unresponsive to other therapy	Renal failure; hepatic disease; hematologic disease	Nephrotoxicity; hepatotoxicity; myelosuppression; platelet dysfunction; hypocalcemia; rebound hypercalcemia	+	Cytotoxic antibiotic; inhibits DNA-dependent RNA synthesis; unpredictable duration of effect; inconvenient administration; limited experience in dogs

Table continued on opposite page

Gallium nitrate	ND (200 mg/m^2 IV every 24 hours for 5 to 7 days, continuous infusion)*	Rapid	6 to 19 days	+ + + +	Moderate to severe hypercalcemia due to glucocorticoid-resistant neoplasia that is unresponsive to other therapy	Renal failure; hematologic disease	Nephrotoxicity; myelosuppression; vomiting pulmonary infiltrates; hypocalcemia	+ +	Experimental antitumor compound; mechanism of action unknown; unpredictable duration of effect; inconvenient administration; experience limited to toxicologic studies in dogs
Prostaglandin synthetase inhibitors									
Aspirin	25 mg/kg every 8 to 12 hours	Rapid	3 to 4 days	+	Rare	Gastroenteritis; thrombocytopenia; platelet dysfunction; renal failure	Vomiting; gastric hemorrhage; gastrointestinal ulceration or perforation; platelet aggregation inhibition; decreased renal blood flow	+ + +	Inhibits PGE$_2$- mediated bone resorption; rarely useful in man; efficacy has not been evaluated in dogs
Indomethacin	ND (0.2 to 0.7 mg/kg PO every 8 hours)*	Rapid	3 to 4 days	+					
Oral phosphate (Neutra-Phos, Willen Drug)	ND (7 to 14 mg/kg every 8 hours)*	Delayed	3 to 6 days	+ + +	Long-term management of chronic hypercalcemia	Renal failure; hyperphosphatemia	Diarrhea; extraskeletal calcification	+ +	Inhibits osteoclastic bone resorption; reduces gastrointestinal calcium absorption; promotes calcium deposition in soft tissues; intravenous phosphate contraindicated; oral phosphate potentially useful for chronic therapy; no reported experience in dogs

Key: OAF = osteoclast activating factor; PGE$_2$ = prostaglandin E$_2$; EHDP = ethane-hydroxydiphosphonate; APD = amino-hydroxy-propylidine-diphosphonate; Cl$_2$MDP = dichloromethylene-diphosphonate; ND = not determined; MRC = Medical Research Council; D5W = 5 per cent dextrose in water.

*Values in parentheses indicate approximate human dosages.

†Approximate time to beneficial therapeutic effect; maximum effect may occur later; immediate = < 2 hours; rapid = 3 to 12 hours; delayed = > 2 days.

‡Percentage of patients expected to show significant decline in serum calcium; + = 0–25%; + + = 26–50%; + + + = 51–75%; + + + + = 76–100%.

§Relative potential of producing adverse effects; + + + + = minimal risk; + + + = generally considered safe; + + = use with caution; + = use with extreme caution.

Table 10. Other Therapeutic Agents That Affect Calcium Distribution

Therapeutic Agent	Approximate Dosage and Route of Administration	Predicted Therapeutic Response: *Onset of Action**	Predicted Therapeutic Response: *Duration of Response*	Predicted Therapeutic Response: *Relative Efficacy†*	Indications	Contraindications	Possible Adverse Effects	Relative Safety‡	Comments
Sodium bicarbonate	Bicarbonate (mEq) = kg body wt × 0.3 × [desired plasma bicarbonate (mEq/L) − measured plasma bicarbonate (mEq/L)] or 1 mEq/kg IV every 10 to 15 min; maximum total dose of 4 mEq/kg	Immediate	1 to 2 hours	+ + + +	Life-threatening hypercalcemic crisis	Alkalosis; congestive heart failure	Alkalosis; hypokalemia; paradoxical CSF acidosis; hypernatremia; ECF hyperosmolality; intracranial hemorrhage; coma; cardiac dysrhythmias	+ +	Decreases both ionized and total calcium in dogs; requires careful monitoring of acid-base status; temporary measure
Sodium EDTA	25 to 75 mg/kg/hour	Immediate	1 to 2 hours	+ + + +	Life-threatening hypercalcemic crisis	Renal failure	Acute renal failure; hypocalcemia	+	Complexes ionized calcium; calcium-EDTA excretion by the kidney; only indicated in emergency situations; temporary measure
Peritoneal dialysis	Low calcium or calcium-free dialysate IP	Rapid	4 to 6 hours	+ + +	Moderate to severe hypercalcemia with concurrent oliguric or anuric renal failure	Few	Peritonitis	+ +	Technically demanding; short duration of response; efficacy has not been evaluated in the treatment of hypercalcemic dogs

*Approximate time to beneficial therapeutic effect; maximum effect may occur later; immediate = <2 hours; rapid = 3 to 12 hours; delayed = >2 days.
†Percentage of patients expected to show significant decline in serum calcium; + + + = 51–75%; + + + + = 76–100%.
‡Relative potential of producing adverse effects; + + = use with caution; + = use with extreme caution.

Table 11. Strategies for Management of Persistent Hypercalcemia

Short-Term Management

For mild hypercalcemia; SCa concentration ≈ 12 to 13.5 mg/dl with minimal renal, cardiac, and/or neurologic dysfunction:

1. Initiate specific therapy for primary disorder.
2. Restore and expand ECF volume with 0.9% sodium chloride IV or alternative fluid that best suits patient's overall needs.

For moderate, severe or rapidly progressing hypercalcemia; SCa concentration greater than ≈ 13.5 mg/dl with evidence of renal, cardiac, and/or neurologic dysfunction that is not immediately life-threatening:

1. Initiate specific therapy for primary disorder.
2. Restore and expand ECF volume with 0.9% sodium chloride IV or alternative fluid that best suits patient's overall needs.
3. Increase urinary Ca excretion using:
   - Furosemide, or
   - Sodium sulfate.
4. Decrease bone resorption if indicated using:
   - Glucocorticoids,
   - Calcitonin,
   - Mithramycin, and/or
   - Diphosphonates.

For hypercalcemic crisis; life-threatening cardiac and/or neurologic dysfunction:

1. Immediately collect blood, serum, EDTA plasma samples for appropriate diagnostic evaluation.
2. Rapidly reduce plasma ionized calcium concentration using:
   - Sodium bicarbonate IV, or
   - Sodium EDTA IV.
3. Initiate therapy listed above for moderate, severe, or rapidly progressing hypercalcemia.
4. Initiate specific therapy for primary disorder.

Long-Term Management

For moderate to severe chronic hypercalcemia; SCa concentration greater than ≈ 13.5 mg/dl with evidence of renal, cardiac, and/or neurologic dysfunction that is not immediately life-threatening:

1. Initiate specific therapy for primary disorder if possible.
2. Decrease bone resporption if indicated using:
   - Glucocorticoids,
   - Calcitonin,
   - Oral phosphate, and/or
   - Diphosphonates.

Key: SCa = serum calcium; ECF = extracellular fluid.

HYPERCALCEMIC CRISES. In the uncommon situation of a hypercalcemic crisis (severe hypercalcemia resulting in life-threatening cardiac or neurologic dysfunction or both), immediate attempts should be made to reduce plasma-ionized calcium with intravenous sodium bicarbonate or sodium EDTA (Tables 10 and 11) (Chew and Meuten, 1982; Henry et al., 1984; Partitt and Kleerekoper, 1980). Both of these agents have extremely short durations of effect and require careful continuous monitoring since they may be associated with significant adverse effects. They should be used only until less hazardous forms of antihypercalcemia therapy can be initiated.

LONG-TERM TREATMENT. Long-term management of hypercalcemia may be required if specific therapy is unavailable because of (1) the nature of the primary disorder, (2) inability to define the exact cause, or (3) contraindications that preclude initiation of specific treatment. In such cases, choice of therapeutic agents is dependent on the etiopathogenesis of hypercalcemia, other concomitant abnormalities, and possible adverse effects associated with prolonged therapy (Tables 9 and 11).

PROGNOSIS

Because of the great diversity of potential causes of hypercalcemia, short- and long-term prognoses for patients with hypercalcemia are variable. The probable outcome and the possibility of recovery are dependent upon the nature of the primary disorder; degree of cardiac, neurologic, and renal dysfunction; significance of concomitant abnormalities; and availability of specific long-term therapy. However, abnormalities caused by hypercalcemia *per se* are potentially reversible if detected early and managed properly.

References and Supplemental Reading

Avioli, L. V.: Calcitonin therapy for bone disease and hypercalcemia. Arch. Intern. Med. 142:2076, 1982.

Bentinck-Smith, J.: A roster of normal values for dogs and cats. *In* Kirk, R. W. (ed.): *Current Veterinary Therapy VIII*. Philadelphia: W. B. Saunders, 1983, pp. 1206–1215.

Blonde, L., Wehmann, R. E., and Steiner, A. L.: Plasma clearance rates and renal clearance of ^{3}H-labeled cyclic AMP and ^{3}H-labeled cyclic GMP in the dog. J. Clin. Invest. 53:163, 1974.

Chew, D. J., and Meuten, D. J.: Disorders of calcium and phosphorus metabolism. Vet. Clin. North Am. 12:411, 1982.

Chew, D. J., and Meuten, D. J.: Primary hyperparathyroidism. *In* Kirk, R. W. (ed.): *Current Veterinary Therapy VIII*. Philadelphia: W. B. Saunders, 1983, pp. 880–884.

Finco, D. R., and Rowland, G. N.: Hypercalcemia secondary to chronic renal failure in the dog: A report of four cases. J.A.V.M.A. 173:990, 1978.

Henry, D. A., Kurokawa, K., and Coburn, J. W.: Hypercalcemia and hypocalcemia. *In* Glassock, R. J. (ed.): *Current Therapy in Nephrology and Hypertension, 1984–1985*. Philadelphia: B. C. Decker, Inc., 1984, pp. 27–38.

Jung, A.: Comparison of two parenteral diphosphonates in hypercalcemia of malignancy. Am. J. Med. 72:221, 1982.

Kiang, D. T., Loken, M. K., and Kennedy, B. J.: Mechanism of the hypocalcemic effect of mithramycin. J. Clin. Endocrin. Metab. 48:341, 1979.

Mallette, L. E., and Tuma, S. N.: A new radioimmunoassay for the midregion of canine parathyroid hormone. Miner. Electrolyte Metab. 10:43, 1984.

Meuten, D. J.: Hypercalcemia. Vet. Clin. North Am. 14:891, 1984.

Meuten, D. J., Kociba, G. J., Capen, C. C., et al.: Hypercalcemia in dogs with lymphosarcoma: Biochemical, ultrastructural, and histomorphometric investigations. Lab. Invest. 49:553, 1983.

Mundy, G. R., Ibbotson, K. J., D'Souza, S. M., et al.: The hypercalcemia of cancer: Clinical implications and pathogenic mechanisms. N. Engl. J. Med. 310:1718, 1984.

Osborne, C. A., and Stevens, J. B.: Hypercalcemic nephropathy. *In* Kirk, R. W. (ed.): *Current Veterinary Therapy VI*. Philadelphia: W. B. Saunders, 1977, pp. 1080–1087.

Partitt, A. M., and Kleerekoper, M.: Clinical disorders of calcium, phosphorus, and magnesium metabolism. *In* Maxwell, M. H., and Kleeman, C. R. (eds.): *Clinical Disorders of Fluid and Electrolyte Metabolism*. New York: McGraw-Hill, 1980, pp. 947–1151.

Peterson, M. E., and Feinman, J. M.: Hypercalcemia associated with hypoadrenocorticism in sixteen dogs. J.A.V.M.A. 181:802, 1982.

Spangler, W. L., Gribble, D. H., and Lee, T. C.: Vitamin D intoxication and the pathogenesis of vitamin D nephropathy in the dog. Am. J. Vet. Res. 40:73, 1979.

Warrell, R. P., Jr., Bockman, R. S., Coonley, C. J., et al.: Gallium nitrate inhibits calcium resorption from bone and is effective treatment for cancer-related hypercalcemia. J. Clin. Invest. 73:1487, 1984.

Weller, R. E., Theilen, G. H., and Madewell, B. R.: Chemotherapeutic responses in dogs with lymphosarcoma and hypercalcemia. J.A.V.M.A. 181:891, 1982.

TREATMENT OF HYPOCALCEMIA

ELIZABETH A. RUSSO, D.V.M.,
and GEORGE E. LEES, D.V.M.
College Station, Texas

Disturbances of calcium homeostasis that produce an abnormally low serum calcium concentration are encountered frequently in veterinary practice. Because of widespread use of serum biochemical test profiles that include measurement of calcium concentration, recognition of hypocalcemia has also become more prevalent. Although severe hypocalcemia is a life-threatening derangement, hypocalcemia does not always require treatment. In fact, treatment of hypocalcemia is contraindicated in some cases. Consequently, consideration of treatment for hypocalcemia must begin with identification of appropriate circumstances for initiating therapy.

Specific therapy for hypocalcemia raises serum calcium concentration either by increasing intestinal calcium absorption or by parenterally administering calcium salts. Generally, parenteral therapy produces a rapid but transient effect and is used for immediate control of hypocalcemic signs. Modification of intestinal calcium absorption produces more sustained effects and is used to maintain adequate serum calcium concentrations in patients that require continued treatment. In either case, efforts to raise serum calcium concentration must be made cautiously. Unnecessary or excessive treatment may cause hypercalcemia, which can be as harmful as hypocalcemia.

GUIDELINES FOR INITIATING THERAPY

In deciding whether or not specific therapy for hypocalcemia is indicated, it is important to recognize that most laboratories routinely measure total serum calcium concentration. Total serum calcium normally includes approximately equal amounts of albumin-bound calcium and ionized calcium plus a small amount of nonionized calcium salts. Only ionized calcium is physiologically active. It is the quantity of ionized calcium in blood that determines whether clinical signs of hypocalcemia will occur. Signs of hypocalcemia usually develop when the concentration of serum ionized calcium is less than 2.5 mg/dl. The corresponding concentration of total calcium at which clinical signs of hypocalcemia will occur is approximately 6 to 7 mg/dl. However, this value represents an estimate influenced by the relative proportions of albumin-bound and ionized calcium. This is affected not only by the concentration of albumin but also by the acid-base status of the patient. Acidosis increases the proportion of ionized calcium, whereas alkalosis increases the proportion of albumin-bound calcium.

Hypocalcemic conditions for which specific therapeutic intervention is not indicated include those characterized by a decrease in total serum calcium but a normal quantity of ionized calcium. If ionized calcium concentrations cannot be determined, decreased total serum calcium with normal ionized calcium may be assumed to exist if hypocalcemia is accompanied by hypoalbuminemia and if signs of hypocalcemia are absent. Recognition of this type of hypocalcemia may be facilitated by adjusting the total serum calcium value for the serum albumin concentration by using the formula

$$\text{Adjusted calcium (mg/dl)} = \text{Measured calcium (mg/dl)} - \text{albumin (gm/dl)} + 3.5$$

Hypoalbuminemia is the primary cause of the decrease in total serum calcium that may accompany malabsorption syndromes, protein-losing enteropathies, nephrotic syndrome, and liver disease.

Specific treatment of hypocalcemia is sometimes contraindicated even when there is decreased concentration of ionized calcium. Slight decreases in serum calcium that are due to some other transient condition (e.g., acute pancreatitis) and are not associated with hypocalcemic signs should not be treated. Likewise, asymptomatic hypocalcemia associated with renal failure should not be treated as long as hyperphosphatemia prevails.

Recognition of clinical signs known to be caused by hypocalcemia is always an indication for immediate parenteral therapy. Clinical signs of hypocalcemia include behavioral aberrations, restlessness, ataxia, paresis, hypersensitivity to light and sound, muscle tremors or fasciculations, tetany, and grand-mal seizures. Signs may occur intermittently with as much as a week elapsing between episodes. Hypocalcemia has been reported to exacerbate congestive heart failure, and a particular type of cataract may develop in animals with chronic hypocalcemia.

Table 1. *Calcium-Containing Solutions Used for Treatment of Symptomatic Hypocalcemia*

Product	Milliequivalents of Calcium per 10 ml	Dose
Calcium gluconate 10%	4.6–4.8	5 to 10 ml (0.5 to 1.5 ml/kg)
Calcium chloride 10%	13.6	1.5 to 3.5 ml
Calcium glycero-phosphate/calcium lactate*	0.8	10 to 30 ml (may be given subcutaneously or intramuscularly)

*Calphosan Solution, Carlton Corporation.

When signs that are suggestive of hypocalcemia occur in postparturient bitches or in patients that have recently received phosphate enemas or have undergone thyroid or parathyroid surgery, a presumptive diagnosis of hypocalcemia and prompt initiation of parenteral therapy are justified. In such cases, blood specimens should be obtained before treatment so that laboratory tests may be subsequently used to confirm the diagnosis of hypocalcemia.

Signs associated with hypocalcemia are not pathognomonic. Even electrocardiographic changes such as prolonged Q-T interval and ST coving are neither specific nor consistent. In the absence of a history suggestive of a condition that produces hypocalcemia, one may be forced to control signs with anticonvulsants or sedatives until a diagnosis of hypocalcemia can be confirmed by laboratory tests.

TREATMENT OF TETANY OR SEIZURES

Several parenteral calcium-containing solutions are available for treatment of clinical signs of hypocalcemia (Table 1). It may be necessary to use parenteral therapy repeatedly until adequate serum calcium levels can be sustained by orally administered maintenance therapy. Calcium-containing solutions are usually given IV by slow infusion over a minimum of 15 minutes. Heart rate should be monitored during the infusion because bradycardia may signal the onset of cardiotoxicity. Electrocardiography may also be used to monitor effects of the calcium infusion on the heart. Elevation of the ST segment or shortening of the Q-T interval indicates that the infusion should be temporarily discontinued and reinitiated at a slower rate. Calcium may also be given in 5 per cent dextrose solutions by slow intravenous infusion. One product may be given by subcutaneous or intramuscular routes as well as intravenously. Slower absorption from these sites decreases the danger of cardiotoxicity. The concentration of calcium in different solutions varies widely. Switching from one product to another

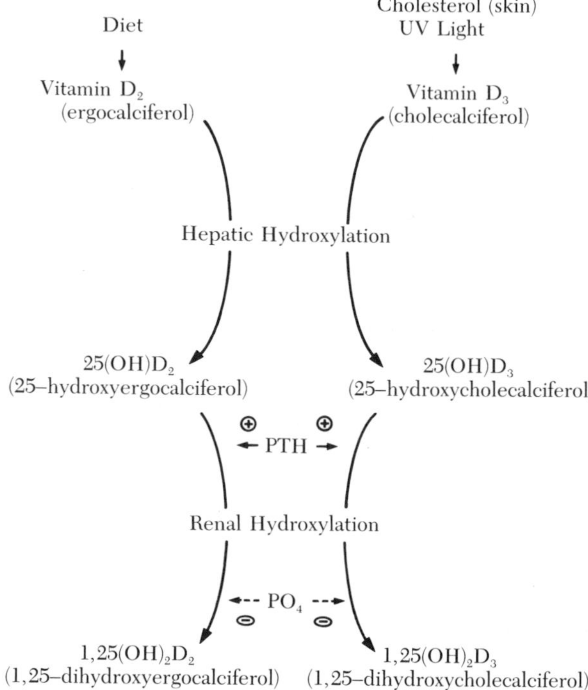

Figure 1. Pathways for activation of vitamin D.

without consideration of the difference in potency could either cause toxicity or lack of expected effect.

Not all clinical signs will abate immediately after administration of an adequate dose of calcium. In particular, nervousness, panting, and behavioral aberrations may persist for a variable period (30 to 60 minutes) after an adequate dose of calcium has been given. If panting is caused partially by hyperthermia associated with hypocalcemic tetany, it may be decreased by bathing the patient in cool water.

MAINTENANCE THERAPY

The necessity for maintenance therapy depends on the cause of hypocalcemia. Recurrence of puerperal tetany may be prevented by weaning the puppies, if that is possible, or by administration of oral calcium supplements. Prednisolone at a dosage of 0.5 mg/kg twice daily has been recommended to prevent recurrence of signs when weaning the litter is not feasible. The mechanism (or mechanisms) by which glucocorticosteroids prevent hypocalcemia is not known. Although after partial parathyroidectomy hypocalcemia may be transient, hypocalcemia due to primary hypoparathyroidism requires maintenance therapy indefinitely.

In hypoparathyroidism, normal serum calcium levels are maintained by administration of a form of vitamin D with or without oral calcium supplementation. In the absence of parathyroid hormone, vitamin D acts primarily by increasing intestinal absorption of calcium. Choosing a regimen of vita-

Table 2. Maintenance Therapy for Hypocalcemia Due to Hypoparathyroidism

Product	Recommended Initial Dosage
Vitamin D_2 (or D_3)	500 to 2000 U/kg/day*
Dihydrotachysterol	0.004 to 0.01 mg/kg/day
Calcium	100 to 500 mg/kg/day in divided doses

*1 mg vitamin D_2 = 40,000 U.

min D and calcium supplementation for maintenance therapy requires consideration of the normal metabolic pathways of vitamin D (Fig. 1). Ergocalciferol (vitamin D_2) is usually derived from the diet, whereas cholecalciferol (vitamin D_3) is synthesized in the skin. They are considered to have equivalent potency. Both are hydroxylated by hepatic microsomal enzymes to the 25-hydroxy form (25-(OH)D). 25-(OH)D is subsequently modified by 1-alpha hydroxylation in the kidneys. The second hydroxylation reaction is facilitated by parathyroid hormone. The most active forms of vitamin D are considered to be the 1,25-dihydroxy forms (1,25-$(OH)_2$D). They are more potent than the 25-hydroxy forms, which are more active than ergocalciferol or cholecalciferol.

In patients with hypoparathyroidism, there is lack of parathyroid-hormone stimulation of renal 1-alpha hydroxylation. Therefore, very high doses of vitamin D_2 or D_3 are needed for treatment of hypocalcemia (Table 2). Hypocalcemia associated with hypoparathyroidism is accompanied by hyperphosphatemia, which also inhibits the renal hydroxylation reaction. Several weeks of therapy are required for the serum calcium concentration to stabilize, but clinical signs of hypocalcemia usually do not occur after the first few days of treatment.

Oral calcium supplements may also be given to some patients (Table 2). In some cases, calcium supplementation may be gradually decreased and eliminated. In others, it may be continued indefinitely. Calcium carbonate contains 40 per cent calcium, calcium lactate contains 13 per cent calcium, and calcium gluconate contains 9 per cent calcium. The goal of therapy is to maintain serum calcium concentration in the low normal range (8.5 to 9.0 mg/dl).

Potential complications of therapy for hypocalcemia include hypercalcemia and nephrocalcinosis. Hypercalcemia may develop during therapy even after serum calcium levels appear to have stabilized. It may also develop without a change in dosage of vitamin D or calcium supplementation. Hypercalcemia may be manifested initially by polyuria and polydipsia, or it may be detected by serial evaluation of serum calcium concentration. These determinations should be made twice weekly at the onset of treatment and gradually decreased in frequency. Eventually such measurements may need to be performed only two to four times a year. If hypercalcemia should develop, all vitamin D and calcium supplementation should be discontinued until serum calcium concentration returns to normal. This may take up to 4 weeks to occur because of vitamin D storage in body fat. Decreases in serum calcium concentration may be hastened by vigorous saline diuresis, furosemide administration, and glucocorticosteroid therapy (consult the article entitled Treatment of Hypercalcemia). When serum calcium concentration has returned to normal, vitamin D therapy may be continued at lower dosages.

In patients with transient hypoparathyroidism (e.g., those with postoperative parathyroid insufficiency), efforts should be made to detect recovery of parathyroid function. If hypercalcemia develops in these patients, vitamin D therapy should be discontinued. It should not be reinstituted unless hypocalcemia (serum calcium below 8 mg/dl) recurs. When postoperative hypoparathyroidism persists for more than 6 to 8 weeks, it is likely that the underlying condition is irreversible.

In humans, nephrocalcinosis associated with deterioration of renal function may develop during treatment of hypocalcemia even when excessive serum calcium levels have not been produced. This is caused by the hypercalciuria that occurs in the absence of parathyroid hormone. This problem has not been reported in dogs treated for hypoparathyroidism, perhaps because they were not followed for an adequate length of time or because their lifespan is shorter.

A number of synthetic hydroxylated vitamin D analogues have been used for treatment of hypocalcemia in humans. These compounds are more potent than vitamin D and therefore raise serum calcium concentration more rapidly. However, their hypercalcemic effects are more rapidly reversible than those of vitamin D. These products are more expensive than vitamin D, and therefore their use may be restricted to patients that are particularly resistant to vitamin D. They may also be used to advantage when there is a narrow therapeutic margin or if several episodes of intoxication have occurred. Among these synthetic vitamin D analogues, only dihydrotachysterol (DHT) has been reported to be used in the dog (Table 2). DHT has been hydroxylated in the liver to form 25-OH-dihydrotachysterol, which, in turn, simulates activity of 1,25-$(OH)_2$D. One DHT product available in liquid form is convenient for accurate dosing of small patients. Other hydroxylated vitamin D analogues vary with respect to their metabolism, relative potency, and time required for reversal of their effects (Table 3). Calcitriol does not require activation; normocalcemia may be restored in less than one week. Because calcitriol is not stored in the body, toxic effects are more short-lived than those associated with any other vitamin D analogue. Cal-

Table 3. Comparison of Vitamin D Analogues

Product	Formula	Activation (Hydroxylation) Required	Relative Potency in Human Hypoparathyroidism*	Time for Reversal of Effect in Man (days)
Ergocalciferol†	Vitamin D_2	Hepatic, then renal hydroxylation	1	17–60
Dihydrotachysterol‡		Hepatic hydroxylation to 25-OH dihydrotachysterol, an analogue of $1,25\text{-}(OH)_2D_3$	3–10	3–14
Calcitriol§	$1,25\text{-}(OH)_2D_3$	No activation required	200–1000	2–10
Alfacalcidiol	$1\text{-}(OH)D_3$	Hepatic conversion to $1,25\text{-}(OH)_2D_3$	100–500	5–10
Calcifediol‖	$25\text{-}(OH)D_3$	Renal hydroxylation	20	7–30

*Numbers based on potency relative to vitamin D.
†Calciferol (50,000 U tabs), Kremers-Urban Co.
‡Dihydrotachysterol U.S.P. (0.125, 0.2, 0.4 mg tabs), Philips Roxane Labs.
‡Hytakerol (0.25 mg/ml), Winthrop Labs.
§Rocaltrol (0.25 μg, 0.5 μg caps), Roche Labs.
‖Calderol (20 μg, 50 μg caps), Upjohn Co.

cifediol does not appear to offer advantages over DHT; its effects persist for a longer period. Alfacalcidiol is not presently available in the United States.

Chlorthalidone (a thiazide diuretic) combined with a salt-restricted diet has been used for treatment of hypocalcemia associated with hypoparathyroidism in humans. This therapeutic strategy maintains adequate serum calcium concentration by decreasing urinary calcium loss and has the advantage of avoiding hypercalciuria and nephrocalcinosis. Use of this approach for treatment of hypocalcemia in animals has not been evaluated.

Use of anticonvulsant drugs in animals that are being treated for hypocalcemia should be discontinued except in refractory cases, because they increase hepatic degradation of vitamin D.

Treatment of hypocalcemia caused by hypoparathyroidism should be individualized with regard to therapeutic regimens and monitoring. Should it be necessary to increase the dosage of vitamin D, increments should not be greater than 15 to 20 per cent. Clients should be educated about the potential dangers of therapy and the necessity for long-term monitoring to ensure desirable results.

References and Supplemental Reading

Camargo, C. A., and Kolb, F. O.: Endocrine disorders. *In* Krupp, M. A., and Chatton, M. J. (eds.): *Current Medical Diagnosis and Treatment.* Los Altos, CA: Lange Medical Publications, 1984, pp. 707–710.
Haussler, M. R., and Cordy, P. E.: Metabolites and analogs of vitamin D. J.A.M.A. 247:841, 1982.
Juan, D.: Vitamin D metabolism. Postgrad. Med. 68:210, 1980.
Lees, G. E.: Hypoparathyroidism. *In* Kirk, R. W. (ed.): *Current Veterinary Therapy VIII.* Philadelphia: W. B. Saunders, 1983, pp. 876–879.

TREATMENT OF HYPERKALEMIA

MICHAEL DUWAYNE WILLARD, D.V.M.
Mississippi State, Mississippi

Hyperkalemia (HK) is caused by aberrations of internal potassium homeostasis (release of intracellular stores into the extracellular fluid), imbalances in external potassium regulation (reduced excretion with or without increased intake), or a combination of both. Medications are an often overlooked but important factor implicated in HK (Table 1). Drug-induced HK is significant because it is avoidable and because it implies an underlying organ dysfunction. Internal homeostatic mechanisms are extremely effective. Drugs usually cannot cause potassium to consistently exceed 5.6 mEq/L in a normal patient, even during sustained IV administration of potassium chloride (KCl), unless the dose exceeds 0.5 mEq/kg/hour. Therefore, when therapeutics cause persistent HK, renal and adrenal disease must be considered. It is not surprising that occult dysfunction of these organs may be uncovered by drugs, since kidney failure and adrenal gland destruction are the best-recognized causes of HK. However, many other spontaneous diseases must also be considered (Table 2).

Table 1. Drugs Associated with Hyperkalemia

Drug	Comments and Mechanism Responsible for Hyperkalemia
Oral or parenteral potassium supplements	Parenteral potassium (as Cl^- or PO_4^{3-} salt) given faster than 0.5 mEq/kg/hr IV increases risk of cardiotoxicity. Any potassium supplement (including slow-release forms) can cause HK if multiple forms of potassium supplementation or other potassium concentration–increasing drugs or diuretics are given or if an occult disease exists.
Oral rehydration solutions	HK may occur if such solutions are used for more than 24 hours.
Enteral feeding solutions	Constant feeding is not physiologically sound. It may cause HK after days or weeks.
Transfusions(?)	RBC breakdown may release enough potassium to cause HK if massive transfusions with aged blood are given.
Antibiotics	The potassium salt of drugs may cause HK when given IV (e.g., potassium penicillin G has 1.7 mEq potassium/10^6 units)
Digitalis (IV or oral)	Severe overdose can inhibit sodium-potassium ATPase.
Succinylcholine	Succinylcholine may result in substantial potassium efflux from muscle cells (especially when repeated or used in patients with intra-abdominal infections, burns, upper motor neuron lesions, or injuries). HK may be inhibited by first using nondepolarizing agents.
Heparin	Inhibits aldosterone biosynthesis.
Captopril	Inhibits angiotensin-converting enzyme.
Nonsteroidal anti-inflammatory drugs	Decreases aldosterone production by impairing renin secretion and decreasing urine flow.
Spironolactone	Inhibits action of aldosterone in renal distal tubule.
Triamterene	Blocks sodium entry and potassium secretion in the renal distal tubule.
Amiloride	Blocks sodium entry into renal distal tubular cell. Risk of HK is increased if amiloride is used with a thiazide diuretic.
Barbiturates, narcotics, and other drugs causing coma	Coma and prolonged recumbency can cause "crush"-type injury to muscle, releasing intracellular potassium.
Beta-blockers	Inhibits β-adrenergic action of epinephrine, which is responsible for its potassium-lowering activity.
Lithium	Perhaps because of increased conductance of potassium across cell membrane, HK tends to be transient.
Fluoride	Interference with enzymatic pathways of carbohydrate metabolism.
o,p'-DDD	Destruction of the adrenal cortex.
Rifampin	Increased metabolism of steroids.

Regardless of cause, clinical signs of HK may be exacerbated by concurrent hyponatremia, hypocalcemia, and acidosis. Muscle weakness and cardiac abnormalities are the most common changes, but nausea, vomiting, ileus, and abdominal pain may also occur. These signs are not always obvious. Mild weakness due to slight increases in potassium (K^+) (e.g., 5.6 mEq/L < K^+ < 7.0 mEq/L) may be confused with lethargy and depression. Severe weakness from greater increases sometimes begins in the rear legs and mimics spinal cord disease. Effects on esophageal muscle may cause megaesophagus with consequent regurgitation.

Cardiac abnormalities detected by physical examination may include bradycardia and a weak femoral pulse. However, an ECG is more likely than the physical examination to detect suggestive arrhythmias and therefore should be performed whenever HK is suspected. An ECG change commonly observed at K^+ concentrations of 6.5 to 7.0 mEq/L is T-wave spiking; however, this change regresses with continued elevation of K^+ concentration. Progressive prolongation of the P-R interval associated with gradual disappearance of the P-wave, diminution and widening of the QRS complex, and bradycardia occur sequentially as the K^+ concentration increases up to 10 to 11 mEq/L (usually a fatal concentration).

Even though ECGs are more readily available than flame photometry, ECGs do not reliably detect HK. Expected changes are often absent if the serum potassium concentration is less than 6.5 mEq/L, and in some instances they may not be detected at 8.5 mEq/L. Bradycardia may be obscured by preterminal ventricular tachycardia. Even when suggestive changes are found by ECG, HK may not be present. Bradycardia does not suggest HK unless QRS and P-wave changes are also present. Hypokalemia can produce enlarged U-waves that mimic tall T-waves; true spiked T-waves can be caused by hypomagnesemia.

Because of these potential errors, a serum potassium determination should always be obtained to confirm that HK is (or was) present. The clinician

Table 2. Causes of Hyperkalemia

Cause	Comments and Mechanism of Hyperkalemia	Criteria for Diagnosis
Iatrogenic Hyperkalemia		
Drug therapy	See Table 1. HK associated with drug therapy often suggests occult adrenal or renal dysfunction	History of drug use; resolution of HK after drug withdrawal
Hyperkalemia Due to Abnormal Internal Potassium Balance		
Acidemia	Primarily occurs when acidosis is due to mineral acids, not organic acids; HK not well-correlated with pH	pH <7.3, $HCO_3^- <15$mEq/L, plus lack of other causes; HK disappears with resolution of acidosis
Tumor lysis syndrome	Massive acute destruction of neoplastic cells, releasing intracellular potassium	History of chemotherapy with subsequent hyperphosphatemia, hypocalcemia, hyperuricemia, and/or renal failure
Rhabdomyolysis	Trauma (due to accidents), persistent recumbency (due to coma, see Table 1); seizures or myopathy causing release of intracellular potassium	Increased CPK, myoglobinuria, and history of injury are expected; if due to coma, may not be suspected initially since limb swelling may be subtle
Hyperthermia	Tissue hypoxia causing potassium release; most noticeable at temperature greater than 45°C	Reversal of HK after body temperature falls
Hyperkalemic periodic paralysis	Rare condition precipitated by exercise, cold, and potassium administration; due to release of intracellular potassium from muscle; myotonia may also occur; high-carbohydrate diet may help prevent it	Elimination of other causes; clinical signs worsen with oral potassium-loading
Hypertonicity	Usually due to hypernatremia or hyperglycemia; a 10 mOsmol/L increase may cause a 0.1 to 0.6 mEq/L increase in potassium; perhaps due to solvent drag from cells that have been glucose primed; usually seen in diabetics, sometimes associated with aldosterone dysfunction; may respond to mineralocorticoids regardless of adrenal function status	Serum potassium concentrations before, during, and after rise in serum osmolality
α-Adrenergic stimulation	Sympathoadrenal activation associated with surgical stress but not anesthesia alone has significant α-stimulation, which impairs potassium uptake by cells; this is particularly important when giving potassium supplements during surgery	α-Blocker will antagonize effect
Burns, infections, high fever (?)	Release of intracellular potassium caused by hypercatabolism, especially when associated with renal disease (?)	Clinical evaluation
Insulin deficiency (?)	Diabetics may have diminished aldosterone responsiveness; this, plus hypertonicity, may be the mechanism of HK (?)	Increased blood glucose; decreased concentrations of plasma immunoreactive insulin
Hyperkalemia Due to Abnormal External Potassium Balance		
Oliguric or anuric renal failure; terminal chronic renal failure	Constellation of causes, including decreased filtration and extraction of potassium from blood, lack of tubular responsiveness to aldosterone, insulin resistance, and catabolic release of potassium from cells	Increased concentrations of serum urea nitrogen, creatinine, and phosphorus; urine production is less than 40 ml/kg/day
Hypoadrenocorticism	Adrenal gland destruction (nonseptic inflammatory, fungal, hemorrhagic); adrenal atrophy from iatrogenic hypoadrenocorticism (not common) or congenital enzyme deficiency (21-hydroxylase)	Inadequate plasma cortisol *AND* aldosterone concentrations after ACTH administration

Table continued on opposite page

Cause	Comments and Mechanism of Hyperkalemia	Criteria for Diagnosis
***Hyperkalemia Due to Abnormal External Potassium Balance* Continued**		
Isolated hypoaldosteronism (18-hydroxylase or 18-dehydrogenase deficiency)	Congenital deficiency leading to adrenal hyperplasia	Normal cortisol response to ACTH; failure of aldosterone concentrations to increase after ACTH administration
Pseudohypoaldosteronism	Failure of renal tubules to respond to aldosterone	Increased plasma aldosterone concentrations; diminished kaliuretic response to exogenous mineralocorticoids and furosemide
Hyporeninemic, hypoaldosteronemic hyperkalemia	Usually occurs in diabetics with marginally low aldosterone concentrations that control sodium but not potassium; may be due to juxtaglomerular apparatus; impaired aldosterone secretion sometimes occurs concurrently	Normal cortisol response to ACTH; low plasma aldosterone and renin values, especially after volume contraction
Ruptured urinary bladder	Potassium not excreted; however, HK usually does not occur until late in course of disease	Urine in abdomen, positive contrast cystography, hyponatremia
Systemic lupus erythematosus	Failure of renal tubules to respond to aldosterone	Positive ANA and LE cell preparation
Renal transplantation	Failure of renal distal tubules to respond to aldosterone	History of renal transplantation
Amyloidosis	Failure of renal distal tubules to respond to aldosterone	Proteinuria, renal biopsy
Obstructive uropathy	Failure of renal distal tubules to respond to aldosterone	Ureterohydronephrosis, history of obstruction

does not have to wait for results before beginning symptomatic therapy when careful evaluation of ECG, history, and physical examination suggests HK (Fig. 1). Without flame photometry, however, an incorrect diagnosis of HK based upon ECG changes may result in iatrogenic morbidity or mortality through continued inappropriate therapy leading to hypokalemia. The only time that laboratory confirmation of HK might not be needed is in the readily diagnosed and clearly defined syndrome of urethral obstruction.

Serum K^+ concentrations determined by flame photometry must be examined carefully for sampling or laboratory errors. Incorrect collection techniques, such as an overly tight tourniquet used for a prolonged time or excessive exertion of the limb during venipuncture, may cause cellular anoxia with excessive leakage of potassium into the sampled blood. Hemolysis due to improper laboratory handling may occur, but this is usually not as significant in dogs and cats as it is in humans. Finally, laboratory error must be considered whenever HK seems unlikely from the history and physical examination. If doubt exists, the patient's serum potassium concentration should be re-evaluated.

When not caused by a sampling or laboratory error, apparent HK may, in fact, be pseudohyperkalemia. This condition is caused by thrombocytosis (i.e., $>750{,}000/mm^3$), extreme leukocytosis (i.e., $>500{,}000/mm^3$), or abnormal white or red blood cells (e.g., abnormal reactive lymphocytes or familial disorders that cause "leaky" membranes). Pseudohyperkalemia occurs as a result of increased release of potassium from these cells during clotting. A simultaneous potassium determination on plasma (avoid potassium EDTA) may aid in detection of this disorder. Although in humans serum and plasma potassium concentrations should normally be within 0.2 to 0.3 mEq/L of each other, the difference in dogs may be slightly greater. If the serum value exceeds the plasma concentration by much more than this range, pseudohyperkalemia should be considered.

Detection of HK in a patient that is not at immediate risk from the cardiotoxic effects of potassium (e.g., $K \leq 7.0$ mEq/L) indicates the need for specific therapy if the cause is known. If the diagnosis is unknown, one may give symptomatic therapy or (preferably) serially monitor the patient's serum potassium concentration while attempts are being made to determine the cause. Diagnostics should commence with a history (including all previous drug therapy) and physical examination if they have not already been obtained. If a well-defined syndrome such as urethral obstruction is present, a confirmatory serum potassium determination may be of therapeutic value. Otherwise, a minimum data base should then be obtained before any therapy commences. This data base should include CBC, serum sodium, serum urea nitrogen, and creatinine concentrations; arterial or venous blood gas determination; urinalysis; and the plasma corti-

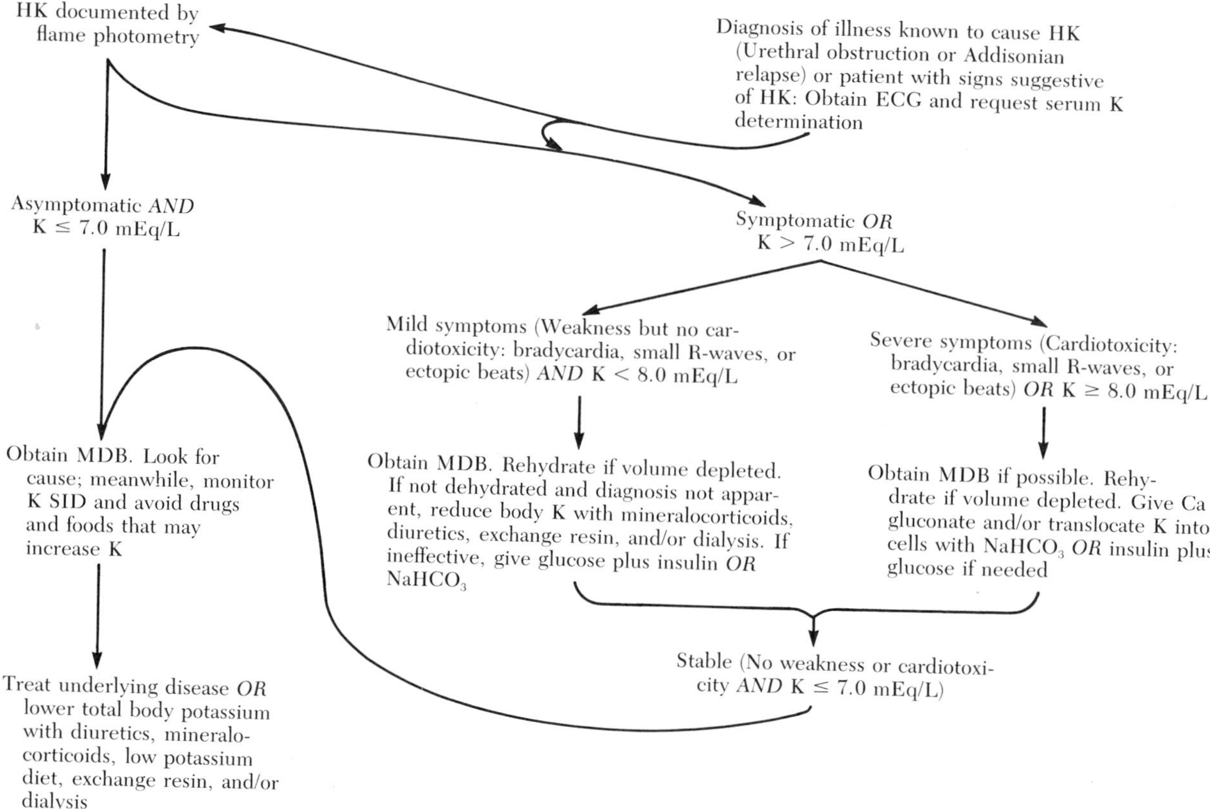

Figure 1. Therapeutic approach to hyperkalemia. MDB = minimum data base.

sol response to ACTH (Fig. 2). An ACTH response test is often important, as hypoadrenocorticism is common in dogs and is often associated with azotemia, isosthenuria, acidemia, or a combination of these conditions. The plasma cortisol response to ACTH is usually necessary for definitive diagnosis in these cases. Interpretation of an ACTH-response test requires careful consideration of prior therapy, since corticosteroids, megestrol, rifampin, ketoconazole, and narcotics may cause this test to inadequately reflect true adrenal function. If there is any confusion after these diagnostic tests are performed, aldosterone concentrations can also be measured, since less common abnormalities affect aldosterone but not cortisol responses to ACTH (Table 2). During this time serum potassium concentrations should be evaluated at least every 24 hours, since they may increase to dangerous levels.

If the concentration of potassium is greater than 7.0 mEq/L or if there is muscular weakness or cardiac arrhythmias, symptomatic therapy should be initiated as soon as possible (Fig. 1). There are four principal types of symptomatic therapy that can be used to treat HK, regardless of its cause.

1. If life-threatening cardiotoxicity is present and immediate results (i.e., within 5 to 15 minutes) are necessary, 10 per cent calcium gluconate (Elkin-Sinn Inc.), not to exceed 0.5 to 1.0 ml/kg, may be given IV over 10 to 15 minutes and repeated as necessary. Greater than expected amounts of calcium may be required if extensive skeletal muscle trauma is present, since the calcium can be taken up by damaged muscle. Calcium ions oppose the cardiotoxic effects of potassium but do not lower the serum concentration of potassium. Since this protection lasts for only 10 to 15 minutes, concurrent therapy should be administered so that the serum potassium concentration is reduced by the time the calcemic effect subsides. Use of the calcium solution in the same syringe or bottle with sodium bicarbonate should be avoided because an insoluble precipitate may form. CAUTION: overzealous administration of calcium may be as life-threatening as HK. Therefore, the heart rate should be monitored during calcium therapy; the calcium infusion should be discontinued if bradycardia occurs or progresses.

2. Rehydration with a potassium-free fluid is indicated whenever dehydration exists. If the patient is hyponatremic or if the sodium status is unknown, a sodium-containing solution is best. If the serum sodium concentration is normal, such solutions are still acceptable, but 5 per cent dextrose in water may also be used (except in patients with diabetes mellitus). In severely dehydrated patients, fluid

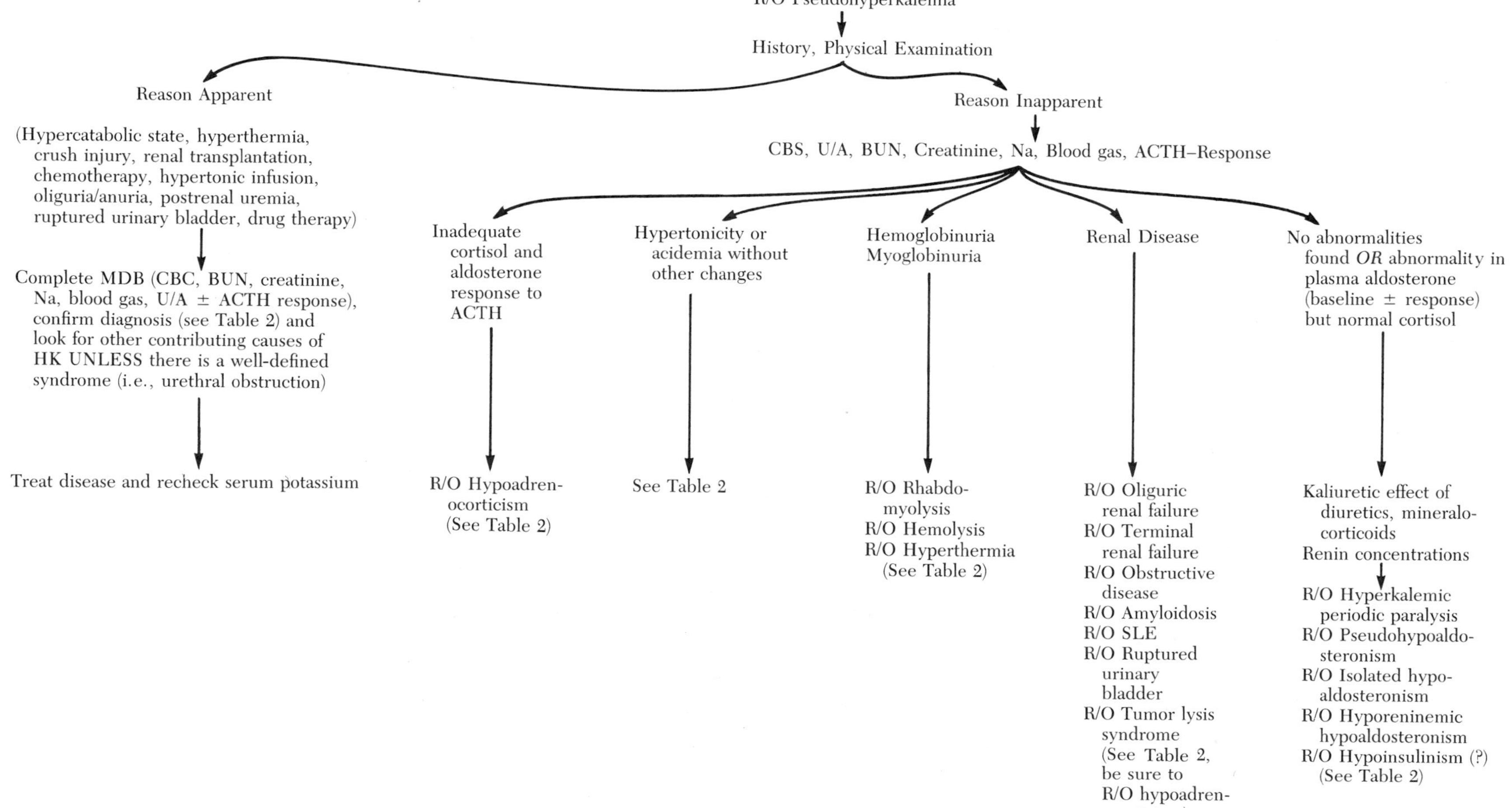

Figure 2. Diagnostic approach to hyperkalemia. R/O = rule out; MDB = minimum data base.

equivalent to 10 per cent of body weight may be given IV over the first 1 to 2 hours (not to exceed 88 ml/kg/hour) unless contraindicated by cardiopulmonary dysfunction. Rehydration dilutes serum potassium and also re-establishes renal blood flow. The consequent increased renal tubular flow augments potassium excretion in the distal tubule and collecting duct, except in some cases of oliguric renal failure.

3. Should aggressive IV fluid therapy be inappropriate or insufficient, sodium bicarbonate will lower serum potassium by increasing the entry of potassium into cells. This effect is caused by pH change and the bicarbonate ion itself. Since many HK patients have metabolic acidosis, sodium bicarbonate is of benefit for treatment of HK and acidosis. If a serum bicarbonate or total carbon dioxide determination is not available, 2 to 3 mEq of $NaHCO_3$/kg body weight given IV over 30 minutes is usually acceptable if the patient has decreased tissue perfusion or renal failure and does not have diabetic ketoacidosis. The potassium-lowering effects of bicarbonate should last a few hours in most patients. However, there is no justification for injudicious use of this potentially dangerous drug. Even a definitive diagnosis of hypoadrenocorticism or acute oliguric renal failure is no guarantee of metabolic acidosis, especially if severe vomiting or fluid therapy has previously occurred. Excessive administration of bicarbonate can cause respiratory arrest due to paradoxical CSF acidosis, hypertonicity resulting in congestive heart failure, shifts in the oxygen-hemoglobin dissociation curve leading to decreased tissue oxygenation, and metabolic alkalosis.

4. Glucose and insulin may be used in place of but usually not in addition to bicarbonate. Insulin-mediated transport of glucose across cell membranes also causes cellular sequestration of plasma potassium. Glucagon or intravenous glucose will stimulate release of endogenous insulin; however, the drop in serum potassium may be only 1.0 to 1.5 mEq/L per hour. Exogenous regular insulin should be given IV when faster results are needed. Except in patients with diabetes mellitus, insulin should not be given without concurrent glucose or glucagon (or both), lest potentially severe hypoglycemia occur. In the cat, regular insulin may be administered IV at 0.5 unit/kg body weight, immediately followed by an IV bolus of 2 gm of dextrose/unit of insulin given. Dogs tend to require more crystalline insulin (i.e., $\geq$ 5 units/kg/hour) in order to reduce the potassium concentration to a level lower than would occur with just IV glucose. Repetition of this therapy may not be associated with further reductions in serum potassium concentration, possibly because body cells "filled" with translocated potassium after the first treatment cannot accept more. Nonetheless, ECG monitoring may document continued decrease of cardiotoxicity. Glucose-insulin therapy is usually safe, although potentially fatal hypophosphatemia is possible in phosphate-depleted patients.

These four methods of therapy are usually sufficient until specific treatment can be initiated to correct the underlying defect. However, should the diagnosis be elusive and additional, interim symptomatic therapy needed, total body potassium can be lowered through other means. Such treatments may last longer than the previously mentioned therapies, but they require periodic monitoring to avoid iatrogenic hypokalemia.

Although usually insufficient by itself, substitution of potassium-poor foods (e.g., fats, breads, and cereals except oatmeal and bran) for those rich in potassium (e.g., milk, salt substitutes, fruits, vegetables, and their juices) avoids further potassium loading. Likewise, diuretics can be used to promote loss of potassium through the kidney. Thiazides are often more useful than the potent loop diuretics; acetazolamide may also be helpful. These agents work by increasing distal renal tubular flow but are usually ineffective in patients with primary renal failure.

Mineralocorticoids are more effective than dietary restriction or diuretics and can be used symptomatically for HK, except in some patients with renal disorders in which the distal tubules are nonresponsive to aldosterone. Desoxycorticosterone acetate (DOCA acetate, Organon) may be given IM at 1 to 5 mg/dog every 24 to 72 hours as needed. Fludrocortisone (Florinef, Squibb) may be given orally at 0.1 to 1.0 mg/dog/day. Although this agent is more convenient, it is less reliable than DOCA acetate. Furthermore, the large quantity of fludrocortisone required to control serum potassium concentrations may induce iatrogenic hyperadrenocorticism.

Potassium exchange resins such as sodium polystyrene sulfonate (Kayexelate, Winthrop-Breon Labs) may be given orally or rectally. Each gram of resin will bind to 1 to 3 mEq of potassium after releasing an equivalent amount of sodium. These resins should not be given concurrently with nonabsorbable cation-donating antacids or laxatives. Two grams of resin/kg body weight (each gram suspended in at least 3 to 4 ml of water) divided into three daily doses is recommended for dogs. If the resin is given orally, a cathartic should also be used to prevent constipation. Cathartics are not used if the resin is given rectally, since the polystyrene must remain in the colon for at least 30 minutes to be effective. If given as a retention enema, the resin should be suspended at the rate of 15 grams in 100 ml of 1 per cent methylcellulose or 10 per cent dextrose. In severe cases of HK, three to four times the normal amount of resin may be given, which is almost as effective as peritoneal dialysis. Exchange resins should be used cautiously in patients with edema, cardiac failure, or oliguria, since they replace potassium with sodium and may cause overhydration. Furthermore, they may cause hypokalemia, hypocalcemia, or hypomagnesemia if used too frequently.

Hemodialysis and peritoneal dialysis are effective although cumbersome. Typically reserved for oliguric renal failure, they may also be used symptomatically to lower the serum potassium concentration. However, peritoneal dialysis will be ineffective if there is hypovolemia or decreased mesenteric blood flow. Hemodialysis reduces serum potassium concentration more rapidly and more effectively. Both of these treatments are usually reserved for cases resistant to other modes of therapy.

References and Supplemental Reading

Batlle, D. C., and Kurtzman, N. A.: Syndromes of aldosterone deficiency and excess. Med. Clin. North Am. 67:879, 1983.

Cohen, L. F., Balow, J. E., Magrath, I. T., et al.: Acute tumor lysis syndrome. Am. J. Med. 68:486, 1980.

Cooperman, L. H.: Succinylcholine-induced hyperkalemia in neuromuscular disease. J.A.M.A. 213:1867, 1970.

Cox, M.: Potassium homeostasis. Med. Clin. North Am. 65:363, 1981.

DeFronzo, R. A.: Hyperkalemia and hyporeninemic hypoaldosteronism. Kidney Int. 17:118, 1980.

DeFronzo, R. A., Bia, M., and Smith, D.: Clinical disorders of hyperkalemia. Annu. Rev. Med. 33:521, 1982.

Grossman, R. A., Hamilton, R. W., Morse, B. M., et al.: Nontraumatic rhabdomyolysis and acute renal failure. N. Engl. J. Med. 291:807, 1974.

Hiatt, N., and Sheinkopf, J. A.: Treatment of experimental hyperkalemia with large doses of insulin. Surg. Gynecol. Obstet. 133:833, 1971.

Lewis, E. D., Griggs, R. C., and Maxley, R. T.: Regulation of plasma potassium in hyperkalemic periodic paralysis. Neurology 29:1131, 1979.

Nanji, A. A.: Drug-induced electrolyte disorders. Drug Intell. Clin. Pharm. 17:175, 1983.

Williams, M. E., Rosa, R. M., Silva, P., et al.: Impairment of extrarenal potassium disposal by α-adrenergic stimulation. N. Engl. J. Med. 311:145, 1984.

TREATMENT OF HYPOKALEMIA

FORD WATSON BELL, D.V.M.,
and CARL A. OSBORNE, D.V.M.
St. Paul, Minnesota

CLINICAL IMPORTANCE OF HYPOKALEMIA

Although profound life-threatening hypokalemia is an uncommon complication in veterinary medicine, varying degrees of lowered serum potassium concentrations occur with sufficient frequency to mandate awareness and understanding of the clinical situations and physiologic mechanisms that predispose an animal to this condition. The problem of depressed serum potassium concentrations may be less of a concern for veterinarians than for physicians, since there are fewer recognized causes of hypokalemia in domestic animals than in humans (Table 1). Most cases of clinically significant hypokalemia in companion animals result from a combination of predisposing factors rather than from a single etiologic entity. For example, anorectic dogs or cats usually maintain normal serum potassium concentrations by releasing intracellular K^+ and activating renal conservation mechanisms. However, institution of parenteral therapy with fluids devoid of potassium or those unable to replace existing K^+ losses (such as physiologic saline or lactated Ringer's) may promote hypokalemia in such patients, as depleting effects of decreased intake are exacerbated by the dilution or diuretic effects of parenteral fluids. Similarly, patients with congestive heart failure who also have relative hypovolemia and compensatory increase in aldosterone secretion may develop subclinical potassium depletion (i.e., lowered total body potassium with normal serum potassium concentration) due to the kaliuretic effects of this mineralocorticoid. Still, hypokalemia may not become clinically manifest until onset of therapy with potassium-losing diuretics (e.g., furosemide). The magnitude of hypokalemia may be enhanced by concomitant use of relatively unpalatable low-salt diets, leading to complete or partial anorexia and decreased potassium intake.

Because potassium ion (K^+) shifts readily from intracellular to extracellular spaces in the face of increased K^+ loss or decreased K^+ intake, serum concentrations are not a consistently reliable index of the true state of body potassium stores. In humans, for example, it has been estimated that a decrement of only 1 mEq/L in normal serum potassium concentrations may represent as much as a 200 to 300 mEq loss to the body (Cohen et al, 1981). In contrast, alterations in potassium balance may be internal in nature (cellular shifts) so that hypokalemia results solely from uptake of potassium into cells without net loss from the body.

Since marginal hypokalemia or potassium deple-

Table 1. Causes of Hypokalemia in Humans, Dogs, and Cats

Cause	Humans	Dogs	Cats
Inadequate Dietary Intake	±	±	±
Gastrointestinal Losses			
Vomiting	+	+	+
Diarrhea	+	+	+
Chronic laxative abuse	+	NR*	NR
Renal Losses			
Diuretics	+	+	+
Mineralocorticoid excess			
Primary aldosteronism	+	NR	NR
Cushing's syndrome	+	−	−
Accelerated hypertension	+	NR	NR
Renal vascular hypertension	+	−	−
Renin-producing neoplasms	+	NR	NR
Licorice excess	+	NR	NR
Adrogenital syndrome	+	NR	NR
Bartter's syndrome (hyperreninism)	+	NR	NR
Renal tubular acidosis	+	?	NR
Metabolic alkalosis	+	+	+
Acute hyperventilation	+	+	+
Starvation	+	?	?
Ureterosigmoidostomy	+	?	?
Antibiotics			
Carbenicillin	+	?	?
Amphotericin	+	+	?
Gentamicin	+	?	?
Diabetic ketoacidosis	+	+	+
Acute leukemia	+	−	−
Cellular shift			
Alkalosis	+	+	+
Insulin administration	+	+	+

*NR = Not reported.

tion may be aggravated by supportive or specific therapy of underlying diseases or associated conditions, it is important to recognize those processes that predispose a patient to subclinical alterations in potassium balance as well as those resulting in clinical abnormalities. Additionally, hypokalemia may complicate a number of common veterinary diseases, and its effects may become particularly apparent at a time when other clinical measurements indicate that the patient is, or should be, improving. For example, the onset of hypokalemia in a dog recovering from diabetic ketoacidosis or a cat with postobstructive diuresis may cause excessive weakness and depression. If electrolyte imbalance is not suspected as a cause of severe muscular weakness, the result may be formulation of an unnecessarily poor prognosis.

INTRACELLULAR VS. EXTRACELLULAR POTASSIUM

Unlike sodium and chloride, which reside primarily in extracellular spaces, the bulk of the body's potassium remains within cells. Therefore, serum potassium concentrations are at best only a rough index of total body potassium balance. Potassium shifts readily between intracellular and extracellular compartments as a result of metabolic alterations and as a consequence of therapeutic manipulations.

ETIOLOGY

Decreased Intake

Since potassium is ubiquitous in biological foodstuffs, it is virtually impossible to consume a diet markedly deficient in potassium content. Only prolonged complete anorexia (starvation) could have a significant effect on body potassium stores in the absence of other potassium-depleting mechanisms. Therefore, inadequate potassium consumption is unlikely to be the primary cause of potassium depletion. However, reduced dietary potassium may predispose an animal to hypokalemia or exacerbate negative potassium balance due to other causes.

Gastrointestinal Losses

The concentration of potassium in canine gastric fluid normally ranges from 10 to 20 mEq/L (Strombeck, 1979). Therefore, vomiting is likely to be associated with some degree of potassium depletion. If vomiting is associated with losses limited to hydrochloric acid–containing gastric secretions without simultaneous loss of alkalinizing duodenal secretions, metabolic alkalosis will ensue. Metabolic alkalosis in turn contributes to potassium loss by enhancing distal tubular secretion of potassium. These losses in gastric secretions and urine are probably aggravated by a shift of extracellular potassium into cells in exchange for hydrogen ions as a result of alkalemia.

Diarrhea, particularly that originating in the large intestine, can result in substantial losses of potassium during a short period. For example, in humans it is known that normal fecal losses range from 5 to 15 mEq/day (Cohen et al., 1981). In contrast, patients with cholera may have fecal losses up to ten times that amount (Watten et al., 1959). Dogs and cats with severe diarrhea may also develop hypokalemia. Therefore, serum potassium concentrations should be regularly monitored during parenteral fluid therapy in such patients.

Potassium may become sequestered in the gastrointestinal tract as a result of obstructive diseases, especially in dogs with gastric outflow obstruction or gastric dilatation-volvulus syndrome (Muir, 1982).

Renal Losses

Varying degrees of hypokalemia may develop in dogs and cats given diuretics to treat disorders associated with body fluid accumulation, particularly congestive heart failure. Furosemide, the diuretic most commonly used by veterinarians, is a potent stimulator of potassium loss in urine. Ethacrynic acid and thiazide diuretics may also cause substantial urinary potassium losses. These drugs exert their kaliuretic effect primarily by increasing tubular flow past the potassium secretory sites, thereby stimulating secretion. Osmotic diuresis induces a similar effect and contributes to loss of potassium in patients with uncontrolled diabetes, postobstructive diuresis, and those treated with mannitol, sodium chloride, or sodium bicarbonate solutions. Acetazolamide, a carbonic anhydrase inhibitor commonly used in the management of canine glaucoma, exerts a diuretic effect proximal to the site of potassium secretion and can thereby augment potassium loss in urine.

All diuretics may stimulate sodium depletion, and thus extracellular fluid depletion as well. As a result, there is a compensatory increase in aldosterone secretion. By stimulating renal conservation of sodium through exchange for potassium, aldosterone can exacerbate the severity of potassium depletion.

Metabolic alkalosis is often associated with hypokalemia; this relationship is discussed later under the heading Metabolic Alkalosis. Acute respiratory alkalosis secondary to hyperventilation, mediated by pain or CNS disturbances, can also induce transient reduction in extracellular potassium levels. The mechanism appears to be a translocation of potassium into cells as a result of increased systemic pH. The resulting increase in cellular potassium probably stimulates its increased secretion by the kidneys.

Metabolic alkalosis in humans is associated with increased renal tubular secretion of potassium. The causative mechanism in this case appears to be related to increased delivery of fluid to the distal tubules.

Although the kidneys are highly efficient in conserving sodium, their ability to conserve potassium is limited. The kidneys regulate total body potassium balance primarily by excretion of the ion. It is not difficult to envision why patients with oliguric renal failure are more likely to develop hyperkalemia than hypokalemia. However, some renal disorders may be associated with depressed serum potassium concentrations. For example, osmotic diuresis occurring during recovery from acute tubular necrosis may result in hypokalemia (Cox, 1981). Also, hypokalemia may be seen in patients with high volume renal failure and in uremic patients undergoing intensive diuresis with hypertonic dextrose or mannitol.

In humans, primary or secondary mineralocorticoid excess is an important cause of hypokalemia. Primary hyperaldosteronism (Conn's syndrome) stems from a solitary adrenal adenoma or bilateral adrenal hyperplasia. Secondary hyperaldosteronism may be due to renin-secreting neoplasms, hyperplasia of the juxtaglomerular apparatus (Bartter's syndrome), and other causes. Irrespective of cause, the common denominator of these disorders is excessive aldosterone secretion. Increased secretion of H^+ and K^+ by the kidneys in response to the persistent influence of aldosterone results in metabolic alkalosis and hypokalemia. Although Cushing's disease is associated with hypokalemia in humans, a comparable finding has not been observed in dogs with Cushing's syndrome.

Ectopic ACTH secretion by various tumors is a recognized cause of hypokalemia in humans. This type of paraneoplastic syndrome has not been recognized in animals.

Cellular Shifts

Persistent alkalosis of any origin is an important cause of depressed serum potassium concentration, because of the intracellular migration of the ion. Administration of insulin or substances stimulating insulin release (dextrose infusion in the nondiabetic patient, for example) will also promote rapid movement of potassium into cells. Hypokalemia caused by shifts of potassium from extracellular fluid to intracellular fluid does not accurately reflect the adequacy of total body potassium stores.

Metabolic Alkalosis

Although the relationship between serum potassium concentrations and acid-base balance is complex, hypokalemia is more apt to be a consequence rather than a cause of metabolic alkalosis (Cohen et al., 1981). However, hypokalemia appears to play a role in maintenance of metabolic alkalosis by two mechanisms. First, hypokalemia causes a reduction in glomerular filtration rate (GFR), thereby reducing glomerular filtration of bicarbonate at a time when serum bicarbonate concentrations are inordinately high. Second, the intracellular acidosis that accompanies hypokalemia (H^+ going into cells; K^+ exiting to maintain serum potassium) is a strong stimulus for tubular bicarbonate reabsorption (Sabatini and Kurtzman, 1984).

Metabolic alkalosis causes hypokalemia by promoting increased reabsorption of the sodium ion (Na^+) in exchange for K^+. It has been proposed that ability of the proximal tubule to reabsorb the bicarbonate ion (HCO_3^-) is temporarily exceeded, resulting in increased delivery of Na^+ and HCO_3^- to the distal tubule. Given the Na^+ avidity that usually accompanies metabolic alkalosis, the increased Na^+ is reabsorbed in exchange for K^+. If fluid and electrolyte losses continue unabated (e.g., persis-

Table 2. Clinical Signs of Hypokalemia

Neuromuscular
Skeletal muscle weakness
Smooth muscle weakness (paralytic ileus and gastric dilatation)

Cardiac
Variable EKG changes; no detectable changes may be noted prior to development of arrhythmias; possible alterations include depression of ST segment, lowered T-wave, prolongation of Q-T interval
A wide range of arrhythmias, including atrial tachycardia, AV dissociation, ventricular tachycardia, and ventricular fibrillation, may occur

Renal
Impaired ability to maximally concentrate urine (humans)

Metabolic
Glucose intolerance secondary to decreased insulin release
Increased renal tubular ammonia production

tent vomiting), Na^+ conservation is further stimulated, resulting in ongoing K^+ loss in the urine.

CLINICAL SIGNS AND LABORATORY EVALUATION

Clinical Signs

Hypokalemia is often an unexpected finding detected during the course of a thorough evaluation of the patient's primary problems. Animals rarely develop signs referable to hypokalemia alone. As previously noted, however, hypokalemia may aggravate or complicate signs of concurrent or associated diseases. When hypokalemia is severe enough to become apparent clinically, the resulting abnormalities fall into four main categories: neuromuscular, cardiac, renal, and metabolic (Table 2). Neuromuscular and cardiac manifestations arise primarily because hypokalemia causes hyperpolarization of resting cell membranes, thereby requiring a greater than normal stimulus to depolarize cells. As a result, impulse conduction and muscle contraction are impeded. Skeletal muscle weakness is usually the earliest manifestation of hypokalemia. In humans, the limb muscles are affected first, whereas the trunk and respiratory muscles become involved later. In addition to effects on transmembrane electrical gradients, potassium deficiency may also decrease blood flow in skeletal muscle, which, in turn, can contribute to ischemia-induced necrosis during extreme muscular exertion.

Hypokalemia also causes smooth muscle dysfunction. Clinical signs are often related to the gastrointestinal tract, usually in the form of paralytic ileus and gastric atony.

Cardiac complications associated with hypokalemia are potentially life-threatening. In the dog and cat, EKG changes are variable and nonspecific. Subtle changes may not be detected before development of hypokalemia-induced arrhythmias. Electrocardiographic changes reported in humans include depression of the ST segment, prolongation of the Q-T interval, and decreased T-wave amplitude. As the severity of hypokalemia increases, a wide range of arrhythmias may develop; they include paroxysmal atrial tachycardia, AV dissociation, ventricular tachycardia, and ventricular fibrillation. Of clinical importance is the fact that hypokalemia predisposes the patient to digitalis toxicity, an interaction that increases the likelihood of arrhythmogenesis. Cardiac patients receiving digitalis are often vulnerable to development of hypokalemia because of concomitant use of diuretics such as furosemide.

The most clinically significant renal manifestation of hypokalemia is an impairment of urine-concentrating ability. Although a number of theories have been proposed to explain this phenomenon, the exact mechanism of this concentrating defect has yet to be elucidated. A reduction in medullary solute content appears to be associated with the underlying abnormality (Peterson, 1984). This condition is well known in human medicine but has not been shown to occur spontaneously in dogs and cats.

Both carbohydrate and protein metabolism are affected by potassium depletion. Potassium deficiency is known to blunt insulin release during hyperglycemia, resulting in glucose intolerance. Restoration of potassium balance is associated with amelioration of glucose intolerance. Hypokalemia also causes increased ammonia production by the kidneys. This phenomenon might be of significance in management of patients with end-stage liver disease, since increased ammonia production could contribute to development of hepatic coma. Patients with advanced liver disease may be predisposed to potassium depletion owing to partial or complete anorexia or to use of furosemide or other potassium-wasting diuretics to manage ascites. Spironolactone is a potassium-sparing diuretic that may be effective in management of ascites in dogs with end-stage liver disease; however, we have had little clinical experience with this drug.

Laboratory Evaluation

Normal serum potassium concentration ranges from about 3.7 mEq/L to 5.8 mEq/L. It is impossible to define a specific serum potassium concentration below which clinical signs of hypokalemia will appear. Animals with markedly reduced serum potassium concentrations may be asymptomatic.

In addition to abnormally low serum potassium, abnormalities in other electrolytes (e.g., hypochloremia) and acid-base status (particularly metabolic

Table 3. Problem-Specific Data Base for Diagnosis of Persistent Hypokalemia

I. History
   A. History of vomiting or diarrhea?
   B. History of diuretic use (furosemide, etc.)?
   C. History of polyuria/polydipsia?
   D. Any significant past medical history (particularly relating to gastrointestinal or renal disease)?
   E. Any current medications (besides diuretics)?

II. Physical examination
   A. Dehydration evident?
   B. Cachexia?

III. Laboratory evaluation
   A. Serum electrolytes
   B. CBC—particularly total plasma protein and erythron
   C. Urinalysis—particularly urine specific gravity, urine pH, and urine glucose
   D. Blood gas
   E. Blood glucose
   F. Abdominal radiographs—especially evidence of gastric outflow obstruction and/or gastric fluid accumulation

alkalosis) may occur. A problem-specific data base for patients with persistent hypokalemia has been developed (Table 3).

MANAGEMENT OF HYPOKALEMIA

Specific Treatment

The most important considerations in managing hypokalemic patients are to identify and treat the underlying cause of depressed serum potassium concentration. Specific therapy for hypokalemia might involve surgery (e.g., removal of gastric foreign body), cessation of medication or reduction of dosage (e.g., diuretics, sodium bicarbonate), or treatment of underlying diseases (e.g., diabetic ketoacidosis). Symptomatic and supportive therapy (see later) are often used in conjunction with specific therapy or as interim measures in absence of an etiologic diagnosis. An algorithm for diagnosis and treatment of persistent hypokalemia has been developed (Fig. 1).

Symptomatic Treatment

Symptomatic treatment may be used to minimize external potassium losses. Such therapy usually is in the form of antiemetics or antidiarrheals.

Supportive Treatment

The object of supportive therapy is to restore and maintain potassium balance until correction of the underlying abnormality can be achieved. Potassium supplements can be given parenterally (IV, SC) or orally.

INTRAVENOUS POTASSIUM SUPPLEMENTATION. Potassium chloride is the parenteral potassium supplement used most commonly in veterinary medicine. It is supplied by several manufacturers in multi-dose vials at 2 mEq/ml. Potassium may be added to IV fluids in variable amounts, depending on the degree of depletion (Table 4). In animals with normal renal function, the rate of parenteral potassium supplementation should not exceed 0.5 mEq/kg/hour. Serum potassium concentrations should be monitored frequently during intravenous potassium therapy so that necessary adjustments in dosage can be made. Intravenous potassium supplementation is normally used until serum potassium is stabilized or until the underlying cause has been eliminated or controlled. Complications of intravenous potassium therapy are usually caused by hyperkalemia (Table 5). Intravenous supplementation should be used with special care in patients with reduced renal function and in patients given potassium-sparing diuretics (e.g., spironolactone).

Potassium supplementation can be used in conjunction with either replacement or maintenance fluid therapy. Physiologic saline (0.9 per cent NaCl), the fluid of choice for patients with metabolic alkalosis and hypochloremia, contains no potassium. Replacement fluids, such as lactated Ringer's and Ringer's solution, typically contain 4 mEq/L of potassium. Maintenance fluids such as Normosol-M in D5-W (CEVA Laboratories) or Plasma-Lyte 56 and 5 per cent Dextrose Injection (Travenol Laboratories) contain 13 mEq/L of potassium.

SUBCUTANEOUS POTASSIUM REPLACEMENT. If intravenous administration is unfeasible or if rapid correction of hypokalemia is unnecessary, potassium chloride may be added to fluids given subcutaneously. Since subcutaneous absorption of potassium is slower, the risk of toxicity is reduced. It has been recommended that the concentration of potassium in subcutaneous fluids not exceed 30 mEq/L.

ORAL POTASSIUM REPLACEMENT. Oral potassium replacement has been used infrequently in veterinary medicine. There are a number of oral products available for human patients, but use of these agents has been limited in companion animals. The newer wax-matrix tablets now in use appear to be associated with a lower incidence of intestinal ulceration in humans than were earlier enteric-coated tablets.

If oral potassium supplementation appears warranted (e.g., hypokalemic patients with high urine output renal failure), potassium gluconate tablets (Kaon, Adria Laboratories) may be given orally at the rate of 2.2 mEq of potassium per 100 calories of required energy intake (Low and Cowgill, 1983). Potassium gluconate elixir (20 mEq/ml) has also been recommended for dogs at a dosage of 5 ml given every 8 to 12 hours. Oral potassium chloride

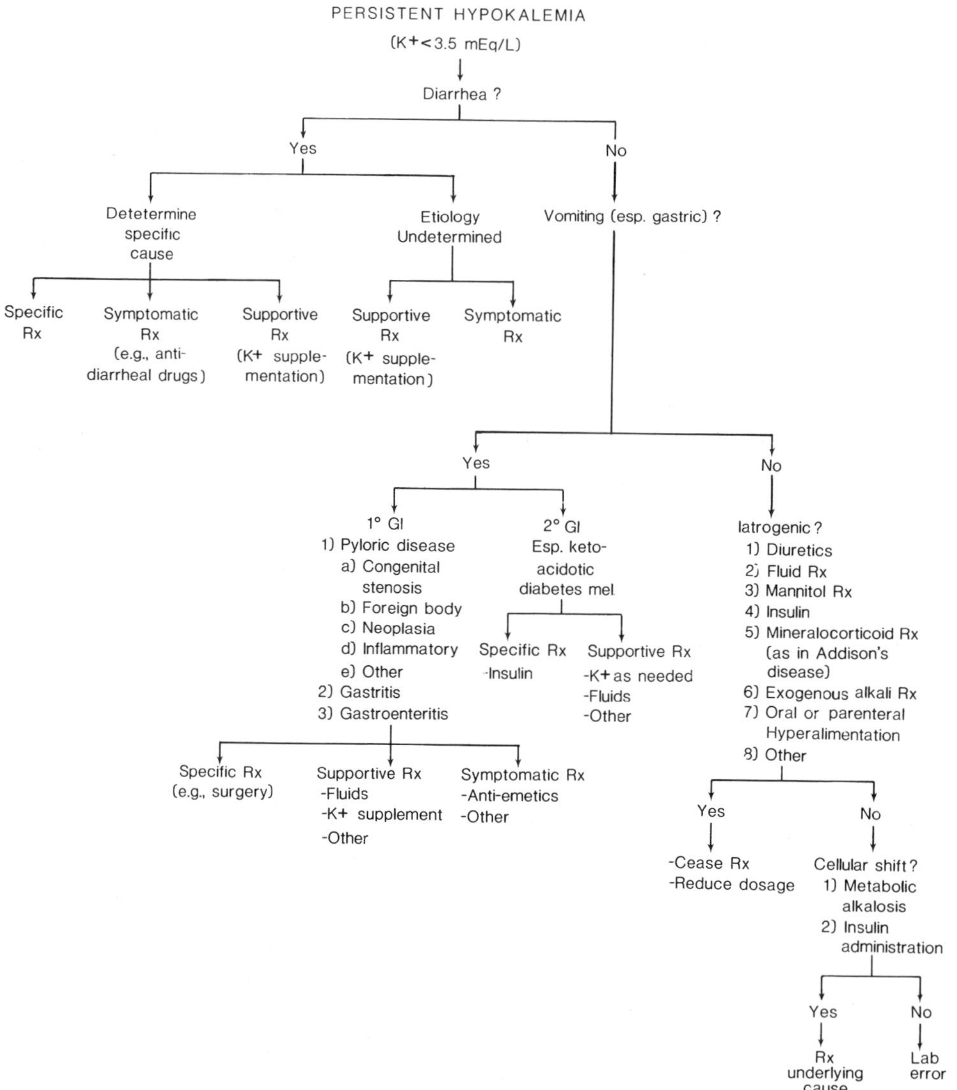

Figure 1. Diagnostic and therapeutic algorithm for persistent hypokalemia.

*Table 4. Guidelines for Intravenous Potassium Supplementation**

Serum Potassium (mEq/L)	mEq KCl to Add per 250 ml of Fluid†	Maximal Infusion Rate (ml/kg/hr)‡
<2.0	20	6
2.1 to 2.5	15	8
2.6 to 3.0	10	12
3.1 to 3.5	7	16

*From Dr. R. C. Scott, Animal Medical Center, New York, N.Y.

†Assume a potassium-free fluid (e.g., 0.9% NaCl). Adjust amount of potassium added according to potassium content of fluid used.

‡Do not exceed 0.5 mEq/kg/hour.

*Table 5. Signs of Iatrogenic Potassium Toxicity**

Physical Signs

Variable and unpredictable; may or may not occur

May include nausea, vomiting, ileus, and abdominal pain

EKG Changes

Degree of hyperkalemia at which EKG changes appear is unpredictable

T-wave spiking seen early: decreasing with continued elevations in serum potassium concentrations

Prolongation of P-R interval; eventual disappearance of P-wave

Widening of QRS complex with decreased amplitudes

Bradycardia

Eventually ventricular fibrillation, asystole, or both may be seen

Laboratory Findings

Serum potassium concentration over 5.8 mEq/L

Clinical signs of hyperkalemia may be aggravated by concurrent hyponatremia, hypocalcemia, and acidosis

*See preceding article, Treatment of Hyperkalemia.

Table 6. Potassium Content of Common Foods (mEq/100 grams)

Bananas	9.5
Beef	9.5 to 11.5
Carrots	8.7
Chicken	9.0
Orange juice	5.1
Peanuts	18.0
Pork	10.0
Potatoes	10.4
Spinach	8.3
Tomatoes	6.3

Adapted from Cohen et al. *in* Brenner and Rector (eds.): *The Kidney*, 2nd ed. Philadelphia: W. B. Saunders, 1981, pp. 908–923.

may be given to dogs at a dose of 1 to 3 gm per day and to cats at 0.2 gm per day (Kirk, 1983). Oral supplementation should be given with appropriate caution, especially in older or debilitated animals. Serum potassium concentration should be evaluated at appropriate intervals.

Mild hypokalemia may be managed conservatively by encouraging consumption of foods high in potassium (Table 6).

Diabetic Ketoacidosis

Patients with diabetic ketoacidosis are particularly prone to develop severe hypokalemia, a phenomenon of therapeutic importance in dogs or cats with this condition. Uncontrolled diabetes mellitus causes potassium loss through the kidneys because of glucosuric osmotic diuresis. Ketoacidosis enhances renal loss and may cause loss due to vomiting as well. Serum potassium concentration is often normal during early stages of the disease because mobilization of intracellular potassium stores maintains normal serum concentrations. Ironically, therapy required to correct fluid imbalances, acidosis, and hyperglycemia may cause significant hypokalemia. Administration of insulin and bicarbonate promotes intracellular uptake of extracellular potassium. Fluid therapy will initially dilute extracellular potassium concentration and may eventually promote renal loss of potassium through diuresis once hydration is restored. Therefore, it is advisable to monitor serum potassium concentrations periodically during intensive therapy of diabetic ketoacidosis and to expect that some form of potassium supplementation will be required.

References and Supplemental Reading

Cohen, J. J., Gennari, F. J., and Harrington, J. T.: Disorders of potassium balance. *In* Brenner, B. M., and Rector, F. C. (eds.): *The Kidney*. Philadelphia: W. B. Saunders, 1981, pp. 908–923.

Cox, M.: Potassium homeostasis. *In* Beck, L. H. (ed.): *The Medical Clinics of North America–Body Fluid and Electrolyte Disorders*. Philadelphia: W. B. Saunders, 1981, pp. 363–384.

Jacobson, H. R., and Seldin, D. W.: On the generation, maintenance, and correction of metabolic alkalosis. Am. J. Phys. 245:F425, 1983.

Kirk, R. W. (ed.): *Current Veterinary Therapy VIII*. Philadelphia: W. B. Saunders, 1983.

Knochel, J. P.: Hypokalemia. *In* Stollerman, G. H. (ed.) *Advances in Internal Medicine*. Vol. 30. Chicago: Year Book Medical Publishers, 1984, pp. 317–335.

Low, D. G., and Cowgill, L. D.: Emergency management of the acute uremic crisis. *In* Kirk, R. W. (ed.): *Current Veterinary Therapy VIII*. Philadelphia: W. B. Saunders, 1983, pp. 989.

Muir, W. W.: Acid-base and electrolyte disturbances in dogs with gastric dilatation-volvulus. J.A.V.M.A. 181:229, 1982.

Peterson, L. N.: Time-dependent changes in inner medullary plasma flow rate during potassium depletion. Kidney Int. 25:899, 1984.

Rose, B. D.: *Clinical Physiology of Acid-Base and Electrolyte Disorders*. New York: McGraw-Hill, 1984.

Sabatini, S., and Kurtzman, N. A.: The maintenance of metabolic alkalosis: Factors which decrease bicarbonate excretion. Kidney Int. 25:357, 1984.

Strombeck, D. R.: *Small Animal Gastroenterology*. Davis, CA: Stonegate Publishing Co., 1979, p. 89.

Watten, R. H., Morgan, F. M., Songkhla, Y. N., et al.: Water and electrolyte studies in cholera. J. Clin. Invest. 38:1879, 1959.

BLOOD SUBSTITUTE THERAPY

CRAIG E. GREENE, D.V.M.

Athens, Georgia

Artificially produced substances that are used to replace blood or its components are defined as blood substitutes. Colloidal compounds such as dextran, hydroxyethyl starch, polyvinylpyrrolidone, and gelatin have been used experimentally and sometimes on a clinical basis to replace blood albumin. Erythrocytes are the only other major component of blood for which adequate substitutes have been developed. The objective of this discussion is to provide an overview of current principles for use of solutions designed to replace erythrocytes in animals. Erythrocyte substitutes may be used in place of blood to correct acute severe hemorrhage or hemolysis (when crystalloids and colloids would be ineffective), and when use of whole blood or packed erythrocytes is unfeasible or contraindicated. Two major forms of erythrocyte substitutes that have been beneficial are hemoglobin solutions and perfluorochemicals. Unfortunately, these compounds are not widely available for use by veterinarians at the present time.

HEMOGLOBIN SOLUTIONS

Hemolysates of whole blood were first proposed as human blood substitutes in the late nineteenth century; however, clinical trials in the early twentieth century revealed that erythrocyte hemolysates were very toxic. It was not until the late 1960s that experimental studies in animals confirmed that erythrocytic stroma within these solutions were responsible for most of the toxicity. Most studies of blood substitutes for animals have been designed to evaluate hemoglobin solutions rather than the newer perfluorochemical compounds.

Hemoglobin is composed of four subunit molecules (a tetrameric arrangement). Erythrocytes protect hemoglobin by maintaining it in a stable structure. In an aqueous medium, hemoglobin is subject to breakdown into a dimeric form, which is more readily excreted than the tetrameric form. Within the erythrocytic membrane, hemoglobin is maintained in the tetrameric form, free from filtration by renal glomeruli, protected from oxidation to methemoglobin, and most efficient in oxygen transport. Unlike fluorochemical blood substitutes, stroma-free hemoglobin (SFH) solutions can transport oxygen in a non-oxygen-enriched atmosphere and are effective osmotic expanders of plasma. Solutions of 7 per cent SFH are comparable in oxygen-carrying capacity to 20 per cent fluorocarbon solutions, and they provide osmotic activity. Since erythrocytic stroma are not present in SFH solutions (as in whole blood), they are not antigenic and thus do not require blood typing or cross-matching before transfusion. Hemoglobin solutions can be stored for longer periods than can whole blood, especially if lyophilized. Crystallized, washed, and sterilized hemoglobin contains fewer contaminants than nonprocessed hemoglobin. If stored at −20°C, it may remain stable for two years.

Research studies of dogs with cardiac bypasses have demonstrated that SFH solutions are of greater therapeutic benefit than albumin. Studies of hemorrhagic shock in dogs revealed that the animals survive with lower hematocrits when SFH solutions are used than they do when whole blood is diluted or mixed with plasma expanders such as dextran.

One disadvantage of unmodified hemoglobin in SFH solutions is that free hemoglobin has a higher oxygen affinity than intact erythrocytes. Increased oxygen affinity impairs release of oxygen to the tissues where it is needed. Since hemoglobin is a colloid, its concentration outside erythrocytes is only 7 gm/dl, as compared with 30 gm/dl within erythrocytes. This difference limits the total amount of oxygen that can be transported by SFH solutions. Furthermore, free hemoglobin is also taken up by the mononuclear-phagocyte system, which limits its life span in the circulation. Large quantities of hemoglobin, especially if given repeatedly, cause blockade of mononuclear clearance mechanisms and increase susceptibility to infections.

Several chemical modifications of the hemoglobin molecule reduce the undesirable properties of free hemoglobin solutions. Macromolecular, intramolecular, and intermolecular modifications have been studied. Macromolecular modifications of hemoglobin have been made by combining it with products such as dextran and inulin. Intra- and intermolecular polymerization of hemoglobin has been accomplished by cross-linking hemoglobin molecules with compounds such as glutaraldehyde. Increasing the molecular size greatly prolongs the intravascular survival of free hemoglobin.

Pyridoxylation of hemoglobin with compounds such as pyridoxal-5-phosphate reduces its oxygen affinity. This modification facilitates release of oxygen to tissues and also reduces formation of methemoglobin. For these reasons, pyridoxylated polymerized hemoglobin has become a common formulation that has been successfully used as an experimental erythrocyte substitute in animals. Use of bovine hemoglobin does not require pyridoxylation because it already functions effectively in the unmodified form. Polymerization of bovine hemoglobin extends its intravascular half-life from 60 minutes to 12 hours.

Unmodified hemoglobin has also been encapsulated within liposomal micelles in an attempt to produce artificial erythrocytes. Liposomes are nontoxic, nonimmunogenic, and have no procoagulant activity. They are also biodegradable but are not taken up by the mononuclear-phagocyte system to any extent. Neohemocytes consist of small volumes of hemoglobins and other solutes that have been placed in microscopic biocompatible liposomal membranes. Neohemocytes readily pass through the lumen of capillaries. Since microencapsulation does not alter the hemoglobin, it should be efficacious in oxygen delivery to the tissues. Use of liposomal-hemoglobin substitutes has been limited to research laboratories.

PERFLUOROCHEMICAL (PFC) COMPOUNDS

Perfluorochemicals are organic compounds that consist of a carbon skeleton in which all hydrogen atoms have been replaced by fluorine. They are excellent gas solvents and dissolve oxygen in solution in proportion to the partial pressure of oxygen to which they are in equilibrium.

PFC compounds are biologically inert. Although they are taken up by the mononuclear-phagocyte system, they persist there for long periods. They are slowly removed by the body through the respiratory tract in expired wastes. PFC compounds are not miscible with water; they must be suspended in emulsions to be soluble in blood. Unfortunately, the micelles suspended in the emulsion must be smaller than 0.1 μm to prevent removal from blood by the mononuclear-phagocyte system. Emulsification also reduces the maximum concentration of oxygen that the PFC can transport.

Because these compounds are very dense, they settle to the bottom of blood samples. They render serum opaque and interfere with laboratory test results obtained by spectrophotometric methods.

Fluosol-DA is a commercially available fluorochemical-based blood substitute that has been licensed for use in Japan for several years (Green Cross Corp., Osaka). It is an emulsion of two compounds, perfluorodecalin and perfluorotripropylamine, placed in a balanced salt solution to which hydroxyethyl starch has been added to provide oncotic properties. An emulsifier consists of Pluronic F68 and egg yolk, with glycerol as a stabilizer. Fluosol-DA has a viscosity that is approximately 50 per cent that of whole blood. Its small micelles provide a large surface area. Uptake and release of oxygen by Fluosol-DA are similar to that by erythrocytes.

Indications and proposed uses of PFCs in human medicine include (1) vehicles for infusion of chemotherapeutic substances, (2) use in emergency surgery or hemorrhagic shock when typed blood is contraindicated or unavailable, (3) local perfusion for oxygenating hypoxic areas, (4) treatment of carbon monoxide toxicity, and (5) a priming solution for transfusion pumps, extracorporeal devices, and organs maintained *ex vivo* for transplantation. Fluosol-DA has been used experimentally in conjunction with mannitol to decrease brain edema in dogs and cats. In other studies, dogs showed less cardiac injury after myocardial ischemia if transfused with Fluosol-DA. Fluosol-DA is thought to be of value in treatment of ischemia because it decreases blood viscosity and increases perfusion and oxygen availability to local tissues.

PFC compounds can deliver soluble oxygen only at a concentration that is three times that of plasma. Since the oxygen-binding action of these compounds follows a nonsigmoidal curve, in most cases patients treated with PFCs must breathe enriched oxygen mixtures. Thus, the patient usually must be anesthetized, intubated, and given 100 per cent oxygen to breathe. Because Fluosol-DA is unstable at room temperature, it must be stored in the frozen state until used. The expense of Fluosol-DA will inhibit its use in animals at the present time.

Potential toxicity of all PFC compounds is that they can become concentrated in tissues containing large numbers of mononuclear cells and other phagocytes. Some compounds have a high vapor pressure and, under certain circumstances, might cause air embolism. PFC compounds activate complement by the alternate pathway. This biologic activity has been suggested as the mechanism responsible for sequestration of leukocytes in lungs after administration of Fluosol-DA. Pulmonary leukostasis results in pulmonary dysfunction, hypoxemia, and neutropenia. Fluosol-DA may also cause coagulation abnormalities as a result of (1) diluting the clotting factors, (2) coagulation activation, and (3) inducing consumptive coagulopathy. As already mentioned, particle size of the micelles is important, since emulsions of small particulate size are associated with decreased removal by the mononuclear-phagocyte system. The small particle size contributes to longer intravascular survival, enhanced oxygen transport, and decreased coagulation abnormalities.

References and Supplemental Reading

Biro, G. P.: Effect of hemodilution with dextran, stroma-free hemoglobin solution and Fluosol-DA on experimental myocardial ischemia in the dog. Bibl. Haematol. 47:54, 1981.

Bolin, R. B., Geyer, R. P., and Nemo, G. J. (eds.): *Advances in Blood Substitute Research*. New York: Alan R. Liss, 1983.

Hauser, C. J., Kaufman, C., Frantz, R., et al.: Use of crystalline hemoglobin as replacement of RBC mass. Arch. Surg. 117:782, 1982.

Hauser C. J., and Shoemaker, W. C.: Hemoglobin solution in the treatment of hemorrhagic shock. Crit. Care Med. 10:283, 1982.

Nunn, G. R., Dance, G., Peters, J., et al.: Effect of fluocarbon exchange transfusion on myocardial infarction size in dogs. Am. J. Cardiol. 52:203, 1983.

Vercellotti, G. M., Hammerschmidt, D. E., Craddock, P. R., et al.: Activation of plasma complement by perfluorocarbon artificial blood: Probable mechanism of adverse pulmonary reactions in treated patients and rationale for corticosteroid prophylaxis. Blood 59:1299, 1982.

THERAPEUTIC HEMAPHERESIS

JEFFREY S. KLAUSNER, D.V.M.,
ELLEN M. POFFENBARGER, D.V.M.
St. Paul, Minnesota

and ROBERT E. MATUS, D.V.M.
New York, New York

Therapeutic procedures for the removal of plasma (plasmapheresis) and cells (cytapheresis) have been used extensively in human medicine in recent years to treat a variety of hematologic, immunologic, and neoplastic disorders. *Apheresis* is derived from the Greek word *aphairesis* meaning *to remove* or *to take away by force.* The recent increase in hemapheresis procedures is related to widespread availability of automated cell separators. Although use of hemapheresis in veterinary medicine has been relatively limited, the numbers of procedures will probably increase as referral centers obtain necessary equipment.

The concept of bloodletting for removal of toxins and restoration of humoral balance predates Hippocrates. Bloodletting reached its peak during the sixteenth and seventeenth centuries, and its use continued until the numerous hazards of the procedure became widely recognized. Plasmapheresis, in which blood removal was followed by return of autologous red blood cells suspended in a replacement salt solution, was first reported in 1914 by Abel and colleagues, who used the procedure to reduce uremic signs in bilaterally nephrectomized dogs (Abel et al., 1914). Manual plasmapheresis was used in 1944 as a means of obtaining plasma for transfusion and in the 1950s and 1960s to treat human patients with myeloma, autoimmune hemolytic anemia, and the hyperviscosity syndrome. Efficient removal of large volumes of plasma became possible in the late 1960s with the advent of automated blood cell separators.

Terminology

Hemapheresis or apheresis includes all procedures for selective removal of any fraction of blood. *Plasma exchange* and *plasmapheresis* are used interchangeably for plasma removal and subsequent return of erythrocytes in a replacement solution. Plasma processing is a procedure in which a substance is selectively removed from plasma before its return to the patient. Removal of blood cells (cytapheresis) can be performed by techniques that permit all white blood cells (leukapheresis), lymphocytes (lymphocytapheresis), platelets (thrombocytapheresis), or red blood cells (erythrocytapheresis) to be removed.

BLOOD SEPARATION

Centrifugal and membrane separation methods are currently available to separate plasma from cellular blood components. In centrifugal systems, blood is withdrawn from the patient through a catheter, mixed with an anticoagulant, and pumped into a centrifuge. Blood components become layered within the centrifuge according to density. Contents of a layer can be continuously or intermittently removed through precisely positioned sampling ports. One or more undesirable components are removed and the remainder is returned to the patient. If plasma is removed, it is replaced with solutions such as fresh frozen plasma or balanced electrolyte solutions.

In membrane systems, movement of plasma through a semipermeable membrane with small pores permits separation of formed elements from plasma. Cytapheresis cannot be performed with membrane systems. However, membrane blood separation techniques require a smaller extracorporeal volume than that needed for centrifugal separation techniques.

THERAPEUTIC PLASMAPHERESIS

Plasmapheresis allows removal of potentially pathogenic materials from blood; these include paraproteins, excess lipids, abnormal metabolites, exogenous poisons and drugs, autoantibodies, immune complexes, and other harmful humoral immunoreactants (Ward, 1985).

The frequency of repeated plasmapheresis is dependent on the disease treated. If the removed material is primarily confined to the vascular space and its rate of synthesis is slow (e.g., IgM paraprotein), the substance may be removed in one or two procedures. If (as in the case of most IgG autoantibodies) the removed substance reappears rapidly by re-equilibration from the extravascular space, plasmapheresis must be repeated frequently. Serial measurement of the plasma concentration of the removed substance is the best method for determining treatment intervals.

Therapeutic plasmapheresis is usually limited to exchange of one plasma volume. The amount of a substance removed from the blood during each procedure progressively decreases as additional plasma is removed because of the continued mixing of the replacement solution with the patient's plasma. A 2-L exchange in a human patient with a plasma volume of 3 L will remove approximately 50 per cent of a circulating substance; a 4-L exchange will remove only an additional 5 per cent (Jones et al., 1981).

Use of cytotoxic drugs in addition to plasmapheresis has been recommended for treatment of patients with elevated titers of autoantibodies or immune complexes (Branda et al., 1975). After plasmapheresis, the concentration of removed antibodies usually rebounds to levels greater than the initial concentration (Terman et al., 1977b). Cytotoxic drugs such as cyclophosphamide and cytosine arabinoside effectively prevent antibody rebound (Terman et al., 1978).

Plasmapheresis is usually well tolerated by humans and dogs; side effects have been reported in approximately 15 per cent of human patients (Ward, 1985). Complications include hypothermia, infection, phlebitis, clotting within the machine, citrate-induced hypocalcemia, and loss of platelets, clotting factors, and antithrombin III. In humans, allergic reactions may also result from use of fresh frozen plasma as a replacement solution.

ON-LINE PLASMA PROCESSING

On-line methods have recently been developed for selective removal of putative toxic substances from plasma. Blood is separated into cellular components and plasma, and plasma is passed through a "purification" device. Selective removal decreases adverse reactions associated with administration of replacement solutions required after removal of large volumes of plasma.

The most common method of on-line processing is to perfuse plasma through columns containing immobilized substances that bind to or inactivate specific plasma constituents. Antigens, antibodies, and enzymes can be incorporated into columns. Examples include columns containing staphylococcal protein A for removal of immunoglobulins and immune complexes (Branda et al., 1984), DNA for removal of anti-DNA antibodies (Terman et al., 1977a), and monoclonal antibodies for removal of specific antigens. A continuous flow immunoadsorption system utilizing protein A bound to sepharose safely reduced circulating IgG concentration by approximately 50 per cent in normal dogs (Branda et al., 1984).

Other experimental methods of on-line plasma processing include (1) cascade filtration, in which plasma is sequentially passed through membrane filters designed to selectively remove plasma components; (2) cryofiltration, in which plasma components are separated by cooling and filtration; and (3) precipitation techniques in which specific plasma components are precipitated and removed by filtration.

CYTAPHERESIS

Leukapheresis is performed to remove an excessive number of cells, to remove abnormal cells, or to modify the immune response. Centrifugal cell separators are designed to remove various cell types from blood based on their differences in cell density.

Patients with myelogenous leukemia and white blood cell counts greater than 70,000/μl are at risk for developing leukostatic syndromes. The large size and relative nondeformity of myeloblasts may block the microcirculation, resulting in organ dysfunction (Ward, 1985). White blood cell counts can be lowered 30 to 50 per cent in a few hours by leukapheresis (Nose, 1982; Lane, 1980). Cytotoxic drugs may take 2 or 3 days to produce a similar effect. Thrombocytapheresis can be used to decrease elevated platelet counts in thrombocythemic patients and thus decrease the risk of thrombosis.

Cytotoxic drugs used to reduce extremely elevated white blood cell counts of leukemic patients may cause adverse reactions because of massive lysis of circulating cells. Disseminated intravascular coagulation, hyperuricemia, and renal failure have been reported in humans (Ward, 1985). Leukapheresis, performed before cytotoxic therapy, may reduce the frequency and severity of these adverse reactions.

Removal of large numbers of lymphocytes by leukapheresis can induce immunosuppression. Peripheral lymphocyte counts may be persistently lowered by 60 per cent (Nose, 1982). Lymphocytapheresis is now being evaluated in humans with immune-mediated disorders such as rheumatoid arthritis.

THERAPEUTIC APPLICATIONS OF PLASMAPHERESIS

More than 70 disorders in man have been treated by apheresis techniques (Kennedy and Domen,

1983). Patients with any disease associated with putative pathogenic substances in the circulation might benefit from plasmapheresis. Unfortunately, definitive therapeutic responses to only a few diseases have been observed. Evaluation of plasmapheresis has been complicated by (1) unavailability of control groups for comparison (many disorders for which plasmapheresis is recommended undergo spontaneous regressions) and (2) concomitant use of other therapy with plasmapheresis.

Hyperviscosity Syndrome

Plasma viscosity may be increased by paraproteins that accumulate in blood. Myeloma, lymphoma, and macroglobulinemia are the most common causes of paraproteinemia in dogs. Increased serum viscosity caused by increased concentration of serum paraprotein decreases perfusion to most organs. Hyperviscosity is often associated with IgM gammopathies because of the large size of IgM molecules, but they may also be associated with IgA gammopathies because of the tendency of IgA to form dimers and trimers. Clinical manifestations of the hyperviscosity syndrome include visual defects, syncope, convulsions, cardiac failure, renal failure, and bleeding.

Although cytotoxic drugs decrease serum paraprotein concentration, their effect is not immediate. Plasmapheresis, on the other hand, rapidly decreases serum paraprotein concentration and serum viscosity. The effectiveness of plasmapheresis is influenced by the distribution of abnormal proteins. If paraproteins such as IGM are primarily confined to the intravascular space, reduction in their concentration can be accomplished by one or two treatments. Additional therapy may be required to remove IgG and IgA paraproteins because they are distributed in intravascular and extravascular spaces. After initial plasmapheresis, chemotherapy is usually required to control production of paraproteins.

Three dogs with IgA myeloma and plasma hyperviscosity were treated with plasmapheresis and chemotherapy (Matus et al., 1983). Twenty-four hours later, clinical signs of hyperviscosity, including epistaxis, weakness, and neurologic signs, had decreased in severity. Plasmapheresis was repeated three times in another dog with IgA myeloma and hyperviscosity syndrome (Shull et al., 1978). After the third treatment, serum viscosity had decreased and clinical signs of hyperviscosity had disappeared. Recently, serum IgA concentrations were reduced in two dogs with IgA myeloma by perfusion of their plasma over sepharose columns containing goat anticanine IgA (Gordon et al., submitted for publication).

Multiple Myeloma

In addition to decreasing plasma viscosity, plasmapheresis may benefit patients with multiple myeloma by removing Bence Jones proteins from the circulation. Bence Jones proteins may obstruct renal tubular lumens with casts, and may have a direct toxic effect on the renal tubules (Misiani et al., 1979). In human patients, plasmapheresis has been shown to remove more than 50 per cent of circulating Bence Jones protein. In addition, the technique has resulted in improvement or stabilization of renal function (Misiani et al., 1979). In 10 dogs with multiple myeloma, treatment with plasmapheresis and alkylating chemotherapy was associated with preservation of renal function (Matus et al., unpublished data).

Immune-Mediated Thrombocytopenia

Plasmapheresis has been recommended for treatment of patients with immune-mediated thrombocytopenia in attempt to decrease their titer of antiplatelet antibodies (Branda et al., 1978). Since a beneficial effect caused by plasmapheresis has not been substantiated in such cases, its use is recommended only for patients that fail to respond to cytotoxic and immunosuppressive chemotherapy.

Autoimmune Hemolytic Anemia

Immune-mediated hemolytic anemia is characterized by destruction of red blood cells, which is mediated by autoantibodies to red blood cell membranes. By decreasing the titer of autoantibody, plasmapheresis may increase survival of the red blood cells. Since the autoantibodies are resynthesized rapidly, however, clinical response is usually transient (Ward, 1985). Plasmapheresis may be utilized as an emergency procedure before cytotoxic therapy has had time to initiate a beneficial response. Temporary stabilization of acute hemolysis occurred in response to plasmapheresis in two dogs with autoimmune hemolytic anemia (Matus et al., 1985).

Systemic Lupus Erythematosus

Systemic lupus erythematosus (SLE) is an immune-mediated disorder characterized by hyperactive B cells and increased circulating immune complexes (CIC) and autoantibodies. Deposition of immune complexes in various tissues is followed by activation of complement and other immune reactants. Plasmapheresis may be of benefit in treatment of SLE by removal of CIC, autoantibodies directed against self-antigens, and circulating factors responsible for defective immunosuppressor activity (Jones et al., 1979). It has been suggested that removal of CIC may "unblock" the reticuloendothelial system and thus enhance removal of remaining immune complexes by tissue macrophages (Jones et al., 1979). In addition, removal of antibodies followed by "antibody rebound" may alter the ratio of antigen to antibody and thus the biologic activity of immune complexes.

Human (Jones et al., 1979) and canine (Matus et al., 1983; in press) SLE patients have benefited from plasmapheresis therapy. Plasmapheresis and immunoadsorption with staphylococcal protein A resulted in clinical improvement and sustained decrease in CIC in a dog that had previously failed to respond to therapy with cyclophosphamide and prednisone (Matus et al., 1983). Intermittent plasmapheresis of dogs with SLE permitted reduction in the dose of corticosteroid and cytotoxic therapy required to control the disease (Matus et al., in press.

Rheumatoid Arthritis

Rheumatoid arthritis (RA) is a progressive, immunologically mediated disorder characterized by shifting lameness and swelling of soft tissues around affected joints. Immune complexes are often identified in joint fluid, synovial membranes, and the circulation. The rationale for use of plasmapheresis to treat rheumatoid arthritis includes the removal of immunoglobulins, CIC, and rheumatoid factor. To date, only marginal benefits of this treatment have been observed in human patients with RA (Ward, 1985). Its use is generally limited to patients who fail to respond to other modes of therapy.

Myasthenia Gravis

Patients with acquired myasthenia gravis (MG) produce IgG antibodies against the nicotinic acetylcholine receptor of skeletal muscles. Blockage of the acetylcholine receptor by antibody results in weakness and quick onset of fatigue. Plasmapheresis has been recommended to decrease antireceptor antibody titers of MG patients. Plasmapheresis has been of temporary benefit to human patients with acute, severe signs of MG, and it was of benefit to human patients with chronic disease if used in conjunction with other therapy (Dau, 1980).

Glomerulonephritis

Antibodies directed against glomerular basement membranes (GBM) and immune complex deposition within glomeruli have been implicated in the pathogenesis of some glomerulopathies. Clinical improvement has been noted in approximately half of the human patients with anti-GBM glomerulonephritis treated with plasmapheresis (Wenz and Barland, 1981). Good results have also been obtained in some humans with immune-complex glomerulonephritis, although favorable responses have been less frequent than those observed in patients with anti-GBM disease (Wenz and Barland, 1981). It is uncertain whether removal of immunoglobulins, immune complexes, or other inflammatory mediators, singly or in combination, contributes to the clinical responses.

Diabetes Mellitus

Plasmapheresis is now being evaluated in human diabetic patients to reduce hypertriglyceridemia and formation of antibodies against islet cells and insulin receptors.

Neoplastic Disorders

Immunoglobulins and CIC may abrogate the immune response to cancer. Plasmapheresis and immunoadsorption of plasma with staphylococcal protein A have been suggested as methods of removing these "blocking" factors. In one report, regression was noted in 35 per cent of human cancer patients treated with plasmapheresis for 3 weeks (Israel et al., 1977). Plasma perfusion over staphylococcal protein A bound to sepharose or silica columns was not associated with clinical response in dogs with various neoplastic disorders (Klausner et al., 1985; Gordon et al., 1983). Further studies are needed to establish the value of plasmapheresis in patients with neoplastic disease.

AVAILABILITY OF HEMAPHERESIS

Hemapheresis and selective plasma absorption are relatively new techniques to veterinary medicine. Additional clinical studies are needed to evaluate their therapeutic potential. At present, plasmapheresis and cytapheresis should be considered when conventional therapy is ineffective or slow to initiate the desired effect. Because hemapheresis procedures require specialized equipment and trained personnel, the technique is presently limited to referral centers. Future advances in technology should increase the availability of these procedures to veterinarians. Centers presently equipped to perform plasmapheresis and cytapheresis include The Animal Medical Center, New York

City; College of Veterinary Medicine, University of Minnesota, St. Paul; College of Veterinary Medicine, University of Georgia, Athens; The Hutchison Cancer Research Center, University of Washington, Seattle; and College of Veterinary Medicine, University of California, Davis.

References and Supplemental Reading

Abel, J. J., Rowntree, L. G., and Turner, B. B.: Plasma removal with return of corpuscles (plasmapheresis). J. Pharmacol. Exp. Ther. 5:625, 1914.

Branda, R. F., Klausner, J. S., Miller, W. J., et al.: Specific removal of antibodies with an immunoadsorption system. Transfusion 24:157, 1984.

Branda, R. F., McCullough, J. J., Tate, D., et al.: Plasma exchange in the treatment of fulminant idiopathic (autoimmune) thrombocytopenia purpura. Lancet 1:688, 1978.

Branda, R. F., Moldow, C. F., McCullough, J. J., et al.: Plasma exchange in the treatment of immune disease. Transfusion 15:570, 1975.

Dau, P. C.: Plasmapheresis therapy in myasthenia gravis. Muscle Nerve 3:468, 1980.

Gordon, B. R., Matus, R. E., Saal, S. D., et al.: Protein A independent tumoricidal responses following extracorporeal perfusion of plasma over *Staphyloccus aureus.* J Natl. Cancer Inst. 70:1127, 1983.

Gordon, B. R., Matus, R. E., Sloan, B. T., et al.: Selective depletion of IgA in dogs using immunoabsorption. Transfusion, submitted for publication.

Israel, L., Edelstein, R., Mannoni, P., et al.: Plasmapheresis in patients with disseminated cancer: Clinical results and correlation with changes in serum protein. Cancer 40:3146, 1977.

Jones, J. V., Clough, J. D., Klinenberg, J. R., et al.: The role of therapeutic plasmapheresis in the rheumatic diseases. J. Lab. Clin. Med. 97:589, 1981.

Jones, J. V., Cumming, R. H., Bacon, P. A., et al.: Evidence for a therapeutic effect of plasmapheresis in patients with systemic lupus erythematosus. Q. J. Med. 192:555, 1979.

Kennedy, M. S., and Domen, R. E.: Therapeutic apheresis: Applications and future directions. Vox Sang. 45:261, 1983.

Klausner, J. S., Miller, W. J., O'Brien, T. D., et al.: Effects of plasma treatment with purified protein A and *Staphylococcus aureus* Cowan I on spontaneous animal neoplasms. Cancer Res., 45:1263, 1985.

Lane, T. A.: Continuous-flow leukapheresis for rapid cytoreduction in leukemia. Transfusion 20:455, 1980.

Matus, R. E., Gordon, B. R., Leifer, C. E., et al.: Plasmapheresis in five dogs with systemic immune mediated disease. J.A.V.M.A., in press (a).

Matus, R. E., Leifer, C. E., Gordon, B. R., et al.: Unpublished data.

Matus, R. E., Leifer, C. E., Gordon, B. R., et al.: Plasmapheresis and chemotherapy of hyperviscosity syndrome associated with monoclonal gammopathy in the dog. J.A.V.M.A. 183:205, 1983.

Matus, R. E., Schrader, L. A., Leifer, C. E., et al.: Plasmapheresis as adjuvant therapy for autoimmune hemolytic anemia in two dogs. J.A.V.M.A. 186:691, 1985.

Matus, R. E., Scott, R. C., Saal, S., et al.: Plasmapheresis-immunoadsorption for treatment of systemic lupus erythematosus in a dog. J.A.V.M.A. 182:499, 1983.

Misani, R., Remuzzi, G., Bertani, T., et al.: Plasmapheresis in the treatment of acute renal failure in multiple myeloma. Am. J. Med. 66:684, 1979.

Nose, Y.: Plasmapheresis and cytapheresis. Trans. Am. Soc. Artif. Intern. Organs 28:631, 1982.

Shull, R. M., Osborne, C. A., Barrett, R. E., et al.: Serum hyperviscosity syndrome associated with IgA multiple myeloma in two dogs. J. Am. Anim. Hosp. Assoc. 14:58, 1978.

Terman, D. S., Garcia-Rinaldi, G., Dannemann, B., et al.: Specific suppression of antibody rebound after extracorporeal immunoadsorption. Clin. Exp. Immunol. 34:32, 1978.

Terman, D. S., Petty, D., Harbeck, R., et al.: Specific removal of DNA antibodies *in vivo* by extracorporeal circulation over DNA immobilized in collodion-charcoal. Clin. Immunol. Immunopathol. 9:90, 1977a.

Terman, D. S., Tavel, T., Petty, D., et al.: Specific removal of antibody by extracorporeal circulation over antigen immobilized in collodion-charcoal. Clin. Exp. Immunol. 28:180, 1977b.

Ward, D.: Therapeutic plasmapheresis and related apheresis techniques. *In* Isselbacher, K. J., Adams, R., Braunwald, E., et al. (eds.): *Harrison's Principles of Internal Medicine, Update V.* New York: McGraw-Hill, 1985, pp. 67–95.

Wenz, B., and Barland, P.: Therapeutic plasmapheresis. Semin. Hematol. 18:147, 1981.

ORGAN TRANSPLANTATION IN DOGS: PRESENT AND FUTURE

DELMAR R. FINCO, D.V.M.,
and JEANNE A. BARSANTI, D.V.M.
Athens, Georgia

Organ or tissue transplantation between different members of the same species is referred to as allogeneic transplantation (allografting). Certain tissues (e.g., cornea) survive allografting because of the lack of vascular connections with the recipient. However, survival of most allografts is jeopardized by immunologic response of the recipient to grafted tissue.

The dog has been used extensively as a research animal for transplantation procedures. This use is advantageous to veterinarians because organ transplantation techniques have been devised, and some characteristics of the dog as an organ or tissue recipient have been uncovered. This discussion will provide a comparative overview of the present state of knowledge about organ transplantation in humans and in dogs, with emphasis on kidney transplantation. We will also speculate on the clinical application of renal transplantation on dogs during the next decade.

IMMUNOLOGIC CONSIDERATIONS IN TRANSPLANTATION

It is well known that grafting an organ from one animal into another of the same species is rarely successful because of immunologic rejection of the donated organ by the recipient. The recipient rejects the transplanted organ by detecting foreign antigen on cell surfaces and mobilizing its immune system to destroy the foreign cells. In the several vertebrates studied, the structure of the most important cell surface antigens is genetically dictated by a single chromosomal complex in each of the donor's cells. This complex is referred to as the major histocompatibility complex and is referred to by the abbreviation HLA in humans. Specific chromosomal sites located in close proximity to one another have been designated as A, B, and C. Since chromosomes are paired, each human has six A, B, and C antigens, three from each parent. The A and B antigens have been serologically defined, and this information is the basis for tissue typing; the C antigen is ignored because of typing difficulties. These antigens (A, B, and C) are designated class 1 antigens and are present on virtually all human cells except erythrocytes, which have their own unique antigenic structure that also must be considered in matching organ donors and recipients.

Tissue typing for human transplantation procedures originally entailed evaluation of just the two A and the two B loci. A zero mismatch indicated identity at all sites. Since such matching was not always possible, transplantations were and still are performed with mismatching at one or more loci. The values of A and B antigen typing were determined retrospectively by compilation of statistics on graft survival in kidney allograft recipients. It was found that such typing was of considerable benefit in predicting graft survival in closely related donors and recipients but of questionable value with unrelated participants. These observations indicated that the A and B antigens were not the exclusive ones involved in histocompatibility. It is likely that in closely related individuals, the A and B loci serve as markers for other undefined antigen determinants common to the individuals because of their location on the same chromosome. In unrelated individuals with fortuitous matchings at A and B loci, the undefined antigenic determinants are probably dissimilar. Additional evidence that the A and B sites were not exclusive for evaluation of histocompatibility was derived from mixed lymphocyte culture reactions (MLC and MLR are both used as abbreviations for this technique). In performing an MLR procedure, lymphocytes are exposed to cells (lymphocytes from another source) and given the opportunity to respond to surface antigens on the other cells. With a two-way test, lymphocytes from each source are allowed to react to one another. With a one-way test the potential organ donor's lymphocytes are rendered incapable of replication by gamma radiation or mitomycin C so that all replication that is detected represents the recipient's reaction against donor antigen. In either test, lymphocyte replication as a response to exposure to foreign antigen is measured by uptake and incorporation of tritiated thymidine into the cell's DNA. Because the results of HLA typing and MLR often did not correlate, it became apparent that determinants for cell antigens other than A and B were significant for histocompatibility.

The genetic basis for the MLR reaction appears to be related to a distinct chromosomal site designated D; serologic tests in humans for D-related (DR) antigens have been devised. These antigens are referred to as class 2 antigens, and they exist on most cells except for erythrocytes, platelets, and T cells. It appears that DR matching, even among nonrelated donors, is of value for kidney graft survival in humans.

This tissue matching system for improving graft survival in humans has developed with considerable effort over about two decades. The techniques for tissue matching have improved but are imperfect, which emphasizes that existing knowledge about transplant antigens and their detection is incomplete. The present success in human transplant programs is as much a matter of efficacy of immunosuppression as it is of tissue matching.

Because dogs have been used experimentally for transplantation and cancer research, considerable effort has been expended in studying canine immunogenetics. Serotyping for cell antigens has been conducted and is referred to as DLA typing. The major histocompatibility complex in the dog appears to have many similarities to human and mouse systems. Likewise, MLR studies can be conducted on dogs. It has been found that DLA typing is helpful but not definitive for matching dogs for organ transplantation and that DLA and MLR results are not always in agreement with one another. For purposes of tissue matching for transplantation, the MLR test may be more reliable than DLA typing.

NATURE OF THE REJECTION RESPONSE IN RECIPIENTS OF KIDNEY ALLOGRAFTS

Graft rejections may occur within minutes to hours of transplantation by what is commonly termed hyperacute rejection. Such rejection is attributed to antibody against allograft antigen in the recipient's blood. Prior blood transfusion (leukocyte antigens) is a common method by which the recipient is sensitized. Hyperacute rejection is characterized by linear deposition of IgG and complement component C3 on glomerular and peritubular capillary walls, platelet aggregation in capillaries, formation of microthrombi, infiltration of polymorphonuclear neutrophils, and cortical necrosis. No satisfactory method exists at present for its treatment.

Acute rejection generally occurs after the first seven to 10 days following transplantation. It may be detected in humans by mild fever, graft tenderness, and a sudden decrease in organ function (e.g., increase in BUN or serum creatinine concentration). Prominent morphologic features are infiltration of the vasculature and interstitium of the transplanted kidney with lymphocytes and interstitial edema. Renal blood flow is decreased. In contrast to the hyperacute rejection phenomenon, which is due to humoral antibody, acute rejection is predominantly related to cellular factors. It often responds well to high doses of corticosteroids.

Chronic rejection refers to subtle, progressive decreases in renal function that occur over months or years. Chronic rejection of kidneys is characterized by narrowing of arteries and thickening of glomerular capillary basement membranes. Because IgM and complement are present in affected vessels, humoral and cellular components to rejection are believed to exist.

IMMUNOSUPPRESSIVE AGENTS

As previously discussed, existing methods for matching organ donors with recipients are not definitive. Even if such methods are developed, it is unlikely that perfect matching can be achieved because of the genetic diversity of a species. Because of these facts, immunosuppression plays a major role in the success of organ transplantation.

Azathioprine has been the major immunosuppressive agent used in allograft recipients since its introduction in 1961. The drug is degraded to 6-mercaptopurine and other metabolites that inhibit synthesis of DNA and RNA. Its effect is quite nonspecific; replication of rapidly dividing cells, including immunoblasts, is inhibited. When used in transplant recipients, azathioprine prevents rejection episodes. However, it is not effective in reversing ongoing rejection. Its lack of efficacy in aborting rejection may be related to a lag of at least 48 hours between administration of the drug and a detectable effect. Azathioprine apparently is well absorbed after oral administration and is metabolized and excreted by the liver. For immunosuppression of canine patients with experimental renal transplants, we have used a dosage of 2.0 mg/kg/day. Because excessive dosage results in leukopenia, WBC counts must be serially performed during its use. The drug should be discontinued when WBC counts of 4000/μl or less are obtained since the patient is vulnerable to fulminating infection. Other abnormalities associated with use of azathioprine are jaundice (hepatic damage), anemia, and poor growth of hair.

Corticosteroids, particularly prednisone, are usually used in conjunction with azathioprine. Corticosteroids induce lymphopenia within hours of administration by interfering with replication of lymphocytes. These drugs block release of interleukin 1 by macrophages, thereby inhibiting interleukin 1–dependent release of interleukin 2. The latter compound appears to be important in replication of activated helper and cytotoxic T cells. Thus, corticosteroids have a predominant effect on cellular immunity. We have used a maintenance dose of prednisone (1.0 mg/kg once daily) in conjunction with azathioprine for immunosuppression of experimental renal allografts in dogs.

Acute allograft rejection in dogs receiving azathioprine and the maintenance dose of prednisone may be reversed with larger doses of corticosteroids. Dexamethasone (2 mg/kg) given IV once daily for two days appeared effective in limited trials, whereas larger doses were associated with gastrointestinal hemorrhage.

Cyclosporine (cyclosporine A) is the most promising immunosuppressive agent introduced since azathioprine. This compound is an endecapeptide produced by two soil fungi. Cyclosporine interferes with activation of lymphocytes on a selective basis. It inhibits both B and T lymphocyte activation. However, its major effect is interference with the function of helper T cells by blocking release of interleukin 2. An important part of the drug's efficacy may be related to its lack of interference with activation and proliferation of suppressor T cells.

Use of cyclosporine as an immunosuppressant has markedly improved one-year survival rates of human recipients of heart and liver transplants. One-year survival of heart transplant recipients improved from 60 to 80 per cent with use of cyclosporine. In those patients with liver transplants, one-year survival improved from 35 to 65 per cent. Results after its use in humans with kidney transplants have not been as impressive, since one-year survival rates are high with conventional therapy (azathioprine, prednisone).

Some complicating factors have been observed after the use of cyclosporine. Because the compound is lipid-soluble, oral administration results in highly variable rates and degrees of absorption, and measurement of blood trough levels by high-pressure liquid chromatography or radioimmunoassay has been used to adjust dosages. Even with the aid of such measurements, establishing doses that provide immunosuppression without toxicity has been difficult. The major side effect from cyclosporine is nephrotoxicity. This problem is particularly vexing in renal transplant patients because differentiating drug toxicity from acute rejection is not easy. Other complications of cyclosporine use in humans include hepatotoxicity, hypertension, gingival hyperplasia, seizures, and hirsutism. There is presently no consensus of opinion on the need for concomitant treatment with corticosteroids and cyclosporine. Trials that should resolve this issue in the near future are under way.

THE TRANSFUSION EFFECT

During course of evaluation of renal transplantation in humans, concern existed that blood transfusion prior to transplantation might expose the recipients to antigens subsequently encountered in the transplanted kidney. Such exposure was assumed to be detrimental to allograft survival. Ironically, when results of transplantation were tabulated in transfused and nontransfused patients, a higher percentage of grafts survived in transfused than in nontransfused recipients. Because the magnitude of the transfusion effect was appreciable, a protocol was developed for deliberate pretransplant transfusion programs in many human organ transplant centers. Experimental studies indicate that the transfusion effect occurs in many species, including the dog. The exact mechanism whereby allograft survival is enhanced by transfusion remains to be established.

Although the transfusion effect is beneficial, transfusions may induce antilymphocyte antibodies in recipients that could lead to hyperacute rejection. For this reason it is necessary to test the recipient's serum against the prospective donor's lymphocytes. Antibody existing in the recipient against a prospective donor's lymphocytes eliminates that donor from consideration, at least as long as the recipient's antibody persists.

ORGAN TRANSPLANTATION IN DOGS: PRESENT AND FUTURE

In dogs, organ transplantation outside of research laboratories is now rare. Several reasons for this exist, including (1) the monetary expense of transplantation, patient monitoring, and immunosuppressive therapy; (2) pessimism about its success; and (3) limited facilities and capabilities for donor-recipient matching.

For several reasons, we anticipate a change in this situation during the next decade, at least with respect to kidney transplantation. Although economic aspects will restrict its application to a select few, our preliminary research experience with renal allografts in siblings makes us optimistic for its success. When azathioprine-prednisone immunosuppression is used, overall one-year survival of sibling allografts is 67 per cent in transfused dogs and 50 per cent in nontransfused dogs. When mortalities unrelated to kidney rejection are not considered, one-year survival is 100 per cent for transfused dogs and 50 per cent for nontransfused dogs.

The overall approach to clinical renal transplantation in dogs during the next decade will probably vary from institution to institution, depending on the emphasis placed on tissue matching, the transfusion reaction, or cyclosporine immunosuppression. Both DLA and MLR procedures are presently available but are relatively expensive. The transfusion effect appears to be sufficiently powerful in dogs to warrant consideration for clinical use, but it should be combined with serologic testing to avoid hyperacute rejection. The efficacy of cyclosporine appears to be so great that its application to canine renal transplantation may overcome problems previously caused by mismatching. Although sibling renal transplantation will probably improve chances of success, the ready availability of nonrelated donors provides veterinarians with an enviable situation, compared with that which exists in humans.

References and Supplemental Reading

Canine Immunogenetics. Transplant. Proc. 7:341, 1975.

Carpenter, C. B., Strom, T. B., and Garovoy, M. R.: Renal transplantation immunobiology. *In* Brenner, B. M., and Rector, F. C. (eds.): *The Kidney*, 2nd ed. Philadelphia: W. B. Saunders, 1981, pp. 2544–2598.

Cohen, D. J., Loertscher, R., Rubin, M. F., et al.: Cyclosporine: A new immunosuppressive agent for organ transplantation. Arch. Intern. Med. 101:667, 1984.

Morris, P. J.: Renal transplantation: Current status. *In* Robinson, R. R. (ed.): *Nephrology*. Vol. 2. New York: Springer-Verlag, 1984, pp. 1627–1643.

Section 2

CHEMICAL AND PHYSICAL DISORDERS

GARY D. OSWEILER, D.V.M.
Consulting Editor

Toxicology 24-Hour Hotline Telephone Number: 217/333-3611

Additional Pertinent Information Found in **Current Veterinary Therapy VIII:**

Case, A. A.: Poisoning and Injury by Plants, p. 145.
Lloyd, W. E.: Sodium Fluoroacetate (Compound 1080) Poisoning, p. 112.
Meerdink, G. L.: Bites and Stings of Venomous Animals, p. 155.
Mercer, H. D., and Stephen, S. P.: Drugs of Abuse, P. 139.
Mull, R. L.: Metaldehyde Poisoning, p. 106.
Oehme, F. W.: Emergency Kit for Treatment of Small Animal Poisoning (Antidotes, Drugs, Equipment), p. 92.
Osweiler, G. D.: Common Poisonings in Small Animal Practice, p. 76.
Osweiler, G. D.: Strychnine Poisoning, p. 98.
Palumbo, N. E., and Perri, S. F.: Toad Poisoning, p. 160.
Robens, J. F.: Carcinogenesis, p. 152.
Schneider, N. R.: Developmental and Genetic Toxicology (Teratogenesis and Mutagenesis), p. 128.

PREVALENCE OF POISONINGS IN SMALL ANIMALS

VAL RICHARD BEASLEY, D.V.M.
Urbana, Illinois

Just as it simplifies matters to know which viruses are most likely to cause clinical infections, it simplifies matters to know which toxicants are likely to cause clinical poisoning in dogs and cats. The frequency of poisoning is a function of the restrictions on activity level and the sensitivity of the animal and on the agent's toxicity, formulation, intended use, and prevalence of access. Plants, compounds, or formulations that are widely available and that have the potential to cause significant toxic effects are more likely to cause clinical poisoning.

There remains a need to better evaluate the total scope and extent of animal poisonings on a national basis. Diagnostic laboratories throughout the country are consulted with regard to toxicoses with potential for quite serious or lethal effects, but many mild or nonlethal toxicoses may not be referred. Moreover, recognition of poisonings is often dependent on the presence or absence of relatively unique features of the disease (such as oxalate nephropathy found on histopathologic examination in ethylene glycol toxicosis) or the availability and dependability of diagnostic tests (such as analytical methods to quantitate lead in the blood or liver and kidney). For many toxicoses, there are few definitive lesions and analytical tests are either unavailable or, because of inadequate background information, results are difficult or impossible to interpret.

Data collected by the National Animal Poison Control Center (NAPCC) have helped to increase our awareness of problems of concern to veterinarians and the public. This information has some epidemiologic bias in that:

1. The telephone number has been publicized primarily among veterinarians.
2. A long-distance call is required, and persons may hesitate to call, depending on their location.
3. Veterinarians, once familiar with a given toxicosis, no longer find it necessary to call.
4. Calls are assessed strictly on the basis of information available over the phone at the time of the call, and most are not confirmed by chemical analysis. A limited number of callbacks are made.

Based on the assurance and degree of exposure, the toxicity of the agent, and the consistency of clinical signs, each call is classified as one of the following: toxicosis, suspected toxicosis, exposure, doubtful toxicosis, information only, residue problem, nutrient deficiency, other disease, or other problems. None of the last four assessment categories accounts for a significant number of calls with regard to small animals. During the past year almost 8000 calls pertaining to dogs and cats were handled, and these have allowed us to compile the data in Tables 1 and 2.

PESTICIDES

Avicides. Although not common, avicide (bird-killing) agents occasionally cause poisoning, and the most prevalent agent causing problems at the present is the convulsant 4-aminopyridine, the active ingredient in Avitrol (Avitrol Corp.). Convulsions induced by 4-aminopyridine are a result of severe, involuntary muscle contractions. Less frequent is poisoning by endrin, an organochlorine avicide and insecticide encountered in Rid-A-Bird. As with other organochlorine insecticides, endrin causes salivation, tremors, falling over backward into seizures, and rapid death. Endrin is even more toxic than most other organochlorine insecticides.

Insecticides. We receive more calls regarding insecticides than any other class of toxicant, and about one third of these are judged to be definite toxicoses and another fifth, suspected toxicoses. Of these calls, more than half are associated with cholinesterase inhibitors of the organophosphate group. During 1984, 206 suspected or actual toxicosis assessments were made by the NAPCC based on calls pertaining to these insecticides in dogs and cats. Chlorpyrifos (dursban; Lorsban, Dow Chemical) is one member of this group that is widely used in agriculture, in the home, and on dogs. Although poisoning may occur in dogs, more often toxicosis and sometimes death results when products in-

Table 1. *Call Distribution by Class and Reason for Canine Calls for 1984*

Class	*Total* No.	*Total* %	*Toxicosis* No.	*Toxicosis* %	*Suspected* No.	*Suspected* %	*Doubtful* No.	*Doubtful* %	*Exposure* No.	*Exposure* %	*Information* No.	*Information* %
Avicide	5	0.1	—	—	1	0.0	—	—	2	0.0	2	0.0
Biotoxin	164	2.9	48	0.8	43	0.7	25	0.4	34	0.6	12	0.2
Construction	214	3.7	30	0.5	31	0.5	31	0.5	118	2.1	4	0.1
Cosmetic	37	0.6	9	0.2	2	0.0	5	0.1	21	0.4	—	—
Fertilizer	115	2.0	15	0.3	17	0.3	17	0.3	60	1.0	6	0.1
Fungicide	19	0.3	3	0.1	7	0.1	5	0.1	3	0.1	1	0.0
Herbicide	195	3.4	25	0.4	57	1.0	59	1.0	28	0.5	26	0.4
Hot-line info.	4	0.1	—	—	—	—	—	—	—	—	4	0.1
Household	384	6.7	69	1.2	63	1.1	41	0.7	207	3.6	4	0.1
Human med.	781	13.6	230	4.0	75	1.3	45	0.8	410	7.1	21	0.4
Insecticide	745	13.0	198	3.4	145	2.5	99	1.7	234	4.1	69	1.2
Metal	119	2.1	17	0.3	24	0.4	25	0.4	36	0.6	16	0.3
Misc. chem.	276	4.8	52	0.9	62	1.1	45	0.8	102	1.8	13	0.2
Molluscacide	26	0.5	9	0.2	8	0.1	2	0.0	4	0.1	3	0.1
Not available	188	3.3	6	0.1	113	2.0	41	0.7	7	0.1	15	0.3
Nutrition ag.	71	1.2	22	0.4	5	0.1	4	0.1	39	0.7	1	0.0
Other	32	0.6	—	—	1	0.0	1	0.0	—	—	25	0.4
Petroleum	96	1.7	29	0.5	14	0.2	7	0.1	42	0.7	4	0.1
Physical	54	0.9	2	0.0	5	0.1	10	0.2	32	0.6	1	0.0
Plant	547	9.5	102	1.8	82	1.4	102	1.8	237	4.1	24	0.4
Rodenticide	1346	23.4	94	1.6	126	2.2	74	1.3	987	17.2	64	1.1
Vet. med.	331	5.8	113	2.0	51	0.9	52	0.9	85	1.5	29	0.5
Totals:	5749	100.00	1073	18.7	932	16.2	690	12.0	2688	46.8	344	6.0

Please note: Percentages are reported as percentage of total number of canine calls received for the stated time period.

Table 2. *Call Distribution by Class and Reason for Feline Calls for 1984*

Class	*Total* No.	*Total* %	*Toxicosis* No.	*Toxicosis* %	*Suspected* No.	*Suspected* %	*Doubtful* No.	*Doubtful* %	*Exposure* No.	*Exposure* %	*Information* No.	*Information* %
Avicide	3	0.2	2	0.1	—	—	1	0.1	—	—	—	—
Biotoxin	36	1.9	7	0.4	5	0.3	10	0.5	7	0.4	6	0.3
Construction	95	5.0	18	0.9	17	0.9	17	0.9	41	2.1	2	0.1
Cosmetic	9	0.5	1	0.1	3	0.2	—	—	2	0.1	3	0.2
Fertilizer	17	0.9	1	0.1	3	0.2	5	0.3	8	0.4	—	—
Fungicide	12	0.6	1	0.1	2	0.1	5	0.3	1	0.1	3	0.2
Herbicide	43	2.3	3	0.2	8	0.4	17	0.9	11	0.6	4	0.2
Hot-line info.	1	0.1	—	—	—	—	—	—	—	—	1	0.1
Household	140	7.3	40	2.1	31	1.6	28	1.5	34	1.8	7	0.4
Human med.	180	9.4	79	4.1	23	1.2	10	0.5	61	3.2	7	0.4
Insecticide	515	27.0	216	11.3	126	6.6	69	3.6	49	2.6	54	2.8
Metal	21	1.1	3	0.2	3	0.2	5	0.3	5	0.3	5	0.3
Misc. chem.	56	2.9	13	0.7	13	0.7	14	0.7	13	0.7	3	0.2
Molluscacide	1	0.1	—	—	—	—	1	0.1	—	—	—	—
Not available	62	3.3	2	0.1	33	1.7	23	1.2	1	0.1	1	0.1
Nutrition ag.	11	0.6	1	0.1	3	0.2	1	0.1	4	0.2	2	0.1
Other	12	0.6	—	—	—	—	—	—	—	—	12	0.6
Petroleum	58	3.0	18	0.9	4	0.2	2	0.1	31	1.6	3	0.2
Physical	14	0.7	—	—	—	—	5	0.3	8	0.4	—	—
Plant	344	18.0	39	2.0	48	2.5	89	4.7	95	5.0	72	3.8
Rodenticide	152	8.0	6	0.3	13	0.7	21	1.1	97	5.1	15	0.8
Vet. med.	125	6.6	43	2.3	30	1.6	16	0.8	21	1.1	15	0.8
Totals:	1907	100.00	493	25.9	365	19.1	339	17.8	489	25.6	215	11.3

Please note: Percentages are reported as percentage of total number of feline calls received for the stated time period.

tended for dogs, especially insecticidal dip solutions, are used on cats. Diazinon (Spectracide, Ciba-Geigy) is another heavily used organophosphate that results in occasional toxicoses. Most species of birds are comparatively sensitive to chlorpyrifos, diazinon, and certain other organophosphates such as monocrotophos (Azodrin, Shell), naled (Dibrom, Chevron), and fenthion. Fenthion (Baytex, Tiguvon, Lysoff, and Spotton [Bayer AG or Mobay]), which is sometimes used as a microfilaricide but is mainly intended for use as a pour-on insecticide for cattle, has caused significant toxicoses in dogs and cats.

Phosmet (Paramite, Prolate, and Imidan [Stauffer]) causes occasional poisoning, primarily in cats. Although very widely used, malathion (Cythion, American Cyanamid) is of somewhat lower toxicity, and only a small fraction of calls were associated with clinical signs. Although tetrachlorvinphos (Rabon, Gardona [Shell]) is of very low toxicity in most species, cats may be somewhat predisposed to toxicosis from this agent.

Carbamate Insecticides. Among the carbamate insecticides, a second group of cholinesterase inhibitors, methomyl (Lannate, Nudrin, and especially Golden Malrin bait [Du Pont, Shell]), stands out as a major cause of poisoning in dogs. Unlike calls concerning heavily used and much safer carbamate product formulations such as those containing propoxur (Baygon, Mobay) and carbaryl (Sevin, Chevron), which were infrequently associated with toxicoses in dogs, most calls pertaining to methomyl were associated with clinically poisoned animals. The high incidence of methomyl toxicosis is probably a result of the inherently high toxicity of methomyl itself and the palatability of the bait materials. Bendiocarb (Ficam, BFC Chemicals) also causes a significant number of toxicoses in dogs. Aldicarb (Temik, Union Carbide) and carbofuran (Furadan, FMC, Bayer AG, or Mobay), although infrequently encountered by dogs and cats, are two of the most highly toxic carbamates and tend to be associated with more serious poisonings. In cats, almost all the carbamates are associated with a significant portion of toxicosis calls.

Organochlorine Insecticides. Because of increased restrictions on their use, organochlorine (chlorinated hydrocarbons) insecticides cause fewer problems than in the past, but certain compounds continue to cause significant problems. Because of its availability for use on animals, lindane (Gamma BHC, Gammex, Isotox, Lintox, and others [Hooker]) continues to cause toxicoses, most of which arise from misuse or extralabel use. Because of the sensitivity of the feline, lindane is not approved for cats, yet almost as much poisoning occurs in cats as in dogs. Aldrin, at one time a major agricultural insecticide, is back on the market, this time for termite control. As with chlordane, another and more widely used termiticide, aldrin causes occasional poisoning. Additional organochlorine insecticides such as endosulfan, endrin, kelthane, and toxaphene occasionally cause toxicoses in small animals. Methoxychlor, which is still fairly widely used, is more readily metabolized and excreted than most organochlorines, and it is therefore one of the most innocuous members of this group, causing few toxicoses.

Pyrethins and Pyrethroids. In most species, pyrethrin and pyrethroid insecticides (pyrethrins, permethrin, allethrin, resmethrin, tetramethrin, and others) are known for their safety and as such they are generally an appropriate choice as pesticides for use on animals. Most preparations contain piperonyl butoxide or other "synergists," which delay the metabolism of these compounds in insects. The synergist thereby increases the insecticide's toxicity to the insect pest, but metabolism and toxicity of the insecticide are similarly affected in the mammalian host. Experience at the NAPCC clearly indicates that both pyrethrins and pyrethroids, primarily in formulations intended for use on animals, are associated with many nonlethal poisonings in cats. These are primarily characterized by salivation, tremors, ataxia, lethargy, and sometimes dyspnea, coma, or rarely death. Dogs are occasionally poisoned as well.

Arsenical Insecticides. Lead arsenate, sodium arsenate, and sodium arsenite are still used as insecticides, most often in powder or liquid sugar baits. In small animals these products are responsible for the majority of arsenic toxicoses. For the sake of comparison it may be noted that, in spite of the much greater use around animals of the carbamate insecticide carbaryl, more cases of arsenic toxicoses were documented by the NAPCC than carbaryl toxicoses. This illustrates the comparatively poor selectivity and continued hazard of arsenic insecticides and calls into question the wisdom of their continued availability.

Boric Acid and Borates. Boric acid may be viewed as innocuous because of use at a 1 per cent concentration in ophthalmic preparations and because of the fact that it may be advertised as a "safe" insecticide. Nevertheless, in 1984, concentrated boric acid used in roach and ant powders resulted in 34 reports to the NAPCC of suspected or actual poisonings of dogs and cats. Animals seem to be exposed most often as a result of walking through or lying in the powder and then licking it from the exposed areas. Clinical toxicosis is evidenced by gastrointestinal irritation, systemic acidosis, and renal damage. The most common clinical complaint was emesis.

Mothballs/Moth Crystals. Most mothballs are naphthalene and most moth crystals are paradichlorobenzene, but either generic chemical may be encountered in either form of product. Naphthalene toxicosis is more of a problem in dogs than in cats and is manifested as a primary problem of gastrointestinal upset and sometimes hemolysis. Paradichlorobenzene toxicosis is less frequent but may be associated with tremors, ataxia, and seizures.

Other Insecticides/Miticides. Amitraz (Mitaban, Upjohn) is not recommended for dogs less than 3 months of age and causes occasionally serious, or even lethal, iatrogenic poisonings. Signs of serious toxicoses, which primarily occur in younger or very debilitated dogs, may include weakness, salivation, ataxia, tremors, dyspnea, coma, and death. It is not unusual for amitraz exposure to cause mild weakness and salivation in healthy, larger dogs, and most such individuals spontaneously recover.

Amdro. Amdro (American Cyanamid), which contains hydramethylnon, is a heavily used fire ant poison; its mechanism of action is poorly understood. The toxicity of Amdro is low, and toxicoses are mild and much less frequent than exposures. The same active ingredient is present in Combat Roach Control System (American Cyanamid).

Citrus Oil Extracts. In an apparent effort to avoid having to satisfy safety regulations, crude citrus oil extracts have been marketed as "pet dips" that "control itching due to" (in small print, followed by) "fleas, ticks, and lice" (in large print) without actually claiming to be insecticidal. Such products were extremely toxic to cats, and ataxia, depression, and death sometimes resulted even when label recommendations were followed. Some such formulations have been withdrawn from the market. These crude products must not, however, be confused with products containing D-limonene (such as those marketed by Pet Chemicals, Inc.). Our experiments with D-limonene dips in cats suggest that cats tolerate 15 times the recommended concentration, although after excessive exposure, toxic effects including significant salivation, hypothermia, and ataxia occur. The latter effects last minutes to several hours, depending on dosage. In addition, scrotal dermatitis may occur after massive overexposure of male cats. Mild, very transient signs sometimes occurred at the recommended concentration.

Rotenone. Although natural in origin, rotenone is toxic not only to insects and fish but also to mammals. Cats were more commonly affected than dogs, and almost all toxicoses were a result of topical exposure to rotenone-containing dips or powders. Most calls regarding rotenone in both dogs and cats were regarded as either toxicosis or suspected toxicosis. Clinical signs were variable but often included emesis, lethargy, tremors, and dyspnea.

Pennyroyal Oil (Ketone pulegone). Each year the NAPCC receives a few calls regarding pennyroyal oil, an aromatic oil sometimes used as an insecticide on small animals. The calls received in 1984 regarding suspected or assured toxicosis consistently involved cats, and each caller described panting, dyspnea, or exaggerated bronchial sounds. These are compatible with reports of pennyroyal oil toxicosis in humans, the effects of which may also include disseminated intravascular coagulation, hepatic necrosis, abortion, and death.

REPELLENTS. Diethyltoluamide (DEET), found in many insect repellent products (such as Off, Deep Woods Off, Cutter Insect Repellent, and others [S. C. Johnson and Son and Cutter]), was associated with seven suspected cases of toxicosis or toxicosis calls in cats and four such calls in dogs. Naturally these occur during warm months and are a result of owner treatment of their pets. In dogs and, especially, cats, primary signs included seizures, tremors, and sometimes emesis. Ataxia or lethargy occasionally occurred.

RODENTICIDES. The rodenticide class is the second most prevalent category of agents associated with calls to the NAPCC for two reasons: (1) Rodenticides are often placed in areas in which both rodents and pet animals are present, and (2) the NAPCC has an agreement with the manufacturers of brodifacoum so that the NAPCC telephone number is on packages containing this common anticoagulant (Talon and Havoc [ICI Americas and others]). Naturally, this causes us to receive a disproportionate number of calls concerning brodifacoum.

Anticoagulant Rodenticides. The vast majority of anticoagulant rodenticide calls, regardless of the agent involved, were for exposure only. In the case of brodifacoum, the number of clinically serious poisonings resulting from exposure was undoubtedly minimized by virtue of access to appropriate antidotal information. It appears that dogs are more sensitive than cats to brodifacoum.

Owing to the extremely wide availability of anticoagulants, a significant number of toxicoses result from their use. Baits that contain bromadiolone, chlorophacinone, pindone, diphacinone, and others are occasionally consumed by small animals. Of these, it appears that diphacinone may cause the greatest number of poisonings (see page 159).

Strychnine. The convulsant strychnine continues to cause toxicosis, but the prevalence of this poisoning may be declining. Nevertheless, strychnine-containing baits are still available over the counter. During 1984, 26 calls pertaining to accidental and malicious poisonings of dogs were received. Only two such calls pertained to cats.

Fluoroacetate (Compound 1080). Fluoroacetate toxicosis is comparatively infrequent at the present time. This is a result of restrictions placed on the use of fluoroacetate-containing baits. Currently, fluoroacetate may be used as a rodenticide only by licensed exterminators. Depending on the outcome of legal battles continuing at the time of this writing, fluoroacetate may eventually be encountered as a result of its use in coyote control in the form of "single lethal dose baits" and less often in toxic collars placed on sacrificial sheep. Because of the body mass of the coyote, the small "single lethal dose baits" contain at least a "single lethal dose" for many less-sensitive but smaller species, including a wide range of wild carnivores and scavengers. There is no evidence that these are less attractive or less hazardous to dogs, cats, foxes, bobcats, and skunks than to coyotes. Veterinarians who practice in areas where poisoning measures are used to control coyotes must be especially aware of the possible use of Compound 1080.

Phosphide Derivatives. Zinc phosphide and occasionally aluminum phosphide seem to be gaining in popularity with exterminators, and as a result, problems are beginning to emerge. Most of the calls regarding zinc phosphide were classified as suspected or assured toxicoses. These agents may cause seizures and serious gastrointestinal and respiratory problems.

Vacor. Vacor has been off the market for several years, and poisoning at present appears to be very rare.

MOLLUSCACIDES. In spite of the success of reformulations that have reduced the palatability of baits to small animals, metaldehyde is still the primary molluscacide causing problems in dogs, mostly in California. Metaldehyde causes acute, often serious, toxicoses initially characterized by tremors, seizures, ataxia, and salivation.

HERBICIDES

Arsenicals. Arsenic-containing herbicides include arsenic trioxide, lead arsenate, dimethylarsenate, monosodium methanearsonate (MSMA, Crystal Chem. Co. and Diamond Shamrock), and others. They are intended for use in killing crabgrass, for controlling growth along fence rows, and as defoliants on crops such as cotton. Recent experience suggests that these agents are not a prevalent cause of poisoning in small animals.

Dipyridyls. Diquat and paraquat occasionally cause poisoning in small animals as a result of exposure to the concentrate or to spray solutions. Toxicoses occurring from contact with the aerosol itself or sprayed plants or fields are not likely.

Phenoxyacetic Acids. Calls regarding the herbicide 2,4-D and other phenoxys such as MCPP (also called Mecoprop [BASF and Bayer AG]) and MCPA (also called Weedone [BASF and Bayer AG]) have been repeatedly associated with a clinical picture in dogs that often includes emesis, diarrhea, salivation, and sometimes lethargy, weakness, and ataxia or tremors. In spite of the large number of calls received by the NAPCC concerning dogs with similar histories, neither the administration of oral doses estimated as somewhat above those likely to be consumed by a dog on treated grass (Yeary, 1984) nor contact with experimentally sprayed grass plots (Arnold et al., 1984) induced clinical toxicosis. Further work is needed to evaluate the apparent correlation between clinical signs and phenoxy herbicide application. For now, it seems appropriate to prevent dogs from contacting phenoxy herbicide-treated lawns for 2 days after spraying and, whether sprays or granular preparations are used, to water the lawn thoroughly and allow it to dry before dogs are given free access to the area. Puddles of spray solution and concentrates may cause more serious toxicoses. Dogs are predisposed to toxicosis from these compounds because of their poor ability to excrete organic acids in the urine.

Triazines. Prometon (Triox, Ciba-Geigy and Chevron) is the triazine herbicide of greatest concern in dogs and cats. Prometon is used agriculturally, but its residential use is greater than that of atrazine, a triazine manufactured in much greater quantity. Triazine poisoning is not common. Among animals significantly exposed, however, clinical toxicosis is likely.

Other Herbicides. Most herbicides are of much lower acute toxicity than most insecticides and rodenticides. Two herbicides, glyphosate (Roundup, Kleenup [Monsanto]) and trifluralin (Treflan, Elanco) are widely used but are rarely associated with toxicosis, perhaps because of their low acute toxicity.

FUNGICIDES. Although the broad category of compounds used as fungicides contains agents that vary widely in toxicity, few clinical poisonings apparently occur in small animals. Highly toxic mercurial fungicides are no longer marketed for use on seed grains.

FERTILIZERS

Fertilizers are commonly encountered by dogs and cats in products intended for agricultural, garden, lawn, and household (houseplant) applications. The receipt of 36 suspected or actual toxicosis calls regarding dogs and cats in 1984 indicates that poisoning, although rarely serious, occurs fairly often, especially as a result of fertilizers intended for use on ornamental plants. Fertilizer ingestion was primarily associated with gastrointestinal upset.

CONSTRUCTION MATERIALS

ADHESIVES. Adhesive exposures are common in small animals, and a wide variety of product formulations are involved. Cyanoacrylate (Superglue, Superglue Corp.; Krazyglue, Krazy Glue Co.) is the adhesive most commonly reported to the NAPCC. The effects are generally minor since the glue rapidly polymerizes and is not absorbed. Careful separation of adhered tissues (e.g., lips, gums, toes) and gentle removal of most of the glue is all that is generally required. Starchy wallpaper pastes are a rare source of rapidly fermented carbohydrates and are associated with gas formation and abdominal pain.

INSULATION. Dogs and, to a lesser degree, cats occasionally chew up and even swallow insulation materials. Styrofoam, vermiculite, and fiberglass are relatively inert, but ingestion may result in irritation of the digestive tract, and the material may act as a foreign body. Usually, the problem is relieved with the help of an oily or saline cathartic. Cellotex fibrous exterior wall sheeting may contain arsenic and might therefore be of greater concern, although we have not encountered problems from this material in small animals.

PAINTS, WOOD PRESERVATIVES, AND PAINT STRIPPERS. Most paints presently marketed for use indoors are either lead free or very low in lead. Lead-based paints are occasionally available for exterior use. Most lead-paint toxicoses result when animals eat lead chips from old peeling paint. Tearing down or refurbishing lead-painted structures often coincides with exposure. Most latex-based paints are of low oral toxicity.

Some stains are formulated with solvent vehicles such as methylene chloride, which can cause toxicoses (see page 201). Volatile fumes from varnishes and paints apparently cause occasional toxicosis or oxygen deprivation in animals confined in areas where such products are used.

In spite of the wide use and notable toxicity of phenolic- (creosote-type) and pentachlorophenol-based wood preservatives, toxicosis in small animals appears to be comparatively uncommon. The few calls pertaining to pentachlorophenol toxicosis in small animals during 1984 primarily concerned dermatitis or cachexia from repeated, low-grade topical exposure.

Other wood preservatives may contain arsenic or chromium and can be quite hazardous. Because of the toxicity of all of the widely used wood preservatives, it is wise to avoid pretreated wood or the use of most wood preservatives inside doghouses and especially whelping boxes.

SOLVENTS. Although paints and wood preservatives cause some poisonings, agents used to thin or remove paint from the skin cause more problems. A common effect is skin irritation. Cats and, to a lesser extent, dogs are extremely susceptible to dermatitis as a result of the use of turpentine (see page 201).

PETROLEUM PRODUCTS

GASOLINE AND KEROSENE. Gasoline toxicoses apparently occur more frequently in cats than in dogs and result from both ingestion and dermal exposures. In calls to the NAPCC, the most commonly mentioned clinical signs were lethargy and stomatitis. Spilled gasoline or gasoline used to remove other substances on the skin causes mild dermatitis, probably from defatting the skin. Perhaps because of the less prevalent use of kerosene, toxicoses are fewer.

OILS AND GREASES. During 1984, 19 calls were received pertaining to suspected or reasonably certain motor oil toxicoses, and at the time of the calls, the most common clinical signs were emesis and lethargy, although seizures were infrequently mentioned.

MISCELLANEOUS CHEMICALS

ANIMAL REPELLENTS. Animal repellents and Mace-type products, which most often contain chloroacetophenone or sometimes capsicum or methylnonyl ketone, obviously cause toxic effects in the targeted pet. As one might expect, dogs are primarily affected, and clinical signs are mainly referable to ocular, facial, or nasopharyngeal irritation. Conjunctivitis or, rarely, more serious ocular damage or dermatitis are the most notable clinical effects.

ANTIFREEZE. Almost all calls regarding antifreeze concerned either suspected or reasonably certain toxicoses rather than reports of exposure or requests for information. Although cats are even more sensitive than dogs, dogs are apparently more commonly poisoned (see page 206). Ethylene glycol is also found in heat-exchange fluids and brake or other hydraulic fluids. Either ethylene or propylene glycol is sometimes used in winterizing water lines and toilets of recreational vehicles, in solar collectors, and in freezing equipment. Propylene glycol is less toxic than ethylene glycol and rarely causes poisoning, but it is not innocuous. Although kidney failure would not be expected with propylene glycol toxicosis, central nervous system depression and acidosis can be significant problems.

Methanol, usually in automobile windshield washer solutions, is infrequently consumed by dogs and cats (see page 201).

HOUSEHOLD CLEANSERS. Ingestion of soaps and anionic or nonionic detergents is a very common cause of poisonings in dogs and, occasionally, cats. In our experience, most affected animals exhibit emesis; lesser numbers become lethargic, and a few become dyspneic or experience diarrhea. Cationic detergents or quaternary ammonium compounds are only occasionally ingested by dogs and cats but, when consumed, are more often associated with serious effects such as significant stomatitis, abdominal pain, serious gastrointestinal irritation, and weakness. Ingestion of ammonia-containing products occasionally results in vomiting in both dogs and cats.

Phenolic-containing cleansers (e.g., Lysol, Lehn and Fink) were associated with more suspected or assured toxicoses in cats than in dogs. Of 11 calls pertaining to phenolic toxicoses, seven included description of oral irritation (manifested by salivation or stomatitis) or gastrointestinal irritation (manifested by vomiting or diarrhea). Surprisingly, in four of the 11 incidents, seizures were described. Ocular irritation was occasionally a primary problem. Similar to phenol toxicoses in prevalence were pine oil (Pine-Sol [American Cyanamid] and others), bleach (hypochlorite), and sodium hydroxide toxicoses. Poisoning from pine oil was primarily characterized by oral or upper gastrointestinal upset and somewhat less often by depression or lethargy. As expected, significant gastrointestinal irritation occurs with all these agents.

POISONOUS GASES. In small animals the primary problem gas is carbon monoxide, and toxicosis is usually due to faulty fossil fuel–dependent space-heating equipment or to automobile exhaust (see page 203).

SALT. Sodium chloride toxicosis occasionally occurs in dogs, primarily as a result of eating rock salt. Occasionally, toxicoses are a result of owners' administering salt or saltwater as an emetic. Because of the potential for serious poisoning, this procedure should be avoided. Most sodium chloride poisonings of dogs do not, however, appear to be life threatening. Free access to water shortly after exposure would be highly recommended. If serious central nervous signs have ensued, however, it would be more appropriate to give small amounts of water periodically in order to avoid aggravating cerebral edema.

COAL TAR. Five calls involved coal-tar poisonings attributable to ingestions of clay pigeons by dogs. Vomiting and lethargy or weakness were most often noted, although one affected dog was in circulatory shock. Rarely, coal-tar toxicosis occurred in dogs as a result of ingestion of shampoos containing these constituents. All such animals should be vigorously treated in an attempt to minimize absorption and resultant massive hepatic necrosis.

MEDICATIONS AND FEED ADDITIVES

ACETAMINOPHEN, ASPIRIN, AND OTHER NONSTEROIDAL ANTI-INFLAMMATORY DRUGS. By far the most common medication causing toxicosis in cats is acetaminophen (e.g., Tylenol, Panadol, Datril [McNeil, Glenbrook, Bristol-Meyers]). Of 66 calls regarding this agent in cats during 9 months of 1984, assessments included 46 reasonably assured toxicoses, five suspected toxicoses, ten exposures (no signs yet), five information calls, and one doubtful toxicosis. Although much less sensitive and less often affected, dogs are also poisoned by acetaminophen. As detailed in another chapter (see page 188), the syndromes are quite different in the two species.

Although quite sensitive to aspirin, cats are apparently much less commonly poisoned by aspirin than by acetaminophen. Calls regarding dogs, however, suggest that aspirin and acetaminophen toxicoses are roughly equal in occurrence. Almost all aspirin toxicoses in either species were characterized by either vomiting or lethargy.

Ingestion of excessive doses of ibuprofen (Advil and Motrin [Upjohn and Whitehall]), mefenamic acid (Ponstel, Parke-Davis), naproxen (Naprosyn, Syntex), phenylbutazone, and other nonsteroidal anti-inflammatory drugs by dogs that eat spilled medications or chew open medicine containers occasionally results in vomiting and, sometimes, severe gastritis and renal damage. Of these agents, ibuprofen was associated with more toxicoses than mefenamic acid. Even fewer naproxen and phenylbutazone toxicoses were reported. Cats are also occasionally poisoned by these drugs.

PARASITICIDES. During 1984, the NAPCC received 31 calls assessed as suspected or reasonably assured ivermectin toxicoses in dogs and only two such calls in cats. Roughly half as many calls pertained to exposure or information only. Ivermectin toxicosis is most serious and by far most common in collies and related herding breeds. Nevertheless, the serious clinical effects of toxicosis, including depression and ataxia (which may be prolonged in duration and quite severe), may occasionally occur in other breeds. In 1984, ivermectin toxicoses reported to the NAPCC included not only collies and related breeds but also two dachshunds, a Newfoundland, a German shepherd, a poodle, and a Dalmatian.

Many of the ivermectin toxicoses were iatrogenic, although with the greater use of oral preparations in horses, owner-administered ivermectin and accidental access to pastes may serve as additional causes of poisoning. Effects compatible with anaphylactoid reactions from rapid microfilaria die-off after ivermectin administration were occasionally documented.

Seven calls were received regarding levamisole in dogs, and of these, all but one were classified as either toxicosis (in four animals) or suspected toxicosis (in two). Signs typically mimic organophosphate toxicosis. Toxicosis from the coadministration of butamisole (Styquin, American Cyanamid) and bunamidine (Scolaban, Burroughs-Wellcome) continues to be an infrequent but serious cause of iatrogenic toxicosis.

Less serious but more common are reactions to the toluene (methylbenzene) in anthelmintics containing toluene and dichlorophene. The latter is not highly absorbed, and toxic effects are primarily due to the toluene present. As many veterinarians know, biting into the liquid contents of such capsules commonly causes profound salivation. Vomiting, mild ataxia, and sometimes diarrhea, all of which are generally transient in character, sometimes occur. Serious reactions are less frequent.

Eight cases of suspected or reasonably certain piperazine toxicosis in dogs and seven cases in cats were reported during 1984. Many of these were associated with overdosage. Disophenol (DNP, American Cyanamid) is a rare cause of poisoning, but the margin of safety is comparatively small and accidental overdoses can be lethal. Vigorous exercise enhances the probability of toxicosis. Effects may include hyperthermia, acidosis, tachypnea, and death, sometimes preceded by terminal seizures. The organophosphate insecticide trichlorfon, used in preparations for bot removal from horses, also causes infrequent poisoning in dogs. Other anthelmintics such as pyrantel pamoate and praziquantel were infrequent causes of toxicosis.

Few calls pertaining to the toxicity of thiacetarsemide (Caparsolate, Abbott) were received. Quinacrine hydrochloride (Atabrine, Winthrop), sometimes used to treat *Giardia* infections, occasionally causes vomiting.

Topical Medications. Benzocaine or other local anesthetics such as dibucaine occasionally cause toxicosis when swallowed. This can result from ingestion of tubes of medication or from application of excessive amounts to the skin, which is then licked clean by the dog or cat. Alternatively, excessive amounts applied by spraying into the mouth to alleviate dental or pharyngeal pain may cause poisoning. At least in dogs, effects are apparently attributable to methemoglobinemia, and cyanosis, tachycardia, weakness, and dyspnea may be encountered.

Dogs also occasionally eat fluorouracil-containing topical medications, which may cause seizures, vomiting, and sometimes death. Zinc oxide in diaper rash ointments for infants is often ingested by dogs. Effects commonly include vomiting and diarrhea. Of 30 calls to the NAPCC, 17 animals were reported to be showing signs compatible with toxicosis. Isopropyl alcohol is occasionally consumed and can cause acute central nervous system depression and possibly an acidosis.

Nutritional Supplements. Mineral supplements, especially those containing ferrous sulfate, cause poisonings occasionally in dogs and less often in cats. Signs are largely characterized by gastrointestinal upset.

Feed Additives. Lasalocid is an ionophore antibiotic feed additive used for chickens (Avitec, Hoffman-LaRoche) and cattle (Bovatec, Hoffman-LaRoche). Poisoning occurs rarely in dogs as a result of eating the concentrated form of Bovatec. Effects of lasalocid poisoning are very characteristic and include salivation, hemoconcentration, extreme and progressive flaccid paralysis with a notable pounding of the heart, and warm extremities in spite of a declining core temperature. Although recumbent and paralyzed, affected dogs tend to remain quite alert and responsive during early stages of poisoning. Over a period of 3 to 15 hours, seriously affected animals develop a respiratory acidosis, and usually respiration ceases before the heart stops. Dogs that live 24 hours usually recover over a period of days to a few weeks.

Urinary Drugs. Toxic doses of methionine preparations (especially Methioform, Vet-A-Mix) are occasionally consumed in great excess by cats and less often by dogs. Toxic effects usually include ataxia, lethargy, and vomiting.

Hormones. Although rare in our experience, poisoning from estrogens must not be overlooked. Estrogens can be toxic to bone marrow, and estradiol cypionate as well as other estrogens can cause serious aplastic anemia and possibly thrombocytopenia.

Central Nervous System Drugs. Primidone causes occasionally serious liver damage in dogs chronically receiving anticonvulsant therapy. Human tranquilizers, however, are a more common cause of calls regarding acute poisonings in dogs. Most episodes of tranquilizer overdose are apparently nonlethal in effect. Of these, thioridazine (Mellaril, Sandoz) may cause poisoning most frequently.

Although amphetamines, barbiturates, LSD, phencyclidine (Sernylan [Parke-Davis], PCP, angel dust), and others occasionally cause poisoning, usually in dogs, much more frequent are calls regarding marijuana toxicosis. During 1984, 22 cells pertained to marijuana toxicosis in dogs and two such calls regarding cats were received. Most affected animals were ataxic and depressed and frequently coma was present.

Cold and Allergy Remedies. Cold and allergy remedies, which often contain adrenergic agents such as phenylpropanolamine, phenylephrine, or pseudoephedrine along with an antihistamine and sometimes other agents, are commonly consumed in excessive amounts by dogs, resulting in toxicosis. Effects are quite variable depending on the dosage and the reaction of the individual animal, but they may include a rapid heart rate (or less often bradycardia) and either excitation and panting or, less often, depression.

Cardiovascular and Pulmonary Drugs. The methylxanthine theophylline (aminophylline, Columbia and Searle) is an occasional cause of poisoning, and about half the calls received were classified as toxicoses, another one-fourth as suspected toxicoses.

BIOTOXINS

Food Poisonings. Chocolate, another agent that contains methylxanthine (theobromine and a lesser amount of caffeine), is a common cause of poisoning and during 1984, 44 calls were received regarding reasonably assured or suspected chocolate toxicoses. Only one fourth as many calls concerned exposure and information combined. No chocolate toxicoses were reported in cats. Most poisonings occur near such holidays as Easter, Halloween, and Christmas (see page 191).

Garbage poisoning continues to be a fairly common occurrence and, although 15 calls specifically related to apparent garbage poisoning of dogs, no suspected or actual garbage toxicoses of cats were documented in 1984. Because of the awareness of veterinarians of appropriate therapy, it is likely that garbage poisonings are vastly underrepresented in these calls. Infrequent food poisonings in dogs or cats also resulted from ingestion of parts of dead animals, bread dough, ethanol-containing beverages, and, especially, "spoiled" dog food. Apparent tremorgenic mycotoxicoses were occasionally suggested in dogs by the presence of tremors or seizures and a history of eating moldy cheese, cream cheese, or other moldy foods.

ZOOTOXINS. Of approximately 30 calls assessed as suspected or assured zootoxin toxicoses, nine were attributable to insect stings or bites, six were associated with snake envenomations, five were attributed to tetrodotoxin in salamanders and a fish, and three were attributed to *Bufo* toad poisoning. Because of the regional awareness of most of these poisonings, these calls do not adequately represent the prevalence of zootoxin problems.

HOUSEPLANTS. Dumbcane (*Dieffenbachia* sp.) and philodendron (*Philodendron* sp.) are members of the *Aracea*, a large group of plants with similar toxic effects (see page 218). Roughly 20 calls pertaining to suspected or reasonably assured toxicoses were received for each species in 1984. Only occasional calls pertained to other members of the group.

The Madagascar dragon tree *(Dracaena marginata)* and other plants identified as *Dracaena* were responsible for nine calls pertaining to suspected or assured toxicoses, all in cats. Most of the cats exhibited vomiting, several experienced reduced activity, and a few developed diarrhea or dyspnea.

Calls pertaining to poinsettia *(Euphorbia pulcherima)* exposures (no signs) were considerably greater than those classified as suspected or assured toxicoses. Of the 16 calls classified as suspected or reasonably certain toxicoses, 13 callers mentioned vomiting. More serious signs such as depression, lethargy, or dyspnea occurred in five of the affected animals, and no deaths were reported.

Ficus plants, principally the fig tree *(Ficus benjamini)*, were associated with five suspected or apparent toxicoses, primarily in cats. Signs were almost entirely limited to vomiting, diarrhea, and salivation. A few calls pertained to English ivy *(Hedera)* toxicoses. Effects were principally vomiting and abdominal pain. *Aloe vera* was responsible for three cases of toxicosis, all associated with gastrointestinal upset.

WILD PLANTS. With regard to toxic constituents from trees, English walnuts *(Juglans regia)* and possibly black walnuts *(Juglans nigra)* that drop to the ground and mold before consumption may act as an occasional cause of poisonings in dogs. Toxicosis may be due to tremorgenic mycotoxins (see page 226). Two calls pertained to toxicosis in dogs due to chokecherry *(Prunus)*, a source of cyanide.

Ingestions of herbaceous parts of pokeweed *(Phytolacca americana)* were associated with four calls classified as toxicosis or suspected toxicosis. Gastrointestinal upset was the most predominant effect. The nightshades (*Solanum* sp.), including European bittersweet *(Solanum dulcamara)*, were responsible for toxicosis or suspected toxicosis calls regarding four dogs and one cat. Reported signs included vomiting, lethargy, and sometimes salivation, tachycardia, mydriasis, and reduced urine output.

Collectively, toxicoses due to mushrooms of unknown identity were responsible for ten suspected or assured toxicosis calls, nine of which occurred in dogs. Vomiting was the most common complaint, followed by depression or lethargy and occasionally salivation or circulatory shock.

ORNAMENTAL PLANTS. Crocus (*Colchicum* sp.) and *Hydrangea* plants were occasionally associated with gastrointestinal upset, but not as often as daffodil (*Narcissus* sp.), for which six suspected or affirmed toxicoses were reported. The latter plant and its bulbs were responsible for a significant incidence of weakness, lethargy, and ataxia.

Ingestion of azalea (*Rhododendron* sp.) and rhododendron (*Rhododendron* sp.) bushes were responsible for five calls regarding probable poisonings in dogs and three in cats. Signs were similar to those described for *Narcissus*; abdominal pain, bradycardia, and coma were occasionally present.

Castor beans *(Ricinus communis)* were responsible for six calls regarding toxicosis, all in dogs. All the dogs exhibited vomiting and additional signs indicating significant or serious toxicosis. These included abdominal pain, diarrhea, lethargy, dehydration, cyanosis, and shock.

Infrequently, Japanese yew (*Taxus* sp.) toxicoses were documented in dogs. At the time of the calls, signs included vomiting and weakness. Such toxicoses could readily become life threatening, and heart block and seizures may be encountered.

MISCELLANEOUS PLANTS. Six cases involving four dogs and two cats pertained to suspected or assured mistletoe *(Phoradendron)* toxicosis. Signs included tremors, vomiting, abdominal pain, and most often depression or lethargy. Mistletoe toxicosis is generally a result of its use in the home at Christmastime, although it grows wild in the far western

United States. The anticipated stimulatory or hallucinogenic effects of catnip (*Nepeta* sp.) were sufficiently bizarre to result in occasional calls from uninitiated persons. Two calls regarding affected dogs indicate that dogs are similarly affected by this plant.

SUSPECTED TOXICOSES WITH UNKNOWN CAUSES

Approximately 115 calls were assessed as suspected toxicoses of unknown cause in dogs, and 35 such calls pertained to cats. This large number is indicative of the difficulty in differentiation of toxicoses on the basis of clinical signs alone. In essentially all such cases, sufficient exposure to a specific toxicant capable of producing the signs observed could not be documented. In addition, even known exposure to a toxicant does not always confirm that toxicosis occurred.

DISCUSSION

Previous attempts to characterize the prevalence of poisoning in small animals should be consulted by the interested reader, especially the chapters entitled Common Poisonings in Small Animal Practice and Potential Sources of Small Animal Poisonings in Current Veterinary Therapy VIII.

As shown in Tables 1 and 2, more than 60 per cent of the calls to the NAPCC in 1984 regarding dogs and 45 per cent of the calls pertaining to cats were classified as either doubtful toxicosis or exposure only. For many exposure calls, therapeutic recommendations are made depending on the degree of exposure and the toxicity of the agent. These often include attempts to minimize the further absorption of toxicants. Experience indicates that more veterinarians need to keep activated charcoal and a saline cathartic such as magnesium sulfate on hand. The use of a combined slurry of activated charcoal (2.2 gm/kg body weight) and a saline cathartic such as magnesium sulfate (Epsom salts, 1.1 gm/kg body weight as a 10 to 20 per cent solution) serves as an essential part of the therapy for a wide range of acute toxicoses, including most of those mentioned here.

References and Supplemental Reading

Arnold, E. K., Beasley, V. R., and Parker, A. J.: Unpublished Data, 1984.

Barton, J., and Oehme, F. W.: The incidence and characteristics of animal poisonings seen in Kansas State University from 1975 to 1980. Vet. Hum. Toxicol. 23:101, 1981.

Humphreys, D. J.: A review of recent trends in animal poisoning. Br. Vet. J. 134:128, 1978.

Maddy, K. T., Peoples, S. A., and Riddle, L. C.: Poisoning in dogs in California with pesticides. Calif. Vet. 31:9, 1977.

Maddy, K. T., and Winter, J.: Poisoning of animals in the Los Angeles area with pesticides during 1977. Vet. Hum. Toxicol. 22:409, 1980.

Osweiler, G. D.: Incidence and diagnostic considerations of major small animal toxicoses. J.A.M.A. 155:2011, 1969.

Osweiler, G. D.: Common poisonings in small animal practice. *In* Kirk, R. W. (ed.): Current Veterinary Therapy VIII. Philadelphia, W.B. Saunders, 1983, pp. 76–82.

Osweiler, G. D.: Potential sources of small animal poisonings. *In* Kirk, R. W. (ed.): Current Veterinary Therapy VIII. Philadelphia, W.B. Saunders, 1983, pp. 93–98.

Yeary, R. A.: Oral intubation of dogs with combinations of fertilizer, herbicide, and insecticide chemicals commonly used on lawns. Am. J. Vet. Res. 45:288, 1984.

INFORMATION RESOURCES FOR TOXICOLOGY

FREDERICK W. OEHME, D.V.M.

Manhattan, Kansas

Compared with other health professionals, veterinary clinicians are uniquely undersupported with technical and information resources. They are usually working alone with one animal technician or assistant and are expected by their clientele to be responsive to questions and to recall veterinary information on the details of conditions affecting all members of the animal kingdom except human beings. The need for scientific information becomes especially critical when the veterinary clinician is confronted with potential problems in specialty areas such as toxicology. The wide variety and increasing number of potentially dangerous chemical exposures, coupled with the variability in potential exposure routes, often provides a complex array of possible diagnoses that must be considered and ruled out in any one animal sickness.

To appropriately evaluate potential toxic chemical exposures, veterinary clinicians require information that is often not common knowledge nor readily available to them. It is therefore useful to have a variety of information resources for toxicology data that may be relied on to assist in evaluating the particular clinical case at hand. These information resources may begin with the most readily available (personal knowledge or reference texts) and extend to sophisticated national and international resources (The National Library of Medicine and various computer data banks).

PERSONAL RESOURCES

Every clinician has a degree of personal professional knowledge and practical experience gained from his or her training and years of clinical practice. For routine poisonings, these resources provide information on the most common poisonings observed in the practice area, the frequency of cases seen in various species, and the likelihood of toxicities occurring from various chemical exposures during certain times of the year. This clinical experience is invaluable and will more often than not provide a rapid probable diagnosis based on the most likely condition to produce the observed clinical syndrome.

This personal body of knowledge is complemented by the veterinarian's own library of notes, continuing education materials from professional meetings, and textbooks and journals providing updated information on the details of common and less frequently seen poisonings. This latter group of written materials is an excellent resource for specifics on antidotes available, management recommendations, specifics of treatment, and special features of diagnosis and confirmatory tests that support the initial clinical impression.

Veterinarians are wise to develop a system of information filing and classification that provides them with the most rapid and direct access to the information required. Notes made at meetings and continuing education material received through the mail and by attendance at continuing education functions should be filed appropriately. Review articles summarizing diagnostic and therapeutic recommendations for poisonings are valuable additions to such a collection. Articles in veterinary journals may be added to such a system to provide rapid retrieval following appropriate categorization. Veterinary textbooks are valuable but expensive additions to such a system. They should be selected carefully and reviewed promptly so that the clinician appreciates the information contained within each book and knows how and where the required specifics may be retrieved. The rapid changes occurring in our veterinary profession require that textbooks be replenished as new editions appear and as more specific and system- or etiologic-oriented volumes are published.

LOCAL INFORMATION RESOURCES

All too often, the clinician's personal information resources lack the details or specifics that might prove crucial for a clinical situation. The next level of inquiry might be to seek consultation with other resources in the local area. Fellow practitioners, who may have experienced similar clinical circumstances as those being observed, can be consulted. Local extension personnel at colleges or universities within the immediate region may also serve as consultants. Specialists at the college or university level may have access to specific details required for the clinician. Colleges of veterinary medicine, departments of veterinary science, and veterinary diagnostic laboratories may have individuals who specialize in toxicologic problems.

Various commercial enterprises within the local area may also be helpful.

Local manufacturers of chemicals, distributors, analytic laboratories, and chemical or industrial firms in the immediate locale may readily have access to necessary information on products used in that area. Compiling a list of such resources, together with telephone numbers and contact persons, will save much time in emergency situations.

Veterinarians who have specialized in toxicology can also be an important information resource. Most veterinary toxicologists are members of the American Academy of Veterinary and Comparative Toxicology (AAVCT) and are located throughout the United States and in several countries. A membership list or names of individuals in a specific locale may be received from the Secretary-Treasurer, Dr. H. D. Mercer, College of Veterinary Medicine, Mississippi State University, Mississippi State, MS 39762 (telephone 601/325–3432).

Details of potential hazardous chemical exposures may also be extrapolated from human experiences and information by contacting local poison control centers. Their addresses and telephone numbers are given in the front portion of local telephone books for easy accessibility. Many poison control centers are affiliated with the American Association of Poison Control Centers (AAPCC). Membership lists or information on the nearest poison control center to a particular practice may be received from the Secretary-Treasurer, Dr. G. Oderda, Maryland Poison Center, 20 North Pine, Baltimore, MD 21201 (telephone 301/528–7604). Poison control centers are staffed 24 hours a day and provide information and advice to all health professionals through a competently trained professional staff.

TELEPHONE RESOURCES

The increasing use of telephones to secure information has reduced the distance between the clinician and information resources. Veterinary clinicians have available to them the University of Illinois National Animal Poison Control Center, which provides a telephone service to answer questions about known or suspected cases of animal poisoning or chemical contamination on a 24-hour basis. The center is located at 2001 South Lincoln Ave., Urbana, IL 61801 (telephone 217/333-3611) and provides a unique emergency telephone service for veterinary toxicology problems.

Manufacturers of chemicals also provide a similar 24-hour-a-day chemical information service for their particular products. Each firm has an emergency number that provides access to specified individuals charged with the responsibility of responding to professional contacts for information about the toxicity or adverse effects of their products. A listing of the manufacturers' emergency telephone numbers for toxicology information was published by *Emergency Medicine* (August 15, 1984). This listing may be secured from a library and should be useful when attempting to receive specific details of a commercial product exposure. Most manufacturers have such emergency numbers available, and practitioners would do well to identify those manufacturers having products readily available to their clients and animals.

REGIONAL AND NATIONAL RESOURCES

On a larger geographic basis, toxicology information is available through various expert groups specializing in toxicology and through national library and computer-based data sources. The previosly mentioned AAVCT could provide individual or group expert opinions in specific animal toxicology situations. The Society of Toxicology (SOT) has a significant veterinary medicine component in its membership and activities. Individuals could be recommended as resources, or in persistent situations such as environmental problems involving animals, expert panels could be convened for consultation purposes. The SOT address is 1133 Fifteenth Street, N.W., Suite 620, Washington, D.C. 20005 (telephone 202/293–5935).

The National Academy of Sciences (2101 Constitution Avenue N.W., Washington, D.C. 20418) has a Board on Toxicology and Environmental Health Hazards that provides expert reports on selected toxicology and environmental health issues. These reports are published as National Academy of Science monographs and serve as excellent resource information since they are compiled by carefully selected experts and are extensively reviewed before release. Similar expert panels are convened by the World Health Organization (WHO, Geneva, Switzerland) to address specific problems and to offer recommendations for dealing with chemical insults or hazards. These expert panel reports are published periodically and are available as resource information through libraries or directly from the World Health Organization.

Perhaps the most exciting recent development for toxicology information resources has been the development of various computerized information services by the National Library of Medicine Toxicology Information Program. The increasing availability of personal computers equipped with modems for telephone hookup and printers for providing hard copy of on-line data gives the veterinary clinician the possibility of direct access to the toxicology information in these specialized information service packages. Toxicology Information Online (TOXLINE) covers the pharmacologic, biochemical, physiologic, environmental, and toxicologic effects of drugs and other chemicals in more than 1,500,000 citations. It is updated monthly. The Toxicology Data Bank (TDB) is a file composed of some 4000 chemical records containing toxicologic, pharmacologic, environmental, occupational, manufacturing, and use information, as well as chemical and physical properties of the chemicals. It is updated quarterly. The Registry of Toxic Effects of Chemical Substances (RTECS) contains basic acute and chronic toxicity data for more than 6700 potentially toxic chemicals. The file is updated quarterly. Chemical Dictionary Online (CHEMLINE) is a chemical dictionary of more than 600,000 unique substances; it is updated every 2 months with chemical names, synonyms, registry numbers, molecular formulas, and related chemical information. These files are available Monday through Friday from 3 AM to 9 PM and Saturday from 8:30 AM to 5 PM (Eastern Standard Time) from the Specialized Information Services of the National Library of Medicine, 8600 Rockville Pike, Bethesda, MD 20209 (telephone 301/496–1131).

The ready availability of these computer-based toxicology information files provides an indication of future directions for toxicology resource data bases. The increasing reliance of veterinary clinicians on rapidly retrievable toxicology information suggests that clinicians will be using their personal and observation skills in working with patients and clients and will be relying more on data retrieval systems for specific toxicologic information.

CONCLUSIONS

Convenience and practicality suggest that local resources for information should be used first in any search for data. Employing local resources also provides the advantage of applying localized experiences and identifying unique characteristics that may play a significant role in the differential diagnosis methodology. Limited local resources, however, might require that regional and even national systems be employed for securing toxicology data. The clinician's experience in using these more diverse systems will allow a wider scope of coverage and considerably more data-base use. Although these regional and national information resources may be more expensive to use than local resources, indications are that the more extensive and diverse nature of centralized toxicology information resources will make their use increasingly popular for veterinary clinicians.

A BRIEF GUIDE TO CLINICAL SIGNS OF TOXICOSIS IN SMALL ANIMALS

GARY D. OSWEILER, D.V.M.
Ames, Iowa

When clinical toxicosis occurs in companion animals, often there is no clear evidence of exposure to a toxicant. Furthermore, many toxicoses present with generalized and poorly defined clinical effects. The clinician may well be able to define which systems are most affected and generally characterize the clinical syndrome, but often a definitive diagnosis is not possible from clinical signs alone.

From veterinary and human forensic experience, we know that circumstantial and historic evidence is invaluable and perhaps the most important single line of evidence to suggest specific synthetic or natural toxicants to be confirmed by chemical analysis. The line of questioning about circumstances and specific chemical exposures depends on knowing what toxicants are commonly and characteristically responsible for generalized or specific clinical responses. For example, the familiar keys to suggest questioning about organophosphate exposure are vomiting, salivation, and muscle tremors. But, what other common toxicants might cause this combination of clinical signs if organophosphates are not the cause?

Since many toxicoses are seen infrequently in clinical practice, a quick reference to clinical effects expected from a variety of relatively common toxicants could be of value in early questioning of clients and in formulating a broader list of toxicologic differential diagnoses. In this regard, a very brief guide to expected clinical effects is offered. As data processing and clinical toxicology become better developed, access to computerized information on a much broader scale may be useful to the veterinary clinician in investigating acute and unfamiliar suspected toxicoses.

NERVOUS SYSTEM

Toxicant-induced seizures are usually generalized, bilateral, symmetric and without local onset. The cause of seizures can seldom be determined by the type of seizure alone. Most probable toxicants that are suggested by neurologic examination can be systematically eliminated or confirmed on a priority basis, depending on the severity of the problem, probability of the cause, available tests, cost, and risk to the patient.

Neurological Toxicants

Excitation or Stimulation of Nervous System
- Amphetamine
- Aminopyridine
- Caffeine
- Cyanide
- Ergot (*Claviceps* sp.)
- Fluoroacetate
- Lead
- Metaldehyde
- Moonseed (*Menispermum canadense*)
- Mycotoxins
- Nicotine
- Organochlorine insecticides
- Organophosphate insecticides
- Phenols and chlorophenols
- Strychnine
- Theobromine
- Theophylline
- Water hemlock (*Cicuta* sp.)

Text continued on opposite page

Neurological Toxicants Continued

Depression, Coma	Organophosphates
Alcohols	Triaryl phosphates
Antihistamines	
Barbiturates	**Autonomic Stimulation**
Carbon monoxide	Atropine
Hydrocarbons, aliphatic	Carbamate insecticides
Hydrocarbons, aromatic	Fly mushroom (*Amanita muscaria*)
Hydrocarbons, halogenated	
Lead	Organophosphate insecticides
Mercury	
Morphine derivatives	
Salicylates	**Behavioral Changes**
Snake venoms	Belladonna alkaloids
	Ergot
Loss of Motor Control	Lead
Botulinum	Lysergic acid diethylamide (LSD)
Buckeye (*Aesculus* sp.)	
Carbon disulfide	Marijuana
Curare	Morning glory
Ergot	Nutmeg
Ethylene glycol	Opium derivatives
Hexachlorophene	Organochlorine insecticides
Lead	Periwinkle
Nicotine	Peyote

ALIMENTARY SYSTEM

There may be a wide variety of toxicants, mechanisms, and manifestations. Effects may be mediated both locally and systemically, resulting in either immediate or delayed effects. Direct irritants affect mainly the upper alimentary tract. Signs often occur in conjunction with dysfunction in other organ systems. Thus vomiting may attend many toxicoses that affect other organs more seriously. The nature and amount of diet as well as speed of oral intake and related factors may influence response to gastrointestinal toxicants.

Gastrointestinal Toxicants

Stomatitis, Pharyngitis	**Gastroenteritis**
Acids and Alkalies	*Amanita* sp.
Aldehydes	Antimony
Chromium salts	Arsenic
Fertilizer	Barium
Mercuric salts	Bismuth
Detergents	Cantharidin
Petroleum distillates	Copper salts
Phenol	Croton oil
	Detergents, soaps, sanitizers
Salivation	Digitalis toxins
Amanita muscaria	Iron
Ammonia	Lead
Cresol	Mercury
Metaldehyde	Mushrooms
Nicotine	Phenoxy herbicides
Organophosphates	Phosphorus
Thallium	Plants (see *Current Veterinary Therapy VII, VIII,* and *IX*)
Dry Mouth	
Amphetamine	Staphylococcus toxin
Antihistamine	Thallium
Atropine	Zinc phosphide
Belladonna	
Opiates	

HEPATOTOXINS

The liver is the major organ of drug metabolism and is a significant avenue for excretion. Because of tremendous hepatic reserve capacity and alterations in other organs induced by toxins, death may occur from other causes before fatal liver failure occurs (e.g., chloroform, arsenic). Liver function tests and clinical signs will not identify a toxic agent but may provide indirect clues to damage compatible with a toxic agent. An animal exposed to a short-term or one-time hepatotoxic incident may regain full liver function if it survives the acute insult. Conversely, continued exposure (days to weeks) to a hepatotoxin may result in fibrosis or even cirrhosis. Hepatotoxicosis typically has a short latent period after hepatotoxic exposure. Liver enlargement often accompanies acute chemical liver injury. Unfortunately, hepatotoxins are easy to suggest but difficult to confirm.

Hepatotoxins

Acetaminophen	Copper
Aflatoxin	Halogenated hydrocarbons
Amanita phalloides	Iron
Blue-green algae	Petroleum distillates
Coal tar derivatives	Phosphorus

NEPHROTOXINS

Acute nephrosis results in similar clinical signs regardless of the cause. Clinical effects may be complicated or obscured by effects of the agent on other systems. Hours to days may be required for manifestation of chemical nephrosis. Depending on the stage of the disease, either oliguria or polyuria may be seen. Once damage has occurred, healing must progress over a period of days to weeks. Therapy must be aimed at determining the potential reversibility of the lesion and keeping the patient alive until recovery can occur.

Nephrotoxins

Inadvertent Nephrotoxins	Thallium
Aldehydes	Turpentine
Amanita mushrooms	Volatile oils (e.g., pennyroyal oil or oil of juniper)
Arsenic	
Bismuth	
Cadmium	**Nephrotoxic Drugs**
Cresols	Acetaminophen
Dichromate	Amphotericin B
Ethylene glycol	Bacitracin
Halogenated hydrocarbons	Gentamicin
Mercury	Kanamycin
Ochratoxin	Neomycin
Oxalates	Polymyxin B
Petroleum distillates	Sulfonamides
Phenols	Vancomycin

BLOOD

A variety of defects may be induced in blood, including hypoxia, hemolysis, aplasia, coagulopathy, and hypocalcemia.

Methemoglobin from nitrites and aniline-based products (e.g., acetaminophen) as well as carboxyhemoglobin induced by carbon monoxide can result in hypoxia. Agents acting directly on the lipid or protein structure of the erythrocyte may result in acute, massive hemolytic crisis with hemoglobinuria and hemoglobin nephrosis (e.g., arsine, snake venoms). Hemolysis can also result from continued oxidative denaturation of hemoglobin with formation of Heinz bodies leading to increased fragility or elevated rate of erythrocyte destruction. Aplastic anemia causes reduced number and function of multipotential stem cells. Anemia is often macrocytic, and reticulocytes are few in number but relatively immature. There is prolonged iron clearance and low red cell iron utilization. Advanced aplastic anemia is usually accompanied by granulocytopenia and thrombocytopenia. Many blood dyscrasias show little dose-response relationship and are based on individual sensitivity.

Blood Toxicants

Methemoglobin	**Aplastic Anemia, Leukopenia, Thrombocytopenia**
Acetaminophen	Arsenicals
Aniline derivatives	Aspirin
Chlorate	Benzene
Copper	Chloramphenicol
Methylene blue	Cytostatic agents
Nitrite	Estrogens
Nitrobenzene	Phenylbutazone
Hemolysis	Toluene
Acetaminophen*	Tricholoroethylene
Aniline	
Arsine	**Coagulopathy (see page 156).**
Chlorates	Aflatoxin
Copper	Aspirin
Methylene blue*	Coumarin rodenticides
Nitrobenzene	Indane-dione rodenticides
Onions	Phosphorus
Snake venoms	Sulfonamides
Turpentine	
Red maple leaves	

*Especially in cats

RESPIRATORY SYSTEM

Exposure to lung-damaging chemicals may be aerogenous or hematogenous. The particulate nature of some toxicants affects toxicity. Excretion mechanisms may also alter effects (e.g., by concentrating volatile chemicals at the pulmonary membranes during expiration). Lung response, to toxicants generally includes irritation, necrosis, fibrosis, or suppressed immunologic function.

Respiratory Toxicants

Air pollutants (nitrogen dioxide, sulfur dioxide)	Gasoline, kerosene
Allergens	Organophosphate insecticides
Ammonia	Ozone
ANTU rodenticide	Paraquat herbicide
Chlorine	Thallium

CARDIOVASCULAR SYSTEM

Effects on the cardiovascular system may be expressed directly or indirectly on heart muscle, coronary vessels, or nervous innervation of the heart. Mechanisms of damage are complex and often interrelated.

Cardiovascular Toxicants

Tachycardia and Arrhythmias	Opiates
Adrenalin	Oleander
Aminophylline	Red squill
Amphetamine	
Aminoglycoside antibiotics	**Myocardial Damage**
Atropine	*Amanita phalloides*
Caffeine	Barium
Cyanide	Carbon monoxide
Dinitrophenol	Oleander
Fluorocarbons	Phosphorus
Nicotine	Thallium
Thallium	
	Vascular Necrosis
Bradycardia	Ergot
Barium	Lead
Cardiac glycosides	Mercury
Digitalis	Selenium
Morphine	

Ocular Toxicants

Mydriasis	Nicotine
Amanita mushrooms	Organophosphates
Atropine	
Beladonna	**Optic Neuropathy**
Methanol	Arsenicals
	Lead
Miosis	Mercury
Heroin	Methanol
Morphine	Thallium
	Vitamin A

General Signs

Fever
- Atropine
- Carbon monoxide
- Dinitrophenol
- Lead
- Metaldehyde
- Organochlorine insecticides
- Oxalates
- Phenols

Hypothermia
- Alcohol
- Arsenic
- Barbiturates
- Heroin
- Morphine

Cyanosis
- Carbon dioxide
- Hydrogen sulfide
- Nitrite
- Paraquat

Pink Skin Color
- Arsenic
- Carbon monoxide
- Cyanide
- Mercury
- Thallium

References and Supplemental Reading

Arena, J. M.: *Poisoning: Toxicology, Symptoms, Treatment*, 4th ed. Springfield: Charles C Thomas, 1979.

Clarke, M. L., Harvey, D. G., and Humphreys, D. J.: *Veterinary Toxicology*, 2nd ed. London: Bailliere Tindall, 1981.

Dresbach, R. H.: *Handbook of Poisoning: Prevention, Diagnosis, and Treatment*, 11th ed. Los Altos: Lange Medical Publications, 1983.

Gosselin, R. E., Smith, R. P., and Hodge, H. C.: *Clinical Toxicology of Commercial Products*, 5th ed. Baltimore: Williams & Wilkins, 1984.

Haddad, L. M., and Winchester, J. F.: *Clinical Management of Poisoning and Drug Overdose*. Philadelphia: W. B. Saunders, 1983.

Kirk, R. W., and Bistner, S. I.: *Handbook of Veterinary Procedures and Emergency Treatment*, 3rd ed. Philadelphia: W. B. Saunders, 1980.

Moeschlin, S.: *Poisoning: Diagnosis and Treatment*. New York: Grune and Stratton, 1965.

Osweiler, G. D., Carson, T. L., Buck, W. D., and Van Gelder, G. A.: *Clinical and Diagnostic Veterinary Toxicology*, 3rd ed. Dubuque: Kendall/Hunt, 1985.

EMERGENCY AND GENERAL TREATMENT OF POISONINGS

E. MURL BAILEY, Jr., D.V.M.
College Station, Texas

Many acutely ill animals are diagnosed as poisoned when no other diagnosis can be readily ascertained. The veterinary clinician should direct efforts toward treating the signs exhibited by the affected animal unless the correct diagnosis is obvious. Pre-existing conditions and the diagnosis should be determined following stabilization of the patient.

Special goals of therapy in cases of intoxication are as follows:

1. Emergency intervention and prevention of further exposure
2. Preventing further absorption
3. Application of specific antidotes
4. Hastening elimination of the absorbed toxicant
5. Supportive measures
6. Client education

PRELIMINARY INSTRUCTIONS TO CLIENTS

Veterinarians are frequently contacted by telephone concerning an intoxicated animal. The preliminary instructions given at this time are very important to the success of subsequent therapeutic measures.

The client should be instructed to protect the affected animal as well as the people in contact with it. This may include keeping the animal warm and avoiding any other stress phenomena. Onlookers should be warned about the condition of the animal, and it may be desirable to muzzle the animal.

If the animal's exposure was topical, the animal owner should be instructed to cleanse the animal's skin or eye with copious amounts of water. The client should also be instructed to be careful to avoid self-exposure to the toxicant and should use some type of protective clothing (e.g., rubber gloves, apron) if available.

In many instances, the client will be concerned about inducing emesis in the animal. The clinician should cite the contraindications to emesis (e.g., central nervous system [CNS] depression; ingestion of petroleum distillates, acids, or alkalis). Emetic preparations and techniques easily available to the lay individuals (e.g., hydrogen peroxide, table salt, copper sulfate, and sticking the finger in the back of the animal's mouth) are generally ineffective and sometimes dangerous. One-half to two teaspoons of syrup of ipecac may be administered if the animal is fully awake.

This article is supported in part by Texas Agricultural Experiment Station, Project No. H-6255.

If the client is very insistent about administering medication, he should be advised to allow the animal to drink as much water as it wants. This will act as a dilutent. In most cases, one may also advise the administration of milk or egg whites. Activated charcoal tablets may also be administered. The client should be cautioned not to administer anything by mouth if the animal is convulsing, depressed, or unconscious.

It is imperative that the client not waste time. The animal should be taken to the veterinarian as soon as possible (or the veternarian should be summoned). The owner should be instructed to bring vomitus or suspected toxic materials or their containers with the animal. The client should be advised to bring the specimens in clean plastic containers or glass jars and should be cautioned not to contaminate the material. In many instances valuable time can be saved by applying the proper therapeutic measure if the suspected intoxicant is known. However, the clinician should not be biased in diagnosis and treatment of an animal based on labels or material brought with the animal. In some cases the signs exhibited by the affected animal do not correspond with suspected ingredients. This suspected material may also be valuable from a medicolegal aspect.

EMERGENCY INTERVENTION

The most important aspect of emergency treatment of intoxications is to ensure adequate physiologic function. All the antidotal procedures available to the clinician will be of no avail if the animal has lost one or all of its vital functions. Emergency intervention may include establishment of a patent airway, artificial respiration, cardiac massage (external or internal), and perhaps the application of defibrillation techniques. Following stabilization of the vital signs, the clinician may proceed with subsequent therapeutic measures.

PREVENTING FURTHER ABSORPTION

Preventing the animal from absorbing additional intoxicant is a major factor in treating cases of intoxication. In many instances intoxication may be prevented in this manner if the animal was actually observed ingesting or coming in contact with suspected material. Removal of the animal from the affected environment is a necessary first step to prevent further absorption. It is hoped that bringing the animal to the veterinary clinic or hospital will suit this purpose. Prevention of absorption may also entail washing the animal's skin to remove the noxious agent. If an external toxicant is involved, caution must be exercised to avoid contamination of persons handling the animal. In addition, the judicious use of emetics, gastric lavage techniques, adsorbents, and cathartics will aid in the prevention of further absorption of toxic materials that are ingested.

INDUCTION OF EMESIS. Emesis may be considered as a method of emptying the stomach of toxic materials. Some commonly available agents are not very reliable, and emesis may be of little value after 4 hours following exposure to a toxicant.

Syrup of ipecac is considered a general emetic. Its mechanism is gastric irritation as well as central stimulation. The dose of ipecac for small animals is 1 to 2 ml/kg, but it is only about 50 per cent effective, and not more than 15 ml (1 tablespoon) should be used with even the largest dog. The dosage may be repeated in 20 minutes if vomiting does not occur. However, if the patient does not vomit, lavage procedure should be instituted to recover the ipecac. Syrup of ipecac can exert a cardiotoxic effect if it is not vomited but absorbed. This agent should never be used when activated charcoal is part of the therapeutic regimen, since it markedly reduces the effectiveness of the charcoal. The drug should not be confused with ipecac fluid extract, which is 14 times stronger than the syrup. Outdated syrup of ipecac should not be used since it becomes ineffective but is still toxic.

Other agents such as copper sulfate, table salt, or hydrogen peroxide have been advocated as locally acting emetics. However, the effectiveness of these agents is highly questionable.

Apomorphine (Eli Lilly & Co.) is the most effective and most reliable emetic available for dogs and cats. Apomorphine is no longer a controlled drug but is not widely available. The effctive dose in most small animals is 0.04 mg/kg IV or 0.08 mg/kg IM or SC. Apomorphine may cause respiratory depression, and protracted emesis may develop following its use. These signs may be effectively controlled with appropriate narcotic antagonists injected IV (naloxone [Narcan, Endo] 0.04 mg/kg; levallorphan [Lorfan, Roche] 0.02 mg/kg; or nalorphine [Nalline, Merck], 0.1 mg/kg). In addition to the general contraindications of emetics, apomorphine may be further contraindicated in cases where additional CNS depression must be avoided. The contraindications for induction of emesis are unconscious or severely depressed animals; ingestion of strong acids or bases; and intoxication by petroleum distillates, tranquilizers, or other antiemetics. If the time interval following exposure to the toxicant is greater than 4 hours, most of the toxicant will have passed the duodenum.

Intoxication with acids or alkalis may be diagnosed when corrosive changes are present in and around the mouth, forepaws, and other areas on the cranial portions of the body. If emesis is induced, caustic agents could cause additional damage to the esophagus and oral cavity. In addition, these agents generally weaken the gastric wall, which could easily be ruptured during forceful emesis.

Activated charcoal may increase the efficacy of emesis. If charcoal is to be used, the clinician should first induce emesis with apomorphine, administer the charcoal, and reinduce emesis with a subsequent IV dose of amomorphine (0.04 mg/kg IV). Syrup of ipecac should never be used if activated charcoal is used, since the agent negates the adsorbent activity of the charcoal.

Any vomitus should be saved for analysis, especially if there are medicolegal considerations. The clinician should conduct treatment accordingly.

Gastric Lavage. Gastric lavage is an emergency procedure that has at times been maligned as being relatively inefficient. Changes in technique (e.g., using a larger tube, more volume, and more frequent lavages) have made this a very reliable procedure when undertaken within 2 hours of exposure to an ingested toxicant.

The animal should be unconscious or under light anesthesia. A cuffed endotracheal tube should be placed within the trachea. The distal end of the tube should extend 2 inches (5 cm) beyond the teeth. This will increase the animal's dead space but is required to prevent any inhalation of lavage fluid. The head and thorax should be lowered slightly but not enough to compromise respiration due to the weight of the abdominal viscera. The stomach tube should be premeasured from the tip of the animal's nose to the xiphoid cartilage. In all cases, as large a stomach tube as possible should be used. A good rule is to use the same size stomach tube as cuffed endotracheal tube (1 mm = 3 French). The volume of water or lavage solution to be used for each washing is 5 to 10 ml/kg body weight. Following infusion of the solution, the fluid should be aspirated from the stomach via the stomach tube with either a large aspirator bulb or a 50-ml syringe. The infusion and aspiration cycle of the lavage solution should be repeated 10 to 15 times. Activated charcoal in the solution will enhance the effectiveness of this procedure.

Some precautions to be taken with this technique are (1) using low pressure to prevent forcing the toxicant into the duodenum, (2) reducing the infused volume in obviously weakened stomachs, and (3) making sure not to force the stomach tube through either the esophagus or the stomach wall.

ADSORBENTS

Activated charcoal is probably the best adsorbing agent available to the practitioner. Although it does not detoxify toxicants, it will effectively prevent absorption of a toxicant if properly used. Activated charcoal can be effectively combined with emetic and gastric lavage techniques.

The proper type of activated charcoal for treatment of intoxications is of vegetable, not mineral or animal, origin. There are several commercial types of activated charcoal available, and these are presented in Table 1. Also available are compressed activated charcoal tablets (5 gm, B. C. Crowley, Co. and Requa Mfg. Co.). These tablets are easier to handle than the powdered charcoal and are apparently as effective.

A bathtub or some other easily cleaned area is the best place to administer activated charcoal to small animals. Activated charcoal is used as follows: (1) Make a slurry of the charcoal with water. The proper dose is 2 to 8 gm/kg body weight in a concentration of 1 gm charcoal/5 to 10 ml water. (2) Administer the charcoal by a stomach tube using either a funnel or a large syringe. (3) A cathartic of sodium sulfate should be administered 30 minutes after administration of the charcoal. This technique may be modified if the charcoal is used in conjunction with emetic or lavage techniques. However, with either technique some charcoal should remain in the stomach and should be followed by a cathartic to prevent desorption of the toxicant. Newer methods suggest the administration of activated charcoal 3 to 4 times a day for 2 to 3 days after occurrence of an intoxication.

Activated charcoal is highly adsorptive for many toxicants, including mercuric chloride, strychnine, other alkaloids (morphine and atropine) barbiturates, and ethylene glycol. It is ineffective against cyanide.

Syrup of ipecac will negate some of the adsorptive characteristics of the activated charcoal. The "universal antidote," consisting of two parts activated charcoal, one part magnesium oxide and one part tannic acid, is very inefficient, since the magnesium oxide and tannic acid decrease the adsorptive capability of the charcoal. Burned or charred toast as described in some emergency texts is highly ineffective as an adsorbing agent.

Cathartics. Sodium sulfate is a more efficient agent for evacuation of the bowel than is magnesium sulfate and is the preferable agent to use, especially with activated charcoal. There is also some danger of CNS depression due to the magnesium ion, although the sodium ion may also precipitate a sodium ion intoxication or water deprivation syndrome. However, either agent may be used in an emergency. The oral dose of sodium sulfate is 1 gm/kg.

Mineral oil or vegetable oils are of value if lipid-

Table 1. *Some Available Activated Charcoal Products**

Commercial Trade Name	Ingredients	Manufacturer or Distributor	Address
Acta-Char	Activated charcoal powder, USP 30 gm in wide-mouth plastic bottle (400-ml capacity)	Med-Corp, Inc.	5310 Harvest Hill Road Dallas, TX 75230
Activated charcoal, USP—Humco	Activated charcoal powder, USP 30 gm in 8-ounce wide-mouth plastic jar (unit dose) 120 gm in 16-ounce wide-mouth glass jar 240 gm in 32-ounce wide-mouth glass jar	Humco Laboratories	1008 Whitaker Texarkana, TX 75504
Activated charcoal, USP—Mallinckrodt	Activated charcoal powder, USP 454 gm (1 pound) in wide-mouth glass jar	Mallinckrodt, Inc.	Box M Paris, KY 40361
Activated charcoal, USP, in liquid base	Activated charcoal, USP, in liquid base containing water and propylene glycol (amount of propylene glycol unspecified) 12.5 gm in 60-ml wide-mouth bottle 25 gm in 120-ml squeeze bottle with spout 50 gm in 240-ml squeeze bottle with spout	Bowman Pharmaceuticals, Inc.	119 Schroyer Ave., S. W. Canton, OH 44702
Bowman Poison-Antidote Kit	1. Activated charcoal, USP, in liquid base containing water and propylene glycol (amount of propylene glycol unspecified) 4 bottles, 12.5 gm each of activated charcoal in liquid base, 60 ml 2. 1 bottle, ipecac syrup, 30 ml	Bowman Pharmaceuticals, Inc.	119 Schroyer Ave., S.W. Canton, OH 44702
Charcoaid	Activated charcoal, USP, 30 gm in sorbitol solution USP, 150 ml, in squeeze bottle with spout	Requa Mfg. Co.	1 Seneca Place Greenwich, CT 06830
Charcolantidote	Activated charcoal powder, USP 15-gm bottle (150-ml capacity) 30-gm bottle (200-ml capacity)	U.S. Products, Inc.	16636 N.W. 54th Ave. Miami Lakes, FL 33014
Insta-Char	Activated charcoal, USP in aqueous suspension (water is the sole liquid ingredient) 15 gm in 120-ml squeeze bottle with spout 50 gm in 250-ml squeeze bottle with spout	Frank W. Kerr Chemical Co.	43155 S.W. Nine Mile Rd. Northville, MI 48167
Liquid-Antidose	Activated charcoal, USP, in liquid base containing carboxymethylcellulose, sodium benzoate (preservative), and water 40 gm in liquid base, 200 ml	U.S. Products	16636 N.W. 54th Ave. Miami Lakes, FL 33014
Norit USP XX	Activated charcoal powder, USP, in bulk 15-kg containers (Norit USP XX is the activated charcoal used in all products listed above)	American Norit Co.	6301 Glidden Way Jacksonville, FL 32201
Toxiban	Granules 47% activated charcoal, 10% kaolin, 42% wetting and dispensing agents, 5 kg-pail Suspension 10.4% activated charcoal, 6.25% kaolin in an aqueous dose; 240-ml bottle	Vet-A-Mix	604 West Thomas Ave. Shenandoah, IA 51601

*Adapted from Anon.: Activated charcoal products for medicinal (antidote) use. Vet. Hum. Tox. 25:294, 1983.

soluble toxicants are involved. Mineral oil (liquid petrolatum) is inert and is unlikely to be absorbed. Vegetable oil, however, is more likely to be absorbed and therefore may be contraindicated. Regardless of the type of oil used, it should be followed by a saline cathartic in 30 to 40 minutes.

A colonic lavage or high enema may be of value to hasten the elimination of toxicants from the gastrointestinal tract. Warm water with castile soap makes an excellent enema solution. Hexachlorophene soaps should be avoided. There are several commercially available enema preparations that act as osmotic agents. Care should be taken to avoid the induction of dehydration and electrolyte imbalances with overzealous treatment (see page 212).

APPLICATION OF ANTIDOTES

LOCALLY ACTING ANTIDOTES. There are numerous locally acting antidotes and therapeutic regimens reported for preventing the absorption of toxicants. The nonspecific antidotal procedures for some of the more common toxicants are described in Table 2.

SPECIFIC ANTIDOTES. There are a few specific antidotal agents available for some of the more common animal toxicants. A list of these specific antidotal procedures is presented in Table 3.

Caution should be exercised with the use of some of the more specific antidotes, since many of these agents are themselves toxic. In certain chronic

Text continued on page 142

Table 2. *Locally Acting Antidotes Against Unabsorbed Poisons and Principles of Treatment*

Poison	Antidote and Dose or Concentration
Acids, corrosive	Weak alkali—magnesium oxide solution (1:25 warm water) internally.
	Never give sodium bicarbonate!
	Milk of magnesia—1 to 15 ml. Flush externally with water. Apply paste of sodium bicarbonate.
Alkali, caustic	Weak acid—vinegar (diluted 1:4), 1%. Acetic acid or lemon juice given orally.
	Diluted albumin (4 to 6 egg whites to 1 quart tepid water or give whole milk) followed by an emetic and then a cathartic, because some compounds are soluble in excess albumin. Local—flush with copious amounts of water and apply vinegar.
Alkaloids	Potassium permanganate (1:5000 to 1:10,000) for lavage or oral administration.
	Tannic acid or strong tea (200 to 500 mg in 30 to 60 ml of water) except in cases of poisoning by cocaine, nicotine, physostigmine, atropine, and morphine.
	Emetic or purgative should be used for prompt removal of tannates.
Arsenic	Sodium thiosulfate—10% solution given orally (0.5 to 3.0 gm for small animals). Followed by lavage or emesis.
	Protein—e.g., evaporated milk, egg whites.
	Tannic acid or strong tea (see specific antidote in Table 3).
Barium salts	Sodium sulfate and magnesium sulfate (20% solution given orally). Dosage: 2 to 25 gm.
Bismuth salts	Acacia or gum arabic as mucilage.
Carbon tetrachloride	Empty stomach; give high-protein and carbohydrate diet; maintain fluid and electrolyte balance.
	Hemodialysis is indicated in anuria. Epinephrine is contraindicated (ventricular fibrillation!).
Copper	Albumin (see Alkali, above).
	Sodium ferrocyanide in water (0.3 to 3.5 gm for small animals). (See specific antidote in Table 3.)
	Magnesium oxide (see Acids, above).
Detergents, anionic (Na, K, NH_4^+ salts)	Milk or water followed by demulcent (oils, acacia, gelatin, starch, egg white)
Detergents, cationic (chlorides, iodides)	Soap (castile) dissolved in 4 times its bulk of hot water.
	Albumin (see Alkali, above).
Fluoride	Calcium (milk, limewater, or powdered chalk mixed with water) given orally.
Formaldehyde	Ammonia water (0.2% orally) or ammonium acetate (1% for lavage).
	Starch—1 part to 15 parts hot water added gradually.
	Gelatin soaked in water for 1/2 hour.
	Albumin (see Alkali, above).
	Sodium thiosulfate (see Arsenic, above).
Iron	Sodium bicarbonate—1% for lavage. (See specific antidote in Table 3.)
Lead	Sodium or magnesium sulfate given orally.
	Sodium ferrocyanide (see Copper, above).
	See specific antidote.
	Albumin (see Alkali, above).
Mercury	Protein—milk, egg whites (see Alkali, above).
	Magnesium oxide (see Acids, above).
	Sodium formaldehyde sulfoxylate—5% solution for lavage.
	Starch (see Formaldehyde, above).
	Activated charcoal—5 to 50 gm. (See specific antidote in Table 3.)
Oxalic acid	Calcium—calcium hydroxide as 0.15% solution.
	Other alkalis are contraindicated because their salts are more soluble.
	Chalk or other calcium salts.
	Magnesium sulfate as cathartic.
	Maintain diuresis to prevent calcium oxalate deposition in kidney.
Petroleum distillates (aliphatic hydrocarbons)	Olive oil, other vegetable oils, or mineral oil given orally. After 1/2 hour, sodium sulfate as cathartic.
	Emesis and lavage are contraindicated for ingested volatile solvents, but petroleum distillates are used as carrier agents for more toxic agents.
Phenol and cresols	Soap-and-water or alcohol lavage of skin.
	Sodium bicarbonate (0.5%) dressings.
	Activated charcoal and/or mineral oil given orally.
Phosphorus	Copper sulfate (0.2 to 0.4% solution) or potassium permanganate (1:5000 solution) for lavage.
	Turpentine (preferably old oxidized) in gelatin capsules or floated on hot water. Give 2 ml 4 times at 15-minute intervals.
	Activated charcoal.
	Do not give vegetable oil cathartic. Remove all fat from diet.
Silver nitrate	Normal saline for lavage.
	Albumin (see Alkali, above).
Unknown (e.g., toxic plants or other materials)	Activated charcoal (replaces universal antidote).
	For small animals—via stomach tube, as a slurry in water. Follow by emetic or cathartic and repeat procedure.

Table 3. Specific Systemic Antidotes and Dosages

Toxic Agent	Systemic Antidote	Dosage and Method for Treatment
Acetaminophen	*N*-acetylcysteine (Mucomyst, Mead Johnson)	150 mg/kg loading dose, orally, or IV then 50 mg/kg every 4 hours for 17 additional doses.
Amphetamines	Chlorpromazine	1 mg/kg IM, IP, IV; administer only half dose if barbiturates have been given: blocks excitation.
Arsenic, mercury and other heavy metals except silver, selenium, and thallium	Dimercaprol (BAL, Hynson, Wescott & Dunning)	10% solution in oil; give small animals 2.5 to 5.0 mg/kg IM (0.025 to 0.05 ml/kg) every 4 hours for 2 days, b.i.d. for the next 10 days or until recovery. NOTE: In severe acute poisoning 5 mg/kg dosage should be given only first day.
	D-Penicillamine (Cuprimine, Merck & Co.)	Developed for chronic mercury poisoning, now seems most promising drug; no reports on dosage in animals. Dosage for humans is 250 mg orally, every 6 hours for 10 days (3 to 4 mg/kg).
Atropine Belladonna alkaloids	Physostigmine salicylate	0.1 to 0.6 mg/kg (do not use neostigmine).
Barbiturates	Doxapram	2% solution: Give small animals 3 to 5 mg/kg IV only (0.14 to 0.25 ml/kg) repeated as necessary.
	NOTE: The above is reliable only when depression is mild; in deeper levels of depression, artificial respiration (and oxygen) is preferable.	
Bromides	Chlorides (sodium or ammonium salts)	0.5 to 1.0 gm daily for several days; hasten excretion.
Carbon monoxide	Oxygen	Pure oxygen at normal or high pressure; artificial respiration; blood transfusion.
Cholinergic agents	Atropine sulfate	0.02 to 0.04 mg/kg, as needed.
Cholinesterase inhibitors	Atropine sulfate	Dosage is 0.2 mg/kg, repeated as needed for atropinization. Treat cyanosis (if present) first. Blocks only muscarinic effects. Atropine in oil may be injected for prolonged effect during the night. <u>Avoid atropine intoxication!</u>
Cholinergic agents and cholinesterase inhibitors (organophosphates, some carbamates; but not carbaryl, dimethan, or carbam piloxime	Pralidoxime chloride (2-PAM)	5% solution; give 20 to 50 mg/kg IM or by slow IV (0.2 to 1.0 mg/kg) injection (maximum dose is 500 mg/min.), repeat as needed. 2-PAM alleviates nicotinic effect and regenerates cholinesterase. Morphine, succinylcholine, and phenothiazine tranquilizers are contraindicated.
Copper	D-Penicillamine (Cuprimine)	Dose for animals not established. Dose for humans is 1 to 4 gm daily in divided doses (250-mg tablets).
Coumarin-derivative anticoagulants	Vitamin K_1 (Aqua-MEPHYTON, Merck & Co.)	5% stable emulsion. 1 mg/kg IV (0.02 ml/kg) in 5% dextrose. Give 5 mg/kg (0.1 ml/kg) IM for 5 days or longer.
	Whole blood or plasma	Blood transfusion, 25 ml/kg.
Curare	Neostigmine methylsulfate	Solution: 1:5000 for 1:2000 (1 ml = 0.2 or 0.5 mg/ml). Dose is 0.005 mg/5 kg, SC. Follow with IV injection of atropine (0.04 mg/kg).
	Edrophonium chloride (Tensilon, Roche)	1% solution; give 0.05 to 1.0 mg/kg IV.
	Artificial respiration	
Cyanide	Methemoglobin (sodium nitrite is used to form methemoglobin)	1% solution of sodium nitrate, dosage is 16 mg/kg IV (1.6 ml/kg) Follow with:
	Sodium thiosulfate	20% solution at dosage of 30 to 40 mg/kg (0.15 to 0.2 ml/kg) IV. If treatment is repeated, use only sodium thiosulfate. NOTE: Both of the above may be given simultaneously as follows: 0.5 ml/kg of combination consisting of 10 gm sodium nitrate, 15 gm sodium thiosulfate distilled water q.s. 250 ml. Dosage may be repeated once. If further treatment is required, give only 20% solution of sodium thiosulfate at level of 0.2 ml/kg.
Digitalis glycosides, oleander, and *Bufo* toads	Potassium chloride	Dog: 0.5 to 2.0 gm, orally in divided doses, or in serious cases, as diluted solution given IV by slow drip (ECG control is essential).

Table continued on opposite page

Table 3. Specific Systemic Antidotes and Dosages Continued

Toxic Agent	Systemic Antidote	Dosage and Method for Treatment
Digitalis glycosides *Continued*	Diphenylhydantoin	25 mg/minute IV until control is established.
	Propranolol (β-blocker)	0.5 to 1.0 mg/kg IV or IM as needed to control cardiac arrhythmias (ECG control is essential).
	Atropine sulfate	0.02 to 0.04 mg/kg as needed for cholinergic control.
Fluoride	Calcium borogluconate	3 to 10 ml of 5 to 10% solution.
Fluoracetate (Compound 1080, Sigma)	Glyceryl monoacetin	0.1 to 0.5 mg/kg IM hourly for several hours (total 2 to 4 mg/kg); or diluted (0.5 to 1.0%) IV (danger of hemolysis). Monoacetin is available only from chemical supply houses.
	Acetamide	Animal may be protected if acetamide is given prior to or simultaneously with Compound 1080 (experimental).
	Phenobarbital or pentobarbital	May protect against lethal dose (experimental).
	NOTE: All treatments are generally unrewarding.	
Hallucinogens (LSD, phencyclidine [PCP])	Diazepam (Valium, Roche)	As needed—avoid respiratory depression (2 to 5 mg/kg).
Heparin	Protamine sulfate	1% solution; give 1.0 to 1.5 mg to antagonize each 1 mg of heparin; slow IV injection. Reduce dose as time increases between heparin injection and start of treatment (after 30 minutes give only 0.5 mg).
Iron salts	Deferoxamine (Desferal, Ciba)	Dose for animals not yet established. Dose for humans is 5 gm of 5% solution given orally, then 20 mg/kg IM every 4 to 6 hours. In case of shock, dose is 40 mg/kg by IV drip over 4-hour period; may be repeated in 6 hours, then 15 mg/kg by drip every 8 hours.
Lead	Calcium disodium edetate (CaEDTA)	Dosage: Maximum safe dose is 75 mg/kg/24 hours (only for severe case). EDTA is available in 20% solution; for IV drip, dilute in 5% glucose to 0.5%; for IM, add procaine to 20% solution to give 0.5% concentration of procaine. BAL is given as 10% solution in oil.
		Treatment:
	EDTA and BAL	1. In severe case (CNS involvement of 100 μg Pb/100 gm whole blood) give 4 mg/kg. BAL only as initial dose; follow after 4 hours, and every 4 hours for 3 to 4 days, with BAL and EDTA (12.5 mg/kg) at separate IM sites; skip 2 or 3 days and then treat again for 3 to 4 days. 2. In subacute case or 100 μg Pb/100 gm whole blood, give only 50 mg EDTA/kg/24 hours for 3 to 5 days.
	Penicillamine (Cuprimine, Merck & Co.)	3. May use after treatments either 1. or 2. with 100 mg/kg/day orally for 1 to 4 weeks.
	Thiamine HCl	Experimental for nervous signs; 5 mg/kg, IV, b.i.d., for 1 to 2 weeks; give slowly and watch for untoward reactions.
Metaldehyde	Diazepam (Valium, Roche)	2 to 5 mg/kg IV to control tremors.
	Triflupromazine	0.2 to 2.0 mg/kg IV.
	Pentobarbital	To effect.
Methanol and ethylene glycol	Ethanol	Give IV, 1.1 gm/kg (4.4 ml/kg) of 25% solution. Give 0.5 gm/kg (2.0 ml/kg) every 4 hours for 4 days. To prevent or correct acidosis use sodium bicarbonate IV, 0.4 gm/kg. Activated charcoal: 5 gm/kg orally if within 4 hours of ingestion.
Methemoglobinemia-producing agents (nitrites, chlorates)	Methylene blue	1% solution (maximum concentration), give by *slow* IV injection, 8.8 mg/kg; (0.9 ml/kg) repeat if necessary. To prevent fall in blood pressure in case of nitrite poisoning, use a sympathomimetic drug (ephedrine or epinephrine).
Morphine and related drugs	Naloxone chloride (Narcan, Endo)	0.1 mg/kg IV. Do not repeat if respiration is not satisfactory.
	Levallorphan tartrate (Lorfan, Roche)	Give IV, 0.1 to 0.5 ml of solution containing 1 mg/ml. NOTE: Use either of the above antidotes only in acute poisoning. Artificial repiration may be indicated. Activated charcoal is also indicated.
Oxalates	Calcium	Treatment: 23% solution of calcium gluconate IV. Give 3 to 20 ml (to control hypocalcemia).
Phenothiazine	Methylamphetamine (Desoxyn, Abbott)	0.1 to 0.2 mg/kg IV; also transfusion. Only available in tablet form.
	Diphenhydramine HCl	For CNS depression, 2 to 5 mg/kg IV for extrapyramidal signs.

Table continued on following page

Table 3. *Specific Systemic Antidotes and Dosages* Continued

Toxic Agent	Systemic Antidote	Dosage and Method for Treatment
Phytotoxins and botulin	Antitoxins not available commercially.	As indicated for specific antitoxins. Examples of phytotoxins: ricin, abrin, robin, crotin.
Plants		Treat signs as necessary.
Red squill	Atropine sulfate, propranolol, potassium chloride	As for digitalis glycosides poisoning, above.
Snake bite Rattlesnake Copperhead Water moccasin	Antivenin (Wyeth) (Trivalent Crotalidae)	Caution: equine origin.
Coral snake	(Wyeth)	Caution: equine origin.
Spider bite Black widow	Antivenin (Merck & Co.)	Caution: equine origin.
	Dantrolene sodium (Dantrium, Norwich-Eaton)	1 mg/kg IV. Followed by 1 mg/kg per os every 4 hours.
Strontium	Calcium salts	Usual dose of calcium borogluconate.
	Ammonium chloride	0.2 to 0.5 gm orally 3 to 4 times daily.
Strychnine and brucine	Pentobarbital	Give IV to effect; higher dose is usually required than that required for anesthesia. Place animal in warm, quiet room.
	Amobarbital	Give by slow IV; inject to effect. Duration of sedation is usually 4 to 6 hours.
	Methocarbamol (Robaxin, Robins)	10% solution; average first dose is 149 mg/kg IV (range: 40 to 300 mg). Repeat half dose as needed.
	Glyceryl quaiacolate (Geocolate, Summit Hill Labs)	110 mg/kg IV, 5% solution. Repeat as necessary.
	Diazepam (Valium, Roche)	2 to 5 mg/kg, control convulsions, induce emesis, then use other agents.
Thallium	Diphenylthiocarbazone	1. Dog: 70 mg/kg orally t.i.d. for 6 days. Hastens elimination but is partially toxic. or
	Prussian blue	2. 0.2 mg/kg orally in 3 divided doses daily.
	Potassium chloride	Give simultaneously with thiocarbazone or Prussian blue, 2 to 6 gm orally daily in divided doses.

metallic intoxications such as lead poisoning, the use of chelating agents has precipitated an acute metallic intoxication. Consequently, the dosage of chelating agents should be reduced in some chronic metal intoxications.

HASTENING ELIMINATION OF ABSORBED TOXICANTS

Absorbed toxicants are generally excreted via the kidneys. Some toxicants may be excreted by other routes (bile-feces, lung, other body secretions). Renal excretion can be manipulated in many instances. Urinary excretion of toxicants may be enhanced by the use of diuretics or altering the pH of the urine.

The use of diuretics to enhance urinary excretion of toxicants requires adequate renal function and hydration of the affected animal. Once these requisites are established, diuretics are indicated. Monitoring of urinary output is essential in these animals, and a minimum urinary flow of 0.1 ml/kg/minute is necessary. The diuretics of choice are mannitol and furosemide (Lasix, Hoechst-Roussel). Both of these agents are very potent diuretics. The dosage for mannitol is 2 gm/kg/hour and for furosemide is 5 mg/kg every 6 to 8 hours. Again, hydration must be maintained for proper renal excretion.

Alteration of urinary pH to expedite the excretion of toxicants and foreign chemicals is a classic pharmacologic technique. The technique relies on the physiochemical phenomenon that ionized compounds do not readily traverse cell membranes and hence are not reabsorbed by the renal tubules. Consequently, acid compounds such as acetylsalicylic acid (aspirin) and some barbiturates remain ionized in alkaline urine, and alkaline compounds such as amphetamines remain ionized in acidic urine. As a result, urinary excretion of many toxic compounds may be enhanced by modifying the urine pH. Urinary acidifying agents include ammonium chloride (200 mg/kg/day in divided doses) and ethylenediamine dihydrochloride (Chlorethamine [Pitman-Moore], 1 to 2 tablets t.i.d. for the average-sized dog). Sodium bicarbonate (5 mEq/kg/hour) may be used as an alkalinizing agent. (There are numerous human preparations available for acidifying or alkalinizing urine).

Peritoneal dialysis is indicated when an intoxicated animal exhibits oliguria or anuria. It is a rather time-consuming but effective technique in many conditions. The process of peritoneal dialysis involves the infusion of 10 to 20 ml/kg of a dialyzing solution into the peritoneal cavity, waiting the prescribed length of time, withdrawing the dialyzing solution, and reinfusing a fresh solution. The infusion and withdrawal cycles should be maintained for 12 to 24 hours or until normal renal function is restored. The pH of the dialyzing solutions may be altered to maintain the ionized state of the offending compound. (For additional information on peritoneal dialysis, see *Current Veterinary Therapy VIII*, pages 1028–1033).

SUPPORTIVE MEASURES

Supportive measures are very important in intoxications. These measures include control of body temperature, maintenance of respiratory and cardiovascular function, control of acid-base imbalances, alleviation of pain, and control of CNS disorders.

BODY TEMPERATURE CONTROL. Hypothermia may be controlled with the use of blankets and by keeping the animal in a warm, draft-free cage. Infrared lamps or heating pads should be used with caution and under constant observation. A pad with circulating warm water may be of greater value and is less dangerous than lamps or conventional heating pads. This type of pain is convenient for both emergency and surgical use (Aquamatic K Pad, American Hospital Supply).

Hyperthermia is controlled through the use of ice bags, cold water baths, cold water enemas, or cold peritoneal dialysis solution. Regardless of the type of temperature control required, it is vitally important that the animal's body temperature be constantly monitored to ensure that overcorrection does not occur.

RESPIRATORY SUPPORT MEASURES. Adequate respiratory support requires the presence of an adequate, patent airway, which may be obtained with either a cuffed endotracheal tube in an unconscious animal or a tracheostomy performed under local anesthesia. An emergency tracheostomy tube may be made from a cuffed endotracheal tube that has been shortened to reduce the dead space.

A respirator such as a Bird Respirator or Ohio Ventilator (Ohio Medical Products) is of great value in cases of respiratory depression; however, an anesthetic machine may be used with manual compression of the bag. A mixture of 50 per cent oxygen and 50 per cent room air is generally adequate unless there is a thickened respiratory membrane, in which case 100 per cent oxyen is necessary.

The use of analeptic drugs in cases of severe respiratory depression or apnea is questionable, owing to the short duration of their effects and to other undesirable side effects. Positive pressure ventilatory support is of greater value.

CARDIOVASCULAR SUPPORT. Cardiovascular support requires the presence of an adequate circulating volume, adequate cardiac performance, adequate tissue perfusion, and adequate acid-base balance. Volume and cardiac activity are of immediate concern; perfusion and acid-base balance, although of no lesser importance, are not of immediate concern.

In the presence of hypovolemia due to loss of both cells and volume, whole blood is the necessary agent. A good rule is to give a sufficient quantity of whole blood to raise the packed cell volume to 75 per cent of the animal's estimated normal level (minimum of 20 ml/kg).

Hypovolemia due to fluid loss alone can be treated with the administration of lactated Ringer's solution or plasma expanders. Central venous pressure should be monitored in these cases to prevent overloading the heart with too much volume too rapidly.

Tissue perfusion should also be monitored periodically to determine the adequacy of the replacement therapy. In some cases it may be necessary to administer massive doses of IV corticosteroids to restore adequate tissue perfusion (dexamethasone [Azium, Schering], 2 to 10 mg/kg). Caution should be exercised in the use of these steroids since hypovolemia may ensue. Therefore, large IV doses of corticosteroids should never be administered unless volume replacement therapy is ongoing.

Cardiac activity can be aided by the application of closed-chest cardiac massage for immediate requirements, but the administration of pharmaceutical agents that can stimulate inotropic and chronotropic activity must also be undertaken in most instances. One of these agents is calcium gluconate, infused very slowly IV. This agent is also reported to be a good nonspecific treatment in many toxicities. Other agents include glucagon, 25 to 50 μg/kg, IV, and digoxin, 0.02 to 0.04 mg/kg, IV. Care must be taken to avoid overdosage with cardioactive agents, since they are highly toxic to the myocardium. The electric activity of the heart should be closely monitored during administration of cardioactive agents.

ACID-BASE IMBALANCE. Control of acid-base balance problems is primarily a matter of physiologically maintaining an animal in a homeostatic condition. The most common acid-base disturbance seen in animals is acidosis, mainly of metabolic origin. However, acidosis or alkalosis may occur in cases of intoxication.

In correcting acidosis not of respiratory origin, sodium bicarbonate, administered IV at a dosage rate of 2 to 4 mEq/kg every 15 minutes, is the drug of choice. Other alkalinizing solutions including 1/6 molar sodium lactate, 16 to 32 ml/kg; lactated Ringer's solution, 120 ml/kg; or tromethamine (THAM) buffer, 300 mg/kg. Bicarbonate is generally the easiest to administer with respect to volume and requires no metabolic conversion. Caution must be exercised with all alkalinizing agents to avoid the induction of alkalosis.

Alkalosis, unless drug-induced, does not generally occur in animals. However, if alkalosis is present, the IV administration of 0.9 per cent sodium chloride (physiologic saline), 10 ml/kg, is usually sufficient for initial therapy. This should be followed by the oral administration of ammonium chloride, 200 mg/kg/day in divided doses. As in the case of acidosis, the clinician should be cautioned about overtreatment of the alkalotic patient.

PAIN CONTROL. Another important supportive measure in cases of intoxications is the control of pain. A minimal dose of morphine (dogs, 1 to 2 mg/kg; cats, 0.1 to 0.2 mg/kg) or meperidine (Demerol, Winthrop) (dogs, 5 to 10 mg/kg; cats, 1 to 2 mg/kg) is indicated in animals showing pain as a result of intoxication.

CENTRAL NERVOUS SYSTEM (CNS) DISORDERS. Management of CNS disorders in cases of intoxication is simple in appearance but complex in actuality. The type of therapy will depend on the presence of depression or hyperactivity. Either disorder can easily be turned into the opposite problem by overzealous therapeutic measures.

CNS Depression. CNS depression can also be considered respiratory depression, since the management of the two conditions is very similar. Although the IV administration of analeptic agents such as doxapram (Dopram, Robins), 3 to 5 mg/kg; or pentylenetetrazol (Metrazol, Knoll), 6 to 10 mg/kg is reported to be efficacious in these conditions, their actions are short-lived, and CNS depression can return if animals are not monitored continuously. Another disadvantage is that analeptics can also induce convulsions. Artificial respiration or respiratory support is of greater value in animals exhibiting CNS depression and is the treatment of choice for most CNS depression syndromes.

CNS Hyperactivity. Cases of CNS hyperactivity including convulsions can be managed by the administration of CNS depressants or tranquilizers. Pentobarbital sodium is generally the agent of choice for convulsions and hyperactivity. Care must be taken, since in many cases a respiratory depressing dose may be required to alleviate the signs. In these cases, respiratory support is mandatory. Inhalant anesthetics have been reported as excellent for long-term management of CNS hyperactivity, but this removes the anesthetic machine from surgery-room use for extended periods. Central-acting skeletal muscle relaxants and minor tranquilizers have been reported for use with convulsant intoxicants. Some of these include methocarbamol (Robaxin, Robins), 110 mg/kg, IV; glyceryl guaiacolate (Gecolate, Summit Hill Labs), 110 mg/kg IV; and diazepam (Valium, Roche), 0.5 to 1.5 mg/kg IV or IM. In other cases of CNS stimulation due to amphetamines and some hallucinogens such as lysergic acid diethylamide (LSD) and phencyclidine, phenothiazine tranquilizers have produced adequate control. Regardless of the regimen of therapy for CNS hyperactivity, the animals should be placed in a quiet, dark room to prevent additional stimulation due to auditory or visual stimuli.

POISON CONTROL CENTERS AND DIAGNOSTIC LABORATORIES

Poison Control Centers and Animal Diagnostic laboratories can be of great value to the clinician in cases of suspected intoxications, especially when labels or containers are presented with the acutely ill animal. *When the suspected compound and the signs exhibited by the animal do not concur, the signs should be treated and the label should be disregarded.*

The diagnosis should be confirmed by chemical analysis, even though this may occur after the fact. An accurate diagnosis, as well as detailed records, may help the veterinarian faced with subsequent cases from the same intoxicant. Detailed records will also be invaluable considerations in any medicolegal proceedings.

References and Supplemental Reading

Doull, J., Klaassen, C. D., and Amdur, M. O. (eds.): *Cassarett and Doulls Toxicology, The Basic Science of Poisons,* 2nd ed. New York: MacMillan, 1980.

Oehme, F. W. (ed.): Symposium in clinical toxocology for the small animal practitioner. Vet. Clin. North Am. 5:737, 1975.

Osweiler, G. D., Carson, T. L., Buck, W. B., and VanGelder, G. A., *Clinical and Diagnostic Veterinary Toxicology,* 3rd ed., Dubuque, IA: Kendall/Hunt, 1984.

LEAD POISONING

DAVID F. KOWALCZYK, V.M.D.
St. Louis, Missouri

Lead poisoning in humans has been recognized for thousands of years and has been implicated in such historic events as the decline of ancient Rome. The association of lead with clinical disease has been extremely difficult to make in the past, owing to the ubiquitous nature of lead in the environment.

Lead poisoning in animals has probably occurred since its recognition in humans, but only in the last 35 years have cases been well documented. Many of these cases were diagnosed postmortem. It was not until 1969 that the significance of lead poisoning in dogs was clearly recognized. Zook and associates (1972) reported that 1 of every 25 dogs less than 6 months of age hospitalized at the Angell Memorial Animal Hospital (Boston) had been poisoned by lead. In 1970, the hospital diagnosed 107 canine cases of lead toxicity.

At the School of Veterinary Medicine in Philadelphia, lead poisoning was rarely diagnosed until the availability of an in-house blood-lead testing service in 1973. It is now the most common toxicity reported in dogs and cats.

The increased incidence of lead poisoning in dogs in the past few years has been the result of intensive screening programs and is not due to an actual increase in exposure to lead. The fault is not with the clinician's ability but with the nonspecific signs displayed during the early stages of lead poisoning (i.e., vomiting and anorexia). The most difficult aspect of lead poisoning is establishing the diagnosis.

ABSORPTION, DISTRIBUTION, AND EXCRETION OF LEAD

The most common route of entry of lead is through the gastrointestinal tract. Inhaled lead particles are cleared by ciliary action and are swallowed. In adult dogs and humans, approximately 10 per cent of ingested lead is absorbed. However, in young animals, as much as 90 per cent can be absorbed. The interaction of many nutritional factors with the bioavailability of lead has been well documented. An enhancement of lead absorption has been demonstrated with dietary deficiencies of calcium, zinc, iron, and protein. Lead dissolves at a much faster rate in an acid environment, such as the stomach, which thus enhances absorption. In bottom-feeding waterfowl, the ingestion of one to three shotgun pellets (which tend to remain in the gizzard) can be lethal.

Once the lead has been absorbed, it is carried by the red blood cells and distributed in the soft tissue. Over 90 per cent of the circulating lead is in the red blood cells. The presence of lead in the liver, kidney, central nervous system, and bone marrow causes the major signs of lead toxicity. Eventually, the lead redistributes to the bone, where it is biologically inert. However, this stored pool of lead may be mobilized if bone demineralization occurs (e.g., in acidosis or calcium deficiency) and can cause toxicity. The penetration of lead across the blood-brain barrier occurs more readily in the immature organism, accounting for the higher incidence of severe neurologic signs in the young animal. Lead can also cross the placenta and enter the mother's milk.

Lead is excreted very slowly from the whole body, predominantly in bile. The enterohepatic circulation of lead in lead poisoning is not known. The elimination of lead through urine is minor unless chelating agents are being used (e.g., calcium disodium edetate [CaEDTA]).

The measurement of blood lead can fluctuate greatly, depending on time of exposure, and it may not reflect tissue lead concentrations or the extent of lead toxicity. This is probably the reason for the poor correlation between blood-lead levels and severity of clinical signs in dogs. Therefore, blood lead should not be the sole criterion in screening animals for lead exposure.

SOURCES OF LEAD

The sources of lead are varied and numerous, the most common being lead-containing paint. Interiors of dwellings painted before 1940 often contain layers of lead-based paint. Leaded paints are sometimes mistakenly used indoor and thus may be accessible to dogs in new as well as old dwellings. Exteriors of buildings (including doghouses) are frequently covered with lead paint, as are fences and painting materials. The lead salts in paint impart a sweet taste; thus their attractiveness to animals. Soil and vegetation may be contaminated with lead as a result of the weathering of lead pigments from painted structures.

Other sources of lead include linoleum, batteries, plumbing materials, putty, lead foil, solder, golf balls, certain roof coverings, lubricants, rug pads, acid (soft) drinking water from lead pipes or improperly glazed ceramic water bowls, and lead weights or objects such as fishing sinkers, drapery weights, and toys. Soil along streets and roadways may contain small amounts of lead from automobile exhaust fumes. Soil contaminated with lead from paint or auto exhausts is not a likely source of poisoning, but it may contribute somewhat to the total body burden of lead. Lead bullets that are present subcutaneously or in muscle tissue usually become encapsulated and biologically inert.

The history may or may not suggest exposure to lead. Recent remodeling of dwellings—especially old dilapidated houses—including removal of old paint, plaster, or linoleum or application of new lead-based paints is a common history. Remember that in cases displaying only mild gastrointestinal signs, the history may be the sole clue.

AGE

Lead poisoning may occur at any age, but most affected dogs are between 2 and 8 months of age. Teething and the bizarre appetites of young dogs result in the gnawing on and ingestion of strange substances.

CLINICAL SIGNS

Clinicals signs of lead poisoning in dogs are associated with the gastrointestinal and nervous systems. Usually both systems are clinically involved, but sometimes only one is. Very often, gastrointestinal signs are present for several days before the dog is examined, and they usually precede the neurologic signs. Such clinical signs in young dogs have led to erroneous diagnosis of canine distemper.

The most common gastrointestinal signs are vomiting, abdominal pain, and anorexia. Diarrhea and constipation are less frequently observed. The presence of abdominal pain or "lead colic" is manifested by whining, restlessness, tensing of abdominal muscles, and crying when the abdomen is palpated. Many gastrointestinal upsets display the foregoing signs, but one should suspect lead toxicity if they persist for more than 3 days. Occasionally, megaesophagus has been associated with lead poisoning and is probably the result of esophageal paralysis.

The most common neurologic signs in order of frequency are convulsions, hysteria (characterized by barking and crying continuously, running in every direction, and indiscriminately biting at animate and inanimate objects), and other behavioral changes. Other neurologic signs are ataxia, blindness, and champing of the jaws. Many dogs with hysteria or convulsions have increased rectal temperatures that decrease after the episode subsides.

The need for recognition of subtle neurologic deficits such as learning impairments, hyperactivity, and loss of visual discrimination during and after exposure to lead has only recently been appreciated. One investigation demonstrated residual neurologic deficits in sheep that were exposed to low levels of lead that never produced toxic blood-lead levels (Van Gelder et al., 1973).

Differential diagnoses, based on history and clinical signs, include canine distemper, epilepsy, intestinal parasitism, hypoglycemia, nonspecific gastrointestinal disturbance, acute pancreatitis, encephalitis, vertebral problems, rabies, and other poisonings. Because of the high incidence of canine distemper in young dogs, the occurrence of convulsions with or without typical signs is usually attributed to canine distemper. However, recent investigations have found many of these cases to be the result of lead poisoning.

LABORATORY FINDINGS

One of the most helpful screening tests for the diagnosis of lead poisoning, without resorting to a quantitative test for lead, is examination of a stained blood smear. Of prime importance is the finding of large numbers of nucleated erythrocytes (5 to 40/100 white blood cells) without evidence of severe anemia-packed cell volume less than 30 per cent. This is considered to be nearly pathognomonic of lead poisoning. The nucleated erythrocytes are a relatively easy cell type to identify regardless of the staining procedure.

Other common abnormalities in red blood cell morphology are anisocytosis, polychromasia, poikilocytosis, target cells, and hypochromasia. The presence of basophilic stippling in red blood cells is another common feature, but detection depends on the staining procedure. One investigation at Angell Memorial Animal Hospital reported basophilic stipping in 94 per cent of lead-poisoned dogs (Zook et al., 1970); however, stippling was found in 42 per cent of dogs with other problems.

Red blood cell abnormalities usually precede clinical signs except in very acute poisoning. Once chelation therapy has been started, these changes disappear quickly.

Moderate numbers of nucleated red blood cells may be found in some dogs with marked and prolonged anemias—e.g., autoimmune hemolytic anemia. Older dogs that have visceral hemangiosarcomas are usually anemic and have numerous nucleated red blood cells but few or no stippled red blood cells.

The leukocyte counts are usually elevated because of a neutrophilic leukocytosis. It is important to correct the white blood cell count for the presence of nucleated erythrocytes; otherwise, exaggerated white blood cell counts will result.

Results of other laboratory tests, such as blood urea nitrogen, creatinine, transaminase, amylase, blood glucose, sedimentation rate, and Coombs' test, are normal. Bone marrow examination discloses an increase of erythroid elements. Elevated reticulocyte counts and the finding of many immature red blood cells in peripheral blood smears indicate early release of erythroid cells from the hyperplastic bone marrow. The urine usually contains granular casts. Often, mild proteinuria and sometimes glycosuria are found. The cerebrospinal fluid may have a normal pressure, protein, and cell content.

Other tests that have become very useful in human lead poisoning are related to detection of abnormalities in heme synthesis. The interference of lead at several enzymatic steps has proved to be a most sensitive indicator of biologic change. The accumulation of various substrates, such as aminolevulinic acid (in urine) and zinc protoporphyrin (in red blood cells), is commonly used as a screening test in high-risk children and lead-exposed workers. These tests reflect the presence and severity of lead poisoning. The substrate levels stay elevated despite fluctuations in blood-lead level. The concentration of zinc protoporphyrin has been shown to increase severalfold in cases of chronic lead poisoning in the horse, cow, and rabbit. However, in experimentally lead-poisoned dogs, the appearance of clinical signs was not well correlated with an increase in zinc protoporphyrin. This suggests that the sensitivity of dogs to lead is not reflected in porphyrin metabolism.

RADIOGRAPHIC FINDINGS

The most helpful radiographic finding is the presence of diffuse radiopaque material in the gastrointestinal tract. This material was found in more than 60 per cent of the cases at the University of Pennsylvania. However, it should be emphasized that it is impossible to differentiate these radiodensities from bone chips or gravel. It is important to radiograph the animal, since chelation therapy has been shown to enhance intestinal absorption of lead.

The metaphyses of long bones may develop lead lines (metaphyseal sclerosis) in immature dogs. These radiopaque bands are best seen just proximal to the open epiphyses of the distal radius, ulna, and metacarpal bones. This is due to the incorporation of lead at the site of endochondral ossification, which stimulates active bone formation, causing a dense zone of mineralized cartilage. The lead lines are mainly the result of new bone formation and not the deposition of lead. Similar radiographic changes are reported in phosphorus and vitamin D intoxication.

The presence of lead lines is a difficult interpretation to make, even for radiologists and, as a diagnostic tool, has not been useful at our hospital.

DIAGNOSIS

Since the clinical signs of lead poisoning are not pathognomonic, a history detailing likelihood of exposure or the finding of many nucleated erythrocytes without anemia may be the first clue. Blood may be taken for lead analysis to confirm the diagnosis, but treatment for lead poisoning should be started.

The analysis of whole blood is the best single index for establishing a definitive diagnosis. Many laboratories can now perform a lead analysis with less than 2 ml of whole, oxalated, or heparinized blood in a clean, lead-free vial. However, it is wise to contact the laboratory personnel directly to find the minimum volume required as it is usually less than the amount stated in their brochure. Versenate (EDTA) anticoagulant interferes with some methods. The finding of 60 μg or more of lead/100 ml of blood (0.6 ppm) is virtually diagnostic of lead poisoning in dogs. Blood-lead values of 30 to 50 μg/100 ml (0.3 to 0.5 ppm) are abnormally high and indicate lead poisoning if associated with typical signs and hematologic findings. Baseline levels for lead range between 5 and 25 μg/100 ml (0.05 to 0.25 ppm). The small difference between background and toxic blood-lead levels make interpretation of this test difficult at the lower levels. The severity of clinical signs may not be correlated with blood-lead content.

For postmortem confirmation, analysis of liver for lead is the best diagnostic test. The upper limit of normal is 3.5 ppm (wet weight); 5 ppm or more is virtually diagnostic. Samples of hair or feces or single specimens of urine for lead analysis are not recommended. Urine specimens taken just before and 24 hours after starting chelation therapy (Ca-EDTA, at the dosage administered for regular treatment) disclose a 10- to 60-fold increase in urine lead output in dogs with lead poisoning. Although this test is reliable, it is expensive and time-consuming, and it is difficult to obtain the specimens.

TREATMENT

The purposes of therapy in lead poisoning are to (1) remove lead, if present, from the gastrointestinal tract so that further absorption is prevented, (2) remove lead from the blood and body tissues rapidly, and (3) alleviate marked neurologic signs.

Lead should be removed from the gastrointestinal tract prior to chelation therapy with enemas and emetics, as chelating agents can enhance the absorption of lead from the intestines. Magnesium sulfate (Epsom salt) is a good choice, since it will precipitate lead (as $PbSO_4$) and prevent further absorption during transit; it also possesses cathartic action. Large objects in the stomach may require surgery.

Many pet birds or waterfowl that have ingested lead objects will retain the lead material in their ventriculus (gizzard) for extended periods, during which time lead is continuously being released and absorbed. A ventriculotomy is often necessary. However, the surgery may be delayed until the bird's condition improves with chelation therapy.

Chelating agents effectively remove heavy metals such as lead by forming nontoxic complexes with the metals that are rapidly excreted via the bile or urine. The chelating agent of choice is CaEDTA, which has been shown to be effective in treating lead poisoning in a wide variety of animals. CaEDTA must be administered as the calcium chelate to prevent hypocalcemia. The need to purchase the calcium disodium salt (Calcium Disodium Versenate, Riker) cannot be overemphasized because the disodium salt (Disodium Versenate, Riker) carries a similar name and is available from the same company. This matter is further complicated by the various abbreviations and names given to CaEDTA. The calcium disodium salt preparation is available for human use as a 20 per cent solution in 5-ml ampules (total of 1 gm) and for horses as a 6.6 per cent solution in 500-ml bottles (Havidote, Haver-Lockhart) (total of 33 gm). The larger volume is more economical in very large dogs. Since no preservatives are added, fractional contents should not be saved for future cases.

CaEDTA is given at the rate of 100 mg/kg body weight daily for 2 to 5 days. The daily dose is divided into four equal portions and administered SC after dilution to a concentration of about 10 mg CaEDTA/ml of 5 per cent dextrose solution. High concentrations of CaEDTA can cause painful reactions at injection sites.

The use of CaEDTA has been extremely effective, with clinical improvement within 24 to 48 hours. Dogs that respond slowly or that have a pretreatment blood-lead level of more than 100 μg/100 ml (1.0 ppm) may need a second 5-day treatment 5 days after completion of the first series. This second treatment prevents recurrence of clinical signs, provided the dog is not allowed to consume more lead after discharge from the hospital. Monitoring blood lead during treatment is not valuable, as the concentration of lead does not correlate with alleviation of clinical signs. There is a rapid drop in blood-lead for 1 to 3 days, depending on the initial concentration, but then it will remain constant in spite of continued therapy and may remain in the toxic range. This is probably due to inability of CaEDTA to cross cell membranes. It is much more important to evaluate the animal's clinical condition than rely on blood-lead values. However, a blood-lead determination 2 to 3 weeks after cessation of chelation therapy can be of benefit in assessing the success of the chelation therapy or in indicating reexposure to lead.

CaEDTA is relatively safe, but continuous therapy should be limited to regimens of 5 days and the daily dose should not exceed 2 gm because of potential nephrotoxicosis. CaEDTA can produce acute necrotizing nephrosis of proximal convoluted tubules that is reversible; however, the renal changes appear to be more severe in rats and human patients. In the dog, CaEDTA causes depression and gastrointestinal signs (e.g., vomiting, diarrhea) that precede the renal changes. Since the gastrointestinal signs of CaEDTA toxicosis are probably similar in most species to those of lead poisoning, only the renal changes were ascribed to CaEDTA toxicosis. The signs of toxicosis are probably related to the chelation of trace metals, most notably zinc. The use of the zinc salt of EDTA (not commercially available) instead of the calcium salt protects the animal from the gastrointestinal effects. Therefore, the dogs with gastrointestinal signs of CaEDTA toxicosis, zinc supplementation may be of benefit.

Penicillamine, an oral chelation agent of proven value in treating lead-poisoned children, offers promise for dogs. Penicillamine, given orally, has a distinct advantage over CaEDTA, which must be repeatedly injected SC, requiring hospitalization. Clinical trials to date indicate that penicillamine is effective in promoting urinary excretion of lead and alleviating clinical signs.

Penicillamine should be given at 110 mg/kg body weight daily for 1- to 2-week courses separated by 1-week intervals. Penicillamine is available as 250-mg scored tablets (Depen Titratabs, Wallace) or in 125-mg capsules (Cupramine, Merck & Co.) The drug should be given to the patient when the stomach is empty to prevent chelation of dietary metals. The daily dose can be divided and given at 6- or 8-hour intervals to prevent some of the adverse effects, such as vomiting, listlessness, and partial anorexia. Antiemetic drugs (e.g., phenothiazines and antihistamines) have been of benefit when given ½ to 1 hour before the dose of penicillamine. Lower doses (33 to 55 mg/kg daily) seem to be better tolerated by the dog and may be just as efficacious in eliminating body stores of lead. The contents of the capsules may be dissolved in fruit juice (penicillamine is stable in acid pH) for ease of administration. At present, penicillamine can be recommended for dogs that are not seriously ill or that do not have marked neurologic disorders or persistent vomiting. If an owner refuses to hospitalize the dog, penicillamine can be prescribed; however, the owner should be warned that side effects may occur and that lead ingested while on treatment is apt to be absorbed more completely than it would be without treatment.

It seems that penicillamine might also be beneficial in combination with CaEDTA. It may be that CaEDTA needs to be given for only a few days, followed by penicillamine. This regimen should assure adequate hydration, promote renal function, and help reduce the care and cost of treatment. Penicillamine might also be useful in treating dogs that recovered slowly from a 5-day course of CaEDTA or that had an initial blood-lead of more than 100 μg/100 ml (1.0 ppm) and therefore should be treated again.

Dimercaprol (BAL; Hynson, Westcott & Dunning) has been used successfully in combination with CaEDTA in children. It has seldom been used in lead-poisoned animals. However, it does offer the advantages of removing lead directly from red blood cells and excreting lead primarily via the bile (important if renal function is compromised).

SUPPORTIVE TREATMENT

The gastrointestinal signs (e.g., vomiting, diarrhea, anorexia) do not usually require specific drug therapy because they subside quickly after chelation therapy. However, the severe neurologic signs (e.g., convulsions) are due to cerebral edema and thus require immediate attention. Mannitol and dexamethasone are the agents of choice. Seizures and hysteria can be controlled with diazepam, pentobarbital, or both, delivered IV. Permanent mental deficiencies and recurrent seizures are common sequelae of lead poisoning in children. Thus, it seems appropriate to treat lead encephalopathy in dogs as well, because these drugs not only appear to speed clinical recovery but may also prevent permanent brain damage.

PROGNOSIS

The prognosis in the majority of lead poisoning cases that undergo chelation therapy is favorable, with a dramatic improvement in 24 to 48 hours. Chelation therapy may thus be used as a diagnostic tool in cases of high suspicion when a blood-lead determination is impractical or delayed. Prognoses in cases treated promptly and adequately depend on the degree and duration of neurologic involvement and, to a lesser extent, the amount of lead found in the blood. Continuous or uncontrolled convulsions warrant an unfavorable prognosis. Dogs with 100 μg or more of lead/100 ml of blood tend to recover slowly, and signs may recur if a second course of therapy is not given. If there are no neurologic signs or if they are mild or readily controlled by ancillary treatment, the prognosis is favorable.

The prognosis in untreated cases that are only displaying gastrointestinal signs may be favorable if further exposure to lead is prevented. If the economic situation does not permit treatment with CaEDTA, a course of oral penicillamine may be advantageous.

PATHOLOGIC FINDINGS

Gross necropsy findings are generally not remarkable; however, careful examination may reveal chips of paint or other lead-containing substances in the gastrointestinal tract. White bands are sometimes found in transversely sectioned metaphyses of immature dogs. Microscopic study may disclose acid-fast intranuclear inclusion bodies in renal proximal tubular cells and less often in hepatocytes. These inclusions are essentially pathognomonic of lead poisoning but are not found in all cases. Lesions in the brain include degenerative changes in small vessels, hemorrhages, laminar necrosis, and proliferation of capillaries and gliosis in chronic encephalopathies.

VETERINARIAN'S OBLIGATION

Animals may manifest signs of toxicity before humans when they are sharing the same environment. Birds have been used for years in mines as sensitive indicators of toxic gas accumulation. In the 1953 mercury poisoning outbreak in Japan, cats were dying a year before the disease was recognized in humans. For detecting lead poisoning, young dogs seem to be the most appropriate animals for screening because they share the same environment and have eating habits (e.g., pica) similar to those of children. A recent study from Illinois indicated that an abnormally high blood-lead level in a family dog increased the probability sixfold of finding a child in the same family with an increased blood-lead level. At the University of Pennsylvania Veterinary School, owners with lead-poisoned dogs were advised to have children between 1 and 5 years of age checked for lead poisoning. A few children had blood-lead levels in the toxic range, even though they were not showing gross clinical signs.

When diagnosing canine lead poisoning to owners with small children, we strongly urge veterinarians to warn the family or family physician adequately. Most urban centers have free clinics for testing children for lead.

LEAD POISONING IN OTHER PETS

Cats are rarely poisoned by lead because, unlike dogs, they are very selective eaters and seldom gnaw on or ingest nonfood substances. Therefore, they are not subject to most sources of lead. Because of their fastidious fur-cleaning habits, however, they may ingest lead-containing dusts or other substances that contaminate their coat.

Parrots may pick at and ingest peeling paint or, if the bars of their cages are painted, they may ingest the paint while clambering about or trimming their beaks. Numerous pet and zoo parrots are known to have died of lead poisoning. In Amazon parrots, hemoglobinuria associated with intravascular hemolysis has been associated with lead poisoning. Any curious pet with indiscriminate eating habits and exposure to lead is a likely candidate for lead intoxication.

References and Supplemental Reading

Calle, P. P., Kowalczyk, D. F., Dein, F. J., and Hartman, F. E.: Effect of hunter's switch from lead to steel shot on potential for oral lead poisoning in ducks. J.A.V.M.A. 181:1299, 1982.

Carson, T. L., Van Gelder, G. A., Buck, W. B., and Hoffman, L. J.: Effects of low level lead ingestion in sheep. Clin. Toxicol 6:389, 1973.

Center, S. A.: Suspected calcium EDTA intoxication in a dog. J.A.V.M.A. 183:884, 1983.

Clarke, E. G. C.: Lead poisoning in small animals. J. Small Anim. Pract. 14:183, 1973.

Finley, M. T., Dieter, M. P., and Locke, L. N.: Lead in tissues of mallard ducks dosed with two types of lead shot. Bull. Environ. Contam. Toxicol. 16:261, 1976.

Galvin, C.: Acute hemorrhagic syndrome of birds. *In* Kirk, R. E. (ed.): *Current Veterinary Therapy VIII*. Philadelphia: W. B. Saunders Co., 1983, pp. 617–619.

Kowalczyk, D. F.: Lead poisoning in dogs at the University of Pennsylvania Veterinary Hospital. J.A.V.M.A. 168:428, 1976.

Kowalczyk, D. F.: Clinical management of lead poisoning J.A.V.M.A. 184:858, 1984.

Pennumarthy, L., Oehme, F. W., and Galitzer, S. J.: Effects of chronic oral lead administration in young beagle dogs. J. Environ. Pathol. Toxicol. 3:465, 1980.

Schunk, K. L.: Lead poisoning in dogs. Small Anim. Vet. Med. Update 8:2, 1978.

Thomas, C. W., Rising, J. L., and Moore, J. K.: Blood lead concentrations of children and dogs from 83 Illinois families. J.A.V.M.A. 169:1237, 1976.

Van Gelder, G. A., Carson, T. L., Smith, R. M., Buck, W. B., and Karas, G. G.: Neurophysiologic and behavioral toxicologic testing to detect subclinical neurologic alterations induced by environmental toxicants. J.A.V.M.A. 163:1033, 1973.

Zook, B. C., Carpenter, J. L., and Leeds, E. B.: Lead poisoning in dogs. J.A.V.M.A. 155:1329, 1969.

Zook, B. C., Kopito, L., Carpenter, J. L., Cramer, D. V., and Schwachman, H.: Lead poisoning in dogs: Analysis of blood, urine, hair, and liver for lead. Am. J. Vet. Res. 33:903, 1972.

Zook, B. C., McConnell, G., and Gilmore, C. E.: Basophilic stippling of erythrocyes in dogs with special reference to lead poisoning. J.A.V.M.A. 157:2092, 1970.

ORGANOPHOSPHATE AND CARBAMATE INSECTICIDE POISONING

THOMAS L. CARSON, D.V.M.

Ames, Iowa

Organophosphate (OP) and carbamate insecticides have been widely employed for control of external parasites on companion animals and livestock, for eradication of insect pests in the home and garden, and as agricultural insecticides for crop production. Some of these compounds can be acutely toxic and may represent a potential hazard to companion animals.

Spilled or improperly stored insecticides, whether in the basement, garage, or farmstead, present a hazard of poisoning to companion animals. Dogs and cats have lapped up liquid concentrates and diluted sprays as well as dry powders and granules intended for home and garden applications. Farm dogs have been poisoned by eating granules of insecticide spilled on the ground or in farm vehicles. Leftover or improperly discarded insecticide preparations have also caused poisoning.

Miscalculation of insecticide concentrations in spraying or dipping procedure for external parasite control have also resulted in toxicosis. Susceptibility differences between species may also exist. For example, cats may be poisoned by some compounds that are used routinely on dogs. Consequently, label directions for the particular preparation should be followed carefully.

Re-treating animals with either dermal or oral OP or carbamate preparations within a few days may result in poisoning of these animals. In addition, some animals may be predisposed to poisoning because of concurrent or previous treatment with some cholinesterase-inhibiting anthelmintics, flea collars, or phenothiazine tranquilizers.

MECHANISM OF ACTION

The OP and carbamate insecticides are discussed together because their mechanisms of action are similar.

Cholinergic nerves utilize acetylcholine as a neurotransmitter substance. Under normal conditions, acetylcholine released at parasympathetic synapses and myoneural junctions is quickly hydrolyzed by cholinesterase enzymes. When the hydrolyzing enzmes are inhibited, the continued presence of acetylcholine maintains a state of nerve stimulation and accounts for the clinical signs observed with poisoning from these insecticides. In general, inhibition of these enzymes by the OP insecticides tends to be irreversible, whereas inhibition by the carbamates is reversible.

CLINICAL SIGNS

Acute clinical poisoning produced by the OP and carbamate insecticides is similar in all species of animals. In general it is characterized by overstimulation of the parasympathetic nervous system and skeletal muscles, with variable involvement of the central nervous system (CNS). Onset of clinical signs in cases of acute poisoning may occur as soon as a few minutes or as late as several hours after exposure.

The earliest signs of acute cholinesterase-inhibitor poisoning in dogs is often increased body stretching, an apparent early indication of skeletal muscle involvement. A state of uneasiness or apprehension may also be observed early in the course of the illness. Increased salivation usually occurs at this time, but excess saliva may not be apparent because the dog is quite efficient at licking its lips and swallowing the excess secretions.

As the condition progresses, increased skeletal muscle tone becomes more pronounced and may be the only clinical sign observed at this time. The affected animal may walk with a stiff-legged gait, and marked muscle tremors may be observed. Urination, defecation, and emesis may also occur.

In advanced toxicosis, slobbering may become evident. The excess saliva, together with increased secretions in the respiratory system, often accounts for coughing and pronounced moist rales. Depending on the severity of the syndrome, dyspnea and cyanosis can follow. Hypermotility of the gastrointestinal tract may result in diarrhea, abdominal cramps, and straining. Excessive lacrimation, sweating, miosis, and urinary incontinence can be observed. Hyperactivity of skeletal muscles is generally followed by muscle paralysis, as the muscles are unable to respond to continued stimulation.

Dogs and cats generally exhibit marked depression of the CNS. Increased CNS stimulation, leading to tonoclonic convulsive seizures, is possible but has been infrequently observed by the author.

Death usually results from hypoxia due to excessive respiratory tract secretions, bronchoconstriction, and erratic, slowed heartbeat. In severe poisoning, death can occur at any time from a few minutes to several hours after the first clinical signs are observed.

NECROPSY LESIONS

Postmortem lesions associated with acute OP or carbamate toxicosis are usually nonspecific. Excessive fluids in the mouth and respiratory tract as well as pulmonary edema may be observed.

DIAGNOSIS

A history of exposure to OP or carbamate insecticides associated with clinical signs of parasympathetic and skeletal muscle stimulation warrants a tentative diagnosis of poisoning with these compounds.

Chemical analyses of animal tissues to detect the presence of these insecticides are usually unrewarding because of the rapid degradation of the OP and carbamate insecticides, resulting in low tissue residue levels. A recent study showed that detecting degradation products of OP insecticides in the urine may help establish a diagnosis. Finding the insecticide in the stomach contents and in the suspect source material can be quite valuable in establishing a diagnosis.

An important part of confirming a diagnosis is to assess the degree of inhibition of cholinesterase enzyme activity in the whole blood or tissue of the affected animal. A reduction of whole blood cholinesterase activity to less than 25 per cent of normal is indicative of excessive exposure to these insecticides. Depending on the specific insecticide involved, blood cholinesterase activity in dogs may remain depressed for several days to several weeks after OP exposure. Some cholinesterase depression is an expected finding after routine application of these types of insecticides to dogs and cats. The variability of cholinesterase enzyme activity levels in clinically normal dogs may make interpretation of laboratory values difficult. In addition, depletion of whole blood cholinesterase activity may not necessarily represent inhibition of cholinesterase at the parasympathetic synapses and myoneural junctions. Therefore, whole blood cholinesterase activity should be viewed only as an indication of the status of the cholinesterase enzymes in the body.

Cholinesterase activity can also be measured in brain tissue. Although the enzyme activity in brain tissue of animals dying from these insecticides will generally be less than 10 per cent of normal activity, there is some variability here too, depending on the specific insecticide. For example, when dogs were dosed with fenthion, brain cholinesterase activity was depressed to 30 per cent of normal but clinical signs of poisoning were not observed (Sundlof et al., 1984).

For best laboratory results, whole blood and brain tissue samples should be well chilled or frozen before submission. A sagittal half of the brain should be submitted, as laboratories vary in the portion of the brain used in the cholinesterase determination. Samples of stomach contents as well as any suspect material should be frozen and submitted to a laboratory for chemical analyses.

TREATMENT

Poisoning of animals by OP and carbamate insecticides represents an emergency because of the rapid progression of the clinical syndrome.

Initial treatment of poisoned animals should involve control of parasympathetic signs by administration of atropine sulfate at a dosage of approximately 0.2 mg/kg body weight. For the fastest response, the initial dose should be divided, with about one fourth of the dose given IV and the balance SC or IM. Atropine sulfate does not counteract the insecticide-enzyme bond but rather blocks the effects of accumulated acetylcholine at the nerve endings. Repeated doses of atropine at approximately one half of the initial dose may be required but should be used *only* to counteract parasympathetic signs. Atropine effects usually persist for 4 to 6 hours. Excessive atropinization should be avoided. Further treatment or handling should be withheld for several minutes or until respiratory distress has been alleviated.

Although a dramatic cessation of parasympathetic signs is generally observed within a few minutes after administration of atropine, skeletal muscle tremors will not be relieved. Some control of these tremors may be achieved by using diphenhydramine (Benadryl, Parke-Davis) at 4 mg/kg body weight, every 8 hours orally (Clemmons et al., 1984).

Clinical OP poisoning may also be complicated by systemic acidosis (Cordoba et al., 1983). IV sodium bicarbonate can be used to counteract the acidosis by an initial dose of 5 mEq/kg body weight. Subsequent doses of 2.5 mEq/kg may be needed every 10 to 20 minutes during the first hour of treatment to help re-establish acid-base equilibrium. As acidosis is controlled, the dosage of atropine often may be reduced.

If vomiting has not already occurred, gastric lavage with 5 per cent bicarbonate water may be of benefit. Orally administered activated charcoal in a water slurry is helpful in reducing absorption after ingestion of these insecticides and may in some cases preclude the need for further atropine therapy.

The oximes, such as pralidoxime chloride (2-PAM; Protopam Chloride, Ayerst), are drugs that act specifically on the OP enzyme complex, reactivating the enzyme. The oximes may supplement atropine therapy when used within the first 24 hours. Pralidoxime chloride should be given either IV or IM at the dosage rate of 20 mg/kg body weight. The oximes are of no benefit in treating carbamate toxicosis.

Dermally exposed animals should be washed with soap and water to prevent continued absorption of these compounds.

Morphine, succinylcholine, and phenothiazine tranquilizers should be avoided in treating OP or carbamate insecticide poisoning.

When OP and carbamate insecticide poisoning are detected early and treated promptly, a favorable prognosis can generally be expected.

References and Supplemental Reading

Clemmons, R. M., Meyer, D. J., Sundlof, S. F., et al.: Correction of organophosphate-induced neuromuscular blockade by diphenhydramine. Am. J. Vet. Res. 45:2167, 1984.

Cordoba, D., Cadavid, S., Angulo, D., et al.: Organophosphate poisoning: Modifications in acid-base equilibrium and use of sodium bicarbonate as an aid in the treatment of toxicity in dogs. Vet. Hum. Toxicol. 25:1, 1983.

Mason, K. V., Ring, J., and Duggan, J.: Fenthion for flea control on dogs under field conditions: Dose response efficacy studies and effect of cholinesterase activity. J. Am. Anim. Hosp. Assoc. 20:591, 1984.

Mount, M. E.: Measurement of dialkyl phosphates in urine as an aid to recognize exposure of organophosphate insecticides. Am. Assoc. Vet. Lab. Diag. 27:383, 1984.

Osweiler, G. D., Carson, T. L., Buck, W. B., et al.: *Clinical and Diagnostic Veterinary Toxicology*, 3rd ed. Dubuque, IA: Kendall/Hunt. 1985.

Sundlof, S. F., Clemmons, R. M., Meyer, D. J., et al.: Cholinesterase activity in plasma, red blood cells, muscle and brain of dogs following repeated exposure to Spotton (fenthion). Vet. Hum. Toxicol. 26:112, 1984.

HERBICIDES

ROGER A. YEARY, D.V.M.
Columbus, Ohio

There are more than 125 chemicals with herbicidal activity in use in the United States (Weed Science Society of America, 1983). Fortunately, most of these chemicals have a relatively low order of mammalian toxicity. They may be used prior to the germination of seeds of undesirable plant species (pre-emergent herbicides) or they may be used to kill unwanted plant species that are actively growing (postemergent herbicides). Some postemergent herbicides are selective for certain plant species, and others are toxic to all vegetation.

Herbicides are commonly formulated as emulsifiable concentrates in solvent carriers. These formulated liquid herbicide products may cause poisoning in animals. Treatment of ingestion of any product containing petroleum distillates should always take into account the potential for aspiration pneumonia. It is quite unlikely that a dog or cat would ingest toxic quantities of herbicides that are formulated as dry granules, usually combined with fertilizers.

The herbicides to which dogs and cats are most likely to be exposed are those used for the control of weeds in lawns. Herbicides most commonly used in lawn care are the pre-emergent herbicides benefin, bensulide, and Dacthal (SOS Biotech) and the postemergent herbicides atrazine, dicamba, 2,4-D, the methane arsenates, and mecoprop. Herbicides for agricultural use include several of those used in lawn care, as well as many others. Because poisoning of pet animals from the agricultural use of herbicides is rare, only a limited few will be discussed here.

Postemergent herbicides that are selectively toxic to plants (e.g., atrazine, dicamba, 2,4-D) are especially unlikely to produce injury to animals by contact with plants after application at correct rates. The approximate residue of herbicide on turf grass immediately following application is as follows:

Application Rate* kg/ha =	lb/A =	mg/ft^2	**Residue PPM** (ppm wet weight basis)
1.12	1	10.4	150
2.24	2	20.8	300
7.84	7	72.8	700–1,000

*Key: ha = hectare; A = acre.

Using 2,4-D as an example, the usual rate of application (1 lb/A) results in a residue of 150 ppm, or about 1.5 mg of 2,4-D in a cupful of fresh grass clippings weighing 8.5 to 10.0 gm. This is a toxicologically insignificant amount, as the no observable effect level (NOEL) in dogs is 500 ppm based on 2-year dietary feeding studies (Hansen et al., 1971). Thus if the diet for a dog consisted solely of grass containing 2,4-D at a concentration of 150 ppm, the dietary intake would be less than the NOEL. In reality, it is unlikely that a dog would consume even a cupful of grass clippings. To translate dietary levels in ppm to dose expressed as mg/kg, divide the dietary level in ppm by 40. Thus 500 ppm corresponds to a daily dietary dose of 12.5 mg/kg (170 mg for a 13.6-kg [30-lb] dog), which may be compared with 1.5 mg per cupful of grass.

Table 1 lists the rate of application and the NOEL for dietary feeding for a number of the herbicides to which dogs are most likely to be exposed. As seen in Table 1, only certain nonselective herbicides such as sodium arsenite may reasonably be expected to result in intoxication from ingestion of treated plants.

Skin contact is unlikely to result in transfer of toxiocologically significant quantities of selective herbicides, since only about 5 per cent of the residue can be dislodged from the plant surface (Thompson et al., 1984).

PRE-EMERGENT HERBICIDES

Pre-emergent herbicides are used in the early spring months prior to germination of weed seeds. The period of use extends from February until the end of May, depending on the climatic region. Poisoning of dogs or cats by benefin, bensulide, or Dacthal has not been reported. The lethal dose for each herbicide for dogs is as follows: benefin, 2000 mg/kg; bensulide, 200 mg/kg; and Dacthal, 250 mg/kg. Treatment of poisoning by benefin or Dacthal would be symptomatic: Prevent absorption, facilitate excretion, and treat the patient, not the poison.

Table 1. *Rate of Application and No Observable Effect Level (NOEL) of Commonly Used Herbicides (in Dogs)*

Common Name	Trade Name	Application Rate (lb/A)*	NOEL (ppm)† or (mg/kg)
Alachlor	Lasso (Monsanto)	1.5–4.0	200
Atrazine	Aatrex (Ciba-Geigy)	2.0	150
Benefin	Balan (Elanco)	1.0	5000
Bensulide	Betasan (Stauffer)	7.5	12
2,4-D		1.0	500
DCPA	Dacthal (SOS Biotech)	10.0	10,000
Dicamba	Banvel (Velsical)	0.06–0.25	50
Glyphosate††	Roundup (Monsanto)	1.0	2000
Oxadiazon	Ronstar (Rhone-Poulenc)	0.75–4.0	72.5
Paraquat††	Ortho Paraquat (Chevron)	0.5–1.0	34
Propachlor	Ramrod (Monsanto)	3.0–6.0	1000
Sodium arsenite††		1.5	50
Trifluralin	Treflan (Elanco)	2.0	10

*Grass residue 1 lb/A is approximately 150 ppm (wet weight basis).
†Concentration in total diet.
††Nonselective.

Bensulide is an inhibitor of acetylcholinesterase in animals. It has weak activity as an insecticide but is an effective pre-emergent herbicide. Figure 1 shows the depression of plasma cholinesterase in dogs given an oral dose of bensulide, 60.9 mg/kg, in a mixture that also contained 2,4-D, 6.5 mg/kg; mecoprop, 3.26 mg/kg; and dicamba 0.55 mg/kg (Yeary, 1984). These dogs were clinically normal. Animals that might be poisoned by bensulide should exhibit the classic cholinergic signs of acetylcholinesterase inhibition. Clinical signs ordinarily do not occur until erythrocyte cholinesterase is significantly depressed (decreased 80 per cent). Atropine should be administered as an antidote at a dose of 0.1 to 1.0 mg/kg. Effectively atropinized dogs will exhibit an unmistakable tachycardia. This should serve as a guide to effective atropinization. It should not be necessary to administer oximes such as pralidoxime (2-PAM) unless there is flaccid paralysis of muscles.

POSTEMERGENT HERBICIDES

The most frequently discussed and misunderstood herbicide is 2,4-D. This herbicide is used to control dandelions in lawns, but it is even more extensively used for weed control in growing wheat and other cereal crops. As discussed previously, it is difficult to conceive that dogs can consume a toxic dose of 2,4-D from ingesting treated grass. However, a dog weighing 20 kg (44 lb) would only have to ingest about 10 ml of a liquid formulation containing 23 per cent of the acid equivalent (2,4-dichlorophenoxyacetic acid) to receive a potentially lethal dose. This formulation can be purchased at garden stores, hardware stores, and discount stores for use by home owners.

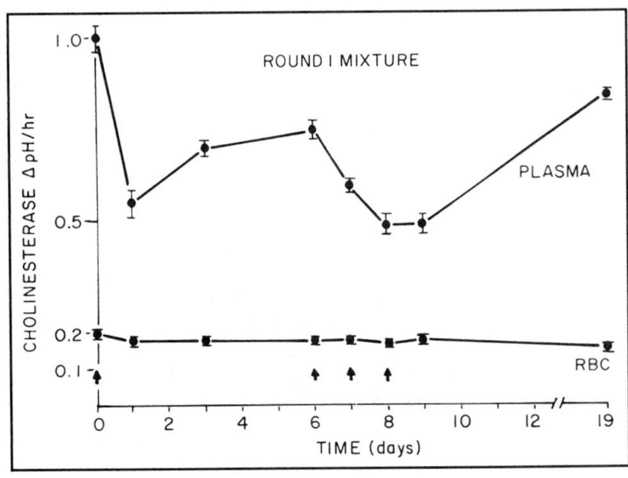

Figure 1. Plasma and erythrocyte cholinesterase (mean ± standard error) for 6 dogs orally intubated with a fertilizer-herbicide mixture used on lawns. Treatment days are indicated by arrows. The mixture contained the herbicide bensulide which was given at a daily dosage of 60.9 mg/kg of body weight. Bensulide is applied to lawns at a rate of 75–120 mg/ft² with a residue on turf of about 700 ppm. (Reprinted with permission from Yeary: Am. J. Vet. Res. 45:288, 1984.)

The effects of acutely lethal doses of 2,4-D in dogs are anorexia, tremors, myotonia, and metabolic acidosis. The LD_{50} for dogs is approximately 100 mg/kg. Concentrated formulations of 2,4-D are irritating and may produce gastroenteritis. Daily oral doses of 20 mg/kg given in gelatin capsules resulted in death within a few weeks. The dogs refused all food and had difficulty swallowing. There was marked weight loss, muscular spasticity, and ataxia. Dogs given 10 mg/kg in gelatin capsules were clinically normal. When fed to dogs for 2 years at a dietary concentration of 500 ppm (12.5 mg/kg), 2,4-D caused no clinical or microscopic pathologic changes. Methods for treating acute poisoning by 2,4-D should include administration of activated charcoal to prevent absorption and alkaline diuresis to promote renal excretion. All salts or esters of 2,4-D are excreted as the acid.

Although less well studied, mecoprop, or MCPP as it is commonly known, is both structurally and toxicologically similar to 2,4-D.

Intoxication of dogs or cats by atrazine or dicamba have not been reported. Atrazine has a low acute toxicity in rodents. The oral LD_{50} values are 3000 mg/kg for rats and 1750 mg/kg for mice. Rodents poisoned by atrazine were initially excited, then depressed, with ataxia and intermittent clonic and tonic seizures. Dicamba is a benzoic acid derivative that may be hepatotoxic at doses greater than 5 mg/kg (250 ppm in diet) during repeated exposures. Based on related compounds such as benzoic acid, one would not expect hepatoxicity from acute exposures of less than 200 mg/kg.

A variety of arsenic-containing herbicides are still in use. Monosodium methane arsenate (MSMA), disodium methane arsenate (DSMA), and the octyldodecyl ammonium salts of methyl arsenic acid are used as selective herbicides for the postemergence control of crabgrass on lawns and for the control of Johnsongrass, nutsedge, foxtail, and other weeds in cotton. Inorganic arsenicals such as arsenic trioxide and arsenic acid are not selective and are used as defoliants prior to harvesting and for control of vegetation along fence rows, for example.

The methane arsenates do not have a high acute toxicity. They are pentavalent forms of arsenic that are considerably less toxic than trivalent forms such as arsenic trioxide and the more soluble and more readily absorbed arsenic acids. Although there are large variations in toxicity of the various arsenicals, the clinical signs of poisoning are similar. Signs of acute arsenic poisoning include anorexia, vomiting, acute abdominal pain, bloody rice water diarrhea, ataxia, and partial paralysis of rear limbs.

Treatment of poisoning by arsenicals tends to be oversimplified. British anti-lewisite (BAL) is effective for the trivalent arsenicals, but it is disappointing for pentavalent arsenicals. The basis for this would appear to be explainable by the observation that trivalent forms of arsenic compete for sulfhydryl groups on enzymes and the pentavalent forms do not. Replacement of fluid loss and prevention of shock is of utmost importance. Gastric lavage or instillation of a 1 per cent solution of sodium thiosulfate or 1 per cent sodium bicarbonate may reduce absorption of inorganic arsenicals if the animal is treated early. Sodium thiosulfate, 1 gm/kg IV, can be used as an alternative to BAL given IM at a dosage of 3 to 7 mg/kg three times daily. Shock and renal failure are common in acute arsenic poisoning, and the prognosis for recovery should be guarded. Judicious use of narcotic analgesics may aid in preventing shock but should not be given if the animal is hypotensive.

NONSELECTIVE HERBICIDES

The inorganic arsenicals, arsenic trioxide and arsenic acid, have been used to control vegetation along fence rows and rights-of-way, but they have largely been replaced with less toxic herbicides such as amitrole, glyphosate, or simazine. Amitrole, or aminotriazole, has unusually low acute toxicity to mammals or fish. Amitrole inhibits several enzymes, including peroxidase, preventing the oxidation of iodine with the subsequent development of toxic goiter. In rats the hyperplastic changes are considered by some pathologists to be neoplastic. Glyphosate is a very popular nonselective herbicide. It is a simple phosphonomethyl derivative of glycine, and poisoning has not been reported. Simazine is chemically similar to atrazine, and poisoning has not been reported for either herbicide.

Paraquat is a nonselective herbicide that kills on contact with plants. In fact, areas where it has been used can be identified because of the visible damage to plant tissue. Concentrated solutions of paraquat are corrosive to the eyes and skin. Acute intoxication occurs with doses of 50 mg/kg and is characterized by hyperexcitability, incoordination, and convulsions. Surviving animals may die 3 to 5 days later from severe pulmonary congestion or may develop pulmonary fibrosis after 7 to 10 days. The lungs of animals dying from paraquat have such severe congestion that they resemble hepatic tissue in color. As little as 0.03 per cent, or 300 ppm, in the diet leads to pulmonary fibrosis. The lung lesions can be prevented experimentally by treatment with selenium and superoxide dismutase (Paloscein, Coopers). Oxygen increases the pulmonary pathology and should be used sparingly in support of paraquat-poisoned animals. Paraquat is a renal tubular toxin, and forced diuresis is an important part of therapy. Because the fatal alteration in the lungs and kidneys may not develop for several days, it is imperative that all animals believed to have ingested paraquat be treated immediately with an adsorbent. Bentonite clay is most effective but is less readily available than activated charcoal. Follow-up should include either an enema or saline cathartic.

References and Supplemental Reading

Hansen, W. H., Quaife, M. L., Habermann, R. T., et al.: Chronic toxicity of 2,4-dichlorophenoxyacetic acid in rats and dogs. Toxicol. Appl. Pharmacol. 20:122, 1971.

Thompson, D. G., Stephenson, G. R., and Sears, M. K.: Persistence distribution and dislodgeable residues of 2,4-D following its application to turfgrass. Pestic. Sci. 15:353, 1984.

Weed Science Society of America: *Herbicide Handbook of the Weed Science Society of America*, 5th ed. Champaign, IL, 1983.

Yeary, R. A.: Oral intubation of dogs with combinations of fertilizer, herbicide and insecticide chemicals commonly used on lawns. Am. J. Vet. Res. 45:288, 1984.

THE ANTICOAGULANT RODENTICIDES

MICHAEL E. MOUNT. D.V.M.,
Davis, California

BENNY J. WOODY, D.V.M.,
Mississippi State, Mississippi

and MICHAEL J. MURPHY, D.V.M.
College Station, Texas

INTRODUCTION

Rodenticides are a common cause of poisoning in companion animals. Of these agents, anticoagulants are of high incidence because of their availability to household owners and their important role in urban and agricultural rodent control programs. In the United States, 95 per cent or more of the rodenticides used in commensal rodent control are the anticoagulant baits (Marsh, 1983).

CLINICAL SIGNS AND DIFFERENTIAL CONSIDERATIONS

A variety of clinical presentations potentially may occur, since the sites of hemorrhage are unlimited. Generally speaking, body cavities are predilection sites for hemorrhage. An animal may be severely poisoned yet appear completely healthy if no site of hemorrhage has been identified.

Clinical evidence of depression, weakness, and pallor are the key clinical signs. Signs of external bleeding (melena, epistaxis, hematemesis, hematuria, gingival bleeding, or profuse bleeding from a small wound) may not be present. In these cases, hemorrhage internally into the peritoneal or pleural cavities, fascial planes, retroperitoneal space, joint spaces, or other "hidden" areas of the body may be present. Signs of nonlocalized pain and fever could easily be confused with trauma-induced injury.

Obvious signs of hemorrhage such as subcutaneous swellings; petechial to ecchymotic hemorrhages of scleral, conjunctival, or mucous membranes; hyphema; and external bleeding may also be readily seen. A venipuncture site may incessantly bleed, and swelling around the site can ensue as a result of hemorrhage unless a pressure bandage is applied. The clinician must quickly consider anticoagulant poisoning, disseminated intravascular coagulopathy (DIC), or autoimmune thrombocytopenia (AITP). Further testing is necessary to differentiate these conditions.

Hemorrhage into vital areas of the body can precipitate a rapid course of events leading to death. The most common cause of acute death is hemorrhage into the pleural cavity, lung parenchyma, or mediastinal spaces, including the pericardial space. Evidence of fluid in the chest should call for emergency protocol and laboratory workup. Hypovolemic shock may develop after rapid blood loss, resulting in an animal that is cold to the touch, semicomatose, and oliguric. Hemorrhage into the restricted cavity of cranium may result in central

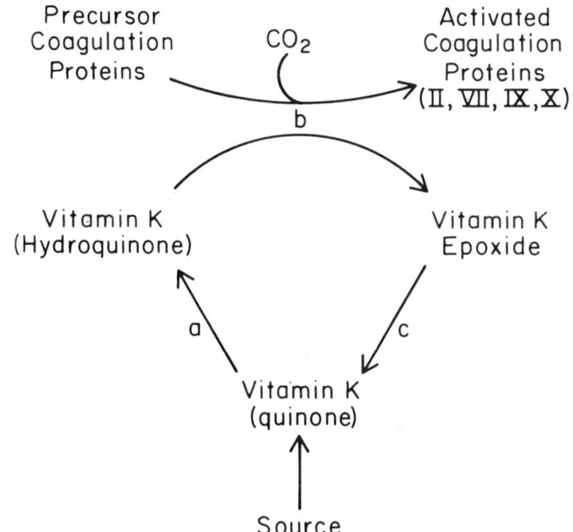

Figure 1. Schematic representation of the vitamin K enzyme complex. Step *a* is a reductase reaction. Step *b* is the simplified and incompletely understood reaction demonstrating carboxylation and epoxidation. Step *c* is the epoxide reductase reaction allowing for regeneration of vitamin K chemically as the quinone. The source becomes an important component when step *c* is inhibited. (Reprinted with permission from Mount et al.: J.A.V.M.A. 180:1354, 1982.)

nervous system manifestations rapidly leading to coma and death.

When unsuspected surgical bleeding occurs, anticoagulant exposure, von Willebrand's disease, hemophilia or other inherited conditions, and drug-induced platelet function antagonism are major diagnostic considerations.

MECHANISM OF ACTION

All the anticoagulants of concern affect the vitamin K enzyme complex (also referred to as the vitamin K epoxide cycle), which is responsible for production of functional vitamin K-dependent Factors II, VII, IX, and X. Vitamin K is responsible for conversion of nonfunctional factors to functional vitamin K–dependent coagulation proteins.

The liver is the site of synthesis of the vitamin K–dependent proteins. Vitamin K is stored in the liver, and two major types are present that can participate in the vitamin K enzyme complex as illustrated in Figure 1. These are the menaquinones, which are produced by bacterial flora in the gastrointestinal tract, and the phylloquinones, which are obtained in the diet via vegetation. One site of the biochemical lesion caused by anticoagulants is the epoxide reductase enzyme (Fig. 1, step c). Inhibition of this enzyme prevents recycling of the epoxide back to vitamin K and results in rapid depletion of body stores of vitamin K. The overall effect observed clinically is reduction in functional coagulation Factors VII, IX, X, and II, whose half-lives in dogs are 6.2, 13.9, 16.5, and 41 hours, respectively. Depletion of these factors prolongs the extrinsic, intrinsic, and common coagulation pathways, leading to coagulopathy.

The mechanism of action is related to therapy. The source of vitamin K becomes extremely important, since recycling of vitamin K by the body is reduced or completely halted; hence, a continuous source of vitamin K is essential. Administration of vitamin K_1 produces a positive biochemical response within 24 hours. This is very rapid when compared with time required for initiating protein synthesis.

ANTICOAGULANTS AND THEIR CLINICAL DIFFERENCES

Eight anticoagulants commonly used in the United States are listed in Tables 1 and 2. Chemically, they form two groups: the hydroxycoumarins and the indanediones. The hydroxycoumarins consist of the "old" (first-generation) and the "new" (second-generation) anticoagulant types. The indanediones are also first-generation anticoagulants. First-generation anticoagulants are those to which resistance was recognized in rodents. The second-generation anticoagulants are those rodenticides effective against warfarin-resistant rodent populations. In addition, single-dose exposure of the second-generation anticoagulants is sufficient to cause fatality, whereas repeated exposure is generally needed for the first-generation anticoagulants.

Although there are currently several anticoagulants in use, the basic biochemical lesion induced results in the same clinical effect. There are no means to clinically differentiate the different anticoagulants, since they all produce the same symptoms. However, the degree and length of coagulopathy are dependent on the chemical group of anticoagulant and the dose consumed.

First-Generation Anticoagulants

COUMARINS. Warfarin and fumarin (or coumafuryl) are in this classification. Historically, these are the most commonly encountered types of anticoagulant poisonings observed by practitioners. Sulfaquinoxaline, a coccidiostat, produces coagulopathy through reduction of the vitamin K–dependent coagulation factors. It is included in some warfarin baits (Prolin, Banarat).

Warfarin has a half-life in dogs of 14.5 hours. Figure 2 illustrates the duration of its toxic effect in dogs after a multiple-dose exposure of four to eight times the LD_{50} as measured by coagulation screening tests (one-stage prothrombin time [OSPT], activated partial thromboplastin time [APTT]). The

Table 1. *Toxicologic Data of the Coumarin Anticoagulants Used in the USA*

	Coumarin Anticoagulants			
	First Generation		Second Generation	
	1†	2‡	3§	4‖
Common or generic names*	Warfarin, coumafene, zoocoumarin	Coumafuryl, fumarin, tomarin	Brodifacoum, volak, BFC	Bromadiolone, bromone
Synonyms or trade names*	Warf 42, Rax, Dethmor, D-Con, Rodex, Tox-Hid, Prolin**, Ratron, others	Ratafin, Fumisol, Rat-a-way, Lurat, Krumkil, others	Talon, Havoc, Weather Block, others	Maki, Contrac, Super Caid, Ratimus, others
ACUTE LETHAL DOSE ESTIMATES (mg/kg body weight)				
Rat	50–100	Similar to warfarin (?)	0.27	1.25
Dog	20–300††	" "	0.25–3.50	11–15
Other	5–30 (cat)	" "	25.0 (?)	>25.0
CHRONIC LETHAL DOSE ESTIMATES (mg/kg body weight; d = days)				
Rat	1/d for 5 d	Similar to warfarin (?)	Similar to acute	Similar to acute (?)
Dog	1–5/d for 5–15 d	" "	" "	" "
Other	1/d for 5 d (cat)	" "	" "	" "
Traditional bait conc. (%)	0.025	0.025	0.005	0.005
Minimal amount that could be potentially lethal using the most toxic estimate above if consumed by a 13.6-kg (30-lb) dog	54.4 gm/d for 5 d (1.9 oz/d)	Similar to warfarin (?) —	68 gm, single dose (2.4 oz)	2992 gm, divided dose (107 oz or 6.7 lb)

*Common names and trade names include those in the USA and in other countries.
†3-("alpha"-Acetonylbenzyl)-4-hydroxycoumarin.
‡3-("alpha"-Acetonylfurfuryl)-4-hydroxycoumarin.
§3-[3-(4′-Bromo[1,1′-biphenyl]-4-yl)-1,2,3,4-tetrahydro-1-naphthalenyl]-4-hydroxy-2H-1-benzopyran-2-one.
‖3-[3-(4′-Bromo[1,1′-biphenyl]-4-yl)-3-hydroxy-1-phenylpropyl]-4-hydroxy-2H-1-benzopyran-2-one *or* 3-["alpha"-(p-[p-bromophenyl)-"beta"-hydroxy-phenethyl]-4-hydroxycoumarin.
**Warfarin plus sulfaquinoxaline.
††5 mg/kg was shown to cause moderate coagulopathic effects.

OSPT and APTT returned slowly to the normal reference range during 6 days of vitamin K_1 administration.

INDANEDIONES. Members of this group include diphacinone, chlorophacinone, valone, and pindone. Diphacinone has a much longer anticoagulant effect than warfarin. The half-life of diphacinone was estimated to be between 4 and 5 days in dogs (Mount, 1984). Blood levels of diphacinone and the measure of the toxic effect are illustrated in Figure 3. Blood levels of diphacinone were detectable throughout the entire course of the coagulative deficits. Therefore, the 5-day treatment of vitamin K_1, which was sufficient to treat warfarin intoxication, was totally unable to correct the toxic effect produced by diphacinone with that vitamin K_1 treatment protocol. This prolonged effect is probably characteristic of the other indanediones.

Second-Generation Anticoagulants

The second-generation coumarins brodifacoum and bromadiolone are members of this group. Brodifacoum is used primarily by pest control professionals but is available over-the-counter as Havoc. The plasma half-life is approximately 6 days in a dog. A marked effect in coagulation was demonstrated (Fig. 4) until therapy corrected the condition. The maximum effect was estimated at between 12 and 15 days, and brodifacoum could still be detected at day 24. The prolonged anticoagulant effect was very obvious at this low exposure level. Standard therapy for warfarin would be insufficient to alleviate the condition.

Bromadiolone is structurally very similar to brodifacoum but is less toxic (Table 1). Similar baits are used as for brodifacoum, but tracking powders are also available. No over-the-counter products are currently available. Figure 5 demonstrates its effect on coagulation in a dog (Woody and Murphy, 1984). No blood concentrations are given, because light sensitivity makes analysis difficult. A prolonged anticoagulant effect of bromadiolone was not demonstrated at the dosages discussed.

Secondary poisoning is a greater hazard from the second-generation anticoagulants, although this may occur with the indanediones and possibly other first-generation chemicals. As much as 100 gm of 0.005 per cent bait may be consumed by a Norway rat,

Table 2. Toxicologic Data of the Indanedione Anticoagulants Used in the USA

	Indanedione Anticoagulants			
	1†	2‡	3§	4‖
Common or generic names	Diphacinone, diphenadione, diphenacin	Chlorophacinone, chlorodiphacinone, chlorophacinon, chlorphenacone chlorphacinone, liphadione	Pindone, pivalyl valone, pivaldione	Valone, isoval, isovaleryl, indanedione
Synonym or trade names	Promar, Diphacin, Ramik, others	Afnor, Caid, Drat, Quick, Raticide-Caid, Ramucide, Ratomet, Raviac, Rozol, Redentin, Ratindan 3, Topitox, others	Pival, Pivalyn, others	PMP, Motomco tracking powder
ACUTE LETHAL DOSE ESTIMATES (mg/kg body weight)				
Rat	1.86–2.88	2.1–20.5	150	Similar to pindone
Dog	0.88–7.5	Similar to diphacinone (?)	4–5 to 75–100	" " (?)
Other	15.0 (cat)	" "	—	" "
CHRONIC LETHAL DOSE ESTIMATES (mg/kg body weight; d = days)				
Rat	—	—	—	—
Dog	0.08 2× for 3 d	0.05/d for 10 d	15–35 divided over several days	Similar to pindone
Traditional bait conc. (%)	0.005	0.005	0.025	Primarily as 0.1–1.0% powder
Minimal amount that could be potentially lethal using the most toxic estimate above if consumed by a 13.6-kg (30-lb) dog	22 gm/d 2× for 3 d (0.77 oz)	13.6 gm/d for 10 d (0.48 oz)	816** gm divided over several days (28.8 oz)**	204†† gm or 20.4‡‡ g (7.2 oz or 0.7 oz)

*Common names and trade names include those in the USA and other countries.
†2-(Diphenylacetyl)-1,3-indanedione.
‡2-[(*p*-Chlorophenyl)phenylacetyl]-1,3-indanedione.
§2-Pivalyl-1,3-indanedione /or/ 2-pivaloylindane-1,3-dione.
‖2-Isovaleryl-1,3-indanedione.
**If using the 4 to 5 mg/kg acute dose estimation, it would be 1/3 this amount.
†† Of 0.1% dust.
‡‡Of 1.0% dust.

providing enough brodifacoum to cause lethal poisoning in a small dog.

TOXICITY

FIRST-GENERATION COUMARINS. A big difference exists between single and repetitive-dose toxicity. The first-generation anticoagulants are usually multiple-dose rodenticides, and companion animals generally require repeated exposure to consume the lethal dose. For warfarin, factors affecting toxicity include the short half-life, the absorptive capacity, and relative lower affinity to the vitamin K enzyme complex. Differences in LD_{50} ranges for warfarin are illustrated in Table 1.

INDANEDIONES. The indanediones also exhibit differences between acute and chronic lethal doses but not as markedly as warfarin. The small differences with diphacinone and possibly other indanediones undoubtedly are related to the extremely long half-life and other factors. Table 2 shows toxicologic estimates for the indanediones.

SECOND-GENERATION COUMARINS. Table 1 compares the toxicologic estimates for the second-generation anticoagulants. A cat LD_{50} value of 25 mg/kg (based on limited data) indicates that cats can tolerate a higher amount of brodifacoum than can dogs.

Bromadiolone at 10 mg/kg in dogs produced an anticoagulant effect for several days, followed by reversal not requiring vitamin K_1 therapy. Death was produced at a 15 mg/kg single-dose exposure.

After only one exposure, clinical signs from second-generation anticoagulants may appear as soon as 1 to 3 days following exposure. Clinical poisoning due to first-generation anticoagulants generally is

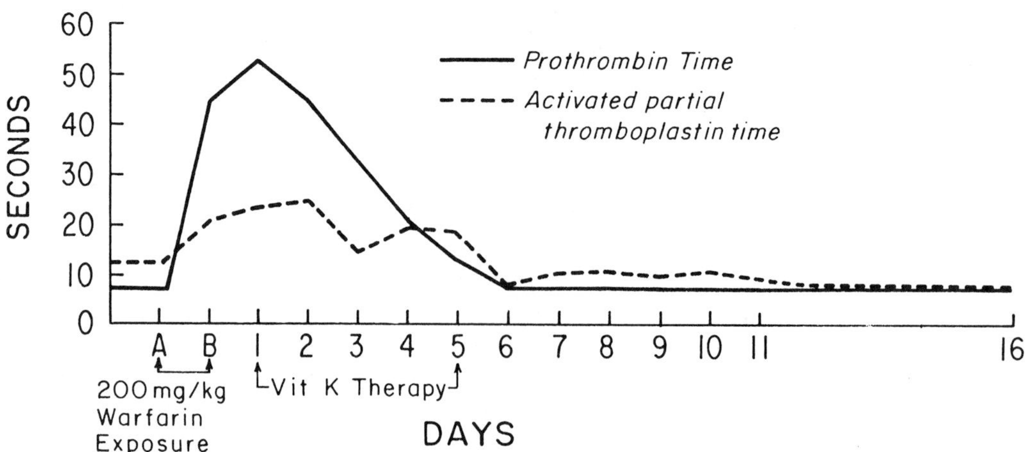

Figure 2. Coagulation changes after a massive multiexposure oral dose of warfarin (days A and B) in a dog. Vitamin K_1 (2.5 mg/kg/day) was given therapeutically for five days. Normalization of coagulation assays occurred by the sixth day after the last dose of warfarin.

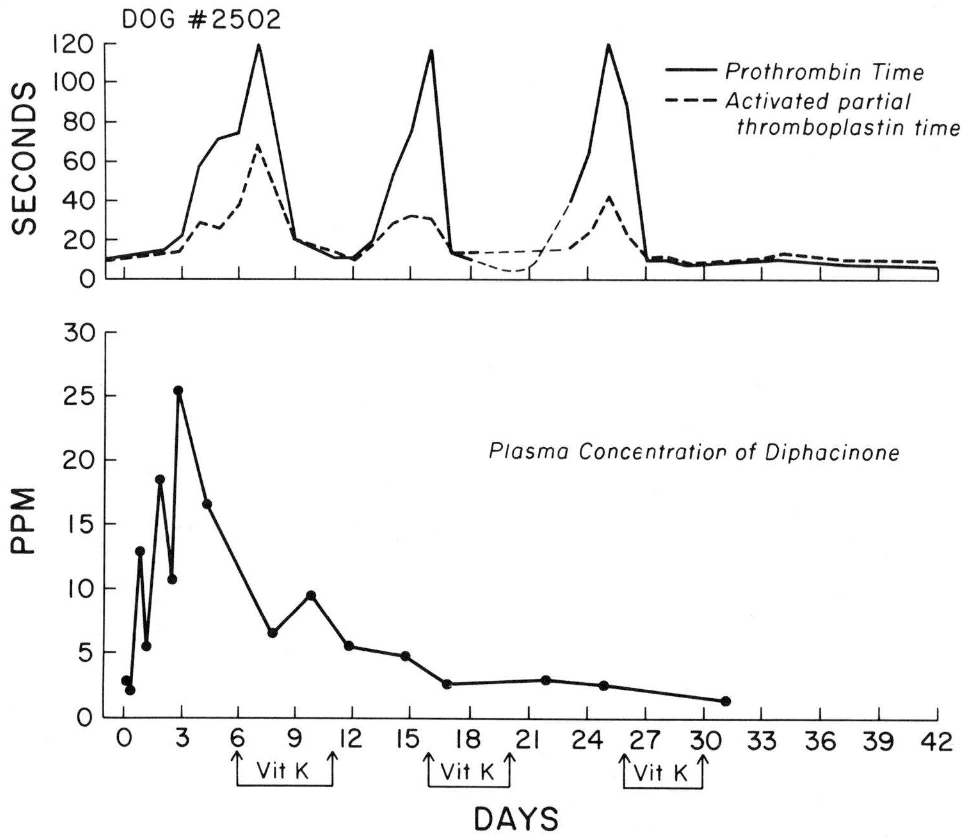

Figure 3. Coagulation changes and concentrations of plasma diphacinone expressed in parts per million (ppm, μg/ml) in a dog exposed to 2.5 mg diphacinone/kg body weight divided over three days (day 0 through day 2). Three 5-day therapeutic regimens of oral vitamin K (2.5 mg/kg/day divided t.i.d.) were required to control the coagulopathy. No diaphacinone was present in the plasma at time 0 but was detectable at approximately 1 ppm concentration on day 31 even though no pathologic effects were present at that time. (Reprinted with permission from Mount et al.: J.A.V.M.A. 180:1354, 1982.)

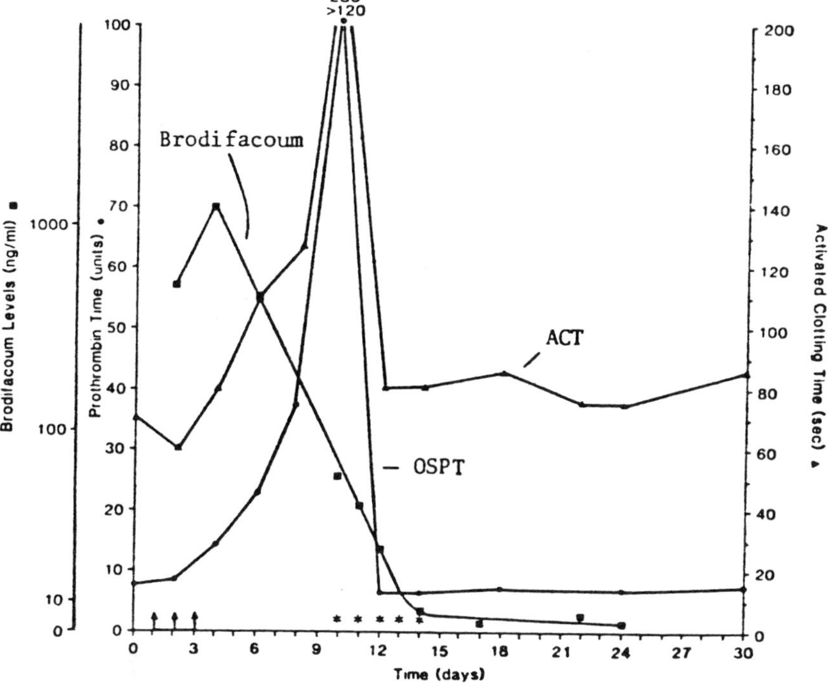

Figure 4. Coagulation changes and concentrations of serum brodifacoum expressed in ng/ml (parts per billion, ppb) in a dog exposed to 0.33 mg brodifacoum/kg body weight each day for three days (arrows). Vitamin K_1 was administered at 2.5 mg/kg divided b.i.d. for five days (days 10 through 14, indicated by *). Brodifacoum was still present in the serum on day 24 even though no pathologic effects were present at that time.

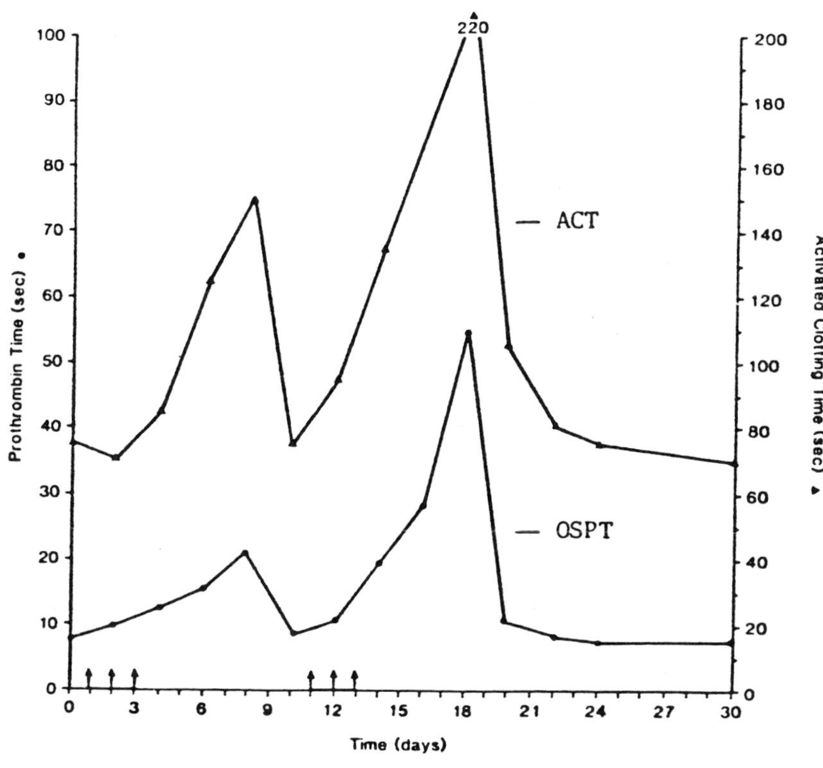

Figure 5. Coagulation changes in a dog exposed to 0.33 mg bromadiolone/kg body weight each day for three days at two different times (see arrows). No vitamin K_1 was administered. The pathologic effects intensified after the second exposure period (days 11 through 13) but coagulation normalized by day 24.

Table 3. *Parenteral and Oral Forms of Vitamin K_1*

Mephyton, oral, 5 mg/tablet (Merck Sharp & Dohme)
Aquamephyton, IV/IM/SC injectable, 10 mg/ml (Merck Sharp & Dohme)
Konakion, IM only, ampule: 0.5 ml, 1 mg; 1 ml, 10 mg (Roche)
Vet-A-K_1, IV/IM/SC injectable, 10 mg/ml (Professional Veterinary Laboratories)

observed 4 to 5 days after an ample single dose or an initial multiple-dose exposure.

Predisposing Factors

Conditions that enhance the toxic effect of the anticoagulants include drugs (long-acting sulfonamides, phenylbutazone, and aspirin) that displace anticoagulant from albumin. Chloramphenicol enhances toxicity by inhibition of microsomal activity. Reduction of circulating coagulation factors, production of endogenous coagulation inhibitors, thrombocytopenia, or vascular injury can reduce hemostatic capability when compounded with the anticoagulant effects. In particular, platelet function is interfered with by aspirin and other nonsteroidal anti-inflammatory drugs. Severe liver disease can result in a decrease in coagulation protein production. Renal disease not only results in a decrease in protein binding capacity associated with uremia but also in loss of albumin, leading to a greater availability of unbound anticoagulant for interaction with the sites of toxic action.

THERAPY

Vitamin K_1 is a very effective antidote. *It must be given for as long as the anticoagulant is present in the body at toxic levels.* This is especially important when a high dose of anticoagulant is consumed and when the anticoagulant is an indanedione or second-generation coumarin. Clinicians should re-evaluate anticoagulant-poisoned animals after discontinuing vitamin K treatment to rule out a longer-acting anticoagulant as the causative agent.

Vitamin K_3 (menadione) is much less expensive than K_1 but is far less effective. Vitamin K_3 should never be used as the sole antidote in an anticoagulant-poisoned animal demonstrating a severe coagulopathy. Vitamin K_1 is available commercially in parenteral or tablet forms (Table 3) (Mount et al., 1982).

VITAMIN K_1 DOSAGE. The great success in treating warfarin poisoning with vitamin K_1 has inspired false confidence in this antidotal protocol. Vitamin K_1 has been recommended at 0.25 to 2.5 mg/kg given in divided doses daily for 5 to 7 days IV, IM, SC, or orally (Szabuniewicz and McCrady, 1977). In the past, an initial IV injection of vitamin K_1 (15 to 75 mg/day) was followed by oral treatment (15 to 75 mg/day) for 4 to 6 days (Buck et al., 1976). Intravenous administration is not recommended because of the risk of anaphylaxis (Mount et al., 1982). These dosage recommendations are sufficient only for first-generation coumarin anticoagulants. The indanediones and second-generation anticoagulants require careful therapeutic protocols. Premature cessation of therapy can quickly precipitate a hemorrhagic crisis (Mount and Feldman, 1983). Vitamin K_1 dosage levels near or below 1 mg/kg body weight (a rough approximation) may provide insufficient protection. Therefore, 5 mg/kg of vitamin K_1 is recommended when known cases of diphacinone poisoning or other long-acting anticoagulants are identified. A loading dose of 5 mg/kg of vitamin K_1 given SC in several sites is recommended. Then follow within 6 to 12 hours with oral administration of 5 mg/kg given divided t.i.d. or b.i.d. for 2 weeks, at which time *coagulation status must be re-evaluated* (as described later). If this is not desirable, maintain the animal for 3 full weeks on vitamin K_1 and restrict activity of the animal for 1 week after the last vitamin K dosage. Re-evaluation of the coagulation status is recommended after 3 weeks of treatment, particularly if excessive exposure to the anticoagulant is suspected.

Where a specific anticoagulant is not identified, give the animal a loading dose of 2.5 mg/kg SC of vitamin K_1 followed with oral administration of 1.0 to 2.5 mg/kg divided t.i.d. or b.i.d. for 5 to 7 days. Re-evaluate as follows: 2 days after the last vitamin K_1 dose, OSPT should be performed. It is desirable to repeat the OSPT in another 2 days if results are normal. If an activated coagulation time (ACT) is performed instead, it is necessary to repeat again in 2 days if no prolongation in the clotting time is observed. Elevation in the assays is evidence that one of the longer-acting anticoagulants is responsible. If the OSPT is significantly elevated 2 days after the last day of therapy, reinstitute vitamin K_1 therapy at 2.5 to 5.0 mg/kg for an additional 2 weeks. If significant prolongation of the OSPT is not evidenced at 2 days but does occur at 4 days after vitamin K_1 therapy, only 1 additional week of vitamin K therapy should suffice. The ACT is not nearly as sensitive as the OSPT, so use it only if the animal is checked a minimum of two times after vitamin K_1 treatment and if the initial assay was within the reference range for healthy animals.

The initial dosage we recommend (5 mg/kg) has been questioned, since adverse effects were observed at dosages similar to ours (Fernandez et al., 1984). Heinz body anemia was observed. This was never observed in 16 dogs given 5 mg of vitamin K/kg orally daily for 21 days (Mount, 1984). Treatment through the entire period with 5 mg/kg is not crucial to control the coagulopathy, since 2.5 mg/kg can maintain recovery if given as long as the toxic effect is present. Therefore, to be cautious, an alternative route would be to administer the preferred dosage (5 mg/kg as loading) for the initial 48 hours followed with 2.5 mg/kg divided daily to the end of the recommended treatment period. However, if the coagulation status of the animal cannot be re-evaluated after termination of therapy, use the 5 mg/kg dosage during the entire treatment period.

OTHER THERAPEUTIC CONSIDERATIONS. When an otherwise healthy animal is seen consuming anticoagulant bait, removal of stomach contents via apomorphine or lavage followed by activated charcoal and a saline cathartic is recommended. The animal should then be placed on vitamin K_1 at 1.0 mg/kg for 5 to 7 days. Re-evaluation is warranted, especially if previous ingestion is suspected. Generally speaking, gentle handling of the patient, administration of electrolytes in balanced solutions, and providing warmth and oxygen are applicable to most cases of coagulopathy. Removal of stomach contents is not recommended in animals presented in a state of coagulopathy.

A dyspneic animal needs special attention to determine the cause. Severe anemia and pulmonary or thoracic hemorrhage need to be considered. Severe anemia associated with dyspnea but without pulmonary or thoracic bleeding is a sound criterion for a whole-blood transfusion (see O'Rourke, 1983).

When dyspnea is related to hemorrhage occurring within the pulmonary or thoracic area, the bleeding sites need to be defined by radiography. If intrapulmonary hemorrhage is recognized, a plasma transfusion is highly recommended at 10 per cent of body blood volume. A dog's blood volume is approximately 90 ml/kg (O'Rourke, 1983); hence, 9 ml/kg body weight is the dose of plasma to be administered IV at the rate of whole blood. The plasma should be warmed, as with whole blood. Plasma may be fresh or stored frozen at temperatures near $-40°C$ for proper preservation.

Plasma transfusions can be very helpful in life-threatening intrapulmonary hemorrhaging crises. Needed coagulation factors are provided that are capable of rapidly supporting hemostasis within the lungs. Vitamin K_1 administration (even IV) is not able to produce effective hemostasis for several hours. In less severe cases, keeping the animal calm and providing an enriched oxygen supply while waiting for the loading dose of vitamin K_1 to generate functional coagulation factors are helpful. More involved procedures are needed if the animal shows no response, which indicates that the blood Po_2 is not corrected by more conservative methods. Infusion of oxygen using positive pressure systems needs to be used in these situations. Narcotics can be used, but the drugs commonly used for treatment of pulmonary edema (aminophylline and furosemide) should be avoided if possible because of impairment of platelet function.

If hemorrhage has occurred into the thoracic cavity, as revealed by fluid line densities on radiographs, drainage of the blood may be necessary. This decision must be made weighing the benefit of improved ventilation against the genuine risk of reinitiating hemorrhage by thoracentesis (Beasley and Buck, 1983).

Symptoms of hypovolemic shock must be taken seriously and treated accordingly. Fluid replacement (including whole blood), steroid stabilization, maintenance of renal output, and possibly respiratory or cardiac support systems and medications are needed (see Haskins, 1983).

Proper management of life-threatening situations, use of vitamin K_1, and proper duration of dosing favor a positive outcome for the patient and the veterinarian. Lack of client compliance in following home vitamin K_1 treatments may result in an "apparent" therapeutic failure in cases of long-acting anticoagulant poisonings. Recognition of this by the veterinarian together with client education will undoubtedly solve these types of "apparent" failures.

DIAGNOSIS

Always obtain blood samples for a coagulation screen prior to administration of vitamin K_1. Dramatic response of the coagulation measurements to proper dosage of vitamin K_1 is highly diagnostic for anticoagulant poisoning.

Coagulation screening (OSPT, APTT, ACT, clotting time tests, or bleeding time) is used to demonstrate a coagulopathy (Green et al., 1979). The OSPT is the most sensitive assay since it is usually more prolonged than the APTT because of the short half-life of Factor VII. The OSPT and APTT are severely prolonged in anticoagulant poisonings. Other assays are highly diagnostic for anticoagulant poisoning. The Thrombotest is an assay sensitive not only to a decrease in concentrations of Factors II, VII, and X but also to the presence of proteins induced by vitamin K absence or antagonism (PIVKA) circulating in the blood. (Further discussion of PIVKA can be found in Section 5.) The Thrombotest was found to be more sensitive than the OSPT (Mount 1984).

Presence of anemia is found on the hemogram. Evidence of a regenerative anemia may be present, but lack of such findings following acute bleeding is not surprising. Prolonged bleeding (approximately 5 days) is required to stimulate regenerative anemia, characterized by a large percentage of reticulocytes and possibly nucleated erythrocytes in the red cell mass. Platelets are not affected unless secondarily because of consumption after extensive blood loss, resulting in a moderate to marked thrombocyto-

Table 4. *Most Common Differential Considerations for Animals Showing Coagulopathy*

	Common Clinical Sign or Problem	Coagulation Screening Assays			Other Tests Showing Significant Changes From Normal Individuals
		OSPT	APTT	ACT	
Anticoagulant	Hemorrhage into body cavities	E*	E	E	Thrombotest Clotting time (CT) Vitamin K response
AITP	Petechia to purpura	N†	N	E	Bleeding time (BT) Clot retraction
	Hemorrhage from body orifices				Thrombocytopenia—marked
DIC	Bleeding associated with a primary disease control	E	E	E	Presence of FDPs BT CT Thrombocytopenia Thrombin test
Abnormal platelet function	Surgical bleeder	N	N	A‡	BT Clot retraction
Inherited disorders:					
Hemophilia	Hemarthrosis Surgical bleeder	N	E	E	Factor VIII activity Factor IX activity
VWD§	Surgical bleeder	N	A	A	BT Factor VIII activity Factor VIII–related antigen

*E = Markedly elevated.
†N = Normal.
‡A = Slight to moderate elevation.
§Von Willebrand's disease.

penia. This will quickly normalize, provided the coagulopathy is corrected.

Monitoring of OSPT prior to and following vitamin K_1 treatment can provide diagnostic information. An obvious response due to therapy can generally be recognized by 12 to 24 hours after administration of the loading dose. Failure to follow the t.i.d. or b.i.d. treatment schedule can result in prolonged OSPT assay times and falsely give the impression that the animal is not responding to treatment. A single dose of vitamin K_1 will lose its effect in lowering the OSPT within about 6 to 12 hours after administration.

Other causes of coagulopathy will not give the degree of responsiveness that is observed in anticoagulant poisoning when vitamin K_1 is given. Therefore, response to vitamin K_1 therapy as measured by the OSPT is diagnostic evidence of anticoagulant poisoning.

Postmortem evidence of anticoagulant poisoning is that of a hemorrhagic diathesis. The most common finding is free blood in the body cavities, especially within the pleural and mediastinal spaces.

Anticoagulant chemical analysis is seldom performed. However, recent developments in the field have provided better assessment of these poisoning cases. The prolonged-acting anticoagulants are excellent candidates for chemical analysis. Figures 3 and 4 show the length of time that diphacinone and brodificoum remain in the blood. The sample recommended is heparinized blood. Separate plasma and freeze it for submission. Serum samples can be used, but partial absorption of anticoagulant onto the clot may occur. Hemolyzed samples require special processing. Liver and heart blood are useful samples to obtain at necropsy.

SUMMARY

1. A variety of clinical presentations may be seen, but depression and pallor are the most universal signs associated with anticoagulant poisoning.
2. There is no means to clinically differentiate on initial presentation the different anticoagulants, since they all produce the same symptomatology. However, the degree and length of coagulopathy are very dependent on the chemical group of the anticoagulant and on the dose consumed.
3. The mechanism of action of anticoagulant toxicity heightens the continual need for a source of vitamin K, since the recycling of vitamin K within the animal's body is reduced or completely halted. Hence the need for a continual source of vitamin K becomes essential as long as the toxic effect of the anticoagulant is present.
4. Vitamin K_1 is the antidote of choice, and therapeutic regimens differ depending on the causative anticoagulant. Make it a rule to re-evaluate anticoagulant-poisoned animals after removal of vitamin K_1 treatment to rule out one of the longer-acting anticoagulants as the causative agent.
5. Always obtain blood sample for a coagulation screen before administering vitamin K_1 in order to use therapy as a diagnostic tool to differentiate

anticoagulant poisoning from other conditions such as DIC and AITP.

References and Supplemental Reading

Beasley, V. R., and Buck, W. B.: Warfarin and other anticoagulant poisonings. *In* Kirk, R. W. (ed.): *Current Veterinary Therapy VIII*. Philadelphia: W. B. Saunders, 1983, pp. 101–107.

Buck, W. B., Osweiler, G. D., and Van Gelder, G. A.: *In Clinical and Diagnostic Veterinary Toxicology*, ed. 2. Dubuque IA: Kendall/Hunt, 1976, pp. 253–256.

Fernandez, F. R., Davies, A. P., Teachout, D. J., et al.: Vitamin K-induced Heinz body formation in dogs. J. Am. Anim. Hosp. Assoc. 20:711, 1984.

Green, R. A., Roudebush, P., and Barton, C. L.: Laboratory evaluation of coagulopathies due to vitamin K antagonism in the dog: Three case reports. J. Am. Anim. Hosp. Assoc. 15:691, 1979.

Haskins, S. C.: Standards and techniques of equipment utilization. *In* Sattler, F. P., Knowles, R. P., and Whittick, W. G. (eds.): *Veterinary Critical Care*. Philadelphia: Lea & Febiger, 1981, pp. 60–110.

Haskins, S. C.: Shock. *In* Kirk, R. W. (ed.): *Current Veterinary Therapy VIII*. Philadelphia: W. B. Saunders, 1983, pp. 2–27.

Marsh, R. E.: Anticoagulant rodenticides—new and old. *In Pest Control Operators' Short Course Manual*. Lexington: University of Kentucky, 1983, pp. 306–314.

Mount, M. E.: Unpublished data. 1984.

Mount, M. E., and Feldman, B. F.: Mechanism of diphacinone rodenticide toxicosis in the dog and its therapeutic implications. Am. J. Vet. Res. 44:2009, 1983.

Mount, M. E., Feldman, B. F., and Buffington, T.: Vitamin K and its therapeutic importance. J.A.V.M.A. 180:1354, 1982.

O'Rourke, L. G.: Practical blood transfusions. *In* Kirk, R. W. (ed.): *Current Veterinary Therapy VIII*. Philadelphia: W. B. Saunders, 1983, pp. 408–411.

Szabuniewicz, M., and McCrady, J. D.: Hemostasis, hemostatic, anticoagulant, and fibrinolytic agents. *In* Jones, L. M., Booth, N. H., and McDonald, L. E. (eds.): *Veterinary Pharmacology and Therapeutics*, ed. 4. Ames IA: Iowa State University Press, 1977, pp. 471–473.

Woody, B. J., and Murphy, M. J.: Unpublished data. 1984.

TOXICOLOGY OF RODENTICIDES AND BIRD TOXICANTS

GARY D. OSWEILER, D.V.M.

Ames, Iowa

Attempts to control rats and mice include limiting access to food and shelter, individual trapping, and use of toxic chemicals for limited or widespread control. Use of rodent poisons by professional and lay people may in some cases place domestic animals at risk. Because rodenticides are designed to kill mammals, exposure of domestic animals and humans may lead to toxicosis in those species. Furthermore, in some cases, consumption of poisoned rodents by carnivores may lead to secondary poisoning, sometimes known as relay toxicity. Examples of rodenticides with high secondary hazard are fluoroacetate and strychnine.

Rodents are exposed to chemical poisons as toxic baits or tracking powders. Use of toxic baits is most common. Rodents come in contact with tracking powders primarily when they walk through them; these substances adhere to the feet and fur and are involuntarily ingested when the animals groom themselves (Marsh, 1983). Exposure to tracking powders by domestic animals appears to be limited. Cats, however, can pick up toxic powders and ingest them during grooming activity. Tracking-powder ingredients include sodium fluosilicate, chlorphenothane (DDT), endrin, lindane, alpha-naphthyl thiourea (ANTU), zinc, phosphide, red squill, and pyriminil. Zinc phosphide is the most recent acute rodenticide available as a tracking powder (Marsh, 1983).

Well-designed baits should be highly attractive to the pest species and should have low potential for ingestion by nontarget species. Colors, odors, or emetic activity may enhance the protective design of baits. Modern rodenticides are often incorporated in paraffinized or microencapsulated forms, which increase their stability under adverse environmental circumstances. They may be distributed in plastic bags, which are not exposed to the environment until opened and consumed by rodents. Bait packets are sometimes designed so that ingestion of several packets by a domestic animal would be necessary.to cause poisoning. Furthermore, use of bait stations allows placing of highly toxic baits in a manner not accessible to domestic animals.

Many chemicals effective in rodent control are moderately or markedly toxic to desirable mammals. Flavors and attractants used to entice rodents may also encourage consumption by wildlife or domestic animals. Careless placement, overuse, and failure to remove poisoned rodents may account for inadvertent exposure in domestic animals. Furthermore, with their reputation for toxicity, rodenticides may occasionally be used for malicious poisoning.

Older rodenticides such as arsenic, cyanide, barium, thallium, and phosphorus are seldom used today and account for only occasional poisoning in companion animals. Recently a wide variety of effective and relatively safe anticoagulant rodenticides have been developed. These constitute by far the greatest volume of rodenticide use in North America (see The Anticoagulant Rodenticides).

Dogs, with their voracious appetites and habit of bolting food, are particularly susceptible to rapid consumption of toxic baits. Cats are much less commonly poisoned.

Except for the anticoagulants and strychnine, few of the available types of rodenticides can be effectively controlled once clinical signs have commenced. Early detection of potential exposure coupled with a program of informing clients about specific hazards of rodenticides appears to be the most effective means of alleviating or preventing rodenticide toxicosis.

ALPHA-CHLORALOSE

Alpha-chloralose is centrally active and has both stimulant and depressant properties. It is used as a rodenticide, as a general anesthetic in laboratory animals, and to immobilize depredating birds (Hayes, 1982). Use in mouse baits is indicated with a warning dye.

Rats, mice, dogs, and cats are approximately equally susceptible. The oral LD_{50} ranges from 100 mg/kg in cats to 600 mg/kg in dogs. Alpha-chloralose selectively depresses neurons of the ascending reticular formation, suppressing the normal arousal response. Small doses increase motor activity, and there are myoclonic movements that may progress to deep anesthesia as dosage increases. Hypothermia may also occur.

Early clinical effects are mild ataxia followed by hyperexcitability. Cats may become aggressive. Early signs progress to posterior weakness, prostration, increased salivation, shallow respiration, weak pulse, and hypothermia. Affected animals appear to lose sensitivity to pain but have increased reactivity to touch, sound, or electrical stimuli.

TREATMENT. Recommended treatment includes restraint to prevent injury, maintenance of normal body temperature, and evacuation of the gastrointestinal tract by appropriate means (see Emergency and General Treatment of Poisonings). Seizures may be controlled by IV or IM use of diazepam. Artificial ventilation in combination with other general toxicologic management is recommended for severe intoxications.

CRIMIDINE

Crimidine (Castrix, Bayer, 2-chloro-4-dimethylamino-6-methylpyrimidine) is a rapidly acting convulsant chemical with no reported age or sex differences in toxicity. Oral LD_{50} in rats and mice are 1.5 mg/kg and 1.2 mg/kg, respectively. Crimidine appears to be an antagonist of vitamin B_6, and clinical signs are central nervous system (CNS) convulsant activity. Toxicosis occurs within 20 to 40 minutes after ingestion but is of short duration because of rapid excretion of the chemical. Twenty lethal doses of crimidine may be eliminated by a dog in 13 hours. Poisoned rats do not pose a secondary poisoning hazard.

Short-acting barbiturates will control seizures. Pyridoxine hydrochloride at 20 mg/kg IV may be an efficient antidote in cases of poisoning (Clark et al., 1981).

NORBORMIDE

Norbormide kills Norway rats in from 15 minutes to 4 hours and has an approximate LD_{50} for rats of 5 mg/kg. It is noncumulative, tolerance does not develop, and it kills rats in one feeding. Use in North America appears very limited. The toxicity of norbormide for dogs and cats is in excess of 1000 mg/kg. Hamsters are relatively susceptible at 140 mg/kg.

Clinical signs described in rats include restlessness, ataxia, posterior weakness, labored breathing, paleness of the extremities, and mild convulsions. Clinical toxicosis in dogs and cats is not likely.

RED SQUILL

Red squill is a red powder obtained from *Urginea maritima* (of the family Liliaceae), which is native to several Mediterranean countries. It is the oldest rodenticidal material known and has a reputation as being safe based on its unpalatable nature and strong emetic action. Red squill is seldom used as a rodenticide in North America.

Acute oral toxicity of red squill is 100 mg/kg in cats and 145 mg/kg in dogs, compared with 490 mg/kg in rats. Red squill contains glycosides of the digitalis type. Overdose produces cardiac and clinical effects similar to digitalis.

Vomiting is an early and characteristic sign. There are convulsions, hyperesthesia, and incoordination. Diarrhea may occur approximately 1 day after emesis and early signs. Death occurs 1 to 3 days after initial ingestion, but recovery is common.

Pathologic changes include gastritis, enteritis, and alimentary mucosal ulceration, as well as congestion of abdominal and thoracic organs. No adequate diagnostic chemical test is available. Diagnosis is based on history of exposure correlated with compatible signs and lesions.

TREATMENT. Specific therapy is not described. General detoxication and supportive therapy should be of value, however (see Emergency and General Treatment of Poisonings). Treat intoxicated animals as for digitalis overdose.

PYRIMINIL

Pyriminil (*N*-3-pyridylmethyl N′-*p*-nitrophenyl urea, Vacor, Rohm & Haas) is a recently developed rodenticide with high toxicity in rats, compared with that in other animals. Pyriminil (2 per cent baits or 10 per cent tracking powders) has been withdrawn from commercial availability. Occasional continuing access to humans or animals may occur for some time to come.

Pyriminil is a nicotinamide antagonist. Cats are more susceptible (62 to 200 mg/kg) than dogs (500 to 1000 mg/kg). The oral LD_{50} in rats is 12 mg/kg.

Clinical signs in dogs may occur from 4 to 8 hours after ingestion of pyriminil. Initial signs are nausea, abdominal pain, vomiting, and depression. Prolonged effects may include anorexia, dilated pupils, dehydration, and lethargy. Breathing is deep and respiratory rate is reduced. Fine to coarse tremors, hind limb weakness, and decreased reflexes occur. Visual problems may develop several days after recovery from acute signs. In the author's experience, one of these signs has been a degree of night blindness in dogs.

TREATMENT. Induction of emesis should be followed by activated charcoal (see Emergency and General Treatment of Poisonings). Injection of 50 to 100 mg nicotinamide IM is recommended. Repeat every 4 hours for up to eight injections, depending on clinical response. Appropriate supportive and symptomatic therapy should be instituted. Nicotinamide (25 to 50 mg/animal) orally should be administered three to five times daily for 7 to 10 days. Owners should watch closely for adverse signs or changes in the animal's health status, particularly during the first week after acute toxicosis.

PHORAZETIM

Phorazetim (Gophacide, Bayer) is an organophosphate compound developed in Germany primarily for control of pocket gophers, but it has occasionally been used in rodent control. It is a powerful cholinergic agent and could potentially cause clinical signs of organophosphate poisoning if consumed by domestic animals. Production has been discontinued, so any hazard of poisoning would be from product currently held by the public. The oral LD_{50} for rats ranges from 3.7 to 7.5 mg/kg body weight.

Treatment of suspected phorazetim toxicosis should involve measures as for other organophosphate compounds (see Organophosphate and Carbamate Insecticide Poisonings).

BARIUM CARBONATE

Barium carbonate is an old rodenticide rarely used or available in North America. It is a weak rodenticide but toxic enough to represent a hazard to domestic animals. Ingestion of barium carbonate causes severe colic, diarrhea, and hemorrhage. Death may result from cardiac arrest.

PHOSPHORUS

Elemental phosphorus is available commercially as both red and white phosphorus. Red phosphorus is used primarily in the manufacture of fertilizers and safety matches; it is generally considered inert and essentially nontoxic. White phosphorus is colorless or pale yellow with a waxy appearance and garlic-like odor. Rodenticides prepared from white phosphorus are generally mixed with a greasy or oily base. Commercially available pastes contain from 1.5 to as much as 5 per cent phosphorus.

Toxicity of white phosphorus is not well documented, but doses of 50 to 100 mg per dog are considered toxic.

Clinical manifestations of phosphorus poisoning are (1) acute initial reaction occurring within hours of ingestion and characterized by gastrointestinal, abdominal, and circulatory signs; (2) an interim or latent phase in which apparent recovery occurs (2 to 3 days after initial signs); (3) recurrence of severe clinical signs characterized by vomiting, hematemesis, icterus, hepatic failure, and CNS dysfunction.

The liver may be enlarged, and icterus is apparent. There may be hypoprothrombinemia and a tendency to bleeding, especially from the gingivae, stomach, intestines, or kidneys. Hypoglycemia may be marked, and liver enzymes are elevated. Oliguria can develop, and urinalysis reveals albuminuria, hematuria, and increased concentrations of amino acids.

TREATMENT. Administer gastric lavage with tap water. Follow with oral mineral oil appropriate to the size of the patient (see Emergency and General Treatment of Poisonings). Monitor for shock, dehydration, pulmonary edema, and hepatic failure. Treat symptomatically as needed.

ALPHA-CHLOROHYDRIN

Alpha-chlorohydrin (3-chloro-1,2-propanediol, Epibloc, Pestcon Systems) has recently been developed as a new rodenticide that kills rats at high dosages but acts as a male antifertility agent at lower doses. It is available only to certified pest control applicators or persons under their direct supervision.

Single lethal doses result in death between 1 and 5 days after ingestion. Cumulative toxicity does not appear to occur. The acute oral LD_{50} is 188 mg/kg for cats and 328 mg/kg for dogs.

Alpha-chlorohydrin is rapidly metabolized and is reportedly degraded in the environment. There appears to be no secondary or cumulative toxicity. There is no evidence of sterility in avian, aquatic, amphibian, or reptilian species treated with alpha-chlorohydrin. Male nontarget species may become reversibly infertile. Normal libido and mating activity are maintained, but eventually testicular atrophy occurs as a result of epididymal blockage.

Toxic doses of alpha-chlorohydrin in rats produced a loss of appetite and body weight, accompanied by dose-related diuresis and increased water intake. Urinary glucose and protein were elevated at dosages above 100 mg/kg body weight. Clinical effects began returning to normal within 7 days after one dose in survivors. Some rats at dosages of 100 to 120 mg/kg developed oliguria or anuria and died.

Descriptions of clinical signs in domestic animals were not found, and no treatment is described.

4-AMINOPYRIDINE

4-Aminopyridine (a bird repellent, Avitrol, Phillips Petroleum) causes birds to become disoriented and have pronounced vocalization known as a distress cry, which induces other members of the flock to avoid places where the distress signals occurred. The baits are usually cracked corn or other grain concentrates ranging from 0.5 per cent to 3.0 per cent 4-aminopyridine.

Although of relatively low lethality for birds, 4-aminopyridine is relatively toxic to mammals. The acute oral LD_{50} for dogs has been estimated at 4 mg/kg body weight. Clinical poisoning incidents have been recorded in horses, cattle, and zoo animals. The toxic dose of 0.5 per cent bait for a 25-kg (55-lb) dog would be 100 mg of 4-aminopyridine, or 200 gm of bait.

4-Aminopyridine enhances transmission at neuromuscular junctions and other synapses. It appears capable of releasing acetylcholine and other synaptic neurotransmitters and is an antagonist to droperidol-fentanyl, ketamine, and xylazine. Experimentally, it has improved neuromuscular function during blockade by botulinum toxin.

Clinical effects in poisoned mammals include hyperexcitability, salivation, tremors, muscle incoordination, seizures, and cardiac or respiratory arrest. Clinical onset is as early as 30 minutes after exposure, and death may occur in 4 hours or less. Tonoclonic seizures may be intermittent with periods of depression, during which the animal may not be roused. Vocalization sometimes occurs. Other clinical signs include muscle tremors, stilted gait, and excitement. Cardiovascular effects are characterized generally by tachycardia and increase in systolic arterial blood pressure. Respiratory rate may also be increased. There may be seizures and cardiorespiratory signs. Other toxicants producing similar clinical signs include amphetamines, caffeine, organochlorine insecticides, acute lead poisoning, nicotine, metaldehyde, tremorgenic mycotoxins, and strychnine. Without history of exposure, many of these, poisonings would be difficult to differentiate clinically from 4-aminopyridine toxicosis. 4-Aminopyridine can be detected in liver and stomach contents by specific chemical methods.

TREATMENT. An accepted treatment for aminopyridine toxicosis in small animals has not been established. If ingestion has occurred recently and the animal is ambulatory, emesis should be initiated using apomorphine or other appropriate measures (see Emergency and General Treatment of Poisonings). If emesis is contraindicated, then gastric lavage should be used. Follow with a slurry of 10 per cent activated charcoal in water at 5 gm charcoal/kg body weight. Thirty minutes later administer sodium sulfate orally at 1 gm/kg body weight.

In addition to oral detoxification, cardiopulmonary support may be required. Propranolol has been considered useful in blocking cardiac effects. A dosage for this purpose has not been established for dogs, but IV administration of 0.1 to 1.0 mg/kg body weight in dogs has suppressed catecholamine-induced arrhythmias.

Seizure control may be needed. Diazepam dosage for control of status epilepticus in dogs and cats is 1 mg/kg body weight IV or orally, and the recommended dosage to control strychnine seizures is 2 to 5 mg/kg IV. If seizure control is attempted for aminopyridine toxicosis, administration of drugs should be carried out with caution and judged according to clinical response. In horses, heavy sedation with xylazine has provided nearly complete relief from excitement and muscle tremors induced by 4-aminopyridine. Although specific therapy using xylazine against 4-aminopyridine seizures appears not to have been developed, use of a standard dosage of xylazine (2.2 mg/kg body weight) IM could be considered if poisoning by aminopyridine has occurred.

3-CHLORO-*p*-TOLUIDINE

3-Chloro-*p*-toluidine (3-CPT, Starlicide) is effective against pests such as starlings, crows, and blackbirds when the oral LD_{50} for these species is less than 4 mg/kg body weight. The acute LD_{50} for rats is 655 mg/kg body weight. Toxic or lethal doses for dogs and cats have not been established. 3-CPT is formulated at 0.1 and 1.0 per cent in baits. Assuming an oral dosage of 665 mg/kg of body weight in dogs and that 10 per cent of the LD_{50} dose may cause lethality, then the lethal dose for a 20-kg (44-lb) dog might be as little as 4 oz of bait. Thus, poisoning from 3-CPT baits is possible but not likely.

Clinical signs include CNS depression, muscular weakness, and cyanosis. 3-CPT is an aniline derivative and may be responsible for development of methemoglobinemia and Heinz bodies in mammals. However, methemoglobinemia is not sufficient to account for lethality. During intoxication, there can be rapid rise in the concentration of uric acid in the blood. Cardiovascular collapse may be a significant factor in lethality.

Gross and microscopic lesions are not consistent, and mild degenerative changes alone do not account for lethality.

TREATMENT. No specific treatment has been established. Recent ingestion of baits should be handled by appropriate oral detoxification procedures similar to those for aminopyridine. Monitor for renal function and blood methemoglobin concentration, using supportive treatment for these complications as needed.

References and Supplemental Reading

Clark, M. L., Harvey, D. G., and Humphreys, D. J.: *Veterinary Toxicology*, 2nd ed. London: Bailliere Tindall, 1981.

Felsenstein, W. C., Smith, R. P., and Gosselin, R. E.: Toxicology studies on the avicide 3-chloro-*p*-toluidine. Toxicol. Appl. Pharmacol. 28:110, 1974.

Hayes, W. J.: *Pesticides Studied in Man*. Baltimore: Williams & Wilkins Co., 1982.

Klein, L., and Hopkins, J.: Behavioral and cardiorespiratory responses to 4-aminopyridine in healthy awake horses. Am. J. Vet. Res. 42:1655, 1981.

Marsh, R. E.: Tracking powders. Pest Control. 50:42, 1983.

Osweiler, G. D., Carson, T. L., Buck, W. B., et al.: *Clinical and Diagnostic Veterinary Toxicology*. Dubuque, IA: Kendall/Hunt, 1985.

Peoples, S. A., and Maddy, K. T.: Poisoning of man and animals due to ingestion of the rodent poison VACOR. Vet. Hum. Toxicol. 21:266, 1979.

Ray, A. C., Dwyer, J. N., Fambro, G. W., et al.: Clinical signs and chemical confirmation of 4-aminopyridine poisoning in horses. J.A.V.M.A. 39:329, 1978.

Spyker, D. A., Lynch, C., Shabanowitz, et al.: Poisoning with 4-aminopyridine: Report of three cases. Clin. Toxicol. 16:487, 1980.

Thomson, W. T.: *Agricultural Chemicals: Book III - Fumigants, Growth Regulators, Repellents, and Rodenticides*. Fresno, CA: Thomson Publications, 1983, pp. 131–154.

ADVERSE DRUG REACTIONS

ARTHUR L. ARONSON, D.V.M.,
and J. EDMOND RIVIERE, D.V.M.
Raleigh, North Carolina

The value and benefit of drugs in modern therapeutics is unquestioned. However, every pharmacologic substance has the potential to affect some individual patient adversely. Although there is no drug that is completely safe, the justification for using a given drug lies in the favorable ratio of anticipated benefits compared with potential risks.

A veterinarian ideally should be able to make a quantitative benefit-risk assessment for each drug that is used clinically. Although adverse drug reactions (ADRs) have been reported for drugs used clinically in veterinary practice, currently there is no detailed information available on their incidence. Thus it is not possible to make a quantitative benefit-risk assessment.

A brief consideration of ADRs will be made in this review, together with listings of selected ADRs in cats and dogs that have been reported to the Center for Veterinary Medicine (CVM, formerly known as the Bureau of Veterinary Medicine) Drug Surveillance Program (Tables 1 and 2). These reports were obtained from CVM memos published since 1975 and updated yearly through 1980. Some additional reports have been obtained and included in the tables.

One might reasonably ask what benefit has resulted from ADR reports. This question was posed to the CVM, and the Center responded by presenting several examples of labeling changes involving the incorporation of additional cautionary statements that clinicians should expect to see in labeling now or in the near future. The inclusion of caution-

Table 1. Adverse Drug Reactions Reported in Cats

Drug	Clinical Signs and Lesions
ANALGESICS	
Acetaminophen	Depression, death
Acetaminophen/codeine	Restlessness, excitement, fear, mydriasis, death
Aspirin	Depression or excitability, ataxia, nystagmus, anorexia, emesis, weight loss, hyperpnea, hepatitis, bone marrow depression, anemia, gastric lesions, death
Phenylbutazone	Inappetence, weight loss, alopecia, dehydration, emesis, severe depression, death
CNS DEPRESSANTS	
Acetylpromazine	Prolonged effect, cardiac arrest, hyperactivity, convulsions, death
Ketamine, ketamine/acetylpromazine	Anoxia, apnea, hypopnea, ineffective and prolonged recovery, tremors, convulsions, excitement, hyperpyrexia, dyspnea, cardiac arrest, bladder and renal hemorrhage, nephrosis, fatty liver, lung edema, deafness, death
Halothane	Cardiac arrest, apnea, shock
Methoxyflurane	Ataxia, death
Thiamylal	Cardiac arrest, respiratory arrest, apnea, prolonged anesthesia, ataxia, shock, death
Xylazine	Prolonged anesthesia, apnea, convulsions
Proparacaine	Mydriasis
ANTIPARASITICS	
Bunamidine	Seizures, coughing, dyspnea, pulmonary congestion, choking, lethargy, pallor, coma, hypersalivation, anorexia, fever, hypothermia, oral lesion, tongue edema, sudden death
n-Butyl chloride	Emesis
Dichlorophene/toluene	Ataxia, twitching, seizures, mydriasis, disorientation, posterior weakness, incoordination, hypersalivation, emesis, hyperpnea, tachycardia, death
Dichlorvos	Death
Glycobiarsol	Emesis, icterus, death
Levamisole	Salivation, excitement, diarrhea, mydriasis
Niclosamide	Depression, ataxia, hypothermia
Piperazine	Emesis, dementia, ataxia, hypermetria, hypersalivation
Praziquantel	Irritation at injection site, lameness, emesis, ataxia, hypothermia
HORMONES	
Megestrol acetate	Polyphagia, hydrometra, uterine rupture
Triamcinolone	Nervousness, hypersalivation, disorientation, syncope
ANTIMICROBIALS	
Ampicillin	Diarrhea
Amoxicillin	Emesis
Amphotericine B	Marked elevation of BUN and serum creatinine following single dose
Cephalexin	Emesis, fever
Chloramphenicol	Anaphylactoid-type reaction, anorexia, ataxia, emesis, depression, diarrhea, neutropenia, death
Gentamicin	Pruritus, alopecia, erythema
Lincomycin	Diarrhea, emesis, collapse and coma following IM injection
Tetracycline	Malignant hyperthermia, emesis, dehydration
Tylosin	Irritation at injection site
Hexachlorophene	Anorexia, ataxia
Miconazole	Erythema, alopecia
Sulfisoxazole	Emesis
Procaine penicillin/dihydrostreptomycin	Ataxia
Trimethoprim/sulfadiazine	Emesis, hypersalivation, mydriasis, ataxia seizures
MISCELLANEOUS	
Bethanechol	Emesis

ary statements on the label, based on drug experience, has positive benefits that include (1) providing information on potential side effects of the drug, thereby enchancing the predictability of a clinician's benefit-risk assessment, and (2) altering the way in which a drug is used to avoid adverse reactions.*

*Clearly, the positive effects of such information are directly dependent on clinicians' periodically reviewing labeling to determine whether new information is included. Most package inserts bear a printing date, which helps determine when revisions have been made.

Two examples can be cited in which a labeling change, brought about by ADR reports, has resulted in fewer reports of ADRs subsequent to the change. The first example involved the concurrent administration of two anthelmintics, bunamidine and butamisole. Toxicity appeared to be enhanced when these two drugs were given simultaneously. This enhanced toxicity was verified by one of the manufacturers. When a contraindication against simultaneous use of bunamidine and butamisole was added to the labeling, the number of adverse reac-

Table 2. Adverse Drug Reactions Reported in Dogs

Drug	Clinical Signs and Lesions
ANALGESICS	
Aspirin	Bleeding disorders
Meclofenamic acid/corticosteroids	Diarrhea, gastrointestinal bleeding, death
Phenylbutazone	Anemia, leukopenia, thrombocytopenia, emesis, hemorrhagic enteritis, epistaxis, elevated liver enzymes, death
CNS DEPRESSANTS	
Acetylpromazine	Atypical behavior, aggression, apprehension, lameness of injected leg, prolonged effect, respiratory distress, bradycardia, pallor, seizures, syncope, weak irregular pulse, urination, defecation
Butorphanol	Sedation, ataxia, salivation, gasping, crying, emesis, depression, anorexia, respiratory and cardiac arrest, anaphylaxis, cyanosis, death
Fetanyl/droperidol	Behavior change, lameness, ataxia, hyperthermia, aggression, seizures, bradycardia, tachycardia, hyperpnea, apnea, tremors, hyperventilation, hyperexcitability, hyperkinesia, nystagmus, cardiac arrest, prolonged recovery, death
Ethylisobutrazine	Hyperexcitability
Halothane	Cardiac arrhythmia, malignant hyperthermia, nystagmus, torticollis, emesis
Ketamine	Convulsions, cyanosis
Lidocaine	Laryngeal and facial edema, respiratory arrest, seizures, ataxia, tremors
Methoxyflurane	Cardiac arrest, hepatitis after 2 weeks, death
Oxymorphone	Bradycardia
Prochlorperazine/isopropamide	Tachycardia
Promazine	Depression, hypotension, hyperthermia, death
Thiamylal	Cardiac arrest, respiratory arrest, prolonged anesthesia, cyanosis, apnea, cardiac arrhythmias, bradycardia, temporary hearing loss, prolonged recovery, death
Thiopental	Cardiac arrest, prolonged recovery, pulmonary edema, slough at injection site, death
Xylazine	Viciousness, bradycardia, cardiac arrest, death
ANTICONVULSANTS	
Phenytoin	Ataxia, hepatotoxicity, leukopenia, emesis, coma, death
Primidone	Liver failure, icterus, emesis, alopecia, polydipsia, polyuria, death
ANTIPARASITICS	
Arecoline/tetrachlorethylene	Mydriasis, ataxia, emesis, diarrhea, severe colic, inability to walk, depression, hypothermia
Bunamidine	Dyspnea, ataxia, emesis, weakness, bloat, gastroenteritis, lung hemorrhage, seizures, sudden death
Butamisole	Dyspnea, ataxia, muscle tremors, collapse, coma, depression, icterus, swelling at injection site, abscess formation, death
n-Butyl chloride	Stupor, ataxia, death
Dichlorophene/toluene	Incoordination, convulsions, emesis, disorientation, mydriasis, lethargy, anorexia, fever, death
Dichlorvos	Diarrhea, emesis, ataxia, tremors, weakness, death
Diethylcarbamazine	Pruritus, weakness, emesis, diarrhea, icterus, anaphylactoid reaction, death
Diethylcarbamazine/styrylpyridinium	Diarrhea, emesis, sterilization, teratogenesis, death
Disophenol	Hyperthermia, hyperventilation, ataxia, collapse, dyspnea, respiratory distress, swelling at injection site, death
Dithiazine iodide	Emesis, diarrhea, depression, apprehension, hyperpyrexia, anorexia, lethargy, death
Glycobiarsol	Emesis
Levamisole	Dyspnea, pulmonary edema, emesis
Mebendazole	Icterus, emesis, anorexia, diarrhea, lethargy, abnormal liver function tests, hepatotoxicity, death
Piperazine	Paralysis, death
Metronidazole	Lethargy, rear limb weakness
Phthalofyne	Hepatitis, splenitis, ataxia, death
Praziquantel	Irritation at injection site, weakness, bradycardia, seizures, emesis, ataxia
Pyrantel pamoate	Emesis
Ronnel	Emesis, twitching, depression
Thenium closylate	Emesis, diarrhea, enteritis, anaphylaxis, hemorrhagic enteritis and liver, seizures, dyspnea, cyanosis, death
Thiacetarsamide	Emesis, icterus, bilirubinuria, elevated liver enzymes, depression, anorexia, cough, renal failure, swelling at injection site, alopecia, dermatitis, bleeding disorders, death
Toluene	Collapse
Trichlorfon	Anorexia, weakness, lethargy
Uredofos	Emesis, diarrhea, death

Table continued on following page

Table 2. Adverse Drug Reactions Reported in Dogs Continued

Drug	Clinical Signs and Lesions
HORMONES	
Betamethasone	Shock, polydipsia, polyuria
Dexamethasone	Polydipsia, polyuria, emesis, diarrhea, bloody diarrhea, melena, panting
Prednisolone	Anorexia, polyphagia, pica, anemia, lethargy, diarrhea, polyuria, elevated liver enzymes
Methylprednisolone	Disorientation, panting
Triamcinolone	Cushing's syndrome, emesis, depression, urticaria, dyspnea, seizures, shock
Estradiol cypionate	Pain at injection site, pyometra
Megestrol acetate	Polyphagia, hydrometra, uterine inertia, uterine rupture, anorexia, depression, death
Mibolerone	Elevated liver function tests, icterus, vaginal discharge, behavioral changes, urinary incontinence
ANTIMICROBIALS	
Amoxicillin	Skin rash, emesis
Ampicillin	Wheals, injection site inflammation, emesis, diarrhea
Bacitracin/polymyxin B/neomycin (ophthalmic)	Eye irritation
Cephalexin	Panting, salivation, hyperexcitability
Chloramphenicol	Emesis, depression, ataxia, diarrhea, death
Gentamicin	Injection site inflammation, edema of lips, eyelids, and vulva; elevated BUN
Hetacillin	Emesis
Lincomycin	Emesis, soft stools, diarrhea, shock after IM injection, death
Nitrofurantoin	Emesis
Potassium penicillin G	Increased respiration and heart rate
Procaine penicillin G	Ataxia, edema, dyspnea
Procaine and benzathine penicillin G	Sterile abscess, anaphylaxis
Sulfachlorpyridazine	Ataxia, hyperirritability
Sulfaguanidine	Keratoconjunctivitis
Sulfamerazine/sulfapyridine	Emesis, dyspnea
Tetracycline	Emesis
Trimethoprim/sulfadiazine	Emesis, diarrhea, anorexia, elevated liver function tests, icterus, hepatitis, bilateral keratoconjunctivitis, swelling and pain at injection site, urticaria, hives, exfoliative dermatitis, fascial swelling, hemolytic anemia, aplastic anemia, polydypsia/polyuria, polyarthritis, seizures
MISCELLANEOUS	
Aminopropazine	Injection site necrosis
Aminophylline	Emesis, anorexia, polyphagia, polydipsia, polyuria, hyperexcitability
Asparaginase	Ataxia, muscle weakness, lethargy
Atropine	Paradoxical bradycardia, heart block
Calcium edetate	Emesis, diarrhea, anorexia, depression
Copper naphthenate (topical)	Skin burns
Dichlorphenamide	Disorientation
Dinoprost tromethamine	Panting, hypersalivation, discomfort, emesis
Digoxin	Emesis, anorexia
Epinephrine/pilocarpine (ophthalmic)	Conjunctivitis
Ibuprofen	Depression, emesis, gastric ulcers, death
Metrizamide	Seizures after myelogram
Neostigmine/physostigmine (ophthalmic)	Emesis, diarrhea, bradycardia, pannus
Neostigmine methylsulfate	Apnea, cardiac arrest, death
Pyridostigmine	Diarrhea, emesis
Sulfurated lime (topical)	Skin burns, edema, dehydration
Theophylline	Diarrhea

tions reported markedly decreased. In the second example, ADR reports indicated that dogs infected with heartworm were experiencing more serious side effects to butamisole. When the labeling was altered to advise against use of butamisole in dogs positive for *Dirofilaria immitis*, the number of ADR reports declined. Unfortunately, more information does not always prevent adverse reactions. Reports of hepatotoxicity associated with mebendazole in dogs have not significantly declined following addition of this information to the label.

Table 3 lists additional cautionary statements that have recently been added or will soon appear in package inserts for amitraz, butorphanol, corticosteroids, fentanyl/droperidol, orgotein, praziquantel, trimethoprim/sulfadiazine, and ivermectin. It is emphasized that ADR reports most often lead to label changes that can be expected to result in more rational use of the product. Only rarely do ADR reports result in a drug's removal from the market. Clearly, the more information that one has about a drug, the more one is able to evaluate anticipated

Table 3. Additions to Cautionary Statements in Drug Labeling

Drug	Cautionary Statements
Amitraz	Concerning dogs: The opportunity for exposure by the oral route should be minimized since ingestion may increase the risk of adversities. Concerning humans: The product as concentrate or diluted may cause eye or skin irritation. Contact with eyes, skin, or clothing should be avoided. If eye contact occurs, it is advised to wash with water for 15 minutes and call a physician immediately.
Butorphanol	Transient sedation and ataxia are being included as adverse reactions.
Corticosteroids	The following warning is being added: Corticosteroids administered to dogs, rabbits, and rodents during pregnancy have resulted in cleft palate in offspring. Corticosteroids administered to dogs during pregnancy have also resulted in other congenital anomalies including deformed forelegs, phocomelia, and anasarca.
Fentanyl/droperidol	Episodic head bobbing reported in Doberman pinschers is being included as an adverse reaction.
Orgotein	Allergic hypersensitivity and systemic anaphylaxis are being included as adverse reactions.
Praziquantel	Local irritation or swelling at the site of SC injection in cats is being added as a cautionary statement.
Trimethoprim/sulfadiazine	The following cautionary statements are being added: Conditions reported following use of trimethoprim/sulfadiazine include polyarthritis, urticaria, facial swelling, fever, hemolytic anemia, polydypsia/polyuria, vomiting, anorexia, diarrhea, seizures, and keratitis sicca. Hepatitis, possibly due to sulfonamide hypersensitivity, has been diagnosed following trimethoprim/sulfadiazine therapy. Individual animal hypersensitivity may result in local or generalized reactions, sometimes fatal.
Ivermectin	On the bases of 88 cases involving 42 deaths in "collie-type" and "non-collie-type" dogs, information is being added to all approved labels cautioning against the use in dogs of ivermectin-containing products approved for species other than dogs and informing the users that severe adverse reactions may occur if such formulations are used.

benefits compared with potential risks in using the product.

WHAT IS AN ADR?

Several definitions of ADRs have been advanced by various groups studying these reactions. It may be useful to consider some of these definitions.

An operational definition used by the Massachusetts General Hospital (Koch-Weser et al., 1969) is "any noxious change in a patient's condition which a physician believes to be due to a drug, which occurs at dosages normally used in man, and which (1) requires treatment, (2) indicates decrease or cessation of therapy with the drug, or (3) suggests that future therapy with the drug carries an unusual risk in this patient." This definition does not include as ADRs any trivial or expected side effects that do not require any change in therapy or noxious events due to deliberate or accidental overdosage.

The World Health Organization definition is similar (Venulet, 1977): "An ADR is one which is noxious and unintended and which occurs at doses used in man for prophylaxis, diagnosis, therapy, or modification of physiological functions."

The CVM definition includes lack of drug efficacy as an ADR: "an unintended change in the structure, function and chemistry of the body including injury, toxicity, sensitivity reaction, or lack of efficacy associated with the clinical use of a drug."

CAUSES OF ADRs. ADRs associated with specific drugs are listed in Tables 1 and 2. Two basic causes of ADRs are *excessive drug use* and *failure to establish a therapeutic endpoint.* It has been shown in several studies that the frequency of ADRs increases as the number of drugs used concurrently in a patient increases. These ADRs may or may not be due to drug interactions. Human patients receive an average of 14 different drugs during a normal stay in the hospital. The isolation and identification of an ADR for a specific drug in this situation is nearly impossible. Also, a toxic endpoint, if not predefined, may occur when toxicity is an extension of the pharmacologic action of a drug. For example, the maximal contractile force obtainable with digitalis glycosides occurs before alterations in cardiac conduction. ADRs to digitalis glycosides could be minimized by selecting improvement in hemodynamics or renal function as the therapeutic endpoint rather than changes in cardiac conduction or the onset of emesis. Failure to establish a therapeutic endpoint also may render it difficult to recognize lack of efficacy, and a useless but potentially toxic drug will continue to be given.

RECOGNITION OF ADRs. There are no unique clinical or laboratory findings that distinguish ADRS from the manifestations of concurrent disease. Thus, an accurate identification of an ADR often is difficult. An alert and suspicious clinician is of the utmost importance. It may be difficult to think of one's treatment as being responsible for the patient's disability. One should expect the unexpected. A suspicious reaction should not be dismissed because it is not described in a pharmacology textbook or on a drug package insert. ADRs may go largely undetected if the clinical signs they induce are indistinguishable from those of common disease syndromes. Drugs that induce a complex of rare clinical signs will attract more attention and will be identified; an example is chloramphenicol-induced aplastic anemia in humans or the teratogenic effects of griseofulvin in queens.

Comparisons of ADR evaluations among experienced observers reveal that the clinical identification of ADRs is complex and subjective. It is difficult to prove a cause-and-effect relationship, and there are differences in the subjective evaluations among individual investigators. The difficulties are compounded when combinations of drugs are administered to a patient.

Nevertheless, everyone does agree that ADRs do occur. The following guidelines may be helpful in identifying a ADR:

1. There is a plausible temporal relationship between administration of the drug and the ADR. Clinical signs develop while the drug is being taken. For example, if a patient goes into anaphylactic shock 10 minutes after the injection of pencillin G, there is a strong likelihood that an ADR occurred. It must be remembered that some ADRs may occur long after the drug is administered. The occurrence of cervical cancer in teenage girls whose mothers took diethylstilbestrol during pregnancy is a case in point.
2. There is improvement in the clinical syndrome when the drug is discontinued.
3. The ADR recurs if the patient is reexposed to the drug.

MINIMIZING ADRs. Information relating to the frequency with which ADRs occur with drugs in clinical use would be most helpful. This would require a drug monitoring and reporting system that would document the frequency, kinds, and causes of ADRs to a specific drug in relation to the total use of the drug. A clinician then would have a basis for determining the possible benefits of a drug compared with its possible harmful effects under a given set of conditions. A study by Ndiritu and Enos (1977) involved a review of 39,541 cases presented to the University of California Veterinary Medical Teaching Hospital. Of these, 130 suspected ADRs were detected and 66 had sufficient data available to specifically identify the drug involved. The following classes of drugs were involved (number of cases): anti-infective agents (21), antineoplastic agents (10), anesthetics and related drugs (20), cardiovascular drugs (2), ophthalmologic preparations (5), and miscellaneous drugs (8). Only four deaths were directly attributed to ADRs. It is worthwhile to emphasize that all drugs possess the potential for producing an ADR and that a drug should not be used unless there is a clearly defined therapeutic objective.

CLASSES OF ADRs

SIDE EFFECTS. Side effects of drugs may be considered ADRs in that they lead to actions that are undesirable but inherent to the drug's action. For example, mydriasis produced when atropine is used as a preanesthetic is undesirable, but it must be accepted along with the desired tachycardia and decreased salivation, since atropine blocks muscarinic receptors nonselectively throughout the body. Similarly, anticancer drugs, by virtue of their ability to affect rapidly proliferating neoplastic tissues, also adversely affect normal tissues with rapid cell turnover, such as in the gastrointestinal mucosa and hematopoietic tissues. For the most part, ADRs related to side effects are predictable and expected, unlike the following classes of ADRs.

DISRUPTION OF CONTROL MECHANISMS. Two classes of drugs have a clearly established potential for disrupting control mechanisms in the body. Suprainfection has been associated with intensive antibacterial drug therapy, particularly when broad-spectrum drugs or combinations of antibacterial drugs are used. Reduced resistance to infection and activation of latent infection have been associated with adrenocorticosteroids, especially during prolonged administration.

DRUG ALLERGY. Certain ADRs have an immunologic basis. These types of reactions require previous exposure and sensitization to the drug. These drugs combine with protein, and antibodies are formed to the drug-protein complex. Subsequent exposure to the drug leads to a typical antigen-antibody reaction with the release of pathologic mediators (histamine, serotonin, bradykinin, and so on), which are responsible for inducing the pathologic effects. Although virtually any body system may be affected, ADRs of this type usually are manifested as abnormalities of the respiratory tract (rhinitis, asthma) and the skin (urticaria, hives) or as generalized systemic reactions (anaphylactic shock, interstitial nephritis). Penicillin and aspirin are examples of drugs that have been implicated in inducing these types of ADRs in humans. Drug allergies, although they undoubtedly occur, are not well documented in domestic animals.

PREDISPOSITION DUE TO PATIENT STATUS. Age, species, and concurrent disease can predispose a patient to an ADR. Very young as well as aged animals are more susceptible to ADRs than are middle-aged animals. Several weeks are required for a neonate to approach the capability of a young adult in drug biotransformation. The dosage schedule for drugs requiring drug biotransformation must be reduced in neonates, particularly if the drug has a high potential for producing toxicity. Chloramphenicol is an example of a drug requiring biotransformation, and it has the potential for producing bone marrow depression. The gray syndrome has resulted when the appropriate reductions in the adult dosage schedule of chloramphenicol were not made for human neonates.

There is very little information available on drug disposition in neonatal dogs and cats. As a consequence, drugs should be used sparingly and with caution in these groups. Another factor predisposing neonates to adverse drug effects is undeveloped renal and hepatic excretory mechanisms. As with drug biotransformation, several weeks are required for the excretory mechanisms of the neonate to become fully functional. Degeneration of organ function resulting in excessive drug accumulation may predispose older animals to ADRs. In humans, the risk of ADRs in patients over 60 years of age is about double that in young adults.

Veterinarians have long recognized that cats are more sensitive to many drugs than is any other species. Some reasons for this include the following:

1. A slower rate of biotransformation for many drugs. Cats also cannot conjugate drugs with glucuronic acid because they have deficient glucuronyl transferase activity, a critical enzyme in this reaction.
2. Cats exhibit unusual receptor-site sensitivity to many drugs. For example, reserpine produces sedation, which persists for a week in cats, whereas a 2-day period of tranquilization is characteristic of other species. Morphine, in high doses, produces excitation in cats, whereas sedation is characteristic in most other species.
3. The red blood cells of cats appear to be more susceptible to oxidative damage. Methemoglobinemia and Heinz bodies result.
4. The grooming habits of cats facilitate the ingestion of any substance falling on their fur. Thus, cats are likely to receive a larger internal dose than would other species of any substance being used in the area in the form of an aerosol or dust.

Concurrent disease can enhance the possibility of ADRs in several ways. Disease conditions characterized by depressed renal or liver function, dehydration, or acidosis may result in higher concentrations of drug in the body than would be expected following conventional drug doses. When the organ (kidney, liver) primarily involved in a drug's elimination is diseased, dosage should be decreased in direct proportion to decreased function (Riviere, 1984). Shifts in the acid balance associated with disease may alter the degree of ionization of the drug; which could affect its partitioning across biologic membranes, its degree of serum or tissue protein binding, or its rate of elimination from the body.

Drug Interactions. An ADR may stem from the concurrent use of another drug. These ADRs may occur either outside or within the body. Other possible interacting "drugs" include food additives, environmental contaminants, insecticides, and other exogenous chemicals or xenobiotics.

The practice of mixing drugs together in the same syringe or infusion solution prior to injection is risky, as the resultant mixture may be incompatible. Some drug incompatibilities include the inactivation of aminoglycoside antibiotics (e.g., gentamicin, kanamycin) by semisynthetic penicillins and the inactivation of penicillin G by solutions of high or low pH or those that contain vitamin B complex vitamins with vitamin C. It should be kept in mind that many drugs can alter the results of laboratory tests. Specimens should be taken for laboratory analysis before drugs are given to the patient.

A number of drug interactions can occur that involve the pharmacokinetic phase of drug action (e.g., absorption, distribution, biotransformation, and excretion) as well as the action at drug receptor sites. Some illustrative examples follow:

Tetracycline reacts with divalent metals to form insoluble complexes. The coadministration of Kaopectate, milk, or iron preparations has been shown to reduce markedly the intestinal absorption of tetracycline. When tetracycline and metal-containing preparations are administered orally, they should be given at least 2 hours apart.

Some drugs are potent inhibitors of the biotransformation of other drugs, including pentobarbital and phenytoin (Dilantin) in several species. Dogs remained anesthetized two times longer and cats three times longer when a therapeutic dose of chloramphenicol was given at the same time as phenobarbital. Signs of phenytoin toxicity (including ataxia, tremors, and incoordination) have been precipitated in dogs when chloramphenicol therapy was instituted to treat a concurrent infection. Signs of toxicity abated when the dosage of phenytoin was reduced by half.

Some drugs are potent stimulators of the biotransformation of other drugs. Phenobarbital has been shown to enhance the biotransformation of many drugs in several species. Phenobarbital has been reported to enhance the rate of biotransformation of digoxin in dogs. If these drugs are given together, more digoxin may be required to digitalize the dog. An ADR from digoxin could arise if the administration of phenobarbital ceased and the dosage of digoxin remained the same.

Finally, some drugs are capable of displacing other drugs from serum albumin binding sites with resultant increased biologic activity of the displaced drug. An example is the displacement of coumarin by some sulfonamide or salicylate, the result being an increased anticoagulant activity.

HUMAN ERRORS. An adverse response resulting from human error perhaps should not be considered an ADR because the reaction may be expected to occur under the circumstances. Nevertheless, some human errors that can result in adverse responses include (1) dosage error due to miscalculation, (2) inappropriate route of administration (for example, a suspension designed for IM or SC administration may produce a fatal embolism if administered IV), and (3) excessive rate of administration by the IV route (for example, meperidine can produce a fatal hypotensive collapse if a therapeutic dose is given by rapid IV administration). Meperidine, as with many drugs that are organic bases, is capable of effecting a rapid release of histamine in the body.

LACK OF EFFICACY. Finally, an ADR may be failure of treatment. This should be regarded as a serious occurrence since a drug was initially given to effect a clinical "cure." If this endpoint is not achieved, then a possible cause should be sought. There are many complicating patient factors that could be responsible. However, it is possible that the drug itself was ineffective or that the drug was dosed in such a manner that effective concentrations at the site of action were not achieved. Reporting this type of ADR could effect a labeling change to alter the approved dosage regimen to one with greater efficacy.

References and Supplemental Reading

Jick, H.: The discovery of drug induced illness. N. Engl. J. Med. 296:481, 1977.

Koch-Weser, J., Sidel, V. W., Sweet, R. H., et al.: Factors determining physical reporting of adverse drug reactions. Comparison of 2000 spontaneous reports with surveillance studies at the Massachusetts General Hospital. N. Engl. J. Med. 280:20, 1969.

Miller, R. R., and Greenblatt, D. T. (eds.): *Drug Effects in Hospitalized Patients*. New York: John Wiley and Sons, 1976.

Ndiritu, C. G., and Enos, L. R.: Adverse reactions to drugs in a veterinary hospital. J.A.V.M.A. 171:335, 1977.

Riviere, J. E.: Calculation of dosage regimens of antimicrobial drugs in animals with renal and hepatic dysfunction. J.A.V.M.A. 185:1094, 1984.

Stowe, C. M.: Antimicrobial drug interactions. J.A.V.M.A. 185:1137, 1984.

Venulet, J.: Methods of monitoring adverse reactions to drugs. Prog. Drug Res. 21:231, 1977.

CLINICAL MANAGEMENT OF ADVERSE DRUG REACTIONS

LLOYD E. DAVIS, D.V.M.
Urbana, Illinois

An essential aspect of the risk-benefit assessment is to consider the possibility that adverse drug reactions (ADRs) might occur. In some cases, these are predictable and avoidable. In others, they cannot be anticipated, but the clinician should be able to recognize them and initiate appropriate action. An ADR has been defined as any response to a drug that is noxious and unintended and that occurs at doses of an appropriately given drug used for prophylaxis, diagnosis, or therapy and occurring within a reasonable time of administration of the drug.

The true incidence of drug-related disorders in veterinary practice is unknown, but it is obvious that such reactions occur, and many of them prove fatal to the affected animals. The incidence of drug-related illness in animals is probably lower than that reported in human medicine. This may be related to shorter duration of therapy and the fact that fewer drugs may be used in a given patient because of the economic constraints of veterinary medical practice. Nevertheless, our modern armamentarium of drugs is very active in modifying physiologic processes, and the risks have increased along with improved efficacy. The frequency of drug-induced disorders in animal patients can probably be reduced by the veterinarian who places the same degree of emphasis on the planning of therapy as the astute clinician normally places on diagnosis.

CLINICAL CONSIDERATIONS

Most drugs that have been evaluated in the target species are relatively safe for their intended use. Inordinate risk has been associated with some drugs that have been evaluated and cleared for use in humans but that have not been studied in the animal species being treated. Examples are acetaminophen in cats, indomethacin and ibuprofen in dogs, and phenylbutazone in ponies, among others. Use of such drugs has resulted in fatal drug reactions. It is generally advisable to employ drugs of a given class that have proved to be relatively safe in veterinary use. *The newest drug available is not always the safest choice for therapy.*

All pharmacologically active compounds present some risk to the patient. However, the therapeutic index will vary considerably among different compounds. Generally, your willingness to accept this risk for your patient should vary in proportion to the severity or seriousness of the disease being treated. A drug with a narrow therapeutic index might be quite acceptable in a life-threatening situation (e.g., IV administration of lidocaine for ventricular tachycardia) or for treating a disease with high mortality (e.g., cytotoxic drugs for lymphosarcoma). There is no justification for administering such drugs to animals with self-limiting disease or for medically trivial purposes. Some of the fatal drug reactions seen resulted from inappropriate or trivial use of the drugs (e.g., anaphylaxis from penicillin given for a viral infection or pancytopenia from an overdose of estrogen administered to a bitch for mismating). Practitioners should be alert to the possibility of adverse reactions occurring with any drug that they use.

It is important to the welfare of an animal treated as an outpatient that the client be properly informed about potential adverse reactions to a drug that has been dispensed. By being properly informed, the owner of the animal can seek help and the drug can be withdrawn or the dosage modified at an early stage if a drug-induced disorder has developed.

FACTORS RELATED TO THE DEVELOPMENT OF ADVERSE DRUG REACTIONS

As each of our patients is a unique being whose exact genome and particular circumstance is unlikely to be duplicated, it is not surprising that there are a number of factors to be considered in the individualization of therapy. These characteristics of the patient, its environment, and nature of the dosage form all need to be considered in relation to the problem of ADRs.

DRUG FACTORS. ADRs in animals may occur in response to components of the dosage form other than the active drug. Considerable morbidity has been seen from propylene glycol used as a vehicle for injectables. When injected IV, propylene glycol causes hemolysis, heart block, and hypotension, and when injected SC, it causes extensive edema by its osmotic effects. Recently, hypersensitivity in one individual after injection of vitamin B_{12} was confirmed to be associated with the benzyl alcohol employed as a preservative.

Many ADRs observed in practice are dose related and are associated with individual variation in pharmacokinetic behavior or individual sensitivity to action of the drug. These incidents can be corrected by modification of the dosage regimen, and they seldom require withdrawal of the drug. Variations in bioavailability, due to the change from one product to another or to change in patient factors, could result in greater plasma concentrations of the drug.

Incorrect route of administration is a frequent cause of ADRs. Barbiturates, chloral hydrate, levarterenol, and other drugs administered SC will cause sloughing of skin. Oral dosage forms given IV may cause sudden death. Particulate suspensions intended for IM administration will cause severe pulmonary embolism and death if administered in the vein.

AGE. The incidence of ADRs is greater in very young (less than 30 days old) and very old animals. This is due to differences in body composition, rate of biotransformation of drugs, alteration in protein binding of drugs, and different sensitivity of some tissues.

HABITUS. Very obese as well as asthenic animals may be more liable to develop adverse reactions to certain drugs. This is frequently due to dosage errors introduced by calculating the dose on the basis of body weight. Drugs with low lipid solubility are not distributed into the excessive volume of adipose tissue. A common example is digoxin toxicity of obese dogs. Digoxin dosage should be predicated on the lean body mass. In contrast, digitoxin that is highly lipid soluble is dosed on the basis of the total weight, as its volume of distribution includes the body fat. Very lean animals such as greyhounds and whippets show prolonged effects of barbiturates and certain other drugs. Severe inanition from starvation or illness may modify the rate of biotransformation of drugs as well as drug distribution.

SEX. ADRs occur more commonly in women than in men. It is unknown whether there is a difference in incidence of drug reactions between the sexes of domesticated animals.

PREGNANCY. Sensitivity to drugs and drug disposition may vary during pregnancy and parturition. Potential adverse effects on the embryo and fetus must be considered when treating animals after breeding and during pregnancy (see References and Supplemental Reading).

SPECIES. The greater occurrence of ADRs in some species compared with others is related to drug disposition factors.

DISEASE. The presence of dysfunctions of various organ systems is an important factor in the occurrence of ADRs. Generally, the pharmacodynamic and pharmacokinetic properties of drugs have been characterized in healthy animals. These properties can be greatly altered by intercurrent or associated disease conditions. Renal diseases may greatly modify elimination rate of a drug by delaying excretion or inhibiting biotransformation. Additionally, uremia may alter receptor sensitivity and change the extent of protein binding of a drug. Hepatic coma may be precipitated by certain drugs administered to animals with hepatitis or cirrhosis.

IMMUNOLOGIC STATUS. Patients with a past history of an allergic reaction to a drug are more likely to suffer a reaction to the same or a similar drug. Atopic individuals are at much greater risk than the general population of suffering adverse reactions to a variety of drugs. Immunodeficient individuals may not respond normally to appropriate antibacterial therapy.

BREED CHARACTERISTICS. A number of congenital disorders occur in various breeds of dogs and other species and may predispose affected individuals to ADRs. For example, latent epilepsy in poodles, German shepherds, Belgian Tervurens, beagles, Welsh corgis, and St. Bernards may become unmasked by corticosteroids. Von Willebrand's disease in cairn terriers, Doberman pinschers, German shepherds, German shorthaired pointers, golden retrievers, miniature schnauzers, poodles, Scottish terriers, Shih Tzus, and Siberian huskies may predispose these animals to bleeding in response to anticoagulants and nonsteroidal anti-inflammatory drugs. The temperaments of different breeds of animals vary considerably and will influence responses to drugs affecting behavior.

PRESENCE OF OTHER DRUGS. The incidence of ADRs increases dramatically with the number of drugs given simultaneously to the same patient.

ENVIRONMENTAL FACTORS. Animals as well as humans live in a much more complex environment now than they did a number of years ago. They are exposed to feed additives, agricultural chemicals, insecticides, atmospheric pollutants, and other chemicals that may modify their response to drugs. These may serve to increase or decrease the liability of developing inappropriate reactions to drugs given therapeutically. Crowding of animals in high-confinement situations may result in unusual responses. The lethal dose of amphetamine in rats was eight times less when animals were caged together than when they were isolated. The significance of this in domesticated animals is unknown, but it may be wise to try to isolate animals that are undergoing drug therapy. Altitude might be another environmental factor to consider, although little definitive information is available. Extremes of ambient temperature (either cold or hot environments) could provoke ADRs that would not occur at neutral temperatures. An example might be the effect of phenothiazine tranquillizers on temperature regulation in which normal control is lost and the patient may quickly develop pyrexia or hypothermia. The optimal environmental temperature for mammals is 23.9°C (75°F), as this requires no expenditure of energy for either heat production or heat loss. It has been observed that after severe trauma, mortality increased 100 per cent at temperatures of 12.8 or 35°C (55 or 95°F) as compared with 23.9°C.

TIMING OF ADRs. ADRs can occur at any time during therapy. Cardiac standstill may occur immediately after administration of quinidine to a patient with complete heart block. Anaphylactic reaction will develop within minutes of administration of the allergen. Reactions to other drugs may require weeks to develop (e.g., reserpine-induced hypotension or exfoliative dermatitis from gold salts). Some may require months (e.g., calcinosis cutis or iatrogenic Cushing's disease from corticosteroids).

ALLERGIC DRUG REACTIONS

Allergic drug reactions, which are also termed hypersensitivity reactions by some authors, are ADRs based on immunologic mechanisms. They are dependent on combination of antigen and antibody. Other types of ADRs due to direct toxicity, drug interactions, and modification of drug disposition by disease are not related to immunologic processes and can generally be anticipated by the clinician and avoided. Allergic reactions in a given patient generally cannot be anticipated by the veterinarian unless the animal has a prior history of allergy to some drug. The clinician should be particularly circumspect about drugs used in atopic individuals, who have a greater tendency to develop allergy to therapeutic agents. The true incidence of allergic reactions to drugs in veterinary practice is unknown. In humans, allergic reactions accounted for 6 to 10 per cent of all drug reactions. A comparatively small number of drugs account for most of the allergic drug reactions that occur in humans. In my experience, allergic reactions in animals have been most frequently associated with penicillin G and cephalosporins. However, I have seen what I presumed to be allergic reactions to acepromazine, aspirin, sulfonamides, nitrofurans, antihistaminic ointments, isoniazid, and worming pastes.

TOXIC DRUG REACTIONS

Direct toxic effects of drugs on organs can occur as an exaggeration of the expected pharmacologic effect or may be associated with actions that are unrelated to any desired therapeutic effect. Often the mechanisms for these effects may be complex and obscure.

Table 1. *Drugs Producing Nephrotoxocity*

ANTIMICROBIAL DRUGS	*ANALGESICS*
Ampicillin, I	Ibuprofen, I
Amphotericin B, T, V	Naproxen, I
Bacitracin, T	Phenacetin, T
Cephaloridine, T	Phenylbutazone, T, V
Colistin, T	Salicylates, T
Gentamicin, T	*ANTINEOPLASTIC DRUGS*
Kanamycin, T	Adriamycin, N
Methicillin, I	Cis-platin, T
Neomycin, T	Cyclophosphamide, T, V
Oxacillin, I	Daunorubicin, N
Penicillin, I, V	Methotrexate, O
Polymyxin B, T	Mithramycin, T
Sulfonamides, O, I	*DIURETICS*
Tetracyclines, T, V	Furosemide, I
Tobramycin, T	Mannitol, T
HEAVY METALS	Thiazides, I, V
Arsenicals, T, N	*MISCELLANEOUS*
Bismuth, T	Captopril, N
Cadmium, T	Dextrans, V
Copper, T	EDTA, T
Gold salts, T, N	Lithium, N
Mercurials, T, N	Penicillamine, N
Uranium, T	Phenazopyridine, T
	Phenindione, I
	Probenecid, N

Key to mechanisms: I = interstitial; N = nephrotic syndrome; O = obstructive; T = tubular; V = vasculitis.
From Davis, L. E.: *Veterinary Clinical Pharmacology*, in preparation.

NEPHROTOXICITY. There are several reasons for the vulnerability of the kidneys to toxic effects of drugs. Of the total cardiac output, 20 to 25 per cent perfuses the kidneys each minute, thereby delivering appreciable amounts of drug over a given period of time. The blood vessels and glomeruli present a large endothelial surface area for contact with drugs, and drugs are concentrated in the tubular fluid by the normal reabsorption of water. Some drugs are also concentrated in epithelial cells of the nephron by active transport from peritubular capillaries. Nephrotoxicity may be manifested as nephrotoxic renal failure, acute glomerulonephritis, interstitial nephritis, lower nephron nephrosis, and nephrotic syndrome. Drugs that are nephrotoxic are listed in Table 1.

HEPATOTOXICITY. The liver is vulnerable to toxic injury because of its strategic location and its central role in the biotransformation of drugs. Drugs administered orally are absorbed into the portal vein and are presented to the liver in relatively high concentrations. If the drug is toxic to tissues or if it is converted to chemically reactive metabolites, hepatotoxicity may be the result. This toxic drug reaction may be classified as hepatocellular or cholestatic depending on the mechanism of injury. Icterus also can be caused by drugs through extrahepatic mechanisms such as intravascular hemolysis or direct yellow discoloration of tissues (quinacrine). Hepatotoxic reactions probably are less common than nephrotoxicity and may be more difficult to recognize as being drug related. They should be suspected in any patient developing icterus, abnormal serum concentrations of transaminases or alkaline phosphatase, or hepatomegaly while receiving a drug. The onset of clinical signs may be abrupt or insidious, and severity may vary from asymptomatic changes in serum enzymes to fulminant hepatic necrosis. Hepatotoxicity is more commonly associated with chronic administration of medication or gross overdosage of certain drugs than with short courses of therapy.

Hepatocellular injury, degeneration, and necrosis result from the cytotoxic effects of the drug or its reactive metabolites on cellular components. Damage also can be mediated by immune mechanisms. This type of reaction is accompanied by marked increase in serum transaminase and bilirubin concentrations and prolonged prothrombin time when there has been extensive necrosis. In less severe injury, the transaminase concentrations will be elevated with no evidence of jaundice. Affected animals will have clinical signs associated with liver failure. Drugs that have caused hepatitis are listed in Table 2. Probably the most significant causes of drug-related hepatotoxicity encountered in veterinary practice are the halogenated anesthetics, acetaminophen, isoniazid, corticosteroids, and anticonvulsants. Certainly, many of the drugs listed could potentially be a problem in animals being treated.

Acetaminophen toxicity generally is seen in ani-

Table 2. *Drugs Causing Hepatotoxicity*

ANESTHETICS	*CARDIOVASCULAR*
Chloroform	Procainamide
Halothane	Quinidine
Methoxyflurane	Warfarin
ANTICONVULSANTS	*ANTINEOPLASTICS*
Carbamazepine	Busulfan
Phenobarbital	Cyclophosphamide
Primidone	L-Asparginase
Valproic acid	6-Mercaptopurine
ANTIMICROBIAL	Methotrexate
Ampicillin	Mithramycin
Carbenicillin	Urethane
Erythromycin estolate	*ENDOCRINE AGENTS*
5-Fluorocytosine	Anabolic steroids (C-17 alkylated)
Griseofulvin	Corticosteroids
Isoniazid	Methimazole
Nitrofurantoin	Propylthiouracil
Quinacrine	*TRANQUILIZERS*
Tetracyclines	Diazepam
Thiabendazole	Haloperidol
ANALGESICS	Phenothiazines
Acetaminophen	*OTHER DRUGS*
Ibuprofen	Cimetidine
Indomethacin	Danthron
Naproxen	Dapsone
Phenylbutazone	Iodochlorhydroxyquin
Salicylates	Nicotinamide
	Stibophen
	Vitamin A

From Davis, L. E.: *Veterinary Clinical Pharmacology*, in preparation.

mals that have accidentally ingested an overdose by eating tablets or capsules that were accessible to them or by the owner's administering the medication. The ADR is being seen more commonly as the drug has become more popular. At lower doses, the primary reaction seen, particularly in cats, is Heinz body anemia. With increased amounts of the drug, hepatotoxicity of the hepatocellular type is seen. Affected animals develop icterus and facial edema and are quite ill. Laboratory values for bilirubin, alanine aminotransferase, and bromsulfonphthalein retention are elevated.

The mechanism for the development of hepatotoxicity has been elucidated by Mitchell and colleagues in a series of elegant experiments. The understanding of this mechanism is essential for the effective treatment of this ADR. At usual doses, acetaminophen is conjugated with glucuronate and sulfate and a portion is oxidized to reactive intermediates. The intermediate is conjugated with glutathione and excreted as the mercapturic acid derivative, which is not biologically active. There is a limited reserve of glutathione available in the liver. As a consequence, with overdosage the supply of glutathione becomes exhausted, the reactive metabolite combines covalently with cellular macromolecules, and the cell dies. Cats have an additional disadvantage in that they have only a limited ability to form glucuronides. After an overdose of acetaminophen, administration of *N*-acetylcysteine can provide sulfhydryl groups and act as a substitute for glutathione within the liver and erythrocyte. This has been shown to be effective in preventing hepatic necrosis and in improving methemoglobinemia and clinical signs of toxicity in cats. The recommended dosage for *N*-acetylcysteine (available commercially as Mucomyst) is 140 mg/kg as an initial dose followed by 70 mg/kg orally every 6 to 8 hours for 4 to 5 days. Acetophenetidin (phenacetin) is metabolized to acetaminophen and presents the same hazard. It may be encountered in a number of over-the-counter analgesic preparations (e.g., A.P.C. Empirin compound, and many sinus remedies).

APLASTIC ANEMIA. Aplastic pancytopenia is an uncommon ADR in animal patients, but when it occurs, its effects are devastating to the victim. True aplastic anemia is characterized by complete failure of hematopoiesis in which the red bone marrow has been replaced by fatty tissue. The affected animal shows signs of pallor of the mucous membranes, weakness, petechiation, hemorrhage, and increased susceptibility to infections. Diagnosis is confirmed by the presence of a hypocellular fatty bone marrow determined by a bone marrow biopsy.

The mechanism by which drugs and certain chemicals produce their toxic effects on the bone marrow is not understood. There appears to be suppression of or damage to pluripotent stem cells in the marrow by either direct toxic or immune-mediated mechanisms. There also is some evidence for individual susceptibility, perhaps a genetically determined predisposition, to the development of aplastic anemia in response to certain drugs. Some agents suppress the bone marrow in all individuals in a predictable dose-related manner. Examples are the effects of ionizing radiation, cytotoxic drugs used in the treatment of cancer, and certain solvents and insecticides. More than 80 drugs have been incriminated as the cause of aplastic anemia in human patients. The reaction occurs infrequently despite widespread use of some of the drugs. In susceptible individuals, pancytopenia may occur with usual doses of the drugs administered for relatively short periods of time.

Table 3. ***Drugs That Have Caused Aplastic Anemia***

ANTINEOPLASTIC	*ENDOCRINE AGENTS*
Busulfan	Estrogens
Cyclophosphamide	Thiouracil
Cytosine arabinoside	Thiocyanate
Methotrexate	Methimazole
Mustargen	Tolbutamide
Vinblastine	*TRANQUILIZERS*
Vincristine	Meprobamate
ANTIMICROBIALS	Phenothiazines
Amphotericin B	*ANTIHISTAMINICS*
Chloramphenicol	Chlorpheniramine
Methicillin	Tripelennamine
Pyrimethamine	*MISCELLANEOUS*
Quinacrine	Benzene
Sulfonamides	Carbamazepine
Tetracyclines	Carbon tetrachloride
ANALGESICS	Chlordane
Phenylbutazone	DDT
Phenacetin	Disophenol
Indomethacin	Gamma-benzene hexachloride
HEAVY METALS	
Organic arsenicals	
Gold salts	
Colloidal silver	

From Davis, L. E.: *Veterinary Clinical Pharmacology*, in preparation.

The drugs that have most frequently been implicated as causes of aplastic anemia in humans are chloramphenicol, phenylbutazone, mephenytoin, trimethadione, organic arsenicals, gold compounds, quinacrine, sulfamethoxypyridazine, and thiouracil. There have been cases documented in the veterinary medical literature involving some of these same drugs (Table 3). Chloramphenicol-induced aplastic anemia is probably very rare among animals. The more usual blood dyscrasia seen with chloramphenicol is dose-related leukopenia, which is reversible on cessation of therapy. Watson and coworkers (1980) described three cases of dyscrasias associated with phenylbutazone in dogs and noted the occurrence of four others. Two of the cases had pancytopenia. The other had nonregenerative anemia and thrombocytopenia. Two of the patients died. These dogs had received usual therapeutic doses of phenylbutazone for periods ranging from 4 to 8 weeks.

A case of erythroid aplasia associated with thiacetarsamide treatment was described in which a dog survived for 7 months before succumbing to the disorder.

Probably the most commonly encountered cause of pancytopenia in dogs is estrogen toxicosis. Dogs are known to be particularly sensitive to the myelotoxic effects of estrogens. After administration of a toxic dose of estrogen, there is an initial leukocytosis and left shift followed by anemia, thrombocytopenia, and granulocytopenia, although any combination of these findings could occur. Several clinical cases have been described. Leukopenia and leukocytosis were seen among the cases; all had thrombocytopenia and anemia. Hemorrhages, petechiation, and the presence of ecchymoses were common. Estradiol cyclopentylpropionate was the most common cause of the marrow failure in these cases. This drug is intended for use in cattle for breeding purposes and should not be administered to dogs.

Drugs may exert direct toxic effects on other organs, and these toxic effects (e.g., retinopathy, ototoxicity, pulmonary infiltrates) are regarded as ADRs.

MEDICATION ERRORS

ADRs that are not related to patient characteristics or to unusual properties of the drug can occur. Relative safety and efficacy of drugs is dependent on an uninterrupted chain from the manufacturer through the distributor, the prescribing veterinarian, and the owner or the veterinary assistant to the patient. In studies of human patients, it was found that between 25 and 59 per cent of these patients committed errors in the self-administration of prescribed medication. In hospitals, it was found that the average nurse made one error for every six medications given. Errors encountered in a veterinary hospital may consist of omission of a dose, miscalculation of dosage, or administration of a wrong drug or improper administration of the drug. Clients may have difficulty in administering a drug to their animal. They may be handicapped or elderly or may not have assistance at home. A frequent cause of ADRs is overzealousness by the owner. Owners who are not sure that the animal swallowed the medication may repeat it to make certain, thereby giving an overdose.

It is important to show a client how to administer medication to the animal and to have them do it while you observe them. For complex management situations, such as control of the diabetic patient, it is useful to have detailed instructions printed that can be provided to the client at the time that the animal is discharged. When dispensing medication, provide complete instructions for use on the package and advise the client about any possible side effects that might be associated with the drug. A small amount of time spent in client education can pay large dividends in terms of safe use of the drug that you prescribed.

MANAGEMENT OF ADRs

Generally, ADRs that are encountered fall into one of two categories. Most are dose related, and the drugs produce their effects either by a direct extension of their expected pharmacologic effects or by organ toxicity. A smaller percentage are idiosyncratic and generally unpredictable. Hence, they constitute an inherent risk of therapy that is unavoidable. The main objectives to pursue in any animal that develops an ADR are to (1) provide life support, (2) stop medication with the drug, (3) enhance elimination of the drug, (4) if continued therapy is required, modify the dosage regimen or change to another drug, and (5) administer drug antagonists or antidotes if available.

As has been discussed previously in this chapter, ADRs vary considerably in their time course. They may range from sudden death from cardiac standstill to a course of weeks to months with certain organ toxicities. Emphasis is placed on the emergency management of acute reactions, as most organ toxicity is managed in the same manner as diseases of those organs from other causes. For example, a patient with acute renal tubular necrosis produced by drugs will be treated in much the same manner as an animal with end-stage renal disease. Similarly, drug-induced bronchoconstriction would be managed as one would approach the patient with asthma.

In the case of sudden collapse after injection of a drug, cardiopulmonary resuscitation should be undertaken if there are signs of cardiac arrest present. These may include cyanosis, poor capillary refill, lack of pulse, and inability to auscultate heart sounds. A patent airway should be established either by positioning the head and extending the tongue or by endotracheal intubation. Ventilation is then established by means of a ventilator or an Ambu bag or by blowing into the endotracheal tube. External cardiac massage should be provided to maintain effective circulation (improvement in color of mucous membranes, palpable peripheral pulse). This may be difficult, if not impossible, to accomplish in large animals. A catheter should be placed into a jugular vein, and saline or Ringer's solution should be infused at a rapid rate. Sodium bicarbonate may be added as needed to correct acidosis. Once clinicians have provided for adequate ventilation and circulation, they should maintain this effort for 5 to 10 minutes before administering emergency drugs. The flaccid, hypoxic heart is fairly unresponsive to drugs. It is better to wait until the myocardium is reoxygenated and acidosis has been corrected before administering catecholamines or calcium salts in an effort to stimulate cardiac contractions. After successful resuscitation, the patient should be observed closely for several hours.

Resuscitation may be more difficult in patients with cardiac arrest attributable to certain drugs than in those cases due to other causes. The drug causing arrest may pharmacologically antagonize efforts to establish autonomous activity of the heart. For example, if quinidine caused arrest of the heart in a patient with complete heart block by extinguishing ventricular pacemakers, the quinidine would also exert depressant effects on excitability and contractility of the myocardium. This may render the heart refractory to treatment.

Acute hypersensitivity reactions can have a rapid onset and must be treated immediately. These include anaphylaxis, angioedema, and urticaria. Anaphylaxis is life-threatening because of profound shock or bronchospasm (depending on species), leading to hypoxia of tissues and cardiac dysrhythmias. Angioedema involving the pharynx, glottis, and larynx may obstruct the airway and cause asphyxia. The immediate course of action is to administer epinephrine IV or IM (*not subcutaneously*). Often it is very difficult to perform a venipuncture under these circumstances because of poor filling of the veins. The adrenergic receptors in the arterioles of skeletal muscle are of the beta type. Consequently, epinephrine will produce vasodilation at the injection site, providing for rapid absorption of the drug into the circulation.

The rationale for administering epinephrine is that it stimulates both alpha- and beta-adrenergic receptors, producing pharmacologic effects that are antagonistic to the effects of many of the mediators of immediate hypersensitivity. Stimulation of alpha receptors will increase blood pressure and decrease blood flow in the skin and mucous membranes. The beta-adrenergic effects increase cardiac output, dilate constricted bronchioles, and inhibit the further release of mediators from mast cells. This comprises definitive therapy for this emergency. Antihistaminics or corticosteroids are not effective in primary treatment of these acute allergic reactions. Antihistaminics will block the H_1 histamine receptors, but histamine is only one among several mediators involved in the pathophysiology of immediate hypersensitivity. The onset of action of corticosteroids is too slow for these drugs to be of value in these circumstances. After initial control of clinical signs with epinephrine, an antihistaminic or glucocorticoid may be useful to prevent a relapse. Generally, though, this is not necessary.

In less urgent situations, stop therapy and allow time for the processes of biotransformation and excretion to remove the drug from the body. Most dose-related effects will abate as the drug is eliminated from the body. An example might be a patient that is comatose from an excessive dose of a depressant. This should not be a cause for undue alarm, as veterinarians induce coma every time they anesthetize a patient. As long as vital functions are maintained, all that is required is supportive care. Fluids should be provided to maintain renal function, hydration, and blood pressure. The eyes should be protected from drying with methylcellulose drops, as tear formation is likely to be inhibited. The patient should be turned regularly to prevent decubitus ulcers and congestion of dependent parts. If pulmonary and renal functions are adequate, the animal should be able to maintain homeostasis.

In some cases, active efforts should be made to enhance elimination of the drug after an overdose. In acute salicylism in cats, the main problems are severe metabolic acidosis with increased anion gap, drug fever, prostration with coma, and gastrointestinal ulceration and bleeding. As the elimination rate of salicylate in cats is slow ($T\frac{1}{2}$ = 38 hours) and dose dependent, one cannot wait for resolution of the problem by normal elimination because the metabolic derangements are so profound that the animal would die before appreciable amounts of the drug had been eliminated. In this situation, we increase the renal clearance of salicylate by maintaining a brisk alkaline diuresis with the IV infusion of mannitol and sodium bicarbonate solutions. Since salicylate is a weak acid (pKa = 3.0), it will be largely ionized in urine at pH of 8.0. This prevents passive reabsorption of the salicylate from the distal tubules and enhances removal of the drug from the blood. The pyrexia is due to uncoupling of oxidative phosphorylation in tissues, resulting in increased heat production. Antipyretic drugs are not indicated under these circumstances. Salicylate toxicity in cats is a serious ADR with high mortality. Successfully treated cases may require a week or more of intensive care before they fully recover.

Sometimes an overdose of a drug may cause nephrotoxicity along with other toxic effects. If acute renal failure has occurred, the only way of enhancing removal of the drug may be by peritoneal dialysis. Not all drugs are readily dialyzable. The extent of protein binding in plasma, the lipid solubility, and the extent of distribution in tissues are factors that affect their ability to be dialyzed.

In a small number of circumstances, antagonists may be available to prevent or mitigate the adverse effects. The administration of acetylcysteine to prevent hepatic necrosis and hemolytic anemia from acetaminophen was discussed earlier. Excessive muscarinic effects of cholinergic drugs can be controlled with atropine. Naloxone will reverse the gastrointestinal and central nervous system effects of opiates, and prazosin will antagonize acute hypertension produced by overdosage of decongestants or appetite suppressants such as phenylpropanolamine.

The most discouraging ADR to manage is aplastic anemia. A high percentage of sufferers will eventually succumb to hemorrhage or overwhelming sepsis. Severe aplastic anemia in humans has been defined by the International Aplastic Anemia Study Group as meeting the following criteria: (1) neutrophil count less than 500/mm^3, (2) platelet count less than 20,000/mm^3, (3) less than 1 per cent reticulocytes, and (4) severe or moderate hypocellularity of bone marrow. Of patients with severe aplastic anemia, 91 per cent died within 4 months of diagnosis.

Blood transfusions may be necessary in animals with symptomatic anemia or bleeding due to thrombocytopenia, but sensitization to the donor cells will eventually develop and render the patient refractory to the benefits of transfusion. Prednisolone (1 mg/kg) may improve capillary integrity in thrombocytopenia, but prolonged therapy was associated with a worse outcome in a large study of aplastic anemia. Anabolic steroids stimulate production of erythrocytes, platelets, and leukocytes by normal bone marrow of animals, but controlled clinical and experimental studies have failed to show efficacy in improving aplastic anemia. This has been the experience noted in case reports of bone marrow failure in animal patients. The most successful approach to the problem in human patients has been by allogeneic bone marrow transplantation after immunosuppression by cyclophosphamide or total-body irradiation combined with cyclophosphamide. Nevertheless, long-term survival was still only 44 per cent. Antimicrobial therapy should not be instituted routinely unless there is documented evidence of an infection. Patients with leukopenia are at increased risk of infection, and indiscriminate exposure to antibiotics may lead to the production of resistant strains of organisms, which would be more difficult to control should sepsis occur.

CONCLUSIONS

ADRs are more easily prevented than treated once they occur. They constitute a major aspect of risk-benefit assessment by the veterinarian. Accordingly, rational use of a drug in practice requires a knowledge of its pharmacologic actions, side effects, and potential risk factors inherent in the patient. Clinicians also must be able to recognize that an ADR has occurred so that they can stop treatment, prevent further damage, and plan a course of action for dealing with the reaction. Therapeutic enthusiasm is difficult to justify in the absence of a diagnosis or when a potent drug is used for trivial medical purposes, as the risks may far outweigh any potential benefits to be gained by therapy.

References and Supplemental Reading

Borda, I. T., Slone, D., and Jick, H.: Assessment of adverse drug reactions within a drug surveillance program. J.A.M.A. 205:99, 1968.

Camitta, B. B., Storb, R., and Thomas, F. D.: Aplastic anemia: Pathogenesis, diagnosis, treatment and prognosis. N. Engl. J. Med. 306:645, 1982.

Cooperative Group for the Study of Aplastic and Refractory Anemia: Androgen therapy of aplastic anemia—a projective study of 352 cases. Scand. J. Haematol. 22:343, 1979.

Davis, L. E.: Adverse effects of drugs on reproduction in dogs and cats. Mod. Vet. Pract. 64:969, 1983.

Davis, L. E.: Hypersensitivity reactions induced by antimicrobial drugs. J.A.V.M.A. 185:1131, 1984.

Mitchell, J. R., Potter, W. Z., Hinson, J. A., et al.: Toxic drug reactions. Handb. Exp. Pharmacol. 28:383, 1975.

Schwark, W. S.: Pharmacologic management of allergic diseases. Vet. Clin. North Am. 4:57, 1974.

Stewart, R. B., and Cluff, L. E.: A review of medication errors and compliance in ambulant patients. Clin. Pharmacol. Ther. 13:463, 1972.

Watson, A. D. J., Wilson J. T., Turner, D. M., et al.: Phenylbutazone-induced blood dyscrasias suspected in three dogs. Vet. Rec. 107:239, 1980.

DRUG-RELATED DIAGNOSTIC ERRORS

LLOYD E. DAVIS, D.V.M.

Urbana, Illinois

There are a number of potential adverse effects of drugs employed in therapy that the veterinary clinician must consider as a part of the medical decision-making process. These include drug toxicity, drug-drug interactions, incompatibilities, and treatment failure. A potentially serious effect of certain drugs is that they may produce clinical signs that mimic those characteristic of various diseases,

Text continued on page 187

Table 1. Drugs That May Modify Results of Blood Chemical Determinations

Test	Elevated Values	Decreased Values
Alkaline phosphatase	Allopurinol, anabolic or androgenic steroids, azathioprine, cephaloridine, clindamycin, corticosteroids, estrogens, erythromycin estolate, gold salts, lincomycin, mithramycin, nitrofurantoin, novobiocin, oxacillin, penicillamine, phenothiazines, phenylbutazone, primidone, procainamide, progestin/estrogen, rifampin, sulfonamides, tetracyclines, tolbutamide	Fluorides, oxalates, phosphates, propranolol, vitamin D
Amylase	Adrenocorticotropic hormone (ACTH), bethanechol, corticosteroids, diatrizoate sodium, furosemide, indomethacin, isoniazid, meperidine, morphine, oxyphenbutazone, pentazocine, phenylbutazone, salicylates, sulfasalazine, tetracyclines, thiazide diuretics	Citrates, fluoride, oxalate
Bilirubin	Acetaminophen, allopurinol, amphotericin B, anabolic/androgenic steroids, azathioprine, barbiturates, carotene, chloroquine, clindamycin, dextran, diazepam, gentamicin, indomethacin, isoniazid, lincomycin, menadione, nitrofurans, novobiocin, oxacillin, phenylbutazone, procainamide, quinacrine, sulfonamides, tetracyclines	Barbiturates, citrate, methylxanthines, salicylates
Calcium	Antacids, anabolic/androgenic steroids, calcium salts, dihydrotachysterol, estrogens, parathormone, potassium, progestins, sodium, thiazide diuretics, vitamin D	Acetazolamide, bromsulphalein (BSP), citrate, corticosteroids, edathamil, fluorides, gentamicin, heparin, insulin, magnesium, methicillin, mithramycin, phosphorus, sulfates
Chloride	Acetazolamide, ammonium chloride, ion exchange resins, oxyphenbutazone, phenylbutazone, triamterene	ACTH, bicarbonate, bromides, corticosteroids, furosemide, glucose influsions, mercurial diuretics, thiazide diuretics, triamterene
Cholesterol	ACTH, anabolic steroids, androgens, bile salts, bilirubin, corticosteroids, ether, iodides, norepinephrine, penicillamine, phenothiazines, progestin/estrogen, salicylates, thiouracil, vitamins A and D	Chlortetracycline, cholestryramine, dextrothyroxin, EDTA, estrogens, glucagon, haloperidol, heparin, kanamycin, neomycin, nitrates, pentylenetetrazol, salicylates, thyroid
Creatinine	Amphotericin B, ascorbic acid, barbiturates, bromsulphalein (BSP), viomycin, colistin, gentamicin, kanamycin, lithium carbonate, methicillin, methramycin, PSP, streptokinase-streptodornase, triamterene	
Glucose	ACTH, arginine, British anti-lewisite (BAL), caffeine, corticosteroids, dextran, D-thyroxine diazoxide, epinephrine, isoniazid, lithium carbonate, morphine, nitrofurantoin, physostigmine, progestin/estrogen, salicylates, thiabendazole, thiazide diuretics, thyroid, triamterene, xylazine	Acetaminophen, anabolic steroids, ascorbic acid, cyproheptadine, dextropropoxyphene, fructose, haloperidol, insulin, phosphorus, potassium chloride, propranolol, reserpine, salicylates, tolbutamide
Lipase	Bethanechol, methacholine, codeine, meperidine, morphine	
Phosphorus	Antacids, heparin, methicillin, vitamin D, tetracyclines	Epinephrine, insulin, mithramycin, parathormone, iodides, isoniazid, nitrate, nitroprusside sodium, phenothiazine, phenylbutazone, progesterone, radiopaque contrast media, salicylates, sulfonamides, thiocyanate, thiopental, thyroid
Potassium	Aminocaproic acid, cephaloridine, copper, epinephrine, heparin, iron, isoniazid, mannitol, methicillin, potassium penicillin G, spironolactone, succinylcholine, triamterene	ACTH, acetazolamide, amphotericin B, furosemide, epinephrine, glucagon, glucose, insulin, laxatives, lithium carbonate, mithramycin, phosphate, polymixin B, salicylates, sulfates, tetracyclines, thiazide diuretics, viomycin
Serum alanine aminotransferase (SGPT)	Acetaminophen, anabolic steroids, androgens, erythromycin, gentamicin, indomethacin, isoniazid, lincomycin, phenothiazines, primidone, progestin/estrogen, triacetyloleandomycin	Salicylates
Serum aspartate aminotransferase (SGOT)	Ampicillin, anabolic steroids, androgens, cephalothin, doxacillin, erythromycin, gentamicin, indomethacin, isoniazid, lincomycin, methotrexate, morphine, nafcillin, oxacillin, phenothiazines, progestin/estrogen, sulfamethoxazole, thiabendazole	Salicylates
Serum urea nitrogen	Amphotericin B, antimony compounds, arsenicals, bactracin, colistimethate, doxapram, fluorides, furosemide, gentamicin, indomethacin, kanamycin, lithium carbonate, mercurials, methicillin, neomycin, nitrofurantoin, polymixin B, propranolol, radiopaque contrast media, salicylates, spectinomycin, streptokinase-streptodornase, tetracyclines, thiazide diuretics, tobramycin, triamterine, vancomycin	Dextrose infusions, phenothiazines
Sodium	Anabolic steroids, calcium, copper, corticosteroids, iron, mannitol, oxyphenbutazone, phenylbutazone, progestin/estrogen, reserpine, saline infusions	Acetazolamide, furosemide, heparin, mercurials, phosphates, spironolactone, sulfates, triamterene

Table 2. *Drugs That May Affect Results of Hematologic Studies*

Test	Effect	Drugs Causing Effect
Coombs	False-positive	Cephalosporins, penicillins
Erythrocyte count, PCV, hemoglobin	Decreased values	Acetaminophen, acetophenetidin, amphotericin B, antimonials, antineoplastic drugs, arsenicals, diiodohydroxyquin, doxapram, estrogens, haloperidol, hydrazine, indomethacin, methylene blue, nitrites, novobiocin, oxyphenbutazone, penicillamine, penicillin, phenytoin, phenylbutazone, primidone, pyrimethamine, sulfonamides, thiocyanates, tripelennamine
Eosinophil count	Elevated values	Ampicillin, barbiturates, cephalosporins, cloxacillin, epinephrine, gold salts, iodides, isoniazid, kanamycin, methicillin, novobiocin, phenothiazines, phenytoin, streptokinase-streptodornase, long-acting sulfonamides, tetracyclines, triamterene, vancomycin, viomycin
	Decreased value	Adrenocorticotropic hormone (ACTH), corticosteroids
Leukocyte count	Elevated value	Corticosteroids, diethylcarbamazine, diphenhydramine, erythromycin, streptomycin, sulfonamides
	Decreased values	Acetaminophen, acetophenetidine, allopurinol, antineoplastic drugs, cephalothin, chloramphenicol, cloxacillin, colistin, diazepam, diiodohydroxyquin, dipyrone, furosemide, gold salts, estrogens, haloperidol, hydralazine, indomethacin, mephenesin, meprobamate, methicillin, methocarbamol, metronidazole, novobiocin, oxacillin, oxazepam, oxyphenbutazone, penicillamine, phenothiazines, phenylbutazone, phenytoin, primidone, procainamide, propylthiouracil, pyrimethamine, quinine, thiabendazole, tripelennamine, vitamin A
Prothrombin time	Elevated values	ACTH, anabolic steroids, anticoagulants, barbiturates, heparin, indomethacin, mefenamic acid, oxyphenbutazone, phenylbutazone, phenytoin, propylthiouracil, quinidine, quinine, salicylates, sulfonamides, thyroid, vitamin A
	Decreased values	Antibiotics, antihistamines, barbiturates, corticosteroids, digitalis, diuretics, griseofulvin, progestin/estrogen, salicylates, sulfonamides, vitamin K, xanthines
Thrombocyte count	Decreased values	Acetazolamide, amphotericin B, antineoplastic drugs, arsenicals, chloramphenicol, chloroquine, estrogens, gold salts, isoniazid, mefenamic acid, oxyphenbutazone, penicillamine, phenylbutazone, pyrimethamine, quinidine, quinine, salicylates, sulfadimethoxine

Table 3. *Drugs Affecting Results of Urinalysis*

Test	Effect	Drugs Causing Effect
Acetone	False-positive	Bromsulphalein (BSP), methionine, phenformin, phenolsulfonphthalein (PSP)
Blood	False-positive	Bromides, copper, formalin, iodides, methenamine, permanganates
Bilirubin	False-positive	Perphenazine, phenazopyridine, phenothiazines
Calcium	Elevated values	Cholestyramine, dihydrotachysterol, parathormone, vitamin D
	Decreased values	Sodium bicarbonate, thiazide diuretics, viomycin
Catecholamines	Increased values	Adrenergic drugs, erythromycin, formalin, methenamine, quinidine, quinine, salicylates, tetracyclines, vitamin B complex
	Decreased values	Hydralazine
Color	Abnormal coloration	Aloe, antipyrine, cascara, chloroquine, danthron, dinitrophenol, dithiazanine, iron-sorbitol, methocarbamol, methylene blue, metronidazole, nitrofurantoin, phenazopyridine, phenothiazine, phenylsalicylate, quinacrine, quinine, riboflavin, sulfasalazine, senna, sulfonamides, triamterene
Creatinine	Increased values	Androgens, corticosteroids, nitrofurans
	Decreased values	Thiazide diuretics
Diagnex blue	False-positive	Aluminum, barium, calcium, iron, kaolin, magnesium, methylene blue, nicotinic acid, phenazopyridine, quinacrine, quinidine, quinine, riboflavin
	False-negative	Caffeine, sodium benzoate
Glucose (Benedict's)	False-positive	Adrenocorticotropic hormone (ACTH), ascorbic acid, aspirin, cephalothin, chloramphenicol, corticosteroids, edathamil, ephedrine, epinephrine, formalin, glucagon, gluconates, hydrogen peroxide, hypochlorites, indomethacin, isoniazid, metaproterenol, morphine, nitrofurans, penicillin, probenecid, phenylbutazone, salicylates, streptomycin, sulfonamides, tetracyclines, thiazide diuretics, xylazine
	False-negative	Ascorbic acid
Hemoglobin	Elevated values	Amphotericin B, bacitracin, corticosteroids, cyclophosphamide, coumarins, gold salts, indomethacin, kanamycin, mephenesin, mercurials, methenamine, methicillin, oxyphenbutazone, phenybutazone, polymixin B, probenecid, sulfonamides, sulfones, thiazide diuretics
Protein	False-positive	Aminophylline, amphotericin B, antimonials, arsenicals, bacitracin, colistimethate, radiopaque media, dihydrotachysterol, dithiazanine, doxapram, edathamil, gentamicin, gold salts, griseofulvin, isoniazid, kanamycin, methenamine, methicillin, neomycin, penicillamine, polymixin B, phenylbutazone, salicylates, sulfonamides, sulfones, tetracyclines, tolbutamide, vitamin D
Urobilinogen	Elevated values	Antipyrine, bromsulphalein (BSP), chlorpromazine,formalin, phenazopyridine, procaine, sulfonamides
	Decreased values	Chloramphenicol

Table 4. *Drugs Affecting Results of Miscellaneous Diagnostic Procedures*

Test	Effect	Drugs Causing Effect
Cerebrospinal fluid protein (Pandy test)	Elevated values	Acetophenetidin, chlorpromazine, salicylates, streptomycin, sulfanilamide
Guaiac test (stool)	False-positive	Bromides, iodides, iron
Color of stool	Abnormal coloration	Antacids, bismuth salts, calomel, dithiazanine, iron, phenazopyridine, salicylates, senna, tetracyclines
Barium series	Delayed gastric emptying	Antacids, bismuth salts, calomel, dithiazanine, iron, phenazopyridine, salicylates, senna, tetracyclines, xylazine
	Accelerated emptying	Cholinergic drugs, anticholinesterases, metoclopramide
Bacteriology, culture and sensitivity	False-negative	Antimicrobials
Bromsulphalein (BSP) clearance	Decreased values	Anabolic steroids, barbiturates, estrogens, morphine, phenazopyridine, probenecid
Serum T_3 and T_4	Increased values	Estrogens, exogenous thyroid hormones
	Decreased values	Androgens, anabolic steroids, dinitrophenol, phenytoin, propylthiouracil, salicylates
Plasma cortisol	Increased values	Exogenous corticosteroids, estrogen, thyroid hormones
	Decreased values	Etomidate, ketoconazole, mitotane
Plasma insulin	Increased values	Exogenous insulin, glucose, glucagon, amino acids, corticosteroids, potassium, calcium, methylxanthines
	Decreased values	Epinephrine, norepinephrine, diazoxide, xylazine

or they may affect results of certain diagnostic procedures so that the data obtained are erroneous. Such information can lead to an incorrect diagnosis. As an accurate diagnosis is a prerequisite to rational drug therapy the error may lead to inappropriate or hazardous therapy. It is important to query the client about any drugs that the patient is receiving or has received. A drug history is an important part of the medical record; drugs should be considered as possible etiologic agents in explaining abnormal physical signs or laboratory values.

Various drugs may cause clinical signs such as mydriasis or miosis, xerostomia or ptyalism, fever or hypothermia, central nervous system stimulation or depression, polyuria or urinary retention, diarrhea or constipation, cardiac dysrhythmias, vomiting, bleeding, dermatitis, weakness, or bronchoconstriction, among others. Such signs in a patient should be interpreted in terms of the drug history. If the signs are associated with primary or side effects of the drug, generally the condition will abate after withdrawal of the drug from the patient. A fairly common and frequently confusing sign is drug-induced fever. This is most commonly associated with disophenol or salicylate overdosage and various antimicrobial drugs. Drug fever from antibiotic therapy is due to hypersensitivity, cannot be anticipated, and can be very misleading. Such fever may lead the clinician to question the original diagnosis of a susceptible bacterial infection, which may be correct, and to pursue another inappropriate course of therapy. Drug fever should be suspected in patients receiving antimicrobial therapy if there is a sustained fever that is not commensurate with other clinical signs. Such individuals will be bright, alert, active, and eating but will remain febrile. Generally, lysis of the fever will occur rapidly after withdrawal of the drug.

Many veterinarians have become overdependent on clinical laboratory data. Uncritical acceptance of such information and failure of careful interpretation can lead to an incorrect diagnosis with the attendant hazards of irrational therapy. Errors may arise from faulty laboratory techniques, equipment failure, or faulty samples that are hemolyzed or lipemic, and other errors may be caused by a particular laboratory unaccustomed to working with specimens from animals.

Drugs may cause spurious results of clinical laboratory and other diagnostic procedures in several different ways. A drug may exert biologic effects in the subject that cause abnormal values of certain tests. Amphotericin B, aminoglycosides, and other drugs that are nephrotoxic may cause elevations of serum urea nitrogen or creatinine values by impairing their excretion. Acetaminophen, methylene blue, and other oxidant drugs can cause hemolytic anemia. Estrogen and antineoplastic drugs may produce pancytopenia by suppressing bone marrow stem cells. Drugs may interfere with results of contrast studies of the gastrointestinal tract by increasing or decreasing the rate of gastric emptying.

Drugs may interfere with the test procedures by their color (dithiazanine, phenazopyridine, carotene), by alterations in pH, or by chemical interference with reactions necessary for the procedure. Some drugs contain the substance being measured (e.g., potassium, iron, iodine, or calcium). Other drugs and their metabolites may be measured by the procedure being used for the measurement of another substance (e.g., a number of glucuronide conjugates will cause false-positive reactions for urinary glucose by Benedict's or Fehling's tests).

A number of drugs and their effects on commonly used diagnostic tests are listed in Tables 1, 2, 3, and 4. If clinicians encounter abnormal laboratory values that are out of proportion to the physical findings, they should first repeat the test to rule out the possibility of laboratory error. If laboratory results are reproducible, the history of exposure to drugs or other chemicals should be reviewed and interpreted in conjunction with tables in this section or references listed at the end of article.

References and Supplemental Reading

Guin, W. (ed.): *Veterinary Values '85*. New York: Ag Resources, 1985, pp. 78–95.

Halsted, J. A., and Halsted, C. H.: *The Laboratory in Clinical Medicine. Interpretation and Application*. Philadelphia: W.B. Saunders, 1981.

Hansten, P. D., and Lybecker, L. A.: Drug effects on laboratory tests. Appendix II. *In* Katzung, B. G. (ed.): *Basic and Clinical Pharmacology*. Los Altos, CA: Lange Medical Publications, 1984, pp. 817–831.

Martin, E. W., Alexander, S. F., Hassan, W. E., Jr., et al.: *Hazards of Medication*. Philadelphia: J.B. Lippincott, 1971, pp. 156–215.

Young, D. S., Pestaner, L. C., and Gidderman, V.: Effects of drugs on clinical laboratory tests. Clin. Chem. 21:1, 1975.

ASPIRIN AND ACETAMINOPHEN

FREDERICK W. OEHME, D.V.M.
Manhattan, Kansas

Owners of companion animals often have considerable sympathy for their pet's injuries and perceived pain. The use of proprietory analgesics is therefore a common event. Further, pet owners frequently use the analgesic that they are taking as "the best one" for their household animal. On occasion, however, owners will assume that the dosage appropriate for themselves or a child is satisfactory for their dog or cat. Further, the frequency of dosing may be similar to that employed for humans.

This situation is further exaggerated when owners have previously administered analgesics to their dogs and now use similar dosage measurements on a family cat. Differences in species metabolism and excretion are not considered, although these are factors that produce life-threatening events if they are ignored. A cat's small size and often deceptively low body weight compared with its abundant fur provide additional risk of overdosing. A cat's decreased ability to conjugate phenolic chemical structures, such as some of the common over-the-counter analgesics, and its therefore reduced capacity for urinary excretion of these metabolites predisposes the cat to high risk when body weight is overestimated, canine or human dosages are used, and the frequency of dosing is similar to that for humans.

The pet owners' sympathetic projection of personal feelings to the pet additionally complicates the analgesic dosing schedule. Owners may assume that the cat is still feeling pain or is "not quite right," and with limited ability to detect improvement in their pet's behavior and activities, may repeat or even increase the analgesic medication dose to promote a more rapid recovery. The owner's personal experience with the common over-the-counter analgesics aspirin and acetaminophen (Tylenol) results in these two compounds being commonly used by owners treating their pets. Aspirin and acetaminophen toxicities are not unusual in companion animals. The risk is especially great when cats are treated, and there has been a significant increase in acetaminophen toxicity due to the increasing popularity of that analgesic.

ASPIRIN

Aspirin, or acetylsalicylic acid, is still the most commonly used anti-inflammatory and pain-relief drug in humans, although its popularity has been eroded because of the recognition of acetaminophen as a similarly effective analgesic without the gastrointestinal irritation properties of aspirin. It is used in companion animals primarily to relieve minor pain and as a nonsteroidal anti-inflammatory treatment for bone and joint diseases. Toxicity in dogs and cats occurs as a result of overdosing, and particularly in cats because of lack of recognition of the extremely long biologic half-life of aspirin in cats (44.6 hours at 25 mg/kg daily) compared with 7.5 hours in dogs at 25 mg/kg every 12 hours. The dose of aspirin required to produce toxicity in cats is greater than 25 mg/kg per day, whereas toxicity would be expected in dogs receiving greater than 50 mg/kg every 8 hours.

Toxic Effects. Dogs and cats exhibit similar signs of toxicity, although the degree of effects are dose dependent and occur more rapidly and with greater frequency in cats. Initial signs, which may develop as soon as 4 to 6 hours after ingestion of a high dose of aspirin, are depression, vomiting, loss of appetite, increased respiratory rate, and elevated body temperature. The vomitus may be blood tinged in 10 to 20 per cent of toxicity cases, because of gastric irritation. The depression leads to muscular weakness and ataxia, with coma and death following in 1 or more days. If animals receive repeated toxic doses of aspirin for several days, the gastric lesions may lead to ulcers and perforation. Anemia may be seen coupled with suppressed bone marrow activity and a toxic hepatitis. Cats are especially prone to bone marrow hypoplasia and the formation of Heinz bodies.

The clinical signs of aspirin toxicity are sufficiently uncharacteristic to make a diagnosis difficult in a presenting animal with no history of aspirin ingestion. Clinicians should elicit from the owner any history of medication given to the patient within 5 days of the initial examination. The acid-base balance disturbances—an initial respiratory alkalosis (recall the early increased frequency of respiration) followed by metabolic acidosis due to the loss of buffering capacity (bicarbonate, sodium, potassium, and water loss) and ketone body formation; increased pyruvic, lactic, and amino acid levels in the circulation; and decreased renal clearance of sulfuric and phosphoric acids—may offer clinical chemistry measurements suggesting the occurrence of aspirin toxicity. The presence of a pre-existing condition that may have led the owner to medicate for pain or swelling should also suggest questioning about owner medication with aspirin. Dogs or cats with chronic aspirin dosing may present with signs of bone marrow depression, anemia, Heinz bodies in the circulating blood, or indications of a toxic hepatitis. These observations should be related to possible aspirin ingestion.

Laboratory tests for plasma aspirin concentrations are routinely offered by most human clinical pathology laboratories, but they may not be readily accessible to the practicing veterinarian. The ferric chloride screening test may therefore be of practical value. A 10 per cent solution of ferric chloride in water is prepared, and urine or serum is tested. One milliliter (20 drops) of the 10 per cent ferric chloride solution is added to 2 ml of urine, or 1 drop of the 10 per cent ferric chloride solution is added to 2 drops of serum placed in a white cup or dish. If aspirin or other salicylates are present, a purple color will result. This test is very sensitive and will also react to sodium, phenyl or methyl salicylates, or phenol derivatives. A positive test should be followed by a determination of the acid-base balance of the blood.

CLINICAL MANAGEMENT. Since there is no specific antidote for aspirin poisoning, the treatment of aspirin toxicity follows the general principles of poisoning management. Unabsorbed aspirin is removed from the stomach by the induction of vomiting or by gastric lavage. Gastric emptying should be performed as long as 6 to 12 hours after aspirin overdoses, since the drug tends to form an insoluble mass in the stomach. Activated charcoal (1 gm/lb body weight, or 2 gm/kg body weight) should be given orally to bind any remaining unabsorbed aspirin in the digestive tract.

Acid-base balance correction is of special importance and should be diligently undertaken in response to the immediate acid-base balance situation of the patient. Repeated evaluations of acid-base balance should be performed, and fluid and electrolyte replacement adjusted accordingly. Alkalinization of the urine with IV sodium bicarbonate will increase urinary excretion of aspirin; this may be enhanced by the concurrent use of diuretics.

In those cases in which the owner is willing, direct removal of the aspirin from the blood may be employed. Peritoneal dialysis is the veterinary complement of the hemodialysis and hemoperfusion techniques used extensively in human aspirin poisoning cases. If patients are seen before severe acid-base disturbances have been established or before bone marrow depression or toxic hepatitis effects are obvious, poisoned pets may be responsive to a thorough and conscientious treatment program. Affected animals in severely dehydrated and comatose conditions are at high risk and do not usually respond to treatment.

ACETAMINOPHEN

The number of acetaminophen-poisoned pets has increased dramatically during the past several years. This is probably due to the increasing acceptance of acetaminophen as an analgesic in humans and the transfer-use of this compound to pets. Unfortunately, cats exhibit the same inability to efficiently metabolize and excrete acetaminophen as they do for other phenolic drugs. One "extra-strength" acetaminophen capsule will produce toxic signs in cats. Two "extra-strength" capsules given within 24 hours to an average-sized cat can cause death. The "regular-strength" capsules, containing 325 mg acetaminophen, will cause clinical toxicity if one is given every 4 hours for two doses. On a body-weight basis, cats are poisoned by as little as 50 to 60 mg/kg orally, whereas dogs usually require 150 mg or more of acetaminophen/kg body weight.

TOXIC EFFECTS. The observed toxicity is due to an active metabolite of acetaminophen that conjugates with glutathione, reducing the hepatic and red blood cell glutathione concentrations. As the glutathione concentrations are decreased, the active metabolite is free to cause cell damage in the liver and other tissues, including red blood cells. (The biochemical mechanism of acetaminophen toxicity is further discussed in the article Clinical Management of Adverse Drug Reactions).

Dogs receiving toxic quantities of acetaminophen will become depressed, lose appetite, and may vomit within hours after receiving the drug. The depression becomes progressive, and abdominal pain is also exhibited. In moderate toxicity, recovery is spontaneous in 48 to 72 hours. With toxicity due to large doses of acetaminophen, methemoglobinemia will develop in a dose-responsive fashion. Cell damage in the liver causes hepatic necrosis and accompanying icterus, weight loss, and eventual death. Some RBCs will undergo hemolysis due to loss of glutathione, and a mild hemoglobinuria may be seen terminally. The clinical syndrome due to large doses of acetaminophen in dogs may result in death within 2 to 5 days after the initiation of clinical signs.

Cats, poisoned by considerably smaller doses of acetaminophen than dogs, develop signs within 1 to 2 hours of dosing. The effects are progressive and initiate with anorexia, salivation, and vomiting. Depression occurs promptly, and methemoglobinemia develops rapidly. RBCs undergo hemolysis, resulting in Heinz body anemia and hemoglobinuria or hematuria. Mucous membranes become brown, and dark, chocolate-colored urine is characteristic. Edema of the face and paws is also seen in a majority of cases. The methemoglobinemia is life-threatening and is the cause of death. Liver necrosis in cats is minimal compared with that seen in dogs, and recovered cats have no aftereffect of liver damage. Clinical signs persist for 12 to 48 hours, depending on the acetaminophen dose received. When the methemoglobin concentration is in excess of 50 per cent, the affected cat may die during normal handling or physical activity. Death due to methemoglobinemia occurs 18 to 36 hours after acetaminophen ingestion.

CLINICAL MANAGEMENT. If accidental overdosage is recognized within hours of the acetaminophen administration, gastric emptying should be performed by the use of emetics and gastric lavage. Activated charcoal, 1 gm/lb body weight or 2 gm/kg body weight, should then be given orally to bind any remaining unabsorbed acetaminophen. However, if more than 4 to 6 hours has passed since the administration of the acetaminophen, the effectiveness of emesis, gastric lavage, and activated charcoal dosing is minimal.

Of most benefit has been the administration of sulfhydryl groups or sulfate donors to substitute for the glutathione that is depleted by the reactive acetaminophen metabolite. *N*-acetylcysteine (Mucomyst, Mead Johnson) is the preferred sulfhydryl donor and is available from pharmacies under the human label. If suspected high doses of acetaminophen have been given or if clinical signs are apparent, the acetylcysteine treatment should be initiated immediately. Acetylcysteine is given orally or IV to dogs and cats at a loading dose of 140 mg/kg body weight as a 5 per cent solution. It is repeated every 4 hours thereafter at a dose of 70 mg/kg (5 per cent solution) for three to five more treatments. If acetylcysteine is not available, sodium sulfate may be used alternatively. It is given IV as a 1.6 per cent solution in water at 50 mg sodium sulfate/kg body weight every 4 hours for a total of six treatments. These treatments have been shown to be effective in cats receiving two- to threefold lethal doses of acetaminophen, but effective recovery requires persistent and conscientious therapy.

Supportive care is also indicated, including giving ascorbic acid (125 mg orally) every 6 hours to combat methemoglobinemia. Drinking water should be available at all times, and parenteral fluid and electrolyte replacement should be given as needed to replace losses due to vomiting and RBC destruction. Physical activity and handling should be limited to reduce the hazard from anoxia. Food may be offered to the patient 24 hours after treatment is started.

With an effective response to treatment, the previously poisoned dog or cat may be appearing and behaving normally 48 hours after the initial therapy. The response may be limited or even ineffectual if severe methemoglobinemia is present or if massive RBC destruction and liver necrosis have already occurred. Whole-blood transfusions may be helpful to replace the hemolyzed RBCs, but the overall clinical effect on a positive outcome is usually transient.

References and Supplemental Reading

Davis, L. E.: Fever, J.A.V.M.A. 175:1210, 1979.

Davis, L. E., and Donnelly, E. J.: Analgesic drugs in the cat. J.A.V.M.A. 153:1161, 1968.

Savides, M. C., and Oehme, F. W.: Acetaminophen and its toxicity. J. Appl. Toxicol. 3:96, 1983.

Savides, M. C., Oehme, F. W. and Leipold, H. W.: Effects of various antidotal treatments on acetaminophen toxicosis and biotransformation in cats. Am. J. Vet. Res. 46:1485, 1985.

Savides, M. C., Oehme, F. W. Nash, S. L., et al.: The toxicity and biotransformation of single doses of acetaminophen in dogs and cats. Toxicol. Appl. Pharmacol. 74:26, 1984.

St. Omer, V. V., and McKnight, E. D. III: Acetylcysteine for treatment of acetaminophen toxicosis in the cat. J.A.V.M.A. 176:911, 1980.

Yeary, R. A., and Brant, R. J.: Aspirin dosages for the dog. J.A.V.M.A. 167:63, 1975.

Yeary, R. A. and Swanson, W.: Aspirin dosages for the cat. J.A.V.M.A. 163:1177, 1973.

METHYLXANTHINE POISONING (CHOCOLATE AND CAFFEINE TOXICOSIS)

STEPHEN B. HOOSER, D.V.M.,
and VAL RICHARD BEASLEY, D.V.M.
Urbana, Illinois

Theobromine, caffeine, and theophylline are naturally occurring methylxanthine compounds that are found in several foods and beverages and in a few veterinary and human medications. Theobromine is present in chocolate, cocoa beans, cocoa bean hulls, cola, and tea. Milk chocolate contains approximately 44 mg of theobromine per ounce, and unsweetened baking chocolate contains approximately 390 mg/oz. Caffeine is present in coffee, tea, chocolate, colas, and human stimulant drugs. Theophylline is found in tea and in veterinary and human medications.

Judging from the number of calls received by the National Animal Poison Control Center (NAPCC), the methylxanthine toxicosis of greatest importance is theobromine (chocolate) poisoning in dogs, followed by toxicosis in dogs due to human stimulants containing caffeine. A number of deaths have been reported in dogs due to chocolate ingestion. However, no deaths due to accidental caffeine consumption have been reported to the NAPCC. The NAPCC has not documented accidental theophylline toxicoses in dogs, and no methylxanthine toxicoses at all have been reported in cats, probably because of the markedly different eating habits of felines. Deaths due to theobromine toxicosis have been reported in horses eating cocoa bean hulls as bedding and in livestock fed cocoa waste in their feed.

The LD_{50} of theobromine in dogs is reported to be between 250 and 500 mg/kg (⅔ to 1⅓ oz of baking chocolate/kg body weight); however, at least one canine death has been reported after exposure to approximately 115 mg/kg. The half-life of theobromine in dogs is very long compared with other species, being approximately 17.5 hours. The LD_{50} of caffeine in dogs is 140 mg/kg and the half-life is about 4.5 hours.

MECHANISMS OF ACTION

The methylxanthines have four primary effects: (1) They inhibit cellular phosphodiesterase, causing an increase in cyclic AMP. This is thought to be the primary effect of the methylxanthines. (2) They cause the release of catecholamines (epinephrine and norepinephrine). (3) The methylxanthines are also competitive antagonists of cellular adenosine receptors. Adenosine has many effects that are the opposite of xanthine effects. (4) They cause an increased entry of calcium and an inhibition of calcium sequestration by the sarcoplasmic reticulum, leading to increased muscular contractility.

CLINICAL AND PATHOLOGIC SIGNS

CAFFEINE. Initial signs of caffeine toxicosis include vomiting, diuresis, restlessness, and hyperactivity; tachycardia and tachypnea are sometimes present. These signs can lead to ataxia, muscle tremors, cyanosis, cardiac arrythmias (including premature ventricular contractions), and seizures. The authors are unaware of deaths due to caffeine ingestion in dogs, although it is possible after large overdoses as a result of cardiovascular collapse or respiratory arrest.

THEOBROMINE. With acute theobromine (chocolate) ingestion in dogs, the predominant signs are vomiting, diarrhea, diuresis (sometimes reported as urinary incontinence), hyperactivity, occasional depression, cardiac arrhythmias (including sinus tachycardia and premature ventricular contractions), hyperthermia, ataxia, muscle tremors, seizures, and coma, sometimes terminating in death. Abdominal pain, hematuria, muscle weakness, bradycardia, and dehydration occasionally are also present.

On postmortem examination, often no lesions are seen other than gastroenteritis and congestion of organs. In one study of chronic theobromine dosing in dogs, a degenerative fibrotic cardiomyopathy was found in the right atrial appendage of several dogs.

DIAGNOSTIC CONSIDERATIONS

The methylxanthines and their metabolites can be measured by high-performance liquid chromatography in serum, plasma, tissue, urine, and stomach contents. They are stable in serum or plasma at room temperature for 7 days, refrigerated for 14 days, and frozen for 4 months. There is very little excretion via the feces; however, they are readily passed in the milk.

TREATMENT

Since there is no specific antidote for methylxanthine poisoning, treatment for poisoning by any of these three methylxanthines is aimed at (1) maintenance of basic life support, (2) prevention of absorption, (3) hastening of elimination, and (4) providing symptomatic treatment of seizures, respiratory difficulties, and potentially life-threatening cardiac arrhythmias.

Initially, the respiratory and cardiovascular status of the patient should be monitored. If necessary, pass an endotracheal tube and supply artificial ventilation. If the animal is in shock, institute IV fluid therapy to support cardiovascular function.

Secondly, if less than 2 hours have elapsed since ingestion, vomiting should be initiated unless the animal is markedly stimulated, comatose, or has lost the postural or gag reflex. In such cases, after administration of agents (if indicated) for seizure control, an endotracheal tube should be put in place, the cuff inflated, and gastric lavage initiated to remove the stomach contents. It should be noted that the chocolate can melt and form a ball in the stomach, and this can be difficult to remove.

Thirdly, to prevent absorption and help increase elimination, give repeated doses of activated charcoal at 0.5 gm/kg PO or by stomach tube every 3 hours for up to 72 hours. It has been shown that continuous dosing of activated charcoal PO can significantly reduce the half-life of methylxanthines in the body. The duration of treatment (72 hours) is often prolonged because of the long half-life of theobromine in dogs. In addition to activated charcoal, an osmotic cathartic (sorbitol) or saline cathartic (sodium or magnesium sulfate) should be given PO or by stomach tube at 0 and 3 hours to hasten evacuation and prevent constipation by the activated charcoal.

Fourth, if the patient is having marked muscle tremors or seizures, diazepam may be given IV at a dosage of 0.5 to 2.0 mg/kg to control the more serious stimulatory effects. If diazepam is unsuccessful, phenobarbital at 6 mg/kg IV twice or four times daily as needed or more frequent doses of a shorter-acting barbiturate may be used.

Fifth, the electrocardiogram of the patient should be monitored. Bradycardias should be treated with atropine at 0.02 mg/kg IV. Frequent premature ventricular contractions in dogs should be treated with lidocaine (without epinephrine) at a dose of 1 to 2 mg/kg as an IV bolus followed by an IV drip of a 0.1 per cent solution at 30 to 50 μg/kg min. If a beta-blocker is indicated (by persistent tachyarrhythmia) metoprolol (Lopressor, Geigy) and propranolol (Inderal, Ayerst) are of equivalent potency so the same dosage can be recommended for either drug. However, metoprolol would be preferable since propranolol has been shown to reduce theophylline clearance in humans. A suggested starting dose for the injectable form of either drug is 0.1 mg/kg, which can be repeated t.i.d., and this may be increased up to 0.3 mg/kg if needed. The dose should be administered at a rate not to exceed 1 mg/2 minutes IV.

Sixth, it may be advantageous to catheterize the urinary bladder to prevent reabsorption of the methylxanthines and their active metabolites from the urine. Studies in dogs have shown that theophylline can be reabsorbed from the urinary bladder. It is reasonable to assume that this occurs with the other xanthines as well.

The ionization characteristics of the methylxanthines do not allow for effective ion trapping in the urine or for peritoneal dialysis, although hemoperfusion is used for theophylline toxicosis in humans.

Owners should be made aware of these potential toxicoses and should keep chocolate and methylxanthine-containing medications away from their pets.

References and Supplemental Reading

Decker, R. A.: Theobromine poisoning in a dog. J.A.V.M.A. 161:198, 1972.

Glauberg, A., and Blumenthal, H. P.: Chocolate toxicosis in a dog. J. Am. Anim. Hosp. Assoc. 19:246, 1983.

Miller, G. E., Radulovic, G. E., et al.: Comparative theobromine metabolism in five mammalian species. Drug Metab. Dispos. 12:154, 1984.

Muir, W. M. and Sams, R.: Clinical pharmacodynamics of beta-adrenoreceptor blocking drugs in veterinary medicine. Comp. Cont. Ed. Pract. Vet. 6:156, 1984.

Radomski, L., Park, G. J., Goldberg, M. J., et al.: A model for the treatment of theophylline overdose with oral activated charcoal. Clin. Pharmacol. Ther. 35:402, 1984.

Rall, T. W.: Central nervous system stimulants, the xanthines. *In* Gilman, A. G., Goodman, C. S., and Gilman, A. (eds.): *The Pharmacological Basis of Therapeutics*. New York: MacMillan, 1980, pp. 592–607.

Wood, J. H., and Leonard, T. W.: Kinetic implications of drug resorption from the bladder. Drug Metab. Rev. 14:407, 1983.

HOUSEHOLD AND COMMERCIAL PRODUCTS

GARY D. OSWEILER, D.V.M.
Ames, Iowa

Hundreds of household and commercial products are available in homes and businesses. Most are relatively safe or largely inaccessible to companion animals. Actual acute poisoning by household and commercial products is often incompletely documented in pets, and information on household products in dogs and cats is often difficult to obtain in veterinary literature.

Household products constitute a significant portion of exposures to or questions about products

Text continued on page 196

Table 1. *Guide to Some Common Household and Commercial Products*

Agent	Major Toxic Components	Toxicity Rating	Clinical Effects	Therapy*
De-icer (automotive)	Ethylene glycol and isopropanol	4	Disorientation, ataxia weakness, vomiting, impaired vision.	Ethanol; volume diuresis. Gastric lavage (see article on ethylene glycol).
Denture cleaners	Sodium perborate	4	Strong direct irritants. Salivation, lacrimination, vomiting. May be CNS depression.	Flush with water. Use demulcents or ointments.
Deodorants	Aluminum chloride, aluminum chlorhydrate	3	Oral irritation or necrosis; hemorrhagic gastroenteritis. Occasionally incoordination and nephrosis.	*Careful* application of emetics or gastric lavage.
Detergents (anionic)	Sulfonated or phosphorylated forms	2–3	Alkaline product. Dermal irritation, vomiting, diarrhea, GI distension. Usually not fatal.	Lavage with water or weak acid (vinegar).
Detergents (cationic)	Quaternary ammonium with alkyl or aryl substituent groups	3–4	Vomiting, depression, collapse, coma. May cause corrosive damage to esophagus.	Milk or activated charcoal orally. Soap is also effective. Treat seizures and respiratory depression as needed.
Drain cleaners	Sodium hydroxide sometimes sodium hypochlorite	NA†	Serious caustic to skin and mucous membranes. Irritation, inflammation, edema, necrosis. Burns on mouth, tongue, pharynx. Liquid cleaners cause esophageal necrosis and stricture.	Flush affected areas with water, milk, or vinegar. DO NOT USE EMETICS OR LAVAGE. Give oral dilute acetic acid or vinegar. Treat for shock and pain. Surgery may be needed in survivors.
Dry-cleaning fluids	1,1,1 Trichloroethane	3	Exposure may be dermal, inhalation, or oral. Anesthesia, depression, disorientation, narcosis. Occasional ventricular fibrillation. Hepatic and/or renal failure.	Artifical respiration. DO NOT USE EMESIS OR LAVAGE. Charcoal for oral exposure. Monitor lungs, use antibiotics and other therapy for hydrocarbon pneumonia.
Fertilizer	Urea and/or ammonium salts. Nitrates, phosphates	2	Urea and nitrate are of low toxicity to monogastric small animals. Urea might release ammonia in cecum and colon of herbivores (e.g., guinea pig, rabbit). Ammonium salts produce GI irritation and systemic acidosis. High concentration of salts mainly causes vomiting and diarrhea. Diuresis may occur.	General therapy with adsorbents (charcoal) and demulcents. Fluids to alter dehydration from diuresis.

Table continued on following page

Table 1. Guide to Some Common Household and Commercial Products Continued

Agent	Major Toxic Components	Toxicity Rating	Clinical Effects	Therapy*
Fireworks	Oxidizing agents (nitrates, chlorates) Metals (mercury, antimony, copper, strontium, barium, phosphorus)	3–4	Abdominal pain, vomiting, bloody feces, rapid shallow respiration. Chlorates may cause methemoglobinemia.	Emesis or gastric lavage. Use methylene blue (not in cats) or ascorbic acid for methemoglobinemia. Treat for specific metal(s) if known.
Fire extinguisher (liquid)	Chlorobromomethane, Methyl bromide	4	Dermal and ocular irritants, Lacrimation, salivation. Metabolized to methanol. Vomiting, impaired vision, dizziness, paresis, coma. Pulmonary edema. Hepatorenal damage, acidosis.	Flush with soap and water. DO NOT USE EMESIS OR LAVAGE. Control pulmonary edema, renal failure, acidosis, and pneumonia.
Fireplace colors	Heavy metal salts: copper, rubidium cesium, lead, arsenic, selenium barium, antimony zinc.	3	Toxicity and signs vary with metal involved. Acute signs usually include gastroenteritis, diarrhea, renal damage.	Control vomiting and diarrhea. Saline cathartics and adsorbents. Specific metal antidotes if possible.
Fluxes (solder)	Acids (hydrochloric, glutamic, salicylic, boric)	3–4	Caustic or corrosive. Irritant to skin, mouth, pharynx. Vomiting, diarrhea, fever, shock.	Mild saline cathartics, oral adsorbents (charcoal), demulcents. Control shock and pain.
Fuels	Petroleum hydrocarbons, ethanol kerosene, gasoline	3	Early CNS depression, disorientation, necrosis. Mucosal irritation. Aspiration or hydrocarbon pneumonia. Hepatorenal damage (see article on volatile hydrocarbons).	Prevent aspiration pneumonia. AVOID GASTRIC LAVAGE OR PROCEED CAUTIOUSLY TO PREVENT ASPIRATION. Monitor and treat for pneumonia.
Furniture polish	Petroleum, hydrocarbons, mineral spirits	3	See Fuels.	See Fuels.
Gasoline	Aliphatic hydrocarbons	3	See Fuels. Benzene content of gasoline may chronically induce bone marrow hypoplasia and anemia.	See Fuels. Supportive therapy for anemia and leukopenia.
Glues and adhesives	Aliphatic or aromatic hydrocarbons (acetone, toluol, toluene, methyl acetate, naptha)	3	Similar to fuels and volatile hydrocarbons. Mucosal irritation, depression, narcosis, pneumonia, hepatorenal damage.	See Fuels article on volatile hydrocarbons.
Laundry bleach	Sodium hypochlorite	3	Irritant and corrosive to mucous membranes and eyes. Inhalation of vapors causes laryngospasm, pharyngeal edema, pulmonary edema. Oral exposure causes vomiting.	Flood skin with water. DO NOT USE EMESIS OR LAVAGE. DO NOT USE ACIDS. Administer oral milk of magnesia or aluminum hydroxide. Oral sodium thiosulfate detoxifies hypochlorite.
Matches	Potassium chloride	2	Gastroenteritis, vomiting. Chlorates may induce methemoglobinemia with cyanosis and hemolysis.	Treat symptomatically. Use methylene blue (except for cats) or ascorbic acid for methemoglobinemia.
Metal cleaners	Acids. Sodium or potassium hydroxide and/or aliphatic hydrocarbons and chlorinated solvents.	3–4	See Acids, Drain cleaners, Fuels, and article on volatile hydrocarbons.	See appropriate section for agent involved.
Oven cleaners	Potassium or sodium hydroxide and petroleum distillates	3	See Drain Cleaners. See Fuels.	See sections for specific agents listed.
Paint and varnish removers	Benzene, methanol, toluene, acetone (10–75 per cent)	3–4	Dermal irritation, depression. Narcosis, pneumonia, hepatorenal damage. See Fuels, article on volatile hydrocarbons.	See Fuels, Dry-cleaning fluids; article on volatile hydrocarbons.

Table continued on opposite page

Table 1. *Guide to Some Common Household and Commercial Products* Continued

Agent	Major Toxic Components	Toxicity Rating	Clinical Effects	Therapy*
Perfumes	Perfume essence comprising various volatile oils, (e.g., savin, rue, tansy, juniper, cedar)	4	Local irritation of skin and mucous membranes. Pneumonitis. Hepatorenal damage with albuminuria, hematuria, and glycosuria. Excitement, ataxia, coma. Volatile odor of oils and breath.	Gastric lavage with weak bicarbonate solution. Prevent aspiration. Saline cathartics and demulcents.
Photographic developer	*p*-Methylaminophenol	4–5	Methemoglobinemia; cyanosis, cardiac and respiratory insufficiency. Ataxia, disorientation, coma.	Gastric lavage, saline catharsis, activated charcoal. Methylene blue (except in cats) or ascorbic acid for methemoglobinemia.
Pine oil disinfectants	Pine oil 5–10 per cent, phenols 2–6 per cent	3	Gastritis, vomiting, diarrhea followed by CNS depression, occasional mild seizures. Phenols may induce nephrosis.	Gastric lavage with cautions to prevent aspiration. Mineral oil or saline cathartic. Monitor pulmonary and renal function.
Radiator cleaners	Oxalic acid (40–100 per cent)	4	Gastroenteritis from acid corrosion. Vomiting, shock. Hypocalcemia seizures. Oxalate-induced renal failure. See article on ethylene glycol.	Oral calcium salts (limewater). Calcium gluconate IV. Treat for shock. Monitor renal function.
Rubbing alcohol	Ethyl alcohol	2–3	Impaired motor coordination, cutaneous hyperemia, vomiting. Progress to peripheral vascular collapse and coma. Hypothermia.	Gastric lavage or emesis. Monitor temperature, cardiac and respiratory function. Alkalinize urine to promote alcohol excretion. Dialysis is useful in severe cases.
Rust removers	Acids (hydrochloric, phosphoric, fluoric, oxalic)	3–4	Direct corrosive and necrotizing action. Dermal exposure most likely. Skin burns, conjunctival edema, and scleral scarring.	Flush with water, clip hair if necessary. Apply bicarbonate paste. DO NOT USE EMESIS OR LAVAGE for oral exposure. Give magnesium hydroxide orally.
Shampoo	Lauryl sulfates and triethanolamine dodecyl sulfate. Usually less than 5 per cent concentration.	2–3	Ocular irritation. Stimulation of mucus production. Ingestion causes diarrhea.	Saline cathartic. Charcoal or kaolin orally.
Shampoo (antidandruff)	Zinc pyridinethione	5	Progressive blindness with retinal detachment and exudative chorioretinitis.	Prompt oral detoxication therapy. No specific antidote.
Shoe polish	Aniline dyes (3 per cent) in some. Small amounts of nitrobenzenes or terpenes	3	Low concentration of these agents reduces toxicity of product. Aniline and nitrobenzene induces methemoglobinemia (see Matches). Probability of poisoning is low.	See Matches for therapy of methemoglobinemia. See also article on volatile hydrocarbons.
Suntan lotion	Alcohol	3	See Rubbing alcohol.	See Rubbing alcohol.
Styptic pencil	Potassium alum sulfate	2	Corrosive due to release of sulfuric acid during hydrolysis of the salt. Oral necrosis from chewing on pencils.	Oral neutralizer should be magnesium oxide or hydroxide. (Do not give bicarbonate orally for acid poisons).
Thawing salt	Calcium chloride	2	Strong local irritant. Erythema, exfoliation of skin. Vomiting and diarrhea, GI ulceration. Dehydration and shock. Considered unpalatable.	Flush affected area with cold water. Orally give water or egg white.

*For specific dosages and supportive therapies, see Emergency and General Treatment of Poisonings, pp. 135–144.
†Not available.

Table 2. Toxicity Ratings

Toxicity Rating	Description	Lethal Dose	Toxic Amount for 20-kg (44-lb) dog
6	Supertoxic	<5 mg/kg	2 to 3 drops
5	Extremely toxic	5–50 mg/kg	1/3 teaspoonful (tsp)
4	Very toxic	50–500 mg/kg	1/3 tsp to 1/3 ounce
3	Moderately toxic	0.5–5 gm/kg	1/3 ounce to 1/2 cup
2	Slightly toxic	5–15 gm/kg	1/2 cup to 1/2 pint
1	Practically nontoxic	>15 gm/kg	>than 1/2 pint

Modified from Gosselin et al.: *Clinical Toxicology of Commercial Products.* 5th Ed. Baltimore. Williams & Wilkins, 1984.

accessible to small animals. Certain items more frequently associated with questions from veterinarians or animal owners are presented in a brief guide to expected effects from agents of real or potential toxicologic concern to pets. Information presented is based on a combination of data from spontaneous animal poisoning, experimental animal studies, and human literature.

When poisoning by a household or commercial product is suspected, an important factor in prognosis and therapy is knowledge of the toxic components. The trade name and ingredients listed on the label are invaluable in order to obtain further help. With this information, a poison control center can provide valuable assistance regarding expected clinical effects and appropriate therapy, which may be adapted to veterinary patients.

Toxicology of household and commercial products is affected by factors other than the active ingredient itself. Toxicity figures for such products must account for the dilution of active ingredient or toxicant in the finished product. For example, if a product contains 10 per cent ethylene glycol (toxic at 3 ml/kg body weight), then the animal must consume 30 ml/kg body weight of the product to obtain a toxic dose. Some commercial products also contain several ingredients that are each toxic to a different degree. Finally, the toxic effects of vehicles, diluents, and drying or curing agents in some products must be considered. Some typical solvents or diluents are listed in Table 1. (See following article on volatile hydrocarbons.)

Toxicity ratings for products in this chapter are based on a standardized classification (Table 2) (Gosselin et al., 1984).

References and Supplemental Reading

Arena, J. M.: *Poisoning: Toxicology, Symptoms, Treatments*, 4th ed. Springfield, IL: Charles C Thomas, 1979.

Clarke, M. L., Harvey, D. G., and Humphreys, D. J.: *Veterinary Toxicology*, 2nd ed. London: Bailliere Tindall, 1981.

Dresibach, R. H.: *Handbook of Poisoning: Prevention, Diagnosis, and Treatment*, 11th ed. Los Altos, CA: Lange Medical Publications, 1983.

Gosselin, R. E., Smith, R. P., and Hodge, H. C.: *Clinical Toxicology of Commercial Products*, 5th ed. Baltimore: Williams & Wilkins, 1984.

Kirk, R. W., and Bistner, S. I.: *Handbook of Veterinary Procedures and Emergency Treatment*, 3rd and 4th ed. Philadelphia: W.B. Saunders, 1980, 1985.

Osweiler, G. D., Carson, T. L., Buck, W. B. et al.: *Clinical and Diagnostic Veterinary Toxicology*, 3rd ed. Dubuque, IA: Kendall/Hunt, 1985.

Sahenk, A., and Mendell, J. R.: Zinc Pyridinethione. *In* Spencer, P. S., and Schaumburg, H. H. (eds.): *Experimental and Clinical Neurotoxicology*. Baltimore: Williams & Williams, 1980, pp. 578–592.

VOLATILE HYDROCARBONS (SOLVENTS, FUELS) AND PETROCHEMICALS

ROBERT W. COPPOCK, D.V.M.,
Vegreville, Alberta, Canada

MICHELLE S. MOSTROM, D.V.M.,
Urbana, Illinois

and DAVID L. SMETZER, D.V.M.
Urbana, Illinois

ROUTES OF EXPOSURE

Dogs, cats, and other small animals are exposed to volatile hydrocarbons and other petrochemicals by the oral, inhalation, and dermal routes. Exposure in dogs is primarily by ingestion, inhalation, and dermal routes, whereas secondary ingestion by grooming is less common. Dogs confined to a garage will drink petroleum hydrocarbons left in open containers. Dogs appear to drink petrochemical substances readily when their feed and water dishes are used as temporary containers. Inhalation exposure generally occurs when the animal has been confined to an unventilated area used for refinishing furniture and automobiles or where a substantial quantity of volatile hydrocarbons has been spilled. Percutaneous exposure generally occurs after exposure has been sufficient to wet the skin. Dogs will attempt to clean themselves, especially their feet, and thereby ingest petrochemicals.

In cats, primary ingestion is uncommon. Because of their exploratory nature, cats fall into open containers or spill petrochemicals on themselves. Additionally, cats are frequently doused with volatile hydrocarbons, especially gasoline. Thus, percutaneous and secondary oral exposure from grooming are the most common. After exposure, cats often hide in small cubbyholes, and significant inhalation exposure can occur. Primary inhalation exposure of cats occurs the same way as with dogs.

Persons who use the volatile hydrocarbons as substances of abuse may include the family pet in such activities. Older members of the family may not be aware that other family members are engaging in such activities.

TOXICITY OF HYDROCARBONS

The nomenclature used by petroleum chemists to classify petroleum hydrocarbons is complex and will not be covered here. However, some generalizations can be made about the toxicity of three large groups of petroleum hydrocarbons: (1) alkanes (paraffins), aliphatic or straight chains; (2) alicyclic or unsaturated cyclic compounds; and (3) aromatics or hydrocarbons that contain unsaturated rings. Each of these groups varies in its toxic effects.

The alkane gases with one or two carbons (C_1 to C_2) are practically nontoxic below their flammability limit and, at higher concentrations, have anesthetic properties. The C_3 to C_5 compounds have increasing narcotic properties, and the branching chain increases the effect. The C_5 alkanes appear to be more neurotoxic than the C_3 and C_5 paraffins. The C_5 to C_9 hydrocarbons have anesthetic and central nervous system (CNS) depressant actions, and the C_5 and C_7 products have neurotoxic properties. The C_6 to C_8 compounds are acutely toxic when aspirated into the lungs and produce cardiac arrest. The C_1 to C_5 alkanes appear to be the most cardiotoxic. The risk of aspiration pneumonia appears to increase up to C_{16} aliphatics. As a general rule, the aliphatics have considerably lower order of hepato-

Table 1. *Petrochemical Products and Principal Paraffins*

Principal Paraffin No. of Carbons	Petrochemical Product
C_1, C_2	Natural gas
C_3, C_4	Liquefied petroleum gas
C_4–C_6	Petroleum ether
C_5–C_7	Petroleum benzine
C_6–C_8	Petroleum naphtha
C_5–C_{10}	Gasoline
C_9–C_{16}	Kerosene, diesel, and heating oils
C_5–C_{16}	Jet and turbine fuels
C_{17} and higher	Lubricants

and nephrotoxicity than the alicyclic and aromatic hydrocarbons. Table 1 is a partial list of petrochemical products and principal paraffins.

The alicyclic and aromatic hydrocarbons are usually more toxic than the aliphatics. Since members of these groups have a large variation in their chemical structure, generalizations are difficult to make. Inhalation of the vapors causes excitement, ataxia, depression, coma, and in some cases death. Ingestion produces severe diarrhea and vascular collapse and may be followed by heart, liver, and brain degeneration. Alicyclic 8- to 12-carbon compounds present marked danger of inhalation pneumonia. The aromatic hydrocarbons have high affinity for nervous tissue and are particularly neurotoxic. Benzene is toxic to the immune and hematopoietic systems.

Regardless of the route of exposure, hydrocarbons with high vapor pressure are eliminated by the lungs. The movement of these gases decreases aeration of the pulmonary alveoli by means of phenomenon essentially the same as the second gas effect of nitrous oxide. Hydrocarbons of lower viscosity have good spreading properties and can easily be aspirated into the lungs during emesis. Also, the lungs appear to have the capacity to transform certain hydrocarbons into highly toxic compounds, and this phenomenon has been referred to as secondary pulmonary toxicity. The alicyclic, aromatic, and halogenated hydrocarbons (Table 2) can depress the myocardium or induce cardiac arrhythmias.

The liver is the principal organ for detoxifying hydrocarbons. As a general rule, the alicyclic and aromatic hydrocarbons are more nephro- and hepatotoxic. Some of these compounds are inherently toxic, and others are metabolized into toxic compounds. It appears that saturation of the hepatic mechanisms to remove hydrocarbons from the blood is important in CNS, pulmonary, and renal toxicity.

Since petrochemicals are manufactured to meet certain industrial standards such as distillation temperature, specific gravity, viscosity, flash point, freezing point, and residue or to perform certain functions, the actual ratio of the three hydrocarbon groups in a particular product varies with the raw

Table 2. *Hydrocarbons That Produce Cardiac Arrhythmias*

High	Intermediate	Low
Benzene	Carbon tetrachloride	Methylchloride
Heptane	Vinyl chloride	Ethylene
Chloroform	Halothane	Ethyl alcohol
Trichloroethylene	Ethane	Acetone
Trichloroethane	Acetylene	Ethylene oxide
Propane	Cyclobutene	Kerosene
Isobutane	Dimethylbutane	Diesel fuel
Isopentane		Xylene
Cyclobutane		Heating oils
Fluorochloromethane		
Toluene		
Gasoline		

material and manufacturing techniques. Additives of hydrocarbon or organometallic composition are often added to a product to enhance desirable or reduce undesirable properties. Some of these additives are toxic. Because of the competitive markets, the majority of manufacturers consider the specific chemical composition of petrochemicals to be trade secrets.

IDENTIFICATION OF THE TOXIC SUBSTANCE

Many of the volatile hydrocarbons have characteristic odors and, thereby, can be identified. If identification is unsuccessful or uncertain, identification of the petrochemical must be established from the patient's history. Books such as *Clinical Toxicology of Commercial Products* (Gosselin et al., 1976) are very helpful references. If these references are unavailable, the local poison control center can be extremely helpful in identifying the ingredients in certain compounds.

TOXICITY AND TREATMENT BY PRODUCTS

KEROSENE

Kerosene (kerosine, coal oil, in the British Isles known as paraffin) is a distillation fraction of crude oil or a condensate from coal gas. The actual chemical composition of kerosene can vary considerably but consists of linear and branched aliphatic, alicyclic, and aromatic hydrocarbons. Kerosene is used as a fuel in lanterns, stoves, and flares; as a degreaser-cleanser for cleaning automotive parts; and as a solvent in insecticides and other commercial products. Deodorized kerosene is sold as water-white kerosene and, after the addition of fragrance, is marketed for decorator lamps. Oil of citronella is often added to white kerosene and burned in lamps as an insect repellent.

TOXICITY. The toxicity of kerosene in small animals has not been well established. Dogs have been exposed to air saturated with white kerosene (generally considered less toxic) for 8 hours and cats to 910 ppm for 6 hours without harmful effects. Kerosene is absorbed percutaneously and is contraindicated for removing tar from dogs because of a high risk of toxicity. The bulk of the aliphatic hydrocarbons in ingested kerosene are not readily absorbed from the intestinal tract. However, certain alicyclic and aromatic hydrocarbon groups are absorbed and can produce CNS and pulmonary pathologic signs. Kerosene does produce emesis, with aspiration pneumonia as a common sequela. Also, kerosene can be cardio- and nephrotoxic.

CLINICAL SIGNS. The clinical signs of kerosene intoxication vary with its chemical composition, the level of exposure, and the duration between exposure and presentation at the hospital. The level of exposure is usually difficult to establish. Clinical signs of kerosene intoxication are ptyalism, emesis, diarrhea, ataxia, dyspnea, coughing, tremors, depression, seizures, and coma. Myocardial depression appears to be more common than cardiac arrhythmias. However, the electrocardiogram should be monitored. Kerosene is irritating to the mouth, eyes, and skin. Additionally, if kerosene was used as a vehicle, the presence of other toxic substances should also be ruled out.

TREATMENT. Any patient known or suspected of being exposed to kerosene should be hospitalized and have radiographs taken of the chest. Follow-up radiographs should be taken as needed, and this may be as frequent as 1- to 2-hour intervals. Cardiac function should be monitored, and cardiac drugs may be indicated (see discussion of gasoline intoxication). Baseline hepatic enzymes and hematologic values should be established. Concern should be given to values that have marked changes even if they are within what is considered the normal range. Comatose patients should be intubated, the pneumatic cuff inflated, and oxygen therapy initiated. If possible, blood oxygen and carbon dioxide levels should be determined. Patients with percutaneous exposure should be bathed with a mild detergent.

Considerable controversy surrounds the following aspects of managing kerosene intoxication: (1) induction of emesis, (2) gastric lavage, (3) administration of mineral oil, (4) administration of prophylactic steroids, and (5) prophylactic use of antibiotics.

Whether or not to induce emesis depends on whether significant pulmonary dysfunction and CNS depression can result from gastrointestinal absorption of kerosene. The liver has excellent capacity to remove toxic hydrocarbons from portal blood. Dogs with cervical esophageal ligation were given orally 20 ml kerosene/kg and no adverse effects were observed at 72 hours. The majority of patients in human and veterinary medicine develop inhalation pneumonia after emesis and, in most cases, hypoxia appears to explain the CNS signs. Conversely, the lungs appear to have the capacity to metabolize certain hydrocarbons found in kerosene to highly pneumotoxic compounds. Certain hydrocarbons found in kerosene, when injected IV, will produce marked CNS effects and pulmonary lesions, and, when these experiments were repeated using the portal vein for hematogenous exposure, no CNS signs and pulmonary lesions were observed. High oral doses of kerosene will produce CNS signs and pulmonary lesions in patients that do not vomit. Thus, the risk and benefits from the induction of emesis appear to depend on dosage and hepatic detoxification. Clinical and experimental evidence supports that, in most cases of kerosene ingestion, the liver is able to remove sufficient hydrocarbons from the portal blood to prevent CNS effects and pulmonary lesions, and, therefore, induction of emesis is contraindicated. If the kerosene contains insecticides and other substances, then induction of emesis should receive thorough risk-versus-benefit considerations.

Cautious gastric lavage has been advocated in the treatment of kerosene poisoning. However, because of problems with restraint, cautious gastric lavage does not exist in veterinary medicine. In the unmedicated patient, gastric lavage often induces emesis. Also, emesis can occur during the induction of narcosis or anesthesia. In the majority of cases of kerosene intoxication, gastric lavage is contraindicated. However, each case must receive prudent management, and, if in your clinical judgment benefits from gastric lavage are greater than the risk, gastric lavage is indicated. In all cases that are lavaged, the trachea should be blocked with a tight-fitting catheter.

Mineral oil PO has been recommended to increase the viscosity of ingested kerosene and prevent the absorption of toxic hydrocarbons. Increasing the viscosity of kerosene should decrease the risk of aspiration pneumonia, and preventing absorption decreases the hepatic detoxification burden. Mineral oil also acts as a cathartic to remove the kerosene from the intestinal tract. Retrospective studies in human medicine have shown that treatment with mineral oil increases the risk of aspiration pneumonia in patients that vomit.

The use of glucocorticoid steroids is controversial. In dogs, long-acting steroids increase the growth of bacteria in the lungs and the time required for resolution of pulmonary damage. However, steroids are beneficial in preventing pulmonary edema and pleural effusion. Again, clinical judgment is necessary in determining if steroids are indicated in kerosene poisoning. Short-acting steroids are considered drugs of choice.

Prophylactic use of antibiotics is finding disfavor in veterinary medicine, primarily because of the massive upset in the normal microbial flora of the body and increased potential for antibiotic resistance. In cases of kerosene intoxication where there is clinical evidence of infection, antibiotics are indicated. A broad-spectrum antibiotic should be used. Additionally, chloramphenicol, due to its partial inhibition of the mixed-function oxidase enzyme system, may be of benefit in preventing the formation of toxic metabolites.

Systematic treatment is indicated. If the patient has CNS signs and myocardial depression, oxygen should be given. Blood gases should be determined, or the mucous membranes should be carefully evaluated for signs of hypoxia. Kerosene hydrocarbons may potentiate many of the CNS drugs, and therefore these drugs should be given in lower doses and administered more frequently. CNS signs can rapidly change, and drugs used to control CNS excitement can complicate CNS depression. Use of epinephrine is contraindicated. Drugs used to control CNS signs can affect cardiac performance. Again, prudent clinical judgment is essential.

All patients with apparent or actual kerosene poisoning should be hospitalized for at least 24 hours and should be free from clinical signs at the time of discharge. The owner should be advised that anorexia often follows kerosene ingestion. Client education to prevent recurrence is essential.

GASOLINE, MOTOR FUELS, AND HEATING OILS

Gasoline is composed of the more volatile groups of aliphatic, alicyclic, and aromatic hydrocarbons. Gasoline can contain 10 to 40 per cent ethyl alcohol, organic lead compounds, alicyclic and aromatic hydrocarbons, and organic magnesium compounds to control rate of combustion. Gasoline is used for motor fuels, cleaning automotive parts, and for solvents. Racing fuels are often a methanol base and may contain nitrobenzene, nitromethane, and castor oil. Fuels used in miniature engines can contain methanol, ethers, nitromethane, and castor oil.

Diesel fuel and home heating oils are manufactured to meet similar industrial standards. Their compositions vary considerably in ratios of aliphatic, alicyclic, and aromatic hydrocarbons. Diesel oils contain additives, such as triazines, to prevent growth of microorganisms.

TOXICITY. The volatile hydrocarbons in gasoline have marked effects on the CNS. These compounds also include cardiac arrhythmias or depress the myocardium. Marked hyper- or hypothermia may also be observed. Gasoline is very irritating to the skin and eyes. Generally, lead intoxication is not a problem. Diesel fuels and home heating oils have essentially the same toxicity as kerosene. In racing fuels, methanol and castor oil appear to be the most toxic constituents. The nitro- compounds may produce hypotension.

CLINICAL SIGNS. Clinical signs of gasoline intoxication are ataxia, emesis, hyperesthesia, seizures, depression, and coma. Cardiac arrhythmias may also be observed, and the electrocardiogram should be monitored. Rapid changes in clinical signs may occur. Hyper- and hypothermia may be observed. Since gasoline is irritating to the mucous membranes, epiphora, ptyalism, emesis, and diarrhea may be observed. Eye irritation from gasoline can result in erosions of the cornea, corneal edema, and photophobia. Clinical signs of diesel oil toxicity are the same as those for kerosene toxicity. (The toxicity of methanol is discussed later.) Castor oil is extremely irritating to the intestinal tract, and violent diarrhea may occur.

TREATMENT. Supportive treatment is essential in gasoline intoxication. Patients with dermal exposure should be bathed with a mild detergent. Patients with marked clinical signs should be given oxygen. As with kerosene intoxication, induction of emesis is generally contraindicated. Gasoline-induced cardiac arrhythmias should be characterized before cardiac drugs are given. Ventricular premature beats and ventricular tachycardia can be controlled with lidocaine and atrial arrhythmias with propranolol or other appropriate drugs, but in atrioventricular block, antiarrhythmic drugs are usually contraindicated (see Section 4 for discussion of cardiac arrhythmias). Body temperature should be monitored and, if necessary, controlled. If there is clinical evidence of keratoconjunctivitis, the eyes should be checked for ulcers by staining with fluorescein. Broad-spectrum antibiotics should be applied topically, and steroids may be indicated (see Section 7).

FURNITURE POLISHES, PAINT AND VARNISH REMOVERS, AND SOLVENTS

Furniture Polishes

Furniture polishes can contain petroleum distillates, mineral seal oil, petroleum naphthas, turpentine, waxes and pine oils. Of these, the volatile hydrocarbons are considered to be the most toxic.

TOXICITY. Mineral seal oil is primarily saturated aliphatic hydrocarbons. It is especially dangerous because aspiration pneumonia may follow ingestion and subsequent emesis. (The toxicity of turpentine and petroleum naphthas are discussed later.)

CLINICAL SIGNS AND TREATMENT. See discussion for kerosene or solvents.

Paint Removers

Flammable paint and varnish removers contain benzene, methanol, acetone, and toluene. Nonflammable ones contain methylene chloride, methanol, and toluene.

Methanol

Methanol (methyl alcohol, wood alcohol, wood spirits, carbinol, methyl hydrate) is used in paint removers, solvents, paints, varnishes, shellacs, and automotive products. Products that contain methanol may also contain ethanol, which delays the onset of clinical signs of methanol intoxication.

TOXICITY. Methanol is readily absorbed from the gastrointestinal tract. Approximately 30 per cent of ingested methanol is excreted by the lungs and 5 per cent by the kidneys. The majority of the ingested dose is metabolized by alcohol dehydrogenase to formaldehyde. Dogs can metabolize approximately 20 per cent of the formaldehyde to formic acid, which is excreted by the kidneys or metabolized to carbon dioxide. Decreased metabolism of lactic acid and metabolites of methanol appear to account for the metabolic acidosis that develops 2 to 12 hours after ingestion. Retinopathy does not appear to be a problem in dogs poisoned with methanol. However, pancreatitis may occur.

CLINICAL SIGNS. The clinical signs of methanol intoxication are ataxia, emesis, dyspnea, motor restlessness, marked abdominal pain, cold extremities, hypothermia, and coma rapidly followed by death. The onset of abdominal pain may be delayed for 3 to 24 hours after ingestion. Clinical pathologic findings are ketonuria, decreased blood pH, methanol in the urine, and an increase in mean corpuscular volume.

TREATMENT. Removal of residual gastric methanol should be instituted by gastric lavage or emesis in the conscious patient. Ethyl alcohol should be given to compete with alcohol dehydrogenase and prevent the formation of toxic metabolites. Body temperature should be maintained. Acidosis should be corrected, and peritoneal dialysis may be of benefit. Treatment with ethyl alcohol and correction of acidosis are discussed in the article on ethylene glycol intoxication. However, unlike ethylene glycol, methanol may potentiate the CNS-depressing effects of ethanol.

Methylene Chloride

Methylene chloride (methylene dichloride, methylene bichloride) is used in paint removers, as a solvent in aerosol products, and in degreasing and cleaning fluids.

TOXICITY. Methylene chloride is metabolized by the mixed-function oxidases to carbon dioxide and carbon monoxide with a concurrent increase in carboxyhemoglobin. Additionally, it can be very irritating to mucous membranes and can damage pancreatic islet cells. The presence of methanol, ethanol, and possibly other hydrocarbons in paint and varnish removers may delay the onset of clinical signs.

CLINICAL SIGNS. Clinical signs are reddening of the mucous membranes, ptyalism, emesis, increased respiratory rate, and dyspnea. If possible, carboxyhemoglobin and blood glucose should be monitored.

TREATMENT. Symptomatic treatment and oxygen therapy generally result in recovery.

Solvents—Toluene, Xylene, and Benzene

Toluene (toluol, methylbenzene, phenylmethane) is an alkylbenzene. Xylene is dimethylbenzene. Benzene is the simplest of aromatic compounds and should not be confused with benzine (hydrocarbon composition similar to gasoline). There has been a move to replace benzene with toluene. These petrochemicals have use as solvents in paints, varnishes, lacquers, glues, and inks and as thinners and cleaners. Toluene appears to be favored as a substance of abuse.

TOXICITY—CLINICAL SIGNS. Benzene and toluene intoxication are similar, but toluene and xylene are not myelotoxic. These solvents are toxic to the CNS, heart, liver, and kidneys. Clinical signs are emesis, ataxia, nervousness, tremors, seizures, coma, and death. Cardiovascular arrhythmias include slowed sinoatrial rate, prolonged P-R interval, and atrioventricular block. Proteinuria and hematuria may be observed along with elevated serum hepatocellular enzymes. These compounds have a oderate risk of causing aspiration pneumonia.

TREATMENT. Treatment of CNS effects is symptomatic and supportive. Emesis and gastric lavage may be beneficial. (The management of cardiac arrhythmias has been discussed under gasoline intoxication.)

Solvents—Turpentine

Turpentine (spirits of turpentine, gum turpentine, oil of turpentine) is a distillate from pine pitch and is composed of terpenes. It is used as a paint solvent, furniture polish, stain remover, and cleaning fluid, as well as in numerous home remedies.

TOXICITY. Turpentine is rapidly absorbed from the gastrointestinal tract, skin, and lungs. This substance is irritating to the skin, eyes, oral membranes, and gastrointestinal and urinary tracts. It induces emesis, but the danger of aspiration pneumonia appears to be less than with kerosene. Turpentine can induce cardiac arrhythmias.

CLINICAL SIGNS. Clinical signs are eye irritation, congestion of the mucous membranes, ptyalism, epiphora, emesis, diarrhea, ataxia, depression, and dyspnea. Cardiac arrhythmias include sinus tachycardia, ventricular premature beats, and idioventricular rhythm. Hematuria, albuminuria, and glycosuria may also be observed.

TREATMENT. See discussions for kerosene and gasoline. In the majority of cases, turpentine intoxication is not fatal.

Solvents—Petroleum Hydrocarbons

Mineral, white, and petroleum spirits; Stoddard solvent; petroleum naphthas; and thinners Nos. 40 to 80 are used as solvents and thinners for paints, varnishes, lacquers, and glues. Additional uses are dry-cleaning fluids, spot removers, degreasing agents, charcoal lighters, and vehicles for pesticides.

TOXICITY. The toxicity of this group of petrochemicals varies considerably depending on the predominate hydrocarbon group. Apparently because of their CNS effects, these hydrocarbons are often used as substances of abuse. Generally, the mineral spirits, petroleum naphthas, and Stoddard solvent have more CNS and cardiotoxicity and fewer gastrointestinal-irritating effects than kerosene. When aspiration occurs, these petrochemicals will produce inhalation pneumonia. Stoddard solvent intoxication mimics that of gasoline, whereas the effects of petroleum spirits and naphthas appear to resemble those of kerosene and gasoline intoxication. Toxicity with some of the thinners mimics that of petroleum spirits, toluene, and benzene.

CLINICAL SIGNS AND TREATMENT. Clinical signs and treatment are similar to those for kerosene, gasoline, toluene, and xylene.

AUTOMOTIVE PRODUCTS

Methanol

Methanol is used in gas-line antifreeze, windshield-washing fluids, emergency heaters (canned heat), and motor fuels. (The toxicity of methanol has been discussed previously.)

Lubricants

Many small animals are exposed to automotive lubricants. Generally, new motor oils have a low order of toxicity. The toxicity of motor oils is often due to the additives, which are antifoaming agents, detergents, and antioxidants. Used motor oils from internal combustion engines that burn leaded gasoline can contain as much as 20,000 ppm lead and numerous other by-products from combustion of fossil fuels. Automatic transmission fluids contain antifoaming agents and corrosion inhibitors. Gear oils and greases may contain antifoaming agents, antioxidants, and lead.

TOXICITY. Most toxicity from automotive lubricants is due to the additives. The detergents in motor oils can be extremely irritating to the gastrointestinal tract. Some of the antifoaming agents, especially the cresyl phosphates, can be toxic to the peripheral nerves and CNS. The antioxidants or rust inhibitors can be very toxic to the CNS. If its composition is unknown, the lubricant should be checked for heavy metals.

CLINICAL SIGNS. Signs of recent motor oil and transmission fluid poisoning are emesis, depression, ataxia, seizures, and, rarely, coma. Marked neurologic signs can develop within 12 to 72 hours. For the antifoaming agents, these can be ataxia and posterior paralysis due to damage of peripheral and spinal nerves. Ataxia, circling, and seizures can develop from certain antioxidants as a result of destruction of nervous tissue in the brain.

TREATMENT. If soiled with oil and grease, the patient should be bathed. Removal of automotive lubricant from the stomach by emesis or lavage should be considered, especially if the exposure has been great. Supportive care and symptomatic treatment are essential. Most cases recover.

SUMMARY

Petrochemical intoxication provides a challenge in diagnosis and medical management. The type of hydrocarbon substance and route and level of exposure should be established. Good clinical judgment is essential in determining if the petrochemical should be removed from the stomach by emesis or gastric lavage. Patients that are soiled with oil, grease, or tar should be bathed with a mild detergent. Acetone has been safely used to remove tar. Supportive care and symptomatic treatment are essential. The pharmacologic effects of the petrochemical must be considered when pharmaceutics are selected for treatment.

Reference and Supplemental Reading

Gosselin, R. E., Hodge, H. C., Smith, R. P., et al.: *Clinical Toxicology of Commercial Products: Acute Poisoning.* Baltimore: Williams & Wilkins, 1976.

TOXIC GASES

THOMAS L. CARSON, D.V.M.

Ames, Iowa

Several toxicants that can represent a health hazard to companion animals exist in a gaseous form. These potentially toxic gases are usually associated with unique environmental or management conditions and are produced from several different sources. Carbon monoxide, a by-product of inefficient combustion of carbonaceous fuels, is potentially lethal to all animals. Nitrogen oxides produced from the fermentation of nitrogenous compounds and the oxides of sulfur associated with industrial air pollution are also of concern. Other important gases associated with the decomposition of urine and feces in closed animal facilities include ammonia, carbon dioxide, methane, and hydrogen sulfide.

Concentrations of toxic gases are usually expressed as parts of the gas per million parts of air by volume (ppm). Sometimes concentrations are expressed as weight of gas per unit volume of air—for example, as micrograms of the gas per cubic meter of air.

CARBON MONOXIDE

Carbon monoxide (CO), an odorless, colorless, poisonous gas that is slightly lighter than air, results from incomplete combustion of hydrocarbon fuels. A common source of CO is the exhaust of gasoline-burning internal combustion engines. Transportation of animals in the trunk of a car with a faulty exhaust system has resulted in poisoning.

Poisoning also occurs when improperly adjusted or improperly vented space heaters or furnaces are operated in tight, often poorly ventilated, buildings. Sometimes fresh-air vents are covered or flue pipes or chimneys become blocked with bird nests or the like, and what was previously a safe operation becomes dangerous.

Carbon monoxide acts by competing with oxygen for binding sites on a variety of proteins, including hemoglobin, with which most of the compound is associated in the body. The affinity of hemoglobin for CO is some 250 times that for oxygen. When CO becomes bonded to the heme group, forming carboxyhemoglobin (COHb), the molecule's oxygen-carrying capacity is reduced. In addition, the oxygen dissociation curve is shifted to the left, meaning that the release of oxygen from hemoglobin to tissues is also impaired. The end result is that CO toxicosis leads to tissue hypoxia. Concentrations of both COHb (expressed in per cent) and CO in the air (expressed in parts per million) can be used to define a toxic dose of carbon monoxide.

Based on blood COHb levels, the following clinical effects can be expected: At 1 to 3 per cent COHb, no effects are observed. At 6 to 8 per cent, the ability to maintain attention is decreased. At 20 per cent, there is definite psychomotor disturbance. At 20 to 40 per cent, lethargy, disturbance in gait, and changes in the electroencephalogram from an arousal to a slow wave, plus spindle pattern, may be observed. Death occurs with 60 to 70 per cent of COHb.

Since CO causes injury by hypoxia, symptoms are referable to tissues with the greatest oxygen consumption—the brain and myocardium.

With sudden high exposures, death may occur very rapidly. Immediate death is most likely cardiac in origin, since myocardial tissue is most sensitive to the hypoxic effects of CO. Cardiac dyfunction usually precedes central nervous system dysfunction. Lower exposures result in drowsiness, disorientation, incoordination, dyspnea, and coma.

At postmortem examination, bronchi are dilated and major blood vessels may be distended. The dilated ventricles of the heart, especially the right, may account for the abrupt rise in central venous pressure sometimes encountered. The blood of animals with a high percentage of COHb may appear bright cherry red, but the finding is somewhat variable.

Histologic changes in the brain as a result of anoxia appear as necrosis in the cortex and white matter of the cerebral hemispheres, the globus pallidus, and the brain stem. Edema, demyelination, and hemorrhage in the brain and necrosis in the Ammon's horn of the hippocampus may occur. The brain lesions may result in permanent damage manifested as deafness in dogs and cats.

Respiratory alkalosis occurs from hyperventilation caused by metabolic acidosis. There is no evidence of carbon dioxide (CO_2) retention.

A diagnosis of CO toxicosis should be entertained when the history suggests exposure to engine exhaust or unvented fuel-burning heaters or when there are clinical signs of acute death or hypoxia.

Exposure to high levels of CO can be confirmed by measuring the CO level in the air or by measuring the percentage of COHb in the blood of the affected animal. Once CO exposure has ceased and the animal is exposed to fresh air, the COHb level may return to normal in as short a time as 3 hours. Therefore, the time of diagnostic sample collection is important when evaluating blood COHb values.

Treatment of acute CO poisoning consists most importantly of removing the affected animal from continued exposure to the gas. Administration of 100 per cent oxygen to accelerate elimination of CO and to improve tissue oxygenation is highly recommended. Oxygen should be given until the COHb level decreases to at least 10 per cent.

Endotracheal intubation and mechanical ventilation are necessary if there is any question about the adequacy of the airway or ventilation, since CO is eliminated from the lungs.

Supportive care should include continuous cardiac monitoring, treatment of arrhythmias, and correction of acid-base and electrolyte abnormalities. Hypotension and severe acidosis should be quickly corrected, since there is a substantial correlation between such abnormalities and white matter degeneration.

Clinical recovery may lag hours or days behind reduction in blood COHb levels. Various neurologic sequelae commonly appear several days to weeks after apparent recovery.

NITROGEN DIOXIDE

Nitrogen oxide is a relatively inert gas produced by high-pressure combustion such as in gasoline engines, from oxidation of atmospheric nitrogen, or from the combustion of nitrogen-containing substances such as explosives, cigarettes, and agricultural wastes. It is further oxidized to nitrogen dioxide (NO_2). Power plants and automobiles are the main sources of this irritating gas. Nitrogen dioxide is also liberated during the rapid decomposition of plant material, as happens in silos. Concentrations as great as 1500 ppm of this gas can be reached during the first 48 hours after filling a silo. Because it is heavier than air, NO_2 may collect in enclosed places.

This yellow-brown gas with a bleach-like smell can injure or kill animals and people. When NO_2 combines with water, it forms nitric acid, which is very corrosive. Progressive weakness, dyspnea, cough, and cyanosis begin 1 to 3 weeks after single or repeated exposure to concentrations of 50 to 300 ppm. Concentrations greater than 300 ppm cause fulminating pulmonary edema or bronchopneumonia; onset is within hours or days.

Humans are able to detect NO_2 at levels as low as 0.1 to 0.2 ppm in the air. Increasing levels of NO_2 affect pulmonary function. Concentrations in the 4- to 5-ppm range for a 10-minute exposure period have their maximum effect of increasing respiratory flow resistance 30 minutes after exposure ceases. The impact of NO_2 exposure is a function of both concentration of gas and length of exposure time. Rats, mice, guinea pigs, rabbits, and dogs have a mortality threshold of between 40 and 50 ppm of NO_2 for a 1-hour exposure.

The extent of pathologic change in the lungs corresponds to exposure dosage. Acute exposures to NO_2 with concentrations of 2 to 3 ppm, which are close to ambient levels, have not resulted in an increase in morphologic abnormalities in dogs.

Treatment of NO_2 exposure consists of providing oxygen to relieve the cyanosis and dyspnea. The pulmonary inflammatory reaction can be reduced by using prednisone or prednisolone orally every 6 hours for several weeks. Additional supportive care includes controlling pulmonary edema and administering broad-spectrum antibiotics for bronchopneumonia. The prognosis should be guarded, as recovery may require from 1 to 6 months. Some emphysematous changes may persist indefinitely.

SULFUR OXIDES

Sulfur dioxide (SO_2), a gas formed in burning coal and oil, is the air pollutant most suspected of affecting pulmonary health. The presence of suspended particles increases lung irritation from SO_2.

A single exposure to 5 ppm SO_2 results in eye irritation and salivation. Hemorrhage and emphysema occur within 24 hours after an 8-hour exposure to 40 ppm SO_2.

At low concentrations, there is eye and nasal irritation. Higher levels produce severe respiratory distress and death. In addition to the mucous membrane irritation of the eye and nose, hemorrhage and emphysema occur in the lungs.

Chronic effects are also possible. Two pigs exposed for a single 8-hour period to 40 ppm SO_2 developed pulmonary fibrosis within 160 days after exposure.

The diagnosis of SO_2 poisoning is based on a history of exposure and the presence of pulmonary changes.

There is no specific treatment. Pulmonary edema can be controlled with prednisolone, and bacterial pneumonia is treated with organism-specific chemotherapy.

AMMONIA

Ammonia (NH_3) is the toxic air pollutant most frequently found in high concentrations in animal facilities. Ammonia production is especially common where excrement can decompose on a solid floor. This gas has a characteristic pungent odor that humans can detect at approximately 10 ppm or even lower. The concentration of NH_3 in enclosed animal facilities usually remains below 30 ppm, even with low ventilation rates, although on occasion it may reach 50 ppm or even higher.

Ammonia is highly soluble in water, and it will react with the moist mucous membranes of the eyes and respiratory passages. Consequently, excessive tearing, shallow breathing, and clear or purulent nasal discharage are common symptoms of NH_3-vapor toxicosis. At concentrations of NH_3 usually found in practical animal environments (less than 100 ppm), the primary effect of this gas is as a chronic stressor. Ammonia may irritate the respiratory mucosa from the nose to the lungs. This irritation may lead to increased secretion of mucus by the respiratory epithelium, shallow breathing, bronchiolar constriction, and hyperplasia of the bronchiolar and alveolar epithelium. No consistent gross or microscopic structural changes tend to be associated with uncomplicated NH_3-vapor toxicosis in animals.

A diagnosis of NH_3-vapor exposure will be primarily based on the history and field observation. Laboratory analysis will be of limited value in cases of inhalation exposures.

The maintenance of adequate ventilation and good sanitary procedures will alleviate the problems associated with high concentrations of NH_3.

Anhydrous NH_3 (gas-NH_3), which is stored, transported, and applied under high pressure is used in large quantities as an agricultural nitrogen fertilizer. This gas presents a potential hazard because the moisture-rich corneal structure of the eye is especially vulnerable to gas-NH_3. Permanent or impaired loss of eyesight, respiratory problems, and skin burns are the result of exposure. First aid for exposure is continuous irrigation of the eyes with water for 15 to 20 minutes.

CARBON DIOXIDE

Carbon dioxide is an odorless gas present in the atmosphere at 300 ppm. It is given off by animals as an end product of energy metabolism and by improperly vented, though properly adjusted, fuel burning heaters. It is also the gas evolved in the greatest quantity by decomposing manure. Despite all of this, its concentration in closed animal facilities rarely even approaches levels that endanger animal health. Carbon dioxide at 5 per cent (50,000 ppm) is well tolerated by animals, producing only an increase in rate and depth of respiration. In the unlikely event that CO_2, which is heavier than air, might collect in a low part of a facility, animals may exhibit anxiety followed by staggering, coma, and finally death as the concentration exceeds 40 per cent.

Diagnosis will usually be based on the clinical history, clinical signs, and lack of other obvious causes. Blood P_{CO_2} can be measured if suitable equipment is available. Samples have to be protected from exposure to the air, even for brief periods of time.

Treatment is simply to provide fresh air. If the respiratory mechanisms are still intact, the body is able to rapidly eliminate the excess CO_2. Chronic damage may result, depending on the severity and duration of apnea.

METHANE

Methane (CH_4), a product of microbial degradation of carbonaceous materials, is not a poisonous gas. It is biologically rather inert and affects animals only by displacing oxygen in a given atmosphere, thereby producing asphyxiation. Under ordinary pressures, a concentration of 87 to 90 per cent CH_4 in a given atmosphere is required before irregularities of respiration and eventual respiratory arrest due to anoxia are produced. Rabbits can breathe a mixture of one part oxygen and four parts CH_4 for extended periods of time without showing ill effects.

Methane, which is lighter than air, is both colorless and odorless. The chief danger inherent in this material is its explosive potential as concentrations of 5 to 15 per cent by volume in air are reached. Its flammability and explosiveness, rather than any toxic effect on living organisms, are the major hazards of this gas.

HYDROGEN SULFIDE

Hydrogen sulfide (H_2S) is a colorless, toxic gas that is heavier than air and has the characteristic odor of rotten eggs. High concentrations of H_2S can occur in natural gas deposits as well as in coal, oil, volcanic gases, and sulfur springs and lakes. This potentially lethal gas is also produced by anaerobic decomposition of sulfur-containing organic matter. This reaction accounts for the hazard of H_2S associated with liquid manure–holding pits in livestock facilities. Less than 10 ppm of H_2S, the level usually found in closed animal facilities, is not toxic. However, when a manure slurry is agitated to resuspend solids prior to being pumped out, it rapidly releases much of the H_2S that may have been retained within it. This release of gas after agitation may produce concentrations of H_2S as great as 1000 ppm or higher within the facility.

Humans can detect the typical odor of H_2S at concentrations as low as 0.025 ppm in air. Exposures to these low concentrations have little or no importance to health, and thus the olfactory response is a safe and useful warning signal. However, at concentrations greater than 200 ppm, H_2S presents a distinct hazard: It exerts a paralyzing effect on the olfactory apparatus, effectively neutralizing the warning signal.

Hydrogen sulfide is an irritant gas. Its direct action on tissues induces local inflammation of the moist membranes of the eyes and respiratory tract. When inhaled, H_2S exerts its irritant action more or less uniformly through the respiratory tract, although the deeper pulmonary structures suffer the greatest damage. Inflammation of the deep lung structures may appear as pulmonary edema. Hydrogen sulfide can also be readily absorbed through the lungs and can produce fatal systemic intoxication if inhaled at sufficiently high concentrations.

At concentrations exceeding 500 ppm, the chemoreceptors of the carotid body are stimulated. The resulting hyperventilation depletes the CO_2 in the blood and leads to respiratory inactivity (apnea). If spontaneous recovery does not occur and artificial respiration is not immediately provided, death from asphyxia is inevitable.

At about 1500 ppm, the reaction is more intense. At 2000 ppm, the respiratory apparatus becomes paralyzed after a breath or two. Generalized convulsions frequently begin at this point.

This form of respiratory failure is not related to the CO_2 content of the blood; instead, H_2S exerts a direct paralyzing effect on the respiratory center. Breathing is usually never reestablished spontaneously after H_2S-induced paralysis of respiration.

If artifical respiration is begun immediately and is continued until the H_2S concentration in the blood decreases as a result of pulmonary excretion, death from asphyxia can be prevented because the heart continues to beat for several minutes. After several minutes, normal respiration is usually reestablished. Victims of acute H_2S poisoning who recover usually do so promptly and completely.

References and Supplemental Reading

Coburn, R. F. (ed.): Biological Effects of Carbon Monoxide. Ann. N.Y. Acad. Sci. 174:369, 1970.

Dreisbach, R. H.: *Handbook of Poisoning*, 11th ed. Los Altos, CA: Lange Medical Publications, 1983.

National Research Council (Committee on Medical and Biological Effects of Environmental Pollutants, Subcommittee on Nitrogen Oxides): *Nitrogen Oxides*. Washington, D.C.: National Academy of Sciences, 1977.

National Research Council (Committee on Medical and Biological Effects of Environmental Pollutants, Subcommittee on Ammonia): *Ammonia*. Baltimore: University Park Press, 1979.

National Research Council (Committee on Medical and Biological Effects of Environmental Pollutants, Subcommittee on Hydrogen Sulfide): *Hydrogen Sulfide*. Baltimore: University Park Press, 1979.

Osweiler, G. D., Carson, T. L., Buck, W. B., et al.: *Clinical and Diagnostic Veterinary Toxicology*, 3rd ed. Dubuque, IA: Kendall/Hunt, 1985, pp. 365–377.

Tintinalli, J. E., Rominger, M., and Kittelson, K.: Carbon monoxide. *In* Haddad, L. M., and Winchester, J. F.: *Clinical Management of Poisoning and Drug Overdose*. Philadelphia: W. B. Saunders, 1983, pp. 748–753.

ETHYLENE GLYCOL (ANTIFREEZE) POISONING

GREGORY F. GRAUER, D.V.M.,
Madison, Wisconsin

and MARY ANNA HULL THRALL, D.V.M.
Fort Collins, Colorado

Antifreeze poisoning is common in small animals because of the compound's widespread availability and sweet taste. Commercial antifreeze solutions contain 95 per cent ethylene glycol, the toxic agent. Ethylene glycol is also a constituent of some color film processing solutions that may be found in home darkrooms. The minimum lethal dose of undiluted ethylene glycol is 4.2 to 6.6 ml/kg for dogs and 1.5 ml/kg for cats. The incidence of poisoning in dogs and cats is similar; however, males of both species are poisoned more frequently than females. Most intoxications take place in the fall, winter, and early spring, reflecting the seasons of peak usage of antifreeze solutions.

Diagnosis of ethylene glycol poisoning may be difficult because the symptoms are nonspecific. Many patients are not correctly diagnosed until the onset of renal failure or at postmortem examination.

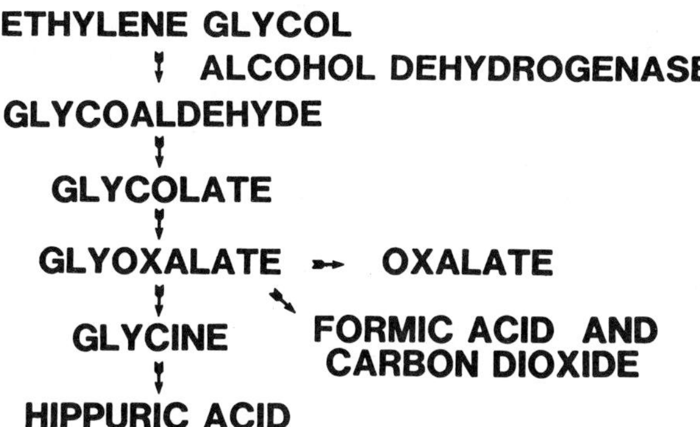

Figure 1. The metabolism pathway of ethylene glycol.

The prognosis for animals poisoned with ethylene glycol depends on the amount ingested and varies inversely with the amount of time between ingestion and treatment. Early diagnosis is imperative in order to treat effectively.

Ethylene glycol is a colorless, odorless, water-soluble liquid that is rapidly absorbed from the gastrointestinal tract and distributed to all body tissues after ingestion. Peak blood concentrations in dogs and cats occur between 1 and 3 hours after ingestion. More than half of the ethylene glycol ingested is excreted unchanged in the urine. Peak urine concentrations occur about 6 hours after ingestion. Serum and urine concentrations of ethylene glycol are usually undetectable 76 hours after ingestion. Renal clearance of ethylene glycol is dependent on glomerular filtration rate and passive distal tubular reabsorption. The proximal tubule is not permeable to ethylene glycol. Renal excretion of the compound is proportional to water excretion.

Metabolism of ethylene glycol occurs primarily in the liver by a series of oxidation reactions (Fig. 1). A liver enzyme, alcohol dehydrogenase, rapidly oxidizes ethylene glycol to glycoaldehyde, which is then oxidized to glycolate by aldehyde dehydrogenase. The glycolate is oxidized to glyoxalate by glycolic acid oxidase or lactic dehydrogenase. The conversion of glycolate to glyoxalate proceeds relatively slowly and is thought to be the rate-limiting step in the metabolism of ethylene glycol. Glyoxalate can enter one of three metabolic pathways. The first is an oxidation reaction that produces formic acid and carbon dioxide. The second is a reversible transamination reaction that forms glycine. Hippuric acid may be produced from the metabolism of glycine. Finally, glyoxalate may be oxidized to oxalate by aldehyde oxidase or lactic dehydrogenase. Oxalate is not readily metabolized and is excreted unchanged in the urine. It is estimated that from 0.25 to 3.7 per cent of the ingested ethylene glycol is converted to oxalate.

Table 1. *Clinical Signs and Stages of Ethylene Glycol Poisoning*

Stage 1—Central nervous system signs
Nausea and vomiting
Mild to moderate neurologic signs—ataxia, depression, and knuckling
Polydipsia and polyuria
Severe neurologic signs—seizures, coma, and death
Stage 2—Cardiopulmonary system signs (often mild or absent in dogs and cats)
Tachypnea
Tachycardia
Stage 3—Renal system signs
Severe depression
Vomiting and diarrhea
Oliguria with isosthenuria
Azotemia or uremia

CLINICAL SIGNS

The clinical syndrome of ethylene glycol poisoning progresses through three stages (Table 1). The clinical signs and their severity are time and dose dependent. Stage 1, associated with central nervous system (CNS) disorders, occurs 30 minutes to 12 hours after ingestion. The clinical signs of this stage are similar to those of acute alcohol intoxication. Nausea and vomiting are common. Neurologic abnormalities can range from mild depression, ataxia, and knuckling to seizures, coma, and death. Severe polydipsia and polyuria occur within 1 hour of ingestion. As depression and ataxia progress, animals usually drink less; however, the polyuria continues, resulting in mild to moderate dehydration. Near the end of stage 1, the clinical signs may abate and animals may appear to have recovered.

Stage 2 takes place 12 to 24 hours after ingestion and involves the cardiopulmonary system. Tachypnea and tachycardia are the prominent clinical features in humans; however, these signs may be mild or absent in dogs and cats. It is common for the first two stages to go unnoticed by pet owners when the amount of ethylene glycol ingested is small or if vomiting has decreased the dose.

Stage 3 is the most commonly observed clinical stage of ethylene glycol poisoning. Characterized by oliguric renal failure, this stage occurs 24 to 72 hours after ingestion in dogs and 12 to 24 hours after ingestion in cats. Signs in both dogs and cats include severe depression, vomiting, diarrhea, azotemia, and minimal urine production. It is important to note that oliguric renal failure is not a characteristic feature of early ethylene glycol intoxication.

PATHOPHYSIOLOGY

Unmetabolized ethylene glycol has approximately the same toxicity as ethanol. CNS dysfunction may be mild or moderate, depending on the dose ingested. Serum hyperosmolality occurs because of the small molecular weight (62 daltons) of ethylene glycol and it stimulates thirst, causing primary polydipsia. Polyuria occurs secondary to the increased water intake and the osmotic diuretic effect of ethylene glycol in the proximal tubule. Urine output of 10 ml/kg/hour (approximately six times the normal urine output) has been observed in dogs within 3 hours of ingestion of commercial antifreeze at a dosage of 10 ml/kg body weight. Vomiting usually occurs soon after ingestion in dogs and cats as a result of gastric irritation or stimulation of the chemoreceptor trigger zone. Metabolites may also activate the emetic center by causing cerebral edema or vestibular dysfunction.

The metabolites of ethylene glycol play the major role in the pathophysiologic effects of the intoxication. Glycoaldehyde is thought to contribute to the CNS dysfunction of ethylene glycol poisoning, because aldehydes depress CNS respiration and serotonin metabolism and alter CNS amine concentrations. Glycoaldehyde does not accumulate in the plasma or tissues, however, because it is rapidly metabolized. The production of glycolate from glycoaldehyde results in a severe metabolic acidosis. This acidosis is partially responsible for the tachypnea and tachycardia observed in stage 2. Glycolate is thought to be the primary toxic metabolite of ethylene glycol. A direct correlation between urine glycolate concentrations and mortality has been observed in rats. Serum glycolate concentrations also correlate with CNS dysfunction. Glyoxalate is the most toxic metabolite on a per-weight basis; however, the half-life of glyoxalate is very short and the compound does not accumulate. Glyoxalate inhibits citric acid cycle enzymes and substrate level phosphorylation in mitochondria.

Oxalate is a highly cytotoxic compound that produces extensive renal damage and acidosis. The percentage of oxalate produced from metabolism of ethylene glycol varies between species. Cats produce relatively large amounts of oxalate, which probably accounts for their increased susceptibility to ethylene glycol poisoning. Oxalate combines with calcium in the bloodstream to form a soluble calcium oxalate complex, which is filtered by glomeruli. As water is reabsorbed by the tubules and the pH of the filtrate decreases, the calcium oxalate precipitates to form crystals within the lumen. These crystals are light yellow; they are arranged in rosettes, prisms, or sheaves and are birefringent when viewed with polarized light. An inflammatory response is not seen in cells adjacent to the crystals. The renal tubular epithelium in contact with the crystals may be normal or degenerative (Fig. 2). Calcium oxalate crystals may be involved in the pathogenesis of the renal damage; however, glycolate and oxalate are thought to play the major role.

Pulmonary edema, congestion, and hyperemia occur during stage 2 of ethylene glycol poisoning. Prolonged CNS depression, such as is possible in stage 1, can cause pulmonary edema and heart failure. The exact pathophysiologic characteristics of stage 2 are not clear, however, and the relationship to the metabolites of ethylene glycol has not been defined.

The kidney damage caused by ethylene glycol metabolites is primarily tubular. Degeneration and necrosis of tubular epithelium occur; however, the tubular basement membranes are usually left intact so that regeneration and repair may occur. Tubular destruction often occurs in the absence of calcium oxalate crystals. Dilated tubules filled with proteinaceous debris are commonly observed. Glomerular changes are usually absent. Severe renal edema accompanies the tubular damage and probably enhances the renal lesions by compromising intrarenal blood flow.

DIAGNOSIS

The nonspecific, multisystemic signs of acute ethylene glycol poisoning make diagnosis difficult. The symptoms of ethylene glycol intoxication can mimic acute gastroenteritis, pancreatitis, diabetic ketoacidosis, acute renal failure from other causes, and primary CNS disorders. In cases in which ingestion of the compound is not witnessed, diagnosis is based on history, clinical signs, and laboratory findings.

The history almost always reveals that the illness had an acute onset. Ataxia, depression, vomiting, polydipsia, and polyuria may be reported by the owner. Male dogs and cats younger than 3 years appear to have an increased incidence, perhaps because of increased inquisitiveness or roaming.

Physical examination findings in the early stages of intoxication include ataxia, depression, dehydration, and possibly tachycardia and tachypnea. Neurologic abnormalities often include knuckling, decreased withdrawal reflexes, and decreased righting ability. Abdominal palpation may be painful as a result of the renal swelling and edema. Hypothermia is occasionally present in animals that are depressed and housed outdoors. Oral ulcers and salivation secondary to uremia are often noted in animals that present in stage 3 of the intoxication. These animals are usually in good flesh and not anemic, helping to rule out chronic renal failure.

Laboratory findings are often the key to making the correct diagnosis. Hyperosmolality is present very early in the disease process. Normal serum osmolality for dogs and cats is 280 to 310 mOsm/kg. In dogs experimentally poisoned with ethylene glycol, serum osmolality was 440 mOsm/kg 3 hours after ingestion. Ethylene glycol ingestion also re-

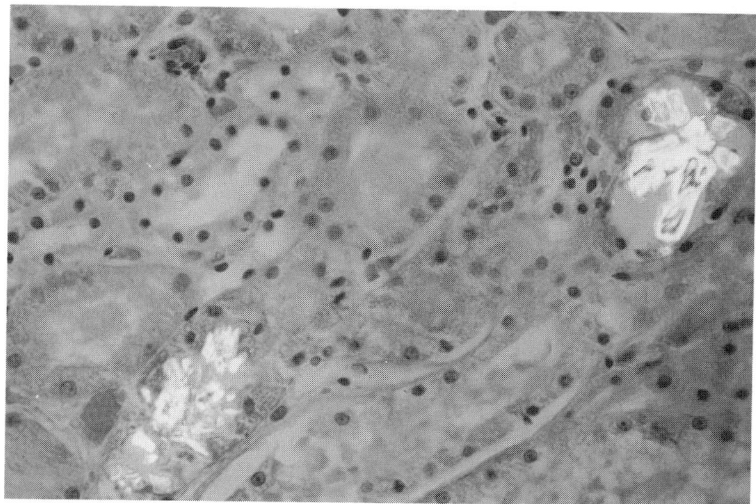

Figure 2. A photomicrograph of a kidney section demonstrating tubular epithelial damage and deposition of calcium oxalate crystals within the tubular lumen (× 400). This photograph was taken with a polarized light source.

sults in an increase in the osmolal gap, or the difference between measured and calculated serum osmolality. The following formula may be used to calculate serum osmolality:

$$\text{mOsm/kg} = 1.86\,(\text{Na} + \text{K}) + (\text{glucose}/18) + (\text{BUN}/2.8) + 9$$

The constant, 9, is added to adjust for unmeasured osmotically active particles in serum, such as phosphate, sulfate, calcium, magnesium, and creatinine. Ethylene glycol increases the osmolal gap significantly, inasmuch as its presence in the serum is not taken into account in the above formula. The normal osmolal gap for dogs and cats is less than 10 mOsm/kg. The average osmolal gap in the experimental dogs cited above was 134 mOsm/kg 3 hours after ingestion. Serum osmolality and the osmolal gap remain significantly elevated 12 hours after ingestion. Serum osmolality can also be used to estimate ethylene glycol serum concentrations by multiplying the osmolal gap by 6.2. For example, if the osmolal gap is 100 mOsm/kg, the predicted ethylene glycol serum level would be 620 mg/dl. Serum osmolality for dogs and cats can be quickly and inexpensively determined at most human hospitals or commercial laboratories either by determining freezing point depression or by vapor pressure osmometry. Many hospitals and commerical laboratories can also determine serum or urine ethylene glycol concentrations quickly enough to be diagnostically useful.

The urine specific gravity of dogs and cats decreases to less than 1.020 within 3 hours of ingestion and remains low throughout the course of the intoxication. Initially, the low specific gravity is due to primary polydipsia and osmotic diuresis; however, as metabolism of ethylene glycol progresses, the isosthenuria is due to renal failure. The inability to maximally concentrate urine in the face of dehydration and serum hyperosmolality demonstrates nephron dysfunction, and its finding warrants consideration of ethylene glycol poisoning. Later, approximately 48 hours after ingestion in dogs and 12 hours in cats, azotemia and hyperphosphatemia occur as a result of tubular damage and consequent decreased glomerular filtration.

Severe metabolic acidosis occurs within 3 hours of ingestion of ethylene glycol. Blood gas analysis reveals decreased blood pH and a base deficit. The P_{CO_2} is usually low as a result of partial respiratory compensation. Acidosis persists throughout the intoxication and is increased by the onset of renal failure. The acidosis is normochloremic, and there is a significant increase in the anion gap as early as 3 hours after ingestion. The anion gap is determined by the following formula:

$$\text{mEq/L} = (\text{Na} + \text{K}) - (\text{HCO}_3 + \text{Cl})$$

The normal anion gap for dogs and cats is 10 to 15 mEq/L. This normal gap is made up of phosphates, sulfates, and negatively charged proteins that are not included in the above equation. The production of glycolate, glyoxalate, and oxalate significantly increases the pool of unmeasured anions and causes the increased anion gap.

Calcium oxalate crystalluria is an important diagnostic finding. These crystals can be seen in the urine of normal dogs and cats; however, their appearance should always arouse suspicion of ethylene glycol poisoning. Calcium oxalate monohydrate crystals are observed most frequently. Monohydrate calcium oxalate can take several forms; most common are six-sided prisms that are morphologically identical to published diagrams of hippuric acid crystals (Fig. 3). Other forms are shaped like hemp seeds or dumbbells (Fig. 4). Calcium oxalate dihydrate crystals (envelope or Maltese-cross forms) (Fig. 5), although more commonly referred to in standard texts on urinalysis, are less frequently

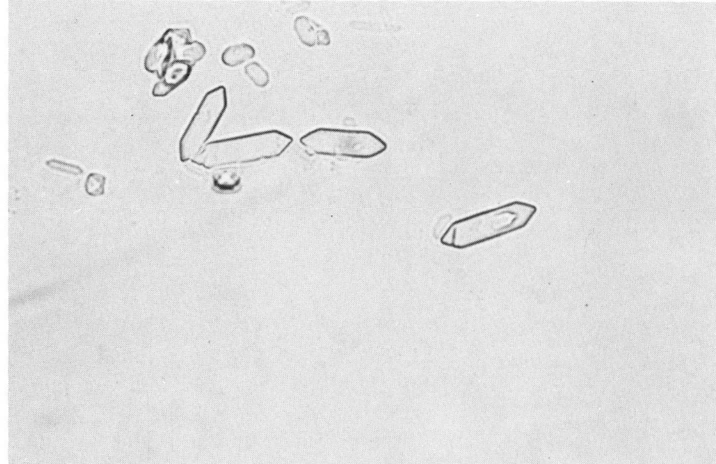

Figure 3. A photomicrograph of monohydrate calcium oxalate crystals in urine sediment (× 400).

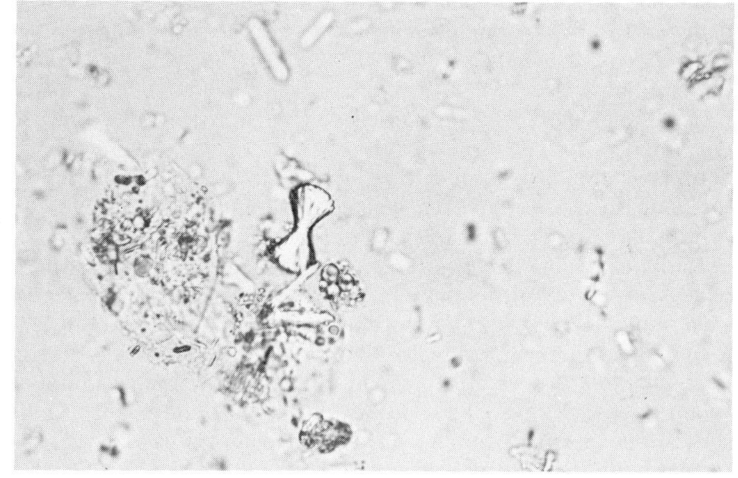

Figure 4. A photomicrograph of dumbbell-shaped calcium oxalate crystals in urine sediment (× 400).

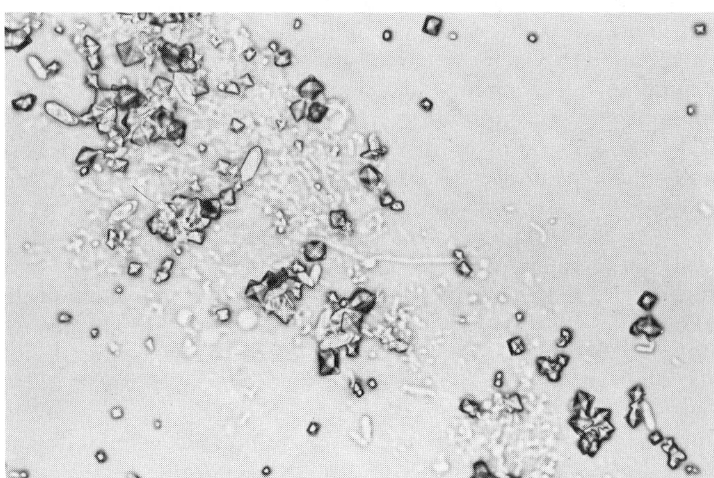

Figure 5. A photomicrograph of urine sediment containing both dihydrate (envelope-shaped) and monohydrate calcium oxalate crystals (× 250).

observed. Both the monohydrate and dihydrate forms are birefringent when viewed with polarized light. Calcium oxalate crystalluria has been observed as early as 5 hours after ingestion in dogs and 3 hours in cats.

Early after ingestion, the urine pH is usually less than 6.5, reflecting the metabolic acidosis. Proteinuria may occur after the onset of tubular damage. Glucosuria is sometimes encountered, either as a result of hyperglycemia or tubular damage. As the renal damage progresses, red and white blood cells, renal epithelial cells, and granular and cellular casts are often seen in the urine sediment.

Other laboratory findings that may be observed in dogs and cats poisoned by ethylene glycol include stress leukograms, hypocalcemia, hyperglycemia, and hyperphosphatemia. Neutrophilia and lymphopenia are probably due to endogenous corticosteroid release secondary to CNS depression, vomiting, and metabolic acidosis. Hypocalcemia is attributable to the precipitation of calcium by oxalate. Clinical signs of hypocalcemia are infrequently observed because of the protective effects of acidosis on ionized calcium concentrations. Hyperglycemia may be the result of inhibition of glycolysis and the Kreb's cycle by aldehydes. Epinephrine, increased endogenous corticosteroids, uremia, and hypocalcemia may also contribute to hyperglycemia. Hypocalcemia can contribute to hyperglycemia by preventing normal insulin release. The hyperglycemia, if of sufficient magnitude, may result in glucosuria before the onset of renal tubular damage. Hyperphosphatemia in dogs (approximately 6.0 mg/dl) has been noted within 1 to 3 hours of ingestion of a commercial antifreeze solution. This was attributed to ingestion of a phosphate rust inhibitor contained in the solution. Phosphorus levels in these dogs slowly returned to normal before the onset of renal azotemia.

TREATMENT

Therapy for ethylene glycol poisoning is aimed at preventing absorption, increasing excretion, and preventing metabolism of the compound. Supportive care to correct fluid, acid-base, and electrolyte imbalances is also necessary. If ingestion of antifreeze is witnessed, vomiting should be induced, unless the animal is severely depressed and there is danger of aspiration. Gastric lavage with activated charcoal is indicated within 1 to 2 hours of ingestion; beyond this time, the procedure is of little benefit.

Intravenous isotonic fluid therapy should be started immediately to correct dehydration. Volume replacement and increased tissue perfusion will also help correct the metabolic acidosis and promote diuresis. The fluid volume administered should be based on the maintenance, deficit, and continuing loss needs of the patient. Overhydration can cause pulmonary edema in animals with oliguric renal failure. Measurement of urine output and central venous pressure is helpful in monitoring fluid therapy. Renal clearance of ethylene glycol varies inversely with tubular water reabsorption; therefore, hydration and diuresis should be maintained during therapy.

Specific therapy to stop the metabolism of ethylene glycol by liver alcohol dehydrogenease is the cornerstone of treatment. In 1965, ethanol was first used as a competitive inhibitor of ethylene glycol in humans. Since ethanol is a better substrate for the enzyme, the metabolism of ethylene glycol is inhibited. Twenty per cent ethanol is administered IV, and a high blood level of approximately 100 mg/dl is maintained until the intact ethylene glycol has been excreted by the kidneys (48 to 72 hours). Therapy with ethanol is usually 100 per cent successful if initiated within 1 hour of ingestion; however, by 4 hours, enough of the ethylene glycol has been metabolized to cause acidosis and cytotoxicity, rendering ethanol therapy much less effective. The suggested dose for dogs is 5.5 ml of 20 per cent ethanol/kg body weight given IV every 4 hours for five treatments and then every 6 hours for four more treatments. The dose for cats is lower: 5 ml of 20 per cent ethanol/kg body weight given IV every 6 hours for five treatments and then every 8 hours for four more treatments. The IV administration of 20 per cent ethanol has several disadvantages. It adds to the CNS depression that is already a feature of the intoxication. Many animals will become comatose during the therapy, complicating their management. Ethanol also enhances the diuresis initiated by ethylene glycol, thereby increasing fluid therapy requirements. Pulmonary edema is common in these comatose patients receiving large volumes of fluid. Finally, ethanol is metabolized rapidly, necessitating frequent treatment with large volumes for 40 to 56 hours.

4-Methylpyrazole, an inhibitor of alcohol dehydrogenase, has been used with excellent results in dogs with experimental ethylene glycol poisoning.* This compound forms an inactive complex with liver alcohol dehydrogenase and nicotinamide adenine dinucleotide by occupying the ethanol binding sites of the enzyme system. Unlike the parent compound pyrazole, 4-methylpyrazole has been associated with no toxic side effects in normal dogs or dogs poisoned with ethylene glycol. 4-Methylpyrazole does not contribute to CNS or to renal concentrating disorders. Treatment with 4-methylpyrazole has been

*Five grams of 4-methylpyrazole (free base, available from Aldrich Chemical Co.) is added to 50 ml of polyethylene glycol (400) and 46 ml of bacteriostatic water to make 100 ml of a 5 per cent solution. This solution should be filtered with a 0.22-μm filter before use.

successful in dogs 8 hours after ingestion of 10 ml of antifreeze/kg body weight. In dogs, the recommended dose of 5 per cent 4-methylpyrazole is 20 mg/kg body weight IV initially, followed by 15 mg/kg IV at 12 and 24 hours, and 5 mg/kg IV 36 hours after the first dose. Treatment of cats with 4-methylpyrazole cannot be recommended at this time because of insufficient data.

In experimental studies, correction of the metabolic acidosis associated with ingestion of ethylene glycol, without any further treatment, significantly increased the recovery rate. If possible, the dose of sodium bicarbonate should be based on serial plasma bicarbonate concentrations using the following formula:

$$\text{Bicarbonate deficit} = 0.5 \times \text{body weight in kg} \times (24 - \text{plasma bicarbonate})$$

For example, a 15-kg (33-lb) dog with a measured plasma bicarbonate of 10 mEq/L would need $0.5 \times 15 \times (24 - 10)$, or 105 mEq of bicarbonate to replace its deficit. Of this, 80 per cent should be administered slowly IV to prevent an overdose. Plasma bicarbonate levels should be monitored every 4 to 6 hours. We have found average bicarbonate levels of 18 mEq/L and 8 mEq/L in experimentally poisoned dogs at 3 and 12 hours after ingestion, respectively. Monitoring the urine pH in response to therapy may also be helpful. It is desirable to maintain the urine pH above 7.0 to 7.5.

In patients that present beyond 24 hours after ingestion or in oliguric renal failure, treatment with ethanol or 4-methylpyrazole is not indicated. Fluid, electrolyte, and acid-base disorders in these patients should be corrected. Establishment of a diuresis, as in any case of acute renal failure, is desirable. Diuretics, especially mannitol, may be beneficial for inducing a diuresis and decreasing renal edema. Diuretics should only be used in patients that are well hydrated.

The tubular damage of ethylene glycol intoxication may be reversible; however, supportive care must maintain the patient during the period of renal regeneration and compensation. Peritoneal dialysis may be useful in this situation.

References and Supplemental Reading

Beasley, V. R., and Buck, W. B.: Acute ethylene glycol toxicosis: A review. Vet. Hum. Toxicol. 22:255, 1980.

Grauer, G. F., and Thrall, M. A.: Ethylene glycol (antifreeze) poisoning in the dog and cat. J. Am. Anim. Hosp. Assoc. 18:492, 1982.

Grauer, G. F., Thrall, M. A., Henre, B. A., et al.: Early clinicopathologic findings in dogs ingesting ethylene glycol. Am. J. Vet. Res. 45:2299, 1984.

Grauer, G. F., Thrall, M. A. Henre, B. A., et al.: Effect of alcohol dehydrogenase inhibitors on the toxicity and pharmacokinetics of ethylene glycol in the dog. Fund. Appl. Toxicol., submitted.

Mueller, D. H.: Epidemiologic considerations of ethylene glycol intoxication in small animals. Vet. Hum. Toxicol. 24:21, 1982.

Oehme, F. W.: Antifreeze (ethylene glycol) poisoning. *In* Kirk, R. W. (ed.): *Current Veterinary Therapy VIII*. Philadelphia: W. B. Saunders, 1983, pp. 114–116.

Thrall, M. A., Grauer, G. F., and Mero, K. N.: Clinicopathologic findings in dogs and cats with ethylene glycol intoxication. J.A.V.M.A. 184:37, 1984.

Thrall, M. A., Grauer, G. F., Mero, K. N., et al.: Ethanol, 1,3-butanediol, pyrazole, and 4-methylpyrazole therapy in dogs with experimental ethylene glycol intoxication. Am. J. Vet. Res., submitted.

Thrall, M. A., Winder, D., and Dial, S. M.: Identification of calcium oxalate monohydrate crystals by X-ray diffraction in urine of ethylene glycol intoxicated dogs. Vet. Pathol., in press.

HYPERTONIC SODIUM PHOSPHATE ENEMA INTOXICATION

CLARKE E. ATKINS, D.V.M.

Madison, Wisconsin

The hypertonic sodium phosphate or Fleet-type (Fleet, Gent-L-Tip) enema (HSPE) has enjoyed increasing popularity as a bowel evacuant prior to radiographic and proctoscopic procedures and as a treatment for constipation. The HSPE can produce serious clinical, biochemical, and acid-base disturbances if used incorrectly—especially in debilitated, very small, or obstipated patients. Clinical intoxi cations have been observed in children, cats, and small dogs.

HSPEs typically contain sodium biphosphate and sodium phosphate equivalent to 2178 mEq sodium and 1756 mEq phosphorus per liter and are packaged in both adult (4-oz) and pediatric (2-oz) dosages in disposable squeeze bottles. There is currently no HSPE marketed specifically for veterinary medicine; however, such products are readily available as over-the-counter preparations for use in the home or in the veterinary clinic. Past recommendations for use in small animal patients have been as follows: mature small animals 25 lb or more, 4 fl oz; smaller animals, 2 to 4 fl oz as directed by the veterinarian. Clinical and experimental evidence suggests that these doses are unsafe in some individuals.

PATHOPHYSIOLOGY

HSPE intoxication, which is in essence sodium and phosphate poisoning, occurs when there is prolonged enema retention, overdosage, colonic dilatation or ulceration, or pre-existing fluid and electrolyte disturbances such as might be seen in renal failure. With large doses, transcolonic fluid transudation into the hypertonic colon can produce hypovolemia and signs of shock. Signs generally are related to electrolyte and acid-base imbalances produced by massive absorption of sodium and phosphate from the colon. The resultant hypernatremia, hyperphosphatemia, hyperosmolality, and hypertonicity are associated with neuromuscular dysfunction. Rapid-onset hypertonicity results in potentially fatal brain shrinkage as intracellular fluid equilibrates with extracellular fluid.

Hypocalcemia and hypomagnesemia secondary to hyperphosphatemia aggravate central nervous system signs, producing tetany and convulsions. Hyperglycemia has been observed in HSPE intoxication in cats and is due to hypertonicity and stress-related catecholamine release, causing diminished pancreatic insulin release and insulin resistance. Hyperglycemia contributes only modestly to the existing hyperosmolality but may promote dehydration via osmotic diuresis. Hypokalemia occasionally results from exchange with colonic sodium or from urinary potassium loss as a cation accompanying excreted phosphate. Significant high-anion-gap metabolic acidosis has been consistent in HSPE intoxication and is due, at least in part, to lactic acid accumulation.

CLINICAL SIGNS

Clinical signs appear rapidly, usually within 30 to 60 minutes of enema administration, but may be delayed depending on dosage, duration of retention, and patient status. Affected animals (most often cats) are somnolent, ataxic, and frequently exhibit tetany or convulsions. Clinically detectable dehydration is not a feature of HSPE intoxication unless present prior to enema administration. Tachycardia, weak pulse, hypothermia, and ashen mucous membranes are noted in some individuals. Vomiting and, less frequently, bloody diarrhea may also be observed. Death has occurred as a result of HSPE intoxication in debilitated cats as well as in one apparently normal experimental cat.

LABORATORY ABNORMALITIES

Hyperglycemia, hyperosmolality, and moderate to severe metabolic acidosis are consistently observed. Hyperglycemia may be extreme (more than 400 mg/dl) and hyperosmolality reaches dangerous levels (more than 340 mOsm/L) in 25 per cent of intoxicated cats. Sixty to 90 per cent of cases suffer hypocalcemia (4.9 mg/dl in one clinical case), mild to moderate hypokalemia, hypernatremia (more than 170 mEq/L in one instance), and moderate to extreme hyperphosphatemia (as much as 60 mEq/L) (Atkins et al., 1984; Schaer et al., 1977). Most important of these abnormalities are hyperosmolality, hypocalcemia, and metabolic acidosis.

Laboratory abnormalities are most extreme 15 minutes to 4 hours after administration and usually return to baseline levels by 24 hours (Fig. 1 and Table 1). It is emphasized that pre-existing conditions or intervening therapies will affect not only

Table 1. *Maximum Deviation from Mean Laboratory Values, Times of Occurrence, and the Durations of These Abnormalities in Experimentally HSPE-Intoxicated Cats Given the High Recommended Dosage (32 ml/kg)*

	Serum Lactate	Plasma Bicarbonate	Serum Sodium	Serum Phosphorus	Calculated Serum Osmolality	Serum Calcium	Serum Potassium	Serum Glucose
Maximum deviation from mean laboratory value	58 mg/dl	13.3 mEq/L	157 mEq/L	15.6 mg/dl	318 mOsm/L	7.3 mg/dl	3.6 mEq/L	204 mg/dl
Time of occurrence after enema administration	15 minutes	15 minutes	30 minutes	30 minutes	30 minutes	45 minutes	60 minutes	4 hours
Time baseline values reattained without treatment	24 hours	24 hours	>24 hours	24 hours	24 hours	24 hours	>24 hours	24 hours
Normal values	(11–14 mg/dl)	(17–24 mEq/L)	(142–155 mEq/L)	(4.5–8.1 mg/dl)	(280–310 mOsm/L)	(7.0–10.2 mg/dl)	(4.0–4.5 mEq/L)	(70–110 mg/dl)

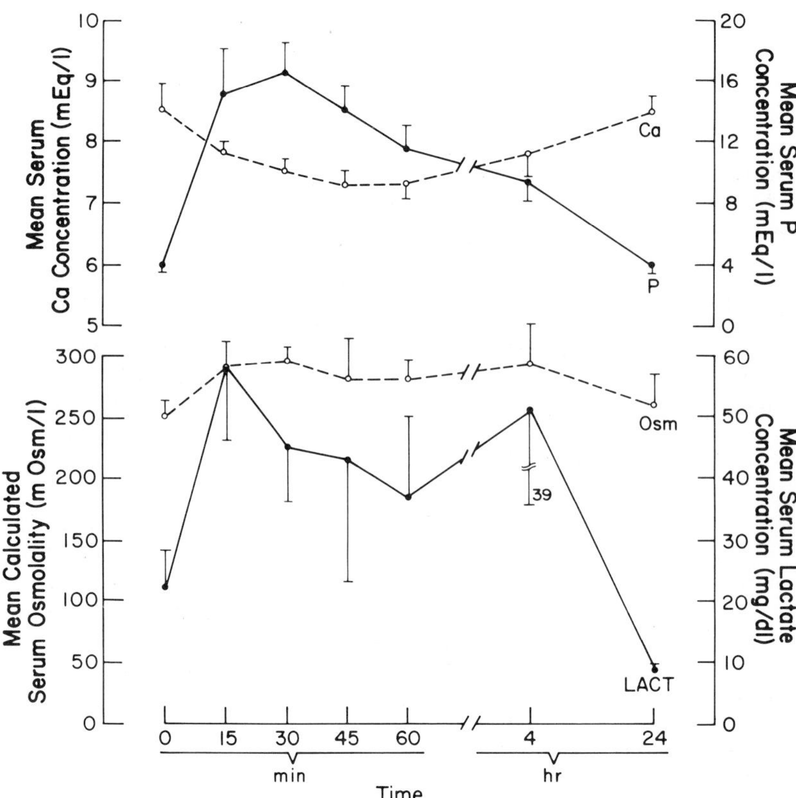

Figure 1. Selected mean (± SEM) laboratory abnormalities associated with high-dose (32 ml/kg) hypertonic sodium phosphate enema given to normal cats.

laboratory values determined on presentation but the duration of such abnormalities as well.

THERAPY

Therapy is complex and is best based on knowledge of the laboratory abnormalities present in the individual patient. However, even without laboratory data, valuable information can be obtained clinically. Blood urea nitrogen (BUN) and blood glucose concentration can be determined with reagent strips; hypokalemia and hypocalcemia may be present if the electrocardiogram (ECG) Q-T interval is greater than 0.16 seconds in cats or greater than 0.22 seconds in dogs. Osmolality can be calculated with minimal laboratory-measured values according to the following formula:

$$\text{Osm} = 1.86\,(\text{Na} + \text{K}) + \frac{\text{blood glucose}}{18} + \frac{\text{BUN}}{2.8}$$

Acid-base status can be assessed by measurement of total serum carbon dioxide. In lieu of these modest measurements, one should assume hypernatremia, hyperphosphatemia, hypocalcemia, hyperglycemia, hyperosmolality, metabolic acidosis, and diminished tissue perfusion. Additionally, hypokalemia, hypomagnesemia, and dehydration with cardiovascular volume contraction may complicate some cases. A therapeutic overview is presented in Table 2.

If tetany exists, 10 per cent calcium gluconate (at approximately 0.5 to 1.5 ml/kg body weight) should be administered slowly IV to effect with continuous ECG monitoring. (Bradycardia or Q-T interval shortening indicates a need to slow or stop infusion.) If the response is poor, magnesium sulfate or anticonvulsant therapy may ameliorate signs of neuromuscular irritability. If calcium therapy has been necessary, subsequent fluids, administered after the cessation of tetany, should contain calcium (7 to 10 mEq/L).

***Table 2.** Overview for Therapy of HSPE Intoxication*

1. Obtain results from blood tests (serum Na, Cl, K, P, Ca, BUN, CO_2, glucose) and electrocardiogram as baseline data *prior* to therapy if clinically appropriate. Assure adequate renal function.
2. Treat tetany or convulsions with calcium gluconate IV.
3. Treat volume contraction and shock, if present, rapidly with 5 per cent dextrose IV, using half the calculated deficit. KCl and Ca gluconate should be added.
4. The rest of the deficit and maintenance fluids can be replaced gradually over 24 to 72 hours as oral water with KCl and Ca gluconate or as 5 per cent dextrose in water IV with KCl and Ca gluconate.

Acidosis, unless very severe (pH less than 7.1, HCO_3 less than 8 to 10 mEq/L in cats), should not be treated with sodium bicarbonate, as this drug is extremely hypertonic. In addition, bicarbonate therapy may aggravate hypokalemia, lactic acidosis, and signs of hypocalcemia; may dimish tissue oxygenation by increasing hemoglobin-oxygen affinity; and may produce rebound metabolic alkalosis, cardiac dysrhythmias, and paradoxical cerebrospinal fluid acidosis. It is suggested that if bicarbonate therapy is necessary, it should be discontinued when the plasma pH reaches 7.2.

The amount of fluid needed to correct hypernatremia can be calculated from the following formula:

$$\text{Fluid deficit in liters} = 0.6 \times \text{kg body weight} \times \left\{\frac{\text{current [Na]}}{\text{normal [Na]}} - 1\right\}$$

if utilized early after HSPE intoxication prior to renal sodium and water loss (Feig, 1981). If laboratory determinations are not available or are delayed, serum sodium should be assumed to be 160 mEq/L. Fluid replacement will help to correct hypernatremia, hyperphosphatemia, acidosis, and hyperglycemia by dilution and increased renal perfusion. Fluid replacement in hypertonic states should be gradual to prevent the development of cerebral edema, unless there are signs of severe volume depletion. Ideally, in these instances, a hypotonic fluid would be administered; however, IV administration of such a fluid may produce localized hemolysis. Instead, in the case of concomitant volume depletion and vascular collapse, IV fluid therapy is indicated using 5 per cent dextrose in water with added potassium chloride (KCl 4 to 5 mEq/L) and calcium gluconate (7 to 10 mEq/L), with initial fluid administration totalling half the calculated deficit or until signs of shock have abated. Insulin therapy for hyperglycemia should be avoided, as rapid reduction in plasma osmolality can produce central nervous system dysfunction secondary to cerebral edema. Edema may occur if the duration of the hyperosmolal state has been long enough (hours to days) to allow the development of "idiogenic osmols," which protect the brain from becoming dehydrated at these times but can cause cerebral edema if serum hyperosmolality is too rapidly corrected by dilution or insulin therapy. During therapy, if improvement in neurologic status is followed by deterioration, the presence of cerebral edema should be assumed. Therapy with mannitol may be necessary. Once vascular collapse has been corrected, the remainder of the calculated fluid deficit, as well as maintenance fluids, should be administered, usually IV, over 24 to 72 hours.

If the animal is not vomiting and can drink or can be safely intubated, oral water with calcium gluconate and KCl added would appear to be the fluid of choice. If oral administration is impossible, an alternative is the use of hypotonic enemas (tap water with KCl and calcium gluconate), which have been successfully employed to treat hypertonicity in humans. The stimulation of insulin release, increase in renal perfusion, correction of acidosis, and dilution of plasma electrolytes will all reduce plasma potassium concentrations, hence KCl should be added to the administered fluid regardless of the route unless anuria or oliguria is present. If medicaments can be administered orally, potassium can be supplemented as KCl tablets or mixed with water at approximately 200 mg daily for cats. Intravenous potassium supplementation is best done cautiously (at a rate no greater than 0.5 mEq/kg/hour) and with knowledge of serum potassium concentration. When rapid volume repletion is not necessary or has been achieved and when hypokalemia is mild, as it typically is in HSPE intoxication, 15 to 20 mEq KCl/L is advisable. Higher concentrations are employed if serum potassium levels are markedly low. Frequent monitoring of serum potassium concentration prior to and during therapy is ideal; if this is impossible, periodic ECG monitoring is useful. In hypokalemia, ST segment changes, depressed T wave amplitude, Q-T prolongation, and less commonly increases in QRS amplitude and duration are noted. Hyperkalemia is typified by peaking of the T wave, shortening of the Q-T interval, and ST segment changes, as well as prolongation of the durations of the P wave, P-R interval, and QRS interval. It is emphasized that complex electrolyte alterations may confuse the issue, as hypocalcemia, which may also be present, produces prolonged S-T and Q-T intervals and tall R waves (Feldman, 1980).

The presence of concurrent renal failure obviously complicates the situation, worsening the prognosis. Peritoneal dialysis may be indicated in such situations. Potassium therapy is inadvisable in the oliguric or anuric patient if measured serum potassium concentrations are unavailable. It is generally not necessary to treat hyperphosphatemia specifically, although this abnormality may be severe and protracted in patients suffering renal failure. Aluminum hydroxide given orally to bind intestinal phosphates, a low-phosphorus diet, and peritoneal dialysis are therapeutic options in such circumstances.

References and Supplemental Reading

Agus, Z. S., and Goldfarb, S.: Clinical disorders of calcium and phosphate. Med. Clin. North Am. 65:385, 1981.

Atkins, C. E., Tyler, R., and Greenlee, P.: Clinical, biochemical acid-base and electrolyte abnormalities following hypertonic sodium phosphate enema administration to normal cats. Am. J. Vet. Res. 46:980, 1985.

Edwards, D. F., Richardson, D. C., and Russell, R. G.: Hypernatremic,

hypertonic dehydration in a dog with diabetes insipidus and gastric dilatation-volvulus. J.A.V.M.A. 182:973, 1983.
Feig, P. U.: Hypernatremia and hypertonic syndromes. Med. Clin. North Am. 65:271, 1981.
Feldman, E. C.: Influence of non-cardiac disease on the heart. *In* Kirk, R. W. (ed.): *Current Veterinary Therapy VII*. Philadelphia: W. B. Saunders, 1980, pp. 340–347.
Haskins, S. C.: Fluid and electrolyte therapy. Comp. Cont. Ed. Pract. Vet.6:244, 1984.
Schaer, M., Cavanaugh, P., Hause, W., et al.: Iatrogenic hyperphosphatemia, hypocalcemia, and hypernatremia in a cat. J. Am. Anim. Hosp. Assoc. 13:39, 1977.

ORNAMENTAL TOXIC PLANTS

LAWRENCE P. RUHR, D.V.M.
Baton Rouge, Louisiana

Poisoning or injury by plants is a potential problem in small animal practice at all times of the year and in all regions of the country. Many of our favorite yard, garden, and household plants are capable of producing illness or death in companion animals. Effects may be minor, such as nausea and vomiting associated with the consumption of lawn grasses in dogs, or death may occur within a few hours of the ingestion of such highly toxic plants as yew and oleander. In most instances, ingestion of the plant is required for poisoning to occur, but some plants produce irritation of the skin or mucous membranes, mechanical injuries, or allergic phenomena without ingestion.

This review will discuss those factors that make a companion animal more likely to experience a plant poisoning, the body systems that are most often affected, the approach to forming a diagnosis, and the treatment of poisoning or injury by plants. A tabular listing of many toxic ornamental plants that the small animal practitioner may encounter is included as a quick reference.

FACTORS INFLUENCING PLANT POISONINGS

Several factors should be considered when evaluating the potential for a plant poisoning. Among these are the individual animal's past history of eating or chewing plants, the age of the animal, other activities or boredom, a change of surroundings, and the normal dietary habits of the pet and owner. Also, factors related to the plant such as its identity, the part consumed, and the amount should all be considered.

Some pets are known by their owners to chew or eat many things, including plants. These animals are more likely to experience poisoning or injury than are animals that have no prior history of this behavior. However, it should be noted that behavioral changes do occur, and other factors may induce this type of activity.

Younger animals with their great curiosity and teething are, much as children, more likely to mouth or ingest poisonous plants than are adult animals. A significant number of pets that ingest poisonous plants are in their first 2 years of life. Clinicians should advise pet owners to "petproof" their home by limiting access to toxic plants.

The activity level that the pet normally maintains can be important in determining access to potentially toxic plants. Additionally, when the activity level is suddenly decreased, the animal may become bored. A bored animal is more likely to investigate and consume plants that had previously been ignored. Confinement to a restricted area of the house or yard is often the prelude to a poisoning.

Much as an area restriction may produce increased interest in familiar plants, moving the pet to new surroundings often is followed by a plant poisoning. When a pet is moved, the new area is investigated by the pet, and the plantings will certainly be of interest. When coupled with the "neurotic" behavior many companion animals exhibit during the stress of a move, the potential for plant poisoning is increased. Although this is most evident with major cross-country moves, some animals respond to as minor a change as moving from one pen to another or the introduction of a single new plant into familiar surroundings.

A final animal factor that contributes to the potential for plant poisonings is the dietary habits of both the pet and the owner. If an animal is a forager or garbage eater, the chances of plant consumption increase. If table or kitchen scraps are fed by the owner, plant material will be more acceptable to the animal. In both of these cases, the potential for plant poisoning is much greater.

When evaluating a potential plant poisoning, it is important to consider several factors related to the plant itself. The first and most obvious is the type of plant. Identifying the plant can be challenging, especially with the numerous horticultural varieties. Help in identification can be sought from county agents, college botany or horticulture departments, toxicologists, florists, and nursery personnel. Many trade books are available with color pictures of flowers and foliage plants. These are recommended for every practice as an aid in identifying ornamental plants. It must be recognized that a solid identification may not be assured, but an interim identification that allows rational decision-making is useful. Samples of the plant, including flowers, fruits, and leaves, should be retained for later identification by pressing and drying or by refrigeration for as long as a week in a closed plastic bag. One problem with identification is the use of common names. Many plants share a common name with one or more taxonomically divergent plants. This can be confusing. Japanese yew *(Taxus* sp.*)* is a highly toxic plant that superficially resembles another plant, *Podocarpus* sp. *Podocarpus* is called Japanese yew in the southern United States and produces only mild gastroenteritis, if any disease. A second problem with common names is the multitude of names that a single plant may have. In many instances, the names are regional, and considerable confusion can result. When possible, the clinician should always attempt to identify the plant by its binomial or scientific nomenclature.

The part of the plant that was ingested is an important consideration. This is well illustrated with several edible plants. Rhubarb is a toxic plant if the leaf blade is consumed, but the petiole is used in pies and other foods. Potato and tomato are two common garden plants that can produce severe gastroenteritis if their foliage is consumed, but the tuber or fruit is a common part of our diets.

Consumption of the plant should be confirmed. The amount of the plant consumed is important, as with any toxicant. Morning glory seeds are relatively small, and seeds missing from a packet could be easily lost rather than consumed. Also, a number of seeds must be consumed and well chewed for a toxic response to be observed even in a small animal, and the ingestion of one or two seeds may not be significant.

One last consideration must be addressed. Much of the information concerning poisonous plants is anecdotal or is based on limited original observations and few reported details other than exposure to a plant and signs in a given body system. Once incorporated into the poisonous plant literature, a plant tends to remain implicated. This may be despite experimental evidence that refutes the original report. Two common ornamentals, philodendron and poinsettia, are in this category of commonly recognized poisonous plants that in all probability do not represent a hazard. In this review and in most other texts, no serious effort has been made to eliminate these reports.

SYSTEMS AFFECTED BY POISONOUS PLANTS

All body systems can be affected by poisonous plants. Many plants affect more than one body system, and the effects observed may vary over the course of the disease. The most commonly affected systems are briefly discussed here. When exposure to a specific plant is encountered, references or resource people should be consulted for more detailed information.

The tables listing plants that affect the different systems in this review are adapted in large part from Clay (1977) and Kunkel (1983). The lists are not exhaustive. Ornamental plants that are often encountered have been included. There are known toxic ornamentals that have not been included. There are also many toxic plants that are as yet unrecognized. With the exception of nettles and some mechanically injurious plants, plants of waste and wild areas and agricultural plants have not been listed. When a possible plant poisoning occurs in a free-roaming pet or a hunting dog, other references should also be consulted. Plants poisonous to farm animals must then be considered and extrapolations made.

The gastrointestinal system is, without question, the system most often affected by plant ingestion. Nonspecific gastroenteritis should always be evaluated with the ingestion of plant materials in mind; it may be due to indigestion, irritation of the gastric mucosa, or highly specific, well-described poisonous principles. Lawn grasses and many other plants that are not part of an animal's normal diet can produce indigestion or simple mechanical irritation of the gastric mucosa. Many spring bulbs such as amaryllis and daffodil or rhizomes such as iris are able to produce salivation, nausea, abdominal pain, vomiting, and diarrhea. Common shrubs or hedges, such as privet, euonymus, holly, box, azalea, and yew are known to produce gastroenteritis. Some such as yew *(Taxus* sp.*)* have other toxic activities that may be even more life-threatening. Table 1 lists by common and scientific name a number of the most widely recognized plants that produce gastroenteritis.

The cardiovascular system is affected by some of the most potent plant toxicants. Foxglove (digitalis), lily of the valley, monkshood, and larkspur all produce bradycardia and arrhythmias. Each is also capable of producing nausea. Table 2 lists some

Table 1. *Plants with Gastrointestinal Effects*

Common Name	Scientific Name	Comments
ALKALOIDS		
Amaryllis	*Amaryllis* sp.	Acute gastric effects with nausea and vomiting.
Daffodil	*Narcissus* sp.	
Hyacinth	*Hyacinthus orientalis,*	
Mushrooms	Many species	
Wisteria	*Wisteria* sp.	
SAPONINS		
English ivy	*Hedera helix*	Acute nausea with vomiting, abdominal pain, and diarrhea.
Buckeye, horse chestnut	*Aesculus* sp.	
Mock orange	*Poncirus* sp.	
Rain tree (monkey pod)	*Samonia samon*	
MISCELLANEOUS PRINCIPLES		
Daphne	*Daphne* sp.	Immediate nausea and vomiting.
Iris, flag	Iris sp.	
Four-o'clock	*Mirabilis jalapa*	
Lords and ladies	*Arum* sp.	
Azalea, rhododendron	*Rhododendron* sp.	Nausea, vomiting, abdominal pain, and diarrhea.
Bird of paradise	*Casesalpinia* sp.	
Common box	*Buxus sempervirens*	
Euonymus	*Euonymus* sp.	
Holly	*Ilex* sp.	
Honeysuckle	*Lonicera* sp.	
Mushrooms	*Amanita* sp.	
Mistletoe	*Phoradendron* sp.	
Privet	*Ligustrum* sp.	
Spurges	*Euphorbia* sp.	
Yellow allamdanda	*Allamanda cathartica*	
Yew	*Taxus* sp.	*Taxus* sp. is highly toxic with cardiovascular collapse and gastroenteritis.
	Podocarpus sp.	*Podocarpus* sp. is only minimally toxic, producing mild gastroenteritis.
TOXALBUMINS		
Black locust	*Robinia pseudoacacia*	Delayed vomiting, abdominal pain, diarrhea with depression or coma.
Castor bean	*Ricinus communis*	
Sandbox tree, monkey pistol	*Hura crepitans*	
SOLANINE GLYCOALKALOIDS		
Ground-cherry	*Physalis* sp.	Delayed vomiting, abdominal pain, diarrhea.
Jasmine	*Cestrum* sp.	
Nightshades	*Solanum* sp.	
Bittersweet, eggplant, Jerusalem cherry, potato		

Table 2. *Plants with Cardiovascular Effects*

Common Name	Scientific Name	Comments
CARDIAC GLYCOSIDES		
Foxglove	*Digitalis purpurea*	Acute nausea and vomiting, bradycardia, and arrhythmias.
Lily of the valley	*Convallaria majalis*	
Oleander	*Nerium* sp.	
Yellow oleander	*Thevetia peruviana*	
ALKALOIDS		
Aconite, monkshood	*Aconitum* sp.	Acute nausea, bradycardia, and arrythmias with collapse.
Larkspur	*Delphinium* sp.	
Yew	*Taxus* sp.	

plants that affect the heart and that companion animals may encounter.

The nervous system is affected by a wide variety of plants in many different ways. Marijuana and morning glory contain hallucinogens. The chinaberry tree produces convulsions. Nightshades, jasmine, and datura all contain atropine or similar compounds. Cyanogenic plants such as hydrangea and the pitted fruits may produce cyanide poisoning. Table 3 is a listing of toxic plants that can cause notable nervous system signs.

Plants may also produce irritation or mechanical injury when pet animals come in contact with them. A number of arums, including dumb cane, caladium, and jack-in-the-pulpit, have insoluble oxalate crystals that can produce significant oral, pharyngeal, and esophageal irritation accompanied by salivation and edema. Several of the nettles produce irritation of the skin or mucous membranes when bioactive amines are literally injected via the hollow hairs on the surface of the plant. These plants often cause a collapse that is more appropriately considered neurologic. Other plants have sharp projections, awns, spines, or thorns that produce mechanical injury. These foreign bodies may migrate a significant distance from the point of entry. Plants producing irritation or mechanical injury are listed in Table 4.

One last group, which is not often a problem in veterinary medicine but is a source of client concern, produces sensitization or allergic reactions. Poison ivy rarely produces clinical problems in pets but may be carried on the fur to a susceptible owner. Other plants also may produce a sensitization reaction in susceptible individuals. Ocular and respiratory irritation from plants that produce hay fever is also occasionally reported in domestic animals. No listing is included for these types of plants because of their low degree of hazard for small companion animals.

DIAGNOSIS AND TREATMENT

Diagnosis of poisoning by plants is often the result of an owner's observation or the recognition of plant materials following gastric evacuation. When the owner comes home to discover a chewed houseplant or actually witnesses the ingestion, the clinician is presented with the need to identify the plant and the amount consumed in order to establish a proper diagnosis. The client can aid in estimating the amount of the plant consumed. After consulting this review, the suggested references, a poison control center, or a toxicologist, the clinician is able to assess the risk or hazard associated with the incident. If the plant is known to be toxic and a significant amount may have been consumed, a rational approach to therapy should be instituted. If no information is found about the plant in question, a period of close observation is indicated.

Therapy for poisonous plant ingestion will, with

Table 3. *Plants with Nervous System Effects*

Common Name	Scientific Name	Comments
NICOTINE-LIKE ACTION		
Cardinal flower	*Lobelia* sp.	Salivation, nausea and vomiting, tachycardia.
Goldenchain tree	*Laburnum anagyroides*	
Kentucky coffee-tree	*Gymnocladus dioica*	
Mescal bean	*Sophora* sp.	
Tobacco, tree tobacco	*Nicotiana* sp.	
ATROPINE-LIKE ACTION		
Jimsonweed, thorn apple, Angel's trumpet	*Datura* sp.	Mydriasis, hyperthermia, and collapse.
Belladonna, deadly nightshade	*Atropa belladonna*	
Jasmine	*Cestrum* sp.	
Henbane	*Hyoscyamus niger*	
Lantana	*Lantana camara*	
CONVULSANTS		
Chinaberry tree	*Melia azedarach*	Convulsions.
Moonseed	*Menispermum canadense*	
Yellow jasmine	*Gelsemium sempervirens*	
Bleeding heart, Dutchman's breeches	*Dicentra* sp.	
HALLUCINOGENS		
Jimsonweed	*Datura* sp.	Depression, aberrant behavior.
Marijuana	*Cannabis sativa*	
Morning glory	*Ipomea* sp.	
Periwinkle	*Vinca rosea*	
CYANOGENIC ACTIVITY		
Apple	*Malus* sp.	Cyanide poisoning with bright red venous blood, dyspnea, and collapse.
Apricot, almond, peach, cherry	*Prunus* sp.	
Elderberry	*Sambucus* sp.	
Hydrangea	*Hydrangea macrophylla*	

Table 4. *Plants Producing Irritation or Mechanical Injury*

Common Name	Scientific Name	Comments
INSOLUBLE OXALATE CRYSTALS		
Caladium	*Caladium* sp.	Oral, pharyngeal, and esophageal irritation with salivation and edema.
Calla lily	*Zantedeschia aethiopica*	
Dumb cane	*Dieffenbachia* sp.	
Elephant's ear	*Colacasia* sp.	
Jack in the pulpit	*Arisaema triphyllum*	
Philodendron	*Philodendron* sp. and many other genera	
AWNS, SPINES, AND THORNS		
Bromegrasses	*Bromus* sp.	Direct puncture wounds; the plant part may remain as a foreign body producing abscesses.
Burdock	*Arctium lappa*	
Barleys	*Hordeum* sp.	
Blackberry	*Rubus* sp.	
Cacti	Many genera	
Carolina nightshade	*Solanum carolinense*	
Cocklebur	*Xanthium* sp.	
Foxtail	*Setaria* sp.	
Goathead	*Tribulus terrestris*	
Needlegrass	*Stipa sp.*	
Pyracantha	*Pyracantha* sp.	
Sandbur	*Cenchrus pauciflorus*	
Triple awn	*Aristida* sp.	
HAIRS THAT INJECT IRRITANTS		
Nettle	*Urtica* sp. *Lasportea canadensis* *Cnidoscolus stimulosus*	Bioactive amines produce salivation, vomiting, arrythmias, dyspnea, and collapse.
IRRITANT SAP OR LATEX		
Pencil cactus, poinsettia, snow-on-the-mountain, spurge, and many others	*Euphorbia* sp.	Irritation generally limited to mucous membranes or gastroenteritis.

few exceptions, be supportive and general. This includes evacuation of the gastrointestinal tract and administration of activated charcoal. Supportive therapy and monitoring should be initiated. (Refer to Emergency and General Treatment of Poisonings for a more detailed discussion.)

CONCLUSIONS

Ornamental plants are found in yards, gardens, and homes in all areas. Pets are exposed to these plants, and clinicians will frequently be presented with questions or potential poisonings. Diagnosis of plant poisoning is difficult and often is made only when an owner observes the ingestion. Nonspecific gastroenteritis should always be investigated with the suspicion that ornamental plant consumption may have been involved. Therapy is general and supportive, and a good prognosis is justified for most patients.

References and Supplemental Reading

Clay, B. R.: Poisoning and injury by plants. *In* Kirk, R. W. (ed.): *Current Veterinary Therapy VI,* Small Animal Practice. Philadelphia: W. B. Saunders, 1977, pp. 179–184.

Fowler, M. E.: *Plant Poisoning in Small Companion Animals.* St. Louis: Ralston Purina, 1980.

Harden, J. W., and Arena, J. M.: *Human Poisoning from Native and Cultivated Plants,* 2nd ed. Durham, NC: Duke University Press, 1974.

Kingsbury, J. M.: *Poisonous Plants of the United States and Canada.* Englewood Cliffs, NJ: Prentice-Hall, 1964.

Kingsbury, J. M.: *Deadly Harvest, A Guide to Common Poisonous Plants.* New York: Holt, Reinhart and Winston, 1965.

Kunkel, D. B.: Poisonous Plants. *In* Haddad, L. M., and Winchester, J. F. (eds.): *Clinical Management of Poisoning and Drug Overdose.* Philadelphia: W. B. Saunders, 1983, pp. 317–335.

Lampe, K. F., and Fagerstrom, R.: *Plant Toxicity and Dermatitis: A Manual for Physicians.* Baltimore: Williams & Wilkins, 1968.

In addition to these references, many state extension services have valuable publications with a regional emphasis.

INTOXICATION DUE TO CONTAMINATED GARBAGE, FOOD, AND WATER

ROBERT W. COPPOCK, D.V.M.,
Vegreville, Alberta

and MICHELLE S. MOSTROM, D.V.M.
Urbana, Illinois

Garbage, food, and water can become contaminated with toxins or toxicogenic microorganisms, with which animals become intoxicated after ingestion. Garbage, especially when high in protein and under favorable conditions of moisture and temperature, is a good substrate for rapid bacterial growth and toxin liberation. Under ideal conditions, pet foods, table scraps, and carrion can have explosive growth of toxicogenic microorganisms, which can colonize the intestinal tract and release toxins after ingestion. Food discarded from the refrigerator can be overgrown with molds and can be a source of mycotoxins. Carrion, garbage, and foodstuffs, under anaerobic conditions and favorable pH, may contain botulism toxins. Ponds, with favorable conditions of temperature, photoperiod, and nutrient balance, can have blooms of blue-green algae that liberate potent toxins.

Garbage frequently contains refuse such as broken glass, meat wrappers, string, plastic items, and bones, which after ingestion may lodge in the oral cavity, throat, or gastrointestinal tract. Splanchnemphraxis from ingestion of these foreign bodies is not uncommon.

Dogs, by virtue of their scavenging habits, generally are more prone to garbage intoxication than are other small animals. Dogs and sometimes cats often experience garbage poisoning after raiding garbage containers, eating road kills, visiting dumps, or spending a night roaming freely. Owners are often unaware or will deny that their pet engages in such activities. Additionally, dogs are often fed foods suspected or known to have caused food poisoning in the family. Owners are often surprised to learn that dogs are susceptible to food poisoning.

Intoxication due to contaminated garbage and water is more common in the summer and in warm climates. Another increase in the incidence of poisoning due to garbage, food, and water occurs during the summer holidays and hunting season and at Thanksgiving and Christmas.

ENTEROTOXIGENIC BACTERIA

Garbage is a good substrate for the growth of bacteria such as *Streptococcus aureus* and *Bacillus subtilis*, which are producers of enterotoxins. *Aeromonas*, a genus of bacteria associated with fish, reptiles, human excreta, and estuarine waters, has been identified as an enterotoxin producer. Its significance in veterinary medicine is not known, but it certainly could account for food poisoning associated with ingestion of fish offal. *Clostridium perfringens* has been reported as one of the most common causes of food poisoning in humans. However, it appears that its significance in small animal medicine is not well established.

Garbage and carrion may also have high bacterial counts of *Escherichia coli* and other gram-negative bacteria, and ingestion of these substances can produce an overgrowth of these organisms in the gut with subsequent release of enterotoxins and endotoxins.

Under anaerobic conditions, carrion and garbage can provide a good substrate for growth of *Clostridium botulinum*.

ENTEROTOXINS

Mechanism of Action. Enterotoxins are substances that produce their biologic effect by (1) changing gut biochemistry, (2) mimicking or antagonizing endogenous hormonal and transmitter substances, and (3) activating autacoids (histamines, kinins, prostaglandins, thromboxanes, and interleukins). All of these factors affect gastroenteric motility, membrane permeability, and nervous system interaction. Certain enterotoxins stimulate the sensory nerves and thereby are potent emetics. Other enterotoxins disrupt normal motility of the gastroenteric tract, possibly prolonging gastric emptying time and decreasing or increasing gut motility. Others alter gastroenteric epithelial biochemistry, resulting in the flow of fluid and electrolytes into the intestinal tract. With some of the enterotoxins, the differentiated enterocytes are permanently damaged and resolution is by necrobiosis, a process that requires approximately 5 days.

CLINICAL SIGNS. The first and most frequent clinical sign of enterotoxicosis is emesis, which generally occurs within 3 hours after exposure. In most cases, vomiting removes the toxins from the gastroenteric tract and complete recovery rapidly follows. However, emesis and retching may persist and may require medical treatment.

Diarrhea, sometimes bloody, is the second clinical sign and generally is observed within 2 to 48 hours after exposure. Spontaneous recovery, within 2 to 48 hours, occurs in most patients. Those patients with persisting diarrhea often require medical treatment. Additionally, since the majority of the patients are indoor pets, diarrhea is intolerable to the owners. Adynamic ileus and gastroplegia can be sequelae to enterotoxicosis. In some cases that have received medical treatment, the remission of clinical signs can be deceiving, as the patient can relapse and can go into shock. This phenomenon may be due to subsequent autointoxication.

Most patients presented to the hospital or clinic have persistent or marked clinical signs. These patients may be acutely ill and may have clinical signs of an acute abdomen. Rebound tenderness over the anterior quadrants of the abdomen is a common finding. The stomach and intestinal tract may be distended with gas, body temperature and white blood cell (WBC) counts can be elevated, and the patient may be dehydrated. Cases with persistent or marked clinical signs should be hospitalized and given immediate attention. Radiographs should be taken to rule out foreign body obstruction, gastric torsion, and other abdominal disorders.

TREATMENT. Treatment of enterotoxicosis has four major objectives: (1) removal of the toxins from the gastroenteric tract, (2) control of emesis, retching, and diarrhea, (3) prevention of adynamic or paralytic ileus and relapse, and (4) client education to prevent recurrence.

Emesis is a natural and generally efficient means of removing ingesta from the stomach. Due to persistent stimulation of the sensory nerves, nonproductive vomiting can persist and can require medical control. However, antiemetics should not be given until the veterinary physician has determined that all toxic ingesta has been removed from the stomach and upper intestinal tract, as pieces of bone and other residual material appear to be residual sources of bacteria or toxins and may explain the relapse phenomenon. Antiemetic drugs such as diphenhydramine (0.5 to 2.0 mg/kg, parenteral), or dimenhydrinate (1.0 to 1.5 mg/kg, parenteral) are preferred to narcotics, especially morphine. Narcotic-induced stasis of the bowel is generally an undesirable side effect.

Cases with gastroplegia, generally characterized by gas distension of the stomach, may be unresponsive to emetics. In these cases, gastric lavage may be beneficial. If large pieces of ingesta cannot be removed, gastrotomy may be indicated.

Diarrhea is due to fluid and electrolyte effusion into the bowel and changes in gut motility. Although unacceptable to the pet's owners, diarrhea is a natural means of purging the intestinal tract of toxic contents. Therefore, the clinician should be satisfied that the offending contents have been removed before administering parasympatholytic drugs such as atropine and scopolamine. Oral treatment with glucose and electrolytes appears to block enterotoxin-induced effusion of electrolytes into the gut. Kaopectate (2 to 5 ml/kg PO every 1 to 6 hours) is generally beneficial and probably adsorbs some of the toxins. Fluid and electrolyte balance of the patient must be monitored as a guide for replacement therapy.

In the majority of cases, antimicrobial chemotherapy should be held in reserve as it prolongs reestablishing normal gut flora. However, antibiotic therapy appears to prevent relapse, so good clinical judgment is essential in prescribing these agents. An antibiotic that has a broad spectrum of activity against gram-negative and gram-positive bacteria is the drug of choice.

Since relapse generally occurs within 48 hours, patients that have clinical signs sufficient to warrant hospitalization should not be discharged until they have been asymptomatic for this period of time. There is no substitute for good clinical judgment in the management of enterotoxicosis.

ENDOTOXINS

In most endotoxicosis cases, the ingesta usually does not contain large quantities of endotoxins. Rather, the ingesta contains large numbers of gram-negative bacteria that have colonized the upper gastrointestinal tract and produced endo- and enterotoxins.

Endotoxins are biologically active through a number of different mechanisms—namely, activation of autacoids, activation of Factor XII, altering capillary permeability, and altering splanchnic and peripheral vascular resistance. There is adherence of the polymorphonuclear leukocytes to the microvessels and concurrent neutropenia. All of these biologic effects can induce shock. Patients that develop anaerobic conditions in the gut may have growth of toxicogenic anaerobic bacteria. This may explain the rapid deterioration of some patients that develop endotoxic shock from eating garbage and carrion.

CLINICAL SIGNS. Clinical features of endotoxicosis vary considerably. There is generally a delay of 5 to 48 hours between exposure and onset of clinical signs. Diarrhea is the most common clinical sign. Emesis may be present but, unlike enterotoxin poisoning, seldom leads to spontaneous recovery. The gastroenteric tract is often distended with gas, and tenderness of the abdomen is a common clinical finding. The patient is generally depressed and in severe cases may be in twilight consciousness. Other clinical features include various degrees of shock, such as increased capillary filling time and cold extremities.

Body temperature may vary from subnormal to 40°C (104°F). Transient leukopenia and neutropenia may be observed and are generally followed by leukocytosis and neutrophilia and the appearance of toxic neutrophils. Moderate hyperglycemia may be observed. The heart rate is often increased. The liver may be enlarged. Oliguria may occur; therefore, urinary output should be established.

TREATMENT. The primary objectives of treatment are to remove the toxic ingesta from the gastroenteric tract, stop the growth of toxicogenic bacteria in the upper bowel, and prevent development of shock. Emesis, gastric lavage, and enemas often are helpful in removing the toxic substances from the gastroenteric tract. Prednisolone succinate (5 to 7 mg/kg IV every 4 hours) or a similar steroid should be given. Broad-spectrum antibiotics, such as chloramphenicol (25 mg/kg IV every 4 hours), effective against gram-negative bacteria, should be prescribed. Aminoglycosides are generally contraindicated as they can depress the myocardium. Alpha-blockers (phenoxybenzamine 0.25 to 0.5 mg/kg every 6 hours) may be beneficial. Fluid volume and electrolyte balance should be maintained. Mannitol (1 to 3 gm/kg in 500 ml IV fluids) should be given at 10 ml/minute to oliguric patients.

In cases of endotoxicosis, relapse can occur and generally is more severe than in enterotoxicosis. Pieces of animal parts in the stomach or intestinal tract can reseed the upper bowel with toxicogenic bacteria and produce this phenomenon. Careful monitoring of these patients should continue for 72 hours after remission of clinical signs.

WATERBORNE TOXINS (ALGAE)

Dogs are subject to intoxication with the toxins produced by blue-green algae, although this type of poisoning is not common. Farm ponds, shallow lakes, sewage lagoons, and other eutrophic bodies of fresh water can, under favorable climatic and nutrient conditions, have rapid growth blooms of blue-green algae and production of algal toxins. Poisoning of dogs and other animals occurs when they ingest the algae-contaminated water. Generally, the contamination of these waters with algal toxins is of short duration. Species of *Anabaena*, *Microcystis*, and *Aphanizomenon* are the most common toxicogenic blue-green algae.

Anatoxin A is produced by species of *Anabaena*. This toxin is rapidly absorbed from the gastroenteric tract and is a potent neuromuscular blocker. Other anatoxins and toxic polypeptides produced by *Anabaena* spp. are hepatotoxic. Also, the genus *Microcystis* produces hepatotoxic polypeptides called microcystins. Many of the microcystinlike toxins are irritating to the gastrointestinal tract. Toxins produced by species of *Aphanizomenon* mimic saxitoxin and microcystins. Saxitoxins inhibit nerve conduction of action potentials and thereby decrease the amount of acetylcholine released at the motor endplate.

CLINICAL SIGNS. Clinical signs of anatoxin A and saxitoxin intoxication (emesis, muscle fasciculations, weakness, convulsions, and paralysis) rapidly follow ingestion. Death may occur within 7 minutes after the onset of clinical signs. The pharmacologic effects of anatoxin A can persist for several days. Other anatoxins and microcystin produce acute hepatocellular necrosis, concurrent increase in serum hepatocellular enzymes, and clinical signs of acute liver disease and intestinal irritation.

TREATMENT. The only known therapy for anatoxin A intoxication is maintenance of respiration and symptomatic treatment. In cases of experimentally induced poisoning, treatment with neostigmine has not been effective. Animals that survive appear to have some resistance to these toxins.

Since saxitoxin blocks the release of acetylcholine, treatment with cholinesterase inhibitors to increase the half-life of acetylcholine may be of benefit. (This treatment is also discussed under Botulism.)

Algal toxins that produce acute liver disease and intestinal irritation should be treated symptomatically.

AUTOINTOXICATION

Autointoxication is a toxicosis produced by microorganisms growing and liberating toxins inside the body. This type of intoxication occurs when (1) large numbers of toxicogenic bacteria are ingested and colonize the gastroenteric tract or (2) ingested food alters the normal microbial flora of the intestinal tract, permitting colonization with toxicogenic bacteria. Some dogs appear to be predisposed to this condition. Autointoxication has also been associated with overeating of foods not normally in the diet; change in brand of pet foods; and ingestion of bones, hoof trimmings, spicy foods, animal and human excreta, and alcoholic beverages. Autointoxication appears to be caused by entero- and endotoxins.

CLINICAL SIGNS. The clinical signs of autointoxication are the same as those of entero- and endotoxins. In most cases of autointoxication, diarrhea lasting 24 to 48 hours is the only clinical sign observed. Acute pancreatitis can be a sequel to autointoxication. The history can be helpful in identifying intemperate or unhealthful eating habits.

TREATMENT. The treatment of autointoxication is the same as for entero- and endotoxins. Dietary planning and client education are important to prevent recurrence. Oral pancreatic enzymes, such as Enzymin (Haver-Lockhart, 1 to 3 tablets with meals), appear to be of benefit.

BOTULISM

The number of confirmed cases of botulism in dogs appears to be limited. In addition to clinical signs, identification of the toxin in serum, vomitus, ingesta, or feces is necessary for confirmation of botulism. Because of the difficulties in establishing a definitive diagnosis, there is reason to suspect that botulism is more common than reported.

The most probable exposure of dogs to botulism is from decaying waterfowl, other carrion, and high-protein garbage incubating under anaerobic conditions.

TOXINS. At least seven antigen types of botulism toxins have been identified. Additionally, these toxins are considered to be among the most potent toxins known. Lethal intraperitoneal dosages in mice range from 0.5 to 2.5 ng/kg. In human medicine, the type of botulism toxin identified varies with geographic location. Type A is most prevalent west of the Mississippi River, type B in the eastern states, and type E in Alaska and the Great Lakes region. Cases of confirmed botulism in dogs have all been due to type C toxin. Since only a few confirmed cases of canine botulism have been reported, it is unknown if this pattern of distribution applies to small animal medicine. Limited clinical evidence suggests that dogs may be considerably less sensitive to botulism than mice, and pups more susceptible than older dogs. After recovery from botulism, dogs have been observed to shed the spores of *C. botulinum* and type C toxin in their feces for at least 114 days.

CLINICAL SIGNS. Botulism toxins act by inhibiting release of acetylcholine from the nerve terminals. Clinical signs of botulism in dogs generally appear 24 to 48 hours after ingestion of the toxin. Vomiting, pain in the anterior portion of the abdomen, salivation, dry eyes, and rear limb weakness usually are the initial clinical signs observed. Also, the deep tendon, withdrawal, gagging, and pupillary reflexes are depressed. Body temperature generally is not elevated. Differential diagnosis of suspected botulism includes tick paralysis, coral snake bites, polyradiculoneuritis, rabies, trauma, algal intoxication, spinal cord disorders, drug intoxication, carbon monoxide poisoning, and myasthenia gravis.

TREATMENT. Treatment should be initiated when botulism is suspected. As much of the offending ingesta as prudently possible should be removed from the gastrointestinal tract with lavage, emetics, enemas, and cathartics. Treatment with an adsorbent such as activated charcoal (Toxiban, Vet-A-Mix, 12 to 24 ml/kg q.i.d.), activated carbons, and Kaopectate (5 ml/kg every 2 to 6 hours) may decrease toxin absorption. Penicillin G (20,000 units/kg IM every 12 hours), ampicillin (16 mg/kg PO or 8 mg/kg IM every 6 hours) should be given to eliminate *C. botulinum* from the intestinal tract. Aminoglycoside antibiotics are contraindicated, as they potentiate the pathophysiologic effects of the toxins.

Botulism antitoxin should be administered. Trivalent antitoxin used in human medicine contains types A, B, and E antitoxins. If available, type C antitoxin should be included in the antitoxin regimen. Since these antitoxins are of noncanine origin, they may produce allergic reactions.

Neuromuscular functioning can be increased by using a therapeutic regimen of acetylcholinesterase inhibitors such as physostigmine and neostigmine. Atropine sulfate or similar drugs should be given as needed to block the muscarinic effects of the acetylcholinesterase inhibitors. This treatment regimen is essentially identical to the management of myasthenia gravis. Symptomatic and supportive treatment and nursing care must be provided during the acute and convalescence phases of botulism intoxication.

MYCOTOXINS

Mycotoxins are the toxic metabolites of toxigenic fungi, the growth of which is influenced by many factors. Of these, three are the most important: substrate, temperature, and moisture. However, the single most important factor is moisture. As a general rule, mycotoxin-contaminated foodstuffs are palatable and do not have a moldy appearance.

Contamination of pet foods with mycotoxins generally occurs by (1) pre-existence in the ingredients used in formulating the feed or (2) production in the finished feeds. Of the ingredients used in pet foods, grains are generally the most common source of mycotoxins. Grain used in pet foods is a source of aflatoxins, trichothecenes, and other mycotoxins that receive considerable attention in large animal practice. Aflatoxin-contaminated corn, purchased on the international market, has just recently been documented as the cause of death in a number of dogs in South Africa. The trichothecenes (toxins in "yellow rain") have been suspected as producing toxicity in dogs. However, well-documented cases of pet poisonings from trichothecenes are not available. Pet foods, especially in self-feeders, have potential for explosive mycotoxin production.

Cryophilic toxigenic fungi grow on refrigerated foodstuffs, such as cheese. Penitrem A–producing species of *Penicillium* are a good example. In the majority of these cases, the food has visible mold growing on it (see article on Mycotoxicosis).

CLINICAL SIGNS. Clinical signs of mycotoxicoses vary with the different mycotoxins. Emesis and diarrhea are a common sign of acute mycotoxicoses. Tremorgens, such as penitrem A, produce clinical signs of ataxia, tremors, and intermittent opisthotonos and seizures, which are not induced by stimulating the patient.

Aflatoxins are potent hepatotoxins. Clinical signs are loss of weight, anorexia, dullness, diarrhea, icterus, melena, polyuria, polydipsia, epistaxis, petechiae of the oral membranes, seizures, prostration, and death. The patient may be tender over the left abdominal quadrant. The patient generally has a normal body temperature and normal WBC count. However, the serum hepatocellular enzymes are usually elevated, and the patient may be anemic.

The trichothecenes mimic parvovirosis and panleukopenia. Depending on which point in the course of the disease the patient is presented, the WBC count may be increased or decreased. Destruction of the bone marrow produces a marked decrease in platelet and red blood cell counts. Emesis, diarrhea that is often bloody, and tonsillitis are common clinical signs observed in dogs experimentally exposed to trichothecenes. Hyperpyrexia may also be observed. Cats are known to be quite sensitive to trichothecenes.

Clinical cases of ochratoxin A intoxication in small animals appear to be rare. Under experimental conditions, clinical signs of anorexia, weight loss, emesis, tenesmus, polydipsia, polyuria, hyperpyrexia (41.1°C, or 107°F), tonsillitis, dehydration, prostration, and death have been reported.

TREATMENT. There is no known specific treatment for mycotoxicoses. All sources of mycotoxins must be removed from the diet. Symptomatic care is indicated. Since aflatoxins and trichothecenes depress native resistance to disease, exposure to infectious diseases should be minimized. As a general rule, steroids, chloramphenicol, and similar drugs are contraindicated. Following recovery, the patient should be revaccinated for the common diseases.

MYCOTOXICOSIS

STEVEN S. NICHOLSON, D.V.M.
Baton Rouge, Louisiana

Mycotoxins are chemicals produced by toxigenic fungi growing in feedstuffs or foods when conditions of moisture and temperature are suitable. Presence of specific toxin-producing fungi in feed or food does not prove toxicity, because conditions may not have been favorable for toxin production. Laboratory analysis to detect a mycotoxin is necessary to confirm that the feed or food is the source. This information—along with history, clinical signs, and lesions compatible with poisoning due to the specific mycotoxin—confirm the diagnosis. Vomitus, urine, and liver, and kidney tissue may be useful for analysis to confirm current exposure.

Naturally occurring conditions caused by mycotoxins are documented in many species, including humans, food animals, horses, dogs, and rabbits. More than a dozen mycotoxins are associated with animal health problems, and specific agents affect specific organs or tissues such as the kidneys, liver, brain, the mucosa of the gastrointestinal tract, and the reproductive system. Signs of clinical illness may be related to acute, subacute, or chronic poisoning. In recent years, secondary mycotoxic diseases associated with lowered resistance to infectious agents and reduced response to vaccines have been recognized.

A specific hepatoxic disease of dogs and swine was recognized in the southeastern states prior to the identification of aflatoxins. Termed "hepatitis X," it was later confirmed to be due to aflatoxin-contaminated peanut meal used in commercial dog food. Clinical signs included anorexia, icterus, dullness, melena, polyuria, polydipsia, and hemorrhagic diathesis. Greene (1977) described disseminated intravascular coagulation as a complication in several Walker hounds with chronic aflatoxicosis from contaminated commercial feed.

Lesions found at necropsy include icterus, hemorrhage, and toxic hepatic damage in aflatoxicosis. Microscopic liver lesions include fibrosis and bile duct proliferation, which are said to be somewhat characteristic but not pathognomonic of subacute or chronic aflatoxicosis.

In addition, aflatoxins are capable of inducing cancer, mutations, and teratogenic changes. Suppressed immune system functions have been demonstrated in some species.

Aflatoxins are produced by *Aspergillus flavus* and *Aspergillus parasiticus* growing in commodities such as corn, cottonseed, and peanuts in the field, in storage, and after processing; they also grow in feed in self-feeders.

Corn and protein meals used in animal food production are potential sources of aflatoxin exposure to dogs, cats, rabbits, and other species. Interstate shipment of foods or feeds is subject to Food and Drug Administration regulations limiting aflatoxin content to less than 20 parts per billion. Dry dog foods produced for local and in-state sales might not be closely monitored for aflatoxin content. This could be of special concern in the Southeast, where corn containing toxic levels of aflatoxin rejected at a grain elevator might be diverted at a low price to another use, such as dog food production.

Dillman (1984) believes that there may be a higher than expected incidence of bile duct carcinoma, hepatocellular cancer, and fibrosis of the liver in large- and giant-breed dogs in the Southeast. These animals, and groups of hounds as well, are often fed a least-cost dry dog food.

Penitrem A, a mycotoxin produced by *Penicillium crustaceum*, a common contaminant of household foodstuffs, has produced acute neurologic signs in dogs after ingestion of moldy cream cheese and moldy walnuts. Arp and Richard (1979) identified *P. crustaceum*, penitrem A, and animal toxicity in moldy cream cheese that was thought to have produced muscle tremors, generalized seizures, intermittent opisthotonos, and ataxia in two garbage-raiding dogs. The cream cheese, which was covered by a blue-green fungal mat, had been removed from the refrigerator and discarded.

In another reported incident, a 6.5-year-old 27.3-kg (60-lb) spayed boxer developed generalized convulsions, ataxia, urination, defecation, polypnea, hyperthermia, and mydriasis 2 to 3 hours after eating moldy walnuts. Richard and coworkers (1981) confirmed the presence of penitrem A and toxicity of the walnuts in laboratory mice.

In dogs, penitrem A toxicosis is dose dependent, and signs vary. An animal can have transitory tremors and ataxia lasting 2 to 4 hours, it can die during seizures, or it can return to normal neurologic function after 1 to 2 days. Pentobarbital sodium controlled seizures in the cases discussed here.

The nephrotoxin ochratoxin A has been reported in corn, Canadian wheat, oats, barley, and rye. Other fungal metabolities with nephrotoxic activity include oxalic acid and citrinin. These mycotoxins have not been reported to be the cause of nephrosis in dogs or cats in the United States.

References and Supplemental Reading

Arp, L. H., and Richard J. L.: Intoxication of dogs with the mycotoxin penitrem A. J.A.V.M.A. 175:565, 1979.

Dillman, R. C.: Personal communication, 1984, North Carolina State University, School of Veterinary Medicine, Raleigh.

Greene, C. E.: Disseminated intravascular coagulation complicating aflatoxicosis in dogs. Cornell Vet. 67:29, 1977.

Richard A. C., Richard, J. L., and Cysweski, S. J.: Implications of mycotoxins in animal disease. J.A.V.M.A. 176:719, 1980.

Richard, J. L., Arp, L. H., and Bacchetti, P.: The mycotoxin penitrem A as a cause of moldy walnut toxicosis in a dog. Calif. Vet. 35:12, 1981.

Section 3

RESPIRATORY DISEASES

BRENDAN C. McKIERNAN, D.V.M.
Consulting Editor

***Additional Pertinent Information Found in* Current Veterinary Therapy VIII:**

Amis, T. C.: Clinical Respiratory Physiology, p. 191.
Bauer, T. G., and Thomas, W. P.: Pulmonary Edema, p. 252.
Burns, M. G.: Pulmonary Thromboembolism, p. 257.
Harvey, C. E., and O'Brien, J. A.: Nasal Aspergillosis-Penicillosis, p. 236.
Haskins, S. E.: Blood Gases and Acid-Base Balance: Clinical Interpretation and Therapeutic Implications, p. 201.
McKiernan, B. C.: Principles of Respiratory Therapy, p. 216.
Roudebush, P.: Diagnostics for Respiratory Diseases, p. 222.

RESPIRATORY IMMUNOLOGY

PETER J. FELSBURG, V.M.D.
Urbana, Illinois

The respiratory tract is in constant contact with the external environment and is therefore a major site of antigenic challenge. This has necessitated the development of an extensive array of nonimmunologic and immunologic pulmonary defense mechanisms that collectively act to cleanse inspired air and inactivate infectious and other potentially injurious agents that are inhaled or aspirated. The defense mechanisms expressed locally in the respiratory tract are not only important in normal host defense against inhaled foreign antigens and in preserving the normal integrity of the lung, but they may also contribute to the pathogenesis of various lung diseases.

In order to understand fully the mode of action of the pulmonary defense mechanisms, it is necessary to review the normal structural and functional relationships between different portions of the respiratory tract. The respiratory tree extends from the nares down to the terminal bronchioles and is primarily involved in air transport. The mucosal surfaces of the nasopharynx, trachea, bronchi, and bronchioles are lined with tightly packed, ciliated, pseudostratified columnar epithelial cells, which undergo a gradual change to cuboidal epithelium in the distal airways. Under this epithelium lies the lamina propria and submucosa, which contains various secretory glands and lymphoid tissue. The lymphoid tissue of the respiratory tract has its highest degree of structural organization in the upper respiratory tract. In addition to the sublingual and palatine tonsils, the regional lymph nodes of the lung—hilar and tracheobronchial lymph nodes—are present. Organized lymphoid nodules are present in association with the mucosa of the major conducting airways. Lymphoid aggregates, lymphocytes, and macrophages are diffusely distributed throughout the submucosa and lamina propria of the respiratory tract.

The peripheral regions of the lung, from the bronchioles out to the alveoli, are primarily involved in gas exchange. The mucosal surface of these regions is made up of a thin epithelial cell layer, which is easily disrupted by minor degrees of local irritation or inflammation. Beneath the epithelial lining is an interstitium consisting of loose connective tissue, pulmonary capillaries, and lymphatic channels. Notably absent from the peripheral regions of the normal lung parenchyma are any organized lymphoid structures. Past the bronchoalveolar junction, the only lymphoid tissue found in the normal lung are small numbers of lymphocytes and macrophages diffusely scattered throughout the interstitium and within the alveolar spaces. The parenchyma of the lung is well endowed with lymphatic vessels, which drain the mucosa and parenchyma of the lower lung to the regional lymph nodes.

NONIMMUNOLOGIC CLEARANCE MECHANISMS

The vast majority of inhaled antigens are efficiently removed from the respiratory tract by nonimmunologic responses, and therefore the antigens are kept from reacting with the specific immunologic components of the respiratory defense system. The intact ciliated epithelium is a barrier that physically prevents entry of antigens through the submucosa of the respiratory tract.

The secretions that line the mucosal surface of the respiratory tract act as a filter to trap most of the inhaled particulate materials and prevent them from either penetrating the respiratory mucosa or gaining access to the distal aspects of the respiratory tract. These secretions contain mucus (produced by the goblet cells in the epithelium and serous and mucous cells in the submucosa) and various enzymes that aid in the neutralization and degradation of inhaled materials. Antigens that are deposited on the mucosal surfaces are mechanically removed by mucociliary clearance and by the sneeze and cough mechanisms. The mucous layer is in continuous flow, moved backward through the nasal cavity and upward from the bronchioles, bronchi, and trachea by ciliary action to the pharynx, where it is normally swallowed and digested in the intestinal tract. The cough reflex provides an important mechanism by which foreign materials can be moved up the respiratory tract and disposed of by either expectoration or swallowing. Stimulation of cough and irritant receptors located throughout the respiratory tract may produce, in addition to a cough, a reflex bronchoconstriction, which aids in preventing a more peripheral deposition of inhaled materials.

Antigens that escape this mucociliary clearance mechanism and gain entrance to the alveoli are phagocytized and digested or degraded by alveolar macrophages.

If any potentially harmful antigens escape these epithelial defense mechanisms and penetrate the epithelium, specific immune responses occur.

IMMUNOLOGIC RESPONSES OF THE RESPIRATORY TRACT

Immunologic responses in the respiratory tract may operate within the lumen, at the mucosal surface, within the submucosa, or within the parenchyma of the lung. Just as the bronchoalveolar junction provides a separation in structure and function, it also provides a separation between the immune reactions of the respiratory tract mucosa and those of the parenchyma. The immune functions expressed at the mucosal surface primarily involve responses that are generated locally by the lymphoid cells in the submucosa. On the other hand, the immune responses expressed in the lung parenchyma depend almost entirely on the recruitment of immunocompetent cells from the systemic immune system into the interstitium and bronchoalveolar spaces.

Mucosal Immunity

The importance of immunologic mechanisms functioning locally in secretions was first recognized when it was shown that the levels of antibodies in mucosal secretions correlated more closely with host resistance to certain infections than did serum antibody titers. It was subsequently shown that a specialized form of IgA, secretory IgA (sIgA), was the predominant immunoglobulin in external secretions, in contrast to serum and internal secretions, in which IgG is the predominant immunoglobulin. The antibody response in external secretions was shown to be regulated independently from antibody responses in serum. These observations are important characteristics of a unique form of local immunity common to mucosal surfaces, which is referred to as the secretory or mucosal immune system. The lymphoid tissue that forms the basis of the mucosal immune system consists of lymphoid nodules and aggregates scattered throughout the system. They are collectively referred to as the mucosal-associated lymphoid tissue. The two major components of this mucosal-associated lymphoid tissue are the gut-associated lymphoid tissue (GALT) and the bronchus-associated lymphoid tissue (BALT). The mucosal immune system contains all the essential components for generating and effecting an immune response—antigen recognition and handling, humoral and cell-mediated immune responses, recruitment of inflammatory cells, and memory.

The respiratory tract, in common with the gastrointestinal (GI) tract, possesses a localized mucosal immune response that can function independently of the systemic immune system. The antigen-sensitive B and T cells of the respiratory tract are distributed either as scattered lymphocytes in the lamina propria of the submucosa or in organized lymphoid nodules in the submucosa, which, as described, have been termed BALT. These lymphoid nodules appear to provide areas of specialized processing for antigens and are the source of IgA precursor cells. They are covered by a specialized nonciliated, flattened lymphoepithelium. These cells are similar to the M cells overlying the Peyer's patches of the GI tract; Peyer's patches have a function similar to that of the lymphoid nodules of the BALT system. This unique epithelial cell provides a mechanism for preferential and controlled antigen uptake—a function central to the role of these nodules in the induction of the secretory immune response. Even though the BALT and GALT are the source of antigen processing and the generation of IgA-committed B cells, there is a marked absence of antibody-producing plasma cells in these tissues. Final differentiation and maturation into antibody-secreting plasma cells apparently takes place after the precommitted IgA B cells leave the BALT or GALT and gain entrance into the systemic circulation. The differentiated IgA-producing plasma cells migrate through the circulation to the mucosal site of origin as well as to other mucosal sites throughout the body. Thus IgA cells derived from GALT will not only end up in the submucosal lining of the GI tract but also migrate to the respiratory tract, lacrimal glands, mammary glands, and urogenital tract. The same is true of IgA cells derived from BALT. These cells will migrate back to the submucosa of the respiratory tract and other mucosal organs as functional IgA-secreting plasma cells.

The secretions of the respiratory tract contain not only sIgA but also IgG and small amounts of IgM and IgE. As in other mucosal secretions, sIgA predominates in the secretions of the upper respiratory tract. The concentration of sIgA decreases toward the periphery of the lower respiratory tract. In the secretions of the terminal bronchioles and alveolar spaces, IgG replaces sIgA as the predominant immunoglobulin.

IgA is produced locally by IgA plasma cells within the lamina propria and submucosa. Inside the plasma cell, two monomeric IgA molecules are joined together by a small glycopeptide called the J chain to form a dimer of two IgA molecules. The dimeric IgA is then secreted and diffuses through the lamina propria to the epithelial cell layer. Because of the tight junctions between epithelial cells, the large dimeric IgA molecule cannot directly gain access to the lumen of the respiratory tract. The epithelial cells themselves aid in the transport of IgA into the lumen by synthesizing a protein called the secretory component. Secretory component is incorporated in the basal and lateral plasma membrane of the epithelial cells and acts as a receptor for the J chain of the dimeric IgA. The complexing of dimeric IgA with secretory component on the cell surface causes endocytosis, which involves the invagination of the cell membrane enclosing the IgA in membrane vesicles. These vesicles are transported across the epithelial cell to its apical membrane, and the dimeric IgA complexed with secretory component is released into the luminal secretions as sIgA by reverse pinocytosis. Secretory component, in addition to facilitating the transport of sIgA, also adds stability to IgA in secretions by protecting it from digestion by proteolytic enzymes released by phagocytic cells and proteases released by certain bacteria.

Any presence of IgM in secretions will occur by a similar process since pentameric IgM also possesses a J chain and will bind secretory component. Serum-derived and any locally produced IgG and IgE enter the lumen of the respiratory tract by passive diffusion between the epithelial cells or by leakage through minor breaks in the mucosal lining. Inflammation will increase the transudation of IgG into the mucosal secretions. The increased concentrations of serum-derived and locally produced IgG in the secretions of the distal respiratory tract probably reflect the physical difference in the mucosal lining—a thin layer of loosely apposed nonciliated epithelium that is easily disrupted by minor irritation.

The presence of sIgA (and other factors) in the secretions of the respiratory tract potentiates the filtering effect of the mucociliary apparatus, and, in combination, they represent the respiratory tract's first line of defense by excluding antigens at the mucosal surface. No concomitant adverse effects are known to be triggered by sIgA antibodies. Compared with IgG and IgM, sIgA interacts with antigens without activating the effector mechanisms of inflammation that are activated in systemic immune responses. If there is an absence of antigen-specific sIgA at the mucosal surface, an excessive antigen exposure that overwhelms the first line of defense, or a prolonged mucosal contact because of an ineffective mucociliary tree, the antigen may penetrate the mucosal surface and encounter a second line of defense in the lamina propria and submucosa. The latter consists of the serum-derived and locally produced IgG and IgM. Immune complexes formed with either IgG or IgM will initiate a local inflammatory reaction by the activation of complement and the attraction of phagocytic cells to the local site. Although this second line of defense may act to localize and prevent dissemination of the antigen, the release of proteolytic and lysosomal enzymes from these cells as they are phagocytizing and degrading the antigen will result in local tissue injury and local clinical disease.

Secretory IgA exhibits a variety of antibody activities against bacteria, viruses, toxins, and other soluble antigens. The dimeric structure of sIgA contains four antigen-binding sites, resulting in an effective cross-linking of antigens. This enables sIgA to be a very efficient agglutinating and neutralizing antibody. The primary biologic function of sIgA is probably to aggregate particulate and soluble antigens and thereby prevent their adherence to the epithelial surface.

It has been shown that the mucosal immune reactions provide a control mechanism to limit the absorption of soluble, nonviable antigens from the GI tract. The mechanism of action here involves the formation of nonabsorbable complexes by sIgA. It has been proposed that a similar mechanism is operable in the respiratory tract to limit the absorption of inhaled, soluble, nonviable antigens (e.g., inhaled allergens).

The presence of local antitoxin antibodies in the respiratory secretions contributes significantly to protection against disease from bacteria that act primarily by secreting exotoxins. Secretory IgA also plays an important role in other respiratory bacterial infections even though it lacks the effector mechanisms of other immunoglobulins for bacterial killing. Normal bacterial killing involves the opsonization of the bacteria, with the subsequent activation of complement. Secretory IgA does not appear to be a very effective opsonizing antibody, nor is it a very effective activator of complement. For bacterial colonization to occur in the respiratory tract, the bacteria must selectively adhere to the epithelial surface (e.g., *Bordetella bronchiseptica*). Normal mucociliary action acts to oppose the colonization of bacteria. The presence of sIgA augments the clearance of bacteria by binding the antigenic determinants of the bacteria, essentially acting as an agglutinating antibody and thereby preventing their adherence and colonization. The sIgA-bacterial complexes are then easily removed by mucociliary action.

A major function of the mucosal immune system is in host resistance to viral infections that gain entrance through the respiratory tract. These include viruses that remain and replicate locally in the respiratory mucosa and viruses that gain entrance through the respiratory epithelium but disseminate to the regional lymph nodes for their primary replication. In the first type of virus, locally produced sIgA plays a major role in not only preventing infection but also in localized clinical disease. The absence of sIgA will permit infection to occur, with the development of localized respiratory disease even in the presence of circulating serum antibody that would help dampen any systemic clinical disease. Any local replication of a virus and the production of a local inflammatory response will destroy the normal integrity of the mucosa, thereby permitting penetration by other antigens. On the other hand, with viruses that initially replicate in the regional lymph nodes, circulating serum antibody is sufficient to prevent infection and systemic clinical disease.

The biologic importance of the dissociation of independently regulated local and systemic immune responses is that natural infection or immunization may stimulate one system without necessarily having an effect on the development of immunity in the other. For example, parenteral immunization against canine parainfluenza virus will prevent the development of clinical signs if dogs are exposed to the virus in the environment, but it will not protect the dog from infection, which results in an asymptomatic carrier for a period of time. On the other hand, intranasal vaccination would result in protection not only from clinical disease but from infection as well. Perhaps a better example is feline rhinotracheitis. Parenteral vaccinations will protect against severe clinical disease but will not protect against infection. This is especially important with this herpesvirus, since infection can result in latent infection and a permanent carrier state. This means that cats vaccinated parenterally against feline rhinotracheitis virus may become infected, develop a latent infection, and become permanent carriers without ever developing clinical disease. These cats are a major reason why certain catteries have problems with chronic, recurrent respiratory infections. Intranasal vaccination will prevent infection, the latent infection, and in turn the carrier state. It will *not*, however, terminate infection in a current carrier. Another advantage of intranasal vaccination is that one does not have to worry about the presence of maternal antibody interfering with the ability to be immunized.

Parenchymal Immune Response

If an antigen escapes the protective mechanism of the mucosal immune system and gains entrance into the distal air spaces of the lower respiratory tract, the antigen may be processed by one of three mechanisms. First, the antigen may be phagocytized by alveolar macrophages and cleared by the mucociliary tree, thus bypassing lymphoid tissue. Second, the antigen may be absorbed into the lymphatics and transported to the regional or systemic lymph nodes and stimulate an immune response. Last, the antigen could be phagocytized and processed by alveolar macrophages in either the bronchoalveolar space or the interstitium and either initiate or amplify a localized immune response.

One of the morphologic features of the lung parenchyma is the lack of organized lymphoid tissue. In addition to the presence of alveolar macrophages, small numbers of B and T lymphocytes are found in the alveolar spaces as well as scattered throughout the interstitium of the lung parenchyma. After intrapulmonary deposition of antigen, both humoral and cell-mediated immune responses can be detected locally in the lung parenchyma. Antibody is derived either by transudation or by local production by antigen-sensitive B cells. The cell-mediated immune reactions are produced by local antigen-sensitive T cells. However, the generation of these antigen-sensitive lymphocytes differs from that of the mucosal immune system. On the initial exposure, the inhaled antigen is absorbed or carried by macrophages into the interstitial spaces and is transported to the regional or systemic lymph nodes, where the immune response begins. The antigen-sensitive B and T cells are then transported back to the lungs through the circulation and are recruited into the interstitium or alveolar spaces, where they can subsequently interact with antigen. This recruitment is enhanced by local inflammation or the persistence of antigen in the lungs.

As mentioned previously, the principal immunoglobulin in the lung periphery is IgG. Thus, the interaction of antibody and antigen in these regions of the lung usually results in the generation of an inflammatory response. In addition, lymphokines released during a local cell-mediated immune reaction primarily act to attract neutrophils and, in particular, to attract, localize, and activate additional macrophages at the site of the lesion. These inflammatory responses represent the mechanism by which antigen is normally eliminated from the lungs. Therefore, unlike the mucosal immune response, most immune reactions occurring in the lung parenchyma will result in transient local tissue injury and local clinical disease due to the release of various proteolytic and lysosomal enzymes from the phagocytic cells.

IMMUNOLOGIC LUNG DISEASE

Although most host immune responses serve a protective function (and form the basis for host defense), occasionally a host immune response may have a deleterious function that results in tissue injury and clinical disease. These deleterious immunologic reactions are called allergies or hypersensitivity reactions. A hypersensitivity reaction can be defined as a specific immunologic reaction whose consequences are detrimental to the host. Hypersensitivity reactions are classified on the basis of the different mechanisms by which immune reactions initiate tissue injury.

TYPE I (ANAPHYLACTIC) REACTIONS. These are

local or systemic immediate hypersensitivity reactions that are initiated by the interaction of antigen and tissue cells passively sensitized with IgE antibody. This antigen-antibody reaction results in the release of pharmacologically active mediators (e.g., histamine, bradykinin, serotonin, slow-reacting substance of anaphylaxis, prostaglandins), which exert their biologic activities on the surrounding target tissue. An example of a type I hypersensitivity reaction in dogs is atopic dermatitis.

TYPE II (CYTOTOXIC) REACTIONS. Type II reactions result from the binding of IgG or IgM antibody to antigenic components of cells or tissue. The consequence of this antigen-antibody reaction to the host is destruction of the cells or tissue by complement or through the inflammatory action of phagocytic cells (primarily neutrophils). Autoimmune hemolytic anemia is an example of a type II hypersensitivity reaction.

TYPE III (IMMUNE COMPLEX) REACTIONS. Type III reactions result from the deposition of circulating antigen-antibody complexes in various tissues or vessels. The binding of complement to these complexes attracts neutrophils into the area, and as they ingest the immune complexes they release various proteolytic and lysosomal enzymes, resulting in damage to the surrounding tissues. Systemic lupus erythematosus is an example of a type III hypersensitivity reaction.

TYPE IV (CELL-MEDIATED) REACTIONS. These reactions result from the interaction of sensitized T lymphocytes with specific antigen. The ensuing cell-mediated immune response is mediated by either direct cytotoxicity or by the release of soluble lymphokines, which act through other mediator cells. Many of the lymphokines have a direct influence on inflammatory cells, particularly macrophages, by recruiting, activating, and keeping them at the local site. In this case, the tissue damage is mediated through the macrophage. An example of a type IV hypersensitivity reaction is allergic contact dermatitis.

Immunologic lung disease is a result of one or more of these hypersensitivity reactions. Damage to the lung tissue is mediated through the various inflammatory reactions associated with the individual hypersensitivity reactions. The accumulation of neutrophils and macrophages represents a normal protective process due to their antimicrobial activities and their ability to degrade various noninfectious agents. As they are performing these protective functions, they also release into the surrounding tissue various mediators that can serve a normal repair function and result in little or no long-term tissue damage. Neutrophils and macrophages release proteolytic enzymes; the most important in the lungs is collagenase, which causes derangement of the interstitial collagen and may thereby injure lung parenchymal cells. The alveolar macrophages help to repair this damage by releasing factors that attract fibroblasts and stimulate their replication, resulting in fibrosis and wound repair. However, if there is persistence of the antigen either through constant antigenic exposure or when the agent is nondegradable, chronic inflammation will result, in which the continuous release of mediators can produce significant tissue damage and clinical disease. This is especially true in the lungs, since changes in the normal structure of the lung parenchyma can lead to interference with gas exchange.

The inflammatory lung diseases discussed below result from immunologic responses to both known and unknown agents and are a consequence of one or a combination of the hypersensitivity reactions. The mention of these human diseases is not intended to be a detailed clinical description of the disease but rather an illustration of how immunologic reactions can contribute to pathologic changes and disease in the lungs. Some of these diseases have been recognized in animals; undoubtedly more will be in the future.

Atopic Respiratory Disease

Atopy is an immediate (type I) hypersensitivity reaction to environmental antigens (allergens) in genetically susceptible animals who produce IgE antibodies to allergens such as pollens, grasses, molds, house dust, animal danders, or food. The most common clinical manifestations of atopy in humans are allergic rhinitis (hay fever) and, less frequently, bronchial asthma. Although atopic disease in dogs and cats is primarily manifested by dermatologic signs, respiratory manifestations are occasionally reported. Allergic rhinitis in dogs may be characterized by profuse watery rhinorrhea, sneezing, and nasal obstruction. Depending on the allergens involved, clinical signs may be seasonal (pollens) or perennial (house dust). A tentative diagnosis of allergic rhinitis can be made by identifying eosinophils in the nasal exudate, observing a favorable response to corticosteroids or antihistamines, or noting clinical improvement when the potential offending allergen is removed. Intradermal skin testing may be beneficial in determining the allergens involved.

Allergic asthma, although rare in animals, has been reported in dogs and cats. This condition is a type I allergic reaction localized in the bronchus. The clinical presentation may consist of wheezing, difficulty in breathing, and coughing.

Chronic bronchitis may also have an allergic (type I) etiology. The disease, as with other type I allergic reactions, may be seasonal or perennial. Chest radiographs may be normal or may reveal a nonspecific bronchial pattern. A diagnosis of chronic allergic bronchitis can be confirmed by the presence of eosinophils in a bacterially sterile bronchial wash and following the elimination of parasitic causes.

Although antigen-antibody interaction is fundamental to the immunopathogenesis of atopic disease, it is not the reaction itself that is responsible for the allergic manifestation. Instead, the allergic reaction is caused by the release or activation of potent pharmacologic agents that mediate the tissue damage.

After the first exposure to an allergen, the animal responds with the production of antibodies of the IgE class. IgE antibodies are called cytotropic antibodies because they have an affinity for binding to membranes of certain mediator cells. In the respiratory tract, the mediator cells are the tissue-fixed mast cells. They are found in the connective tissue beneath the basement membrane of the mucosal lining of the airways, near blood vessels in the submucosa, scattered throughout muscle bundles, and in the intra-alveolar septa. IgE is produced by plasma cells in the lamina propria and submucosa of the mucosal lining of the respiratory tract. The IgE binds to the mast cells through receptors for IgE on their surface. Once IgE is fixed to mast cells, the animal is considered sensitized. The receptors for IgE on the mast cells do not discriminate between allergen specificities. For this reason, a single mast cell may have IgE antibodies to many different allergens on its surface.

Once an animal has become sensitized, subsequent encounters with that allergen will result in a localized anaphylactic reaction. This occurs when the allergen combines with two allergen-specific IgE molecules on the surface of the mast cell, forming a bridge. It is imperative that these molecules be physically close enough to allow this bridging to occur. The bridging causes a physical distortion of the antibody molecules, initiating a series of enzymatic events and resulting in degranulation of the mast cell and the release of pharmacologic mediators, which exert their effects on adjacent target tissue. The two major mediators of clinical disease in allergic rhinitis appear to be histamine and bradykinin. Both cause contraction of smooth muscles, increased vascular permeability, and increased secretion by nasal and bronchial mucous glands. Slow-reacting substance of anaphylaxis (SRS-A), which causes a prolonged constrictive effect on smooth muscles, is probably the principal mediator of the prolonged bronchospasm in bronchitis and asthma. Another important mediator is eosinophil chemotactic factor of anaphylaxis (ECF-A). It causes an influx of eosinophils into the area of allergic inflammation. Eosinophils contain enzymes that degrade histamine and SRS-A and are capable of phagocytizing IgE-containing immune complexes and intact mast cell granules. As such, they exert a negative feedback control on type I reactions by limiting the amount of mediator and removing the IgE-allergen complexes by phagocytosis.

Allergic Bronchopulmonary Aspergillosis

Allergic bronchopulmonary aspergillosis (ABPA) is an uncommon human syndrome that is due to multiple immunologic reactions against *Aspergillus fumigatus* that colonizes the mucous secretions of the bronchopulmonary tree without invading the tissue. Release of antigenic materials during its colonization is responsible for sensitization of the host. Four dogs have been recently diagnosed with ABPA at the University of Illinois Veterinary Medicine Teaching Hospital.

Initially, the clinical presentation is that of atopic or allergic asthma, which may include intolerance to exercise, wheezing, dyspnea, cough, peripheral eosinophilia, and sputum production. Chest radiographs reveal ill-defined pulmonary infiltrates. Atelectasis and pneumonia may occur, especially in the dependent lobes. The lesions may disappear, only to recur at a different location. As the disease progresses, signs of bronchiectasis involving the proximal airways and pulmonary fibrosis will develop.

The immunologic pathogenesis in ABPA involves a combination of type I and type III hypersensitivity reactions. The initial clinical signs of asthma and eosinophilia are due to a typical IgE-mediated allergic reaction. As the disease progresses, patients develop precipitating IgG antibodies to *Aspergillus*. Immune complexes involving IgG antibodies produce inflammatory injury to the walls of the major bronchi, resulting in proximal bronchiectasis.

Hypersensitivity Pneumonitis (Extrinsic Allergic Alveolitis)

Hypersensitivity pneumonitis (HP) is a diffuse inflammatory disease of the distal portions of the lungs following inhalation of a variety of organic dusts by sensitized hosts. The disease primarily affects the alveolar and interstitial tissues. The acute form of the disease is characterized by fever, dry cough, and dyspnea 4 to 6 hours after exposure of a sensitized animal to the antigen; it lasts approximately 12 hours, providing there is no additional exposure. Chest radiographs may be normal at this stage or may demonstrate the presence of infiltrates or nodules. The chronic form of the disease can result from either repeated or chronic exposure to the antigen. These patients present with clinical signs of chronic respiratory failure and pulmonary fibrosis. The pathologic condition of the lung at this stage of the disease is typical of interstitial fibrosis with granuloma formation.

HP differs from type I hypersensitivities in that it is not associated with IgE and it affects the terminal airways and lung parenchyma rather than the larger airways. The immunopathogenesis of this disease appears to involve both type III and type IV hypersensitivity reactions. Evidence for the involvement of a type III hypersensitivity reaction is the presence of high levels of complement-fixing, precipitating IgG antibodies and the time course of clinical reactivity following antigenic challenge. The development of interstitial fibrosis and granuloma formation in the chronic form of the disease strongly suggest that type IV reactions are also important in HP.

Idiopathic Interstitial Pulmonary Fibrosis

Idiopathic pulmonary fibrosis is a progressive interstitial lung disease of unknown cause. It starts as an alveolitis and progresses to interstitial fibrosis. The major clinical sign is dyspnea progressing to respiratory failure. Chest radiographs reveal diffuse interstitial infiltrates, which are most prominent in the dependent lung.

Tissue damage is a result of a chronic inflammatory reaction involving both neutrophils and macrophages. The alveolitis alters the lung parenchymal cells and mediates the interstitial fibrosis, which is caused both by derangement of interstitial collagen due to proteolytic enzymes released by the inflammatory cells and by increased lung fibroblast production or activity, which is mediated by macrophages. The stimulus for this chronic inflammatory reaction remains to be determined; however, circumstantial evidence suggests that immunologic mechanisms are involved. Patients with idiopathic interstitial pulmonary fibrosis have a high incidence of autoantibodies, elevated levels of serum immunoglobulins, elevated levels of IgG in bronchial secretions, and elevated levels of circulating immune complexes.

Sarcoidosis

Sarcoidosis is a systemic granulomatous disease of unknown cause involving the mediastinal lymph nodes and the interstitium of the lungs. The acute respiratory form of the disease consists of bilateral hilar lymphadenopathy and varying degrees of pulmonary infiltration. Progressive pulmonary fibrosis is characteristic of the chronic form of the disease in the lungs. Depending on the stage of the disease, radiographic findings vary from bilateral hilar lymphadenopathy to extensive pulmonary infiltrates with fibrosis.

The chronic inflammatory reaction involves primarily T lymphocytes and macrophages (type IV hypersensitivity reaction). The stimulus for the activation of the T cells is unknown, but their activation apparently plays an important role in the activation of the macrophages.

Pulmonary Infiltrates with Eosinophils

Pulmonary infiltrates with eosinophils (PIE) is characterized by diffuse inflammatory infiltrates in the lungs and a pronounced peripheral eosinophilia. In severe cases, dogs will have dyspnea and an intolerance to exercise and may have a chronic cough. Radiographs will exhibit the presence of diffuse interstitial infiltrates, and bronchial washes may contain numerous eosinophils, but on occasion eosinophils will only be seen on cytologic inspection of fine-needle lung aspirates.

This syndrome is usually associated with type I, IgE-mediated allergic reactions and allergic bronchopulmonary aspergillosis; it can also be a consequence of parasitic infections of the lungs (e.g., helminth and microfilarial infestations).

References and Supplemental Reading

Bienenstock, J. (ed.): *Immunology of the Lung and Upper Respiratory Tract.* New York: McGraw-Hill, 1984.

Tizard, I. *An Introduction to Veterinary Immunology.* Philadelphia: W. B. Saunders, 1982.

Wilkie, B. N.: Respiratory tract immune response to microbial pathogens. J.A.V.M.A. 181:1074, 1982.

RESPONSE OF THE LUNG TO INJURY

WANDA M. HASCHEK, B.V.Sc.
Urbana, Illinois

The lungs are exposed to a wide variety of potentially injurious agents. Infectious and noninfectious agents can reach the lungs through the airways after inhalation or through the bloodstream after ingestion, parenteral administration, or spread from other organs in the body. A variety of pulmonary defense mechanisms exist, such as mucociliary clearance and the alveolar macrophage system, which prevent contact of the injurious agent with vulnerable tissues. However, all too frequently these defenses are inadequate, and pulmonary injury occurs.

Recognition and understanding of the normal structure and function of the lungs and trachea are essential to the interpretation of the response to pulmonary injury. There is considerable variation in the gross and microscopic anatomy of the lungs between species; however, gaseous exchange and other functions are identical.

LUNG MORPHOLOGY

Gross Anatomy

The gross anatomy of the trachea and lungs of dogs and cats are very similar to each other. The trachea is virtually circular on cross section at each end, and the intervening portion is slightly flattened dorsally. The trachea bifurcates opposite the fifth rib into right and left principal bronchi, which further divide into lobar bronchi before entering the lungs.

The right lung is larger than the left and consists of four lobes. These lobes (and their old synonyms) are the cranial (anterior or apical), middle (or cardiac), caudal (posterior or diaphragmatic), and an accessory (intermediate or mediastinal). The left lung consists of two lobes, a cranial (anterior or apical) and a caudal (posterior or diaphragmatic). The left cranial lobe grossly is deeply divided by a fissure into a cranial and a caudal segment. Anatomically, these segments do not constitute lobes because their bronchi arise directly from the same principal bronchus. However, they function as lobes because they are surrounded almost completely by visceral pleura.

Table 1. *Comparative Pulmonary Anatomy*

Species	Secondary Lobulation	Pleura	Muscular Layer of Pulmonary Blood Vessels
Dogs, cats, rhesus monkeys	Absent	Thin	Thin
Horses, humans	Incomplete	Thick	Thin
Cattle, sheep, pigs	Present	Thick	Thick

Lobar (or secondary) bronchi divide into segmental (or tertiary) bronchi. Segmental bronchi and the pulmonary parenchyma they ventilate are known as bronchopulmonary segments. The segmental bronchi undergo further branching and a decrease in diameter, to the level of the bronchioles. The bronchioles branch into the terminal bronchioles and further into well-developed respiratory bronchioles, which are characterized by alveoli that open directly into their lumina. These respiratory bronchioles lead to alveolar ducts, which in turn lead to multiple alveolar sacs and thus to the alveoli, the smallest units of the respiratory system. The functional unit of the lungs is the acinus, which consists of the respiratory bronchiole and associated parenchymal unit. Many lung diseases, particularly those of aerogenous origin, affect acinar units.

Circulation of blood through the lungs is achieved through two separate systems, the pulmonary and bronchial. The pulmonary artery carrying venous blood from the right heart supplies the distal portion of the respiratory bronchioles, the alveolar ducts, and alveoli, as well as the pleura. The bronchial arteries are derived from the aorta and carry oxygenated blood. They supply the bronchi and terminate in the distal airways. The pulmonary veins course through the lung parenchyma alongside the bronchi and pulmonary arteries. Dog and cat lungs, unlike those of other common domestic animals and humans, are not subdivided into secondary lobules (Table 1) and do not have interlobular bronchial arteries. The nonlobulated lung allows for better collateral ventilation, which appears to occur through the respiratory bronchioles and alveolar ducts, which anastomose between adjacent lung segments. Unlike most domestic species, cats and dogs do not have bronchial artery–pulmonary artery anastomosis and, therefore, poorly tolerate distal occlusion of the bronchial artery. The muscular layer of the pulmonary arteries and veins, as well as the pleura, are thin in dogs and cats, as compared with other species (Table 1).

Lymphatic drainage from the lungs is accomplished through a subpleural network that is joined by perivascular and peribronchial lymphatics. Afferent lymphatic vessels from the lungs drain into the tracheobronchial lymph nodes and subsequently into the mediastinal lymph nodes.

Microscopic Anatomy

The cartilaginous support of the airways in dogs is fairly similar to that in humans but unlike that in rodents. The trachea is lined by pseudostratified columnar ciliated epithelium consisting primarily of ciliated cells, mucous cells, and basal cells with occasional brush cells and APUD (amine precursor uptake and decarboxylation) endocrine cells. Serous and mucous glands are present within the connective tissue of the submucosa. The C-shaped tracheal rings are composed of hyaline cartilage, which may ossify in older animals.

The bronchi and larger bronchioles are similar in histologic structure to the trachea, except that the cartilaginous structures are in the form of plates, rather than rings, and gradually decrease in size and number with decreasing bronchial diameter. The cartilaginous elements end when the diameter of the terminal bronchioles is equal to or less than 1 mm. There is a complete ring of smooth muscle encircling bronchi and bronchioles, extending to the level of the respiratory bronchiole. In larger airways, it is interposed as a layer between the cartilaginous plates and the mucosa. Bronchial glands are very abundant within the submucosa of cats but are inconspicuous in dogs.

The epithelium becomes flatter, and the number of mucous cells gradually decreases as the bronchial diameter becomes smaller. At the level of the terminal bronchiole, the mucous and basal cells disappear and the epithelium changes into simple columnar ciliated epithelium, and nonciliated bronchiolar epithelial (Clara) cells replace the mucous cells. The epithelium of the most distal airways consists almost entirely of Clara cells (see Nonciliated Bronchiolar Epithelial [Clara] Cells). In the respiratory bronchioles, the epithelium becomes cuboidal and finally merges with the alveolar epithelium. The latter epithelium consists of flat, thin, type I cells (membranous pneumocytes) and cuboidal type II cells (granular pneumocytes).

FUNCTIONAL CONSIDERATIONS

Collateral ventilation is a function of the degree of lung lobulation and affects the response to mechanical airway obstruction. Collateral ventilation in dogs (compared, for example, with that of pigs), allows maintenance of ventilation distal to small-airway obstruction. However, this is not true in larger airways, since collateral ventilation does not occur between lobes.

There are significant lobar variations in the ability of collateral ventilation to maintain tidal volume, with greatest capacity in the caudal lobes. This may partially explain why the incidence of atelectasis and pneumonia is least in the caudal lobes. However, drainage of secretions to the more ventral regions of the lungs may also play an important part. Failure to maintain adequate ventilation subsequent to airway obstruction may lead to alveolar hypoxia or atelectasis. Hypoxia may, among other things, suppress pulmonary macrophage function and allow development of pneumonia in air spaces with long collateral time constants (time required for 63 per cent pressure equilibration between an isolated segment and the remainder of the lung). The good collateral ventilation of a dog's lungs may allow the spread of inflammatory processes throughout a lobe, resulting in lobar pneumonia.

CELLS OF THE LUNG

Ciliated cells are the most abundant of all airway epithelial cells and, together with the epithelial mucous (goblet) cells, make up the bulk of the tracheobronchial epithelium. Ciliated epithelial cells and mucus-producing cells play an important role in the defense mechanism of the airways, as well as the upper respiratory tract, by contributing directly to the mucociliary transport system. This system combines mucus secretion and ciliary action to remove foreign particles, including viruses and bacteria, from the airway. In the terminal bronchioles, the mucous cells are gradually replaced by Clara cells, which are able to detoxify or activate foreign substances (xenobiotics).

In the alveoli, the major cell types are the epithelial type I and II cells and the pulmonary endothelial cells. These cells are frequently damaged during exposure to toxic or infectious agents. The major pulmonary defense in these distal regions of the lung is the alveolar macrophage system.

Ciliated and Mucous Epithelial Cells

BIOLOGY. Ciliated cells of the airway epithelium are columnar, with cilia extending from the luminal surface. The structure of cilia is basically the same in all species. The coordinated beat of the cilia transports mucus toward the pharynx, where it is swallowed. The physical nature of the mucous layer and the amount of mucus present can influence the efficacy of mucociliary clearance. Ciliary activity may be altered by histamine and serotonin, as well as by such factors as humidity, temperature, osmolarity, and pH.

The epithelial mucous cells, together with serous cells, contribute to the secretion of airway mucus. Serous cells produce a secretion of lower viscosity than that of mucous cells and, after exposure to certain irritants, may transform into mucous cells. Mucous and serous cells are found most frequently in the submucosal glands and epithelium of the trachea and large airways. The major source of mucus secretions appears to be the submucosal glands. Cholinergic, alpha-adrenergic, and beta-adrenergic stimulation increase secretion from the submucosal glands.

Secretion of mucus glycoproteins may be altered by chemical mediators, including histamine, prostaglandins, cyclic adenosine monophosphate (AMP) and guanosine monophosphate (GMP), and calcium ions. Some of these mediators may be released in response to airway damage or antigen challenge and may thus be associated with respiratory disease. (Refer to Respiratory Immunology for additional information on the inflammatory mediators in lung disease.)

Clinical Relevance. The airway epithelium is continually shed and regenerated from basal cells in the large airways and from Clara cells in terminal bronchioles. Damage to ciliated epithelial cells such as loss of cilia, ciliostasis, and cell destruction can be caused by pathogens such as *Mycoplasma*, *Bordetella*, and influenza virus; by air pollutants such as nitrogen dioxide, sulfur dioxide, and ozone; and even by hyperoxia. The end result of this damage is an impairment of mucociliary clearance.

Influenza virus and many of the paramyxoviruses enter the cell by way of attachment to the cilia, which subsequently slough from the surface, leaving only irregular microvilli. In contrast, bacteria that attach to cilia (e.g., *Bordetella* spp.) do not enter the cell but release toxins that cause cell degeneration and necrosis.

Structural defects are found in cilia from patients with (1) Kartagener's syndrome, characterized by the association of bronchiectasis, sinusitis, and *situs inversus*; (2) the "immotile cilia syndrome," in patients without *situs inversus*; and (3) in "primary ciliary dyskinesis," in which cilia are motile but the motion is abnormal. The clinical manifestations of these syndromes include productive cough, sinusitis, otitis, and bronchiectasis. Recurrent respiratory infections may be associated with impaired ciliary structure and function.

The principal causes of chronic bronchitis are believed to be exposure to airborne pollutants, such as irritant gases, and bacterial infection. Chronic bronchitis in dogs may be associated with *Bordetella bronchiseptica*, in which chronic cough is the major clinical manifestation. Early bronchitis is associated with loss of cilia, epithelial mucous cell hyperplasia, and hypertrophy of submucosal glands. In chronic bronchitis, dramatically increased numbers of mucous cells are seen in large, as well as small, peripheral airways. Patients with chronic bronchitis may produce 3 to 30 times the normal amount of mucus during exacerbations. Excess mucus has an irritant effect on sensory nerve endings, often inducing the cough reflex. Release of acetylcholine from irritated synapses of the autonomic innervation present in bronchiolar epithelium causes bronchiolar constriction and mucus secretion. In addition, serum proteins present in airway exudate of patients with chronic bronchitis, as well as in those with asthma and cystic fibrosis, appear to stimulate mucus secretion. It has been suggested that mucus secreted into small airways might interfere with the surfactant layer in the bronchioles and therefore cause airway collapse. In advanced cases, damage to bronchioles and alveoli may occur and can lead to the development of emphysema.

In allergic bronchitis ("feline asthma" in cats), mucus secretion is also increased and mucus viscosity may be altered. In cats, there is hyperplasia of bronchial glands and smooth muscle hypertrophy, with eosinophilic infiltration of bronchial walls. In chronic or severe asthma, the plugging of airways with thick, viscous mucus is a serious problem. This may be associated with structural changes in airways similar to those described for chronic bronchitis, as well as impairment of mucociliary transport. Release of mast cell mediators can further increase mucus glycoprotein secretion. Prostaglandins and arachidonic acid and its lipoxygenase products also appear to stimulate mucus secretion. It is therefore possible that drugs that can inhibit lipoxygenase may be effective in treating excessive mucus secretion. Drugs that increase mucus transport, such as beta-adrenergic agonists, theoretically may be of therapeutic value.

Nonciliated Bronchiolar Epithelial (Clara) Cells

Biology. Clara cells are columnar in shape and are found in large numbers in the bronchioles of dogs and cats. Although the basic morphologic features of Clara cells are similar in many species, their ultrastructure shows a great deal of interspecies variation. Unlike those in rats, mice, and rabbits, Clara cells in dogs and cats contain little smooth endoplasmic reticulum (SER). Ovoid membrane-bound granules, numerous in Clara cells of most species, appear to be absent in cats and rare in dogs.

The Clara cells appear to have a diverse range of functions. They are the progenitor cells for the bronchiolar epithelium after injury and differentiate into ciliated cells. Clara cells may also transform into mucus-secreting cells after continued airway irritation. They are also secretory cells, as evidenced by the presence of granules; however, the exact nature and function of the secreted material are not known. Clara cells may play a major role in the metabolism of exogenous agents. SER in quantity has been associated with detoxification or activation of xenobiotics via the cytochrome P_{450} mixed-function oxidase system. Metabolites so formed may be more active than their parent compound and may be carcinogenic, mutagenic, or highly toxic.

CLINICAL RELEVANCE. The relationship of the Clara cell to pulmonary function in both health and disease still remains to be determined. Since little SER is present in the Clara cells of dogs and cats, xenobiotic metabolism is not considered to be a major function in these species.

Alveolar Epithelial Cells

BIOLOGY. Alveolar type I cells are attenuated, highly differentiated cells that do not divide; they cover approximately 90 per cent of the alveolar surface. Since this cell has few organelles and a large surface area, it is highly susceptible to injury by a variety of agents. The main function of the type I cell is in gas exchange and the maintenance of a barrier to prevent leakage of fluid and proteins across the alveolar wall into the air spaces.

The type II cells are cuboidal in shape and contain characteristic lamellar bodies in which surfactant is stored. The role of the type II cell is to maintain alveolar stability and normal pulmonary function through the production of surfactant. The principal role of surfactant is to create a low surface tension during the expiratory phase of respiration and thus prevent alveolar collapse and atelectasis. Hormones such as corticosteroids and thyroid hormone appear to exert a strong influence on surfactant synthesis and production, and both adrenergic and cholinergic agents stimulate surfactant secretion. Hyperventilation appears to be a major physiologic stimulus for the secretion of surfactant. The type II cell is also the progenitor or stem cell for the alveolar epithelium and is able to proliferate and differentiate into type I cells. This occurs during lung development, after pneumonectomy, and after diffuse lung injury. Other postulated activities include defense of the lungs against oxidant injury by the enzyme superoxide dismutase, metabolism of some xenobiotic substances, and participation in fluid and electrolyte transport.

CLINICAL RELEVANCE. Type I cells are selectively damaged by such chemical toxins as paraquat and butylated hydroxytoluene and by viruses such as feline calicivirus. Paraquat also causes necrosis of type II epithelial cells. Necrosis is rapidly followed by type II cell division and repopulation of the alveolar surface. Type II cells then transform into type I cells, thus resulting in regeneration of the gas-exchanging alveolar surface. Interference with this normal sequence of events may lead to the development of pulmonary fibrosis.

Surfactant deficiency is a major factor in the neonatal respiratory distress syndrome, whereas deficient or altered surfactant lipids may play a role in the adult respiratory distress syndrome.

Endothelial Cells

BIOLOGY. The pulmonary capillary endothelium is a continuous, highly attenuated cell layer between the blood and lung tissue. It forms a barrier that prevents leakage of excess water and macromolecules into the pulmonary interstitium. It also functions in the transport of respiratory gases, water, and solutes and selectively processes a wide range of substances including vasoactive amines, prostaglandins, adenine nucleotides, peptides, lipids, hormones, and drugs. Pulmonary endothelial cells may determine the quantities of such substances entering the systemic circulation and may therefore influence activities of other organs in addition to those of the lung itself. The implications of these activities have yet to be investigated.

CLINICAL RELEVANCE. The pulmonary endothelium is susceptible to injury by a large number of toxic agents including endotoxins, hyperoxia, and chemotherapeutic agents such as bleomycin, as well as infectious agents such as *Ehrlichia canis* and microfilaria of *Dirofilaria immitis*. Injury may alter the biochemical activities of the pulmonary endothelium, affect intercellular junctions, or cause severe damage resulting in necrosis. Such injury may contribute to the development of pulmonary edema. Necrosis is normally followed by proliferation of the remaining endothelial cells, and interference with this process can also lead to fibrosis. Immune-mediated diseases such as anaphylaxis or immune complex disease may be initiated in the lungs by agents such as influenza and cytomegalovirus, which unmask receptors for the third component of complement, or the Fc portion of immunoglobin G, which are present on endothelial cells.

Alveolar Macrophages

BIOLOGY. Alveolar macrophages vary in morphology and state of activation. They are generally large, mononuclear phagocytic cells with numerous lysosomes and a well-developed rough endoplasmic reticulum. Alveolar macrophages are derived from monocytes that emigrate from the bone marrow and travel through the blood to the pulmonary interstitium, where they may divide, depending on available stimuli. The alveolar macrophages may either remain in the interstitium or migrate into the alveoli, from which they are usually cleared by mucociliary transport.

The alveolar macrophages participate in lung defense, inflammation, and immune responses. They are the first line of defense against inhaled particles, both infectious and noninfectious, which reach the alveoli. The alveolar macrophages attempt to phagocytize, digest, and export these particles from the lungs. Xenobiotics are also metabolically detoxified to some extent by the alveolar macrophages. The role of alveolar macrophages in inflammation and the immune response includes presentation of antigens to lymphocytes, release of factors that attract other inflammatory cells, and response to immunologic signals from sensitized lymphocytes (see also Respiratory Immunology).

CLINICAL RELEVANCE. During normal phagocytosis, a variety of enzymes with proteolytic, elastolytic, and inflammatory properties may be released into the cytoplasm or extracellular milieu. These enzymes, which are also released after cell death, are associated with inflammation, fibrosis, and emphysema.

In addition, increased susceptibility to respiratory infection occurs if the functions of the alveolar macrophages are compromised. In viral infection, phagocytosis and intracellular killing of bacteria are inhibited, and oxidant injury by gases such as oxygen, nitrogen dioxide, and ozone also depresses phagocytosis by alveolar macrophages.

RESPONSE TO INJURY

Although it would be of great diagnostic convenience if a characteristic type of response would be elicited by a particular agent, the lung responds in a similar way to a wide variety of infectious and toxic agents. The response does vary to some degree depending on the nature of the agent and on the severity and persistence of injury, as well as on the particular cell type affected and the reparative mechanisms initiated by the injury. Although the type of inflammatory reaction present may allow one to narrow the list of differential diagnoses, there is often little etiologic specificity in the histologic picture unless one can recognize the presence of specific viral inclusion bodies or of causative agents, such as fungal elements, themselves.

Airway Response

Injury to airways may nonspecifically affect all epithelial cells or be limited to a single cell type (Fig. 1). The acute response to severe injury, such as that caused by chemical agents or necrotizing viruses (e.g., herpesvirus and certain adeno- and myxoviruses), is nonspecific necrosis and sloughing

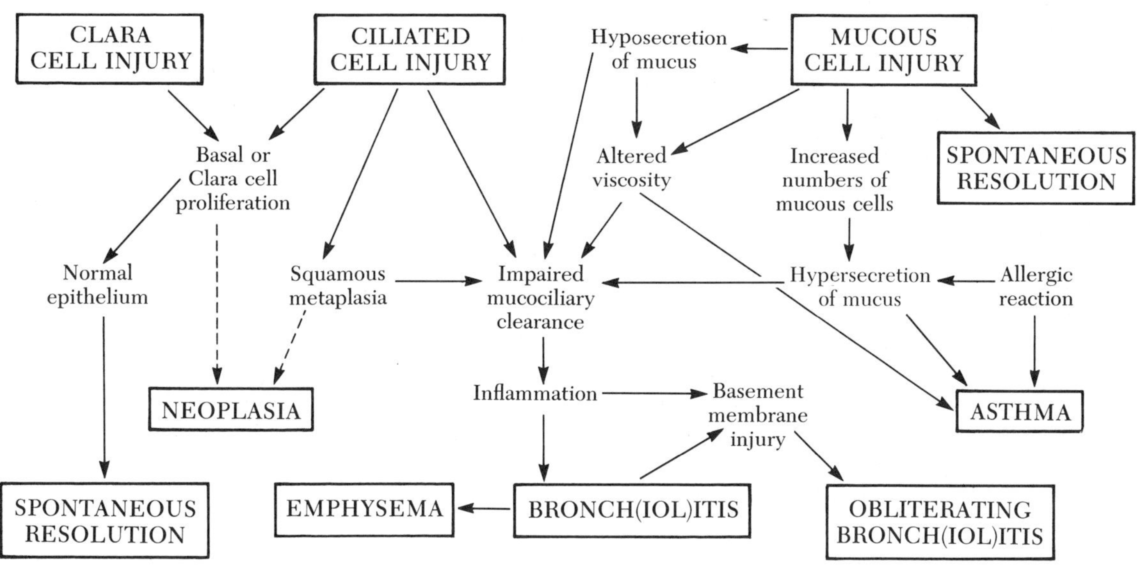

Figure 1. Airway injury: Injury to bronchi or bronchioles may lead to mucous cell injury or irritation with resultant hypersection of mucus or change in its viscosity. Injury to ciliated cells may result in impaired mucociliary clearance either directly or through squamous metaplasia. Spontaneous resolution may occur after Clara or basal cell proliferation, otherwise bronch(iol)itis, and even obliterating bronch(iol)itis, may occur if basement membrane has been damaged. If damage to alveoli follows, emphysema may develop. Solid line indicates proven progression; dashed line indicates unproven progression. (Adapted from Pickrell *in* Pickrell: *Lung Connective Tissue: Location, Metabolism, and Response to Injury.* Boca Raton, FL: CRC Press, 1981.)

of epithelium, resulting in severe necrotizing bronchitis and bronchiolitis. This leads to impairment of mucociliary clearance and inflammation. Inflammation may be confined to the airway wall or may spill over into the lumen. Neutrophils predominate in the early stages of inflammation, whereas mononuclear cells are prominent in later stages. Eosinophils may be associated with some allergic or parasitic conditions.

If the basement membrane is not damaged and the injurious agent does not persist, the epithelium may regenerate within a few days by basal cell or Clara cell proliferation. If the basement membrane is damaged, fibroblast precursors may migrate from the ulcerated airway wall into the lumen, particularly when a fibrinous exudate is present. Organization can occur within 7 to 10 days, resulting in obliterating bronchiolitis. If severe inflammation is present as well as basement membrane damage, bronchiectasis or abscess formation may occur.

Epithelial hyperplasia may be a feature in bronchitis, particularly with some adenovirus infections. Increased numbers of mucous cells in larger airways and mucous cell metaplasia from Clara cells in smaller airways may occur if continued irritation is present. The result is an overproduction of mucus in the larger airways and replacement of the normal watery bronchiolar secretion by mucus in the smaller airways. If spontaneous resolution does not take place, there may be narrowing or plugging of airways with consequent reduction of pulmonary function and predisposition to bronchopneumonia. Retrograde flow of mucus may lead to alveolar injury.

Damage to ciliated cells can alter normal clearance mechanisms and consequently mucus viscosity. Debris can accumulate and incite an inflammatory response. If clearance is impaired sufficiently and spontaneous resolution does not take place, obstruction of airways with concomitant bronchoconstriction and hypoxic vasoconstriction may occur and lead to alveolar injury and emphysema. If the damage is severe enough to cause necrosis of ciliated cells, proliferation of basal or Clara cells, depending on location within the airways, will occur. These cells will then transform into ciliated cells, and a normal epithelium will be restored. In the event of continued irritation, basal cells do not transform into ciliated cells but form a squamous epithelium (squamous metaplasia). Both squamous metaplasia and uncontrolled cell proliferation may potentially be followed by neoplasia.

Alveolar Response

Alveolar damage may occur to either endothelial or epithelial cells (Fig. 2). Endothelial cells are injured or die, exposing basement membrane and resulting in increased vascular permeability. Platelets may adhere to the vessel wall, resulting in complement activation, coagulation, and fibrinolysis before the basement membrane is repopulated. Increased vascular permeability allows the leakage of fluid into interstitial spaces and lymphatics. When epithelial cell junctions are damaged or when lymphatic drainage is overwhelmed and interstitial hydrostatic pressure rises, fluid can pour out into the alveolar spaces and result in alveolar edema. If damage is more severe, edema may be followed by interstitial inflammation.

Epithelial damage usually involves type I cells. Necrosis and sloughing of type I cells is accompanied by the acute exudative phase of inflammation. If the injury is not too severe and the basement membrane remains intact, type II cells will start to proliferate within 12 to 24 hours. Within the next few days, the exudative phase develops (characterized by fibrin, neutrophils, and edema), only to be replaced by a proliferative phase during which type II cells may line alveoli, and the inflammatory component will be composed of increasing numbers of mononuclear cells and macrophages. Resolution may occur by transformation of type II cells into type I cells and subsidence of the inflammatory component. However, if alveolar epithelium has been denuded and the basement membrane has been damaged, fibroblast precursors move rapidly into the alveolar space and, particularly in the presence of fibrin, will result in intra-alveolar fibrosis. Similarly, fibrosis may be a consequence of severe endothelial cell damage. Interstitial fibrosis may occur after distortion of the normal cell-cell contacts by inflammation or edema. Fibroblast proliferation can be noted within 72 hours after initial injury, and by 14 days dramatic fibrosis may be evident. In areas of such scarring, atypical type II cells may persist and neoplasia, so-called scar cancer, may result.

Continued inflammation of the alveolar wall implies persistence of the causative agent or injurious mechanisms and is an important feature of chronic interstitial pneumonia. The characteristic components of chronic alveolar irritation are proliferation and persistence of type II epithelial cells, interstitial thickening by fibrosis, and accumulation of mononuclear cells. Intra-alveolar exudate, when present, is usually composed of macrophages.

PNEUMONIA

Interstitial Pneumonia

Interstitial pneumonia results from diffuse or patchy damage to alveolar septa caused by a bloodborne insult in most instances, although inhalation

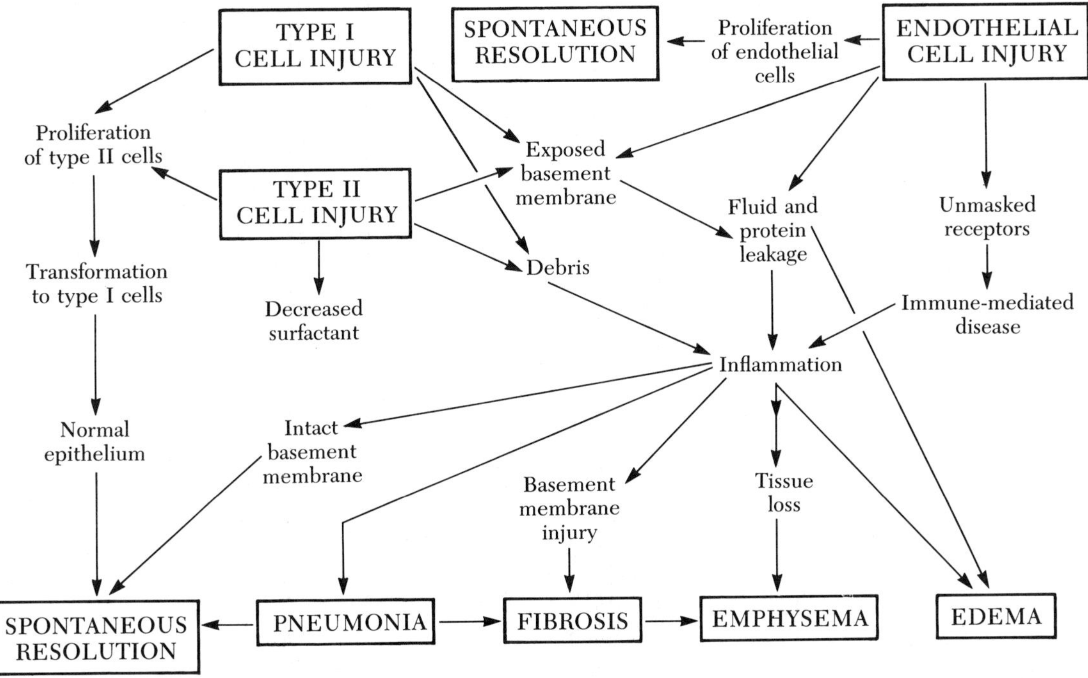

Figure 2. Alveolar Injury: If the basement membrane remains intact, damage to either the endothelium or epithelium is repaired by proliferation of endothelial or type II epithelial cells, respectively. Cellular damage with exposure of basement membrane results in increased permeability allowing fluid and protein leakage and ultimately inflammation. Cellular debris and immune-mediated disease may also initiate inflammation. Spontaneous resolution or, alternatively, scarring and fibrosis may occur if basement membrane is damaged. Severe tissue loss may progress to emphysema. (Adapted from Pickrell *in* Pickrell: *Lung Connective Tissue: Location, Metabolism, and Response to Injury.* Boca Raton, FL: CRC Press, 1981.)

of widely distributed irritants, such as oxygen, may also be responsible. Grossly, lesions of interstitial pneumonia are widely distributed throughout the lungs, often with greater involvement of the dorsocaudal areas.

In the acute phase, injury occurs to the capillary endothelial or alveolar epithelial cells, with subsequent flooding of alveoli with serofibrinous exudate. Occasionally, hyaline membranes composed of fibrin, serum proteins, and cell debris line the airspaces. This is followed by leukocytic infiltration of both alveolar lumina and interstitium. (Clinically, in human medicine, this stage of the disease is frequently referred to as the respiratory distress syndrome.) If the animal survives, the interstitial components soon predominate.

The central features of chronic interstitial pneumonia are intra-alveolar accumulation of various mononuclear cells (mostly macrophages), proliferation and persistence of alveolar type II cells, and interstitial thickening by accumulations of lymphoid cells and fibrous tissue.

Most of the recognized spontaneous interstitial pneumonias in animals are caused by infectious agents, chemical toxins (particularly those entering by the digestive tract), and allergic reactions. Systemic infections such as canine distemper, feline infectious peritonitis, toxoplasmosis, and canine ehrlichiosis may result in acute interstitial pneumonia. Noninfectious acute interstitial pneumonia may be encountered following hyperoxia and after the ingestion of paraquat in dogs, and it may progress to the chronic form if unresolved. Other causes of chronic interstitial pneumonia include histoplasmosis and the chronic hypersensitivity reaction, which may affect dogs with dirofilariasis.

In many cases, it is impossible to determine the causative agent from the histologic changes in the lung; however, in a small percentage of cases, identifying features may be present. These include characteristic inclusion bodies in viral infections such as canine distemper and adenovirus; the presence of the causative agent such as *Histoplasma* or *Toxoplasma*; a characteristic type of tissue response such as the severe necrosis frequently associated with toxoplasmosis; or the presence of multinucleated giant cells frequently associated with paramyxoviruses such as canine distemper.

Bronchopneumonia

Most inhaled viruses such as adeno-, myxo-, and caliciviruses can infect both airway and alveolar epithelium and thus produce lesions involving bronchioles and the adjacent alveolar parenchyma. This histologic orientation of inflammation around small airways is characteristically referred to as bronchopneumonia, although the term *broncho-interstitial* pneumonia has also been used. The term *interstitial pneumonia* is frequently retained for these viral infections, since interstitial accumulation of lymphocytes, plasma cells, and macrophages rapidly becomes the predominant feature.

Viral infection paves the way for bacterial disease, so that in many cases (e.g., in canine distemper), bacteria-induced bronchopneumonia becomes a feature of the typical syndrome produced by that virus. In many cases, the primary mechanism by which viruses increase susceptibility to bacterial infection appears to be by decreasing the bactericidal mechanisms of the lung as a result of a dysfunction in intracellular processing within the alveolar macrophage. Other contributing factors may be the destruction of ciliated cells, with resulting impairment of mucociliary clearance, and the presence of edema fluid, which may allow sufficiently rapid bacterial multiplication to overcome ingestion by alveolar macrophages.

Severe bronchopneumonia in animals is primarily due to gram-negative bacteria such as *Escherichia coli, Klebsiella, Pseudomonas, Pasteurella,* and *Bordetella* or exogenous material such as feed or medication, which enters the lungs by aspiration. The resulting inflammation is oriented around small airways, and the gross pattern generally has a cranioventral distribution. The pattern of inflammation depends on the type and virulence of the bacteria involved. Typically the pneumonia progresses through hyperemia, serous exudate, and cellular infiltrate, which is characterized by intense exudation of inflammatory cells (primarily neutrophils) into the alveoli and airways. Resolution of the bronchopneumonia depends on the extent of damage to the alveolar and airway walls and the persistence of the invading organisms. Complications of bronchopneumonia include bronchiectasis, abscess formation, fibrosis, and pyothorax.

CONCLUSION

The lungs are continuously exposed to a large variety of potentially injurious agents, both infectious and noninfectious. Pulmonary defense depends on mucociliary clearance and the function of alveolar macrophages to prevent injury from occurring in most cases. If injury does take place, an inflammatory response occurs and repair mechanisms are activated. When damage is severe or the agent persists, permanent damage such as fibrosis or emphysema may result. Fortunately, in the majority of cases, the injury is adequately repaired and inflammation is resolved.

From a diagnostic standpoint, it would be very convenient if each causative agent would incite a characteristic reaction. Unfortunately, the lungs, like many other organs, can respond to injury in only a limited number of ways, and only a few generalities are possible. A list of differential diagnoses may be made based on the species affected, clinical data, and, if the animal dies, on the pattern of gross and microscopic changes present. However, in many cases, a definitive diagnosis depends on the microscopic identification of the specific etiologic agent or specific agent-induced changes.

References and Supplemental Reading

Chevile, N. F.: *Cell Pathology*, 2nd ed. Ames: Iowa State University Press, 1983, pp. 530–558.

Dungworth, D. L.: Interstitial pulmonary disease. Adv. Vet. Sci. Comp. Med. 26:173, 1982.

Gail, D. B., and Lenfant, C. J. M.: Cells of the lung: Biology and clinical implications. Am. Rev. Respir. Dis. 127:366, 1983.

Pickrell, J. A.: Sequence of events in pulmonary injury. *In*: Pickrell, J. A. (ed.): *Lung Connective Tissue: Location, Metabolism, and Response to Injury*. Boca Raton, FL: CRC Press, 1981, pp. 123–130.

Plopper, C. G., Mariassay, A. T., and Hill, L. H.: Ultrastructure of the nonciliated bronchiolar epithelial (Clara) cell of mammalian lung. II. A comparison of horse, steer, sheep, dog, and cat. Exp. Lung Res. 1:155, 1980.

Robinson, N. E.: Some functional consequences of species differences in lung anatomy. Adv. Vet. Sci. Comp. Med. 26:1, 1982.

TRACHEOBRONCHIAL CYTOLOGY

WALTER E. HOFFMANN, D.V.M.,
Urbana, Illinois

and MAXEY L. WELLMAN, D.V.M.
Columbus, Ohio

Cytology is becoming an increasingly valuable tool in the diagnosis of disease in veterinary medicine and will continue to gain importance as more veterinarians make use of this technique. Its use should be encouraged, as it can be an efficient and practical means of helping to establish a diagnosis. Cytology often can rule out several possible causes while lending support to others, and it is invaluable in leading the veterinarian to appropriate therapy. It might be reasoned that each one of us who has looked at a cell through a microscope is a cytologist. There is no reason, therefore, to avoid using and improving these skills. "Look and you shall see, don't look and you never will" (Perman et al., 1979).

These comments are especially appropriate when considering tracheobronchial cytology. Specimens for tracheobronchial cytology may be obtained in an atraumatic manner. Microscopic examination provides an immediate description of the disease process and, in many cases, establishes a cause for that disease, which in turn suggests a specific treatment.

TECHNIQUES AND INDICATIONS FOR THE COLLECTION OF SPECIMENS

Cytologic specimens taken for the purpose of establishing an etiologic diagnosis in respiratory disease are likely to be of diagnostic value only when appropriate sampling techniques are used. These techniques include transtracheal aspiration, bronchial washing, bronchial brushing, and percutaneous transthoracic aspiration of the lung. The techniques and indications for each of these procedures are described in *Current Veterinary Therapy VIII*, but it should be emphasized that no single technique is suitable for obtaining specimens of diagnostic value in *all* forms of respiratory disease.

SAMPLE HANDLING

Processing of samples for tracheobronchial cytology is dependent on collection techniques used. The cellularity of samples collected in saline (transtracheal aspiration and bronchial wash) is quite variable. Direct smears should be made from these samples and used to estimate cellularity. However, for samples containing low numbers of cells, cell concentration techniques prior to slide preparation enable the visualization of larger numbers of cells. These concentration techniques include slow centrifugation (1500 to 2000 rpm) to sediment the cells or cytocentrifugation. After slow centrifugation, the supernate is decanted and sedimented cells are gently resuspended in the remaining drops of saline. A drop of these cells may be dispersed between two microscope slides or coverslips, resulting in a monolayer of cells with a minimal amount of cell damage. Cytocentrifuge preparations of cells are ideal but require a centrifuge, not readily available to most veterinarians.

Bronchial brushings and lung aspirates contain variable numbers of cells, which are often present in a very small amount of material. Bronchial brushings can be gently rolled onto the surface of a microscope slide, whereas lung aspirates can be prepared by the microscope slide dispersion technique described above.

Prepared slides should be air dried and stained. Either a Romanovsky's stain (Wright's, Wright's-Giemsa, or one of the rapid stains*) or new methylene blue can be used on air-dried specimens. The Romanovsky's stains combine the advantages of a relatively easy technique and, because of their routine use in staining blood smears, familiar staining characteristics. The Papanicolaou's stain is not suitable for air-dried slides but can be used after wet fixation in 95 per cent ethanol.

NORMAL PULMONARY CYTOLOGY

(For a discussion of the normal cells in the respiratory tract, see Response of the Lungs to Injury.)

---

*Dif-Quik (Harleco) or Camco Quik (Cambridge Chemical Products)

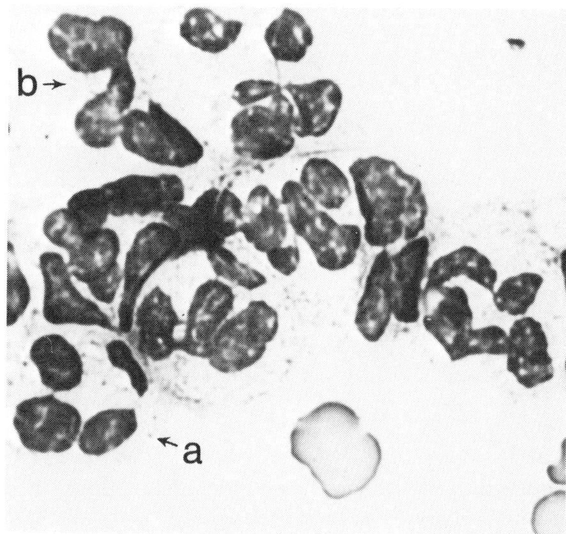

Figure 1. Concentrated preparation of cells obtained by tracheal wash. Hypersegmented neutrophil (*a*) and ragged-appearing or lysed neutrophil (*b*) (×1200).

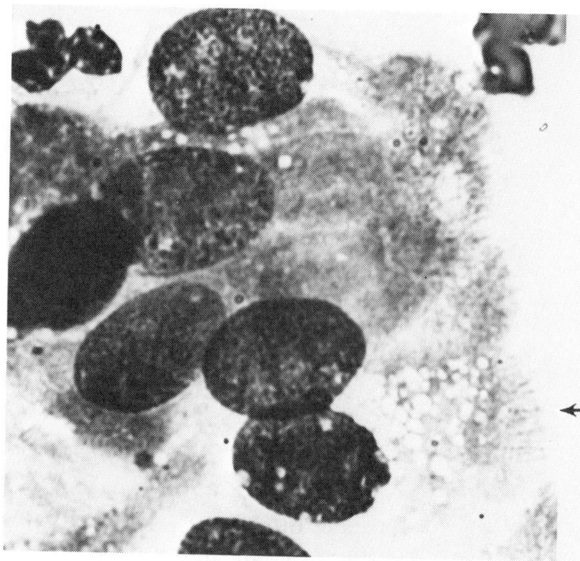

Figure 3. Ciliated epithelial cells obtained by bronchial brushing. Note cilia at arrow (×1200).

The cells observed in a transtracheal aspiration and bronchial wash from normal animals include a few to moderate numbers of neutrophils, epithelial cells, and goblet cells; a few alveolar macrophages; and a rare lymphocyte or eosinophil. This mixed cell population reflects the removal of foreign material, the sloughed macrophages and epithelial cells, and neutrophils by the mucociliary blanket.

The neutrophils obtained by transtracheal aspiration have been subjected to a series of environmental changes and may exhibit a more ragged appearance than peripheral blood neutrophils (Fig. 1).

Alveolar macrophages are identified by their round to oval appearance; large size (greater than 10 μm); and round, eccentrically located nucleus. These cells are classified as differentiated (activated) alveolar macrophages (Fig. 2) if they are even larger in size and have abundant cytoplasm and numerous cytoplasmic vacuoles. Generally the macrophages from the normal animals are of the undifferentiated type with few or no vacuoles.

Respiratory epithelial cells can be easily identified by their columnar to cuboidal shape, prominent cilia, granular-appearing chromatin, basally located nucleus, and prominent nucleoli (Fig. 3). Cyto-

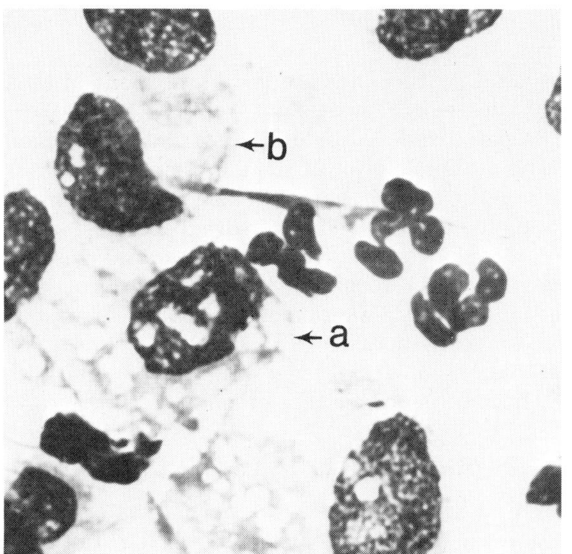

Figure 2. Slide made from lung aspirate demonstrating differentiated macrophage (*a*) and undifferentiated macrophage (*b*) in the presence of three neutrophils (×1200).

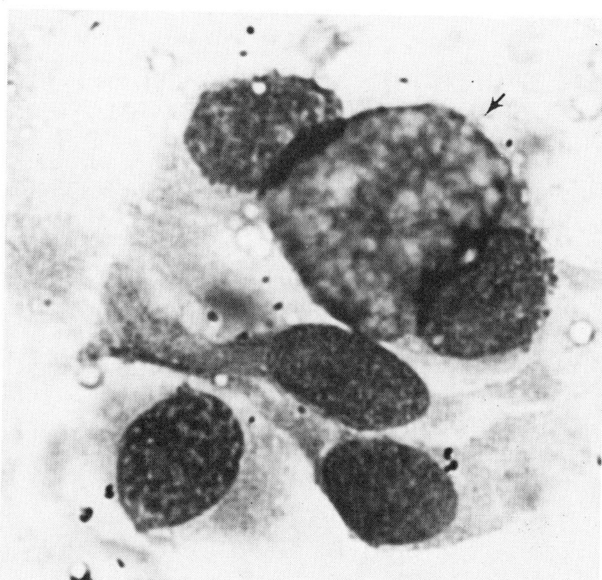

Figure 4. Slide made from bronchial brushing demonstrating a goblet cell (arrow) and several epithelial cells (×1200).

plasmic vacuolation may often be present. It should be expected that many of these cells may no longer be intact and that all identifying characteristics may not be visible. Goblet cells also are columnar in shape with a basally located nucleus (Fig. 4). However, goblet cells do not have cilia and contain characteristic large vacuoles that hold mucin.

Bronchial brushing is more likely to yield entire sheets of the ciliated bronchial epithelial cells. Aspiration of the lung results in a lower number but more diversified population of cells. The aspiration technique results in passage of the needle through a highly vascular organ, and some amount of blood is therefore to be expected, but the predominant cells from the lung itself will be the ciliated epithelial cells. The observation of cilia is undisputed identification of these cells and assurance that a specimen from the lung was truly obtained.

ABNORMAL FINDINGS AND INTERPRETATION

Abnormal findings in a cytologic preparation from the trachea or lung can include increased numbers of a specific cell, the presence of infectious or parasitic organisms, and atypical cells. Increases in neutrophil numbers indicate an inflammatory condition, and these are the most commonly seen increased cell type. Evidence of neutrophil degeneration, including karyolysis (nuclear swelling), is indicative of a toxic environment and suggests a septic process as the cause of the inflammation. Hypersegmentation and pyknosis (nuclear condensation) of neutrophils (Fig. 1) are indicative of a relatively nontoxic environment and suggest a nonseptic inflammatory condition. Care must be taken in assessing the condition of neutrophils obtained by tracheal wash, since this process can result in artifactual changes in neutrophil morphology.

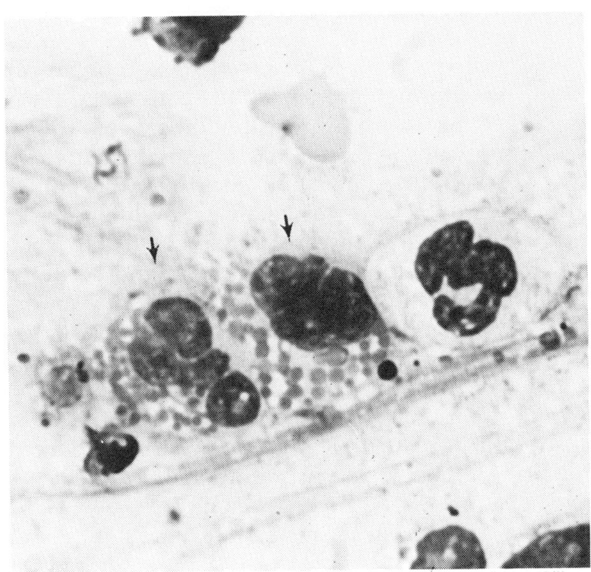

Figure 5. Slide made from bronchial brushing demonstrating two eosinophils (arrows) and a neutrophil (×1200).

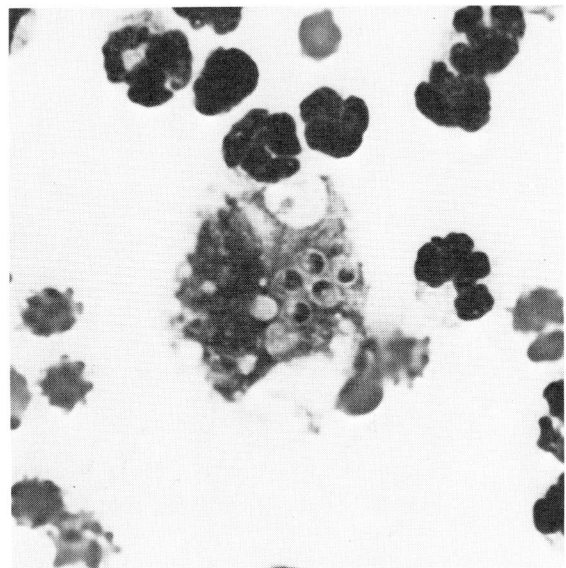

Figure 6. Several encapsulated *Histoplasma* organisms in large macrophage in center of picture. Note size of organisms compared with neutrophil and crenated red blood cells on slide (×1200).

Eosinophils also are often found in increased numbers. These cells are recognized by their segmented nucleus and orange-red granules on a Wright's stained smear (Fig. 5). As with neutrophils, eosinophils also can be injured during collection and processing, resulting in the release of their granules. Care must be taken to ensure that these cells do not go unnoticed. Increases in eosinophils occur in hypersensitivity reactions, which can be a result of parasitic infection or inhaled allergens. It is unusual to demonstrate the cause on the smear.

Increased numbers of goblet cells are generally seen on smears from animals with a history of chronic cough or chronic pulmonary disease. They are accompanied by abundant extracellular mucus. Spiral-shaped molds (Curschmann's spirals) suggest chronic obstruction of lower airways.

A cell sometimes seen and referred to as a globule leukocyte contains large metachromatic granules similar to the mast cell. These cells may represent a later stage in the life cycle of the mast cell and are involved in immunologic reactions in tissue. The presence of these cells is not diagnostic of any specific cause, and they have been observed with fungal infections and parasitic and neoplastic diseases of the lungs. These cells are not consistently present in any of these conditions, however.

Increased numbers of alveolar macrophages, especially activated macrophages, suggest a subacute to chronic inflammatory condition. They are more often seen in samples collected by fine-needle lung

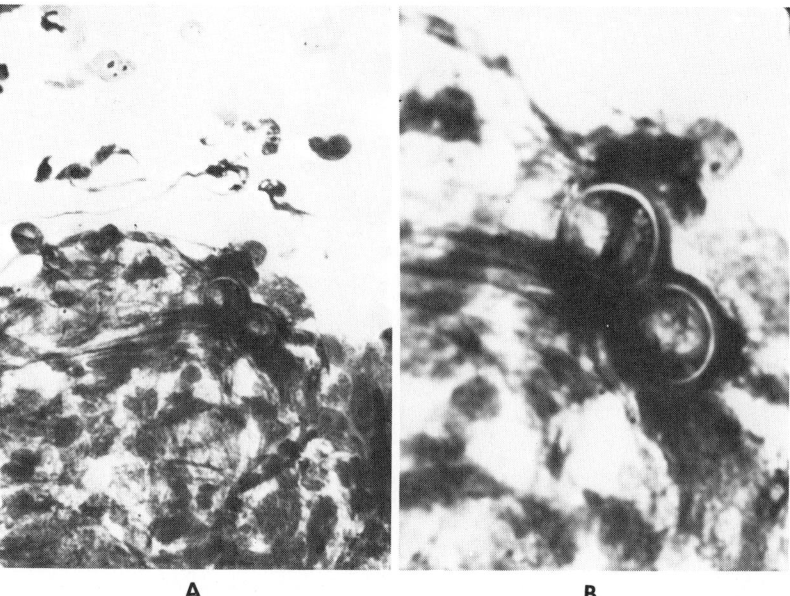

Figure 7. *A*, note encapsulated *Blastomyses* organism giving appearance of figure eight in thick area of smear made from bronchial brushing (×500). *B*, higher magnification of the same field; organism is surrounded by nuclear debris from lysed cells (×1200).

aspiration or transtracheal aspirate or bronchial wash than in those samples taken by bronchial brushing. Activated alveolar macrophages may contain mucus, carbon, hemosiderin, fungal organisms, and occasionally whole cells.

Bacteria can be seen at 1000-power magnification. Observation of a few organisms does not imply a pathologic process. Evidence of neutrophils in large numbers implies an inflammatory process, and the presence of bacteria within neutrophils strongly suggests that a bacterial cause exists. Not all bacteria will stain with the Romanovsky's stain, and identification of type of bacteria cannot be made with this stain; therefore, it is suggested that a Gram stain and culture be made to identify the specific organism involved (see also Bacteriology of the Lower Respiratory Tract).

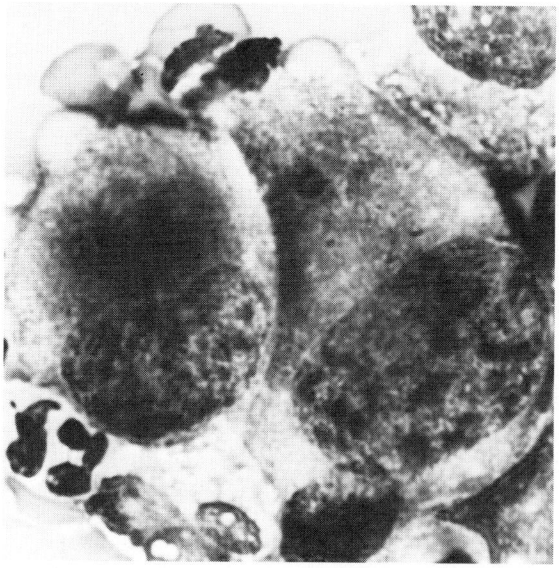

Several fungal organisms can occur in respiratory cytologic samples. These include *Histoplasma capsulatum*, *Blastomyces dermatitis*, *Cryptococcus neoformans*, and *Coccidioides immitis*. The prevalence of these organisms is highly correlated with geographic exposure. With a Romanovsky's stain, these organisms are recognized primarily by their nonstaining capsule and their size. *Histoplasma* organisms (Fig. 6) are approximately 2 μm in diameter; have a thin, nonstaining capsule and stained cytoplasm; and usually are found within macrophages. *Blastomyces* organisms (Fig. 7) are approximately 8 to 15 μm in diameter; have a well-defined, thick, double-walled capsule with a well-stained organism within the capsule; and are often seen as the budding yeast form with a broad budding base. *Cryptococcus* organisms are 8 to 15 μm in diameter; have a less well defined but very thick, unstained capsule; and have a very narrow budding base. *Coccidioides* organisms are larger (20 to 60 μm), are often surrounded by neutrophils, and occur in animals with a history of exposure in the southwestern United States. Recognition of the latter three types of organisms can generally be made by scanning the thicker part of the smears with 100 × magnification, but confirmation and identification will require greater magnification. Visualization of the *Histoplasma* organism requires 400 to 1000 × magnification. These mycoses cannot always be diagnosed with tracheal washings or brushings and may require lung aspirates of lesions identified on thoracic radiographs or cytology specimens collected from other affected organs.

Figure 8. Neoplastic cells obtained by bronchial brushing. Note large size of cells compared with neutrophil and variation in nuclear size between the two cells (×1200).

The use of the techniques described above for diagnosis of metazoan parasitic diseases involving the respiratory tract is less rewarding. The smear may reveal an eosinophilic infiltrate with no evidence of the parasite, its eggs, or larvae. Fecal samples should be checked for evidence of enteric parasites, whose larval migration through the lungs may result in clinical respiratory disease (see *Current Veterinary Therapy VII and VIII* for a detailed description of the more common metazoan respiratory parasites). Identification of microfilaria as being derived from *Dirofilaria immitis* may suggest that the lung disease is a result of this organism.

Neoplastic cells present in the lung or trachea can be a result of either primary or metastatic neoplasms (Fig. 8). Criteria by which cells can be identified as neoplastic include variation in cell size; variation in nuclear to cytoplasmic ratio; variation in size, shape, and number of nuclei and nucleoli; finely stippled chromatin; unusually basophilic cytoplasm; and abnormal mitotic figures. Although not all of these criteria will be present in each case, sufficient numbers should be evident to ensure that the process is neoplastic and not hyperplastic. It should be emphasized that this differentiation cannot always be made cytologically, especially with well-differentiated tumors. Histologic examination of the lesion usually can resolve the problem. The most commonly seen primary neoplasm in the lungs is the adenocarcinoma, which may have additional criteria such as abnormal cellular adhesions or altered mitotic activity, resulting in multinucleated cells and cells of extremely large size.

Metastatic tumors include both carcinomas and sarcomas. Depending on location, these may be diagnosed by transtracheal aspiration, bronchial wash, or brushing. Greater success will be attained with lung aspirates guided by visualization of the lesion on radiographs or directly through fluoroscopy. Although neoplastic cells can often be recognized as such, it is often difficult to identify the specific neoplastic cell type. Histopathologic study of the lesion is usually required to determine the cell of origin.

References and Supplemental Reading

Breeze, R. G., and Wheeldon, E. G.: State of the art: The cells of the pulmonary airways. Am. Rev. Respir. Dis. 116:705, 1977.

Greenlee, P. G., and Roszel, J. F.: Feline bronchial cytology: Histologic/cytologic correlation in 22 cats. Vet. Pathol. 21:308, 1984.

Perman, V., Alsaker, R. D., and Riis, R. C.: *Cytology of the Dog and Cat.* South Bend, IN: American Animal Hospital Association, 1979.

Rebar, A. H., DeNichola, D. B., and Muggenburg, B. A.: Bronchopulmonary lavage cytology in the dog: Normal findings. Vet. Pathol. 17:294, 1980.

BACTERIOLOGY OF THE LOWER RESPIRATORY TRACT

DWIGHT C. HIRSH, D.V.M.
Davis, California

Infectious disease of the lower respiratory tract leads to significant mortality unless prompt therapeutic intervention is instigated. Use of an antimicrobial drug that is effective against the agent of infection is crucial. The susceptibility of the agent to antimicrobial drugs will not be known for 48 hours after collection of the sample, too long to be of use in the formulation of the initial treatment plan. The purpose of the discussion that follows is to outline a rational approach to the selection of an antimicrobial drug in the initial treatment of bacterial disease of the lungs.

DETERMINING AN INFECTIOUS CAUSE

The lower respiratory tract is the most difficult of the organ systems to culture bacteriologically. Unless precautions are taken, representative samples should not be obtained from the respiratory system by any transoral approach because of the potential for contamination by indigenous oral flora. Suitable methods used to sample the respiratory tract include transtracheal aspiration technique and bronchoscopic wash (or brush). In very rare cases, percutaneous transthoracic lung aspiration may be indicated. By using these techniques, the oral cavity is bypassed and a representative specimen from the respiratory tract is obtained, and therefore the validity of a properly taken sample is not compromised. Though the normal lower respiratory tract may not be sterile, the number of microorganisms found is low (i.e., less than 10^4/gm of lung tissue).

Whether or not an infectious agent is involved must be determined in order to form a rational basis for the use of an antimicrobial drug. Observation of the contents of a stained direct smear and bacteriologic culture of the sample are two ways in which this determination can be accomplished. Ideally, both should be performed.

Observing bacteria in the direct smear is the quickest and easiest way to determine whether the process is infectious. What stain is used is immaterial. Most practices will have one stain at their disposal for routine hematology, usually a Romanovsky's-type stain (e.g., Wright's stain). The presence (or absence) of bacteria and the shape of the organisms will form the basis for a rational choice of antimicrobial agent.

Approximately one third of tracheal washes from dogs with bacterial pneumonia will contain sufficient numbers of bacteria to be seen in stained smears prepared from pellets obtained after centrifugation (in centrifuge or cytofuge). Noting the shape of the bacteria is crucial. Cocci are either *Staphylococcus* or *Streptococcus*. Rods are almost always gram-negative. The most common isolates obtained from transtracheal aspirates of dogs with suspected bacterial pneumonia presented at the Veterinary Medical Teaching Hospital, University of California, are shown in Table 1.

Table 1. *Bacterial Agents Isolated from the Lower Respiratory Tract of Dogs (n = 105) with Bacterial Pneumonia**

Bacterial Agents		No. of Isolates (%)
Members of family Enterobacteriaceae		46 (44)
Escherichia coli	30 (29)	
Klebsiella pneumoniae	16 (15)	
Pasteurella multocida		28 (27)
Pasteurella spp.		7 (7)
Anaerobic bacteria		19 (18)
Bordetella bronchiseptica		16 (15)
Pseudomonas aeruginosa		6 (6)
Other gram-negative rods		13 (12)
Streptococcus		24 (23)
S. canis	12 (11)	
beta streptococci	5 (5)	
alpha/gamma steptococci	4 (4)	
other streptococci	3 (3)	
Coagulase-positive *Staphylococcus*		9 (9)
Mycoplasma spp.		5 (5)

*Veterinary Medical Teaching Hospital, University of California, 1982–1984.

SELECTING AN ANTIMICROBIAL AGENT

Once the presence of bacterial forms and their shape are noted, a choice of antimicrobial agent can be made. If rod-shaped forms are seen, it must be assumed that a member of the family Enterobacteriaceae is present, because they are the most frequently isolated. The members of this family are also the most unpredictable with respect to susceptibility to antimicrobial agents. The one drug preparation that is active against most of the gram-negative rods that are commonly isolated, except for *Klebsiella pneumoniae*, is trimethoprim-sulfonamide (Tables 2 and 3). If the presence of *K. pneumoniae* is a distinct possibility, then the broadest coverage can be obtained with a combination of a cephalosporin and trimethoprim-sulfonamide. If coccal forms are seen, then the presence of *Staphylococcus* or *Streptococcus* is possible. A cephalosporin or trimethoprim-sulfonamide is a reasonable choice in these cases. Mixed infections account for 42 per cent of positive cases (Table 4).

In order to confirm whether the correct choice of an antimicrobial agent has been made, the sample must be subjected to bacteriologic culture. A susceptibility test should be run on any isolate whose susceptibility to a particular antimicrobial cannot be predicted. Of the frequently encountered causes of bacterial pneumonia, these are the members of the family Enterobacteriaceae, in particular *Escherichia coli* and *K. pneumoniae*. All of the others are predictably susceptible to certain antimicrobial agents (Tables 2 and 3).

To determine as quickly as possible whether the isolate is a member of the family Enterobacteriaceae, certain methods are available to the clinician. If the sample containing the isolate is sent to a commercial or diagnostic laboratory, this determination will be made by the use of the oxidase test. This test is run on an isolate (obtained 24 hours after submission of the sample), and the results are available at this time. All members of the family Enterobacteriaceae are oxidase-negative, whereas *Bordetella bronchiseptica*, *Pasteurella* spp. (*Pasteurella multocida* is the most commonly encountered), and *Pseudomonas aeruginosa* are oxidase-positive. The microbiologist at the diagnostic or the commercial laboratory should be able to give a clue as to the identity of the isolate so that a determination whether to change or continue with the therapy started 24 hours previously can be made.

The same answers can be obtained in the practice laboratory if the sample is inoculated onto a bi-plate containing blood agar on one side and MacConkey agar on the other. How the isolate appears the next day will allow the clinician to make a rational decision in the therapeutic strategy for the case. Briefly, members of the family Enterobacteriaceae and *P. aeruginosa* grow on the blood agar and the MacConkey agar to the same size after 24 hours'

Table 2. *Antimicrobial Susceptibility of Common Isolates from the Lower Respiratory Tract of the Dog*

Bacterial Isolate (Antimicrobials)	Minimal Inhibitory Concentration (μ/ml)*			Approximate MIC Correlate Susceptible
	Range	50%	90%	
E. coli (n = 25)				
Amikacin	<2–4	<2	4	<16
Ampicillin	<0.1–>64	37	60	<8
Carbenicillin	4–>256	150	256	<16
Cephalothin	2–>64	4.5	20	<8
Erythromycin	8–>16	13	16	<2
Gentamicin	<0.25–4	0.33	1.2	<4
Penicillin	16–>32	23	30	<2
Tetracycline	4–>64	45	62	<4
Trimethoprim-sulfonamide†	<0.25–>8	<0.25	5	<2
K. pneumoniae (n = 13)				
Amikacin	NA	<2	<2	<16
Ampicillin	8–>64	47	66	<8
Carbenicillin	64–>256	190	260	<16
Cephalothin	2–16	3.2	10	<8
Erythromycin	1–>16	11	15	<2
Gentamicin	0.25–8	2.3	7	<4
Penicillin	16–>32	2	29	<2
Tetracycline	4–>32	10	23	<4
Trimethoprim-sulfonamide†	<0.2–>8	1.3	6.6	<2
B. bronchiseptica (n = 15)				
Amikacin	<2–16	2.8	7.9	<16
Ampicillin	2–32	<2	9.6	<8
Carbenicillin	2–32	13	30	<16
Cephalothin	8–>64	13	30	<8
Erythromycin	0.5–>16	1.3	7	<2
Gentamicin	0.5–32	0.62	2.3	<4
Penicillin	16–>32	13	35	<2
Tetracycline	<0.5–32	0.7	1.7	<4
Trimethoprim-sulfonamide†	<0.25–4	<0.25	0.7	<2

* = 50 per cent and 90 per cent MIC required to inhibit 50 per cent and 90 per cent of the isolates, respectively.
† = Value expressed is for trimethoprim concentration. Trimethoprim and sulfonamide are formulated in a 1:20 ratio.

incubation. *Pseudomonas* will have a characteristic odor (described as "tortillalike"). *Pasteurella* will not grow on MacConkey agar. *Bordetella* will grow on blood and MacConkey agar, but after 24 hours of incubation, the colonies are very small (less than 1 mm in diameter), especially on the MacConkey agar. *Staphylococcus* and *Streptococcus* will not grow on MacConkey agar and will have characteristic pigmentation (*Staphylococcus* is white), hemolytic pattern (complete hemolysis around a streptococcal colony, usually two zones around a staphylococcal colony), or size (streptococcal colonies are less than 1 mm in diameter).

In summary, the use of clinical microbiology as a guide to initial therapy of diseases of the lower respiratory tract starts with the examination of stained direct smears for infectious forms. Depending on the shape of the agent—rod or coccus—a rational choice of an antimicrobial drug can be made. The results of culture and, if necessary, susceptibility testing may further guide the treatment strategy.

Table 3. *Antimicrobial Susceptibility of Common Isolates from the Lower Respiratory Tract of the Dog*

Bacterial Isolate (Antimicrobials)	Percent Susceptible
Anaerobic species (n = 14)	
Ampicillin	93
Cephalothin	93
Penicillin	86
Tetracycline	93
Trimethoprim-sulfonamide	100
P. multocida (n = 9)	
Ampicillin	100
Cephalothin	100
Erythromycin	33
Gentamicin	89
Penicillin	93
Tetracycline	88

Table 4. *Number of Isolates Per Positive Sample*

No. of Isolates	Frequency (%)
1	57 (58)
2	23 (23)
3	11 (11)
≥4	7 (7)

References and Supplemental Reading

Creighton, S. R., and Wilkins, R. J.: Transtracheal aspiration biopsy: Technique and cytologic evaluation. J. Am. Anim. Hosp. Assoc. 10:219, 1974.

English, P. B.: Plasma concentration and disposition of antimicrobial agents in the dog. Aust. Vet. J. 60:353, 1983.

Lindsey, J. O., and Pierce, A. K.: An examination of the microbiologic flora or normal lung of the dog. Am. Rev. Respir. Dis. 117:501, 1978.

van der Waaij, D.: *Antibiotic Choice: The Importance of Colonization Resistance.* New York: Research Studies Press, 1983, pp. 33–35.

THORACIC RADIOGRAPHY

S. K. KNELLER, D.V.M.

Urbana, Illinois

POSITIONING AND TECHNIQUE

Ideal radiographs reveal normal and abnormal structures, whereas poor radiographs yield erroneous information. The most common error found on poor-quality thoracic radiographs is due to motion of the animal during exposure. This may result from either voluntary motion by the animal resisting its restraint or involuntary motion from cardiac and respiratory activity. An extremely short exposure time is the best method of overcoming motion of either type. Guidelines are available in various texts for decreasing motion artifacts. With equipment of extremely low milliamperage, the combination of high-speed film and high-speed or rare earth screens may be an advantage in stopping motion, but radiographic mottle or unsharpness may be observed. Newer rare earth systems can offer the speed without the mottle.

Another common error when radiographing the thorax is not including the entire thorax on the film. This limits the diagnostic value of the radiographs. A simple rule is "the thorax is inside the rib cage." If you include all the ribs, you will x-ray the whole thorax. If you have to squeeze it on a film, be *sure* that the first rib is on the film. The caudal limit of the thorax is normally at the bow of the tenth rib.

Rotation is another positioning problem in thoracic radiography. One rule that helps considerably when trying to get the thorax straight is to "*get the entire animal straight.*" All of the parts are connected, and the position of one influences that of another.

When lateral radiographs are made, the forelimbs should be pulled well forward and off the thorax. Care should be taken, however, not to apply unusual stress (stretching), which may cause compression of the thorax, distorting the shape of the structures and compressing the lungs (Fig. 1). The spine and sternum should be parallel to the table. The head should be held in an "alert" position, as flexion of the head and neck often causes a confusing deviation of the thoracic trachea (Fig. 2). The beam should be centered on the fifth intercostal space (caudal edge of the scapula). Equally important as knowing how to position animals is being able to recognize a malpositioned radiograph, which often influences the interpretation. On the lateral thoracic radiograph, three bony structures aid in recognizing malpositioning: (1) The costochondral junctions of one side should be at the same level as those on the other side; (2) the dorsal arches of the ribs should be superimposed on one another (or at least at the same level); and (3) the shape of thoracic vertebral bodies should be "recognizable," and their lateral margins should be superimposed to produce one shadow in the path of the central ray.

On ventrodorsal (VD) radiographs, the sternum

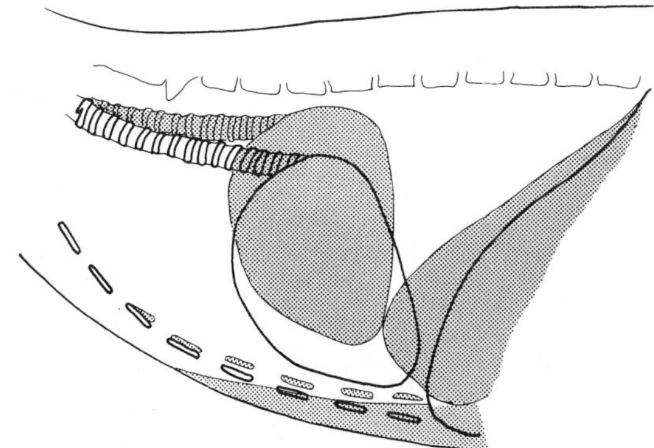

Figure 1. Displacement of thoracic structures due to extreme tension during radiography (lateral view). *Shaded* outlines of the heart, trachea, sternum, and diaphragm indicate displacement, which compresses the lungs and changes relationship of structures. These changes also occur with over-stretching on the VD or DV views but are more difficult to recognize.

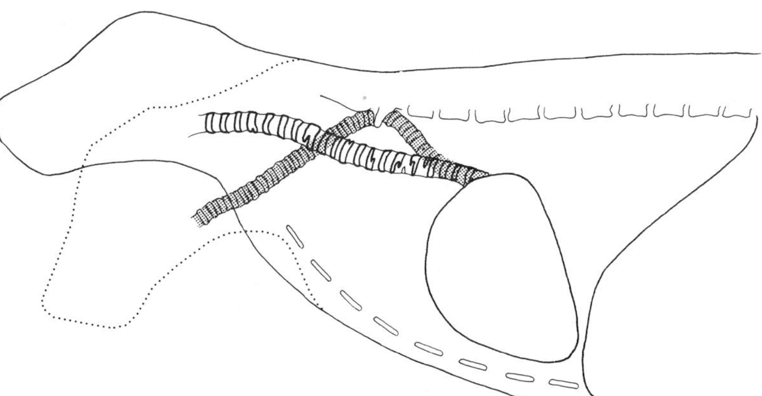

Figure 2. Effect of position of head and neck on tracheal alignment. Flexing the neck (dotted line) may cause an intrathoracic bowing of the trachea (shaded outline). Positioning is exaggerated for emphasis.

should be the most dorsal structure and on the midline, and the ribs should be symmetric. The animal should be aligned with the beam. Some breeds (pointers, setters, and hounds) may be difficult to align because of anatomic asymmetry of the sternum. Dogs with a deep, thin chest may be easier to position dorsoventral (DV) than VD. Long-haired dogs are difficult to position and often require palpation to determine if they are straight. The beam again should be centered at the fifth intercostal space (caudal edge of scapula).

When a thoracic radiograph is made with good positioning, the sternum is superimposed over the spinal column and, of course, the entire lung field is on the film. The ribs on one side are the same length (vertebra to inside bow of rib) as those on the other side. If the ribs are not the same length, the sternum is rotated toward the side of the "longest" rib. Both cranial and caudal ribs should be inspected, as one end of the thorax may be rotated while the other is aligned properly.

When the medical condition of the animal makes dorsal recumbency (i.e., a VD radiograph) inadvisable, the sternum may be placed on the table for a DV view. Care must be taken to make sure that the entire thorax is on the film, because there is a tendency to misjudge the location of the thorax in this position. This can be done with the same guidelines as for the VD view. Some cardiologists believe that the DV view should be used when evaluating the heart.

GROSS PULMONARY ANATOMY

For the purposes of radiography, there are seven lung "lobes" (regions) in dogs and cats. These lobes are divided into right and left sides by the mediastinum, which contains the trachea, esophagus, great vessels, lymph nodes, thymus, and nerves. Each lung has a cranial, a middle, and a caudal segment (the left "middle" lobe is actually the caudal portion of the cranial lobe). An accessory lobe is present on the right side and is separated from the rest of the right lung by the caudal vena cava (Fig. 3). It should be noted that the cranial and caudal lobes of each side meet dorsally over the tracheal bifurcation. The middle and accessory lobes lie against most of the heart, with the cranial lobes against the craniolateral edges of the heart. The accessory lobe is the only lobe routinely touching both the heart and the diaphragm. It contacts the center (dome) of the ventral diaphragm. In some animals, the right middle lobe also contacts the diaphragm ventrally. The caudal lobes are in contact with the crura of the diaphragm, the thoracic wall, and the accessory and middle lobes. These contact points are helpful when using the silhouette sign to localize disease.

On the lateral view, the cranial mediastinum is seen as a soft tissue density containing the trachea; it extends from the heart to the thoracic inlet and its ventral borders are near the costochondral junction of the first rib. On the VD view, it is a narrow soft tissue density between the right and left cranial lobes. On a well-positioned VD or DV view, the cranial mediastinum will be superimposed on the spine. The cranial mediastinum should be about the same width as the vertebrae or slightly wider, depending on breed and body condition (amount of fat). The trachea can be seen in the mediastinum under normal conditions because it contains air, but other mediastinal structures, which are of soft tissue and fat density, blend together. The aortic arch and thoracic aorta can sometimes be seen leaving the other structures and passing between the right and left caudal lobes. The ventral portion of the cranial mediastinum can be seen on the VD or DV view as an oblique soft tissue density extending from the right near the first rib to the left border of the heart.

Within the lung field, vessels and bronchi may be seen as tubular structures that radiate from the center of the thorax and taper toward the periphery (Fig. 4). They differ in that the bronchi contain air and the vessels contain fluid. As these structures taper, they become increasingly difficult to visual-

RADIOGRAPHIC CANINE LUNG ANATOMY

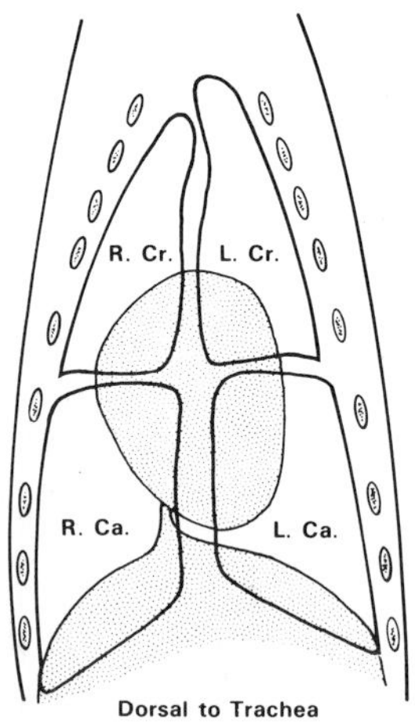

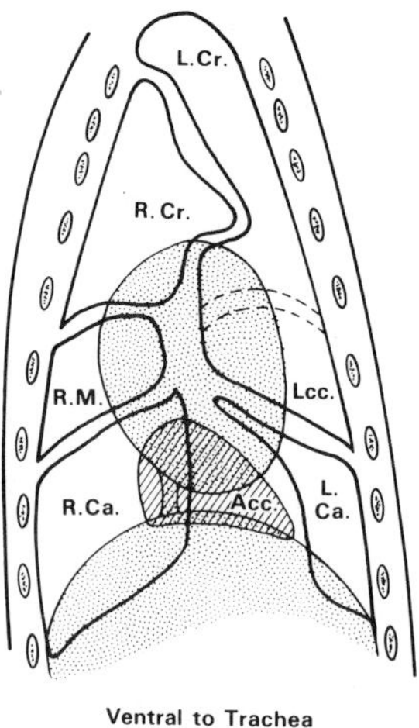

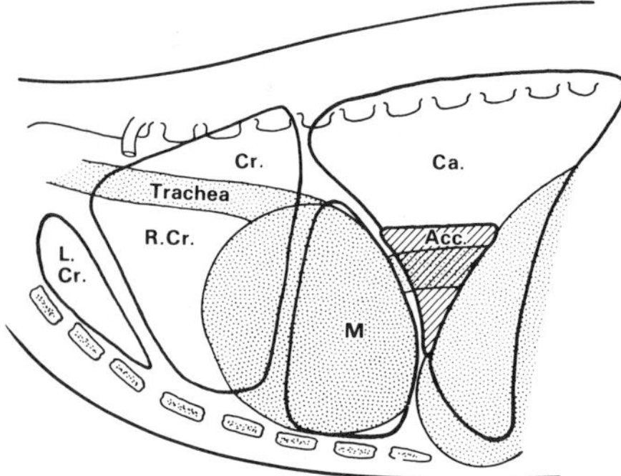

Figure 3. Radiographic anatomy. Knowing the divisions between lung sections is helpful in evaluating for pleural as well as parenchymal lung disease.

ize. Because they are more dense (because of their fluid content), the vessels can be seen farther out into the lung field than the bronchi. The major vessels and bronchi to each lobe maintain a consistent relationship, allowing one to distinguish artery from vein. In the cranial lobes, on the lateral view, there is a dorsoventral relationship of the artery, bronchus and vein. On the VD view, caudal lobe structures can be seen and, from lateral to medial, are in the same artery-bronchus-vein relationship. Precise differentiation of artery and vein is difficult in other areas because of the superimposition of numerous vascular and bronchial structures. In attempting to identify a medium- to large-size vessel, one should try to determine if its origin at the heart is the left atrium (pulmonary veins) or cranial to the tracheal bifurcation (pulmonary arteries).

Age Variation

In immature animals, the thymus is often seen. On the VD view it may appear in the cranial mediastinum as a triangular structure (sail sign) on the left side just cranial to the heart. On the lateral view, especially in kittens, the mediastinum may extend to the sternum, masking the cranial border of the heart because of the large thymus (Fig. 5).

In animals 5 to 6 years of age and older, the vessels are often more prominent than in younger animals. The walls of the bronchi and trachea may become mineralized with age. Miliary mineral densities are often found scattered in the lungs of older animals. In some older animals, the pleura becomes thickened, resulting in thin fissure lines on radiographs. This may be a result of previous or present pleural disease.

Breed Variation

The considerable variations in chest shape may influence the evaluation of the lungs. Dogs with deep, narrow thoraces often have lungs that appear more black on radiographs than do the lungs of heavier-bodied breeds. Chondrodystrophic breeds such as English bulldogs, dachshunds, and basset hounds have an irregular margin of the lateral thoracic wall on the VD view, because of the conformation of their rib cage. (This sometimes

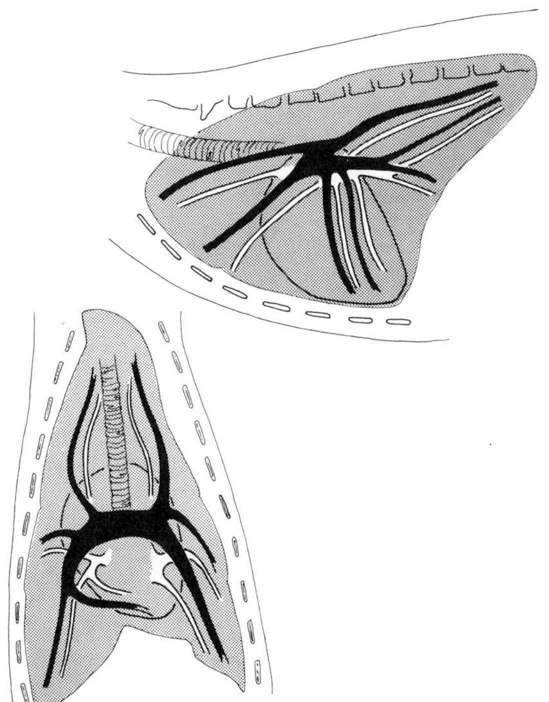

Figure 4. Radiographic anatomy of pulmonary arteries and veins. Arteries (black) and veins (white) are located on either side of the corresponding bronchi and must be distinguished from bronchial walls.

looks like fluid separating the lungs from the thoracic wall.) Calcification of the bronchial wall occurs at an earlier age in these dogs. On a VD view, the trachea of a chondrodystrophic dog often curves to the right in the cranial mediastinum.

The cat thorax varies from that of dogs in some respects on the lateral view. Pulmonary vessels are more visible in cats, and the caudodorsal margin of the lung lobes is deviated slightly ventral from the spine by heavy sublumbar muscles. This should not be mistaken for lung retraction due to pleural fluid.

Physiologic Variation

Animals that have been in lateral recumbency for a period of time may have partial collapse of the lung lobes on the dependent side. This may be recognized by increased lung density and shifting of the heart and mediastinum in that direction. This can happen very rapidly in older animals (6 to 7 years and older) or animals with lung disease. If these animals are anesthetized for thoracic radiography, a VD view should be made before the lateral view and with minimal delay to avoid collapse of dependent lung lobes, which may compromise accurate evaluation.

Obesity causes considerable anatomic variation. Fat is deposited in the mediastinum, in the pericardium, and along the thoracic wall. In contrast to the appearance of the lungs, fat may appear quite dense, making the mediastinum appear enlarged.

ROENTGEN SIGNS OF THE THORAX

Like any clinical sign, a roentgen sign is an abnormal finding. Just as cough is a sign of tracheobronchial irritation, increased density in the lung field is a roentgen sign of abnormal fluid or cellular material in the lung.

Most roentgen signs are not specific for a single diagnosis. However, only a certain group of diseases is likely to produce increased lung density with a given pattern. Because no one can memorize the radiographic appearance of every thoracic disease and some thoracic diseases may have varied radiographic appearances, the roentgen-sign approach is very important. Rather than looking for specific abnormalities to support what we think *may* be the diagnosis, we look at the entire radiograph, list the abnormalities found, and proceed to determine the cause of the observed abnormalities. By using this systematic approach, fewer lesions are overlooked and more diagnoses are made.

When interpreting any radiograph, one must be sure that the entire radiograph has been evaluated.

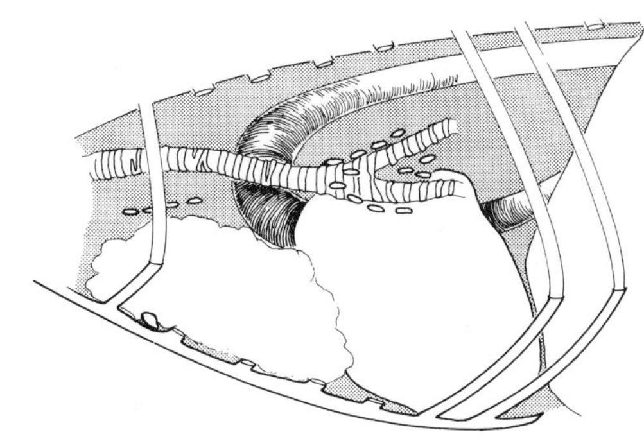

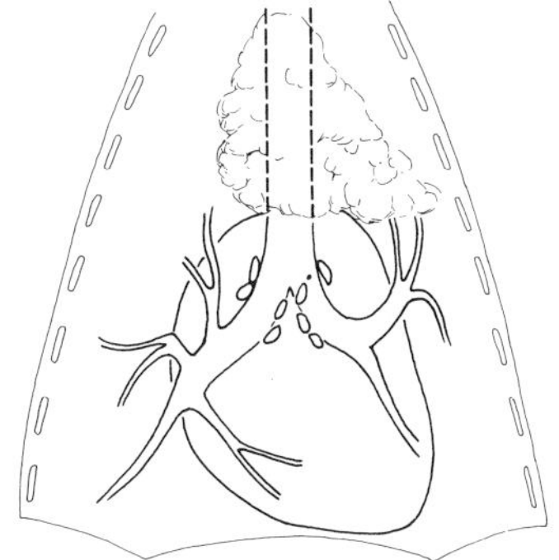

Figure 5. Location of thymus and intrathoracic lymph nodes. The thymus in the young animal is in the cranioventral mediastinal. Small, white, oval structures represent the tracheobronchial lymph nodes at the tracheal bifurcation, the cranial mediastinal nodes beneath the trachea, and the sternal lymph node dorsal to the second sternebrae.

To do this, a systematic method must be followed to avoid overlooking an area or a significant change. The order in which areas are inspected is not as important as the consistency. There are five areas that should be inspected separately: (1) the thoracic wall, (2) the pleural cavity, (3) the mediastinum, (4) the heart, and (5) the lung fields. In the lung fields, the vessels, bronchi, and lung parenchyma should be inspected in a systematic matter by looking for abnormal densities or abnormal appearance of normal structures. One method of examining the lung parenchyma is to check each lobe separately. Always remember to look for abnormalities in density as well as in shape, size, contour, and margination.

Extrapulmonary Evaluation

The structures bordering the thorax, including the skin and subcutaneous tissues surrounding the thorax, the spine, sternum, ribs, and the diaphragm, should not be overlooked. They should all be evaluated for abnormalities of density, size, shape, position, and margination. Density changes in the subcutaneous tissues can give hints regarding the nature of the thoracic disease. Anomalies of the spine, sternum, diaphragm, or rib cage might alter the size and shape of the thoracic cavity or impair respiration and thereby be linked with respiratory difficulty. Loss of visualization of part or all of the diaphragm is possible with diaphragmatic hernia or pleural fluid or lung disease. Diaphragmatic position varies with patient positioning, fullness of the stomach, degree of abdominal distension (e.g., fat accumulation, organ enlargement), and the respiratory cycle. Extreme inspiratory efforts will result in a caudally displaced diaphragm that appears flattened. Focal soft tissue masses on the diaphragm extending into the thoracic cavity might include hiatal hernias or portions of liver or spleen trapped in a small tear in the diaphragm. Focal lesions may occur on the thoracic wall in the extrapleural tissue and project into the thoracic cavity on the radiograph. These lesions include hematomas, abscesses, and neoplastic masses. They are characterized by a well-defined, convex contour facing the lungs and having tapering edges. The tapering effect is the result of lifting of the parietal pleura by the mass.

The pleural cavity is a potential space between the lungs and thoracic wall, between the lungs and mediastinum, and between lobes of the lungs. It is lined by the thin membrane, which is not seen radiographically unless thickened by disease or possibly by aging in some dogs. Normally, individual lobes cannot be distinguished or outlined. If the lung margins can be seen, something is abnormal. The lobes may be outlined by a gas density (e.g., pneumothorax) or by a fluid density (e.g., hydrothorax—pleural effusion). The lungs retract from the thoracic wall because of the presence of either gas or fluid in the pleural space. With pneumothorax, the lungs appear more radiodense (more white) than normal because of (1) contrast with surrounding pleural gas density and (2) loss of intrapulmonary air as the lung collapses. A third reason for increased lung density might be pulmonary contusion (hemorrhage) secondary to trauma (the most common cause of pneumothorax). With pleural effusion, the lung lobes are outlined by a fluid density that allows identification of individual lobes because of the visibility of the interlobar fissures. With large volumes of fluid, the lung lobes collapse significantly and the smaller cranial and middle lobes may become completely obscured.

The volume of air or fluid present in the pleural cavity will greatly affect the ability to detect it radiographically. In a small breed of dog, as much as 50 ml of pleural fluid may not be visible radiographically, and in a medium-size to large breed of dog, as much as 100 ml may not be detected. The smallest volume that can be detected radiographically is roughly 11 ml/kg. Films taken on expiration are helpful when attempting to identify small volumes of fluid or air in the pleural cavity. To identify air, a DV view is preferred over a VD because the air will rise to the highest and widest portion of the pleural cavity and be more likely to be projected on the radiograph. For fluid, the opposite is true. A small amount can more easily be distinguished on a VD view, as it will gravitate to the wider portion of the dorsal cavity, which will be dependent on a VD view (Fig. 6). On the DV view, however, widening of the caudal ventral mediastinum may be seen because of fluid accumulation in the adjacent pleural cavity.

Older dogs and cats often have thickened pleural membranes as a result of a buildup of connective tissue during the years. This may be seen radiographically as interlobar fissure lines of thin fluid densities and is impossible to distinguish from a small volume of pleural fluid. However, the patient's age may suggest pleural thickening as a more likely diagnosis. Figure 3 shows the normal location of pleural fissure lines.

Roentgen Signs of Pneumothorax

1. Air density in the pleural space.
2. Retraction of the lung lobes resulting in increased lung density.
3. Loss of contact between the heart and sternum on a recumbent lateral view (the heart falls away from the sternum because of collapse of the lung lobes).

Causes of Pneumothorax

1. Penetrating wounds of the chest wall.
2. Lung laceration with or without rib fracture.
3. Rupture of a major bronchus.
4. Rupture of a congenital lung cyst or acquired bulla.

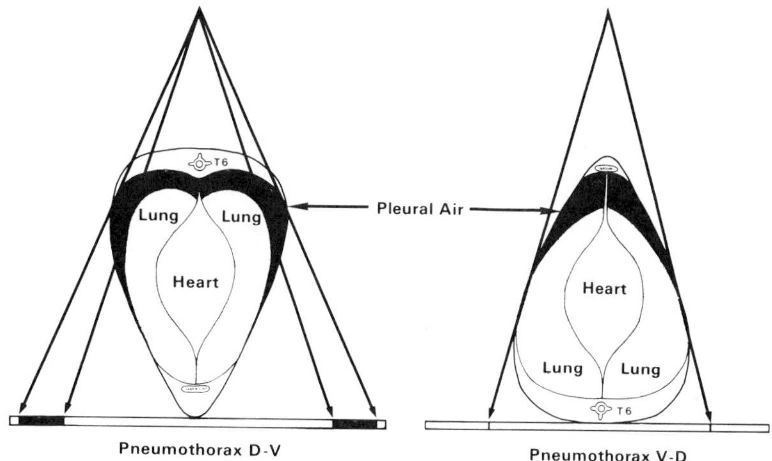

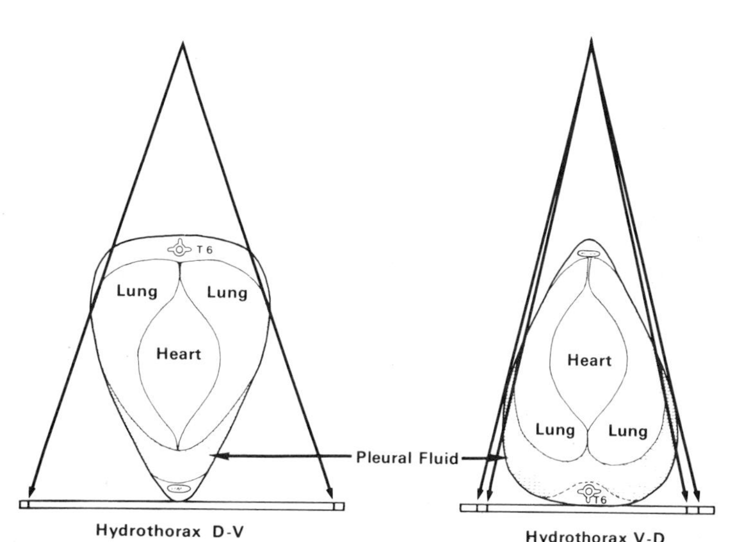

Figure 6. Effect of position on the demonstration of free pleural fluid and gas during thoracic radiography. Gas (black), which rises, is more visible along lateral margins of lungs on the DV view (top left), whereas fluid (white), which seeks the lowest level, is more visible on VD view (lower right).

ROENTGEN SIGNS OF PLEURAL FLUID

1. Soft tissue density in the ventral thorax, with a scalloped appearance of the ventral margin of lung lobes (lateral view).

2. Obscured cardiac shadow (silhouette sign between the heart and fluid, which are in contact), especially on a VD or DV view but also on a lateral if there is sufficient fluid.

3. Apparent widening of the mediastinum on a VD or DV view because of gravitation of fluid.

4. Retraction of the lung borders from the thoracic wall, with wedge-shaped, fluid-dense interlobar fissures visible. With a small volume of fluid, the fissure lines are thin and not wedged.

5. Loss of the diaphragmatic line (silhouette sign between the diaphragm and fluid, which are in contact).

Abnormal accumulation of fluid in the pleural cavity may be due to transudates (hydrothorax), blood, chyle, or inflammatory exudates. Aspirating the fluid provides a sample for diagnosis and also clears the thorax for further radiography. Large effusions, which are diagnosed by auscultation and percussion, should be drained prior to thoracic radiography.

Evaluation of Mediastinum

According to Suter and Head (1975, p. 767), "The canine or feline mediastinum is a compartmentalized partition separating right and left pleural cavities. It contains the thymus, heart, trachea, esophagus, several large vessels, lymph nodes, and nerves. It consists of two pleural layers and a scanty amount of interstitial tissue between them (mediastinum proper)."

The mediastinum is an extension of the extrapleural space and may communicate with the subcutaneous tissues through the deeper fascia of the neck and with the retroperitoneal space through the aortic and esophageal hiatuses. The mediastinum does not normally provide a tight seal between the two sides of the pleural cavity. Therefore, unilateral pleural disease is uncommon in dogs and cats and requires some pre-existing abnormalities such as fibrinous deposits, adhesions, or scars in order to impair the passage of air or fluid between the two sides. Only a few mediastinal structures can be identified on normal survey radiographs. These are the trachea, heart, aorta, thymus (young animals only), and caudal vena cava. Occasionally a small amount of swallowed air may be visualized in the esophagus. To simplify identification or localization of normal mediastinal structures or abnormal masses, it is advantageous to think of the mediastinum as divided into regions.

In normal animals, the two halves of the thorax appear symmetric on a well-positioned VD or DV view; the mediastinum separates them in the middle. After an evaluation is made for poor positioning technique, any asymmetry in size of the right and left halves of the lung field should prompt one to evaluate for possible shifting of the mediastinum. Mediastinal shift is the result of an uneven inflation of the two halves of the lungs. It is most easily recognized by looking at the position of the trachea and heart on the VD or DV view. Some possible causes of mediastinal shift are listed below:

MECHANICAL DISPLACEMENT

1. Adhesions of lung or mediastinum to thoracic wall (infection, trauma, surgery).
2. Masses (diaphragmatic hernia, lung tumor, pleural or extrapleural masses, abscesses, granulomas, lung cysts).

UNILATERAL LOSS OF LUNG VOLUME OR PRESSURE DIFFERENTIAL

1. Lung collapse (obstruction of airway, recumbency, postinfection).
2. Unilateral tension pneumothorax or hydrothorax.

Air collecting in the mediastinal space will contrast with the soft tissue structures and render them visible on the radiograph (pneumomediastinum). The structures in the cranial mediastinum (cranial vena cava, main branches of the aorta, azygos vein, esophagus, outer wall of trachea) are particularly well visualized by a pneumomediastinum. Migration of air to the subcutaneous tissues of the neck and trunk from the mediastinum can appear quite dramatic, although it is rarely a cause of respiratory difficulty. Pneumothorax often occurs concurrent with pneumomediastinum (or secondary to it) and can be a source of dyspnea.

Increased mediastinal size and space-occupying lesions can be subclassified into diffuse infiltrations and focal masses. Focal masses can be further subcategorized according to the mediastinal region they occupy to aid in determining their origin. It is not uncommon to have a mediastinal mass and fluid together, or mediastinal disease concurrent with pleural or parenchymal lung disease. The pleural or parenchymal disease may obscure mediastinal disease. Accumulations of pleural fluid along the midline on the VD or DV radiographs can also mimic mediastinal enlargement.

Diffuse widening may involve one or more of the cranial, hilar, or caudal portions of the mediastinum. The cranial mediastinum may normally be wider in brachycephalic breeds and often is prominent in obese animals because of fat accumulation. Pathologic widening may be caused by the following:

1. Mediastinitis—neck wounds, esophageal puncture due to foreign bodies, caustic agents, secondary to pleural disease.
2. Tumor infiltrate.
3. Edema—obstruction to venous return to the right atrium by a focal mass or right heart failure.
4. Hemorrhage—rupture of an artery or a vein in the mediastinum.
5. Megaesophagus—vascular ring anomaly or other cause of esophageal enlargement. The mediastinum may have less subject density because of esophageal gas accumulation.

The regional approach should be used to narrow the possible causes of a focal space-occupying mass in the mediastinum. As in identifying abdominal masses, a key is to look for displacement of adjacent structures. The most visible structure to evaluate is the trachea. Remember that, on the VD or DV view, the trachea may normally curve slightly to the right starting at the level of the first rib and return to midline at the base of the heart. This curve is accentuated in brachycephalic breeds. On the lateral view, the trachea diverges from the spine as it courses from the thoracic inlet to the carina. At the carina, it takes a slight ventral bend as it splits into the principal bronchi. The position of the head and neck will greatly affect tracheal positioning, so be sure to assess this before diagnosing pathologic tracheal deviation (see Fig. 2). A swallow of barium (esophagram) may be helpful in determining esophageal displacement or obstruction by a mediastinal mass. All areas of the mediastinum may be enlarged by abscess, hematoma, granuloma, or lipoma formation. The following is a partial list of differential diagnoses for focal mediastinal masses, by regions:

1. Cranial (ventral to the trachea)—lymphadenopathy, lymphoma, thymoma, or normal thymus in young animals; prominent aortic arch, esophageal diverticulum.
2. Cranial (dorsal to the trachea)—neurogenic tumors, paraspinal tumors, esophageal enlargement.
3. Perihilar—heart base tumor, lymphadenopathy (fungal disease), lymphoma, esophageal enlargement, enlarged pulmonary arteries or aorta, paraspinal tumors, enlarged left or right atrium.
4. Caudal—esophageal enlargement, hiatal her-

nia, neurogenic tumor, paraspinal tumors, diaphragmatic hernia.

Pulmonary Evaluation

Dogs and cats have two lungs with a total of six lobes: The right lung has four, the left has only two. They must be thought of as such in considering disease of vascular or bronchial origin, whereas the concept of seven regions described earlier is important in considering pleural and some parenchymal pathologic conditions. The major components of the lungs that should be evaluated are the (1) vasculature, (2) bronchi, (3) interstitium, and (4) alveoli. The overall density of the lungs and contrast between air and fluid densities depend on the ratio between the air content of the alveoli and bronchial tree and the fluid or cellular content of the vessels, interstitium, and alveoli. Any process that alters the normal ratio between these two components will alter the overall density of the lungs. Both pathologic and physiologic alterations can lead to changes in lung density; they may occur concurrently and lead to confusion in interpretation. The degree of lung inflation at the time of radiography is the single most important factor modifying the naturally occurring lung density. There is a considerable variation in density between inspiratory and expiratory radiographs. The decreased volume of air in the lungs and overall decreased size of the thoracic cavity on expiration produces a significant increase in overall lung density that may be mistaken for disease. Features to evaluate on the *lateral* view when distinguishing inspiratory from expiratory radiographs are as follows (Fig. 7):

1. Overall lung density—more dense on expiration, less dense on inspiration.
2. Triangular area of accessory lung lobe—more black and larger on inspiration, more dense and smaller on expiration.
3. Contact between heart and diaphragm—minimal or none on inspiration, moderate contact on expiration (affected by body type and obesity).
4. Diaphragm—flattened on inspiration, rounded (convex cranially) on expiration.

Besides the phase of respiration, another major physiologic factor affecting lung density is the animal's age. As described previously, these changes must not be confused with pathologic conditions.

The lungs are commonly thought of as divided into regions for interpretation, and the four components (vessels, bronchi, alveoli, interstitium) are evaluated in each region. The regions are (1) hilar, (2) middle, and (3) peripheral, dividing the lung approximately into thirds starting from the hilus and expanding outward concentrically. The lung regions and their approximate location are outlined in Figure 8. In the hilar region, the large pulmonary arteries and veins and major bronchi are present, along with the heart and tracheobronchial nodes. The tracheobronchial nodes will not be visible *per se* unless pathologically enlarged or calcified. There is little actual lung tissue (alveoli and interstitium) visible in the hilar region, although some lung densities from the middle and peripheral zones may be superimposed on the hilus on either the VD or lateral view. A second view taken 90 degrees to the first may show the density in question to be outside the hilar zone. The middle zone of the lung contains medium-sized pulmonary arteries and veins and medium-sized bronchi. In the peripheral zone, with high-quality radiographs one can usually visualize some small vessels (usually arteries) contrasted by the air-filled alveoli. The bronchial walls are usually too thin to see in this region. A faint background density of interstitial tissue may be seen in older animals.

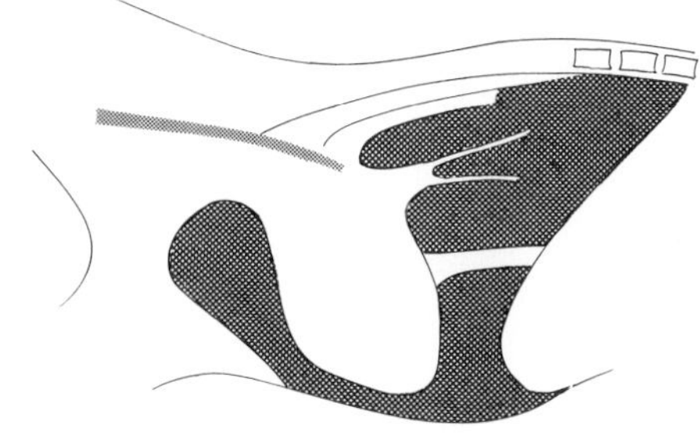

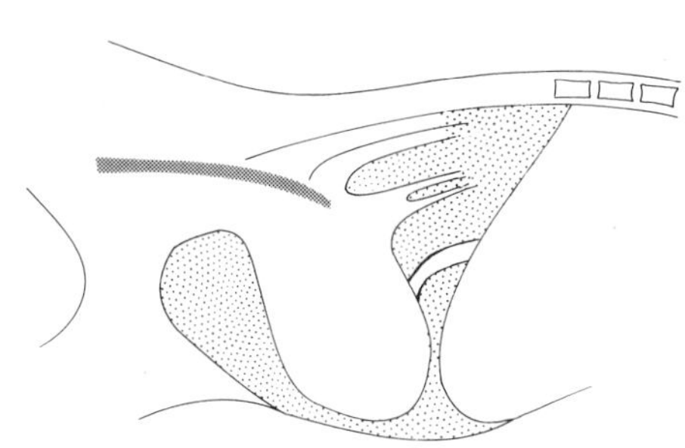

Figure 7. Effect of phase of respiration on lung evaluation. Compared with radiographs made during inspiration (top), on expiration (bottom), the thorax and thoracic structures are more compressed, resulting in less air and more soft tissue density in the lungs.

VASCULATURE

The vasculature that is visualized radiographically consists of pulmonary arteries and veins. The bronchial branches of the bronchoesophageal system are present but are not identifiable *per se*. They contribute to the overall background density, or what

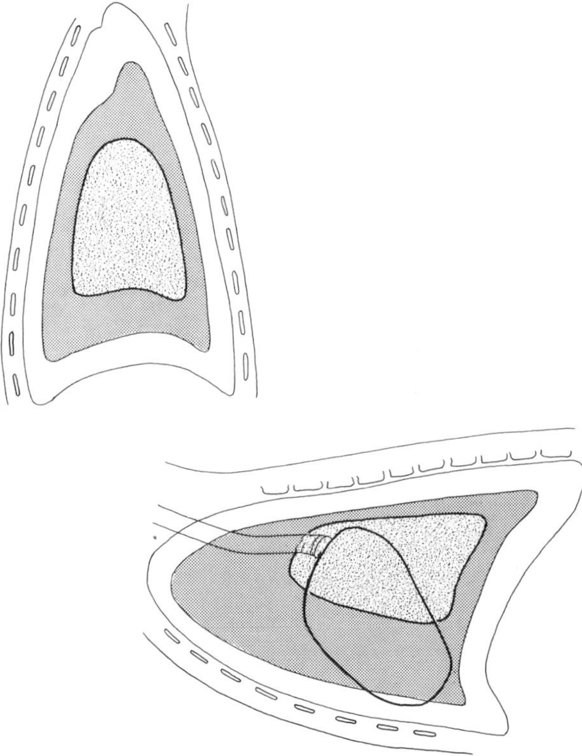

Figure 8. Regions of the lung. Lungs are divided into regions based on size and visibility of bronchi and pulmonary vessels. Large structures in the hilar region are quite visible, tapering in the middle region to barely perceptible size in the peripheral region.

will be referred to as the interstitial pattern. The major pulmonary arteries and veins are identifiable in the hilar and middle lung regions as tubular or linear soft tissue densities that gradually taper and branch as they course to the periphery. A blood vessel viewed on end will appear as a circular soft tissue density and must be distinguished from nodular lung densities such as metastases. An end-on vessel will be associated with an underlying linear-appearing vessel of the same or larger diameter. An end-on vessel will be quite radiodense, as it is a tube; therefore, viewed on end, its thickness is greater than its diameter. End-on vessels are also commonly associated with end-on bronchi. In the hilar region, arteries and veins tend to run in pairs on either side of their associated bronchus. In the middle region, the arteries tend to stay with the bronchi but the veins may not. The distinction between arteries and veins is important when evaluating cardiopulmonary disease (see Fig. 4). The artery and vein of a given pair should be roughly the same size. Disease can cause a significant difference in the size of paired vessels. Distended veins indicate either a delay in passage of blood through the left side of the heart (causing back-up into the pulmonary veins) or overcirculation. This occurs in left heart failure (e.g., mitral insufficiency or stenosis and patent ductus arteriosus [PDA]). Distended pulmonary arteries indicate overcirculation of the lung either from a left-to-right shunting congenital lesion (PDA, ventricular septal defect) or enlargement due to heartworm disease. Viewed on end, grossly enlarged arteries may appear as large interstitial nodules of metastatic neoplasia. The criteria previously mentioned for differentiation should be evaluated. Assessing vessel size is a very subjective evaluation. As a starting point, compare the vessels at the junction of the hilar and middle regions with the diameter of the dorsal third of the third rib. The diameter of the vessels should be no greater than the third rib at that point. A decreased visibility of pulmonary vascular structures (hypovascularity) may occur in cases of shock or pulmonic stenosis. Although hypovascularity is considered by many to be typical of pulmonic stenosis, this author has observed normal vascularity in at least half of these cases. Hyperinflation of the lungs may produce a hyperlucent-appearing lung field and create a hypovascular appearance. The same thing might occur with overexposure of the radiograph. Pathologic causes of hyperlucent lung fields would include emphysema (or air trapping) or any condition causing prolonged, accentuated inspiratory efforts. Decreased visibility of vessels may occur with increased lung density because of the silhouetting effect of interstitial or alveolar density (edema).

THE BRONCHI

Bronchi appear as tubular air-filled structures with thin walls. The walls may or may not be calcified in older dogs and chondrodystrophic breeds. The bronchi taper and branch in a manner similar to the vessels as they course to the periphery and are closely associated with an artery and vein, as previously mentioned. The bronchi taper slightly, so that at any one point the walls may appear parallel. In young, normal dogs and cats, the bronchial walls are difficult to visualize except for the major bronchi in the hilar region. The walls should be thin with sharp margins. Seen on end, bronchi appear as ring-shaped soft tissue structures with dark centers, often referred to as "doughnuts." The linear presentation of bronchi with their thin parallel walls has been referred to as "tram lines." The increased number and visibility of doughnuts and tram lines is referred to radiographically as a *bronchial pattern* and may be the result of acute or chronic thickening of the bronchial walls. This pattern may represent bronchial wall calcification, inflammation in and around the bronchus, hyperplasia of the mucous glands, or build-up of connective tissue in and around the bronchus. In any case, the bronchial wall, or doughnut, will appear thicker, somewhat fuzzy, and the lumen may be smaller. In contrast, a normal bronchial wall will appear thin and well defined. Bronchial lumina may become dilated and irregular with chronic bronchial wall disease such as chronic bronchitis and bronchiectasis. With bronchiectasis, the bronchial walls lose their parallel relationship and do not taper as they normally should but appear sacculated as a result of irregular dilatations in the wall. There often is a consolidation of lung tissue ventral or distal to the bronchiectatic bronchus because of lack of the normal mucociliary transport past the diseased segment. This accounts for the concurrent appearance of interstitial and alveolar fluid densities with bronchial disease, often masking the bronchial pattern.

THE INTERSTITIUM

The interstitium refers to the connective tissue, smooth muscle, and fine vasculature of the interalveolar septa and the peribronchial and perivascular tissues. An increased interstitial density (interstitial pattern) occurs when there is an accumulation of fluid, cellular material, or both in these areas. Interstitial fluid or cellular material reduces the air content of the lungs by compressing alveoli rather than filling them up. Less air in the alveoli means that the lungs appear more dense (whiter) on the radiograph. It is important to assess the phase of respiration for this reason (Fig. 7). Interstitial patterns may be structured (nodular), unstructured (hazy or reticular), or a combination of the two. They can also be described by distribution (symmetric and generalized, symmetric and regional, nonsymmetric—patchy, and either localized or generalized).

Structured or nodular densities usually result from accumulation of cellular material in the interstitium. These nodules may be of varying sizes, solid or cavitated, solitary or multiple; if multiple, they may be similar or dissimilar in size. Nodules smaller than about 3 mm cannot be discerned and tend to result in a miliary or unstructured type of density pattern. Nodules 3 to 10 mm in diameter may be visualized as such on well-exposed radiographs taken at peak inspiration with no respiratory motion. Usually nodules greater than 1 cm in diameter are easily seen if the technique is satisfactory and motion is not present. Inflammatory nodules tend to be poorly defined (they have hazy margins), whereas noninflammatory nodules are well defined. The more chronic a process is, the better defined its margins become as the nodule organizes and fluid around the nodule decreases. Some chronic processes undergo mineralization, giving the nodules a bone-density appearance.

INFLAMMATORY NODULAR DENSITIES. These lesions include granuloma or abscess (often accompanied by bronchial pattern).

Mycoses may assume the following forms:

1. Acute blastomycosis, histoplasmosis, or coccidiomycosis—numerous small- to medium-sized nodules (2 cm or less), poorly defined and distributed in a regional (hilar or middle or both) or generalized and symmetric fashion.
2. Chronic (usually histoplasmosis)—few to many small- to medium-sized, well-defined nodules; same distribution as acute forms; may be calcified (also may have calcified tracheobronchial lymph nodes).

Parasitic diseases include the following:

1. Paragonimus—few to many medium-sized nodules (about 1 cm in diameter), which may be poorly or well defined depending on the reaction of the surrounding lung tissue. They may be solid or may have an eccentrically placed gas density if the cyst has opened to the bronchus. Their location is usually in the caudal lobes.
2. Aelurostrongylus—multiple small (2 to 5 mm in diameter), poorly defined nodules, mainly in the caudal lobes. These tend to coalesce into large patchy densities in heavy infestations (southeastern United States).

Foreign bodies (migrating plant awns, others) are usually solitary, medium-sized (1 to 3 cm in diameter), hazy nodules, commonly located in accessory or caudal lobes.

NONINFLAMMATORY NODULAR DENSITIES. These lesions may assume the following forms:

1. Metastatic neoplasia—few to many small- to large-sized nodules, usually well defined and generalized in distribution. Varying-sized nodules are commonly seen because of multiple metastases occurring at different times.
2. Primary neoplasia—solitary, usually large when detected, well defined, more common in the right caudal or accessory lobe, but any lobe may be affected.
3. Fibrous or calcified nodules found in older patients; small, usually scattered, multiple, and well defined (common in old collies).
4. Differentials—end-on vessels, overlying nipples or other subcutaneous masses.

Unstructured interstitial densities can be either fluid or cellular material in the interstitial spaces, causing an increased density having no distinct form or definable margin. The appearance of this pattern has been described as lacy, fuzzy, or hazy. The addition of this type of density to the lung field decreases the visibility of structured densities (both normal and abnormal) such as vessels, bronchi, or nodular densities. The outlines or margins of these structures will appear smudged. The vessels are usually the easiest structures to evaluate in this way. As more and more interstitial fluid or cellular material accumulates, the structured densities become less defined and begin to fade into the background density. At some point, the fluid or cellular material spills over from the interstitium to the

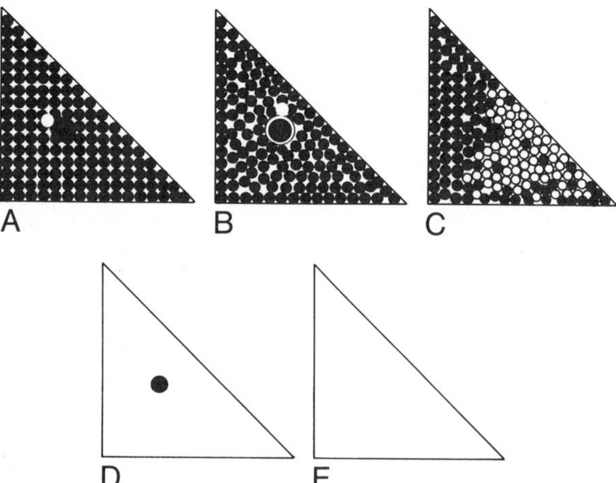

Figure 9. Air bronchogram and silhouette sign (cross-sectional view). *A*, Normal lung: the end-on vessel (white circle) is easy to see because its soft tissue density is surrounded by air. The bronchus (large black circle) is difficult to see because it is filled with and surrounded by air. Its thin wall absorbs very little radiation. *B*, Bronchial thickening or peribronchial infiltration: here the bronchial wall is thick enough to absorb sufficient radiation for differentiation from alveolar density. *C*, Alveolar disease: white circles are alveoli filled with fluid or cellular material. The vessel cannot be differentiated because it has a soft tissue density and is situated adjacent to the soft tissue of the diseased alveoli. The bronchus is seen because it contains air and is now surrounded by soft tissue. *D*, All the alveoli are filled with soft tissue density, whereas the bronchus contains air, resulting in a clear air bronchogram. Notice that thickness in the bronchial wall cannot be seen because the soft tissue of the thickened wall would be touching the soft tissue of the diseased alveoli, causing a silhouette sign. *E*, Here even the bronchus is filled with soft tissue density, and all structures of the lung section are of the same radiographic density (e.g., a completely consolidated lobe).

alveoli. As alveoli fill up, the area takes on a solid soft tissue density and obscures the interstitial pattern. Etiologic classification of unstructured interstitial patterns is best based on distribution. Since the alveolar pattern is basically an extension of the interstitial pattern, the distribution of alveolar densities has a similar interpretation. A combined outline for both patterns will follow a description of the alveolar pattern.

THE ALVEOLI

The alveoli make up the vast majority of the lung volume. They normally contain air, which provides a good contrast to the soft tissue structures they surround (vessels, bronchial walls). Alveolar diseases are conditions in which the alveoli are filled with a fluid density (exudate or transudate) or in which the alveoli are collapsed (atelectasis). The canine and feline lung lobes are nonsegmented and alveolar septa are thin; therefore, alveolar fluid tends to spread easily and has a poorly defined margin on the radiograph until it reaches the edge of a lung lobe. Flooding of a few alveoli is not discernible radiographically and tends to be classified as an unstructured interstitial pattern. As a large group of alveoli become filled with fluid, a solid soft tissue density area can be recognized and an alveolar pattern diagnosed. The periphery of these lesions will appear hazy or fluffy except at lung lobe borders. The radiographic hallmark of alveolar disease is the *air bronchogram sign.* This occurs when the alveoli surrounding a bronchus are nearly completely filled with a fluid density while the bronchial lumen still contains air. The resulting appearance is that of a radiolucent (black), linear (often branching) structure within an area of solid fluid density. Because of overlying structures, the air bronchogram may be recognized as a sign of alveolar disease before the solid soft tissue density is recognized. The bronchial walls and accompanying artery and vein are not seen, as they are masked by the alveolar fluid density in contact with them. If bronchial walls can be recognized, the air bronchogram sign is not present, *although there is a place in the phase of alveolar filling in which there may be an "almost" or "partial" air bronchogram.* This would also indicate alveolar disease, confirmed by the bronchial lumen's appearing blacker than surrounding lung. When two structures or tissues

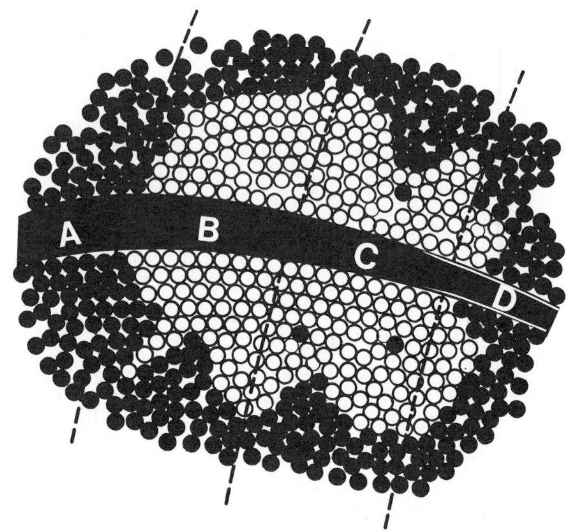

Figure 10. Air bronchogram and silhouette sign (sagittal view). *A*, Normal lung: The bronchus is difficult to differentiate from the alveoli because they all have thin walls and all contain air, thus they have the same radiographic density. *B*, Alveolar disease: alveoli are now filled with material of soft tissue density and are a different density than the air in the bronchus, resulting in an air brochogram. *C*, Alveolar disease and bronchial disease: bronchial walls are thickened at the right side of this section but difficult to see because the soft tissue of the thick wall produces silhouette sign with the soft tissue density of the diseased alveoli. Radiographically, *B* and *C* would appear the same. *D*, Normal alveoli and diseased bronchus: here the thickened bronchial walls can be easily seen because the soft tissue density contrasts with the air density in the alveoli and bronchus.

of the same radiographic density lie in contact with one another, their opposing margins will not be visible (*silhouette sign*). This explains why bronchial walls and adjacent vessels will not be visible with the air bronchogram sign (Figs. 9 and 10). It also explains why the heart is not visible when there are large accumulations of pleural fluid.

In some cases, the lung lobe or multiple lobes may have a solid soft tissue density with no air bronchograms visible. This indicates complete absence of air in the lobe, including the bronchial lumen, because of flooding of the bronchus, chronic atelectasis, or replacement of lung parenchyma (primary or metastatic tumor involving the entire lobe) or because of obstruction of the major bronchus due to compression by a mass at the hilus, torsion, or a foreign object in the bronchus. Small segments of lung parenchyma may develop discrete localized soft tissue density due to foreign body obstruction of a segmental bronchus. These lesions differ from nodular lesions in that the shape is that of the obstructed segment.

DISTRIBUTION PATTERNS FOR ALVEOLAR AND UNSTRUCTURED INTERSTITIAL (UI) DENSITIES

GENERALIZED AND SYMMETRIC DENSITIES

1. Mycotic pneumonia:
   Severe active blastomycosis: mainly UI ± alveolar
   Histoplasmosis: nodular + UI ± alveolar (often with increased bronchial pattern)
2. Severe edema:
   Cardiogenic (left heart failure): UI ± alveolar
   Electric shock: UI ± alveolar
   Toxemias: UI ± alveolar
3. Allergic reactions: UI ± alveolar (may or may not have increased bronchial pattern)
4. Chronic fibrosis ("old dog lung"): UI ± nodules

GENERALIZED AND NONSYMMETRIC (PATCHY)

1. Severe contusion: UI + alveolar
2. Severe bacterial pneumonia: UI + alveolar (often have increased bronchial pattern)
3. Early pneumonias: UI
4. Allergic pneumonitis or pulmonary infiltrate with eosinophilia (PIE): UI ± alveolar (may or may not have increased bronchial pattern)
5. Disseminated intravascular coagulopathy: UI + alveolar
6. Miliary or septal spread of pulmonary metastases (uncommon): UI + alveolar ± nodules

GENERALIZED AND REGIONAL (USUALLY HILAR ± MIDDLE REGIONS) (FIG. 8)

1. Systemic edema (earlier or less severe cases of left heart failure, electric shock, toxemia): UI ± alveolar

NONSYMMETRIC (PATCHY) AND LOCALIZED

1. Contusion: UI ± alveolar
2. Bacterial or aspiration pneumonia (usually ventral): UI + alveolar (often have increased bronchial pattern)
3. Heartworm thromboembolism (usually caudal): UI + alveolar (superimposed over increased vessel size)
4. Lung collapse
   Recumbency (anesthesia): UI + alveolar
   Airway obstruction: UI + alveolar (may have a "solid" lobe)

One should remember that most lung diseases produce a mixture of radiographic patterns (e.g., bronchial-interstitial or interstitial-alveolar) because of the contiguous nature of the various structures and their simultaneous involvement in a disease process. Many diseases start with bronchial or vascular involvement, which spreads to the interstitium and finally involves the alveoli. As healing occurs, the process is reversed. A residual interstitial density often remains after resolution of pulmonary disease as a result of scar tissue formation. When several patterns are present simultaneously, one should classify the disease based on the predominant pattern, keeping in mind the significance of the lesser pattern or patterns that may be present. Since roentgen signs rarely are specific for a histopathologic diagnosis, one must use the predominant radiographic pattern and distribution of disease to formulate a working list of likely causes and use additional clinical data to arrive at a final diagnosis.

References and Supplemental Reading

Reif, J. S., and Rhodes, W. H.: The lungs of aged dogs. A radiographic-morphologic correlation. J. Am. Vet. Radiol. Soc. 7:5, 1966.

Suter, P. F., and Head, J. R.: Mediastinal, Pleural and Extrapleural Diseases. *In* Ettinger, S. J. (ed.): *Textbook of Veterinary Internal Medicine*. Philadelphia: W. B. Saunders, 1975, pp. 767–806.

Suter, P. F., and Lord, P. F.: *Thoracic Radiography. A Text Atlas of Thoracic Diseases of the Dog and Cat.* Davis, CA: Stonegate Publishing, 1984.

Ticer, J. W.: *Radiographic Technique in Veterinary Practice*, 2nd ed. Philadelphia: W. B. Saunders, 1984.

TRACHEOTOMY AND TRACHEOSTOMY

COLIN E. HARVEY, B.V.Sc.
Philadelphia, Pennsylvania

DEFINITIONS

TRACHEOTOMY. Literally, a tracheotomy is an incision into the trachea. In the following discussion, *tracheotomy* will be used to refer to incision into the trachea and placement of a tube for temporary bypass of the upper airway.

TRACHEOSTOMY. A tracheostomy forms a new opening into the tracheal lumen. In the following discussion, *tracheostomy* will be used to refer to the creation of a permanent new opening through the skin into the tracheal lumen. The opening does not require the presence of a tube to maintain an airway opening.

INDICATIONS AND DISADVANTAGES

Tracheotomy most often is used to temporarily bypass upper airway obstruction, either as an aid in the management of acute airway obstructive episodes or to permit unobstructed access for surgical manipulation and prevent postoperative airway obstruction. Tracheotomy is also useful for reducing anatomic dead space and providing access for oxygen enrichment, for administering intratracheal medications, or for employing suctioning devices in animals with severe bronchopneumonia. Combined with light sedation, placement of a cuffed tube through a tracheotomy incision provides an option for medium- to long-term, controlled or assisted positive pressure ventilation. By using a tube placed through a tracheotomy incision, the need for heavy sedation or anesthesia to prevent chewing on the tube is avoided (see also Short-Term Ventilator Support).

Tracheostomy is indicated as a "salvage" treatment for animals with severe upper airway obstruction that cannot be treated by more conservative surgical means. Animals with severe laryngeal collapse or with laryngeal malignancies are examples.

Both tracheotomy and tracheostomy bypass the upper airway and the filtration, humidification, and warming of inspired air that occurs there. These two procedures also interfere with the efficiency of the normal cough reflex, because closure of the glottis (Valsalva maneuver) and thus the build-up of expiratory pressure prior to the explosive expulsion of debris from the airway are prevented. Both procedures also break the continuity of the normal mucociliary clearance of particulate matter from the lungs and lower airway. These two factors result in a considerable buildup of viscid lower airway secretions during the first days after an upper airway bypass. Cleansing of the tube is essential in order to prevent obstruction in an animal with a tracheotomy tube in place. Animals with a permanent tracheostomy go through an accommodation phase of increased secretions that accumulate around the tracheostomy opening. Secretions typically catch and dry out on the sutures, making the 1 to 2 weeks until suture removal an awkward period that requires frequent and gentle removal of secretions. A low-humidity environment was found to be beneficial in laboratory dogs in the first several days after tracheostomy. Animals with a tracheostomy are unable to prevent entry of fluid into their trachea, and they therefore cannot be permitted to swim and must be bathed with care.

TRACHEOTOMY

Equipment

The two types of tracheotomy tubes most commonly used in small animal practice are the double-lumen metal or plastic tube and the rubber or soft plastic T tube. The double-lumen tube is preferred because it can be placed through a between-ring incision and because the inner tube can easily be removed for cleaning while the outer tube remains in place to provide an airway. The advantage of the T tube is that it permits passage of air both through the tube opening and through the animal's own airway (larynx), although this can also be achieved with the double-lumen tube by using a tube size that is smaller than the lumen of the trachea. Neither of these tubes can be used for positive pressure ventilation, as they do not have a cuff included in their design. Tubes with one or multiple cuffs and a built-in ventilator adaptor are used for long-term ventilatory support in humans. An oral endotracheal tube passed through a tracheotomy opening will provide the same option for veterinary patients at minimal cost. Wire-reinforced endotracheal tubes have the advantage of not kinking when flexed at a sharp angle. These tubes, however, do not include the low-compliance cuff, which is used in humans to avoid tracheal epithelial necrosis and subsequent stenosis (a significant and real complication of positive pressure ventilation performed through a tracheotomy tube). (Tubes suitable for controlled or positive pressure ventilation are discussed in Short-Term Ventilatory Support.)

The size of the tube used depends on the size of the animal. Using a double-lumen tube that is smaller than the tracheal lumen is possible only in dogs weighing more than about 10 kg (22 lb). For a cat or very small dog, size 0 or 00 is necessary. A 10-kg dog can manage with a size 2 or 3 tube, and a large or giant breed of dog can manage with a size 6 or 7 metal double-lumen tube, provided that the animals are not exercised or excited. Both metal (Pilling Co.) and PVC (Shiley Laboratories) tubes are available. Except in the very small sizes, these tubes come as a set consisting of an outer tube with fixation flanges, an inner cannula that locks in place inside the outer tube by twisting the key on the outer tube, and an obturator that is used to assist the smooth placement of the tube.

Technique

A hasty emergency tracheotomy rarely is necessary in dogs with upper airway obstruction, as passage of an endotracheal tube under sedation or thiopental anesthesia is almost always possible. Oral endotracheal intubation enables the animal to be ventilated while being unhurriedly prepared for the tracheotomy. Tracheotomy with local anesthesia and minimal chemical restraint may be necessary in dogs with severe bronchopneumonia.

The ventral neck area is clipped and prepared for surgery. A midline incision is made in the skin caudal to the cricoid cartilage, the subcutaneous tissues are divided, and the sternohyoid muscles are separated on the midline to expose the trachea. The recurrent laryngeal nerves are usually located on either side of the trachea and are subsequently avoided.

I prefer to make a between-ring incision, as the tracheal rings will spring back to their normal shape after removal of the tube, collapse of one or more rings is avoided, and healing is rapid. The incision is made with a scalpel midventrally and is enlarged with a hemostat until it is approximately one-third the circumference of the trachea. The tube is inserted with the obturator in place, depressing the tracheal ring cranial to the incision. The obturator is then removed and the inner cannula inserted. To prevent its dislodgement, the tube's swivel neck plate is secured to the animal by skin sutures or a length of umbilical tape placed around the neck. The incision is not closed unless there is a considerable length extending above or below the tube.

Management

Animals (particularly cats and small dogs) with a tracheotomy tube in place require almost constant care because of the potential for obstruction. The tube must be periodically cleared of secretions (about once every 30 minutes initially, and increasing in frequency if necessary). With a double-lumen tube, this can be done by the owner at home if the technique is explained correctly. Regular suctioning of the lower airway through the tube is not necessary unless the animal appears to be obstructed or auscultation reveals copious, coarse crackles. The routine use of *N*-acetylcysteine, a mucolytic drug that can be administered directly into the trachea, is not indicated, as acetylcysteine irritates the airway epithelium and is likely to increase the amount of secretions. If secretions are copious and a sample obtained from the trachea is liquified when mixed with acetylcysteine *in vitro*, one to five drops of acetylcysteine mixed with 2 to 10 ml of saline (depending on the size of the animal) can be given 5 to 10 minutes prior to suctioning the airway. (The technique for airway suctioning through a tracheotomy tube is described in Short-Term Ventilatory Support.)

Antibiotics are no longer used routinely at the Veterinary Hospital, University of Pennsylvania simply because a tracheotomy tube is in place, although a suitable antibiotic should obviously be given to an animal with a severe productive bronchopneumonia. The intubated lower airway quickly becomes colonized by bacteria, and routine antibiotic therapy merely results in the selective growth of resistant species.

The most helpful maneuver for an animal with a tracheotomy tube in place is to remove it as soon as possible. When using a T tube or a double-lumen tube smaller than the lumen of the trachea, the exterior end of the tube can be occluded with adhesive tape; if the animal is able to breathe comfortably for 10 minutes with the tube occluded, it usually can be safely removed. For smaller animals in which this maneuver is not an option, the tube is removed when clinical experience suggests that this is appropriate or the animal is sedated or anesthetized so that the upper airway can be examined. The incision is not closed after removal of the tube; it heals by granulation-contraction.

Complications

Complications due to tracheotomy itself are rare in dogs and cats. Plugged or dislodged tubes can result in airway obstruction and asphyxiation. Subcutaneous emphysema or infection may result if the incision is closed or covered with a dressing after removal of the tube. Laryngeal paralysis is possible if the recurrent laryngeal nerves are not protected and preserved during the procedure.

TRACHEOSTOMY

Technique

The trachea is exposed as for tracheotomy, although the approach incision should be about 1 cm longer at either end. Before the incision is made into the tracheal lumen, the trachea at the tracheostomy site is undermined, and the separated sternohyoid muscles are sutured together dorsal to the trachea with two horizontal absorbable mattress sutures. This causes the trachea to be elevated ventrally.

A standard tracheotomy incision is made at the middle of the proposed tracheostomy site. Two additional ventrolateral incisions in the trachea are made to form an H, with the horizontal bar of the H being the original between-ring incision. The side incisions are made through two or three rings, both cranial and caudal to the initial incision. This forms two ventral flaps that will be sutured to the edges of the original skin incision. Tracheostomy openings will decrease to about 50 per cent of their original size as a result of contraction during healing, so the opening must be made large enough to accommodate this contracture. A minimum distance of 3 cm between flaps is suggested for smaller animals and 4 to 5 cm for medium or large dogs. Before the sutures are placed, any exposed cartilage edges are trimmed with fine scissors. Simple interrupted or continuous sutures of synthetic absorbable material are used to appose the skin and tracheal mucosal edges accurately. Any excess length of skin incision is closed with skin sutures.

Care and Prognosis

Initially there will be some accumulation of blood around the sutures. This will be followed by accumulation of mucopurulent debris. These secretions stick to the sutures and must periodically be gently cleaned off to avoid obstruction. This problem is less severe if continuous sutures are used. Once the sutures are removed or absorbed, there is less tendency for the secretions to accumulate, although this may continue in long-haired animals. Periodic clipping of the hair around the opening in these animals is helpful. Some animals learn to clear secretions from their tracheostomy opening during normal grooming; others will require assistance from their owners once or twice a day for the duration of the animal's life. One reason for the initial accumulation of secretions is that the tracheal mucosa at the site of the stoma responds to the changed conditions by undergoing squamous metaplasia, although the normal ciliated mucosa becomes re-established within several weeks.

To date, no detailed clinical reports of long-term follow-up results in a series of animals are available, although present clinical experience indicates that the procedure is practical in all but cats and very small dogs. These animals may even benefit from the procedure once management techniques to carry the patient through the initial accommodation phase have been worked out. If the entire upper airway is bypassed, brain temperature in dogs does increase with increasing ambient temperature because the panting mechanism has been bypassed; however, this has not resulted in any clinically obvious effects.

References and Supplemental Reading

Dalgard, D. W., Marshall, P. M., Fitzgerald G. H., and Rendon, F.: Surgical technique for a permanent tracheostomy in beagle dogs. Lab. Anim. Sci. 29:367, 1979.

Harvey, C. E., and Goldschmidt, M. H.: Healing following short duration transverse incision tracheotomy in the dog. Vet. Surg. 11:77, 1982.

Harvey, C. E., and O'Brien, J. A.: Upper airway obstruction surgery: 6. Tracheotomy—analysis of 89 episodes in dogs and cats. J. Am. Anim. Hosp. Assoc. 18:563, 1982.

Hedlund, C. S., Tangner, C. H., Montgomery, D. L., et al.: A procedure for permanent tracheostomy and its effects on tracheal mucosa. Vet. Surg. 11:13, 1982.

LARYNGEAL DISEASES OF DOGS AND CATS

A. J. VENKER-VAN HAAGEN, D.V.M.
Utrecht, The Netherlands

HISTORY

In laryngeal diseases of dogs and cats, one or more of the following characteristic symptoms will typically be the reason why veterinary assistance is sought:

1. A raw, dry *cough* usually occurs during both the day and the night. (Fits of coughing are sometimes interrupted by a few swallowing attempts.)
2. *Stridor* (an inspiratory or expiratory wheeze) may be heard either only with exertion or continuously during normal breathing. Its sound is soft and rasping if the obstruction is mild or a high-toned wheeze when the obstruction becomes severe.
3. *Dyspnea* occurring at intervals (spasm) is a less-common symptom but is sometimes a complication in chronic laryngitis. A persistent obstruction may cause dyspnea either during exertion or continuously, according to the severity of the obstruction. A severe obstruction causes respiratory distress and may be associated with cyanosis and vomiting. The occurrence of these symptoms indicates that the obstruction may be life-threatening.
4. A *change of voice* is not a very common symptom in laryngeal diseases in dogs and cats, in contrast to those in humans, and when it occurs it most often indicates severe alterations in the larynx, usually involving the vocal folds. Purring can become a very unpleasant sensation to a cat, and it is frequently interrupted by swallowing movements.
5. *Painful swallowing* indicates that laryngeal irritation is present and is spreading to the pharyngeal area.

CLINICAL EXAMINATION

The procedure for examining a patient with laryngeal dysfunction depends largely on the degree to which respiration is impaired. If the patient is not in respiratory distress, a thorough clinical examination of the respiratory and cardiovascular systems is indicated. This should be followed by radiography and then laryngoscopy and, possibly, electromyography. If the patient is in severe respiratory distress, the clinical examination is reduced to a minimum and often does not exceed listening to the stridor to determine its origin. Laryngoscopy under anesthesia follows immediately. In this situation and in cases in which immediate intubation is necessary, the following procedure is the least dangerous in dogs: The dog is calmed as much as possible and is gently placed in a sitting position so that the front leg can be supported for intravenous administration of a barbiturate anesthetic. Less than one tenth of the normal dose will be sufficient to induce the dog to lie on its side and accept without resistance the opening of the mouth for intubation. A laryngoscope and several *small*-sized endotracheal tubes must be available. After intubation, the lungs are inflated once or twice by blowing on the tube. As soon as respiration and circulation are restored, more barbiturate is administered to facilitate adequate laryngoscopic examination or tracheostomy.

When there are no signs of life-threatening respiratory distress, the first step in clinical examination is listening to the patient's spontaneously produced coughs and the occurrence of stridorous breathing. When, according to the owner, sounds are only produced in certain circumstances, the owner is requested to assist with the examination by reproducing these circumstances (running, pulling on the leash, inducing purring). In listening to a stridor, not only the sound and its continuity are important, but also its occurrence during inspiration alone or during both inspiration and expiration. The latter is indicative of a more severe obstruction.

Palpation of the larynx can reveal information about the degree of irritation of the laryngeal mucosa. In severe irritation, a harsh, dry cough is produced immediately when the larynx is touched. Palpation can also reveal a change in location of the larynx or a deformation. Exogenous deformation, such as may result from metastatic involvement of the superficial retropharyngeal lymph nodes, is as important as endogenous deformation due to neoplastic involvement of the larynx itself. Severe alterations can result in attachment to surrounding structures so that the larynx is found to be immobile. The cartilages of the larynx can become indurated by ossification in cases of chronic laryngitis, to the extent that the larynx feels as hard as a stone.

A lateral *radiograph* can be helpful in detecting

ossification and tumor growth. Even moderate respiratory distress can influence the configuration of air pockets in and around the laryngeal structures, and care must be taken not to confuse the interpretation of these radiographs.

For further examination, the patient must be anesthetized. If a dog is suspected of having laryngeal paralysis, barbiturate anesthetic is administered intravenously just until there is a loss of resistance to opening the mouth. Laryngeal movements are then observed with the aid of a *laryngoscope*. If necessary, xylocaine spray is used to suppress reflex swallowing. In cats, laryngeal movements are also observed when there is just loss of resistance to opening the mouth during the induction of anesthesia with ketamine hydrochloride (Ketaset, Bristol) and xylazine hydrochloride (Rompun, Chemagro) administered intramuscularly. The use of xylocaine spray is indispensable in cats.

When clinical signs and laryngoscopy confirm a diagnosis of laryngeal paralysis, *electromyography* of the intrinsic laryngeal muscles should be performed. Anesthesia does not interfere with the detection of denervation potentials, pseudomyotonia, or myotonia. When the detection of normal action potentials is also of importance, a superficial level of anesthesia is required. After the initial dose of barbiturate anesthetic has been administered, the dog is placed in dorsal recumbency. The needle electrode is introduced orally, and its tip is inserted through the laryngeal mucosa into the intrinsic laryngeal muscles in a sequential fashion. During the electromyographic recordings, the preferred level of anesthesia is the one at which spontaneous movements of the vocal folds can be observed, if such movements are present. Electromyography should not be attempted in cats, because severe edema usually develops after any manipulation of the cat's laryngeal mucosa, and the insertion of the needle electrode through the laryngeal mucosa causes a severe traumatic reaction. For similar reasons, laryngeal electromyography should be considered with great caution in very young puppies; the resulting edema may cause a major obstruction to airflow because of the very small size of the larynx.

Congenital Laryngeal Malformation

Congenital malformations of the laryngeal structures are recognized occasionally in dogs and cats. Malformations can affect all three parts of the laryngeal cavity: the vestibule, the glottis, and the infraglottic cavity. In most cases, stenosis occurs and stridorous breathing and dyspnea are the major signs. Laryngoscopy provides the necessary detailed information to establish the diagnosis. All visible structures of the larynx should be evaluated, because there are usually multiple malformations.

Surgical correction should be considered only when the results can be expected to allow the patient to develop normally and live with minimal respiratory distress. Minor abnormalities discovered in young animals can diminish during maturation, and an attempt at surgical correction at an early age could have an adverse influence on the development of the larynx. In serious obstructive malformations, euthanasia is justified.

Brachycephalic dogs, and in particular the English bulldog and the Pekingese, are frequently afflicted with inadequate development of the cartilaginous structures of the larynx, leading to various degrees of obstructive malformation. Laryngeal collapse, eversion of the lateral ventricles, and insufficient abduction of the vocal folds are all phenomena of the same underlying malformation. Since these dogs often have one or more additional malformations causing obstruction of the airway (including stenosis of the nares, a relatively elongated soft palate, and stenosis of the trachea), surgical correction should be attempted only when satisfactory improvement in the total airflow in the upper airways can be achieved. This realistic philosophy all but completely eliminates the indications for surgical treatment. The disablement is quite variable from dog to dog and is considerably influenced by the demands imposed on the dog by the owner.

Inflammation

Acute inflammation of the laryngeal mucous membranes is characterized by a raw, dry cough. When spontaneous coughing is absent during the initial examination, palpation of the larynx will immediately evoke a short cough, often followed by short swallowing movements. The patient may exhibit uneasiness or anxiety during this examination.

Canine infectious tracheobronchitis (kennel cough), a viral or bacterial inflammation of the laryngeal, tracheal, and, sometimes, bronchial mucosa, is the most common cause of acute laryngeal inflammation in dogs. In cats, viral rhinotracheitis and calicivirus may also affect the laryngeal mucosa, but the symptoms of laryngitis never dominate the complex of symptoms in these diseases. Acute laryngitis can occur in a dog after a day of continuous barking and panting and in both dogs and cats after intubation for anesthesia or after inhalation of caustic gases.

However alarming the discomfort of the patient is, acute laryngitis is seldom life-threatening, because profuse local edema and laryngospasm are infrequent complications. Therapy consists of strict rest and avoidance of excitement. Pediatric cough syrups, containing only an expectorant, are usually very effective. If syrups containing ephedrine are used, care should be taken to specify the maximum daily dose based on the ephedrine content. There is no indication for treatment with corticosteroids, and if there is no fever there is no indication for antibiotic therapy.

Edema of the laryngeal mucosa and submucosa can occur in all three parts of the laryngeal cavity. In all cases, the symptoms are alarming, consisting of acute inspiratory and expiratory stridorous breathing and respiratory distress. Because of the unpredictable progress of the disease, the patient should be placed under continuous observation and preparations should be made for immediate intubation, if necessary, followed by tracheotomy. Further treatment consists of calming the patient, administering a sedative if necessary (avoid morphine derivatives), and administering a corticosteroid intravenously. Tracheotomy provides relief to the patient and should also be considered in the early stage of the developing edema. The prognosis is generally good when care is taken to maintain homeostasis, because in most cases edema is caused by a transient affliction such as an insect bite or local trauma.

An *abscess* in the larynx is a rare finding but can be caused by a penetrating foreign body such as a needle, fish bone, or stick. According to the location and size of the abscess, the symptoms are those of an obstructive laryngeal disease. Symptoms can develop during a period of days or weeks. The abscess should be opened and drained under general anesthesia, while care is taken to prevent exudate from being aspirated into the trachea. The exudate should be cultured, but antibiotic therapy can be started immediately and changed later if required by the results of sensitivity testing. In most cases, healing is prompt.

Chronic laryngeal inflammation is a rarity in cats but a rather common disease in dogs, to which the following discussion refers. In the *mild* form of the disease, a short, raw, dry cough is produced frequently, several times a day. Other than the apparent recurrent irritation of the laryngeal mucosa, however, there are no symptoms of laryngeal dysfunction such as stridor, dyspnea, or loss of endurance. The voice of the dog is normal, but barking may be interrupted by a cough, after which barking is resumed.

Palpation of the larynx may elicit elaborate, noisy, raw coughs, but there are no signs of pain or anxiety. Lateral radiographs do not provide conclusive information. Laryngoscopy reveals that the laryngeal mucosa is red and thickened. The vocal folds are also more voluminous and dark red. The laryngeal movements are normal. These laryngeal changes occur without involvement of the pharynx, trachea, or bronchi.

The results of treatment are usually disappointing. The cause of the disease is speculative, but dogs in the habit of continuous barking and panting are certainly candidates for the disease.

In the *severe* form of chronic laryngeal inflammation, there are definite hyperplastic changes associated with occasional or continuous laryngeal dysfunction or pain. In these cases, laryngeal spasm can occur during exertion or excitement. However alarming the symptoms are, death caused by asphyxia seldom occurs. Treatment consists of avoiding the precipitating exertion or excitement. This disorder often occurs in (over)trained dogs under training conditions. Unfortunately, the only effective treatment in such cases is complete and permanent cessation of the training. Medical treatment and periods of rest never result in the complete restoration of the dog's ability.

Hyperplasia of the vocal folds results in hoarseness and stridorous breathing. Palpation of the larynx evokes painful swallowing attempts and gives the impression that the larynx is a solid mass. The radiographic density of the laryngeal cartilages is increased, and there are foci of even greater density, caused by ossification. Laryngoscopy reveals that the surface of the epiglottis is irregular, and sometimes there are yellow patches. There is a striking redness and hypervascularization of the laryngeal mucosa. Treatment consists of administering corticosteroids and analgesics, but the prognosis is poor. The cause is unknown.

Tumors

Primary laryngeal tumors occur occasionally in dogs and cats. The most common is squamous cell carcinoma, but other tumors such as rhabdomyosarcoma have been reported. Squamous cell carcinomas often invade very rapidly and are often inoperable by the time the veterinarian is consulted. Sometimes, however, when the tumor originates in one of the vocal folds and has not yet spread (evaluation by laryngoscopy), surgical removal is still possible, with a satisfactory long-term prognosis. Surgery should be performed as soon as possible. For careful removal of one vocal fold with the tumor, the midline ventral approach through the thyroid cartilage is the most secure, since it allows sufficient exposure for careful preparation. Tracheostomy is performed, and the anesthetic gases are administered through an endotracheal tube introduced into the stoma. After surgery, the endotracheal tube is replaced by a tracheal cannula, which remains in place for about 5 days. When radiation is available, it should be considered as a complementary treatment in these cases.

Laryngeal Paralysis

Laryngeal paralysis is a complete or partial loss of function of the larynx. The paralysis can be neurologic, muscular, neuromuscular, or ankylotic. The severity of the clinical symptoms is correlated with the severity of dysfunction. The diagnosis is made by laryngoscopy and electromyography of the intrinsic laryngeal muscles.

Laryngeal paralysis of *neurologic* origin can be complete or partial. When caused by trauma to the neck, one or both recurrent laryngeal nerves may be interrupted. Interruption of one recurrent laryngeal nerve does not usually lead to clinical signs unless the animal is exerted. The abduction of the normal vocal fold together with the position of the paralyzed vocal fold guarantees sufficient air passage through the glottis. Vocal ability is sufficient or normal, since the nonparalyzed vocal fold passes through the midline during adduction and touches the paralyzed vocal fold. Interruption of both recurrent laryngeal nerves causes both severe dyspnea and vocal insufficiency. Vocal impairment may be limited to hoarseness, since the stretching of the vocal folds, a function of the cricothyroid muscles (innervated by the cranial laryngeal nerves), is undisturbed. More frequently, laryngeal paralysis is presented as a slowly progressive disease characterized by increasing stridor and decreasing endurance over a period of several months. In these cases, the loss of the voice is seldom mentioned spontaneously in the case history but is to be expected. In the Netherlands, this disease occurs most frequently in the Bouvier des Flandres, in which signs first appear at the age of 3 to 8 months. It is also common in Leonbergers, in which signs first appear at the age of 2 to 4 years. Laryngeal paralysis also occurs in older dogs of several breeds; the most frequently affected in the Netherlands are Irish setters and German pointers.

Laryngeal paralysis caused by a *muscular* disease is rare but has been diagnosed in bull terriers and in dogs of various other breeds. Laryngeal paralysis is never the sole disorder in such cases but rather is one aspect of a polymyositis or generalized muscular disease. Similarly, the *neuromuscular* disease myasthenia gravis may involve the intrinsic laryngeal muscles in some cases.

Laryngeal paralysis caused by *ankylosis* of the cricoarytenoid articulations is a rare disorder. Electromyography reveals normal motor unit potentials in the intrinsic laryngeal muscles of a paralyzed larynx. Older dogs with a long case history of recurrent or continuous laryngitis are prone to develop this disorder.

Except for muscular laryngeal paralysis, which should be treated according to the diagnosis of the muscular disease, laryngeal paralysis should be treated surgically if the dyspnea prevents the dog or cat from living an acceptable life.

Whenever there is a sudden increase in the frequency with which laryngeal paralysis is diagnosed in a breed or a closed population, investigation of the possible hereditary transmission of the disease should be given urgent consideration. Investigations of the pathogenesis of laryngeal paralysis in the Bouvier have demonstrated that in this breed the disease is a neurogenic degenerative disease, which is by definition a hereditary disorder. Elimination of the disease by selective breeding is possible once its hereditary basis is established.

In our experience, the surgical technique of choice in bilateral obstructive laryngeal paralysis is the lateralization of one vocal fold. Tracheostomy is performed, and the anesthetic gases are administered through an endotracheal tube inserted into the stoma. One side of the larynx is exposed by a ventral paramedian incision of the skin. After a 1-cm-long transection of the thyropharyngeus muscle is made, the dorsal edge of the thyroid cartilage is lifted and its attachment to the cricoid cartilage is severed. The arytenoid cartilage is disconnected from the cricoid cartilage, and the ligamental connection between the two arytenoid cartilages is also severed. The arytenoid cartilage is then fixed to the caudodorsal edge of the thyroid cartilage with stainless steel wire. The manipulation of the arytenoid cartilage and the point of its fixation must be guided by laryngoscopy. The success of the surgery is adequate in most cases, but there is a permanently open glottis. Laryngeal function is disturbed with regard to vocalization, prevention of inspiration of foreign material, the closing reflex in coughing, and adaptation to increased exertion and activity at higher temperatures.

Trauma

Accidental trauma to the larynx causes a life-threatening situation when hemorrhage and edema prevent normal airflow. The animal should be anesthetized immediately by intravenously administered short-acting barbiturate (in dogs) or by intramuscularly administered ketamine and xylazine hydrochloride (in cats). After intubation, blood should be removed from the trachea and major bronchi by aspiration through the endotracheal tube. A tracheotomy is then performed, and the patient is allowed to awaken. In most cases, full evaluation of the more permanent damage caused by the trauma is not possible until the hemorrhage and edema have subsided, sometimes many days later.

Iatrogenic trauma includes the complications after laryngeal surgery but also paralysis caused by surgical damage to the laryngeal nerves. One of the most feared complications is *laryngeal webbing* after surgical trauma to the vocal folds. Webbing is the development of obstructive scar tissue in the glottis, and it occurs most frequently between the vocal folds. It results in a serious narrowing of the glottis. In many cases, removal of the web does not result in normal laryngeal movements because of more extensively distributed scar tissue. Webbing occurs when the mucosa of the lower portions of both vocal folds is removed at the same time (e.g., in surgical debarking of dogs) or as a result of rough handling of tissues in opening the thyroid cartilage on the ventral midline. The disablement of the patient can be very serious and permanent. Any laryngeal surgery can cause the development of scar tissue and, consequently, strictures and fixation. The larynx should therefore always be manipulated with great care.

References and Supplemental Reading

Venker-van Haagen, A. J.: Laryngeal paralysis in young Bouviers. *In* Kirk, R. W. (ed.): *Current Veterinary Therapy VII*. Philadelphia: W. B. Saunders, 1979, pp. 290–291.

Venker-van Haagen, A. J.: Investigations on the pathogenesis of hereditary laryngeal paralysis in the Bouvier. Thesis, State University Utrecht, Utrecht, The Netherlands, 1980.

SHORT-TERM VENTILATORY SUPPORT

PETER J. PASCOE, B.V.Sc.
Guelph, Ontario, Canada

Except during procedures for which a patient is anesthetized, it may be difficult to predict the length of time that ventilatory support may be required, and therefore it is imperative to aim for optimal conditions. It is axiomatic that ventilatory support requires intensive management of the patient. The animal is attached to a machine that is programmed to function in a certain way. The machine could break down, it could deliver the wrong mixture of gas, or the tubing might become plugged or kinked. In a conscious animal, there is the further risk that the tubing connected to the airway could be dislodged, twisted, or even bitten off. Ventilated animals need close and continuous supervision; if it is not worthwhile providing this, then ventilatory support should not be instituted. In using the term *support*, one should recognize that this form of therapy does *not* cure the underlying condition, and, since it is an invasive technique, it can be associated with significant complications.

INDICATIONS FOR VENTILATORY SUPPORT

There are two main indications for ventilatory support: (1) acute brain swelling and (2) respiratory insufficiency. Acute brain swelling may cause respiratory depression, but even if it does not, ventilatory support is indicated. Intracranial pressure is a function of the volume of liquid (blood and cerebrospinal fluid) and the volume of solid (brain tissue) in the cranial vault. If the intracranial pressure increases enough, venous and cerebrospinal fluid outflow from the cranial vault will cease and the pressure will rise precipitously. When the brain tissue swells (i.e., cerebral edema), one mechanism of maintaining an acceptable intracranial pressure is to reduce the amount of liquid in the cranium. Cerebral blood flow is controlled, to a large extent, by the arterial partial pressure of carbon dioxide (Pa_{CO_2}), so a reduction in the latter will decrease flow to the brain and subsequently reduce the intracranial pressure. In clinical use, Pa_{CO_2} should be reduced to 20 to 30 mm Hg by hyperventilating the patient, and it should be maintained at this level. A reduction below 20 mm Hg is contraindicated, as it may reduce blood flow so much that the delivery of oxygen to the brain is impaired.

Respiration includes ventilation, gas exchange, and transport of gas to and from the tissues. An insufficiency in any of these areas may require ventilatory support. The decision as to when an animal needs supportive therapy is not an easy one to make if the judgment is based purely on clinical signs. As an example, cyanosis is an indication of gross hypoxemia and can be seen when there is 85 per cent hemoglobin saturation or less (i.e., when the Pa_{O_2} is 50 to 60 mm Hg). However, if circulation is poor, desaturation in the capillaries may occur because more oxygen is extracted as the blood slowly passes through the tissues. If the animal is anemic, cyanosis may not be seen at all, even though there is significant desaturation. (Five gm of desaturated hemoglobin per 100 ml of blood is required to produce detectable cyanosis.) In addition, the interpretation of cyanosis varies with differing lighting conditions and mucous membrane pigments. Another example of the difficulty in decision-making based solely on clinical signs is hypoventilation, which can manifest itself in several different forms. An animal with head trauma may have a slow, shallow respiratory pattern due to depression of the respiratory center. There may be an exaggerated respiratory effort with paradoxical chest wall movement and stridor if the trauma has produced upper airway obstruction, or there may be rapid, shallow respiration with exaggerated effort and open-mouth breathing if the head trauma has produced neurogenic pulmonary edema. So the clinical questions are as follows:

1. Is there an obvious reduction in ventilation?
2. Is there excessive effort required to achieve ventilation?
3. Does the animal show signs of "air hunger"—open-mouth breathing, distressed facial expression, cyanosis, or a gasping ventilatory pattern?

If the answer to any of these questions is *yes*, ventilatory support should be considered. Before proceeding, one must determine if some other therapy will be effective. If the animal is in extreme distress, one may want to institute ventilatory support in order to buy time to deal with the underlying causes. In humans, the criteria used for the institution of ventilatory support involve measurement of vital capacity, inspiratory force, minute ventilation, and arterial blood gases. The first two measurements require patient cooperation and so are difficult to apply to dogs and cats. Minute ventilation can be measured by using a respirometer, but blood gas values are the best objective measure of ventilation. From these numbers, one can discern whether the animal is hypoxic or hypercarbic and can monitor the therapy much more effectively. If the Pa_{O_2} is less than 60 mm Hg or the Pa_{CO_2} is greater than 55 mm Hg, ventilatory support should be considered.

Having established that the patient has signs of respiratory insufficiency, the possible cause or causes should be identified. This is necessary because there are many treatable problems that do not require artificial ventilation. A dog that has received an overdose of opiate drugs can be given a competitive reversing agent (e.g., naloxone), which will decrease the respiratory depression. On the other hand, the condition of a dog that has eaten a bottle of barbiturate sleeping tablets cannot be reversed, and the animal will need ventilatory support and further therapy in order to allow it to clear the drugs by using its own metabolism. A cat or dog with an air- or fluid-filled pleural space can show significant improvement in ventilation once the air or fluid is removed. In diseases in which there is a decreased area for oxygen uptake (e.g., pneumonia), raising the inspired concentration of oxygen (fraction of inspired oxygen [FI_{O_2}]) may be the only therapy required to relieve the animal's distress. One can then proceed to institute specific treatment for the underlying condition.

A decision chart for the institution of ventilatory support is presented in Figure 1. Dogs or cats with clinical evidence of brain swelling should be ventilated to help reduce intracranial pressure. The patient with obvious hypoventilation as encountered in drug overdose, severe metabolic disease, cranial trauma, spinal cord damage, polyradiculoneuritis, or muscle weakness will also need ventilatory support if the underlying problem cannot be reversed immediately. In a dyspneic animal, one has to differentiate between airway obstruction, pleural effusions (fluid or air), pulmonary damage, and cardiac disease involving right-to-left shunt. With the presence of crackles, increased bronchovesicular sounds, or upper airway obstruction, oxygen therapy should be instituted. If this raises the Pa_{O_2} above 60 mm Hg, then ventilatory support is not needed. If the animal shows little improvement and the Pa_{O_2} remains below 60 mm Hg, then ventilatory support is indicated. In those patients with reduced lung or heart sounds, indicative of fluid or air within the thorax, oxygen therapy after complete thoracocentesis will improve the condition significantly. If the animal does not respond and its Pa_{O_2} level remains low, then ventilatory support may be necessary.

Animals with a cardiovascular defect that produces a significant right-to-left shunt (venous admixture) will not be greatly improved by ventilation. Raising the FI_{O_2} may give some marginal improvement, but the only effective way of treating the hypoxemia in these cases is to deal with the underlying cause.

Pulmonary edema produces a decreased area for gas exchange. Initially, this occurs because of small airway closure. As the syndrome progresses, it leads to alveolar flooding, which will gradually extend up into the larger airways. Artificial ventilation will not reverse this process, but it is part of the therapeutic armamentarium used to treat the condition. The goals of artificial ventilation in pulmonary edema are to keep the small airways open and improve the area for gas exchange. This can be done by applying positive end-expiratory pressure (PEEP) or continuous positive airway pressure (CPAP). Experimen-

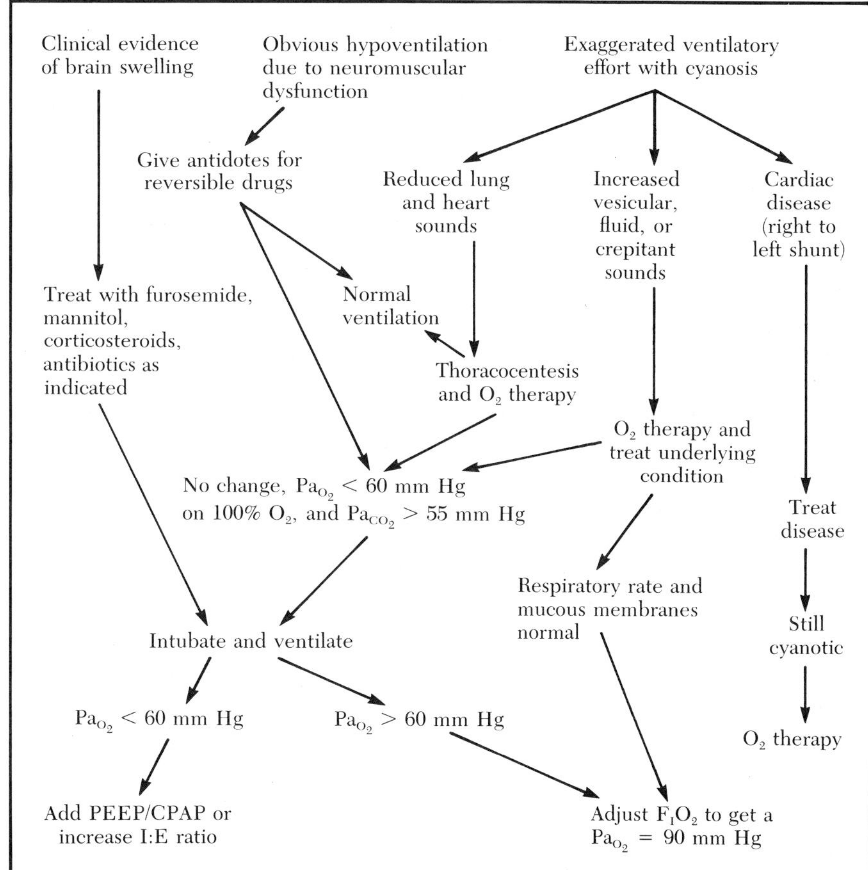

Figure 1. Decision chart for the institution of ventilatory support.

tally, it has been shown that PEEP does not decrease extravascular water in edematous lungs. (In some experiments, it has actually led to an increase.) The effect of PEEP is to redistribute this water away from the alveoli to the cuffs around the extra-alveolar vessels, and this is accompanied by a significant improvement in lung mechanics. Whether one adds controlled positive pressure ventilation to this maneuver will depend on how well the patient tolerates the PEEP/CPAP.

There are very few absolute contraindications to ventilatory support. Previous authors have stated that a closed pneumothorax is a contraindication, but this is only the case if one cannot drain the thorax. Initially, removal of air from the pleural space can be achieved with the most basic equipment (a needle, a three-way stopcock, and a syringe). If there is a continuing leak, a chest drain should be inserted and suction applied to remove the air. Animals with pulmonary contusions may require ventilatory support, but this should be avoided in these cases if at all possible. The author has seen two traumatized dogs in which intermittent positive pressure ventilation (IPPV) has caused further pulmonary hemorrhage, which contributed to their deaths. An animal with a "whiplash" tracheal separation should not be put on a ventilator until one can secure the distal part of the airway.

EQUIPMENT

In order to provide ventilatory support in animals, the following equipment is needed: endotracheal tubes, suction catheters and a vacuum (suction) pump, an oxygen supply and a controlled method of adjusting the $F_{I_{O2}}$, a ventilator, and a method for humidifying the gas supplied to the patient.

Most endotracheal tubes supplied for veterinary use are made of a durable material (e.g., rubber, plastic, or silicone), and the cuff is made of a relatively thick piece of the same material. The economics of veterinary practice necessitate that these tubes be reusable. During long-term intubation, these tubes may exert pressure on the laryngeal mucosa and lead to ulceration. Rubber tubes are harder than silicone tubes and are therefore more likely to induce this kind of damage. Movement of the tube within the larynx will also damage the mucosa, so very heavy sedation is necessary. Further complications may arise if there are residual chemical irritants on the tubes from inadequate rinsing or aeration after sterilization. Figure 2 shows the cuff on a standard type of endotracheal tube. This is known as a high-pressure, low-volume cuff, and it may require pressures as high as 180 to 250 mm Hg to prevent leakage around the cuff. When this pressure is applied to the tracheal mucosa for short periods of time, as during routine surgery, no permanent damage results; but as the time is extended (longer than 12 hours), the tracheal mucosa begins to necrose. After several days, there is total destruction of the tracheal mucosa, with exposure of the cartilaginous rings. This may lead to tracheal stenosis or tracheoesophageal fistulation as a serious complication of the prolonged intubation.

Low-pressure, high-volume cuffs (Fig. 2) have now been developed, and these are much less likely to damage the mucosa. They require pressures in the range of 30 to 40 mm Hg to prevent leaking of air around the tube and to prevent aspiration of fluid from the pharynx. As can be seen in Figure 2, the material used to make these cuffs is thin and is easily damaged, so they are not as durable as the standard tubes. Nevertheless, if one is expecting to ventilate an animal for more than 12 hours, a low-pressure, high-volume cuffed endotracheal or tracheostomy tube is recommended.

Endotracheal intubation with a cuffed endotracheal tube will block the mucociliary clearance of the airway. In order to prevent accumulation of secretions, the airway must be suctioned. To do this, one needs a catheter that is made of a soft material, has an external device allowing one to control the suction, and has holes in the end and sides of the catheter to minimize the chances of sucking up pieces of tracheal mucosa (Fig. 3). The catheter should be sterile, and its external diameter should be less than half of the diameter of the airway. If it is larger than this, it will increase the resistance to gas flow into the lungs, raising the risk of atelectasis when suction is applied.

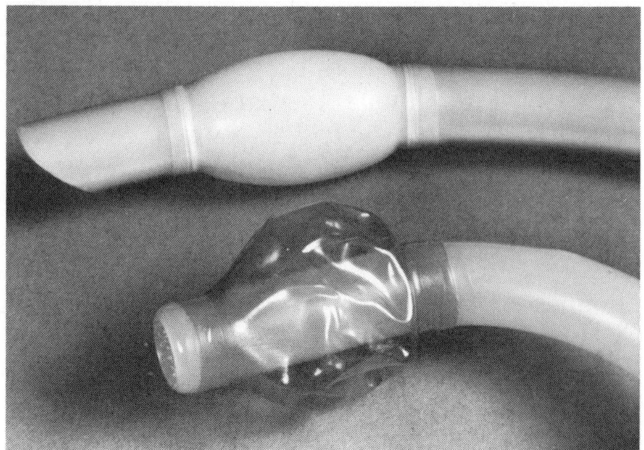

Figure 2. Endotracheal tube cuffs. Top: high pressure, low volume endotracheal tube cuff. Bottom: low pressure, high residual volume endotracheal tube cuff.

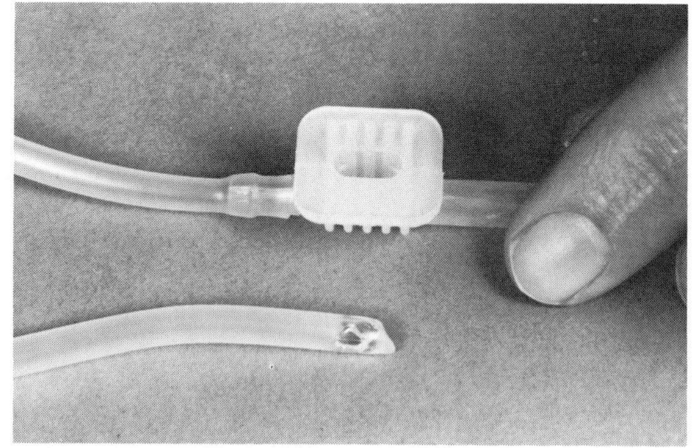

Figure 3. Tracheal suction catheter; note the thumb vent to control suction application and the side hole in the end of the catheter.

When contemplating ventilatory support, one should be aware of the risks of oxygen toxicity. When dogs are exposed to 100 per cent oxygen at one atmosphere pressure, the average survival time is approximately 50 hours. Some dogs have died in less than 30 hours, and functional and physical changes occur in the lung after the first 12 hours. As with most drugs, oxygen toxicity is dose related: 80 per cent oxygen exposure took 5 to 7 days to kill dogs, and those exposed to 50 per cent showed some functional changes (pulmonary hypertension); but all dogs survived a 35-day exposure, and there was no permanent damage. This evidence implies that one should not leave a dog on 100 per cent oxygen for more than 12 hours unless concentrations of that order are required to maintain an acceptable Pa_{O_2} level. In order to reduce the concentration of oxygen, another gas should be added, and ideally this should be nitrogen, although entrainment of room air will also work. One should be able to check the concentration in the delivered gas to ensure that the correct FI_{O_2} is used. An oxygen meter may be used, or a sample of the gas mixture can be taken and run through a blood gas machine. The easiest gas to use on most veterinary anesthetic machines is nitrous oxide, which is acceptable for short-term use but is also toxic and should only be used at 30 per cent or less for no longer than 24 hours.

IPPV can be provided in many ways, and the equipment may be very simple or extremely complex. For the very short term, hand ventilation can be achieved by using an Ambu bag or an anesthetic circuit with a rebreathing bag. There is always a tendency to hyperventilate with these manual techniques, and there may be a lot of variation between the tidal volume (V_T) of the breaths delivered. Nevertheless, ventilating by hand does give some information about airway resistance and lung compliance. Since we do not have any easy method for measuring these conditions, it is useful to apply periodic manual ventilation to obtain a subjective evaluation of the change in the mechanical characteristics of the lungs.

Mechanical ventilators are of two types: constant flow generators and constant pressure generators. These machines are cycled by introducing a limiting factor such as V_T, pressure, or time. In North America, most ventilators are of the constant flow variety, and either pressure or V_T is the limiting factor. These machines produce a uniform flow of gas, and the airway pressure gradually rises as the lung is inflated. The constant pressure generators, which are used extensively in the United Kingdom, give a constant airway pressure, but the flow gradually reduces as the pressure from the lungs approaches the pressure generated by the ventilator (these ventilators cannot be pressure cycled). For the constant flow generator, the two most common methods of cycling, pressure and volume, each have their advantages and disadvantages. A *volume-limited ventilator* will deliver the preset volume regardless of changes in resistance or compliance. (On most of these machines there is an upper limit of pressure delivered, for safety purposes, but this is much higher than needed for normal ventilation.) A *pressure-limited ventilator*, on the other hand, is very dependent on changes in compliance or resistance. For example, if compliance decreases (the lungs become "stiffer"), the preset pressure will be reached before the estimated V_T is reached. The disadvantage of the volume-limited machine is that if there is a leak in the circuit, the animal may end up receiving only a small part of the required breath, whereas the pressure-limited ventilator will deliver gas until the pressure is reached. As long as the leak is minor, a pressure-limited machine will give a reasonable V_T to the animal, and the longer time taken to reach the preset pressure may indicate to the person monitoring the machine that there is an equipment problem.

Although it is not possible to discuss here each individual machine, the end point for the animal is the same for all conventional machines. The variables that one wants to control are as follows:

1. Number of breaths per minute. On some machines this is labeled as respiratory rate, and on others it may be defined as expiratory pause or expiratory time. For the latter, if one increases the expiratory pause (i.e., the time between breaths), then one will reduce the respiratory rate.

2. Tidal volume. On volume-limited machines, this is set either directly as a V_T or indirectly by setting the minute volume (in this case, V_T is found by dividing the minute volume by the rate). On pressure-limited ventilators, one does not have a direct measure of V_T. A peak pressure of 12 to 20 cm H_2O will give normal V_T in the normal lung, but much higher pressures may be required in a compromised animal. Volumes may be measured with a spirometer.

3. Inspiratory flow rate. This controls the rate of inflation of the lungs. A long, slow inflation will allow adequate time for gas exchange, but the applied pressure in the thorax will impede venous return to the heart and hence reduce cardiac output. A very rapid inflation will produce less effect on cardiac output but may not allow time for adequate gas exchange. Thus, the setting that is used is a compromise between these two factors, and in most instances one would aim to deliver the inspiratory portion 0.1 to 2 seconds.

4. Trigger effort. This control is present on many ventilators, and it determines the negative pressure that the patient must generate to cycle the ventilator. If this is at its most sensitive setting, then the slightest change in airway pressure will trigger the ventilator. On some machines, this is so sensitive that it will respond to the heartbeat! The purpose of this control is to allow one to select an assisted (i.e., the animal sets the respiratory rate) or a controlled (i.e., the machine determines the frequency of breathing) mode of ventilation.

5. Expiratory flow rate. The controls described above are the most important ones. If there is a control for expiratory flow rate, it should generally be set to allow for passive expiration. If a longer time is required for gas exchange, then the flow rate can be retarded. It should never be used to pull gas out of (create negative airway pressure in) the animal, because this will promote atelectasis and airway closure.

A ventilator can be attached to the patient directly or through an anesthetic machine. Most ventilators designed for intensive care will be connected directly to the patient. If an anesthetic machine with a circle system is used, care must be taken to change the soda lime before it becomes exhausted.

PEEP and CPAP have already been mentioned, but the technical differences should be explained. With PEEP, the patient exhales through a resistance. Thus, during spontaneous ventilation, the upper airway pressure must fall below atmospheric pressure during inspiration even though it is maintained above this level until the beginning of the next inspiration. CPAP, on the other hand, maintains the airway pressure above atmospheric throughout the breath (as long as the flow delivered during inspiration exceeds the peak inspiratory flow generated by the animal). When controlled IPPV is used, CPAP and PEEP amount to the same thing, since inspiration is produced by positive pressure from the machine rather than negative pressure from the animal (Fig. 4). In practice, it is easy to apply PEEP to a spontaneously breathing animal. The patient is connected to a nonrebreathing circuit such as a Bain's circuit, and then the expiratory

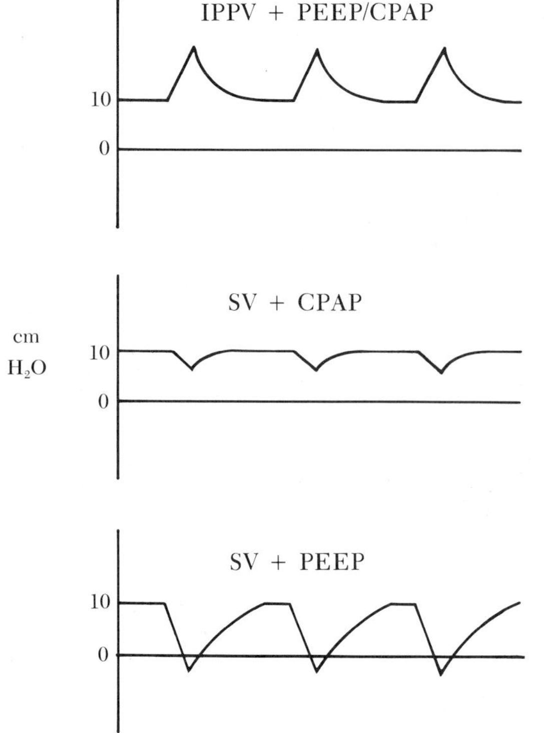

Figure 4. Pressure/time traces for intermittent positive pressure ventilation (IPPV) or spontaneous ventilation (SV) with application of positive end expiratory pressure (PEEP) or continuous positive airway pressure (CPAP).

limb is submerged under water to the level of PEEP required (i.e., if one wants 10 cm H_2O PEEP, the end of the circuit is 10 cm below the surface of the water). This system could be made to deliver CPAP simply by raising the flow rate to a level close to the peak inspiratory flow. However, for a 20-kg (44-lb) dog, this represents a flow of 15 to 18 L/minute, and so it is not a cheap way to produce this effect. Some modern ventilators have PEEP/CPAP controls on them, and on some it is possible to program them to deliver PEEP or CPAP during spontaneous or controlled ventilation.

Intermittent mandatory ventilation (IMV) involves the use of a ventilator to provide a certain minute volume while allowing the patient to breathe spontaneously in between the delivery of positive pressure breaths. The appeal of this technique is that it allows the patient to control respiration but ensures that eucapnia is maintained. It requires sophisticated equipment, and to date many of the expected advantages of the technique have not been substantiated, so its applicability in veterinary patients would appear to be limited.

Recently, considerable interest has been shown in techniques of high-frequency ventilation. These use ventilatory rates of 60 to 1800 *per minute.* These high frequencies use very small volumes, and there is no clear understanding as to how they work; however, they can produce adequate gas exchange in what appears to be a totally apneic animal. The main advantage with this system is the use of lower peak airway pressures, thus reducing the negative effects on the venous return and reducing the risks of barotrauma associated with conventional techniques. Humidification of the gas appears to be a problem. The methods have not yet fully evolved, but this may become a very useful method for critically ill animals in the future.

Humidification of the inspired gases is important, because the use of an endotracheal tube (or tracheotomy tube) bypasses the nasopharynx, where air is humidified during spontaneous breathing, and also because compressed gases are dry. The aim is to ensure that air entering the endotracheal tube has a water content of 30 mg/L. Bubbling the gas through cold water will only add about half this amount. In order to carry this amount of water as vapor, the gas must be saturated at 30°C, which is likely to give the patient an excessive heat load. This problem is overcome by nebulizing water into tiny droplets, thus making it easy to exceed the water vapor capacity for any given temperature of the inspired gas. (A full description of the care and use of this equipment can be found in Haskins, 1984.)

TECHNIQUE

Having decided to provide ventilatory support, one must next choose between an oral endotracheal tube or a tracheotomy tube. To use the orotracheal route, the animal will almost certainly require anesthesia or heavy sedation if it is not already comatose. Having to keep an animal sedated or anesthetized for long periods of time will depress some immunologic responses as well as remove the cough reflex and increase the risks of atelectasis and lung congestion. Once a tracheotomy has been performed, it is often feasible to ventilate the animal without anesthetizing it, and with careful management awake patients have been ventilated for considerable periods of time. Occasionally, the animal will not tolerate the ventilation or physical restraint, and it will become necessary to use some form of chemical sedation.

There are very few reports in the literature of anesthesia or sedation of pet dogs and cats for intensive therapy. What is needed is a drug or combination of drugs that produces minimal cardiovascular depression while producing sufficient respiratory depression to prevent the animal from fighting the ventilator. In theory, the opioid drugs fit this description but, in the author's experience, have not been found to be sufficient when used alone. Combining opioids with benzodiazepines improves the chemical restraint, but this is still not enough for many cases. Some practitioners use an opioid combined with a muscle relaxant such as pancuronium. With this combination, it is rather difficult to ascertain the level of consciousness of the animal. Dogs will tolerate fairly high doses of opioids, but since there is a narrow margin between sedation and central excitation in cats, this technique is not recommended. A major advantage with the opioid-relaxant combination is that both drugs are reversible. In cats, the use of the steroid anesthetic Saffan* (where available) has been recommended and appears to be quite successful. Since it is metabolized quickly, cats will still recover rapidly at the end of the period of sedation. This steroid anesthetic is not yet available in the United States, so a combination of an opiate and a barbiturate is probably the best alternative. The author has successfully used combinations of opioids and pentobarbital for sedation and restraint for periods in excess of 48 hours. A recent report described a combination of guaifenesin, xylazine, and ketamine for anesthetizing dogs (Benson et al., 1985). This combination appears to produce a smooth anesthetic period with a rapid recovery, and although it has not been used for prolonged restraint, its use should be investigated.

Inhalant agents such as halothane, methoxyflurane, enflurane, or isoflurane have been used to achieve short periods of restraint through anesthesia (less than 12 hours), and if one is ventilating from an anesthetic machine, this would work for even greater periods of time. This technique will probably mean using nitrous oxide as well, but it should be noted that it can produce myeloid suppression when given for prolonged periods. Most ventilators used for intensive care are not designed to deliver inhalant agents, so injectable drugs are indicated in this situation.

Initial dosages of drugs for chemical restraint while ventilating dogs are presented in Table 1. It should be emphasized that these drugs *must* be given to effect. There is a great deal of difference between the requirements of a dog with acute brain swelling and that of a previously healthy animal with aspiration pneumonia. If the drugs are set up in an intravenous drip, then great care should be taken to monitor the level of sedation they produce in the animal.

Once the animal is intubated, the normal clearance of material from the airway has been bypassed and the clinician has to keep the airway clear. To do this, the mucociliary blanket must be correctly hydrated. If it is dry, then the cilia will cease to function; if it is overhydrated, the viscoelastic properties of the mucus are altered and the ciliary movement becomes less effective. The gases entering the airway must be humidified, and the patient should have sufficient fluid intake to maintain normal production of lower airway secretions. Once this fluid reaches the upper airway in the intubated patient, it can only be removed by suction. This fluid should be removed whenever it is present, and it can be detected by auscultating the upper airways. Suctioning is a traumatic procedure, and its use at arbitrarily fixed intervals (e.g., every 30 minutes) should be avoided. It is better to apply suction only as it is indicated. The technique for suctioning the airways is as follows:

1. Auscultate to verify the presence of fluid in the upper airways (e.g., coarse crackles on inspiration and expiration).
2. Assemble the equipment: suction apparatus (set at medium to low pressure), sterile suction catheter, sterile saline or water for rinsing the catheter, anesthetic machine or resuscitator bag with an oxygen source, and sterile saline in a syringe.
3. Preoxygenate the patient with 100 per cent oxygen, and hyperinflate lungs (four to five breaths are sufficient).
4. Put on sterile gloves.
5. Introduce the catheter gently as far as needed (to the fourth intercostal space).
6. Apply suction (by closing the thumb hole—Fig. 2) while rotating and pulling the catheter up the airway. Do not apply suction for more than 10 seconds at a time.
7. Repeat if necessary, being as gentle as possible,

Table 1. *Chemical Restraint for Ventilatory Support in Dogs*

Drugs	Concentration	Dosage
Oxymorphone	1.5 mg/ml	0.2 mg/kg (up to 4.5 mg) IV; 0.1 to 0.2 mg/kg every 1 to 1½ hours
+		
Pancuronium	2.0 mg/ml	0.1 mg/kg IV; 0.05 mg/kg every hour thereafter
Oxymorphone	1.5 mg/ml	0.2 mg/kg (up to 4.5 mg) IV; 0.1 mg/kg every 2 hours thereafter
+		
Pentobarbital	65 mg/ml	4 mg/kg initially IV; 2 to 4 mg/kg/hour thereafter
Guaifenesin	50 mg/ml	0.55 ml/kg bolus initially followed by 2.2 ml/kg/hour thereafter
+		
Ketamine	1 mg/ml	
+		
Xylazine	0.25 mg/ml	

*Alfaxalone and alfadolone acetate; manufactured in Great Britain by Glaxo Laboratories.

and rinse the catheter if it becomes plugged with mucus or blood.

8. If the secretions are very viscid, inject saline at 1 ml/10 kg into the airway, ventilate for two or three breaths, then repeat the suctioning.

9. Once suctioning is complete, hyperinflate the lungs two or three times before reconnecting the ventilator.

In order to assist with airway drainage and to prevent congestion and atelectasis, the animal should be placed on a slight incline with the head down and should be turned over every hour. Percussion (coupage) of the chest wall has been advocated to help move secretions. The hands should be cupped slightly, and the chest is lightly thumped as rapidly as possible for about 5 minutes on each side, three or four times per day. The intent of coupage is to vibrate the chest without producing too much trauma to the chest wall. This is probably helpful, but higher-frequency chest wall vibration (15 Hz) produces a marked increase in mucociliary clearance (340 per cent increase over baseline). Vibrations at these frequencies require specialized equipment.

The ventilator should be set up to provide the best gas exchange for the condition of the patient. Controlled ventilation is more efficient in this regard than assisted ventilation. Initially the ventilator should be programmed to deliver a V_T of about 20 ml/kg with 8 to 12 breaths/minute and an inspiratory-to-expiratory ratio (I:E ratio) of 1:2 or 1:3 (i.e., with an I:E ratio of 1:2 and 10 breaths a minute, each breath takes 6 seconds, so inspiration occurs in 2 seconds and the expiration/pause phase takes 4 seconds). This should result in a Pa_{CO_2} of 40 mm Hg; adjustments in the delivered volume should be made to maintain this value or to lower the Pa_{CO_2} to 20 to 30 mm Hg in the case of an increased intracranial pressure. Using these larger tidal volumes, the author has not found it necessary to "sigh" animals that are ventilated. If the animal still appears to be hypoxemic or an arterial blood gas still gives a Pa_{CO_2} below 60 mm Hg on 100 per cent oxygen, then one should try adding PEEP/CPAP. If this is not available, then the I:E ratio should be changed to prolong inspiration. This allows greater time for gas exchange. When adding PEEP/CPAP, one should ideally ascertain the best amount ("optimal") for that animal. This is done by using 100 per cent oxygen and then adding PEEP/CPAP in increasing amounts (5 cm H_2O, then 10 cm H_2O, then 15 cm H_2O), allowing about 20 minutes at each setting and checking the blood gas values. The best PEEP/CPAP is the one that produces the highest Pa_{O_2}.

When IPPV is instituted, the generation of inspiration changes from a negative intrathoracic pressure to a positive one. This produces a significant difference in venous return. With spontaneous respiration, venous return is augmented during inspiration; but with IPPV, the positive pressure generated tends to collapse the great veins and inhibit venous return (Fig. 4). In a normal animal, the autonomic response to this is to increase venous tone, thus raising the right atrial filling pressure. With hypovolemia, the animal may be at the limit of compensation, and so the end result will be a significant reduction in cardiac output. The simplest manifestation of this is the cyclical change in pulse pressure associated with ventilation. If the pulse feels strong and then gets weak or disappears just after the end of the inspiratory phase, then the animal may be hypovolemic. If one can monitor the arterial pressure by using a transducer attached to a direct arterial line, the flattening of the pulse contour can be seen very easily. If this phenomenon is detected when IPPV is instituted, the volume deficit should be corrected before PEEP/CPAP is added. The exception to this rule is the animal with limited cardiac reserve or with pulmonary edema. In the latter case, we have already established that IPPV with PEEP/CPAP is only a supportive measure and will not reduce the edema. If the pulmonary edema is due to left ventricular failure, then increasing the contractility of the left ventricle will aid in removing the fluid. If the condition is caused by increased capillary permeability, therapy should be directed toward fluid restriction and reduction of pulmonary arterial pressure. As the blood volume is reduced, the effects of PEEP/CPAP will be exacerbated, and so the only method of compensating for this is to increase cardiac output using positive inotropic drugs. With pulmonary edema from both cardiogenic and increased capillary permeability, volume restriction and cardiac support are indicated. Dopamine and dobutamine are the ionotropic drugs of choice for this support.

Once the initial support has been instituted, the animal has to be monitored continuously. Ideally, this monitoring should include (in order of increasing sophistication) mucous membrane color and hydration, auscultation of the chest and airways, pulse rate and character, the adequacy of ventilation (visual inspection), the demeanor or responsiveness of the patient, body weight (to determine fluid balance), urine output, radiographic assessment of the thorax, electrocardiogram, central venous pressure, arterial blood pressure, blood gases, electrolytes, pulmonary arterial pressure, pulmonary wedge pressure, and cardiac output. Although the progress of therapy can be determined crudely by clinical assessment, the measurement of blood gases provides the best objective assessment of therapeutic efficacy. If we are going to have to support a small animal for longer than 24 hours, this becomes a serious problem in terms of the amount of blood removed for each sample. Great care should be taken to ensure that one does not produce an anemic animal by sampling too frequently. In order to facilitate arterial blood gas sampling, it is almost essential to place an arterial catheter to avoid making multiple or serial arterial punctures.

Animals that are weak or debilitated before ventilatory support is started may need nutritional support in order to make them strong enough to fight infection and to eventually be weaned from the ventilator. This can be provided fairly readily by oral supplementation if the animal is awake, but consideration should be given to using intravenous hyperalimentation for any patient that is comatose or anesthetized for more than 24 hours.

Weaning the patient from the ventilator should be considered as soon as possible. Ventilation is an invasive procedure that may have serious complications that increase with the duration of therapy. In cases of primary hypoventilation (e.g., barbiturate overdose, coonhound paralysis), the patient should be assessed for signs of fighting the ventilator. In the animal in which there is interference with gas exchange, one wants to be able to maintain a Pa_{O_2} greater than 60 mm Hg with an FI_{O_2} of 20 to 25 per cent. If the animal has been on PEEP/CPAP, then the FI_{O_2} is reduced first; if blood gases remain stable, then the PEEP/CPAP may be gradually reduced while the response of the animal is monitored.

For an animal to breathe spontaneously, it must have a potent respiratory drive and be strong enough to maintain its own ventilation. This is produced by reducing ventilation, thus allowing carbon dioxide to build up, and by awakening the animal. A conscious animal will tend to breathe at a lower Pa_{CO_2}. Once a decision has been reached to wean the animal, any reversible drugs used to produce sedation should be antagonized and ventilatory rate reduced to two to four breaths per minute. This can be continued safely for 10 to 15 minutes, during which time the animal should show spontaneous respiratory movements. If ventilatory efforts are weak or nonexistent, then the ventilatory support should be reinstituted. If the ventilator is removed, it is prudent to make further assessment of the respiration before the endotracheal, or tracheotomy, tube is taken out. The respiration should be deep and even, and there should be no evidence of fatigue. Fifteen to 20 minutes after the start of spontaneous respiration, an arterial blood gas sample will provide a definitive measurement of the adequacy of ventilation. Depending on the original problem, the animal should be monitored for several hours in order to ensure that there is no further need for ventilatory support.

COMPLICATIONS

As already stated, ventilatory support may be lifesaving, but it carries many potential risks with it. The presence of an endotracheal tube interferes with mucociliary transport, and the use of heavy sedation or opiates will prevent the animal from coughing. Both of these mechanisms are important in the pulmonary defense against infection. The use of positive pressure to inflate the lungs may damage the lungs, leading to a pneumothorax (barotrauma). This is an unlikely complication in the normal lung, but it may occur when the lung has already been traumatized. The effect of the airway pressure on venous return to the heart has been mentioned, but the effect of IPPV on the splanchnic organs is also significant. There is a significant increase in splanchnic vascular resistance and a reduction in portal venous flow, and so the liver is more susceptible to ischemia from arterial hypotension. The urine output falls by as much as 40 per cent on 10 cm H_2O PEEP, indicating that renal function is also adversely affected.

SUMMARY

Ventilatory support is indicated whenever there is a ventilatory insufficiency or an acute brain swelling. Its use requires careful preparation, attention to details, and knowledge of the expected outcome of the therapeutic maneuvers. Continuous monitoring must be available, and the animal should be weaned as soon as possible to reduce the risks of pulmonary infection, pulmonary barotrauma, and the adverse effects on other body systems.

References and Supplemental Reading

Benson, G. J., Thurmon, J. C., and Tranquilli, W. J.: Intravenous infusion of glyceryl guaicolate, ketamine, and xylazine in dogs: Cardiopulmonary responses. Vet. Surg. 14:71, 1985.

Haskins, S. C.: Management of pulmonary disease in the critical patient. *In* Zaslow, I. M. (ed.): *Veterinary Trauma and Critical Care.* Philadelphia: Lea & Febiger, 1984, pp. 339–384.

Hedley-Whyte, J., Burgess III, G. E., Feeley, T. W., et al.: *Applied Physiology of Respiratory Care.* Boston: Little, Brown & Co., 1976.

Martz, K. V., Joiner, J. W., and Sheperd, R. M.: *Management of the Ventilator Patient System. A Team Approach,* 2nd ed. St. Louis: C. V. Mosby, 1984.

Watson, C. B.: High Frequency Ventilation (HFV). Anesthesiol. Rev. 11:15, 1984.

Weisman, I. M., Rinaldo, J. E., Rogers, R. M., et al.: Intermittent mandatory ventilation. Am. Rev. Respir. Dis. 127:641, 1983.

BRONCHODILATOR THERAPY

MARK G. PAPICH, D.V.M.
Saskatoon, Saskatchewan

Bronchodilator therapy can be useful as an adjunct to the treatment of cardiopulmonary diseases in small animals. Chronic tracheobronchitis, collapsing trachea, allergic bronchitis, and pulmonary edema are all diseases for which bronchodilator therapy has been used. Drugs used in bronchodilator therapy are the methylxanthines (e.g., theophylline), corticosteroids, adrenergic agents, and anticholinergic agents.* Traditional textbooks of veterinary pharmacology contain little information pertaining to the clinical pharmacology of these agents, and only recently have textbooks of small animal medicine addressed this area.

BRONCHOCONSTRICTION

Several distinct mechanisms contribute to the pathogenesis of increased airway resistance in small animals. Primary tracheobronchitis may result from viral, bacterial, or fungal infection or chemical or thromboembolic injury. Inflammatory cells and mediators enter the respiratory mucosa and lamina propria. Edema of the mucosa, increased secretion of the glandular epithelium, and bronchial smooth muscle constriction and thickening can result. These factors lead to increased airway resistance and therefore an increased work of breathing.

Tracheobronchitis may be a secondary condition. In dogs, the most frequent cause of this is a collapsing trachea. Whether this condition is primary or secondary, if the correct therapy is not given the affected animal may develop chronic tracheobronchitis.

Pulmonary edema results from both cardiac and noncardiac conditions. Cardiogenic pulmonary edema is the result of increased pulmonary venous pressure, which leads to accumulation of fluid in the terminal airways and interstitial spaces. Noncardiogenic pulmonary edema may result from increased permeability of alveolar epithelium and capillary endothelium as the result of inflammatory causes. Small airway constriction is a consequence of interstitial edema and the accumulation of fluid.

Allergic tracheobronchitis may occur in both cats and dogs. True asthma, as seen in humans, is probably rare in dogs. Allergic bronchitis in cats, characterized by an acute respiratory distress syndrome, has been called "feline asthma," but the exact cause of the disease has not been defined. Bronchial constriction and obstruction as it occurs in allergic tracheobronchitis is related to increased bronchial smooth muscle contraction caused by mediators released from sensitized mast cells, including histamine, serotonin, prostaglandins ($PGF_{2\alpha}$, PGD_2), and leukotrienes LTC and LTD (components of the slow-reacting substance of anaphylaxis [SRS-A]) (Fig. 1) (Wasserman et al., 1980). Inflammatory mediators activated during episodes of allergic bronchitis (e.g., vasoactive amines, complement, kinins, and white blood cell products) also contribute to increased airway resistance by increasing capillary permeability, granulocyte chemotaxis, and secretions—all of which lead to edema of the bronchioles and mucus secretion into the airways.

It is not known which mediator or mechanism is the dominant factor in each situation. The functional decrease in airway diameter that occurs most likely results from a combination of processes. Species differences are also known to exist. For example, histamine H_1 receptors are thought to play a minor role in the pathophysiology of feline asthma in comparison with its role in asthma in other species (Eyre, 1973).

BRONCHODILATING DRUGS

Adrenergic Drugs

The pathogenesis of bronchoconstrictive diseases may involve (1) insufficient beta-receptor activity, (2) increased alpha-receptor activity, or (3) increased cholinergic activity (Lockey and Buckantz, 1979). It is not firmly established which process may be predominant in domestic animals. It is known, however, that increased beta-receptor activity decreases airway resistance and leads to clinical improvement.

Adrenergic receptors may be classified into alpha (α) or beta (β) types. Alpha-receptors are present on vascular and bronchial smooth muscle and on mast cells. Stimulation of α-receptors leads to sys-

*Many doses cited are outside the range approved by the FDA, and most are not approved for use in dogs and cats.

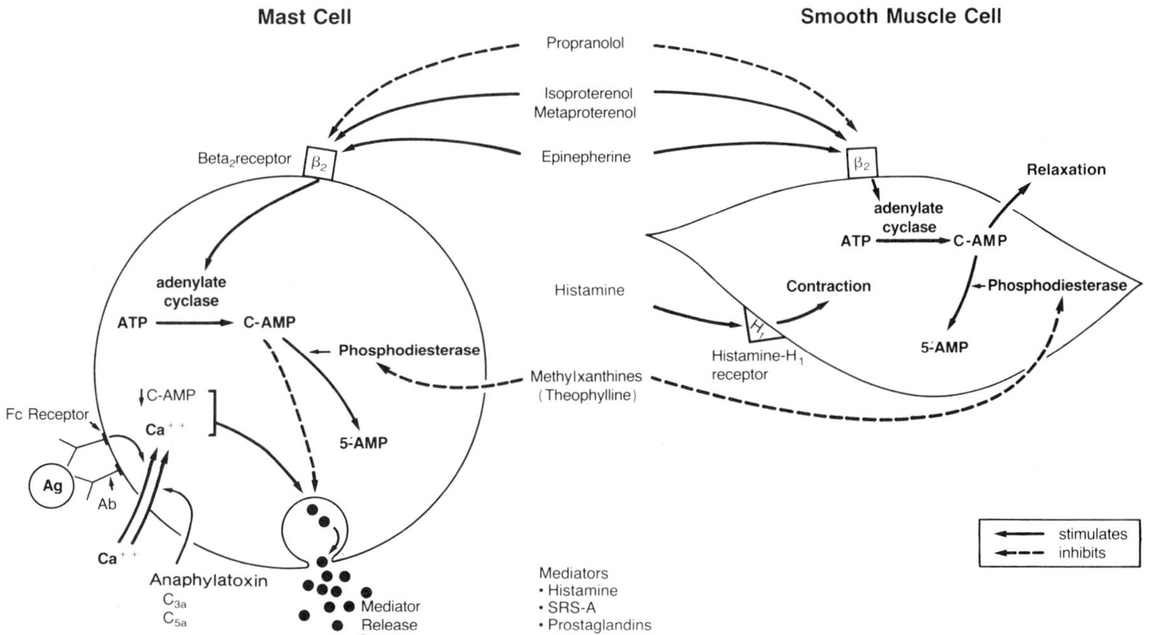

Figure 1. Mast cell on left and smooth muscle cell on right. Binding of antigen (Ag) to immunoglobulin molecules (Ab) on mast cell surface, and anaphylatoxins stimulate influx of calcium (Ca^{++}) and release of mast cell mediators: histamine, slow-reacting substance of anaphylaxis (SRS-A), and prostaglandins (PG-D_2 and PG-F_2). Mast cell mediators (histamine shown here) stimulate the smooth muscle cell to contract. Stimulation of β_2 receptors and inhibition of phosphodiesterase increase intracellular cyclic AMP (C-AMP), inhibit mast cell degranulation, and promote smooth muscle relaxation.

temic vasoconstriction and increased blood pressure and also acts to increase bronchial smooth muscle constriction and facilitate the release of mediators from pulmonary mast cells. Presumably, this effect is mediated through the formation of cyclic guanosine monophosphate (GMP) from guanosine triphosphate (GTP). Activation of α-receptors will also lead to constriction of blood vessels of the respiratory mucosa and decrease secretion of fluids into the airways.

Beta-receptors may be classified as β_1 or β_2. Beta$_1$-receptors are primarily located in the heart, and their stimulation leads to an increase in cardiac rate, contractility, and conduction velocity. Beta$_2$-receptors are found in many tissues. For this discussion, the important locations are the bronchial smooth muscle and pulmonary mast cells. Stimulation of β_2-receptors leads to increased activity of the enzyme adenylate cyclase in the cell membrane (Fig. 1). Increased adenylate cyclase activity generates increased intracellular cyclic adenosine monophosphate (cAMP), which subsequently relaxes bronchial smooth muscle cells and inhibits release of mediators from mast cells (Adams, 1984). Both effects are beneficial when dealing with bronchoconstrictive pulmonary disease.

The adrenergic drugs available vary in their specificity for α-, β_1-, and β_2-receptors. The specificity for a particular receptor is relative and usually dose dependent. It is most beneficial to use a drug with primarily β_2-receptor activity in bronchodilator therapy; however, since some overlap occurs, α-, β_1-, and β_2-receptor activation may occur as well. One must be knowledgeable of the potential side effects that may occur from activation of these other receptors.

Specific drugs available are listed in Table 1. In a patient that presents with acute respiratory distress or anaphylaxis, epinephrine is the drug of choice. As well as the beneficial β_2 stimulation in anaphylaxis, epinephrine also has cardiac-stimulating β_1 activity and α-receptor vasoconstricting ability, which will improve systemic blood pressure. For longer-term therapy, β_2-selective agents should be employed, since a drug with equipotent β_1 and β_2 activities (isoproterenol) may lead to undesirable tachycardia and arrhythmias.

Adverse effects of β_2-adrenergic agents result from dose-related sympathetic stimulation and include skeletal muscle tremors, nervousness, fatigue, and tachycardia. Doses are listed in Table 1 for dogs and cats. Doses have not been critically evaluated in these species, and in most cases the dose represents an extrapolation from human medicine.

Formulations are available for injection, and parenteral administration is useful in an acute situation. Beta$_2$ stimulation dilates muscular blood vessels and facilitates intramuscular absorption. Oral or inhaled dosage forms must be used for longer-term therapy. For obvious reasons, portable nebulizers that deliver a measured amount of drug to the respiratory mucosa through inhalation are im-

Table 1. *Adrenergic Drugs*

Drug*	Adrenergic Receptor Affinity† α	β_1	β_2	Dosage Form	Dose§
Epinephrine (Adrenaline, Parke-Davis)	+	+ +	+	Injectable	20 μg/kg of 1:10,000 solution
Ephedrine	+ +	+ +	+ +	25 and 50 mg capsules and tablets	Dog: 5–15 mg PO Cat: 2–5 mg PO
Isoproterenol (Isuprel HCl, Elkins-Sinn; Isuprel Compound Elixir, Winthop-Breon)		+ +	+ + +	Inhaled; oral compound elixir; injectable (20-ml ampules)	Isuprel HCl: 0.1–0.2 mg every 6 hours IM, SC Isuprel Elixir: 0.44 ml/kg every 6–12 hours PO
Isoetharine (Bronkosol, Winthrop-Breon)			+ +	Inhaled	0.5–1.0 ml, 1:3 with saline by aerosol
Metaproterenol (Alupent, Boehringer Ingelheim; Metaprel, Dorsey)			+ +	Inhaled; oral syrup, 10- and 20-mg tablets	0.5 mg/kg every 6 hours
Terbutaline (Brethine, Geigy; Bricanyl, Merrill Dow)			+ +	Injectable (2-ml ampules); 2.5- and 5.0-mg tablets	Dog: 2.5 mg PO every 8 hours Cat: 1.25 mg PO every 12 hours
Albuterol‡ (Proventil, Schering; Ventolin, Glaxo)			+ +	Inhaled; oral	

*Proprietary name in parentheses.
†Receptor affinity: + to + + + denotes an increase in receptor affinity.
‡Also known as salbutamol.
§Use caution with doses and modify to individual animal as appropriate.
Key: PO = oral; IM = intramuscular; SC = subcutaneous

practical to use in veterinary medicine. In a hospital setting, however, drugs may be nebulized through a face mask or endotracheal tube. The use of the aerosol has the advantage of delivering the greatest amount of drug to the airways for local effect with the least chance for systemic toxicity. Local administration of the drug by aerosolization prevents any first-pass metabolism by the liver that might occur after oral absorption. Particle size is important if aerosol therapy is considered. Optimal particle size is 2 to 5 μm, as smaller particles may be exhaled and larger particles are deposited in the upper airways or pharynx. As much as 80 to 90 per cent of the total dose of an aerosol may be deposited in the mouth or pharynx (Ruffin et al., 1978), and the beneficial effect of the drug through topical or gastric absorption after swallowing is minimal. The oral dosage forms are generally well absorbed and are available as tablets, capsules, or syrup.

Anticholinergic Drugs

There is evidence that cholinergic mechanisms (vagally mediated) may be responsible for increased airway resistance in certain conditions. The vagus nerve provides parasympathetic innervation to smooth muscle of the airways, and stimulation of the vagus motor nerve of laboratory animals may produce bronchial narrowing. This effect is stimulated by acetylcholinesterase inhibitors and blocked by atropine (Gross and Skorodin, 1984). Therapy with antimuscarinic drugs has proved useful in treating the bronchoconstriction of emphysema (Gross and Skorodin, 1984). In diseases such as asthma, additional bronchoconstrictive forces play a central role, and antimuscarinic agents have only moderate activity as bronchodilating agents. Antimuscarinic agents (e.g., atropine) administered parenterally or orally will produce systemic effects. Side effects (xerostomia, tachycardia, cycloplegia) make this group of drugs undesirable for long-term therapy. Antimuscarinic agents will reduce the volume of bronchial secretions, which may be an undesirable effect in patients in which an increase in viscosity of bronchial secretions (e.g., chronic bronchitis) may obstruct the airways.

Quaternary ammonium compounds are poorly absorbed from mucosal surfaces and do not readily enter the central nervous system. Nebulization of quaternary ammonium derivatives of atropine, such as ipratropium bromide or atropine methonitrate, provide local anticholinergic effects without systemic effects.

If systemic administration is considered, atropine may be administered at a dose of 0.02 to 0.04 mg/kg

Table 2. Beneficial Effects of Theophylline

1. Smooth muscle relaxation—bronchodilation
2. Inhibition of release of mast cell mediators
3. Improvement in right and left ventricular performance
4. Improvement in contractile strength of respiratory muscles
5. Diuretic
6. Increased mucociliary clearance

for a duration of effect of 1.0 to 1.5 hours. Glycopyrrolate (Robinul-V, Robins), an atropinelike anticholinergic, has a slower onset but a longer duration of action, 4 to 6 hours. It produces less tachycardia and does not enter the central nervous system as readily as atropine. The suggested dose of glycopyrrolate is 0.01 to 0.02 mg/kg.

The clinical effectiveness of anticholinergics as bronchodilators has not been evaluated to any great extent in small animal medicine. Atropine and belladonna extracts have been given to horses for relief of obstructive pulmonary disease ("heaves"). The response of human patients to these drugs may vary.

Methylxanthines

The methylxanthines are the cornerstone of bronchodilator therapy in small animals. These drugs appear to have good clinical efficacy, and recent pharmacokinetic studies provide accurate dosing information for dogs and cats (McKiernan et al., 1981, 1983). Theophylline, caffeine, theobromine, and dyphylline are all methylxanthines. Theophylline and theophylline compounds are the most widely used members of this family of drugs.

The beneficial effects of theophylline in the management of pulmonary disease are listed in Table 2. There is at present a controversy as to which of these effects is most important. Relaxation of bronchial smooth muscle plays an important role in decreased airway resistance due to smooth muscle contraction. Bronchoconstriction caused by mediators released from mast cells may be relieved or prevented by the inhibition of mast cell degranulation. Recent evidence indicates that therapeutic doses of theophylline improve respiratory muscle contractility, increasing the contractile force of the diaphragm by as much as 15 to 20 per cent (Murciano et al., 1984). A mechanism other than bronchodilation therefore may account, at least in part, for the therapeutic efficacy of theophylline in obstructive pulmonary diseases.

Theophylline is frequently used in conjunction with other drugs in the treatment of cardiogenic pulmonary disease. In addition to increasing airway diameter, theophylline also improves both right and left ventricular performance through positive inotropic and chronotropic effects and the subsequent increase in cardiac output. Improvement may be partly due to the vasodilating properties of theophylline through smooth muscle relaxation. The diuretic properties of theophylline are considered to be of low potency, and tolerance may develop with repeated use.

MECHANISM OF ACTION. The smooth muscle–relaxing properties of the methylxanthines are due to inhibition of the enzyme phosphodiesterase (Fig. 1). Phosphodiesterase is responsible for the breakdown of cAMP into 5′-AMP. Inhibition of the enzyme increases intracellular cAMP. Although methylxanthines and β_2-adrenergic agents act by different mechanisms, both increase intracellular cAMP, which relaxes smooth muscles of the respiratory tree, vessels, and other organs. In mast cells, an increase in intracellular cAMP inhibits release of mast-cell products (Fig. 1). Blockade of adenosine receptors may also play a role in the action of xanthines. Adenosine serves as an autacoid to stimulate contraction of smooth muscle through a potentiation of the actions of norepinephrine, and it may also stimulate the release of mediators from mast cells.

Cardiovascular effects of methylxanthines are due to an increase in the influx of calcium into myocardial cells, thus increasing the strength of contraction. This effect is probably mediated by increased intracellular cAMP, although a cardiac-stimulating increase in the release of catecholamines also has been postulated. Other cardiac effects result from an improvement in coronary arterial blood flow due to the vasodilation and a direct action on the sinus node and atrioventricular pacemaker cells. The improvement in respiratory muscle contractility and capacity for muscular work is probably due to a facilitation of the influx of calcium into the muscle cell.

PRODUCTS AVAILABLE. Theophylline has been formulated for intramuscular, intravenous, and rectal use and as elixirs, aqueous solutions, tablets, and capsules for oral administration. Theophylline is only slightly soluble in water and when given orally may cause gastric irritation, nausea, and vomiting. "Salts" of theophylline have been formulated that are more water soluble, better tolerated orally, and more readily absorbed. Theophylline salts dissociate to yield the parent drug in biologic fluids. The most widely used formulation is theophylline ethylenediamine (aminophylline), which is 78 to 86 per cent theophylline; thus, 100 mg of aminophylline will contain approximately 80 mg of theophylline. Other salts of theophylline are listed in Table 3. It is important to note that, when a particular product is prescribed, the dose should be based on the theophylline content. No one salt of theophylline offers a distinct advantage over another as long as equivalent doses of theophylline are administered.

There are sustained-release (slow-release) theo-

Table 3. *Equivalency of Formulations of Theophylline Derivatives and Salts Compared with Parent Theophylline*

Formulation or Salt	Trade Name	Per Cent Theophylline
Theophylline base and theophylline elixir	Various	100 per cent
Theophylline monohydrate	—	90 per cent
Theophylline ethylenediamine (aminophylline)	Various	78–86 per cent
Choline theophylline (oxtriphylline)	Choledyl (Parke-Davis)	65 per cent
Theophylline sodium glycinate (Sandoz)	Synophylate (Central Pharm.)	50 per cent
Theophylline calcium salicylate	Quadrinal (Knoll)	48 per cent

Modified from McKiernan, B. C.: Lower respiratory tract diseases. *In* Ettinger, S. J. (ed.): *Textbook of Veterinary Internal Medicine,* 2nd ed. Philadelphia: W. B. Saunders, 1983, p. 824.

phylline products available (e.g., Slo-Phyllin [Rorer], Theo-Dur [Key], Theobid [Glaxo]). Since theophylline requires frequent dosing to maintain therapeutic plasma concentrations in the dog, sustained-release products offer the advantage of less frequent dosing, improved compliance, and less fluctuation in blood concentrations. Slow-release products may vary in their extent and duration of absorption, and variations may occur among individuals, which may necessitate monitoring blood concentrations during long-term therapy. Slow-release products should not be crushed, dissolved, or chewed when administered. Further studies with sustained-release products in dogs and cats will determine accurate dosing information.

DOSAGE. Pharmacokinetic studies of theophylline have been performed in dogs and cats (McKiernan et al., 1981; 1983). The comparative pharmacokinetics of theophylline in dogs, cats, and humans are listed in Table 4. The oral absorption and bioavailability of the products studied is excellent in all species (greater than 90 per cent). The elimination half-life in dogs is slightly shorter than in cats, necessitating more frequent dosing.

Theophylline is dependent on hepatic metabolism for its elimination. Only 10 per cent of a dose is excreted unchanged in the urine; the rest is converted to metabolites by hepatic microsomal enzymes (Brashear et al., 1980). Diseases that affect the liver (hepatic cirrhosis and hepatic congestion) may decrease the clearance of theophylline. In hepatectomized dogs, the elimination half-life increased 348 per cent and clearance decreased by 70 per cent in comparison with control dogs (Brashear et al., 1980).

Drugs may also influence the hepatic clearance of theophylline. Phenobarbital and phenytoin may induce hepatic microsomal enzymes and increase clearance. Other drugs, such as cimetidine, erythromycin, and propranolol may decrease clearance by 30 to 50 per cent. In human patients, the dose is often adjusted up or down to compensate for drug interactions when theophylline is used in conjunction with drugs that alter hepatic metabolism (Jonkman and Upton, 1984). For precise dosing in small animals, patients should be observed for signs of toxicity or lack of therapeutic effect when theophylline is used in combination with drugs known to alter hepatic metabolism or when hepatic disease exists. Plasma concentration determinations can also be made to assist in adjusting the dosage.

Human studies indicate that plasma or serum concentrations should be kept within the therapeutic range of 10 to 20 μg/ml, although some benefit may accrue at concentrations as low as 5 μg/ml. Recommended starting doses of theophylline are 9 mg/kg every 6 to 8 hours for dogs and 4 mg/kg every 8 to 12 hours for cats. (An equivalent dose of aminophylline would be 11 mg/kg for dogs and 5 mg/kg for cats.) A loading dose can be calculated based on pharmacokinetic information and the following relationship: Dose = desired plasma concentration × volume of distribution. For example, if we wish to reach a plasma concentration of 15

Table 4. *Comparative Pharmacokinetics of Theophylline**

Species	Peak Concentration After Oral Administration (Hours)	Elimination Half-Life (Hours)	Volume of Distribution (L/kg)	Per Cent Bioavailability	Recommended Theophylline Dose
Humans	0.5–2.0	9.0	0.5	96 per cent	4 mg/kg every 6 hours
Dogs	1.5	5.7	0.82	91 per cent	9 mg/kg every 6–8 hours
Cats	1.5	7.8	0.46	96 per cent	4 mg/kg every 8–12 hours

*This table documents regular release formulations of theophylline.
Data from McKiernan et al., 1981; McKiernan et al., 1983; Ogilvie, 1978.

μg/ml in a dog (volume of distribution = 0.82 L/kg) the loading dose is (0.82 L/kg) × (15 μg/ml) = 12.3 mg/kg. Repeated administration can then be given at the recommended dosage.

In addition to oral administration, intramuscular and intravenous dosage forms are also available. Intramuscular administration is not recommended, because the injections are painful and plasma concentrations attained are low. Intravenous administration should be injected slowly over several minutes. In most patients, oral absorption is complete and rapid, and parenteral administration is rarely necessary (Ogilvie, 1978).

TOXICITY. Toxicities, which are often an extension of the pharmacologic effects, may develop at increased plasma concentrations of theophylline. There is a paucity of clinical toxicologic information in the literature for small animals. In humans, toxicity is rare at plasma concentrations of less than 25 μg/ml, whereas at higher concentrations adverse cardiac and neurologic signs may be seen. Minor reactions include restlessness, tachycardia, nausea, and vomiting. More severe signs may include cardiac arrhythmias, tremors, seizures, and tachypnea. Occasionally, serious side effects may occur before minor side effects are seen. In dogs given theophylline, the threshold for ventricular fibrillation was decreased by 30 to 40 per cent in normal dogs and by 60 per cent in dogs with respiratory failure (Mungall, 1983).

THERAPEUTIC MONITORING. Some veterinary hospitals and most human hospitals are able to measure serum or plasma concentrations of theophylline to assess dosage. There is considerable biologic variability in the dog and cat (McKiernan et al., 1981; 1983), and it is advised that the dosage regimen be individually adjusted in critically ill animals. When obtaining a blood sample for theophylline assay, one should obtain a peak concentration, which occurs 1.5 to 2.0 hours after oral administration. It is essential that plasma measurements not be made until steady-state (plateau) concentrations are reached, which requires 4 to 5 drug half-lives (e.g., 23 to 28 hours in the dog, with a half-life of 5.7 hours). If steady state has not been reached when blood samples are taken, valid dose adjustments cannot be made. If the plasma concentration is less than 10 μg/ml and a desired therapeutic effect has not been attained, increase the dose by 25 per cent and reassess the patient. If the plasma concentration is greater than 20 μg/ml, the dose should be decreased by 25 per cent or the dosing interval lengthened. If the plasma concentration is greater than 25 μg/ml and toxic signs are observed, immediately discontinue administration for at least two dosing intervals and resume dosing at a dose that is 25 to 50 per cent lower.

Corticosteroids

For many years, corticosteroids have been used to treat asthma in humans, but the exact mechanism of action remains unknown. An often suggested mode of action is sensitization of β-adrenergic receptors on bronchial smooth muscle by corticosteroids. They may also act synergistically with methylxanthines. Most likely, the benefit of corticosteroids is derived from their anti-inflammatory effects. Corticosteroids inhibit release of mediators from sensitized mast cells and reduce the subsequent inflammation induced by inflammatory mediators. Steroid-induced impairment of leukocyte migration and improvement of capillary integrity in inflamed tissues may prevent the edema and congestion in respiratory tissues that lead to narrowing of airways. Other mediators such as prostaglandins ($PGF_{2\alpha}$, PGD_2) (Wasserman et al., 1980) mediate bronchoconstriction, and a beneficial effect of corticosteroids may be the inhibition of prostaglandin synthesis, although there is no evidence that other prostaglandin synthesis inhibitors (nonsteroidal anti-inflammatory drugs) are useful in bronchoconstrictive diseases.

Recommended anti-inflammatory doses of prednisone and prednisolone are 0.5 to 1.0 mg/kg/day for dogs and 1 to 2 mg/kg/day for cats. Cats with feline asthma often respond quite well to corticosteroids, and a commonly used dose is 2 mg/kg of methylprednisolone acetate (Depo-Medrol, Upjohn). The use of corticosteroids for treatment of chronic bronchitis is quite controversial, and until there is evidence that supports its efficacy for this condition, its routine use cannot be recommended.

Cromolyn Sodium

Cromolyn sodium, or disodium cromoglycate (Intal, Fisons), has been used in human patients to prevent bronchospasm from inhaled allergens and excercise-induced bronchoconstriction and also in horses for obstructive pulmonary disease. Cromolyn acts by inhibiting antigen-induced release of anaphylactic mediators from sensitized mast cells. The exact cellular mechanism is not understood, but it appears to prevent calcium influx into mast cells.

Cromolyn must be given prophylactically to be effective. Because of poor oral absorption (less than 10 per cent), it must be administered by inhalation. The short half-life (45 to 90 minutes in animals) necessitates prophylactic administration four to five times daily to prevent bronchoconstriction. These properties make it unlikely that cromolyn will gain acceptance for bronchodilator therapy in small animals.

DISEASE CONDITIONS

In summary, bronchodilator therapy in small animals may be useful in the management of several disease conditions. Cats with asthma will benefit most from theophylline therapy or corticosteroids. For an acute presentation, both drugs may be used concurrently.

In dogs, theophylline is the most widely used bronchodilator. Collapsing trachea, tracheobronchitis, allergic bronchitis, or pulmonary disease secondary to heart failure may all benefit from bronchodilator therapy. Intrathoracic collapsing trachea can be relieved with theophylline administration in many cases. Dilation of the airways relieves tracheal narrowing and reduces intrathoracic pressure on expiration. Theophylline may improve pulmonary disease that is secondary to heart failure by bronchial smooth muscle relaxation and by the beneficial effects on the failing heart, as well as by the diuretic and vasodilator actions. A potential risk in these cases, however, is the increased chance of cardiac arrhythmias. In obstructive diseases of the airways, theophylline and adrenergic agents may improve the condition of the patient when used alone or in combination. Their effects may be synergistic.

In thoracic restrictive diseases such as excessive obesity or thoracic masses (tumors), some airway obstruction may be improved through bronchodilator therapy. Theophylline treatment may improve contractility of the respiratory muscles. Increased respiratory muscle contractility may also help in neuromuscular diseases such as polyradiculoneuritis (coonhound paralysis), myasthenia gravis, and spinal cord injury.

Pulmonary function tests are not performed on cats and dogs as easily as they are on humans; therefore, the efficacy of bronchodilator agents is often a subjective evaluation by the owner and veterinarian. Nevertheless, if bronchodilator therapy appears to be unsuccessful, the following conditions should be considered:

1. Misdiagnosis
2. Bronchial obstruction due to inspissated mucus plugs or foreign body
3. Concurrent infection
4. Subtherapeutic blood concentrations of drug (theophylline)
5. Theophylline hypersensitivity

References and Supplemental Reading

Adams, H. R.: New perspectives in cardiopulmonary therapeutics: Receptor-selective adrenergic agents. J.A.V.M.A. 185:966, 1984.

Brashear, R. E., Nelson, R. L., Gilick, M. R., et al.: The role of the liver in theophylline elimination. Lung 158:101, 1980.

Eyre, P.: Histamine H_2-receptors in the sheep bronchus and cat trachea: The action of burimamide. Br. J. Pharmacol. 48:321, 1973.

Gross, N. J., and Skorodin, M. S.: Anticholinergic antimuscarinic bronchodilators. Am. Rev. Respir. Dis. 129:856, 1984.

Jonkman, J. H. G., and Upton, R. A.: Pharmacokinetic drug interactions with theophylline. Clin. Pharmacokinet. 9:309, 1984.

Lockey, R. F., and Bukantz, S. C.: Allergy and asthma. *In* Sodeman, W. A., and Sodeman, T. M. (eds.): *Pathologic Physiology*, 6th ed. Philadelphia: W. B. Saunders, 1979, pp. 507–527.

McKiernan, B. C., Neff-Davis, C. A., Koritz, G. D., et al.: Pharmacokinetic studies of theophylline in dogs. J. Vet. Pharmacol. Ther. 4:103, 1981.

McKiernan, B. C., Koritz, G. D., Davis, L. E., et al.: Pharmacokinetic studies of theophylline in cats. J. Vet. Pharmacol. Ther. 6:99, 1983.

Mungall, D.: Theophylline. *In* Mungall, D. (ed.): *Applied Clinical Pharmacokinetics*. New York: Raven Press, 1983, pp. 127–152.

Murciano, D., Aubier, M., Lecocguic, Y., et al.: Effects of theophylline on diaphragmatic strength and fatigue in patients with chronic obstructive pulmonary disease. N. Engl. J. Med. 311:349, 1984.

Ogilvie, R. I.: Clinical pharmacokinetics of theophylline. Clin. Pharmacokinet. 3:267, 1978.

Ruffin, R. E., Montgomery, J. M., and Newhouse, M. T.: Site of beta-adrenergic receptors in the respiratory tract. Chest 74:256, 1978.

Wasserman, M., Griffin, R. L., and Marsalisi, F. B.: Potent bronchoconstrictor effects of aerosolized prostaglandin D_2 in dogs. Prostaglandins 20:703, 1980.

PULMONARY HYPERSENSITIVITIES

KATHLEEN E. NOONE, V.M.D.
New York, New York

The causes and mechanisms of pulmonary hypersensitivities are poorly understood in both human and veterinary medicine. Essentially, hypersensitivity reactions represent an excessive immune reaction to a substance that is usually innocuous in most individuals. Type I (immediate hypersensitivity) is probably the most common mechanism of immune injury. Type III and IV involvement has also been suggested, but it is not fully understood why sensitization occurs. Type II is rarely involved in pulmonary disease. (See Pulmonary Immunology for a detailed discussion of these reactions.) Suspected and known causes of pulmonary hypersensitivities in humans and animals include fungi, molds, spores, drugs, bacteria, and parasites (Wessels et al., 1973). Clinical syndromes of allergic asthma, bronchitis, and pneumonitis are the most common hypersensitivity reactions, but even in these conditions, the inciting material is seldom determined.

EOSINOPHILS AND PULMONARY INFILTRATION WITH EOSINOPHILIA

Pulmonary infiltration with blood eosinophilia (PIE) is defined as the presence of both pulmonary-associated (as evidenced by radiographic infiltrates) and peripheral eosinophilia. This combination characterizes most pulmonary hypersensitivities. However, eosinophilic infiltrates can be limited to the airways (allergic bronchitis or asthma) or the alveoli (allergic pneumonitis, parasitic pneumonia, immune-mediated occult dirofilariasis) or can be present in varying degrees in both structures.

In 1952, an attempt was made to classify eosinophilic lung disease in humans into five categories based on clinical and radiographic features and the duration of illness (Crofton et al., 1952). Crofton's classification is as follows:

1. *Simple pulmonary eosinophilia* (Löffler's syndrome)

   Transient and mild clinical signs of 2 to 4 weeks' duration

   May not require therapy

   Examples: migrating ascarids, ancyclostoma, drugs, unknown causes

2. *Prolonged pulmonary eosinophilia*

   Severe clinical signs, prolonged course (2 to 6 months or longer)

   Requires therapy

   Examples: parasites, fungi, viruses, bacteria, external antigens, unknown causes

3. *Pulmonary eosinophilia with asthma*

   Both alveoli and airways involved

   Frequently associated with *Aspergillus*

4. *Tropical pulmonary eosinophilia*

   May have prolonged clinical signs

   Responds to diethylcarbamazine

   Examples: reaction to the filaria of *Dirofilaria immitis*

5. *Polyarteritis nodosa*

   Severe signs, hemoptysis, usually fatal

   Pulmonary vasculature and other organs involved

   Unknown causes

Crofton acknowledges, however, that this grouping is artificial and can be obscure because of overlapping characteristics of the groups. Furthermore, it is limited since it is not based on or suggestive of cause or pathogenesis. The term PIE is all that is suggested for use at present in veterinary medicine.

The single most important conclusion to be drawn, however, is that PIE should be viewed as a spectrum of hypersensitivity reactions that range from mild to severe, transient to chronic, self-limiting to sometimes fatal.

Obviously, the determination of the role that eosinophils play is critical to the understanding of PIE. However, the eosinophils themselves, the reactions they participate in, the factors that provoke their infiltration, and their functional mecha-

The author wishes to thank Dr. Karen Feibusch for invaluable assistance in the preparation of this manuscript.

nisms are some of the more poorly understood areas of inflammation in general. Eosinophils are produced in the bone marrow, transiently circulate in the blood, and localize in the skin or subepithelial stroma of the respiratory, gastrointestinal, and urogenital tracts. Their production in the bone marrow is partially regulated by soluble factors released by sensitized T cells. Activation of this pathway results in peripheral eosinophilia.

In immediate hypersensitivity reactions, initial exposure to an allergen provokes mechanisms that ultimately result in the production of IgE antibodies, which bind to mast cells or basophils. The host is then said to be sensitized to this specific foreign substance (or substances). With re-exposure, the allergen combines with the IgE on the mast cell surface and causes degranulation. Mast cell granules contain many vasoactive factors, mediators of inflammation, and substances that are chemotactic for eosinophils. Eosinophilic chemotactic factors of anaphylaxis (ECF-A), certain products of complement, arachidonic acid, specific products of sensitized lymphocytes, antigen-antibody complexes—all are chemotactic for eosinophils (Weller and Goetzl, 1980). Some of these are also eosinophilopoietic, inducing an increased bone marrow production to meet the demand at peripheral tissue. Eosinophils help regulate the immediate type I hypersensitivity reaction. They can have a beneficial role since they (1) inhibit mast cell mediator release from granules, (2) degrade mast cell mediators of inflammation, (3) phagocytize mast cell granules and IgE-antigen complexes, and (4) release *major-basic protein*, which neutralizes heparin released from mast cells (Schatz et al., 1981). In essence, they modulate the reaction by dampening the effect of mast cell products. However, eosinophils can also have detrimental effects on the lungs. Major-basic protein injures the respiratory epithelial cells, resulting in necrosis, sloughing of the epithelium, and, most importantly, disruption of the mucociliary apparatus, a vital defense mechanism of the lungs.

Essentially, then, a hypersensitivity reaction represents an exposure to a protein, host sensitization, and an inflammatory reaction mediated by mast cells and controlled by eosinophils. The lungs are especially vulnerable to immediate hypersensitivities, since they are continuously exposed to foreign material and have abundant mast cells in their epithelium. When a hypersensitivity reaction occurs, it is a function of immunologic characteristics of the host combined with physical and biochemical characteristics of the inducing antigen following prior exposure history (sensitization).

Helmintic parasites typically cause a blood and tissue eosinophilia. The increased tissue and blood eosinophilia is part of the inflammatory response to migrations of these parasites. Some helminths release factors that are chemotactic for eosinophils. The strongest eosinophil response generally occurs during the pulmonary migration phase.

Evaluation and Diagnostic Plan

In the presence of radiographic pulmonary changes, parasitic hypersensitivities can be suspected when parasitic ova or larvae are detected in either fecal or tracheal wash specimens; they can also be determined by serologic testing (occult heartworm cases). Drug exposure can best be assessed by history. Testing for hypersensitivities caused by a variety of fungi, spores, bacteria, or other allergens is presently not available, requiring a diagnosis by elimination. A fairly complete diagnostic workup for suspected cases would include a complete white cell count and differential, heartworm check, serological tests for heartworm, thoracic radiograph, fecal analysis, tracheal wash, and intradermal skin testing.

Necessary historic information includes time spent outdoors, past and present geographic locations, environmental influences, and use of medication. Young patients who spend large amounts of time outdoors in areas endemic to *Dirofilaria, Aelurostrongylus, Capillaria,* and *Paragonimus* should have fecal analysis and heartworm checks. The drug history is important because certain drugs may provoke a pulmonary hypersensitivity, whereas glucocorticoids decrease blood eosinophil counts and may mask a possible PIE syndrome.

Most animals are presented for evaluation of a chronic cough, which may be either productive or nonproductive, mild or severe, progressive or nonprogressive. Weight loss, exercise intolerance, dyspnea, and, occasionally, hemoptysis have also been reported.

Physical examination usually reveals an animal with a normal resting respiratory rate, which may become tachypneic with exercise or stress. Others have moderate to severe dyspnea and cyanosis at rest. Dyspnea of this degree implies massive parenchymal disease, bronchoconstriction, pneumothorax, or secondary pneumonia. Auscultation reveals lung sounds that vary from bronchovesicular to crackles and areas of diminished or absent breath sounds.

Hematologic changes consistent with a hypersensitivity reaction include a mild leukocytosis, eosinophilia, and, occasionally, a basophilia. A microfilaria test should be performed on all dogs and cats in endemic heartworm areas if there is an eosinophilia, and especially if there is a concurrent basophilia. Serologic testing for heartworms should be performed if clinical signs, hematologic tests, and thoracic radiographs are consistent with heartworm disease even though microfilaria testing is negative.

Thoracic radiographs are essential in the assessment of pulmonary disease and may help confirm the diagnosis of a parasitic hypersensitivity. Parasitic pulmonary disease may cause increased linear or nodular interstitial markings or large solid to cavitated parenchymal densities. In rare cases, there is an associated pneumothorax or pneumonia. Heartworm disease typically creates changes in the pulmonary vasculature and may cause right-sided cardiac enlargement. Nonparasitic forms of pulmonary hypersensitivities have no definitive radiographic features; however, common findings include irregular alveolar infiltrates and increased bronchial markings.

All animals with an eosinophilia should have multiple fecal analyses performed. The fecal analysis may reveal the presence of *Toxocara* or *Ancyclostoma* ova or *Strongyloides stercoralis* larvae, which can have a pulmonary migration phase as part of their life cycles. It may also reveal *Paragonimus* or *Filaroides* larvae, or *Capillaria* or *Aelurostrongylus* ova, which are coughed up from the lungs or airways, swallowed, and passed in the stool. The Baermann technique should be used to detect larval stages in feces.

If the history, radiographs, fecal analyses, and hematologic and serologic tests do not establish the specific cause of the pulmonary disease, a tracheal wash should be performed and the sample submitted for cytologic analysis and culture. The cytologic examination may reveal larva or ova that were overlooked in the fecal analysis. Large numbers of eosinophils without ova or larvae suggest a diagnosis of asthma, allergic bronchitis, or allergic pneumonitis. Rarely, chronic bacterial or fungal infections (*Histoplasma, Aspergillus*) may produce an eosinophilic response.

Skin testing with suspected allergens is indicated if no cause is determined and a seasonal or environmental influence is evident from the history. Unfortunately, the allergens identified by the intradermal testing may not be the same as those causing the pulmonary hypersensitivity. A possible reason for this disparity in dogs may be the difference of mast cell distribution between the lungs and skin.

FELINE BRONCHIAL ASTHMA

Asthma is a reversible airway obstruction provoked by a hyperreactivity to stimuli innocuous to normal individuals. Bronchoconstriction, excessive mucus production, and cellular debris contribute to airway obstruction. In humans, asthma assumes three forms: intrinsic, extrinsic, and mixed. Intrinsic asthma is nonimmunologically based and is induced by exercise or infection. Extrinsic asthma is immunologically based (IgE) and is caused by the inhalation of specific allergens in sensitized patients. Mixed asthma occurs in patients with allergic asthma in whom infections also precipitate the attacks. Stress, exercise, air pollution, aspirin, body position, and ambient temperature variation can all be involved in provoking an asthma attack. In veterinary medicine, it is not known which form of asthma occurs. IgE, used to distinguish intrinsic from extrinsic asthma in humans, is difficult to isolate, and interpretation is questionable because of frequent parasite problems. Furthermore, feline asthma shares characteristics of all three groups. Extrinsic asthma in humans usually starts during childhood and tends to be familial, implying a genetic predisposition. In cats, asthma usually has its onset at a young age (1 to 3 years) and is most common in Siamese and Himalayans at our institution. Genetic studies are presently not available on these cats. Seasonal worsening during fall and spring may indicate an allergic reaction to environmental allergens in cats (extrinsic asthma). A few cats with asthma have simultaneous bronchial infections, which may suggest the mixed form of asthma. The role of stress and exercise is difficult to evaluate in cats because they have a sedentary life-style.

Asthma differs from other pulmonary hypersensitivities in that the reaction principally involves the airways and not the parenchyma. The lung tissue can secondarily become emphysematous, a consequence of trapping air peripherally. Unlike other airway diseases (chronic bronchitis or bronchiectasis), asthma is a reversible airway obstruction occurring only when the inciting cause stimulates the tracheobronchial tract. Hence, asthmatic cats have paroxysmal clinical signs.

The pathogenesis of asthma is thought to have two bases: immunologic or neurologic (Middleton et al., 1981). Allergic asthma, a type I (immediate hypersensitivity) reaction, involves mast cells, IgE, allergens, and eosinophils. The products of mast cells provoke an eosinophilic infiltration and cause bronchial smooth muscle contraction, mucus gland hypersecretion, increased capillary permeability, and granulocyte chemotaxis. The result is airway obstruction due to bronchoconstriction, mucus plugs, edema fluid, and cellular debris. Bronchial glands are more abundant in cats than in other species, making asthma a more serious problem. Eosinophils dampen mast cell reactions but also release major-basic protein, which can denude the respiratory epithelium to the level of the basement membrane, resulting in loss of the mucociliary apparatus. This loss impairs clearance of mucus from lower airways, further aggravating the obstruction. The neurologic basis of asthma is thought to be a cholinergic, β_2-adrenergic, or α-adrenergic imbalance. This theory explains asthma caused by stress, infection, exercise, or air pollutants. Cholinergic stimulation of bronchial smooth muscle causes an intracellular elevation of cyclic guanosine monophosphate (cGMP) and results in bronchoconstriction. Alpha-adrenergic stimulation lowers intracellular cyclic adenosine monophosphate (cAMP) and also produces bronchoconstriction. Beta$_2$-adrenergic stimulation causes bronchodilation by increasing intracellular cAMP. Hence, any factor that blocks β_2-adrenergics or stimulates α-adrenergics or cholinergics can precipitate bronchoconstriction and cause asthma. Infections are thought to do the former. Bronchodilator therapy is aimed at increasing cAMP levels by either increasing its formation or decreasing its rate of degradation. Beta$_2$-adrenergics, and possibly glucocorticoids, stimulate adenylcyclase conversion of adenosine triphosphate (ATP) to cAMP, whereas methylxanthines (theophylline) decrease phosphodiesterase conversion of cAMP to 5′AMP (see also Bronchodilator Therapy).

History is highly variable in feline asthma cases but usually involves a chronic, paroxysmal cough. Most cats are normal between events; however, some are slightly tachypneic or wheezy. Occasionally, exercise or handling precipitates a coughing spell and the acute onset of abnormal lung sounds.

The asthmatic cat may be clinically normal when seen or may be in status asthmaticus, a state of respiratory failure and acidosis. Coughing, gagging, wheezing, and mild forms of tachypnea and cyanosis are the most common physical findings. Less common but more serious are severe dyspnea and cyanosis, open-mouth breathing, gasping, aerophagia, and frantic behavior. When these clinical signs are present, emergency therapy is required to save the animal.

The diagnosis of feline bronchial asthma is based on hematologic tests, radiographs, and cytologic results of a tracheal wash. The most common hematologic finding is a peripheral eosinophilia that is variable in degree and may be absent if the cat is stressed or has recently been given steroids. The radiographic features most consistent with asthma are bronchial wall thickening (due to smooth muscle hypertrophy, bronchial gland hyperplasia, edema, and cellular infiltrates), aerophagia, and an increased vascular pattern. Other changes include diaphragmatic flattening, peripheral hyperlucency, alveolar infiltrates, and an expanded thoracic size. If the radiographs and hematologic changes are consistent with asthma and the fecal analysis is negative for parasites, a tracheal wash should be performed to confirm the diagnosis and to obtain cultures. Tracheal wash cytologic testing reveals thick mucus strands, eosinophils, and the absence of larvae or ova. Hyperplastic bronchial epithelium and occasional mast cells within thick mucus are also consistent with a diagnosis of asthma. Culture results vary; however, respiratory pathogens (*Klebsiella* spp., *Pseudomonas* spp., *Escherichia coli*) may be isolated with concurrent infection.

Therapy is dictated by the severity of clinical signs at presentation (Table 1). All cats with even slight respiratory distress should be handled without causing additional stress. All cats with severe respiratory distress should be placed in oxygen and given only parenteral medication. Although IV administration delivers the most rapid distribution to tissue, the stress of restraint may be too great and therefore IM or SC injections are preferred. All emergency cases should be given glucocorticoids, a bronchodilator, and a sympathomimetic drug. Most cats respond in about 30 minutes. Cats presented in status asthmaticus can be hypothermic and cyanotic, with a respiratory pattern and auscultatory findings that mimic cardiomyopathy and pleural effusion. Because sympathomimetic drugs are contraindicated in most cases of heart failure yet essential in status asthmaticus therapy, cats who present in this manner should be given epinephrine with caution, unless they are known asthmatic patients. Cats who are only mildly tachypneic usually respond to glucocorticoids and bronchodilator therapy alone.

Long-term management requires close client communication and a commitment on the part of the owner. The client must be aware that asthma is a state of airway hypersensitivity and that medication and perhaps occasional hospitalizations will be needed in an attempt to control (but not cure) the condition. Most cats respond well to oral prednisone and a bronchodilator (aminophylline or terbutaline). Bronchodilators can be given on a daily basis or, alternatively, can be used only during periods of exacerbation. The advantage of concurrent bronchodilator therapy is that a lower dose of glucocorticoids is required to control the asthma. The dose of glucocorticoids needed for control is highly variable. Usually, cats can be managed with prednisone (5

Table 1. *Therapeutics for Use in Feline Asthma*

Agent	Dose
Oxygen	
Glucocorticoids	
Prednisolone sodium succinate*	Emergency, 50–100 mg IV
Dexamethasone sodium phosphate†	Emergency, 1 mg/kg IV
Prednisone	Nonemergency—5 mg PO, t.i.d. and then rapidly decrease to alternate day use (or stop completely)
Methylprednisolone acetate‡	1.0–2.0 mg/kg IM
Bronchodilators	
Epinephrine§	0.1 ml (0.1 mg) of a 1:1000 dilution, SC, IV
Terbutaline‖	2.5 mg PO, t.i.d.
Aminophylline (various)	25 mg PO, b.i.d. or t.i.d.

*Solu-Delta Cortef, Upjohn.
†Tech America Group.
‡Depo-Medrol, Upjohn.
§Adrenalin chloride solution 1:1000, Parke-Davis.
‖Brethine, Geigy.

mg PO b.i.d. or t.i.d.) during attacks and then rapidly tapered over 2 to 5 days to 2.5 or 5 mg daily or every other day. If the clinical signs are controlled with low-dose steroids (2.5 mg every other day), steroids can be stopped as they may not be needed. Unfortunately, some cats require high levels of steroids daily; however, attempts to taper the dose should still be made. Those cats who are difficult to pill or need daily medication that owners are unwilling or unable to give can be treated with long-acting steroid injections (methylprednisolone acetate, 10 to 20 mg IM). This method, although convenient, should be avoided as a frequent, long-term method of control because of the potential for inducing adrenal-hypothalamic axis suppression.

CANINE HEARTWORM PNEUMONITIS

The infection of dogs with adult heartworms does not always have an associated microfilaremia. Infections that are prepatent, infections that have sexually incompetent or unisex parasites, as well as those with immune destruction of the microfilariae within the pulmonary vasculature may, in the author's experience, account for as much as 70 per cent of all heartworm infections. Of these, fewer than one fourth are the result of immune destruction. A pulmonary hypersensitivity can occur when host sensitization develops against filarial antigen during the prepatent phase (4 to 7 months after infection). These antibodies do not interfere with microfilaria production and are thought to be consumed at the time of patency. Dogs can also become sensitized against microfilaria. In such instances, excessive microfilaria-specific antibodies are produced and a pulmonary hypersensitivity results. This antibody, in combination with eosinophils and neutrophils, traps and immobilizes the microfilariae within the pulmonary microvasculature, causing a hypersensitivity pneumonitis. It is the reaction of the host against the parasite, not the mere physical presence of the worm, that determines severity of disease. Pulmonary damage induced by host-parasite reactions includes infarction, hemorrhage, and inflammation. Eosinophilic lung injury is extensive in these cases because of the intense host-parasite reaction.

Dogs with heartworm-induced pulmonary hypersensitivity are presented for chronic cough, dyspnea, hemoptysis, or exercise intolerance. Results of the physical examination are variable, ranging from a clinically normal dog to one with cyanosis, tachypnea, crackles, and a split second heart sound. Radiographic findings are also variable. Pulmonary artery tortuosity and blunting, especially of the caudal lobe vessels, and right-sided cardiac enlargement may be present but obscured by massive alveolar infiltrates. These parenchymal changes represent areas of eosinophilic infiltrates, microfilaria-associated granulomas, hemorrhage, and infarction. Hematologic changes include a variable degree of eosinophilia and basophilia, a mild leukocytosis, and occasionally an anemia. If the radiographic, clinical, and hematologic findings are suggestive of heartworm disease yet no microfilariae are detected, serologic confirmation is indicated. Serologic findings consistent with immune-mediated occult heartworm disease include positive indirect immunofluorescence assay (IFA) for microfilarial antibody and positive enzyme-linked immunosorbent assay (ELISA) tests for adult antibodies. Cross-reactivity with intestinal or other pulmonary parasites causes false-positive results with some of these tests, and considerable experience is required for proper interpretation. Newer ELISA tests for adult antigen are currently being evaluated.

Dogs with a severe cough, hemoptysis, or extensive parenchymal involvement should be treated with glucocorticoids prior to adulticide therapy (prednisolone at 1 to 2 mg/kg body weight PO, divided b.i.d. and tapered over a 10- to 14-day period). On re-evaluation, if there has been significant improvement of the cough and regression of the alveolar and interstitial infiltrate, adulticide therapy can be initiated. Thiacetarsamide sodium (2.2 mg/kg body weight IV b.i.d. for 2 days) is the recommended therapy. Dogs undergoing therapy should be monitored in a standard manner with a pre- and posturinalysis and serum biochemistries.

Glucocorticoids protect adult heartworms against thiacetarsamide, thus the two drugs should not be used simultaneously. Steroids also lead to an increase in intimal proliferation and therefore greater vascular obstruction. This effect may complicate the post-adulticide therapy period, when severe pulmonary hypertension and worm embolization occur. Hence, the use of steroids after adulticide therapy is reserved for dogs that have severe acute emboli and fever. Routine, low-dose aspirin therapy (10 mg/kg daily) has been shown to help minimize the endothelial changes in dogs after heartworm treatment.

FELINE HEARTWORM DISEASE

Feline heartworm disease, caused by *Dirofilaria immitis*, is being recognized more and more. Cats are an aberrant host, hence less than 20 per cent of infections have circulating microfilariae. It has been stated that a shorter prepatent period, the fewer microfilariae produced, the fewer adults, and a shorter development and length of survival make diagnosis more difficult in cats than in dogs (Dillon, 1984). In addition, other common feline pulmonary diseases such as asthma and parasites have clinical features similar to those of heartworm disease; they include chronic cough, steroid responsiveness, and eosinophilia.

Most cats with signs of feline heartworm disease develop a chronic cough with or without respiratory difficulty. Some cats present only for chronic vomiting and show no signs of respiratory disease. Other cats present with anorexia or weight loss. Rarely, peracute death occurs from infections.

Results of the physical examination are variable, depending on severity of the disease. The cat may be clinically normal or may have tachypnea, cyanosis, or crackles when examined.

The radiographic feature most consistent with feline heartworm disease is enlarged caudal lobe pulmonary arteries, which are seen best on the ventrodorsal view. Patchy alveolar infiltrates, similar to those seen in canine heartworm disease, may also be present. A peripheral eosinophilia is usually present 4 to 7 months after infection but thereafter is an inconsistent finding. This same trend is seen in the cytologic results of a tracheal wash (Dillon, 1984). The absence of eosinophilia from lungs or blood, therefore, does not rule out the diagnosis of feline heartworm disease. A Knott test should be performed if radiologic and clinical pathologic findings are suggestive of heartworms. Less than 20 per cent of cats are positive, and definitive diagnosis of most cases requires serologic testing or angiography. Nonselective angiograms accentuate the tortuous and blunted pulmonary arteries and may reveal worm emboli. There are many serologic tests available; however, only those ELISA tests specifically adapted for cats should be used.

Glucocorticoids may be required prior to adulticide therapy if severe eosinophilic pneumonitis is radiographically evident (prednisolone at 1 to 2 mg/kg body weight PO divided b.i.d. and tapered over a 10- to 14-day period). Thiacetarsamide sodium, 2.2 mg/kg IV twice daily for 2 days, is usually safe. The risk of therapy is pulmonary embolization, a much more severe problem in cats than in dogs. Embolization usually occurs within the first 2 weeks after therapy (Dillon, 1984), and these cases should be closely watched during this time. Treatment with steroids and fluids is indicated if embolization should occur. The routine use of aspirin in cats with heartworms has not been evaluated.

PARASITIC PULMONARY HYPERSENSITIVITIES

Parasitic infections of the respiratory tract of dogs and cats may produce a peripheral or pulmonary eosinophilia. The eosinophil count is highest during stages of parasitic migration through tissues. The accumulation of eosinophils in the lungs is attributed to both endogenous substances secreted by some parasites and, more important, to selective eosinophil chemotactic factors released during the immediate and delayed hypersensitivity reactions of the host toward the invading helminths. There are two categories of parasites affecting the respiratory tract: migrating intestinal parasites and resident pulmonary parasites.

Intestinal parasites known to migrate through the lungs are *Toxocara* spp., *Strongyloides stercoralis*, and *Ancylostoma* spp. Most of these parasitic migrations produce either subclinical or mild and transient signs. The diagnosis of pulmonary hypersensitivity secondary to their presence is difficult to confirm for several reasons: Eggs or larvae are inconsistently found in fecal specimens; a peripheral eosinophilia is an inconsistent finding; and there are no definitive radiographic features. Negative fecal results may occur because pulmonary migration usually takes place during the prepatent stage and because standard flotation techniques often will not reveal parasitic larvae. For example, isolation of *Strongyloides* larvae requires the Baermann technique. A tracheal wash to detect larval forms may occasionally confirm the diagnosis but is reserved for cases with severe respiratory distress. As most hypersensitivity reactions are mild and only transiently clinical, treatment with anthelmintics or steroids is usually not required.

There are many parasites of the respiratory system of cats and dogs. Some reside in the trachea and bronchi (*Capillaria aerophilia*, *Oslerus [Filaroides] osleri*, and *Crenosoma vulpis*), whereas others inhabit terminal bronchioli and alveoli (*Paragonimus* spp., *Aelurostrongylus abstrusus*, *Andersonstrongylus [Filaroides] milksi*).

Many infections are asymptomatic or self-limiting, diagnosed only by the presence of ova or larvae in routine fecal analyses. Other animals are presented for chronic cough or mild tachypnea, with or without weight loss and anorexia. A complete white cell count and differential, thoracic radiographs, and fecal analysis should be performed to evaluate the cause of respiratory signs. A tracheal wash for culture and cytologic examination is indicated if the diagnosis cannot be established by these methods. Study of tracheal washes provides a diagnostic advantage over fecal analysis in that ova or larvae concentrate in bronchial secretions and are more easily observed.

The goal of therapy is twofold: elimination of the parasite and suppression of the hypersensitivity reaction. Anthelmintics that have been used include levamisole, albendazole, fenbendazole, and thiabendazole (Pechman, 1984; Ford, 1984; Barsanti and Prestwood, 1983). The use of glucocorticoids to suppress the inflammation associated with the parasite (e.g., prednisolone, 1 to 2 mg/kg body weight PO divided into two to three doses) dramatically improves the clinical signs prior to parasite elimination.

PULMONARY HYPERSENSITIVITIES CAUSED BY DRUGS

In humans, many drugs can cause various pulmonary abnormalities, including edema, fibrosis, bronchoconstriction, and hypertension. The following are some of the few drugs that are known to cause PIE in humans (Weg, 1982):

1. Carbamazepine
2. Chlorpropamide
3. Imipramine
4. Mephenesin carbamate
5. Para-aminosalicylate
6. Penicillin
7. Sulfa drugs
8. Tetracycline

Type I allergic reaction is the suspected mechanism of most drug hypersensitivities. In humans, the clinical course can be transient and mild, responding to drug withdrawal alone, or prolonged and severe, requiring steroids and supportive care. In veterinary medicine, drug-induced pulmonary hypersensitivities are rare and are poorly documented.

ALLERGIC BRONCHITIS AND ALLERGIC PNEUMONITIS

Little work has been undertaken in small animal medicine on hypersensitivity reactions to inhaled allergens. In humans, repeated inhalation of certain actinomycetes and fungus-laden organic dusts or foreign animal proteins can cause allergic tissue injury of the lungs (Wessels et al., 1973). Types I, III, and IV immune mechanisms are thought to be involved; however, types I and IV are the best documented. Known allergens and the diseases they cause in humans are listed below (Weg, 1982).

1. *Microsporum faeni* and *Thermoactinomyces vulgaris*—farmer's lung
2. *Alternaria*—pulp worker's disease
3. *Aspergillus clavatus*—malt worker's disease
4. *Aspergillus fumigatus*—mill worker's disease
5. *Penicillium casei*—cheese washer's lung
6. *Aspergillus versicolor*—dog's house disease
7. Cork dust
8. Coffee bean dust
9. Bird sera, protein, and droppings

Experiments using foreign soluble antigens demonstrate that previously sensitized guinea pigs, rabbits, rats, monkeys, and horses develop pulmonary hypersensitivity reactions on re-exposure (Wessels et al., 1973). Certain naturally occurring diseases of cattle and horses (e.g., fog fever and heaves, respectively) have clinical signs similar to those of hypersensitivity pneumonitis of humans. These signs include a cough and increased respiratory effort. Exposure to the allergens acutely worsens the condition.

The role of inhaled allergens in small animal pulmonary hypersensitivity is at present unknown. *M. faeni* and *T. vulgaris* can grow in many warm, damp places (hot-air furnaces, air conditioners, humidifiers, and fireplace flues) and may possibly lead to exposure (Weg, 1982). These organisms may be responsible for cases of suspected pulmonary hypersensitivity that defy etiologic diagnosis. The inhalation of *Aspergillus*, *Toxoplasma* oocysts, or ascarid eggs may also cause a pulmonary hypersensitivity in sensitized animals. The effect of air pollutants, cigarette smoke, and other aerosolized substances needs further investigation, although a detailed history may suggest a possible role of these agents.

Most inhaled allergens in dogs produce dermatologic manifestations. Intradermal skin testing identifies many of these offending allergens. It is possible that these same allergens induce variable degrees of pulmonary hypersensitivity with or without clinical evidence of skin disease. Therefore, skin testing for suspected pulmonary allergens may be advisable. It is important to recognize that only type I hypersensitivities will be detected if the skin test is read immediately.

Animals with allergic bronchitis or pneumonitis usually have a chronic cough that worsens during exercise and excitement. If exercise intolerance is reported, it is more characteristic of allergic pneumonitis than bronchitis. Most affected dogs are young adults or middle-aged. These problems are more common in small breeds, especially terriers, at our institution.

Results of physical examination of most animals with allergic bronchitis or pneumonitis are abnormal. Tachypnea, mild to moderate cyanosis, dyspnea, and abnormal lung sounds are the most common findings. Crackles and wheezes are often heard throughout the lung fields, especially after a cough. A variable peripheral eosinophilia (4 to 50 per cent) and abnormal thoracic radiographs may be found. Allergic bronchitis is characterized radiographically by increased interstitial and peribronchial markings. Changes consistent with allergic pneumonitis include ill-defined (and variable) patchy alveolar infiltrates. These infiltrates are thought to be eosinophils.

Animals with eosinophilic bronchitis or pneumonitis will not improve unless treated with glucocorticoids. The only exception occurs when the identification of a specific allergen is possible, with subsequent prevention of re-exposure or successful hyposensitization therapy. This situation, however, rarely occurs. Prednisone should be started at 1 to 2 mg/kg divided twice or three times daily. Every 7 to 10 days the total daily dose of steroids should be lowered by one fourth to one half, provided that the clinical signs are controlled. After 3 to 4 weeks, alternate-day or every-third-day steroid therapy can be tried. Some well-controlled animals can be taken off steroids or be given a low dose during periods of exacerbation.

This disease complex is frequently controllable but rarely curable. The owners must be apprised of this fact from the onset to ensure client compliance for long-term management of the pet's illness. In dogs, when tracheal collapse is also present, the cough may be much more difficult to control, and the judicious use of cough suppressants is indicated. Bronchodilators should also be considered if bronchoconstriction is suspected, especially in cases only partially responsive to glucocorticoids and cough suppressants.

References and Supplemental Reading

Barsanti, J. A. and Prestwood, A. K.: Parasitic diseases of the respiratory tract. *In* Kirk, R. (ed.): *Current Veterinary Therapy VIII*. Philadelphia: W. B. Saunders, 1983, pp. 241–246.

Crofton, J. W., Livingston, J. L., Oswald, N. C., et al.: Pulmonary eosinophilia. Thorax 7:1, 1952.

Dillon, R.: Feline dirofilariasis. Vet. Clin. North Am. 14:1185, 1984.

Ford, R. B.: Infectious respiratory disease. Vet. Clin. North Am. 14:985, 1984.

Middleton, E., Atkins, F. M., Fanning, M., et al.: Cellular mechanisms in the pathogenesis and pathophysiology of asthma. Med. Clin. North Am. 65:1013, 1981.

Pechman, R. D.: New knowledge of feline bronchopulmonary disease. Vet. Clin. North Am. 14:1007, 1984.

Schatz, M., Wasserman, S., and Patterson, R.: Eosinophils and immunologic lung disease. Med. Clin. North Am. 65:1055, 1981.

Weg, J. G.: Chronic noninfectious parenchymal diseases. *In* Guenter, C. A., et al. (eds.): *Pulmonary Medicine*. Philadelphia: J. B. Lippincott, 1982, pp. 607–661.

Weller, P. F., and Goetzl, E. J.: The human eosinophil. Roles in host defense and tissue injury. Am. J. Pathol. 100:791, 1980.

Wessels, F., Salvaggio, J., and Lopez, M.: Animal models of hypersensitivity pneumonitis. J. Am. Anim. Hosp. Assoc. 9:588, 1973.

PYOTHORAX

TIMOTHY BAUER, D.V.M.
Seattle, Washington

Pyothorax, or empyema, is the accumulation of infected material and fluid within the pleural space. Causative agents may reach the pleural space by three routes: (1) as a result of systemic sepsis, infection reaches the pleura by either lymphatics or blood; (2) as a result of spread from an adjacent structure: pneumonia with bronchopleural communication and parapneumonic spread, rupture of the esophagus, mediastinitis, or subphrenic infection; or (3) by direct introduction of organisms as a result of penetrating trauma, thoracocentesis, or surgery.

There is normally a small amount of fluid present in the pleural space. This fluid grossly resembles serum and has a protein content of approximately 1.5 gm/dl. There exists a precarious balance between hydrostatic and oncotic forces within the pleurae (Starling's forces).

Hydrostatic and oncotic pressures within the systemic circulation, pulmonary circulation, and the intrapleural space collectively produce a water gradient of approximately 9 cm, which favors transudation of fluid from the parietal pleura into the pleural space. These same forces provide a gradient of approximately 10 cm of water, favoring absorption of this fluid into the visceral pleura's vasculature (the pulmonary capillaries and lymphatics). The result of this is the continual net flow of fluid from parietal to visceral pleura. This delicate balance can be interrupted by any disorder that alters (1) oncotic pressure, (2) systemic or pulmonary capillary pressure, (3) lymphatic competence, (4) capillary permeability, or (5) effective surface area.

In the case of pyothorax, aberrations of all these factors probably play a role in the accumulation of the large effusions encountered in this disorder. Inflammation produces an increase in regional blood flow, resulting in capillary hypertension. Increased capillary permeability results in colloid flux toward the pleural space, causing a rise in pleural oncotic pressure. With loss of favorable oncotic gradient, fluid removal must be maintained by regional lymphatics, the effectiveness of which may be compromised by fibrosis or obstruction with cellular and infectious debris.

The clinical recognition of pyothorax begins with the detection of physical findings compatible with loss of lung volume and is confirmed by the observation of a pleural effusion on chest radiographs. Laboratory examination of the effusion is the only definitive means of making the diagnosis; thus thoracocentesis is required. Presence of organisms on Gram or acid-fast stains and their subsequent growth in culture media are an absolute requirement for both diagnosis and definitive therapy.

CLINICAL PRESENTATION

Fever, anorexia, weight loss, and shortness of breath are the chief signs associated with pyothorax. An infectious prodrome may have been noted days to weeks prior to the owner's seeking medical help. The subacute or acute nature of the process may be marked by a prior history of surgery, hospitalization for a seemingly unrelated illness, or having been away from home for several days.

In the author's experience with 42 canine and feline cases of pyothorax, the patient populations differ in age and sex distribution. Feline patients are largely domestic long- and short-hairs, and few purebreds are affected. They have a mean age of 5.6 years, with equal distribution between the sexes. Canine patients have a mean age of 3.6 years, and males outnumber the females 2:1. Labradors, shepherds, and golden retrievers were the most frequently affected breeds, although hounds, terriers, Dalmatians, and spaniels also had a significant incidence. It should be noted that breed incidence as well as causative organisms will vary in different geographic regions of the country.

None of these patients had any documentation of a pre-existing debilitating disease such as neoplasia, immunologic disorders, or chronic lung disease. All had clinical signs referable to loss of lung volume secondary to a large pleural effusion.

The mean hematocrit at the time of admission was 26 per cent for cats and 37 per cent for dogs. There was no demonstrable fall in hematocrit over the period of hospitalization; however, those patients with chronic disease may develop a normocytic, normochromic anemia. No incidence of hemolytic anemia was observed. The mean leukocyte count was 27,000/ml in feline patients and 32,000/ml in canine patients, ranging from 5,900 to 76,000 (feline) and 10,400 to 51,300 (canine). A low or normal leukocyte count is found with some frequency and has no correlation with severity. Leukocyte counts return to normal in an average of 14 days (feline) and 9 days (canine) with appropriate therapy. It should be noted that some feline patients may initially show a profound leukocytosis after initial pleural drainage. Results of routine clinical chemistry evaluation (SMA 1260) and urinalysis for the most part are unremarkable. Mild prerenal azotemia may be present in those patients with altered volume status. Serum globulin levels are elevated more frequently in canine patients (mean of 5.2 gm/dl).

RADIOGRAPHIC FINDINGS

In all cases, a moderate to large pleural effusion is present, obscuring the cardiac silhouette and a large portion of the pulmonary and pleural detail. In most cases, the effusions are bilateral; however, in a significant number (12 per cent), the exudate is unilateral because of pleural and mediastinal involvement. Although large amounts of free pleural gas are rarely present, pyopneumothorax is a frequent finding when standing or horizontal beam lateral views are obtained in patients with anaerobic infection or necrotizing pneumonia. On immediate postdrainage films, approximately 50 per cent of feline patients and 70 per cent of canine patients had pulmonary infiltrates or identifiable consolidation, most frequently involving the left cranial lobe in both feline and canine patients. Most of these findings are absent on subsequent (48 to 72 hours) radiographs.

MICROBIOLOGY

The Gram stain is the most important tool for rapid assessment of microorganisms in pleural fluid. Specimens collected by transtracheal aspiration may also be of value in the early assessment.

Both cats and dogs with pyothoraces have a high incidence of anaerobic infection, either as a sole pathogen or in combination with aerobic organisms. For this reason, it is of extreme importance to submit both aerobic and anaerobic cultures. Anaerobes are capable of creating a fetid odor; this is mainly due to the volatile amines, short-chain fatty acids, and organic acids they produce. The absence of a fetid smell, however, does not rule out the presence of anaerobes. The morphology of anaerobes as seen on Gram stains may set them apart from aerobic organisms.

The list of causative organisms overlaps in the two species. In general, feline patients tend to have a higher incidence of pure anaerobic infection and fewer enteric infections. Table 1 lists the organisms encountered in order of their apparent frequency.

TREATMENT

Tube thoracostomy should be performed as soon as the diagnosis is made. Chest tube drainage is best accomplished by continuous water seal suction at approximately 20 cm of water. Only a small number of patients require bilateral chest tube placement as a result of persistent loculation of fluid or a complete mediastinum, which prevents adequate evacuation of both hemithoraces with a single chest tube. The use of continuous water seal suction is ideal and is the key to the complete and rapid

Table 1. Organisms Cultured from Pleural Fluid of 42 Pyothoraces*

Cats	Dogs
Bacteroides	*Fusobacterium*
Mycoplasma	*Actinomycetes*
Actinomycetes	*Corynebacterium*
Peptostreptococcus	*Streptococcus*
Streptococcus	*Bacteroides*
Pasteurella	*Pasteurella*
Fusobacterium	*Escherichia coli*
	Klebsiella
	Peptostreptococcus
	Coccidiodes immitis

*Listed in order of apparent frequency. Order and organisms may vary by geographic location.

removal of infected pleural exudate. Tube thoracostomy without continuous water seal drainage is less than an ideal means of pleural drainage. Continuous removal facilitates a more complete and rapid resolution of the pyothorax. As is true with treatment of any abscess cavity, medical resolution cannot take place without complete drainage of the infected material. Patients will not improve clinically until effective drainage is established.

The total amount of fluid removed from each patient was 2850 ± 1700 ml (canine) and 490 ± 75 ml (feline). The average amount of fluid removed in the first 24 hours was 320 ± 75 ml (feline) and 1510 ± 831 ml (canine), followed by a decline until chest tube removal. The criteria for discontinuing drainage are (1) chest radiographs showing complete chest evacuation for 48 hours, (2) negative Gram stain, and (3) production of less than 50 ml of nonpurulent fluid in 24 hours in canine patients, 15 ml in feline patients. Premature chest tube removal may necessitate a second tube placement. Average length of drainage was 4.1 ± 1.3 days (cats) and 5.4 ± 1.4 days (dogs), with hospital discharge 24 hours after removal of the chest tube.

After volume restoration, tube thoracostomy is performed without general anesthesia in all patients. In those patients who appear anxious or uncooperative, low-dose narcotic sedation prior to the procedure may be used.* The area should be surgically prepared and a 2 per cent lidocaine block employed. Placement of the chest tube is similar in all patients. A small skin incision is made over the last rib in the middle to dorsal half of the thorax. The chest tube (Argyle trochar chest catheter, Sherwood Medical) is advanced subcutaneously to the level of the seventh or eighth intercostal space, where it is introduced into the chest. A pursestring suture is placed at the entrance wound, and the tube is affixed to the skin by means of two butterfly bandages sutured to the skin.

Cytologic examination of the pleural fluid should be undertaken frequently to assess the effectiveness of antimicrobial therapy. Gram stains may be evaluated every 48 hours throughout the course of drainage. Gram stains frequently fail to reveal any bacteria after an average of 2.5 days. Serial cultures are obtained only when (1) patients continue to produce an infected effusion despite antimicrobial therapy and (2) a change is noted in organism morphology on Gram stain. In a few cases, a new organism may be obtained on subsequent culture that was not isolated at the time of primary bacteriologic workup.

In most patients, therapy should be initiated with moderately high doses of a parenteral synthetic penicillin. An oral agent can be substituted as the clinical condition improves. Duration of treatment depends chiefly on clinical impression and response to therapy. The author arbitrarily uses 3 months of oral therapy after complete tube drainage.

Penicillin remains the drug of choice for all forms of anaerobic pleuropulmonary infection. *Bacteroides fragilis* is present in 15 per cent of feline isolates and in a smaller percentage of canine patients. *B. fragilis* has generally been shown to be penicillin resistant *in vitro*; for this reason, either chloramphenicol or clindamycin is employed when it is isolated.

In community-acquired infection, there is a high probability that the causative organisms will be sensitive to ampicillin. As such, unless hospital-acquired infection is known to exist or the Gram stain suggests otherwise, patients should be started on a synthetic penicillin. For canine patients, the author has employed ampicillin at an average dose of 1 gm every 4 hours for the first 48 hours, then every 6 hours for the remainder of the first week. At discharge, the dosage is decreased to every 8 hours. Feline patients are treated with an average dose of 250 mg on the same schedule.

Hospital-acquired infection is less predictable and, under most circumstances, should not be treated with a single agent. While cultures are pending, treatment with a combination of cephalosporin and aminoglycoside is suggested.

DISCUSSION

The established diagnosis of pyothorax constitutes a medical emergency that should be treated without delay. Tube thoracostomy should be performed to achieve effective drainage of infected material. Chest tube size should be governed by the size of the intercostal space (typically 26 French for dogs and 16 French for cats). This procedure is associated

**Editor's note*: Extreme caution must be used with any sedation or anesthesia in these patients. Respiratory reserve is usually minimal, and any decrease in respiratory effort or drive as the result of sedation may be fatal.

with a low rate of complications, none of which have proved fatal in the author's experience.

Neither proteolytic enzymes nor pleural space lavage need to be used, as excellent results in both drainage and pleural space sterilization have been obtained without their use. There is no convincing evidence that enzymes adequately lyse established fibrin plaque. They may be of use in maintaining the patency of small chest tubes; however, this problem is alleviated by the use of the largest possible tube and frequent "stripping" of the water seal tubing.

Radiographs taken immediately (1 to 8 hours) after tube thoracostomy and drainage need not reflect the ultimate adequacy of drainage or the presence of pneumonic disease. At this stage of therapy, pneumonic consolidation, pulmonary edema, and pleural features cannot be adequately differentiated from localized effusion or postcollapse atelectasis. Patchy densities are frequently observed that disappear on subsequent examinations; therefore, 24-hour studies are preferable when chest tube position and adequacy of drainage are evaluated. During the initial phase of treatment, auscultation and percussion are valuable indices of drainage and lung re-expansion. Should physical findings dictate ineffective drainage, an earlier radiograph may be obtained.

Pyothorax, regardless of cause, in the immunologically competent patient appears to be a readily treatable disease if treated early and vigorously, as described in this text. Previous case reviews show a mortality rate of 42 to 80 per cent when therapy consisted of thoracocentesis and antibiotic therapy alone. In the 42 pyothorax cases reported in this series, only one dog and no cats died, and as such the diagnosis warrants a good prognosis.

Patients were restored to the former state of health without functional limitation. Post-treatment chest radiographs should have no significant radiographic change.

If allowed to persist untreated or if treated only with antibiotic therapy, the disorder may progress to the chronic stage. The consequences of improper or late management are costly and often result in pulmonary dysfunction and limitation if the patient survives. It is the author's belief that thoracocentesis or tube thoracostomy without continuous water seal drainage should seldom, if ever, be employed as a sole means of pleural space evacuation. Successful treatment requires prompt and thorough removal of infected material from the pleural space, the most satisfactory means being tube thoracostomy with continuous water seal drainage, and long-term antibiotic therapy.

References and Supplemental Reading

Clinical Aspects of Chest Drainage. St. Louis: Argyle Division of Sherwood Medical.

Pidgeon, G.: Feline pyothorax. Calif. Vet. 32:11, 1978.

Robertson, S.: Thoracic empyema in the dog: A report of twenty-two cases. J. Small Anim. Pract. 24:103, 1983.

CHYLOTHORAX

NEIL K. HARPSTER, V.M.D.

Jamaica Plain, Massachusetts

The accumulation in the pleural cavities of lymph fluid, which contains a high concentration of suspended chylomicrons and other lipid by-products of small bowel digestive processes, is referred to as chylothorax. In most, if not all, instances this accumulation results from a disruption in continuity of the thoracic duct, the main lymphatic vessel responsible for draining lymph fluid from posterior portions of the body. The thoracic duct originates in a subdiaphragmatic position at the cisterna chyli and courses the entire length of the thorax, where it joins the venous system, either at the junction of the left jugular vein with the cranial vena cava or by multiple venous communications in the cranial thorax.

The principal function of lymph in the thoracic duct is transport of ingested fats. As much as 95 per cent of the thoracic duct lymph volume arises from the liver and intestinal lymphatics, and the majority of the remaining volume comes from other intra-abdominal and intrathoracic sources. The amount of lymph contributed by the extremities is negligible under normal circumstances.

The composition of thoracic duct lymph is greatly influenced by the relationship between sampling time and the postprandial state; both the volume and fat content increase after a fatty meal. It has been suggested that fatty acids having fewer than 10 carbon atoms in the chain are absorbed by intestinal capillaries, whereas all other lipids resulting from triglyceride digestion (e.g., long-chain fatty acids, monoglycerides, diglycerides, triglycerides) are absorbed by intestinal lymphatics. It is the high lipid content of intestinal lymph that gives both thoracic duct lymph and chylous thoracic fluid their typical gross appearance. Other constituents of thoracic duct fluid include protein (total protein ranges from 2.20 to 5.98 gm/100 ml, with nearly equal concentrations of albumin and globulin), electrolytes, antibodies, and enzymes. Most of these other substances are in concentrations similar to those found in plasma. The concentration of fat-soluble vitamins is directly related to the amount ingested. Lymphocytes are the predominant cellular element, whereas the red cell count rarely exceeds 50 cells/mm.^{3}

ETIOLOGIC CONSIDERATIONS

The human medical literature addresses the classification of chylothorax according to the following categories: congenital, surgical trauma, nonsurgical trauma, neoplasia, and indeterminant. Congenital anomalies involving the thoracic lymphatic system range from atresia to complete absence of the thoracic duct and include both multiple peripheral lymphatic channels that fail to communicate with larger lymphatics and fistulas between the thoracic duct and pleural space due to incomplete communication of segmental components of the embryonic duct. Chylothorax has been recognized to occur after almost every known type of thoracic operation. However, those cardiovascular procedures involving mobilization of the aortic arch (e.g., repair of aortic coarctation, Blalock-Taussig shunt, repair of vascular ring anomalies, and closure of patent ductus arteriosus) are most likely to be associated with this complication. Penetrating wounds of the ventral neck, thorax, or cranial abdomen can interrupt continuity of the thoracic duct or a major lymphatic branch at any site along its course. Blunt chest and abdominal trauma can also be responsible, with physical forces probably being similar to those in traumatic rupture of the diaphragm. Trivial chest trauma, such as rapid changes in intrathoracic pressure associated with coughing or vomiting, has also been cited as a cause. This is most likely to occur in the postprandial state, when increased pressure and distension of the thoracic duct are observed. Lymphoma is the most common malignant tumor responsible for the development of chylothorax, with compression or obstruction of the thoracic duct as the inciting cause. Metastatic carcinomas are less frequently accountable and are generally the result of mediastinal involvement. Malignant cells have been observed in the thoracic duct lymph of patients with primary abdominal carcinomas, but primary lung tumors are more often the reason. Tumors involving the thoracic duct itself (e.g., lymphangiomyoma) have also been reported, although they are quite rare. Other recognized causes of chylothorax in humans include tuberculosis, filariasis, and thrombosis of the subclavian vein.

The causes of chylothorax in small companion animals are less well defined. No single large series of cases has been reported. Identified causes have included congenital anomalies and nonpenetrating chest trauma in dogs; whereas nonpenetrating chest trauma, dirofilariasis, and cardiomyopathy are reported causes in cats. In both species, rapid changes in intrathoracic pressure as a result of coughing or vomiting have been considered responsible in some cases, as has lung lobe torsion and lobectomy in dogs. However, in most patients, a cause cannot be established.

The clinical summaries of a series of dogs and cats with chylothorax are tabulated in Tables 1 and 2. The causative factors are further categorized in Table 3. As reported previously, the most common causes in dogs include the following: no inciting cause defined, major trauma, and trivial chest trauma associated with coughing or vomiting. The two dogs in which severe coughing was believed to be responsible were both kenneled 7 to 10 days before the onset of the initial clinical signs (e.g., coughing), and infectious tracheobronchitis was considered to be the inciting cause. Other explanations for the development of chylothorax are also provided by this group of cases, including some previously unreported causes, thus enlarging the number of differential diagnoses to be considered. Both anterior thoracic masses and generalized heart failure serve to elevate thoracic duct pressure by either obstruction or increased venous pressure, respectively. Distension of the thoracic duct (which results from the pressure) is then at increased risk to rupture, either spontaneously or secondarily to trivial chest trauma (e.g., coughing, vomiting). An intravenous catheter was responsible for cranial vena cava thrombosis and chylothorax in a single dog (Case 14, Table 1). In most of the cats in this series (Table 3), the causes of chylothorax were similar to those reported previously, and no definable inciting cause, major trauma, or cardiomyopathy was responsible in 64.7 per cent of the cases reviewed. Only anterior mediastinal masses and trivial chest trauma appear to be significant but infrequent or previously unreported associations. Transtracheal aspirates in three of the cats with long-standing coughs demonstrated either an eosinophilic or mononuclear inflammatory reaction. Chronic allergic bronchitis was thought to be responsible for the disorder in these cats. A thymoma

Table 1. *Clinical Summaries of 27 Dogs with Chylothorax**

Case No. and Breed	Age (yr)	Sex	Clinical Signs: Predominant	Duration (Days)	Radiographic Findings	Associated Conditions	Management
1. Labrador retriever	12	FS	Cough	14	BPE	None	Euthanasia
2. Borzoi	2	M	Vomiting/retching	4	BPE	Gastric volvulus	Thoracic duct (TD) ligation
3. Shepherd X	8	FS	Tachypnea	42	BPE	None	Thoracentesis, medical treatment, TD ligation
4. Bull mastiff	6	F	Episodic dyspnea	320	BPE	Pleuritis, unknown cause	TD ligation
5. Labrador X	8	M	Cough, dyspnea	21	BPE	None	TD ligation (twice)
6. Great Dane	10	F	Weakness, lethargy	5	BPE; cardiomegaly; mass on rib	Cardiomyopathy, osteosarcoma left first rib	Euthanasia
7. Dachshund	5	FS	Fever, lame left foreleg, tachypnea	27	BPE; anterior mediastinal mass	Lymphoma	Euthanasia
8. German Shepherd	4	M	Nocturnal dyspnea	14	BPE	None	TD ligation
9. German Shepherd	8	FS	Dyspnea	3	BPE	None	TD ligation
10. Afghan	12	M	Cough Dyspnea	58 14	BPE; cardiomegaly	Cardiomyopathy	Thoracentesis, medical treatment of heart disease
11. Samoyed	1	F	Heavy breathing	90	BPE	None	TD ligation
12. Collie X	1	FS	Polypnea after AA	2	BPE	Blunt chest trauma	TD ligation
13. Miniature poodle	2	M	Dyspnea	60	BPE	None	TD ligation
14. Dachshund	9	FS	Dyspnea	2	BPE	Idiopathic thrombocytopenic purpura; cranial vena cava thrombosis	Died acutely
15. Doberman	9	F	Dyspnea	3	BPE; cardiomegaly	Cardiomyopathy	Thoracentesis, medical treatment, euthanasia
16. Shepherd X	6	M	Dyspnea 5½ mo after AA	6	BPE	? Blunt chest trauma	Thoracentesis, medical treatment, euthanasia
17. Borzoi	5	F	Dyspnea	10	BPE; consolidated right upper and middle lung lobes	Lung lobe torsion; pleuritis unknown cause	Thoracentesis, lobectomy
18. Doberman	4	FS	Dyspnea	14	BPE	AA 2 yr previously	Chest tube, TD ligation (twice)
19. Husky	4	M	Heavy breathing; exercise intolerance	4	BPE	None	Repeated thoracentesis
20. Shepherd/wolf	7	FS	Cough, choking, blood in mouth	1	BPE	None	TD ligation
21. Dachshund	2	M	Dyspnea	2	BPE	None	Thoracentesis
22. Shetland sheepdog	2	FS	Hacking cough Dyspnea	5 1	BPE	Infectious tracheobronchitis	TD ligation
23. Afghan	1	M	Cough Heavy breathing	120 8	BPE; healed rib fracture	AA 6 mo previously	TD ligation
24. Shetland sheepdog	1	M	Cough, retching	10	BPE	None	TD ligation, reoccurrence postop, medical treatment, died 5 mo later
25. Doberman	6	F	Heavy breathing, choking	30	BPE	None	TD ligation
26. Afghan	3	M	Heavy breathing Anorexia	30 3	BPE	None	TD ligation (twice)
27. West Highland white terrier	7	M	Cough Dyspnea	26 7	BPE	Infectious tracheobronchitis	TD ligation, died 48 hr postop

*Cases seen at Angell Memorial during a 17-year period.
Key: AA = automobile accident; BPE = bilateral pleural effusion; F = female; FS = female, spayed; M = male; TD = thoracic duct; X = cross.

was the anterior mediastinal mass in two cats, and a histologic diagnosis was not established in the remaining cat.

PATHOLOGIC PHYSIOLOGY

The rapid accumulation of sizable quantities of any pleural effusion has immediate effects on mechanical lung function. This is particularly appropriate for chylothorax, as the basal rate of flow through the thoracic duct has been reported at 1.38 ml/kg body weight every hour and is substantially increased after ingestion of food and water. The result is compression of functional lung tissue, which may lead to acute ventilatory failure due to alveolar hypoventilation (i.e., atelectasis) and reduced vital capacity. In the acute setting, blood gases will demonstrate the typical findings of alveolar hypoventilation—acidosis, hypoxemia, and hypercapnia. These events can rapidly lead to shock and death if allowed to progress unattended.

Table 2. *Clinical Summaries of 17 Cats with Chylothorax**

Case No. and Breed	Age (yr)	Sex	Clinical Signs Predominant	Duration (Days)	Radiographic Findings	Associated Conditions	Management
1. Siamese	4	MC	Dyspnea, decreased appetite	10	BPE; cardiomegaly	Cardiomyopathy	TD ligation, euthanasia
2. DSH, orange tiger	14	MC	Dyspnea	2	BPE; anterior mediastinal mass	Anterior mediastinal mass	Thoracentesis; euthanasia
3. DLH, tabby	8	FS	Cough	120	Right-sided effusion	Allergic bronchitis	Chest tube
4. Siamese X	4	FS	Cough Dyspnea	180 7	BPE	? Pulmonary disease	Attempted TD ligation; died at surgery
5. Persian	1	M	Cough Dyspnea	42 28	BPE	Mononuclear bronchitis	TD ligation
6. DLH, black/white	10	MC	Cough Dyspnea	14 7	BPE	Fell from tree 7 wk previously	TD ligation
7. Siamese	16	FS	Cough	21	BPE; anterior mediastinal mass	Cystic thymoma	Multiple thoracentesis
8. DSH, black/white	2	M	Dyspnea, paralyzed hind legs	1	BPE; suggestive of restrictive pleuritis	Car accident, blunt chest trauma, spinal injury	Euthanasia
9. DSH, black/white	12	MC	Dyspnea	14	BPE	None	Chest tube 3 wks; euthanasia
10. DSH, black/white	7	FS	Dyspnea	1	BPE	None	Euthanasia
11. DSH, brown, tabby	7	MC	Heavy breathing	120	BPE; cardiomegaly	Cardiomyopathy	Thoracentesis, treatment for heart disease
12. Siamese	5	MC	Cough Dyspnea	49 37	BPE	None	TD ligation (twice)
13. Siamese	5	MC	Cough Dyspnea	14 7	BPE	None	Thoracentesis
14. Himalayan	2	MC	Dyspnea	2	BPE	None	Chest tube 5 days
15. DSH, gray tiger	6	MC	Lethargy, dyspnea	7 1	BPE; anterior mediastinal mass	Thymoma	Euthanasia
16. DLH, cream/sable	1	MC	Dyspnea	1	BPE	Cardiomyopathy	Chest tube 7 days
17. DSH, gray/white	14	MC	Dyspnea	3	BPE	Cardiomyopathy	Thoracentesis, treatment for heart disease

*Cases seen at Angell Memorial during a period of 10 years.
Key: BPE = bilateral pleural effusion; DLH = domestic longhair; DSH = domestic shorthair; FS = female, spayed; M = male; MC = male, castrated; TD = thoracic duct; X = cross.

The long-term effects of chylothorax on lung function are less well established. Most reports in the medical literature consider chyle a nonirritating substance and prolonged exposure of the pleural surfaces of little consequence. However, in cats, and less commonly in dogs, chronic chylothorax can result in severe restrictive pleuritis due to fibrous lung encapsulation (see Complications). Chyle is considered bacteriostatic owing to its lecithin content, presence of free fatty acids, or both. Thus, reports of infection or pyothorax as complications of chylothorax are rare.

The long-term metabolic effects of chylothorax can be life-threatening because of the need for frequent thoracic drainage. Fat is the most conspicuous component of chyle, but the loss of fat is less detrimental than the loss of proteins and fat-soluble vitamins. Total body loss of water and electrolytes can also lead to severe deficits if adequate replacement is not maintained. Finally, loss of lymphocytes and circulating antibody levels may lead to a lowered resistance to infections.

PATIENT EVALUATION

The presenting complaints in dogs and cats with chylothorax do not differ significantly from those accompanying other causes of pleural effusion.

Table 3. *Etiologic Factors Responsible for Chylothorax in the Dog and Cat*

Etiologic Factors	Canine (n = 27) Number	(%)	Feline (n = 17) Number	(%)
Idiopathic, spontaneous	14	(51.9)	5	(29.4)
Blunt chest trauma	4	(14.8)	2	(11.8)
Trivial chest trauma (coughing, vomiting)	3	(11.1)	3	(17.6)
Anterior mediastinal tumors				
Cardiomyopathy	2	(7.4)	3	(17.6)
Lung lobe torsion	2	(7.4)	4	(23.5)
Cranial vena cava thrombosis	1	(3.7)		
	1	(3.7)		

Rapid heavy breathing is the prominent clinical sign, which may be present for varying periods of time before veterinary attention is sought (Tables 1 and 2). Postponement of veterinary care is enhanced by the otherwise normal action of the pet. Less frequently, cough is a significant part of the clinical picture. This may precede the onset of breathing abnormalities by days, weeks, or even months, suggesting its role in the development of the chylothorax. However, the author has seen several cats in which the cough developed only after the accumulation of a significant pleural effusion; therefore, it is not totally clear in these cases whether the cough is a cause or a consequence of the chylothorax. Far less commonly, lethargy and anorexia are reported on presentation. These may be the result of pulmonary dysfunction due to severe pleural effusion, a primary disease process that is responsible for the chylothorax, or some other unrelated condition.

On physical examination, rapid, exaggerated respiratory movements at rest are the most pronounced abnormality. The animal tends to be quieter than expected and prefers a standing or sitting position (orthopnea). Visible mucous membranes may be pink or mildly cyanotic. Capillary refill time is usually normal. On thoracic percussion, there is dullness ventrally. Thoracic auscultation reveals diminished heart sounds bilaterally and absence of lung sounds ventrally. Lung sounds are frequently increased dorsally. When substantial quantities of pleural fluid are present, the liver is usually palpable as a result of posterior movement of the diaphragm. Rarely, fluid is also present in the abdomen because of the concomitant development of chyloabdomen.

DIAGNOSTIC PROCEDURES

Data base evaluation of the patient with chylothorax starts with thoracic radiographs or thoracocentesis to confirm the presence of pleural effusion. When breathing is severely impaired, a single exposure taken in the animal's most comfortable position will suffice, as the stress of exacting radiographic positions in two views causes further compromise of ventilation and may be life-threatening. Placing the animal in an oxygen cage for 10 to 15 minutes before the radiographic procedure and providing supplemental oxygen by face mask during the procedure may reduce these risks. The presence of a diffuse, hazy density ventrally causing indistinct cardiac borders along with small, round lung lobes dorsally and a diffuse homogenous pattern that obliterates all intrathoracic detail are the expected radiographic findings of most pleural effusions in the lateral and ventrodorsal projections, respectively. With lesser degrees of pleural effusion, interlobar fissure lines and blunting of the costophrenic angles will be seen in the ventrodorsal view.

Once the presence of pleural effusion is confirmed (by either physical examination or thoracic radiography), thoracentesis should be performed. This will provide an immediate improvement in the animal's ventilatory ability, as well as a sample for fluid analysis. The author prefers tapping dogs in a standing position. Cats are tapped in sternal recumbency, and cranial portions of the body are elevated. In both species, either the seventh or eighth intercostal space is entered at or just below the costochondral junction, after instillation of a 2 per cent mepivacaine hydrochloride solution (Carbocaine, Sterling). In dogs 9.0 kg (20 lb) or larger, a Duke's trocar is used, which additionally requires a 6- to 8-mm skin incision to permit its introduction. This system allows drainage of both pleural cavities from a unilateral entry into the chest. Some care must be used to prevent excessive introduction of air during inspiration. However, the ingress of some air during the procedure seems to increase the quantity of fluid that can be removed. In dogs and cats weighing less than 9.0 kg, a ¾-inch (19-mm), 21-gauge butterfly system (Medi-Wing Infusion Set, Sherwood Medical) is preferred and seems well tolerated even without the routine use of a local anesthetic block. Both sides of the thorax should be tapped, using this latter system, in order to remove as much fluid as possible. When the chest has been sufficiently drained, thoracic radiographs are repeated in both views to allow evaluation of the lungs and to reveal the presence of any abnormalities.

A definitive diagnosis of chylothorax relies on proper evaluation of the thoracic fluid that is removed. Grossly, chyle is white and opaque, having a homogeneous consistency, although varying numbers of red blood cells may impart a pink or red color to the fluid. Its gross appearance may be confused with chest fluids having large numbers of white blood cells (e.g., neoplastic processes, infections) and those containing increased concentrations of cholesterol (termed *chyliform* or *pseudochylous* effusions). Pseudochylous thoracic effusions appear to be quite rare in dogs and cats. Differentiation of these various fluids of similar gross appearance requires cytologic examination and measurement of the lipid composition (Tables 4 and 5). Finally, it should be understood that the gross appearance of chylous effusions is not always characteristic. It can be significantly altered by the presence of other intrathoracic disease processes, such as neoplasia, inflammation, and venous congestion (e.g., heart failure, lung lobe torsion), as well as by fat content of the diet and the fasting state. Under these circumstances, the diagnosis may initially be missed because appropriate laboratory evaluation of the fluid has not been carried out.

Table 4. *Fluid Analysis Characteristics of Chylous Pleural Effusions in the Dog and Cat**

Analysis	Canine (n = 27)	Feline (n = 17)
Gross appearance	Opaque, white to red. Supernatant white, opaque after centrifugation.	Opaque, white to red. Supernatant white, opaque after centrifugation.
Specific gravity	1.026 (1.014–1.046)	1.032 (1.019–1.050)
Total protein	3.8 (2.0–7.9)	5.0 (2.6–10.3)
WBC count	5,220 (880–23,870)	7,987 (1,650–24,420)
RBC count	130,000 (7,200–1,070,000)	55,625 (8,000–200,000)
Mononuclear cells	16% (0–60)	8% (0–30)
Lymphocytes	43% (1–98)	70% (22–97)
Neutrophils	41% (0–91)	22% (3–75)

*Results are reported as mean and range (in parentheses).

Thoracic fluid that is milky or opalescent strongly suggests chylothorax and should be subjected to the following laboratory procedures: centrifugation, white cell count and differential white cell count, lipophilic staining of the supernatant or an ether clearing procedure, Gram stain and bacteriologic culture, and lipid analysis. As discussed previously, white, opaque pleural effusions may be the result of chyle, a purulent or highly cellular exudate, or the presence of a chyliform effusion. Centrifugation will result in clearing of the supernatant in the cellular exudate, whereas the chylous and chyliform effusions remain opaque. Cytologic examination of a chylous effusion will establish the presence of either a modified transudate or aseptic exudate (Table 4), but this finding alone is not distinguishing nor diagnostic of a chylous effusion. The use of both lipophilic stains (e.g., Sudan III, Sudan IV, oil red 0) to identify the presence of chylomicra in the fluid and the process of clearing the supernatant after alkalinization of the fluid and the addition of an equal volume of ether usually confirm the presence of chyle. However, neither of these procedures provides consistent results. Bacteriologic cultures of chylous thoracic effusions are rarely positive but should be performed routinely and, particularly, if repeated chest taps or chest tube drainage has been carried out in the past.

Table 5. *Comparison of Pleural Fluid Triglyceride and Cholesterol Levels in Dogs and Cats with Chylous and Nonchylous Effusions*

Categories	Triglyceride Levels* Mean (Range)	Cholesterol Levels* Mean (Range)
Canine		
Chylous effusions (n = 8)	766 (133–1386)	144 (72–187)
Nonchylous effusions (n = 3)†	31 (2–46)	91 (78–103)
Feline		
Chylous effusions (n = 8)	1317 (142–2460)	107 (49–189)
Nonchylous effusions (n = 5)‡	40 (10–108)	81 (55–113)

*Reported in mg/dl.

†Includes 1 dog with lymphoma and pleural fluid from two dogs after successful thoracic duct ligation.

‡Includes four cats with cardiomyopathy and pleural fluid from one cat after successful thoracic duct ligation.

The wide variation in the fluid analysis measurements (Table 4) is not a result of blood contamination, as the values for specific gravity, total protein, or white blood cell count were unrelated to the total red blood cell count of the fluid. Nor were the cell types present influenced by the quantity of red blood cells in the fluid. More likely, these variations are an effect of the duration of the chylothorax and the response of the pleural cavity to its presence. This could certainly explain the higher values for specific gravity, total protein, and white blood cell count in cats, as the pleural cavity in this species does seem more reactive to chyle than in dogs (see Complications). However, this theory does not account for the greater percentage of lymphocytes found in the pleural fluid of cats with chylothorax, which suggests less influence by pleural inflammation. Other unexplained factors must be responsible for these differences.

The most definitive laboratory procedures for the identification of chylothorax and differentiation between chylous and chyliform effusions is lipid analysis of the fluid. Chylous effusions contain chylomicra and high concentrations of triglycerides, whereas the concentration of cholesterol approximates that of the serum. Chyliform effusions are usually of long-standing duration, which for unexplained reasons results in cholesterol accumulation. Thus, they are characterized by cholesterol levels that exceed that of the serum, whereas triglyceride levels are comparable to or below those found in the serum. It has been reported that triglyceride values greater than 110 mg/dl are highly suggestive of a chylous effusion. Table 5 summarizes the results of lipid analyses performed in dogs and cats with pleural effusions.

MANAGEMENT

The optimal management of chylothorax in humans begins with the placement of a chest tube into the side of the chest in which the lymph fluid is leaking. This can be established easily in patients with unilateral effusion, but it requires lymphangiography when bilateral effusion is present. Constant maintenance of negative pressure on the chest tube by an underwater sealed system is preferable to intermittent aspiration, as it maintains more fully expanded lungs, thereby enhancing the formation

Table 6. *Summary of Management Methods and Success Rate in the Dog and Cat with Chylothorax*

Method of Management	Canine (n = 23) Number (% success)	Feline (n = 14) Number (% success)
Thoracentesis, plus diet and medical management	8 (37.5)*	5 (0.0)
Chest tube, plus diet and medical management	1 (0.0)†	5 (40.0)‡
Thoracic duct ligation		
Single operation	14 (78.6)	5 (40.0)
Two or more operations	3 (66.7)	1 (0.0)

*Two dogs subsequently had thoracic duct ligation.
†Thoracic duct ligation carried out after 2 weeks.
‡Two cats eventually had thoracic duct ligation.

of adhesions at the site of the fistula. The chest tube is left in place for a minimum of 7 to 10 days and up to a maximum of 4 weeks, depending on the patient's condition and the ability to maintain an adequate homeostatic balance during this period. Parenteral hyperalimentation is preferred to the ingestion of a low-fat diet during this period of conservative management, as even the oral intake of water increases thoracic duct flow. Adequate maintenance of body fluid, serum proteins, vitamins, minerals, and daily caloric needs must be carried out. Surgical intervention is usually not considered for 2 to 4 weeks, but when large quantities of pleural fluid are removed daily (making satisfactory support of the patient difficult) it may be performed earlier. The nonsurgical methods described are effective in approximately 50 per cent of human patients.

Our approach to the management of chylothorax in companion animals would be considered aggressive by human medical standards. Surgical intervention is entertained earlier and frequently is used as the primary approach. The reasons for this are numerous: (1) expense of maintaining satisfactory long-term conservative management; (2) problems encountered in the proper and safe care of chest tubes, intravenous catheters, and nutritional support of our patients for a prolonged period; (3) the unpredictable outcome encountered with conservative methods; and (4) the superior results realized by thoracic duct ligation.

Our experience in the management of 37 dogs and cats with chylothorax is summarized in Table 6. The results obtained by conservative, nonsurgical methods, including multiple thoracentesis and chest tube drainage, were poor: only 5 of 19 (26.3 per cent) showed a satisfactory response. However, none of these animals was managed by the optimal methods that are recommended for humans. All were permitted free access to water and were fed either a low-fat prescription diet (r/d Prescription Diet, Hill's Pet Products) or an alternative low-fat human-type diet to which a medium-chain triglyceride supplement (MCT Oil, Mead Johnson) was added. Both fat- and water-soluble vitamins were administered parenterally, and exercise restriction was enforced. All animals were maintained on this program for at least 1 week, at which time thoracic duct ligation was carried out or euthanasia performed for financial reasons.

Thoracic duct ligation is routinely approached from a right eighth, ninth, or tenth intercostal space thoracotomy. The author has not found a significant difference in accessibility to the thoracic duct by any of these approaches and prefers the eighth space as it enhances visual inspection of the anterior thorax and permits removal of twisted lung lobes, when present, from a single incision. Visualization of the thoracic duct is improved by feeding heavy cream 3 to 4 hours prior to surgery. In the past, we injected lymphangiographic dyes into the esophageal wall at surgery, and these were also very useful in outlining the thoracic duct. Unfortunately, these dyes are no longer commercially available. At the present time, we are mixing a lipophilic dye (Sudan Black B, Harleco) with heavy cream (250 mg/1 oz) and administering 1 to 2 oz orally or by stomach tube 3 to 4 hours before surgery.

After thoracotomy, the diaphragmatic lung lobe is retracted cranially and the mediastinal pleura is incised between the aorta and azygos vein from the tenth to the twelfth intercostal spaces. All mediastinal tissue is bluntly dissected away from the aorta and thoracic vertebral bodies to the left mediastinal pleura and is doubly ligated en mass in the tenth, eleventh, and twelfth intercostal spaces with 2-0 braided silk. The right mediastinal pleura is then closed with 3-0 surgical gut, and the dorsal mediastinal pleura is abraded with surgical gauze from the diaphragm to the base of the heart. The thorax is closed routinely after placement of a drainage tube.

Postoperatively, the chest tube is maintained for a minimum of 48 hours or until its use can no longer be justified. A high-fat diet is fed to evaluate the success of surgery, and a fluid sample is removed 48 hours after surgery for measurement of triglyceride levels.

Reasons for the differences in surgical success between dogs and cats are unclear (Table 6). Surgical procedures in both have been carried out in a similar manner. Variations in the position or course of the thoracic duct and its radicles in cats could be one explanation, although lymphangiographic studies have not been reported in this species. Further studies are warranted to evaluate this.

COMPLICATIONS

In addition to the ventilation abnormalities associated with chylothorax during its acute development and the substantial loss of fluids, proteins, and lipid nutrients (including fat-soluble vitamins) during its conservative management, other major complications are commonly recognized. These may result in chronic pulmonary dysfunction or may be responsible for the development of acute breathing difficulty.

Lung Lobe Torsion

Torsion of a lung lobe has been reported as a cause of chylothorax but is also a well-recognized complication of chylothorax and other causes of pleural effusion. It is far more likely to occur in deep-chested breeds than in other dogs, and it has not been reported in cats. The right cranial and middle lobes are at greatest risk because of their increased mobility due to an absence of pleural attachments. Rarely, the left cranial lobe may become twisted.

Lung lobe torsion results in acute interruption of blood flow to the affected lobe, which then becomes nonfunctional. Initially, passive congestion and then necrosis and inflammation lead to the rapid development of pleural effusion. When both lung lobe torsion and chylothorax occur concurrently, gross characteristics of the pleural fluid may be sufficiently altered to make recognition of the chylothorax difficult. The routine measurement of triglyceride levels in all pleural fluids will eliminate this potential error.

Radiographically, a dense lung lobe occupying an abnormal position will be seen after thoracentesis. An air bronchogram will be visible for 1 to 2 days after the torsion, making recognition of the dense structure as a lung lobe easily accomplished, but the air pattern is frequently missing after this period. Bronchoscopy utilizing flexible fiberoptic equipment or bronchography will establish the diagnosis beyond question. Treatment of choice is surgical excision of the affected lung lobe. At surgery, a dense, nonfunctional lung lobe is found. Thoracic duct ligation should be carried out simultaneously, if the presence of chylothorax has been established by pleural fluid analysis.

Pleural Fibrosis

Although chyle is considered to be a relatively inert, nonirritating substance, it unquestionably causes a pleural reaction in some dogs and in most cats. This reaction involves all pleural surfaces in a fairly equal distribution. It consists of the deposition of collagenous connective tissue and fibrin over the parietal and visceral surfaces in a diffuse or multifocal pattern, which eventually organizes to form fibrous connective tissue. The major consequences of this complication include severe atelectasis and alveolar fibrosis, both of which contribute to pulmonary dysfunction.

Management is directed at the surgical decortication of all involved lung lobes. The author has usually limited this to a one-sided approach with reasonably good results, and this is carried out at the time of thoracic duct ligation. At surgery, pleural fibrosis is characterized by a pale white, opaque parietal pleura that is thickened and that prevents normal lung expansion. Similar changes may be seen on the visceral pleura. The fibrous capsule is peeled away from all accessible lung lobes, back to and including the hilus. This is not easily accomplished, and the pleura and the most superficial alveoli are inadvertently removed in some areas. Postoperatively, continuous negative intrathoracic pressure is maintained by attachment of a chest tube to an underwater sealed system in order to promote maximal lung expansion. This is continued for 2 to 4 days or until all surgically induced lung leaks have sealed. Corticosteroids (e.g., prednisone, 0.5 mg/kg, divided b.i.d.) are begun immediately after surgery and are continued for 2 to 4 weeks at a progressively decreasing dosage.

Postoperatively, thoracic radiographs will demonstrate some degree of persisting atelectasis, characterized by incomplete lung expansion and rounding of lung margins. Further improvement in lung expansion will be seen radiographically over a 2- to 3-month period, at which time maximum pulmonary function is realized. If severe atelectasis of left lung lobes persists, decortication of these lobes should also be considered.

Intrathoracic Infections

Infections involving the chest cavity and other intrathoracic structures are rare complications of chylothorax and its management. Pleural infections are usually the result of nonsterile chest tapping procedures or the inadvertent contamination of chest tubes. Pulmonary infections are of increased risk due to atelectasis and reduced mucociliary function. Pleural infections are managed by culturing of the chest fluid and the removal of all existing chest tubes. If pleural effusion persists, a chest tube should be placed aseptically into the opposite side of the chest to allow complete drainage. Antibiotic therapy is instituted based on susceptibility tests performed on the chest fluid.

Pulmonary infections are usually associated with a fever and a cough. Radiographic recognition may be difficult when varying degrees of atelectasis are present. Management includes transtracheal aspiration for cytologic examination and culture and the initiation of antibiotic therapy based on these findings. Adequate hydration, bronchodilators, and nebulization therapy are useful ancillary measures.

References and Supplemental Reading

Bessone, L. H., Ferguson, T. B., and Burford, T. H.: Chylothorax. Ann. Thorac. Surg. 12:527, 1971.

Birchard, S. J., Cantwell, H. D., and Bright, R. M.: Lymphangiography and ligation of the canine thoracic duct: A study in normal dogs and three dogs with chylothorax. J. Am. Anim. Hosp. Assoc. 18:769, 1982.

Bradley, R., and DeYoung, D. W.: Chylothorax with concurrent chyloabdomen in a dog. V.M./S.A.C. 72:1024, 1977.

Donahue, J. M., Kneller, S. K., and Thompson, P. E.: Chylothorax subsequent to infections of cats with *Dirofilaria immitis*. J.A.V.M.A. 164:1107, 1974.

Gilmore, C. E.: Characteristics of some abnormal chest fluids. Small Anim. Clin. 2:334, 1962.

Light, R. W.: Pleural effusions. Med. Clin. North Am. 61:1339, 1977.

Lord, P. F., Grenier, T. P., Greene, R. W., et al.: Lung lobe torsion in the dog. J. Am. Anim. Hosp. Assoc. 9:473, 1973.

Meincke, J. E., Hobbie, W. V., and Barto, L. R.: Traumatic chylothorax with associated diaphragmatic hernia in the cat. J.A.V.M.A. 155:15, 1969.

Patterson, D. F., and Munson, T. O.: Traumatic chylothorax in small animals treated by ligation of the thoracic duct. J.A.V.M.A. 133:452, 1958.

Roy, P. H., Carr, D. T., and Payne, W. S.: The problem of chylothorax. Mayo Clin. Proc. 42:457, 1967.

Stoats, B. A., Ellefson, R. D., Budahn, L. L., et al.: The lipoprotein profile of chylous and nonchylous pleural effusions. Mayo Clin. Proc. 55:700, 1980.

Suter, P. F. and Greene, R. W.: Chylothorax in a dog with abnormal termination of the thoracic duct. J.A.V.M.A. 159:302, 1971.

Wilkins, R. J.: Clinical pathology of feline cardiac disease. Vet. Clin. North Am. 7:285, 1977.

TRACHEAL COLLAPSE

HARMON C. LEONARD, D.V.M.
Salida, Colorado

With rare exceptions, dogs that suffer from a flattened or collapsed trachea are the toy and other small breeds of dogs. Tracheal collapse, as the condition is commonly called, usually appears at middle age and may be progressive. The cause is speculative. Among the causes considered are neurologic deficiency of the trachealis muscle, change in the organic matrix of the cartilage, genetic and nutritional factors, small airway disease, and a physiologic phenomenon referred to as flow limitation.

In considering a course of treatment for the respiratory distress associated with tracheal collapse, a thorough examination is essential. The patient should be examined for cardiac, laryngeal, and other pulmonary abnormalities. An electrocardiogram, thoracic radiographs, and a clinical pathologic examination (including a hemogram, heartworm and fecal check, selected blood chemistries, and a complete urinalysis) may be indicated. Clinically, the animal will have a chronic, dry, easily induced cough. It may be described as a "goose honk" cough if there is extensive collapse, or more commonly an "end-expiratory collapse" will be heard as the intrathoracic trachea collapses. In the more severe cases, the dog will tire easily, may be cyanotic, and may experience syncopal episodes. Palpation of the cervical trachea may reveal a flattened or flaccid trachea. The degree of respiratory distress is usually an indication of the extent or degree of collapse as well as the duration of the problem. Those affected for an extended period often show evidence of small airway disease (e.g., expiratory prolongation, wheezing, and air trapping).

Radiographic examination is widely used to confirm the diagnosis. However, if the dog is in severe distress at the time of the initial examination, a conservative approach should be used.

Medical management consists of restricting activities, and low-dose sedation may be indicated in excitable dogs (promazine, phenobarbital). Antitussives (Hycodan, Endo; Torbutrol, Bristol), bronchodilators (Theofed, National Pharm.), and short-term glucocorticoid therapy have been used to manage tracheal collapse cases medically. Weight reduction is a critical factor in these patients. Primary or secondary cardiac disease should be treated when present, but as a large percentage of middle-aged and older small-breed dogs have some degree of mitral insufficiency (*without* failure), care must be taken not to overtreat these patients.

Unless the condition deteriorates, the owner is instructed to return the animal in 10 to 14 days for a re-evaluation. Patients that are showing satisfactory response will have their level of medication modified to minimal requirements. Many dogs with tracheal collapse will live a relatively normal life with this course of medical management.

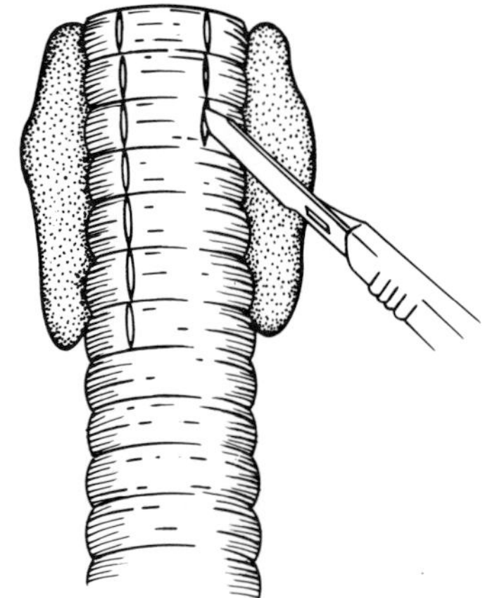

Figure 1. Placement of shallow incisions for repair of flattened trachea.

RADIOGRAPHIC DIAGNOSIS

Patients who have not responded to the treatment described should be examined further to rule out other cardiopulmonary diseases. Radiography is used both as a diagnostic tool to *confirm* the diagnosis of tracheal collapse and to rule out other concurrent cardiopulmonary diseases. Lateral radiographs should be taken during both inspiration and expiration in order to demonstrate the dynamic collapse. A ventrodorsal (VD) radiograph should also be routinely obtained.

The radiographs will reveal the portion of the trachea that is narrowed (cervical, thoracic inlet, intrathoracic or even main stem bronchi). The section at the thoracic inlet is most consistently restricted in animals with a flattened trachea. Tracheal collapse occasionally involves the entire trachea.

Fluoroscopy, if available, should be used to completely demonstrate the tracheal changes that are present during the respiratory cycle.

SURGICAL PROCEDURES

Surgical procedures that have been used to relieve the distress associated with a flattened trachea include cuffing the trachea with prosthetic rings, plicating the trachealis muscle, and chondrotomy.

Chondrotomy of the tracheal rings in the flattened portion of the trachea is a relatively simple and effective procedure in the author's experience. Anesthesia is induced, and the dog is intubated and maintained on inhalation anesthesia. During the anesthetic induction, the larynx should be examined with a laryngoscope. Laryngeal collapse, if noted, may be secondary to changes in the laryngeal cartilages or due to the effect of prolonged (and increased) inspiratory pressures associated with cervical tracheal collapse. The prognosis should be guarded if laryngeal collapse is present.

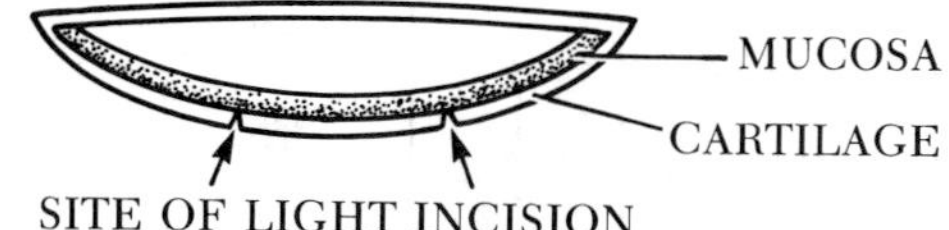

Figure 2. When incisions are made in a flattened trachea, the cartilage and mucosal lining should not be cut through.

If an endoscope is available, a view of the trachea during respiration gives a dramatic insight regarding the location and severity of tracheal collapse.

The patient is placed in dorsal recumbency, and the ventral cervical region is prepared for surgery. A tightly rolled towel is placed under the neck to elevate the surgical site. A ventral midline incision is made from the larynx to the thoracic inlet. The trachea is exposed and the sternohyoideus and sternomastoideus muscles are separated on the midline. The fascia is gently stripped from the tracheal rings. Starting at the first flattened tracheal ring, two very shallow incisions are made into the cartilage at 4 o'clock and 8 o'clock (Fig. 1). Care should be taken not to incise through the cartilage and inadvertently into the mucosal lining of the trachea (Fig. 2). Cutting through the mucosal lining may result in subcutaneous emphysema. Gentle pressure on the trachea with the fingers will "break" the cartilage at the points of the incisions (Fig. 3). Each exposed flattened cartilage should be incised. At the thoracic inlet, gentle cranial traction on the trachea will allow exposure of two or three of the intrathoracic tracheal rings, which should also be incised. The contraction of the trachealis muscle will cause the shape of the tracheal lumen to become roughly trapezoidal (Fig. 3). The sternohyoideus and sternomastoideus muscles are reapposed with 3-0 catgut, and the skin incision is closed with appropriate sutures.

In the author's experience, approximately 10 per cent of the dogs presented as surgical candidates will have collapsed tracheal rings as opposed to flattened rings. The collapsed rings are soft, flaccid, and lack rigidity, but because of the abnormal cartilage, they do not respond well to chondrotomy. As this change extends intrathoracically, it is difficult to treat by either cuffing or plication. These patients are critical, and the owner should be advised that the prognosis is guarded. Have a frank

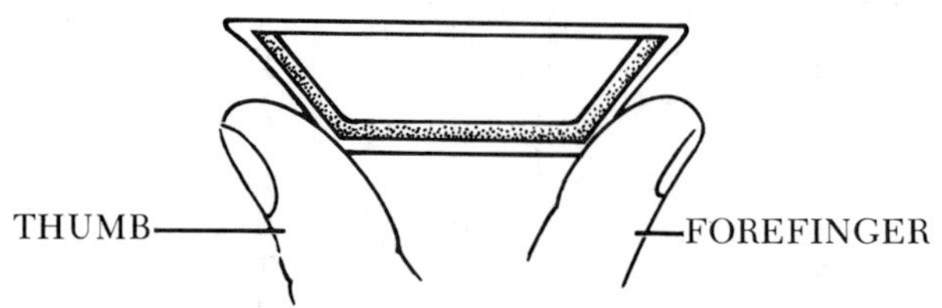

Figure 3. After light incisions are made, gentle pressure will allow the trachea to assume a trapezoidal shape.

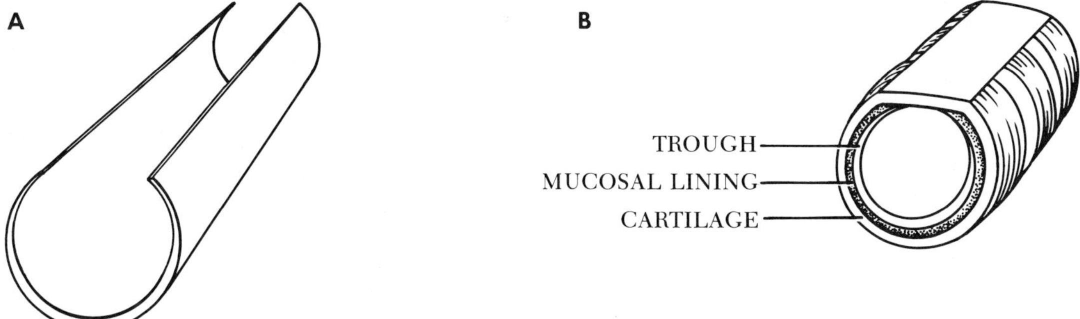

Figure 4. *A*, Trough shaped for tracheal prosthesis. *B*, Trough in place.

discussion with the owner before considering the possibility of surgical treatment.

The flaccid condition of the matrix of the tracheal cartilages may also involve the laryngeal cartilages. Collapse of these cartilages will cause additional inspiratory stress.

A decision regarding which procedure to use should be made at the time of surgical exposure of the trachea. If the tracheal cartilages are translucent and the markings of the endotracheal tube can be seen clearly through the matrix of the cartilage, the use of a tracheal prosthesis should be considered.

An internal Silastic prosthesis has been used successfully by the author for collapsed trachea. A Silastic tube one-fourth inch in diameter is slipped over a wooden dowel pin. With a bench grinder, using a fine-grained wheel, the external wall of the tube is ground thin on only that portion that is to come in contact with the lateral walls of the trachea. The tube is cut from the dowel, and 25 per cent of the thinned portion is removed, producing a trough (Fig. 4*A*). The open area of the trough will approximate the trachealis muscle (Fig. 4*B*). The length of the prosthesis to be used should be determined from tracheal measurements taken from the animal's radiographs.

The animal is anesthetized, and the trachea is approached surgically as described above. The annular ligament is cut between the fifth and sixth rings, and the endotracheal tube is withdrawn to a point anterior to the site of the incision. The sterilized prosthesis is inserted into the trachea. The distal end of the prosthesis should extend through the thoracic inlet to relieve any collapse at that site, but not far enough to reach the carina when the neck is flexed. The proximal end of the prosthesis is drawn forward so that the end lies two rings anterior to the incision in the trachea. The prosthesis is anchored in place by using two nonabsorbable sutures attached to cartilages distal to the incision. These sutures should be snug but not tight enough to cause necrosis of the cartilage. The incision through the annular ligament is closed with 3-0 chromic gut. The muscles and the skin incision are closed in a routine manner.

Postoperative care should consist of cage confinement and administration of a broad-spectrum antibiotic, prednisolone, and an antitussive as needed. If a concurrent infectious tracheobronchitis is thought to be present, a culture may be taken during surgery and appropriate antibiotics chosen based on sensitivity test results.

The tracheal prosthesis has limitations, and its use should be confined to those patients in which more standard treatments have failed and whose owners have decided on last-resort measures.

References and Supplemental Reading

Bojrab, M. J.: Collapsed tracheal rings. *In* Bojrab, M. J. (ed.): *Current Techniques in Small Animal Surgery.* Philadelphia: Lea & Febiger, 1975, pp. 189–191.

Hobson, H. P.: Total ring prosthesis for surgical correction of collapsed trachea. J. Am. Anim. Hosp. Assoc. 12:822, 1976.

Knowles, R., and Snyder, C. C.: Proceedings of the 34th Annual Meeting of AAHA. New York, 1967, p. 246.

Leonard, H. C.: Surgical correction of collapsed trachea in dogs. J.A.V.M.A. 158:598, 1971.

Leonard, H. C., and Wright, J. J.: An interluminal prosthetic dilator for tracheal collapse in the dog. J. Am. Anim. Hosp. Assoc. 14:464, 1978.

CHRONIC BRONCHITIS IN DOGS

TERENCE C. AMIS, B.V.Sc.
Davis, California

In recent years, our understanding of the causes and pathogenesis of acute infectious tracheobronchitis of dogs has improved considerably, whereas chronic noninfectious canine respiratory disease has received much less attention. The differential diagnosis and clinical management of chronic cough in dogs remains a particular challenge to the veterinary clinician.

One of the more common causes for chronic cough in dogs, especially middle-aged and old animals, is chronic bronchitis. The importance of this disease in humans is well recognized, and its pathology, pathogenesis, pathophysiology, epidemiology, and clinical management have been studied extensively. Despite this, the natural history of chronic bronchitis in humans and its relationship to emphysema and airway obstruction continue to remain unclear.

It is only in the past 10 years that naturally occurring chronic bronchitis of dogs has been defined as a clinical entity, and although the pathology of the condition has been described in detail, few clinical studies have been reported.

DEFINITION

In humans, chronic bronchitis refers to a condition of chronic hypersecretion of bronchial mucus. In 1974, Wheeldon and colleagues adapted this definition by defining naturally occurring chronic bronchitis of dogs as a condition of chronic or recurrent excessive mucus secretion in the bronchial tree not attributable to other lung disease and manifested clinically by coughing occurring on most days of at least two consecutive months in the preceding year.

A diagnosis of chronic bronchitis requires the fulfillment of three criteria: (1) chronic cough, (2) evidence of excessive mucus secretion, and (3) exclusion of other chronic respiratory disease (e.g., pulmonary neoplasia, parasitism, tuberculosis, fungal pneumonia).

PATHOLOGY

The main feature of chronic bronchitis found at postmortem examination is excessive amounts of viscid mucus or mucopus in the tracheobronchial tree. Thick mucus plugs may occlude smaller bronchi. The viscous nature of the mucus results from the presence of decreased amounts of epithelial sulfomucins and increased amounts of epithelial sialomucins. The bronchial mucosa often appears hyperemic, thickened, and edematous. Polypoid proliferations may project into the bronchial lumen. In approximately 25 per cent of the cases, patchy pneumonic lesions are present. Some dogs have dorsoventral flattening of the trachea and principal bronchi, typical of tracheal collapse.

Microscopically, bronchial walls are thickened and the mucosa is folded and irregular. Large numbers of neutrophils and macrophages are found in the bronchial mucus. Fibrosis, edema, and cellular infiltration of the lamina propria by lymphocytes, plasma cells, macrophages, and neutrophils may be present. There is focal ulceration of bronchial epithelium, combined with loss of cilia and squamous metaplasia at other sites.

The main histopathologic feature is a significant increase in the proportion of bronchial wall occupied by mucous glands, which are increased in both number and size, and an increased number of epithelial goblet cells.

Emphysema, characterized by destruction of interalveolar septae and an increase in size of air spaces distal to terminal bronchioles, is frequently encountered but is usually confined to small rims of pale, distended lung tissue around the edges of lobes. Emphysema in association with canine chronic bronchitis appears to be a much less important lesion than it is in humans.

In severe cases, hypertrophy of the smooth muscle in the wall of the small pulmonary arteries has been described.

ETIOLOGY

Although the cause of canine chronic bronchitis is unknown, it is widely assumed to be multifactorial in nature and associated with chronic exposure to inhaled irritants. In humans, cigarette smoking and exposure to atmospheric pollutants are the chief causes. Previous episodes of viral bronchitis, especially in childhood, and superimposed bacterial infections may also be involved. Genetic factors are important in the development of human emphysema (e.g., α_1-antitrypsin deficiency); their role in chronic bronchitis of dogs is unknown.

Chronic exposure of dogs to sulfur dioxide gas (500 to 600 ppm, 2 hours per day twice a week for 4 to 5 months) produces a syndrome of chronic cough, hypersecretion of bronchial mucus, and pathologic changes in the bronchial tree typical of naturally occurring chronic bronchitis. The significance of passive cigarette smoking in pet dogs remains speculative and awaits a controlled epidemiologic study. Some investigators have suggested an increased incidence of chronic respiratory disease in urban dog populations, but the evidence for this is not extensive or well controlled, and chronic bronchitis does occur in nonurban dog populations.

Acute infectious tracheobronchitis in young dogs may initiate the persistent inflammatory changes and disruption of normal tracheobronchial defense mechanisms typical of chronic bronchitis. The most common bacterial isolate from the bronchial tree of dogs with chronic bronchitis is *Bordetella bronchiseptica*, an organism that is an important component in the acute infectious canine tracheobronchitis complex.

PATHOGENESIS

It is generally assumed that the development of chronic bronchitis represents the result of a vicious cycle of airway damage and patient response. In health, the airways are protected by a set of pulmonary defense mechanisms, including normal ciliary action, a normal quantity and quality of mucus secretion, efficient collateral ventilation, and an efficient cough mechanism. Sustained injury to the bronchial epithelium associated with persistent infection or chronic inhalation of airborne irritants stimulates transformation of the ciliary epithelium, hyperplasia and hypertrophy of mucus-secreting structures, and hyperemia and cellular infiltration of the bronchial mucosa. With chronicity, these changes may impede normal defense mechanisms and improve the environment for bacterial colonization.

Edema and cellular infiltration of airway walls, increased amounts of tenacious mucus, localized endobronchial narrowing associated with fibrosis and polyp formation, spasticity of bronchial smooth muscle, collapse of larger bronchi associated with inflammatory weakening of bronchial walls, mucus plugging of smaller bronchi, obliterative inflammation of bronchioles, development of emphysema, and flooding of alveoli with mucus all contribute to a decrease in the efficiency of normal pulmonary defense mechanisms and promote the development of functional obstruction to intrapulmonary gas flow.

PATHOPHYSIOLOGY

Chronic bronchitis is defined solely in terms of mucus hypersecretion and not in terms of the development of any particular functional abnormality. However, the most common functional sequela is the development of airflow obstruction.

Since in life it is difficult to separate effects of chronic bronchitis and emphysema, the term *chronic obstructive pulmonary disease* (COPD) was introduced to describe human patients with chronic, minimally reversible airflow obstruction not explained by any specific or infiltrative lung disease. The term *minimally reversible* differentiates COPD from asthma, although the exact level of reversibility (response to bronchodilator administration) required to establish a diagnosis of asthma in humans still remains in dispute.

The diagnosis of COPD in humans depends on quantitative documentation of airflow obstruction through pulmonary function testing. In clinical veterinary medicine, pulmonary function tests are not widely available and airway obstruction is usually determined on the basis of clinical and radiographic findings. An exception is COPD of horses, in which pulmonary function testing has been used to demonstrate the nature, severity, and level of reversibility of airflow obstruction. Such studies of naturally occurring chronic bronchitis in dogs have yet to be performed, and much of our present knowledge in this area derives from experimental studies performed on dogs chronically exposed to inhaled irritants.

Increased airway resistance and a reduction in maximum expiratory flow rates are characteristic findings in COPD. Dogs chronically exposed to sulfur dioxide increase pulmonary resistance by 200 per cent or more above pre-exposure values. The predominant site of irreversible airflow obstruction in humans lies in peripheral airways less than 3 mm in diameter. Mucus hypersecretion in these airways leads to mucus plugging and displacement of the surfactant layer, allowing them to close more easily. Small airways may also be blocked by inflammatory exudate and become distorted, stenosed, and even obliterated. Recent evidence in dogs suggests that airway inflammation *per se* rather than hypertrophy of bronchial mucous glands or epithelial thickening is responsible for the development of chronic airflow obstruction.

In considering the role of small airway disease in the development of chronic airflow obstruction, it should be remembered that only a relatively small percentage of total airway resistance is contributed by the small airways. Despite the fact that airways decrease in diameter toward the alveoli, the vast increase in number of airways dramatically increases the total cross-sectional area available for gas flow. Disease of the small airways must be relatively extensive before airway resistance will be increased sufficiently enough to produce clinical signs. This is particularly so in poorly lobulated species, such as dogs, which have extensive interconnections between lung units on both an alveolar (via pores of Kohn) and bronchiolar level. Collateral ventilation through these channels allows alveoli subtended by obstructed bronchioles to continue to be ventilated.

Collateral ventilation will also modify the development of gas trapping in COPD. Processes that decrease the elasticity of the lung (e.g., emphysema) or increase the resistance of small airways (e.g., inflammation, mucus) promote premature closure of small airways during expiration, a process that tends to trap gas in the lungs. In advanced disease situations, gas trapping may occur during tidal breathing, resulting in the clinically described barrel-chested appearance of some COPD patients. Hyperinflation and airway closure at functional residual capacity have been confirmed in dogs with experimentally induced chronic bronchitis.

Large airway function may also be abnormal in COPD. Reactive large airway narrowing (bronchoconstriction) is thought to explain the partial reversibility of airway obstruction in nonemphysematous humans who smoke. Although bronchial hyperreactivity is well documented in chronic bronchitis of humans, recent studies suggest that dogs chronically exposed to inhaled sulfur dioxide have decreased airway reactivity as judged by challenge with inhaled histamine. Airway hyperreactivity therefore might not be as significant a component of airway obstruction in dogs with chronic bronchitis as it is in humans.

An important cause of expiratory flow limitation is dynamic compression of airways. During a forced expiration, gas flows out of the lungs because of the difference between alveolar pressure and atmospheric pressure. Alveolar pressure is the sum of pleural pressure and the elastic recoil pressure of the lungs. Since during expiration airway pressure falls from alveolus to mouth, a point is reached at which airway pressure is equal to pleural pressure. This is known as the equal pressure point, which represents that site along the airways where the elastic pressure generated by the lungs has been dissipated. From this point forward, within the thorax, there will be a net pressure tending to compress the airways; they will narrow, thus limiting bulk gas flow. Outside the thorax, the pressure surrounding the trachea is atmospheric; intraluminal pressure remains greater than atmospheric, so no tendency to collapse exists. On inspiration, the lowered pleural pressure tends to hold intrathoracic airways open and extrathoracic airways tend to be narrowed because of negative intraluminal pressures.

In COPD, increased airway resistance results in the early formation of the equal pressure point in more peripheral airways. Loss of rigidity of airway walls promotes airway collapse and impedes expiratory gas flow.

In toy breeds, this situation is commonly aggravated by a predisposition to weakness of the cartilaginous rings of the trachea and major bronchi. Tracheobronchial collapse occurring during expiration, and particularly during cough, impedes not only expiratory gas flow but also the efficient clearance of mucus from the bronchial tree.

The lesions of chronic bronchitis result in increased inhomogeneity in the distribution of ventilation within the lung. The development of ventilation-to-perfusion ratio ($\dot{V}A/\dot{Q}$) inequalities causes hypoxemia and widening of the alveolar-to-arterial difference for oxygen ($PA_{O_2} - Pa_{O_2}$). Chronic hypoxemia stimulates erythropoesis, resulting in polycythemia. Hypoventilation (elevated Pa_{CO_2}) is usually not a feature of arterial blood gas analysis in chronic bronchitis until the disease is in advanced stages. Increased airway resistance leads to an increase in the work of breathing. When the amount of work involved in maintaining a normal level of alveolar ventilation becomes too large, Pa_{CO_2} rises and respiratory acidosis develops.

Lung regions with impaired ventilation (and therefore a low alveolar partial pressure of oxygen, or Pa_{O_2}) also have reduced perfusion. This pulmonary hypoxic vasoconstrictor response, together with the loss of pulmonary capillary beds associated with emphysema, tends to raise pulmonary vascular resistance and pulmonary artery pressure. Chronically elevated levels of pulmonary vascular resistance may precipitate right heart failure (cor pulmonale).

CLINICAL FEATURES

SIGNALMENT. Chronic bronchitis is a disease of adult dogs. It is rarely encountered in animals less than 3 to 5 years of age, and it is more commonly encountered in small breeds. There is no sex predilection.

CLINICAL SIGNS. The main clinical sign associated with chronic bronchitis is a chronic, intractable cough. The onset of coughing is usually insidious. Often animals have been treated repeatedly, resulting in varying periods of remission followed by exacerbations, which may be associated with changes in weather.

Coughing may be unproductive, resonant, dry, harsh, and hacking, occurring in paroxysms, and is easily elicited by tracheal palpation, excitement, or exercise. At other times, owners report a nocturnal or early morning productive moist cough followed by gagging (retching). Dogs rarely expectorate, but when sputum is produced, it may vary in character from clear frothy mucus to greenish or brownish mucopus.

Affected animals are often obese. Except during severe exacerbations or episodes of bronchopneumonia, signs of systemic illness are not a feature of chronic bronchitis. Exercise tolerance may be limited by coughing bouts and severe airway obstruction. Some dogs experience paroxysmal bouts of coughing, leading to cyanosis and collapse. Body temperature is usually normal but may be elevated if there is associated bronchopneumonia.

Depending on the degree of airway obstruction, lung sounds may vary from normal through accentuated bronchovesicular sounds to paninspiratory coarse crackles and high-pitched, polyphonic, expiratory wheezes. An end-expiratory click or snap may be heard during coughing or forced expiratory efforts in dogs with intrathoracic tracheal collapse. In dogs with little airway obstruction, respiratory rate and pattern of breathing remain normal. In those with more severe obstruction, hyperinflation, pronounced expiratory respiratory effort (expiratory respiratory distress), and a prolonged expiratory phase of respiration may be noted.

DIAGNOSTIC TECHNIQUES

RADIOLOGY. In nonobstructive chronic bronchitis, the chest radiograph may be normal or may show evidence of bronchial wall thickening, indicated by "doughnut" shadows (end-on view of bronchi with thickened walls) and "tram lines" (tubular shadows associated with a longitudinal sectional view of bronchi with thickened walls). There is usually a generalized increase in airway-oriented interstitial density. It is important not to confuse the increased visibility of calcified bronchial cartilage in elderly dogs with the changes of chronic bronchitis. Interpretation of an increased bronchial pattern is most reliable in dogs between the ages of 3 and 5 years. In older dogs, these findings are apt to be equivocal unless changes are marked.

The main radiographic feature of airway obstruction is pulmonary hyperinflation. This is reflected by hyperlucency and enlargement of the lung fields, with caudal displacement (flattening) of the diaphragm. At end inspiration, the phrenicolumbar recess may be at the twelfth or thirteenth thoracic vertebra instead of the tenth or eleventh as seen in normal animals. Comparison of inspiratory and expiratory films aids significantly in detecting intrapulmonary gas trapping and in the demonstration of expiratory collapse of the intrathoracic trachea and bronchi. Fluoroscopic examination performed during a cough or forced expiratory effort helps to confirm tracheobronchial collapse. Patchy alveolar infiltrates are indicative of superimposed bronchopneumonia. Chest radiography is an indispensable component of the clinical investigation of dogs with chronic bronchitis because of the importance of ruling out other specific respiratory diseases.

CLINICAL PATHOLOGY. The hemogram is often normal, although increased white blood cell counts may be associated with episodes of bronchopneumonia. Polycythemia usually reflects chronic hypoxemia. Increased numbers of circulating eosinophils suggest parasitic or allergic respiratory disease.

Arterial blood gas analyses are often normal. In more advanced cases, hypoxemia, widening of the difference between PA_{O_2} and Pa_{O_2}, and metabolic acidosis will be encountered. Elevation of the Pa_{CO_2} is indicative of hypoventilation and represents the onset of ventilatory failure associated with increased work of breathing.

TRACHEOBRONCHIAL CYTOLOGY. Samples of bronchial mucus obtained via transtracheal aspiration or at bronchoscopy may only contain excess amounts of mucus and normal bronchial epithelial cells. In other cases, increased numbers of macrophages, goblet cells, hyperplastic epithelial cells, neutrophils, and lymphocytes are present. Purulent material with a large number of polymorphonuclear cells and bacteria may be found during exacerbations associated with bronchial infection. Large numbers of eosinophils are indicative of parasitic or allergic disease.

BACTERIAL CULTURE. Transtracheal aspirates or bronchial brushings can be sterile or may contain a number of different bacterial species. *Streptococcus* spp., *Pasteurella* spp., *Escherichia coli*, *Pseudomonas* spp., and *Klebsiella* spp. have all been isolated from dogs with chronic bronchitis. However, the most common bacterial isolate is *Bordetella bronchiseptica*. It is tempting to postulate a causative role for these bacteria in younger dogs with a previous history of acute-onset infectious tracheobronchitis from which recovery has never been complete.

BRONCHOSCOPY. The main feature of the bronchoscopic examination of dogs with chronic bronchitis is diffuse airway inflammation with hypersecretion and thick, tenacious mucus found in sticky strands or small plaque-like accumulations. Mucus plugs occur in smaller airways. Roughening and hyperemia of the bronchial mucosa is evident. Polypoid or nodular projections into the bronchial lumen occur in some animals. Tracheobronchial collapse may be evident.

OTHER DIAGNOSTIC TECHNIQUES. Fecal samples should be examined for evidence of parasitic (primary or migratory) respiratory disease. Blood samples should be taken to rule out heartworm disease.

Skin testing for allergic respiratory disease has not been widely employed in dogs but may prove useful to help confirm a diagnosis in cases characterized by eosinophilic infiltrates in bronchial mucus samples.

DIFFERENTIAL DIAGNOSIS

Chronic cough is a nonspecific clinical sign associated with many respiratory diseases, particularly those primarily involving the airways. It is important to rule out specific causes for chronic cough before a diagnosis of chronic bronchitis is made.

The main conditions to be ruled out include cardiac disease, chronic pneumonia, pulmonary neoplasia, tuberculosis, foreign body bronchitis, dirofilariasis, pulmonary parasitism (e.g., *Filaroides* spp.), and fungal disease. Eosinophilic or allergic bronchitis is usually classified separately from chronic bronchitis, since the presumed causes differ. Bronchiectasis may arise as a complication of chronic bronchitis but can be encountered as a seemingly primary occurrence.

THERAPY

Structural alterations in airway anatomy associated with chronic bronchitis are not readily reversible. Emphysema is a permanent change, as is structural weakness of airway walls associated with tracheobronchial collapse. Cessation of exposure to initiating factors may lead to a reduction in inflammatory changes and the return of airway wall anatomy toward normal. However, since these factors are usually not identified, exposure probably continues in most clinical cases. True cure of chronic bronchitis is rarely achieved.

Therapeutic strategies, however, can be devised to alleviate clinical signs and control exacerbations. Since animals present at different stages of the disease process and with varying degrees of functional abnormality, which may or may not be complicated by superimposed bacterial infection, it is difficult to design a therapeutic plan applicable to all situations. Instead, the approaches described below need to be applied on the basis of an assessment of the nature and severity of each individual animal's problems.

In the design of a therapeutic program for the management of chronic bronchitis, the following goals need to be considered: (1) client education, (2) avoidance of exacerbating factors, (3) control of infection, (4) promotion of bronchial hygiene, (5) relief of airway obstruction, (6) judicious control of cough, and (7) support of gas exchange.

CLIENT EDUCATION. The essentially incurable nature of chronic bronchitis and the goal of any prescribed therapy should be clearly communicated to the owner. Clients need to understand the natural history of this disease and their role in its control. This is perhaps the single most important service the veterinary clinician can provide in the management of dogs with chronic bronchitis.

AVOIDANCE OF EXACERBATING FACTORS. Whenever possible, owners should avoid exposing affected animals to inhaled irritants. Although the role of passive smoking is speculative, some animals may benefit from reduced exposure to this potential causative factor.

A number of dogs with chronic bronchitis suffer from paroxysmal coughing bouts associated with stress or excitement. Avoidance of such situations may be useful. Since exacerbations of the disease occur more commonly in the winter months, owners should be informed of the importance of maintaining a warm environment.

CONTROL OF INFECTION. Rational use of antimicrobials in the management of chronic bronchitis should ideally be based on demonstrated bronchial infection through bacterial culture. Material for culture must be obtained from the lower airways and *not* from the pharynx.

Many animals with chronic bronchitis do not have continuously superimposed bacterial infections. However, the development of episodes of infection and disease exacerbation are common. Lethargy, inappetence, fever, alterations in the hemogram, and radiographic signs of bronchopneumonia should alert the clinician to the potential presence of a bacterial infection. Prompt and effective treatment of bacterial infection with adequate systemic levels of an appropriate antibiotic is important in minimizing further damage to the bronchial tree. Ampicillin, trimethoprim-sulfonamide combinations, the cephalosporins, and the aminoglycosides have all been used for this purpose.

Administration of antibiotics by inhaled aerosol is widely regarded as not efficacious, although some reports suggest that aerosolized aminoglycosides may reduce airway colonization by *B. bronchiseptica*.

PROMOTION OF BRONCHIAL HYGIENE. Measures to promote removal of accumulating airway secretions are an important component of any therapeutic plan for the clinical management of chronic bronchitis. The following are some of the approaches that are available:

Aerosol Therapy. Inhaled water deposited in the bronchial tree helps to liquefy thickened secretions. In the hospital, this is usually accomplished with a nebulizer and an enclosed cage. A bland aerosol (0.45 to 0.9 per cent saline) administered for 15 to 30 minutes three or four times daily is usually recommended. The effectiveness of aerosolized mucolytic substances (e.g., *N*-acetylcysteine) remains controversial and is not recommended.

At home, aerosol or humidity therapy is most easily achieved by exposing the animal to steam generated by a hot shower in the bathroom. Care should be taken that the patient does not overheat. Cold or hot room vaporizers are used by some owners.

Chest Physiotherapy. Liquefaction of bronchial

secretions will not aid in bronchial hygiene unless other mechanical events subsequently remove secretions from the bronchial tree. Chest physiotherapy regimens induce vibrations in airway walls, thus dislodging mucus that may then be removed by coughing.

Chest percussion is most easily achieved by using the cupped hand to induce vibrations in the patient's thoracic wall. Chest physiotherapy should be applied three to four times daily for 5 to 10 minutes and is most effective after aerosol administration. Successful treatment is noted by the induction of a bout of productive coughing.

Light exercise after aerosol therapy aids in dislodging bronchial mucus and promotes an increase in lung volume associated with the standing posture. This helps to open small airways, particularly in dependent lung zones.

Postural drainage as employed on human patients is difficult to apply to canine patients but can be achieved in some cooperative animals. Drainage into central airways will need to be followed by coughing to achieve effective removal of mucus from the bronchial tree.

Expectorants. Expectorant drugs supposedly stimulate increased secretion of less viscous bronchial mucus. Two groups of drugs have been employed for this purpose, the saline expectorants (ammonium chloride, potassium iodide, and sodium or potassium citrate) and guaifenesin, which reflexly stimulate respiratory tract secretion through stimulation of receptors in the gastric mucosa, and the volatile oils (terpin hydrate, eucalyptus, and pine oil), which directly stimulate tracheobronchial secretions when inhaled as a vapor. The efficacy of these drugs is questionable.

Relief of Airway Obstruction

Bronchodilators. Drugs used to relieve spasm of bronchial smooth muscle fall into three main categories: the β-adrenergic agonists (e.g., isoproterenol, epinephrine, metaproterenol, salbutamol, and terbutaline), the xanthines (theophylline and its various salts), and the anticholinergic drugs (e.g., atropine). For bronchodilation purposes, inhaled selective β_2-agonists such as salbutamol are widely used in therapy of COPD and asthma in humans. In animals, the ease of oral dosage associated with the xanthines has made drugs such as aminophylline the most popular choice (see also Bronchodilator Therapy).

The use of bronchodilating drugs in the treatment of chronic bronchitis of dogs is predicated on the assumption that bronchoconstriction is present and is a significant component of any airway obstruction. Many dogs with chronic bronchitis do not exhibit signs of airway obstruction. It is difficult, without the benefit of pulmonary function tests (e.g., a measurement of airway resistance), to confirm the presence and reversibility of bronchoconstriction. The presence of expiratory respiratory distress, wheeze, and hyperinflation is usually assumed to indicate underlying bronchoconstriction but may in fact be caused by structural alterations in airway anatomy. The role of airway inflammation in the development of airway obstruction in dogs with chronic bronchitis and the demonstrated lack of airway hyperreactivity in dogs chronically exposed to sulfur dioxide may indicate that bronchoconstriction is not as important a component of airway obstruction as was previously assumed.

In subjects with associated bronchopneumonia and alveolar filling, the vasodilatory properties of some bronchodilators may tend to relieve pulmonary hypoxic vasoconstriction and increase blood flow through poorly ventilated lung units, thus actually exacerbating $\dot{V}A/\dot{Q}$ mismatch and worsening hypoxemia.

Until pulmonary function tests are readily available, dogs showing clinical signs of airway obstruction should at least have the benefit of a bronchodilator trial. The usefulness of this regimen will need to be judged in terms of clinical improvement.

Corticosteroids. Anti-inflammatory drugs might be expected to alleviate chronic airflow limitation caused by airway inflammation and bronchoconstriction. Since inflammation appears to play an important role in the development of airway obstruction in canine chronic bronchitis, corticosteroid therapy may be beneficial to some animals.

Patients without significant bronchopneumonia and not responding well to other measures may benefit from a 10- to 14-day corticosteroid trial. If improvement results, a longer course of the drug should be considered. Some animals may require prolonged alternate-day therapy. Inhaled corticosteroids have proved useful in the treatment of COPD in humans but are not applicable in dogs.

Weight Loss. Many dogs with chronic bronchitis are obese. The presence of abdominal fat imposes a restrictive defect on the respiratory system and thus reduces lung volume. Low lung volume predisposes animals to small airway closure. Weight loss may help to increase lung volume and improve the distribution of gas flow in the lungs. Weight loss will also tend to reduce stress on the cardiopulmonary system and promote increased exercise ability. Significant improvement has been observed in cases of chronic bronchitis with weight loss alone.

Judicious Control of Cough. Cough is an important pulmonary defense mechanism. This is particularly so in chronic bronchitis, in which effective removal of airway secretions is of great importance. Coughing should not be indiscriminately suppressed, especially in the face of bronchial infection.

Some dogs with chronic bronchitis experience paroxysmal bouts of severe nonproductive cough. This harsh, hacking cough is exhausting to the animal and distressing to the owner. Severe, protracted, recurrent coughing may promote weakness and collapse of airway walls. Complete tracheobronchial collapse during forceful expiratory efforts contributes to ineffectiveness of the cough and promotes retention of secretions.

In this situation, antitussive medications are used to break the cough cycle and allow both animal and owner to rest. Administration of such medications should be restricted to periods of cough exacerbation. Their continual use will result in further retention of bronchial mucus.

For the expressed purpose of controlling severe bouts of coughing, the narcotic cough suppressants (codeine, hydrocodone bitartrate) have the additional effect of sedation. This can be particularly useful in the management of excitable breeds of toy dogs.

SUPPORT OF GAS EXCHANGE. All the approaches described aid in supporting gas exchange by better matching ventilation to perfusion within the lung. In advanced cases and during exacerbations, hypoxemia may be so severe as to require correction by oxygen therapy.

Oxygen therapy (usually administered in an oxygen cage) is used to temporarily support a patient while other measures are employed to correct the underlying problem. In chronic bronchitis, this particularly applies to measures aimed at the control of infection and the promotion of removal of bronchial secretion.

Retention of carbon dioxide (elevated Pa_{CO_2}) is evidence of alveolar hypoventilation and suggests the onset of ventilatory failure. Human COPD patients with chronic carbon dioxide retention may hypoventilate to an even greater degree when supplemental oxygen is administered (presumably because of the removal of the hypoxic drive stimulus). Oxygen must be administered to such patients in as low a concentration as is possible, while maintaining a reasonable Pa_{O_2}.

Human COPD patients with chronic hypoxemia benefit from continuous (home) oxygen therapy. This is not practical in most veterinary situations.

COMPLICATIONS

The development of bacterial bronchopneumonia is the most common complication associated with chronic bronchitis. Other complications include bronchiectasis and cardiac disease.

Chronic inflammatory changes cause the development of irreversible dilation of airways (bronchiectasis) in some chronic bronchitis sufferers. Such animals accumulate large amounts of inspissated mucopus in the airways and are subject to repeated (if not continual) bacterial infection.

The increased incidence of cardiac valvular disease in older dogs may complicate the management of dogs with chronic bronchitis. Right heart failure as a consequence of increased pulmonary vascular resistance can develop as a direct complication of chronic bronchitis (see Cor Pulmonale).

PROGNOSIS

Chronic bronchitis is essentially incurable; it is a chronic, progressive, debilitating disease marked by periods of exacerbation. However, except during such periods, most dogs with chronic bronchitis are affected only by recurrent coughing. Many live for a number of years with their disease. The prognosis is improved when infection can be controlled and exposure to environmental respiratory irritants reduced.

References and Supplemental Reading

Chakrin, L. W., and Saunders, L. Z.: Experimental chronic bronchitis—Pathology in the dog. Lab. Invest. 30:145, 1974.

Done, S. H.: Canine tracheal collapse—Aetiology, pathology, diagnosis and treatment. Vet. Annu. 18:255, 1978.

McKiernan, B. C.: Principles of respiratory therapy. *In* Kirk, R. W. (ed.): *Current Veterinary Therapy VIII*. Philadelphia: W. B. Saunders, 1983, pp. 216–221.

McKiernan, B. C.: Therapeutic strategies involving antimicrobial treatment of the lower respiratory tract in small animals. J.A.V.M.A. 185:1155, 1984.

O'Brien, J: Chronic bronchitis in the dog. Vet. Annu. 14:125, 1973.

Pirie, H. M., and Wheeldon, E. B.: Chronic bronchitis in the dog. Adv. Vet. Sci. Comp. Med. 20:253, 1976.

Seltzer, J., Scanlon, P. D., Drazen, J. M., et al.: Morphologic correlation of physiologic changes caused by SO_2-induced bronchitis in dogs. Am. Rev. Respir. Dis. 129:790, 1984.

Suter, P. F.: Lower airway and pulmonary parenchymal diseases. *In* Suter, P. F. (ed.): *Thoracic Radiography-Thoracic Diseases of the Dog and Cat*. Wettswil, Switzerland: P. F. Suter, 1984, pp. 520–537.

Wheeldon, E. B., Pirie, H. M., Fisher, E. W., et al.: Chronic bronchitis in the dog. Vet. Rec. 94:466, 1974.

Wheeldon, E. B., Pirie, H. M., Fisher, E. W., et al.: Chronic respiratory disease in the dog. J. Small Anim. Pract. 18:229, 1977.

COR PULMONALE

PHILIP R. FOX, D.V.M.
New York, New York

Cor pulmonale is a secondary form of right heart disease and, potentially, right ventricular failure. It is precipitated by acute or chronic pressure overload due to pulmonary arterial hypertension. The use of the term *cor pulmonale* varies among clinicians and may refer to (1) increased pulmonary vascular resistance or pulmonary arterial pressure due to primary lung disease, (2) right ventricular hypertrophy secondary to long-standing pulmonary hypertension, or (3) the clinical syndrome of right-sided congestive heart failure resulting from previously mentioned abnormalities. The term *pulmonary heart disease* has been applied to describe cardiac effects due to abnormalities in pulmonary circulation. Although pulmonary hypertension invariably precedes cor pulmonale, it is not a synonym for cor pulmonale. If pulmonary hypertension is secondary to either congenital heart disease or primary disorders of the left heart, a diagnosis of cor pulmonale is automatically ruled out.

PATHOPHYSIOLOGY

There are several unique and different properties of the pulmonary circulation in comparison with the systemic circulation. The entire right ventricular cardiac output is ejected into a single pair of organs, the lungs. Resistance and, consequently, perfusion pressure in the pulmonary circuit is much lower than in the systemic circuit. Under normal conditions, the autonomic nervous system does not significantly influence pulmonary arteriolar resistance. Moreover, the pulmonary capillary bed has a vast reserve capacity. New channels may be recruited to lower the resistance to flow (in response to an increase in cardiac output) without increasing pulmonary perfusion pressure. A reduction of at least 50 per cent of the pulmonary vascular capacity is necessary to cause pulmonary hypertension. A number of disorders can contribute to this process.

Pulmonary arteriolar vasoconstriction resulting in pulmonary pressure elevation occurs consistently and normally in response to regional hypoxia. Alveolar hypoventilation and hypoxemia may result from respiratory disease. In older dogs, chronic obstructive pulmonary disease (COPD)* may be the predominant disorder associated with cor pulmonale. In addition, the contributing and complicating factor of obesity (pickwickian syndrome) is common in these animals and adversely affects mechanical respiration. Vasoactive chemicals can also cause pulmonary vasoconstriction (i.e., serotonin released from degranulated platelets in pulmonary thrombosis). Whatever the cause, alveolar hypoxia may result in local hypoxemia, hypercapnia, and acidosis, which then stimulates pulmonary vasoconstriction.

Decreased pulmonary vascular patency may occur by mechanical obstruction from thromboembolism. Clinical recognition is often difficult, but thromboembolism has been reported in dogs with hyperadrenocorticism, endocarditis, renal amyloidosis, and nephrotic syndrome. Additional associations include dogs and cats with membranous glomerulonephropathy, in experimentally induced hypothyroidism in dogs fed high-fat, high-cholesterol diets, and in feline cardiomyopathy. (Pulmonary thromboembolism is further discussed in *Current Veterinary Therapy VIII.*)

Factors associated with thrombosis include (1) chronic endothelial injury (e.g., mechanical, infectious, chemical), which promotes activation of clotting mechanisms; (2) turbulence, stasis, or disrupted pulmonary blood flow (promoting localized concentration of activated procoagulants); and (3) "hypercoagulable state" due to decreased anticoagulant or increased clot-promoting factors. Resultant decreased pulmonary blood flow and increased pulmonary vascular resistance, in concert with hypoxemia and pulmonary vasoconstriction, lead to pulmonary hypertension, right ventricular dilation and hypertrophy, and, potentially, right-sided congestive heart failure.

Heartworm infection can cause pulmonary artery disease and cor pulmonale. Simple pulmonary artery obstruction by heartworms does not cause pulmonary hypertension. The addition of intralum-

**Editor's note:* COPD is a term applied to the clinical syndrome that is produced by multiple pathologic conditions, including chronic bronchitis or bronchiolitis and emphysema. In dogs and cats, it may be clinically recognized by the presence of a chronic cough, an expiratory effort or prolongation, expiratory wheezes, and, occasionally, air trapping as detected on a thoracic radiograph.

inal pulmonary arterial lesions (intimal proliferative response to live worms and thromboembolism of dead parasites) is required for significant impedance to occur. With a heavy infection and progressive vascular disease, pulmonary vascular resistance increases and pulmonary hypertension develops. Right-sided congestive heart failure, when it occurs, usually develops gradually.

Regardless of the cause of cor pulmonale, right ventricular dilation and hypertrophy occur in response to pulmonary hypertension. Right heart failure is more likely to occur when underlying cardiac disease is already present. However, right-sided congestive heart failure is an uncommon sequela and not an integral aspect of cor pulmonale.

DIAGNOSIS

Chronic cor pulmonale may become evident in two different clinical presentations: (1) animals in which it appears late in the course of severe respiratory disease (e.g., chronic obstructive lung disease) and (2) animals in which it displays a relatively early onset with respect to the underlying disease process (e.g., pickwickian syndrome, thoracic deformities).

Since the common denominator of cor pulmonale is significant pulmonary hypertension, clinical diagnosis depends on the ease or difficulty by which pulmonary hypertension is diagnosed. Since direct measurement of pulmonary artery pressure is not routinely available in clinical practice, we must depend on its indirect recognition as inferred by historic, clinical, electrocardiographic, radiographic, and clinical pathologic features.

History. Chronic respiratory disease may be associated with chronic cor pulmonale. The signalment may be that of an old, small (miniature or toy) breed of dog or a brachycephalic breed, which may be predisposed to tracheal collapse, COPD, and atrioventricular valvular insufficiency. Often, indoor nonworking pets are part of a socioeconomic environment that predisposes to a lack of exercise, overfeeding, and obesity. Consideration of the animal's initial and current origin with attention to geographic regions with warm climates (i.e., increasing risk for heartworm infection) or regions endemic for systemic mycoses (i.e., river valleys for histoplasmosis or southwestern United States for coccidioidomycosis) can suggest epidemiologic predisposition for respiratory diseases. Working or hunting dogs in these situations may be at higher risk for chronic lung disease. In addition, pets with prior histories of smoke inhalation or bacterial pneumonia may be predisposed to long-term respiratory sequelae (e.g., chronic bronchitis, pulmonary fibrosis, bronchiectasis).

Clients may describe minimally progressive chronic coughing and wheezing of months to years in duration. These signs may worsen subacutely or may change from intermittent to continuous, being exacerbated by infection or other illness. As a result, dyspnea, weakness, and, infrequently, syncope may develop. Hemoptysis occurs frequently in dogs with advanced pulmonary vascular disease. Weight loss may accompany chronic congestive heart failure or may be a sign of an underlying systemic disease.

In cats with chronic heartworm infection, vomiting or respiratory signs (coughing or dyspnea) may be reported, although most cats are asymptomatic.

Physical Examination. With severe chronic cor pulmonale, tachypnea, weakness, exercise intolerance, exertional dyspnea, coughing, and wheezing with excitement or exertion may be observed. Orthopnea (positional dyspnea: open-mouth breathing, abducted forelegs, and reluctance to sit or lie down) and cyanotic mucous membranes may accompany advanced disease. Thoracic auscultation may reveal abnormal lung sounds consistent with the specific underlying respiratory disorder. These sounds may include crackles (discontinuous or intermittent sounds heard mostly during inspiration), rhonchi, and wheezes (continuous, often musical whistling sounds heard mostly during expiration), pleural friction rubs, silent areas, or increased bronchovesicular sounds. Tachycardia or gallop rhythm may accompany congestive heart failure. Systolic murmurs of mitral or tricuspid insufficiency may be auscultated if endocardiosis (chronic valvular-myocardial heart disease) is present. A murmur of tricuspid insufficiency and, rarely, pulmonic insufficiency from valve orifice dilation due to compensatory right heart dilation may be heard. If severe cardiac rotation is present, the murmur of tricuspid insufficiency may be prominent at the left sternal border. Accentuation or, less commonly, splitting of the second heart sound may be evident. Evaluation of the jugular pulse may show giant "a" waves (right atrium contracting against increased resistance to right ventricular filling) and prominent "v" waves (if tricuspid insufficiency is present). If overt right-sided congestive heart failure is present, then there may be jugular venous enlargement, hepatosplenomegaly, and pleural, pericardial, or abdominal effusion.

Radiography. Dogs with chronic cor pulmonale associated with respiratory disease may display radiographic changes compatible with those underlying diseases (e.g., collapsed trachea, pulmonary fibrosis, atelectasis, chronic airway disease). Cardiac changes are the most consistent radiographic sign of chronic cor pulmonale and include enlargement of the right ventricle (RV), right atrium (RA), and pulmonary artery (PA) segment. If right-sided congestive heart failure is present, then extracardiac signs include dilation of the caudal vena cava, hepatosplenomegaly, and pleural, pericardial, or abdominal effusion. Dogs affected with heartworm disease may have additional pulmonary vascular changes more specific and sensitive than RV and PA enlargement (the inverted D-shaped heart is a late and inconsistent feature of heartworm disease). Changes in right caudal pulmonary arteries may represent the earliest radiographic abnormalities of canine heartworm disease and are best evaluated in the dorsoventral view. Enlarged, tortuous, pruned pulmonary arteries may be evident. Parenchymal lung disease is suggested by focal, poorly defined areas of consolidation (if pulmonary infarction is present) or greater than normal radiolucency in peripheral lung lobes (if thromboembolism occurs without pulmonary infarction).

In feline heartworm disease, the most distinctive radiographic sign is enlarged PAs with ill-defined margins that are most prominent in the caudal lung lobes on the ventrodorsal view. Blunting and tortuosity of the PAs, an enlarged main PA segment, and RV enlargement are not classic features of feline dirofilariasis.

With pulmonary thromboembolism, there may be no radiographic pulmonary parenchymal changes. Increased radiolucency in obstructed lobes due to decreased vascular filling and hyperperfused areas can occur, although these changes are often obscure.

Pulmonary angiography offers a means of definitive diagnosis of suspected thromboembolism. It may be performed nonselectively, which is relatively safe, easy, and inexpensive. Selective pulmonary arteriography is more definitive but less suitable for clinical settings. Angiography will display intraluminal filling defects (e.g., clear "blocks" or "cutoffs" in pulmonary arterial opacification).

Nuclear medicine imaging techniques (perfusion and ventilation lung scanning) are useful but restricted in availability (see page 11). They may assume greater utility in the future.

ELECTROCARDIOGRAPHY. Electrocardiographic changes are inconsistent and variable in cor pulmonale. Sensitivity and specificity of electrocardiography for right-axis deviation (greater than 105 degrees in the frontal plane) is low. P pulmonale (increased P-wave amplitude) may occur with chronic cor pulmonale in the dog. Rightward deviation of the mean electric axis (S waves in leads I, II, III, aVF) can occur, and secondary depolarization changes involving the S-T segment and T wave may be observed. With canine heartworm disease, the electrocardiogram is usually unremarkable. Right ventricular enlargement patterns may be seen with advanced, severe heartworm disease, often accompanied by right-sided heart failure. In feline dirofilariasis, a right-axis deviation of more than 120 degrees in the frontal plan is rare.

ECHOCARDIOGRAPHY. Chronic heartworm infection and cor pulmonale may display RV dilation, well-visualized wide excursions of the tricuspid valve, and paradoxical septal motion. Specific assessment of RV free-wall measurements may be difficult. The sensitivity and specificity of echocardiographic evaluation of cor pulmonale requires further clarification.

CLINICAL PATHOLOGY. Biochemical and hematologic measurements may be unremarkable or may reflect underlying systemic disease processes associated with cor pulmonale. Dogs with heartworm disease may have mild normochromic, normocytic anemias (PCV less than 40), progressing to a more severe macrocytic anemia if liver failure develops. Monocytosis, basophilia, and, especially, eosinophilia may be present. Demonstration of microfilaremia is more commonly definitive. In cats, concentration techniques are recommended but are rarely positive. When microfilaremia cannot be demonstrated in clinically suspicious animals, occult dirofilariasis can be tested for by immunodiagnostic, serodiagnostic, or enzyme-linked immunosorbent assay (ELISA) techniques.

If pulmonary thromboembolism is present, elevated serum fibrinolytic split products, prolonged prothrombin time, and partial thromboplastin time may also be present. Evaluation of blood gas, if available, may display hypoxemia (Pa_{O_2} less than 80 mmHg), acidosis (pH less than 7.4), and hypercapnia (Pa_{CO_2} greater than 40 mmHg).

Acute cor pulmonale is often associated with pulmonary thromboembolism. Historic and physical examination findings are not consistent or accurate enough to suggest pathognomonic diagnostic criteria. Severe, intractable dyspnea (often inappropriate for the degree of radiographic involvement) that is unresponsive to therapy may be the most consistent clinical sign. Other signs such as cyanosis, weakness, syncope, or accentuated or split second heart sounds may sometimes be recorded. Coughing and hemoptysis are rarely evident. Sudden death may occur.

Thoracic radiography may be unremarkable or may display increased radiolucency with normal to reduced lung volume (as a result of hypoperfusion of obstructed lung lobes) and hyperlucency of unobstructed, hyperperfused areas. Abnormalities associated with specific underlying associated disease processes may cause changes in clinical pathologic conditions or in the results of special diagnostic techniques (e.g., echocardiography, angiography, bronchoscopy, aspiration cytology).

PRINCIPLES OF MANAGEMENT

General Measures

Since cor pulmonale is a result of pulmonary hypertension, therapeutic strategies should strive to decrease right ventricular work load by decreasing PA hypertension. This generally requires relieving arterial hypoxemia. Ultimately, clinical improvement depends on success in alleviating respiratory failure.

Therapeutic approaches must be individualized with respect to the cause and severity of the underlying pulmonary disorder. Cor pulmonale with underlying pulmonary disease processes that are reversible are often responsive to therapy. Respiratory tract infections may aggravate $\dot{V}/\dot{Q}$ imbalance in bronchitis, for example, but may be reversed with appropriate therapy. Even diseases causing anatomic pulmonary arterial occlusion may have a reversible component contributing to pulmonary hypertension.

Improvement in respiratory gas exchange is central to management of cor pulmonale, since hypoxemia and respiratory acidosis are important causes of pulmonary vasospasm in many cases. In pets affected with pulmonary thromboembolism and heartworm disease, additional symptomatic and specific therapy may be initiated.

Treatment of Acute Cor Pulmonale

OXYGEN. Relief of acute hypoxemia and hypercapnia is important. Improvement of respiratory gas exchange with supplemental oxygen helps to reverse hypoxemia and respiratory acidosis. Oxygen therapy cages (which should also control temperature and humidity) are available commercially and can deliver an oxygen-enriched mixture of 35 to 50 per cent. This low concentration of oxygen delivery is important to avoid blunting the respiratory drive. Face masks provide a less ideal method of oxygen delivery since they involve some restraint and are less well tolerated. Administration should be monitored by observing ventilation and, if available, arterial blood gas analyses.

BRONCHODILATORS. These agents have value by improving reversible airway obstruction, thereby improving pulmonary gas exchange. Theophylline compounds (which also slightly augment ventricular function) are most commonly employed. Theophylline is potentially arrhythmogenic in a severely hypoxic myocardium.

ANTIBIOTICS. Antibiotics should be considered if a bacterial infectious component is thought to have contributed to decompensation of the underlying respiratory disorder. Chloramphenicol or a cephalosporin is frequently chosen in such cases. More specific agents may be employed as directed by cytologis examination or culture and sensitivity of specimens from the lower respiratory tract.

CORTICOSTEROIDS. Indiscriminate use of these drugs is not justified. Their value must be determined by their likely effect on the underlying abnormalities in ventilatory function. Studies in humans have suggested that pulmonary function improves more rapidly in COPD patients with bronchitis who do not have pneumonia.

It has been demonstrated that prednisolone increases the percentage of surviving female heartworms after thiacetarsamide therapy, thereby decreasing efficacy of this adulticidal drug. Therefore, prednisolone should be reserved in heartworm disease for dogs with extensive pretreatment lung disease or who develop lung disease after adulticidal therapy with thiacetarsamide.

CARDIAC DRUGS. If right ventricular heart failure occurs, certain measures should be initiated. These include the following:

(1) Strict cage rest. Rest intervals of at least 2 weeks before and 4 weeks after adulticide therapy are recommended for heartworm-infected dogs in right-sided heart failure.

(2) Furosemide and sodium-restricted diets are recommended with cage rest for animals in states of decompensated heart failure.

(3) Digitalization is controversial. It is used primarily for its inotropic effects on the failing right ventricle, and the dose should be modified to account for azotemia, hypoxemia, acidosis, or electrolyte imbalances, which could predispose to digitalis-induced arrhythmias.

VASODILATOR THERAPY. Use of vasodilators to reduce pulmonary arterial hypertension and right ventricular afterload by lowering pulmonary vascular resistance has currently provided unpredictable and poorly monitored responses. Many factors may contribute to lack of success, such as the presence of fixed vascular obstructive disease instead of active vasoconstriction, profound disease progression, or adverse nonpulmonary vascular side effects (e.g., systemic hypotension). They should be used very cautiously, if at all, at present.

SODIUM THIACETARSAMIDE. When cor pulmonale results from heartworm infection, adulticide therapy may alleviate the problem. Dogs with decompensated right-sided heart failure should be given strict cage rest for 2 weeks prior to adulticide therapy. Furosemide and dietary sodium restriction should be initiated and digitalization contemplated. Complications of thiacetarsamide may be associated with pulmonary thromboembolism commencing 7 to 10 days after adulticide treatment. This may cause a sharp rise in pulmonary arterial pressure and can produce clinical signs of right-sided heart failure. Appropriate supportive therapy may be necessary.

ASPIRIN. In thiacetarsamide-treated heartworm-infected dogs, low-dose aspirin therapy (10 mg/kg daily) has been shown to improve pulmonary arterial blood flow and reduce pulmonary parenchymal and vascular wall injury. This may be mediated by aspirin's effect of decreasing platelet adhesion to damaged vascular surfaces and eventually reducing myointimal proliferation. Its use has also been recommended (1¼ grain every second or third day) for spontaneous thromboembolism associated with feline cardiomyopathy. Unfortunately, aspirin can cause vasoconstriction and increased pulmonary vascular resistance in some animals.

ANTITHROMBOTIC THERAPY. When pulmonary thromboembolism is diagnosed, anticoagulation therapy may be indicated. Heparin is the drug of choice and is initially administered intravenously and titrated to increase activated clotting time (ACT) 2 to 3 times normal and activated partial thromboplastin time (APTT) 1½ to 2½ times normal. Antiplatelet drugs (e.g., aspirin) or various heparin dosage regimens can be utilized for longer periods, depending on the status of the problem.

Treatment of Chronic Cor Pulmonale

The primary goal in managing chronic cor pulmonale is to achieve therapeutic reversal of acute, precipitating factors. This may restore for a time RV function and PA pressures until new causes of decompensation occur or until inexorable pulmonary disease develops. Early recognition and treatment of respiratory infections is more rational than long-term prophylactic use of antibiotics. Weight loss should be promoted for obese animals. Dietary sodium restriction and perhaps diuretics may be indicated for chronic right heart congestive failure.

PROGNOSIS

For animals with cor pulmonale, prognosis is linked to that of the underlying pulmonary disorder. If existing mechanisms of circulating disorders are controlled, these diseases may potentially be reversible. When cor pulmonale is secondary to the gradual obliteration of pulmonary arteries by intrinsic disease or interstitial fibrosis, the prognosis is poor. If right-sided congestive heart failure develops, the prognosis is guarded. Alternatively, when reversible disease is causative or contributory (e.g., bronchitis) and the proper therapy instituted, the prognosis is favorable.

References and Supplemental Reading

Albert, R. K., Martin, T. R., and Lewis, S. W.: Controlled clinical trial of methyl-prednisolone in patients with chronic bronchitis and acute respiratory insufficiency. Ann. Intern. Med. 92:753, 1980.

Burns, M. G.: Pulmonary thromboembolism. *In* Kirk, R. W. (ed.): *Current Veterinary Therapy VIII*. Philadelphia: W. B. Saunders, 1983, pp. 257–265.

Burns, M. G., Kelly, A. B., Hornof, W. J., et al.: Pulmonary artery thrombosis in three dogs with hyperadrenocorticism. J.A.V.M.A. 178:388, 1981.

Dillon, R.: Feline dirofilariasis. *Vet. Clin. North Am.* 14:1185, 1984.

Fishman, A. P.: Cor pulmonale—general aspects. *In* Fishman, A. P. (ed.): *Pulmonary Diseases and Disorders*. New York: McGraw-Hill, 1980, p. 853.

Keith, J. C., Jr., Rawlings, C. A., and Schaub, R. G.: Pulmonary thromboembolism during therapy of dirofilariasis with thiacetarsamide: Modification with aspirin or prednisolone. Am. J. Vet. Res. 44:1278, 1983.

Knight, D. H.: Heartworm disease. *In* Ettinger, S. J. (ed.): *Textbook of Veterinary Internal Medicine*, 2nd ed. Philadelphia: W. B. Saunders, 1983, pp. 1097–1124.

Lombard, C. W., and Buergelt, C. D.: Echocardiographic and clinical findings in dogs with heartworm-induced cor-pulmonale. Comp. Cont. Ed. Pract. Vet. 5:971, 1983.

Matthay, R. A., and Matthay, M. A.: Pulmonary thromboembolism and other pulmonary vascular diseases. *In* George, R. B., Light, R. W., and Matthay, R. A. (eds.): *Chest Medicine*. New York: Churchill Livingstone, 1983, p. 323.

Rawlings, C. A.: Acute response of pulmonary blood flow and right ventricular function to *Dirofilaria immitis* adults and microfilaria. Am. J. Vet. Res. 41:244, 1980.

Rawlings, C. A., Keith, J. C., Losonsky, J. M., et al: An aspirin-prednisolone combination to modify postadulticide lung disease in heartworm-infected dogs. Am. J. Vet. Res. 45:2371, 1984.

Schaub, R. G., Keith, J. C., Jr., Rawlings, C. A.: Effect of acetylsalicylic acid on vascular damage and myointimal proliferation in canine pulmonary arteries subjected to chronic injury by *Dirofilaria immitis*. Am. J. Vet. Res. 44:449, 1983.

Spaulding, G., and Owens, J.: Cor pulmonale. *In Manual of Small Animal Cardiology*. New York: Churchill Livingstone, 1984, p. 167.

Welch, M. H.: Obstructive Diseases. *In* Guenter, C. A., and Welch, M. H. (eds.): *Pulmonary Medicine*, 2nd ed. Philadelphia: J. B. Lippincott, 1982, p. 664.

Section 4

CARDIOVASCULAR DISEASES

JOHN D. BONAGURA, D.V.M.
Consulting Editor

***Additional Pertinent Information Found in* Current Veterinary Therapy VIII:**

Bonagura, J. D.: Therapy of Cardiac Arrhythmias, p. 360.
Harpster, N. K.: Boxer Cardiomyopathy, p. 329.
Haskins, S. C.: Cardiopulmonary Resuscitation, p. 377.
Helphrey, M. L., and Schollmeyer, M.: Pacemaker Therapy, p. 373.
Keene, B. W., and Bonagura, J. D.: Valvular Heart Disease, p. 311.
Kittleson, M.: Concepts and Therapeutic Strategies in the Management of Heart Failure, p. 279.
Thomas, W. P.: Congenital Heart Disease, p. 301.

***Additional Pertinent Information Found in* Current Veterinary Therapy VII:**

Feldman, E. C.: Influence of Non-cardiac Disease on the Heart, p. 340.
Horn, B. R., and Ansfield, A. H.: Cardiopulmonary Resuscitation for People, p. 293.
Staaden, R.: Cardiovascular System of the Racing Dog, p. 347.
Suter, P. F.: Diseases of Peripheral Lymphatics: Lymphedema, p. 337.

TREATMENT OF HEART DISEASE: AN OVERVIEW

JOHN D. BONAGURA, D.V.M.,
and ROBERT L. HAMLIN, D.V.M.
Columbus, Ohio

The type and cause of heart disease must be identified before appropriate treatment can be administered. The following chapters detail therapy for specific cardiovascular disorders in small animals. Each contributor has included pertinent aspects of pathophysiology and diagnosis, since these are the basis of therapy. The purpose of this article is to provide an overview of heart disease, to summarize principles of diagnosis, and to offer a general perspective of therapy. The reader may find the tables useful when managing patients with heart disease.

GENERAL CAUSES AND TYPES OF HEART DISEASE

The numerous and diverse causes of heart disease can be recalled using the mnemonic DAMN IT (Table 1). A list of potential anatomic lesions of the cardiovascular system is less extensive, owing to the limited responses afforded the heart, pericardium, and blood vessels (Table 2). Specific locations for these cardiovascular lesions are the pericardium, myocardium, cardiac valves and endocardium, specialized impulse-forming and conduction system, and blood vessels. Anatomic lesions are manifested functionally in the patient as low cardiac output, weakness, tiring, congestive heart failure, hypoxia, arrhythmia, limb ischemia, or secondary organ dysfunction of the lungs, kidneys, or brain.

Examples abound. Obstructive cardiac lesions such as congenital subaortic and pulmonic stenosis cause exertional syncope, arrhythmias, and sudden death. Cyanotic heart disease (e.g., tetralogy of Fallot) leads to incapacitating hypoxia and polycythemia. Volume overloading, as with patent ductus arteriosus or mitral regurgitation, and cardiac muscle failure caused by dilated cardiomyopathy are likely to cause congestive heart failure with pulmonary edema. Cardiac arrhythmias, such as atrial fibrillation or ventricular tachycardia, cause syncope or precipitate heart failure in pets with cardiomyopathy or valvular heart disease. These functional disturbances and their causes can be grouped on the basis of the pathophysiologic cause of heart failure (Table 3). There are important therapeutic implications in such a classification (Table 4).

DIAGNOSIS OF HEART DISEASE

The diagnosis of heart disease is often simple, yet the clinical significance of a murmur or cardiac abnormality can be perplexing to the clinician. Noncardiac conditions can mimic heart disease. The problems of cough, tiring, dyspnea, auscultable respiratory crackling, and right-sided heart enlargement (cor pulmonale) are as common to bronchopulmonary disease as they are to heart failure. Pleural effusion in cats has many potential causes, including cardiomyopathy, lymphosarcoma, trauma, and infection. Accordingly, the veterinarian needs a suitable data base to identify, diagnose, and assess heart disease in a patient. Table 5 lists some of these important diagnostic evaluations.

There are common pitfalls of diagnosis. One is not obtaining an adequate data base owing to economic considerations or to hasty conclusions. Another is excessive dependence on a single diagnostic test. Electrocardiography, for example, is mandatory for evaluation of cardiac rhythm, but it is inappropriate for assessment of myocardial function or quantitation of heart failure. There are also species differences with which to contend. When pleural effusion is caused by congestive heart failure (CHF) in dogs, the effusion usually occurs with ascites; however, pleural effusion is often encountered without significant ascites in cats with cardiomyopathy. Such simple diagnostic clues as elevated jugular venous pressure or enlarged pulmonary veins (on x-ray films) are often overlooked, even though these findings may signify CHF. Difficulties can arise in separating heart disease causing CHF with secondary pulmonary dysfunction from primary respiratory disorders. This problem is encountered by practicing veterinarians and cardiologists alike. Certain diagnostic dilemmas can be resolved by reviewing lists of differential considerations and by completing a thorough and systematic evaluation (Table 5). When therapy (e.g., diuretics) fails to provide anticipated relief from heart disease, the diagnosis (and patient) should be reconsidered.

Table 1. *Causes of Cardiovascular Disease*

Principal Causes	Examples
Degeneration	Endocardiosis (mitral valve insufficiency)
Disease of other organs	Kidneys (hypertension) Lungs (hypoxia, cor pulmonale) Thyroid (cardiomyopathy) Brain (arrhythmias)
Dysautonomia	Abnormal sympathetic or parasympathetic tone, arrhythmia, gastric dilation Brain-heart syndrome
Anomalies	Patent ductus arteriosus Atrioventricular septal defects Subaortic stenosis Pulmonic stenosis Mitral and tricuspid valve dysplasia Tetralogy of Fallot Endocardial fibroelastosis Vascular anomalies
Anemia	Chronic blood loss (hookworms)
Metabolic disease	Thyrotoxicosis (cardiomyopathy) Hypothyroidism (atherosclerosis) Pancreatitis (cardiac arrhythmias) Electrolyte disorders (arrhythmias)
Nutritional deficiencies	Vitamin E and selenium
Neoplasia	Heart base tumors (aortic body tumor, ectopic thyroid carcinoma) Hemangiosarcoma Lymphosarcoma Pericardial mesothelioma
Inflammation	
Infective	Infective pericarditis Bacterial endocarditis Suppurative myocarditis Dirofilariasis
Noninfective	Feline cardiomyopathy Boxer dog myocarditis
Immune-mediated	?
Idiopathic heart disease	Cardiomyopathy Nonsuppurative myocarditis Sanguineous pericarditis
Ischemia	Coronary occlusion, shock, arteriosclerosis
Iatrogenic injury	Drugs (digitalis, anesthetics) Overinfusion of fluids Surgery
Trauma	Traumatic myocarditis Rupture of the heart or blood vessels Arteriovenous fistula
Toxins	Drugs, anesthetics, doxorubicin, sodium iodide

Table 2. *Anatomic Cardiovascular Lesions*

Region of Injury	Examples
Pericardium	Pericardial effusion: Idiopathic hemorrhage or pericarditis Bacterial/granulomatous pericarditis Cardiac/heart base tumors Hemorrhage: ruptured atrium Constrictive pericarditis Intrapericardial mass
Myocardium	Cardiomyopathy: dilated, restrictive, hypertrophic Excessive moderator bands Myocarditis (e.g., parvovirus) Myocardial degeneration, fibrosis, infarction, hemorrhage, and neoplasia
Endocardium and valves	Endocardiosis (degenerative) Endocarditis (bacterial) Ruptured chordae tendineae
Impulse-forming and conduction system	Degeneration, hemorrhage, infarction, or inflammation leading to arrhythmias and conduction disturbances
Blood vessels	Arteriosclerosis Atherosclerosis Thrombosis (e.g., feline cardiomyopathy, endocarditis) Pulmonary embolism Dirofilariasis (arteritis) Vasculitis Arteriovenous fistula Phlebitis Rupture
Cardiac and vascular anomalies	Many (see Table 1)

THERAPY OF HEART FAILURE

The principal goals of therapy for heart failure are to (1) normalize the cardiac rhythm, (2) adjust the fluid compartments and venous pressures to maintain blood flow but prevent congestion, (3) improve tissue circulation, and (4) maintain tissue oxygenation. These objectives can only be attained by an understanding of the hemodynamic failings of heart disease and by an appreciation of how drug therapy modifies cardiac, circulatory, pulmonary, renal, and hormonal activities. When an asymptomatic patient has compensated well for heart disease, therapy is unnecessary—unless the underlying condition can be cured (i.e., heartworm disease or a potentially serious arrhythmia). However, if animals with heart disease develop such clinical signs of heart failure as low cardiac output (weakness) or congestion (pulmonary edema, pleural effusion, ascites), therapy is required. Heart failure evokes a number of neurohumoral and cardiorenal responses; these are double-edged swords that both support the blood pressure and vital circulations and lead

Table 3. *Heart Failure—A Pathophysiologic Classification*

Myocardial failure (muscle failure)
- Dilated cardiomyopathy
- Myocardial ischemia/infarction
- Necrotizing myocarditis (parvovirus)
- Drug toxicity (anesthetics, doxorubicin)
- Chronic volume or pressure overload
- Hypoxia

Hemodynamic overload
- Volume overload
  - Congenital heart disease (patent ductus arteriosus, atrioventricular septal defects)
  - Valvular insufficiency
- Pressure overload
  - Subaortic stenosis
  - Systemic hypertension
  - Pulmonic stenosis
  - Tetralogy of Fallot (+ shunt)
  - Heartworm disease
  - Cor pulmonale
- High-output states
  - Chronic anemia
  - Thyrotoxicosis
  - Arteriovenous fistula

Compliance failure
- Pericardial tamponade/constrictive pericarditis
- Hypertrophic cardiomyopathy
- Restrictive cardiomyopathy

Arrhythmia

to clinical signs. These mechanisms—and treatments to counteract them—are described below.

Activation of the sympathetic nervous system, formation of angiotensin II, and release of vasopressin result in elevated systemic vascular resistance; increased left ventricular afterload; redistribution of blood flow away from the skin, kidneys, muscles, and gut; and augmentation of myocardial contractility and heart rate. The tachycardia of sympathetic stimulation taxes the heart and can be blunted with β-adrenoceptor blockers such as propranolol, nadolol, atenolol, and pindolol (see Beta-Blocking Therapy in Dogs and Cats); however, these agents can further reduce myocardial contractility. The peripheral vasoconstriction of heart failure supports blood pressure but is also believed to diminish left ventricular stroke volume. This has prompted the use of drugs that directly dilate arterioles (see discussion of hydralazine in Vasodilator Therapy), that block vascular sympathetic α-receptors (e.g., prazosin, also in Vasodilator Therapy), or that inhibit the renin-angiotensin system (see Captopril Therapy in Dogs with Heart Failure).

Heart failure is also characterized by renal retention of sodium and water, sympathetic-induced venoconstriction, elevated venous and ventricular filling pressures, and congestion. Intrinsic alterations in renal blood flow and the hormones vasopressin (antidiuretic hormone) and aldosterone act in concert to cause sodium and water retention by the kidneys. It has long been recognized that such diuretics as furosemide (Lasix, Hoechst) and hydrochlorothiazide improve CHF by preventing this sodium retention. Novel agents such as the angiotensin-converting enzyme inhibitors captopril and

Table 4. *Treatment of Heart Failure: Principles of Therapy*

Cause of Heart Failure	Methods
Myocardial failure	Remove offending agent (e.g., drug) Positive inotropic drugs (digitalis, dopamine, dobutamine, amrinone, milrinone) Diuretics and sodium-restricted diet Exercise restriction Vasodilators, captopril
Hemodynamic overload*	
Congenital shunts	
Patent ductus arteriosus	Rest, furosemide, surgery
Ventricular septal defect	Pulmonary artery band, surgery, CMT†
Atrial septal defect	Surgery, CMT
Mitral regurgitation	Diuretics and sodium restricted diet, rest Vasodilators, captopril, with or without digitalis (see text)
Tricuspid regurgitation	CMT
Aortic regurgitation	Treat endocarditis if present Diuretics, sodium restricted diet, rest Vasodilators or captopril with caution
Pressure overloads*	
Pulmonic stenosis	Surgery, CMT if CHF‡
Subaortic stenosis	(?) Surgery, β-blockers Subacute bacterial endocarditis prophylaxis
Tetralogy of Fallot	Palliative shunt, phlebotomy, β-blocker, surgery
Heartworm disease	Chemotherapy (sodium thiacetarsemide), aspirin, corticosteroids, CMT if CHF, oxygen
Compliance failure	
Pericardial disease	Pericardiocentesis, surgery, antibiotics, glucocorticoids, furosemide and venodilators if CHF is present
Hypertrophic and restrictive cardiomyopathy	Diuretics, β-blockers, aspirin, captopril

*Whenever possible, specific therapy (e.g., surgery) is the treatment of choice.

†CMT = Conventional medical therapy, which consists of digitalis, furosemide, sodium-restricted diet, rest, and antiarrhythmic drugs if indicated.

‡CHF = Congestive heart failure.

Table 5. Diagnostic Tests

History	Signs of disease, current and past medications, response to therapy, signs of drug toxicosis
Physical examination	Heart rate and rhythm, mucous membranes, arterial pulse, jugular venous pressure, precordial impulse, auscultation (heart, lungs, and thorax), palpation (ascites, hepatomegaly, edema), examination for obstructive airway disease
Electrocardiogram	Heart rate, cardiac rhythm, beneficial or toxic response to drug therapy, cardiac chamber enlargement patterns, evidence of pericardial effusion or myocardial ischemia
Thoracic x-ray films	Heart size and specific chamber enlargement, abnormalities of aorta or main pulmonary artery, vena caval distension (right-sided CHF), pulmonary vascular dynamics (left-sided CHF, pulmonary hypertension, heartworm disease, overcirculation or undercirculation), pulmonary density changes (edema vs. pulmonary parenchymal disease), tracheobronchial abnormalities (collapse, compression, bronchitis), pleural effusion, mediastinal mass Nonselective angiocardiography
Hematologic and laboratory tests	Heartworm tests, complete blood count, biochemical profile (renal function, electrolytes), serum thyroxine, analysis of pleural and peritoneal effusions, blood culture
Tests for respiratory disease	Inspiratory/expiratory lateral x-ray films, transtracheal aspiration cytology and culture, fine-needle lung aspirate, thoracocentesis, laryngoscopy, and bronchoscopy
Special tests (by referral)	Echocardiography, cardiac catheterization and angiocardiography, second opinion

enalapril, and diuretic-aldosterone antagonists with spironolactone (Aldactazide, Searle) may prevent further sodium retention in severe CHF. The congested state can also be improved by drugs that venodilate to lower pulmonary venous pressures. For this reason, nitroglycerine ointment (see Vasodilator Therapy) has gained popularity in the treatment of fulminant left-sided CHF.

Cardiac *muscle* dysfunction is difficult to measure in clinical practice. The radiographic finding of cardiomegaly cannot always be equated with decreased muscle contractility. Volume overloads imposed by congenital cardiac shunts or by atrioventricular valve incompetence may cause dramatic cardiomegaly, yet ventricular muscle function may be preserved. A similar point can be made for CHF associated with reduced ventricular compliance—again, myocardial contractility is normal. But the situation is very different with dilated cardiomyopathy or with severe and chronic hemodynamic overload, in which myocardial contractility is subnormal and the administration of inotropic drugs such as digitalis, dobutamine, dopamine, amrinone, or milrinone generally is indicated (see Positive Inotropic Drugs in Heart Failure). Insofar as the failing ventricle is concerned, therapeutic support can be provided by giving drugs that either increase the inherent contractile force (such as inotropic drugs) or that reduce the ventricular afterload (such as arterial vasodilators). The judicious use of diuretics is also required to reduce venous congestion but maintain optimal ventricular filling.

The dog with dilated cardiomyopathy, atrial fibrillation, and frequent premature ventricular complexes is a prime example of the important relationship between cardiac output and cardiac rate and rhythm. Regular and coordinated ventricular contractions promote adequate cardiac filling and optimal ventricular ejection. Dogs with underlying valvular or myocardial disease tolerate arrhythmias poorly. Supraventricular tachyarrhythmias (e.g., atrial fibrillation and flutter) result in a loss of atrioventricular synchronization and shortened ventricular filling time. Slowing the ventricular rate with digitalis and beta-blockers is central to the management of CHF in such animals (see Beta-Blocking Therapy in Dogs and Cats). Ventricular ectopia not only lowers stroke volume, but it may be hemodynamically and electrically destabilizing and can cause syncope or sudden death. Antiarrhythmic drug therapy (see accompanying article in this section) is therefore an important adjunct in the treatment of heart failure.

SPECIFIC CAUSES OF HEART FAILURE

Dilated cardiomyopathy (see Canine Myocardial Diseases) is the prototype of *myocardial failure* in veterinary medicine (Table 2). Necrotizing myocarditis initiated by canine parvovirus and doxorubicin-induced cardiomyopathy are other examples of muscle failure. Treatment of this group focuses on conventional methods: digitalis and furosemide administration, sodium restriction, and rest. The advent of new inotropic drugs such as dobutamine-dopamine and amrinone-milrinone offers the clinician a chance to treat these conditions more aggressively. Severe or refractory cases are often treated with vasodilators, captopril, or antiarrhythmic drugs including propranolol and procainamide. All of these methods of treatment are discussed in other articles in this section.

Hemodynamic overloads (Table 4) essentially pose "plumbing" problems to the heart. The ideal solution to such problems as heartworm disease, congenital malformations, and valvular heart disease is specific curative chemotherapy or surgery. In reality, only a few of these disorders—heartworm disease and patent ductus arteriosus are two examples—can be definitively managed. When heart failure supervenes, the clinician is forced to manage the hemodynamic consequences of the lesion.

What therapy should be given for hemodynamic overloads (Table 4)? The issue of inotropic support in these cases is unresolved. Muscle dysfunction is generally a late finding in valvular heart disease; thus, many clinicians withhold digitalis unless there is an atrial arrhythmia, biventricular heart failure, or refractory CHF. Diuretics and sodium restriction are mainstays of treatment for these problems. Afterload reducers such as hydralazine or prazosin may be advantageous by reducing the degree of mitral valve regurgitation or the volume of shunt flow through a congenital left-to-right shunt. Captopril provides relief for some dogs with refractory edema or ascites. Special therapy is applicable to congenital heart diseases (Table 4), bacterial endocarditis, and dirofilariasis (see articles in this section).

Ventricular *diastolic dysfunction* results in inadequate cardiac filling. Disorders such as pericardial disease and hypertrophic cardiomyopathy therefore pose different therapeutic concerns. Pericardiocentesis is the treatment of choice for initial stabilization of pets with cardiac tamponade (Table 4). Subsequent therapy is individualized for the situation (see Pericardial Disease). Inotropes have no known role here, but low doses of furosemide combined with vasodilators such as nitroglycerin ointment can quickly reduce the degree of congestion. Both sinus tachycardia and atrial arrhythmias result in elevations of pulmonary venous pressure in cats with hypertrophic cardiomyopathy (see Feline Myocardial Diseases). Since propranolol and other β-blockers slow the heart rate, they have been advocated for long-term treatment of cats with this condition. Propranolol also causes bronchoconstriction and vasoconstriction, so it should be withheld when there is severe pulmonary edema or pleural effusion or when there is aortic thrombosis.

Heart failure is frequently amenable to medical therapy, and many pets are returned to a comfortable state. Clients may be eager to understand more about the disorder that affects their companion animal, and they frequently cooperate by providing exemplary home care. In order to provide excellent medical care and client education, veterinarians should be familiar with the causes and clinical syndromes of heart failure in companion animals. Furthermore, clinicians should understand the clinical pharmacology and toxicity of the myriad drugs available for treatment of heart failure. The upcoming chapters are designed to assist clinicians in their efforts.

POSITIVE INOTROPIC DRUGS IN HEART FAILURE

MARK D. KITTLESON, D.V.M.,
Davis, California

and GRANT G. KNOWLEN, D.V.M.
Pullman, Washington

Heart failure is the end result of many types of cardiovascular disease. Clinically, it presents as pulmonary or systemic venous congestion or both, with or without edema or poor perfusion. A depression in cardiac contractility is a common underlying cause of heart failure. However, not all cases of heart failure have significant myocardial failure (i.e., a depression in myocardial contractility). As examples, many dogs with mitral regurgitation appear not to have a clinically significant depression of cardiac contractility, especially in the early stages of heart failure. Cardiac contractility is usually not decreased in hypertrophic cardiomyopathy, a common cardiac disease causing heart failure in cats. Other diseases in dogs and cats are always accompanied by a depression in cardiac contractility when heart failure is present, such as in congestive (dilated) cardiomyopathy.

A positive inotropic drug by definition increases cardiac contractility. If one is committed to treating cardiac diseases on a logical rather than empirical basis, positive inotropic drugs should only be administered to patients that have clinically significant myocardial failure and not to all patients with heart failure. Evaluation of cardiac function is usually not possible in a veterinary practice; however, the more common causes of heart failure in veterinary medicine present in a relatively uniform fashion. Therefore, as long as a diagnosis of the underlying disease can be established, a logical therapeutic plan can be formulated. Differentiating between underlying diseases is crucial in some situations. The classic example is distinguishing hypertrophic from congestive cardiomyopathy in cats. In hypertrophic cardiomyopathy, positive inotropic agents are contraindicated, but in congestive cardiomyopathy they are the primary mode of therapy.

Positive inotropic agents are not always effective in patients with myocardial failure. Usually a drug has been identified as a positive inotropic agent by testing it in a normal animal. Clinicians must realize that the ability of a drug to increase contractility in a normal animal does not necessarily equate with an ability to increase contractility in an animal with myocardial failure. Diseased cells may or may not respond to the influence of a positive inotropic drug, depending on the method by which the drug increases contractility, the potency of the drug, the type of defect resulting in a loss of contractility, the severity of the defect present in the cell, and the number of cells involved (i.e., the percentage of the myocardial mass involved).

The use of positive inotropic agents in myocardial failure is predicated on the existence of a contractile reserve. In cases of severe myocardial failure, this reserve may be so small that a clinically significant response cannot be produced. Drug potency may also be a factor, and a drug with a lesser potency may not elicit a response. To be clinically meaningful, an increase in contractility brought about by a drug in a patient with myocardial failure must be large enough to increase cardiac output at rest to a point that clinical signs are alleviated (i.e., it improves the *quality* of the patient's life) and must be sustained over months to increase survival time (i.e., it improves the *quantity* of life).

Positive inotropic agents exert their effect by increasing the amount of calcium available for the contractile proteins, the amount of calcium bound by intracellular structures, or the sensitivity of contractile proteins to calcium. Those drugs that are thought to act by increasing intracellular calcium binding (catecholamines, amrinone, milrinone) are more potent and probably more effective than those drugs that nonspecifically increase cellular calcium concentrations (digitalis glycosides). In myocardial failure, one of the primary cellular defects thought to be present is a decrease in calcium binding by intracellular proteins. A drug that has the potential for reversing this calcium-binding deficit should be more effective than a drug that cannot directly counteract the problem.

Positive inotropes do not directly improve cellular oxygenation or result in salvage of dying cells. In normal hearts, they increase myocardial oxygen consumption by increasing contractility. In hearts with myocardial failure, however, they tend to decrease myocardial oxygen consumption through a reduction in diastolic and systolic left ventricular volumes and thus a reduction in systolic myocardial wall stress (afterload). This may prolong the life of dying cells. However, long-term success with positive inotropic agents can occur only if cells in the myocardium remain viable and responsive to the drug. A disease process that results in continued myocardial destruction ultimately results in refractory myocardial failure and death. In diseases such as congestive cardiomyopathy, it appears that continued destruction of the myocardium occurs either directly from the myocardial disease or indirectly from a prolonged increase in myocardial oxygen consumption. Positive inotropic drug administration, in those patients that do respond, can prolong life but only for a relatively short time.

The number of positive inotropic drugs available for chronic use is small but should increase in the near future. The digitalis glycosides have been the only practical agents available for long-term oral use. Recently, a new class of drugs has been identified that is active orally and is more potent than the digitalis glycosides. These drugs are bipyridine derivatives (amrinone, milrinone), and they are very promising drugs for the chronic treatment of myocardial failure.

CATECHOLAMINES

The catecholamines are a group of drugs used primarily for *short-term* inotropic support of failing myocardium. The endogenous and most synthetic catecholamines have extremely short half-lives and so are useful only when administered as IV boluses or by constant-rate infusion. This limits these drugs to short-term administration. Recently, several catecholamines that can be used orally have been synthesized; however, their use in long-term treatment of myocardial failure is not established.

Catecholamines exert their effects by stimulating adrenergic receptors located throughout the body. The cardiovascular effects are the result of stimulation of β_1- and α-receptors in the heart; β_2-, α_1-, α_2-, and dopaminergic receptors in the peripheral vasculature; and α_2-receptors in the brain stem. The positive inotropic effect is exerted through β_1- and α-receptor stimulation. Stimulation of β_1-receptors activates adenyl cyclase, which converts adenosine triphosphate (ATP) to 3′5′-cyclic adenosine monophosphate (cAMP). Cyclic AMP activates protein kinases, which phosphorylate various intracellular proteins (including the sarcoplasmic reticulum), resulting in enhanced transport of intracellular calcium. It is this enhanced transport of calcium that results in the increase in contractility. Stimulation of β_1-receptors also increases heart rate. Cardiac α-receptor stimulation also increases contractility by increasing calcium movement into the cell. Myocardial α-receptor stimulation decreases heart rate.

In the peripheral vasculature, β_2- and dopaminergic-receptor stimulation results in arteriolar *dilation*, and α_1- and α_2-receptor stimulation causes arteriolar *constriction*. Alpha$_1$-receptors are thought to mediate vasoconstriction in areas that are heavily innervated, and α_2-receptors mediate vasoconstriction in areas that are sparsely innervated. Alpha$_1$-receptors are located on vascular smooth muscle within the area of the nerve synapse (intrasynaptic), whereas α_2-receptors are located some distance from the synapse (extrasynaptic). Alpha$_2$-receptors are also located proximal to synapses (presynaptic) on sympathetic nerve fibers. Stimulation of these presynaptic receptors inhibits the release of norepinephrine.

Stimulation of α_2-receptors in the brain stem results in a reduction in sympathetic outflow and an increase in vagal tone. The net result is a decrease in heart rate, contractility, and systemic vascular resistance. The catecholamines differ in their ability to stimulate α-, β-, and dopaminergic receptors, and many of these effects are dose-dependent.

Epinephrine

Epinephrine increases contractility and stimulates α_1-, α_2-, and β_2-receptors peripherally. In the periphery, α-receptor stimulation is stronger than β_2-stimulation, resulting in predominant arteriolar constriction. The increase in cardiac output that occurs with β_1-stimulation and the systemic arteriolar constriction combine to produce an increase in systemic arterial blood pressure and, subsequently, an increase in afterload. Epinephrine is also very dysrhythmogenic. These two factors make epinephrine a poor choice for treating myocardial failure except in the extreme situation of cardiac arrest. In cardiac arrest, epinephrine is used to increase the perfusion pressure of cardiac compressions, to increase the efficacy of defibrillation in ventricular fibrillation, and to correct asystole and severe bradyarrhythmias (idioventricular rhythms). Dosage is 5 μg/kg (1 ml of a 1:10,000 dilution per 10 kg) IV or intratracheally every 5 minutes in cardiac arrest. It can also be administered as a constant infusion at 0.04 μg/kg/min (0.6 mg or 6 ml of 1:10,000 dilution in 500 ml of normal saline infused at 2 ml/kg/hour).

Isoproterenol

Isoproterenol is a synthetic β-receptor agonist. It increases contractility more than the other catecholamines and increases heart rate while decreasing blood pressure because of its β_2-receptor activity. Its use in heart failure is extremely limited because of its positive chronotropic effect (i.e., its ability to increase heart rate) and its potential to precipitate malignant ventricular dysrhythmias. Infusion rates are from 0.045 to 0.09 μg/kg/min.

Norepinephrine

The administration of norepinephrine is generally contraindicated in heart failure because the predominant α-receptor stimulation in arteriolar smooth muscle results in an increase in systemic arterial blood pressure, increased cardiac afterload, and decreased cardiac output. Norepinephrine is also a β_1-receptor agonist, so it increases contractility, but it is only administered as a last resort to heart failure patients that are in cardiogenic shock when blood pressure can no longer be maintained at levels compatible with life.

Dopamine

Dopamine is an endogenous precursor of norepinephrine. It stimulates β_1-receptors, stimulates the release of norepinephrine, especially at higher infusion rates, and stimulates dopaminergic receptors. Dopaminergic receptors are predominantly found in renal, mesenteric, coronary, and cerebral arterioles, where they mediate vasodilation. Infusion rates of 2 to 10 μg/kg/min produce an increase in cardiac output secondary to an increase in contractility, with little change in heart rate or blood pressure. Dopamine infusion results in preferential blood flow to kidneys, mesentery, and heart. Infusion rates greater than 10 μg/kg/min may cause α-stimulation and vasoconstriction and an increase in blood pressure through the stimulation of norepinephrine release.

Dobutamine

Dobutamine is a synthetic catecholamine that predominantly stimulates β_1-receptors. It also stimulates β_2- and α_1-receptors peripherally, but the stimulation is mild and balanced so that changes in systemic arterial blood pressure usually do not develop. Heart rate changes are generally not clinically significant when the infusion rate is kept between 5 and 20 μg/kg/min. Higher infusion rates may result in an increase in heart rate.

Indications for the use of dobutamine are acute myocardial depression, short-term stabilization of chronic heart failure, and possibly long-term stabilization of chronic heart failure. There is evidence in humans to suggest that prolonged (72 hours) administration of dobutamine to patients with chronic myocardial failure results in improved myocardial ultrastructure and prolonged improvement in hemodynamics. Usually catecholamines are ineffective after as little as 8 hours of administration because of desensitization of myocardial β_1-receptors. The chronic intermittent administration of repeated, brief infusions of dobutamine has also been reported to produce long-term improvements in human heart failure patients.

PIRBUTEROL

Pirbuterol is a synthetic β-receptor agonist that is effective after oral administration. It is predominantly a β_2-receptor agonist, although it does stimulate β_1-receptors. In heart failure, its major beneficial effect probably is arteriolar dilation and reduction of afterload. Pirbuterol has not been studied in veterinary patients with heart failure. In humans, its usefulness appears to be limited by side effects and desensitization of β-receptor function, with an attenuation of the hemodynamic effects over time.

PRENALTEROL

Prenalterol is a relatively specific β_1-agonist that can be administered orally or intravenously. When administered acutely to humans with myocardial failure, it increases contractility and cardiac output, decreases pulmonary capillary pressure, and does not change heart rate or systemic arterial blood pressure. With continued administration, the beneficial effect, however, is gone within 3 months, either because of β-receptor desensitization or because of continued myocardial deterioration. Prenalterol has not been studied in veterinary patients with heart failure.

DIGITALIS GLYCOSIDES

Digoxin and digitoxin are used clinically in heart-failure patients for long-term inotropic support of failing myocardium and for heart rate control. They have the negative features of having a low toxic:therapeutic ratio, relative impotency (33 per cent increase in contractility in normal hearts versus 100 per cent increase with dobutamine), and the ability to produce arrhythmias and lethal toxic effects. Considerable controversy exists in human medicine about the effectiveness of the cardiac glycosides in patients with heart failure. In veterinary medicine, it has been demonstrated that some dogs with congestive cardiomyopathy respond well to the positive inotropic effects of digoxin but the majority do not. Those dogs that do respond usually live longer than nonresponders, averaging 10 months survival for responders and 6 weeks for nonresponders.

The digitalis glycosides increase calcium influx nonspecifically into myocardial cells. This nonspecific increase can result in increased inotropy if the intracellular structures that bind calcium are healthy. If they are not healthy, contractility will not be increased and, instead, the myocardial cells may become overloaded with calcium. Calcium overload causes electric instability of myocardial cells, which may result in premature depolarizations. Myocardial cells that are failing are already overloaded with calcium, thus making the cells more susceptible to the toxic effects of digitalis. Because of this increased susceptibility, it is the authors' opinion that digitalis should not be administered in loading doses to patients with myocardial failure. Loading doses frequently result in mildly to moderately toxic serum concentrations that can be lethal to patients with myocardial failure.

Large dogs are the predominant type that develops severe myocardial failure (e.g., congestive cardiomyopathy). They require less digoxin per kilogram body weight than do small dogs. It appears that a dose based on body surface area is more appropriate. It is recommended that digoxin be administered at a dose of 0.22 mg/m^2 of body surface area twice daily. This dose consistently results in serum concentrations of digoxin within the therapeutic range of 1.0 to 2.5 ng/ml. The dose for digitoxin is 0.03 to 0.04 mg/kg twice or three times daily. Tincture of digitoxin is the only form of digitoxin that has been proved effective in dogs. However, it usually is not practical for use in large dogs because the largest capsule marketed is 0.25 mg.

Digitalis intoxication should be avoided. Mild intoxication causes nausea, anorexia, vomiting, and diarrhea. Treatment consists of withdrawal of the drug. Moderate to severe intoxication causes cardiac dysrhythmias. Ventricular tachydysrhythmias are among the most common and the most lethal. Antidysrhythmic drugs should be used in an attempt to control ventricular dysrhythmias caused by digitalis intoxication. Phenytoin and lidocaine are the most effective agents. Oral phenytoin (35 mg/kg t.i.d.) may be administered prophylactically to dogs with myocardial failure in an attempt to prevent dysrhythmia formation. Propranolol and procainamide can also be used to treat digitalis-induced ventricular dysrhythmias. Administration of quinidine and verapamil are contraindicated in digitalis intoxication because they increase serum digoxin concentrations and may potentiate the myocardial toxicity of digoxin. Quinidine may also displace digoxin from myocardial binding sites, making the drug less effective.

For a more detailed description of digitalis pharmacokinetics, pharmacodynamics, and toxicity see *Current Veterinary Therapy VIII*, Drugs Used in the Management of Heart Failure. See Canine Myocardial Diseases for use in dilated cardiomyopathy of dogs and Feline Myocardial Diseases for the use of digoxin in cats.

AMRINONE

Amrinone (Inocor, Sterling) is a new nonadrenergic, nonglycoside-positive inotropic drug with positive inotropic capabilities similar to those of the catecholamines and mild to moderate arteriolar dilating properties. Amrinone is the first drug of its kind to be marketed for human use. Milrinone, a more potent derivative of amrinone, will probably be marketed in the near future for human and veterinary use. The mechanism of action of these drugs is unknown, but myocardial phosphodiesterase inhibition does occur and may explain the positive inotropic effects of these drugs. Phosphodiesterase breaks down intracellular cAMP, and inhibition of this enzyme causes increased intracellular concentrations of cAMP. The cAMP increases contractility by stimulating protein kinases within the cell, so phosphodiesterase inhibitors cause an increase in contractility in a manner similar to catecholamines. The major difference is that phosphodiesterase inhibition does not affect β-receptors. Hence, phosphodiesterase inhibitors do not lead to receptor desensitization, found with β-receptor agonists. Amrinone, although it is active after oral administration, is marketed only for IV use. The IV preparation is expensive, is not licensed for use in dogs or cats, and has not been studied in dogs or cats with naturally occurring myocardial failure. However, the drug has been studied in normal dogs and cats. Preliminary recommendations regarding clinical use can be made.

A bolus injection of 1.0 to 3.0 mg/kg of amrinone causes an immediate 60 to 100 per cent increase in cardiac contractile force, a 10 to 30 per cent decrease in systemic arterial blood pressure, and a 5 to 15 per cent increase in heart rate in normal anesthetized dogs. The positive inotropic effect peaks at 5 minutes, is about 50 per cent of peak at 10 minutes, and is gone after 20 to 30 minutes. Constant infusion rates of 30 to 100 μg/kg/min increase contractile force 40 to 80 per cent, increase heart rate 10 to 30 per cent, and decrease systemic arterial blood pressure 10 to 20 per cent in normal, unanesthetized dogs. Peak effect occurs 60 minutes after the start of infusion. Effect is approximately 50 per cent of peak 30 minutes after an infusion is started. In anesthetized dogs with drug-induced myocardial failure, the IV infusion of amrinone results in an increase in myocardial contractile force of 40 to 200 per cent, an 80 per cent increase in cardiac output, and a decrease in central venous pressure. Amrinone has been administered to normal anesthetized cats as a constant-rate infusion (30 μg/kg/min). Its administration increases dP/dt max (an index of left ventricular contractility) 40 per cent. Peak effect occurs 90 minutes after starting the infusion.

In humans with myocardial failure, amrinone administration results in improved left ventricular performance as evidenced by increased cardiac output and decreased pulmonary capillary pressures. Renal blood flow and glomerular filtration rate increase. Blood flow to skeletal muscle also increases during exercise, since maximum oxygen uptake increases during exercise. The effect of the drug appears to be sustained over months of therapy, since withdrawal of the drug from human patients after 10 months of therapy results in cardiac decompensation.

The administration of IV amrinone is indicated in dogs and possibly cats with acute or chronic myocardial depression. In animals with chronic myocardial failure, IV amrinone can only be used for short-term stabilization of the patient. Based on the pharmacodynamic information, the dose in dogs is 1 to 3 mg/kg as an IV bolus followed by a constant infusion at 30 to 100 μg/kg/minute. One-half the initial bolus may need to be administered 20 to 30 minutes after starting the infusion. The dose in cats is probably similar, although the half-life of the drug may be longer.

Studies to date have indicated that amrinone is very safe. It has a very large therapeutic range and a large toxic:therapeutic ratio. Possible side effects are an increase in heart rate and the formation of ventricular dysrhythmias. If possible, electrocardiographic monitoring should be performed when the drug is first administered.

MILRINONE

Milrinone, a methylcarbonitrile derivative of amrinone, is 20 to 30 times more potent than its parent compound. It is active after IV and oral administration. It has cardiovascular effects similar to amrinone in dogs and cats, but the dosage is reduced because of the increased potency. Milrinone, like amrinone, is relatively safe when compared with the cardiac glycosides and the catecholamines. It also has a wide therapeutic range and a large toxic:therapeutic ratio. The only adverse effect, encountered in fewer than 5 per cent of dogs with myocardial failure, has been ventricular dysrhythmia formation. Milrinone is still an experimental drug, but it should be marketed for oral veterinary use in the near future.

Intravenous milrinone produces cardiovascular effects similar to those of amrinone when administered to anesthetized dogs as a bolus at a dose of 30 to 300 μg/kg. Constant infusions of 1 to 10 μg/kg/min to conscious dogs have effects similar to those of amrinone. Peak effect occurs 30 minutes after starting the infusion. The effect is about 50 per cent of peak 1 hour after discontinuing the infusion and is gone after 90 minutes. A constant IV infusion of milrinone to cats at a rate of 1 μg/kg/min increases left ventricular contractile force 40 per cent, which is greater than that in dogs. This suggests that cats may require a smaller dose than dogs.

Oral administration of milrinone has been studied in normal conscious dogs and in conscious dogs with congestive cardiomyopathy. In normal dogs, oral doses of 0.1 to 1.0 mg/kg increase cardiac contractile force 35 to 100 per cent. The effect is present within 15 to 30 minutes and lasts at least 4 hours. In dogs with myocardial failure, we have demonstrated that a dose of at least 0.5 mg/kg is needed to effect a cardiovascular response. Doses as large as 1.0 mg/kg have been administered, but with no further increase in contractility when compared with a dose of 0.5 mg/kg. A starting dose of 0.75 mg/kg is recommended, however, since some dogs do not respond to a 0.5 mg/kg dose, and this increased dose is not associated with any toxic effects.

In our study, milrinone increased left ventricular shortening fraction, a correlate of ejection fraction, from an average of 20 to 30 per cent (normal shortening fraction is greater than 30 per cent) in 14 dogs with myocardial failure. Heart rate did not change. Clinical improvement was apparent in most dogs. There was no evidence of tachyphylaxis to the drug, since the cardiovascular effects of milrinone persisted for at least 4 weeks with continued administration. Average survival time for dogs with congestive cardiomyopathy was approximately 6 months. This is comparable to the survival time we have noted previously in dogs with congestive cardiomyopathy that responded to digoxin. However, in our group of dogs treated with milrinone, all dogs responded to the drug, and only 40 per cent of the dogs we studied after digoxin administration responded. The two groups were not comparable, however, because the dogs treated with milrinone were all in relatively early stages of heart failure and were clinically stable, whereas the dogs that received digoxin were in various stages of heart failure and most were clinically unstable. Preliminary evidence from a large group of dogs treated with milrinone suggests that approximately 70 per cent of dogs with myocardial failure respond to the positive inotropic effects of milrinone. Of the dogs that we have studied after milrinone administration, those with right ventricular myocardial failure have survived much longer than those with left ventricular myocardial failure.

The half-life of milrinone in dogs is 2 to 3 hours, compared with 1.5 to 2.0 hours in humans. In our study, dogs with myocardial failure had cardiovascular effects for as long as 12 hours, but they were quite attenuated by this time. The positive inotropic effect was 75 per cent of maximum 5 to 7 hours after administration, 45 per cent 8 to 10 hours after administration, and 35 per cent 12 hours after administration. In canine patients, milrinone may be effective when dosed at 12-hour intervals, but intervals of 8 hours or even 6 hours may be required in dogs with severe myocardial failure or dogs with minimal or attenuated responses to milrinone. The half-life and duration of effect of milrinone are unknown in cats.

Because of its safety, potency, and response rate, milrinone is a very promising drug for the treatment of myocardial failure in dogs and cats.

References and Supplemental Reading

Baim, D. S., McDowell, A. V., Cherniles, J., et al.: Evaluation of a new bipyridine inotropic agent—milrinone—in patients with severe congestive heart failure. N. Engl. J. Med. 309:748, 1983.

Jentzer, J. H., LeJemtel, T. H., Sonnenblick, E. H., et al.: Beneficial effect of amrinone on myocardial oxygen consumption during acute left ventricular failure in dogs. Am. J. Cardiol. 48:75, 1981.

Kittleson, M. D.: Drugs used in the management of heart failure. *In* Kirk, R. W. (ed.): *Current Veterinary Therapy VIII.* Philadelphia: W. B. Saunders, 1983, pp. 285–296.

Kittleson, M. D.: Concepts and therapeutic strategies in the management of heart failure. *In* Kirk, R. W. (ed.): *Current Veterinary Therapy VIII.* Philadelphia: W. B. Saunders, 1983, pp. 279–284.

Kittleson, M. D.: Dobutamine. J.A.V.M.A. 177:642, 1980.

Kittleson, M. D., Pipers, F. W., Knauer, K. W., et al.: Echocardiographic and clinical effects of milrinone in dogs with myocardial failure. Am. J. Vet. Res. 46:1659, 1985.

LeJemtel, T. H., Keung, E., Ribner, H. S., et al.: Sustained beneficial effects of oral amrinone on cardiac and renal function in patients with severe congestive heart failure. Am. J. Cardiol. 45:123, 1980.

VASODILATOR THERAPY

JOHN D. BONAGURA, D.V.M.,
and WILLIAM MUIR, D.V.M.
Columbus, Ohio

Heart failure is characterized by a reduction in cardiac output and by compensatory mechanisms that increase heart rate and systemic vascular resistance. Peripheral vasoconstriction assists in maintaining mean arterial blood pressure (ABP) as shown by the following relationship (Fig. 1):

$$\text{Mean ABP} \propto \text{cardiac output} \times \text{peripheral resistance}$$

Maintenance of ABP is necessary to satisfy perfusion requirements of the myocardium and brain; however, peripheral vasoconstriction redistributes blood flow away from other tissues, promoting skeletal muscle weakness and renal retention of sodium and water. Recent evidence suggests that systemic vasoconstriction may also aggravate heart failure by increasing left ventricular work and reducing stroke volume (Fig. 2).

Ventricular stroke volume is determined by heart rate, myocardial contractility, method of ventricular electric activation (synergy), and by the *loading* conditions imposed on the heart (Fig. 1). *Preload,* which is related to cardiac filling and ventricular size, is often increased in heart failure. Ventricular afterload impedes left ventricular output and contributes to overall myocardial oxygen demands (Fig. 2). *Afterload* is difficult to define clinically, but it is increased by high peripheral vascular resistance and by ventricular dilatation. Afterload is estimated by measuring the mean ABP (since this depends in part on vascular resistance).

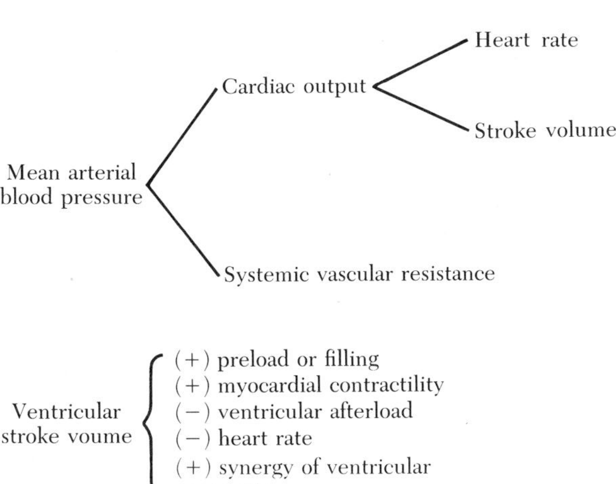

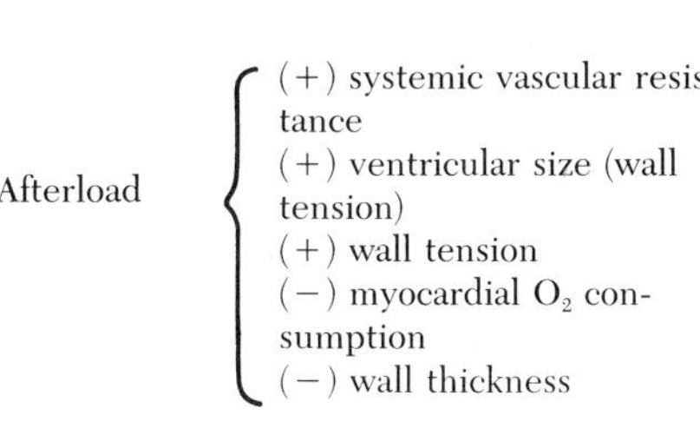

Figure 1. Important hemodynamic relationships.

Why do vasoconstriction and increased ventricular afterload occur in heart failure? The answer to this question is complex, and a number of factors are implicated in the vasoconstriction of heart failure (Table 1). Heart failure increases adrenergic tone, which stimulates sympathetic α_1-receptors, causing vasoconstriction. This action is potentiated in congestive heart failure by "waterlogging" of blood vessels or by perivascular edema: These are the so-called vascular stiffness factors. Some stages of heart failure are characterized by increased plasma concentrations of angiotensin II and of arginine vasopressin. Both of these peptides are potent vasoconstrictors. Venoconstriction is also precipitated by heart failure, owing to increased sympathetic tone and to vascular stiffness factors. These result in elevated central venous pressure and predispose the patient to edema.

Clinicians have attempted to counteract the deleterious effects of vasoconstriction by administering vasodilator drugs. Because the causes of vasoconstriction are multifactorial (Fig. 2), a variety of agents have been employed by clinicians, including direct-acting arteriolar and venodilator drugs, α-adrenergic blockers, and drugs that inhibit the renin-angiotensin system. Each group of drugs has theoretic merits and practical disadvantages; these are outlined below. The predominant site of vascular action also differs among the various drugs (Table 2). Accordingly, the terms arterial vasodilator, venodilator, or "balanced" (arterial and venous)

Table 1. *Causes of Increased Vascular Resistance*

Sympathetic-induced vasoconstriction
Renin-angiotensin system
Arginine vasopressin
Vascular stiffness factors
Rebound from vasodilator drugs

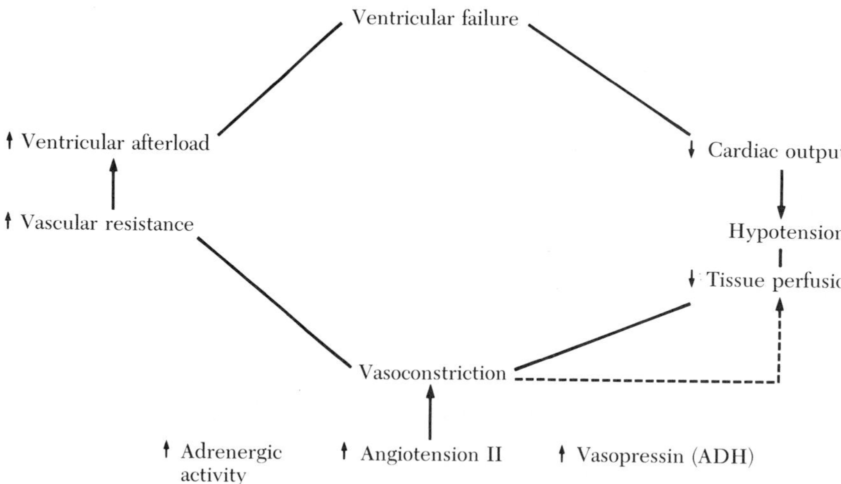

Figure 2. Consequences of vasoconstriction in heart failure.

vasodilator have developed. Arteriolar vasodilators reduce afterload and myocardial oxygen demand and increase stroke volume. Venodilators dilate systemic capacitance veins, lower venous pressures, and reduce edema. Balanced vasodilators should do both. There is a great need for objective studies that critically assess vasodilator therapy in dogs and in cats. Until such studies are completed, vasodilator therapy must be considered to be a "clinical trial."

EFFECTS OF VASODILATORS IN HEART FAILURE

Venodilators

Congestive heart failure (CHF) is associated with increased venous pressures caused by ventricular failure, renal retention of sodium and water, and systemic venoconstriction. Venous pressure is highest behind the failing ventricle, and this pressure is the cause of edema and serous cavity effusions that characterize the CHF state. The administration of drugs that dilate systemic veins (e.g., the nitrates) leads to a reduction in venous pressure. Agents such as isosorbide dinitrate and topical nitroglycerin ointment act directly on vascular smooth muscle to produce venodilation. Although these effects are greater on systemic than on pulmonary veins, venodilation serves to translocate blood from the pulmonary vascular bed and into the systemic venous system. This reduces pulmonary venous pressure and helps to prevent the formation of pulmonary edema.

Table 2. Commonly Used Vasodilator Drugs—Indications and Mechanisms of Action

Drug	Principal Dilator Effect	Indications
Nitroglycerin ointment	Venous*	CHF
Isosorbide dinitrate	Venous*	CHF Mitral regurgitation
Sodium nitroprusside	Arterial and venous	Low-output failure CHF
Hydralazine	Arterial	Low-output failure Mitral regurgitation ? Pulmonary hypertension
Prazosin	Arterial and venous	Low-output failure CHF Mitral regurgitation
Captopril	Arterial and (?) venous	Low-output failure CHF Mitral regurgitation

* = Systemic capacitance veins.
(?) = Uncertain in dogs.

Hypotension occurs when venodilators are administered to normal animals. This is attributed to a concomitant arteriolar dilator effect and to pooling of blood in the capacitance veins. Venodilator-induced hypotension may be less likely in animals with heart disease when venous pressures are high and systemic vascular resistance is increased. It is important to recognize that venodilators will diminish venous return and lower preload; therefore, these drugs must be administered only to patients who demonstrate objective signs of pulmonary venous congestion. Following venodilation, venous return may still be sufficient in such patients. Since potent diuretics enhance the action of venodilators by decreasing plasma volume, the combined use of venodilators and diuretics can decrease cardiac output and cause hypotension.

Arterial Vasodilators

Arteriolar or balanced vasodilators reduce systemic vascular resistance and decrease ventricular afterload. Provided that ventricular filling (preload) is maintained, stroke volume and cardiac output increase. Heart rate usually increases to maintain mean ABP (Fig. 1). The net effects may be improved organ and skeletal muscle perfusion and increased exercise tolerance. Arterial vasodilators also reduce the magnitude of mitral regurgitation by facilitating forward flow from the left ventricle. The patient with a low cardiac output, dilated left ventricle, and mitral regurgitation is most likely to benefit from arteriolar dilator therapy.

Problems arise when arterial dilation is excessive, since symptomatic hypotension may result. Lethargy, weakness, and syncope are clinical features of hypotension in dogs. Reduced coronary perfusion and severe reflex tachycardia are additional consequences of hypotension, and these complications can aggravate cardiac failure. Vasodilation provokes other physiologic responses, including activation of the sympathetic nervous and the renin-angiotension systems. As the drug effect dissipates, these responses lead to rebound vasoconstriction and to renal retention of sodium and water. Drug-induced compensatory reactions are particularly prominent with hydralazine and can be the cause of "drug failure" in some animals. Thus, arterial vasodilators can improve ventricular performance but also can induce serious adverse effects related to hypotension.

CLINICAL USE OF VASODILATORS

Patient Selection

Candidates for vasodilator therapy usually fall into one of three categories: venous congestion with pulmonary edema, reduced cardiac output, or both. Animals with severe congestion due to elevated venous pressures are candidates for venodilation with drugs such as nitroglycerin. Before administering venodilator drugs (Table 3), the clinician should objectively determine that CHF is evident based on physical examination (e.g., auscultation, jugular venous distension) and thoracic radiography (e.g., pulmonary edema). A dog with a dilated left ventricle, venous congestion, increased vascular resistance with low cardiac output, and mitral regurgitation is the *best candidate* for arterial vasodilation. Arterial vasodilation is contraindicated in hypovolemia or hypotension, and it must be monitored by ABP determination in dogs with cardiogenic shock.

Three different cases can be used to illustrate the types of patients that may respond to vasodilator drugs. The first example is a dog or cat with *fulminant pulmonary edema*, in which the principal therapeutic goals are to reduce venous pressure and increase tissue oxygenation. Intravenous furosemide and topical nitroglycerin act in concert to reduce venous pressure and lessen the formation of edema. A second case involves dogs with *severe mitral regurgitation* causing heart failure that is progressively less responsive to diuretics. Here, an arterial dilator such as hydralazine, prazosin, or captopril can be given to reduce mitral regurgitant fraction. The giant breed of dog with *severe CHF* due to dilated cardiomyopathy represents a third candidate for vasodilator therapy. When conventional therapy of digitalis, furosemide, and rest fails to reduce signs of heart failure, vasodilators such as hydralazine, prazosin, or captopril may increase cardiac output and enhance exercise capacity. Captopril offers the added benefit of lowering serum aldosterone and limiting sodium and water retention by the kidneys.

Administration of Vasodilator Drugs

Physicians monitor the results of vasodilator therapy in human patients by measuring venous pressures, cardiac output, ABP, and clinical status. Owing to a number of technical and economic limitations, detailed invasive hemodynamic monitoring is not widely employed in veterinary medicine. Even the determination of ABP can be difficult or impossible to attain. Accordingly, the veterinarian must depend on clinical and subjective criteria to assess vasodilator therapy.

Effective vasodilation results in controlled hypotension with decreased afterload, mild reductions in mean ABP, and corresponding increases in cardiac output. Examination of the patient will usually document the development of vasodilation and increased blood flow, and these important clinical findings are summarized in Table 4. When signs of moderate to severe hypotension occur, the drug should be terminated or the dosage reduced. The clinical criteria employed here to monitor therapy are somewhat crude, but they may be useful when objective measures such as blood pressure cannot be obtained. Serial mixed venous oxygen samples (tensions) may also be helpful in monitoring the effects of vasodilator therapy, as venous Po_2 may correspond to directional changes in cardiac output; that is, if mixed venous Po_2 values increase, the cardiac output may be increasing. To summarize, clinical findings, blood pressure (and other hemodynamic measurements), and venous Po_2 are used to monitor vasodilation.

Our method of initiating oral vasodilator therapy is to hospitalize the patient, perform baseline evaluations (Table 4), select an appropriate vasodilator and dose, and administer *one-half* of the calculated drug dose. The animal is examined for drug effects at 1, 2, and 3 hours after administration of either hydralazine, prazosin, or captopril. If insignificant changes are observed, the animal is given a full

Table 3. *Vasodilator Drugs*

Drug	Proprietary Preparation	Approximate Dose*	Adverse Effects
Nitroglycerin ointment 2%	Nitrol: (Kremers-Urban)	¼–1 inch cutaneously every 6–8 hours (dogs) ¼ inch every 6–8 hours (cats)	Hypotension, rash
Isosorbide dinitrate	Isordil: 5, 10-mg tablets (Ives)	0.5–2.0 mg/kg PO every 8 hours (dogs)	Hypotension
Sodium nitroprusside	Nipride: 50-mg vials (Roche)	5–15 μg/kg/minute IV (dogs)	Hypotension, tachycardia, cyanide poisoning
Hydralazine	Apresoline: 10-, 25-, 50-mg tablets (Ciba)	0.5–2.0 mg/kg PO every 12 hours (dogs) 2.5 mg PO every 12 hours (cats)	Hypotension, tachycardia, syncope, sodium retention, GI
Prazosin	Minipress: 1-, 2-, 5-mg capsules (Pfizer)	0.5–2.0 mg PO every 8–12 hours (dogs)	Hypotension, syncope
Captopril	Capoten: 25-, 50-mg tablets (Squibb)	0.5–2.0 mg/kg PO every 8–12 hours (dogs) ⅛–¼ of a 25-mg tab every 8–12 hours (cats)	Hypotension, GI, hyperkalemia, (?) renal failure

*See text for details
Key: GI = gastrointestinal disturbances including anorexia and emesis; (?) = relationship uncertain

dose of the drug 8 to 12 hours later and is again reexamined for drug effects or for hypotension.

It is important to monitor vasodilator therapy, and for some patients it is information relayed to the veterinarian by the client that is most helpful in determining the ultimate benefits, if any, of vasodilation. A client's identification of improved level of activity, reduction in episodes of coughing, and abatement of dyspnea would suggest that drug therapy is appropriate and helpful. Lack of response can be due to many factors, including inadequate dose, improper patient selection and evaluation, loss of vascular responsiveness, or development of compensatory reactions such as rebound vasoconstriction and renal retention of sodium and water. When the history suggests drug-induced hypotension (e.g., the client notes tachycardia, weakness, or syncope) or gastrointestinal side effects (which are common), the vasodilator must be discontinued or the dosage reduced.

Table 4. *Evaluation of Vasodilator Therapy*

Patient Variable	Therapeutic Response	Signs of Hypotension
Heart rate	Decreased, no change, or increased by 10–30 bpm	Tachycardia
Arterial pulse pressure	Increased intensity	Weaker or thready
Capillary refill time	Decreased	Prolonged
Attitude	Still alert	Depressed, comatose
Exercise tolerance	Improved or maintained	Weak, ataxic, syncopal
Mean arterial blood pressure (measured)	Reduced by 10–30 mm Hg	Moderate to severe hypotension
Arterial pulse pressure (systolic–diastolic)	Increased	—
Serial venous Po_2	Increased from baseline	—
Venous congestion, pulmonary edema	Reduced congestion, less dyspnea	—

SPECIFIC VASODILATOR DRUGS

Nitrates

The nitrates are both arterio- and venodilators when administered intravenously; however, when applied cutaneously or given orally, the effect on capacitance veins predominates. *Sodium nitroprusside* is usually administered intravenously, and this drug is so potent that it may be dangerous to use without direct measurement of ABP and ventricular filling pressure. *Nitroglycerin* ointment, the preparation most often used for dogs and cats, appears to be well tolerated and useful in the management of severe CHF. The long-term value of nitroglycerin is unresolved, and some cardiologists are reluctant to use the drug except for acute cases of pulmonary edema. However, if appropriate precautions are taken to prevent the client's skin from contacting the drug, the ointment can be prescribed for the home care of chronic debilitating edema. Nitroglycerin ointment is also valuable when clients have difficulty administering oral medications. The benefits of nitrate therapy should be assessed both in the hospital and at home, and the veterinarian and client should be convinced that administration of the drug is clinically useful. The ointment is measured (by the 1/4 inch) using supplied dose papers, and it is usually rubbed onto the skin over the thorax, groin, or inside of the ears. Another nitrate, *isosorbide dinitrate*, has been recommended for use by some clinicians. This drug is given orally. When hypotension occurs in animals receiving nitrates, the drug dosage must be reduced, and it may also be necessary to decrease the daily dosage of furosemide. Since the nitrates are less likely to increase cardiac output when given topically or orally, inotropic or arterial vasodilator therapy may be required to increase forward blood flow.

Hydralazine

Hydralazine is a potent direct-acting arteriolar vasodilator that has been used with some success in dogs and less frequently in cats. This drug can induce severe hypotension, and the veterinarian and client must work together to establish an effective and safe dose. The duration of action of hydralazine in dogs is about 12 hours, so the drug is generally given twice daily. Rebound increases in renin-angiotensin-aldosterone can be expected with hydralazine, and concurrent dietary sodium restriction and diuretic therapy are essential. Hydralazine can be combined with nitroglycerin to attain a more balanced effect. This drug should not be given to dogs demonstrating signs of hypovolemia or hypotension.

Prazosin

Prazosin is an α_1-adrenoceptor-blocking agent that is effective in reducing mean ABP in renal hypertensive dogs. When compared with hydralazine, prazosin causes less reflex tachycardia and less activation of the renin-angiotensin system. Unfortunately, it is difficult to assess clinically the relative importance of sympathetic vasoconstriction in chronic heart failure. Furthermore, reports of effects on humans suggest that tachyphylaxis may develop. However, other reports have indicated that prazosin improves exercise tolerance in humans when given on a chronic basis, and this anticipated benefit has been extrapolated to dogs. The first dose of prazosin may cause pronounced hypotension owing to sudden adrenergic blockage. Prazosin capsules are less versatile than the tablet forms of hydralazine or captopril because they must be divided for administration to small patients (i.e., less than 5 kg). The clinical importance of the venodilator effect of prazosin in dogs with CHF has yet to be assessed. Some dogs appear to respond well to prazosin, and this drug can be considered for use in dogs that do not respond well to other agents, such as hydralazine.

Captopril

Captopril (Capoten, Squibb) and the experimental drug enalapril are inhibitors of the enzyme that converts angiotensin I to the active peptide angiotensin II. These drugs appear to be effective in the treatment of advanced heart failure in dogs. Arterial vasodilation, possibly venodilation, and decreased retention of sodium and water occur after administration of these drugs. (Captopril is discussed in detail in Captopril Therapy in Dogs with Heart Failure.)

References and Supplemental Reading

Cavero, I.: Cardiovascular effects of prazosin in dogs. Clin. Sci. 51:609s, 1976.

Kittleson, M. D., Eyster, G. E., Olivier, N. B., et al.: Oral hydralazine therapy for chronic mitral regurgitation in the dog. J.A.V.M.A. 182:1205, 1983.

Kittleson, M. D., and Hamlin, R. L.: Hydralazine pharmacodynamics in the dog. Am. J. Vet. Res. 44:1501, 1983.

Kittleson, M. D., Johnson, L. E., and Oliver, N. B.: Acute hemodynamic effects of hydralazine in dogs with chronic mitral regurgitation. J.A.V.M.A. 187:258, 1985.

Knowlen, G. G., Kittleson, M. D., Nachreiner, R. F., et al.: Comparison of plasma aldosterone concentration among clinical status groups of dogs with chronic heart failure. J.A.V.M.A. 183:991, 1983.

Koch-Weser, J.: Medical Intelligence. N. Engl. J. Med. 295:320, 1976.

Macho, P., and Vatner, S. F.: Effects of prazosin on coronary and left ventricular dynamics in conscious dogs. Circulation 65:1186, 1982.

Massingham, R., and Hayden, M. L.: A comparison of the effect of prazosin and hydralazine on blood pressure, heart rate, and plasma renin activity in conscious renal hypertensive dogs. Am. J. Pharmacol. 30:121, 1975.

Miller, R. R., Palomo, A. R., Brandon, T. A., et al.: Combined vasodilator and inotropic therapy of heart failure: Experimental and clinical concepts. Am. Heart J. 102:500, 1981.

Miller, R. R., Fennell, W. H., Young, J. B., et al.: Differential systemic arterial and venous actions and consequent cardiac effects of vasodilator drugs. Prog. Cardiovasc. Dis. 24:353, 1982.

Packer, M., and Le Jemtel, T. H.: Physiologic and pharmacologic determinants of vasodilator response: A conceptual framework for rational drug therapy for chronic heart failure. Prog. Cardiovasc. Dis. 24:275, 1982.

Pagani, M., Vatner, S. F., and Braunwald, E.: Hemodynamic effects of intravenous sodium nitroprusside in the conscious dog. Circulation 57:144, 1978.

Riegger, G. A. J., Liebau, G., Holzschuh, M., et al.: Role of the renin-angiotensin system in the development of congestive heart failure in the dog as assessed by chronic converting-enzyme blockade. Am. J. Cardiol. 53:614, 1984.

Zelis, R.: Mechanisms of vasodilation. Am. J. Med. 74(6B):3, 1983.

Zelis, R., and Flaim, S. F.: Alterations in vasomotor tone in congestive heart failure. Prog. Cardiovasc. Dis. 24:437, 1982.

CAPTOPRIL THERAPY IN DOGS WITH HEART FAILURE

GRANT G. KNOWLEN, D.V.M.,
Pullman, Washington

and MARK D. KITTLESON, D.V.M.
Davis, California

Captopril is an orally active inhibitor of angiotensin-converting enzyme (ACE) in dogs (Freeman et al., 1979). Captopril has the structure shown in Figure 1 and the chemical name of 1-[3-mercapto-2-methyl-1-oxopropanoyl]-L-proline (Singhvi et al., 1981). As an inhibitor of ACE (also called kininase II and peptidyldipeptide carboxyhydrolase), captopril has proved effective in the therapy of diseases characterized by hyper-reninemia, hypernatremia, hypokalemia, hyperaldosteronemia, and hypertension (Heel et al., 1980). Hyperaldosteronemia is a feature of congestive heart failure in dogs (Knowlen et al., 1983).

THE RENIN-ANGIOTENSIN-ALDOSTERONE SYSTEM

Since ACE is an integral component of the renin-angiotensin-aldosterone system (RAAS), an understanding of this system and its activation in heart failure is a prerequisite to the rational use of captopril in the therapy of heart failure.

The RAAS involves a series of hormones and enzymes, beginning with the production of the prohormone renin substrate (angiotensinogen) in the liver (Fig. 2). Renin substrate is a glycoprotein, of which there are several forms. Renin is responsible for separating the decapeptide angiotensin I from the various forms of renin substrate (Skeggs et al., 1980). However, the structure of the angiotensin I cleaved from each form is the same.

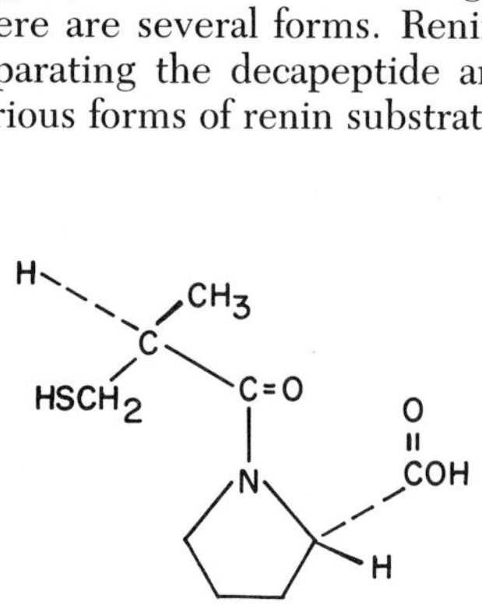

H, CH3, C, HSCH2, C=O, N, O, COH, H

Figure 1. Chemical structure of captopril (1-[(2S)-3-mercapto-2-methyl-1-oxopropyl]-L-proline). (Modified from Singhvi et al., 1981.)

Renin is produced in the granular cells of the juxtaglomerular apparatus of the kidney and is the rate-limiting component in the RAAS cascade. The release of renin is closely regulated by four complementary mechanisms. Decreases in afferent renal artery pressure cause an increase in the rate of renin release via an intrarenal baroreceptor mechanism. Increases in renal nerve traffic (i.e., increased tone in the sympathetic nervous system) result in an increase in the rate of renin release. Changes, probably decreases, in the quantity of sodium or chloride or both flowing past the macula densa in the distal tubule cause an increase in the rate of renin release. Finally, increased levels of the octapeptide angiotensin II have a negative feedback effect on the rate of renin release, causing a decrease in the amount of circulating renin activity (Zehr et al., 1980).

The angiotensin I produced by the action of renin on renin substrate has no intrinsic activity *in vivo* and is rapidly converted into angiotensin II by the action of ACE. ACE removes two amino acids from the carboxyl terminal end of angiotensin I to produce the octapeptide angiotensin II (Matthews and Johnston, 1979). ACE, although present in plasma, is found primarily on the luminal surface of pulmonary endothelial cells and in renal endothelial cells (Knowlen et al., 1983). Angiotensin II is the most potent vasopressor substance in the body. It is also the primary stimulus for the release of aldosterone from the adrenal gland zona glomerulosa and is a strong stimulus for the release of antidiuretic hormone (ADH) from the posterior pituitary (Blair-West et al., 1972; Vander, 1980).

Angiotensin I can also be converted to des Asp-angiotensin I, an inactive compound, by the aminopeptidase angiotensinase A. This compound is converted to angiotensin III by ACE. Another pathway for the formation of angiotensin III is the direct conversion of angiotensin II to angiotensin III by angiotensinase A (Fig. 3). Angiotensin III, although

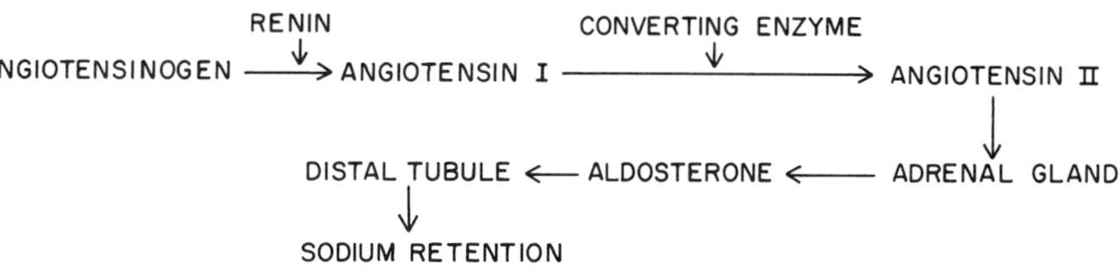

Figure 2. Components of the RAAS and their relationships. (Modified from Knowlton et al., 1983; Matthews and Johnston, 1979.)

retaining similar potency to angiotensin II to stimulate aldosterone release, retains only about 50 per cent of the vasopressor activity of angiotensin II (Vander, 1980).

As previously mentioned, the primary stimulus for the release of aldosterone is the circulating level of angiotensin II. Hyponatremia is also a strong stimulus for the release of aldosterone, as is hyperkalemia. Increases in circulating adrenocorticotropic hormone will also stimulate the release of aldosterone, although this mechanism assumes a minimal role in relation to the other three primary stimuli (Blair-West et al., 1972; Vander, 1980).

Aldosterone is the primary mineralocorticoid present in the body. The effect of aldosterone is primarily in the cells of the distal tubules and collecting ducts of the kidney, where it is responsible for regulating the retention or loss of approximately 2 per cent of the filtered load of sodium (Blair-West et al., 1972). The action of this steroid hormone is to activate a sodium-potassium pump to cause the absorption of sodium from the tubular fluid and the excretion of potassium into the tubular fluid. Concurrently, the presence of ADH is necessary for water to follow the absorbed sodium into the circulation from the distal tubules and collecting ducts (Vander, 1980).

Activation of the RAAS (i.e., increased serum concentrations of the components or end products) results when total body sodium is depleted, total body potassium is increased, renal nerve traffic is increased, or renal artery pressure is decreased. Decreases in renal artery pressure and increases in sympathetic tone, although characteristic of many other diseases, are thought to be the primary stimuli provided to the RAAS in heart failure (Fig. 4) (Ayers et al., 1972). The electrolyte abnormalities, although not generally present in the initial stages of heart failure, can still increase circulating aldosterone by direct stimulation of the adrenal cortex.

We assume that heart failure initially starts as forward failure; that is, a decrease in blood flow into the systemic arterial circulation. This decrease in cardiac output results in an initial decrease in renal artery pressure and an initial decrease in aortic body and carotid sinus baroreceptor activity. The decrease in renal artery pressure is sensed by an intrarenal baroreceptor mechanism in the area of the granular cells of the juxtaglomerular apparatus, causing the release of renin. Since normal aortic body and carotid sinus baroreceptor tone is inhibitory to sympathetic outflow from the central nervous system (CNS), a decrease in efferent traffic from these receptors results in an increase in efferent sympathetic traffic from the CNS and subsequently an increase in renal nerve traffic (Ayers et al., 1972).

The initial decreases in renal artery pressure and flow cause constriction of the efferent renal arteries, thus preserving the glomerular filtration rate (GFR) but significantly increasing the filtration fraction (FF) in the glomerulus. This preservation of GFR and increase in FF result in a decrease in efferent renal artery hydrostatic pressure and increase in oncotic pressure. The net result of the change in efferent artery fluid composition and quantity is the absorption of more sodium and water from the proximal tubule, with subsequently less sodium and chloride being presented to the distal tubule. This provides the third stimulus for an increased rate of renin release in heart failure.

Since renin is the rate-limiting component of the RAAS, there is then adequate stimulus for the formation of angiotensin II. This causes systemic vasoconstriction to aid in returning arterial pressure to normal and as a strong stimulus for the release of aldosterone and ADH, which will cause volume

THE RENIN-ANGIOTENSIN-ALDOSTERONE-SYSTEM (RAAS)

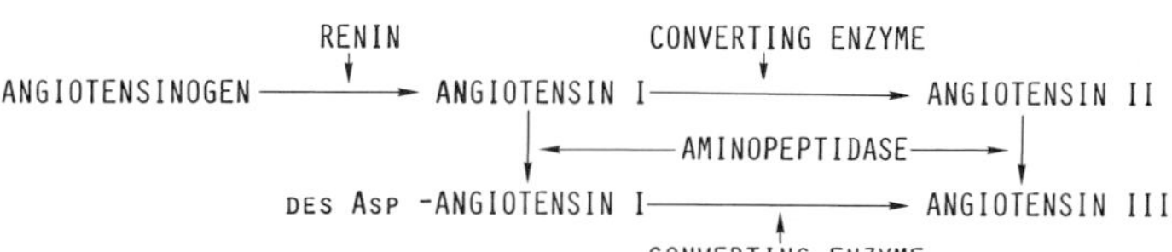

Figure 3. The formation of angiotensin III and its relationship to angiotensin I and II. (Modified from Blair-West et al., 1972.)

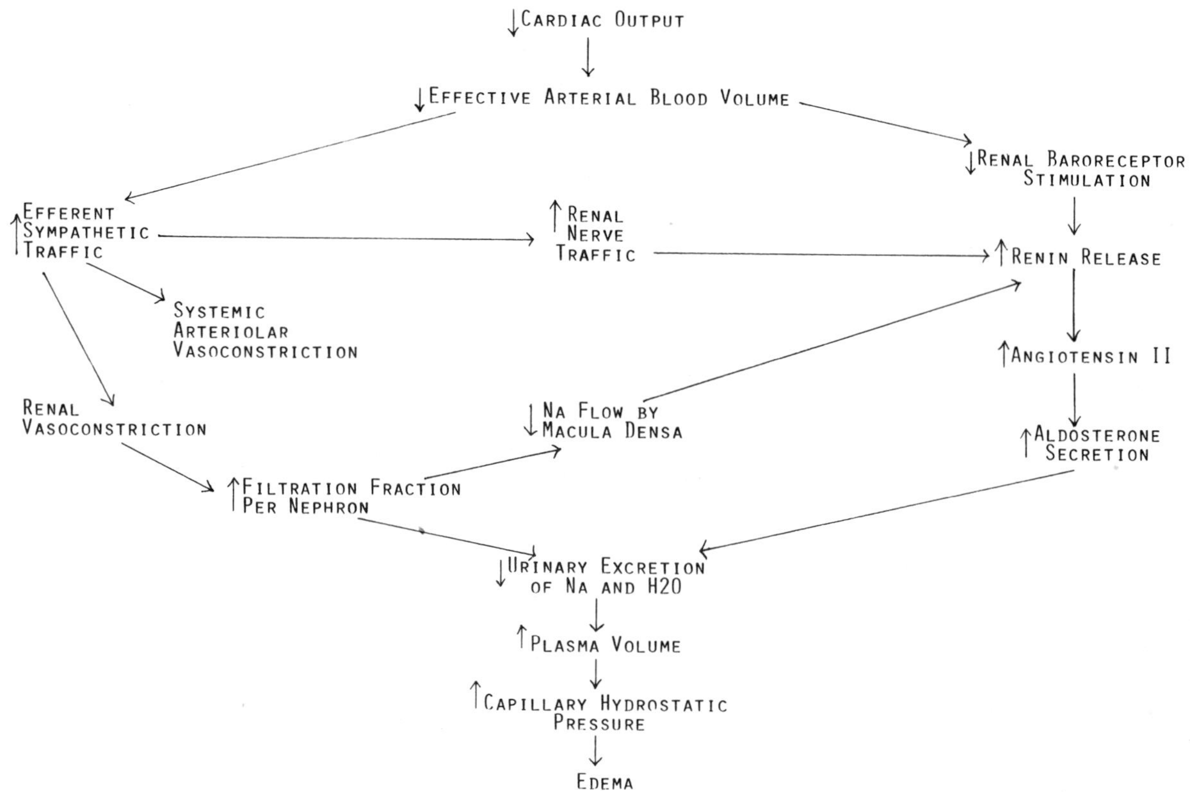

Figure 4. Activation of the RAAS in heart failure.

expansion and an increase in cardiac output through an increase in end-diastolic volume and the Frank-Starling mechanism (Ayers et al., 1972). The cardiovascular system then stabilizes at some new level of cardiac output and venous pressure, albeit with an increased total body water and sodium, an increased intravascular volume, and a decreased cardiovascular reserve capacity. Stabilization of the patient's cardiovascular status removes the stimuli for RAAS activation, and the plasma concentrations of the components of the system return to normal. However, if the patient is unable to stabilize, such that the cardiac output continues to decrease, then greater intracardiac volumes and venous pressures are required to maintain a life-sustaining cardiac output. Activation of the RAAS becomes necessary to continuously expand the vascular compartment. The continued RAAS activation and resultant increased intravascular volume create more severe backward heart failure, further activation of the system, congestion, and eventual death of the patient from severe heart failure (Ayers et al., 1972).

CAPTOPRIL: MECHANISM OF ACTION

Captopril is a direct inhibitor of ACE (Fig. 5) and can be used to provide improvement in those clinical signs attributable to activation of the RAAS (Ayers et al., 1972). ACE is responsible for cleaving the amino acids histidine and leucine from the carboxyl terminal of the decapeptide angiotensin I to create the octapeptide angiotensin II. ACE is also responsible for the inactivation of bradykinin and kallidin by the removal of two amino acids (Fig. 6) (Matthews and Johnston, 1979).

Blocking the formation of angiotensin II by administering captopril has three beneficial effects in patients with heart failure. First, since angiotensin II is a very potent vasoconstrictor, decreasing plasma concentrations of this compound results in arteriolar dilation and venodilation. Second, plasma aldosterone concentration is decreased (Fig. 4), resulting in less sodium retention. Third, plasma ADH decreases, resulting in the patient's losing water commensurate with sodium loss. The net

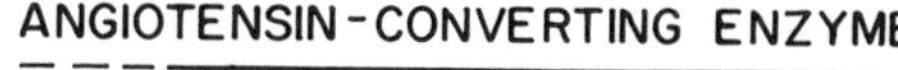

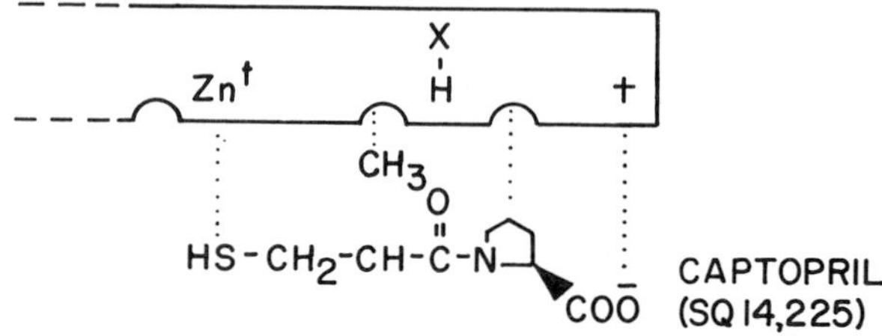

Figure 5. Proposed sites of bonding between angiotensin converting enzyme and captopril. (Modified from Ayers et al., 1972.)

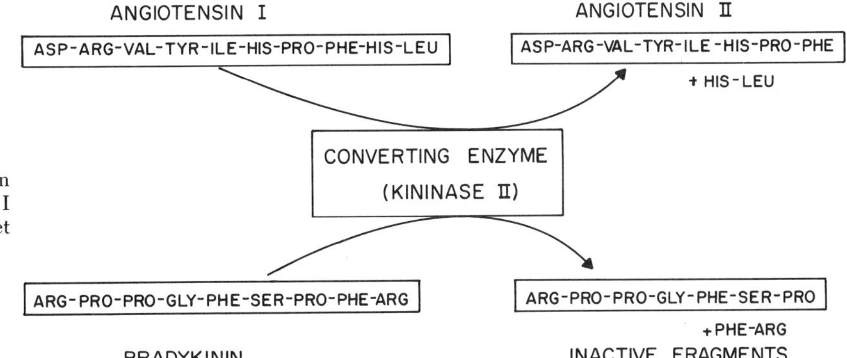

Figure 6. The reaction of angiotensin converting enzyme with angiotensin I and bradykinin. (Modified from Zehr et al., 1980.)

effects are decreased venous and diastolic intracardiac pressures with a resultant decrease in edema formation, and a decrease in afterload with a resultant increase in cardiac output (Romankiewicz et al., 1983).

There are other beneficial effects to blocking the action of ACE. Since bradykinin and kallidin are potent vasodepressor substances, preventing their breakdown and allowing plasma levels of these hormones to increase will also result in vasodilation. Captopril, aside from its effects on angiotensin and kinins, stimulates (either directly or indirectly) increased production of the vasodepressor prostaglandin PGE_2 and possibly PGI_2 (Romankiewicz et al., 1983). Angiotensin II and bradykinin are both known to stimulate increased formation of PGE_2. Since bradykinin is found in increased concentrations in patients treated with captopril, an indirect route of stimulation is likely. However, captopril may also directly increase the formation of prostaglandins by influencing the activity of phospholipase (Swartz et al., 1980).

To summarize, captopril increases plasma concentrations of angiotensin I; decreases concentrations of angiotensin II; increases concentrations of bradykinin, kallidin, and PGE_2; decreases concentrations of aldosterone; possibly decreases concentrations of ADH; increases sodium loss; increases potassium retention; increases water loss; and dilates arterioles and systemic veins. Captopril by itself does not change the heart rate, but administration of this compound may cause heart rate changes by reflex baroreceptor mechanisms. Left ventricular stroke volume index increases as a result of arteriolar dilation and the resultant decrease in systolic wall stress (afterload). End-diastolic wall stress (preload) decreases as a consequence of venodilation. Coronary blood flow is increased with the administration of an effective dose of captopril, and myocardial oxygen consumption is decreased, resulting in more effective work for any given level of energy consumption (Heel et al., 1980; Romankiewicz et al., 1983). These properties make captopril a beneficial drug in severe heart failure.

The increases in renal blood flow that result from an increased cardiac output and vasodilation result in little change in GFR but do result in a decrease in FF (Romankiewicz et al., 1983). This change aids in the excretion of extra sodium and water accumulated in the body during the initial phases of heart failure and assists in preventing the further accumulation of salt and water in a patient that is not able to compensate well.

PHARMACODYNAMICS OF CAPTOPRIL

In humans, approximately 70 per cent of an orally administered dose of captopril is absorbed within 1 hour when the subjects are fasted. Absorption is decreased by 35 to 40 per cent in nonfasted hypertensive humans, but this has been shown not to interfere with the clinical effect of the drug (Izumi et al., 1983). Similar data are not available for dogs. In dogs, 40 per cent of captopril is bound to protein in plasma, and it is uniformly distributed throughout the body, although it is not known to cross the blood-brain barrier (Wong et al., 1981). The primary route of excretion of captopril and its metabolites in dogs is through renal tubular secretion in parallel with the rate of creatinine clearance. Approximately 50 per cent of an IV dose is secreted as metabolites (Singhvi et al., 1981). Although it is presumed that metabolism occurs in the liver, biliary excretion of captopril has been found to be negligible in dogs. The half-life of captopril is approximately 2.8 hours in dogs, compared with 1.7 hours in humans (Table 1) (Singhvi et al., 1981).

CLINICAL ADMINISTRATION

Captopril is used as a vasodilator and as an adjunct to diuretics to decrease plasma volume. Vasodila-

Table 1. Pharmacokinetic Data for Captopril in Dogs

Pharmacokinetic Trait	Mean + SD
Steady-state blood level, μg/ml	0.19 ± 0.02
Body clearance, ml/kg/hour	605 ± 103
Renal clearance, ml/kg/hour	341 ± 91
Biliary clearance, ml/kg/hour	0.45 ± 0.08
Creatinine clearance, ml/kg/hour	253 ± 94
Renal clearance/body clearance	0.56 ± 0.11
Renal clearance/creatinine clearance	1.40 ± 0.15
Net tubular secretion, %*	28 ± 7
Apparent volume of distribution, L/kg	2.45 ± 0.28
Volume of central compartment, L/kg	0.49 ± 0.13
Half-life (T½), hour	2.77 ± 0.51

*Represents minimum net tubular secretion, as protein binding was assumed to be zero.

Modified from Singhvi et al.: J. Pharm. Sci. 70:1108, 1981.

tors, as a general rule, are indicated at that point in therapy when traditional therapeutic modalities (i.e., positive inotropes or diuretics or both) are no longer able to prevent the progression of heart failure or alleviate the existing signs and symptoms of heart failure (see Vasodilator Therapy) (Kittleson, 1983). Since captopril can cause vasodilation and volume contraction simultaneously, a clinician must be very cautious about administering this drug concurrently with other drugs, such as hydralazine or prazosin, that also have vasodilative properties. Care must be taken to correctly assess electrolyte balance in a patient before administering captopril. Patients with hyponatremia secondary to the inappropriately high levels of ADH seen in severe heart failure can have their problem exacerbated, as can patients that are hyperkalemic or on the verge of hyperkalemia secondary to the use of potassium-sparing diuretics or the exogenous administration of potassium supplements.

Since the clearance of captopril and its metabolites parallels creatinine clearance, patients with reduced creatinine clearance should have their dose of captopril reduced accordingly (Singhvi et al., 1981). Indications or suspicions of reduced renal function can be gained from determinations of serum urea nitrogen and creatinine, urinalysis, and a determination of creatinine clearance.

In adult humans, doses as small as 0.15 mg/kg t.i.d. are effective, although the recommended beginning dose is approximately 0.32 mg/kg t.i.d. (i.e., 25 mg t.i.d. for an average 70-kg adult) (Cody et al., 1982). Because of the half-life of captopril in humans and dogs, one would probably choose a more frequent dosing interval than three times daily. However, the biologic effect of the drug appears to be present for at least 6 hours in humans. This duration of effect, combined with the larger doses, allows less frequent dosing (Cody et al., 1982). In our clinical experience with dogs, we have used captopril at a beginning dose of 1 mg/kg t.i.d. If the patient appears unresponsive at this dose level, we have used 2 mg/kg t.i.d. and achieved the desired effect of vasodilation, afterload reduction, and sodium and water loss (Fig. 7) (Knowlen et al., 1983).

We have encountered at least two cases of induced glomerular lesions and renal failure resulting in death concurrent with the use of captopril at a dose level of 3 mg/kg t.i.d. We have also noted renal failure in a patient with captopril administered at 3 mg/kg b.i.d.; the problem did not resolve after administration of the drug was discontinued. These findings are not inconsistent with reports in humans and provide further impetus for proper prior assessment and monitoring of renal function in patients given captopril (Chrysant et al., 1983). It is our firm recommendation, based on the foregoing, that a dose of captopril in a dog should not exceed 2 mg/kg t.i.d. We have found that a large number of dogs will respond adequately to a dose of 1 mg/kg t.i.d., and some to lower doses than this.

In humans, other adverse side effects reported are hypotension, cutaneous rash and pruritus, mild gastrointestinal upset, neutropenia, and altered taste sensation (Romankiewicz et al., 1983). Vomiting and diarrhea are the only other side effects we have encountered in dogs. The abundant reports of protein-losing renal disease and the increased incidence of glomerular lesions in human patients placed on captopril therapy suggest that veterinar-

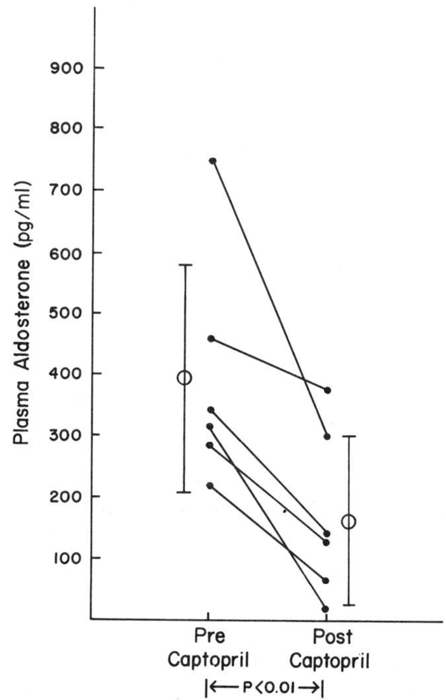

Figure 7. Plasma aldosterone concentrations in six dogs with heart failure before and after treatment with captopril. The response of each patient is represented by the connected points. Statistical analysis was by Student's t test for paired data. Note that plasma aldosterone levels declined in each case. Vertical bars are mean ± SD.

ians should pay particular attention to the possibility of these complications when using captopril in dogs. We have documented severe hypotension in one dog who received a combination of hydralazine and captopril. We recommend caution if this combination of drugs is used.

Captopril may also prove to be of benefit in the treatment of certain forms of renal hypertension in dogs, as well as in the treatment of other diseases (e.g., neoplasia characterized by the presence of hyperaldosteronemia). We presently have no experience with the use of captopril in the treatment of disease other than heart failure in dogs.

We have clinical experience with captopril in two types of cardiac disease causing heart failure—congestive cardiomyopathy and mitral regurgitation. Clinical response to captopril has been variable in each condition. In dogs with congestive cardiomyopathy, we have observed responses ranging from spectacular to dismal. In those dogs that have responded, we have documented a decrease in edema formation and improvement in peripheral perfusion (increased cardiac output or increased venous oxygen tension). A favorable response to the drug has not always been equated with prolonged survival, since some responsive dogs have died within the first several days to several weeks after captopril therapy was initiated. Dogs with mitral regurgitation have also had variable responses. In some, pulmonary edema has improved and the venous oxygen tension has increased. In others, edema has improved but the venous oxygen tension has decreased. The variable response may be attributed to the balance between venodilation and arteriolar dilation. In those dogs that have predominant arteriolar dilation, one would expect forward cardiac output to increase and, with it, venous oxygen tension. Dogs that respond with predominant venodilation may have a decrease in forward cardiac output as a result of the decrease in preload.

References and Supplemental Reading

Ayers, C. R., Bowden, R. E., and Schrank, J. P.: Mechanisms of sodium retention in congestive heart failure. Adv. Exp. Med. Biol. 17:227, 1972.

Blair-West, J. R., Coghlan, J. P., Denton, D. A., et al.: The role of the renin-angiotensin system in control of aldosterone secretion. Adv. Exp. Med. Biol. 17:167, 1972.

Chrysant, S. G., Dunn, M., Marples, D., et al.: Severe reversible azotemia from captopril therapy, report of three cases and review of the literature. Arch. Intern. Med. 143:437, 1983.

Cody, R. J., Schaer, G. L., Covit, A. B., et al.: Captopril kinetics in chronic congestive heart failure. Clin. Pharmacol. Ther. 32:721, 1982.

Cushman, D. W., Ondetti, M. A., Cheung, H. S., et al.: Inhibitors of angiotensin-converting enzyme. Adv. Exp. Med. Biol. 130:199, 1980.

Freeman, R. H., Davis, J. O., Williams, G. M., et al.: Effects of the oral converting enzyme inhibitor, SQ 14225, in a model of low cardiac output in dogs. Circ. Res. 45:540, 1979.

Heel, R. C., Brogden, R. N., Speight, T. M., et al.: Captopril: A preliminary review of its pharmacological properties and therapeutic efficacy. Drugs 20:409, 1980.

Izumi, Y., Honda, M., Hatano, M., et al.: Influence of food on the clinical effect of angiotensin I converting enzyme inhibitor (SQ 14225). Tohoku J. Exp. Med. 139:279, 1983.

Kittleson, M. D.: Drugs used in the management of heart failure. *In* Kirk, R. W. (ed.): *Current Veterinary Therapy VIII*. Philadelphia: W. B. Saunders, 1983, pp. 285–296.

Knowlen, G. G., Kittleson, M. D., Nachreiner, R. F., et al.: The relationship of plasma aldosterone concentration to the clinical status group of dogs with heart failure. J.A.V.M.A. 183:991, 1983.

Matthews, P. G., and Johnston, C. I.: Responses of the renin-angiotensin system and kallikrein-kinin system to sodium and converting enzyme inhibitor (SQ 14225). Adv. Exp. Med. Biol. 120A:447, 1979.

Romankiewicz, J. A., Brogden, R. N., Heel, R. C., et al.: Captopril: An update review of its pharmacological properties and therapeutic efficacy in congestive heart failure. Drugs 25:6, 1983.

Singhvi, S. M., Peterson, A. E., Ross, J. J., et al.: Pharmacokinetics of captopril in dogs and monkeys. J. Pharm. Sci. 70:1108, 1981.

Skeggs, L. T., Dorer, F. E., Levine, M., et al.: The biochemistry of the renin-angiotensin system. Adv. Exp. Med. Biol. 130:1, 1980.

Swartz, S. L., Williams, G. H., Hollenberg, N. K., et al.: Captopril-induced changes in prostaglandin production. J. Clin. Invest. 65:1257, 1980.

Vander, A. J.: *Renal Physiology*, New York: McGraw-Hill, 1980.

Wong, K. K., Lan, S., and Migdalof, B. H.: *In vitro* biotransformations of (14C)captopril in the blood of rats, dogs, and humans. Biochem. Pharmacol. 30:2643, 1981.

Zehr, J. E., Kurz, K. D., Seymour, A. A., et al.: Mechanisms controlling renin release. Adv. Exp. Med. Biol. 130:135, 1980.

CALCIUM ANTAGONISTS

BRUCE W. KEENE, D.V.M.,
Madison, Wisconsin

and ROBERT L. HAMLIN, D.V.M.
Columbus, Ohio

Calcium antagonists are a chemically diverse group of agents with a wide spectrum of therapeutic indications. They are known by a variety of synonyms, such as calcium-inhibitory compounds, calcium-channel blockers, or slow-channel inhibitors—names that reflect their common property of impeding the flow or action of calcium entering the cell through the slow calcium channel. Three of these drugs are currently available in the United States, and this discussion will be limited to the current and potential therapeutic applications of verapamil, nifedipine, and diltiazem to veterinary medicine.

In order to understand the pharmacologic actions of calcium antagonists, it is essential to understand the role of calcium in the regulation of the contractile machinery of the heart and of smooth muscle in peripheral arteries, as well as some of the differences between heart muscle and arterial smooth muscle. Alterations in the intracellular concentration of calcium ions regulates the degree of shortening and force of contraction of cardiac muscle cells in response to varying hemodynamic loads. Changes in both force of contraction and length are triggered and regulated by the concentration of calcium in the sarcoplasmic reticulum, T tubules, and mitochondria. Calcium serves as the essential link between the electric depolarization of the surface membrane and the mechanical contraction of the myofibril (excitation-contraction coupling, or ECC). With the entry of calcium ions into the cell, adenosine triphosphatase (ATPase) catalyzes the conversion of adenosine triphosphate (ATP) to adenosine diphosphate (ADP), and the energy liberated is used for contraction. In mammalian heart muscle, ECC is thought to be accomplished by the binding of calcium ions to troponin C, which, by way of a complex series of protein interactions, moves tropomyosin to a position that permits the actin-myosin interaction (systolic contraction). Falling concentrations of calcium ions allow this sequence to be reversed (diastolic relaxation).

Although the concentration of calcium also regulates contraction-relaxation cycles in arterial smooth muscle, it is now apparent that the mechanism of contractile protein regulation is different between heart muscle and smooth muscle. In smooth muscle, the primary regulatory step initiating actin-myosin interactions appears to involve calcium–calmodulin-dependent phosphorylation of myosin light chains. Calmodulin is a calcium-binding protein serving this regulatory function in many biologic systems. Another prominent difference between cardiac and smooth muscle is that arterial smooth muscle, like sinoatrial (SA) and atrioventricular (AV) nodal tissue, is depolarized primarily by a calcium-dependent slow channel rather than the sodium-dependent fast channel depolarization characteristic of cardiac muscle and Purkinje's fibers. Although a detailed discussion of the mechanoregulatory and electrophysiologic mechanisms of the action of calcium ions is beyond the scope of this text, it is important to realize that these properties form the basis for the structure-activity relationships of the calcium antagonists and that the tissue differences briefly mentioned here are responsible in part for the different spectra of activity encountered with the three calcium antagonists to be discussed. In summary, calcium ions are important in the depolarization of some tissue (nodal and arterial smooth muscle) and in almost all contractile processes, although different regulatory mechanisms probably apply.

Calcium antagonists then might be expected to delay or abolish depolarization in tissues in which calcium-dependent slow channel activity is important, and to weaken or abolish contractile activity, resulting in negative inotropy (in the heart) and vasodilation (of the arteries). These are indeed the basic actions of all calcium antagonists; however, the relative potency and specificity of a particular compound for a particular action (e.g., vasodilation) varies greatly. Thus, although all are relatively potent coronary vasodilators in both dogs and humans, verapamil has valuable properties as an antiarrhythmic drug, nifedipine is primarily a vasodilator, and diltiazem is intermediate in its activity.

VERAPAMIL

Verapamil (Isoptin, Knoll; Calan, Searle), a papaverine derivative, is the calcium antagonist that has been studied most extensively in both dogs and humans. In humans, it is used primarily as an antiarrhythmic agent and coronary vasodilator. In veterinary medicine, verapamil has found only limited applications as an antiarrhythmic, and, although potential may exist for broader application (e.g., in hypertrophic or obstructive cardiomyopathy, hypertension, and postresuscitation management of cardiac arrest), much work is needed to establish its safety and efficacy in clinical settings.

Electrophysiologically, verapamil has a potent and specific action on the AV node, increasing the effective and functional refractory periods, thus causing AV conduction delay or block. This action may be quite useful in supraventricular tachycardias such as atrial fibrillation or flutter, in which the rapid response to impulses arriving in the ventricles via the AV conduction system may decrease cardiac output and increase myocardial oxygen demand. Verapamil thus reduces the ventricular response to atrial fibrillation and flutter and is also useful for the suppression of re-entrant supraventricular tachycardia.

Hemodynamically, verapamil has complex effects that reflect both direct actions and neurohumoral responses in the intact animal. Verapamil in intact animals has a much more potent negative inotropic effect than either nifedipine or diltiazem, and it must be used with extreme caution in the presence of congestive heart failure. Part of the negative inotropic effect may be mitigated by concurrent reductions in heart rate and afterload due to its vasodilator effect. As a consequence of these potentially deleterious hemodynamic effects, verapamil must be used only in closely monitored situations, and preferably not in animals with congestive heart failure unless tachycardia contributes substantially to the failure. In treating supraventricular tachycardia in dogs, the dose we have used is 0.05 mg/kg, IV, administered slowly over 5 minutes. This may be repeated in one-half hour if the rhythm disturbance is not improved or alleviated and if no adverse hemodynamic effects are seen. The half-life of IV verapamil is approximately 2½ hours in dogs (Keefe and Kates, 1982). It is metabolized to inactive metabolites in the liver, and excretion is primarily renal. In humans, there is an important digoxin-verapamil interaction, resulting in elevated digoxin levels most likely due to reduced renal clearance. This interaction has not yet been clarified in dogs; however, caution is urged. *Contraindications* to verapamil therapy include sick sinus syndrome, digitalis toxicity, pre-existing β-blockade, AV block, and myocardial failure.

Until further research is completed, we recommend that verapamil be used at the present time primarily in the setting of supraventricular tachycardia (see Antiarrhythmic Drugs and Management of Cardiac Arrhythmias) unresponsive to a vagal maneuver and occurring in patients without severe myocardial failure. If toxic effects are seen, IV calcium gluconate (1 ml of the 10 per cent solution per 10 kg body weight) is valuable in managing exacerbations of heart failure; however, it appears to be ineffective against excessive AV block. Atropine (0.02 mg/kg, IV) or β-agonists (especially isoproterenol, dripped to effect) have been recommended to combat this complication in humans. Oral administration has been advocated in humans when reduction of the ventricular rate is not urgent, as the drug has milder side effects and toxicity may be less likely by this route. A dose of 0.1 to 0.2 mg/kg PO has been used in a small number of dogs.

NIFEDIPINE

Of the three compounds discussed here, nifedipine (Procardia, Pfizer) produces the most peripheral arterial dilation and has the least effect on the AV conduction time. In a conscious animal, the P-R interval is not affected by nifedipine, and this drug has no value in reducing the ventricular response to atrial tachyarrhythmias.

Graded doses of IV nifedipine in a conscious dog produce a linear reduction in arterial blood pressure with concurrent increases in heart rate and cardiac output (up to a dose of 0.1 mg/kg IV, after which severe hypotension ensues and cardiac output falls). In preliminary observations, oral dosing in conscious animals produced a short-lived tachycardia with variable, mild increases in cardiac output and variable but mild reductions in systemic arterial pressure. Although nifedipine exerts a potent *in vitro* negative inotropic effect, *in vivo*, at reasonable doses (<0.1 mg/kg IV) in the intact dog it provides a positive inotropic response, mediated over reflex pathways. It appears that the tachycardia that occurs with nifedipine administration in conscious, intact dogs—which is greater with nifedipine than with verapamil or diltiazem—is caused primarily by sympathetic activation. The milder positive chronotropic response to verapamil in conscious dogs is thought to be due mostly to vagal withdrawal, and diltiazem, which has the least effect on heart rate when given in equihypotensive doses, is thought to induce a small, balanced reflex.

Whether nifedipine will find clinical use in dogs

as an antihypertensive or vasodilator will depend on further studies to quantitate its effects, particularly in animals with heart failure. Nifedipine does not appear to alter pulmonary vascular resistance in healthy dogs, so it is unlikely to be useful in the pulmonary hypertension of heartworm disease. The heart rate response, as well as the short half-life (1 hour IV) and even shorter duration of oral effects, may prevent nifedipine from realizing a therapeutic niche in veterinary medicine (Hamann and McAllister, 1983). At the present time, nifedipine should be considered as a potent vasodilator for investigational use only. Its final status awaits further controlled studies.

DILTIAZEM

Diltiazem (Cardizem, Marion) is a benzothiazipine derivative that was developed in Japan in the early 1970s and, like the other compounds discussed, is a potent coronary vasodilator. Diltiazem does prolong AV node conduction time (though not as much as verapamil) and may be a useful antiarrhythmic. In addition, it is the least potent *in vitro* negative inotrope of the three combinations discussed. It is a peripheral arterial dilator, although its effect is not as marked as nifedipine. Like verapamil and nifedipine, diltiazem has a relatively short serum half-life (2.24 hours following IV administration). After oral administration in dogs, peak plasma levels occurred between 30 minutes and 1 hour, bioavailability is 50 to 75 per cent (increasing with increasing doses, suggesting a saturable first-pass effect mechanism), and there is a secondary serum concentration peak at 3 to 4 hours after dosing, indicating enterohepatic recycling (Wiens et al., 1984). Diltiazem is metabolized by the liver and eliminated by both biliary and renal excretion in dogs. Because of its unique spectrum of action, having "intermediate" AV nodal (antiarrhythmic) and peripheral vascular effects with minimal negative inotropic properties, diltiazem may have an important therapeutic application in the treatment of canine dilative cardiomyopathy. In this setting, diltiazem could be potentially useful to replace a β-blocker in slowing the rate of ventricular response to atrial fibrillation. The potential advantages of diltiazem include decreasing the peripheral vascular resistance and afterload (as opposed to most β-blockers, which actually increase peripheral vascular resistance), slowing of conduction through the AV node, and minimal cardiodepressant activity. It must be emphasized that (to our knowledge) diltiazem has not yet been used in this setting and is not approved for use in cardiomyopathy or antiarrhythmic therapy in humans. At the present time, diltiazem must be described as a promising drug that cannot be recommended for any clinical veterinary application, pending further investigation. In humans, diltiazem has been shown to have moderate beneficial effects in pulmonary hypertension in addition to its other uses, an application that is also potentially useful in dogs.

SUMMARY

The calcium antagonists are an interesting group of drugs with a variety of potential applications in veterinary medicine. Verapamil is the only one in clinical veterinary use, and this use is restricted at this writing to the treatment of selected supraventricular tachycardias. Of the other two drugs, diltiazem appears to have the best chance for future clinical use in veterinary medicine. Because of their hemodynamic and electrophysiologic pitfalls, as well as the lack of clinical experience and testing, all of these drugs at the present time should be used only in carefully monitored, controlled situations pending the results of future and current investigations. In the future, development of anticalmodulin agents and other novel compounds sharing the basic property of calcium antagonism may expand the potential uses and usefulness of these drugs.

References and Supplemental Reading

Hamann, S. R., and McAllister, R. G., Jr.: Plasma concentrations and hemodynamic effects of nifedipine: A study in anesthetized dogs. J. Cardiovasc. Pharmacol. 5:920, 1983.

Keefe, D. L., and Kates, R. E.: Myocardial disposition and cardiac pharmacodynamics of verapamil in the dog. J. Pharmacol. Exp. Ther. 220:91, 1982.

Piepho, R. W., Bloedow, D. C., and Lacz, J. P.: Pharmacokinetics of diltiazem in selected animal species and human beings. Am. J. Cardiol. 49:525, 1982.

Singh, B. N., and Opie, L. H.: Calcium-antagonists. *In* Opie, L. H. (ed.): *Drugs for the Heart* (American edition). New York: Grune & Stratton, 1984, pp 39–64.

Wiens, R. E., Runser, D. J., Lacz, J. P., and Dimmit, D. C.: Quantitation of diltiazem and desacetyldiltiazem in dog plasma by high-performance liquid chromatography. J. Pharm. Sci. 73:688, 1984.

BETA-BLOCKING THERAPY IN DOGS AND CATS

WILLIAM MUIR, D.V.M.
Columbus, Ohio

The autonomic nervous system plays a vital role in regulating and maintaining normal cardiovascular function. Activation of the adrenergic division of the autonomic nervous system results in the release of the neurotransmitters norepinephrine and epinephrine. The systemic effects of these neurotransmitters are dependent on the distribution and density of α- and β-adrenoceptors. Both α- and β-adrenoceptors are classified into α_1 and α_2 and β_1 and β_2 subtypes based on receptor demand for a particular chemical stimulus. Postsynaptic α-adrenoceptors are primarily involved in regulating vascular tone; their stimulation results in vasoconstriction. Postsynaptic β-adrenoceptors are located in the heart, bronchi, and gut. Stimulation of postsynaptic β_1-adrenoceptors increases cardiac rate and contractility, whereas stimulation of β_2-adrenoceptors produces bronchodilation, vasodilation, and hyperglycemia. Adrenergic activity and the release of norepinephrine and epinephrine reflexly increase in dogs and cats with cardiovascular disease in order to maintain cardiac output and arterial blood pressure. Sustained stimulation of α- and β-adrenoceptors, however, can predispose the patient to tachyarrhythmias, increased myocardial metabolism and oxygen consumption, and hypertension. These responses are potentially deleterious to the animal if atrial fibrillation or ventricular arrhythmias develop and when myocardial oxygen demands exceed the ability of the heart to deliver adequate quantities of oxygenated blood.

CLINICAL PHARMACOLOGY OF BETA-ADRENOCEPTOR-BLOCKING DRUGS

Beta-adrenoceptor-blocking drugs (β-blockers) compete with norepinephrine and epinephrine for β-adrenoceptors, thereby diminishing or abolishing their effects. Beta-blockers exhibit a variety of therapeutic and potentially deleterious effects (Muir and Sams, 1984). The β-blockers available for clinical use include propranolol, nadolol, timolol, pindolol, metoprolol, and atenolol (Muir and Sams, 1984). Differences in their therapeutic efficacy are the result of several important pharmacologic properties, including β-adrenoceptor selectivity (cardioselectivity), membrane-stabilizing (local anesthetic) activity, and intrinsic sympathomimetic activity. Most β-blockers are nonselective and produce both β_1 and β_2 blockade. Only metoprolol and atenolol exhibit preferential affinity for β_1-adrenoceptors, although some β_2-blocking activity is retained. Most, if not all, of the therapeutic effects observed during β-blocking therapy are due to β_1-adrenoceptor blockade. Blockade of β_2-adrenoceptors causes unpleasant and potentially deleterious side effects. Bronchoconstriction and vasocontriction are produced by β_2-blocking drugs. Bronchoconstriction could produce respiratory distress in patients with obstructive small airways disease (e.g., asthma).

Membrane-stabilizing, local anesthetic, or quinidinelike effects are produced by several β-blockers but are of questionable clinical importance. This property is known to cause a reduction in cardiac impulse and atrioventricular conduction, a decrease in spontaneous firing rate, and increases in fibrillatory threshold. Electrophysiologically, these effects could be responsible for antiarrhythmic activity and bradycardia. Membrane-stabilizing effects occur independently of β-blocking activity and are observed at drug plasma concentrations of 50 to 100 times those recommended clinically. This implies that most, if not all, of the antiarrhythmic effects of β-blockers are due to β_1-adrenoceptor blockade only.

Some β-blockers cause stimulation (partial agonism) of the β-receptor before producing blockade. This effect has been termed intrinsic sympathomimetic activity (ISA). The clinical relevance of this pharmacologic property is that β-blockers possessing ISA are postulated to protect patients against heart failure, severe bradycardia, bronchoconstriction, and depression of atrioventricular conduction. Pindolol is the only commercially available β-blocking drug demonstrating ISA. The clinical use of β-blocking drugs possessing ISA does not limit their clinical use as antiarrhythmic drugs, although their potential benefits in limiting bronchoconstriction and peripheral vascular constriction have yet to be determined. Table 1 summarizes the comparative β_1-blocking potency, β_1-selectivity, and ISA of the currently available β-blocking drugs.

***Table 1.** Pharmacologic Properties of Beta-Blockers*

Drug	Relative Potency	Cardioselectivity	Membrane Stabilization	Intrinsic Sympathomimetic Activity
Propranolol	1.0	No	Yes	No
Nadolol	1.0	No	Yes	No
Timolol	8.0	No	No	No
Pindolol	5.0	No	No	Yes
Metoprolol	1.0	Yes	No	No
Atenolol	1.0	Yes	No	No

CLINICAL CONSIDERATIONS FOR THE USE OF BETA-BLOCKERS

Beta-blocking drugs are used clinically to slow sinus rate, eliminate supraventricular and ventricular arrhythmias, slow ventricular response during atrial fibrillation and flutter, and decrease myocardial oxygen consumption in dogs and cats with cardiovascular disease (Table 2). An as yet controversial therapeutic use of β-blockers in animals is to reduce afterload. Beta-blockers reduce plasma renin activity, thereby decreasing arterial blood pressure (afterload) and sodium and water retention.

The dose and choice of a β-blocker should be determined by the severity and type of cardiovascular disease, existing disease in other organ systems (e.g., lung, kidney), concurrent drug administration, and the veterinarian's experience with the various β-blocking drugs available. Hemodynamic derangements caused by factors other than increased sympathetic tone, such as fever, hypokalemia, organic heart disease, and inflammatory processes, do not respond significantly to β-blocking therapy. Beta-blockers must be used cautiously in patients with long-standing congenital or acquired heart disease in which cardiac output has become heart-rate dependent. Decreases in heart rate could result in cardiogenic shock unless appropriate intravenous or oral inotropic support is initiated. Drugs that produce both β_1- and β_2-blocking activity (Table 1) can produce serious respiratory complications in patients with bronchitis, pulmonary infections, pulmonary fibrosis, asthma, or heartworm disease. The presence of renal disease can result in drug accumulation and prolong the effect of those β-blocking drugs dependent on renal excretion for their elimination. Dosages of β-blocking drugs that decrease cardiac output and liver blood flow decrease the clearance of several β-blockers and potentially prolong the duration of action of drugs metabolized by the liver (such as lidocaine). Concurrent acute or chronic inflammatory disease may require increases in the dosage of β-blockers that are highly protein bound (e.g., propranolol). Inflammatory disease increases plasma concentrations of β_1-acid glycoprotein, thereby increasing propranolol protein binding and decreasing its biologic effect. Table 2 lists the route of elimination, presence of active metabolites, bioavailability, and dosage schedule for β-blockers in dogs and cats.

***Table 2.** Therapeutic Uses of Beta-Blocking Drugs*

Indications
- Cardiac arrhythmias
  - Sinus tachycardia
  - Supraventricular tachycardia
  - Premature flutter or fibrillation
  - Atrial flutter or fibrillation
  - Premature ventricular depolarizations
- Hypertrophic cardiomyopathy
- Hypertrophic obstructive heart disease (tetralogy of Fallot, aortic or pulmonic stenosis)
- Hyperthyroidism
- Pheochromocytoma

Potential contraindications
- Obstructive airway disease
- Uncompensated congestive heart failure
- Bradycardia
- Impaired atrioventricular conduction
- Hypoglycemia

PROPRANOLOL THERAPY IN DOGS AND CATS

Propranolol is the β-blocking drug most frequently used in dogs and cats. Propranolol blocks both β_1- and β_2-adrenoceptors, does not demonstrate ISA, and is metabolized by the liver (Tables 1 and 3). Propranolol is used to treat sinus tachycardia, tachyarrhythmias, hypertrophic and obstructive cardiomyopathy, hypertension, hyperthyroidism, and pheochromocytoma. Like all β-blocking drugs, propranolol's effects are dependent on the prevailing sympathetic tone and its plasma drug concentration. Therapeutic plasma concentrations (25 to 100 ng/ml) of propranolol decrease sinus rate, ventricular rate during atrial fibrillation, and the frequency of atrial or ventricular premature depolarizations. Paroxysmal atrial or junctional tachycardia may respond favorably to propranolol. Propranolol is rarely capable of converting atrial fibrillation to sinus rhythm, although ventricular rate almost always decreases during therapy. Decreases in heart rate increase the time for ventricular filling and reduce myocardial oxygen consumption. Combined with proper inotropic therapy, propranolol's effects may improve cardiac output, help to prevent myocardial ischemia, and prevent the development of other cardiac arrhythmias. Propranolol is also useful in the treatment of arrhythmias caused by therapeutic or toxic concentrations of digitalis glycosides. The antiarrhythmic effects of quinidine, procainamide, and lidocaine are enhanced by simultaneous propranolol therapy, thereby emphasizing the sig-

Table 3. Properties of Beta-Blocking Drugs in Dogs

Drug	Route of Elimination	Presence of Active Metabolites	Oral Bioavailability	Oral Dosage Schedule
Propranolol (Inderal, Ayerst)	Hepatic metabolism	Yes	Low, variable	5–80 mg t.i.d., dogs (0.21–1 mg/kg t.i.d.) 2–15 mg t.i.d., cats
Nadolol (Corgard, Squibb)	Renal excretion	No	Good	5–40 mg b.i.d. or t.i.d., dogs (0.1–1 mg/kg once daily or t.i.d.)
Timolol (Blocadren, Merck, Sharp & Dohme)	Hepatic metabolism	No	Low, variable	0.5–5 mg t.i.d., dogs
Pindolol (Visken, Sandoz)	Hepatic metabolism and renal excretion	No	Good	1–3 mg t.i.d., dogs
Metoprolol (Lopressor, Geigy)	Hepatic metabolism	Yes	Low	5–60 mg t.i.d., dogs 2–15 mg t.i.d., cats
Atenolol (Tenormin, Stuart)	Renal excretion	No	Good	10–20 mg b.i.d., dogs

nificant role of sympathetic tone in arrhythmia production.

Hypertrophic forms of cardiac disease with or without outflow obstruction are treated with propranolol. Tetralogy of Fallot, pulmonic and aortic stenosis, and idiopathic hypertrophic cardiomyopathy of dogs and cats have all been successfully managed with propranolol. Blockade of β_1-adrenoceptors decreases heart rate and myocardial oxygen consumption, improves myocardial filling and perfusion, and potentially decreases afterload. The last effect is mediated by the β_1-blocking effects, which decrease cardiac contractility, and by the β_2-blocking effects, which decrease plasma renin activity and cause a reduction in sodium ion and water retention. Propranolol produces variable effects on pressure gradients induced by hypertrophied, hyperdynamic ventricles or fixed obstructions; the results depend on the relative degree of cardiac hypocontractile versus peripheral vascular effects produced. Functional cardiomyopathy and cardiac arrhythmias associated with hyperthyroidism are successfully managed with propranolol, since β-blockers interfere with the conversion of thyroxine to triiodothyronine and reduce sympathetic hyperactivity associated with hyperthyroidism (see Hyperthyroid Heart Disease in Cats).

CHOOSING A BETA-BLOCKER AND ITS DOSAGE

Regardless of the type of cardiovascular disease being treated, all β-blockers decrease cardiac contractility. This pharmacologic effect could produce disastrous effects in patients with severely compromised myocardial function or in patients with heart failure in which cardiac output has become heart-rate dependent. Intermittent short-term or chronic inotropic therapy therefore may be necessary in order to initiate or maintain β-blocking therapy.

The choice of a β-blocker and the initial dose are often difficult to determine. Inability to ascertain the patient's prevailing sympathetic tone, wide variations in patient response, β_1 versus β_2 effects, previous experience, and marked variability in the rate of drug elimination suggest that caution be used in determining dose rates. Specific β_1-blockers such as metoprolol and atenolol may be preferred in patients with pulmonary disease. Nadolol may be chosen in preference to propranolol if a long duration of drug therapy and infrequent dosing are desired. Beta-blocking therapy is usually established by initiating a dose at the low end of the dosage range and gradually increasing this dose until the desired effect is achieved (Table 3). Heart failure and atrial fibrillation with a rapid ventricular response (greater than 200 bpm) during digitalis therapy are usually treated with an initial dose of propranolol of 0.2 mg/kg t.i.d. for 1 day. This dose is doubled daily or increased daily by 0.2-mg/kg increments with comprehensive monitoring of heart rate and circulatory status until heart rate decreases or signs of pulmonary congestion or cardiac decompensation occur. Propranolol generally produces significant reductions in heart rate without compromising cardiovascular status when combined with adequate inotropic and diuretic therapy. Maximum oral propranolol dosages rarely exceed 80 mg t.i.d. in large dogs and 10 mg t.i.d. in cats. Periodic adjustments in propranolol therapy may be required in order to maintain a therapeutic effect and avoid toxicity if cardiac output and liver blood flow change appreciably. Concurrent acute or chronic inflammatory diseases, as previously stated, may require increased propranolol dosages until the inflammatory process is eliminated.

Beta-blocking therapy may have to be continued

indefinitely in patients with chronic heart disease in order to regulate ventricular rate, prevent cardiac arrhythmias, and minimize myocardial oxygen consumption. Sudden withdrawal of chronic β-blocking therapy should be avoided and could produce hypersensitivity to the endogenous release of norepinephrine and epinephrine, resulting in persistent tachycardia, cardiac arrhythmias, and hypertension. Beta-blocking therapy should be terminated by gradually decreasing the oral dosage in a stepwise manner over several days while frequently monitoring heart rate and rhythm. Therapeutic failures during β-blocking therapy are indicative of severe heart failure, electrolyte and acid-base imbalances, or inappropriate drug administration.

ADVERSE SIDE EFFECTS OF BETA-BLOCKERS

Most of the adverse side effects associated with β-blocking therapy are due to excessive blockade of β_1- or β_2-adrenoceptors and appear to be independent of dose. The explanation for this latter observation reflects the wide interpatient variability in oral bioavailability and the rate of elimination of β-blocking drugs. Adverse reactions occur most frequently in aged patients with chronic heart failure or in patients with acute decompensating heart disease. Clinically relevant adverse side effects include depression, lethargy, bradycardia, impaired atrioventricular conduction, congestive heart failure, bronchoconstriction, and hypoglycemia. Diarrhea and syncope have been observed in dogs receiving propranolol and other β-blockers. The simultaneous administration of negative inotropes (e.g., anesthetics, calcium-channel entry blockers) and hypoglycemics (insulin) may exacerbate the adverse actions of β-blockers. Non-receptor-related adverse effects such as gastrointestinal discomfort, rash, and fever occur infrequently and are poorly documented in dogs and cats. Beta-blocking therapy should be decreased or withdrawn if adverse side effects occur or are suspected. Bronchoconstriction can be treated with terbutaline sulfate (2 to 5 mg PO b.i.d.) or oxtriphylline (4 to 8 mg PO t.i.d.). The acute onset of congestive heart failure will respond to dobutamine (1 to 5 μg/kg/minute IV), furosemide (1.0 mg/kg IM), and oxygen therapy. Glycopyrrolate (0.01 mg/kg IM) and dopamine (1 to 5 μg/kg/minute IV) can be used to treat bradycardia, and dextrose (5 per cent dextrose in water) can be used as temporary therapy for hypoglycemia. In conclusion, β-blocking therapy should not be instituted without careful evaluation of the patient's current physical status and consideration of the pharmacologic effects of concurrent drug administration.

Reference and Supplemental Reading

Muir, W. W., and Sams, R. S.: Clinical pharmacodynamics and pharmacokinetics of beta-adrenoceptor blocking drugs in veterinary medicine. Compend. Cont. Ed. Pract. Vet. 6:156, 1984.

ANTIARRHYTHMIC DRUGS AND MANAGEMENT OF CARDIAC ARRHYTHMIAS

LARRY PATRICK TILLEY, D.V.M.,
and MICHAEL S. MILLER, V.M.D.
Roslyn, New York

An arrhythmia can be defined as an abnormality in the rate, regularity, or site of origin of the cardiac impulse or a disturbance in conduction of the impulse such that the normal sequence of activation of the atria and ventricles is altered. During normal sinus rhythm, the cardiac impulse originates in the sinoatrial (SA) node and spreads in an orderly fashion throughout the atria, through the atrioventricular (AV) node and His-Purkinje system, and throughout the ventricles.

Abnormalities of impulse formation or impulse conduction are the basic mechanisms that underlie the arrhythmias. Arrhythmias, from the viewpoint of the electrophysiologist, arise also from alterations

Table 1. Classification of Common Arrhythmias

Site	Tachycardia*	Bradycardia†
Sinus node	Sinus tachycardia	Sinus bradycardia SA arrest and/or block
Atrium	Atrial premature complexes Atrial fibrillation Atrial flutter Atrial tachycardia	
AV junction	Junctional premature complexes	2° AV block (Mobitz type 1)
	Junctional tachycardia Supraventricular, re-entrant, tachycardia	3° AV block (proximal)
His-Purkinje fibers	Ventricular premature complexes	2° AV block (Mobitz type 2)
Ventricles	Ventricular tachycardia Ventricular fibrillation	3°AV block (distal)

*Abnormalities of impulse formation.

†Abnormalities of impulse conduction, except sinus bradycardia. Pre-excitation syndrome (WPW), sick sinus syndrome, and atrial standstill (sinoventricular rhythm) are three abnormalities that represent mixed disturbance of impulse formation and conduction.

in either automaticity or conductivity or both. Table 1 shows the classification of common arrhythmias in dogs and cats, based on disturbances in impulse formation and conduction as well as heart rate.

A knowledge of the anatomic and physiologic properties of the unique impulse-forming and impulse-conducting system of the atria, the AV junction, and the ventricles is essential for the accurate analysis of cardiac arrhythmias (Fig. 1).

Activation of heart muscle results from spontaneous discharge in a pacemaker and conduction of this impulse from cell to cell. The physiologic pacemaker is located in the SA node. The rate and rhythm of the heart are controlled by the SA node; hence the normal cardiac rhythm is termed sinoatrial or sinus rhythm (Fig. 1). The impulse originating there is propagated through the atria via internodal tracts leading from the AV node. After a delay at the AV node, the impulse travels down the bundle of His, the bundle branches and their subsidiaries, and the Purkinje fiber system (which eventually comes in contact with the ventricular myocardium). The heart has many potential pacemaking cells. The SA node has the fastest inherent discharge rate, whereas the cells in the rest of the conduction system exhibit a slower rate of impulse formation. The more distal a potential pacemaker is from the SA node, the slower is its inherent discharge rate. The normal pacemaker is under the influence of the autonomic nervous system. Its rate is constantly adjusted by autonomic impulses according to need.

CLINICAL CONSEQUENCES OF AN ARRHYTHMIA

The various rhythm disturbances affect a dog's normal hemodynamics by (1) changing the heart rate (tachycardia, bradycardia), (2) altering the regularity of the heartbeats, (3) changing the time relationship of atrial and ventricular contractions, (4) losing the atrial assistance and regularity of the ventricles in atrial fibrillation, (5) creating a loss of synchrony in ventricular contractions, and (6) causing a change in cardiac contractility independent of ventricular filling. All these hemodynamic effects are more prominent if myocardial function is impaired by heart disease. For example, ventricular tachycardia in a normal heart may cause no major hemodynamic problems, whereas its occurrence in an animal with a diseased heart will usually cause congestive heart failure.

Ventricular premature complexes (VPCs) can have a major effect on cardiac output. The premature beats cause the ventricle to contract too soon, before the chamber has had time to adequately fill with blood. The blood pressure drops when the premature beat occurs. If these beats become frequent, clinical signs can occur. An occasional VPC can reduce coronary blood flow by 12 per cent, whereas ventricular tachycardia can reduce coronary blood flow by as much as 60 per cent. Clinical signs in dogs with such a cardiac arrhythmia can include weakness, lethargy, lack of tolerance to exercise, ataxia, dyspnea, fainting, personality changes, seizures, and even sudden death.

Diminished cardiac output reduces perfusion of the brain, kidneys, liver, and myocardium, which in turn causes changes in animal behavior. Eventually, oliguria may occur as the body attempts to conserve sodium and water, and pulmonary gas exchange at the alveolar level is compromised because the excess fluid backs up. Tissue hypoxia from poor coronary circulation can cause the animal to develop additional and more serious arrhythmias.

In a given animal, some techniques during the physical examination may be helpful in diagnosing an arrhythmia even before an electrocardiogram (ECG) is obtained. These include examination for the presence of a jugular pulse and auscultation of the heart simultaneously with palpation of the femoral pulse. Jugular pulsations occur when an arrhythmia causes the right atrium to contract on a closed AV valve, thus forcing the blood backward into the jugular vein. The heart rate on auscultation should be routinely correlated with the femoral pulse. A pulse deficit is a sign that an abnormality of rhythm is present. A pulse deficit is often found with premature cardiac impulses and atrial fibrillation.

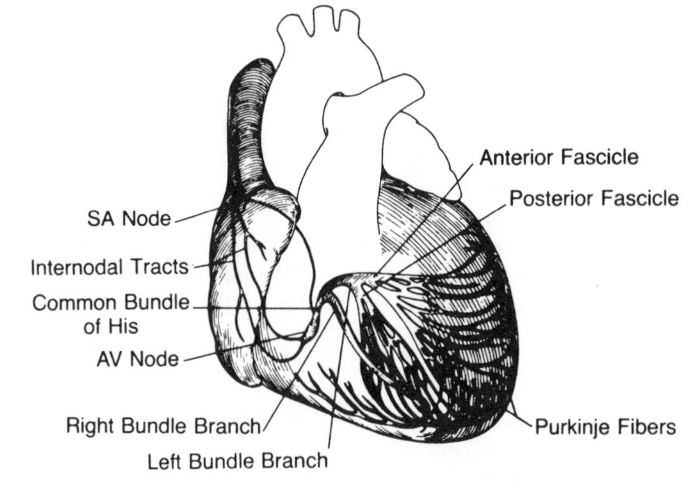

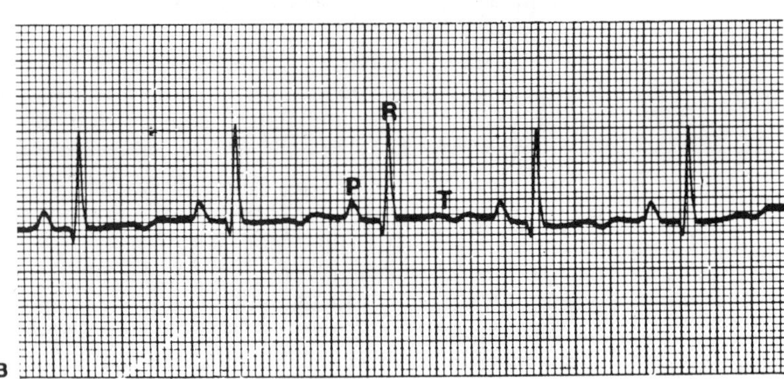

Figure 1. *A*, impulse-forming and impulse-conducting system of the heart. (From DeSanctis, R. W. *in* Rubenstein, E. (ed.): Scientific American Medicine. New York: Scientific American, 1984. © 1984 Scientific American *Medicine*. All rights reserved.) *B*, the normal lead II electrocardiogram shows a normal cardiac rhythm, termed sinoatrial or sinus rhythm.

The heart sounds heard on auscultation are caused by the abrupt acceleration or deceleration of the blood; the first sound is due to closure of the mitral and tricuspid valves, the second to closure of the aortic and pulmonic valves. These sounds may vary in intensity or rhythm or may have extra sounds in the presence of various arrhythmias. For example, atrial fibrillation has a rapid irregular rhythm with variable intensity of the heart sounds. A third heart sound is not uncommon and is usually the result of rapid ventricular filling of a dilated, failing ventricle.

CAUSES OF ARRHYTHMIAS

It is important that the cause of an arrhythmia be established, since such information may affect the approach to a case as well as the interpretation, prognosis, and therapy. The possible sources of arrhythmias in dogs can be divided into three basic categories: (1) autonomic nervous system, (2) cardiac sources, and (3) extracardiac disorders. Some of the more common causes of arrhythmias in dogs and in cats are listed in Tables 2 and 3, respectively.

In many cases, there is a disorder that can be corrected to cure the arrhythmia without the need for antiarrhythmic drugs or pacemakers. The clinician not only must treat the ECG as a source of highly specific and sensitive diagnostic information but must also consider it a source of clues as to what is happening in the patient. Atrial tachycardia with AV block may accompany digitalis toxicity. Atrioventricular block may indicate an irreversible anatomic lesion in the conduction system or may represent reversible changes produced by drugs or electrolytes. Ventricular arrhythmias may be compatible with cardiac irritability produced by myocardial hypoxia, neurogenic factors, electrolyte imbalances, sepsis, or other metabolic disorders.

RECOGNITION OF ARRHYTHMIAS

Some tests useful in the diagnostic evaluation of arrhythmias include (1) ECG, (2) exercise testing, (3) electrophysiologic studies, and (4) 24-hour Holter ECG. An ECG is a test that is easy and inexpensive to obtain, and it also provides information that determines the source of the rhythm and the frequency with which the impulse arises. The ECG recording of the arrhythmia can often be used to select the most appropriate therapy. In some cases, exercise testing can be beneficial by inducing an otherwise intermittent arrhythmia. Electrophysiologic studies as well as other advanced techniques are often used to clarify the origin and extent of heart disease.

The ECG must be evaluated in conjunction with a complete data base. The ideal data base for the cardiovascular system consists of history, physical examination, thoracic radiographs, and laboratory profile. The history is a record of age, breed, weight, medication (especially digitalis), and associated diseases. The laboratory examination includes thoracic radiography and an analysis of blood, urine, and extravascular fluids.

With the foregoing general knowledge of the normal anatomic and physiologic properties of the impulse-forming and impulse-conducting system of the heart (Fig. 1) and through the use of a systematic approach to interpretation of the ECG strip, accurate diagnosis of arrhythmias can be greatly simplified. The reader is encouraged to refer to the supplemental reading list at the end of this chapter. A systematic method for an accurate ECG analysis of a rhythm strip (usually lead II) for arrhythmias includes the following steps:

Table 2. *Causes of Arrhythmias in Dogs*

Autonomic Nervous System

Respiratory influences on vagal tone (called sinus arrhythmia)—a normal variation

Severe respiratory disorders or gastrointestinal disease (parasympathetic influence)—bradycardia, SA arrest

Excitement, exercise, pain, or fever (sympathetic influence on the SA node)—sinus tachycardia, AV junctional and ventricular tachycardia

Organic brain disease causing sympathetic or vagal stimulation

Cardiac Sources

Heredity (believed to be genetic)—AV block, WPW syndrome, His bundle degeneration (sudden death syndrome in Dobermans), persistent atrial standstill, sick sinus syndrome, SA arrest (congenital deafness in dalmatians), stenosis of the His bundle (AV block and SA arrest in pugs)

Acquired damage to the conduction system—hypertrophic cardiomyopathy, degenerative myocardial disease (microscopic intramural myocardial infarction, MIMI), AV bundle degeneration (sudden death, personality changes), neoplasia, surgical interruption

Diseases of the atria—atrial arrhythmias occurring in mitral valvular disease (congenital or acquired) (mitral valve leaflet as site of ectopic impulses), neoplasia, dilated cardiomyopathy with secondary atrial dilatation

Diseases of the ventricles—myocarditis (many causes, often not proved conclusively), cardiomyopathy, neoplasia, trauma, myocardial ischemia secondary to heart failure

Extracardiac Sources

Hypoxia

Disturbances of the acid-base balance

Electrolyte imbalance (especially hyperkalemia associated with uremia and adrenocortical insufficiency)

Hypothermia

Drugs, e.g., digoxin, thiamylal sodium, and atropine

Endocrine diseases—hyperthyroidism, hypothyroidism, pheochromocytoma, diabetes mellitus, Addison's disease

Mechanical stimulation—faulty placement of the IV fluid catheter in either the right atrium or the right ventricle, cardiac catheterization procedures

From Tilley, L. P. (ed.): *Essentials of Canine and Feline Electrocardiography. Interpretation and Management.* 2nd ed. Philadelphia: Lea & Febiger, 1985, with permission.

Table 3. *Causes of Arrhythmias in Cats*

Autonomic Nervous System

Excitement, exercise, pain, or fever (sympathetic influence)—sinus tachycardia, junctional and ventricular arrhythmias

Respiratory influences on vagal tone (not as pronounced in the cat as in the dog; thus, marked sinus arrhythmias rare)

Organic brain disease causing sympathetic or vagal stimulation

Cardiac sympathetic neural discharge as a possible mechanism for digitalis-induced arrhythmias

Cardiac Sources

Heredity (rare)

Acquired damage to the conduction system—hypertrophic cardiomyopathy (high predilection for the conduction system), neoplasia

Diseases of the atria—atrial arrhythmias occurring in neoplasia, hypertrophic cardiomyopathy, and in various congenital heart defects with secondary left atrial enlargement

Diseases of the ventricles—myocarditis (many causes); neoplasia, myocardial ischemia secondary to heart failure in cardiomyopathy

Extracardiac Sources

Hypoxia

Disturbances of the acid-base balance

Electrolyte imbalance (particularly hyperkalemia associated with urethral obstruction)

Drugs, e.g., digoxin, halothane (accelerated junctional rhythm and AV block), propylene glycol diluent (used in both IV diazepam and phenytoin sodium), ketamine hydrochloride (increased heart rate), propranolol (AV block, SA arrest, and severe bradycardia), lidocaine (severe bradycardia)

Endocrine diseases—hyperthyroidism, diabetes mellitus

Mechanical stimulation—faulty placement of the venous catheter tip in either the right atrium or the right ventricle, cardiac catheterization procedures

From Tilley, L. P. (ed.): *Essentials of Canine and Feline Electrocardiography. Interpretation and Management.* 2nd ed. Philadelphia: Lea & Febiger, 1985, with permission.

1. General inspection of the ECG. A determination should be made as to whether an arrhythmia, if present, is occasional, frequent, or continuous; regular or irregular; and repetitive or occurring with various combinations. The heart rate should be classified as rapid (tachycardia), slow (bradycardia), or normal.

2. Identification of P waves. This should include a determination of whether the atrial activity is uniform or regular. A lead (usually lead II) should be selected that illustrates discrete P waves. The direction and shape of the P wave can also help to analyze an arrhythmia. A normal P wave (positive and rounded, as in lead II) in most cases indicates that the impulse is originating in the SA node. The absence of P waves usually signifies atrial fibrillation, atrial standstill, atrial activity of low voltage in the respective lead, or buried P waves in the T waves or the QRS complexes of AV junctional rhythms. In various supraventricular tachycardias,

the P wave can be superimposed on a portion of the QRS complex, S-T segment, or T wave of the preceding cardiac cycle.

3. Recognition of QRS complexes. The QRS complexes should be characterized as to their morphology, uniformity, and regularity. A QRS complex of normal width and morphology and also identical to those recorded before an arrhythmia indicates a normal activation of the ventricles. Such complexes may be the result of an impulse formed in the SA node or an abnormal impulse originating anywhere above the bundle of His. Normal-appearing QRS complexes can be categorized as "supraventricular." Wide QRS complexes with various configurations may indicate an ectopic pacemaker below the bundle of His (ventricular) or a lesion in the intraventricular conduction system.

4. Relationship between P waves and QRS complexes. The time from the onset of the P wave to the onset of the QRS complex is called the P-R interval and is a measure of AV conduction. The P-R intervals are essentially constant in normal sinus rhythm. P waves may precede normal QRS complexes by different time spans. An abnormally long P-R interval usually indicates an AV conduction delay or first-degree heart block.

An abnormally short P-R interval may be seen in conditions such as accessory conduction around the AV node or in AV junctional rhythms in which the P wave is positioned close to the QRS complex. When all P waves are not followed by QRS complexes, an AV block has occurred. By establishing the relationship of the P wave and QRS complex, the clinician can determine the dominant rhythm. From different portions of the heart, impulses may originate at rates faster than, slower than, or the same as the normal sinus rate. Arrhythmias with rates slower than the sinus rate usually occur because of SA nodal depression, allowing "escape" of other pacemakers from its influences. These slow cardiac rhythms are called passive or escape rhythms. Abnormalities of impulse formation, which usually exceed the SA node rate, may be intermittent or persistent, repetitive, or occurring in varying combinations.

CLASSIFICATION OF THE ARRHYTHMIA

By following the preceding four steps, the clinician can usually identify rhythm disorders, leading to the final interpretation of the arrhythmia. Classification of the arrhythmia can be determined by asking the following questions:

1. What is the dominant rhythm? The dominant rhythm in most common arrhythmias is sinus, with normal impulses from the SA node. An ectopic rhythm may also be dominant, as in atrial tachycardia. Occasionally, the dominant rhythm will change from the SA node to an ectopic focus (atrial, AV junction, or ventricular).

2. Is the arrhythmia an abnormality of impulse formation or of impulse conduction or both? What is the site of this abnormality?

With these basic questions answered, the final classification of the arrhythmia can be made. Once an arrhythmia is diagnosed, the following questions should be answered:

1. What is the likely cause of the rhythm or conduction disturbance?

2. How will the ECG abnormality affect hemodynamics (blood pressure and flow)? If cardiac output and tissue perfusion are not impaired, the animal may require no treatment even though the arrhythmia persists. But arrhythmias that impair cardiac output should be treated.

3. How can progressive complications be anticipated and prevented?

4. What is the best therapeutic regimen? First, the relative risks of the arrhythmia and that of the treatment must be compared. Several approaches to therapy are possible, as outlined in Table 4. The

Table 4. *Methods Available for the Termination of Arrhythmias*

Physiologic Maneuvers
Ocular pressure
Carotid sinus pressure (massage)
Diving reflex
Alteration of Receptors
α- and β-adrenergic
Dopaminergic
Histaminic (H_1, H_2)
Purinergic
Correction of Acid-Base, Electrolyte, and Fluid Disorders
Oxygen Therapy
DC Cardioversion
Atrial and Ventricular Pacing
Drug Therapy
Vagomimetics
Anticholinergics
Sympathomimetics
α- and β-adrenergic blocking agents
Antiarrhythmic drugs
Calcium-channel blocking agents
Inotropic agents
Other Therapy
Blood transfusion
Rest
Surgery
Corticosteroids
Antibiotics
Analgesics

From Tilley, L. P. (ed.): *Essentials of Canine and Feline Electrocardiography. Interpretation and Management.* 2nd ed. Philadelphia: Lea & Febiger, 1985, with permission.

general categories include (1) drugs, (2) physiologic maneuvers, (3) cardioversion, (4) pacemakers, and (5) a combination of drugs and other treatment. *Drug therapy is the most common approach to arrhythmias and will be the focus of this chapter.*

The following specific bradyarrhythmias with heart rates of less than 60 beats per minute (bpm) (less than 120 bpm in cats) often must be treated expeditiously, especially if the animal has signs of decreased cardiac output: sinus bradycardia, SA arrest or block, advanced AV block (second- and third-degree AV block), junctional and ventricular escape rhythms, and ventricular asystole.

The following specific tachyarrhythmias with heart rates greater than 180 bpm (greater than 240 bpm in cats) may need to be treated if the animal has signs and symptoms of decreased cardiac output: sinus tachycardia, paroxysmal atrial tachycardia, atrial flutter, atrial fibrillation, paroxysmal AV junctional tachycardia, and ventricular tachycardia.

DRUGS USED TO TREAT ARRHYTHMIAS

As previously discussed, arrhythmias result from abnormalties of impulse formation or impulse conduction. Cardiac arrhythmias and conduction disturbances occur in every region of the heart and are caused by numerous diseases. In the final analysis, however, all arrhythmias and conduction disturbances, regardless of their pathologic cause, result from critical alterations in the electric activity of myocardial cells. The electric activity causing these abnormalities may result from changes in ionic mechanisms responsible for generation of normal transmembrane action potentials.

A classification of some antiarrhythmic drugs used in humans is based on how these drugs influence membrane ionic currents, cardiac excitability, conduction, and refractiveness (Table 5). Class I drugs interfere with fast-current sodium channels. Class II drugs are β-adrenoreceptor blockers. Class III drugs prolong the action potential duration. Class IV drugs are calcium-channel blockers. Class I drugs have recently been subdivided into three subclassifications. Class IA drugs have a moderate effect on conduction velocity and prolong repolarization. Class IB drugs have mild effects on conduction velocity and shorten repolarization. Class IC drugs markedly depress conduction velocity but have little or no effect on repolarization.

Based on the proper ECG diagnosis and the establishment of the cause, the majority of cardiac arrhythmias in dogs can be managed with drugs listed in Table 5. It is very important, however, to determine whether the dog is receiving other cardiac drugs, especially digitalis. Digitalis can cause almost every arrhythmia reported. Antiarrhythmic drugs are often more effective when the underlying

Table 5. *Classification of Antiarrhythmic Drugs*

Class IA	Quinidine Procainamide Disopyramide
Class IB	Lidocaine Tocainide* Mexiletine* Phenytoin
Class IC	Encainide* Flecainide* Lorcainide*
Class II	β-adrenergic-blocking agents Propranolol
Class III	Bretylium Amiodarone* Bethanidine* Clofilium* Meobentine* Sotalol†
Class IV	Calcium-channel blocking agents Verapamil Diltiazem

*Investigational drugs.
†Also a β-adrenergic blocking agent.

cause of the arrhythmia is treated. For example, the correction of hypoxia or acid-base and electrolyte imbalances may eliminate the arrhythmia or make the antiarrhythmic drug more effective. The treatment of congestive heart failure will often terminate the existing arrhythmia. Drugs that affect the central nervous system, such as phenytoin (diphenylhydantoin) and diazepam, can be useful for digitalis-induced and excitement-induced arrhythmias. Propranolol has been advised for preventing neurogenic arrhythmias secondary to increased sympathetic activity during naturally elicited emotional behavior.

Table 6 summarizes the indications, adverse effects, and dosages for the antiarrhythmic drugs used in dogs and cats. The clinician should also be familiar with the modes of action, contraindications, and side effects of these drugs. (Further information can be found in the Supplemental Readings.)

Specific treatment for many arrhythmias in cats is rarely required. In most cases, arrhythmias disappear when the underlying disease is controlled. For example, the correction of hyperkalemia in urethral obstruction and normalization of acid-base status and intravascular fluid volume may eliminate the associated arrhythmias. When drugs are indicated, propranolol and digoxin are the two agents used most often in the treatment of arrhythmias in cats. Other antiarrhythmic drugs used in dogs—quinidine, procainamide, lidocaine, and phenytoin (diphenylhydantoin)—have not been used extensively in cats. Information is not available concerning the kinetics of absorption after either oral or intramuscular administration of quinidine and pro-

Text continued on page 354

Table 6. *Drugs Used in the Therapy of Cardiac Arrhythmias*

Generic Name	Commonly Used Preparations	Indications	Adverse Effects	Approximate Dosage*
		Antibradyarrhythmic Agents		
Atropine	Atropine sulfate USP 0.4 mg/ml	Sinus bradycardia, sinoatrial arrest, incomplete AV block	Sinus tachycardia, ectopic complexes, ocular, gastrointestinal, and pulmonary side effects, paradoxic vagomimetic effects	0.01–0.2 mg/kg IV, IM 0.02–0.04 mg/kg SC (dog and cat)
Glycopyrrolate	Robinul (Robins) injection 0.2 mg/ml	Sinus bradycardia, sinoatrial arrest	As per atropine	0.005–.01 mg/kg IV, IM 0.01–0.02 mg/kg SC (dog and cat)
Isopropamide	Darbid (Smith Kline) 5-mg tablets	Incomplete AV block, sinoatrial arrest	As per atropine, keratoconjunctivitis sicca	2.5–5 mg b.i.d.–t.i.d.
Isoproterenol	Isuprel HCl (Breon) injection 0.2 mg/ml; 1- and 5-ml ampules Proternol (Key) 20-, 40-mg tablets Isuprel glossets, 10 mg	Sinoatrial arrest, sinus bradycardia, complete AV block	CNS stimulation, ectopic complexes Tachycardia, emesis	0.4 mg in 250 ml D5W, drip slowly to effect. Proternol—10–20 mg every 4–6 hours, Isuprel glossets—5–10 mg sublingual or per rectum every 4–6 hours
		Antitachyarrhythmic Agents		
Digitoxin	Crystodigin (Lilly) 0.2 mg/ml 0.1-, 0.2-mg tablets Foxalin (Standex) 0.1, 0.25, 0.5 mg	Supraventricular premature complexes, supraventricular tachycardia, atrial flutter/fibrillation	Anorexia, depression, vomiting, diarrhea, AV block, ectopia, junctional tachycardia	Oral maintenance: 0.04 to 0.1 mg/kg divided b.i.d. to t.i.d. Rapid IV digitalization: 0.01 to 0.03 mg/kg; administer ½ of calculated dose IV, wait 30 to 60 minutes and administer ¼ of dose, wait 30 to 60 minutes and administer remaining dose if necessary.
Digoxin	Lanoxin (Burroughs Wellcome) elixir 0.05 mg/ml, 0.125-, 0.25-, 0.5-mg tablets Cardoxin (Vita Elixir) elixirs 0.05, 0.15 mg/ml	Same as digitoxin	Same as digitoxin	Oral maintenance: 0.01 to 0.02 mg/kg divided b.i.d. Rapid IV digitalization: 0.01–0.02 mg/kg IV as per digitoxin. Rapid oral digitalization: 0.02 to 0.06 mg/kg divided b.i.d. for one day. Cat: 0.007–0.015 mg/kg divided b.i.d.

		***Antitachyarrhythmic Agents** Continued*		
Lidocaine HCl	Xylocaine (without epinephrine) (Astra) 2% (20 mg/ml)	Ventricular premature complexes, ventricular tachycardia	CNS excitation, seizures, tremors, emesis (treat with diazepam), other rhythm disturbances	2–4 mg/kg IV slowly, repeat to maximum of 8 mg/kg. For the cat: 0.25–1 mg/kg IV over 5 minutes. Constant-rate infusion† for the dog: 25–75 μg/kg/min.
Procainamide	Pronestyl (Squibb) injection of 100 or 500 mg/ml, 250- and 500-mg tablets Procan (Parke-Davis) sustained release (SR) 250, 500 mg	Ventricular premature complexes, ventricular tachycardia	Weakness, hypotension, decreased contractility, anorexia, vomiting, diarrhea, widening of QRS and QT interval, AV block	6–8 mg/kg IV over 5 min; CRI: 25–40 μg/kg/min, 6–20 mg/kg IM every 4–6 hours. Tablets—8–20 mg/kg every 6 hours Procan SR—8–20 mg/kg every 6–8 hours
Propranolol HCl	Inderal (Ayerst) 1 mg/ml vials, 10-, 20-, 40-, 80-mg tablets	Supraventricular premature complexes and tachyarrhythmias, atrial fibrillation, ventricular premature complexes	Decreased contractility, bronchoconstriction, loss of compensatory mechanisms	0.04–0.06 mg/kg IV slowly 0.2–1.0 mg/kg orally t.i.d. (dog and cat)
Quinidine sulfate, gluconate, and polygalacturonate	Quinidine gluconate USP injection 80 mg/ml Quinidine sulfate tablets USP 200 mg, Quinidex (sustained-release) (Robins) tablets, 300 mg Quinaglute Dura-tabs (quinidine gluconate) (Berlex) 324 mg Cardioquin (Purdue Frederick) tablets (quinidine polygalacturonate) 275 mg	Ventricular premature complexes, ventricular tachycardia, acute atrial fibrillation, refractory supraventricular tachycardias	As per procainamide, drug interaction with digoxin; urine retention	6–20 mg/kg IM, every 6 hours 6–16 mg/kg orally every 6 hours Quinaglute Dura-tabs (quinidine gluconate) and Cardioquin tablets (quinidine polygalacturonate) 8–20 mg/kg every 6–8 hours

*All dosages are for the *dog* unless otherwise noted.

†Formula for CRI: Body weight (in Kg) × dose (in μg/kg/min) × 0.36 = total dose in mg to administer IV over 6 hours
e.g., 20-kg dog, 50-μg/kg/min infusion
e.g., (20) (50) (.36) = 360 mg over 6 hours

From Bonagura, J. D., and Muir, W. W. *in* Tilley, L. P. (ed.): *Essentials of Canine and Feline Electrocardiography. Interpretation and Management.* 2nd ed. Philadelphia: Lea & Febiger, 1985, with permission.

cainamide. Phenytoin should not be used in cats despite its efficacy in dogs and humans. Lidocaine, when used as an antiarrhythmic drug, has been shown to be dangerous in cats, unless low dosages and slow rates of infusion are given. The majority of the adverse reactions are neurotoxic and cardiovascular, including conduction disturbances, bradyarrhythmias, and sinus arrest.

Propranolol is presently our antiarrhythmic drug of choice in cats because of its broad antiarrhythmic effects. Propranolol works primarily by blocking the β-adrenergic receptors (see Beta-Blocking Therapy in Dogs and Cats). Propranolol may be beneficial in atrial tachycardia, atrial flutter, Wolff-Parkinson-White (WPW) syndrome, and ventricular arrhythmias. It also has an additive effect with digitalis in slowing AV conduction, especially for atrial fibrillation. Propranolol has been advised for tachyarrhythmias in hyperthyroidism. Propranolol is contraindicated in asthma, bradycardia, AV block, and some types of cardiac failure. The drug can depress myocardial performance and accentuate cardiac failure.

Of the forms of digitalis, digoxin alone has been used in cats. The clinical use of digoxin in cats falls primarily into two categories: (1) for control of ventricular rate in atrial fibrillation, atrial tachycardia, and atrial flutter and (2) for the inotropic effect in the improvement of cardiac performance in dilated cardiomyopathy. Manifestations of digoxin toxicity include effects on the heart and effects on the gastrointestinal system.

On a more practical basis, the antiarrhythmic agents used in dogs and cats can be divided into those drugs for tachyarrhythmias and those drugs for bradyarrhythmias. Most commonly used antitachyarrhythmic agents include cardiac glycosides, quinidine, lidocaine, procainamide, and propranolol. The investigational drugs listed in Table 5 are antitachyarrhythmic agents.

Antibradyarrhythmic agents include atropine sulfate, glycopyrrolate, isoproterenol, isopropamide, and epinephrine. These drugs are useful when artificial pacemakers are not immediately available.

In the treatment of certain arrhythmias, several drug groups are contraindicated. Digoxin is contraindicated in advanced AV block, when there are frequent VPCs and ventricular tachycardia. Drugs that increase heart rate are contraindicated in congestive heart failure and with certain ectopic arrhythmias. Atropine can lower the ventricular fibrillation threshold and predispose the animal to sympathetic-induced arrhythmias. The majority of drugs used to treat arrhythmias are contraindicated in advanced AV block and in severe congestive heart failure because of their negative inotropic effects.

With this general overview of arrhythmia analysis and management in mind, we can proceed to a discussion of general guidelines for the treatment of common arrhythmias. For ECG features of each arrhythmia as well as associated conditions, the reader is encouraged to refer to the Supplemental Reading list. Figure 2 provides examples of common arrhythmias recorded in dogs and cats.

BRADYARRHYTHMIAS

Sinus bradycardia is a regular sinus rhythm, with a heart rate less than 70 bpm (less than 60 bpm in large breeds and less than 160 bpm in cats). Associated conditions are often systemic noncardiac disorders. Sinus bradycardia usually indicates a serious underlying disorder that needs immediate attention. The underlying condition should always be treated. If clinical signs such as weakness or syncope develop, parenteral atropine or glycopyrrolate should be used. Sympathomimetic agents such as epinephrine, isoproterenol, or dopamine may be needed in emergencies such as cardiac arrest. Artificial pacing is sometimes necessary if there is no response to drug therapy.

Sinus arrest is the failure of impulses to be formed within the SA node owing to depressed automaticity in the node, whereas *sinoatrial block* is a disturbance of conduction from a regularly fired SA node. The failure of the SA node to discharge on time can cause fainting or even sudden death. Asymptomatic sinus arrest or SA block does not require therapy. If the animal is symptomatic, the underlying cause should be treated, any causative drugs (digoxin, propranolol) discontinued, and atropine, glycopyrrolate, isoproterenol, or isopropamide administered. An artificial demand pacemaker is needed in selected cases.

Second-degree AV block and *third-degree AV block* are characterized by a failure or disturbance of AV conduction. Third-degree AV block occurs when there is no AV conduction, whereas second-degree AV block is represented by intermittent failure of AV conduction. Clinical signs can include syncope and sometimes congestive heart failure. Digitalis toxicity often causes AV block. If weakness or syncope is evident, then atropine, dopamine, isoproteronol, or a temporary or permanent cardiac pacemaker is required. For third-degree AV block, treatment with drugs is usually of no value. Artificial pacing is usually necessary, especially in symptomatic animals. An IV isoproterenol or dopamine infusion may be useful to stimulate escape foci until pacing can be established. Ventricular antiarrhythmic agents are extremely dangerous and contraindicated because they tend to suppress escape foci.

Atrial standstill is a life-threatening abnormality associated with hyperkalemia (Addison's disease, acute renal failure, urinary obstruction, ruptured bladder, and diabetic ketoacidosis). No P waves are seen, the QRS complexes are normal or bizarre (depending on the intraventricular conduction), and T waves may be peaked. Since the SA node continues to fire and may be conducted, the rhythm is better termed sinoventricular. *Persistent atrial standstill* is a disorder commonly reported in English springer spaniels and some cats with dilated cardiomyopathy. There is degeneration and fibrosis of the atrial myocardial cells, and a junctional or ventricular escape rhythm supervenes.

If hyperkalemia is suspected, emergency treatment should be directed to transferring extracellular potassium into the body cells. Lowering the serum potassium can be done with fluid therapy (saline for Addison's disease), sodium bicarbonate (1 to 2 mEq/kg body weight IV), regular insulin for emergency treatment (0.5 to 1 unit/kg body weight with 2 gm dextrose/unit insulin), and soluble IV glucocorticoids (for Addison's disease). The ECG is monitored throughout treatment. Ideally, electrolytes are measured every 4 to 8 hours.

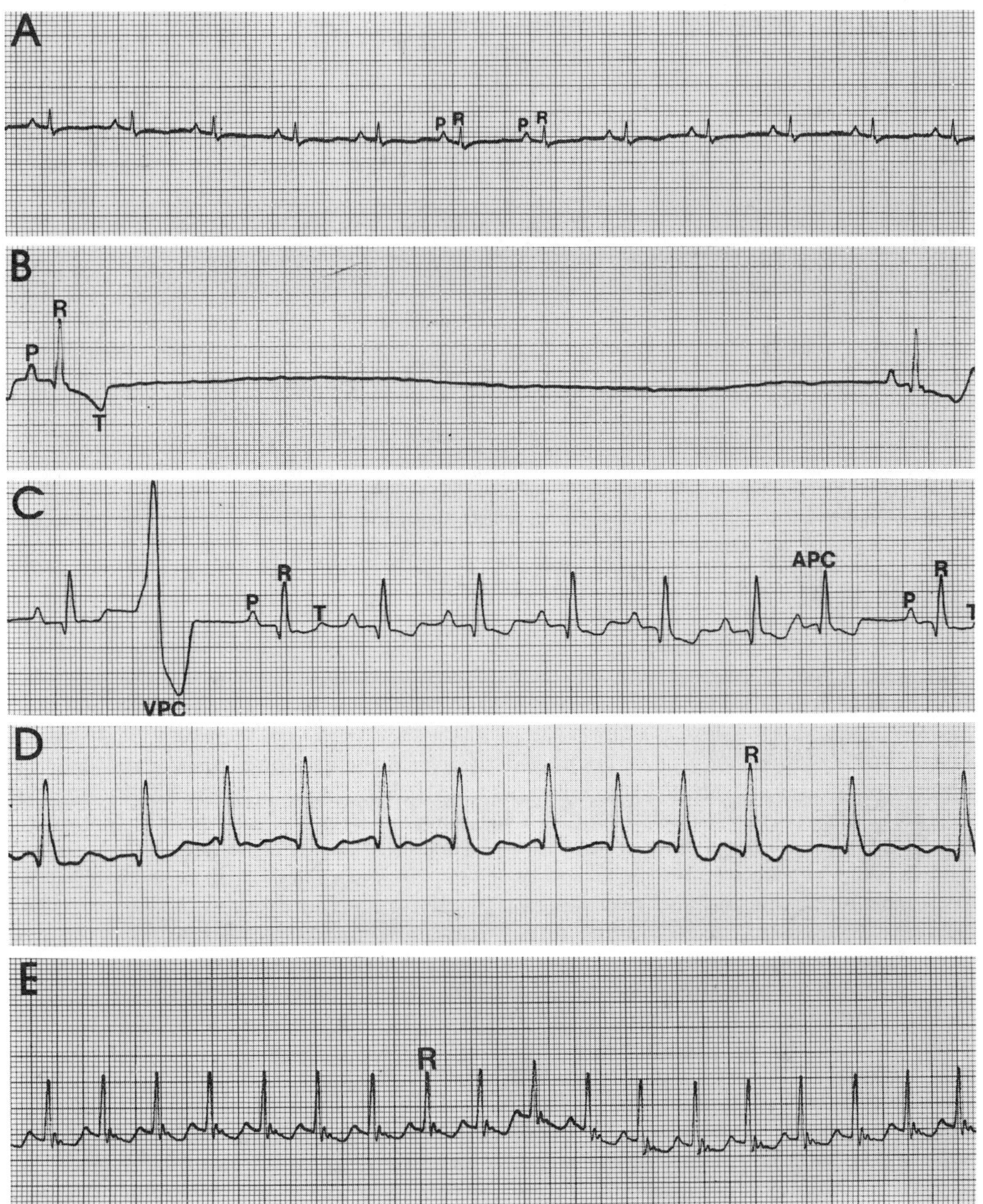

Figure 2. Common arrhythmias in the dog and cat. Lead II rhythm strips, paper speed of 50 mm/sec; 1 cm = 1 mv. *A*, normal sinus rhythm, cat; *B*, sinoatrial block (sick sinus syndrome), miniature schnauzer; *C*, atrial and ventricular premature complexes, dog; *D*, atrial fibrillation, dog; *E*, supraventricular tachycardia, cat with hyperthyroidism; *F*, ventricular tachycardia, dog; *G*, ventricular fibrillation, dog; *H*, second-degree AV block, dog; *I*, complete AV block, dog.

Illustration continued on following page

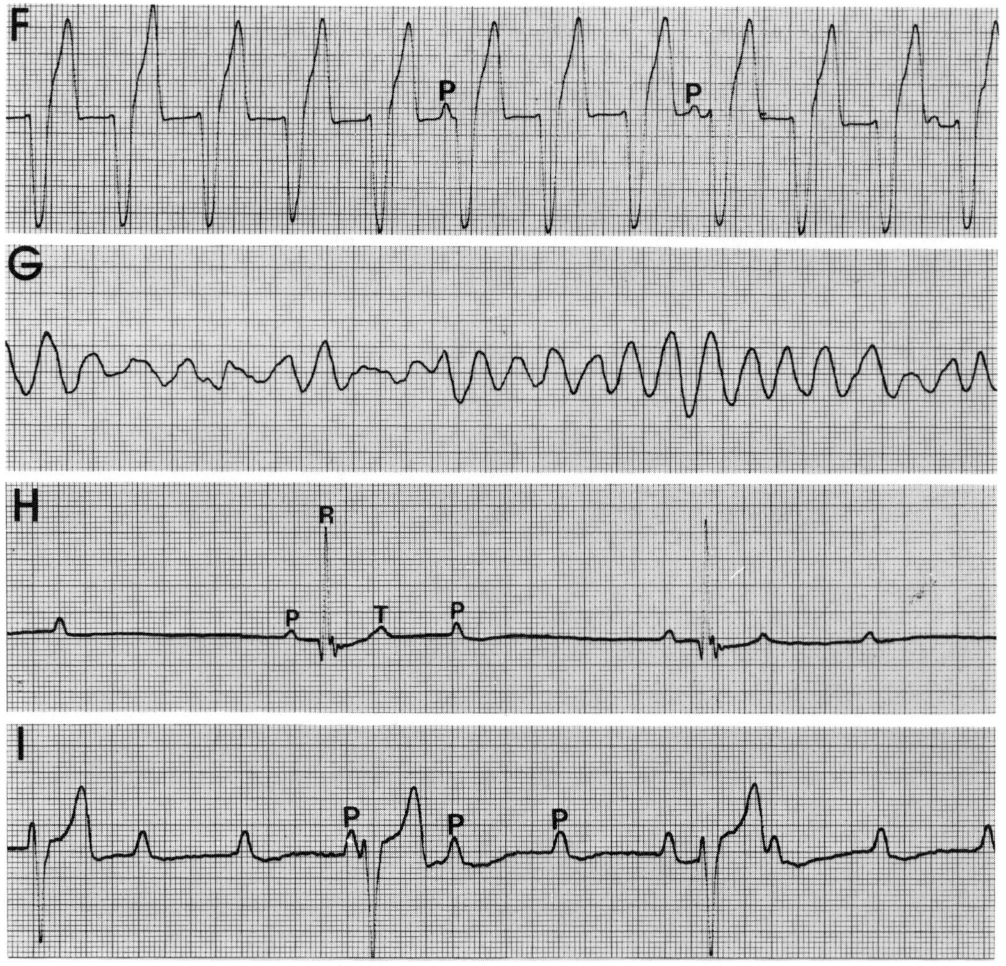

Figure 2. *Continued*

TACHYARRHYTHMIAS

Atrial Arrhythmias

Atrial premature complexes arise from ectopic sites in the atria. The impulses spread through the atria to the AV node, and they may or may not reach the ventricles. They are frequently caused by cardiac disease and atrial dilation and may lead to atrial tachycardia, atrial flutter, or atrial fibrillation. An atrial premature complex usually has an abnormal premature P wave followed by a normal QRS complex. Infrequent atrial premature complexes can be normal and do not require treatment. If this arrhythmia is associated with congestive heart failure, then digoxin and diuretic therapy are given. If the premature complexes are correlated with a poor hemodynamic status without congestive heart failure, then digoxin, propranolol, or occasionally quinidine or procainamide should be considered. Animals not responding to digitalization may benefit from the addition of propranolol.

Atrial tachycardia is a rapid regular rhythm originating from an atrial focus outside the SA node. Three or more consecutive atrial premature complexes are considered to be atrial tachycardia.

Atrial tachycardia is usually due to severe underlying cardiac disease, especially those conditions causing atrial enlargement. This arrhythmia may also be secondary to digitalis toxicity. In cats, the arrhythmia can be associated with hypertrophic cardiomyopathy, hyperthyroidism, and other types of systemic disease. Atrial (supraventricular) tachycardia can be associated with WPW syndrome.

Atrial tachycardia causes weakness, hypotension, and syncope. Immediate treatment is often required; however, it is important to distinguish atrial tachycardia from sinus tachycardia. Vagal maneuvers (ocular pressure or carotid sinus pressure) may terminate re-entrant atrial tachycardia. A vagal maneuver may also cause temporary AV block, as well as help in identifying atrial flutter waves. Edrophonium chloride (1 to 5 mg IV), for its vagal effects, is sometimes indicated if the usual methods of treatment fail to slow the heart rate. Intravenous digoxin may slow the ventricular response and improve the clinical status. Digoxin is contraindicated in hypertrophic cardiomyopathy unless the arrhythmia is absolutely uncontrollable. If digoxin is ineffective, IV propranolol or verapamil may convert atrial tachycardia to sinus rhythm. Both of these drugs are relatively contraindicated in the presence of heart failure. Quinidine gluconate, verapamil, lidocaine, or procainamide can be tried in dogs with refractory atrial tachycardia. Electrical cardioversion or intracardiac pacing may be attempted if the animal is critical and the arrhythmia uncontrollable. A thump delivered to the chest with a clenched fist can possibly be used to correct atrial tachycardia, especially in an emergency when resuscitative drugs and equipment are not available.

Atrial flutter is basically not different from atrial tachycardia, except for the atrial rate and the presence of flutter waves in atrial flutter. Atrial flutter usually occurs at rates greater than 300 bpm. The term *supraventricular tachycardia* is used when atrial flutter cannot be differentiated from atrial tachycardia. Atrial flutter is associated with the same conditions that cause the other atrial arrhythmias. The therapeutic approach for atrial flutter is similar to that described for atrial tachycardia and atrial fibrillation. The urgency of therapy depends on AV conduction and the ventricular rate, since fast ventricular rates usually cause hypotension or heart failure. Digoxin is usually the drug of choice for atrial flutter.

Atrial fibrillation is common in dogs, most often associated with severe underlying heart disease. The loss of the "atrial kick" combined with the rapid heart rate may substantially reduce cardiac output and cause congestive heart failure. A high number of disorganized atrial impulses bombarding the AV node are responsible for this arrhythmia. The ventricular rate is rapid and irregular. Instead of P waves, small or large oscillations (f waves) are present. Atrial fibrillation is rare in cats and is primarily associated with hypertrophic cardiomyopathy.

Underlying congestive heart failure must first be controlled. Digoxin is the initial drug of choice to slow the ventricular response. After approximately 2 to 3 days, propranolol may be added to further control the ventricular rate. The propranolol dose is increased slowly until the ventricular rate is adequately controlled. The lowest possible dose of propranolol will lessen the negative inotropic effects. Most giant breeds of dogs require a maintenance dose of between 20 and 40 mg of propranolol every 8 hours to maintain the rate below 140 to 160 bpm. In the future, longer-acting β-adrenergic–blocking agents such as nadolol (see Beta-blocking Therapy in Dogs and Cats) may be substituted for propranolol. Verapamil may represent another drug for slowing the ventricular rate. The antiarrhythmic drug quinidine may be useful in dogs in select situations for converting atrial fibrillation to normal sinus rhythm. Quinidine is usually effective if there is a normal-size heart and a lack of congestive heart failure. Lidocaine should not be used, since it may increase AV conduction and lead to an even more rapid ventricular response.

Ventricular Arrhythmias

Ventricular premature complexes (VPCs) are impulses that arise from an ectopic focus within the ventricles. They spread through both ventricles with delay, causing a bizarre, widened QRS complex. VPCs are the most frequent type of abnormal rhythm in dogs and cats. Physical examination usually reveals a pulse deficit during a VPC, as the cardiac output is temporarily decreased. A reduction in cardiac output is of greater significance when the animal has pre-existing heart disease or repetitive VPCs. There are numerous causes of VPCs, including primary cardiac diseases, secondary cardiac diseases, and drugs.

VPCs do not always require antiarrhythmic therapy. A medical data base including a thoracic radiograph, complete blood count and blood chemistry screen, and urinalysis is essential to rule out the secondary causes of VPCs. Specific supportive therapy may be required. Underlying congestive heart failure should be controlled with inotropic agents, diuretics, and vasodilator therapy. Indications for aggressive treatment include (1) frequent VPCs, greater than 20 to 30 bpm, (2) repetitive complexes or runs of VPCs, (3) multiform (multifocal) QRS configurations, (4) R on T phenomenon (vulnerable period for development of ventricular fibrillation), in which the VPC occurs during the Q-T interval of the previous complex, and (5) clinical signs of poor cardiac output (e.g., weakness, dyspnea, and syncope). Ventricular escape complexes should not be treated, as they represent a safety mechanism for maintaining cardiac output.

Antiarrhythmic drugs commonly used to control VPCs include intravenous lidocaine and parenteral or oral procainamide, quinidine, disopyramide, propranolol, and phenytoin (for digitalis-induced VPCs). Specific therapeutic guidelines are similar to those for ventricular tachycardia outlined below. New antiarrhythmic agents that are being investigated for VPCs include aprindine and amiodarone. VPCs rarely require aggressive treatment in cats, since they tend to decrease and often disappear spontaneously. Propranolol administered intravenously in small increments may decrease ventricular ectopic activity.

Ventricular tachycardia implies a series of repetitive VPCs that are usually of sudden onset. It may be intermittent (three or more VPCs in a row) or persistent (all complexes originating in the ventricles). Ventricular tachycardia is generally considered one of the most serious of all tachyarrhythmias. It is often associated with severe underlying cardiac disease. Ventricular tachycardia can be life-threatening; animals present with hypotension, syncope, seizures, shock, or congestive heart failure. Some animals with ventricular tachycardia may show no clinical signs, especially if there is no other underlying primary cardiac disease. This arrhythmia can be electrically unstable and may lead to ventricular fibrillation and sudden death.

Antiarrhythmic therapy is required in most animals with ventricular tachycardia. Exceptions include animals with severe acid-base or electrolyte imbalances, which may respond to specific electrolyte and fluid therapy. Antiarrhythmic therapy is not required in complete heart block, in which the ventricular rhythm may be an escape mechanism.

Lidocaine hydrochloride without epinephrine (2 to 3 mg/kg) via slow IV administration is the initial treatment of choice in dogs. Lidocaine must be used with extreme caution in cats (0.5 mg/kg slowly IV) since they are particularly susceptible to its neurotoxic effects. Hypotension may also occur if the bolus is given too rapidly in dogs or cats. The lidocaine bolus may have to be repeated several times at 10- to 15-minute intervals. A maximum total dose of 8 mg/kg over 10 minutes is advised in dogs. Since the therapeutic effects of lidocaine are short-lived, a constant-rate infusion for 1 to 3 days may be required for a continued antiarrhythmic effect. Alternately, intramuscular or oral therapy with procainamide or quinidine may be started and the lidocaine infusion slowly reduced over a 24- to 48-hour period. Synchronized electrical cardioversion is indicated when the animal is in a hemodynamic crisis and when lidocaine fails.

When treatment with lidocaine is not indicated or practical, quinidine or procainamide may be used to control the arrhythmia. An initial loading dose of 12 to 20 mg/kg, IM, followed by repeat doses of 4- to 6-hour intervals at 6 to 12 mg/kg may be effective. Oral quinidine or procainamide can be given as a maintenance dose once the arrhythmia is initially controlled. Other antiarrhythmic drugs that may be useful include disopyramide, propranolol, phenytoin, and aprindine.

The ECG must be monitored at frequent intervals. If the arrhythmia increases in severity, inadequate drug dosage as well as possible drug toxicity must be considered. Procainamide or quinidine toxicity can sometimes induce multiform ventricular tachycardia. Combinations of drugs such as procainamide and quinidine, procainamide and propranolol, or adding diazepam may be indicated if the arrhythmia is refractory.

Many animals with controlled ventricular arrhythmias only require therapy for 1 to 3 weeks. If ventricular ectopic activity is low on recheck ECGs, the daily drug dosage should not be changed unless there are associated clinical signs. If weekly checkups show no evidence of recurrent ventricular ectopic activity, the medication can be discontinued. The ECG should be re-evaluated in 1 to 2 days. Another approach is to decrease the dose by 50 per cent and then evaluate the ECG in a few days.

MANAGEMENT OF CARDIAC ARRHYTHMIAS WITH CARDIAC ARREST

Cardiac arrest is an emergency in which there is a sudden lack of effective myocardial contractions. The ventricles are unable to pump enough blood to maintain perfusion of the body's vital organs. Cardiac arrest can be correlated by ECG with (1) ventricular flutter or fibrillation, (2) ventricular asystole, or (3) electric-mechanical dissociation. Many factors can predispose an animal to cardiac arrest, including a wide variety of chronic and acute cardiovascular conditions. Pertinent references should be consulted for further information (see *Current Veterinary Therapy VIII*).

To effectively manage a cardiac arrest, the clinician must follow seven steps, but before these are done, the diagnosis of cardiac arrest must be established and a decision made as to whether the animal should be resuscitated. Necessary equipment and drugs should be organized and set up in advance to be ready for emergencies. Drug dosages and protocols should be posted in plain view.

Seven Steps in Resuscitation

The first five steps in the management of cardiac arrest represent the "A-B-C-D-E" of resuscitation. The sixth step is treating the arrhythmia. The seventh and final step is managing the animal after resuscitation.

Step 1. A—Airway
Step 2. B—Breathing
Step 3. C—Cardiac massage or circulation
Step 4. D—Drug therapy

Rapid establishment of an airway, positive pressure ventilation, oxygen, and an IV line are important aspects of cardiac resuscitation. The objectives of drug therapy during cardiac arrest are, first, to increase blood flow to the coronary arteries and brain, and second, to minimize the adverse effects of metabolic acidosis secondary to inadequate tissue perfusion.

The essential drugs used in cardiac arrest include oxygen, sodium bicarbonate, epinephrine, atropine sulfate, lidocaine, and calcium chloride. Other useful drugs include vasoactive drugs (e.g., levarterenol), corticosteroids, dopamine, diuretics, and procainamide. Sodium bicarbonate is used to prevent metabolic acidosis from lowering the threshold of the heart to ventricular fibrillation. Lidocaine has been shown to increase the threshold for ventricular fibrillation.

Step 5. E—Electrocardiogram

An ECG should be obtained to diagnose the arrhythmia responsible for the cardiac arrest—usually this is ventricular fibrillation or ventricular asystole.

Ventricular asystole represents no impulses generated from atrial or ventricular pacemakers. There is no cardiac rate or ventricular rhythm. Treatment involves the use of sodium bicarbonate, epinephrine, calcium chloride, atropine sulfate, and dopamine hydrochloride. Direct-current shock may convert asystole to ventricular fibrillation.

Ventricular fibrillation is the most common rhythm in cardiac arrest and is the arrhythmia most likely to respond to therapy. Electrical defibrillation is the initial treatment of choice. If defibrillation is unsuccessful, the animal should receive sodium bicarbonate, epinephrine, and lidocaine therapy. This should be followed by a second attempt at defibrillation. Other antiarrhythmic agents such as procainamide may also be used. Before further defibrillation attempts, the protocol should be proper oxygenation, correction of severe acidosis and electrolyte abnormalities, and attempts to determine and correct any other possible underlying cause. An effective method may be by pharmacologic defibrillation, a mixture of 1.0 mEq potassium/kg body weight and 6.0 mg acetylcholine/kg body weight by intracardiac injection.

Step 6. Treatment of arrhythmia

Step 7. Postcardiac resuscitation support

Sick Sinus Syndrome

Sick sinus syndrome is a term given to a number of ECG abnormalities of the SA node, including (in both dogs and humans) severe sinus bradycardia and severe SA block or sinus arrest. Many cases with these ECG abnormalities have recurrent episodes of supraventricular tachycardias in addition to an underlying slow SA rhythm. The clinical manifestations of the sick sinus syndrome are quite variable. Heart rates may be so slow as to reduce cardiac output and cause cardiac failure, but the most common clinical signs are syncope and weakness. Miniature schnauzers appear to be genetically prone to sick sinus syndrome.

If the animal is asymptomatic or has only minimal clinical signs, treatment is not necessary. Drug therapy (e.g., atropine) alone is usually unsuccessful since the drug for treatment of the tachyarrhythmia component (digoxin or propranolol) is harmful to or aggravates the bradyarrhythmia component and vice versa. There is usually a lack of long-term therapeutic effect of pharmacologic agents (e.g., atropine or propantheline) used for the bradyarrhythmia. The treatment of choice is a permanent ventricular demand artificial pacemaker. After implantation of the pacemaker, antiarrhythmic agents can be safely used if required. The drugs indicated are similar to the recommendations for the various tachyarrhythmias not associated with sick sinus syndrome.

Ventricular Pre-excitation (WPW Syndrome)

Ventricular pre-excitation occurs when impulses originating in the SA node or atrium activate a portion of the ventricles prematurely through an accessory pathway. SA impulses are able to reach the ventricles initially without going through the AV node. The WPW syndrome consists of ventricular pre-excitation with episodes of paroxysmal supraventricular tachycardia. The paroxysmal tachycardias associated with ventricular pre-excitation (WPW syndrome) can be explained by a re-entry mechanism. An impulse traveling to the ventricles through the AV junction may turn around and reenter the atria through the accessory pathway. A reciprocal rhythm or electric circuit is thus established. This ECG abnormality is associated with hypertrophic cardiomyopathy, congenital cardiac disease, and in some animals as an isolated congenital defect.

Ventricular pre-excitation without tachycardia does not require therapy. The WPW syndrome with atrial tachycardia, atrial flutter, or atrial fibrillation may require conversion. Ocular or carotid sinus pressure can sometimes be effective. Cardiac drugs, including propranolol, digitalis, lidocaine, quinidine, and procainamide, have been used. Calcium blocking agents (see Calcium Antagonists) can be effective. Encainide or amiodarone, new cardiac drugs, may be effective.

Some of the cardiac drugs listed previously can also be dangerous—for example, the use of digitalis for the treatment of atrial fibrillation in WPW syndrome. Digitalis glycosides may actually shorten the antegrade refractory period of the accessory pathway. Verapamil and propranolol would also be contraindicated, since they too reduce the refractoriness of the accessory pathway. The treatment of choice in such cases is either lidocaine or procainamide. Propranolol and digitalis glycosides are the drugs of choice in the therapy of regular reciprocating supraventricular tachycardia. The safest policy is to give neither digoxin nor verapamil to animals with WPW syndrome without a prior electrophysiologic evaluation of the risk of anterograde conduction.

References and Supplemental Reading

Miller, M. S.: Treatment of cardiac arrhythmias and conduction disturbances. *In* Tilley, L. P., and Owens, J.: *Manual of Small Animal Cardiology*. New York: Churchill Livingstone, 1985, p. 333.

Rosen, M. R., and Hoffman, B. F.: *Cardiac Therapy*. Boston: Martinus Nijhoff Publishers, 1983.

Somberg, J. C.: New directions in antiarrhythmic drug therapy. Am. J. Cardiol. 54:83, 1984.

Tilley, L. P. (ed.): *Essentials of Canine and Feline Electrocardiography. Interpretation and Management*. 2nd ed. Philadelphia: Lea & Febiger, 1985.

SYSTEMIC HYPERTENSION

LARRY D. COWGILL, D.V.M.,
Davis, California

and ANDREW J. KALLET, D.V.M.
Corte Madera, California

Systemic hypertension is a disease of considerable public awareness and clinical concern in human medicine but only recently has been recognized as a significant entity in companion animals (Cowgill and Kallet, 1983; Spangler et al., 1977; Welser et al., 1977). The clinician of companion animals is now obliged to recognize and manage arterial hypertension in both its silent and overt forms to ameliorate its destructive effect on susceptible target organs.

INCIDENCE AND SIGNIFICANCE

In surveys of clinically normal research dogs in controlled environments, the incidence of spontaneous arterial hypertension is less than 1 or 2 per cent. If these surveys are representative of the canine population, then primary hypertension is much less significant in dogs than in humans. The incidence of secondary hypertension has been examined in greater detail in dogs. *Renal disease* is the most frequent disorder associated with hypertension and has been documented to occur in 50 to 93 per cent of cases. This broad range undoubtedly reflects differences in the extent and nature of the associated renal diseases in the individual surveys, but it nevertheless confirms the significance of systemic hypertension in canine patients with renal injury. In our experience, greater than 60 per cent of dogs with renal disease manifest sustained hypertension independent of the severity or the nature of the renal lesion. On the other hand, 80 per cent of dogs with glomerular diseases are hypertensive and represent a significant risk population. Hyperadrenocorticism, diabetes mellitus, polycythemia, hypothyroidism, and pheochromocytoma are additional causes of hypertension in dogs.

Numerous epidemiologic surveys clearly document the morbid consequences of sustained hypertension in humans. Cardiac enlargement, heart failure, vascular disease, stroke, and renal failure represent the principal complications. The pathologic significance of hypertension in companion animals is not known, but the development and progression of renal and cardiovascular insufficiency is circumstantially evident. Necrosis, sclerosis, fibrinoid lesions, hyalinization, and capillary occlusion have been described in glomeruli of hypertensive dogs. Similarly, fibrinoid lesions, hyalinization, and myoarteritis have been observed in renal arterioles, promoting tubular degeneration and interstitial fibrosis.

Left ventricular hypertrophy is a consistent feature of renal insufficiency and is attributed in part to sustained hypertension in both humans and dogs. Cardiovascular stress induced by hypertension may cause ventricular dilatation, reduce cardiac reserve, and predispose the myocardium to ischemia and arrhythmias.

Retinal hemorrhage and detachments are less frequent but overt manifestations of hypertension that require immediate medical intervention. Hypertensive retinopathy or acute onset of blindness secondary to retinal detachment or hemorrhage may be the only sign of hypertension in lieu of routine blood pressure measurements. A comprehensive classification system for canine hypertensive retinopathy has not been established despite the development of characteristic retinal changes. Increased vascular tortuosity is an early lesion, but it progresses with the extent and severity of the hypertension to accelerated retinal hemorrhage, swelling of the optic nerve head, perivasculitis, and diffuse intraocular hemorrhage. The presence of these changes documents the clinical relevance of the hypertension.

There is little information available about companion animals to directly correlate hypertension-induced changes in renal, cardiac, or other target organ morphology with changes in their respective organ function. Until this information is available, it is reasonable to regard sustained arterial hypertension as a harmful and organ-destructive process, as confirmed in humans. The resultant arteriosclerosis, glomerular and tubular atrophy, and nephrosclerosis should be regarded as significant factors eroding residual renal mass, cardiac reserve, and other target organ function.

DIAGNOSIS

Animals at high risk for the development of arterial hypertension or those presented for acute blindness, ocular hemorrhage, retinal detachment, epistaxis, or abnormal neurologic function should have blood pressure measurements included in their diagnostic plan.

Systemic hypertension is diagnosed by measurement of a sustained and reproducible increase in systolic or diastolic arterial pressure in a patient not otherwise stressed, excited, or apprehensive. Arterial pressures can be obtained by a variety of direct or indirect techniques. Direct measurements are easily performed on dogs and tolerant cats by percutaneous puncture of the femoral artery with 25- to 23-gauge needles connected to appropriate pressure-sensing and recording equipment (Cowgill and Kallet, 1983; Kittleson and Olivier, 1983). This technique provides accurate, sensitive, and reproducible results. Indirect and noninvasive measurements of systemic blood pressure can be obtained in either dogs or cats by ultrasonic Doppler or, in dogs, by oscillometric techniques. Both techniques use inflatable cuffs to generate the blood pressure information. The size and placement of the cuff are critical for consistent and reliable measurements, but with experience and careful technique, accurate results are obtainable (Weiser et al., 1977; Spangler et al., 1977; Kittleson and Olivier, 1983). Indirect techniques eliminate pain-induced artifacts and are noninvasive. They offer ease and convenience for routine and sequential measurements of arterial blood pressure in clinical settings.

In our normal hospital population using a direct technique, average femoral arterial pressure in conscious dogs was 148 ± 16 mm Hg systolic, 87 ± 8 mm Hg diastolic, and 102 ± 9 mm Hg mean. These values are consistent with others reported in conscious or slightly sedated dogs, recorded with both direct and ultrasonic Doppler techniques (Spangler et al. 1977; Weiser et al., 1977; Kittleson and Olivier, 1983). Arterial hypertension is arbitrarily defined as when systolic or diastolic pressures are sustained in excess of 180 mm Hg and 95 mm Hg, respectively.

Normal values for arterial pressure in cats are less readily available. Measurements in unanesthetized cats using direct techniques yield values higher than those reported for dogs. In a study of 10 conscious cats, femoral arterial pressures were 171 ± 22 mm Hg systolic, 123 ± 17 mm Hg diastolic, and 149 ± 24 mm Hg mean (Gordon and Goldblatt, 1967). When the same cats were evaluated under anesthesia, the pressures were 5 to 10 mm Hg lower, documenting the influence of restraint, apprehension, and the tenacity of cats. The diagnosis of hypertension in cats, therefore, represents a more formidable problem and must be made cautiously in the absence of overt clinical signs. Systolic pressures greater than 200 mm Hg and diastolic pressures greater than 145 mm Hg in tolerant cats are surely abnormal and serve as guidelines for therapeutic intervention.

All animals in which arterial hypertension is documented should be given a thorough clinical evaluation to determine if it is primary or secondary in origin. The workup should include a complete history and physical examination, a complete blood count and biochemical profile (including blood urea nitrogen or plasma creatinine), and a urinalysis. Abnormalities in the screening profile must be pursued until a specific diagnosis is identified. Excretory urography, renal ultrasonography, arteriography or scintigraphy, or renal biopsy may be required to document a renal basis for the hypertension. Testing for hyperadrenocorticism, hyperthyroidism, hypothyroidism, primary hyperaldosteronism, pheochromocytoma, or diabetes mellitus may be required before primary or essential hypertension is diagnosed. All documented or suspected hypertensive patients should have a thorough ophthalmoscopic evaluation. Also, a cardiac ultrasound examination should be performed if the equipment is available to document the presence and extent of left ventricular hypertrophy.

TREATMENT OF ARTERIAL HYPERTENSION

Therapy for arterial hypertension should be formulated with an understanding of the benefits of therapy, patient risks, and pathogenesis of the disease. These concerns are ill defined in veterinary patients, and insights from human medicine must be applied until more appropriate information is available. Recent studies clearly document the reduced morbidity and mortality in humans when all degrees of hypertension are properly managed. The lack of significant coronary artery disease, risk factors related to lifestyle, and shorter life span may not allow the full pathologic expression of hypertension in companion animals. However, the available veterinary literature documents sufficient similarities in target organ susceptibility to warrant therapy when hypertension is diagnosed. At the present time, we recommend treatment of all animals whose sustained arterial pressures exceed the normal limits defined above. Since most patients have secondary hypertension, an aggressive therapeutic effort must be directed at the primary disease also.

Arterial hypertension develops when normal vasopressor and volume controls are deregulated, leading to an increase in cardiac output or peripheral vascular resistance. Logically, the management of arterial hypertension should abate the specific disturbances involved in its pathogenesis, but the underlying mechanisms are rarely identifiable or so compounded that a more generic therapeutic approach is required. Antihypertensive therapy thus consists of dietary salt restriction and a stratified drug protocol commensurate with the severity of the hypertension.

Dietary Sodium

The role of dietary sodium as a risk factor for the development of primary hypertension in a normal population is controversial. Its role in the development of hypertension in humans with renal insufficiency and its contribution to the maintenance of hypertension of other causes is firmly established, however. Consequently, moderate to strict reduction of dietary sodium intake is a mainstay of management strategies. This recommendation is particularly appropriate in dogs, in which renal disease is the most prevalent risk factor. Commercial dog foods contain sodium in amounts of approximately 0.5 per cent (dry food), 0.7 per cent (semimoist food), or 1.0 per cent (canned food), which are far in excess of the sodium requirements of dogs (Lewis and Morris, 1983). In hypertensive dogs, sodium intake should be reduced to 0.1 to 0.3 per cent of the diet to counter the tendency for sodium retention and expansion of extracellular fluid volume. A variety of the canine and feline prescription diets contain this amount of sodium in a range of protein contents that will meet the nitrogen requirements of normal, proteinuric, or azotemic animals. Animals with normal renal function should accommodate the dietary change readily, but the transition from a high- to low-sodium diet should be made gradually in patients with moderate or advanced renal insufficiency. The two diets can be mixed proportionally to effect a gradual reduction of the high-salt diet over a 2- to 4-week period. The patient should be closely monitored during this time for evidence of dehydration or progressive azotemia, and the sodium restriction should be stopped or tapered if these signs develop. Some reduction in renal function may be evident transiently in animals with renal insufficiency as the new sodium balance is established and blood pressure is controlled. In this case, careful monitoring of plasma creatinine is essential to prevent progression of renal damage. Because of the overriding significance of sodium balance and vascular volume in the pathogenesis of renal parenchymal hypertension, the use of salt supplementation to promote an increase in water turnover is strictly contraindicated. Salt supplementation will exaggerate the hypertension and accelerate renal deterioration.

Salt restriction alone will produce mild reductions in blood pressure. In mild cases of hypertension, this may be sufficient to regulate arterial pressure. In more severe cases, salt restriction is inadequate and the addition of drug therapy is required for pressor control.

Drug Therapy

Classic drug therapy for hypertension in humans consists of diuretics, sympatholytic agents, and vasodilators administered in sequence to provide pressor control. These drugs are targeted to counteract the volume overload and vasoconstriction perpetuating the hypertension, regardless of the underlying cause. Current drug strategies are empirical and are inadequately tested in dogs; however, similarities in the pathogenesis of canine and human hypertension warrant a treatment program similar to that used for humans.

Diuretics

Thiazide diuretics are used for the initial pharmacologic management of hypertension and should be initiated in all patients refractory to dietary salt restriction. These drugs provide mild natriuresis, reduction in exchangeable sodium and intravascular volume, and decreased peripheral vascular resistance. They potentiate the effects of salt restriction and prevent the salt retention inherent with other antihypertensive drugs. Either chlorothiazide (Diuril, Merck Sharp & Dohme) at 20 to 40 mg/kg every 12 to 24 hours or hydrochlorothiazide (Hydrodiuril, Merck Sharp & Dohme) at 2 to 4 mg/kg every 12 to 24 hours should be given in combination with dietary salt restriction. Blood pressure should be reassessed within 2 to 4 weeks of initiating therapy to ensure pressor control or the need for dosage modification.

Animals with moderate to advanced renal insufficiency (plasma creatinine greater than 4 mg/dl) may fail to respond to even maximal doses of thiazide diuretics. In these patients, furosemide

(Lasix, Hoechst-Roussel) given at 2 to 4 mg/kg every 12 to 24 hours should be substituted for the thiazides. Diuretic-induced potassium depletion, hypokalemia, and excessive extracellular fluid volume contraction are the most notable complications of diuretic use. Excessive volume contraction is more likely to occur when diuretic therapy is combined with strict sodium limitation and is corrected by appropriate lowering of the diuretic dose or moderation of the salt restriction. Hypokalemia is uncommon but can be controlled by dosage modification, addition of other antihypertensive drugs, or dietary potassium supplementation.

Adrenergic Inhibitors

If arterial pressure is not controlled by sodium restriction combined with diuretic administration, adrenergic inhibitors are added to the therapeutic regimen. These drugs act either centrally to decrease sympathetic outflow and catecholamine release or peripherally to block α- or β-adrenergic receptors and thus modulate the activity of the adrenergic nervous system.

In recent years, β-adrenergic antagonists have become popular as second-stage antihypertensive medications (see Beta-Blocking Therapy in Dogs and Cats). Their mechanism of action is complex and incompletely understood. No single mechanism adequately or completely explains their antihypertensive properties, but reductions in cardiac output, suppression of renin secretion, interference with central sympathetic outflow, and presynaptic blockade of neurotransmitter release have been proposed. Beta-blockers may be used as single agents in mild forms of hypertension but are most effective when combined with diuretics or other antihypertensive drugs. Propranolol (Inderal, Ayerst) is the prototype drug in this class. It is usually incorporated into the treatment regimen after salt restriction and diuretic therapy have been used, but propranolol may be included in the initial therapy of patients with severe hypertension. It is administered at a dosage of 5 to 20 mg each 8 to 12 hours in proportion to the patient's size but may be increased two- or threefold if the initial dose is ineffective. Serious side effects are uncommon. It must be used judiciously, however, in patients with pre-existing cardiac or pulmonary disease, because hypotension, bradyarrythmias, bronchospasm, and congestive heart failure may develop.

Prazosin (Minipress, Pfizer) is an α-adrenergic receptor antagonist that offers special hemodynamic properties and few side effects. It preferentially blocks postsynaptic adrenergic receptors on the vascular wall to produce vasodilation. The selectivity of its actions to the α_1-receptor prevents feedback release of norepinephrine and the attendant tachycardia and renin stimulation characteristic of nonspecific α-adrenergic receptor antagonists. Prazosin is indicated in both moderate and severe hypertension when diuretics or combination antihypertensive therapy is ineffective. The pharmacokinetics of prazosin and its toxicity have not been characterized for veterinary patients. However, this drug is being used with increasing frequency for the management of congestive heart failure in dogs. Therapy should be initiated at a dosage of 0.25 to 0.5 mg each 8 to 12 hours for small dogs and 1 to 2 mg each 8 to 12 hours in dogs heavier than 15 kg (33 lb). It should be routinely combined with a diuretic to prevent fluid retention. Prazosin may produce hypotension, ataxia, and syncope when first administered ("first-dose" effect), but these signs usually abate with continued therapy or dose reductions. At present, we use prazosin as a third-choice drug following diuretics and β-adrenergic antagonists; however, this order is by convention, and perhaps prazosin is more fitting as a second-choice drug after diuretics. Prazosin therapy, in our experience, is more effective than propranolol.

Centrally acting adrenergic inhibitors have gained widespread use and have demonstrated efficacy as antihypertensives in humans. Clonidine (Catapres, Boehringer Ingelheim) and methyldopa (Aldomet, Merck Sharp & Dohme), the prototype drugs in this class, are effective and relatively free of overt side effects. Experience with these drugs in veterinary patients is too limited to provide specific recommendations, but they should be applicable to hypertensive states in dogs. Both drugs decrease cardiac output and peripherial vascular resistance as their major actions. Neither drug alters renal blood flow, and both are suitable for patients with renal insufficiency. Salt and fluid retention are major side effects that obligate their combination with a diuretic for long-term pressor control. Sedation is also frequently experienced in humans.

Vasodilators

Vasodilators represent the third traditional category of pharmaceuticals used to treat hypertension (see Vasodilator Therapy). Their use is generally reserved for patients refractory to other antihypertensive measures or those with severe elevations of blood pressure and accelerated target organ deterioration. Hydralazine, the prototype drug, works through direct but unknown intracellular mechanisms to relax arterioles and small arteries and reduce peripheral vascular resistance. In conjunction with its antihypertensive actions, hydralazine promotes reflex sympathetic increases in heart rate and cardiac output that require simultaneous β-adrenergic blockade and enhanced renin release and fluid retention that mandates simultaneous diuretic therapy. Hydralazine (Apresoline, Ciba) is given at a dosage of 1 to 2 mg/kg every 12 hours. Side effects include hypotension, nausea, fluid retention, and tachycardia. A lupus-like syndrome has also been described in humans.

A new generation of drugs that specifically inhibit angiotensin-converting enzyme (captopril, see Captopril Therapy in Dogs with Heart Failure), or block calcium channels (verapamil, see Calcium Antagonists) is reported to have effective vasodilatory properties in human patients with severe and refractory hypertension. These drugs offer new directions for therapy and may be of future importance in veterinary patients.

Hypertensive emergencies are rarely encountered but may be induced by the pressor episodes of pheochromocytoma, acute renal failure, or acute glomerulonephritis. Signs of retinal detachment or hemorrhage, encephalopathy, intracranial hemorrhage, or acute heart failure are indications for rapid correction of hypertension. IV injections of 0.25-mg boluses of acepromazine can be tried initially. If ineffective, the boluses may be repeated up to a maximum of 3.0 mg. If the response is inadequate, sodium nitroprusside (Nipride, Roche) can be infused by continuous IV drip at a rate of approximately 3 μg/kg/min. Dosages as large as 10 μg/kg/min may be used in refractory patients. In patients receiving antihypertensive therapy, a lower dosage may be effective.

References and Supplemental Reading

Cowgill, L. D., and Kallet, A. J.: Recognition and management of hypertension in the dog. *In* Kirk, R. W. (ed.): *Current Veterinary Therapy VIII*. Philadelphia: W. B. Saunders, 1983, pp. 1025–1028.

Gordon, D. B., and Goldblatt, H.: Direct percutaneous determination of systemic blood pressure and production of renal hypertension in the cat. Proc. Soc. Exp. Biol. Med. 125:177, 1967.

Kittleson, M. D., and Olivier, N. B.: Measurement of systemic arterial blood pressure. Vet. Clin. North Am. [Small Anim. Pract.] 13:321, 1983.

Lewis, L., and Morris, M. L., Jr.: *Small Animal Clinical Nutrition*. Topeka, KS: Mark Morris Associates, 1983, pp. 10–34.

Spangler, W. L., Gribble, D. H., and Weiser, M. G.: Canine hypertension: A review. J.A.V.M.A. 170:995, 1977.

Weiser, M. G., Spangler, W. L., and Gribble, D. H.: Blood pressure measurement in the dog. J.A.V.M.A. 171:364, 1977.

PERICARDIAL DISEASE

WILLIAM P. THOMAS, D.V.M.,
Davis, California

and JOHN R. REED, D.V.M.
Sacramento, California

Pericardial disorders constitute a small but important percentage of the cardiac diseases of dogs and cats. Pericardial effusion sufficient to cause cardiac tamponade is one of the more frequent causes of right heart failure in dogs. Clinically apparent pericardial disease is rare in cats. Most of the information that follows has therefore been derived from studies in dogs, but the principles of diagnosis and treatment are probably applicable to cats. Although the clinical signs of pericardial disease may simulate other cardiac and noncardiac disorders, the combined findings from physical examination and routine diagnostic tests are usually sufficiently distinctive to allow a tentative or definitive diagnosis to be made. Because pericardial disease may produce dramatic and life-threatening clinical signs, and because treatment of pericardial disease is very different from most other types of cardiac disease, it is important to understand the pathophysiology and clinical features of the common pericardial disorders.

Conditions reported to cause pericardial disease in dogs and cats are listed in Table 1. Pericardial effusion is by far the most common of the major categories, accounting for more than 90 per cent of the pericardial disorders encountered clinically or at necropsy. In dogs, pericardial effusion is most often hemorrhagic or serosanguineous, occurring secondary to cardiovascular neoplasms, especially right atrial hemangiosarcomas and heart-base tumors, and as an idiopathic hemorrhagic effusion, which may be self-limiting or recurrent. Hydropericardium (transudate or modified transudate) from the causes listed is common but is usually of small volume, and it rarely causes cardiac tamponade or clinical signs. The other causes of hemorrhagic and

Table 1. Pericardial Diseases of Dogs and Cats

Congenital disorders
Pericardial defects*
Peritoneopericardial hernia*
Pericardial cyst (?)
Acquired disorders
Pericardial effusion
Transudate (hydropericardium)*
Congestive heart failure
Hypoalbuminemia
Peritoneopericardial hernia
Exudate (pericarditis)
Infection—bacterial, fungal
Sterile—idiopathic, uremia, other infectious diseases
Hemorrhage (hemopericardium)
Neoplasia—hemangiosarcoma, heart-base tumor, mesothelioma, lymphosarcoma, other
Trauma—iatrogenic, external
Coagulation disorder
Cardiac rupture, especially left atrium
Idiopathic
Constrictive pericardial disease
Idiopathic
Infection—bacterial, fungal
Pericardial foreign body
Neoplasia
Pericardial mass lesion (with or without effusion or fibrosis)
Pericardial cyst
Neoplasm (see above)
Granuloma—actinomycosis, coccidioidomycosis

*Conditions that rarely compromise cardiac function.

exudative effusions are uncommon. Although classified for convenience, it is important to realize that considerable overlap exists between categories of pericardial effusion. For example, heart-base tumors and idiopathic pericarditis occasionally produce serous effusions with little blood, and pericardial masses usually coexist with pericardial effusion or fibrosis. Since recent work indicates that physical, chemical, and cytologic analysis of pericardial fluid is of *limited* diagnostic value in dogs, other diagnostic techniques must be employed to distinguish neoplastic from non-neoplastic effusions. The following discussion presents a pathophysiologic, diagnostic, and therapeutic approach to the most commonly acquired pericardial diseases in dogs and cats.

The most important physiologic effect of pericardial disease is reduction of ventricular compliance and limitation of diastolic ventricular volume. Depending on the rate of development and the ability of the pericardium to expand, variable volumes of pericardial fluid can accumulate before a marked increase in pericardial pressure and ventricular compression occur. Rapid development of pericardial effusion, sudden hemorrhage, or the coexistence of pericardial fibrosis allows cardiac compression to occur from smaller pericardial fluid volumes. For this reason, pericardial effusion volumes in dogs with cardiac tamponade (compression) vary widely, from as little as 150 ml to as much as 1800 ml in a large dog. Clinical signs are related to decreased left ventricular output (weakness, fatigue, hypotension, syncope) and systemic venous hypertension (jugular vein distension, hepatomegaly, ascites). Pericardial fibrosis (constrictive pericarditis) causes a similar restriction of ventricular filling but tends to occur gradually, with signs of systemic venous congestion and edema predominating. Although pericardial masses may produce clinical signs by space occupation and displacement, compression, or invasion of adjacent structures (e.g., cranial vena caval obstruction by a heart-base tumor), most masses cause pericardial effusion or fibrosis with signs identical to those of other origins. Importantly, in most cases myocardial contractility is unaffected by pericardial disease, with cardiac output limited by the decreased diastolic ventricular volume. Accordingly, inotropic therapy with digitalis glycosides is of little benefit and is not indicated in most patients with pericardial disease. Drugs that decrease ventricular afterload (arteriolar vasodilators) or preload (diuretics and venous vasodilators) are also of limited benefit if the pericardial disorder is not remedied. These drugs can cause hypotension or further reduction of ventricular filling and cardiac output, resulting in further fatigue, weakness, or collapse in dogs with cardiac tamponade. They should be used cautiously or not at all in such patients.

PERICARDIAL EFFUSION/TAMPONADE

Although a patient's history and signs depend partly on the cause of the disorder, most pericardial effusions in dogs are either neoplastic (mostly right atrial hemangiosarcomas or heart-base tumors) or idiopathic and hemorrhagic, and the signs are similar in most cases. The few available reports indicate that neoplastic and infectious causes are most common in cats.

Diagnosis

Pericardial effusion is most commonly diagnosed in large dogs older than 6 years, and males are more frequently affected than females. German shepherds appear to be particularly predisposed to both neoplastic and idiopathic hemorrhagic effusions. In most cases, no pre-existing conditions (except congenital pericardial disorders) predispose these dogs to pericardial effusion. With effusions that are small or develop gradually, pericardial pressure and ventricular diastolic pressure may be minimally elevated, resulting in little cardiac compression and no signs observable by the owner. Signs of illness develop when a critical pericardial volume and pressure are reached at the limit of pericardial distensibility. To the pet owner, this may appear to occur suddenly. Rapidly developing cardiac tamponade caused by left atrial perforation secondary to chronic mitral regurgitation; traumatic laceration or rupture of a coronary artery, great vessel, atrium, or ventricle; or sudden bleeding from a neoplasm, especially a hemangiosarcoma, can cause acute hypotension, weakness, dyspnea, collapse (cardiogenic shock), and sudden death. Most effusions, however, accumulate gradually, allowing development of the syndrome of cardiac tamponade over several days to a few weeks. Owners most commonly complain that the pet exhibits lethargy, fatigue or weakness, tachypnea, cough, abdominal enlargement, and syncope.

Small pericardial effusions may not be detectable by routine examination. The findings of physical examination are abnormal in most dogs and cats with cardiac tamponade, although abnormalities may be subtle. Larger effusions often result in diminished intensity of heart sounds and precordial impulse. In most patients, other auscultable abnormalities (murmurs, gallops, arrhythmias) are absent. Since soft heart sounds occur with other thoracic disorders and in many normal animals, diminished heart sounds are most significant when accompanied by physical signs of cardiac tamponade. These include a resting sinus tachycardia, systemic venous hypertension (visible or palpable jugular vein distention, central venous pressure greater than 12 cm H_2O), diminished cardiac output (palpably diminished femoral artery pulse, prolonged capillary refill time), and right heart failure (hepatomegaly, ascites). The presence of pulsus paradoxus, an abnormal respiratory variation in arterial pressure characterized by an exaggerated (greater than 10 mm Hg) fall in arterial pressure during inspiration, is highly suggestive of cardiac tamponade and is often palpable or recordable by direct arterial puncture in dogs with nearly normal respirations. If necessary, the dog's mouth should be held closed to encourage slower breathing and facilitate the cardiovascular examination. Central venous pressure can be measured directly by means of an 18- to 20-gauge, 15- to 25-cm jugular vein catheter connected to a water manometer. The triad of diminished heart sounds, diminished arterial pulses, and systemic venous distention is strongly suggestive of pericardial effusion with tamponade.

Although there are no pathognomonic electrocardiographic (ECG) features of pericardial effusion, several findings support the clinical diagnosis. Diminished QRS voltages are the most common finding. In dogs, QRS complex amplitudes less than 1.0 mV in all limb and thoracic leads are considered diminished. The normally low-voltage ECG complexes in cats make detection of diminished complexes nearly impossible. Nonspecific S-T segment deviation is seen occasionally. Electric alternans, mainly of the QRS complexes, is often detected in one or more leads in carefully recorded tracings from dogs. Although not a highly sensitive indicator, this finding is considered strongly suggestive of pericardial effusion in the appropriate clinical setting. Sinus rhythm is usually present; other arrhythmias occur infrequently.

As pericardial effusion accumulates and distends the pericardial sac, the radiographic cardiac silhouette becomes enlarged and spherical in shape, with loss of chamber contours. Although small effusions may cause no recognizable radiographic changes, in most cases of cardiac tamponade the heart is round in both views. Other findings, such as widening of the caudal vena cava, are variable and nonspecific. Pleural effusion from congestive heart failure frequently obscures the cardiac silhouette, preventing recognition of the typical spherical cardiac shadow unless the pleural space is drained by thoracentesis. Occasionally, a heart-base tumor may cause a visible soft tissue shadow or dorsal tracheal displacement over the cranial heart base. When the diagnosis remains in doubt after survey radiography, fluoroscopy can be useful in demonstrating markedly reduced motion of all but the heart-base region of the enlarged cardiac silhouette. Although rarely required, venous angiography can outline normal or small cardiac chambers displaced dorsally within the globular cardiac silhouette. Angiography may also outline intracardiac portions of atrial or heart-base tumors, displacement or distortion of normal structures by pericardial masses, or vascular blushing of heart-base tumors.

The most sensitive and specific technique for detecting pericardial effusion is echocardiography, which can identify even small, subclinical effusions. By M-mode or two-dimensional echocardiographic techniques, pericardial effusion appears as an echo-free space on both sides of the heart, between the pericardium and right and left ventricular walls. M-mode tracings usually cannot be used to distinguish idiopathic from neoplastic effusions. The two-dimensional technique, because of its ability to display anatomically familiar cardiac tomograms in real time, can detect and localize cardiac and pericardial masses in most cases and can usually distinguish soft tissue masses arising from the right atrium (hemangiosarcomas) versus those originating from the region of the ascending aorta (heart-base tumors). It is therefore the preferred method for distinguishing neoplastic from non-neoplastic effusions and for making recommendations regarding therapy.

The definitive diagnosis and *initial treatment* of pericardial effusion is by *pericardiocentesis*. The authors prefer the following technique: The patient, unsedated if possible, is restrained in left lateral recumbency on the x-ray table, ECG leads are attached, and the area over the right third through seventh intercostal spaces from the sternum to the costochondral junctions is clipped and surgically prepared. The right side is preferred to minimize the risk of puncturing a large extramural coronary artery. A 14- or 16-gauge 15- to 20-cm over-the-needle intravascular catheter (Angiocath, Deseret) is prepared by cutting two or three smooth side holes near the tip with a scalpel blade and attaching a 3-ml syringe to the needle. Lidocaine (1 to 2 ml) can be infiltrated into the intercostal muscles at the puncture site, if desired, and a small stab incision made through the skin. The exact site of entry is best determined from survey radiographs or echocardiograms but is usually between the fourth and sixth ribs just lateral to the sternum and near the cranial border of a rib. During continuous ECG monitoring, the needle-catheter is slowly inserted straight through the chest wall toward the heart while intermittent suction is applied to the syringe. When pericardial fluid is obtained, the catheter is carefully advanced over the needle into the pericardial sac. Intravenous extension tubing is attached to the catheter, and as much fluid as possible is removed by syringe. Sterile fluid samples are collected for chemical and cytologic analysis, but bacteriologic culture is performed only if cytologic results indicate possible infection. In dogs, the fluid usually appears hemorrhagic or serosanguineous. If there is doubt about the origin of a hemorrhagic fluid (pericardial versus intracardiac), samples of fluid and peripheral blood are centrifuged in microhematocrit tubes. In most cases, pericardial fluid does not clot, has a packed cell volume (PCV) different from that of blood, and has xanthochromic serum. If possible, we prefer not to alter the animal's position during the procedure to minimize the chance of catheter dislodgment.

Immediately after drainage, a single left lateral radiograph is obtained to check technique, positioning, and the presence of pleural leakage of pericardial fluid. Pneumopericardiography is then performed by injection of carbon dioxide (room air is satisfactory) equivalent to ⅔ to ¾ of the pericardial fluid volume removed, and radiographs are immediately obtained in right lateral, left lateral, dorsoventral, and ventrodorsal positions. The lateral views are most informative, and it is essential that both be obtained. The dorsoventral view, although less informative than the lateral views, is superior to the ventrodorsal view for outlining atrial and heart-base lesions. Although we consider two-dimensional echocardiography to be the superior technique for identification and localization of cardiac and pericardial masses, pneumopericardiography accurately outlines most cardiac masses, is practical to perform, and allows differentiation of neoplastic from idiopathic, hemorrhagic effusions in approximately 75 to 80 per cent of cases. Confidence in the study requires good technique (complete pericardial drainage, adequate gas volume, multiple views) and knowledge of the appearance of normal cardiac structures in each view (Thomas et al., 1984). If the study is adequate, residual gas is withdrawn (only if room air was used) and the pericardial catheter is removed. Maintenance of an indwelling pericardial catheter is probably only indicated for continuous or frequent drainage of infectious pericarditis.

Laboratory analysis of pericardial fluid will correctly identify chylous and infectious (bacterial) effusions. However, although heart-base tumors tend to produce effusions that are more serous than those caused by hemangiosarcoma and idiopathic pericarditis, reliable differentiation of these disorders is prevented by wide variability and overlapping ranges of protein content, red cell, and nucleated cell counts. Difficulty in identifying neoplastic cells versus reactive mesothelial cells also prevents reliable diagnosis from exfoliative cytology. The authors base most diagnoses, prognoses, and therapeutic recommendations on the results of pneumopericardiography and echocardiography (and, rarely, angiocardiography).

Therapy

A summary of our approach to the diagnosis and treatment of the most common types of neoplastic and idiopathic effusions in dogs is presented in flowchart form in Figure 1. If a mass lesion is identified as the cause of the effusion, three options are available. The most aggressive approach includes thoracotomy, parietal pericardiectomy, and attempted removal of the mass. We have had excellent surgical success with non-neoplastic masses (cysts, abscesses), limited success with heart-base tumors, and very poor results with hemangiosarcomas, which have usually metastasized by the time of surgery. We therefore advocate a more conservative approach to all but very small right atrial or right auricular masses. Although parietal pericardiectomy in all cases has been advocated by others, if no mass lesion is identified we recommend a conservative approach involving initial pericardiocentesis, follow-up examination for recurrence of effusion (radiography, echocardiography), and one or two additional pericardiocenteses, if necessary. In our experience, approximately 50 per cent of dogs with idiopathic hemorrhagic pericardial effusion will recover after one or two pericardiocenteses. The remaining 50 per cent recur within a few days, a few weeks, or as long as 4 to 5 years later. Although there are no data available from dogs and cats, the use of intrapericardial, parenteral, or oral corticosteroid treatment in anti-inflammatory doses for recurrent idiopathic pericarditis in human patients has been recommended by some authorities and should be considered for recurrent

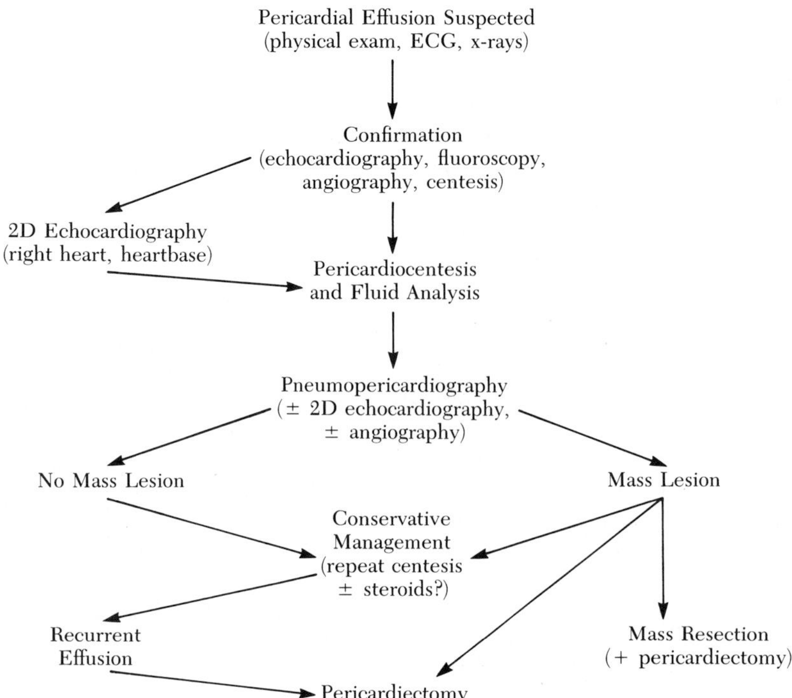

Figure 1. Flow chart of a diagnostic and therapeutic approach to pericardial effusion in the dog.

idiopathic effusions in dogs and cats. Idiopathic effusions and those caused by heart-base tumors usually develop gradually enough that a diagnosis can be made or recurrent effusion recognized prior to the development of life-threatening cardiac tamponade. In contrast, bleeding from right atrial hemangiosarcomas can be sudden, causing acute cardiac tamponade that requires emergency pericardiocentesis.

In animals with recurrent effusion that is idiopathic or secondary to a nonresectable heart-base tumor, subtotal parietal pericardiectomy ventral to the phrenic nerves is recommended. This can be performed by lateral thoracotomy or median sternotomy, depending on whether a mass lesion is to be removed. Partial pericardiectomy (pericardial window technique) is not recommended. Visceral (epicardial) pericardiectomy is unnecessary in most dogs. The results of parietal pericardiectomy are excellent in dogs with recurrent idiopathic effusions. Although the benefit is temporary, we have also had gratifying results in dogs with nonresectable heart-base tumors. These tumors, which are most often histologically identified as chemoreceptor tumors (chemodectoma, nonchromaffin paraganglioma) or thyroid carcinoma, tend to be slow growing, locally invasive, but slow to metastasize to other sites. Comfortable survival for as long as 3 years by dogs with heart-base tumors has been achieved by subtotal parietal pericardiectomy without tumor resection, making this a reasonable option for such patients. Because of the metastatic behavior and the potential for sudden bleeding of hemangiosarcomas, the authors have been reluctant to recommend pericardiectomy alone in affected dogs.

Results of other types of cancer therapy in dogs and cats with neoplastic pericardial effusions have not been reported. The authors have no experience with chemotherapy or immunotherapy in such patients. Radiotherapy of heart-base tumors has been attempted by others, but the results, although promising, have not been reported. In most veterinary hospitals, therapy of idiopathic and neoplastic pericardial effusions in dogs and cats is currently limited to pericardiocentesis, parietal pericardiectomy, and mass removal in some cases.

CONSTRICTIVE PERICARDIAL DISEASE

Restriction of diastolic ventricular compliance and filling is occasionally caused by pericardial fibrosis alone (constrictive pericarditis) or a combination of fibrosis and a small pericardial effusion (effusive-constrictive pericarditis). The authors have encountered dogs with pericardial constriction secondary to recurrent idiopathic, hemorrhagic effusion, presence of a metallic foreign body, infections (actinomycosis, coccidioidomycosis), and neoplasms (heart-base tumor, mesothelioma); it also occurs as a primary idiopathic disorder. Most commonly affected have been dogs of large breeds, both sexes, and older than 4 years. We have not diagnosed antemortem constrictive pericarditis in a cat.

The clinical signs of pericardial constriction are similar to pericardial effusion with tamponade. Owners' most frequent complaints are of abdominal enlargement, dyspnea or tachypnea, weakness or syncope, exertional fatigue, and weight loss, developing over several days to several months. Most dogs have no history of prior pericardial or other cardiovascular disorders. Occasional cases have been misdiagnosed as primary abdominal or liver disease and may have been subjected to exploratory laparotomy. Physical examination consistently reveals ascites and jugular venous distention or pulse. Diminished audible heart sounds are found in most dogs, and diminished arterial pulse strength in about half of the cases. Third and fourth heart sounds are not audible in most cases. In many of these dogs, pericardial effusion may be suspected on the basis of the history and physical examination.

Electrocardiograms show prolonged P-wave duration (greater than 45 msec) in most cases and diminished QRS voltages in about half of the dogs. Sinus rhythm is typical, but there is increased susceptibility to supraventricular tachycardia or atrial fibrillation. Thoracic radiographs most often show variable pleural effusion, mild to moderate cardiomegaly, variable degrees of rounding of the cardiac silhouette in one or both views, and widening of the caudal vena cava. Fluoroscopy shows diminished motion of the cardiac borders in most dogs, whereas angiocardiography is often normal or shows only dilation of the atria and vena cava and increased endocardial-pericardial distance along the border of the opacified right atrium or ventricle. Central venous pressure is consistently elevated above 8 mm Hg (10 cm H_2O) unless diuretic therapy has been aggressive. Echocardiograms will detect any pericardial effusion, but pericardial thickening is usually not recognizable.

In summary, constrictive pericardial disease should be considered in a dog or cat with signs of right heart failure (jugular distention, ascites, pleural effusion) not caused by other congenital, valvular, or myocardial disorders, especially when mild cardiomegaly, small ECG complexes, and increased duration of P waves are present. Reliable preoperative diagnosis of pericardial constriction requires simultaneous catheterization of the right and left hearts to demonstrate elevation and equilibration of atrial and ventricular diastolic pressures. The diagnosis is therefore difficult to establish in most veterinary practices. It is confirmed by surgical demonstration of pericardial fibrosis with little or no effusion and by relief of signs following pericardiectomy. Fibrosis is limited to the parietal pericardium in most cases, allowing adequate surgical treatment by simple subtotal parietal pericardiectomy without epicardial stripping, which is technically more difficult and is associated with a higher operative and postoperative mortality. Nevertheless, the authors recommend a median sternotomy surgical approach to maximize the surgeon's ability to examine both sides of the heart in case dissection of epipericardial adhesions or epicardial stripping is required. The most common postoperative complication has been pulmonary thromboembolism, but parietal pericardiectomy has been successful in about 75 per cent of dogs in which it has been performed.

PERICARDIAL MASS LESIONS

Most masses within the pericardial sac, including neoplasms, granulomas, cysts, and liver segments (peritoneopericardial hernia) cause pericardial effusion and are diagnosed by echocardiography, pneumopericardiography, or angiocardiography during evaluation of pericardial effusion. Occasionally, such lesions are suspected from abnormalities of the cardiac silhouette on survey thoracic radiographs obtained for other reasons or because of cardiac abnormalities detected on physical examination (muffling or displacement of heart sounds, jugular vein distention, heart murmur) or ECG (axis deviation, diminished voltages). In the absence of pericardial effusion, the diagnosis of a cardiac or pericardial mass requires special diagnostic studies. Two-dimensional echocardiography is the most sensitive and specific technique for outlining neoplasms, cysts, abscesses, and hernias involving the pericardial sac. Angiocardiography will usually outline intracardiac masses and can outline pericardial masses that are large enough to displace the wall of an opacified chamber or great vessel or produce a soft tissue shadow between an opacified structure and the border of the cardiac silhouette. Pneumopericardiography is also useful if there is enough pericardial effusion to allow insertion of a pericardial catheter. Treatment requires surgical exploration. Although a guarded prognosis is warranted in patients with intrapericardial tumors and infectious granulomas, most pericardial cysts, pericardial abscesses, and peritoneopericardial hernias can be resected or repaired and carry a favorable long-term prognosis.

References and Supplemental Reading

Berg, R. J., and Wingfield, W.: Pericardial effusion in the dog: A review of 42 cases. J. Am. Anim. Hosp. Assoc. 20:721, 1984.

Gibbs, C., Gaskell, C. J., Darke, P. G. G., et al.: Idiopathic pericardial haemorrhage in dogs: A review of fourteen cases. J. Small Anim. Pract. 23:483, 1982.

Lorell, B. H., and Braunwald, E.: Pericardial disease. *In* Braunwald, E. (ed.): *Heart Disease. A Textbook of Cardiovascular Medicine*, 2nd ed. Philadelphia: W. B. Saunders, 1984, pp. 1470–1527.

Owens, J. M.: Pericardial effusion in the cat. Vet. Clin. North Am. 7:373, 1977.

Sisson, D., Thomas, W. P., Ruehl, W. W., et al.: Diagnostic value of pericardial fluid analysis in the dog. J.A.V.M.A. 184:51, 1984.

Thomas, W. P.: Pericardial disease. *In* Ettinger, S. J. (ed.): *Textbook of Veterinary Internal Medicine*, 2nd ed. Philadelphia: W. B. Saunders, 1983, pp. 1080–1097.
Thomas, W. P., Reed, J. R., Bauer, T. G., et al: Constrictive pericardial disease in the dog. J.A.V.M.A. 184:546, 1984.
Thomas, W. P., Reed, J. R., and Gomez, J. A.: Diagnostic pneumopericardiography in dogs with spontaneous pericardial effusion. Vet. Radiol. 25:2, 1984.
Tilley, L. P., Bond, B., Patnaik, A. K., et al.: Cardiovascular tumors in the cat. J. Am. Anim. Hosp. Assoc. 17:1009, 1981.
Wagner, S. D., and Breznock, E. M.: Surgical management of pericardial and intramyocardial diseases including chemodectomas. *In* Bojrab, M. J. (ed.): *Current Techniques in Small Animal Surgery*, 2nd ed. Philadelphia: Lea & Febiger, 1983, pp. 470–475.

CANINE MYOCARDIAL DISEASES

WENDY A. WARE, D.V.M.,
and JOHN D. BONAGURA, D.V.M.
Columbus, Ohio

Heart muscle disease is commonly encountered in clinical practice. Myocardial disorders of dogs are the result of infection, idiopathic degeneration, trauma, neoplasia, inflammation, toxicosis, ischemia, and multisystemic disorders. The term *cardiomyopathy* has evolved to describe certain syndromes of myocardial dysfunction characterized by either reduced contractility, altered ventricular filling, cardiac dysrhythmia, or a combination of these problems. Both idiopathic (primary) and definable (secondary) cardiomyopathies have been described in dogs. These conditions are associated with clinical signs ranging from apparent good health to problems of mild disability, syncope, congestive heart failure, and sudden death. That myocardial injury may be overshadowed by disruptions in other body systems is axiomatic, for cardiac disease may be evident only at necropsy. Cardiac manifestations of multisystemic disorders are common, however, and the contribution of cardiac failure or arrhythmias to the overall status of the patient is being increasingly recognized by astute clinicians. The purpose of this chapter is to define the causes, diagnoses, and therapy of myocardial diseases in dogs.

TYPES OF CANINE MYOCARDIAL DISEASE

Primary Myocardial Disease

DILATED (CONGESTIVE) CARDIOMYOPATHY

Dilated cardiomyopathy is characterized by dilation and decreased contractile activity of the left and possibly the right ventricles. Atrial dilation is usually present. Large and giant breeds of dogs are most commonly affected, although smaller breeds can occasionally be involved. Doberman pinschers, Great Danes, Saint Bernards, Irish wolfhounds, boxers, Old English sheepdogs, and other large purebred and mixed-breed dogs are frequently affected. Dilated cardiomyopathy has also been reported in English cocker spaniels, schnauzers, and other smaller breeds. Males are affected about four times as often as females, and the average age of onset for both sexes is 4 to 6 years. Some dogs are affected at an early age (2 years or younger), but others are older.

The presenting signs often include weakness and lethargy, dyspnea, exercise intolerance, cough, anorexia, weight loss (which is often rapid in onset), abdominal distension (ascites), and syncope (Table 1). The cough is frequently nocturnal and may be described by the owner as gagging or choking. Other dogs with dilated cardiomyopathy are asymptomatic or simply appear off par to the observant owner.

Physical examination may reveal mucous membranes that are pale from decreased perfusion and peripheral vasoconstriction. Capillary refill time may be prolonged. Weight loss is usually accentuated along the dorsal midline, and some patients exhibit cardiac cachexia. Increased respiratory efforts may be present. Thoracic auscultation usually

Table 1. *Common Historic and Physical Findings in Dilated Cardiomyopathy*

Large dogs	Abdominal distension
Male > female	Syncope
Middle-aged	Increased bronchovesicular sounds/crackles
Weakness/lethargy	S_3 gallop
Dyspnea	Irregular cardiac rhythm
Exercise intolerance	Poor pulses/pulse deficits
Cough	AV valve insufficiency murmur
Anorexia	Hepatosplenomegaly/ascites
Weight loss	

reveals increased bronchovesicular sounds with or without fine inspiratory crackles. Percussion of the thorax may suggest pleural effusion. Jugular venous distension or pulsations are often noted, especially if right heart failure or tricuspid valve insufficiency is present. Hepatomegaly or splenomegaly may be detected by abdominal palpation, although with severe right heart failure, marked ascites may preclude adequate palpation.

Careful cardiac auscultation is essential. The heart sounds may be muffled secondary to decreased contractile strength or pleural effusion. A striking finding that is present in many patients is the rapid and irregular (rate and intensity) heart sounds of atrial fibrillation. Such dogs have pulse deficits with extremely irregular and weak femoral pulses. If the ventricular response is very fast (greater than 200 bpm), the rhythm may sound somewhat regular. Sinus tachycardia may be the predominant heart rhythm, particularly in Doberman pinschers and smaller dogs. Premature beats occur often and may be atrial or ventricular in origin. Apical systolic murmurs of moderate intensity (I–III/VI) can be heard in many dogs with dilated cardiomyopathy. These usually are caused by mitral or tricuspid insufficiency secondary to atrioventricular (AV) valve annulus dilation, altered ventricular geometry, papillary muscle dysfunction, or degenerative valve disease (endocardiosis). The majority of dogs with dilated cardiomyopathy, however, do not have severe endocardiosis. An S_3 gallop is usually present but may be difficult to identify when atrial fibrillation is present.

Radiographs characteristically show generalized cardiomegaly, although left ventricular and left atrial enlargement may predominate (Fig. 1). Cardiomegaly in some dogs may be so severe as to suggest a large pericardial effusion. Doberman pinschers often appear to have only left atrial enlargement without marked cardiomegaly (see below). Evidence of pulmonary venous congestion and increased pulmonary interstitial and alveolar densities, especially in the hilar and dorsocaudal regions, are suggestive of lung edema. If right heart failure is also present, pleural effusion, distension of the caudal vena cava, hepatomegaly, and ascites can be found.

When atrial fibrillation is the cardiac rhythm, the *electrocardiogram* (ECG) will show no P waves, a rapid undulating baseline (fibrillation waves), and a fast heart rate (often greater than 200 bpm) with irregularly spaced QRS complexes (Fig. 2). The QRS complexes may indicate left ventricular dilation by their height (R_{II} greater than 3.0 mV), or the complexes may be small (less than 1 mV), suggesting pleural effusion or concurrent hypothyroidism. Often the QRS complex is widened (greater than 0.06 seconds duration) with a "sloppy" R wave descent and ST-T coving; these suggest myocardial disease. Dogs in sinus rhythm often have widened and notched P waves (greater than 0.04 to 0.05 sec), indicating left atrial enlargement. These dogs may later develop atrial premature complexes or atrial fibrillation. Ventricular premature complexes (either unifocal or multiform) have been observed with sinus rhythm or atrial fibrillation.

Echocardiography is very helpful in determining the cardiac chamber dimensions and myocardial contractility of these dogs and for differentiating pericardial effusion from cardiomegaly. Dogs with dilated cardiomyopathy have the diagnostic features of significantly decreased fractional shortening (con-

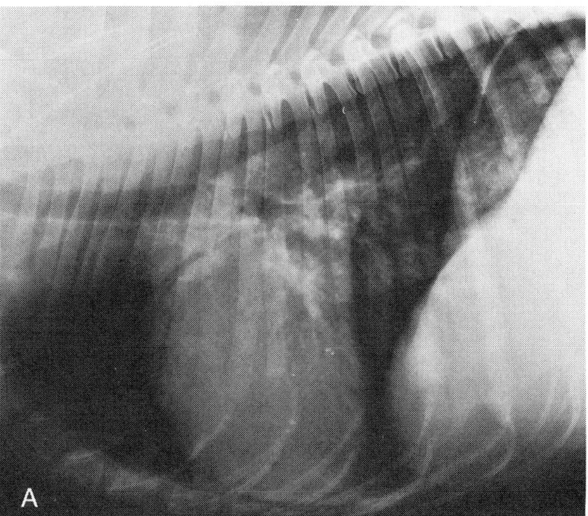

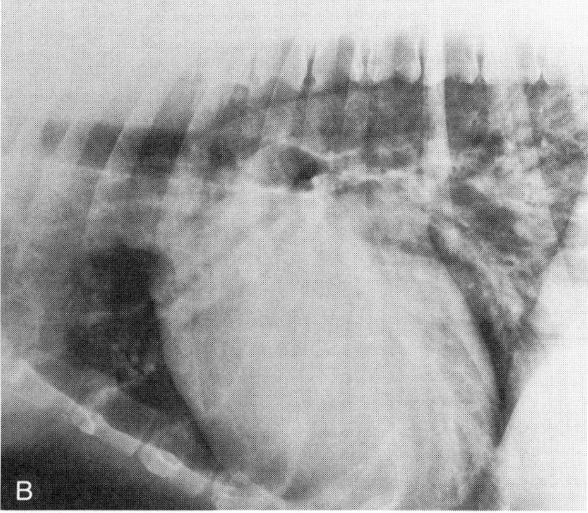

Figure 1. *A*, chest radiograph of a Doberman pinscher with dilated cardiomyopathy taken after diuretic therapy. Note the prominent left atrium. There is pulmonary venous congestion and mild hilar edema. *B*, chest radiograph of a Great Dane with dilated cardiomyopathy and congestive heart failure. Note the generalized cardiomegaly, pulmonary venous congestion, and pulmonary interstitial and alveolar edema.

tractility) of the left ventricle and left ventricular and atrial dilatation.

Clinical laboratory findings are usually noncontributory, although azotemia from decreased renal perfusion and mild increases in liver enzymes secondary to passive hepatic congestion may be found. Severe heart failure is also associated with hypoproteinemia and dilutional hyponatremia. Hypothyroidism, with hypercholesterolemia, has been found in some dogs with dilated cardiomyopathy.

The principal functional defect of dilated cardiomyopathy is *decreased systolic pump* function. As ventricular contractility deteriorates, cardiac output falls. There is also evidence of increased diastolic stiffness in dilated myopathic ventricles, and this contributes to increasing end-diastolic pressure and to venous congestion. As the ventricles dilate, papillary muscle atrophy may occur. Changes in ventricular size and geometry and papillary muscle function can lead to poor apposition of AV valve leaflets in systole, with resulting valve insufficiency. Some dogs also have degenerative valve disease, which causes further regurgitation of blood into the atria. All of these factors contribute to diminished forward pumping ability of the dilated ventricle, atrial dilation, and venous congestion.

Sympathetic, hormonal, and renal compensatory mechanisms are responsible for driving the tachycardia, increasing peripheral vascular resistance, and augmenting pulmonary venous pressure. With decreased forward flow, coronary perfusion may be compromised, leading to myocardial ischemia. The enlarging atria are predisposed to atrial arrhythmias, notably atrial tachycardia and fibrillation. Normally, atrial contraction contributes a significant volume of blood at end diastole, especially at faster heart rates. The loss of the atrial "kick" in atrial fibrillation can cause marked declines in cardiac output. The reduced forward flow may lead to signs of low-output heart failure as well as to congestive signs. The development of atrial fibrillation in dogs with dilated cardiomyopathy is one of the factors that leads to acute clinical decompensation.

At necropsy, dilation of all cardiac chambers with thickening of the subendocardium is common. Papillary muscles appear flat and atrophic. Dilation of

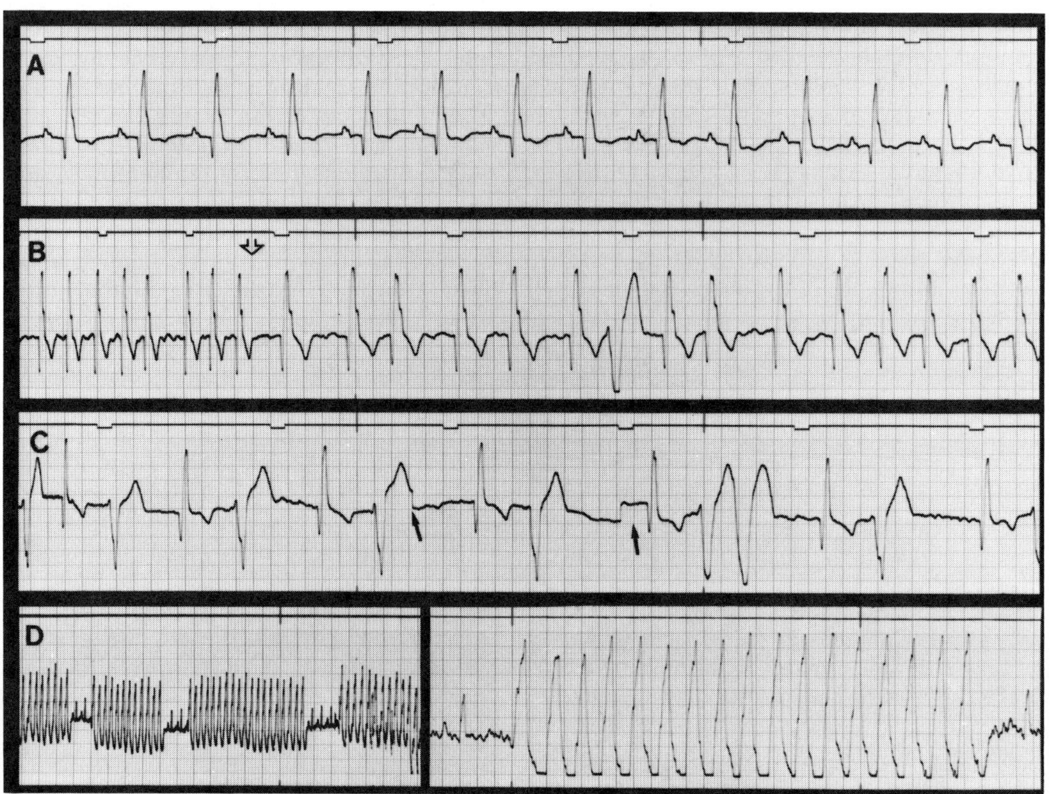

Figure 2. *A*, electrocardiogram (lead aVF) from a Doberman pinscher with dilated cardiomyopathy in sinus rhythm. The P-waves and QRS complexes are widened and sloppy. Note the slurred R wave descent. Paper speed 50 mm/sec, 1 cm = 1 mV. *B*, atrial fibrillation in a Doberman with dilated cardiomyopathy (lead aVF). Observe the irregular R-R intervals and undulating baseline with no P-waves. One VPC is present. The paper speed changes from 25 mm/sec to 50 mm/sec (open arrow), 1 cm = 1 mV. *C*, atrial fibrillation in an Old English sheepdog with dilated cardiomyopathy (lead II). Frequent VPCs (mostly in bigeminal distribution) are seen. Digoxin toxicity should be ruled out in this patient. Paper speed 50 mm/sec, 0.5 cm = 1 mV (calibration marks indicated by arrows). *D*, paroxysmal ventricular tachycardia of boxer cardiomyopathy (lead II). Note the upright configuration of the VPCs. Left panel is at 10 mm/sec, right panel at 50 mm/sec, 1 cm = 1 mV.

the AV valve annulus is common. Multiple small, pale areas of myocardial necrosis may be found, especially in the subendocardium. Histopathologically, scattered areas of myocardial necrosis, degeneration, and fibrosis may be seen, especially in the left ventricle. Inflammatory cell infiltrates and myocardial hypertrophy are inconsistent features of this disease.

The *prognosis* for dogs with dilated cardiomyopathy is generally guarded. Most dogs do not survive beyond 3 months after diagnosis; however, when the initial response to treatment is good, about 25 to 35 per cent of affected dogs will live longer than 6 months. Some dogs have done well for over 2 years.

BOXER CARDIOMYOPATHY

A type of primary myocardial disease that is different from dilated cardiomyopathy of other large dogs has been recognized in boxers. The cause of this disease is not known at present, but an inherited component has been suggested. Male boxers with this disease outnumber females. In Harpster's report, the mean age of onset was 8.5 years, with a range of 1 to 15 years.

Affected dogs usually are presented with a history of *syncope* and episodic *weakness*. Left heart failure or biventricular heart failure can occur as with dilated cardiomyopathy described above; however, many boxers are asymptomatic at the time of initial diagnosis. The most consistent clinical finding is the observation of a cardiac arrhythmia. This may be the only clinical sign in the asymptomatic dog. Signs of heart failure such as pulmonary edema, ascites, hepatomegaly, and pleural effusion may be noted.

The ECG usually documents an underlying sinus rhythm, although atrial fibrillation or other atrial tachyarrhythmias can occur. Ventricular premature complexes (VPCs) are characteristic (Fig. 2*D*) and occur singly, in pairs, in short runs, or in sustained ventricular tachycardia. Most of the VPCs appear to have a left bundle branch configuration (upright in leads II and aVF). Some boxers have multiform VPCs, and symptomatic (fainting) dogs are usually experiencing paroxysmal or sustained ventricular tachycardia. The sinus P-QRS-T complexes may be normal or show evidence of chamber enlargement. Radiographically, the heart and lungs may be normal or enlarged. If advanced muscle disease is present, generalized cardiomegaly and heart failure are found. Echocardiographically, these dogs may have normal to increased ventricular dimensions and normal to decreased contractility. Laboratory findings are usually normal. Mildly affected dogs and those with a history of syncope or weakness may proceed to develop congestive heart failure at a later time. Ventricular arrhythmias can be quite refractory to antiarrhythmic therapy. Many of these dogs die suddenly, presumably from an arrhythmia leading to ventricular fibrillation.

Necropsy descriptions of affected boxer hearts have noted mild left-sided dilation, degenerative AV valve changes, and occasional fibrotic areas in the myocardium and endocardium. Histologically, more extensive lesions are found in these dogs than in those with dilated cardiomyopathy. The most common findings are atrophy of myofibers, fibrosis, and fatty infiltration. Focal areas of myocytolysis, necrosis, hemorrhage, and mononuclear cell infiltration occur with regularity (Harpster, 1983). The prognosis for these dogs, especially if heart failure is present, is poor. Asymptomatic cases or dogs with easily controlled arrhythmias have a more optimistic future, but the chance of developing serious and refractory arrhythmias, congestive heart failure, or sudden death is high.

DOBERMAN PINSCHER CARDIOMYOPATHY

Dilated cardiomyopathy in many Doberman pinschers is clinically similar to the "classic" idiopathic cardiomyopathy encountered in large breeds. However, a number of affected dogs have primary myocardial disease with pronounced ventricular arrhythmias. Most of these dogs also have severely compromised ventricular contractility. The history and physical findings observed with these dogs are similar to those already described for dilated myopathy, but an acute onset of fulminant *pulmonary edema* is common (often with hemoptysis). Some of these dogs exhibit cardiogenic shock from low output, as well as congestive heart failure. Radiographically, the heart shadow may not appear to be greatly enlarged and only the left atrium may seem dilated (Fig. 1A). Pulmonary edema may be severe and diffuse, prompting a misdiagnosis of pulmonary neoplasia or pneumonia, particularly if the accompanying pulmonary venous dilation is overlooked. The ECG may show atrial fibrillation or sinus rhythm. Paroxysmal or sustained ventricular tachycardia, fusion complexes, and multiform VPCs all can occur. Fractional shortening measured by echocardiography is often less than 10 per cent (normal is greater than 28 per cent). Necropsy findings include ventricular dilation, atrial dilation, myocardial fibrosis, fatty infiltration, and myocytic degeneration. The prognosis for these dogs is guarded to grave, depending on the severity of the heart failure. Sudden death can occur.

HYPERTROPHIC CARDIOMYOPATHY

In contrast to its occurrence in cats, idiopathic hypertrophic cardiomyopathy is infrequently encountered in dogs. (Hypertrophy secondary to hypertension associated with renal disease is more common.) Again, males are involved more frequently than females. In one retrospective study (Liu et al., 1979), the mean age at death was 6 years although the range was from 1 to 13 years. German shepherds may be predisposed to hypertrophic cardiomyopathy. Most but not all of the reported dogs were of large breeds.

Signs of heart failure or syncope occur prior to death in some cases, but most dogs have no historic cardiac signs. *Sudden death* may be the first and only indication of heart disease. Complete heart block and other conduction abnormalities (first-degree AV block and fascicular blocks) have also been reported. Because of the infrequent recognition of this disease, little is known about the clinical course; however, it should be suspected in dogs with ejection murmurs and a history of syncope. Echocardiography appears to be the best way to diagnose the condition.

Severely reduced diastolic compliance may play a role in cases that develop left-sided heart failure (see Feline Myocardial Diseases). Myocardial ischemia secondary to severe hypertrophy and possibly reduced coronary perfusion associated with hypotensive episodes may lead to arrhythmias and death. The significance of dynamic left ventricular outflow obstruction is unresolved. Postmortem studies have shown increased heart weight as compared with those of normal dogs and increased septal and left ventricular free-wall thickness. Most affected dogs have asymmetric hypertrophy of the ventricular septum but, according to Liu, only 20 per cent have the marked myocardial cell disorganization characteristic of the human disease.

Secondary Myocardial Disease

INFECTIVE MYOCARDITIS

Many infectious agents can attack heart muscle. Some infections cause significant heart failure and arrhythmias, whereas others are clinically silent. Involvement of other organ systems may mask myocarditis, and evidence of infective myocarditis may only appear as the animal is recovering from the acute phase of the disease. Myocardial function may be permanently (and progressively) compromised even after recovery from acute myocarditis. Persistent cardiac arrhythmias may be sequelae to infection.

Viral Myocarditis

Except for canine parvovirus myocarditis, clinically significant viral myocarditis is rare in dogs. *Parvovirus myocarditis* has been encountered mostly in 4- to 8-week-old puppies. Usually this necrotizing infection has a peracute clinical onset, causing sudden death in apparently normal pups. Signs of respiratory distress may occur just prior to death. Milder forms of the disease occur and cause heart failure, arrhythmias, and death in puppies from 10 weeks to 6 months old. Pups with chronic myocarditis show increased pulmonary densities, cardiomegaly, pleural effusion, ascites, and hepatomegaly. Systolic murmurs, gallops, and arrhythmias are sometimes auscultated. At postmortem, cardiomegaly, pale streaks in the myocardium, and gross evidence of heart failure are common. Histologically, the left ventricular myocardium is most severely affected, with diffuse infiltrates of lymphocytes and plasma cells. Interstitial fibrosis, degenerative changes in myocytes, and basophilic intranuclear inclusion bodies all can be noted. The diagnosis can be confirmed by serologic and histopathologic tests.

Canine distemper virus can experimentally cause myocarditis in young puppies. Clinical infections are usually masked by the multisystemic signs of distemper. The histologic changes in canine distemper myocarditis are very mild compared with the inflammation caused by parvovirus.

Bacterial Myocarditis

Focal, suppurative myocarditis or abscessation can occur following bacteremia, bacterial endocarditis, or pericarditis. Hematogenous dissemination of bacteria can result from localized infection elsewhere in the body. Clinically affected dogs may show lethargy and weight loss. Fever may be present but is an inconsistent finding. Murmurs are usually not noted unless valvular endocarditis or an underlying cardiac defect exists. Arrhythmias or conduction disturbances are often detected on the ECG and form the basis for a tentative diagnosis. Serial blood cultures may be helpful in isolating the causative organism.

Protozoal Myocarditis

Chagas' disease, or trypanosomiasis, has been reported to affect young dogs in southern and western portions of the United States (Texas, Louisiana). The protozoan *Trypanosoma cruzi* is carried by various blood-sucking insects of the family Reduviidae. Amastigotes of *T. cruzi* invade the myocardium, causing disruption and necrosis of myocardial fibers and a mononuclear cellular infiltrate. Pulmonary edema, hepatosplenomegaly, and visceral lymphadenopathy may occur. Clinically, affected dogs have lethargy, depression, and possibly heart failure, arrhythmias, and sudden death. Various tachyarrhythmias have been reported, and AV conduction delay secondary to inflammation and fibrosis in the AV node and bundle of His has been produced experimentally. Serologic tests, as well as blood culture techniques, have been used to diagnose some cases antemortem. The disease also affects humans.

Rarely, toxoplasmosis (*Toxoplasma gondii*) infections can cause clinical myocarditis, particularly in immunosuppressed patients. The toxoplasma organism, after initial infection, encysts in various body tissues, including the heart. These cysts may rupture, expelling bradyzoites that cause hypersensitivity reactions and tissue necrosis. Immunocompromised dogs with chronic toxoplasmosis may be at risk for developing active disease, including significant myocarditis, chorioretinitis, pneumonia, or encephalitis.

Other Infective Myocarditites

Fungi (*Aspergillus, Cryptococcus*), algae (*Prototheca*), and rickettsiae may affect the myocardium secondary to causing systemic disease. Often, affected animals are immunosuppressed. The rickettsiae responsible for spotted fever (see Rocky Mountain Spotted Fever and Ehrlichiosis) can induce myocarditis and serious ventricular arrhythmias in dogs.

INFILTRATIVE MYOCARDIOPATHIES

Tumors can invade the heart; examples include right atrial hemangiosarcoma, aortic or carotid body tumors, ectopic thyroid carcinomas, and other sarcomas. Occasionally, metastatic tumors infiltrate the myocardium. Generally the location of the tumor determines the clinical signs, and right heart failure (inflow obstruction), arrhythmias, conduction blocks (AV block), and pericardial effusion (see Pericardial Disease) are observed most commonly. Amyloidosis of the myocardium is quite rare in dogs and, when it occurs, is usually overshadowed by signs of infiltration in other organs, especially the kidney.

TOXIC MYOCARDIOPATHIES

Various substances have the potential for significant depression of myocardial function. These include the "myocardial depressant factors" of shock, acute pancreatitis, and the gastric dilatation-volvulus complex. Electrolyte abnormalities, especially hypocalcemia, hypophosphatemia, and hyperkalemia, can cause deterioration of cardiac cell function and lead to death from heart failure.

Doxorubicin (Adriamycin, Adria Labs) is a commonly used drug in the chemotherapy of various neoplasms; it has both acute and chronic effects on the myocardium. The acute effects of decreased left ventricular filling and decreased cardiac output appear to be mediated by histamine and secondary catecholamine release. With chronic administration (cumulative doses as low as 100 mg/m^2 but usually greater than 160 mg/m^2), a progressive myocardial degeneration develops with a clinical picture similar to dilated cardiomyopathy of large dogs. This cardiomyopathy can be difficult to manage and may continue to worsen despite cessation of doxorubicin therapy. Other toxic effects of doxorubicin include bundle branch blocks, infranodal AV conduction blocks, and ventricular arrhythmias.

Ethyl alcohol, especially when administered IV in the therapy of ethylene glycol intoxication, can cause severe myocardial depression and death. Dilution to at least 20 per cent should be used, and the drug should be administered slowly. Anesthetic drugs similarly can cause significant myocardial depression. Other toxins, including cobalt and certain plants (taxus, foxglove, buttercups, and black locust), can all cause myocardial depression if ingested in sufficient quantities.

Certain metabolic diseases interfere with myocardial function. These include the *endocrinopathies* diabetes mellitus (leading to vascular abnormalities) and hypothyroidism (leading to decreased myocardial contractility and possibly to coronary atherosclerosis and its sequelae). *Chronic uremia* may have deleterious effects on the heart, as can renal glomerular disease that causes hypertension and secondary myocardial hypertrophy. It is not known if nutritional deficiencies (vitamin E, selenium) play a role in the myocardiopathies of dogs.

OTHER CAUSES OF MYOCARDIAL DYSFUNCTION

Although the type of major coronary artery disease so prevalent in humans is infrequent in dogs, intramyocardial coronary artery disease may be more common than generally recognized. Chronic degenerative valve disease (endocardiosis) has been associated with hyalinization of vessels and microscopic intramural myocardial infarctions (MIMI). Severe hypothyroidism may lead to atherosclerotic lesions and myocardial hypoxia.

The authors have recognized occasional canine cases of acute *myocardial infarction*, characterized by acute onset of depression, pulmonary edema and dyspnea, and dramatic ST-T changes in the ECG (greater than 5 mm S-T segment deviation). Myocardial infarctions can also result from emboli of septic, neoplastic, or thrombotic diseases.

Genetic diseases such as *muscular dystrophy* of the fasciohumoral type (springer spaniels) may cause atrial standstill and heart failure. *Traumatic myocarditis* either from penetrating wounds or blunt trauma can result in persistent sinus tachycardia, S-T segment deviation, serious ventricular arrhythmias, myocardial dysfunction, and death. The "brain-heart" syndrome of myocardial and subendocardial hemorrhage and necrosis subsequent to excess adrenergic stimulation is caused by brain injury and can lead to significant ventricular arrhythmias. Immunologic mechanisms may play a role in some types of myocarditis (English bulldogs?), and there is some evidence that idiopathic dilated cardiomyopathy may have an autoimmune component.

TREATMENT OF CANINE MYOCARDIAL DISEASES

THERAPY OF DILATED CARDIOMYOPATHY

Goals of therapy include management of congestive heart failure, enhancement of cardiac contractility and cardiac output, reduction of heart rate if atrial fibrillation is present, and control of cardiac arrhythmias.

Initial Therapy

Most dogs are presented with some degree of congestive heart failure. The clinician must assess the severity of the failure and treat with appropriate aggressiveness, realizing that the clinical condition of an individual patient is not static and can deteriorate rapidly. Frequent evaluation of lung sounds, respiration rate and character, pulses, heart rate and rhythm, peripheral perfusion, rectal temperature, hydration, body weight, and mentation are necessary to manage the dog properly.

In some cases, the clinician should postpone certain diagnostic tests (e.g., radiographs, blood studies) until the condition of the dog is no longer critical. In those cases, IV or IM furosemide (Lasix [Hoechst-Roussel] 2 to 4 mg/kg), 2 per cent nitroglycerin ointment (Nitrol [Rorer], Nitro-Bid [Marion] ¼ to 1 inch cutaneously every 6 to 8 hours), aminophylline (4 to 8 mg/kg IM), oxygen therapy (40 to 50 per cent), and cage rest with or without morphine (0.2 to 0.3 mg/kg SC or IM) may help stabilize the dog and allow further diagnostic tests (Table 2).

The therapy of dilated cardiomyopathy includes inotropic support and generally involves digitalization. Digoxin (Lanoxin [Burroughs Wellcome] or Cardoxin [RAFA]) is most often used at a maintenance dose of 0.01 to 0.015 mg/kg PO divided twice daily. Some large dogs (especially Doberman pinschers) are very sensitive to this drug and develop toxicity at surprisingly low doses. We generally do not use maintenance doses of more than 0.5 mg/day in any large dog, and we use less in Dobermans (0.375 mg/day or less). When atrial fibrillation results in a heart rate of greater than 230 bpm, IV digitalization (0.01 to 0.02 mg/kg in 2 to 4 divided doses, given over 4 hours) or twice the oral maintenance dose of digoxin is given the first day to achieve effective blood levels more quickly. Electrolyte levels and blood urea nitrogen (BUN)/creatinine should be monitored periodically, as hypokalemia and azotemia can predispose to digoxin toxicity. If occasional isolated VPCs are present, the ECG should be carefully monitored for worsening of the arrhythmia as the patient becomes digitalized. If multiple VPCs (greater than 25/min) or repetitive VPCs (ventricular tachycardia) are diagnosed, digitalis glycosides are withheld until the VPCs are controlled with antiarrhythmic drugs. If a ventricular antiarrhythmic drug is needed and will be used with digoxin, it is best to use lidocaine (see Antiarrhythmic Drugs and Management of Cardiac Arrhythmias) or procainamide (6 to 20 mg/kg every 6 to 8 hours IM or PO) and to avoid quinidine, which can increase serum digoxin levels. Serum digoxin concentrations are helpful in assessing therapeutic

Table 2. *Therapy of Dilated Cardiomyopathy*

Initial therapy	
Diuretic drug	Furosemide*
Oxygen and cage rest	
Inotropic support	Digoxin* Dobutamine or dopamine Amrinone or milrinone
Vasodilator	Nitroglycerin
Bronchodilator	Aminophylline
Other therapy	Morphine
Maintenance therapy	
Diuretics	Furosemide* Hydrochlorothiazide Spironolactone
Inotropic support	Digoxin* or digitoxin Milrinone
Low-sodium diet*	
Exercise restriction*	
Vasodilators	Hydralazine Prazosin Captopril
For atrial fibrillation, when the ventricular rate is not controlled by digoxin:	
Beta blocker	Propranolol,* nadolol, or atenolol
Ventricular arrhythmias	
	Procainamide* Propranolol Quinidine Tocainide

*Most commonly used treatments; see text for drug dosages and details.

efficacy. Samples are drawn after 5 to 7 days of therapy from 8 to 12 hours after the previous oral dose. Therapeutic serum digoxin levels range from 1.0 to 2.4 ng/ml.

Digoxin may also be helpful in controlling supraventricular arrhythmias and slowing the ventricular response in atrial fibrillation (see below). Digitoxin may be used, especially if significant renal disease is present. Digitoxin (0.04 to 0.08 mg/kg divided b.i.d. or t.i.d.) has a lesser parasympathetic effect than digoxin and may not be as effective for supraventricular arrhythmias. Therapeutic serum concentrations of digitoxin are 15 to 35 ng/ml.

Dogs with extremely poor myocardial contractility, cardiogenic shock, or fulminant congestive heart failure may benefit from an IV infusion of dobutamine at 2 to 5 μg/kg/min or dopamine at 2 to 8 μg/kg/min administered for 2 days (see Positive Inotropic Drugs in Heart Failure). During this time, the animal must be carefully observed for increasing tachycardia or arrhythmias (increasing VPCs). The IV drip rate must be constantly monitored and discontinued or reduced if arrhythmias occur. Other inotropic agents that have been used include the recently released human drug amrinone (Inocor [Sterling] 0.5 to 1 mg/kg IV every 6 hours for 1 to 2 days) and its chemical relative milrinone (still experimental, but given PO at 0.5 to 1 mg/kg b.i.d. or t.i.d.).

Diuretics are used to prevent excess fluid accumulation. Furosemide is most often used (1 to 4 mg/kg once daily to t.i.d., PO, SC, IM, or IV). For maintenance dosing, it is best to use the lowest effective dose that can be administered orally at a consistent time interval. The diuretic dose and frequency of administration can then be increased when necessary. Hypokalemia and alkalosis can occur but are uncommon unless the patient's appetite is poor or digitalis toxicity (vomiting) has occurred. Potassium supplements are used only if serum levels are low (less than 3.5 mEq/L). Alternatively, hydrochlorothiazide with spironolactone (1 mg/kg once daily, Aldactazide 50 mg [combined]) can be given in place of one of the daily furosemide doses. This combination serves to spare potassium.

Important adjuncts to therapy are exercise restriction and a low-sodium diet. A commercial prescription low-salt diet is available in both canned and dry forms (h/d, Hills), and some clients are willing to make a home diet for their pet. Bronchodilator therapy may be helpful in cases of severe pulmonary edema and wheezing from bronchoconstriction. Aminophylline has transient diuretic properties and is also a mild inotropic agent as well as a bronchodilator. The usual dose is 4 to 8 mg/kg IV or IM or 6 to 10 mg/kg PO every 8 hours. Chronic bronchodilator therapy is not typically administered at our hospital.

Ancillary Therapy

Because of poor cardiac contractile force, low cardiac output may be a problem in these dogs. Arterial or mixed arterial/venous vasodilators, used judiciously, may be helpful for improving cardiac output and exercise tolerance and for decreasing congestion (see Vasodilator Therapy). The clinician must be aware of the propensity of these agents to cause hypotension and reflex tachycardia if not carefully titrated to individual needs. When starting vasodilator therapy, we usually give half of a maintenance dose and then monitor the animal for adverse effects of worsening tachycardia, weakened pulses, decreasing blood pressure, or lethargy. If this initial dose is well tolerated, the full maintenance dose is given and the monitoring is repeated. It is advisable to begin vasodilator therapy in the hospital. Dosages may be slowly and carefully increased if necessary.

Hydralazine (Apresoline, Ciba) is a pure arterial vasodilator. The usual initial dose is 0.5 to 1 mg/kg twice daily, PO. Mixed vasodilators that have been used include prazosin (Minipress, Pfizer) at 1 to 2 mg PO twice or three times daily or captopril (Capoten, Squibb) at 0.25 to 1 mg/kg three times daily. Captopril is an angiotensin-converting enzyme inhibitor that theoretically has the dual benefits of causing vasodilation as well as reducing aldosterone secretion and the tendency to retain sodium and water (see Captopril Therapy in Dogs with Heart Failure).

Fluid therapy (either SC or IV) may be needed in nonalimentative dogs, especially after aggressive diuresis. Lactated Ringer's solution, IV 5 per cent dextrose with potassium chloride added (12 mEq/500 ml), or a solution of 0.45 sodium chloride with 2.5 per cent dextrose with potassium chloride added may be used at conservative dosages, such as 20 to 40 ml/kg/day. The clinician must assess each case individually and monitor body weight, serum creatinine, serum sodium and potassium levels, plasma protein, and oral fluid intake to direct fluid therapy.

Control of Atrial Fibrillation

Dogs with dilated cardiomyopathy and atrial fibrillation usually cannot be converted to sustained sinus rhythm because of the severity of their underlying atrial disease. The goal of therapy then is to reduce the ventricular rate to a level at which the ventricles have sufficient time to fill without the "atrial kick."

Digoxin, by slowing conduction through the AV node, is helpful in this regard. Most dogs are "slowly" digitalized by using a maintenance dose schedule (0.01 to 0.15 mg/kg divided b.i.d.). Dogs with initial heart rates of greater than 230 bpm are given a loading dose (twice the oral maintenance dose or an IV loading dose of 0.01 to 0.02 mg/kg divided in 2 to 4 doses over 4 hours). Some dogs, when fully digitalized after 3 to 5 days of therapy, have heart rates less than 150 bpm. Most dogs, however, exhibit uncontrolled rapid ventricular rates despite therapeutic digoxin levels. It is in these dogs that β-blockade is useful (see Beta-Blocking Therapy in Dogs and Cats).

Propranolol (Inderal, Ayerst) is the most commonly used β-blocker for this purpose. Like other β-blockers, it is a negative inotropic agent and is not used before the dog is digitalized (for at least 1½ to 2 days). Propranolol, being a nonspecific β-blocker, also causes bronchoconstriction and is best used after pulmonary edema and heart failure have been controlled. The usual oral starting dose is 0.6 mg/kg divided three times daily. The total daily dose is then increased over several days (using 0.6-mg/kg/day increments) until the heart rate is controlled at 100 to 140 bpm at rest. Maximum recommended dose is 1 mg/kg three times daily.

There is now a long-acting form of propranolol (Inderal-LA, Ayerst), which may require dosing only once or twice a day, but more experience is needed with this formulation. Nadolol (Corgard, Squibb) may be used instead of propranolol at an initial dose of 0.1 mg/kg twice daily and then titrated to effect. Other more heart-specific β-blockers, such as atenolol, may become more popular in the future.

Management of Other Arrhythmias

Ventricular arrhythmias can be persistent, but if they are few in number (less than 20/minute), unifocal, and do not occur on the preceding T wave, they are simply monitored with serial ECGs. Propranolol, if given for atrial fibrillation, may be helpful in suppressing ventricular ectopia. When ventricular arrhythmias warrant further treatment, IV lidocaine may be used and then IM or PO preparations of procainamide (see Antiarrhythmic Drugs and Management of Cardiac Arrhythmias).

Chronic Management Considerations

Many dogs can be maintained with digoxin, furosemide, low-sodium diet, restricted exercise, and a β-blocker such as propranolol (if needed for atrial fibrillation). Client education is important, particularly regarding the understanding of adverse drug effects. The client should understand which and how much medication is given, since medication orders are often changed by phone conversation. Owners should be taught how to take their dog's resting heart rate (by chest palpation), especially in patients with atrial fibrillation or in dogs given vasodilators. Patients should be re-evaluated periodically (initially every week and then every 1 to 3 months depending on their condition), and body weight, serum electrolytes, BUN or creatinine, ECG, and pulmonary status should be monitored. Vasodilator drugs are often used in the treatment of chronic heart failure. When pulmonary edema or ascites is refractory to diuretics and digitalis, captopril (Capoten, 0.25 to 1 mg/kg t.i.d.) is prescribed. Fatigue and weakness due to low cardiac output might be improved by therapy with hydralazine (0.5 to 2 mg/kg b.i.d.) or prazosin (1 to 2 mg b.i.d.), but these drugs should be used with caution (see Vasodilator Therapy). As time goes by, medication adjustments are made on an individual basis.

Table 3. *Therapy of Boxer Cardiomyopathy*

For congestive heart failure (see Table 2)	
Avoid digitalis glycosides in dogs with frequent VPCs	
For ventricular arrhythmias	
Lidocaine:	2 to 4 mg/kg IV, repeated up to maximum of 8 mg/kg over 10 minutes Constant-rate infusion, 25 to 75 μg/kg/min
Procainamide:	6 to 8 mg/kg IV over 5 minutes (beware hypotension) or 8 to 20 mg/kg q.i.d. IM, PO or Procan SR, 8 to 20 mg/kg t.i.d. PO
Quinidine:	6 to 20 mg/kg q.i.d. IM (gluconate) or PO (many preparations)
Propranolol:	0.2 to 1.0 mg/kg t.i.d. PO
For persistent supraventricular arrhythmias	
Digoxin:	0.01 to 0.02 mg/kg divided b.i.d. PO
Propranolol	(If adequate myocardial function or simultaneous digoxin): 0.02 to 0.06 mg/kg IV, slowly 0.2 to 1.0 mg/kg t.i.d. PO

THERAPY OF BOXER CARDIOMYOPATHY

The key to therapy of this condition involves management of dysrhythmias as well as congestive heart failure when present (Table 3). Initially, hospitalization with frequent ECG monitoring is required. Lidocaine boluses (2 to 4 mg/kg slowly IV) followed by constant-rate lidocaine infusions (25 to 75 μg/kg/minute) or parenteral procainamide (Pronestyl, Squibb), 6 to 8 mg/kg IV over 5 minutes or 8 to 20 mg/kg IM (and later PO) four times daily are our initial treatments of choice. Quinidine, 6 to 20 mg/kg IM or PO, is an alternative for ventricular arrhythmias. Supraventricular tachycardias are less common but are treated in the same way as atrial fibrillation, described above. If congestive heart failure is present, then management with diuretics, low-salt diet, rest, and oxygen is indicated. Caution must be used when administering digoxin, since it may exacerbate ventricular arrhythmias. Digoxin is avoided in patients with complex (repetitive, multiform) VPCs.

Long-term control of ventricular arrhythmias is

attempted by using procainamide (Pronestyl, Squibb) or sustained-release procainamide (Procan SR, Parke-Davis) at a dose of 10 to 20 mg/kg three times daily. Often a β-blocker (Inderal, 0.5 to 1 mg/kg PO t.i.d.) must be added to the procainamide in order to control the arrhythmia. Quinidine preparations (see page 353) are a reasonable substitute for procainamide when the latter drug is ineffective or causes severe side effects. Tocainide, a newly released antiarrhythmic drug, may hold promise for refractory cases that previously responded to lidocaine. Prednisolone (1 mg/kg b.i.d. for 10 days) is given to boxers that will not respond to any antiarrhythmic treatment. Refractory cases do occur. Client education about the possibility of sudden death despite treatment is important (see *Current Veterinary Therapy VIII* for further information).

THERAPY OF CARDIOMYOPATHY IN DOBERMAN PINSCHERS

Our experience is that Doberman pinschers as a breed have the worst cases of cardiomyopathy. Extremely poor myocardial function can result in signs of severe congestive failure and low-output cardiovascular shock. Atrial fibrillation with a rapid ventricular response is typical. Intractable ventricular arrhythmias can complicate therapy, and positive inotropic agents may aggravate ventricular arrhythmias.

Aggressive diuretic therapy must be tempered with an awareness of peripheral perfusion, renal function, and systemic blood pressure. Often IV fluid therapy is necessary in conjunction with diuretics and venodilators such as nitroglycerin. Rapid PO or IV digitalization or preferably a 24- to 48-hour infusion of dobutamine or dopamine is usually indicated. The recently released amrinone (Inocor, Sterling-Winthrop) may be used (as an experimental treatment) at a dose of 0.5 to 1 mg/kg IV every 6 hours for 24 hours. Antiarrhythmic therapy (lidocaine, procainamide) is often needed. The therapeutic considerations outlined above under dilated cardiomyopathy and boxer cardiomyopathy apply here as well.

THERAPY OF HYPERTROPHIC CARDIOMYOPATHY

If the diagnosis of hypertrophic cardiomyopathy is made antemortem, administration of β-blockers such as propranolol (0.5 to 1 mg/kg t.i.d.) may be helpful in reducing myocardial oxygen consumption; reducing heart rate, allowing for increased diastolic filling; and protecting from arrhythmias induced by increased sympathetic activity. In those cases with signs of left heart failure, diuretic therapy might be helpful but digoxin is contraindicated. In human patients with hypertrophic cardiomyopathy and outflow obstruction caused by asymmetric septal hypertrophy, the decrease in contractility caused by propranolol can reduce the outflow obstruction. Currently, therapy with calcium-channel blockers such as verapamil is under investigation. It appears that verapamil (see Calcium Antagonists) may be helpful in reducing outflow obstruction, although in some human patients it has worsened the obstruction. Little is known about the effects of verapamil in dogs with hypertrophic cardiomyopathy, but the drug would be contraindicated in cases with AV conduction disturbances. Marked exercise restriction is also advised, as well as screening for hypertensive renal disease, thyrotoxicosis, and pheochromocytoma.

THERAPY OF OTHER MYOCARDIAL DISEASES

Dogs with clinical signs of myocarditis (arrhythmias, fever, sudden onset of heart failure) should be evaluated with a general data base. This should include (1) a complete blood count to screen for changes suggesting bacterial or viral infection; (2) a serum chemistry profile to assess electrolytes, renal function, cholesterol, blood sugar, and pancreatic and liver enzymes (these findings may suggest an underlying metabolic or endocrine cause of myocardial disease); (3) an ECG to define the arrhythmia; (4) chest and abdominal radiographs to evaluate cardiac size and shape, lung patterns, and evidence of masses, infection, or trauma; and (5) echocardiography, when possible, to assess myocardial function and to reveal intracardiac or pericardial masses or vegetative lesions.

When fever is present or if a bacterial cause of myocarditis is suspected, two to four blood cultures taken at 30-minute intervals may reveal the causative organism. Serologic tests for toxoplasmosis or spotted fever, especially a rising titer on paired samples, could be diagnostic.

Therapy of secondary cardiomyopathies should be individualized. The underlying condition should be sought and treated, and the cardiac manifestations managed as necessary. Since arrhythmias are the major clinical manifestation of myocardial injury, these must be defined and controlled (see Antiarrhythmic Drugs and Management of Cardiac Arrhythmias). When heart failure occurs, treatment with furosemide and digitalis may stabilize the patient and offer the heart time to heal. Some cases of neonatal myocarditis have resolved after 2 to 8 weeks of medical therapy. The role of corticosteroids in cases of myocarditis is unresolved, but they may be helpful in postviral and traumatic myocarditis. Myocardial disease associated with sinoatrial or AV nodal disease is treated with surgical implantation of a pacemaker.

References and Supplemental Reading

Bonagura, J. D.: Therapy of cardiac arrhythmias. *In* Kirk, R. W. (ed.): *Current Veterinary Therapy VIII*. Philadelphia: W. B. Saunders, 1983, pp. 360–372.

Harpster, N. K.: Boxer cardiomyopathy. *In* Kirk, R. W. (ed.): *Current Veterinary Therapy VIII*. Philadelphia: W. B. Saunders, 1983, pp. 329–337.

Kittleson, M.: Drugs used in the management of heart failure. *In* Kirk, R. W. (ed.): *Current Veterinary Therapy VIII*. Philadelphia: W. B. Saunders, 1983, pp. 285–296.

Liu, S. K., Maron, B. J., and Tilley, L. P.: Canine hypertrophic cardiomyopathy. J.A.V.M.A. 174:708, 1979.

Mulvey, J. J., Bech-Nielsen, S., Haskins, M. E., et al.: Myocarditis induced by parvoviral infection in weanling pups in the United States. J.A.V.M.A. 177:695, 1980.

Sisson, D., and Thomas, W. P.: Dynamic subaortic stenosis in a dog with congenital heart disease. J. Am. Anim. Hosp. Assoc. 20:657, 1984.

Tilley, L. P., Liu, S. K., and Fox, P. R.: Myocardial disease. *In* Ettinger, S. J. (ed): *Textbook of Veterinary Internal Medicine*, 2nd ed. Philadelphia: W. B. Saunders, 1983, pp. 1029–1052.

Van Vleet, J. F., Ferrans, V. J., and Weirich, W. E.: Pathologic alterations in congestive cardiomyopathy of dogs. Am. J. Vet. Res. 42:416, 1981.

William, G. D., Adams, L. G., Yaeger, R. G., et al.: Naturally occurring trypanosomiasis (Chagas' disease) in dogs. J.A.V.M.A. 171:171, 1977.

Wood, G. L.: Canine myocardial diseases. *In* Kirk, R. W. (ed.): *Current Veterinary Therapy VIII*. Philadelphia: W. B. Saunders, 1983, pp. 321–329.

FELINE MYOCARDIAL DISEASES

NEIL K. HARPSTER, V.M.D.
Jamaica Plain, Massachusetts

Unquestionably, some of the nearly exponential increase in feline myocardial diseases during the past 20 years is the result of an increase in the popularity of the domestic cat as a companion animal, particularly in the urban setting, and the planned breeding of the species for pets. Genetics, however, does not appear to be as strong an influence as the population size itself. Most likely, other ill-defined environmental factors play a more significant and perhaps a major role.

Much credit for our current level of understanding of feline myocardial diseases goes to the staff members at the Animal Medical Center in New York City. Through their investigative efforts and reports of their findings, the feline myocardial diseases have evolved from a veterinary medical enigma to a well-defined clinical entity.

PRIMARY MYOCARDIAL DISORDERS

This group of diseases of undefined origin constitutes, by far, a predominance of the myocardial disorders recognized in domestic cats. It comprises three well-recognized forms that differ considerably in their effects, primarily on left ventricular hemodynamics and performance, although the right ventricle may rarely be singularly affected. In *hypertrophic cardiomyopathy*, the major hemodynamic abnormality emanates from an interference with left ventricular diastolic filling. This is primarily the result of left ventricular hypertrophy, which substantially reduces the left ventricular cavity diastolic dimensions and contributes a stiffness factor of undefined magnitude that further interferes with diastolic filling. Myocardial fibrosis probably confers additional stiffness to the left ventricle in some cats. The effects of these alterations are increased left ventricular end-diastolic pressure (LVEDP), increased left atrial pressure, and reduced stroke volume, which is further depressed when rapid heart rates or arrhythmias cause shortening of the diastolic period. Additional consequences recognized in cats with hypertrophic cardiomyopathy include (1) left ventricular outflow obstruction in a small percentage of affected cats due to excessive septal hypertrophy and (2) mitral valve incompetence, most likely the result of altered geometry of the left ventricular chamber and either relative excessive length or abnormal orientation of chordae structures.

Dilatative cardiomyopathy most certainly represents a heterogeneous condition that could be the end stage of a variety of cardiac conditions. However, in cats, as in other species with this disorder, the primary hemodynamic alteration is the result of depressed ventricular myocardial contractility. The left ventricular cavity is typically dilated, with flattening and reduced size of the papillary muscles and thinning of the ventricular walls. The LVEDP is usually elevated but cardiac output is reduced, the consequences of depressed ventricular contractility. Left atrial pressure increases in response to the elevation in LVEDP and the presence of secondary mitral valve incompetence; this latter complication is the result of left ventricular annular ring dilatation and the effects of altered ventricular geometry on position of chordae structures.

In *restrictive cardiomyopathy*, hemodynamic abnormalities consist of alterations in both diastolic filling and left ventricular contractility, although it is not unanimously agreed that any interference with the effectiveness of ventricular systolic function exists. This form of cardiomyopathy is characterized by the patchy or diffuse deposition of fibrous tissue in an endocardial position, subendocardial position, or both. The left ventricle tends to be most severely affected, as in other forms of cardiomyopathy. An elevation in the LVEDP is most likely a combined effect of reduced ventricular compliance (interference to left ventricular filling imposed by the fibrous tissue, resulting in ventricular stiffness) and varying degrees of depression of left ventricular contractility. Papillary muscle fibrosis and alterations in left ventricular chamber geometry are contributory factors to the development of secondary mitral valve incompetence. It has not been established whether depressed myocardial contractility in restrictive cardiomyopathy is a sequel to decreased ventricular compliance, which can interfere with both ventricular relaxation and systolic contraction (Starling's law), or whether other undefined factors play a role.

Hypertrophic Feline Cardiomyopathy

In hypertrophic feline cardiomyopathy (HFCM), cardiac hypertrophy occurs in the absence of any defined increase in cardiac work, thus fulfilling the criteria for a primary myocardial disorder. Although genetic influences have been proposed as a cause for this disease in a selected group of cats and a similar disease in humans has been demonstrated to have strong inheritable ties, proof is lacking that genetic factors are responsible in most affected cats. Difficulties in identifying the parentage of affected cats and the lack of breeding studies leave this question unresolved at present. We have observed the occurrence of HFCM in unrelated cats from the same household, suggesting the possibility of infectious agents or other environmental influences as etiologic agents.

Although HFCM may occur in cats of any age, it is found most commonly in young and middle-aged cats (Table 1). Male predominance has been observed in all statistical reports of this disorder, and the male incidence ranges from 70 to 85 per cent. Clinical signs are usually a result of either acute left-sided heart failure or thromboembolic episodes of the systemic circulation, although arrhythmia-induced syncopal episodes are responsible in a few affected cats (see later section on complications). Premonitory signs are frequently absent up until the time of an acute crisis.

There are no distinct findings that permit the unequivocal diagnosis of HFCM or allow its differentiation from other recognized forms of feline cardiomyopathy on physical examination. Frequent physical findings include systolic or holosystolic murmurs over the left and right cardiac apices; irregularities in cardiac rhythm; diastolic gallop rhythms; polypnea and dyspnea with inspiratory crackles; mild hepatomegaly; and lameness, paresis, or paralysis affecting one or more limbs and accompanied by decreased skin temperature and cyanotic toe pads. In most affected cats, body condition is excellent, evidence suggesting the absence of long-standing symptomatic disease. Murmurs or gallops loudest over the left or right cardiac apex and cardiac arrhythmias are occasionally found in asymptomatic cats on routine physical examination, and these can serve as markers for the presence of early or mild stages of HFCM.

Thoracic radiography in HFCM usually demonstrates the presence of mild to moderate left or biventricular enlargement based on tracheal elevation, an increased area of cardiac sternal contact, or both. There may also be evidence of left atrial enlargement. This is seen on the lateral view as a loss of caudal waist, whereas on the ventrodorsal projection it is characterized by a convex prominence along the left cardiac border from the 1 to 3 o'clock position. When left heart failure is present, pulmonary vessels tend to be prominent and are accompanied by pulmonary edema. In mild heart failure, pulmonary edema may be seen as fluffy interstitial and aveolar densities distributed along the course of pulmonary vessels. However, when heart failure is severe, diffuse alveolar densities with air bronchgrams are observed and are frequently accompanied by mild bilateral pleural effusion and hepatomegaly.

Electrocardiographic (ECG) abnormalities are present in approximately 70 per cent of cats with HFCM (Table 2). Prolongation of the P waves (greater than 0.04 sec) and QRS interval (greater than 0.04 sec) in lead II and increased amplitude of P_{II} (greater than 0.2 mV) are common findings. Arrhythmias have been observed in more than half of affected cats, with ventricular exceeding supraventricular by a ratio of approximately 3 to 1. Ventricular premature beats are most common, with supraventricular premature beats, paroxysmal ventricular tachycardia, paroxysmal supraventricular tachycardia, and accelerated idioventricular rhythm found in a progressive decreasing order of frequency. Atrial fibrillation, conduction abnormalities associated with the pre-excitation syndrome (i.e., Wolff-Parkinson-White [WPW] syndrome), and other intraventricular conduction abnormalities are infrequently observed. One distinguishing ECG finding in approximately 40 per cent of cats with HFCM is the presence of left-axis deviation in the frontal plane (Fig. 1). This pattern is characterized by progressive decrease in R wave amplitudes ac-

*Table 1. Distinguishing Clinical Features of the Various Recognized Forms of Feline Cardiomyopathy**

Criteria	Hypertrophic (31)†	Restrictive (11)	Dilatative (31)
Average age (range)	4.86 (8 mo–14 yr)	11.27 (7–19 yr)	7.81 (5 mo–14 yr)
M:F ratio (% male)	6.75 (87.1)	1.20 (54.5)	0.72 (41.9)
Breed predilection: No.(%)			
Domestic shorthair	21(67.7)	7(63.3)	13(41.9)
Domestic longhair	9(29.0)	1(9.1)	5(16.1)
Siamese	—	1(9.1)	10(32.3)
Burmese	—	—	2(6.4)
Persian	1(3.2)	2(18.2)	1(3.2)
Clinical signs: No.(%)			
Dyspnea	15(48.4)	7(63.6)	21(67.7)
Arterial embolism			
1. Initial (1st admission)	5(16.1)	—	4(12.9)
2. Late complication	—	1(9.1)	2(6.5)
Lethargy/anorexia	6(19.4)	2(18.2)	5(16.1)
Syncopal episodes	—	—	1(6.5)
Abdominal enlargement	—	2(18.2)	—
Cough	2(6.5)	—	—
Asymptomatic	3(9.7)	—	—
Cardiovascular findings: No.(%)			
Murmur cardiac apex			
Greater over left apex	13(41.9)	1(9.1)	7(22.6)
Greater over right apex	4(12.9)	1(9.1)	1(3.2)
left = right	4(12.9)	—	1(3.2)
Total	21(67.7)	2(18.2)	9(29.0)
Diastolic gallop rhythm	12(38.7)	3(27.2)	21(67.7)
Arrhythmias	8(25.8)	6(54.5)	10(32.3)
Hepatomegaly	6(19.4)	3(27.3)	9(29.0)
Ascites	—	2(18.2)	1(3.2)

*Values are based on the analysis of clinical data from 73 consecutive cats over a 3½-year period in which a diagnosis was based on nonselective angiocardiography.

†Numbers in parentheses identify the number of cats in each group.

companied by a progressive increase in S wave depth in leads I through III (Fig. 1). S waves are usually absent in lead I. The frontal plane mean electric axis ranges from 0 degrees counterclockwise to −60 degrees. It needs to be clarified whether this ECG pattern is the effect of severe left ventricular predominance alone or represents left anterior fascicular block, as has been suggested by some reports.

Congestive heart failure in HFCM is managed initially by the use of diuretics. Furosemide, 4.4 mg/kg IV, is administered, followed by subsequent doses at 2.2 mg/kg twice or three times daily by PO or SC routes. A quiet, oxygen-enriched environment affords additional benefits in the presence of severe pulmonary edema. This is best accomplished in an oxygen cage, which will deliver and maintain oxygen concentrations of 40 to 50 per cent. The cat should be left undisturbed except for examination and treatment, both of which should be carried out in a gentle and expedient manner. By these approaches, the heart failure is normally stabilized within 24 to 48 hours, at which time diagnostic procedures can be carried out to identify the form of cardiomyopathy that is present (see Differentiation of the Various Forms of Cardiomyopathy). Once a diagnosis of HFCM is confirmed by appropriate studies and heart failure is controlled, propranolol (Inderal, Ayerst; 2.5 mg b.i.d. or t.i.d. for cats less than 4.5 kg and 5.0 mg b.i.d. or t.i.d. for cats more than 4.5 kg) is added to the therapeutic regimen, along with aspirin or an aspirin-Maalox combination drug (Ascriptin, Rorer) at 2.5 grains twice weekly. At this point, the furosemide can safely be reduced to a maintenance dose of 1.0 to 2.0 mg/kg daily in a single dose or divided twice daily.

Both acetylsalicylic acid (i.e., aspirin) and propranolol have antithrombogenic properties that are believed to be beneficial in the prevention of thromboembolism in feline cardiomyopathy. Propranolol provides the additional benefit of slowing the heart rate, thereby enhancing left ventricular filling and coronary blood flow, decreasing cardiac work and myocardial oxygen requirements, and reducing cardiac automaticity (which provides an antiarrhythmic effect).

The prognosis with HFCM is better than with the other forms of cardiomyopathy, provided com-

Table 2. Comparison of the ECG Findings in 73 Cats with Cardiomyopathy

Criteria	Hypertrophic (31)* No.(%)	Restrictive (11) No.(%)	Dilatative (31) No.(%)
P wave (lead II)			
>0.04 sec	3(9.7)	3(27.3)	6(19.4)
≥0.2 mV	6(19.4)	1(9.1)	2(6.5)
QRS interval 0.04 sec.	11(35.5)	6(54.5)	22(71.0)
LVH pattern†	12(38.7)	3(27.3)	12(38.7)
Arrhythmias			
1. Supraventricular			
Premature beats	4(12.9)	3(27.3)	3(9.7)
Paroxysmal tachycardia	1(3.2)	—	1(3.2)
Atrial fibrillation	1(3.2)	2(18.2)	—
2. Ventricular			
Premature beats	11(35.5)	5(54.5)	15(48.4)
Paroxysmal tachycardia‡	4(12.9)	2(18.2)	4(12.9)
Accelerated idioventricular rhythm	1(3.2)	1(9.1)	2(6.5)
3. Total (all types)	17(54.8)	7(63.6)	18(61.3)
Conduction disturbances			
Left axis deviation§	8(25.8)	—	—
Left anterior fascicular block§	4(12.9)	1(9.1)	—
Sinoatrial block	—	1(9.1)	1(3.2)
Left bundle branch block	—	—	1(3.2)
Right bundle branch block	—	—	1(3.2)
Other intraventricular	2(6.5)	1(9.1)	1(3.2)
Pre-excitation syndrome	1(3.2)	—	1(3.2)
Total (all types)	15(48.4)	3(27.3)	5(16.1)

*Numbers in parentheses denote the number of cats in each group.

†LVH pattern is based on the presence of increased R wave amplitude in one or more of the following leads: lead II >0.9 mV; lead V4 >1.0 mV; lead V6 >0.6 mV; lead base/apex >1.0 mV.

‡Based on the presence of two or more repetitive ventricular premature beats.

§ECG differentiation between these two categories was based on the duration of the QRS interval (left axis deviation ≤0.04 sec; left anterior fascicular block >0.04 sec).

plications from thromboembolism can be avoided. A significant number of affected cats will live for more than 3 years with proper management. Chronic management incorporates the use of propranolol, diuretics (either furosemide or hydrochlorothiazide-spironolactone combination diuretics [Aldactazide, Searle] at 1 to 2 mg/kg daily), and aspirin. Periodic re-examination should be carried out, with particular attention to the heart rate and frequency of arrhythmias. The dosage of propranolol should be adjusted to maintain the heart rate under 180/min in the examination room.

Dilatative Feline Cardiomyopathy

The left ventricular and less commonly recognized biventricular dilatation associated with depressed contractility in dilatative feline cardiomyopathy (DFCM) are unaccompanied by other cardiac or systemic abnormalities, thereby fulfilling the accepted criteria for a primary myocardial disorder. Genetic influences are suspected to be responsible in a limited number of affected cats, notably members of the Siamese and Burmese breeds, based on the high incidence of this disease in these breeds and the small, embryonal size of myocardial fibers seen histologically in some of these cats. In most affected cats, however, genetic factors are impossible to evaluate. Since myocardial fibers appear normal in size histologically, other undefined causative factors are more likely responsible.

Although cats of all ages may be affected, DFCM predominates in middle-aged and older cats (Table 1). Although a male predominance has been reported, we have observed a fairly equal sex distribution during the past 5 years. Clinical signs tend to be gradual in onset, with lethargy, decreased activity, and a reduced appetite frequently preceding overt manifestations of cardiac dysfunction by 7

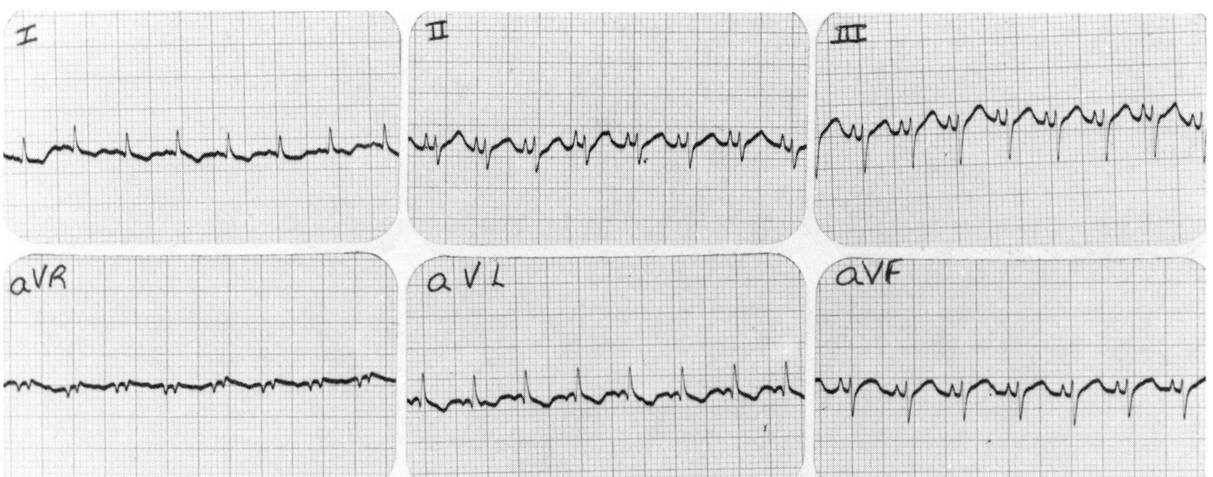

Figure 1. Bipolar and unipolar limb leads recorded on a one-year-old, male, blotched tabby DSH cat with hypertrophic feline cardiomyopathy. Notice the progressive decrease in R wave amplitude and increase in S wave depth in leads I through III. This finding, characteristic of left axis deviation, or "left anterior fascicular block," is found primarily in cats with HFCM. (Frontal plane mean electrical axis is −45.5°.) Notice also the QR complexes in lead aVL, which is another expected finding. P waves in lead II are prominent, suggesting atrial enlargement. There is prolongation of the QRS interval (0.06 second). 1.0 mV = 1.0 cm.

to 10 days or longer. However, most cats are not presented for veterinary attention until difficulty in breathing is observed.

On physical examination, hypothermia (rectal temperature less than 36.4°C [98°F]), lethargy, poor body condition with reduced skin turgor, cool extremities, and weak femoral pulses are distinguishing features of cats with DFCM. Polypnea and dyspnea of varying severity are accompanied by harsh bronchovesicular sounds dorsally and absence of lung sounds ventrally on auscultation. Thoracic percussion supports the presence of dullness ventrally. A diastolic gallop rhythm is the most common finding on cardiac auscultation, and it may be accompanied by holosystolic murmurs over the cardiac apices bilaterally and by irregularities in cardiac rhythm. The liver can usually be felt behind the costal arch. Jugular venous distension is not uncommon. Visible mucous membranes are cyanotic, with prolonged capillary refill time due to the combined effects of impaired ventilation and reduced peripheral circulation.

In the initial thoracic radiographs, most normal thoracic detail is obliterated by the presence of bilateral pleural effusion. Once this has been eliminated, varying degrees of generalized cardiac enlargement are observed, with tracheal elevation, some rounding of the cardiac silhouette in both views, and mild to moderate left atrial enlargement. The postcava is frequently widened, and the liver can be seen extending behind the costal arch. Main pulmonary vessels are somewhat distended, but lung fields are clear. Pulmonary edema is usually absent on radiographic examination.

Electrocardiographic findings in DFCM are not significantly different from those described for HFCM, except for the absence of left-axis deviation or left anterior fascicular block and a greater number of cats with prolongation of the QRS interval (Table 2). Alterations in P wave morphology in lead II are seen more commonly as prolongation (greater than 0.04 seconds) than as the increase in amplitude found in cats with the hypertrophic form. Cardiac arrhythmias are present in more than 60 per cent of affected cats, with ventricular origins predominating.

Initial management of cats with DFCM usually requires thoracentesis to resolve the hypoventilation and atelectasis caused by the pleural effusion. The author prefers a 3/4-inch-long, 21-gauge butterfly system (Medi-Wing, Sherwood Medical), which can usually be accomplished without sedation. When this has been completed, the cat in most instances is sufficiently stable to proceed with diagnostic procedures to identify the existing form of cardiomyopathy (see Differentiation of the Various Forms of Cardiomyopathy). Once a diagnosis of DFCM has been confirmed, therapy is initiated with digoxin elixir (Lanoxin, Burroughs Wellcome; 0.007 to 0.008 mg/kg/day divided b.i.d.), low doses of furosemide (1.0 to 2.0 mg/kg/day divided b.i.d.), and low maintenance levels of sodium-free fluids (5 per cent dextrose in water, 20 to 40 ml/kg/day divided b.i.d. or t.i.d., to which 20 mEq potassium chloride is added for each 500 ml of fluids). Urine production must be monitored closely, and thoracic radiographs taken every 2 days to evaluate the need for additional thoracentesis. After 2 days on this regimen, the Lanoxin elixir is reduced to a maintenance dose of 0.002 to 0.004 mg/kg/day divided twice daily.

Most cats with DFCM are not responsive to the therapeutic regimen previously described. We have noted transient improvement in some cats during the IV administration of both dobutamine hydrochloride (Dobutrex, Lilly) and dopamine hydrochloride (Inotropin, Arnar-Stone; 5 to 10 μg;/kg/minute). However, the response to these inotropic agents is frequently short-lived and is often complicated by adverse reactions (e.g., seizures, cardiac arrhythmias, sudden death secondary to ventricular fibrillation). Those cats that show an initial response may be improved further by the addition of a vasodilator drug. Nitroglycerin ointments have been advocated in this setting, although our results with these agents have not been good. We have had a favorable response to the use of hydralazine (0.5 to 0.8 mg/kg b.i.d.) in a small group of cats.

The long-term prognosis in most cats with DFCM is dismal. Most are resistant to any method of therapy and cannot be stabilized despite heroic attempts. An occasional cat can be managed successfully for 6 to 12 months, and rarely for longer than 2 years. M-mode echocardiography is a useful prognostic tool for differentiating between the responders and the nonresponders at the time of presentation. Intermittent administration of aspirin is included in the therapeutic protocol of cats that are successfully managed (e.g., 2.5 grains twice weekly). High doses of diuretics (e.g., furosemide or hydrochlorothiazide-spironolactone combination at 4 to 8 mg/kg/day divided b.i.d.) are frequently required to maintain these cats free of thoracic fluid accumulations.

Restrictive Feline Cardiomyopathy

As previously discussed, restrictive cardiomyopathy implies the presence of focal or diffuse endocardial and subendocardial fibrosis that impedes left ventricular relaxation, thereby resulting in fixed diastolic dimensions and the development of elevated LVEDP. However, since these functional alterations are not novel to the restrictive form and meaningful criteria for the diagnosis of this form of cardiomyopathy by M-mode echocardiography have not been defined, the author prefers the term *intermediate feline cardiomyopathy* (IFCM).

The characteristic changes seen at postmortem examination in IFCM are unique to this form and serve to differentiate it from the other forms discussed. The lesions suggest an inflammatory response in the past, although causative factors responsible for these changes have not been identified. Thus, it is not surprising that a breed predilection has not been observed in cats with IFCM, making genetic influences unlikely. The absence of a significant sex prevalence and the advanced age of the affected cats (Table 1) also dictate against the role of inheritable factors. If these conclusions are correct, then IFCM may represent a secondary form of cardiomyopathy of undefined cause.

Clinical signs in IFCM are not distinct but may encompass any of those described for both the hypertrophic and dilatative forms. The onset may be sudden or gradual, and acute left ventricular failure, biventricular failure, abdominal enlargement, or thromboembolic episodes are responsible in most affected cats. A variable period of lethargy and decreased appetite frequently precedes the development of overt signs related to heart failure.

In the examination room, polypnea and dyspnea or abdominal enlargement are the usual abnormalities noted on cursory inspection. Affected cats are generally bright but thin, and the rectal temperature ranges from normal to subnormal but not below 37.7°C (99.5°F). Cardiac arrhythmia is the most common abnormality noted on thoracic auscultation, but diastolic gallop rhythms and heart murmurs may also be present. Lung abnormalities will depend on the mechanism of the heart failure. Bilateral hilar rales are found with acute left heart failure, whereas ventral dullness is the predominant finding in the presence of biventricular failure. Of the two cats with ascites that we examined, neither had significant quantities of pleural effusion on presentation (Table 1). The liver can frequently be palpated caudal to the costal arch, and femoral pulses tend to be weak.

In thoracic radiography, there is considerable disparity in cardiac size and rounding of the silhouette in both views. The trachea is elevated over the heart base, and moderate left atrial enlargement is seen as loss of caudal waist on the lateral view and a left auricular appendage bulge at the 1 to 3 o'clock position on the ventrodorsal view. The effects of heart failure are evidenced by the presence of pulmonary vascular prominence and either pulmonary edema or bilateral pleural effusion. The liver usually extends behind the costal arch a variable distance.

Electrocardiographic abnormalities in IFCM tend to be less characteristic and distinct than those seen with the other forms of cardiomyopathy. Evidence of left atrial enlargement is seen as prolongation of the P wave in lead II without an increase in amplitude, whereas ventricular enlargement is characterized by increased duration of the QRS interval without either left-axis deviation or an increase in R wave amplitudes. Notching and slurring of the QRS complexes and the presence of multi-waveform QRS complexes are common findings. Cardiac arrhythmias are also frequent, and both supraventricular and ventricular arrhythmias are present in fairly equal numbers (Table 2).

Initial approaches to stabilization of cats with IFCM depend on the nature of the heart failure that exists. When pulmonary edema results from left ventricular failure, the use of furosemide (2 to 4 mg/kg IV), oxygen therapy, and bronchodilators (aminophylline, 6 to 10 mg/kg IM or slowly IV) are indicated, whereas pleural effusion secondary to biventricular failure addresses the need for thoracentesis. In the rare cat presented with isolated ascites, peritoneocentesis and fluid analysis should be carried out to eliminate other potential causes. Once cardiopulmonary function has been stabilized, specific diagnostic procedures can be performed to define the form of cardiomyopathy (see Differentiation of the Various Forms of Cardiomyopathy). Cats with IFCM are managed similarly to those with the dilatative form; digitalis glycosides and diuretics are the basic therapeutic agents.

The long-term prognosis in IFCM is guarded, with survival times ranging between those of the hypertrophic and dilatative forms. Most cats can be successfully managed for 6 to 12 months, and survival for as long as 3 years has been realized. Long-term management consists initially of digoxin elixir (0.002 to 0.004 mg/kg/day divided b.i.d.). With time, heart function further deteriorates and additional therapeutic measures are needed. Options available include higher doses of diuretics and the use of vasodilator agents (e.g., hydralazine, 0.5 to 0.8 mg/kg b.i.d.). A low-salt diet may also be of considerable benefit. Chronic management should include the use of low-dose, intermittent aspirin (2.5 grains twice weekly) in an attempt to prevent endocardial thrombosis.

DIFFERENTIATION OF THE VARIOUS FORMS OF CARDIOMYOPATHY

From the information provided in Tables 1 and 2, it would seem logical to conclude that definition of the form of cardiomyopathy in some cats should be possible on the basis of patient statistics and noninvasive, inexpensive diagnostic procedures. In part this is true, as we have never seen a Siamese or Burmese cat with HFCM. However, with this exception, none of the other measurements listed permits clear differentiation of the three forms recognized. A QRS pattern of left-axis deviation or left anterior hemiblock is strongly suggestive of HFCM but can also be found rarely in IFCM and with some frequency in hyperthyroidism, making this finding less useful. Although other criteria may also prove helpful (e.g., the presence of hypothermia and large pleural effusion providing strong evidence for DFCM), in most cats, other diagnostic tests are required for confirmation.

M-Mode Echocardiography

Echocardiography, or cardiac ultrasonography, is a relatively new diagnostic tool. From a rather inauspicious beginning in human medicine in the late 1960s, it has developed into the state of the art in noninvasive cardiac diagnostics and has been found to have significant clinical application in cats and other mammalian species. Initial clinical applications involved the use of single-dimensional echocardiography (M-mode echocardiography). This has now been replaced, in part, by the two-dimensional echocardiography, which provides additional information by recording cardiac structures in two planes.

It should be noted at the outset of this discussion

Table 3. *Differentiating Features of the Various Forms of Feline Cardiomyopathy on M-mode Echocardiography*

Criteria	HFCM	IFCM	DFCM	Normal Mean	Values SD	Reported* Range
LVFW thickness (mm)	Inc	N to Dec	Dec	3.13	1.08	2.05–4.21
LVEDD (cm)	Dec	N to Inc	Inc	1.28	0.17	1.12–1.45
LVESD (cm)	Dec	N to Inc	Inc	0.83	0.15	0.68–0.99
Fractional shortening (%ΔD)	Inc	N to Dec	Dec	34.5	12.6	21.9–47.1
D-E amplitude (mm)	Dec	N to Inc	N to Inc	4.63	1.08	3.55–5.71
E point septal separation (mm)	Overlapping	0.0 to 3.0	>3.0		N.R.	
LA dimension (cm)	Inc	Inc	Inc	0.98	0.17	0.82–1.15
Aortic root dimension (cm) (end-systole)	N	Usually N	Dec	0.92	0.15	0.78–1.07
Aortic amplitude	N	N to Dec	Dec		N.R.	
LA/Ao ratio	Inc	Inc	Inc	1.09	0.27	0.82–1.36

*Reported by Soderberg, et al.: J. Am. Vet. Radiol. Soc. 24:66, 1983.

Abbreviations: LVFW = left ventricular free wall; LVEDD = left ventricular end-diastolic dimension; LVESD = left ventricular end-systolic dimension; LA = left atrial; LA/Ao = left atrial to aortic root; Inc = increased over normal values; N = normal; Dec = decreased.

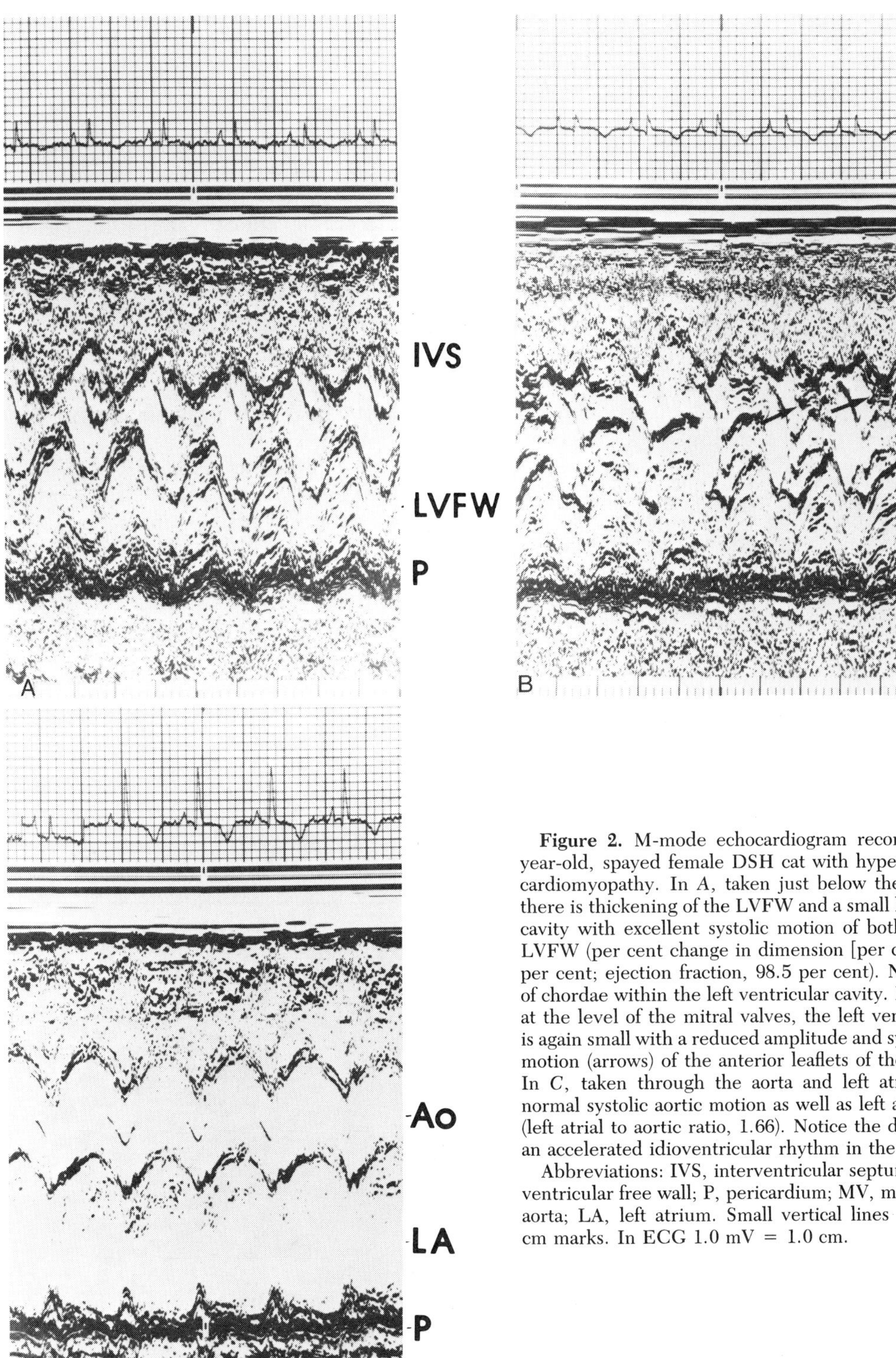

Figure 2. M-mode echocardiogram recorded on an 8-year-old, spayed female DSH cat with hypertrophic feline cardiomyopathy. In *A*, taken just below the mitral valve, there is thickening of the LVFW and a small left ventricular cavity with excellent systolic motion of both the IVS and LVFW (per cent change in dimension [per cent ΔD], 77.6 per cent; ejection fraction, 98.5 per cent). Notice portions of chordae within the left ventricular cavity. In *B*, recorded at the level of the mitral valves, the left ventricular cavity is again small with a reduced amplitude and systolic anterior motion (arrows) of the anterior leaflets of the mitral valve. In *C*, taken through the aorta and left atrium, there is normal systolic aortic motion as well as left atrial dilatation (left atrial to aortic ratio, 1.66). Notice the development of an accelerated idioventricular rhythm in the ECG.

Abbreviations: IVS, interventricular septum; LVFW, left ventricular free wall; P, pericardium; MV, mitral valve; Ao, aorta; LA, left atrium. Small vertical lines represent 1.0-cm marks. In ECG 1.0 mV = 1.0 cm.

that M-mode echocardiography is not a panacea for the diagnosis of feline cardiomyopathy. Inherent problems are encountered with some degree of frequency, the greatest of which is a lack of cooperation by the patient. Other problems confronted include limited accessibility to the heart around overlying lung tissue, particularly in cats without significant cardiomegaly, and poor near-field imaging detail owing to equipment focusing limitations. Because of greater anatomic separation of intracardiac structures in DFCM, this form is far more easily recognized by M-mode echocardiography than the other forms. We have come to use M-mode echocardiography as a screening procedure to identify those cats with DFCM, in which nonselective angiocardiography is of some risk. When echocardiographic findings do not demonstrate those findings considered typical of HFCM or IFCM (Table 3), then nonselective angiocardiography is carried out to establish a definitive diagnosis.

Thickening of the septal and left ventricular free walls, reduction in both the end-diastolic (LVEDD) and end-systolic (LVESD) left ventricular chamber dimensions, maintenance of good septal and left ventricular free-wall (LVFW) systolic motion, and left atrial enlargement are the expected M-mode echocardiographic findings in HFCM (Fig. 2). These changes result in increased values of calculated indices pertaining to left ventricular functions (e.g., fractional shortening [per cent ΔD] greater than 60 per cent; ejection fraction greater than 90 per cent). Calculated values for the velocity of circumferential fiber shortening are also increased (greater than 4.0 circumferences/sec). Another distinguishing feature in HFCM is the presence of systolic anterior motion (SAM) of the anterior leaflet of the mitral valve. However, this has been recognized in less than 50 per cent of the cats studied.

The echocardiographic features of IFCM are less distinct and have not been well characterized. Part of this stems from the less frequent occurrence of this form of cardiomyopathy. The greatest problems lie in differentiating IFCM from the normal feline heart and from other types of heart disease. The septum and LVFW are usually of normal thickness, with mild to moderate increase in LVEDD and LVESD and normal to slightly depressed systolic motion of the septum and LVFW (Fig. 3). As a consequence of these changes, there is a modest decrease in the calculated indices for left ventricular function (e.g., per cent ΔD and ejection fraction), whereas the velocity of circumferential fiber shortening rate tends to remain normal (Table 3).

Thinning of the septal and LVFW, marked increase in both the LVEDD and LVESD, and depressed systolic motion of the septum and LVFW are the typical findings that characterize DFCM. The left ventricular functional indices, per cent ΔD and ejection fraction, and the circumferential fiber shortening rate are all depressed. The mitral valves appear suspended in a large left ventricular cavity and frequently assume a double diamond configuration (Fig. 4).

Left atrial enlargement (i.e., based on a left atrial dimension to aortic root dimension ratio [LA/Ao ratio] of greater than 1.36) is common to all forms of feline cardiomyopathy, although absolute values tend to be greater in the hypertrophic and intermediate (restrictive) forms. However, calculated values for the LA/Ao ratio are comparable in all forms because of the reduced size of the aortic root dimension found in cats with DFCM. Aortic amplitude (i.e., movement to the right during ventricular systole) remains normal in HFCM but is consistently reduced in the other forms.

Nonselective Angiocardiography

This diagnostic procedure is ideally suited to cats with cardiomyopathy, as its small size permits the rapid administration of a sufficient volume of contrast medium for adequate visualization of intracardiac structures. The absence of shunts avoids the superimposition of right- and left-sided structures encountered with certain congenital cardiac defects; furthermore, the various forms of cardiomyopathy are sufficiently distinct to allow their clear definition by this study. Nonselective angiocardiography is an easily performed, low-risk procedure. Superior studies are obtained when special radiographic equipment is available that will permit frequent, multiple radiographic exposures, such as a rapid film cassette changer or 70-mm and 105-mm rapid-sequence spot films. The standard protocol we use for nonselective angiocardiography is summarized in Table 4. When special radiographic equipment is not available, diagnostic studies can be accomplished in most cats with a single, properly timed radiographic exposure in the lateral view. A good starting point is to make an exposure 6 to 8 seconds after complete injection of the contrast medium. If this timing does not provide an adequate study, additional injections of contrast medium with changes in the timing sequence can be made, up to a total volume of 6.6 ml/kg.

Inherent complications have been recognized in a small percentage of cats immediately after nonselective angiocardiography. In those with reasonably normal cardiac performance, vomiting may occur within 1 minute after the injection as a result of stimulation of emetic centers in the brain. It is largely abrogated under the influence of ketamine hydrochloride, so it rarely occurs when our routine protocol is followed (Table 4). Of greater consequence is the development of marked bradycardia and rarely cardiac arrest in cats with DFCM. This latter complication can be avoided in most cats by

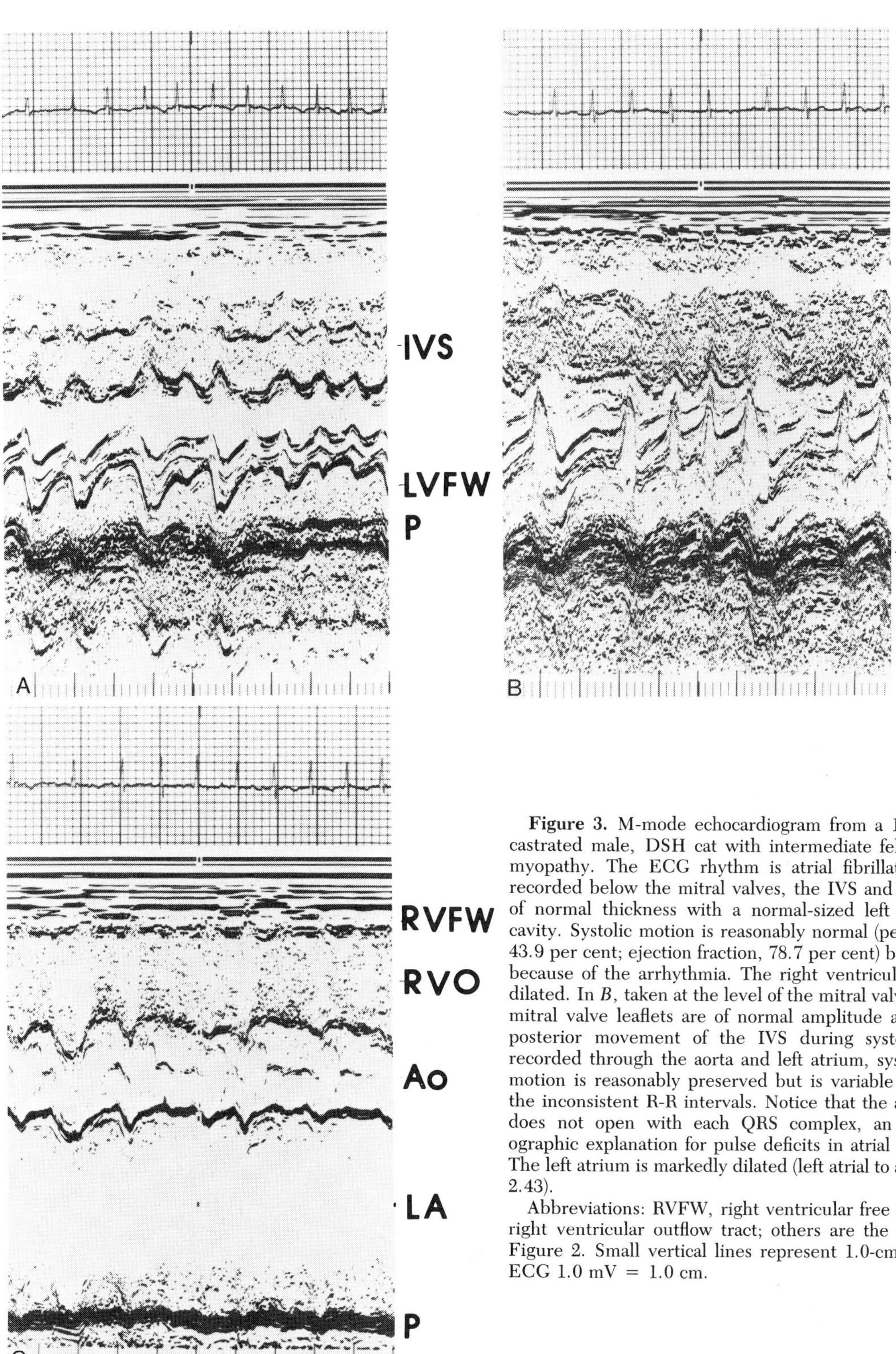

Figure 3. M-mode echocardiogram from a 10-year-old, castrated male, DSH cat with intermediate feline cardiomyopathy. The ECG rhythm is atrial fibrillation. In *A*, recorded below the mitral valves, the IVS and LVFW are of normal thickness with a normal-sized left ventricular cavity. Systolic motion is reasonably normal (per cent ΔD, 43.9 per cent; ejection fraction, 78.7 per cent) but is erratic because of the arrhythmia. The right ventricular cavity is dilated. In *B*, taken at the level of the mitral valve, anterior mitral valve leaflets are of normal amplitude and overlap posterior movement of the IVS during systole. In *C*, recorded through the aorta and left atrium, systolic aortic motion is reasonably preserved but is variable because of the inconsistent R-R intervals. Notice that the aortic valve does not open with each QRS complex, an echocardiographic explanation for pulse deficits in atrial fibrillation. The left atrium is markedly dilated (left atrial to aortic ratio, 2.43).

Abbreviations: RVFW, right ventricular free wall; RVO, right ventricular outflow tract; others are the same as in Figure 2. Small vertical lines represent 1.0-cm marks. In ECG 1.0 mV = 1.0 cm.

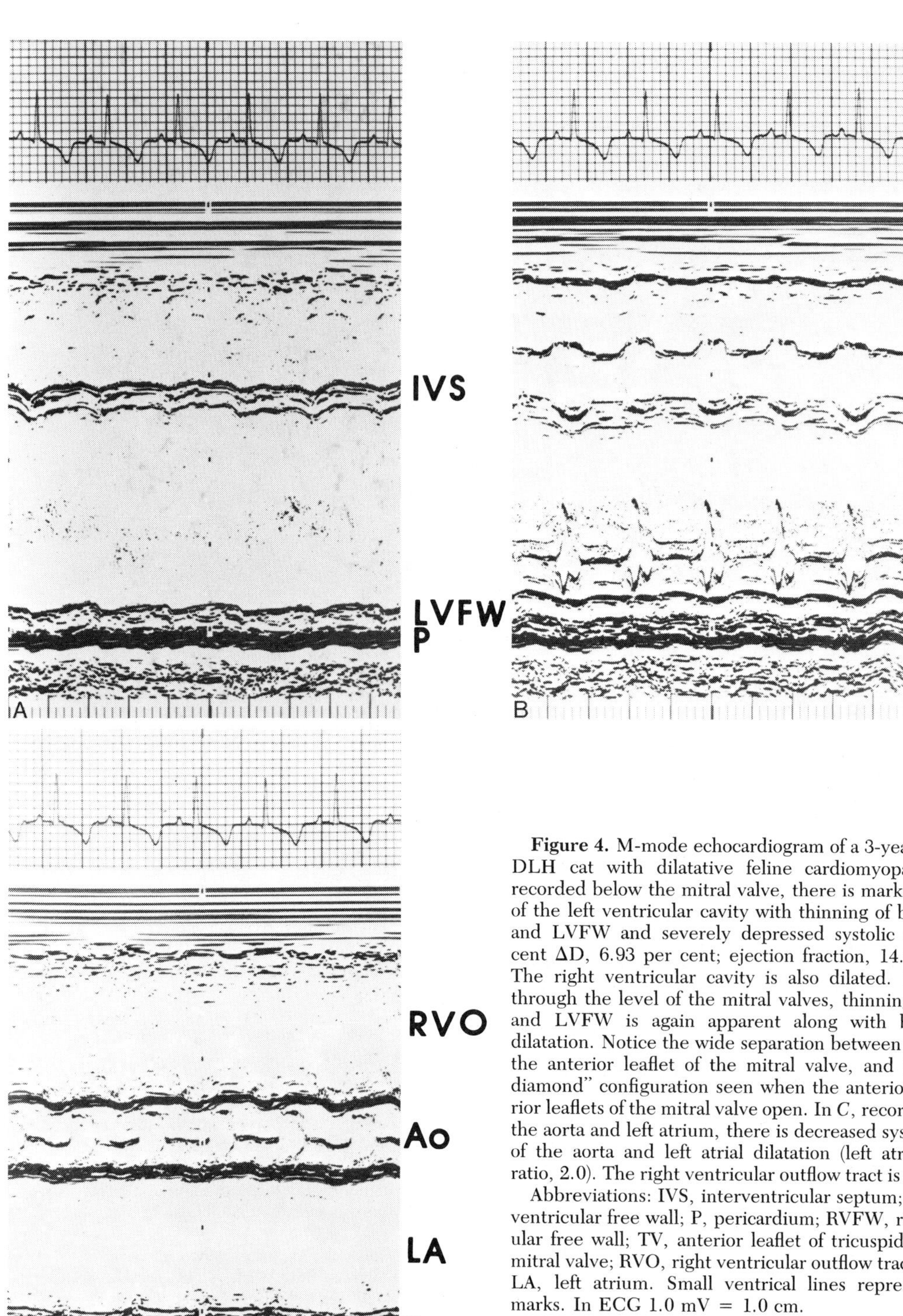

Figure 4. M-mode echocardiogram of a 3-year-old, male, DLH cat with dilatative feline cardiomyopathy. In *A*, recorded below the mitral valve, there is marked dilatation of the left ventricular cavity with thinning of both the IVS and LVFW and severely depressed systolic motion (per cent ΔD, 6.93 per cent; ejection fraction, 14.9 per cent). The right ventricular cavity is also dilated. In *B*, taken through the level of the mitral valves, thinning of the IVS and LVFW is again apparent along with biventricular dilatation. Notice the wide separation between the IVS and the anterior leaflet of the mitral valve, and the "double diamond" configuration seen when the anterior and posterior leaflets of the mitral valve open. In *C*, recorded through the aorta and left atrium, there is decreased systolic motion of the aorta and left atrial dilatation (left atrial to aortic ratio, 2.0). The right ventricular outflow tract is also dilated.

Abbreviations: IVS, interventricular septum; LVFW, left ventricular free wall; P, pericardium; RVFW, right ventricular free wall; TV, anterior leaflet of tricuspid valve; MV, mitral valve; RVO, right ventricular outflow tract; Ao, aorta; LA, left atrium. Small ventrical lines represent 1.0-cm marks. In ECG 1.0 mV = 1.0 cm.

Table 4. *Standard Protocol for Performing Nonselective Angiocardiography in Cats*

No food or water for 12 hours before the procedure.

Administer sedation 5 to 10 min prior to the procedure to minimize stress and improve cooperation.

1. Diazepam: 1.0 mg/kg IV
2. Ketamine hydrochloride: 1 to 2 mg/kg IV

Place a 20-gauge, 1-inch (2.54-cm) polyethylene cannula in a cephalic vein and tape or bandage it in place.

Restrain the cat on the x-ray table in lateral recumbency.

Inject 1 to 2 ml/kg of radiopaque contrast media (Hypaque 50 or Renografin 60) into the IV cannula as rapidly as possible.

Starting at the end of the injection, take three to four exposures per second for 10 secs using either a rapid film or cassette changer or 70-mm rapid-sequence spot films.

Additional studies may be performed, but total volume of contrast medium should not exceed 6.6 ml/kg.

postponing the study until cardiovascular stability is attained. Lower volumes of contrast media also seem preventive. Epinephrine (0.05 mg) and atropine (0.2 mg) should be available for treatment of severe bradycardia after angiography.

Thickening of the left ventricular posterior wall, a small diastolic left ventricular chamber with prominent papillary muscles, and nearly complete ejection of contrast media during left ventricular systole are the typical findings in HFCM (Fig. 5). Circulation time is normal, based on the disappearance of contrast media within 8 to 12 seconds. Left atrial enlargement is another common feature, frequently accompanied by pulmonary venous distension, whereas the aorta is of normal diameter.

A filling defect involving the left ventricular apex is the most common feature of nonselective angiocardiography in IFCM (Fig. 6). The left ventricular posterior wall is normal or slightly decreased in thickness; the left ventricular cavity is more rounded than expected with little increase in size; papillary muscles are seen well and are normal to decreased in size; and there is usually a modest decrease in ejection fraction, based on comparisons of the left ventricular end-diastolic and end-systolic chamber dimensions. Left atrial enlargement and pulmonary venous distension are routinely present, whereas the aortic diameter is of normal size.

An enlarged, thin-walled left ventricle and marked reduction in ejection fraction are the characteristic findings in DFCM (Fig. 7). Papillary muscles are difficult to detect, but when this is possible they are seen as thin bands arising in a basilar position. Left atrial enlargement and pulmonary venous distension are other expected findings, although these changes seem less impressive than in the hypertrophic or restrictive forms. The aorta was decreased in diameter in most of the cats studied.

A summary of the pertinent findings on nonselective angiocardiography in the various forms of cardiomyopathy in the cat is presented in Table 5.

Data Base Evaluation

The basic approach in the evaluation of cats with cardiomyopathy has been discussed previously. These are summarized in Table 6. Routine abdominal radiographs are probably less important in cats than in dogs with heart disease, as their small size lends itself well to physical examination. However, abdominal radiographs can be justified for the detection of small peritoneal effusions and nephrocalcinosis. Complete laboratory testing is imperative in defining the presence of concurrent disease and in helping to make wise choices in drug and dose therapy in the initial and long-term management of affected cats. Because of the high incidence of hyperthyroidism and its similarity in many aspects to the hypertrophic and intermediate forms of cardiomyopathy, thyroid tests should be performed on all cats 8 years of age and older.

Although it is not obligatory to perform specific diagnostic tests to define the form of cardiomyopathy, the information yielded unquestionably permits the institution of optimal therapy and probably improves the long-term prognosis. When equipment is not available to diagnose the type of cardiomyopathy, it is probably better to use nonspecific therapeutic approaches (e.g., diuretics, aspirin) than to assume the underlying form and institute therapy that may prove detrimental.

Recognized Complications of Feline Cardiomyopathy

Complications are commonplace in feline cardiomyopathy and can contribute significantly to confusing the clinical picture and altering the prognosis. Congestive heart failure, the most frequently recognized complication, has already been thoroughly discussed. Intracardiac thrombosis with arterial embolization is another complication that occurs with a high degree of frequency. Far less commonly, syncopal episodes, chylothorax, and chronic anemia play a significant role in the clinical picture.

THROMBOEMBOLIC EPISODES

Intracardiac thrombus formation has a predilection to develop in the left auricular appendage between pectinate muscles. Much less frequently, it may form in the left ventricular apex, particularly

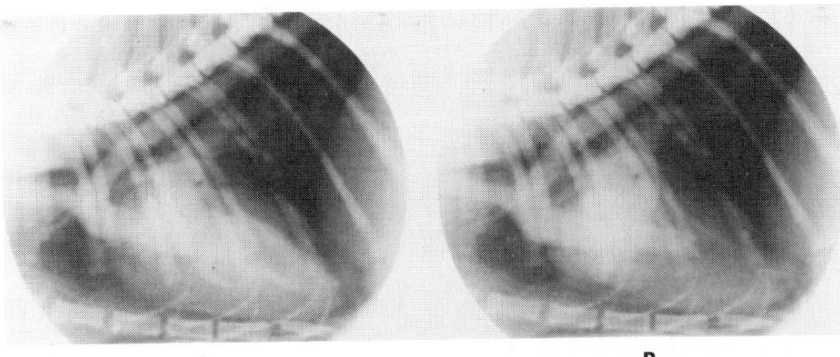

Figure 5. A nonselective angiocardiogram of an adult, castrated male, DLH cat with hypertrophic feline cardiomyopathy. In *A*, during diastole, notice thickening of the left ventricular posterior wall. The left ventricular cavity is irregular in shape with filling defects, the result of prominent anterior and posterior papillary muscles. In *B*, during systole, all dye is ejected from the left ventricular cavity except for a small amount remaining immediately below the aortic and mitral valves. Notice that the aorta is of normal diameter.

in cats with HFCM having partial left ventricular outflow obstruction, and in the right side of the heart. Initiating factors in the evolution of endocardial thrombosis in feline cardiomyopathy probably include focal endocardial inflammation (i.e., the nidus for deposition of platelets and other factors in the clotting mechanism) and static blood flow. The presence of intracardiac thrombosis is recognized clinically in most cats by the occurrence of systemic arterial embolization, usually to a limb or limbs, which results in acute lameness or dysfunction of the affected limbs. To a far lesser extent, large left atrial thrombi (i.e., a "ball thrombus") may develop, resulting in interference with left atrial emptying and poor, unexplained response to therapy for congestive heart failure.

Emboli arising from thrombi in the left side of the heart can be carried to any site supplied by the systemic circulation, where they cause partial or complete obstruction to blood flow. Organs having large circulatory volumes (e.g., heart, kidneys) are at increased risk of occlusion by small blood clots, whereas large blood clots have a propensity to lodge at the aortic bifurcation. Clinical recognition of this complication is difficult, except when vascular obstruction to a limb results in impaired circulation. Because of the high incidence of aortic bifurcation occlusion and its characteristic presenting signs, the following paragraphs will deal with this syndrome and its management.

Acute onset of hind limb dysfunction with neurologic deficits, pain, absence of femoral pulses, and decreased skin temperature distally are the expected findings with vascular occlusion at the aortic bifurcation. Neurologic abnormalities can range from mild ataxia to dropped hock, proprioception deficits, and complete flaccid paralysis, depending on the severity of the ischemia. (It has been well established experimentally that this syndrome is partly related to associated interference with collateral blood flow, as ligation of the aorta at its bifurcation does not result in the signs seen clinically.

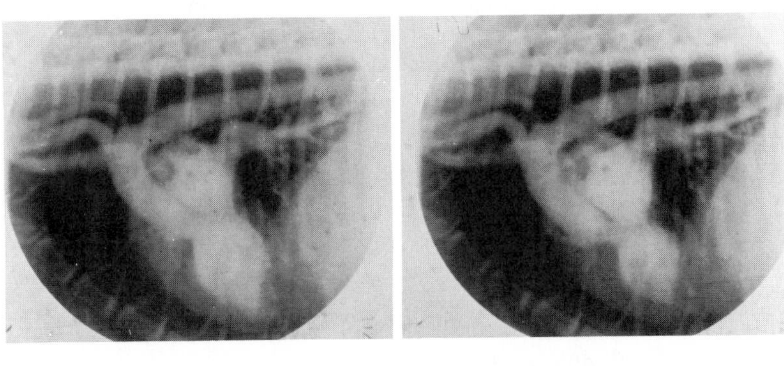

Figure 6. A nonselective angiocardiogram of a 14-year-old, spayed female Persian cat with intermediate feline cardiomyopathy. In *A*, during diastole, the left ventricular posterior wall is of normal thickness. The apex of the left ventricular cavity is misshapen, owing to an apparent filling abnormality. Papillary muscles are poorly seen. The aortic outflow area seems slightly narrowed. In *B*, during systole, a fairly normal ejection fraction can be observed. However, the left ventricular apex retains its abnormal shape, and narrowing of the outflow tract is accentuated. Filling defects in the left ventricle represent papillary muscles. Notice the aorta is of normal diameter.

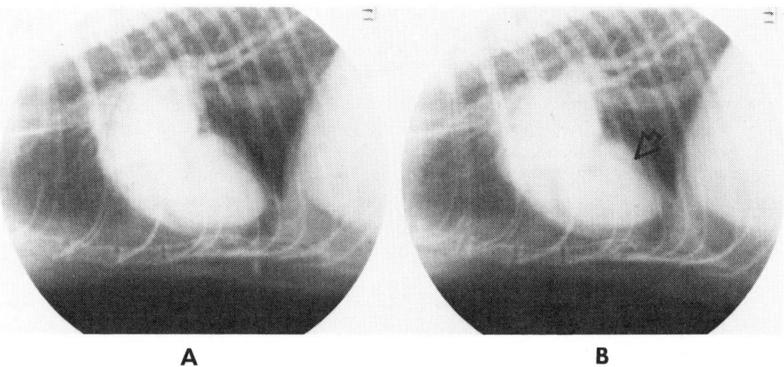

Figure 7. A nonselective angiocardiogram of an 8-year-old, spayed female Siamese cat with dilatative feline cardiomyopathy. In *A*, during diastole, the left ventricular posterior wall is thin and poorly seen. No filling defects can be seen in the left ventricular cavity and papillary muscles are not apparent. Poor visualization of the cranial border of the left ventricle is caused by the retention of dye in the right atrium and right ventricle, the result of poor circulation. In *B*, during systole, the left ventricular posterior wall remains thin. The ejection fraction is reduced. A thin filling defect over the posterior portion of the left ventricular cavity represents the posterior papillary muscle (arrow). Notice the small diameter of the aorta and the widened posterior vena cava.

Local release of some vasoactive substance, possibly serotonin or thromboxane, has been suggested as the cause.) Clinical recognition of this syndrome is usually made easily, based on the abnormal findings described. When the status of the femoral pulses is uncertain, the absence of external iliac pulses bilaterally, on rectal examination will confirm the diagnosis.

Acute management of aortic bifurcation occlusion is directed at prevention of clot propagation and improvement in collateral blood flow. After determining the baseline clotting time, 220 units/kg of heparin USP is given IV. Three hours later, maintenance heparin therapy is begun at 66 units/kg four times daily SC and is adjusted to maintain the clotting time to between two and two and one-half times the baseline level. The hematocrit should also be monitored two to three times daily to evaluate for spontaneous hemorrhage. Our attempts to improve collateral blood flow have involved the use of acepromazine maleate (Prom Ace, Fort Dodge; 0.2 to 0.4 mg/kg t.i.d. SC), and more recently hydralazine (Apresoline, Ciba; 0.5 to 0.8 mg/kg PO t.i.d.). Although some cats have shown improvement on both these regimens, the clinical efficacy of these agents has not been established. The use of serotonin antagonists and thrombolytic agents is another possible method of managing this problem and deserves clinical evaluation. Surgical intervention is not considered unless medical therapy has not resulted in some improvement within 24 to 48 hours. (The earliest indications of improvement detected clinically are increased temperature of affected limbs and return of femoral pulses. Neurologic deficits are the last to recover.) During this period of medical evaluation, any existing heart failure should be controlled, cardiac arrhythmias stabilized, and diagnostic procedures performed to define the underlying form of cardiomyopathy.

Surgical intervention (i.e., embolectomy) is indicated when status of the hind limb has not improved after 24 to 48 hours of adequate medical therapy or earlier when aortic occlusion occurs at or proximal to the origin of the renal arteries. This latter complication is associated with a rapidly increasing azotemia, but it must be confirmed by aortography in order to fulfill the criteria as defined. (Aortography is carried out as the procedure for nonselective angiocardiography [Table 5], with the x-ray beam centered over the abdomen. A radiographic exposure taken 8 to 10 seconds after the injection of contrast media should result in good visualization of the aorta and its branches in most cats.) We have attempted removal of the clot with an embolectomy catheter introduced through the femoral artery, but with poor results. Thus, exploratory laparotomy with incision in the aorta made directly over the embolus is the procedure of choice when surgery is indicated. Sodium bicarbonate is administered IV during surgery (10 to 20 ml/kg of 5 per cent dextrose in water to which 44.6 mEq of sodium bicarbonate has been added) to counteract the acidic metabolites that are released into the systemic circulation when circulation to the ischemic limbs is re-established.

Postoperative problems following embolectomy encompass cardiac arrhythmias, low cardiac output syndrome, and sudden death. Knowledge of the existing form of cardiomyopathy prior to surgery is helpful in managing these complications. However, even with this information, nearly 50 per cent of cats will succumb within the first 24 hours. In light of the poor long-term prognosis in cats with DFCM and their poor surgical risk, embolectomy should be discouraged. After successful medical or surgical management of aortic bifurcation occlusion, weeks or even months may pass before neurologic function returns to normal.

Chronic management of recurring thromboem-

***Table 5.** Differentiating Features of the Various Forms of Feline Cardiomyopathy on Nonselective Angiocardiography**

Criteria	HFCM	IFCM	DFCM
Left ventricle diastolic characteristics	Small, thickened posterior wall; prominent papillary muscles	Normal to slightly small; posterior wall normal to slightly thin; filling defect apex; papillary muscle visible	Enlarged, rounded; thinning of posterior wall; papillary muscle not seen
Systolic features	Minuscule; dye present in base only below aortic and mitral valves; marked thickening of posterior wall	Retains same shape as diastolic chamber; filling defect apex; posterior wall normal to slightly thin; papillary muscle seems small	Remains rounded with little change in size; posterior wall thin; may see tiny papillary muscle midchamber or closer to base
Ejection fraction (est.)	Increased	Decreased	Markedly decreased
Left atrium†			
Size	Enlarged	Enlarged	Enlarged
Other features	Rounded, enlarged pulmonary veins	Rounded, enlarged pulmonary veins	Rounded, enlarged pulmonary veins
Aorta			
Size	Normal	Normal to slightly small	Reduced
Estimate of circulation rate	Normal	Slightly reduced	Markedly reduced; slow clearing of right side; filling of caudal vena cava

*It may be difficult to differentiate between HFCM and forms of heart disease associated with a hyperdynamic left ventricle, such as hyperthyroidism and primary mitral valve incompetence.

†There are no discerning features in the left atrium between the various forms.

bolic episodes has been discouraging over the years. Despite the routine advocation of aspirin for the prevention of this complication in cats with cardiomyopathy, aspirin seems totally ineffective in the prevention of recurring episodes. In a number of cats, we evaluated the efficacy of subcutaneous heparin in the outpatient setting. Although the cats were free of thromboembolic episodes for the 2- or 3-month period heparin was administered, all developed recurrent episodes when heparin therapy was stopped. At the present time, we are evaluating the use of warfarin sodium (Coumadin, Endo; 0.08 to 0.1 mg/kg once daily or adjusted to maintain the prothrombin time between 15 and 20 seconds). Although too few cats have been managed to determine the clinical effectiveness of warfarin sodium, the initial results are encouraging.

CARDIOVASCULAR SYNCOPAL EPISODES

Syncopal episodes are a well-recognized but infrequent complication of cardiomyopathy; they are the predominant clinical sign in less than 1 per cent of cats with this disease. The typical episode is characterized by acute weakness or collapse of brief duration (e.g., usually less than 30 seconds), which may be accompanied by vocalization, urination, and defecation. Consciousness is normally maintained, although the client may have difficulty determining the conscious state. A variable period of lethargy and weakness usually follows the acute episode. Between episodes, the cat may behave perfectly normally or may be less active and have a depressed appetite.

Cardiac arrhythmias are the usual cause of syncopal episodes, but transient strokes should be considered if any neurologic abnormalities are found. Metabolic derangements such as hypoglycemia, hypocalcemia, and severe anemia as well as primary neurologic disease must be entertained as possible causes and ruled out. Bradyarrhythmias (e.g., paroxysmal third-degree atrioventricular [AV] block, sinus arrest) are more commonly responsible

***Table 6.** Data Base Evaluation in Feline Cardiomyopathy*

1. Comprehensive history
2. Complete examination
3. Thoracic and abdominal radiographs
4. Electrocardiogram
5. Complete laboratory testing
   A. Complete blood count, SMA profile, urinalysis
   B. T_3T_4 levels in cats 8 years or older
6. Diagnostic procedure to establish form
   A. Echocardiography
      1. M-mode
      2. 2-Dimensional
   B. Nonselective angiocardiography

than tachyarrhythmias (e.g., paroxysmal atrial and ventricular tachycardia), but both mechanisms have been observed. Paroxysmal supraventricular tachycardia as a sequela to pre-excitation syndrome (i.e., WPW syndrome) has been reported as a cause of syncope in the veterinary literature.

Unlike the arrhythmias affecting most cats with cardiomyopathy (which tend to decrease in frequency or disappear with definitive management of the heart disease), those responsible for syncopal episodes demand specific therapy for the arrhythmias. However, the first course of action is still a complete data base evaluation for feline cardiomyopathy (Table 6), unless the arrhythmia is life-threatening and commands immediate action.

The bradyarrhythmias are difficult to manage medically. They are usually the effect of a permanent organic pathologic disorder (e.g., fibrosis) that is distributed along conduction pathways, and failure to improve conduction will allow clinical signs to persist. Although trial therapy with parasympatholytic agents (e.g., atropine sulfate [Lilly], 0.04 to 0.06 mg/kg t.i.d. or q.i.d.; propantheline bromide [Pro-Banthine, Searle], 0.8 to 1.6 mg/kg t.i.d.) and sympathomimetic agents (isoproterenol [Proternol, Key Pharmaceuticals], 0.8 to 1.6 mg/kg t.i.d. or q.i.d.; ephedrine sulfate, 2 to 3 mg/kg t.i.d.) can be tried, the results generally are ineffective. Permanent pacemaker therapy provides the most consistent long-term benefits, although the cost of this approach is frequently prohibitive.

Syncopal episodes as a result of tachyarrhythmias in HFCM may be totally controlled by the use of propranolol (2.5 to 5.0 mg b.i.d. or t.i.d.) alone. When this proves ineffective, the addition of either procainamide (7 to 14 mg/kg t.i.d. or q.i.d.) or quinidine sulfate (5 to 10 mg/kg t.i.d.) may be of benefit. The use of propranolol should be avoided in both IFCM and DFCM until digitalization is completed, and even then must be used with proper precautions. Because of its profound effect on myocardial contractility, propranolol should be reserved for use in those cats with IFCM and DFCM that do not show an adequate response to the other antiarrhythmic agents.

CHYLOTHORAX

A cause for the development of chylothorax during the chronic management of cats with cardiomyopathy has not been defined. As its occurrence seems to be limited to those with either IFCM or DFCM that have experienced one or more bouts of biventricular failure accompanied by pleural effusion, high systemic venous pressure and, thereby, high thoracic duct pressure may play a role. Management of these cats has been approached by repeated thoracocentesis or short-term placement of a chest tube, diet restrictions, and vigorous therapy for heart failure because of the high risk involved in surgical intervention. The results with these approaches have not been satisfactory.

CHRONIC ANEMIA

Anemia of a severity that requires specific treatment is a rare complication in feline cardiomyopathy. It is characterized by a low reticulocyte count and hypoplastic bone marrow. Although a specific cause for its development has not been defined, renal dysfunction may be a factor in some cats. Its presence increases cardiac work and may be responsible for a less than adequate response to therapy for congestive heart failure.

Medical management consists of the administration of anabolic steroids (stanozolol [Winstrol V, Winthrop], 2 mg PO daily; nandrolone decanoate [Deca-Durabolin, Organon], 50 mg IM weekly), and in some cats this alone is effective. Blood transfusions should be used when the hematocrit falls below 20 per cent. Good stability of the heart failure and slow administration of transfusions are important in preventing untoward problems.

EXCESSIVE LEFT VENTRICULAR MODERATOR BANDS

This unique endomyocardial disorder is discussed separately to emphasize its distinct features. It is characterized by the presence of an exorbitant number of moderator bands within the left ventricle, usually extending from the posterior or anterior papillary muscles, or both, to the ventricular septum. The effects of this abnormal anatomic arrangement are reported to be interference with left ventricular filling due to restrictions imposed on left ventricular diastolic dimensions, resulting in elevated left ventricular end-diastolic pressure and eventual congestive heart failure.

Left ventricular excessive moderator bands (LVEMB) most likely is a genetically influenced anomaly of low incidence, although a role by infectious agents during early cardiac development must also be considered. We too have observed this clinical entity, but far less frequently than the 7.05 per cent reported in a survey of cats with heart disease. It has a modest male predominance and results in clinical signs in young to middle-aged cats.

The clinical features of LVEMB are indistinct from those described for the various forms of cardiomyopathy. Lethargy, rapid breathing, anorexia, emesis, acute onset of lameness or paresis, and syncopal episodes are the usual reasons for presentation. On physical examination, hypothermia, dyspnea, heart murmurs, diastolic gallop rhythms, and mild to moderate hepatomegaly are commonly found. Cardiomegaly accompanied by pulmonary edema, pleural effusion, or both are the expected findings on thoracic radiography. Atrioventricular (AV) and intraventricular conduction disturbances are the most common ECG abnormalities reported, with right bundle branch block, left anterior fascicular block, and varying degrees of AV block, including third-degree AV block, being found in a decreasing order of frequency.

The greatest challenge lies in differentiating LVEMB from the various other recognized forms of cardiomyopathy. This has so far not been accomplished by either noninvasive studies or angiocardiography. Echocardiography is a possible answer to this dilemma, but the findings in this condition have not been reported. Two-dimensional echocardiography would seem to offer the greatest promise, as the tunnel-vision imaging encountered with M-mode echocardiography would appear to make distinct visualization of surplus moderator bands a great problem and differentiation between these and normal chordae structures especially difficult.

Specific methods for managing cats with LVEMB have not been defined. However, until improved diagnostic procedures become available, meaningful treatment and prognostic data are difficult to formulate. At the present time, since LVEMB may be accompanied by either left ventricular hypertrophy or dilatation, it would seem logical to approach it therapeutically by following the same general guidelines used for feline cardiomyopathy. When diagnostic studies demonstrate a small left ventricular cavity and thickening of the left ventricular posterior wall, the use of propranolol would be indicated along with diuretic therapy; however, if the left ventricle is dilated and thin-walled, the use of digitalis glycosides should be considered. Intermittent aspirin therapy should be used in all affected cats because of the incidence of thromboembolism.

The finding of left ventricular hypertrophy in some and dilatation in other individual cats with LVEMB raises some questions as to the true functional significance of the excessive moderator bands found. Since the histologic changes in the myocardium are similar to those seen in various forms of feline cardiomyopathy, it is conceivable that the moderator bands represent an incidental finding in a group of cats with cardiomyopathy. It will be necessary to gather additional clinical data to resolve these questions.

SECONDARY MYOCARDIAL DISEASES

The secondary feline myocardial diseases consist of a varied but limited group of myocardial diseases of known cause. This assortment of diseases, certain congenital cardiovascular anomalies, and pericardial diseases make up the great majority of conditions that will need to be differentiated from the primary myocardial diseases (i.e., idiopathic cardiomyopathy). Of the *congenital diseases,* aortic stenosis (both valvular and subvalvular) and mitral valve dysplasia present the most common challenges in differentiation—the former because of similarities to HFCM found on both echocardiography and nonselective angiocardiography, and the latter owing to the presence of a murmur of mitral valve incompetence. Persistent presence of common AV canal frequently results in findings identical to those in mitral valve dysplasia, but it is usually accompanied by greater degrees of biventricular enlargement, as well as cardiac decompensation at a younger age. The pericardial diseases, which are relatively rare in cats, offer less difficulty in distinction from cardiomyopathy, particularly when echocardiographic equipment is available to demonstrate the presence of pericardial fluid. The minimal amount or absence of fluid in most cats with congenital peritoneopericardial diaphragmatic hernia will create greater problems in differentiation, and either an upper gastrointestinal contrast study or nonselective angiocardiography is often required to make a definitive diagnosis.

In the paragraphs that follow, the secondary myocardial diseases will be categorized and discussed on the basis of etiologic factors that are responsible. It should be understood that these are based on our present level of knowledge. Rare causes or those of questionable significance will be omitted, as their role has not been sufficiently established. It is anticipated that the importance of the secondary myocardial diseases will increase in feline cardiology as they become better defined.

Infectious Myocarditis

Myocarditis is a well-recognized complication of a variety of infectious diseases in humans. Similar associations have been reported in cats, but with much less frequency. Systemic signs usually predominate in early stages of these diseases (i.e., fever, lethargy, depressed appetite), and myocardial involvement may be absent or overlooked only to become manifest at a later date. The early signs of myocarditis are relatively nonspecific and are frequently unrecognized. Tachycardia, cardiac enlargement, heart murmurs, arrhythmias, and overt heart failure constitute later but more specific evidence of myocarditis. Thromboembolic episodes may contribute to the clinical picture. If diligently sought, ECG abnormalities are frequently found to be present, with arrhythmias, conduction disturbances, and ST-T repolarization abnormalities predominating.

Myocardial injury in myocarditis may be the result of a variety of contributing factors. Myocardial cell damage or death is frequently responsible in bacterial and fungal infections, as a result of either a direct effect of the organism or elaborated toxins. However, in viral and certain parasitic infections, immune-mediated allergic or hypersensitivity reactions are thought to be accountable.

Viral agents are a commonly mentioned but infrequently proven cause of myocardial disease in cats. These infectious agents have been suggested as responsible for various forms of feline cardiomyopathy and endomyocardial disease in the kitten mortality complex. However, to the present time, only feline coronaviral disease (i.e., feline infectious peritonitis virus) has been demonstrated to result in cardiac manifestations, and this involvement is generally limited to the pericardial and epicardial surfaces. Less commonly, myocardial performance may be affected by extension of the inflammation into superficial portions of the myocardium or due to the development of constrictive pericarditis. These manifestations of feline coronaviral disease are usually accompanied by significant systemic signs (e.g., fever, lethargy, anorexia), which are helpful in distinguishing it from feline cardiomyopathy. Pericardiocentesis with demonstration of a pale yellow, viscid fluid having a high specific gravity (greater than 1.017) and high protein content (greater than 4.0 gm/L) will be necessary to establish a diagnosis.

Bacterial myocarditis in cats is generally a sequela of endocarditis, in which the mitral valve is most commonly affected. Myocardial involvement may arise either by direct extension from infected valve tissue or by way of septic emboli that lodge in the coronary arteries. Systemic signs (e.g., fever, lethargy, anorexia) predominate in the clinical picture because of spread of infection and septic emboli to many body organs. Early recognition may prove difficult before the development of distinct cardiac abnormalities.

Early diagnosis of bacterial endomyocarditis usually depends on clinical suspicions and a well-organized protocol for managing cats with a fever of undetermined origin. Recent infections or nonsterile surgery provide additional clinical clues to its existence. Cats that are immunosuppressed because of either natural (e.g., positive feline leukemia virus status) or iatrogenic (e.g., those receiving chemotherapeutic agents) causes are at increased risk. The following findings are strongly suggestive of bacterial endomyocarditis: fever; elevated white count accompanied by an absolute neutrophilia, with or without a left shift; heart murmur of recent origin; cardiac arrhythmias; and evidence of systemic thromboembolic disease. However, positive blood cultures are an absolute prerequisite to establishing an indisputable diagnosis. The reader should refer to Bacterial Endocarditis (in this section) for further information regarding the diagnosis, clinical course, and management of this disease.

Only bacterial endomyocarditis and cardiomyopathy are common causes of thromboembolism in cats. Differentiation between these two diseases can usually be made based on the absence of a fever and a normal white blood count in feline cardiomyopathy. Heart murmurs and arrhythmias are common to both. When evidence of thromboembolism is lacking, only positive blood cultures will clearly separate bacterial endomyocarditis from other causes of myocarditis.

Protozoan myocarditis may occur rarely in cats as a result of infection by *Toxoplasma gondii*, an obligate intracellular parasite. Far more commonly, active infections are associated with signs related to the central nervous, visual, respiratory, and gastrointestinal systems, whereas myocardial involvement is clinically silent and is identified only at postmortem examination. When myocardial involvement is recognized clinically, it is difficult to differentiate from other causes of myocarditis.

Toxoplasma myocarditis is characterized by tachycardia, arrhythmias, and S-T segment repolarization changes. Although congestive heart failure has not been recognized in cats, it is a reported complication in humans. Blood cultures will be negative but should be performed because of similarities between this disease and bacterial endomyocarditis. The diagnosis is established by a high serum antibody titer or, preferably, a rising titer over a 2- to 3-week period. Treatment includes the administration of sulfadiazine (60 mg/kg/day divided q.i.d.) and a single dose of pyrimethamine (Daraprim, Burroughs Wellcome; 0.5 to 1.0 mg/kg). These two drugs act synergistically to inhibit folate metabolism, and the administration of folinic acid (Leucovorin Calcium Injection, Lederle; 1.0 mg/kg/day) is recommended to prevent toxic side effects.

OTHER RECOGNIZED MYOCARDIAL DISORDERS

Hyperthyroidism is a fairly recent disease entity recognized in domestic cats. It is caused by the benign hyperplasia of normal thyroid tissue, which has been histologically identified as multinodular thyroid adenomas or thyroid adenomatous goiter. Noncardiac signs dominate the clinical picture because of the effect of the hypermetabolic state on other body organ functions. However, on physical examination, cardiac abnormalities are frequently the most significant findings. Tachycardia, heart murmurs of greatest intensity over the left or right cardiac apex, and arrhythmias are the most commonly observed abnormalities. Congestive heart failure is an unusual complication. Varying degrees of cardiomegaly are seen in thoracic radiographs, and ECG abnormalities include sinus tachycardia (greater than 200/min); increased R wave amplitudes; occasional deep S waves in leads II, III, and aVF; prolonged QRS intervals, shortened Q-T intervals; and a variety of cardiac arrhythmias with supraventricular arrhythmias (e.g., atrial premature beats, atrial tachycardia) predominating. Both nonselective angiocardiography and M-mode echocardiography demonstrate a hyperdynamic left ventricle with or without moderate thickening of the left ventricular posterior wall. A diagnosis is established by the presence of increased serum concentrations of triiodothyronine (T_3), thyroxine (T_4), or both in affected cats. The reader should refer to Hyperthyroid Heart Disease in Cats for further information regarding clinical signs, diagnostic procedures, and the management of this condition.

Differentiation of thyroid adenomatous goiter from HFCM and primary mitral valve incompetence is most difficult based on the use of noninvasive and invasive cardiovascular studies alone. Increased ejection fractions (greater than 85 per cent) and velocity of circumferential fiber shortening (greater than 4.50 circumferences/sec) are common to all; and although differences in the left ventricular posterior wall thickness may exist, these are frequently subtle changes that are difficult to recognize. These similarities emphasize the importance of performing serum T_3 and T_4 levels in all cats that are suspected of having cardiac disease and are older than 7 years.

Other reported causes of myocardial disease in cats are far less clearly defined. Potentially *toxic agents*, such as digitalis glycosides, propranolol, anesthetics, and sedatives, can unquestionably have profound deleterious effects on myocardial performance when administered in excessive doses. Profound bradyarrhythmias, including idioventricular rhythms, are well-recognized complications of prolonged *urethral obstruction* as a result of the development of hyperkalemia and metabolic acidosis. *Systemic hypertension* has been suggested as a complication of renal dysfunction that can lead to cardiac hypertrophy and arrhythmias, particularly in cats with pre-existing cardiac disease. *Diabetes mellitus* may have a similar effect on the systemic blood pressure in some cats. Finally, the role of *nutritional deficiencies* as a cause of myocardial disease in cats has not been adequately investigated. Thiamine deficiency, especially, is a possible culprit, as it is a well-proven cause of central nervous system abnormalities in this species.

CONCLUSIONS

Myocardial disease is a well-recognized clinical entity in domestic cats. Over a span of 15 years it has evolved from a medical curiosity to a major cause of illness and death. During this period, substantial advancements have been made in our understanding of these diseases and their management. However, frustrations flourish because of our inability to identify specific causes. At the present time, nearly 80 per cent of cats evaluated for heart disease are diagnosed as having one of the recognized forms of cardiomyopathy, and hyperthyroidism and congenital heart disease account for most of the others.

References and Supplemental Reading

Butler, H. C.: An investigation into the relationship of an aortic embolism to posterior paralysis in the cat. J. Small Anim. Pract. 12:141, 1971.

Holzworth, J., Theran, P., Carpenter, J. L., et al.: Hyperthyroidism in the cat: Ten cases. J.A.V.M.A. 176:345, 1980.

Liu, S.-K.: Acquired cardiac lesions leading to congestive heart failure in the cat. Am. J. Vet. Res. 31:2071, 1970.

Liu, S.-K., Fox, P. R., and Tilley, L. P.: Excessive left ventricular moderator bands in the cat. J.A.V.M.A. 180:1215, 1982.

Liu, S.-K., Tashjian, R. J., and Patnaik, A. K.: Congestive heart failure in the cat. J.A.V.M.A. 156:1319, 1970.

Lord, P. F., Wood, A., Tilley, L. P., et al.: Radiographic and hemodynamic evaluation of cardiomyopathy and thromboembolism in the cat. J.A.V.M.A. 164:154, 1974.

Ogburn, P. N.: Ventricular pre-excitation (Wolff-Parkinson-White syndrome) in a cat. J. Am. Anim. Hosp. Assoc. 13:171, 1977.

Peterson, M. E., Keene, B., Ferguson, D. C., et al.: Electrocardiographic findings in 45 cats with hyperthyroidism. J.A.V.M.A. 180:934, 1982.

Petrak, M., and Carpenter, J. L.: Feline toxoplasmosis. J.A.V.M.A. 146:728, 1965.

Pipers, F. S., and Hamlin, R. L.: Clinical use of echocardiography in the domestic cat. J.A.V.M.A. 176:57, 1980.

Schaub, R. G., Meyers, K. M., Sande, R. D., et al.: Inhibition of feline collateral vessel development following experimental thrombolic occlusion. Circ. Res. 39:736, 1976.

Schlant, R. C.: Physiology of idiopathic cardiomyopathies. Cardiovasc. Clin. 4:61, 1972.

Soderberg, S. F., Boon, J. A., Wingfield, W. E., et al.: M-mode echocardiography as a diagnostic aid for feline cardiomyopathy. J. Am. Vet. Radiol. Soc. 24:66, 1983.

Tilley, L. P.: *Essentials of Canine and Feline Electrocardiography*, 1st ed. St. Louis: C. V. Mosby, 1979.

Tilley, L. P., Liu, S.-K., Gilbertson, S. R., et al.: Primary myocardial disease in the cat. Am. J. Pathol. 87:493, 1977.

Wenger, N. K.: Infectious myocarditis. Cardiovasc. Clin. 4:167, 1972.

HYPERTHYROID HEART DISEASE IN CATS

BETSY R. BOND, D.V.M.
New York, New York

Hyperthyroidism in cats is caused by overproduction of thyroxine (T_4) and triiodothyronine (T_3), usually by a benign adenoma of one or both thyroid lobes. It is a multisystemic disorder affecting primarily energy metabolism and the cardiovascular system. A typical cat with hyperthyroidism displays hyperexcitability and weight loss, although depression and anorexia also are encountered.

A form of reversible cardiomyopathy is common in feline hyperthyroidism. Affected cats most commonly develop hypertrophic cardiomyopathy, which may or may not be associated with congestive heart failure. Therefore, serum concentrations of T_4 should be determined in all elderly cats with cardiac abnormalities, especially if other clinical signs compatible with hyperthyroidism are present. In cats in which the congestive heart failure persists despite correction of the hyperthyroid state, it is possible that pre-existing primary cardiac disease is also present. Although the prognosis for hyperthyroid cats that have developed overt congestive heart failure is guarded, all cardiac medications can eventually be discontinued in many cats after successful therapy for hyperthyroidism.

PATHOPHYSIOLOGY OF HYPERTHYROID HEART DISEASE

Hyperthyroidism causes a high-output, or hyperkinetic, circulatory state. There is an increase in cardiac output secondary to increased metabolic demands and decreased peripheral vascular resistance. Effects of hyperthyroidism on the heart are mediated through direct action of thyroid hormone and the effects of catecholamines.

It has been reported that thyroid hormone exerts its direct effect on the heart by increasing protein synthesis at the level of the cell nucleus. This leads to cardiac hypertrophy and hypercontractility. Thyroid hormone also exerts a direct effect on the sinoatrial (SA) node, leading to sinus tachycardia. The interaction of thyroid hormone and the sympathoadrenal system also contributes to cardiac changes. Catecholamines contribute to the development of additional cardiovascular changes; thus, a β-adrenergic blocker frequently is administered, along with antithyroid medication, to cats with hyperthyroid heart disease.

Changes in cardiac function caused by hyperthyroidism include marked increases in cardiac output, heart rate, left ventricular ejection fraction, and pulse pressure and a decrease in circulation time. Myocardial oxygen consumption and blood volume also are increased, both of which can lead to heart failure. Left ventricular ejection fraction is maximum with thyrotoxicosis and cannot increase during exercise.

DIAGNOSIS OF HYPERTHYROIDISM

History and Physical Examination

Weight loss, hyperactivity, polydipsia and polyuria, vomiting, diarrhea, and increased fecal volume are associated with feline hyperthyroidism. Apathetic hyperthyroidism, characterized by anorexia, lethargy, and weakness, can be misdiagnosed because of its resemblance to other metabolic diseases. Most affected cats are old (mean age of 12 to 13 years); there is no breed or sex predilection. Signs of heart failure in hyperthyroid cats are the same as in cats with cardiomyopathy, i.e., lethargy, anorexia, and dyspnea.

Physical examination of cats with hyperthyroid heart disease reveals cachexia, nervousness, and hyperexcitability, although cats that develop cardiac problems early in the course of hyperthyroidism might not have these typical signs. Careful palpation of the cervical area usually reveals a thyroid nodule. Cardiac abnormalities include tachycardia, a systolic murmur of moderate intensity near the left sternal border, a strong pulse, and a prominent apex beat that is easily palpated over the thorax. Cats with less severe disease might only have a systolic murmur or tachycardia. Cats in heart failure are dyspneic and often have pleural effusion (decreased heart and lung sounds) and pulmonary edema (pulmonary crackles).

Table 1. ECG Changes in Cats with Hyperthyroidism

Tachycardia
Increased R wave amplitude (lead II)
Prolonged QRS duration
Shortened Q-T interval
Atrial premature complexes
Left anterior fascicular block
Ventricular premature complexes
Right bundle branch block
First-degree atrioventricular block
Second-degree atrioventricular block with ventricular escape complexes
Atrial tachycardia
Ventricular tachycardia and bigeminy
Ventricular pre-excitation

Electrocardiography

Sinus tachycardia and increased R wave amplitude in lead II (greater than 1 mV.) are the most common changes seen on the electrocardiogram (ECG) of cats with hyperthyroid heart disease. Various atrial and ventricular arrhythmias and intraventricular conduction disturbances also are observed (Table 1). In almost all cats that return to euthyroidism, the ECG returns to normal.

Radiography

Approximately 50 per cent of all cats with hyperthyroidism have mild to moderate cardiomegaly, as revealed by thoracic radiographs. Of these, a small percentage have extracardiac features of heart failure• including pleural effusion, pulmonary edema, or both. Unless primary cardiomyopathy and hyperthyroidism are concurrent, follow-up radiographs taken several months after initiation of therapy show a return of the cardiac silhouette to normal.

Additional Studies

There is a high incidence of *echocardiographic* changes in hyperthyroid cats. The most common of these are left ventricular hypertrophy, aortic root and left atrial enlargement, and increased shortening fraction and velocity of circumferential fiber shortening. After therapy, these abnormalities disappear.

Definitive diagnosis of hyperthyroidism is based on serum biochemical testing with demonstration of elevated serum T_4 and T_3 concentrations (see Feline Hyperthyroidism). In addition, elevations in liver enzymes frequently are encountered. *Radionuclide scanning* with radioactive iodide (^{131}I) or technetium ($^{99m}TcO_4$) has also proved valuable in the diagnosis and preoperative workup of hyperthyroid cats. The procedure reveals whether one or both thyroid glands are affected, locates ectopic thyroid tissue, and can detect metastasis of a functioning thyroid carcinoma.

THERAPY

The choice of therapeutic regimen for a cat with thyrotoxic heart disease depends on the patient's metabolic and cardiovascular status, the availability of facilities, and the owner's wishes. Three methods of treatment are available: (1) long-term administration of oral antithyroid drugs, (2) surgical removal of one or both thyroid lobes and (3) radioactive iodine therapy. Radioactive iodine therapy is safe, simple, and effective, but its use is severely limited because of the lack of widespread availability of computerized nuclear medicine facilities for veterinary use and because of radiation safety requirements. Surgery is currently the treatment of choice, but the risk of anesthesia precludes its use in some cats with severe myocardial dysfunction. Oral antithyroid drugs can be used preoperatively to reduce the risk of anesthetic complications associated with hyperthyroidism, and, in cats that cannot undergo surgery, long-term therapy is indicated. The primary goal of therapy is to return thyroid concentrations to normal and reverse the metabolic and cardiovascular consequences of thyrotoxicosis. Secondary goals include controlling congestive heart failure, correcting cardiac arrhythmias, and blocking the effects of excess catecholamines.

Antithyroid Drugs

Propylthiouracil (PTU) or methimazole (Tapazole, Lilly) inhibits the synthesis of thyroid hormone but does not affect the iodide pump or release of preformed thyroid hormone from the follicles. Thus, 1 to 4 weeks might be required to lower thyroid hormone concentrations to normal.

Initial loading dosages are 50 mg for PTU and 5 mg for methimazole; both drugs are given orally every 8 hours. Thyroid hormone concentrations are remeasured at 14 days, at which time a thyroid scan can be performed if surgery is planned. Cats unable to undergo surgery are given a daily maintenance dose of 100 to 200 mg PTU or 10 to 20 mg methimazole. Thyroid hormone concentrations are determined every 7 to 14 days, and the dosage is adjusted as needed.

Vomiting, lethargy, and anorexia are the most common side effects of antithyroid drug therapy. Serious complications include acute immune-mediated hemolytic anemia, neutropenia, and thrombocytopenia. Methimazole appears to cause fewer side effects than PTU.

Surgery

Successful surgical removal of one or both thyroid lobes depends as much on preoperative therapy as on the surgical procedure itself. A thyroid scan indicates if unilateral or bilateral thyroidectomy is necessary and if ectopic thyroid tissue is present. The administration of propranolol (see below) to control the effects of catecholamines and antithyroid drugs to lower T_4 concentrations to normal substantially decreases the anesthetic risk. Heart failure, when present, should be resolved by administration of diuretics and, possibly, digitalis.

CONGESTIVE HEART FAILURE AND HYPERTHYROIDISM

The dilemma facing the clinician treating a cat with hyperthyroid congestive heart failure is whether or not to take the risk of performing surgery. Echocardiography has proved invaluable by providing objective criteria by which to judge the functional status of the myocardium. In the absence of echocardiography, subjective evidence of severe myocardial impairment includes hypothermia, weak pulses, slow capillary refill time, and a weak left ventricular apex beat. Affected cats are treated with digoxin (Lanoxin, Burroughs Wellcome), furosemide (Lasix, Hoechst-Roussel), and, sometimes, vasodilators (see Vasodilator Therapy). The dosage schedule for digoxin is as follows: for cats weighing 1.9 to 3.2 kg (about 4 to 7 lb), ¼ of a 0.125-mg tablet every second to third day; for cats weighing 3.2 to 6.0 kg (about 7 to 13 lb), ¼ tablet daily; for cats weighing more than 6 kg, ¼ tablet daily to twice daily. Furosemide is administered at the lowest effective oral dosage, usually 1 to 2 mg/kg, once or twice daily. Oxygen therapy and thoracentesis might be required in severe or acute cases of heart failure.

Propranolol is a β-adrenergic blocking drug that has definite indications in hyperthyroid cats that do *not* have congestive heart failure. Clinical signs that improve with propranolol therapy include tachycardia, tremor, restlessness, and anxiety. Propranolol has no significant effect on oxygen consumption or contractility in hyperthyroidism. All cats with tachycardia (heart rate greater than 200 bpm at rest), tall R waves in lead II, or ventricular or atrial arrhythmias should be treated with propranolol as well as with antithyroid medications. The oral maintenance dosage for propranolol is 2.5 mg (for cats weighing less than 6 kg) or 5 mg (for those weighing more than 6 kg), twice to three times daily.

Side effects of propranolol therapy are uncommon but might develop. Lethargy, weakness, and bradycardia are cardiac manifestations of overdosage. Propranolol is contraindicated in cats with asthma, chronic lung disease, or bradycardia, and in most cats with uncontrolled congestive heart failure.

Cats in high-output heart failure may respond to furosemide and methimazole, and such cats are good candidates for surgery. Propranolol (Inderal, Ayerst) is indicated in this setting if heart failure is associated with extreme tachycardia or results from frequent extrasystoles. It should be administered with caution, however, because of its negative inotropic effects (see Beta-blocking Therapy in Dogs and Cats).

In the treatment of thyrotoxic cats with heart failure, all cats should be considered for surgery, following a period of stabilization, except those cats in obvious low-output failure. Therapeutic recommendations are as follows:

1. All cats are treated with furosemide; mild cases of right-sided failure or pulmonary edema may only require administration of a diuretic.
2. Digoxin, with or without a vasodilator, might be needed for more severe, right-sided heart failure.
3. Propranolol is used, with caution, in cats with heart failure secondary to tachyarrhythmia, and the drug is not given until congestive heart failure has been resolved.
4. Methimazole or PTU is used in all cases.
5. Surgery is performed as soon as the heart failure is resolved and T_4 concentrations are normal.
6. Cardiac medications frequently can be discontinued after surgery.

Long-term results of surgery or radioactive iodine therapy are generally excellent. Occasionally, cats need supplementation with thyroxine after treatment (see Feline Hyperthyroidism), but only for 3 to 4 months. Cats with no cardiac abnormalities or very mild cardiac changes have the best prognosis, although even cats with congestive heart failure can be cured. If low-output heart failure is present, the prognosis is very guarded. Cardiac medications are continued for 1 to 2 months after surgery. Electrocardiograms and thoracic radiographs are taken every 1 to 2 weeks for the first 1 to 2 months after cessation of cardiac drugs to ensure that heart failure is not returning. Serum T_4 concentrations should be monitored every 6 months to 1 year, even after bilateral thyroidectomy or radioactive iodine therapy, since a small number of cats regenerate residual, adenomatous thyroid tissue and suffer a relapse of hyperthyroidism.

References and Supplemental Reading

Birchard, S. J., Peterson, M. E., and Jacobson, A.: Surgical treatment of feline hyperthyroidism: Results of 85 cases. J. Am. Anim. Hosp. Assoc. 20:705, 1984.

Klein, I., and Levey, G. S.: New perspectives on thyroid hormone, catecholamines, and the heart. Am. J. Med. 76:167, 1984.

Liu, S.-K., Peterson, M. E., and Fox, P. R.: Hypertrophic cardiomyopathy and hyperthyroidism in the cat. J.A.V.M.A. 185:52, 1984.
Peterson, M. E.: Propylthiouracil in the treatment of feline hyperthyroidism. J.A.V.M.A. 179:485, 1981.
Peterson, M. E.: Treatment of canine and feline hypoparathyroidism. J.A.V.M.A. 181:1434, 1982.
Peterson, M. E., and Becker, D. V.: Radionuclide thyroid imaging in 135 cats with hyperthyroidism. Vet. Radiol. 25:23, 1984.
Peterson, M. E., Hurvitz, A. I., Leib, M. S., et al.: Propylthiouracil-associated hemolytic anemia, thrombocytopenia, and antinuclear antibodies in cats with hyperthyroidism. J.A.V.M.A. 184:806, 1984.
Peterson, M. E., Keene, B., Ferguson, D. C., et al.: Electrocardiographic findings in 45 cats with hyperthyroidism. J.A.V.M.A. 120:934, 1982.
Peterson, M. E., Kintzer, P. P., Cavanaugh, P. G., et al.: Feline hyperthyroidism: Pretreatment clinical and laboratory evaluation of 131 cases. J.A.V.M.A. 183:103, 1983.
Turrel, J. M., Feldman, E. C., Hays, M., et al.: Radioactive iodine therapy in cats with hyperthyroidism. J.A.V.M.A. 184:554, 1984.

BACTERIAL ENDOCARDITIS

DAVID SISSON, D.V.M.,
Pullman, Washington

and WILLIAM P. THOMAS, D.V.M.
Davis, California

Bacterial infection of the heart valves or mural endocardium is a life-threatening disorder resulting in serious cardiac and extracardiac sequelae. Although the clinical incidence of bacterial endocarditis in dogs and cats is unknown, reports of prevalence at necropsy in dogs vary from 0.06 to 6.6 per cent. Large male dogs older than 4 years are most frequently affected, and German shepherds and boxers may be at increased risk. No relationship between myxomatous degeneration of the mitral valve and bacterial endocarditis has been established in dogs. However, a strong association between congenital discrete subaortic stenosis and bacterial endocarditis of the aortic valve has been reported. Because the paucity of clinical reports of bacterial endocarditis in cats precludes review of its clinical features, the following discussion summarizes experience reported in dogs and humans.

ETIOLOGY AND PATHOGENESIS

Although a wide variety of gram-positive and gram-negative organisms have been reported to cause infective endocarditis, *Streptococcus* spp., *Staphylococcus aureus*, *Pseudomonas aeruginosa*, *Corynebacterium* spp., *Erysipelothrix rhusiopathiae*, *Escherichia coli*, and *Aerobacter aerogenes* are the most commonly reported isolates in dogs. Although species of *Streptococcus* have historically been reported as the most commonly cultured organisms, recent investigators have reported more variable culture results. The cause of this disparity is unknown, although all investigators have not used uniform criteria for confirming the diagnosis. In humans, bacterial endocarditis has been classified as either acute or subacute based on the usual clinical course associated with particular organisms. Although similar patterns in dogs have not been documented, the differing pathogenesis of these two subclassifications is illustrative of the mechanisms probably operating in bacterial endocarditis in dogs and cats.

A transient or persistent bacteremia is an absolute requirement for the establishment of either form of infection. In acute bacterial endocarditis, bacteremia is often associated with active infection at a site remote from the heart (skin, prostate, gingiva, bone, lung). The causative organisms in the subacute form are usually part of the indigenous flora that gain entrance to the circulation as a result of trauma (surgery, dental manipulation). In both forms of endocarditis, there may be no identifiable predisposing infection or portal of entry. There is substantial evidence that intermittent transient bacteremia is a common normal occurrence, and additional mechanisms have been suggested to explain the initiation of cardiac infection. Central to the theorized pathogenesis of acute endocarditis is the ability of certain bacteria (*Staphylococcus, Pseudomonas* spp.) to adhere to the surfaces of the valve leaflets. Additional requirements proposed for the development of subacute bacterial endocarditis include the following: (1) the presence of a previously damaged valve or jet lesion, (2) formation of a sterile platelet-fibrin thrombus, and (3) increased size of the inoculum due to clumping caused by agglutinating antibody directed against the infecting organism. It is certain that additional factors modifying host resistance (concurrent illness, immunosuppression) and degree of exposure (e.g., in-dwelling catheters) also play important roles in the establishment of infection. Once a cardiac infection is established, the ensuing clinical course depends on the site and severity of the local infection (and thereby the virulence of the organism); extension of infection into the myocardium, pericardium, or aortic root; and involvement of other organ systems as a result of metastatic infection, embolization, generalized sepsis, or immune-mediated disorders.

The basic lesion of bacterial endocarditis is a vegetation that usually is located on the mitral, aortic, or both valves in dogs and cats. Primary involvement of the mural endocardium or the valves on the right side of the heart is uncommon. Explanations for this pattern of distribution based on hemodynamic stresses and the Venturi effect have been suggested but offer little explanation for the differing sites of infection observed in other species. Fresh vegetations are friable and consist of a large inner layer of platelets, fibrin, red and white blood cells, and some bacteria; a middle layer of bacteria; and an outer fibrin layer. The less friable, older vegetation is covered by a layer of fibrous tissue with varying amounts of necrosis, phagocytosis, hyalinization, and calcification. Valve dysfunction occurs most commonly as a result of necrosis, perforation, or prolapse. Stenosis of the valve by large vegetations is rare. Congestive heart failure occurs more commonly with aortic than mitral valve endocarditis. Extension of infection into the valve annulus, pericardium, or myocardium may result in abscess formation, aortoatrial shunt, purulent pericarditis, myocarditis, arrhythmias, or destruction of the conduction system. Because of the location of the infection and friable structure of the vegetations, peripheral arterial embolization is common. Although the heart, brain, intestine, or other organs may be affected, the kidney and spleen are the most common sites of infarction at necropsy. The significance of some findings is uncertain. It is difficult to discern if areas of infection remote from the heart (diskospondylitis, septic arthritis) are primary or secondary lesions. The frequency and clinical importance of myocarditis, polyarthritis, and glomerulonephritis due to the deposition of immune complexes is uncertain. Clearly, bacterial endocarditis is best described as a broad group of clinical presentations, with cardiac infection as the common denominator.

CLINICAL MANIFESTATIONS AND DIAGNOSIS

Bacterial endocarditis has been called the "great imitator" because of the many organ systems that may be involved and the variety of clinical signs that may result. Early signs are nonspecific and reflect the presence of infection and extracardiac disorders more often than they suggest a cardiovascular disease. Lethargy, weight loss, and anorexia are common, along with persistent or intermittent signs of secondarily affected organs or body regions such as lameness, vomiting, diarrhea, hemi- or paraparesis, seizures, and hematuria. Congestive heart failure develops in most dogs with aortic valve endocarditis and in many dogs with mitral valve endocarditis. Syncope may occur as a result of tachyarrhythmias or heart block with or without heart failure. Cardiac signs may not be manifest or may occur alone or together with ophthalmic, central nervous system, orthopedic, renal, or peripheral vascular disorders. The physical findings of fever, an organic heart murmur, and evidence of peripheral embolization warrant a presumptive diagnosis of endocarditis. Unfortunately, any or all of these signs may be absent in a given patient. The recognition and interpretation of abnormal heart sounds in this clinical setting is essential. The sudden development of an organic heart murmur suggests bacterial endocarditis but must be distinguished from physiologic murmurs due to infection (fever) or anemia and murmurs of other acquired heart diseases. The murmur of mitral regurgitation due to myxomatous degeneration is so common in older, small dogs that it is a poor indicator of bacterial endocarditis. This murmur may also change in character and intensity as a result of changes in preload and afterload in the absence of endocarditis. In contrast, the development of a diastolic murmur together with exaggerated (bounding) arterial pulses strongly suggests aortic valve insufficiency due to bacterial endocarditis. Arrhythmias may be heard in as many as 50 to 75 per cent of affected dogs, and a third heart sound (protodiastolic gallop) may be present as congestive heart failure develops. With the exception of petechiae of the mucous membranes and ocular fundus, the peripheral stigmata of endocarditis in humans (subungual splinter hemorrhages, Osler's nodes, Janeway's lesions, clubbing) are usually absent or undetected in dogs and cats. Bacterial endocarditis should be considered in any patient with an unexplained fever, organ involvement compatible with embolic phenomena, polyarthritis, and new cardiac abnormalities or multisystem disease.

The diverse clinical features and systemic manifestations of bacterial endocarditis mandate thorough laboratory examination, including hematologic evaluation, a complete serum chemistry profile, and urinalysis. Normocytic, normochromic anemia (usually mild) and leukocytosis due to neutrophilia and monocytosis are common but variable findings. Elevation of the erythrocyte sedimentation rate is inconsistently observed in affected dogs. Serum chemistry abnormalities usually reflect extracardiac organ involvement due to metastatic infection, embolization (infarction), immune-mediated damage, or congestive heart failure (particularly elevations of the blood urea nitrogen). Pyuria, hematuria, and proteinuria may be due to pyelonephritis, glomerulonephritis, or renal infarction. Urine cultures are frequently negative or misleading and should not be substituted for properly performed blood cultures. Confusion with immune-mediated diseases often prompts immunologic testing. Antinuclear antibody, Coombs', and rheumatoid factor tests may be positive in dogs with bacterial endocarditis and must be interpreted cautiously with consideration of all other clinical and laboratory data. Depending on the pathogenesis (infective versus immune-mediated), septic or nonseptic inflammatory fluids may be obtained from joints or the central nervous system.

Overt cardiac manifestations (murmurs, arrhythmias) or suspicion of endocarditis warrants electrocardiographic, radiographic, and echocardiographic evaluation. Electrocardiography is useful in the identification of premature depolarizations, paroxysmal or sustained tachycardias, and conduction disturbances such as bundle branch block and second- and third-degree heart block. Left atrial and ventricular enlargement accompanying hemodynamically advanced lesions or ischemic S-T deviation due to coronary artery embolism or heart failure may also be detected. Radiography allows evaluation of heart size and detects signs of left heart failure but is not specifically diagnostic for endocarditis. The value of M-mode and two-dimensional echocardiography in the diagnosis of endocarditis resides in their ability to noninvasively image internal cardiac structures and to detect vegetative lesions and hemodynamic abnormalities resulting from valvular infection. Vegetative lesions as small as 2 mm in diameter may be detected, and cardiac complications such as dilation, aortic root abscess, flail valve leaflets, and ruptured chordae tendineae may be visualized. Aortic regurgitation may also be detected indirectly by noting abnormal mitral valve motion, including diastolic fluttering or premature closure. Although aortic valve vegetations are usually readily imaged, difficulty in distinguishing small vegetations from acquired degenerative (myxomatous) lesions may be a significant limitation to the echocardiographic evaluation of mitral valve endocarditis in dogs.

Blood culture is the most important diagnostic procedure indicated in a patient suspected of having bacterial endocarditis. Bacteremia is continuous in this condition, so that culturing need not coincide with fluctuations in body temperature. A minimum of three sets (two bottles each) of blood cultures within a 24-hour period should be obtained. In extremely ill animals, these cultures may be obtained within a few hours. A positive blood culture (preferably two or more) should be expected in 75 per cent of dogs with bacterial endocarditis. The causes of culture-negative endocarditis include (1) recent antibiotic therapy (common in dogs and cats); (2) fastidious, slow-growing bacteria; (3) nonbacterial (i.e., fungal) endocarditis (rare); (4) right-sided endocarditis (rare); and (5) noninfective endocarditis. In these cases, a presumptive diagnosis must be based on the combination of history, physical findings, laboratory evaluation, and echocardiographic evaluation. It may be particularly difficult to distinguish bacterial endocarditis of the mitral valve from acquired mitral regurgitation and bacteremia without a cardiac infection. In this setting, the authors institute therapy for endocarditis in the absence of a definitive diagnosis.

In summary, a definitive clinical diagnosis of bacterial endocarditis requires a positive blood culture combined with clinical and laboratory evidence of cardiac involvement (new or progressive murmur, echocardiographic vegetations) or embolic phenomena. In the absence of a positive blood culture, a presumptive diagnosis can be made when there is clinical and laboratory evidence of systemic infection (fever, leukocytosis) combined with cardiac and embolic signs.

MANAGEMENT

The medical management of bacterial endocarditis requires treatment of the underlying infection and of the resulting cardiac and extracardiac complications. Treatment must be intensive, aggressive, and carefully monitored and is therefore likely to be comparatively expensive. Since there have been no studies on the efficacy of antimicrobial therapy in this condition in animals, the following principles of treatment are adapted from clinical experience and from recommendations for the management of human infective endocarditis, with modifications for organisms most commonly encountered in dogs.

1. *Establish a microbiologic diagnosis by blood culture.* In most animals, the 3 to 24 hours required to obtain three blood cultures will not alter the disease course significantly. Only in patients with acute endocarditis and severe septicemia should antibiotic treatment be initiated before initial microbiologic examination is completed. If an organism is identified, antimicrobial sensitivity testing using a disk or, preferably, a broth dilution technique to determine minimum inhibitory concentrations (MIC) or, preferably, minimum bactericidal concentrations (MBC) should be performed. If cultures are negative, broad-spectrum combination bactericidal antibiotic therapy is advised because of the diversity of organisms commonly cultured in dogs.

2. *Administer bactericidal antibiotics parenterally (IV) in bactericidal doses.* Drugs capable of

penetrating fibrin are preferred, but results of sensitivity testing are most important. Antibiotics that can be given safely at doses resulting in serum concentrations greater than the MBC should be used. Ideally, drugs should be administered IV for as long as 4 to 6 weeks, depending on the infecting organisms. In veterinary practice, however, drugs are usually administered IV for 7 to 10 days in the hospital and are continued PO for several weeks at home. Since data in dogs and cats are limited, the following empirical regimens for treating humans with bacterial endocarditis are probably applicable for dogs and cats: For penicillin-sensitive *Streptococcus* spp.: sodium penicillin G up to 50,000 units/kg four times daily; or ampicillin 30 mg/kg three times daily for 4 weeks; or alternatively, penicillin G or ampicillin and dihydrostreptomycin 10 mg/kg three times daily for 2 weeks. For enterococcal group D *Streptococcus:* penicillin or ampicillin and an aminoglycoside such as gentamicin 2 to 3 mg/kg three times daily for 2 weeks (follow renal function closely) or amikacin 5 mg/kg three times daily for 2 to 3 weeks. For *Staphylococcus:* penicillin or ampicillin if penicillin sensitive; or oxacillin 50 to 60 mg/kg three times daily; nafcillin 10 to 20 mg/kg four times daily; or cephalothin 15 to 25 mg/kg three times daily for 4 to 6 weeks in penicillinase-producing isolates. For *Pseudomonas aeruginosa:* carbenicillin 100 mg/kg four times daily or ticarcillin 40 to 50 mg/kg four times daily and an aminoglycoside for 2 weeks. If therapy of greater than 2 weeks is required, then amikacin should be used and renal function followed carefully. Treatment of other gram-negative organisms should be based on the results of sensitivity testing. Anaerobic isolates are usually sensitive to penicillin or ampicillin. In culture-negative endocarditis or when culture results are pending in acute endocarditis, an aminoglycoside together with penicillin, ampicillin, oxacillin, or nafcillin is used. When prolonged aminoglycoside therapy is anticipated and renal function is compromised, the authors prefer amikacin to other aminoglycosides for susceptible isolates. Caution must be exercised when using drugs with dosage-dependent toxicities, particularly the aminoglycosides. Drug interactions that may potentiate toxicity must be considered. In particular, urine output, urine sediment, and serum creatinine concentration should be monitored when furosemide and aminoglycosides are used concurrently.

3. *Perform frequent examinations and follow-up blood cultures.* Patients should be examined daily for changes in heart sounds, cardiac rhythm, arterial pulse pressure, or signs of new systemic complications. To assess the efficacy of therapy and detect relapses, blood cultures should be obtained 2 days after starting antibiotic therapy and 1 and 2 months following completion of therapy.

4. *Treat predisposing conditions and complications.* The animal should be carefully examined for a portal of entry of the infection, which may then be eliminated. Although rarely proved by microbiologic examination, concurrent conditions reported to occur in dogs and cats with endocarditis include abscesses, periodontal disease, prostatitis, urinary tract infections, pneumonia, diskospondylitis, and other infections. Surgical drainage should be considered when possible.

The most common cardiac complications requiring medical therapy are congestive heart failure and arrhythmias. Congestive heart failure is the most common cause of death in dogs with endocarditis, especially of the aortic valve. Administration of cardiac glycosides, diuretics, and arterial or mixed vasodilators is indicated (see Positive Inotropic Drugs in Heart Failure; Vasodilator Therapy). However, because valve replacement surgery is unavailable to most veterinary patients, the development of heart failure unresponsive to routine medical therapy warrants a grave prognosis. Serious tachyarrhythmias require specific antiarrhythmic medication (see Antiarrhythmic Drugs and and Management of Cardiac Arrhythmias), and high-grade atrioventricular block may require pacemaker therapy.

The inability to replace infected valves that have large friable vegetations makes prevention of systemic embolization and infarction difficult. Anticoagulation is usually contraindicated because it has not been shown to significantly reduce embolic complications, and serious bleeding episodes may occur. The site of embolization and resulting impairment of the target organ may determine the prognosis in some patients. The development of septic shock or renal failure requires aggressive therapy, which will complicate coexisting heart failure. Thus, the prognosis is dependent on the virulence of the infecting organism, the hemodynamic consequences of valvular damage, the presence of heart failure, and the severity of extracardiac complications such as renal failure, sepsis, or systemic embolization. Successful treatment is usually dependent on diagnosis prior to these complications, requiring a high index of suspicion in patients with unexplained fever accompanied by other signs. Once treatment is begun, there should be *no therapeutic compromises*, even when there is early improvement in clinical and laboratory abnormalities.

PREVENTION

Successful prophylaxis of bacterial endocarditis requires (1) identification of susceptible individuals, (2) knowledge of what procedures or circumstances are associated with transient bacteremia, and (3) documentation of an effective prophylactic protocol specific for the procedure or circumstance. Because little information about this type of prophylaxis in animals is available, the authors' recommendations are based on limited studies in experimental animals and on a report demonstrating bacteremia resulting from dental manipulations in dogs. In dogs and cats with pre-existing valvular heart disease, particularly discrete fibrous subaortic stenosis, ampicillin (20 mg/kg) and gentamicin (3 mg/kg) are given 1 hour before and for 24 hours after the procedure.

References and Supplemental Reading

Black, A. P., Crichlow, A. M., and Saunders, J. R.: Bacteremia during ultrasonic teeth cleaning and extraction in the dog. J. Am. Anim. Hosp. Assoc. 16:611, 1980.

Bonagura, J. D.: Bacterial endocarditis. *In* Ettinger, S. J. (ed.): *Textbook of Veterinary Internal Medicine.* Philadelphia: W. B. Saunders, 1983, pp. 1052–1062.

Calvert, C. A.: Valvular bacterial endocarditis in the dog. J.A.V.M.A. 180:1080, 1982.

Garvey, M. S., and Aucoin, D. P.: Therapeutic strategies involving antimicrobial treatment of disseminated bacterial infection in small animals. J.A.V.M.A. 185:1185, 1984.

Lowbard, C. W., and Buergelt, C. D.: Vegetative bacterial endocarditis in dogs; echocardiographic diagnosis and clinical signs. J. Small. Anim. Pract. 24:325, 1983.

Shouse, C. L., and Meier, H.: Acute vegetative endocarditis in the dog and cat. J.A.V.M.A. 129:278, 1956.

Sisson, D., and Thomas, W. P.: Endocarditis of the aortic valve in the dog. J.A.V.M.A. 184:570, 1984.

Weinstein, L.: Infective endocarditis. *In* Braunwald, E. (ed.): *Heart Disease.* Philadelphia: W. B. Saunders, 1984, pp. 1136–1182.

Wilson, W. R. et al.: Symposium on infective endocarditis. Mayo Clin. Proc. 57:3, 1982.

THERAPY OF CANINE HEARTWORM DISEASE

CLAY A. CALVERT, D.V.M.,
and CLARENCE A. RAWLINGS, D.V.M.
Athens, Georgia

EPIZOOTIOLOGY

Dirofilaria immitis, or heartworm, is found in most temperate and tropical areas of the world, particularly the coastal regions of the oceans, including the Indian and Mediterranean. In the United States, *D. immitis* has been endemic along the southeastern coastlands for more than a half century. The incidence of heartworm infection in previously nonendemic areas is increasing, probably as a result of the movement of infected dogs. Heartworm disease is now commonly recognized in most midwestern states and is spreading westward even to the west coast. For a more detailed discussion of the epizootiology of *D. immitis*, the reader is referred to chapters on heartworm disease in the *Textbook of Veterinary Internal Medicine* (Ettinger, 1983) and *Current Veterinary Therapy VIII* (Kirk, 1983).

PATHOPHYSIOLOGY

The time course and severity of pulmonary arterial disease depend on the adult worm burden, duration of infection, and host-parasite interaction. Pulmonary hypertension is not due to the physical obstruction of the arteries by adult *D. immitis* but results from vascular lesions incited by the presence of adult worms in the immediate vicinity.

Immature adult heartworms reach the pulmonary arteries, particularly those of the caudal lung lobes, between 90 and 100 days after infection. These worms develop to adult size during the next 3 to 6 months. When the number of adult worms exceeds 25 in a 25-kg (55-lb) dog, heartworms are commonly found in the right ventricle as well as in the pulmonary arteries. Dogs with more than 50 worms commonly have some in the right atrium, and if there are 75 to 100 or more worms, the caudal vena cava may become obstructed.

The disease of the pulmonary arteries results from endothelial damage caused by adjacent adult worms. Endothelial cells swell, develop wider intercellular junctions, have activated leukocytes adhering to them, and slough longitudinal strips within 3 days of the presence of adult worms in the arteries. Activated platelets adhere to focal areas of exposed subendothelium and appear to release a trophic factor—platelet-derived growth factor. Intimal smooth muscle cells beneath these activated platelets multiply rapidly and migrate toward the surface. These cells and the collagen that they produce result in the pathognomonic villus proliferation from the pulmonary arterial surface. The de-endothelialized areas of the villi eventually develop an endothelium-like covering. Villi develop within 3 weeks of heartworm infestation and progressively increase in size and severity. Villi are distributed throughout the pulmonary arterial tree, from the pulmonary valves to arteries as small as can accommodate a heartworm. Smaller pulmonary arteries also have medial hyperplasia that tends to obstruct their lumina to blood flow.

All large arteries (especially the caudal lobar arteries) dilate, become tortuous, develop aneurysms, and lose their normal tapering arborization. Linear lucencies of adult heartworms may be seen by angiography, and small arterial disease is recognized as an abrupt pruning of peripheral arteries. Flow of contrast media may be negligible or delayed through these lung regions, with poor small vessel circulation. Alveolar consolidation is present radiographically as a focal area surrounding the caudal lobar arteries. This consolidation is due to focal edema and inflammation, which are extensions of changes occurring on the endothelium. These lung changes probably involve bronchioles sufficiently to initiate the cough reflex.

Morphologic changes in the small pulmonary arteries increase pulmonary arterial resistance and pressure, leading to increased right ventricular afterload. Pulmonary hypertension develops within a few months of adult heartworm infestation and is produced by the morphologic changes. Clinical signs of exercise intolerance occur when the right ventricle can no longer increase its output on demand because of pulmonary hypertension and the inability to collaterally recruit and dilate small pulmonary arteries.

Although considerable morphologic changes are initiated by the presence of live heartworms, this host-parasite interaction is less severe than those changes initiated by the death of the heartworms. Extensive pulmonary changes are produced when heartworms die either as a result of adulticide treatments or following a natural life course. These changes are most obvious during the first 3 to 6 weeks after heartworm death; subsequently, the disease processes begin to reverse to preinfection normalcy. The death of heartworms eliminates their protective mechanisms against the host defense responses. Severe thrombosis and a granulomatous inflammatory response are initiated. The most characteristic response of the arterial wall lining is an exaggerated development of the same myointimal proliferation into rugose villi as is produced in response to live heartworms. These arterial walls have areas with focal loss of endothelium and an increased protein permeability. Coagulation is initiated, and coagulation fibrinolysis may be severe enough to initiate either a local or systemic disseminated intravascular coagulopathy (DIC). The villus proliferation and thrombosis are typically so severe that flow is obstructed through the caudal lobar and intermediate arteries. Flow obstruction increases pressure sufficiently to distend the large pulmonary arteries and increases right ventricular afterload. The characteristic radiographic sign of worm embolism after therapy with an adulticide is the development of a focal area of increased alveolar density in the caudal and accessory lung lobes. These alveolar changes frequently involve whole lobes. The density may be produced by either edema or blood. Auscultatory crackles are usually evident at this time. The caudal airways of some dogs may fill with blood, and coughing and hemoptysis may occur. The radiographic and arteriographic changes produced by dead heartworms begin to resolve within 3 to 4 weeks after adulticide treatment.

Resolution of the changes on the surface of the proximal pulmonary arteries can be detected as early as 6 weeks after adulticide treatment. The villi are either markedly reduced in size or absent. The cellular axis remains disoriented, and there is a swirling appearance to the endothelium. Villi are uncommon findings in arteries 1 year after treatment. Pulmonary hypertension, a reflection of small arterial disease, can revert to normal pulmonary artery pressure as soon as 6 months after successful adulticide treatment. The larger arteries decrease in size and tortuosity as the hypertension resolves. The aneurysms and dilation in the small arteries also tend to resolve less completely. The parenchymal lesions about these arteries should be markedly resolved within 2 to 3 months after adulticide treatment.

CLINICAL STAGES OF HEARTWORM DISEASE

If appropriate client education is practiced and annual microfilariae tests are performed, most heartworm-infected dogs will be asymptomatic at the time of diagnosis, and the treatment success rate should be virtually 100 per cent. However, if, for whatever reasons, heartworm infection remains undiagnosed for 2 or more years, clinical signs will often be apparent (Table 1).

Coughing and exercise intolerance are usually associated with moderate to severe pulmonary arterial disease. However, pulmonary infiltrates with eosinophilia, as in allergic pneumonitis or eosinophilic granulomatosis, produce severe clinical signs, usually with radiographic evidence of only mild to moderate pulmonary arterial enlargement. Dyspnea and hemoptysis are always associated with either severe pulmonary arterial disease, pulmonary

Table 1. Clinical Signs Associated with Complicated Heartworm Disease

Clinical Signs	Usual Associations
Cough, weight loss, dyspnea	Moderate to severe radiographic abnormalities Pulmonary infiltrates of eosinophils (PIE) syndrome
Hemoptysis	Severe radiographic abnormalities Pulmonary thromboembolism Disseminated intravascular coagulopathy
Ascites	Severe radiographic abnormalities ECG evidence of right ventricular hypertrophy
Shock syndrome	Vena cava syndrome Pulmonary thromboembolism Severe pulmonary hypertension

thromboembolism, pulmonary infiltrates with eosinophilia, or the caval syndrome. Weight loss of 10 per cent or greater is associated with advanced disease with severe pulmonary hypertension, and right-sided congestive heart failure is often present or imminent.

As a general rule, most dogs with clinical signs of advanced heartworm disease have immune-mediated occult infections. Severe pulmonary hypertension is usually present, although allergic pneumonitis and pulmonary eosinophilic granulomatosis are usually not associated with severe pulmonary arterial enlargement. In some endemic areas, the caval syndrome is a common cause of a shock syndrome. Regardless of the severity of clinical signs, most dogs with heartworm disease can be effectively treated. The time commitment, cost, and effort required for the successful management of advanced disease are factors that may be more limiting than the disease itself.

OCCULT HEARTWORM INFECTIONS

Strictly speaking, the term *occult heartworm infection* or disease refers to the presence of adult *D. immitis* in dogs in which an immune-mediated or hypersensitivity reaction in the pulmonary capillaries has entrapped and killed the microfilariae. However, the term has also been loosely applied to several circumstances in which microfilaremia is not present or detected. The incidence of heartworm infections without circulating microfilariae has been reported to be 10 to 67 per cent. In the United States, this incidence is usually between 15 and 40 per cent (Otto, 1978; Wong et al., 1973).

The presence of adult *D. immitis* organisms without circulating microfilariae may be the result of several circumstances: (1) prepatent infections, (2) unisexual infections, (3) drug-induced changes, and (4) immune-mediated factors. The incidence of each of these circumstances among infected dogs without microfilaremia is unknown, but each represents a diagnostic challenge to the clinician. Young adults (fifth-stage larvae, L_5) may be found in the right ventricle and pulmonary arteries as early as 2 months after L_3 infection, and angiographically detectable abnormalities subsequently develop within 1 month. Heavy infections (more than 40 worms) may produce radiographically detectable abnormalities within 4 to 5 months of L_3 infection. Since patency seldom is reached in less than 6 months and may occasionally require 9 months, it is possible, although unlikely, that clinical and radiographic abnormalities may be detected 1 to 2 months prior to microfilaremia. The index of suspicion of prepatent infections is increased with the use of some serologic tests.

Occasionally, so-called occult infections may result from drug therapy. Levamisole, when used as a microfilaricide, may on occasion reduce the fecundity of or sterilize adult female worms that survive adulticide therapy. Assuming that most male and some female worms have been killed, the clinical and radiographic signs of heartworm disease will improve over a period of several months but may not totally resolve. Serologic tests for adult worms would remain positive. Another way that occult infections can result from drug therapy occurs if all male worms are killed but some females survive. Microfilaremia will recur soon after microfilaricide and may persist for months. Eventually, however, microfilariae will cease to be produced. Thus, repeated courses of microfilaricide without repeated attempts at adulticide may eventually result in the absence of microfilariae but the presence of adult females. This scenario should suggest the presence of a post-thiacetarsamide infection consisting of females only.

Perhaps the most common circumstance in which adult *D. immitis* heartworms are present without circulating microfilariae is the true occult infection resulting from host immune responses. Immune-mediated host hypersensitization with a state of antimicrofilarial antibody excess results in microfilarial entrapment within the pulmonary capillaries. Antibody-dependent leukocyte activation and adhesion to microfilariae promote this entrapment. IgG is important in this reaction, and it was recently reported that the IgM class of antibody is involved in microfilarial opsonization. This process is enhanced by a source of complement and neutrophils are the predominant effector cells (El-Sadr et al., 1983).

Occasionally, eosinophils as well as neutrophils are particularly numerous around the entrapped microfilariae. This may result in the allergic pneumonitis syndrome encountered in some occult infections. Subsequently, the dead microfilariae become engulfed in a granulomatous inflammatory response composed of mononuclear and giant cells (El-Sadr et al., 1983). In some such instances, severe pulmonary eosinophilic granulomas may develop.

In general, the incidence of severe pulmonary arterial disease and hypertension is greater with immune-mediated occult than with microfilaremic infections. At the University of Georgia Veterinary Teaching Hospital (UGVTH), approximately 70 to 80 per cent of all instances of severe pulmonary hypertension (cor pulmonale) are associated with occult disease. Apparently, the hypersensitivity, immune-mediated, and granulomatous reactions are more severe and produce accelerated endothelial damage and myointimal proliferation. The mean, median, and range of ages of dogs with occult infections, including severe pulmonary disease, seen at the UGVTH are not different from those of dogs with microfilaremic infections.

Pneumonitis Associated with Occult Heartworm Disease

Although most heartworm-infected dogs manifesting severe clinical signs have advanced pulmonary arterial disease, such is not always the case. Nine of 67 (13 per cent) consecutive cases of occult heartworm disease seen at the UGVTH had signs of moderate to severe respiratory disease but only mild enlargement of the lobar pulmonary arteries.

Consistent and progressive clinical signs were coughing, dyspnea, crackles, and exercise intolerance. Cyanosis was detected in four dogs. Eosinophilia and hyerglobulinemia were consistent findings, and basophilia was present in seven of nine dogs. Serologic tests for adult and microfilarial antigens were positive. Eosinophils, nondegenerate neutrophils, and macrophages were seen in transtracheal lavage specimens. The thoracic radiographic appearance of this syndrome is a mixed linear interstitial and alveolar pattern, which is most obvious in the caudal lung fields. The infiltrates frequently obscure the appearance of the lobar pulmonary arteries, which are not severely enlarged.

Prednisone at dosages of 1 to 2 mg/kg daily results in clinical improvement beginning within 12 to 24 hours, and both clinical and radiographic abnormalities are largely eliminated within 2 to 3 days. Prednisone therapy is stopped after 3 to 5 days, and adulticide therapy is given immediately. Relapse of the clinical signs of this allergic or immune-mediated syndrome has not been observed.

SEVERE PULMONARY HYPERTENSION

Although severe pulmonary hypertension develops in less than 10 per cent of heartworm-infected dogs by the time of diagnosis, in endemic areas this incidence rate produces a significant number of severely affected dogs. At the UGVTH, occult infections account for approximately 70 per cent of such cases.

At the time of diagnosis, dogs with the most severe pulmonary hypertension variably exhibit exercise intolerance, coughing, dyspnea, syncope, weight loss, hemoptysis and, in approximately 50 to 60 per cent of affected dogs, ascites. There is radiographic evidence of severe pulmonary arterial disease and right ventricular enlargement. Pleural effusion is notably absent. The electrocardiograms (ECGs) from approximately 80 per cent of these dogs reflect right ventricular hypertrophy. Ninety per cent of heartworm-infected dogs with definitive ECG evidence of right ventricular hypertrophy also exhibit ascites. Dogs with ECG evidence of right ventricular hypertrophy but lacking ascites usually develop clinical signs of right-sided congestive heart failure within 2 to 3 months.

The recommended *treatment* for heartworm disease with concomitant severe pulmonary artery disease or heart failure is as follows:

1. Cage rest for 1 to 2 weeks prior to adulticide and for 4 weeks after adulticide
2. Aspirin therapy for the above duration
3. Cortocisteroid hormones when indicated
4. Adulticide therapy not sooner than following 1 week of cage rest and after resolution of pulmonary parenchymal disease, if present
5. Judicious dosages of furosemide (Lasix, Hoechst-Roussel) and a low-sodium diet for those dogs with ascites

The survival rate of 63 dogs with severe pulmonary hypertension, including 38 dogs with ascites and 25 dogs without ascites, was 85 per cent. The presence of right-sided congestive heart failure did not seem to worsen the prognosis compared with dogs showing similar radiographic abnormalities but lacking ascites. Most dogs dying of severe disease do so 10 to 14 days after administration of thiacetarsamide, with signs and laboratory data consistent with DIC. Dogs older than approximately 12 years have a worse prognosis but constitute a small proportion of the total. The survival rate of 26 dogs not treated with the above method was 65 per cent. Digitalis glycosides are, in the authors' experience, not indicated, do not alter the survival statistics, and frequently complicate therapy as a result of intercurrent digoxin intoxication.

During the course of hospitalization, it is advised that careful observation be made for thrombocytopenia and DIC. Thrombocytopenia is a consistent abnormality that develops 7 to 14 days after adulticide and may be severe. Gastrointestinal bleeding secondary to aspirin therapy is to be expected but is usually not severe. Because of the prolonged period of hospitalization, the clients' costs are rather high, but it is the authors' experience that sufficient observation, detection of early signs of complications, and adequate restriction of activity are not likely to be provided in the home environment.

MINIMUM DATA BASE

There is no one minimum data base that should be recommended prior to heartworm treatment. Factors such as age, clinical signs, possible duration of infection, and microfilarial status influence the extent of the data base.

Asymptomatic dogs younger than approximately 5 years that have been tested yearly for microfilaremia require only a complete blood count, blood urea nitrogen (BUN), and urinalysis. Older dogs, symptomatic dogs, and those with suspected occult infections require an extended data base including a serum chemistry profile. Thoracic radiographs are indicated for symptomatic dogs, dogs not tested yearly for microfilaremia, older dogs, and dogs suspected of having occult infections. Liver function tests, such as sulfobromophthalein (BSP) retention, are indicated only when hypoalbuminemia, icterus, or ascites is present. An ECG is useful only when an arrhythmia, severe thoracic radiographic abnormalities, or ascites is present. A transtracheal lavage may be performed in affected dogs that are coughing, especially if a concomitant fever or an inflammatory leukogram is present.

Table 2. *Hematologic Abnormalities Associated with 193 Dogs with Heartworm Disease Seen at the UGVTH*

Abnormality	Incidence (%)
Anemia (PCV < 38%)	
Asymptomatic to moderately symptomatic	10
Severe pulmonary hypertension	60
Neutrophilia	
Asyptomatic to moderately symptomatic	20
Severe pulmonary hypertension	80
Eosinophilia	
Microfilaremic	80
Occult	90
Basophilia	
Microfilaremic	50
Occult	70
Liver enzyme elevations	10
Decreased BSP Clearance	
Asymptomatic	5
Mildly to moderately symptomatic	20
Severe pulmonary hypertension	50
Azoteinuria (BUN > 30/dl)	5
Proteinuria (≥ 2+)	
Asymptomatic	10
Symptomatic	30
Metabolic acidosis arterial pH < 7.31)	15
Hypoxia (P_{AO_2} < 85)	30

CLINICAL PATHOLOGY

Abnormalities of the complete blood count and serum chemistries are sporadic and variable. Most asymptomatic dogs have no significant hematologic abnormalities other than possible eosinophilia or basophilia. A mild normochromic, normocytic anemia may occur in symptomatic dogs (Table 2).

Most severely affected dogs are anemic, but severe anemia is commonly associated only with the caval syndrome or DIC. Anemia associated with the latter is regenerative, and evidence of erythrocyte fragmentation is present.

With chronicity, there is a trend toward lymphopenia and a left shift of the leukogram. There is little correlation between neutrophilia and mild to moderate clinical signs, but most dogs with severe pulmonary hypertension have a neutrophilia, frequently exceeding 25,000 to 30,000/mm^3, usually with a marked left shift and monocytosis.

Eosinophil and basophil counts vary widely, but eosinophilia is most notable when young adult worms reach the heart and again when the first microfilariae appear. Basophilia, when present, is usually associated with eosinophilia, and as a general rule, both are more pronounced in occult, symptomatic infections. In endemic areas, eosinophilia and basophilia are of limited diagnostic importance because of the prevalence of endo- and ectoparasites and *Dipetalonema reconditum* infections.

Elevations of the serum alkaline phosphatase (SAP) or serum glutamic pyruvate transaminase (SGPT) are unusual in asymptomatic dogs. The presence of twofold or greater elevations of liver enzymes does not appear to correlate with either the severity of heartworm disease or the likelihood of adverse reactions to thiacetarsamide. BSP retention of 8 to 15 per cent (normal is less than 5 per cent) at 30 minutes is observed in some symptomatic dogs and is most common in dogs with right-sided congestive heart failure.

Proteinuria is common in symptomatic infections and usually is the result of immune complex glomerulopathy. In most instances, proteinuria is of little prognostic significance and resolves within several months of effective heartworm therapy. However, severe proteinuria, particularly when associated with hypoalbuminemia, suggests the possibility of a severe glomerulopathy and is an indication for quantitation of 24-hour urine protein loss. Amyloidosis or severe glomerulonephritis can be associated with renal failure and the nephrotic syndrome, and renal biopsy is required for a definitive diagnosis. Fortunately, severe, irreversible glomerulopathies are uncommonly associated with heartworm disease.

Arterial blood gases are normal in most heartworm-infected dogs. A mild, compensated metabolic acidosis occurs in some dogs, and mild hypoxia affects approximately one third of dogs with moderate to severe pulmonary arterial disease. Some dogs with hypoxia have a metabolic acidosis, probably due to lactic acidosis.

DIAGNOSIS OF HEARTWORM INFECTION

Laboratory Tests

The usual and most definitive means of diagnosing heartworm infection is the identification of *D. immitis* microfilariae in the peripheral blood. Techniques of microfilaria detection include the direct blood smear, hematocrit tube, Knott concentration, and filter tests. Positive results indicate the need, in most circumstances, to treat with thiacetarsamide. A negative test result indicates that the dog may be placed on a prophylactic drug and may indicate that existing clinical abnormalities are due to some other cause, but it does not absolutely rule out the possibility of heartworm infection. Since the microfilariae of *D. reconditum* produce a degree of eosinophilia and basophilia equal to or exceeding that resulting from *D. immitis* infection and because *D. reconditum* infection produces no known pathologic condition, the differentiation of these two microfilariae is important.

In addition to a 10 to 67 per cent incidence of heartworm disease without circulating microfilariae, microfilariae may be present in the absence of adult worms in the following circumstances: after adulticide treatment, prior to or following ineffective microfilaricide treatment, when adult worms die of natural causes, as a result of transfusion of contaminated blood, as a result of transplacental transfer, and in dogs infected with *D. reconditum. D. immitis* microfilariae may survive for 2 years after the death of adult worms.

The direct blood smear is a reasonably accurate test for microfilaremia if the microfilariae count is high. The microscope used for the evaluation should be fitted with a micronometer. The microfilariae of *D. immitis* have a median length of 323.8 ± 9.5 μm, whereas those of *D. reconditum* measure 277.2 ± 9.2 μm. A drop of 0.04 per cent ammonium hydroxide or 2 per cent saponin may be used to lyse the erythrocytes, enabling better visualization. The dimensions of microfilariae identified by concentration techniques differ according to the effects of formalin or lysing solutions. The absence of microfilariae on a direct smear is meaningless, since infections with fewer than 1000 microfilariae/ml of blood are likely to be overlooked. In general, the direct blood smear is 10 to 50 per cent less accurate than concentration tests. When samples are procured for a concentration test, one to two drops of blood are often retained for a direct smear that can be examined prior to the concentration test.

The hematocrit capillary tube test, although a rapid, inexpensive test, has the limitation of inaccuracy when the microfilaria count is low. After centrifugation, the buffy coat region is examined under the low-power objective. The light from the microscope causes microfilariae to enter the plasma. Those of *D. immitis* are less active than those of *D. reconditum* and tend to collect in the dependent half of the hematocrit tube, whereas the latter tend to be dispersed throughout the plasma.

The modified Knott test is performed by mixing 1 ml of venous blood with 10 ml of 2 per cent buffered formalin, and the mixture is centrifuged at 1500 rpm for 3 to 5 minutes. The supernatant is decanted, and the sediment is mixed with an equal volume of 1:1000 new methylene blue. The sediment is then examined under the low-power objective. Microfilariae of *D. immitis* detected by this technique measure between 279 and 324 μm in length, whereas those of *D. reconditum* measure between 213 and 270 μm in length. Microfilariae measuring 275 to 290 μm should be identified by other criteria. Microfilariae of *D. immitis* are wider (6.1 to 7.2 μm), compared with those of *D. reconditum* (4.7 to 5.8 μm) when measured at a standard location such as the anal pore. The microfilariae of *D. immitis* have a tapered head and relatively straight tail, whereas the head of *D. reconditum* is blunt and often has a tail hook of greater than 180 degrees relative to the longitudinal axis. The tail morphology tends to be altered by filter tests.

Commercially available filter test kits utilize 1 ml of EDTA or heparin-anticoagulated venous blood mixed with 10 ml of a lysate. The mixture is filtered through a chamber, and the filter is removed and placed on a microscope slide, stained, and examined under low power. With filter tests the lengths of *D. immitis* microfilariae are 234 to 286 μm, whereas those of *D. reconditum* are 213 to 240 μm.

Many studies have determined that the concentration tests are more accurate than the direct blood smear, particularly when the microfilaria counts are low. In general, the modified Knott test and the commonly used filter tests are equally reliable. Errors in technique may result in inaccuracy of any test for microfilariae. Improper cleaning of test tubes containing microfilariae could result in a subsequent false-positive Knott test. Contamination of the lysate with microfilariae-containing blood and improper cleaning of filter chambers has resulted in a false-positive incidence as high as 24 per cent (Jackson, 1978; Noyes, 1978). Improper filter placement may result in loss of microfilariae.

The microfilaria count in the peripheral blood

bears no direct relationship to either the numbers of adult worms present or the severity of cardiopulmonary disease. The numbers of circulating microfilariae are affected by the season, time of day, ambient temperature, stage of infection, host immune response, and drug therapy. Microfilariae are first detected 5.5 to 7 months after L_3 infection, and their population increases for the next 2 to 5 months before a decline begins. Microfilaria counts tend to be higher between 4 and 10 PM, during warmer periods, and when the intermediate host (mosquito) population is greatest.

The diagnosis of heartworm infection in the absence of microfilaremia requires the use of serologic or immunodiagnostic tests or thoracic radiographs. Infected dogs that are asymptomatic or exhibit only a cough or mild exercise intolerance may not have obvious diagnostic radiographic abnormalities. However, most dogs with more severe signs can be accurately diagnosed by thoracic radiography. Occasionally, confusion arises when a dog previously treated for heartworm disease continues to have clinical signs consistent with heartworm infection, including radiographic abnormalities. Rarely, dogs can exhibit clinical and radiographic signs of a moderate to severe degree, even though all adult worms have died of natural causes.

Immunodiagnostic tests depend on the isolation of either a specific antigen or antibody. Because of variations in specificity of test reagents, procedures and results vary from one laboratory to another. The host immune response varies during the evolution of heartworm infection, a fact that alters test results. Furthermore, cross-reactivity with intestinal nematodes and *D. reconditum* must be considered when certain test results are interpreted.

The indirect fluorescent antibody (IFA) test using microfilarial cuticular antigen currently is the test of choice for the diagnosis of true occult heartworm disease (i.e., immune-mediated occult infection) (Wong et al., 1983). This test should not be confused with IFA tests intended for the detection of antibodies to adult worms. The IFA test is consistently negative in uninfected dogs, during prepatent infections, and during microfilaremia. A positive IFA test can be expected in 80 to 90 per cent of naturally occurring occult infections. False-positive results are theoretically possible if adult worms have died of natural or drug-induced causes. The duration of positive IFA reactivity following the cessation of production and elimination of microfilariae may be as long as 1 year. A false-negative rate of 14 to 20 per cent occurs with the IFA test. Cross-reactivity to intestinal nematodes and the microfilariae of *D. reconditum* does not occur, because the IFA test detects antibodies to surface or cuticle *D. immitis* microfilarial antigens. The IFA test will be negative in prepatent and unisex infections, since microfilariae are not produced under these circumstances. Obviously, one cannot be certain that suspected heartworm disease in the absence of circulating microfilariae would be due to immune reactions, unisex infection, or prepatency.

The enzyme-linked immunosorbent assay (ELISA) and IFA tests for *adult* heartworms are useful for the diagnosis of adult heartworm infection when microfilaremia is absent and to determine the efficacy of thiacetarsamide. For detection of adult worms, somatic antigens are used, and specificity of the tests is related to the purification of the antigen.

A positive ELISA for adult antigens can arise as early as 10 weeks following L_3 infection (i.e., during prepatency). Titers remain elevated throughout infection but often decline at 6 to 7 months after L_3 infection. Titers tend to rise and peak 4 weeks after administration of thiacetarsamide and then decrease to nondetectable levels after 6 months if eradication of adult worms is complete, although the time required to reach a negative titer is variable (Knight et al., 1983).

False-positive ELISA and IFA tests for adult worms have been observed in dogs known to have never been infected with heartworms. Cross-reactivity with ascarids and *D. reconditum* is common. Cross-reactivity with *D. reconditum* is of particular concern, since their microfilariae counts are low and often not detected on concentration tests. Furthermore, the eosinophilia and basophilia produced by *D. reconditum* are as great as or greater than those of *D. immitis*. ELISA and IFA tests are usually positive in dogs known to be free of *D. immitis* but in the prepatent stages of *D. reconditum* infection.

A positive ELISA or IFA may occur with prepatent *D. immitis* infections after approximately day 70. The efficacy of thiacetarsamide against migrating larvae between 70 and 100 days is unknown. However, it is known that thiacetarsamide will kill only approximately 50 per cent of male and 20 per cent of female larvae at approximately 110 days after infection. Thus, thiacetarsamide treatment administered during prepatency on the basis of an ELISA or IFA test may not eradicate the infection. Subsequently, microfilaremia would probably develop. If this microfilaremia were detected within the ensuing 5 to 6 months, thiacetarsamide given at that time would still be unlikely to eradicate all worms. Additionally, a positive ELISA or IFA titer may persist after effective eradication of larvae by drugs such as ivermectin. Apparently, the extreme sensitivity of these tests detects lingering low concentration of antibody (McCall, 1985).

ELISA and IFA titers should decrease following effective thiacetarsamide treatment, and with complete eradication the titer is often negative by 6 months after treatment. If ELISA titers are compared before treatment and 4 weeks after treatment, a rise in the second titer is expected if adult worms have been killed. In order to confirm complete eradication, a third titer could be measured at 6 months after thiacetarsamide. If that titer were high, incomplete kill would be likely. If the titer were low, subsequent titers could be measured at monthly intervals to detect a delayed adulticide effect (Knight et al., 1983). A negative ELISA or IFA test almost eliminates the possibility of heartworm infection. The ELISA and IFA tests for adult *D. immitis* have very similar sensitivity and specificity, and both tests share the same shortcomings.

A test for the detection of adult *D. immitis* antigens is superior to the ELISA and IFA tests for antibodies to adult antigens. The test is sensitive, specific, and should replace tests designed to detect antibodies to adult antigens. The antigen test is also accurate in the diagnosis of heartworm infections in cats.

Radiography

Thoracic radiographs are most useful in assessing the severity of heartworm disease. However, thoracic radiographs are not an obligate component of the minimum data base. Young asymptomatic dogs that have been tested for microfilariae on a yearly basis are unlikely to have severe pulmonary disease. However, thoracic radiographs should always be procured when microfilaremia is detected in older or symptomatic dogs, when the duration of infection is unknown, or if occult infection is suspected.

Since the primary pathologic condition of heartworm disease is within the pulmonary arteries, a careful assessment of their size, tortuosity, and associated parenchymal lung disease is critical to the accurate assessment of pulmonary arterial function and the likelihood of severe obstructive lung disease occuring after adulticide.

At the UGVTH, 86 per cent of 200 dogs seen consecutively with heartworm disease and microfilaremia had radiographic abnormalities consistent with dirofilariasis. One third of these dogs had some degree of enlargement of the right ventricle, main pulmonary artery, and right cranial lobar pulmonary artery. Sixty per cent of all dogs had right ventricular enlargement, but severe enlargement was present in only 20 per cent. Two thirds of the dogs had main pulmonary artery enlargement. In general, the severity of radiographic abnormalities is greater with time or occult infections, and approximately 70 to 80 per cent of all examples of severe pulmonary abnormalities occur with occult infections.

The radiographic abnormalities associated with heartworm disease are related to both the adult worm burden and duration of infection or host-parasite interactions. That is, some dogs with severe pulmonary disease and occult infections have a relatively low adult worm burden. The caudal lobar pulmonary arteries, particularly the right, are the first to become abnormal, and they usually manifest the more severe abnormalities. The absence of detectable enlargement of the right cranial lobar pulmonary artery is a poor indicator of the absence of heartworm infection. Enlargement of the caudal lobar pulmonary arteries occurs earlier but is best evaluated by the dorsoventral position.

By the time that right ventricular hypertrophy can be diagnosed by ECG, 50 per cent of affected dogs have obvious pulmonary artery tortuosity and 75 per cent have parenchymal lung disease. Thus, thoracic radiographs are a far more sensitive indicator of moderate to severe pulmonary arterial disease than is the ECG. When the ECG contains no evidence of right ventricular hypertrophy, radiographic evidence of right ventricular enlargement is detected in approximately one third of the dogs, although severe enlargement is not seen.

Thoracic radiographs are also essential in the diagnosis of heartworm-associated pneumonitis, pulmonary eosinophilic granulomas, and both pre- and postadulticide thromboembolic disease with parenchymal lung involvement.

Electrocardiography

The ECG of most dogs with heartworm infection is normal. Of 276 ECGs evaluated at the UGVTH, disturbances of the cardiac rhythm were detected in only 15 dogs (6 per cent). Clinical right-sided congestive heart failure is rarely present when the ECG contains no criteria of right ventricular hypertrophy. Radiographic evidence of severe right ventricular enlargement occurs weeks or months prior to the development of conclusive ECG evidence of right ventricular hypertrophy.

There is a significant association between the presence of three or more ECG criteria of right ventricular hypertrophy and the presence of clinical right-sided congestive heart failure. Ascites was present in 42 of 53 dogs (80 per cent) with three or more criteria of right ventricular hypertrophy. No such association existed when there were fewer than three criteria present. Of those dogs without ascites but having conclusive ECG evidence of right ventricular hypertrophy, ascites usually developed within 2 to 3 months unless adulticide was accomplished or restricted activity was enforced. The presence of ascites in the absence of ECG evidence of right ventricular hypertrophy suggests a separate problem, and cytologic analysis of the effusion is indicated. In all instances of conclusive ECG evidence of right ventricular hypertrophy, there are severe pulmonary arterial and right ventricular abnormalities present on thoracic radiographs.

ADULTICIDE THERAPY

Thiacetarsamide is the only drug approved by the United States Food and Drug Administration (FDA) for the treatment of adult *D. immitis*. Although thiacetarsamide is generally considered to be an effective treatment, not all heartworms are killed in every dog. The rate of kill of adult worms varies widely among individual dogs; nonetheless, it has been demonstrated that improvement in pulmonary function occurs even when there is incomplete clearance of adult worms (Rawlings, 1980).

Thiacetarsamide should be refrigerated and administered at a dosage of 2.2 mg/kg IV, twice daily (0.22 ml/kg of 1% solution) for 2 days at dosage intervals of 8 to 16 hours. This regimen has been recommended for nearly two decades, and no other regimen has been proved superior. Adult worms begin to die within a few days and continue to die over a 3-week period. The above dosage schedule given for 3 days produces similar efficacy, but increased severity of pulmonary embolism has been reported (McCall et al., 1981). This may be due to a more rapid kill rate resulting from the additional dosages.

Since no component of the minimum data base is predictive of acute reactions to thiacetarsamide, it is imperative that each patient be evaluated prior to each injection. At the UGVTH, a urine specimen is examined for bilirubinuria, and the patient is fed one-half hour before each injection. Injections are given either directly through a 20- to 22-gauge needle or a butterfly needle set into as peripheral a vein as possible. Because of the local vascular damage produced by thiacetarsamide, consecutive injections should not be given in the same vein, and the third and fourth injections should be given at more proximal sites. In no instance should thiacetarsamide be injected if there is any possibility that drug extravasation might occur.

In general, it has been shown that 90 per cent or more of mature male heartworms are killed by the recommended treatment protocol. Female worms, on the other hand, are more difficult to eradicate. Probably 70 per cent or more of female worms 20 months of age or older will be killed. Young female worms 4 to 12 months of age are difficult to kill. Presumably, dogs with natural infections have worms of various ages as a result of multiple infections. It is unlikely that all female worms will be eradicated by one adulticide treatment regimen, and a second course of therapy 1 year later may be required.

MICROFILARICIDE THERAPY

Approximately 4 weeks after thiacetarsamide therapy, treatment of microfilariae is indicated in virtually all microfilaremic dogs. On rare occasions, microfilariae are not detected 4 to 6 weeks following adulticide therapy in dogs that were previously microfilaremic. Whether or not these isolated instances are sampling artifacts is not known. The reader is referred to chapters on heartworm disease in the *Textbook of Veterinary Internal Medicine* (Ettinger, 1983) and *Current Veterinary Therapy VIII* (Kirk, 1983) for detailed discussions on the use of dithiazanine, levamisole, and fenthion as microfilaricides. Although the authors do not necessarily advocate the routine use of ivermectin, a discussion on the subject is appropriate because of its increasing use by clinicians.

Ivermectin, one of the avermectin compounds produced by the actinomycete *Streptomyces avermitilis*, has shown good microfilaricide activity. One oral dose of ivermectin given 4 weeks after adulticide will eradicate most microfilariae from the blood of most dogs within 3 weeks. In fact, microfilaria counts usually decrease drastically within the first few hours after treatment, and most dogs will be cleared of microfilariae within 1 week. Since adult *D. immmitis* may live and produce microfilariae for 3 weeks after thiacetarsamide treatment, some microfilariae may escape if ivermectin is given sooner than 4 weeks after thiacetarsamide.

Although higher dosages of ivermectin may have slightly greater efficacy, one oral 50-μg/kg dose (0.05 mg/kg) is usually adequate. Ivermectin, when given as a microfilaricide, also kills the L_3 and L_4 larvae up to 2 months after infection. Thus the potential problem of reinfection occurring before prophylaxis can be instituted is eliminated as long as ivermectin is given within 2 months of adulticide. Ivermectin should not be given to dogs by injection and should not be administered by any route to collies and, possibly, Shetland sheepdogs. At higher dosages, adverse reactions of variable severity occur at an incidence of 10 to 15 per cent (Jackson and Seymour, 1981). At a dose of 50 μg/kg, reactions occur in less than 5 per cent of treated dogs (Jackson, 1984). Ivermectin (Ivomec, Merck, Sharp and Dohme) can be diluted 1:10 with propylene glycol (1 ml of Ivomec plus 9 ml of propylene glycol) and administered at an oral dose of 1 ml/20 kg (0.05 mg/kg). Ivomec should be administered in the morning, and the dog observed for adverse reactions during the day (Jackson, 1984).

A microfilaria concentration test is performed 4 weeks after ivermectin administration. If negative, heartworm prophylaxis is begun. If positive, ivermectin is repeated at 50 μg/kg (0.05 mg/kg). If adulticide has been incomplete, microfilaremia usually persists and diethylcarbamazine should not be administered, but a second course of thiacetarsamide is indicated. Since female *D. immitis* heartworms up to 12 to 18 months of age are not likely to be killed by thiacetarsamide, microfilaremia may persist for several months or longer. If a second course of thiacetarsamide and microfilaricide does not clear the microfilaremia, the best alternative is to wait 1 year and repeat the entire treatment when the suspected surviving female worms are older. If persistent microfilaremia occurs and it is suspected that resistant female worms are present, ivermectin may be administered orally at a dose of 2 to 10 μg/kg (0.002 to 0.01 mg/kg) on a once-monthly basis as a prophylactic measure. At this dosage of 10 μg/kg, ivermectin may kill the L_4 stage 4 to 8 weeks after infection, thus compensating for clients who neglect a monthly dosage.*

Regardless of the microfilaricide that is chosen, it should be appreciated that microfilaremia usually recurs within days or a few weeks if gravid female worms survive thiacetarsamide therapy. If dithiazanine or levamisole is administered as the microfilaricide and a concentration test is performed and found negative immediately at the end of the treatment schedule, a concentration test should be repeated in several weeks in order to detect the possible re-emergence of microfilariae. This is one possible explanation for the apparent success of treatment followed by the detection of microfilariae 1 year later when diethylcarbamazine has been faithfully administered. Since a concentration test is performed 4 weeks after ivermectin or fenthion is given, if microfilaremia is to recur, it will likely do so by the time of testing.

There is little evidence to support the practice of administering a microfilaricide prior to thiacetarsamide therapy. The success rate of conventional therapy is very high in asymptomatic and mildly symptomatic dogs. At the UGVTH, there has been no apparent benefit of administering a microfilaricide prior to thiacetarsamide in dogs with advanced heartworm disease. That is, there have been no observed differences in survival rates or the incidence of adverse reactions. There is no proven correlation between the presence of microfilariae and the incidence of adverse reactions to thiacetarsamide.

THE ROLE OF ASPIRIN IN HEARTWORM DISEASE THERAPY

Aspirin has been shown to reduce pulmonary arterial disease in experimental infections and to be beneficial to dogs with severe natural disease. Heartworm disease produces pulmonary hypertension, which becomes progressively more severe, eventually leading to right-sided congestive heart failure. Platelet adhesion to pulmonary arterial endothelium results in myointimal proliferation, which leads to villous endarteritis. Aspirin, 5 mg/kg daily, decreases the severity of myointimal proliferation, probably through the inhibition of platelet-derived growth factor release from platelets. Furthermore, aspirin probably allows for some regression of preexisting lesions.

Aspirin appears to be clinically useful as a preadulticide therapy for dogs with severe clinical signs and radiographic evidence of severe pulmonary arterial disease. Most often such affected dogs have occult infections. Aspirin may retard the progression of pulmonary hypertension and may allow some resolution of disease.

Death of adult heartworms, either as a result of natural death or chemotherapy, produces a rapid increase in pulmonary endothelial damage, myointimal proliferation, granulomatous inflammation, and thromboembolism. In addition to pre-adulticide benefit, aspirin therapy continued through and following adulticide treatment has been shown to result in improved pulmonary artery blood flow and slightly less parenchymal disease. Platelet adhesion, thromboembolism, and myointimal proliferation in response to endothelial damage are significantly reduced.

Although aspirin therapy may be beneficial both before and after adulticide, at the UGVTH aspirin is routinely prescribed only for those dogs with *moderate to severe* disease, that is, dogs with exercise intolerance, coughing, weight loss, radiographic evidence of moderate to severe pulmonary arterial disease, ECG evidence of right ventricular hypertrophy, or ascites.

Aspirin is given for 7 to 14 days prior to adulticide and for 21 to 28 days after adulticide. Aspirin is not prescribed for dogs exhibiting hemoptysis or biochemical eividence of DIC, including dogs with platelet counts less than 50,000/mm^3.

Gastrointestinal bleeding occurs with aspirin treatment and may, on occasion, be severe. Therefore, the packed cell volume is measured every few days, and cimetidine (Tagamet, SmithKline Beckman; 30 mg/kg daily in 3 divided doses) is prescribed if ulcers are suspected. Vomiting, but not melena, may be a sign of early, severe gastrointestinal bleeding. In the face of clinical evidence of significant gastrointestinal bleeding, aspirin treatment is temporarily withdrawn and protectants or emollients are administered.

THE ROLE OF CORTICOSTEROIDS IN HEARTWORM DISEASE THERAPY

Preadulticide corticosteroid treatment should be reserved for dogs with allergic pneumonitis, eosinophilic granulomas, or moderate to severe parenchymal and alveolar disease resulting from pulmo-

---

*Editor's Note: It must be emphasized that ivermectin does *not* have FDA approval for use against canine heartworms. The comments here refer to experimental trials only.

nary arterial thromboembolism. Corticosteroids have been shown to markedly reduce the parenchymal lung disease associated with these disorders.

Corticosteroids also significantly reduce parenchymal lung disease resulting from adulticide therapy. Intimal damage from live and dead heartworms leads to increased vascular permeability and periarterial edema and inflammation. Such changes are most severe in the dorsocaudal areas of the caudal lung lobes, especially the right lobe. The lung parenchyma surrounding these areas is less severely affected in corticosteroid-treated dogs compared with untreated dogs. However, corticosteroid-treated dogs have decreased arterial blood flow and increased intimal disease compared with untreated dogs. Thrombosis and obstruction to pulmonary blood flow are more severe in corticosteroid-treated dogs and may be the result of delayed clearance of dead heartworms because of suppression of the inflammatory response and phagocytosis.

Thus, postadulticide corticosteroid use should be reserved for dogs with documented severe alveolar disease. Such parenchymal disease may be suspected 7 to 14 days after thiacetarsamide treatment, or later, in dogs that exhibit fever, coughing, crackles, dyspnea, or hemoptysis. Thoracic radiographs should be performed to document the presence and severity of alveolar disease, and only those dogs severely affected should then be given corticosteroids.

An additional, although less important, adverse affect of corticosteroids may be their interference with adulticide. Corticosteroids given during the first week after thiacetarsamide may slightly decrease the kill rate of young female heartworms.

INDICATIONS TO ABORT ADULTICIDE THERAPY

Attempts have been made to identify factors associated with adverse reactions to thiacetarsamide therapy. Acute adverse reactions, most often vomiting, anorexia, bilirubinuria, and icterus, occur with an overall frequency of approximately 15 to 30 per cent. These reactions are most often associated with either the first or second dose of thiacetarsamide.

Factors such as age, breed, or sex of affected dogs; the presence or absence of clinical signs; lung sounds; cough; weight loss; heart murmur; and abormalities in complete blood count, serum biochemistry, ECG, and radiographs are not predictive of acute adverse reactions.

Vomiting is the most common adverse reaction to thiacetarsamide and, when present, usually occurs after the first or second injection. One or two vomiting episodes following an injection are not an indication to stop therapy unless anorexia, depression, or other signs coexist. Vomiting may be centrally mediated through stimulation of the chemoreceptor trigger zone and vomiting center. Persistent or numerous vomiting episodes are always associated with anorexia, depression, or other signs and are an indication to stop therapy. Dogs that eat readily one-half hour prior to therapy and do not appear ill seldom have been experiencing multiple vomiting episodes.

Bilirubinuria is the earliest detectable sign of hepatotoxicity. However, this condition alone is not an indication to stop therapy unless other signs are also present. Gross bilirubinuria may occur after any of the four injections. When gross bilirubinuria occurs after the first or second injection, therapy is usually aborted and is always stopped if additional signs are observed. Gross bilirubinuria after the third injection is not an indication to stop therapy unless additional adverse signs are also present. Icterus is always an indication to abort therapy, but it rarely occurs in the absence of other signs.

Pretreatment elevations of serum liver enzyme activity or elevations occurring during the course of adulticide are commonplace and are not indications to delay or stop therapy. At the UGVTH, up to 10-fold increases in pretreatment liver enzyme levels have not been associated with an increased incidence of acute adverse reactions when compared with normal enzyme levels. After one or more injections of thiacetarsamide, liver enzyme elevations may occur but do not correlate with adverse reactions. In short, far too much emphasis is placed on the value of liver enzymes in the evaluation of heartworm disease. Evidence of reduced hepatic function, such as increased BSP retention of 5 to 10 per cent at 30 minutes, has not been associated with adverse reactions. In most instances of increased liver enzyme levels or BSP retention, values were normal, near normal, or not more abnormal 6 weeks after thiacetarsamide treatment.

Whether or not acute, adverse reactions to thiacetarsamide are more likely in azotemic patients is unclear, since the drug is seldom administered to azotemic patients. Preadulticide azotemia is an uncommon complication of heartworm disease. Azotemia should be diagnosed as either renal or prerenal, and if prerenal, fluid therapy is indicated and will usually return the BUN to normal. The cause of renal azotemia must be accurately determined. The long-term prognosis is guarded if azotemia is due to a glomerulopathy or tubular disease. If the azotemia is moderate to severe in degree, heartworm therapy is given only after the client is advised of a poor prognosis and after renal function is improved as much as possible by IV fluid therapy. Mild renal azotemia (BUN less than 50 mg/dl) is more readily corrected with fluid therapy, and renal function usually improves after successful completion of heartworm therapy. Azotemia diagnosed during or following adulticide therapy is usually either prerenal owing to repeated vomiting and dehydration or is the result of an inadequate pretreatment assessment of renal function. Prerenal azotemia is readily corrected by either IV or SC fluid administration.

If adulticide therapy is aborted because of acute adverse reactions to thiacetarsamide, re-treatment after 4 weeks is seldom associated with further complications. No specific treatment is necessary following adverse reactions, although the feeding of a high-carbohydrate, low-fat diet seems prudent. So-called liver-sparing drugs such as inositol, choline, and methionine are of no value; neither are vitamin C or corticosteroid hormones.

PRE-ADULTICIDE PULMONARY THROMBOEMBOLISM

Occasionally, dogs with advanced disease with radiographic evidence of moderate to severe pulmonary arterial enlargement will experience acute pulmonary thromboembolism. This syndrome is characterized by the acute onset of fever, dyspnea, tachycardia, hypotension, pale mucous membranes, weakness, and possibly coughing and hemoptysis. Crackles may be auscultated, and radiographs may reveal focal areas of variable-sized alveolar densities, usually in the caudal or accessory lung lobes. The alveolar densities may be the result of plasma leakage through damaged vessels or blood. If extensive hemorrhage finds access to the distal bronchioles, hemoptysis is likely.

Cage confinement, corticosteroid hormones, bronchodilators, judicious fluid therapy, and oxygen are the appropriate treatments. Aspirin (5 mg/kg once daily) may be given if the platelet count exceeds 50,000/mm^3 and there is no hemoptysis or DIC. Marked clinical improvement usually occurs within 1 to 2 days of diagnosis, but continued cage confinement and supportive care for 7 to 14 days are warranted. The platelet count and activated clotting time should be monitored.

POST-THIACETARSAMIDE THROMBOEMBOLIC COMPLICATIONS

Pulmonary arterial thromboembolism is the most common and most serious complication of effective adulticide treatment. Adult worms begin to die within several days and continue to die over a 3-week period. All affected dogs will experience some degree of pulmonary obstructive lung disease, most notably in the caudal lung lobes. Although it is difficult to predict severe complications, dogs with pre-existing radiographic evidence of pulmonary embolism, periarterial granulomas, or severe pulmonary arterial enlargement and tortuosity are at greatest risk. In general, dogs with occult infections tend to have more severe pulmonary disease.

Signs of thromboembolic disease begin 5 to 7 days after thiacetarsamide treatment is finished and are most severe at 10 to 14 days. Early clinical signs are fever, anorexia, and lethargy, and coughing frequently begins or worsens. High fevers, dyspnea, and hemoptysis are associated with severe pre-existing pulmonary disease. Dogs with few or no clinical signs and radiographic evidence of mild pulmonary disease seldom experience severe complications. Low-grade fever, coughing, and lethargy often occur, and strict restriction of exercise is adequate therapy. Corticosteroid hormones will reduce the febrile and inflammatory responses, but one may wish to avoid their use until 1 week after thiacetarsamide in order to avoid minor interference with the killing of female worms.

Severe reactions should not be totally unexpected if an appropriate pretreatment clinical evaluation and minimum data base have been performed and accurately assessed. With advanced disease, severe reactions may be avoided or eliminated by cage confinement and aspirin therapy instituted at the time of diagnosis and continued for 3 or more weeks. Severe coughing, dyspnea, or hemoptysis is treated with corticosteroids, bronchodilators, and cage confinement. Antibiotics, generally cephalosporins or chloramphenicol, are often prescribed empirically.

Thrombocytopenia is to be expected and persists from 5 to 21 days after adulticide, the nadir of the platelet count usually occurs at 10 to 14 days. Low-grade local coagulopathy or DIC usually occurs in dogs with advanced disease, but specific therapy is usually not indicated. Aspirin therapy probably should be curtailed if the platelet count decreases below 50,000/mm^3 or if hemoptysis occurs. Vincristine (Oncovin, Lilly; 0.4 mg/m^2 IV) may be given when the platelet count is monitored and found to be approaching 50,000/mm^3. Within 2 to 3 days of one dose of vincristine, the platelet count will exceed 150,000/mm^3 and will remain in a safe range until the danger period has elapsed.

Most dogs that die of severe pulmonary thromboembolism do so between 10 and 14 days after thiacetarsamide therapy. Such dogs can be recognized by pretreatment thoracic radiographs as being at increased risk. Thrombocytopenic and other evidence of DIC is usually present prior to death.

DISSEMINATED INTRAVASCULAR COAGULOPATHY

DIC may be associated with the caval syndrome and possibly with severe diethylcarbamazine reactions. However, DIC occurs most often 5 to 14 days, or occasionally later, after adulticide. The presence and severity of this complication can be estimated by the platelet count and activated clotting time. The activated clotting time becomes progressively prolonged and the platelet count decreases as the process progresses. Chronic or low-grade DIC is characterized by thrombocytopenia with a normal activated clotting time and other coagulation tests. Affected dogs usually have radiographic and clinical evidence of severe pulmonary disease and may exhibit epistaxis, hemoptysis, petechial hemorrhages, or hemolytic serum. Acute and end-stage DIC are categorized by thrombocytopenia and different degrees of abnormalities of the activated clotting time and other coagulation tests. The severity of pre-existing abnormalities is similar to that associated with chronic DIC, but severe hemorrhage, hemorrhagic effusions, and hemolysis are present.

Dogs with heartworm disease and low-grade or chronic DIC have a guarded prognosis but usually survive with appropriate supportive care. Cage confinement, aspirin therapy, and close monitoring of the platelet count and activated clotting time are usually all that are required. Aspirin therapy is temporarily stopped if the platelet count decreases below 50,000/mm^3 and vincristine is given. Low-dose heparin (200 units/kg SC t.i.d.) may also be prescribed for chronic or low-grade DIC, but most dogs recover without its use.

The prognosis for dogs with acute and end-stage DIC is poor. Higher doses of heparin (500 units/kg SC t.i.d.) are given for the former, and low-dose heparin and clotting factor replacement are given for the latter. In the authors' experience, the mortality rate associated with acute and end-stage DIC approaches 100 per cent.

ADVERSE REACTIONS TO MICROFILARICIDES

The most common adverse effects associated with dithiazanine and levamisole are vomiting and anorexia. The incidence of these reactions can be reduced by dividing the daily dosage and feeding a small meal prior to each dose. In fact, levamisole should not be administered on an empty stomach. The dosage of levamisole (11 mg/kg) must be adhered to because of its low therapeutic index; doses exceeding 15 mg/kg are associated with an increased incidence of toxicity. If levamisole treatment is not stopped when adverse signs begin, more severe toxicity characterized by panting, nervousness, trembling, gait abnormalities, and seizures may develop. The recommended dosages of 4.5 to 5.5 mg/kg of dithiazanine are often insufficient, and higher dosages are associated with a higher incidence of gastrointestinal disturbances and lethargy.

Adverse reactions to ivermectin (50 μg/kg) occur at a rate of less than 5 per cent. Most reactions occur within 1 to 4 hours and are of a mild nature. Vomiting, trembling, and lethargy may occur, and tachycardia, hypotension, tachypnea, and collapse occasionally develop. When evidence of shock is present, IV fluids and soluble glucocorticoids are indicated. Fatalities are rare when careful observation and appropriate therapy are provided. Some dogs do not undergo any acute reactions but experience mild listlessness for 1 or 2 days after ivermectin administration (Jackson, 1984). Acute reactions are most common when microfilaria counts are relatively high (greater than 10,000/ml) and all or most of the microfilariae are killed within 24 hours.

ADVERSE REACTIONS TO DIETHYLCARBAMAZINE

Diethylcarbamazine should not be administered to dogs with circulating microfilariae. Adverse reactions are likely to occur within 1 hour and vary in degree from mild to severe, with an associated mortality rate as high as 20 to 25 per cent (Palumbo et al., 1978; Atwell and Boreham, 1983). The dose of diethylcarbamazine and the microfilariae count do not correlate with the incidence or severity of reactions.

Anorexia, fever, lethargy, salivation, vomiting, diarrhea, and abdominal discomfort are commonly observed clinical signs. Tachycardia, pale mucous membranes, hypotension, dyspnea, and collapse are signs occurring with severe reactions. Associated changes are hemoconcentration, an initial leukopenia followed within 6 hours by neutrophilia, thrombocytopenia, and eosinophilia. Thrombocytopenia, hypofibrinogenemia, and fibrin degradation products may be seen with severe reactions and indicate the presence of DIC (Palumbo et al., 1978).

Hepatic venule and vein constriction in response to some humoral factors produces hepatic congestion, pooling of blood in the splanchnic veins, poor intestinal perfusion, and decreased circulating blood volume. Elevation of SGPT occurs within a few hours and SAP within 24 hours, probably as a result of hepatic congestion and hypoxia (Atwell and Boreham, 1983). The mediators of the reaction are not clearly defined, but the presence of gravid worms, microfilariae, and diethylcarbamazine are required.

HEARTWORM INFECTION PREVENTION

Diethylcarbamazine, ivermectin, and thiacetarsamide are the three drugs best suited to the killing of the tissue-migrating larvae of *D. immitis*. Of these, diethylcarbamazine and ivermectin are the most useful. Diethylcarbamazine probably exerts its effects at the L_3 and early L_4 stages. The effect of ivermectin on L_3 of *D. immitis* is unknown. Although levamisole and fenthion have activity against the tissue-migrating larvae, they offer no advantage and some disadvantages when compared with diethylcarbamazine and ivermectin.

Diethylcarbamazine, given at an approximate dose of 5.0 to 7.0 mg/kg once daily is highly efficacious. Despite the short half-life of this drug, a margin of safety exists so that alternate-day administration is usually effective, although not recommended. Prophylaxis should begin before infection is likely and should continue for 60 days after the mosquito season. In many regions, this means that diethylcarbamazine is administered continuously.

Diethylcarbamazine must not be given to microfilaremic dogs until adulticide and microfilaricide are first completed. An exception to this rule is that if microfilaremia is detected in dogs receiving diethylcarbamazine, the drug should be continued during thiacetarsamide and microfilaricide treatment. Diethylcarbamazine may be instituted or continued in occult infections in order to provide protection against reinfection. If diethylcarbamazine treatment is stopped for more than a few days in microfilaremic dogs, it should not be reinstituted until microfilaricide is complete. One negative concentration test for microfilariae following microfilaricide treatment is sufficient justification for prescribing diethylcarbamazine, providing it is instituted within a few days. A disadvantage of diethylcarbamazine is the recommendation for daily administration. Although most clients are willing to begin diethylcarbamazine prophylaxis, many do not continue long-term treatment.

Ivermectin, at a dose of 2 to 5 μg/kg (0.002 to 0.005 mg/kg) PO once monthly is an effective prophylaxis. Although monthly administration is convenient and may persuade some clients to continue prophylaxis, it is also likely that some clients will forget to administer the drug unless reminded. Although diethylcarbamazine cannot be prescribed for dogs with microfilaremia, ivermectin may be administered as a prophylaxis to dogs that are microfilaremic. Thus, the possibility of reinfection occurring between thiacetarsamide treatment and microfilaricide is decreased. *Ivermectin has not been approved for use in dogs*, and whether or not it will ever supplant diethylcarbamazine as a preventative drug remains to be seen. Although the dose of 2 to 5 μg/kg is effective on a monthly basis, higher dosages have been shown to be effective on a bimonthly basis. Thus, a higher dosage, such as 10 μg/kg monthly, could be prescribed and effective prophylaxis maintained even if a client failed to administer occasional doses.

Thiacetarsamide is effective against some of the tissue-migrating larvae and thus when administered at 6-month intervals may prevent adult heartworm infection. For those clients who, for whatever reasons, cannot or will not administer daily diethylcarbamazine, thiacetarsamide may be used as a prophylactic treatment. However, for these clients it would seem that monthly or bimonthly ivermectin administration would be a better choice.

References and Supplemental Reading

Atwell, R. B., and Boreham, P. F. L.: Studies on the adverse reactions following diethylcarbamazine to microfilaria-positive dogs. In Otto, G. F. (ed.): *Proceedings of the Heartworm Symposium, 1983.* Edwardsville, KS: Veterinary Medicine Publishing Co., 1983, pp. 105–109.

El-Sadr, W., Masamichi, A., and Greene, B. M.: Mechanism of killing microfilariae of *Dirofilaria immitis. In* Otto, G. F. (ed.): *Proceedings of the Heartworm Symposium, 1983.* Edwardsville, KS: Veterinary Medicine Publishing Co., 1983, pp. 94–104.

Ettinger, S. J. (ed.): *Textbook of Veterinary Internal Medicine.* 2nd ed. Philadelphia: W. B. Saunders, 1983.

Jackson, R. F.: Studies on the filter techniques for the detection and identification of canine microfilariae. *In* Otto, G. F. (ed.): *Proceedings of the Heartworm Symposium, 1977.* Bonner Springs, KS: Veterinary Medicine Publishing Co., 1978, pp. 38–44.

Jackson, R. F.: Ivermectin. Am. Heartworm Soc. Bull. 10:9, 1984.

Jackson, R. F., and Seymour, W. G.: Efficacy of avermectins against microfilariae of *Dirofilaria immitis. In* Otto, G. F. (ed.): *Proceedings of the Heartworm Symposium, 1980.* Edwardsville, KS: Veterinary Medicine Publishing Co., 1981, pp. 131–136.

Kirk, R. W. (ed.): *Current Veterinary Therapy VIII.* Philadelphia: W. B. Saunders, 1983.

Knight, D. G., Grieve, R. B., and Glickman, L. T.: Measurement of antibody to *Dirofilaria immitis* as an indication of infection status following adulticide administration in dogs. *In* Otto, G. F. (ed.): *Proceedings of the Heartworm Symposium, 1983.* Edwardsville, KS: Veterinary Medicine Publishing Co., 1983, pp, 48–52.

McCall, J. W., Lewis, R. E., Rawlings, C. A., et al.: Re-evaluation of thiacetarsamide as an adulticide agent against *Dirofilaria immitis* in dogs. *In* Otto, G. F. (ed.): *Proceedings of the Heartworm Symposium, 1980.* Edwardsville, KS: Veterinary Medicine Publishing Co., 1981, pp. 141–145.

McCall, J.: Personal communication, University of Georgia, 1985.

Noyes, J. D.: Comparison of Knott and filter techniques. *In* Otto, G. F. (ed.): *Proceedings of the Heartworm Symposium, 1977.* Bonner Springs, KS: Veterinary Medicine Publishing Co., 1978, pp. 34–37.

Otto, G. F.: The significance of microfilaremia in the diagnosis of heartworm infection. *Proceedings of the Heartworm Symposium, 1977.* Bonner Springs, KS: Veterinary Medicine Publishing Co., 1978, p. 22.

Palumbo, N. E., Peri, S. F., Desowitz, R. S., et al.: Preliminary observations on adverse reactions to diethylcarbamazine in dogs infected with *Dirofilaria immitis. In* Otto, G. F. (ed.): *Proceedings of the Heartworm Symposium, 1977.* Bonner Springs, KS: Veterinary Medicine Publishing Co., 1978, pp. 97–103.

Rawlings, C. A.: Cardiopulmonary function in the dog with *Dirofilaria immitis* infection: During infection and after infection. Am. J. Vet. Res. 41:319, 1980.

Wong, M., Suter, P. F., Rhode, E. A., et al.: Dirofilariasis without circulating microfilariae. J.A.V.M.A. 163:133, 1973.

Wong, M., Thomas, W. P., Ewert, A., et al.: Serodiagnosis of dirofilariasis by IFA and ELISA tests: Comparison with necropsy examination. *In* Otto, G. F. (ed.): *Proceedings of the Heartworm Symposium, 1983,* Edwardsville, KS: Veterinary Medicine Publishing Co., 1983, pp. 88–93.

FELINE HEARTWORM DISEASE

RAY DILLON, D.V.M.
Auburn, Alabama

Dirofilaria immitis infection in cats has been recognized as a clinical problem with an apparent increasing incidence and awareness (Calvert and Mandell, 1982; Dillon, 1984). Heartworm disease in cats has been reported worldwide and is consistently diagnosed in heartworm endemic areas (Otto, 1972). The increased awareness of the disease by clinicians has made antemortem diagnosis of the disease more common. The frequency of heartworm infection in cats generally correlates with the dog population of the area, but at a lower incidence.

Experimental production of heartworm disease is more difficult in cats than in dogs (Donahue, 1975), and the percentage of infective larvae (L_3) developing into adult worms is significantly less in cats (1 to 25 per cent) than in dogs (40 to 90 per cent). Experimentally (Donahoe, 1975; Fowler et al., 1972; Wong et al., 1983), when adequate infective larvae are used, the percentage of infective larvae developing to adult *D. immitis* is low, but the percentage of cats from which adult worms are recovered is high (66 to 90 per cent). Thus, the cat at risk would be one in a heavily endemic area where repeated bites by infected mosquitoes would be common.

Correspondingly, the worm burden is less in cats (range usually 1 to 9 worms) than in dogs, but as many as 19 adults have been experimentally induced in a cat. Although the adult worms reach significant size in cats (female, greater than 21 cm; male, greater than 12 cm), the development seems to be slower in cats than in dogs. Once infected by adult heartworms by either infective larvae (L_3) or transplantation (from superinfected dogs), the natural resistance of the cat induces a shortened period of patency and a lower concentration of, or absent, microfilariae. Microfilaremia is uncommon (fewer than 20 per cent of cases) and inconsistent or transient when present. Infective larvae developed in about 1 per cent of *Anopheles* and *Aedea* mosquitoes that fed on cats with patent infections (Donahoe, 1975).

Evidence tends to support the premise that adult heartworms in cats have a relatively short life span (probably less than 2 years) compared with that in dogs (approximately 5 years) (Donahoe, 1975; Grieve et al., 1981; Wong et al., 1983). A shortened longevity would contribute to an underestimation of the incidence of heartworm disease in cats based on routine necropsy examination of the general population. A gradual decrease in the number of adult worms found in the heart has been noted when cats are chronologically studied (Dillon, 1985; Donahoe, 1975; Wong et al., 1983).

Thus, the cat is a susceptible but resistant host for *D. immitis*, with probably a more transitory disease than in the dog. The current uncertainty centers on the difficulty in diagnosis because of the occult nature of the infection and the problems associated with postadulticide thromboembolization.

PATHOLOGY

The pathologic condition in cats is identical to that in dogs. Muscular hypertrophy, villous endarteritis, and cellular infiltrates of the adventitia are typically more severe in the caudal pulmonary arteries. The host's response to the parasite is intense, as demonstrated by enlarged pulmonary arteries within 1 week of transplantation (Dillon, 1985). Embolization of pulmonary arteries is a major contributing factor to initiation of clinical signs. Although pulmonary hypertension does on occasion occur, right-axis deviation in the electrocardiogram (ECG), radiographic evidence of right-sided hypertrophy, and right-sided heart failure are infrequent, indicating that severe cor pulmonale is uncommon in cats with heartworm.

CLINICAL DISEASE

Experimentally, there is not an age predilection to *D. immitis* infection in cats, and a wide age range of clinically infected cats is reported (1 to 17 years) (Calvert and Mandell, 1982; Dillon et al., 1982). Indoor and outdoor cats are represented, but outdoor cats seem to be overrepresented. The higher incidence in males compared with females may represent a sex susceptibility or, more probably, an increased risk of exposure. Feline leukemia virus (FeLV) infection is not a predisposing factor, and heartworms are not a common incidental finding at necropsy of cats with FeLV (Dillon, 1985).

Table 1. *Clinical Signs Associated with Feline Dirofilariasis*

Acute	Chronic
Collapse	Coughing
Dyspnea	Vomiting
Convulsions	Dyspnea
Vomiting/diarrhea	Lethargy
Blindness	Anorexia
Tachycardia	Weight loss
Syncope	

Clinical Signs

Infected cats may die acutely, may exhibit chronic signs, or may be asymptomatic (Table 1). From evidence of cardiopulmonary changes and experimental studies, most cats even with severe heartworm disease are asymptomatic. In the acute cases, death may be so rapid as to preclude diagnosis or treatment. Sudden death has been attributed to circulatory collapse and respiratory failure from acute pulmonary arterial infarction (Dillon, 1984). Acute collapse may occur with or without previous clinical signs. Cats that die from heartworms can be clinically normal 1 hour before death. All cats with peracute death should be examined for heartworm disease. In acute cases, as few as two worms have been found, accompanied by severe pulmonary congestion, infarction, and edema. In the acute syndrome, the worms do not always form emboli in the pulmonary arteries.

The most common historic complaints in cats with clinical signs are coughing, dyspnea, vomiting, lethargy, anorexia, and weight loss. Vomiting or respiratory signs are the predominant clinical complaint in chronic cases. It seems to be unusual for an infected cat to have both respiratory signs and vomiting. The vomiting tends to be sporadic and can be related to eating. The vomitus generally contains food or foam and is rarely stained with bile. Retching and severe paroxysmal vomiting are a rare historic finding. Heartworm disease in endemic areas should be included in the differential diagnosis of chronic emesis in cats.

The respiratory complaints most common are coughing and intermittent dyspnea. Hemoptysis is occasionally noted. The coughing can occur in severe paroxysmal attacks. Periods of normalcy (days) often elapse between episodes. Based on historic data, the coughing is usually temporarily responsive to corticosteroids, and exacerbation is seen during therapy (Dillon et al., 1982). The dyspnea may represent acute emboli. Occlusion of a caudal pulmonary artery is, on occasion, accompanied by a radiographic appearance of lung lobe consolidation and the development of acute dyspnea.

The nonspecific clinical signs of heartworm disease are consistent with many feline diseases. Anorexia or lethargy can be the only presenting sign in heartworm-infected cats. Heartworm disease is often an incidental finding on thoracic radiographs during a diagnostic screening. Cats with worms found in abnormal locations may have signs attributable to obstructed blood flow or a local pathologic condition. Neurologic signs can occur in infected cats with or without worms in the central nervous system (Otto, 1974).

DIAGNOSIS

Diagnostic testing for feline dirofilariasis is outlined in Table 2.

Physical Examination

Findings from the physical examination are usually normal in *D. immitis*–infected cats. A systolic murmur and occasionally a gallop rhythm may be present but as a general rule are uncommon. Harsh, "dry" lung sounds are the most frequent abnormal finding and can be present in cats without other respiratory signs. Ascites, exercise intolerance, and signs of right-sided heart failure are rare. There does not seem to be a correlation between the clinical signs, physical findings, and radiographic findings.

Clinical Pathology

Routine complete blood counts may demonstrate mild anemia (hematocrit 23 to 33 per cent) and, occasionally, nucleated erythrocytes, eosinophilia, and basophilia. The anemia is present in about one third of the infected cats and, as in heartworm-infected dogs, is nonregenerative. Peripheral eosinophilia, present in about one third of cats at diagnosis, is an inconsistent finding even on serial samples in the same cat and is dependent on the stage of infective larvae. The eosinophilia occurs 4 to 7 months after infection and intermittently thereafter (Donahoe et al., 1976; Donahoe, 1975). The absence of eosinophilia does not rule out a diagnosis of heartworm infection. As in dogs, the presence of basophilia is highly suggestive of heartworm disease. Blood chemistries and urinalysis are usually normal. Although hyperglobulinemia does occur in

Table 2. *Diagnostic Testing for Suspected Feline Dirofilariasis*

1. Complete blood count	6. IFA—microfilarial antibody
2. Knott's test	7. ELISA—adult antibody
3. Thoracic radiographs	8. ELISA—adult antigen
4. Fecal examination	9. Tracheal wash
5. ECG	10. Arteriogram

some affected cats (Calvert and Mandell, 1982), it is not consistent or predictable and should not be used to rule out feline heartworm disease (Dillon, 1984). Normal serum globulins and normal electrophoresis are found in cats that are heartworm positive based on Knott tests, immunofluorescent antibody (IFA) tests, or enzyme-linked immunosorbent assay (ELISA) tests.

Although experimentally infected cats usually produce a transient microfilaremia if both sexes are present, the condition seems to be of short duration and of low numbers. Thus a positive blood test for microfilariae is unlikely but diagnostic when present. The odds are increased by repeated testing (3 to 4 tests) and using larger quantities of blood (5 ml) for each test. Concentration tests such as Knott tests or Millipore filter techniques are better. Even with repetitive testing, occult heartworms represent more than 80 per cent of feline heartworm disease.

Serology

A positive IFA test (which detects antibodies to microfilarial *cuticular* antigen) is diagnostic (in about 33 per cent of the cases), but the presence of sterile worms, worms of only one sex, or the absence of host response to antigen will not produce a diagnostic titer (Dillon et al., 1982). Use of the somatic IFA test (which detects antibodies to microfilarial somatic antigen) is nonspecific (Wong et al., 1983). The term ELISA simply denotes a method of analysis, and antigen preparation, antibody sources, and techniques can vary between diagnostic laboratories. An ELISA test (which detects antibodies to adult heartworm antigen) shows promise, but false-positives related to cross-reactivity remain a potential complication (Greive et al., 1981; Wong et al., 1983). The use of this ELISA (adapted from the canine ELISA) (Greive et al., 1981; Green et al., 1983) in cats to confirm a clinical diagnosis has been very helpful. However, the canine methods for antibody detection *cannot* be used for cat sera. Initial studies of cats in which the adult parasite has been eliminated naturally or after adulticide treatment reveal that a negative ELISA titer develops several months after the adult is no longer present.

Results of an ELISA for the detection of adult antigen in circulation (Filarochek, Mallinckrodt) are

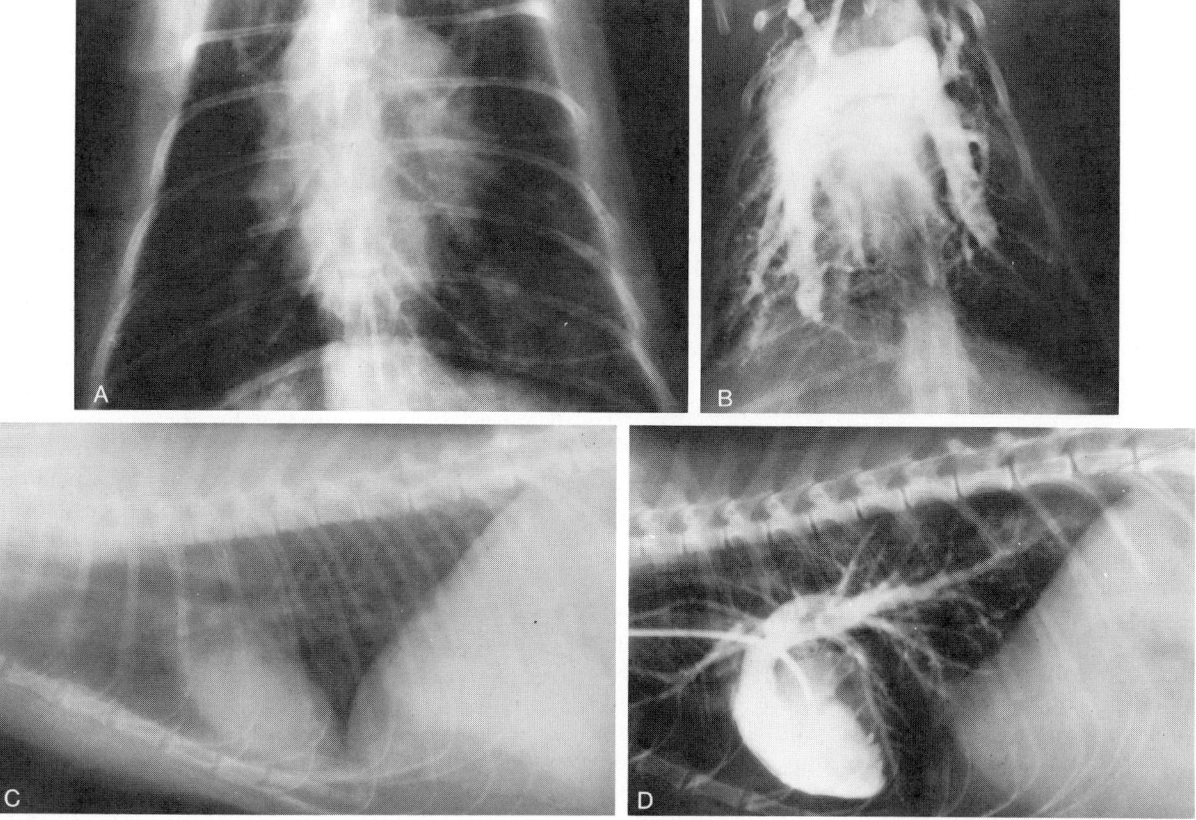

Figure 1. *A*, ventrodorsal radiograph of cat infected with heartworms, showing marked prominence of the caudal pulmonary arteries. Severe radiographic changes are typical of the vascular lesions without cardiac changes. *B*, ventrodorsal radiographs taken 4 seconds after contrast, illustrating the blunting of the pulmonary arteries. *C*, lateral radiographs of cat with increased densities, especially in the caudal lung lobes. *D*, lateral radiographs taken 4 seconds after contrast, illustrating the blunting and embolization of the caudal arteries. Linear filling defects can be observed; these represent adult heartworms.

positive in many cats with heartworms. This monoclonal-antibody method can be used on any species of animal (dog, cat, ferret). Since the antigen being detected seems to be derived primarily from the adult female reproductive tract, tests of cats with sexually immature worms or cats with a low worm burden are negative. Thus, it would be prudent at this time to consider a positive test diagnostic, but a negative test does not rule out heartworms,. With the high incidence of occult disease in cats, this ELISA-antigen test should be a valuable asset when *positive*. When the adult worms are eliminated, results of the ELISA antigen test become negative.

Electrocardiogram

Although subtle signs of right ventricular enlargement are occasionally noted (with unipolar chest leads), a right-axis vector (greater than 120 degrees) on a standard six-lead ECG is rare. Ectopic ventricular beats and other arrhythmias have been seen rarely after adulticide therapy in otherwise asymptomatic cats.

Radiographs

Radiographs offer one of the best screening tests for feline heartworms. The pulmonary parenchymal changes are nonspecific and can change rapidly in infected cats. The lung changes include diffuse or coalescing infiltrates, perivascular densities, and lung atelectasis. The most distinctive radiographic sign is enlarged pulmonary arteries with ill-defined margins. This is most prominent in the caudal lung lobes on the ventrodorsal (VD) view. Blunting and tortuosity of the pulmonary arteries are occasionally seen, but not as commonly as in dogs. An enlarged main pulmonary arterial segment extending beyond the cardiac border on the VD or dorsoventral (DV) view is *not* a classic feature of feline heartworm disease. Arteriograms as a diagnostic tool may demonstrate the enlarged pulmonary arteries and embolus. A nonspecific angiocardiogram is a simple and safe method of confirming a tentative diagnosis of heartworms. A radiographic exposure 5 to 6 seconds after injection of 4 to 6 ml of contrast material (an intravenous iodide) into the cephalic or jugular vein will provide good imaging of right-sided outflow in either the VD or lateral views. The classic lesions of enlarged caudal pulmonary arteries with blunting and pruning of vessels is best observed on a VD view. Linear filling defects may be seen in the arteries, confirming the presence of worms. There does not seem to be a correlation between the severity of lesion based on angiocardiogram and the severity of clinical signs or post-adulticide reaction.

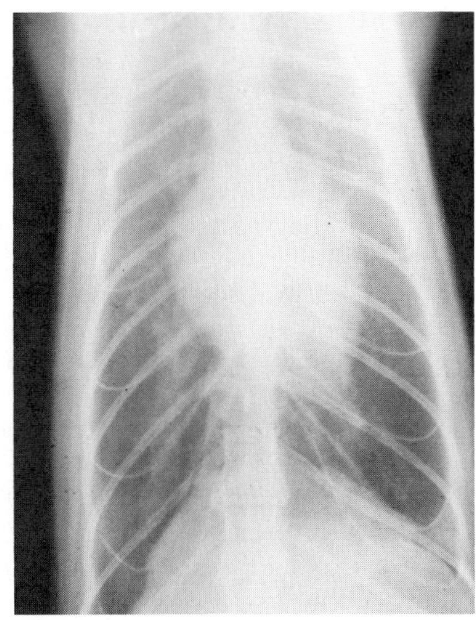

Figure 2. When present, marked prominence of the caudal pulmonary artery is diagnostic. This cat has a very distinct right caudal lobar artery.

Tracheal Cytology

The finding of eosinophils on a tracheal wash is common in heartworm disease, asthma, and the parasitic lung diseases. *Aelurostrongylus abstrusus* larvae or *Paragonimus kellicotti* eggs can be recovered in the latter. In feline heartworm disease, the greatest number of eosinophils on the wash seems to occur 4 to 7 months after L_3 infection and often may not be present when adult worms are present. Tracheal washes typical of chronic inflammation may be present after the eosinophilic reaction resolves. Careful fecal examination should be performed before the tracheal wash. Fecal flotation and direct smears may reveal the large operculated egg of *P. kellicotti* or the larvae of *A. abstrusus*.

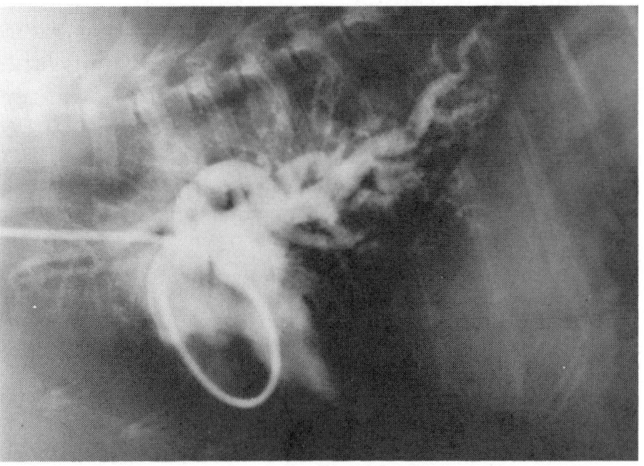

Figure 3. The severity of the reaction does not indicate the prognosis. This cat was asymptomatic and dirofilariasis was an incidental finding. Radiographically, the disease is severe and right ventricular pressure and pulmonary arterial pressures (mean, 38 mm Hg) were elevated.

DIFFERENTIAL DIAGNOSIS

In cats with respiratory signs, heartworm disease must be differentiated from *A. abstrusus* or *P. kellicotti* infection, asthma, and cardiomyopathy. Although each disease, in various stages, can mimic the clinical and radiographic pulmonary parenchymal changes of dirofilariasis, the pulmonary arterial changes of heartworm disease are unique and can be enhanced by contrast procedures. The peripheral eosinophilia, eosinophilic tracheal cytology, and chronic cough of feline heartworms can be mistakenly diagnosed as bronchial asthma. However, an apparent higher incidence of asthma has not been reported in areas endemic to heartworm. The enlarged pulmonary arteries and muscular hypertrophy of *A. abstrusus* and *Toxocara cati* infection is clinically uncommon.

THERAPY

Treatment of feline heartworm cases with IV thiacetarsamide sodium (2.2 mg/kg b.i.d. for 2 days) is safely tolerated by cats and does not produce immediate complications of hepatotoxicity or renal toxicity. Clinical signs tend to improve after therapy. However, chronically anorexic cats may have to receive hyperalimentation. Dithiazanine iodide (Dizan, Elanco; 6 to 10 mg/kg PO for 7 days) and levamisole hydrochloride (10 mg/kg PO for 7 days) have both been used successfully as a microfilariacide. (The latter drug does not have FDA approval for this use.)

Complications after therapy are related to embolization. Sudden death can occur, especially within the first 10 days after adulticide therapy. Although severe thrombocytopenia has not been noted, embolization can induce severe infarction, hemoptysis, and dyspnea. Embolization most often affects the caudal lung lobes, and thoracic radiographs may demonstrate a consolidated lung lobe. Oxygen therapy is indicated if hypoxemia or cyanosis occurs. High doses of corticosteroids (2.2 to 4.4 mg/kg of prednisolone t.i.d.) with careful IV fluid therapy (lactated Ringer's) will often support the cat through the crisis. The peracute nature of the postadulticide reaction requires the cat to be under constant attention, especially during the first 2 weeks (Dillon, 1985). The clinical and radiographic signs of acute embolization can resolve over 1 to 2 days. However, death can occur before therapy can be instituted. The client should be aware that the risk of complications in cats seem to be more severe than in dogs. Currently, in an asymptomatic cat with an incidental diagnosis of heartworms, the severity of the postadulticidal reaction poses a dilemma for the veterinarian, and the risk of complications probably is greater than for the spontaneous disease. Although heartworms may not live as long in cats as in dogs, clinical signs and even death (although unlikely) are a potential risk.

The efficacy of thiacetarsamide cannot be evaluated in cats because of the occult nature of the disease. However, of cats that have had microfilariae, repeated attempts to eliminate microfilariae failed and repeated adulticidal therapy was required. Problems associated with drug efficacy have been alluded to in microfilaremic cats. Current research seems to indicate that the adulticide is effective, and clinical signs usually abate during the initial weeks after thiacetarsamide therapy.

Due to the relative resistance of cats to infective larvae and, perhaps, the resistance of cats to mosquito bites, it is not currently recommended that diethylcarbamazine be used to prevent heartworms in cats.

References and Supplemental Reading

Calvert, C. A., and Mandell, C. P.: Diagnosis and management of feline heartworm disease. J.A.V.M.A. 180:550, 1982.

Dillon, A. R.: Feline heartworm disease: Clinical evaluation. *In* Otto, G. F. (ed.): *Proceedings of the Heartworm Symposium*, 1984. Vol. 83. Edwardsville, KS: Veterinary Medicine Publishing Co., 1984, pp. 31–33.

Dillon, A. R.: Feline Heartworm Disease: Grace Kemper Research Project, 1985, in progress.

Dillon, A. R., Sakas, P. S., Buxton, B. A., et al.: Indirect immunofluorescence testing for diagnosis of occult *Dirofilaria immitis* infection in three cats. J.A.V.M.A. 180:80, 1982.

Donahoe, J. M.: Experimental infection of cats with *D. immitis*. J. Parasitol. 61:599, 1975.

Donahoe, J. M., Kneller, S. K., and Lewis, R. E.: Hematologic and radiographic changes in cats after inoculation with infective larvae of *D. immitis*. J.A.V.M.A. 168:413, 1976.

Fowler, J. L., Matsuda, K., and Fernan, R. C.: Experimental infection of the domestic cat with *D. immitis*. J.A.V.M.A. 8:79, 1972.

Greive, R. B., Mika-Johnson, M., Jacobson, R. H., et al.: Enzyme-linked immunosorbent assay for measurement of antibody responses to *Dirofilaria immitis* in experimentally infected dogs. Am. J. Vet. Res. 42:66, 1981.

Green, B. J., Lord, P. F., and Greive, R. B.: Occult feline dirofilariasis confirmed by angiography and serology. J. Am. Anim. Hosp. Assoc. 19:847, 1983.

Otto, G. F.: Epizootiology of canine heartworm disease. *In* Bradley, R. W. (ed.): *Canine Heartworm Disease—Current Knowledge*. Gainesville Department of Veterinary Science, Institute of Food and Agricultural Science, University of Florida, 1972.

Otto, G. F.: Occurrence of the heartworm in unusual locations and in unusual hosts. *In* Morgan, H. C., Jackson, R. F., and Otto, G. F. (eds.): *Proceedings of the Heartworm Symposium*, 1974. Edwardsville, KS: Veterinary Medicine Publishing Co., 1974, pp. 6–13.

Wong, M. M., Pedersen, N. C., and Cullen, J.: Dirofilariasis in cats. J. Am. Anim. Hosp. Assoc. 19:855, 1983.

Section 5

IMMUNOLOGY, ONCOLOGY, AND HEMATOLOGY

BRUCE R. MADEWELL, V.M.D.
Consulting Editor

Immunology

Oncology

Hematology

Additional Pertinent Information Found in Current Veterinary Therapy VIII:

Additional Pertinent Information Found in Current Veterinary Therapy VII:

Immunology

DIAGNOSIS OF IMMUNE-MEDIATED DISEASES AND INTERPRETATION OF IMMUNOLOGIC TESTS

N. T. GORMAN, B.V.Sc.,
Cambridge, England

and L. L. WERNER, D.V.M.
Davis, California

Immune-mediated diseases arise when the immune response is directed against host cells. In considering both the causes and clinical manifestations of these diseases, it is important to divide them into (1) primary immune-mediated diseases and (2) secondary immune-mediated diseases.

Primary immune-mediated disease results from a clear autoimmune response against self-antigens. The term *primary* is probably an oversimplification in that it implies that there is no inciting agent and the disease can therefore only be a failure in immunoregulation. There is, however, an increasing awareness that infectious agents are responsible for triggering many of the so-called primary immune-mediated diseases, but the agent itself is frequently not directly involved in the immunopathology. In contrast, secondary immune-mediated diseases are clearly associated either with a concurrent disease state, parasitism (e.g., *Hemobartonella felis*), neoplasia (e.g., lymphoma), viral infection (FeLV), or drug administration (e.g., propylthiouracil, sulfadiazine). The basis of treatment of primary immune-mediated disease is suppression of the autoimmune response. In secondary immune-mediated disease, suppression of the immune response may or may not be required. However, treatment of the underlying disease is of paramount importance.

PRIMARY IMMUNE-MEDIATED DISEASES OR AUTOIMMUNE DISEASES

General Considerations

Autoimmune diseases appear without a known cause, often have a fluctuating course, can result in the demise of the animal, and can even disappear either after or without treatment. The ability of veterinarians to recognize and treat autoimmune diseases in the dog and cat has increased markedly over the past decade. It is not unreasonable to suggest that as further autoimmune diseases are documented in human medicine, the recognition of autoimmune diseases in veterinary medicine will similarly increase.

Most autoimmune diseases are associated with autoantibody production. These antibodies can either be restricted to an organ-specific antigen (e.g., thyroglobulin) or can react to an antigen common to many organs (e.g., DNA). Although there are well-documented experimental autoimmune diseases (such as allergic encephalomyelitis or allergic orchitis) that are mediated by cellular effector mechanisms, it is noteworthy that there are no spontaneous autoimmune diseases that have been shown to be the direct result of cell-mediated responses alone. In the spectrum of autoantibodies in the autoimmune diseases it would appear that there are two broad categories of autoantibodies: those that are produced against antigens such as erythrocytes, lymphocytes, platelets, DNA, and immunoglobulin, and those that are produced against very selected antigens such as acetylcholine receptors or TSH receptors. In the first group it is common for there to be more than one autoantibody present in the disease. In the second group there is often only one autoantibody associated with the disease process. It is difficult to accept that the mechanism or mechanisms involved in the production of both groups of autoantibodies are identical. Indeed, there is increasing and persuasive evidence that a single process is not responsible. The discussion that follows proposes that there are various levels of failure in immunoregulation that give rise to the production of autoantibodies.

FAILURE OF IMMUNOREGULATION

The immunologic basis and the immunopathology of autoimmune disease is now relatively well understood. It was originally considered that all autoreactive cells were deleted early in development, thereby obviating the risk of immune responses against self-antigens. Recent advances have shown this to be a false premise. The ability to recognize antigen is dependent upon antigen-specific receptors on lymphocytes. Antigen receptors are expressed on the surface of B and T cells. The B cell antigen receptor is surface immunoglobulin. The T cell receptor is a molecule comprising two chains, both of which bear similarities to the domain structure of immunoglobulins. The T cell receptor has a greater number of antigen-binding sites and is, overall, larger than the antigen-combining site of immunoglobulin molecules. Receptors on both B and T cells are the end result of a random series of genetic recombinations. This process takes place in the total absence of antigen, and as a result many clones, each with a different specificity, are produced. In this way the immune system has the capacity to produce sufficient clones of cells that among them have the ability to recognize any antigen. An inevitable consequence of this is that receptors will be produced that are directed against self- or autoantigens. It is now quite clear that autoreactive B cells and T cells are present in each individual and the potential to develop autoimmune disease is therefore universal. The mere fact that the level of autoimmune disease is not higher is a tribute to the control of the normal immune system.

There are built-in controlling influences that prevent the expansion of these autoreactive cells. Firstly, there is clonal abortion of autoreactive cells in the developing thymus. Secondly, contact of early (pre-B) cells with self-antigens results in the capping and loss of antigen receptors and the consequent clonal abortion of that cell clone. The mechanisms of clonal abortion are clearly imperfect and consequently autoreactive T cell and B cell clones escape and are present in the normal animal. It appears that autoreactive T cell clones are less prevalent than autoreactive B cell clones because of the greater level of clonal abortion of autoreactive clones in the thymus early in life. In contrast, the pool of B cells is replenished throughout life, and autoreactive B cells are continually produced. This can be demonstrated relatively easily by nonspecific mitogen stimulation of lymphocytes. In such experiments autoantibodies to common antigens are produced. Therefore, control mechanisms must exist that act upon the autoreactive clones that escape clonal abortion.

The expansion of autoreactive B clones and the production of autoantibodies are prevented by various immunoregulatory systems. These include a network of antigen-specific T helper/inducer cells (Th) and antigen-specific T suppressor cells (Ts) and are best appreciated by considering a normal antibody response. In a specific antibody response it is mandatory that the antigen be processed by an antigen-presenting cell (usually a macrophage) and then recognized by the appropriate antigen-specific Th cell. The Th cell provides the helper stimulus for the B cell expansion and, as a result, an antibody response is generated. A prerequisite for these cellular interactions is that antigen is recognized in association with a class II major histocompatability complex (MHC) antigen.

Antibody responses are controlled in two principal ways. Firstly, there is the success of the immune response, i.e., removal of the antigen. Secondly, there is the influence of antigen-specific suppressor cells (Ts cells). Ts cells act by suppressing the antigen-specific Th cells, thereby removing the helper stimulus for B cell expansion. Ts cells are also antigen-specific, and therefore the suppression is quite specific. The cellular interactions between the Th cell, B cell, and Ts cell are mediated by the recognition of class II MHC antigens expressed on these cells and by a number of soluble mediators.

As stated above, there is a continual production of autoreactive B cell clones *in vivo*. The expansion of these clones is prevented by sustained T cell suppression and by failure of Th cells to recognize the autoantigen. The Ts cells act predominantly on the autoantigen-specific Th cells and in so doing prevent Th–B cell cooperation. In addition, the Th cells have a restricted capacity to recognize the autoantigens, as many are expressed on cells that are devoid of class II MHC antigens. As such the cells are protected, because the Th cells are unable to recognize antigen in isolation; therefore, the autoreactive Th cell–B cell cooperation does not occur.

Autoimmune diseases arise when the various levels of immunoregulation are circumvented. This can occur under the following circumstances:

POLYCLONAL B CELL ACTIVATION. There are a number of antigens and adjuvants that nonspecifically stimulate B cell proliferation in the absence of antigen-specific Th cells. If some of the stimulated B cell clones happen to be autoreactive, then autoantibodies will be produced. A good example of polyclonal activation is the production of autoantibodies following certain viral and parasitic infections, e.g., leishmaniasis, herpesvirus, feline infectious peritonitis, or leukemia virus infections.

FAILURE OF TS FUNCTION. It is clear that any defect in Ts function will enable autoreactive Th cells to expand and provide the stimulus for autoreactive B cell clonal expansion. There is evidence that certain strains of experimental animals have severe Ts cell dysfunction. In some circumstances this can be an inherited trait, and in others it would appear as though it were acquired. The factors associated with this acquired trait are multiple and include hormonal influences, retrovirus infection, and age. A reduction in the number of circulating Ts cells, which is a common finding, would accompany such defects. Examples of these defects are seen in systemic lupus erythematosus and polymyositis.

BYPASS OF TS FUNCTION. Ts function operates by suppressing autoreactive Th cell clones. It is, however, possible for an alternative Th cell (i.e., one that is not an autoreactive Th cell) to provide the helper stimulus for autoreactive B cell clones to expand. This can occur when an antigen, be it a drug, virus, or toxin, is associated with the self-antigen. The Th cell to the modified self-antigen provides the stimulus for the autoreactive B cell clones.

INCREASED AUTOREACTIVE TH FUNCTION. In order for Th cells to recognize an antigen, there has to be an association with a class II MHC molecule. It is well known that there are many autoantibodies produced against cells on which there is no expression of class II antigens. This point begs the question: What are the cell interactions involved in these cases? Firstly, cell-free self-antigen can become associated with a class II molecule on a local or distant antigen-presenting cell, e.g., DNA absorbed onto a macrophage. Secondly, an intriguing idea has been proposed that suggests that cells can become dedifferentiated and express class II MHC antigens in addition to normal class I MHC antigens. It has been demonstrated that after injury by either an infectious or toxic agent, many cells will express class II MHC antigens; these cells include endothelial, glial, and epithelial cells. One of the actions of interferon on cells is to induce the expression of class II MHC antigens on many cell types, and this may in part explain the production of autoantibodies after certain viral infections.

As previously stated, the generation of antigen receptors on both B and T cells is the end result of a random series of genetic recombinations that occur in the absence of antigen. It is therefore not surprising that antigen receptors will be produced that react to the unique determinants expressed in immunoglobulin molecules. These unique determinants are called idiotopes and are isolated in the variable portion of the molecule. An individual immunoglobulin molecule can be defined as expressing an idiotype (i.e., the sum of the idiotopes) that is unique to that particular molecule. It is now quite clear that a T cell receptor also contains unique determinants (i.e., idiotopes) and has an idiotype.

There is overwhelming evidence showing that *in vivo* there is a constant series of antibody responses to the idiotypes expressed on immunoglobulin molecules and on T cells (i.e., idiotype–anti-idiotype).

Increasing attention has been given to the role of idiotype–anti-idiotype interactions as a level of control of the normal immune response. The implications of this system are complex in that for every idiotype there is an anti-idiotype and for every anti-idiotype there is an anti-(anti-idiotype) and so on. It is possible to argue that this idiotypic network can generate autoantibodies not as a defect in B cell control but as a normal consequence of the system. Autoantibodies can be generated within the idiotype network in two principal ways: anti-idiotype antibodies and cross-reacting idiotypes.

ANTI-IDIOTYPE ANTIBODIES. The mechanism whereby idiotype–anti-idiotype interactions generate an autoimmune response can readily be illustrated by the receptor-hormone interaction. An antihormone antibody will naturally bind to the hormone. Therefore, the hormone not only can bind to the cell surface receptor but also can bind to the antibody-combining site. It can be proposed that the antibody and the receptor have similar binding sites. The extension of this argument is that the anti-idiotype antibody will be an image of the hormone molecule itself and as such will bind to the cell surface receptor. The consequence of this is that the anti-idiotype antibody has the capacity to interfere with normal hormone receptor function. The very nature of the mechanism involved makes the process a very selective one. This principle has recently been used to explain the association between certain viruses and diseases (e.g., coxsackie and diabetes mellitus in humans).

CROSS-REACTING IDIOTYPES. The antigens expressed on various bacteria, viruses, and other microorganisms have long been believed to cross react with host cell antigens. The evidence in direct support of this argument has not always been compelling. The idiotype–anti-idiotype network can explain some of these findings. An antibody response to a bacterial antigen can result in the production of an autoantibody that could be responsible for an autoimmune disease. If the autoreactive cell had cell surface receptors that expressed an idiotype that mimicked the bacterial antigen, antigen-specific Th would help not only expansion of the antibacterial antibody but also expansion of the autoreactive antibody cells. Secondly, it is known that antibody molecules can express cross-reacting idiotypes. It can therefore be suggested that if an antibody response to a bacterial antigen stimulates antibodies that share a cross-reactive idiotype with an autoreactive clone, then appropriate Th help for the autoreactive clone will be provided.

In summary, the potential to develop autoimmune disease is present in all individuals. This potential is usually not realized because of the control of autoreactive cells. In circumstances in which these mechanisms are bypassed or fail, autoreactive cells proliferate and autoimmune disease ensues. In the majority of cases the immune system fails to regain control unless treatment is instigated.

BASIC IMMUNOPATHOLOGIC MECHANISMS

There are four types of immunopathologic mechanisms, three of which are important in immune-mediated diseases. These have been described in other comprehensive reviews and therefore will not be described in detail. Their salient features are listed in Table 1.

DIAGNOSIS OF IMMUNE-MEDIATED DISEASES

The immune-mediated diseases commonly seen in dogs and cats are shown in Table 2 along with the major immunopathologic mechanisms that are involved in each disease. There has been a tendency to overclassify the immune-mediated diseases into organ-specific and non-organ-specific diseases. There are a limited number of diseases (e.g., myasthenia gravis) that fall into an organ-based classification such that both the immunologic abnormality and the clinical presentation are restricted to a single organ system. However, there are many immune-mediated diseases that either have multiple immunologic abnormalities with only one major organ system affected or have restricted immunologic abnormalities that involve several organ systems. This makes the simple organ-based and non-organ-based concept somewhat untenable. Emphasis should be given to the underlying immunologic abnormalities.

The clinical presentations of immune-mediated disorders are varied and challenging to the clinician. This is largely due to the facts that these disorders often have clinical signs compatible with other common diseases (e.g., neoplasms, toxins, infections) and that there is often secondary or concurrent disease that masks the underlying immunopathology. More importantly, it should not be overlooked that immune-mediated disease can commonly manifest itself secondary to an underlying infectious or

Table 1. *Basic Immunopathologic Mechanisms Involved in Immune-Mediated Diseases*

Type	Mechanism	Result	Example
1	Antigen interaction with IgE bound to mast cells	Anaphylaxis	Allergic disease (not autoantibodies)
	Release of histamine and other vasoactive substances	Local or systemic angioedema	
2	Antigen expressed on a cell surface	Cell lysis	AIHA
	Antigen bound to a cell surface	Removal of cells	IMT
	Antigen closely associated with a cell surface	Membrane disruption	Pemphigus
	Antigen-antibody interaction with either complement activation or removal of cell by phagocytic cells		Pemphigoid
3	Antibody and extracellular antigen, which forms an immune complex	Deposition of immune complexes at basement membranes	SLE, rheumatoid arthritis
	Activation of complement and release of phlogistic agents	Local arthus or systemic serum sickness–like reactions	Glomerulonephritis
4	Sensitized T cell reaction against antigen	Lymphocytic and monocytic infiltrate	Thyroiditis?
		Cell lysis, tissue damage	

neoplastic condition. It is therefore mandatory that an evaluation of a patient include a thorough history, physical, and laboratory examination.

The specific clinical presentations of the various immune-mediated diseases are presented in detail elsewhere in this text. The major purpose of this section is to review briefly the immunodiagnostic tests that are available and the indications for use in clinical practice.

Immunodiagnostic Tests

Immunodiagnostic laboratory services have become more widely available to the veterinary practitioner for routine use. A full appreciation of the indications, the type of sample required, and the significance of the result will maximize the value of immunologic tests for both the clinician and the patient. Many commercial and human hospital laboratories offer a variety of immunologic tests that

Table 2. *Immune-Mediated Diseases in the Dog and Cat*

Disease	Type of Immunologic Injury (Table 1)
Systemic lupus erythematosus (SLE)	2, 3, 4
Sjorgen's syndrome (SS)	2, 3
Polymyositis (PM)	2
Systemic immune complex (non-SLE) vasculitis	3
Autoimmune hemolytic anemia (AIHA)	2
Immune-mediated thrombocytopenia (IMTP)	2
Immune-mediated neutropenia	2
Rheumatoid arthritis	2, 3, 4
Nonerosive polyarthritis	3
Myasthenia gravis	2
Feline chronic progressive polyarthritis	
Canine familial dermatomyositis	3, 4?
Pemphigus pemphigoid complex	2
Discoid lupus erythematosus	3
Glomerulonephritis	3
Thyroiditis	2, 4
Eosinophilic myositis	2

may or may not employ reagents and techniques appropriate for a particular animal species. Knowledge of test methods and species criteria is therefore an important prerequisite for selecting a laboratory to perform these services. Table 3 highlights the important aspects of the commonly available immunodiagnostic tests for dogs and cats. Although guidelines for sample specifications and interpretation of results are provided, the laboratory service enlisted should always be consulted as well.

COOMBS' TEST. The direct Coombs' antiglobulin test remains the most readily available and reliable test for diagnosis of autoimmune hemolytic anemia (AIHA). However, a simple and extremely useful "test" in *any* anemic patient is to observe the blood sample in the anticoagulant tube for presence of autoagglutination. This should be done immediately upon drawing the sample and also after cooling to refrigeration temperature (4°C). The finding of autoagglutination at body temperature or colder is virtually diagnostic for AIHA, and the Coombs' test is then redundant or unnecessary. Rouleau formation is macroscopically indistinguishable from true agglutination. Therefore, if clumping of red cells is present, a small amount of the blood should be mixed in equal amounts with physiologic saline (1:4 for cats) and re-examined, again at both temperatures, macroscopically and under low-power microscopy. Saline mixing will disperse rouleau formation but not autoagglutination. If the red cells agglutinate only at low temperature, warming the sample back to body temperature will disperse the agglutination, indicating the presence of an anti-RBC antibody with optimal binding activity in colder temperatures (cold agglutinins).

Most forms of AIHA will require the direct Coombs' antiglobulin test to detect the presence of autoantibodies (nonagglutinating types) on the patient's red cells. Coombs' reagents are readily available for dogs and cats, but not all labs utilize antisera that detect autoantibodies of *both* IgG *and* IgM class in addition to the third component of complement (C3). IgG autoantibody is more common than IgM in canine AIHA, whereas both IgG and IgM are prevalent in feline cases. IgA autoantibody is quite rare. Detection of RBC membrane–bound complement (C3) is an important feature of the Coombs' test, since it can often be detected in cases that are negative for IgG or IgM because of weak binding affinity or cold temperature dependency of the autoantibody. The conventional incubation temperature for the Coombs' test is 37°C. Since many domestic animals have low titers of cold-acting nonagglutinating anti-RBC antibody (nonpathogenic), a Coombs' test performed under cold conditions (4°C) is not valid. Demonstration of cold agglutinins, as described above, or high titers of cold-acting antibody as demonstrated by the indirect Coombs' test (4°C) are the only reliable means of establishing a diagnosis of cold-acting AIHA.

The most common causes of false negative Coombs' test results are failure to utilize serial dilutions of the Coombs' antiserum, the use of non-species-specific antiserum, and the use of antiserum that detects only one class of immunoglobulin. Corticosteroid therapy does not significantly alter Coombs' test results until substantial increases in hematocrit are achieved, indicating disease remission. The most common cause of false positive results in the Coombs' test is prior blood transfusion. Incompatible RBCs can react with pre-existing isoantibody in the patient or "immunize" the patient to produce antibody. Both are readily detectable in the Coombs' test even when clinical evidence of transfusion incompatibility is lacking. Occasionally, false positive results for the Coombs' test occur in conjunction with infectious or neoplastic diseases, probably because of adherence of circulating immune complexes on red cell membranes. This may or may not be associated with progressive immune-mediated hemolytic anemia.

The indirect Coombs' test, using a serum sample from the patient, is not as reliable in animals as it is in humans because of a high incidence of false positive and false negative results when donor red cells that are nonidentical with the patient blood type are used in the test. Newer tests, using enzyme-linked immunosorbent (ELISA) and staphylococcal protein A techniques, are currently being evaluated.

ANTINUCLEAR ANTIBODY (ANA) TEST. Presence of two or more of the following clinical signs of systemic lupus erythematosus (SLE) is an indication for an ANA test: nonseptic polyarthritis, myositis, proteinuria (glomerulonephritis), dermatitis favor-

Table 3. Immunodiagnostic Tests

Test and Sample Requirements	Indications	Method	Disease	Interpretation	Laboratory Sources*
Direct Coombs' Test 1 ml whole blood in EDTA; mail on ice; do *not* freeze	Progressive, regenerative, hemolytic anemias; distal extremity dermatoses; anemia with hepatosplenomegaly; *not* a screening test for autoimmune disorders without anemia	Direct hemagglutination for detection of Ig or C3 on patient RBCs incubated with serial dilutions of species-specific antisera to IgG, IgM, or C3	Autoimmune hemolytic anemia (AIHA); cold agglutinin disease (distal extremity dermatoses)	Agglutination at one or more serial dilutions of Coombs' antiserum is significant; prior transfusion may cause false-positive results; see text for further details	1, 2, 3, 4, 5, 6, 7
Indirect Coombs' Test 1 to 2 ml frozen serum; mail on ice	As above	Indirect hemagglutination for detection of circulating autoantibody; dilutions of patient serum are incubated with donor RBC suspension; if no agglutination is observed, a direct Coombs' test is then performed	As above	Titers ≥1:164 are significant; isoantibody to major blood group antigens or prior blood transfusion may give false-positive results; false-negative results can occur if patient RBC autoantigen differs from that represented in donor RBC pool	5
Antinuclear Antibody Test (ANA) 1 to 2 ml frozen serum; mail on ice	Polysystemic, noninfectious, inflammatory disorders; autoimmune hemolytic anemia; immune-mediated thrombocytopenia; unexplained leukopenia; fever of undetermined origin	Indirect immunofluorescence for detection of circulating ANA, using nuclear substrate and fluorescein-conjugated anti-Ig (species-specific) under fluorescent microscopy	Systemic lupus erythematosus (SLE)	Significant titer levels vary with substrate and laboratory controls: ≥1:20 for mouse liver; ≥1:80 for Vero cell line, ≥1:40 for HeLa cell line	1, 2, 3, 4, 5, 7
LE Cell Test 5 to 10 ml whole clotted or heparinized blood; deliver to lab within several hours	As above	Sample is processed through wire mesh or agitated with glass beads, stained, and examined for presence of large intracytoplasmic, homogeneous, inclusions within PMNs	SLE	Presence of 3 or more LE cells is considered significant; tart cells are sometimes falsely interpreted as LE cells; corticosteroids interfere with the LE cell phenomenon	2, 3, 4, 5, 6
Platelet Factor 3 Test (PF-3) 3 ml citrated plasma fresh frozen and mailed (express) on dry ice	Idiopathic thrombocytopenia	Detects antiplatelet antibody in a clotting test system using patient plasma and donor platelets; PF-3 released from antibody-coated platelets results in shortened clotting time compared with controls	Immune-mediated thrombocytopenia (IMT); SLE with thrombocytopenia; Evans's syndrome (AIHA & IMT)	Steroids may interefere; false-positive results can occur owing to platelet activation from improper handling of samples; *use* Vacutainer collection system	1, 2, 6
Rheumatoid Factor Test (RF) 1 to 2 ml frozen serum; mail on ice	Progressive, erosive, nonseptic, polyarthritis	Indirect hemagglutination test; detection of autoantibody (RF) to IgG using rabbit IgG–sensitized sheep RBCs and serial dilutions of patient's serum	Rheumatoid Arthritis (RA)	Serum titers ≥1:16 are significant; serum RF can be present in other inflammatory disorders; 25 to 40% of canine RA cases are RF negative	1, 2, 3, 4, 5
Immunoelectrophoresis (IEP) 1 to 3 ml frozen serum; mail on ice	Qualitative screening test for hypoglobulinemia and for monoclonal immunoglobulin class identification	Double immunodiffusion with electrophoresis of patient serum to separate out Ig classes; polyvalent (all classes) or monospecific (single Ig class) antisera can be used (species-specific)	Multiple myeloma; lymphosarcoma (B cell origin); benign monoclonal gammopathy	Monoclonal precipitin pattern shows restricted electrophoretic band by using dilutions of patient serum compared with control serum	2, 3, 4, 6, 7
			Waldenstrom's macroglobulinemia	Restricted electrophoretic pattern for IgM	
			Hypoglobulinemia (all classes)	Decreased or absent precipitin bands for IgG, IgM, and IgA	
			Selective Ig deficiency	Decreased or absent precipitin band for single Ig class	
Immunoglobulin Quantitation 1 to 3 ml frozen serum; mail on ice	Quantitative evaluations for hypoglobulinemia, selective Ig deficiency, and monoclonal hyperglobulinemias	Radial immunodiffusion (RID), rocket immunoelectrophoresis, ELISA, or nephelometry, using species-specific monovalent antiserum	As above	Quantitative excess or deficiency of single or multiple Ig classes	1, 2, 3, 4
Tissue-fixed Ig/C3 Skin, kidney or other organ biopsies fixed in Michel's preservative (2-wk limit for processing) or snap frozen in liquid nitrogen and mailed express on dry ice	Vesiculobullous skin disorders; protein-losing glomerulonephropathy; detection of immune complex vasculitis	Direct immunofluorescence using fluorescein-labeled antisera (species-specific)	SLE	Ig or C3 deposits at cutaneous dermoepidermal junction; granular Ig or C3 deposits along glomerular basement membrane	1, 2, 7
			Immune-complex glomerulonephritis	Same as for lupus nephritis	
			Pemphigus var.	Intercellular Ig deposits	
			Bullous pemphigoid	Linear Ig or C3 deposits along dermoepidermal junction	
			Pemphigus erythematosus	Ig or C3 deposits consistent with both lupus and pemphigus	
			Immune-complex vasculitis	Ig or C3 deposits in vessel walls	

*Laboratory sources: 1. Veterinary Reference Laboratory, (800)527–7673, Laboratories located in Anaheim and San Leandro, CA; Dallas, TX. Pick-up services in many major US cities. 2. Convet, 1676 1st Avenue, New York, NY 10128, (212)534–4900. 3. Omni Diagnostics, 701 Bedford Road, Bedford Hills, NY 10507, (914)241–1999. 4. University of Tennessee, Department of Pathobiology, Immunology Laboratory, PO Box 1071, Knoxville, TN 37901, (615)546–9230. 5. University of Miami School of Medicine, Division of Comparative Pathology, PO Box 016960, Miami, FL 33101, (305)547–6594. 6. Wadsworth Center for Laboratories and Research, New York State Department of Health, Albany, NY 12201, (518)869–4507. 7. University of Florida, College of Veterinary Medicine, Clinical Immunology Laboratory, J-126, JHMHC, Gainesville, FL 32610, (904)392–4751.

ing distribution to the head and mucous membrane regions, progressive hemolytic anemia (Coombs' positive), leukopenia, thrombocytopenia, antibiotic nonresponsive fever, myocarditis, serositis, and unexplained neurologic disease.

Antinuclear antibody is a broad and general term that encompasses a whole range of antibodies that bind to the components of the nucleus. Many different methods are used to detect ANA in the patient's serum. The latex particle agglutination test is not as widely used in dogs and cats as is indirect immunofluorescence utilizing a tissue culture cell line (such as HeLa or Vero cells) or mouse liver frozen sections. The significance of the various patterns of immunofluorescence in the nucleus and on the nuclear membrane has not been fully evaluated in dogs and cats. Whether these patterns have any relevance to the progression of the disease (as they do in man) is unknown. Serum samples are screened at a low dilution (usually 1:10) and if positive, an endpoint positive titer is established. Since low titers of ANA can be found in a number of infectious, inflammatory, and neoplastic disorders, the level of significance of a particular ANA titer must be established according to laboratory controls and compatible clinicopathologic criteria for SLE.

The ANA test is positive in 75 to 90 per cent of dogs with classic SLE. Probable SLE is the diagnosis applied to ANA-negative cases that demonstrate two or more major signs or ANA-positive cases showing only one major sign compatible with SLE. In any event, it is important to remember that immune complex disorders can arise from a multitude of exogenous antigens (chronic antigenic stimulation), and although the disorders are "lupus-like," ANA will not be detected in most cases. There is considerable refinement in the techniques used to detect antinuclear antibody activity in humans. These include the Farr immunoassay, counterimmunoelectrophoresis, and immunoprecipitation. These tests allow for identification of autoantibodies to the precise nuclear and cytoplasmic antigens involved. This has enabled a better understanding of SLE and the overlap syndromes, and it is important that a similar trend be followed in veterinary clinical immunology.

Lupus Erythematosus (LE) Cell Test. The LE preparation test is not as sensitive as the ANA, in that LE cells may not be found in every case of SLE, or it may require multiple samples to demonstrate them. LE cells are neutrophils that have phagocytized nuclear material that has been opsonized by antinuclear protein antibody. Since these cells are produced more readily by *in vitro* manipulations and are rarely seen *in vivo*, it is useless to try to detect LE cells in a peripheral blood smear. LE cells are rarely found in joint fluid smears from patients with polyarthritis but are highly supportive of a diagnosis of SLE when present. The one advantage to this test is that any hematologic laboratory can provide this service, and no specialized reagents for animal species are required. A negative LE cell test does not rule out SLE. A minimum of three to four LE cells is considered diagnostic. Rare LE cells (fewer than three) can be seen in a variety of other diseases besides SLE. Tart cells, i.e., neutrophils that have phagocytized *intact* nuclei, should not be mistaken for LE cells.

Platelet Factor 3 (PF-3). This test detects autoantibody (against platelets) in the patient's plasma and is indicated in conditions involving thrombocytopenia when the cause is not apparent. Immune-mediated thrombocytopenia (IMT) is sometimes seen in conjunction with Coombs' positive anemias and SLE. Thus, a Coombs' test and an ANA test are also indicated when significant anemia is encountered with IMT. PF-3 testing is not widely available because it has been repeatedly found to be a relatively difficult test to standardize and interpret.

Other methods of detecting platelet autoantibody, including immunofluorescence and an ELISA test, have very limited availability at this time. However, it is more likely that these tests will eventually provide a very useful and reproducible assay system for detecting anti-platelet antibodies.

Rheumatoid Factor (RF) Test. The most commonly used RF test for the dog utilizes sheep red blood cells (SRBC) coated with rabbit antibody (IgG) to SRBC. This is called the Rabbit Rose-Waaller test and is available through human hospital or commercial laboratories. Rheumatoid factor refers to autoantibody against the dog's own IgG. This autoantibody is usually IgG (in dogs) but may be IgM. Only 40 to 75 per cent of canine patients with rheumatoid arthritis (RA) will have a positive RF test. Therefore, a negative test does not rule out RA. Most often a titer of 1:16 or greater is significant; lesser titers are seen in some normal patients and in those with a variety of other illnesses and arthropathies. IgG-coated latex or bentonite particles are also used to detect RF. Dogs with progressive erosive arthropathy should also be screened for ANA, since some cases of canine SLE manifest a more destructive form of arthritis than is usual for SLE.

Direct Immunofluorescence Assay (DIFA). DIFA has become extremely popular and useful in veterinary medicine with the increased recognition of autoimmune skin diseases, particularly in dogs and cats. Biopsies of skin lesions must be either snap frozen in liquid nitrogen and mailed on dry ice or, more conveniently, preserved in Michel's medium (provided by the laboratory), which will keep the tissue-fixed immunoglobulin viable for up to 2 weeks. The tissue submitted should be taken from only freshly erupting lesions to avoid frustrating negative results when clinical suspicion is high. Tissue sample sizes in the range of 4 to 8 mm are best, and they should always include a margin of uninvolved skin as well. Biopsies are sectioned and fluorescein conjugated anti-Ig or anti-C3 is used to detect the presence of autoantibody or immune complexes. Other tissues can be examined as well; most commonly, renal tissue is taken in suspected glomerulonephritis. The indirect IFA test detects autoantibodies (against tissue antigens) in the serum. Since indirect IFA tests are rarely positive (compared with DIFA) in autoimmune skin diseases of the dog and cat, they are not routinely used as a screening test.

Methods for detecting immunoglobulin or C3 deposits in formalin-preserved biopsies have many advantages over direct immunofluorescence but are as yet less widely available. Such tests utilize enzyme-labeled antisera or staphylococcal protein A to detect tissue-fixed immunoglobulin or complement.

The significance of positive immunofluorescence is dependent upon obtaining the correct sample and the quality of the reagents that are used. If appropriate attention is given to these points, then positive results are most informative. There is nothing more dispiriting than obtaining equivocal results because of operator or reagent error. There is little doubt that this immunodiagnostic tool should be used not only in the commonly recognized autoimmune diseases of small animals but also in those in which there is already a precedent in other species (e.g., endocrinopathies, polyendocrinopathies, coeliac disease).

IMMUNOGLOBULIN QUANTITATION. The most commonly employed method of quantitating specific immunoglobulin classes is a single radial immunodiffusion (RID). In this test, monospecific antiserum is incorporated into agar gel during the liquid phase. After gel solidification, wells are made, and serial dilutions of patient and standard control sera are added. Following incubation, the diameters of the resultant precipitin rings are measured. A standard curve constructed from the known control sera is used to determine the protein content of the patient sample.

Rocket electrophoresis (single immunoelectrodiffusion) incorporates electrophoresis of patient serum dilutions added to wells in agar impregnated with monospecific antiserum. The resultant length of the rocket-shaped precipitin patterns is measured and compared with a known standard.

The above assays are now being replaced by ELISAs. These have many advantages over other assays in that they are highly sensitive, reproducible, and economical on time as well as expense. Whilst these assays are not widely available, it is to be expected that they will have replaced the conventional assays in the near future.

The significance of immunoglobulin levels in immune-mediated disease relative to other disease processes is unclear. The elevated levels sometimes recorded reflect an inflammatory reaction rather than a specific disease. It should not be overlooked that a minute quantity of autoantibody can produce a devastating effect without contributing to an increase in the total immunoglobulin level. A much more informative determination would be the quantitation of antigen-specific antibody. This would indicate whether or not autoantibodies were involved. With the advent of more sensitive assays, this could be done.

IMMUNOELECTROPHORESIS (IEP)

Immunoelectrophoresis employs electrophoretic separation of patient and control sera placed in separate gel agar wells. After separation, nonspecific or polyvalent antiserum to Ig classes is added to a central trough placed between sample wells and allowed to diffuse overnight. The resultant precipitin band is a qualitative assessment of the Ig present in the patient serum compared with that in a normal control. It is also semiquantitative in that the density of the precipitin can be compared with that of the control sample. Moreover, in the case of monoclonal hyperglobulinemia, the Ig precipitin can be demonstrated in dilutions of the patient serum (1:20 to 1:40) that are higher than those of control serum. Table 3 shows the diseases associated with abnormal IEP patterns that are recognized in the dog and cat. IEP is not a useful adjunct to diagnosis of diseases associated with polyclonal hyperglobulinemias, in which multiple Ig classes are elevated in association with chronic inflammatory, infectious, or neoplastic disorders.

Serum immunoelectrophoresis has been a useful aid in the characterization of both hyper- and hypoglobulinemic states. It is a qualitative means of identifying the specific immunoglobulin classes that appear deficient or excessive on the basis of total serum globulin levels and serum protein electrophoresis. Thus, the latter two biochemical determinations are prerequisite to the performance of the IEP and the quantitative immunoglobulin assessments discussed previously. The class- and subclass-specific ELISAs will soon replace the limited usefulness of immunoelectrophoresis.

HEMOLYTIC COMPLEMENT (CH_{50})

Complement levels are relatively constant within an individual, although there is a wide range between individuals. The level that is determined is dependent upon *in vivo* production, *in vivo* consumption, and the sensitivity of the *in vitro* assay. The measurement of complement function is a most useful adjunct to diagnosis. In many immune-mediated diseases, particularly immune complex disease, the CH_{50} is considerably reduced because of activation and consumption at the site of immune complex deposition. Hypocomplementemia is, however, not unique to immune-mediated disease and is found in a wide range of infectious and noninfectious diseases and in neoplasia.

There are a limited number of laboratories that measure serum complement levels. When it is possible, the determination should be made on the day the sample is taken. In circumstances in which this is not possible, serum samples stored at −90°C should be sent to the laboratory. Incorrect handling and storage of serum samples will result in erroneous and confusing results. The quantitation of each complement component is of considerable use in human studies, for instance, many patients with an inherited deficiency of C2 will develop SLE. In dogs and cats, there are assays for certain complement components but these tests are restricted to a few noncommercial laboratories.

IMMUNE COMPLEXES. The involvement of immune complexes in immune-mediated disease is considerable, and measurement of the circulating complexes can be helpful, not only in the diagnosis but also in the monitoring of animals on treatment. There is a wide range of tests that will give accurate quantitation of immune complexes, although these are often technically capricious. The availability of such tests in practice is limited unless there is a nearby medical center. In all assays monospecific canine and feline reagents have to be used in order to obtain useful results.

LYMPHOCYTE FUNCTIONAL STUDIES. The section on the cause of immune-mediated diseases highlighted the central role of T and B cell function. In many species it is now possible to examine carefully not only the number of lymphocytes but also the various types (Th, Ts, Tc) and the functional capacity of each population. It is well recognized that T cell function is severely compromised in autoimmune disease, and in humans the level of dysfunction can be quantitatively and qualitatively examined. At this time there are a very restricted number of assays available to examine this point in both the dog and cat. These mainly revolve around various forms of nonspecific blastogenesis studies and leukocyte migration assays. Although neither are complicated to perform, they pose difficulties in interpretation and significance. It is hoped that the increased availability of monospecific reagents to identify lymphocytes in the dog and cat will overcome the current problems in identifying the various cell populations and performing appropriate functional studies. In addition, it is hoped that by the next edition of this text, more informative information will be available on cellular function in immune-mediated diseases.

References and Supplemental Reading

Cook, A., Lydyard, P. M., and Roitt, I. M.: Mechanisms of autoimmunity: a role for cross reactive idiotypes. Immunol. Today 4:170, 1983.

Fauci, A. S.: Vasculitis. J. Allergy Clin. Immun. 72:211, 1983.

Gosslein, S. J., Capen, C. C., Marini, S. L., et al.: Autoimmune lymphocytic thyroiditis in dogs. Vet. Immunol. Immunopathol. 3:185, 1982.

Jain, N. C., and Switzer, J. W.: Autoimmune thrombocytopenia in dogs and cats. Vet. Clin. North Am. (Small Anim. Pract.) 2:421, 1981.

Koller, L. D.: Chemical-induced immunomodulation. J.A.V.M.A. 181:1102, 1982.

Lennon, V. A., Palmer, A. C., Pflufelder, C., and Indieri, R. J.: Myasthenia gravis in dogs: Acetylcholine receptor with and without antireceptor autoantibodies. *In* Rose, N. R., Bigazzi, P. E., and Warner, N. L. (eds.): Genetic Control of Autoimmune Disease. Amsterdam: Elsevier, 1978.

Pedersen, N. C., Pool, R. R., and Morgan, J. P.: Joint diseases of dogs and cats. *In* Ettinger, S. J. (ed.): *Textbook of Veterinary Internal Medicine: Diseases of The Dog and Cat,* 2nd ed. Philadelphia: W. B. Saunders, 1983, pp. 2187–2235.

Schultz, R. D., and Adams, L. S.: Methods for detecting humoral and cellular immunity. Vet. Clin. North Am. (Small Anim. Pract.) 14:1039, 1978.

Scott, D. W., Walton, D. K., Manning, T. O., et al.: Canine lupus erythematosus I: Systemic lupus erythematosus. J. Am. Anim. Hosp. Assoc. 19:461, 1983.

Siskind, G. W.: Immunological tolerance. *In* Paul, W. E. (ed.): *Fundamental Immunology.* New York: Raven Press, 1984, pp. 537–558.

Tan, E. M.: Autoantibodies to nuclear antigens: Their biology and medicine. Adv. Immunol. 33:167, 1982.

Tan, E. W., Cohen, A. S., Frioes, J. F., et al.: Revised criteria for the classification of systemic lupus erythematosus. Arthritis Rheum. 25:1271, 1983.

Werner, L. L., and Gorman, N. T.: Immune mediated disorders of cats. Vet. Clin. North Am. (Small Anim. Pract.) 14:1039, 1984.

FELINE ACQUIRED IMMUNODEFICIENCY SYNDROME (FAIDS) INDUCED BY THE FELINE LEUKEMIA VIRUS

JENNIFER L. ROJKO, D.V.M.,
and LAWRENCE E. MATHES, PH.D.
Columbus, Ohio

The profound depression of the immune system that accompanies persistent infection with the feline leukemia virus (FeLV) has been the subject of intense clinical and experimental research lately for several good reasons. First, immunosuppression is the most frequent and most devastating manifestation of FeLV viremia in clinical and experimental studies (for review, see Rojko and Olsen, 1984). Second, the syndrome of acquired T-lymphocyte defects and secondary diseases so resembles the human acquired immunodeficiency syndrome (AIDS) in progressive clinical deterioration despite conventional therapy and in probable cause and pathogenesis that it has been termed the feline acquired immunodeficiency syndrome (FAIDS). FAIDS and its simian counterpart, the simian acquired immunodeficiency syndrome (SAIDS), therefore represent naturally occurring and experimentally reproducible animal models in which the pathogenesis, cellular mechanisms, and nonconventional therapy of retrovirus-induced ablation of specific immune function may be studied. It is the intent of this article to consider the clinicopathologic presentation of cats with FAIDS in the context of recent information regarding the interactions between FeLV and target lymphocytes, marrow cells, and macrophages. It is hoped that understanding of these interactions will enable the development of new therapeutic regimens leading to the permanent reversal of FeLV viremia and protection from FeLV-related diseases.

CLINICAL PRESENTATION

The hallmark of FAIDS in pet cats is an increased susceptibility to opportunistic or otherwise innocuous pathogens. As viruses seem to be a particular nemesis for cats, it is not surprising that viremic cats succumb to infectious peritonitis (corona) virus (FIPV) and have chronic or recurrent herpetic rhinitis and sinusitis. Persistent rhinitis, either bacterial or herpetic, occurs in a high proportion of viremic cats and a moderate proportion of latently infected cats in multiple cat households with an adequate vaccination program. Lastly, there are sporadic reports of a panleukopenia-like syndrome in cats vaccinated with modified live panleukopenia virus (FPLV) vaccines. Clearly, studies to document the effect of concurrent infections with FPLV, FIPV, and FeLV are needed.

Viremic cats also display unusual sensitivity to nonviral opportunists and may die of antibiotic-unresponsive enteritis, gingivitis, stomatitis (noma), dermatitis, pneumonia, or septicemia of bacterial origin or may develop fatal hemotropic hemobartonellosis or systemic toxoplasmosis (Cotter et al., 1975). Cats that develop opportunistic infection may appear healthy, but often even healthy viremic pet cats demonstrate lymphopenia, persistent or cyclic neutropenia, or fluctuating levels of serum complement and immune complexes. Whether these hematologic and serologic alterations are the consequence of direct virus replication or of antiviral host activity is not known at present. Alternatively, the immunosuppression may be so severe that the animal dies of "fading kitten disease," manifest by thymic atrophy and lymphoid depletion at postmortem. The antiparallel or precedent to lymphoid depletion associated with FeLV immunosuppression is the marked mandibular lymphadenopathy seen in preneoplastic adult cats with chronic FeLV

Supported by NIH NCI RO1 CA-35747-02 and NCI Contract No. FOD-0634. J.L.R. is a Scholar of the Leukemia Society of America, Inc.

infection. This disease is not yet well understood but is sometimes seen after experimental inoculation of FeLV, and it may well mimic the persistent lymphadenopathy that precedes AIDS in humans as part of the AIDS-related complex (ARC) of diseases (Ioachim et al., 1983). In both FAIDS and AIDS, it is likely that the lymphadenopathy represents excessive but ineffective stimulation of the lymphoid system in an attempt to escape persistent retrovirus infection. Other FeLV-associated diseases also reflect overstimulation of the immune system and include membranous glomerulonephritis, circulating immune complexes, and hypocomplementemia (Hardy, 1982). Lastly, cats with FAIDS also are unfortunate in that they experience functional attrition of two other life-sustaining systems: erythropoiesis and fertility. For further discussion of the effects of FeLV on hemopoiesis, see Hematologic Consequences of Feline Leukemia Virus Infection.

PATHOGENESIS OF FeLV INFECTION

Sequence of Viral Replication

Although the likely effectors of FeLV immunosuppression are the viral envelope protein (p15E) and FeLV-containing immune complexes (Hardy, 1982; Mathes et al., 1978), the immunosuppression probably is a consequence of direct interaction between replication-competent (infectious) FeLV and lymphocytes, macrophages, and bone marrow cells. To understand these interactions, it is useful to recapitulate the scheme of FeLV replication in the cat after experimental FeLV inoculation by using the oronasal route to simulate natural exposure. FeLV first enters the cat by way of tonsillar lymphocytes and macrophages in the posterior oropharynx; the virus then repopulates the draining submandibular lymph nodes and enters the recirculating lymphocyte pool for hematogenous distribution to the sites of secondary virus replication and amplification. The secondary and most significant sites of virus amplification are in the B-lymphocyte areas of the visceral lymphoid tissue, Peyer's patches and spleen, the rapidly dividing precursor cells in the bone marrow (principally myelomonocytic precursors), and intestine (crypt epithelia). By 4 to 6 weeks after exposure to a single bolus of oronasal virus, the cat either becomes persistently viremic or becomes latently infected. Progression or regression depends upon the cat's state of immune competence at the time of initial exposure and at the time of virus regression (4 to 6 weeks after exposure in most cats). However, many cats retain latent bone marrow or lymph node infections for months (30 to 50 per cent of regressor cats) to years (10 to 40 per cent of regressor cats, depending on the strain of virus used). In latently infected cats, reactivation of FeLV by stress, complement depletion, or intercurrent viral or bacterial infection can precipitate viremia or nonproducer lymphoma or anemia. Although the immunologic defects experienced by the latently infected cat are minimal compared with those of viremic cats, they are not insignificant compared with those unexposed cats (see below).

In multiple cat households, 15 to 30 per cent of the cats exposed to FeLV become persistently viremic. In the laboratory, only 15 per cent of cats older than 4 months of age develop chronic productive infections, as compared with 100 per cent of neonates and 85 per cent of weanlings. Productive infection implies persistent viral replication in B-lymphocytes in the nodes, spleen, and Peyer's patches, in myelomonocytic precursors and megakaryocytes in the bone marrow, and in multiple mucosal epithelia, which fosters virus dissemination to the environment by means of saliva and urine. Relevant to immunosuppression, persistent virus replication creates high titers of FeLV (10^4 to 10^5 infectious particles/ml) released into the plasma and even higher titers (10^5 to 10^6 infectious particles/ml) released locally in the nodes, spleen, and bone marrow. Administration of various corticosteroids (especially repository preparations of methylprednisolone acetate) will increase the output of FeLV by macrophages five- to 100-fold and by bone marrow cells three- to fivefold.

Relevance

The significance of these findings is that the reversal of FeLV immunosuppression is likely to require reversal of viremia and cessation of production of FeLV by B cells and macrophages. Furthermore, corticosteroid therapy of immunosuppressed animals is likely to worsen, rather than alleviate, the immune dysfunction. Corticosteroids themselves dampen T cell, especially helper T cell, function and aggravate virus production by non-T cells. The more virus produced, the greater the level of immunosuppression generated.

CHARACTERISTICS OF THE IMMUNOSUPPRESSION

Immunologic Factors

The primary problem is that the T cell, particularly the helper T cell, fails to function in viremic cats. It is now known that T cells have to be activated to acquire function. Activation requires a stimulus (either a T-dependent antigen or a nonspecific inducer called a mitogen, because it triggers mitosis) and the release of soluble mediators by other T cells and macrophages. In T cell failure induced by FeLV, there is a direct failure of some stimuli to elicit primary activation. More importantly, there is a failure of the stimulus to elicit the production of a soluble mediator known as T cell growth factor (interleukin-2). T cell growth factor is absolutely necessary to sustain T cell activation, to recruit other lymphocytes into the activation process, and to provide enough cells to ward off potential pathogens, kill virally infected cells or tumor cells, and help B cells in the production of immunoglobulin G (IgG). In this regard, it appears that B cells from viremic cats can still produce immunoglobulin M (IgM) antibody in response to T-independent antigens and, hence, a primary B cell defect is not likely. In viremic cats, the antigen-specific, helper T cells needed to allow the cat to switch from IgM to IgG production and thus make an anamnestic response, do not work (Trainin et al., 1983).

Causes of the Immunosuppression

FeLV is immunosuppressive for many reasons. A component protein of the viral envelope that has a mass of 15,000 daltons and is designated p15E is directly immunosuppressive. In the laboratory, p15E added to cultures of lymphocytes from nonviremic cats or healthy humans will directly abrogate lymphocyte function. Furthermore, when p15E is administered to cats concurrently with the commercially available FeLV vaccine, p15E will prevent the development of a protective antibody response to feline oncornavirus-associated cell membrane antigen (FOCMA).

Other less well-characterized immunosuppressive factors also are important clinically. Viremic cats have high levels of circulating immune complexes containing FeLV proteins and antiviral antibodies. Viremic cats also have low or fluctuating levels of serum complement. That this is relevant mechanistically is suggested by our recent demonstration that experimental complement depletion of FeLV-immune cats will cause transient re-expression of viremia *in vivo*. Furthermore, removal of circulating immunosuppressive immune complexes (see below) may sometimes cause reversal of viremia and remission of lymphoma.

THERAPEUTIC CONSIDERATIONS

Reversal of viremia is of paramount importance and is at present not very successful. The most promising treatment protocols include extracorporeal removal of immune complexes and treatment with staphylococcal protein A, monoclonal antibodies to FeLV, and, possibly, macrophage stimulants. In extracorporeal removal of immune complexes, viremic cat plasma is passed over sterile columns of staphylococcal protein A. Protein A has an affinity for IgG, and immune complexes containing IgG are removed. The cleaned plasma is returned to the cat and the procedure is repeated at weekly or biweekly intervals (Jones et al., 1980). Reversal of viremia after weeks to months is concordant with the appearance of complement-dependent antibodies that lyse lymphoma cells. More recently, 7 per cent of viremic cats injected with staphylococcal protein A have shown regression of FeLV (Liu et al., 1984). Many additional viremic cats show partial remission of tumors and partial regression of lymphomas. The 7 per cent that actually abort viremia have increased levels of circulating interferon and complement-dependent antibodies that lyse tumor cells.

Passive antibody therapy using polyclonal anti-FeLV or anti-FOCMA antibodies does not have wide clinical application despite some documented success in regression of lymphoma and viremia. The problems include expense of antibody production, anaphylactic reactions to antisera produced in heterologous species, and antibody therapy that is most effective at preventing rather than reversing viremia. Experimentally, single dose antibody therapy only works if given within the first week of FeLV infection, and cats with chronic viremias have very poor responses to antibody therapy. The recent development of several highly specific monoclonal antibodies with FeLV-neutralizing capability may lead to more clinically useful treatment regimens.

Lastly, although there is some suggestion that macrophage stimulants may encourage cat macrophages to fight viremia, there is yet no proven evidence that they do.

Other therapeutic considerations concern management of the viremic cat. There is some controversy regarding the vaccination of viremic cats. Vaccination with the commercially available FeLV vaccine will NOT lead to reversal of viremia nor will it cause remission of disease. Furthermore, as FeLV-positive cats are unable to mount anamnestic antibody responses to T cell–dependent antigens, one is forced to question the efficacy and safety of modified live viral vaccines in viremic cats. Experiments to determine the value of multivalent feline vaccines currently are in progress.

It would perhaps be appropriate to conclude with the statement that viremia need not be reversed if it can be prevented. The commercially available FeLV vaccine has been shown to be safe and efficacious in experimental and clinical trials. Whether vaccination will reduce the number and duration of latent FeLV infections remains to be determined.

References and Supplemental Reading

Cotter, S. M., Hardy, W. D. H., Jr., and Essex, M.: Association of feline leukemia virus with lymphosarcoma and other disorders in the cat. J.A.V.M.A. 166:449, 1975.

Hardy, W. D. H., Jr.: Immunopathology induced by the feline leukemia virus. Springer Semin. Immunopathol. 1985:75, 1982.

Ioachim, H. L., Lerner, C. W., and Tapper, M. L.: Lymphadenopathies in homosexual men: Relationships with the acquired immunodeficiency syndrome. J.A.M.A. 250:1306, 1983.

Jones, F. R., Yoshida, L. H., Ladiges, W. C., et al.: Treatment of feline leukemia and reversal of FeLV by *ex vivo* removal of IgG. Cancer 46:675, 1980.

Liu, W. R., Good, R. A., Trang, L. Q., et al.: Remission of leukemia and loss of feline leukemia virus in cats injected with *Staphylococcus* protein A: Association with increased circulating interferon and complement-dependent cytotoxic antibody. Proc. Natl. Acad. Sci. USA 81:6471, 1984.

Mathes, L. E., Olsen, R. G., Hebebrand, L. C., et al.: Abrogation of lymphocyte blastogenesis by a feline leukemia virus protein. Nature 274:687, 1978.

Rojko, J. L., and Olsen, R. G.: Immunobiology of the feline leukemia virus. Adv. Vet. Immunol. Immunopathol. 6:107, 1984.

Trainin, Z., Wernicke, D., Ungar-Waron, H., et al.: Suppression of the humoral antibody response in natural retrovirus infections. Science 220:858, 1983.

IMMUNODEFICIENCY

PETER J. FELSBURG, V.M.D.
Urbana, Illinois

The body's immune system is multicellular and composed of two main components—one concerned with nonspecific immune responses and one concerned with specific immune responses. The cells involved in the nonspecific immune response are phagocytic cells, primarily neutrophils and monocytes (macrophages), which are responsible for the nonspecific engulfment (phagocytosis), digestion, and elimination of foreign substances from the body. The cells of the specific component of the immune system are the lymphocytes. They interact with antigens in a highly specific manner that exhibits not only specificity but also memory to individual antigens. This part of the immune system is divided into two different functional components—the humoral (B cell) and cell-mediated (T cell) immune systems. The primary function of the humoral immune system is the production of antibodies against foreign antigens. The cell-mediated immune system has many functions, including the production of soluble substances called lymphokines, which exert their influence on the cells of the nonspecific component of the immune system, and the destruction of virus-infected and tumor cells by cytotoxic (killing) mechanisms. In addition, the T cell system, through helper T cells and suppressor T cells, regulates antibody production by turning on and off the B cell system.

Immunodeficiency disease results from abnormalities in one or more of the components of the immune system. The major clinical manifestation of immunodeficiency is an increased susceptibility to infection. Table 1 lists clinical observations that should suggest a possible immunologic defect. In most immunodeficient animals, an increased frequency of infection occurs with one or more of the other conditions. The type of infection involved and the clinical signs are influenced by the severity of the defect and which part of the immune system is affected. Defects in the B cell system usually predispose an animal to increased susceptibility to bacterial infection. Animals with a defective cell-mediated immunity are more susceptible to fungal, protozoal, and viral infections. Disorders of the phagocytic system are associated with superficial skin infections or systemic infections with pyogenic organisms. Some of the common clinical findings of immunodeficiencies are summarized in Table 2. These clinical findings are not specific for any one particular immunodeficiency but are common to immunodeficiencies in general.

Immunodeficiencies can be classified as either primary (congenital) or secondary (acquired). Primary immunodeficiencies are congenital diseases in which the inherited defects in the immune system predispose the animal to increased susceptibility to infections. Secondary immunodeficiencies, on the other hand, are alterations in immunologic function and increase susceptibility to infection as a result of some underlying disease process. Animals with secondary immunodeficiencies initially have an intact immune system but, during or following the

Table 1. *Conditions Suggesting an Immunodeficiency*

Increased frequency of infection
Increased severity of infection
Chronic or prolonged infection
Incomplete clearing between episodes of infection
Incomplete or no response to treatment
Infection with usually nonpathogenic organisms

***Table 2.** Clinical Features Associated with Immunodeficiencies*

Recurrent or chronic respiratory infections
Repeated bacterial infections
Chronic otitis
Chronic diarrhea
Recurrent abscesses
Skin lesions—chronic dermatitis or pyoderma
Recurrent or chronic fungal infections
Recurrent or chronic viral infections
Growth failure
Adverse reactions to modified live virus vaccination

primary disease, their immune response becomes transiently or permanently impaired. Differentiation between a primary and secondary immunodeficiency is important from the standpoint of treatment and prognosis.

DIAGNOSIS OF IMMUNODEFICIENCY DISEASE

Although the clinical history and findings may be suggestive of an immunodeficiency, the diagnosis must be established by appropriate laboratory tests. The tests requested depend upon the part of the immune system that is suspected of being deficient.

A complete blood count, differential, and evaluation of cellular morphology are often helpful in the diagnosis of a disorder of T cells or neutrophils. A marked, persistent lymphopenia (less than 1000/mm^3) is present in many T cell deficiencies. If a lymphopenia is suspected, several counts over a period of several weeks are indicated to rule out a transient lymphopenia. A cyclic neutropenia or a persistent leukocytosis with a shift to the left and hypersegmented mature neutrophils suggest a neutrophil disorder.

The best screening test of the humoral immune system is the quantitation of the serum immunoglobulins (IgG, IgM, and IgA). It is important that one not overemphasize the significance of low values for immunoglobulins, especially in young animals. Serum immunoglobulin concentrations are greatly influenced by the age of the animal and do not reach normal adult concentrations in dogs until approximately six months of age. Unfortunately, the only published normal values for serum immunoglobulin concentrations in dogs are for normal adults, and it is these values that most laboratories use as normal measurements. For dogs younger than six months of age, results of this test *must* be compared with age-matched controls. Until published normal values for all age groups are available, it is important for each laboratory to establish its own values. Immunoglobulin concentrations below the 95 per cent confidence intervals for that age group are suggestive of a humoral or B cell deficiency. If the immunoglobulin concentrations are extremely low compared with those of animals of comparable age, a diagnosis of a humoral immunodeficiency can usually be made. Ambiguous immunoglobulin levels can be resolved by functional studies. The easiest of these is to determine if the animal has produced antibodies to a previously administered vaccine (e.g., canine parvovirus or canine distemper virus). Alternatively, one can immunize the animal and determine whether it produces a primary and secondary antibody response after immunization (*do not* use a modified-live virus vaccine in a patient suspected of having an immunodeficiency). These functional tests take a considerable period of time and only evaluate the antibody response to the antigen that was used in the immunization. A new *in vitro* test of B cell function has been developed that evaluates the functional capability of all the B cells independent of antigen specificity.

The principal laboratory test to evaluate T cell function is the lymphocyte transformation test. This test measures the functional capability of T lymphocytes to proliferate after stimulation. This test is an *in vitro* correlate of an *in vivo* process, which regularly occurs when an antigen interacts with specifically sensitized T lymphocytes in the host. This test is commonly performed by using T cell mitogens, which activate T cells regardless of their specificity. The results of this test *must* be compared with the 95 per cent confidence intervals of age-matched controls established by the laboratory performing the test. It is important for the laboratory to incorporate both optimal and suboptimal concentrations of the antigen or mitogen or both in the test to properly evaluate the patient's response. Patients with T cell deficiencies will demonstrate an absence of response or a markedly depressed response to nonspecific stimulation with T cell mitogens and to specific antigens. To make a diagnosis of a T cell deficiency based upon this test, it is important that the patient be tested on at least two occasions to rule out a transient T cell suppression due to a concurrent viral infection.

Neutrophil function can be best evaluated by bactericidal assays. These are *in vitro* tests that measure the end product of neutrophil function—the ability to kill bacteria. In these assays, neutrophils from normal animals will kill over 95 per cent of the bacteria. It is important that a control animal be tested at the same time the patient is being evaluated. A defect in phagocytosis also will result in an abnormal bactericidal assay.

PRIMARY IMMUNODEFICIENCIES

There are approximately 30 primary immunodeficiencies that have been documented in humans. The study of primary immunodeficiency diseases in dogs and cats is still in its infancy. The following primary immunodeficiency diseases are congenital disorders of the specific (lymphocytic) and nonspecific (phagocytic) components of the immune system that have been described in the dog and are associated with increased susceptibility to infections. To date, no primary immunodeficiencies with associated increased susceptibility to infections have been documented in the cat.

Combined Immunodeficiency

Combined immunodeficiency (CID) is probably the most severe of all the primary immunodeficiencies. CID is characterized by deficiencies of both the B and T cell systems associated with lymphoid hypoplasia and thymic dysplasia. Since both components of the immune system are deficient, clinical signs occur early in infancy, and affected individuals are susceptible to a wide spectrum of microbial agents, both bacterial and viral. Human patients rarely survive past the first year. Foals with CID rarely survive more than several months before succumbing to overwhelming infections. CID is an inherited disorder with an autosomal recessive mode of inheritance in foals and both a sex-linked and autosomal recessive mode of inheritance in humans.

A sex-linked form of CID has been recently documented in the dog (Felsburg et al., 1982). These dogs present as early as three weeks of age with clinical signs that include pyoderma, otitis, and gingivostomatitis. These infections, usually of bacterial origin, have been completely unresponsive to antibiotic therapy. A universal finding in the affected dogs has been a failure to thrive (stunted growth). All affected puppies have died before 4 months of age from viral infections, primarily distemper. Several affected puppies vaccinated with a modified live distemper vaccine died 2 to 3 weeks later of distemper induced by the vaccine. Farrow and colleagues (1972) reported on six male miniature dachshunds that died of *Pneumocystis carinii* pneumonia between 9 and 12 months of age. *Pneumocystis carinii* pneumonia is a common sequela in human cases of CID. Unfortunately, no immunologic studies were performed on these dogs; however, they may represent the first cases of canine CID.

Laboratory findings usually reveal a marked lymphopenia and hypoglobulinemia. When compared with age-matched normal dogs, these dogs have a marked absence of a T cell response and a marked deficiency of IgG and IgA. IgM concentrations vary; they can either be markedly deficient or normal (this is also seen in humans with CID).

Selective IgA Deficiency

Selective IgA deficiency is the most common primary immunodeficiency in humans. The prevalence in the "normal" population is approximately 1:600. Although many of these IgA-deficient individuals appear healthy, studies of individual patients as well as extensive studies of large numbers of patients suggest that IgA deficiency predisposes these people to a wide variety of diseases. Young patients with undetectable or low IgA are predisposed to chronic, recurrent infections of the upper respiratory tract, gastrointestinal tract, and skin. This is not surprising, since secretory IgA plays a major role in the local immune response of mucosal surfaces. IgA-deficient individuals are at greater risk of developing allergies and autoimmune diseases, especially rheumatoid arthritis, systemic lupus erythematosus, and autoimmune thyroiditis. Convulsive episodes of unexplained cause have also been associated with selective IgA deficiency. A transient form of IgA deficiency has been reported in humans in which the affected children develop normal levels of IgA during adolescence and lose their tendency to contract recurrent respiratory infections.

This condition has been recently documented in the dog (Felsburg et al., 1985). The clinical presentation in young dogs consists of recurrent upper respiratory tract (URT) infections, otitis, and chronic dermatitis. As in humans, there does not appear to be a difference in the clinical manifestations between dogs with undetectable IgA and dogs with low IgA levels. In spite of intranasal vaccination with an effective bivalent vaccine, these dogs develop mild, recurrent URT infections due primarily to *Bordetella bronchiseptica* and canine parainfluenza virus. Several dogs have also experienced episodes of convulsions. There is some evidence to suggest that IgA-deficient dogs may be more susceptible to gastrointestinal parasitic infections, especially giardiasis. The infections are usually not severe or life-threatening. There is a possibility that some of these dogs may have a transient IgA deficiency and will outgrow their tendency for recurrent infections as they become adults.

Screening of large populations of clinically normal adult dogs has revealed IgA deficiencies in apparently "healthy" adults, just as is seen in humans. Unfortunately, their clinical history as young dogs is unknown. A large number of these "healthy" IgA-deficient dogs possess autoantibodies but no autoimmune disease. Prospective studies are needed to determine whether these dogs will go on to develop autoimmune disease, as will humans. Recent epidemiologic studies have shown that puppies born of "healthy" IgA-deficient dams are at much higher risk of developing upper respiratory and gastrointestinal infections than are puppies born of dams with normal concentrations of IgA.

The only abnormal laboratory finding is an absence or markedly low concentration of IgA when compared with values in age-matched normal dogs. The immunologic defect appears to be in the maturation and differentiation of the IgA B cells.

Transient Hypogammaglobulinemia of Infancy

Transient hypogammaglobulinemia of infancy is a self-limiting immunoglobulin deficiency resulting from an abnormally prolonged delay in the onset of immunoglobulin synthesis by the neonate and young puppy. The puppies show a normal decline in maternal antibody over the first weeks of life, but they fail to synthesize their own immunoglobulins until much later than normal. This disorder is characterized by an increased susceptibility to infection after the disappearance of maternal antibody until the affected puppy's own B cell system is fully operational.

These puppies present with chronic or recurrent bacterial infections of the respiratory tract and skin that start around 2 to 3 months of age, following the disappearance of maternal antibody. Spontaneous recovery occurs as the levels of immunoglobulins become normal around 5 to 6 months of age (Felsburg et al., manuscript in preparation).

The only significant laboratory finding is low levels of immunoglobulins, when compared with those of dogs of comparable age, that occur after the disappearance of maternal antibody and persist until the puppies are 5 to 7 months of age. It is essential to monitor the immunoglobulin concentrations of puppies diagnosed as immunoglobulin deficient in order to determine whether it is a permanent or transient defect.

Cyclic Neutropenia

Neutropenia is the most common disorder of the polymorphonuclear phagocytic system in humans. Neutropenia results in increased susceptibility to severe bacterial infections and a poor response to antibiotic therapy. Neutropenia can either be congenital or acquired.

A congenital form of neutropenia has been documented in the dog (Lund et al., 1967). It is characterized by cyclic fluctuations of peripheral blood neutrophils and has been designated cyclic neutropenia after a similar condition in humans. It was originally reported in gray collies and has been shown to be inherited as an autosomal recessive trait. The disease is characterized by a cyclic neutropenia generally occurring every 8 to 12 days and lasting for 2 to 4 days. Clinical signs are only present during the neutropenia and consist of fever, malaise, oral ulcers, skin lesions, arthralgia alone or in combination. During the marked neutropenia, potential life-threatening infections occur. Infections are less severe if a monocytosis occurs during the period of neutropenia. The infections usually clear when the neutrophils return to normal levels.

There does not appear to be a functional defect in the neutrophils, but infections occur because of a lack of sufficient numbers of functional neutrophils. The defect appears to be at the level of the hematopoietic stem cell. No other immunologic abnormalities have been documented in these dogs.

The laboratory diagnosis is based upon the presence of the cyclic neutropenia.

Canine Granulocytopathy Syndrome

This disease is a congenital disorder of neutrophil function that is characterized by recurrent life-threatening bacterial infections (Renshaw et al., 1975). These dogs present with a neutrophilia, but, unlike their condition in cyclic neutropenia, these neutrophils are defective in their ability to kill phagocytocized bacteria. The defect is inherited as an autosomal recessive trait.

Clinically, these dogs present at a young age with a history of recurrent episodes of infections with pyogenic bacteria that respond poorly to routine antibiotic therapy. Suppurative skin lesions, gingivitis, and marked lymphadenopathy are common clinical findings. In advanced states, osteomyelitis may be observed.

Hematologic findings consist of a persistent leukocytosis with a regenerative left shift. Mature neutrophils exhibit prominent nuclear hypersegmentation. These dogs apparently have competent humoral and cell-mediated immune systems. The only functional defect appears to be related to an inability of the neutrophils to kill bacteria, as determined by bactericidal assays. This defect is intrinsic to the neutrophil, since serum from these dogs possesses normal opsonizing antibodies for neutrophils from normal dogs.

SECONDARY IMMUNODEFICIENCIES

Secondary or acquired immunodeficiencies are by far the most commonly encountered immunodeficiencies in humans and animals. As mentioned previously, these disorders are secondary to some other underlying disease process. Conditions that have been associated with secondary immunodeficiencies are various infectious diseases, malignancy, autoimmune diseases, endocrine disorders, malnutrition, immunosuppressive therapy, and failure to receive colostrum. Since many of these conditions are mentioned in detail in other sections, they will only be mentioned briefly in this section.

Acquired immunodeficiency in the dog has been reported in canine distemper infections, canine parvovirus infections, malnutrition, canine demodicosis, various neoplastic diseases, growth hormone deficiency, and invasive aspergillosis. We have also seen secondary immunodeficiencies associated with diabetes, systemic lupus erythematosus, and zinc deficiency. The dogs with zinc deficiency present with moderate to severe skin infections and a marked T cell deficiency. The skin infections clear and the T cell defect is corrected after zinc replacement therapy.

Secondary immunodeficiencies in the cat have been associated with both feline leukemia and feline panleukopenia virus infections.

MANAGEMENT OF ANIMALS WITH IMMUNODEFICIENCY DISEASES

Successful management of patients with immunodeficiency diseases depends upon whether the deficiency is primary or secondary, and which part or parts of the immune system are affected.

Secondary immunodeficiencies are treated with symptomatic therapy such as antibiotics to control infections while attempts are made to cure or treat the underlying disease process. Once the underlying disease is cured, the immunodeficiency should be resolved.

Primary immunodeficiencies pose a very special problem to the clinician and clinical immunologist. Since these are newly recognized diseases in the dog, our experience in treating them is limited. Nevertheless, we can draw upon the knowledge gained over the past 30 years in treating human primary immunodeficiencies. Antibiotics are lifesaving in the treatment of the infectious episodes of patients with immunodeficiencies.

Humoral immune or B cell deficiencies with normal T cell function are the easiest to manage. Aggressive antibiotic therapy should be first used in an attempt to control infections. In cases in which this approach is insufficient, patients may be given gamma globulin preparations to replace the immunoglobulins that they are lacking. In humans, monthly intramuscular injections of gamma globulin at a dosage of 100 mg/kg is sufficient to keep patients symptom-free. If gamma globulin preparations are not available, plasma transfusions at a dosage of 20 ml/kg/month may be employed. The exception to the use of gamma globulin or plasma is selective IgA deficiency. IgA-deficient patients cannot be given preparations that contain IgA, since many will have an anaphylactic reaction to it. In addition, serum IgA probably plays a very minor role in host defense. What really has to be replaced is secretory IgA, and at this time there is no practical way of passively administering secretory IgA. These patients have to be treated symptomatically.

At this time, there is *no practical* way of treating a T cell deficiency other than by symptomatic therapy. Nonspecific immunostimulators have yet to be shown by well-controlled studies to be of any benefit in treating T cell deficiencies in the dog. *Do not* use modified-live virus vaccine in animals with a T cell deficiency or a combined immunodeficiency. These animals may develop infections from the vaccine itself.

Patients with a neutrophil defect should be treated aggressively with a broad-spectrum *bactericidal* antibiotic. If the defect is primary or permanent, it is important to initiate therapy with high doses of a bactericidal antibiotic to treat even mild infections.

Most life-threatening infections associated with immunoglobulin deficiencies or neutrophil defects result from delay in diagnosis or treatment. Depending upon the severity of the deficiency, continuous antibiotic therapy may be required to control infections.

When the clinician deals with animals with primary immunodeficiencies, perhaps the best reason for understanding why the patient has an increased susceptibility to infection is to be able to advise the client on the prognosis for a cure or successful management of the case. (Some patients may not get better no matter how *you or another veterinarian* treat them.) Knowledge that a patient has a primary immunodeficiency will also permit the clinician to give advice on future breeding programs.

CONCLUSIONS

Our knowledge of primary immunodeficiency diseases in dogs and cats is at the stage at which knowledge of such diseases in humans was 25 to 30 years ago. As clinical immunology evolves as a discipline in veterinary medicine and as clinicians become aware that such diseases exist, many of the same immunodeficiencies that have been documented in humans will probably be found in the dog and cat. Since these diseases are of genetic origin, it is conceivable that the incidence of primary immunodeficiencies will be higher in dogs and cats because of the practice of inbreeding. As the number of diagnosed cases of primary immunodeficiencies increases, so will our knowledge of how to treat these diseases. The ultimate goal is to define the basic immunologic defect in these patients in order to develop specific methods of immunologic intervention for potential cures.

References and Supplemental Reading

Ammann, A. J., and Fudenberg, H. H.: Immunodeficiency Diseases. *In* Fudenberg, H. H., Stites, D. P., Caldwell, J. L., et al. (eds): *Basic and Clinical Immunology*, 3rd ed. Los Altos, CA: Lange, 1980, pp. 409–441.

Cockerell, G. L.: Naturally occurring acquired immunodeficiency diseases of the dog and cat. Vet. Clin. North Am. 8:613, 1978.

Farrow, B. R. H., Watson, A. D. J., Hartley, W. J., et al.: Pneumocystis pneumonia in the dog. J. Comp. Pathol. 82:447, 1972.

Felsburg, P. J., and Jezyk, P. F.: A canine model for combined immunodeficiency. Clin. Res. 30:347, 1982.

Felsburg, P. J., Glickman, L. T., and Jezyk, P. F.: Selective IgA deficiency in the dog. Clin Immunol. Immunopathol. 36:297, 1985.

Lund, J. E., Padgett, G. A., and Ott, R. L.: Cyclic neutropenia in grey collie dogs. Blood 29:452, 1967.

Olsen, R. G., and Krakowka, S.: Immune dysfunctions associated with viral infections. Comp. Cont. Ed. Pract. Vet. 6:422, 1984.

Renshaw, H. W., Chatburn, C., Bryan, G. M., et al.: Canine granulocytopathy syndrome: Neutrophil dysfunction in a dog with recurrent infections. J.A.V.M.A. 166:443, 1975.

ALLERGIC DRUG REACTIONS

JEFF R. WILCKE, D.V.M.
Blacksburg, Virginia

An allergic drug reaction is the direct result of interaction between a drug molecule, acting as an antigen, and one or more components of the patient's immune system. Immune system components that initiate an allergic drug reaction may include lymphocytes sensitized to the drug, antibodies specific for it, or both. As a consequence, true allergic drug reactions generally occur after immunologic induction and should be differentiated from nonspecific activation of the complement cascade, changes in rates of prostaglandin synthesis, suppression of regulatory components (suppressor T-cells) of the immune system, and nonspecific release of inflammatory mediators. These latter reactions occur immediately at the first administration of the drug, and their severity depends on the dose of drug given.

DRUG INTERACTION WITH THE IMMUNE SYSTEM: HAPTEN IMMUNOLOGY

A hapten is a substance that, although not immunogenic itself, may induce an immune reaction when it is combined with some macromolecule. Macromolecules involved are usually tissue proteins (as are most true antigens) but may also include nucleic acids and lipids. Immune reactivity of these hapten-macromolecule complexes generally requires that a stable bond be formed. The necessary stability is associated with covalent bonding, coordination, and in rare instances multiple salt linkages. The reversible ionic and hydrogen bondings that most drugs undergo with serum albumin and carrier globulins are generally ineffective for immune stimulation. It would appear, however, that the stability of the bond is more important than any special chemical or physical property of the bond itself. Polynucleotides forming large numbers of ionic bonds with proteins can stimulate immune reactions. The summation of the forces generated by the bonds formed results in a reasonably stable complex.

Generally, a drug's ability to combine with macromolecules—its reactivity—is directly proportional to the potential for allergic drug reactions. When the parent drug does not readily combine with proteins, the reactive molecule may be a hepatic metabolite rather than the parent drug itself. In penicillin hypersensitivity (human), the best studied example of an immune-mediated drug reaction, antibodies have been demonstrated to the penicilloyl group, penicillinate (and its oxidation products), penicillamine, penamaldoyl, penicilloaldehyde, and polymers of 6-aminopenicillanic acid. The reactive component may also be a contaminant of the manufacturing process, as can be the case in allergic reactions to aspirin. Aspiroyl anhydrides contaminating certain commercial aspirin preparations have been shown to produce an immune response in guinea pigs. Antiaspiroyl antibodies have been detected in human patients, although the vast majority of acute reactions to aspirin appear to involve other mechanisms (Parker, 1981). Enzymatic coupling of drugs to macromolecules may also occur, as can be demonstrated with isoniazid or hydralazine linked to albumin or nucleohistones by epidermal transglutamase (Buxman, 1979). Clinical evidence for immune disease caused by antigens created in this way is lacking, however.

Any amino acid residue (part of some protein) that can assume a charge is a candidate for combination with a reactive drug. Antibodies formed recognize the drug combined with the protein molecule. Once formed, the antibody may also combine with the drug even when the macromolecule portion of the full antigenic determinent is lacking.

Further, once antibodies specific for the hapten are elaborated, complexes of the drug and macromolecules other than the original protein may participate. In some cases, the antibody is specific for the drug molecule and nearby amino acid side-chains so that the antibody will combine only with the drug-protein complex. These reactions will subside when the drug is discontinued. If, however, enough amino acid residues are involved, the antibody can combine with the protein even after the drug is gone. The exact nature of the hapten-macromolecule-antibody interaction will determine the duration and nature of therapy. Unfortunately, except by therapeutic trial, it is impossible to determine whether therapy will continue for life or simply until the drug has been eliminated from the body.

Reactions other than molecular bonding of the drug to a macromolecule may result in the production of immunogenicity. Ions of heavy metals such as nickel, cadmium, and silver may produce contact dermatitis, probably through the formation of coordination complexes with proteins. Drug molecules may also polymerize to form large complexes capable of stimulating the immune system. Antibodies to polymers of 6-aminopenicillanic acid can be demonstrated in some human patients allergic to penicillin.

DIAGNOSIS OF DRUG ALLERGY

Definitive diagnosis of immune-mediated drug reactions requires the demonstration of drug-sensitized lymphocytes or drug-specific antibodies. Unfortunately, a diagnosis by *in vitro* testing is rarely possible. It is generally difficult to duplicate the conditions that result in stimulation of the immune system in the patient. The offending drug molecule or metabolite as well as the specific macromolecule and conditions for complex formation are often unknown. Likewise, skin testing is often unrewarding, because the drug molecule, metabolite, or contaminant may be unknown or unavailable. Even when skin testing is performed with drug products known to be immunogenic, there may be false positive reactions. False positive reactions occur when pharmacologic mediators are released in response to nonspecific irritants.

Provocative studies with low doses of the suspect drug can be used to support the diagnosis of an allergic drug reaction, but they are not conclusive. There are obvious reasons for concern about instituting a diagnostic procedure, the positive result of which is the induction of a disease. In human patients with a history of penicillin allergy but no recent exposure, the rate of adverse response to intentional, controlled test exposures is approximately 35 per cent. Of these, 10 per cent developed anaphylaxis and 10 per cent of those suffering anaphylaxis died despite prompt and aggressive medical therapy (Patterson, 1982). A recent report of two cases of immune-mediated polyarthritis in dogs included challenge studies (Werner, 1983). This report provides one of the very few well-documented examples of drug-induced immune disease in veterinary patients.

The clinical diagnosis of allergic drug reactions depends first on awareness on the part of the clinician of the potential for such reactions. New clinical signs that appear during the course of therapy should be evaluated by the following criteria: the reaction should (1) not resemble the pharmacologic actions of the drug; (2) be elicited by minute amounts of the drug; (3) occur only after an induction period of at least 5 to 7 days after primary exposure to the drug; (4) include classic signs of allergic reactions such as anaphylaxis, urticaria, asthma, and serum sickness; and (5) recur promptly upon re-exposure to small amounts of the drug.

Reaction: Type I Hypersensitivity

Type I, or immediate, hypersensitivity reactions are initiated when molecules of IgE, bound to basophils or tissue mast cells, are cross-linked by a di- or polyvalent antigen. Cross-linking of the IgE molecule causes the mast cell to degranulate and release vasoactive and immunoregulatory substances. Histamine, slow-reacting substance of anaphylaxis (SRS-A), eosinophil chemotactic factor of anaphylaxis (ECF-A), and prostaglandin and related lipid substances are among the mediators of the type I reaction.

The clinical manifestations of immediate hypersensitivity classically include anaphylaxis, urticaria, and angioedema. Clinical signs associated with anaphylaxis include systemic hypotension and possible circulatory collapse in all animals, varying degrees of bronchoconstriction, and disruption of gastrointestinal motility and secretion, depending on the species involved (see Table 1). Type I reactions have also been implicated in "mixed-type" hypersensitivity reactions, such as that occurring in chronic obstructive pulmonary disease.

Although reports in the literature of anaphylaxis in veterinary patients are scarce, it is a potential outcome of the administration of a substantial list of drugs. Penicillin is the best known and probably most common cause. Veterinarians and veterinary technicians should be prepared for type I hypersensitivity reactions when foreign antisera, blood products, L-asparaginase, vaccines, and venoms are administered. Other agents associated with these reactions in human beings include most antimicrobials, the polypeptide hormones (ACTH, TSH, insulin), iron dextran, methylergonovine maleate, and nitrofurantoin. Diagnostic agents such as sulfobro-

Table 1. Characteristics of Anaphylaxis in Various Species

Species	Main Stock (Target) Organ	Clinical Signs	Pathologic Features	Immunologic Mediators
Guinea pig	Lungs (bronchi)	Cough, cyanosis, dyspnea, convulsions	Emphysema	Histamine, prostaglandin SRS-A, kinins, thromboxane b2
Rat	Intestinal vessels	Cyanosis, scratching, collapse	Congestion, hemorrhage	Serotonin, histamine, SRS-A
Rabbit	Pulmonary artery	Cyanosis, dyspnea, collapse	Right heart dilatation	Histamine, serotonin, kinins
Dog	Hepatic veins	Vomiting, diarrhea, dyspnea, collapse	Visceral/hepatic engorgment, visceral hemorrhage	Histamine, kinins, SRS-A
Cat	Lungs (bronchi), Pulmonary vessels	Pruritus, vomiting, dyspnea	Pulmonary edema, emphysema, hemorrhage	Histamine, SRS-A, PGF2a

Adapted from Davis: J.A.V.M.A. 185:1131, 1984.

mophthalein sodium (BSP) and allergen extracts may also be involved.

Emergency treatment of anaphylaxis is first directed at hypotension associated with profound vasodilation. Large volumes of fluids (crystalloid) should be administered rapidly. Epinephrine or norepinephrine should be given to increase vascular tone and counteract other effects of vasoactive substances derived from the immune system. Aminophylline, glucocorticoids, and antihistamines may be indicated to counter the actions of other immune mediators and decrease associated tissue damage, but they are of secondary importance to aggressive fluid therapy and epinephrine. The value of these drugs will vary, depending on the species involved. Indirect blood pressure monitoring is helpful in determining the rate of drug administration and evaluating the progress of therapy. Therapy of urticarial reactions and angioedema is essentially the same as for anaphylaxis, although high rates of fluid administration are rarely necessary. These reactions are often self-limiting and have begun to resolve by the time veterinary care can be provided.

Reaction: Type II Hypersensitivity

Type II, or cytotoxic, hypersensitivity reactions result when the drug molecule binds to proteins, glycoproteins, lipids, or phospholipids of cell surfaces. IgG and IgM antibodies, elaborated in response to the altered antigenic nature of cell components, bind to cells and cause the activation of the complement cascade. The result is cell lysis and cell phagocytosis by macrophages.

A number of cell lines may be involved in cytotoxic reactions mediated by the immune system. The best recognized case is immune-mediated hemolytic anemia associated with penicillin treatment in humans. Cytotoxic reactions have also been associated with thrombocytopenias and neutropenias. Generally, the process is limited to one or, at most, two cell lines. It is possible, however, for stem cells to be involved; this results in diseases that represent decreases in cell production. Organ-specific damage occurs when a drug binds (specifically) to cell types within the organ. The disease may also be limited to a single organ when reactive metabolites are responsible for binding and are produced only in the target organ.

Cytotoxic reactions mediated by the immune system are well recognized in veterinary medicine but the association between the immune reaction and the administration of a drug has rarely been made. Cytotoxic drug reactions known or thought to have an immune basis in humans include polymyositis and hemorrhagic alveolitis induced by penicillamine; hemolytic anemia by alpha-methyldopa; systemic lupus erythematosus by hydralazine, procainamide, and isoniazid; hepatitis by oxyphenisatin, venocuran, and halothane; scleroderma by vinyl chloride; tubular nephropathy by penicillin; antifactor VIII antibodies by penicillin; thrombocytopenia by quinine and quinidine; and angioblastic lymphadenopathy by penicillin and other drugs.

Therapy for cytotoxic reactions should be based on the administration of large doses of corticosteroids (2 mg/kg of prednisolone or prednisone, b.i.d.). Once the disease is in remission, the total amount of steroid used may be decreased to a maintenance level. Because these reactions may persist even in the absence of the offending drug, there may be need for lifelong therapy. Adjunctive immunosuppressive therapy may be necessary in cases in which control is difficult to achieve. Cyclophosphamide or azathioprine may be combined with the glucocorticoids for both induction and maintenance regimes. In immune-mediated thrombocytopenia, vincristine may be beneficial because it possesses thrombocytogenic activity. Splenectomy is advocated by many authors, as a last resort, for refractory cases. Adjunctive blood transfusions may be indicated or specifically contraindicated. In the case of immune-mediated hemolytic anemia, the transfusion may be lifesaving or it may induce a massive hemolytic crisis. Thrombocytopenia, on the other hand, can be safely treated with platelet-rich plasma.

Reaction: Type III Hypersensitivity

Type III reactions begin with the formation of soluble immune complexes. These complexes are composed of variable ratios of antigen and its specific IgG or, possibly, IgM antibody, along with complement components and other plasma proteins. Vasculitis is induced through the deposition of these immune complexes in blood vessels and the activation of complement. Because the immune complexes are soluble and tissues are injured as "innocent bystanders," the clinical signs associated with type III reactions tend to be generalized unless the total amount of antigen is small. The reaction is characterized by fever and rash and may include purpura or urticaria. Lymphadenopathy, arthralgia, and renal dysfunction may appear if drug therapy continues for an extended period. When IgE antibody is involved there is release of vasoactive substances from mast cells, which is likely to be responsible for urticarial reactions. When antibody is in excess of antigen, the reaction is a localized, "arthus-type" reaction such as hypersensitivity pneumonitis, which results from the inhalation of antigenic materials (as could occur during nebulization therapy).

A number of drugs have been associated with serum sickness in humans. These drugs include penicillin, sulfonamides, thiouracil, cholecystographic dyes, hydantoins, aminosalicylic acid, and streptomycin. Serum sickness–like disease in two dogs associated with the administration of sulfadiazine and trimethoprim has recently been reported. The course of the disease in each of the dogs included a period of sensitization and prompt recovery when the medication was discontinued. The immune basis of the clinical signs was not confirmed by finding antibodies to either drug, but challange of the dogs by readministration of the drugs caused an exacerbation of clinical signs.

Circulating immune complexes are probably also associated with drug-induced systemic lupus seen in human patients. For the purpose of this article, drug-induced disease that resembles systemic lupus will be referred to as "lupuslike" to distinguish it from autoimmune systemic lupus. Lupuslike syndromes have been induced by hydralazine, procainamide, phenytoin, isoniazid, propylthiouracil, and chlorpromazine. Although clinical evidence for lupuslike diseases caused by drugs in veterinary patients is lacking, antinuclear antibody induction by hydralazine has been reported in beagles.

Resolution of type III hypersensitivity reactions generally comes when the offending medication is withdrawn. Systemic glucocorticoids may be indicated to relieve clinical signs, but they are rarely required. In systemic lupus the reaction is mixed (type II and III) and certainly requires anti-immunologic therapy.

Reaction: Type IV Hypersensitivity

The release of lymphokines by T-lymphocytes, in response to immune complexes or to antigens interacting with the lymphocyte surface, is responsible for type IV hypersensitivity. The reaction is also referred to as delayed hypersensitivity because the clinical signs result from the accumulation of lymphocytes, macrophages, and other cells in response to these lymphokines over a period of 24 to 72 hours. Contact dermatitis is the disease most often associated with type IV hypersensitivity. It has been associated with heavy metals, aniline dyes, organophosphate insecticides, and neomycin. When topical medication is employed to treat inflammatory skin conditions, the appearance of contact dermatitis may be taken for an exacerbation of the disease condition. Whichever is the actual case, the therapeutic regime is likely to change. If the signs are those of contact dermatitis, they will subside if the offending agent has been withdrawn.

Treatment of contact dermatitis is best accomplished by avoidance of the offending agent. Systemic glucocorticoids may be useful on a short-term basis to control acute inflammatory signs. If several drugs are employed topically, they should be discontinued. Drugs can be reinstituted individually, if necessary, in order to identify the offending agent.

ADVERSE DRUG REACTIONS RESEMBLING ALLERGY

Drug reactions associated with nonspecific release of immunologic mediators and direct tissue toxicity may mimic true hypersensitivity. Although these reactions may be controlled by certain immune system components (degranulation of mast cells in response to the administration of morphine or large volumes of hypertonic solutions), they are not initiated by antigen combining with sensitized lymphocytes or specific antibodies.

Acute collapse has been observed after the administration of certain vehicles and drugs. The cardiovascular effects of chloramphenicol, aminoglycosides, polymyxins, tetracyclines, and propylene glycol (which include arrhythmias, hypotension, momentary cardiac standstill, and decreased pulmonary blood flow) can be confused with anaphylaxis (Adams, 1975). Intravascular precipitation of a water-insoluble drug after IV administration may cause acute collapse. Drug precipitates will become trapped in pulmonary arterioles and produce embolism.

Nonimmunologic acute hemolytic reactions may occur after the administration of hypotonic solutions and certain organic vehicles. In these situations the effects are generally transient, and persistent anemia seldom develops. Oxidant drugs may cause hemolytic anemia accompanied by methemoglobinemia and formation of Heinz bodies. Examples of oxidant drugs include acetaminophen, methylene blue, sulfonamides, quinacrine, nitrofurans, neoarsphenamine, and nalidixic acid.

Aspirin sensitivity in humans is thought to be mediated through blockade of the cyclo-oxygenase pathway in all but a few cases. Metabolites of arachidonic acid are then shunted to the lipoxygenase pathway, which generates slow-reacting substance of anaphylaxis (SRS-A). Most aspirin-sensitive patients cannot tolerate indomethacin or other blockers of the cyclo-oxygenase pathway, but acetominophen can be substituted for aspirin. In rare cases of true aspirin hypersensitivity, structurally unrelated nonsteroidal anti-inflammatory drugs can be substituted.

Finally, drug fever may be produced either as the result of drug allergy or by mechanisms that are not immune-mediated. Immune-mediated drug fever is initiated by the elaboration of lymphokines by sensitized lymphocytes which, in turn, stimulate the release of endogenous pyrogens from neutrophils. Drugs such as amphotericin B, however, may cause fever by disrupting cell membranes, which release pyrogens into the circulation. Certain drugs, in overdose, may increase the body temperature by uncoupling oxidative phosphorylation in tissues. Energy derived from metabolism is then dissipated as heat rather than trapped in high-energy phosphate bonds. The latter mechanism is responsible for drug fever associated with salicylate and disophenol toxicoses.

References and Supplemental Reading

Adams, H. R.: Acute adverse effects of antibiotics. J.A.V.M.A. 166:983, 1975.

Buxman, M. M.: The role of enzymatic coupling of drugs to proteins in induction of drug specific antibodies. J. Invest. Dermatol. 73:250, 1979.

Davis, L. E.: Hypersensitivity reactions induced by antimicrobial drugs. J.A.V.M.A. 185:1131, 1984.

Halliwell, R. E.: Autoimmune diseases in domestic animals. J.A.V.M.A. 181:1088, 1982.

Parker, C. W.: Hapten immunology and allergic reactions in humans. Arthritis Rheum. 24:1024, 1981.

Patterson, R., and Anderson, J.: Allergic reactions to drugs and biologic agents. J.A.M.A. 248:2637, 1982.

Werner, L. L., and Bright, J. M.: Drug-induced immune hypersensitivity disorders in two dogs treated with trimethoprim sulfadiazine: Case reports and drug challenge studies. J.A.A.H.A. 19:783, 1983.

Oncology

IMMUNODIAGNOSIS OF FELINE LEUKEMIA VIRUS INFECTION

HANS LUTZ, Dr. med. vet.,
Zürich, Switzerland

and NIELS C. PEDERSEN, D.V.M.
Davis, California

Feline leukemia virus (FeLV), a member of the Retroviridae family, is spread horizontally from cat to cat. It is an important infectious agent that is responsible for a wide variety of diseases in cats, including anemias, secondary infections due to FeLV-induced immunosuppression, and several forms of neoplastic diseases.

Cats are usually infected from close intimate contact with asymptomatic FeLV-carriers (through bites, mutual grooming, and sharing litter boxes and food containers). The virus can also be transmitted by using blood-contaminated needles and instruments and by blood transfusions. About 20 per cent of the kittens of carrier queens will be born with the infection and carry it into later life. The remaining kittens will die while still in the uterus or will be born dead or in a greatly weakened state. The main source of the virus is saliva, which may have up to 10^6 virus particles per milliliter. The virus may also be shed in feces and urine.

The infection begins in the lymphoid tissue near the point of entry (Rojko et al., 1979). It then travels to distant lymphoid tissues through a few infected blood mononuclear cells. The infection can be halted at this point or proceed to involve the bone marrow. Once the rapidly dividing bone marrow cells are infected, viremia develops and leukocytes and platelets loaded with viral antigen enter the blood stream. As a consequence of this viremia, FeLV starts to replicate in different organs, including salivary glands, intestinal mucosa, and the epithelium of the urinary bladder. Virus shedding begins at this point. Persistently viremic animals may remain clinically asymptomatic for weeks or years. Eventually, however, they develop any number of FeLV-associated diseases.

The incidence of persistent viremia is variable. In households with only one or two cats, the frequency of persistent infection is low, perhaps 1 to 5 per cent. Under crowded conditions, as in catteries where some cats may live under social stress and where repeated or continuous exposure to FeLV takes place, more than 30 per cent of the animals may be persistently viremic (Hardy et al., 1976). Kittens younger than 12 to 16 weeks are more susceptible than older cats to the infection.

It is important to note that an efficient immune reaction may terminate the infection at any stage, even if a cat has been viremic for several weeks. A successful immune response usually results in the development of virus-neutralizing antibodies (Lutz et al., 1980a).

DETECTION OF FeLV INFECTION

There are three procedures that are used currently for the routine diagnosis of FeLV infection: (1) isolation of infectious virus from the blood, (2) detection of FeLV antigens present in peripheral blood leukocytes and platelets by the indirect immunofluorescent assay (IFA), and (3) detection of the major FeLV core protein in the serum or plasma by the enzyme-linked immunosorbent assay (ELISA).

Virus Isolation

The virus isolation procedure is used mostly in Great Britain for research and routine diagnosis of FeLV infection (Jarrett et al., 1982) and in a few specialized laboratories in other countries. In this technique, a serum or plasma sample to be tested is added to cells of a monolayer cell culture that latently harbors the genome of a sarcomavirus. If FeLV is present, it infects these cells, the sarcomavirus genome is expressed, and the infected cells become malignantly transformed. Foci of transformed cells can be demonstrated microscopically a few days later.

The IFA Procedure

In this technique, which was developed by Hardy and coworkers (1973), the group-specific antigens (gsa) of FeLV are demonstrated in the cytoplasm of leukocytes and platelets in the peripheral blood. Ideally, three smears are prepared from fresh blood, which are then air-dried and sent to a clinical pathology laboratory experienced with the test. Smears prepared from older blood samples anticoagulated with EDTA, partially clotted blood, or leukopenic and thrombocytopenic samples are less suited for diagnosis.

The smears are acetone-fixed in the laboratory and incubated with a rabbit or goat hyperimmune serum specific for FeLV gsa. After nonbound gsa-specific immune serum has been removed, bound antibody is revealed by a second incubation with a fluorescein-labeled immunoglobulin conjugate directed against the gsa-specific antibody and subsequent examination in a fluorescent microscope. Detection of fluorescence in the cytoplasm of leukocytes and in the platelets is diagnostic for FeLV infection.

The ELISA Procedure

The ELISA is the most widely used technique for detection of FeLV infection. It is usually based on the use of monoclonal antibodies to the major viral core protein (FeLV-p27) (Lutz et al., 1983a). Test kits using these antibodies are available at this time from several commercial companies (Leukassay-F, Pitman-Moore; Diasystems-FeLV, Tech-America). The test kits permit serum of plasma samples to be tested within 30 minutes in the practitioner's office. An aliquot of serum or plasma is added to a test plate well to which a monoclonal antibody specific for FeLV-p27 is coated. Together with the sample a small amount of conjugate solution is added to the well. This conjugate solution contains monoclonal antibodies (labeled with an enzyme) that are also specific for FeLV-p27. However, the enzyme-labeled antibodies recognize antigenic determinants distinct from those to which the immobilized antibody is directed. If FeLV-p27

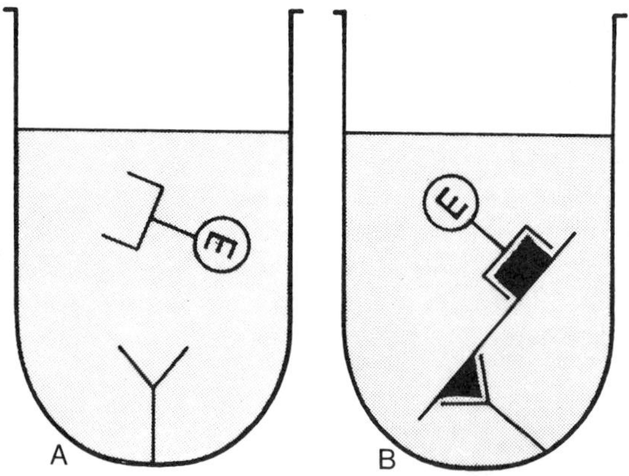

Figure 1. Principle of the ELISA. *A*: One monoclonal antibody (the catching antibody) is coated to the surface of the well. The enzyme-conjugated antibodies in solution are directed against antigenic determinants distinct from that to which the catching antibody is directed. *B*: If p27 antigen is present in the serum sample added to the well, it will serve as a link between the catching and the enzyme-conjugated antibody. After the unbound conjugate is washed out, the enzyme activity bound to the surface of the well is demonstrated by adding an appropriate substrate. Under the influence of the enzyme, the substrate will change its color, indicating the presence of FeLV antigen.

is present in the sample, it will serve to link the first antibody coated to the well and the enzyme-labeled antibodies (Fig. 1). After unbound enzyme-antibody conjugate is removed in a washing step, a solution with colorless substrate is added to the well. If FeLV-p27 was present in the sample, the enzyme-conjugate will be immobilized to the well and convert the sustrate to a colored form. Therefore, any color development distinctly darker than that of the negative control serum indicates the presence of FeLV in the serum or plasma sample.

Detection of Antibodies to FeLV and the Feline Oncornavirus-Associated Cell Membrane Antigen (FOCMA)

In many research laboratories the immune response of cats to FeLV and FOCMA has been investigated. As the cell-mediated immune response is technically difficult to assess, most investigations have dealt with the study of humoral antibodies. Of great biological importance are virus-neutralizing antibodies (VNA). VNA are directed against the major component of the virus envelope, a glycoprotein of 70,000 molecular weight (FeLV-gp70). High titers of VNA protect a cat against FeLV infection by coating the infecting FeLV with antibodies and thereby making it impossible for the virus to become attached to the cell surface receptors and to infect the host cells. Serum samples are tested for VNA by measuring their ability to inhibit the infection of FeLV on monolayer cell cultures. Infection of the monolayer can be measured by induction of foci, IFA staining, or by FeLV-p27 expression by ELISA.

Antibodies to FeLV can also be tested by an ELISA procedure that is somewhat different from the ELISA antigen detection test described earlier. Purified FeLV is coated to the surface of test-plate wells. The serum to be tested is added for a certain time until antibodies bind to the FeLV antigens. After unbound antibodies are removed in a washing step, an immunoglobulin-enzyme conjugate is added that specifically binds to the immobilized cat antibody. After an additional washing, substrate solution can be added. The development of a colored reaction product indicates that anti-FeLV antibodies are present in the cat's serum. It is important to note that antibodies detected by this ELISA procedure are not necessarily virus-neutralizing (Lutz et al., 1980a).

Antibodies to FOCMA are found in the serum of many cats that have had contact with FeLV. These antibodies are detected with an IFA procedure using living FL74 cells, a cat lymphoma cell producing FeLV of the subtypes A, B, and C. Detection of fluorescing cell membranes or patches on the membrane are indicative of FOCMA-specific antibodies. The nature of FOCMA was investigated for many years. It is now clear that a wide variety of different antigens present on the FL74 cell membrane contribute to FOCMA. The most important of these antigens is a protein that is very similar or identical to FeLV-gp70 of subtype C FeLV (VedBrat et al., 1983). High titers of antibodies specific for FOCMA, however, may protect cats against the development of lymphosarcomas (Essex et al., 1971). This protection is not complete and does not extend to other FeLV-related diseases.

INTERPRETATION OF FeLV TEST RESULTS

To understand FeLV test results, much may be learned from studying the experimental disease. When the course of the infection was studied by using ELISA and IFA for the detection of FeLV-p27 in the serum and gsa in leukocytes and when antibodies to FeLV and FOCMA were measured, it was found that the course of infection could be classified into four categories (Lutz et al., 1983b).

Cats in category 1 developed a persistent viremia that was characterized by positive ELISA and IFA test results. Viremia started several weeks after exposure and lasted for months to years. Usually, the ELISA was positive 1 to 2 weeks before gsa was detected in the leukocytes and platelets by IFA. Very low antibody titers to FeLV were detected and FOCMA antibodies were either low or not demonstrable.

Category 2 was characterized by a transient

viremia that lasted between 2 and 8 weeks. The ELISA was positive 1 to 2 weeks before the IFA in most animals and remained positive for a week or more after the IFA test became negative. After the transient viremia, high titers of antibody to FeLV and FOCMA were found.

In category 3, ELISA and IFA were never positive. From the fact that high antibody titers to FeLV and FOCMA were detected, it was concluded that these animals became immune to the virus without ever going through a viremic stage.

Category 4 was characterized by persistent antigenemia as detected by ELISA. The IFA, however, was never positive or was positive for only 1 or 2 weeks. In several cats in this category high antibody titers to FeLV and FOCMA were detected. In some of these animals virus isolation was attempted and infectious FeLV was found in several organs, including the salivary gland and urinary bladder. From these observations it was concluded that cats belonging to category 4 were silent shedders of FeLV if tested only by the IFA procedure. Fortunately, only about 5 per cent of infected cats end up in this category. Although not every cat belonging to category 4 may shed amounts of FeLV as large as those shed by IFA-positive cats, prudence suggests that every ELISA-positive cat be considered a health hazard to other cats.

How can these data help in the interpretation of FeLV test results in individual cats? A cat with a negative ELISA can be considered free of FeLV. If the cat is sick with FeLV-related symptoms such as anemia, leukopenia, secondary infections, or tumors, a positive ELISA result should not pose a problem for interpretation. An asymptomatic cat with a positive ELISA result may either be persistently viremic, transiently viremic, or belonging to category 4. In this case, the cat should be isolated from other cats and retested after 12 to 16 weeks. If the cat then shows a negative test, it was transiently viremic at the first test. The animal may now be considered recovered from the infection and does not pose a health hazard to other cats. If the cat remains ELISA-positive at the second test, it may be persistently viremic or belong to category 4.

A positive IFA result in most cases is indicative of persistent viremia. The probability that a transient viremia may be detected by IFA is relatively small because FeLV antigen–carrying leukocytes and platelets only appear for a few days, if at all, in the blood. A negative IFA result indicates that the cat is not viremic in the leukocytes and platelets. A negative IFA test does not exclude an occasional transient infection or a cat in category 4.

It is important to note that some cats that have been exposed to FeLV and overcome viremia (category 2 and 3) may remain latently infected for months or possibly years (Rojko et al., 1982; Madewell et al., 1983; Pedersen et al., 1984). This latent infection is not detected by ELISA, IFA, or virus isolation from blood. It is diagnosed in research laboratories only by culturing bone marrow cells *in vitro* for many weeks and monitoring the culture fluids for virus elaboration. It is possible to reactivate the infection in some cats within the first few months after recovery by injecting them with corticosteroids (Pedersen et al., 1984; Rojko et al., 1982).

COMPARISON OF ELISA AND IFA PROCEDURES

There is some difference of opinion on the relative accuracy of ELISA and IFA test procedures. When both tests are performed accurately, the correlation between them is about 95 per cent (Lutz et al., 1980b). The 5 per cent difference is made up largely of cats in categories 3 or 4 that are detected only by ELISA. The advantages of the ELISA are its greater sensitivity and the ease with which it can be conducted. It also lends itself to in-house use. A disadvantage of the procedure is that false positives can result when the test is improperly run. Most false positives are associated with improper or too hasty washing of the reaction wells at the end of the incubation steps, and with the use of whole blood or badly hemolyzed serum. The latter type of samples tend to be more difficult to wash from the wells and are more likely, therefore, to be falsely positive under improper washing conditions. The IFA procedure, if properly run, does not yield false positives. It does, however, yield a small number of false negatives (cats in categories 2 or 4, or cats with low leukocyte and platelet numbers). Overall, both procedures will yield comparable results. It is important that veterinarians using these procedures utilize laboratories that are well qualified to run them. In the case of in-house ELISA testing, care should be taken to follow test instructions, carefully wash out wells, and avoid whenever possible the use of whole blood or badly hemolyzed serum (regardless of test-kit instructions).

In conclusion, a positive result by any test (ELISA, IFA, or virus isolation) is indicative of FeLV infection. A positive test, however, does not allow prediction of the outcome of the infection and does not diagnose the type of FeLV-related disease from which the cat is suffering.

References and Supplemental Reading

Essex, M., Klein, G., Snyder, S., and Hanold, J. B.: Correlation between humoral antibody and regression of tumors induced by feline sarcoma virus. Nature 233:195, 1971.

Hardy, W. D., Jr., Hirshaut, Y., and Hess, P.: Detection of the feline leukemia virus and other mammalian oncornaviruses by immunofluorescence. Bibl. Haematol. 39:778, 1973.

Hardy, W. D., Jr., Hess, P. W., MacEwen, E. G., et al.: Biology of feline leukemia virus in the natural environment. Cancer Res. 36:582, 1976.

Jarrett, O., Golder, M. C., and Weijer, K.: A comparison of three methods of feline leukaemia virus diagnosis. Vet. Rec. 110:325, 1982.

Lutz, H., Pedersen, N. C., Higgins, J., et al.: Humoral immune reactivity to feline leukemia virus and associated antigens in cats naturally infected with feline leukemia virus. Cancer Res. 40:3642, 1980a.

Lutz, H., Pedersen, N. C., Harris, C. W., et al.: Detection of feline leukemia virus infection. Feline Pract. 10:13, 1980b.

Lutz, H., Pedersen, N. C., Durbin, R., et al.: Monoclonal antibodies to three epitopic regions of feline leukemia virus p27 and their use in enzyme-linked immunosorbent assay of p27. J. Immunol. Methods 56:208, 1983a.

Lutz, H., Pedersen, N. C., and Theilen, G. H.: The course of feline leukemia virus infection and its detection by ELISA and monoclonal antibodies. Am. J. Vet. Res. 44:2054, 1983b.

Madewell, B. R., and Jarrett, O.: Recovery of feline leukaemia virus from non-viraemic cats. Vet. Rec. 112:339, 1983.

Pedersen, N. C., Johnson, L., and Theilen, G. H.: Biological behavior of tumors and associated retroviremia in cats inoculated with Snyder-Theilen fibrosarcoma virus and the phenomenon of tumor recurrence after primary regression. Infect. Immun. 43:631, 1984.

Rojko, J. L., Hoover, E. A., Mathes, L. E., et al.: Pathogenesis of experimental feline leukemia virus infection. J. Natl. Cancer Inst. 63:759, 1979.

Rojko, J. L., Hoover, E. A., Quackenbush, S. L., et al.: Reactivation of latent feline leukemia virus infection. Nature 298:385, 1982.

VedBrat, S., Rasheed, S., Lutz, H., et al.: Feline oncornavirus-associated cell membrane antigen: A viral and not a cellularly coded transformation-specific antigen of cat lymphomas. Virology 124:445, 1983.

ONCOLOGIC EMERGENCIES

URS GIGER, Dr. med. vet.,
Philadelphia, Pennsylvania

and N. T. GORMAN, B.V.Sc.
Cambridge, England

It is common for cancer patients to present as emergency cases, and since the management of cancer in small animals has improved in recent years, the early detection and appropriate management of these oncologic emergencies is of increasing importance. The aim of this review is to define the common oncologic emergencies and their treatment.

Oncologic emergencies can be conveniently classified into three groups according to the underlying pathophysiologic mechanisms: (1) *local tumor invasion* of vital organs resulting in either mechanical compression, obstruction, or organ destruction; (2) *systemic effects of the tumor* such as hematologic, metabolic, and endocrine disturbances; and (3) complications of *cancer therapy* including chemotherapy, surgery, and radiation therapy. A classification of oncologic emergencies according to the end organ involved has previously been described (Giger and Gorman, 1984a, b, and c).

Table 1 outlines the *clinical approach* to oncologic emergencies. The precise clinical manifestations vary according to which end organ or organs the tumor invades and the pathophysiologic mechanisms involved. Some tumors cause acute complications with very specific clinical signs (e.g., local tumor invasion that obstructs the airway or compresses the spinal cord). In contrast, there are many tumors that cause acute complications with nonspecific clinical signs such as lethargy, dehydration, and anorexia. These signal the need for emergency laboratory tests to identify certain life-threatening systemic problems that may be associated with the tumor. In emergency cases in which there is a previously diagnosed tumor, it is essential to assess whether the acute problems are a result of the

Table 1. *Clinical Approach to Oncologic Emergencies*

1. Identify emergency problem or problems
   - History of previously diagnosed cancer and therapy
   - Chemotherapy protocol currently used
   - Clinical signs (dehydration, hemorrhage, effusion, infection, neurologic abnormalities)
   - Emergency laboratory tests (blood and urine analyses, electrocardiography, radiography)
2. Provide immediate support and monitor patient
   - Use general intensive care protocols
   - Apply recommendations outlined in this article
3. Collect baseline data and samples for tumor diagnosis
   - Biopsy, touch preparation, or fine-needle aspirate of possible tumor tissue for histopathologic or cytologic examinations
   - Routine blood, urine, and radiographic tests
   - Bacterial culture of urine, exudate, or blood if infection is suspected
4. Define prognosis with and without cancer treatment
   - Determine expected life span and quality of life
   - Estimate costs for cancer therapy

Modified from Giger and Gorman: Comp. Cont. Ed. Pract. Vet. 6:689, 805, 873, 1984a.

tumor itself, the cancer therapy, or a concurrent non-oncologic disease process.

LOCAL TUMOR INVASION OF VITAL ORGANS

The local growth of a tumor and the inflammatory response and hemorrhage frequently associated with it can mechanically obstruct and compress vital organs or, in extreme cases, can destroy organs. This can lead to acute and life-threatening complications, even though the underlying neoplastic disease process is chronic in nature. These oncologic emergencies can be divided into neurologic, cardiopulmonary, gastrointestinal, and urologic complications, depending on which organ is invaded or affected (Table 2).

Neurologic Complications

INCREASED INTRACRANIAL PRESSURE AND BRAIN HERNIATION. In small animals, primary brain tumors occur more often than metastatic brain tumors. The most frequent canine brain tumors are meningiomas, gliomas, undifferentiated sarcomas, pituitary adenomas, and plexus papillomas. In contrast, the most commonly reported feline brain tumors are meningiomas and lymphomas. Brain tumors cause focal irritation and destruction of neural tissue that can lead to local cranial nerve deficits and focal seizures. The intracranial tumor mass and associated inflammation, edema, hemorrhage, and obstruction of cerebrospinal fluid pathways increases intracranial pressure, resulting in behavioral changes, dementia, and generalized seizures. A final sequela is often brain herniation through the foramen magnum or under the falx cerebri or the bony tentorium cerebelli. This causes progressive neural dysfunction, resulting in tetraplegia, coma, apnea, and death.

Table 2. *Acute Complications Due to Local Tumor Invasion*

Neurologic	Increased intracranial pressure and brain herniation Spinal cord compression and invasion
Cardiopulmonary	Upper airway obstruction Superior vena cava syndrome Pleural effusion Pericardial effusion and cardiac tamponade
Gastroenterologic	Gastrointestinal obstruction Gastrointestinal perforation Intra-abdominal hemorrhage Intraluminal gastrointestinal hemorrhage
Urologic	Postrenal obstruction with azotemia Hematuria

Clinically localizing a tumor mass in the brain is difficult. Computerized tomography is the most accurate method; however, neurologic examinations, electroencephalographic tracings, and cerebrospinal fluid analyses and pressure measurements are helpful in some cases. The collection of cerebrospinal fluid can, however, cause lethal brain herniation after the sudden lowering of intracranial pressure. It is important to note that symmetrical and generalized neurologic clinical signs are frequently associated with the systemic effects of cancer, such as hypoglycemia and thrombocytopenia.

The prognosis for animals with brain tumors is generally poor, although surgical removal of some tumors (such as meningiomas) has been successful, particularly in the cat. Palliative measurements include administrating intravenous anticonvulsive agents to control the seizures, intravenous dexamethasone to decrease edema and inflammation, and, in the case of brain herniation, slow intravenous infusion of mannitol.

SPINAL CORD COMPRESSION. Extradural spinal cord compression resulting from vertebral body tumors (multiple myeloma, osteosarcoma) or metastases from mammary, prostate, pulmonary, and renal carcinomas are common in the dog. Epidural lymphomas occur frequently in the cat; however, intramedullary and intradural spinal tumors (meningioma and neurofibroma) are relatively rare in small animals. The thoracolumbar area is the most common site of compression and invasion.

The spinal cord lesion is localized by neurologic examination, radiography, and myelography. Prognosis is from guarded to poor, depending upon the degree of loss in spinal cord functioning (i.e., whether there is paresis or paralysis) and the duration of dysfunction. In any case, intravenous dexamethasone is administered immediately to decrease the edema and inflammation associated with the tumor. The clinician may also consider surgical decompression, removal of the tumor mass, or chemotherapy in treatment of lymphoma or multiple myeloma.

Cardiopulmonary Emergencies

UPPER AIRWAY OBSTRUCTION. Squamous cell carcinoma of the larynx and lymphoma of the tonsils often cause intraluminal airway obstruction. Extraluminal masses, such as lymphomas of the mandibular lymph nodes and mediastinum and tumors of the thyroid gland or thymus, can compress the upper airways and result in respiratory distress. In addition, the tumor-associated inflammatory reaction, which includes edema, hemorrhage, and accumulation of secretions and debris, can further occlude the airway. Simple palpation of laryngeal masses may increase the edema and induce laryngeal spasms. Manipulation of masses associated with the trachea can suddenly cause tracheal collapse and obstructive airway disease. Clinical signs include dyspnea, stridor, and cyanosis. In a severely dyspneic animal with a high tracheal obstruction, the tumor may be surgically debulked or a low tracheostomy tube inserted prior to definitive treatment with surgery, radiotherapy, or chemotherapy alone or in combination. Chemotherapy for lymphoma can reduce the size of the tumor within days.

SUPERIOR VENA CAVA SYNDROME. The superior vena cava syndrome occurs rarely in small animals and is associated with tumors in the cranial thorax that obstruct venous return from the head, neck, and forelimbs. The superior vena cava is vulnerable to compression by bronchogenic carcinoma, lymphoma, thymoma, and mediastinal metastases. Clinical signs include cervicofacial and forelimb edema, venous distention, and dyspnea. Radiotherapy for prompt reduction of the tumor mass is the preferred treatment in humans and, if available, should be used in animals. Chemotherapy can be most helpful in responsive tumors, such as lymphoma.

PLEURAL EFFUSION. Mediastinal tumors (particularly lymphoma), mesotheliomas, and metastatic carcinomas with implants on the pleural surface can cause malignant pleural effusions. Pleural effusion can also develop subsequent to the tumor's obstruction or disruption of lymphatic or venous drainage. Diagnostic studies of the pleural fluid include measurements of protein and triglyceride concentrations, bacterial culture, differential cell count, and cytologic tests. It is preferable to remove large amounts of fluids with a uni- or bilateral chest tube that allows effective drainage for several days.

PERICARDIAL EFFUSION AND CARDIAC TAMPONADE. Hemangiosarcoma of the right atrium, heart base tumors, lymphoma, and metastases to the heart may result in malignant or acute hemorrhagic (cardiac tamponade) pericardial effusions. Clinical features of cardiac tamponade include dyspnea, pale mucous membranes, hypotension, tachycardia, venous distention, paradoxical pulse, and distant heart sounds (low voltage and electrical alternans on ECG). Thoracic radiographs typically show a global heart, but echocardiography is the most reliable diagnostic technique and is of great help in guiding a needle into the effusion. Pericardiocentesis can temporarily relieve the clinical signs; however, hemorrhagic effusions portend a grave prognosis.

Gastrointestinal Emergencies

GASTROINTESTINAL OBSTRUCTION OR PERFORATION. Bowel obstruction occurs with intraluminal intestinal tumors or with compression or constrictive adhesions from intra-abdominal masses. The common clinical signs are vomiting and the existence of an abdominal mass. Plain and contrast radiography will usually show an obstructive bowel pattern and may delineate the abdominal mass. Gastrointestinal perforation can ensue from ulcerative gastric or intestinal tumors. Diagnostic features of a perforation include abdominal pain, pneumoperitoneum, and septic peritonitis. An emergency laparotomy is required to relieve the obstruction or remove the perforated bowel. In addition, the frequently associated metabolic imbalances must be corrected.

INTRA-ABDOMINAL HEMORRHAGE. Splenic and hepatic hemangioma and hemangiosarcoma are the most common tumors that cause extraluminal bleeding. Acute intra-abdominal hemorrhage leads to abdominal distention, dyspnea, hypovolemia, and anemia. A splenic or hepatic mass can often be palpated, and a peritoneal tap will demonstrate free blood. These patients require blood transfusion and exploratory laparotomy with splenectomy or partial hepatectomy to remove the tumor mass.

INTRALUMINAL GASTROINTESTINAL HEMORRHAGE. Acute blood loss from gastrointestinal ulcers can occur with intestinal lymphoma and leiomyosarcomas, gastric and colonic carcinomas, and metastatic tumors. Gastric ulcers may also result from mast cell tumors that release histamine and from gastrin-secreting pancreatic tumors. Hematemesis and melena are characteristic of upper gastrointestinal bleeding. In an effort to reduce hemorrhage from gastroduodenal ulcers, the clinician may administer antacids and cimetidine. Hematochezia is more typical of colonic bleeding but may come from the upper tract if there is brisk blood loss. Endoscopy and contrast radiography may aid in localizing the gastrointestinal ulcer, but surgery is usually needed for diagnosis and treatment. In cases of extreme blood loss, whole blood transfusions might be necessary.

Urologic Emergencies

POSTRENAL OBSTRUCTION WITH AZOTEMIA. Postrenal azotemia can result from either bilateral compression of the ureters, caused by any advanced pelvic or retroperitoneal tumor (e.g., lymphoma), or an outlet obstruction of the bladder and urethra, caused by papillomatous bladder tumors, urethral tumors, or prostatic carcinomas. In addition, tumor-associated urinary tract infections may eventually lead to urinary calculus formation and secondary obstruction. Postrenal obstructions cause abdominal pain, stranguria, ruptured bladder, and acute renal failure with anuria. Diagnostic studies include urinary catheterization, abdominal and rectal palpation, and abdominal radiography and a cystogram. Although urethral catheterization provides immediate relief in most cases of distal obstruction, surgical intervention may be indicated. Furthermore, appropriate fluid therapy is necessary to restore or preserve renal function.

HEMATURIA. Massive hematuria can occur with renal tumors, transitional cell carcinoma of the bladder, and prostatic tumors. Hypovolemia as well as acute blood loss may ensue and necessitate blood or plasma transfusions as well as surgical corrections. Hematuria in cancer patients treated with cyclophosphamide is due to drug-induced hemorrhagic cystitis.

Table 4. *Various Anemias Associated with Neoplasia*

Blood loss anemia (vascular destruction, thrombocytopenia, DIC)
Myelophthisic anemia (hematogenous tumors and metastatic carcinomas)
Anemia of chronic inflammatory disease
Microangiopathic anemia (e.g., hemangiosarcoma)
Hypersplenism with anemia (rare)
Immune-mediated anemia (hematogenous malignancies)
Dyserythropoietic and megalobastic anemia
Feline leukemia virus–related anemia (common)
Blood parasite–associated anemia (*Haemobartonella, Babesia, Ehrlichia*)

SYSTEMIC EFFECTS OF TUMORS

Oncologic emergencies arising from the systemic effects of cancer are summarized in Table 3. The decreased or increased production of either blood cells or serum proteins results in a number of hematologic complications. Metabolic and endocrine derangements are frequently observed with tumors arising from endocrine glands; however, various nonendocrine tumors also produce and release active substances ("ectopic hormones") into the circulation that lead to serious metabolic disturbances. The systemic effects of these "ectopic hormones" are known as paraneoplastic syndromes. The clinical signs of these disturbances are generally nonspecific; therefore, laboratory tests are often needed to reach a diagnosis.

Hematologic Emergencies

LEUKOPENIA AND INFECTION. Leukopenia, including neutropenia and lymphopenia, results from invasion of the bone marrow by the tumor (myelophthisis) and decreased survival of circulating white blood cells. However, leukopenia is most commonly secondary to the myelosuppressive effect of chemotherapeutic agents. The major consequence of leukopenia is the enhanced risk of severe infection. The incidence of infection is inversely related to the number of circulating granulocytes and also correlates with the duration of granulocytopenia. This means that risk for infection increases when the granulocyte count drops below 3000/μl for a prolonged time. Other contributing factors include (1) skin and mucous membrane wounds, (2) indwelling catheters, (3) immunosuppression, (4) tumor necrosis, and (5) malnutrition.

Table 3. *Emergencies Associated with the Systemic Effects of Tumors*

Hematologic Complications	
Leukopenia and infection	
Anemia	
Thrombocytopenia	
Disseminated intravascular coagulation	
Hyperviscosity:	Monoclonal gammopathy
	Erythrocytosis
	Polycythemia vera
	Leukocytosis
Metabolic and Endocrine Complications	
Dehydration	
Hypercalcemia	
Hypoglycemia	
Hyperthyroidism	
Hyponatremia	
Hypergastrinemia	
Hyperhistaminemia	

Most primary infections are endogenous in origin and more than half of them are caused by gram-negative bacteria, such as *Escherichia coli, Pseudomonas aeruginosa*, and *Klebsiella pneumonia. Staphylococcus aureus, Bacteroides* spp., fungal (*Candida* spp.), and polymicrobial infections are also common.

The diagnosis of infection can be difficult. The lack of granulocytes means that the common clinical signs of a localized infection may be absent. The most consistent sign of infection is *fever* unrelated to either a blood transfusion or drug reaction. Gram-negative bacteria can also precipitate endotoxemic shock. The clinician should obtain samples of blood, urine, and tissue from any obvious site of infection for appropriate culture.

Leukopenic cancer patients with infection require immediate treatment. Initially, a broad-spectrum antibiotic that is bactericidal rather than bacteriostatic should be administered intravenously. Typically, cephalosporin or ampicillin in combination with gentamicin are used. Antibiotic therapy is adjusted according to drug susceptibility and continued for at least a week or until 4 days after the fever and leukopenia are brought under control.

ANEMIA. Anemia in cancer patients is usually normocytic and normochromic, but megaloblastic and microcytic anemias can occur. The different types of anemia associated with neoplasia are summarized in Table 4. Diagnostic tests to define the cause for the anemia, its form, and its severity include a complete blood cell count, reticulocyte and platelet counts, clotting profile, and blood smears for detection of poikilocytosis and blood parasites. A bone marrow aspirate or core biopsy is warranted in nonregenerative anemias, and whenever hemolysis is suspected, a Coombs' test is indicated. The emergency treatment includes a transfusion of cross-matched and typed blood, surgical control of overt hemorrhage, and administration of immunosuppressive drugs to inhibit erythrocyte destruction.

THROMBOCYTOPENIA. Thrombocytopenia can arise either from decreased production or increased consumption of platelets. Platelet production is often decreased in hemopoietic neoplasms because of infiltration of the bone marrow. In addition, platelet production can be affected by many chemotherapeutic agents that directly affect the megakaryocytes. An increase in platelet consumption may be immunologically mediated or a result of disseminated intravascular coagulation (see below).

Laboratory tests for evaluation of thrombocytopenia include measurement of platelet factor 3 levels and a bone marrow aspirate or core to estimate the number of megakaryocytes and to detect the existence of any antibody against megakaryocytes and platelets. Administration of fresh platelet concentrates or fresh whole blood are warranted if an animal is actively bleeding from severe thrombocytopenia. One unit of fresh blood increases the platelet count above the critical level of 20,000/μl for a few days in a mid-sized dog. Corticosteroids and other immunosuppressive drugs are indicated in immune-mediated thrombocytopenia.

DISSEMINATED INTRAVASCULAR COAGULATION (DIC). DIC in cancer patients may be initiated by (1) the tumor's release of thromboplastic substances into the blood stream; (2) damage to small vessels within the tumor, exposing subendothelial collagen; (3) the production by the tumor of proteolytic enzymes; and (4) bacterial sepsis. Laboratory data and clinical findings vary, reflecting the dynamic balance between hypercoagulation and fibrinolysis. However, fibrin split products should be present.

The hypercoagulable form of DIC is associated with arterial thromboemboli and is seen with many solid tumors; it should be treated with subcutaneous heparin. The hemorrhagic form of DIC is most often seen with hematogenous tumors, hemangiosarcoma, and inflammatory mammary tumors. Here, the prognosis is usually very poor. Surgical control of bleeding and replacement of clotting factors and platelets can sometimes be helpful.

HYPERVISCOSITY. An enhanced resistance of blood flow is caused by an increase in blood elements. Acute complications to hyperviscosity include thromboembolism and hemorrhagic complications as well as neurologic and ocular disorders. Monoclonal gammopathy accompanies multiple myeloma, Waldenström's macroglobulinemia, and, occasionally, lymphocytic leukemia. The viscosity of serum depends on both the concentration and structure (polymerization) of the individual paraprotein (IgM, IgG, IgA).

Erythrocytosis (PCV > 60 per cent) associated with renal and liver tumors may result from tumor cells producing erythropoietin or erythropoietin-stimulating factor. The erythrocytosis may also result from renal hypoxia that induces erythropoietin activation. Polycythemia vera is a myeloproliferative disorder with panhyperplasia of the bone marrow, extramedullary hematopoiesis, and normal erythropoietin levels. Phlebotomy of 20 to 30 ml blood/kg with appropriate fluid replacement (or plasmapheresis in serum hyperviscosity) alleviates the symptoms of hyperviscosity; however, treatment of the underlying neoplastic diseases has to be attempted after emergency care.

Leukocytosis (WBC > 100,000/μl) can be associated with leukemia. Although severely leukemic patients are at risk for death from leukostatic thrombi, some patients with chronic lymphocytic leukemia have counts exceeding 150,000/μl for several months without showing clinical signs. After a bone marrow aspirate has been collected, dexamethasone, hydroxyurea, or doxorubicin (Adriamycin, Adria) should be administered to decrease the number of circulating neoplastic cells.

Metabolic and Endocrine Emergencies

DEHYDRATION. Volume depletion frequently occurs in cancer patients because of decreased fluid intake, prolonged vomiting and diarrhea, kidney disease, and metabolic complications associated with malignant diseases. Fluid replacement and correction of electrolytes can rapidly improve the patient's condition.

HYPERCALCEMIA. Hypercalcemia (serum calcium > 12.0 gm/dl) is the most common paraneoplastic syndrome and occurs with various tumors. Hematogenous malignancies such as lymphoma and multiple myeloma invade the bone. The lymphokine, osteoclast activating factor (OAF), and prostaglandins may accelerate bone resorption and lead to hypercalcemia. Carcinomas of mammary glands, exocrine pancreas, lungs, and nasal cavities often metastasize to bone and hypercalcemia develops. In older female dogs, hypercalcemia associated with adenocarcinomas derived from apocrine glands of the anal sac is caused by excessive concentration of serum 1,25-dihydroxyvitamin D. Finally, parathyroid gland adenomas or adenocarcinomas produce a primary hyperparathyroidism that can precipitate hypercalcemia.

The gastrointestinal signs of hypercalcemia include anorexia, vomiting, constipation, and pancreatitis. The neuromuscular effects are lethargy, weakness, and coma. Cardiac arrhythmias and renal failure due to nephrocalcinosis are undoubtedly the most serious complications in hypercalcemic patients. Hypercalcemia should be treated immediately with intravenous normal saline to restore vascular volume and increase glomerular calcium excretion. Furosemide can be used in a rehydrated animal to further enhance calciuresis. Corticosteroids are effective in hematogenous malignancies but are unpredictable in other cases.

HYPOGLYCEMIA. A fasting hypoglycemia with concomitant elevated serum insulin levels is diagnostic for pancreatic islet cell tumors (adenocarcinomas). Hypoglycemia also occurs occasionally with extrapancreatic malignancies, such as large abdominal or thoracic tumors, hepatoma, massive hepatic metastases, and even lymphoma. The factors thought to induce hypoglycemia in these patients include (1) impaired hepatic gluconeogenesis; (2) increased glucose utilization by tumor cells; (3) lack of counter regulatory hormones; and (4) production of insulinlike growth factors by tumor tissue.

The clinical signs of hypoglycemia reflect the severity and rapidity of the decline in blood glucose level. Intermittent weakness, muscle tremor, behavioral changes, syncope, seizures, and coma are typically seen. Emergency treatment involves an intravenous bolus of 50 per cent dextrose followed by 5 to 10 per cent dextrose infusion. Some patients may prove unresponsive, owing to advanced nerve damage with edema. They require additional therapy as outlined under neurologic complications.

HYPERTHYROIDISM. Functional thyroid gland adenomas commonly occur in older cats but are rarely seen in dogs. Hyperthyroid cats typically have a history of hyperactivity, weight loss, polyphagia, and increased defecation and urination. Some animals may present in an advanced hypermetabolic state, which causes hyperthermia, tachypnea, tachyarrhythmia, and signs of congestive heart failure (including pulmonary edema, pleural effusion, and shock). This fulminant presentation is called thyrotoxic storm in humans. Unilateral or bilateral thyroid gland enlargement, elevated serum T3/T4 levels, or the presence of both are diagnostic.

Initial treatment involves administration of propranolol (to counter the cardiac effects of excessive thyroid hormone) and prednisone, propylthiouracil, and sodium iodine to suppress further release and production of thyroid hormones. In certain cases, thoracocentesis, diuretics, and oxygen may be required.

HYPONATREMIA. The rare syndrome of inappropriate antidiuretic hormone secretion occurs with small cell carcinoma of the lung and some other tumors. These patients have hyponatremia with hypo-osmolality and an expanded extracellular fluid volume. This causes edema in the absence of a maximally diluted urine. Hyponatremia is corrected by restricting fluid intake. Occasionally, administration of furosemide, hypertonic saline, and glucocorticosteroids is needed.

HYPERGASTRINEMIA AND HYPERHISTAMINEMIA. The secretion of gastrin by pancreatic tumors, known as Zollinger-Ellison syndrome, and the release of histamine by mast cell tumor degranulation promote gastric acid secretion and can lead to gastroduodenal ulcers. Vomiting, acute intraluminal bleeding, and gastric perforations can all ensue. Cimetidine blocks the histamine H_2 receptors and thereby reduces the secretion of gastric acid and the related complications. In addition, mast cell degranulation may precipitate an anaphylactoid reaction and shock that requires treatment with fluids, corticosteroids, and antihistamines.

COMPLICATIONS RELATED TO CANCER THERAPY

Oncologic emergencies may be caused or aggravated by various modalities of cancer treatment. Surgical methods can lead to acute complications, as shown in Table 5. Radiotherapy may result in extensive tissue necrosis and myelosuppression, thereby predisposing a cancer patient to infection. Chemotherapy-related complications, however, are undoubtedly the most common.

Chemotherapy-Related Emergencies

Because cancer chemotherapy is not directed solely against neoplastic cells and the drugs are usually given at the highest dose a patient can tolerate, substantial host toxicity may result. The common serious complications associated with chemotherapy in small animals are summarized in Table 6. The toxicity from drugs with extremely short half-lives is usually dose-related, predictable, and reversible. The toxicity of other agents is a function of the total cumulative dose; these complications are less predictable and are usually irreversible.

The complications of chemotherapy can also be

Table 5. *Surgery-Related Emergencies in Cancer Patients*

Bleeding from surgical site due to underlying abnormality in hemostasis
Suture dehiscence and poor wound healing caused by tumor infiltration or chemotherapy
Infections ensuing disruption of mechanical barriers
Mast cell degranulation after tumor debulking
Hypocalcemia resulting from (inadvertent) removal of or damage to parathyroid gland
Adrenal insufficiency as a consequence of adrenalectomy or hypophysectomy

Table 6. Chemotherapy-Related Emergencies

Chemotherapeutic Agent (Trade Name)	Allergic Reaction	Myelosuppression	Gastroenteric Toxicity	Other Common Side Effects and Comments
L-Asparaginase	Common	Occasional	Common	Pancreatitis, hepatotoxicity
Bleomycin	Common	—	—	Pulmonary fibrosis
Bulsulfan	—	—	—	Pulmonary fibrosis
Chlorambucil	—	Occasional	Occasional	—
Cisplatin	Occasional	Occasional	Common	Nephropathy
Corticosteroid	—	—	Common	Cushing's syndrome
Cyclophosphamide	Occasional	Common	Occasional	Hemorrhagic cystitis (dog), secondary bladder tumor
Cytarabine	Occasional	Occasional	—	—
Dacarbazine (DTIC)	—	—	Common	—
Doxorubicin	Common	Common	Occasional	Cardiotoxicity, phlebitis
5-Fluorouracil	—	—	Common	Neuropathy, stomatitis
Hydroxyurea	—	Occasional	—	Megaloblastic anemia
Melphalan	Occasional	Occasional	—	—
Mercaptopurine	—	Common	—	Nephropathy
Methotrexate	Occasional	Common	Common	Nephro-, hepato-, neuropathy
Mitotane (*o,p′*-DDD)	—	—	Common	Adrenal insufficiency, Nelson's syndrome
Nitrogen mustard	Common (man)	—	—	(Protect yourself adequately)
Propylthiouracil	Common (cat)	—	Occasional	Coombs'-positive anemia, thrombocytopenia
Streptozocin	—	—	Common	Nephropathy
Vinblastine	—	Occasional	Common	Phlebitis, neuropathy (peripheral)
Vincristine	Occasional	Occasional	Common	Phlebitis, neuropathy (peripheral)

classified according to how long after administration of the drug they occur.

1. *Immediate side effects* begin within the first day after administration and include anorexia, vomiting, phlebitis, skin rash, drug fever, and anaphylaxis.

2. *Early side effects* begin within days to weeks and include leukopenia, thrombocytopenia, anemia, renal failure, stomatitis, and diarrhea.

3. *Delayed effects*, such as cardiomyopathy induced by doxorubicin, pulmonary fibrosis seen with bleomycin, and secondary bladder tumor (a complication of cyclophosphamide), occur within weeks to months.

There is an increased morbidity when chemotherapeutic agents are used in (1) animals with poor bone marrow function and reserve, (2) severely emaciated patients (cancer cachexia), and (3) animals with underlying infection and other concomitant medical problems. The early detection of serious complications depends upon the serial assessment of minimal data (physical examination, complete blood cell and platelet count, serum creatinine content, and urinalysis). There are no known antidotes for the currently used chemotherapeutic agents; however, in most situations, discontinuation of the offending drug and immediate symptomatic medical care will control the problems.

MYELOSUPPRESSION. Most chemotherapeutic agents have acute, dose-related, and self-limiting effects on the bone marrow; however, a few drugs (BCNU, estrogens) cause prolonged myelosuppression. The myelosuppressive effect of drugs used in combination is usually noncumulative, presumably because they act on the same dividing cell population while the resting stem cells are protected. Clinically, bone marrow failure usually occurs 5 to 10 days after drug administration. It is characterized by leukopenia, thrombocytopenia, and, later, anemia alone or in combination with the associated bone marrow hypoplasia. Drug-induced myelosuppression has been classified according to the peripheral blood picture into (1) *grade 1 toxicity*, with 3000 to 4000 WBC/μl and 80 to 120,000 platelets/μl, and (2) *grade 2 toxicity*, with a WBC and platelet count of less than 3000/μl and 80,000/μl, respectively. With grade 2 toxicity, myelosuppressive drugs have to be discontinued, at least until a grade 1 toxicity is reached. With a grade 1 toxicity, the drug dose has to be reduced by at least 50 per cent. The management of cytopenias has been discussed previously in the section on hematologic emergencies.

ANOREXIA AND VOMITING. Chemotherapy-induced anorexia and vomiting are usually temporary phenomena lasting a few hours; when dehydration and metabolic disturbances ensue, the clinician must institute supportive care with intravenous fluids, electrolytes, and antiemetics. Antiemetics, such as subcutaneous prochlorperazine, lingual haloperidol, and parenteral metaclopramide are effective in controlling drug-induced vomiting.

PHLEBITIS. Vinca alkaloids, vincristine and vinblastine, and doxorubicin hydrochloride are commonly used vasosclerotic chemotherapeutic agents. In the case of an accidental, perivascular injection, the injection site should be infiltrated immediately with sterile saline and dexamethasone. Hot compresses and dimethylsulfoxide can also be applied topically to prevent a devastating necrotizing phlebitis.

CARDIOTOXICITY. Doxorubicin hydrochloride (Adriamycin) can cause immediate, early, and delayed effects on the heart. Nonspecific, acute cardiac arrhythmias can occur during intravenous injection or within two weeks after infusion. Arrhythmias develop more often in patients with an underlying heart disease and are usually transient; however, sudden deaths from severe arrhythmias have been reported. The delayed drug reaction that depends on the cumulative dose of doxorubicin can eventually trigger the development of cardiomyopathy. This serious toxicity usually occurs after 250 mg/m^2 have been given to a patient. It appears irreversible and unresponsive to conventional cardiac treatment.

HEMORRHAGIC CYSTITIS. Metabolites of cyclophosphamide commonly induce a hemorrhagic cystitis in the dog. This urologic complication can occur at any time after administration of cyclophosphamide, but it is most often seen after prolonged oral dosage or high intravenous drug doses. Cyclophosphamide should be discontinued after clinical signs become obvious (micro- or macroscopic hematuria). Severe hemorrhagic cystitis can lead to massive blood loss and warrant lavage of the bladder with cold saline solution, the use of antispasmotics, and blood transfusions. The previously advocated lavage with formalin, however, is generally restricted for severe, refractory cases, because it may precipitate bladder rupture and fatal systemic toxicity.

TUMOR LYSIS SYNDROME. Effective chemotherapy of malignancies may result in the massive release into the blood of potassium, phosphate, and other breakdown products of dying tumor cells. In addition, hypocalcemia may occur with hyperphosphatemia. Cardiac arrhythmias from hyperkalemia and hypocalcemia can be life-threatening. The tumor lysis syndrome occurs with lymphoproliferative diseases and develops within hours to a few days of treatment for the underlying neoplasm. Vigorous intravenous hydration with half-normal saline is required. Calcium gluconate is administered by very slow intravenous injection in order to control the hypocalcemia- and hyperkalemia-related arrhythmias.

In summary, oncologic emergencies are common in small animals and can be caused by local and systemic effects of the tumor as well as by cancer therapy. Early recognition of the various complications associated with malignancies as well as immediate and appropriate management are important.

References and Supplemental Reading

DeVita, V. T., Hellman, S., and Rosenberg, S. A. (eds.): *Cancer, Principles and Practice of Oncology.* Chapter 42, Oncologic Emergencies, Philadelphia: J. B. Lippincott, 1982, pp. 1582–1627.

Feldman, B. F.: Disseminated intravascular coagulation. Comp. Cont. Ed. Pract. Vet. 3:46, 1981.

Giger, U., and Gorman, N. T.: Oncologic emergencies in small animals. Part I. Chemotherapy-related and hematolgic emergencies. Comp. Cont. Ed. Pract. Vet. 6:689, 1984a.

Giger, U., and Gorman, N. T.: Oncologic emergencies in small animals. Part II. Metabolic and endocrine emergencies. Comp. Cont. Ed. Pract. Vet. 6:805, 1984b.

Giger, U., and Gorman, N. T.: Oncologic emergencies in small animals. Part III. Emergencies related to organ systems. Comp. Cont. Ed. Pract. Vet. 6:873, 1984c.

Klastersky, J., and Staguet, M. D. (eds.): *Medical Complications in Cancer Patients.* New York: Raven Press, 1981.

Madewell, B. R.: Adverse effects of chemotherapy. *In* Kirk, R. W. (ed.): *Current Veterinary Therapy VIII.* Philadelphia: W. B. Saunders, 1983, pp. 419–423.

Perry, M. C., and Yarbro, J. W. (eds.): *Toxicity of Chemotherapy.* New York: Grune & Stratton, 1984.

Portlock, C. S., and Goffinet, D. R. (eds.): *Manual of Clinical Problems in Oncology.* Boston: Little, Brown, 1980.

Theilen, G. H., and Madewell, B. R. (eds.): *Veterinary Cancer Medicine.* Philadelphia: Lea & Febiger, 1979.

Weller, R. E.: Paraneoplastic disorders in companion animals. Comp. Cont. Ed. Pract. Vet. 4:423, 1982.

Yarbro, J. W., and Bernstein, R. S. (eds.): *Oncologic Emergencies.* New York: Grune & Stratton, 1981.

PRECANCER

BRUCE R. MADEWELL, V.M.D.
Davis, California

The natural history of disease, unaffected by treatment, is variable, and it is often difficult to determine when a disease begins or when an animal has or does not have disease. Chronic diseases such as cancer may extend over time through a sequence of stages, and their evolution may be extremely long; factors favoring the development of chronic disease are often present early in life, antedating the appearance of clinical manifestations by many years. Precancer is a consistent antecedent of many invasive neoplasms; clinical and experimental studies have shown that carcinogenesis begins long before it becomes apparent to conventional morphologic observation.

The progression of a neoplastic disease encompasses several stages, namely: (1) the stage of susceptibility, (2) the stage of preclinical disease, and (3) the stage of clinical disease. This categorization is relevant in terms of developing strategies for therapeutic intervention. The stage of susceptibility includes those factors that favor the occurrence of the disease—the so-called risk factors. Risk factors may be either immutable or subject to change. For example, host factors including age, breed, family, or sex may influence risk for neoplastic disease but cannot be changed for a particular individual. Extrinsic or environmental factors, on the other hand, such as dietary habit or sunlight exposure, can often be modified to influence risk. Not all animals possessing a given risk factor will necessarily develop that disease, however, and the absence of risk factors will not always ensure absence of the disease.

At the preclinical stage, there is no overt disease, but the interaction of factors leading to clinical disease have started to occur. The changes are not yet manifest through conventional morphologic observation. During this often long period, precursor lesions are influenced by one or more promotional events specific to particular sites; in the absence of these influences, they may remain static or even regress. Finally, however, at the stage of clinical disease, sufficient end-organ changes have occurred so that there are recognizable signs of disease. For cancer, clinical disease is characterized by a specific histologic type, as well as a site and evidence of spread, i.e., the clinical stage. This categorization of disease stages does not imply, however, that progression to invasive cancer will always occur for any given lesion; an animal fortunate enough to survive into old age possesses numerous neoplastic lesions in the form of benign lesions of the skin, mammary gland, prostate gland, and other organs. There has been little questioning of the meaning of these lesions or their pathogenic relationship to clinical cancer; their clinical diagnostic significance alone has been the subject of study.

The term precancer is used by clinical oncologists to embrace those cellular events recognizable by histopathology, cytopathology, or cytogenetics which range from the beginning of an abnormality and extend to the boundary of invasive cancer. From a molecular viewpoint, however, the criteria for the cancer phenotype may be extended well beyond those observations based on morphologic characteristics. The induction of the aggregate phenotype that is referred to as the malignant cell is an extremely complicated process that includes, in its broadest sense, intracellular change or injury and a process by which the altered cell remains viable and is given the momentum to express the aberrant phenotype in a significant manner.

Numerous examples of morphologic (architectural and nuclear) changes preceding the development of frank malignancy have been recorded in human medicine. Many of these changes have been studied in detail in experimental systems, but few convincing precancers have been described for spontaneous tumors in domestic animals. The intent of the remainder of this article is to list defined precancerous conditions in human medicine and to review those entities that have been addressed in the veterinary literature.

PRECANCEROUS CONDITIONS

Human cervical cancer is antedated by a host of dysplastic changes as well as carcinoma *in situ*. For mammary gland neoplasms, atypical hyperplasias and a group of arbitrarily defined, *in situ* carcinomas may precede mammary cancer. Premalignant lesions of the oral cavity include leukoplakia, erythroplasia, and palatal keratosis. In the lungs, dysplasia of the basal cells of the bronchi and of the Clara or mucus-producing cells may precede proximal and peripheral carcinomas, respectively. Gastric precancerous processes are recognized morphologically as chronic gastritis, intestinal metaplasia, and dysplasia. An adenoma-carcinoma sequence has been identified for large bowel neoplasms, particularly for patients with familial polyposis, and carcinoma *in situ* has been a demonstrated antecedent to urinary bladder cancer in some patients.

Other sites and precancer-cancer associations include esophageal dysplasia and cancer of the esophagus, hepatic adenoma and hepatocellular cancer, pancreatic dysplasia and cancer of the pancreas, endometrial hyperplasia and cancer of the endometrium, dysplasia nevi and malignant melanoma, actinic keratosis and basal cell skin cancer, and preleukemia, or hemopoietic dysplasia.

Preneoplastic conditions that have been recognized morphologically and studied in some detail in companion animals include premalignant changes in the mammary gland, actinic keratosis and squamous cell carcinoma of the skin, and the syndrome of preleukemia. Individual case reports suggest that precancers may precede the development of oral neoplasms, and a transformation of benign papilloma to invasive carcinoma has been described.

Premalignant Changes in the Mammary Gland

Despite the high incidence rate for spontaneous dysplastic and neoplastic mammary lesions in the bitch, the pathogenesis of these diseases remains incompletely characterized. The developmental sequence of mammary neoplasia has been extensively studied and partially characterized in rodents. In rats and mice, local hyperplasias designated as hyperplastic alveolar nodules have been recognized unequivocally as preneoplastic. A myriad of similar atypical nodules categorized as inflammatory or hyperplastic (and, particularly, diffuse epithelial hyperplasias) have been recognized in the canine mammary gland. These lesions are seen more commonly in the caudal mammary glands and may be associated with the relatively high incidence of mammary tumors in the dog. Nonpalpable (1 to 4mm) nodules have been recognized in bitches as young as 2 to 4 years of age, and they may appear after the first or second estrous cycle. The age of onset of palpable, clinically apparent tumors is 6 to 8 years. If there is, indeed, an association between dysplastic lesions of the canine mammary gland and true neoplasms, then the cause or causes of those lesions must also be operative early in development. The finding that dysplastic lesions are often multifocal within a gland (as well as within an animal) supports the concept of multifocal origin of these neoplasms. Recognition of morphologic changes, including duct epithelial proliferation with moderate and marked atypia, and the coexistence of *in situ* carcinoma with invasive cancer supports the concept of a multistage progression for mammary carcinogenesis in the bitch.

Sunlight–Skin Cancer Association

After hemolymphatic neoplasms, tumors of the skin are the second most frequently recognized neoplasms in domestic cats. Although few risk factors have been established for most tumors of domestic animals, lack of pigment on nose, ears, and eyelids and exposure to sunlight are known to increase risk for squamous cell carcinoma in the cat. The importance of sunlight exposure in the genesis of squamous cell carcinoma in domestic cats is emphasized by the fact that there is a 76 per cent average probability for sunshine (sunrise to sunset) in a 12-month period in the central valley of California—a figure common to most of the arid and semiarid regions of the western United States. The annual incidence rate for cutaneous squamous cell carcinoma in white cats in California was estimated at 26.9 cases per 100,000 cats, whereas by contrast, the annual incidence rate for oral carcinomas in white cats was 9.0 cases per 100,000 cats.

The carcinogenic effect of ultraviolet rays in the range of 290 to 320 nm is well established in experimental animals. There are presumed to be genetic influences on carcinogenesis, but whether the differences are a function of morphologic characteristics (such as distribution of keratin or melanin) or related to more subtle influences (e.g., DNA repair or immune response) is unknown.

Direct photosensitivity disorders can be divided into two types: (1) immediate or acute sunburn reactions and (2) delayed or chronic sun damage (senile degeneration, premalignant, and malignant lesions). Both types of disorders are due to direct effects of sunlight on the skin. The damage has been attributed to the UVB spectrum, which penetrates the epidermis and causes detrimental photochemical changes to viable cells, but longer wavelengths (UVA) may augment the effects of UVB exposure.

The principal sunlight-induced premalignant lesion is actinic or solar keratosis (hyperkeratosis arising on exposed skin), and at least in humans, approximately 25 per cent of the individuals with multiple actinic keratoses have been reported to develop squamous cell carcinomas in one or more of the precancerous lesions. Malignancy developing in an actinic keratosis usually presents as a shallow central ulceration covered by a crust with a widely elevated and indurated border. It is generally felt that squamous cell carcinomas arising in sun-damaged skin are less apt to metastasize than those arising in other sites.

Another syndrome of sunlight-associated skin cancer has been recognized in dogs. Tumors develop in lightly pigmented glabrous skin of the flank or ventral abdomen after chronic sunlight exposure and long periods of dermatosis. Although any lightly pigmented breed of dog is at risk, tumors have been recognized most often in beagles, dalmations, whippets, and white bull terriers. Microscopic examination of tissues from affected dogs reveal a progressive development of epithelial hyperplasia through stages of solar keratosis-like lesions to invasive and metastatic squamous cell carcinoma.

Preleukemia

Preleukemic syndromes are a group of acquired bone marrow disorders characterized by progressive impairment in the maturation of hematopoietic cells. The preleukemic syndromes provide a clinical setting for evaluation of the evolution of relatively benign to frankly malignant neoplasms. Other terms used to describe these syndromes include hematopoietic dysplasia, refractory anemia with excess of myeloblasts, subacute myeloid leukemia, and myelodysplastic and dysmyelopoietic syndromes. The preleukemic syndromes are characterized clinically by refractory cytopenias and an indolent clinical course complicated by infection or hemorrhage, defective myeloid maturation sequences in marrow, and, ultimately, an acute blast transformation. These preleukemic syndromes have been recognized in several dogs and cats. The syndromes preceded the development of acute myelogenous or myelomonocytic leukemias by several months, and they were characterized by hematologic abnormalities including anemia, neutropenia, and thrombocytopenia. Bone marrow abnormalities included evidence of diserythropoiesis, disorderly myelopoiesis, and high numbers of megakaryocytes. The natural argument when viewing those reported cases of preleukemia in veterinary medicine is, however, that the animals studied were, in fact, already leukemic during their "preleukemic" phase.

Other Precancers

Other infrequently documented precancer-cancer sequences in small domestic animals include both the progression of canine oral papilloma to carcinoma and a large bowel carcinoma in a dog arising in a colorectal polyp. The pathologic changes in dogs with infection of *Spirocerca lupi* include, among other changes, a reactive granuloma that develops around the parasite. The fibroblasts in the inflammatory lesions may be quite metaplastic and appear transitional between granuloma and sarcoma; definitive neoplastic transformation does occur in some cases, and associated neoplasms include fibrosarcoma and osteosarcoma, some of which ultimately metastasize.

Endometrial carcinoma is rarely described in the dog or cat, although endometrial hyperplasia occurs often in rabbits as well as in other laboratory rodents and in humans. Relationships have been described between endometrial hyperplasia and endometrial carcinoma; in the rabbit, endometrial carcinoma is commonly encountered, and there are morphologic signs of an evolutionary scale from endometrial hyperplasia to malignant anaplastic carcinoma. The tumors can show progression, which is characterized by increasing anaplasia. In both human patients and rabbits, there are signs indicating relationships between endometrial carcinoma and sex hormones, notably estrogens. In the bitch, cystic endometrial hyperplasia may be a stimulus for polyp formation; focal hyperplasia elicits a response from connective tissue surrounding the cystic glands. Progressive elevation of the mucosa, vascularization, and organization leads to solitary or multiple polyps. Hormonal stimulation of the cystic glands may cause further endometrial proliferation. No evidence has been found, however, that endometrial polyps are preneoplastic changes of the canine or feline uterus.

THERAPY

Knowledge of the progression of precancerous lesions in veterinary practice is incomplete, and definitive statements regarding strategies for therapeutic intervention cannot be made. Pragmatic practitioners should include in the decision regarding a proper course of action a consideration of the alternatives of observation, local destruction of the lesion, or more extensive excision.

For lesions of the mammary gland, local excision (segmental resection or "lumpectomy") for lesions that appear benign may be warranted; if the histologic diagnosis confirms malignancy, then no harm will have resulted from the local excision if that biopsy is followed promptly by more aggressive definitive mastectomy. Other methods for therapeutic intervention, such as hormonal or immunologic modes of therapy for preneoplastic lesions of the mammary gland, have not been adequately tested in the bitch or queen in veterinary practice.

Preventive measures for dogs and cats at risk for sunlight-associated neoplasms include the use of PABA-containing sunscreen lotions for protection from sunlight and restriction of the animal's exposure to direct (overhead) sunlight. For premalignant changes in the skin of dogs, the topical application of dinitrochlorobenzene (DNCB) 1:100 in a lanolin-water cream topically every 7 days to the affected area will induce a delayed hypersensitivity reaction and effect control of premalignant (solar keratosis) lesions. The person applying the medication must avoid direct skin contact with DNCB, and after its application the animal must be restrained by use of collars or bandages from licking the lesion. A mild to marked inflammatory reaction will result from drug application, followed by regression of small lesions. Alternatively, the topical application of 5-fluorouracil 5 per cent cream topically every 48 hours will also cause regression and control of premalignant lesions. The drug will induce a mild to marked inflammatory reaction characterized by erythema, vesiculation, ulceration, and possibly necrosis, which will repair itself after cessation of drug treatment. The drug causes local pain after application, and the dog must not lick the medication. Also, rubber gloves must be worn by the veterinarian or owner to avoid direct skin contact when applying the drug. Treatment methods for established tumors may be modified for preneoplastic changes, and they include surgical excision, local radiofrequency hyperthermia, external beam irradiation (i.e., orthovoltage [x] irradiation, or ^{90}Sr irradiation), and cryosurgery. An alternative to cytotoxic methods of treating cancer is chemoprevention, i.e., the pharmacologic enhancement of cellular self-repair mechanisms to prevent cancer. Chemoprevention of sunlight-associated skin cancer by using retinoids (synthetic derivatives of vitamin A) is now being evaluated in veterinary and human medicine, and it is based on the ability of those compounds to reverse metaplastic changes in epithelium. Vitamin A and retinoids do promote cellular differentiation, but whether a daily low dose of a retinoid such as isotretinoin (13-*cis*-retinoic acid) would reduce the risk for cancer awaits the results of clinical trial.

For preleukemic syndromes, efforts to treat either the preleukemic or leukemic phases of these disorders with chemotherapy have been largely unsuccessful in human patients, and other contradictory methods of therapy have included the use of vitamins, corticosteroids, splenectomy, supportive therapy with blood products, or even no therapy. The use of agents aimed at forcing maturation of leukemia cells has been proposed in human practice, and some success attained in clearing blood and bone marrow of blast cells was reported in patients given low doses of cytosine arabinoside; these methods have yet to be evaluated critically in veterinary clinical practice. A low-dose regimen of cytosine arabinoside for dogs or cats would be 5 to 10 mg/m^2 body surface area, given twice daily, subcutaneously or by continuous intravenous infusion.

References and Supplemental Reading

Becker, F. F.: Recent concepts of initiation and promotion in carcinogenesis. Am. J. Pathol. 105:3, 1981.

Cameron, A. M., and Faulkin, L. J.: Hyperplastic and inflammatory nodules in the canine mammary gland. J. Natl. Cancer Inst. 47:1277, 1971.

Couto, C. G., and Kallett, A. J.: Preleukemic syndrome in a dog. J.A.V.M.A. 184:1389, 1984.

DeCosse, J. J.: Precancer—An overview. Cancer Surv. 2:348, 1983.

Dicken, C. M.: Retinoids: A review. J. Am. Acad. Dermatol. 11:541, 1984.

Dorn, C. R., Taylor, D. O. N., and Schneider, R. S.: Sunlight exposure and risk of developing cutaneous and oral squamous cell carcinomas in white cats. J. Natl. Cancer Inst. 46:1073, 1971.

Elsinghorst, Th. A. M., Timmermans, H. J. F., and Hendriks, H. C. Ch. J. M.: Comparative pathology of endometrial carcinoma. Vet. Quart. 6:200, 1984.

Forbes, P. D.: Photocarcinogenesis: An overview. J. Invest. Dermatol. 77:139, 1981.

Freinkel, R. K., et al: Consensus conference: Precursors to malignant melanoma. J. Am. Med. Assoc. 251:1864–1866, 1984.

Gelberg, H. B., and McEntee, K.: Hyperplastic endometrial polyps in the dog and the cat. Vet. Pathol. 21:570, 1984.

Gilbertson, S. R., Kurzman, I. D., Zachrau, R. E., et al.: Canine mammary epithelial neoplasms: Biologic implications of morphologic characteristics assessed in 232 dogs. Vet. Pathol. 20:127, 1983.

Greenberg, P. L.: The smoldering myeloid leukemic states: Clinical and biologic features. Blood 61:1035, 1983.

Gullino, P. M.: Considerations on the preneoplastic lesions of the mammary gland. Am. J. Pathol. 89:413, 1977.

Jehn, U., DeBock, R. De., and Haanen, C.: Clinical trial of low-dose ara-c in the treatment of acute leukemia and myelodysplasia. Blut 48:255, 1984.

Koeffler, H. P., and Golde, D. W.: Human preleukemia. Ann. Intern. Med. 93:347, 1980.

Madewell, B. R., Conroy, J. D., and Hodgkins, E. M.: Sunlight-skin cancer association in the dog: A report of three cases. J. Cutan. Pathol. 8:434, 1981.

Madewell, B. R., Jain, N. C., and Weller, R. E.: Hematologic abnormalities preceding myeloid leukemia in three cats. Vet. Pathol. 16:510, 1979.

Marks, P. A., and Rifkind, R. A.: Differentiation modifiers. Cancer 54:2766, 1984.

Mausner, J. S. and Kramer, S.: *Epidemiology—An Introductory Text.* Philadelphia, W.B. Saunders, 1985.

Rywlin, A. M.: Terminology of premalignant lesions in light of the multistep theory of carcinogenesis. Hum. Pathol. 15:806, 1984.

Warner, M. R.: Age incidence and site distribution of mammary dysplasias in young beagle bitches. J. Natl. Cancer Inst. 57:57, 1976.

Watrach, A. M., Small, E., and Case, M. T.: Canine papilloma: Progression of oral papilloma to carcinoma. J. Natl. Cancer Inst. 45:915, 1970.

Wisch, J. S., Griffin, J. D., and Kufe, K. W.: Response of preleukemic syndromes to continuous infusion of low-dose cytarabine. N. Engl. J. Med. 309:1599, 1983.

INFECTIOUS COMPLICATIONS OF CANCER

DWIGHT C. HIRSH, D.V.M.
Davis, California

Animals with cancer have an increased risk of developing infectious disease. More often than not, the agents responsible are bacterial. The reasons for this occurrence are many and varied, but the three most common are (1) immunosuppression induced by the cancer itself, (2) the immunosuppressive and cytotoxic effects of the drugs used to treat the cancer, and (3) the microbiological effects of antimicrobial agents sometimes used to protect the patient from the deleterious consequences of the first two.

The degree of immunosuppression induced by the cancerous state depends upon the type of neoplasm. For example, solid malignancies have less suppressive effect than those of the myeloid system. The immunosuppressive effect may involve the lymphoid system, leading to abnormalities (hyporesponsiveness) of the humoral as well as the cell-mediated compartments of the immune system. In addition, and perhaps more importantly, animals with certain tumors will have a granulocytopenia. This state, in addition to the deranged immune system, leaves the patient vulnerable to disease that may be produced by microorganisms in the environment.

Drugs used to treat some cancers will adversely affect the defense systems of the host. The systems affected are at two levels. The first are the mucosal barriers. Disruption of these barriers, especially those lining the alimentary canal, leads to the passage of bacteria, normally excluded by the barrier, into the circulation of the patient. A second effect of drugs used to treat cancer is on the immune system.

At some time in the treatment of a patient with cancer, antimicrobial drugs will probably be given. There are many reasons for this, including the perceived need to "cover and protect" the granulocytopenic patient, to treat a real or imagined infectious process, or to "cover and protect" the patient given immunosuppressive or cytotoxic drugs. Antimicrobic drugs will affect the microbiologic flora of the patient and, depending upon the magnitude of the effect, may place the patient in jeopardy. Certain antimicrobics will upset the homeostatic mechanisms operative in and on the surface of the alimentary canal and will lead to overgrowth and translocation of microorganisms. Translocation will occur in the normal animal if overgrowth of certain taxa of microorganisms (e.g., members of the family Enterobacteriaceae) is allowed. In the animal with both a damaged mucosal barrier and a depressed host defense system, translocation may have disastrous consequences.

The microorganisms that produce disease in the cancer patient are almost always those that occupy the alimentary canal of the patient. For this reason it is important that precautions be taken to ensure that the flora remain as stable as possible, since the normal flora is defined and already known to you. This knowledge encompasses not only the species of bacteria that might produce disease in the patient, but also the antimicrobial agent that will be effective in treating such disease. If the normal flora is changed in some way, especially by antimicrobial agents, then the nature of an infectious process will be unknown to the clinician who, as a consequence, will be forced to use very broad-spectrum antimicrobics. These antimicrobics are usually more toxic and more expensive than others that might have been indicated if the patient had had a relatively normal bacterial flora.

The microorganisms responsible for infectious disease of animals with cancer usually belong to the family Enterobacteriaceae. In our experience, *Escherichia coli* and *Klebsiella pneumoniae* are the two most common.

Early determination of the presence of an infectious process demands the utmost in clinical prowess when the clinician is confronted with any ill patient. In the case of the cancer patient, there is greater risk of mortality the longer the diagnosis of infectious complication is delayed.

The cardinal sign of infectious process in the cancer patient is fever. This is especially true if the patient is granulocytopenic; in this case, if fever is present, the patient should be considered septic until proven otherwise.

When fever is present, the site of the infection should be determined, for it is from here that the agent will be isolated. Once the agent is isolated, a rational choice of antimicrobic can be made. However, since isolation of the infectious agent and subsequent susceptibility testing take time, other procedures must be performed in addition to bacterial and fungal culture techniques. The most useful technique is the direct smear. Examination of the contents of the direct smear will provide two very important answers. First, and most important, is confirmation that an infectious process is present. Second, the shape of the microorganism will give a clue as to the identity of the agent, allowing the choice, with some degree of confidence, of an antimicrobial drug for treatment.

How the bacteria are revealed is not important. Most reference laboratories will use the Gram stain. In practice, a Romanovsky-type stain (Wright's and Giemsa are examples) is just as useful. Rods are almost always members of the family Enterobacteriaceae; cocci are almost always *Staphylococcus* or *Streptococcus*.

Once the sample is obtained from the suspected focus, it should always be subjected to culture techniques, even if no bacteria are seen in the direct smear, because approximately 10^6 bacteria per milliliter of sample are needed for one bacterium to be seen in one field under oil-immersion magnifications. In other words, there could be 10,000 organisms/ml, and the observer would only see one of them after examining 10 to 100 oil-immersion fields.

All the preliminary isolation and identification procedures can be performed in the office laboratory. The important determinations are whether bacteria are present and whether the isolate is a member of the family Enterobacteriacae (gram-negative or rod-shaped) or *Staphyloccocus* or *Streptococcus* (gram-positive or coccal-shaped). The best and most efficient way of accomplishing this is to inoculate a bi-plate containing blood agar on one side and MacConkey agar on the other. Only certain gram-negative organisms, most notably members of the family Enterobacteriacae and those of the genus *Pseudomonas*, will grow on the bile-containing MacConkey agar. If these organisms are isolated, then they may be sent to the reference laboratory for susceptibility testing. Colonial morphology as well as the catalase test will identify *Staphyococcus* and *Streptoccoccus*, the former being a white, pigmented colony that is catalase positive and around which there are usually two zones of hemolysis.

If no infectious locus is discovered, then blood must be cultured.

The bacteriologic culture of blood is more an art than a science, since there are numerous variables to deal with in order to successfully isolate an organism from the blood. The most important factors include the amount of blood collected, the medium inoculated, the timing and frequency of collection, and the conditions of incubation of the inoculated medium.

Table 1. *Effect of Certain Antimicrobial Agents on Normal Flora of Host*

Drug	Effect
Doxycycline	Little
Cephradine	Little
Trimethoprim and sulfonamide	Little
Amoxicillin	Some
Cephalexin	Some
Ampicillin	Great
Cloxacillin	Great
Tetracycline	Great
Chloramphenicol	Great

Modified from van der Waaij and Verhoef: *New Criteria for Antimicrobial Therapy: Maintenance of Digestive Tract Colonization Resistance.* Amsterdam: Excerpta Medica, 1979.

There may be fewer than 10 bacteria/ml of bacteremic blood. Therefore, as much blood as possible should be collected for analysis. Because components of the blood (e.g., granulocytes, complement proteins, and, if present, antimicrobial agents) might suppress or even prohibit growth of bacteria inoculated into the medium, the collected blood must be diluted 1:10 with bacteriologic medium.

Most commercially available blood culture bottles contain a tryptic digest of protein. Studies have shown that an additive such as the anticoagulant sodium polyanetholsulfonate (SPS) increases the chances of isolating any bacteria by acting as an anticoagulant, inactivating aminoglycoside antibiotics (if present), interfering with complement activity, and interfering with phagocytosis by WBC in the collected specimen.

Bacteremia may be continuous or sporadic, depending on the source of the bacteria. If the bacteremia is continuous, as in bacterial endocarditis, the timing of the collection of the blood sample is not critical. But if entry of bacteria into the bloodstream is sporadic, the timing of sample collection is important. Maximal efficiency of recovery of bacteria has been demonstrated when three to four samples are collected, spaced no less than 1 hour apart, within a 24-hour period. If there is periodic fever, most efficient recovery of bacteria will be made just before the fever reaches maximum.

Obligate aerobes (e.g., *Pseudomonas* spp.) as well as obligate anaerobes (e.g., *Bacteroides* spp.) may be in the bloodstream. For this reason, the conditions of incubation of inoculated blood culture bottles are important. Uninoculated, commercially available blood culture bottles are anaerobic. Two bottles are injected through the stopper with blood obtained from the patient. One of them is then rendered aerobic by the process of "venting," which consists of allowing air to enter the bottle through a sterile hypodermic needle containing sterile cotton in the hub.

The inoculated bottles are incubated at 37°C. After 24 hours of incubation, aliquots taken from

***Table 2.** Effect of Polymyxin B-Neomycin* on the Concentration of Gram-Negative Enteric Bacteria in the Feces of the Dog†*

No. of Bacteria/gm Feces	Days of Treatment
10^7	1
10^6	3
10^3	5
10^2	7
<10	9

*Polymyxin B is given at 20 mg/kg body weight orally; neomycin at 200 mg/kg body weight, divided in two doses, orally.

†Modified from Heidt in van der Waaji and Verhoef: *New Criteria for Antimicrobial Therapy: Maintenance of Digestive Tract Colonization Resistance.* Amsterdam: Excerpta Medica, 1979, pp. 54–62.

the bottles are examined for the presence of bacteria after they have been stained and subcultured to appropriate media. In the practice laboratory, these aliquots can be subcultured to the bi-plates described above. These bi-plates can be incubated at 37°C in air. The presence of anaerobic bacteria can be inferred if bacteria are seen in the direct smear of the aliquot but fail to grow an isolate on inoculated medium.

The choice of an antimicrobial agent for treatment of a real or perceived infectious process should be made carefully. As alluded to above, certain antimicrobials have a great deal of influence upon the normal flora; others, very little (Table 1). As a consequence, the patient may be placed at greater risk from the treatment than from the infectious process. If bacteria are seen in the direct smear, then their shape will determine which drugs might be most useful. If cocci are seen, the possibilities are *Staphylococcus* or *Streptococcus*. Most staphylococci are resistant to penicillin (and also ampicillin and amoxicillin), but they are susceptible to the penicillinase-resistant penicillins (methicillin, nafcillin, oxacillin, cloxacillin, and dicloxacillin) and to the cephalosporins. The streptococci (especially the beta-hemolytic strains, the most commonly isolated in our experience) are susceptible to all of the penicillins, including the penicillinase-resistant, and the cephalosporins. If a choice between streptococci and staphylococci cannot be made with certainty, then *Staphylococcus* should be the presumptive identification until confirmation is made in the laboratory. In this situation, a cephalosporin (cephalexin, for example) would be the preferred choice. If there are clues that *Streptococcus* is present (i.e., chains of cocci), then a penicillin (ampicillin or amoxicillin) is the drug of choice.

If rods are seen in the direct smear, then a member of the family Enterobacteriaceae must be presumed to be present until proven otherwise. Though any of the family may be present, *E. coli* and *K. pneumoniae* are the two most common. Since most strains of *E. coli* and *K. pneumoniae* are resistant to ampicillin and kanamycin (chloramphenicol is bacteriostatic and is not indicated for the granulocytopenic patient and, in addition, greatly disturbs the normal flora), neither of these drugs should be considered without susceptibility test results. Approximately one half of the isolates of *K. pneumoniae* are resistant to the combination of trimethoprim and sulfonamide, so this preparation is not indicated in the absence of knowledge of the genus of the infecting microorganism. This leaves the combination of a cephalosporin (e.g., cephalexin) for almost all strains of *K. pneumoniae* and some strains of *E. coli*, together with gentamicin for all strains of *E. coli* and *K. pneumoniae*. Some in-hospital strains of enterics are resistant to gentamicin. In such instances, amikacin is a reasonable alternative.

Treatment of the febrile, granulocytopenic patient without certain knowledge of the basis of the fever entails the assumption that a member of the family Enterobacteriaceae is present and treated accordingly. The cephalosporin-aminoglycoside combination will be effective against most other agents (including *Staphylococcus* and *Streptococcus*) involved with infectious disease in the cancer patient.

If the patient is seen to be at risk for the development of an infectious process, then certain steps can be taken to minimize the risk. Since it has been shown that the source of microorganisms that produce infectious disease is most often the alimentary tract of the patient, a reduction in the number of potential pathogens (*E. coli* and *K. pneumoniae*) can be attempted. This is done in human hospitals by giving patients nonabsorbable antimicrobics orally. Examples of these agents are polymyxin and neomycin. This combination reduces the numbers of enterics in the tract to almost zero (Table 2).

Another, perhaps more reasonable approach would be to use an antimicrobial agent that has little effect upon the normal flora and, at the same time, has broad activity against the target microorganism. One such preparation is a combination of trimethoprim and sulfonamide. Since the normal flora is left almost totally intact, the risk of overgrowth or increase in the number of members of the family Enterobacteriaceae is minimized.

References and Supplemental Reading

Brown, A. E.: Neutropenia, fever, and infection. Am. J. Med. 76:421, 1984.

Hirsh, D. C., Jang, S. S., and Biberstein, E. L.: Blood culture of the canine patient. J.A.V.M.A. 184:175, 1984.

Pizzo, P. A., Commers, J., Cotton, D., et al.: Approaching the controversies in antibacterial management of cancer patients. Am. J. Med. 76:436, 1984.

van der Waaij, D.: *Antibiotic Choice: The Importance of Colonization Resistance.* New York: Research Studies Press, 1983, pp. 33–55.

van der Waaij, D., Verhoef, J.: *New Criteria for Antimicrobial Therapy: Maintenance of Digestive Tract Colonization Resistance.* Amsterdam: Excerpta Medica, 1979.

CHEMOTHERAPEUTIC AGENTS AVAILABLE FOR CANCER TREATMENT

DENNIS W. MACY, D.V.M.
Fort Collins, Colorado

Cancer chemotherapy has become an established part of small animal medical practice in the past 15 years. In 1971, *Current Veterinary Therapy IV* described combination chemotherapy for canine lymphosarcoma. The fifth edition of this volume (1974) described therapies for monoclonal gammopathies, myeloproliferative disorders, polycythemia, and lymphosarcoma. *Current Veterinary Therapy VI* (1977) described methods of treatment for polycythemia, gammopathies, and feline and canine lymphomas, and it contains a section on the principles of cancer chemotherapy. The seventh edition (1980) again had sections on the principles of chemotherapy and treatment of canine lymphosarcoma. More recently, in *Current Veterinary Therapy VIII* (1983), an entire section was devoted to oncology; specific topics addressed chemotherapy of transmissible venereal tumors, solid tissue tumors, and adverse effects of chemotherapeutic agents in veterinary patients. It would be redundant to repeat much of the information contained in these previous discussions, and the reader is therefore referred to these sections for general principles of chemotherapy, specific protocols for tumor treatment, and a discussion of patient-related toxicity.

Several recent developments in the storage and safe handling of cancer chemotherapy agents are worthy of discussion. Cancer chemotherapy can be expensive and frequently is the primary reason given by clients either for not attempting therapy or for discontinuing therapy once it is initiated. The expense associated with chemotherapy often centers around the drugs, which are packaged in dose quantities based on human body size. Once reconstituted, many of these drugs have a limited shelf life, and clients many times have been forced to pay the same cost for drugs to treat a cat as they would for drugs to treat a human patient. The unused reconstituted drug is then discarded because of the unlikelihood of another patient requiring the same drug in the near future. The commonly used chemotherapeutic agent, vincristine, now comes in a multiple-dose vial, which has made the use of this particularly expensive agent more economical for clinical veterinary practice.

With the recent widespread use of the stem cell assay in human medicine, very small amounts of chemotherapeutic agents were needed, and thus laboratories utilizing this technique on human cells were faced with a problem similar to that of the veterinarian in clinical practice who was trying to treat small animals. Utilizing known sensitive cell lines, researchers reconstituted chemotherapeutic agents, froze them in small aliquots for varying periods of time, and retested the sensitivities of the cell line to these agents to determine how their potency had changed by freezing or storage.

The following antineoplastic agents have been evaluated for potency for the prescribed time periods. In many cases, the potency may be longer than the period in which it has been tested.

Cyclophosphamide (Cytoxan)—longer than 6 months frozen
Doxorubricin (Adriamycin)—longer than 6 months frozen
Bleomycin—at least 3 weeks frozen
Cisplatin—at least 3 weeks frozen
5-FU(fluorouracil)—at least 3 weeks frozen

Based on these findings, it is no longer necessary to throw away all reconstituted drugs, and clinicians may, within these rough guidelines, expect drug efficacy similar to that of freshly reconstituted agents. Readers should be aware that this method of preservation of drugs is not endorsed by their manufacturers or by the FDA, and that none of the 30 commercially available antineoplastic drugs has FDA approval for use in the treatment of cancer in domestic animals. Another economic problem fre-

Text continued on page 470

Table 1. *Cancer Chemotherapeutic Agents Used in Veterinary Practice*

Agent	Price: *Unit*	Price: *Cost (In US Dollars)*	Route of Administration	Dosage	Patient Toxicity	General Hazard	Effect on Skin	Manufacturer's Advice on Handling Precautions	Action on Contamination
Alkylating Agents									
Cyclophosphamide (Cytoxan) Mead Johnson 25, 50 mg tablets 100, 200, 500 mg vials	25 mg tablet 50 mg tablet 100 mg vial	0.57 1.12 52.50	Oral, mornings IV slow	2.2 mg/kg 3 to 4 days/week 10 mg/kg, weekly	Bone marrow depression, cystitis, transitional carcinoma	Pro-drug, requires metabolism in liver before becoming cytotoxic, carcinogenic, and teratogenic	Irritation is rare	No special precaution	Wash thoroughly with water
Chlorambucil (Leukeran) Burroughs Wellcome 2 mg tablets	2 mg tablet	0.30	Oral	0.1 to 0.2 mg/kg, daily	Bone marrow depression	NA	NA	NA	NA
Melphalan (Alkeran) Burroughs Wellcome 2 mg tablets	2 mg tablet	0.63	Oral	0.1 mg/kg, daily for 10 days, then 0.05 to 0.1 mg/kg, daily	Bone marrow depression	Carcinogenic, mutagenic	Not a skin irritant	Gloves and dye shield	Solution of 3% sodium carbonate should be used if spilled
Busulfan (Myleran) Burroughs Wellcome 2 mg tablet	2 mg tablet	0.38	Oral	0.1 mg/kg, daily	Bone marrow depression, pulmonary fibrosis	NA	NA	NA	NA
Thiotepa Lederle 15 mg vial	15 mg vial	21.68	IV or intracavitary	Maximum systemic dosage, 9 mg/m^2; intracavitary, bladder: 5 to 10 mg diluted in 30 mls, allow contact 30 min, repeat weekly	Bone marrow depression	NA	NA	NA	NA
Cisplatin (Platinol) Bristol-Myers 10 to 50 mg vials	10 mg vial 50 mg vial	25.67 119.98	IV	30 to 50 mg/m^2 every 3 weeks; pretreat with fluids 12 hours, 60 mls/kg, administer mannitol 0.5 gm/kg 30 min before drug therapy; slow drip 1 to 6 hours, follow with 12 hours fluid diuresis 60 ml/kg	Bone marrow depression, nephrotoxicity, local irritation	Carcinogenicity, mutagenicity, and teratogenicity suspected	Potentially allergenic	Gloves and mask necessary only if spilled	Wash thoroughly with water
Antimetabolites									
Methotrexate Lederle 2.5 mg tablets 25 to 50 mg vials	2.5 mg tablet 25 mg vial	0.56 6.65	Oral IV	2.5 mg/m^2, daily 0.3 to 0.8 mg/kg, weekly	Bone marrow depression	Teratogenic, carcinogenic, mutagenic	Irritant	Gloves	Wash with water, apply a bland cream for transient stinging, for systemic absorption of significant quantities, give calcium folinate (leucovorin); cover
6-Mercaptopurine (6-MP, Purinethol) Burroughs Wellcome 50 mg tablets	50 mg	0.62	Oral	2 mg/kg, daily	Bone marrow depression	NA	NA	NA	NA

Azathioprine (Imuran) Burroughs Wellcome 25 and 50 mg	50 mg	0.50	Oral	2.2 mg/kg, daily (dog)	Bone marrow depression	NA	NA	NA	Wash off quickly with water
5-Fluorouracil (5-FU) Roche 500 mg vials	500 mg vial	1.31	IV	5 to 10 mg/kg, weekly	Do not use in cats; bone marrow depression, CNS signs	Cytostatic	Minor local inflammation if skin is broken	No special precautions, but avoid contact with skin and mucous membranes	Flush affected parts with copious amounts of water
6-Thioguanine (6-TG) Burroughs Wellcome 40 mg tablets	40 mg	0.90	Oral	1 mg/kg, daily	Bone marrow depression	NA	NA	NA	NA
Cytosine arabinoside (Ara-C, Cytosar) Upjohn 100 to 500 mg vials	100 mg 500 mg	6.73 26.75	IV SC	100 mg/m², daily for 4 days; repeat cycle at 3-week intervals 30 mg/kg, weekly	Bone marrow depression	Teratogenic; causes corneal speckling if applied to eyes for several days	Not absorbed through intact skin	No special precautions	Wash thoroughly with water
Antibiotics									
Bleomycin (Blenoxane) Bristol-Myers 15 unit vials	15 unit vial	121.94	IV, SC, IM	10 mg/m² weekly, to maximum of 200 mg/m²	Pulmonary fibrosis	Cytostatic	Locally toxic, allergenic	Gloves and mask	Rinse thoroughly with water, then wash with soap and water
Doxorubicin (Adriamycin) Adria Labs 10 to 50 mg vials	10 mg	28.34	IV	30 mg/m²; repeat every 3 weeks to maximum cumulative dose of 200 mg/m²	Bone marrow depression, cardiomyopathy	Antimitotic, cytotoxic	Irritant	Gloves	Wash copiously with soap and water
Plant Alkaloids									
Vincristine (Oncovin) Lilly 1 to 5 mg vials	1 mg vial	29.54		0.5 to 0.8 mg/m², weekly, or 0.02 mg/kg, weekly	Locally irritating, peripheral neuropathy	Suspected to be teratogenic	Irritant	Gloves	As for vinblastine
Vinblastine (Velban) Lilly 10 mg vial	10 mg	30.48	IV	3 mg/m²; weekly, or 0.1 to 0.4 mg/kg, weekly	Bone marrow depression, peripheral neuropathy	Suspected to be teratogenic	Irritant	Gloves	Wash thoroughly and immediately with large amounts of water, if accidental injection into subcutaneous tissues, apply heparin cream to affected area
Miscellaneous Agents									
L-Asparaginase (Elspar) Merck, Sharp & Dohme 10,000 and 50,000 unit vials	10,000 unit vial	27.98	IV, IP, IM	400 units/kg, weekly	ANA phylaxis	Cytostatic	Not a skin irritant	No special precautions	Wash with water
Hydroxyurea (Hydrea) Squibb 500 mg tablets	500 mg	0.67	Oral	80 mg/kg every 3 days or 40 mg/kg, daily	Bone marrow depression				

Table 2. *Precautions to be Taken on Spillage of Antineoplastic Drugs*

1. Put on protective gloves
2. Wear a face mask and eye protection if there is a powder spill.
3. Place spilled materials in a polyethylene bag.
4. Wipe up remains with a damp cloth or cotton and place in bag.
5. Seal bag, place in second bag, and seal.
6. Label bag, stating contents, and mark it *DANGER*.
7. Wash contaminated surfaces with copious amounts of water; wash exposed skin areas with soap and water.
8. Wash eyes copiously with water or isotonic saline; seek ophthalmological advice if eye irritation continues.
9. Dispose of washing materials used in steps 3 to 6 above; send waste for disposal by incineration.
10. Take precautions to prevent further spillage.

quently encountered by the veterinarian is estimating cost of therapy. In Table 1 a list of wholesale prices of individual drugs is included so that the veterinarian may get a rough idea of the potential cost of a proposed treatment protocol.

Cancer chemotherapy employs some of the most toxic pharmaceutical agents available in modern medicine. A detailed discussion of the adverse effects associated with the use of these drugs in domestic animals is contained in *Current Veterinary Therapy VIII*. Despite the fact that some of these agents have been used in humans for 25 years, it has only been in the last several years that concern for potential health risks to persons preparing and administering these drugs has been appreciated. A limited number of studies have reported persons working in oncology units or pharmacies have mutagenic substances in their urine that are not present in the urine of individuals working in other portions of hospitals. In addition, there have been reports of acute toxicities including nausea, headache, dizziness, lightheadedness, and dermatitides in personnel working with these drugs (including one who worked in a veterinary facility). The specific long-term risks of low-level exposure to these agents are yet to be defined, but most believe that the evidence to date justifies precautionary measures in handling these materials. Because these reports have appeared in a relatively short period of time, the guidelines for handling, preparation, storage, and disposal of these agents are not universal and vary between institutions.

In light of the relatively infrequent use of these agents in most veterinary practices (compared with human hospitals), the following recommendations appear to be reasonable safety measures (Table 2). Informed consent should be obtained from all employees handling cytotoxic agents. Since most private practices and some institutions will not have the recommended biological safety cabinets available for drug preparation, pregnant workers should not handle cytotoxic agents. Persons handling cytotoxic agents should wear gloves, masks (optimally, a NIOSH-approved respiratory mask), long-sleeved lab coats or disposable gowns, and eye protection. Drugs should be mixed in an uncongested area over a plastic-backed absorbable pad. Syringes and IV sets with Luer-lock fittings should be used both in the preparation and in the administration of cytotoxic agents. Techniques that avoid the generation of pressure differences between the inside and outside of rubber-capped vials should be employed. This may be accomplished by adequately venting air before diluent is added. Special needles are available for this purpose (Millex-F6 Filter Unit, Millipore Corp.). Practitioners who pulverize alkylating agents such as cyclophosphamide or melphalan in order to produce smaller-sized capsules should be especially careful to avoid aerosolization of these agents. Needles, syringes, and IV sets should be disposed of in a manner that avoids subsequent human contact. These recommendations are reasonable even if you are a heavy smoker, eat meat, and drink polluted water with your bourbon.

References and Supplemental Reading

Jeffrey, L. P.: *Consensus Responses to Unresolved Questions Concerning Cytotoxic Agents.* Providence, RI: National Study Commission on Cytotoxic Exposure, Rhode Island Hospital Department of Pharmacy, 1984.

Solimando, D. A., Jr.: Preparation of antineoplastic drugs: A review. Am. J. Intrav. Ther. Clin. Nutr. 10:16, 1983.

Davis, M. R.: Guidelines for safe handling of cytotoxic drugs in pharmacy departments and hospital wards. Hosp. Pharm. 16:17, 1981.

Rosenthal, R. C., and Kingston, R. E.: Nitrogen mustard: Human exposure and toxicity in a veterinary hospital. J. Am. Anim. Hosp. Assoc. 20:821, 1984.

Franco, R. S., Miller, T. J., Kraft, T. J., et al.: Stability of antineoplastic activity after freezing and storage of chemotherapeutic agents to use in the human tumor stem cell assay. Am. Assoc. Cancer Res. Abs. 24:5, 1983.

Yang, L. Y., and Drewinko, B.: The stability of the lethal efficacy of antitumor drugs. Am. Assoc. Cancer Res. Abs. 24:315, 1983.

DRUG RESISTANCE IN CANCER CHEMOTHERAPY

ROBERT C. ROSENTHAL, D.V.M.
Madison, Wisconsin

Chemotherapy has assumed an important role in combined-modality cancer treatment. Anticancer drug therapy may precede, follow, or be used concurrently with surgery, radiation therapy, immunotherapy, or hyperthermia. Combination chemotherapies designed on the rational basis of selecting drugs that have different dose-limiting toxicities and attack the cell cycle at different phases have not, however, resulted in improved cure rates. Likewise, protocols based on tumor growth kinetic analysis have not improved cure rates from chemotherapy. In the long run, the major problem confronting the chemotherapist has been drug resistance. To compound the problem further, drug resistance may be temporary or permanent.

Temporary drug resistance is based on pharmacologic or kinetic considerations. Pharmacologic resistance may be related to (1) the inaccessibility of some agents to some body compartments or (2) the nature of the blood supply in a tumor and poor diffusion of drug to the neoplastic cells. Kinetically, growth fraction decreases with increased mass and distance from the blood supply. Late in the natural course of a tumor, most cells are in a resting (G_0) phase and are thus resistant to drugs that are only effective against actively cycling cells. In neither of these situations are the cancer cells inherently resistant to the drugs.

Permanent drug resistance is a greater problem. Important aspects of the problem of emerging permanent drug resistance relate to the natural history of tumor growth and the ability to detect a neoplasm clinically. Consider a tumor arising from a single transformed cell. This cell undergoes 30 doublings to become a mass of approximately 1 gm (10^9 cells), generally considered the smallest clinically detectable mass. The mass will increase to 10 gm (10^{10} cells) after another 3.25 doublings. At this point it is more likely to be detected, but the metastatic process may already have begun.

Once metastases have been established, localized forms of therapy (surgery, radiation) will be ineffective; systemic therapy will be required. The next 6.75 doublings will result in a tumor mass of 10^{12} cells, about 1 kg of tumor, the maximum compatible with life in most instances. Of a total of 40 doublings in the natural history of a tumor, 30 or more occur before any mass is detected. Therefore, every malignant tumor noted clinically is late in its course. The genetic instability of cancer cells and the selection of variant subpopulations are hallmarks of tumor progression. The result is that the tumor mass is heterogenous in several characteristics, including resistance to drugs.

It was demonstrated experimentally over 40 years ago that microbial drug resistance develops spontaneously, not as the result of drug treatment. Similarly, cancer cells develop resistance spontaneously. With time, both the number and proportion of resistant cells increase regardless of the mutation rate. Once resistance emerges, the probability of attaining cure falls rapidly from 95 per cent to 5 per cent in just 1.77 logs of growth (5.9 doublings).

Spontaneous drug resistance in the cancer cell may occur by several mechanisms relating to the presence of the active form of the drug in a cancer cell or by other biochemical responses of the cell to avoid drug toxicity. A cancer cell may develop resistance to a drug by more than one mechanism.

Antineoplastic drugs act intracellularly. If they are unable to gain access to or remain within the cancer cell, their cytotoxic effect will be decreased. Resistance to methotrexate or nitrogen mustard may be based on decreased carrier-mediated transport into the cell; resistance to doxorubicin may be based on increased removal of the drug from the cancer cell. Cytosine arabinoside may bind less avidly to membrane sites, thus decreasing uptake.

Resistance related to decreased uptake may be overcome by giving greater amounts of the drug. The resultant increases in serum concentrations might alter uptake kinetics sufficiently to allow the drug to enter the cell efficiently. Of course, this tactic carries with it the probability of increased toxicity and cannot always be employed.

Once within the cancer cell, some anticancer drugs need to be activated. Defective drug activation occurs in neoplastic cells that have decreased concentrations of deoxycytidine kinase, leading to resistance to cytosine arabinoside. Decreased amounts of enzymes in other systems lead to defective activation of other drugs; for example, decreases in uridine kinase, uridine phosphorylase, and orotic acid phosphoribosyltransferase will decrease the activation of 5-fluorouracil. Both 6-mercaptopurine and 6-thioguanine are ineffectively activated in the presence of decreased concentrations of hypoxanthine-guanine phosphoribosyltransferase. Doxorubicin is ineffectively activated in the presence of decreased concentrations of cytochrome P_{450}. Resistance to methotrexate has been associated with defective polyglutamation. The polyglutamated form of methotrexate is retained in the cell for long periods of time even in the absence of extracellular drug, thus increasing the effective contact time between the drug and the cancer cell.

It is also reasonable to anticipate that increased drug inactivation in the cancer cell will lead to resistance. Within the resistant cancer cell, increased concentrations of alkaline phosphatase inactivate 6-mercaptopurine and 6-thioguanine. Increased concentrations of cytidine deaminase in resistant cancer cells favor a pathway for cytosine arabinoside, which yields the inactive product ara-U rather than the active product ara-CTP. Doxorubicin and alkylating agents are inactivated by increased concentrations of glutathione in resistant cancer cells. Bleomycin is inactivated by increased concentrations of hydrolases, and *cis*-platinum is inactivated by increased concentrations of metallothionein. Alterations in both activation and inactivation of anticancer drugs decrease the cytotoxicity by decreasing the intracellular concentration of active drug.

Some cancer cells acquire resistance through other intracellular responses. Enhanced DNA repair related to the increased excision of damaged bases or increased ligation of intact DNA segments (or both conditions) has been associated with resistance to alkylating agents, doxorubicin, and *cis*-platinum. By gene amplification, neoplastic cells are able to increase the amount of an intracellular target and thus diminish the efficacy of an anticancer drug. By producing increased amounts of dihydrofolate reductase, the enzyme inhibited by methotrexate, neoplastic cells may gain resistance. Similarly, increased concentrations of thymidylate synthetase produced by neoplastic cells have been associated with resistance to 5-fluorouracil.

The neoplastic cell may not necessarily produce greater concentrations of intracellular products but may alter the targets slightly. Altered dihydrofolate reductase effectively reduces folate cofactors from di- to tetrahydrofolate forms but is not successfully inhibited by methotrexate. Altered thymidylate synthetase is not inhibited by 5-fluorouracil, thus allowing pyrimidine synthesis to proceed unimpeded. Alterations in tubulin and membrane lipids are associated with resistance to vincristine and doxorubicin, respectively. These structural components are vital for successful cell replication. Altered steroid receptors provide a means of resistance to steroids in cases in which these drugs have an antineoplastic effect.

Pleiotropic drug resistance (PDR) may develop after exposure to a single dose of an antitumor antibiotic or a plant alkaloid, usually doxorubicin or vincristine. Tumor cells that develop PDR become cross-resistant to unrelated compounds, even those that have different mechanisms of action. Such resistant cells have high concentrations of enzymes important in membrane glycoprotein synthesis and low concentrations of enzymes that catabolize membrane glycoproteins. The membranes of cells with PDR are characterized by the presence of a specific moiety called *P-glycoprotein*. This component seems to provide these cells a degree of impenetrability like that offered by the glycoprotein capsules of antibiotic-resistant bacteria. In the future, it may be possible to overcome PDR by directing monoclonal antibodies tagged with cellular toxins to specific antigenic determinants of P-glycoprotein.

The concept of drug resistance is an important one for the chemotherapist to understand, as it carries with it implications for therapy. By reducing a tumor mass by cytotoxic means, it is theoretically possible to "turn back the resistance clock" by removing a large mass of cells and leaving a small, nonresistant population. It is also apparent that early treatment, even in the face of a theoretically late disease, is beneficial. *There is nothing to be gained from a "wait and see" approach.* Additionally, it is clear that the best chance of cure accompanies the first therapy. It is well recognized that second and third therapies tend to be less effective in inducing and maintaining remissions. In responsive diseases such as lymphosarcoma, the use of alternating combinations of non-cross-resistant drugs may help delay this emergence of resistance and result in longer first remissions and survivals. On the other hand, maintenance therapy has not been proven to be beneficial, and its role remains undefined. Such therapy may theoretically encourage the emergence of highly resistant clones. Clearly, the question of drug resistance must be kept in mind when cancer therapy is designed.

References and Supplemental Reading

Curt, G. A., Clendeninn, N. J., and Chabner, B. A.: Drug resistance in cancer. Cancer Treat. Rep. 68:87, 1984.

DeVita, V. T.: The relationship between tumor mass and resistance to chemotherapy. Cancer 51:1209, 1983.

Fidler, I. J., and Hart, I. R.: Biological diversity in metastatic neoplasms: Origins and implications. Science 217:998, 1982.

Goldie, J. H.: New thoughts on resistance to chemotherapy. Hosp. Pract. 18:165, 1983.

Goldie, J. H., Coldman, A. J., and Gudauskas, G. A.: Rationale for the use of alternating non-cross-resistant chemotherapy. Cancer Treat. Rep. 66:439, 1982.

Osieka, R.: Primary and acquired resistance to antineoplastic chemotherapy: A preclinical and clinical study. Cancer 54 (suppl.) 6:1168, 1984.

CANINE EXTRANODAL LYMPHOMAS

C. GUILLERMO COUTO, D.V.M.
Columbus, Ohio

Lymphomas (lymphosarcomas, malignant lymphomas) are thought to arise in a uni- or multifocal manner from nodal tissues with subsequent spread to other nodal or visceral sites. Ten to 20 per cent of human lymphomas appear to have an extranodal origin, however, and are referred to as primary extranodal lymphomas (ENL) (Rudders et al., 1978). Secondary extranodal involvement in human lymphomas is also common. The prevalence of ENL in dogs appears to range between 7 and 14 per cent when cutaneous and alimentary forms are included (Theilen and Madewell, 1979; Priester, 1980). Since lymphocytes are ubiquitous and circulate freely throughout the body, virtually any organ can give raise to ENL. However, this atypical form of presentation is more commonly seen in skin, the alimentary tract, mucocutaneous regions, eyes, kidneys, and the central nervous system (CNS). Lymphomatous involvement of endocrine glands, muscle, bone, lungs, and pharynx, among others, have also been documented.

Clinical manifestations of ENL are extremely variable and usually result from replacement of the affected organ or tissue by neoplastic lymphoid cells. Therefore, either a space-occupying lesion or parenchymal organ dysfunction are common findings in patients with ENL.

Hematologic and biochemical abnormalities in dogs with ENL are variable and nonspecific, usually stemming from organ infiltration (eg., azotemia in renal involvement) or tumor necrosis (e.g., neutrophilia and monocytosis in ulcerated superficial neoplasms). Radiographic changes in dogs with ENL are nonspecific.

A definitive diagnosis of lymphoma is usually obtained by examining a cytologic specimen obtained by fine needle aspiration. This technique is highly reliable and devoid of significant complications. When superficial masses (e.g., cutaneous or mucocutaneous) are aspirated, surgical preparation of the area is generally not necessary; however, when aspiration involves intra-abdominal or intrathoracic organs, the skin should be clipped, shaved, and prepared aseptically. A 22-gauge needle attached to a 12-cc syringe is adequate in most instances. Aspiration is begun once the needle penetrates the mass, and the suction is released before the needle is withdrawn. The amount of cells present in the hub of the needle is usually adequate to obtain two to four good-quality smears. Specimens can be stained with new methylene blue, Giemsa, or Wright's stains. Cytologic features of ENL are similar to those of nodal lymphomas. However, the interpretation of samples from cutaneous or mucocutaneous lesions should include other "round cell" neoplasms such as transmissible venereal tumor, mast cell tumor, amelanotic melanoma, histiocytoma, and basal cell tumor in the differential diagnoses. The cytologic characteristics of these neoplasms have been described elsewhere (Duncan and Prasse, 1979).

Depending upon the location of ENL, biopsies can be taken by using a wide variety of techniques and instrumentation; biopsy of ENL will be discussed individually in each section. Histologically, lymphomas are usually composed of immature lymphoid cells with a diffuse distribution. Several histologic categories have been described following Rappaport's classification. Most of the canine ENLs diagnosed at the Veterinary Teaching Hospital, The Ohio State University (VTH-OSU), appear to be "histiocytic" or lymphocytic, poorly differentiated; this is in agreement with human ENLs, in which these two histologic types predominate (Rudders et al., 1978). Since the Rappaport classification of lymphomas is not widely used by veterinary pathologists, some ENLs are still reported according to their former nomenclature, "reticulum cell sarcoma."

The organ distribution of canine ENL is depicted

in Tables 1 and 2. Gastrointestinal, cutaneous, neural, and mucocutaneous forms will be discussed in detail.

GASTROINTESTINAL LYMPHOMA

The gastrointestinal (GI) tract is the most common site of presentation of ENL in dogs; it represents approximately 2 to 7 per cent of all lymphomas. Most ENLs in the GI tract arise from the gut-associated lymphoid tissue and are thus composed primarily of B-lymphocytes.

Twenty-three dogs with GI-ENL were diagnosed at the VTH-OSU during a 13-year period. Ages at presentation ranged between 1 and 13 years, with a median of 6.5 years, and males outnumbered females (male:female ratio = 4.75:1). No breed appeared to be overrepresented.

Clinical signs on presentation included vomiting or diarrhea (20 dogs), with blood present in the vomitus or in the stool in 11 dogs, anorexia and weight loss (16 dogs), and tenesmus (one dog). The duration of signs ranged between 3 days and 6 months, and 18 dogs had previously been treated symptomatically. Physical findings were nonspecific, including emaciation (nine dogs), presence of mid- or cranial abdominal masses (six dogs), abdominal pain (five dogs), pyrexia (four dogs), hepatomegaly (two dogs), pallor (one dog), and icterus (one dog).

Hematologic changes included anemia (six dogs), hypoproteinemia (13 dogs), microcytosis (three dogs), neutrophilic leukocytosis (13 dogs), left shift (six dogs), monocytosis (eight dogs), and lymphopenia (14 dogs). Serum biochemical abnormalities were dominated by hypoproteinemia (11 of 15 dogs evaluated) and hypoalbuminemia (7 of 10 dogs evaluated). Radiographic changes were present in 13 out of 23 dogs, and included the appearance of an intra-abdominal mass (three dogs), splenomegaly (three dogs), hepatomegaly (three dogs), microhepatia (two dogs), thickened gastric wall (one dog), irregular colonic wall (one dog), and changes compatible with peritonitis (one dog). Positive contrast upper GI studies were helpful in identifying the lesion or lesions in 13 of 14 dogs for which the procedure was done. Irregularities in the gastric (seven dogs) or small intestinal wall (seven dogs) and lymphadenopathy (two dogs) were common findings. A histologic diagnosis was obtained by exploratory laparotomy in 14 cases, gastroscopy in one case, proctoscopy in three cases, and necropsy in the remaining five. The distribution of the neoplasm was determined during laparotomy or necropsy (Table 3). Since this was retrospective study, it was difficult to evaluate response to therapy.

Table 1. *Organ Distribution of Canine ENL*

Organ/Tissue	Number	Per Cent
All lymphomas	1,452	100
Alimentary	26	1.8
Skin	20	1.4
Endocrine	13	0.9
Liver	7	0.5
Kidney	6	0.4
Eye	5	0.35
Pleura/Mediastinum	4	0.3
Oropharynx	4	0.3
Spinal cord	3	0.2
Nose/sinuses	3	0.2
Mouth	2	0.1
Meninges/brain	1	0.06

Modified from Priester and McKay: *Natl. Cancer Inst. Monograph No. 54*, 1980, pp. 31–43; 59–71.

Table 2. *Clinicopathologic Types in 144 Lymphomas*

Clinicopathologic Type	Number	Per Cent
Multicentric	121	84.0
Alimentary*	10	6.9
Cutaneous*	9	6.3
Mediastinal	3	2.2
Miscellaneous*	1	0.6

*Extranodal lymphoma

From Theilen and Madewell: *Veterinary Cancer Medicine.* Philadelphia: Lea & Febiger, 1979, pp. 204–288.

Surgical excision for GI-ENL is indicated only when intestinal obstructions, perforations, or solitary masses are present, or when it is used as a means of obtaining a tissue specimen. Dehiscence of the affected gut with subsequent peritonitis is a possible postoperative complication. Surgical excision is the primary treatment of choice in human gastric lymphomas, and prolonged survival times often ensue. Similarly, complete excision of solitary, localized GI lymphomas in the dog may result in prolonged remission and survival times.

Combination chemotherapy with various agents is used for treatment of diffuse GI lymphomas. Different drug combinations are outlined in Table 4. Although definitive data are not available, there is preliminary evidence that protocols such as CHOP (see Table 4) using doxorubicin (Adriamycin, Adria) are more effective in inducing remission in diffuse GI lymphomas than are COAP or COP protocols (Table 4). Drug combinations including

Table 3. *Organ Involvement in 23 Dogs with GI-ENL*

Organ(s)	Number	Per Cent
Stomach alone	3	13
Stomach and small intestine	8	35
Small intestine alone	7	30
Small and large intestines	2	8.7
Large intestine alone	1	4.6
Stomach, small and large intestine	2	8.7

***Table 4.** Combination Chemotherapy Protocols Used in the Treatment of Canine Lymphomas*

1. COAP*	
Cyclophosphamide (Cytoxan, Mead Johnson)	50 mg/m² BSA, PO, every other day
Vincristine (Oncovin, Lilly)	0.5 mg/m² BSA, IV, once a week
Cytosine arabinoside (Cytosar, Upjohn)	100 mg/m² BSA, IV or SC, once a day for 4 days
Prednisone	50 mg/m² BSA, PO, every day for a week; then 25 mg/m² BSA, PO, every other day
2. COP	
Cyclophosphamide (Cytoxan)	200 to 300 mg/m² BSA, IV, once every 3 weeks
Vincristine (Oncovin)	0.75 mg/m² BSA, IV, once a week
Prednisone	25 mg/m² BSA, PO, every other day
3. CHOP†	
Cyclophosphamide (Cytoxan)	100 to 200 mg/m² BSA, IV, on day 1 of the cycle
Doxorubicin (Adriamycin, Adria)	30 mg/m² BSA, IV, on day 1 of the cycle
Vincristine (Oncovin)	0.75 mg/m² BSA, IV, on days 8 and 15 of the cycle
Prednisone	25 mg/m² BSA, PO, every other day

*This protocol is used during 8 weeks to induce remission. Once remission is attained, the same protocol can be used every other week for 6 cycles, then every 3 weeks for 6 additional cycles. Administration of this drug combination once every 4 weeks may suffice to maintain remission.

†Cycle is repeated every 3 weeks.

Key: BSA, body surface area; IV, intravenously; PO, orally; SC, subcutaneously.

doxorubicin are considerably myelosuppressive, so the use of prophylactic antimicrobial therapy is recommended; sulfadiazine-trimethoprim (Tribrissen, Wellcome Animal Health) at a dose of 13 mg/kg, PO, is given twice a day.

CUTANEOUS LYMPHOMAS

Cutaneous lymphomas are almost as prevalent as GI forms in the dog. Three different forms of primary cutaneous lymphomas have been identified on the basis of morphology and pathogenesis: (1) *Mycosis fungoides*, a T-cell neoplasm with defined histologic characteristics (i.e., Pautrier microabscesses); (2) *Woringer-Kolopp disease* (or pagetoid reticulosis), another epidermotropic T-cell lymphoma that primarily differs from mycosis fungoides in that it lacks formation of Pautrier microabscesses; and (3) *"histiocytic" lymphomas*, composed mainly of large histiocyte-like cells, which in most cases are of B-cell origin. The third form is usually a cutaneous manifestation of multicentric lymphomas (i.e., secondary extranodal involvement). Cutaneous lymphomas will be discussed in the Dermatology section.

NEURAL LYMPHOMAS

Neoplastic lymphoid cells may infiltrate different neuroanatomic structures and result in a wide variety of clinicopathologic manifestations. Isolated peripheral or cranial nerves can be involved by a lymphomatous process, causing local or regional neurologic dysfunction; although the prevalence of this form is unknown, only a few cases have been documented.

Central nervous system lymphomas are apparently more common than peripheral forms. They can affect any neuroanatomic structure, including the meninges. *Epidural lymphomas* usually cause spinal cord compression of acute onset, resulting in paralysis or paresis caudal to the lesion. Most epidural lymphomas reported in the veterinary literature affect the thoracolumbar spine. As with other meningeal neoplasms, pain is a consistent finding. A confirmation of the neuroanatomic diagnosis is usually obtained by means of a myelogram. Accurate localization of the lesion is vital for diagnostic and therapeutic purposes. Surgical exploration of the affected area usually provides a diagnostic tissue sample; moreover, complete excision of the mass may result in transient improvement of the clinical signs owing to decompression. Effective tumor debulking should be followed by systemic anticancer chemotherapy, as outlined in Table 4. Localized epidural masses can be irradiated by teletherapy. Total dosages of 3,000 to 4,000 rad delivered three times a week (Monday, Wednesday, and Friday) in 300- to 500-rad fractions usually result in complete tumor remission and palliation of clinical signs. However, if prolonged survivals are attained, irreversible radiation-induced myelopathy may occur 3 to 6 months after therapy.

Lymphomas affecting the *neuropil*, the *leptomeninges*, or both areas usually cause seizures and clinical signs compatible with multifocal CNS involvement. Eight such cases were described in one report (Couto et al., 1984). One dog was considered to have primary CNS lymphoma, while the other seven showed CNS signs and lesions either simultaneously with the development of multicentric lymphoma or late in the course of therapy for multicentric lymphoma (CNS relapse). A diagnosis was obtained by identifying high numbers of abnormal lymphoid cells (range of 100 to 8,500 WBC/μl; normal values are fewer than 5 WBC/μl) in cerebrospinal fluid (CSF) in seven dogs from which CSF was collected; the CSF protein concentration was elevated in six of seven dogs (range of 34.2 to 310 mg/dl; normal is less than 20 mg/dl). In the remaining dog, the diagnosis was confirmed on necropsy.

Two of the dogs were treated with systemic anticancer chemotherapy using the COAP protocol (Table 4, No. 1). The cytosine arabinoside (Cytosar, Upjohn) was administered as a continuous intravenous drip during 96 hours in order to attain therapeutic concentrations in the CSF. Both dogs showed rapid remission of clinical signs, and in one dog for which a CSF analysis was repeated, the WBC count decreased from 830 to 15 cells/μl. Four dogs were treated with intrathecal chemotherapy and craniospinal irradiation. Cytosine arabinoside was used intrathecally at a dose of 20 mg/m^2 of body surface area (BSA) by bolus injection after an equal volume of CSF was withdrawn. The total dose was diluted to 2 to 4 ml in lactated Ringer's solution and was injected twice weekly for a total of six treatments. Irradiation (^{60}Co teletherapy) of the craniospinal axis was delivered in six fractions of 500 rad each, three times a week (Monday, Wednesday, and Friday). Rapid resolution of the clinical signs occurred after one to three treatments in three of four dogs. In one dog, a tentorial herniation due to high CSF pressure occurred after the first CSF tap. Despite the prompt response to treatment in five of six dogs, none of them lived for more than 3 months after therapy for the CNS lymphoma was instituted.

MUCOCUTANEOUS LYMPHOMAS

Mucocutaneous junctions are often infiltrated by neoplastic lymphoid cells. The orolabial tissues seem to be affected more often than other mucocutaneous areas, although involvement of the preputial, anal, and ocular areas have been identified.

Mucocutaneous lymphomas can mimic a wide variety of disorders, including immune-mediated diseases (e.g., pemphigus vulgaris, pemphigus erythematosus, bullous pemphigoid, systemic lupus erythematosus), bacterial pyodermas, drug eruptions, dermatomycoses, granulomatous dermatitis, mast cell tumors, transmissible venereal tumors, and histiocytomas. The primary and secondary lesions are extremely variable, ranging from papules and pustules to plaque-like lesions, with or without erythema or pruritus. When mycosis fungoides affects mucocutaneous regions, pruritus is usually an important component of the disease.

Tissue samples should be obtained before corticosteroid therapy is instituted, since steroids may distort the morphology of neoplastic lymphoid cells, compromising their identification. Fine needle aspirates or Baker's biopsy punch samples (Baker-Cummins) are usually sufficient to obtain a diagnosis. Cytologic specimens may be diagnostic; however, in order to characterize the tumor histologically (e.g., mycosis fungoides versus "histiocytic" lymphoma), it is necessary to obtain a core or punch biopsy. As with most ENLs, mucocutaneous lymphomas are primarily of the diffuse, "histiocytic" type (i.e., diffuse, large cell lymphomas). Although most cases appear to be primary ENL (the neoplastic process confined to one mucocutaneous region), multiple mucocutaneous forms have been identified (e.g., oral, preputial, and perianal). Isolated cases of mucocutaneous involvement in dogs with multicentric lymphomas have also been recognized.

The therapeutic approach for primary mucocutaneous lymphomas is similar to the other forms previously described. Solitary masses can be surgically excised or irradiated, thus achieving local control of the disease. Cases with widespread mucocutaneous involvement are given systemic chemotherapy. As in the case of gastrointestinal lymphoma, there are preliminary data to show that dogs with mucocutaneous involvement respond better to drug combinations that include doxorubicin. In two dogs, the addition of methotrexate (2.5 mg/m^2 BSA, PO, twice to three times a week) to the COAP protocol resulted in complete tumor remission. Initial response to therapy is excellent, but survival times are often shorter than for dogs with the multicentric form of lymphoma.

GENERAL APPROACH TO THE DOG WITH ENL

Extranodal lymphomas should be approached like any other neoplasm; after a complete history and physical examination, thoracic and abdominal radiographs are helpful in determining the extension of the neoplasm. A complete blood count, platelet count, and serum biochemical analysis may disclose the presence of a paraneoplastic syndrome (e.g., hypercalcemia, monoclonal gammopathy, immune-mediated thrombocytopenia), reveal the presence of circulating blast cells, or suggest that the patient's bone marrow is infiltrated with neoplastic cells (e.g., pancytopenia, leukoerythroblastic reaction). A confirmation of the diagnosis is usually obtained by cytologic or histopathologic evaluation of each affected area. In the presence of a confirmed ENL, a bone marrow aspirate for cytologic evaluation should be obtained to rule out tumor involvement of this organ.

Once all these data have been collected, the tumor should be *staged* according to the World Health Organization recommendations. However, staging ENL poses a problem from the prognostic viewpoint, since all cases with extranodal involvement are classified as stage V. In theory, tumors in a high stage (e.g., stage V) should bear a worse prognosis than a lower stage (e.g., stage III). This does not seem to be the case for ENL, for dogs with solitary masses that are completely excised usually have longer survival times than dogs with generalized lymph node involvement (stage III). Therefore, the current staging system does not seem to be appropriate for ENL.

After a diagnosis has been obtained, the clinician will face different therapeutic options:

1. For solitary gastrointestinal, cutaneous, or mucocutaneous lymphomas, surgical excision of the mass should be followed by low-grade chemotherapy. Protocol No. 1 (Table 4) can be used every second or third week; since aggressive therapy may not be necessary, cytosine arabinoside can be left out of the protocol. Another method that has been used to induce remission is a combination of chlorambucil (Leukeran, Burroughs Wellcome) at a dosage of 2 mg/m² BSA, PO, every other day; methotrexate (Methotrexate, Lederle) at a dosage of 2.5 mg/m² BSA, PO, two or three times a week; and prednisone (20 mg/m² BSA, PO, every other day). The patients should be evaluated every 4 to 6 weeks; particular attention should be paid to the primary tumor site, lymph nodes, liver, and spleen. A complete blood count, platelet count, and serum biochemical profile should be obtained at the time of each examination.

2. For multifocal ENL, surgery is recommended only as a means of obtaining a tissue sample or when gastrointestinal masses are causing an obstruction or perforation. Intensive chemotherapy (Table 4) is given in an attempt to induce complete tumor remission (disappearance of tumor masses). After 6 to 10 weeks of *induction chemotherapy*, the patient is treated with a *maintenance drug* combination (e.g., chlorambucil, methotrexate, and prednisone) only if the patient is considered to be in complete remission. If complete remission is not achieved, *intensification* with agents such as L-asparaginase (Elspar, Merck, Sharp & Dohme) at a dosage of 10,000 to 20,000 IU/m² BSA, subcutaneously (single dose) should be used before the dog is started on maintenance therapy.

3. For CNS lymphomas, craniospinal irradiation constitutes a safe and effective way of achieving tumor cytoreduction and thus decreasing CSF pressure. Intrathecal cytosine arabinoside, at the dosage described under Neural Lymphomas, may be useful in inducing remission. A risk, however, is that collection of CSF before the injection may cause a tentorial herniation if the intracranial pressure is markedly elevated.

4. Occasionally, solitary ENL (e.g., epidural masses) can be effectively treated with external beam irradiation as described above. Adjuvant chemotherapy should also be used in those cases.

References and Supplemental Reading

Couto, C. G., Cullen, J., Pedroia, V., et al.: Central nervous system lymphosarcoma in the dog. J.A.V.M.A. 184:809, 1984.

Duncan, J. R., and Prasse, K. W.: Cytology of canine round cell tumors. Vet. Pathol. 16:673, 1979.

Priester, W. A., and McKay, F. W.: The occurrence of tumors in domestic animals. *Natl. Cancer Inst. Monograph No. 54,* 1980, pp. 31–43; 59–71.

Rudders, R. A., Ross, M. E., and DeLellis, R. A.: Primary extranodal lymphoma: Response to treatment and factors influencing prognosis. Cancer 42:406, 1978.

Theilen, G. H., and Madewell, B. R.: Leukemia-sarcoma disease complex. *In* Theilen, G. H., and Madewell, B. R.: *Veterinary Cancer Medicine.* Philadelphia: Lea & Febiger, 1979, pp. 204–288.

FELINE MAMMARY HYPERTROPHY-FIBROADENOMA COMPLEX

DAVID W. HAYDEN, D.V.M.,
and KENNETH H. JOHNSON, D.V.M.
St. Paul, Minnesota

Feline mammary hypertrophy (FMH) is a benign condition, seen predominantly in young, sexually intact female cats in which one or more mammary glands show abnormally rapid growth and subsequent enlargement. Pregnant, neutered, and non-neutered cats that have been given progestins also are affected. Synonyms for FMH include fibroepithelial hyperplasia, fibroadenomatous hyperplasia, fibroadenomatosis, total or partial fibroadenomatous change, and fibroadenoma. The latter term arose largely because of morphologic similarities between FMH and certain mammary tumors found in rats and women. Current evidence indicates that FMH represents a hormone-dependent or hormone-responsive non-neoplastic proliferation of mammary duct epithelium and stroma. Clinical awareness of

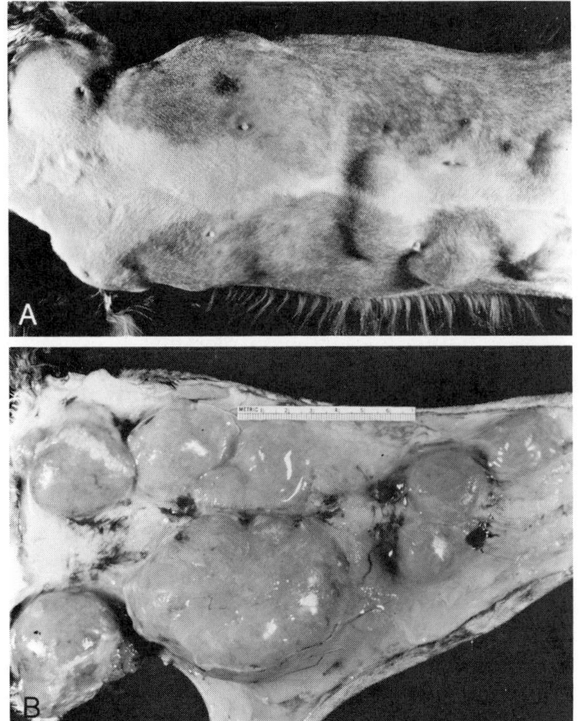

Figure 1. *A*, mammary hypertrophy in an 8-month-old, nonpregnant, female cat. The left thoracic gland (top) is greatly enlarged. *B*, area shown in *A*, viewed from the subcutaneous surface. The axillary (left), thoracic, and abdominal mammary glands are asymmetrically enlarged.

this condition is important because of (1) its association with both natural and synthetic progestational substances and (2) the need to distinguish it from mammary carcinoma, which is a more common condition in cats.

CLINICOPATHOLOGIC FINDINGS

Mammary hypertrophy usually occurs in female cats aged two years and younger (range is 3 months to over 10 years) that are having estrous cycles; there is no apparent breed predilection. All mammary glands may be symmetrically enlarged or, alternatively, only a few glands may be involved (Fig. 1). Multiple lesions can occur in mammary glands, making it possible to have more swellings than there are glands. Affected glands vary considerably in size (from 2 or 3 cm to about 10 cm in diameter), and in some instances, the overlying skin is tense, erythematous, and necrotic. Milk secretion is uncommon. Enlarged glands that are soft on palpation consist of glistening, pinkish-white to cream-colored tissue with the consistency of fat, whereas palpably firm lesions are meaty or shiny white and more difficult to cut. The sectioned surface is often finely lobulated and may contain yellowish-red areas and small cysts. The entire mass may be partially or completely surrounded by mammary duct walls and may or may not exhibit fluid accumulation.

Microscopically, FMH is characterized by concomitant proliferation of mammary duct epithelium and stroma, which often assumes a distinct lobular pattern of growth. The complexity of tubular development and the degree of involvement of preexistent mammary lobules varies between lesions. Generally, more than 50 per cent of the lesion consists of stroma, although both epithelial and mesenchymal cells commonly display mitotic activity. The stroma is edematous and loosely organized in some hypertrophied glands, yet it is collagenous and compact in others. Both pericanalicular and intracanalicular growth patterns are encountered. Hemorrhages and focal areas of coagulation necrosis occur about 5 per cent of the time.

HORMONAL RELATIONSHIPS

Clinical reproductive histories indicate that FMH occurs (1) in the luteal phase of the estrous cycle, (2) in the early stages of pregnancy, and (3) after administration of progestins.

Corpora lutea are present when the ovaries of estrous-cycling cats with mammary hypertrophy are examined. Mammary hypertrophy often occurs 2 to 4 weeks after estrus, which coincides with follicular luteinization and increased serum progesterone levels. In normal cats, serum progesterone increases rapidly to peak at approximately 24 ng/ml (if the cat is not pregnant) and 35 ng/ml (if it is pregnant) by day 21. Progesterone values as high as 20.5 ng/ml have been recorded in a nonpregnant cat with mammary hypertrophy (Hayden, unpublished data).

Pregnant cats that develop mammary hypertrophy usually do so during the first 4 to 5 weeks of the gestation period. Abortion results in complete resolution of these lesions. Thus, during pregnancy, FMH appears to represent an exaggerated response of the prelactational mammary tissue to progesterone.

Mammary hypertrophy in neutered male and female cats given the synthetic progestins megestrol acetate (Ovaban, Schering) and medroxyprogesterone acetate (Depo-Provera, Upjohn) provides strong circumstantial evidence to implicate progesterone in the pathogenesis of this condition. It would appear, however, that FMH is a relatively uncommon sequela to the administration of these agents, which are used to suppress estrus and to treat a variety of dermatologic and behavioral problems in cats. Approximately 3 per cent of the cats treated for skin disorders at the University of Minnesota developed mammary hypertrophy when given megestrol acetate at a dosage of 5 mg daily for 1 week followed by 5 mg/week for up to 2 years (McKeever, 1984). Progestins, given at various total dosages, usually require months (to years) to produce mammary hypertrophy in cats. For example, in one neutered male, 2.5 mg of megestrol acetate daily for 60 days was sufficient to cause enlargement of one gland. Also, a single 100-mg dose of medroxyprogesterone acetate, given parenterally to prevent urine spraying, caused hypertrophy of one mammary gland in a neutered male four months after treatment. Studies of these cats and other such reports give the impression that synthetic progestins usually affect only one or two glands rather than the entire mammary system of neutered male and female cats. In addition, long-term administration of progestins has been associated with mammary cancer in cats (Hernandez et al., 1975; Tomlinson et al., 1984).

The presence of progesterone receptors (PR) but no estrogen receptors (ER) in cats with mammary hypertrophy (Hayden et al., 1981) and mammary carcinomas (Johnston et al., 1984) supports the observation that progesterone has a role in the genesis of these conditions. Whether treatment with progesterone or synthetic progestins increases the number of cytoplasmic PRs, as occurs in the uterus and mammary gland of beagles, is not known. The PR-positive and ER-negative status of FMH and mammary carcinoma is puzzling, since induction of PR in most mammalian tissues is regulated by estrogen. Furthermore, oral therapy with tamoxifen (Nolvadex, Stuart Pharmaceuticals), an anti-estrogen, caused no tumor regression when used in three cats with mammary carcinomas (Johnston et al., 1984). The value of additive or ablative endocrine therapy in ER-negative, PR-positive feline mammary tumors awaits further study.

It is also feasible that progestins may act directly or indirectly by modifying the actions of other hormones that influence the mammary gland. Competition by progestins for glucocorticoid binding sites has been demonstrated in mammary carcinoma and in lactating mammary glands. Since glucocorticoids are involved in mammary gland maturation, it seems plausible that progestins may affect mammary tumor growth by altering glucocorticoid activity. For example, megestrol acetate, which appears to have a long metabolic half-life in the cat, causes significant suppression of adrenal cortical function when administered at the "recommended dose" (Chastain et al., 1981). In dogs, medroxyprogesterone acetate has similar glucocorticoid activity, and it also stimulates secretion of growth hormone (Concannon et al., 1980). One effect of growth hormone in dogs is an increased incidence of mammary nodules. In addition, medroxyprogesterone acetate has potent androgenic properties, suggesting that the effects of some progestins may be mediated by way of the androgen receptor (Janne et al., 1978). Thus, it appears that progesterone, alone or in combination with other hormones, is the pivotal factor in the pathogenesis of FMH.

This scenario would not be complete without mentioning the rare occurrence of mammary hypertrophy in neutered female cats with no history of progestin therapy. In one cat, a two-and-one-half-year-old female that was neutered at 6 months of age, the entire mammary chain was involved (Seiler et al., 1979). In another cat, a 7-month-old female, ovariohysterectomy caused regression of diffuse mammary hypertrophy only to be followed three months after surgery by re-enlargement of the posterior pairs of mammary glands with galactorrhea (McKeever, 1984). Possibly unknown sources of endogenous progestogens or other hormonal inter-relationships were involved, but these were not substantiated by hormonal assay in either cat.

DIAGNOSIS AND THERAPY

Diagnosis of FMH is based on signalment, age of the patient, sexual status, and reproductive history (including treatment with progestins). Differentiation of FMH from mammary carcinoma is essential, as the latter has a dismal prognosis and occurs in older cats. These conditions are readily distinguished by microscopic evaluation of mammary tissue obtained by surgical biopsy or surgical excision. The value of aspiration cytology or tissue-core needle biopsy as a means to diagnose FMH needs to be determined.

Therapy consists of removing the inciting cause (i.e., source of progesterone), the mammary swellings, or both. In young, estrous-cycling females, ovariohysterectomy usually effects complete remission, but spontaneous resolution of mammary hypertrophy is also known to occur. Mastectomy may be required for some hypertrophied mammary glands. For neutered male or female cats on progestins, mastectomy and drug withdrawal are the treatment of choice. Certain luteolytic agents might theoretically provide an alternative to ovariectomy for valuable breeding cats.

References and Supplemental Reading

Allen, H. L.: Feline mammary hypertrophy. Vet. Pathol. 109:501, 1973.

Chastain, C. B., Graham, C. L., and Nichols, C. E.: Adrenocortical suppression in cats given megestrol acetate. Am. J. Vet. Res. 42:2029, 1981.

Concannon, P., Altszuler, N., Hampshire, J., et al.: Growth hormone, prolactin and cortisol in dogs developing mammary nodules and an acromegaly-like appearance during treatment with medroxyprogesterone acetate. Endocrinology 106:1173, 1980.

Dorn, A. S., Legendre, A. M., and McGavin, M. D.: Mammary hyperplasia in a male cat receiving progesterone. J.A.V.M.A. 182:621, 1983.

Hayden, D. W., Johnston, S. D., Kiang, D. T., et al.: Feline mammary hypertrophy/fibroadenoma complex: Clinical and hormonal aspects. Am. J. Vet. Res. 42:1699–1703, 1981.

Hayden, D. W., Johnson, K. H., and Ghobrial, H. K.: Ultrastructure of feline mammary hypertrophy. Vet. Pathol. 20:254, 1983.

Hernandez, F. J., Fernandez, B. B., Chertack, M. C., et al.: Feline mammary carcinoma and progestogens. Feline Pract. 5:45, 1975.

Hinton, M., and Gaskell, C. J.: Non-neoplastic mammary hypertrophy in the cat associated either with pregnancy or with oral progestagen therapy. Vet. Rec. 100:277, 1977.

Janne, O., Kontula, K., Vihko, R., et al.: Progesterone receptor and regulation of progestin action in mammalian tissues. Med. Biol. 56:225, 1978.

Johnston, S. D., Hayden, D. W., Kiang, D. T., et al.: Progesterone receptors in feline mammary adenocarcinomas. Am. J. Vet. Res. 45:379, 1984.

Mandelli, G., and Finazzi, M.: Histopathologische befunde bei dem milchdrüsen-hypertrophie-fibroadenomkomplex der katze. D.T.W. 90:482, 1983.

McKeever, P. J.: Personal communication, 1984.

Seiler, R. J., Kelly, W. R., Menrath, V. H., et al.: Total fibroadenomatous change of the mammary glands of two spayed cats. Feline Pract. 9:25, 1979.

Tomlinson, M. J., Barteaux, L., Ferns, L. E., et al.: Feline mammary carcinoma: A retrospective evaluation of 17 cases. Can. Vet. J. 25:435, 1984.

THE MANAGEMENT OF CANINE MAMMARY TUMORS

ANDREW S. LOAR, D.V.M.
Hermosa Beach, California

The most common tumor in the female dog is of mammary gland origin. Likewise in this species, malignant mammary tumors are by far the leading form of cancer. In dogs of both sexes, only the skin shows a higher reported occurrence rate of neoplastic disease. However, virtually every published review during the past two decades has lamented the limited accumulated knowledge regarding the biologic behavior, significant prognostic features, and optimal therapeutic management of these neoplasms. One explanation for this is that most dogs with mammary tumors are treated by the general practitioner rather than at referral centers, and thus large amounts of data concerning disease outcome are seldom available or reported. Secondly, mammary neoplasms exhibit considerable variety in their historical, clinical, and histologic appearance. For these reasons, prediction of both tumor behavior and response to therapy in a dog with a mammary neoplasm may be extremely difficult and subjective. Nonetheless, an accurate prognosis is valuable to the clinician in selecting the most appropriate treatment. Certain characteristics of canine mammary gland tumors are of proven, or suspected, prognostic significance and are discussed herein. Surgical, adjunctive, and palliative therapies will be described and are recommended based on the prognosis for each stage of tumor.

The approximate median age of dogs with mammary tumors is 10 to 11 years. The reported ages range from 2 to 20 years; however, mammary neoplasia in bitches younger than five years is extremely uncommon. Although most studies of breed predilection have not examined the prevalance of various breeds in the population, cocker spaniels, poodles, and fox and Boston terriers appear to have a higher risk for the development of mammary tumors than other pure-bred or cross-bred dogs; chihuahuas and boxers are reported to be at a decreased risk. Some oncologists have observed that mammary cancer in the German shepherd shows a more malignant behavior than in other breeds. These tumors are very rare in male dogs, accounting for about 1 per cent of all reported mammary neoplasms. Similar to the case in humans, most mammary tumors in the male dog are aggressive cancers.

BIOLOGIC BEHAVIOR AND CLINICAL FEATURES

The tumor characteristics that are most important to the clinician are those associated with an unfavorable prognosis. Certainly, histologic features of malignancy correlate with a poor long-term prognosis; however, other clinical factors also have significant impact on the disease outcome. These include the mode and rate of growth of the tumor, the total volume of tumor at the time of presentation, and the involvement of regional or distant lymph nodes.

The rate of tumor growth and duration of clinical

signs frequently can be determined by a careful history. Animals with mammary cancer are often presented with a complaint of rapid increase in tumor size. Generally, the duration of disease prior to surgical removal of the tumor is longer for benign tumors than for carcinomas; the reported median interval is of 8 to 12 months and 4 to 6 months, respectively (Fidler and Brodey, 1967). However, other studies have found no correlation between duration of signs and prognosis. Rapid growth, or regrowth, usually indicates an aggressive malignancy and is considered a negative prognostic finding. An exception to this occurs when a benign lesion results in the rapid development of a large, fluid-filled cyst or hematoma. Another special problem is that of sessile, presumably benign nodules transforming after several months or years into invasive, rapidly growing cancers. This is not an infrequent event, nor is it predictable. Likewise, biopsies of small, slow growing nodules may reveal foci of malignant cells. These observations emphasize two principles in the management of mammary tumors. First, postponement of surgical excision of a tumor should not be based on the clinical appearance or history of the mass. Second, to provide the most accurate prognosis, all tumors should be submitted for histologic examination.

The mode of growth of a neoplasm is often an indicator of its relative invasiveness. Well-circumscribed, also called expansive, lesions are more readily excised and thus have a better prognosis than those with less distinct borders. Gross infiltration of the skin, either with or without ulceration, or of tissues deep to the mammary glands suggests an aggressive tumor and a high postoperative recurrence rate. Often, however, assessment for degree of invasiveness is most reliable when based on microscopic examination of biopsy sections (see the following discussion of histopathology).

Enlargement of regional lymph nodes secondary to neoplastic infiltration implies a high metastatic potential for the tumor. Nevertheless, Misdorp and Hart (1979) found that the presence or lack of nodal or lymphatic vessel involvement was not associated with significant differences in survival in dogs whose mammary cancers were treated by surgical excision. In profound contrast, Gilbertson and his colleagues (1983) showed that microscopic evidence of tumor invasion into lymph nodes or vessels was highly significant and correlated with a 95 per cent recurrence rate. This author believes that management recommendations should be offered based on the latter study and emphasizes the importance of gross as well as microscopic evaluation of lymphatic structures, particularly the lymph nodes draining the excised tumor. In addition to tumor cell infiltration, gross lymphadenopathy may occur because of inflammation or other causes of reactive hyperplasia.

An uncommon clinical presentation of mammary neoplasia is the inflammatory carcinoma. This rapidly fulminating condition carries a grave short-term prognosis, and it has been recently described in the dog (Susaneck et al., 1983). Animals with inflammatory carcinoma typically show multiple gland involvement, often with both mammary chains affected. The tumor is frequently warm and painful and may be hyperemic. In addition, edema is commonly manifest in the mammary glands, overlying skin, and the nearest limb. Laboratory analysis may reveal anemia and, occasionally, disseminated intravascular coagulation; the latter problem increases the risks of subsequent surgical intervention. Nearly all dogs with this condition have systemic metastatic disease at the time of presentation. Metastasis to regional and distant nodes, as well as to the lungs, has been reported. Surgical resection is seldom complete, and frequently it is followed by rapid recurrence. Adjuvant therapy, discussed later in this article, is unlikely to control tumor progression.

The value of the clinical characteristics described above is that they provide the clinician a subjective, relative prognosis for each patient. If several clinical features could be collected and then developed into a system capable of predicting tumor behavior in a quantitative fashion, then this system could be useful in comparing results of various treatments. This is the concept of a clinical staging system. The stage of a tumor represents the extent of disease involvement, and it is calculated by choosing the clinical characteristics that are of the most prognostic significance. The clinical characteristics that show the highest influence on disease outcome include the total volume of the primary tumor, the degree of local invasion, the number and extent of regional lymph node involvement, and the presence of distant metastatic disease. This Tumor-Node-Metastasis (TNM) system has been developed for staging most of the common neoplasms of companion animals and was offered to veterinary clinicians in 1980 by the World Health Organization (WHO).

The WHO staging protocol for canine mammary tumors (Table 1) classifies four stages of mammary cancer. Although several studies have examined the prognostic significance of selected clinical factors, none of the reports in the literature have used this staging protocol in an attempt to correlate the stage of disease with a specific prognosis. The author has recently retrospectively evaluated 204 dogs presented to the Animal Medical Center (AMC) in New York for treatment of mammary tumors. At initial examination, no animals showed evidence of distant metastatic disease (i.e., no stage IV tumors). The goal of therapy was to render the dogs free of all gross disease; in each case this was achieved by mastectomy or by modified or complete unilateral radical mastectomy. All dogs were monitored for clinical evidence of disease recurrence for at least 2

*Table 1. Clinical Staging System for Canine Mammary Tumors**

Stage Grouping	T	N	M
I	T_1	N_0 (−) or any N a(−)	M_0
II	T_0	N_1 (+)	M_0
	T_1	N_1 (+)	M_0
	T_2	N_0 (+) or N_1 a(+)	M_0
III	T_3	Any N	M_0
	Any T	Any N b	M_0
IV	Any T	Any N	M_1

*Modified from Owen, L. N. (ed.): *The TNM Classification of Tumours in Domestic Animals.* Geneva: World Health Organization, 1980.

KEY: T (Primary Tumor): T_0 = no evidence of tumor; T_1 = tumor less than 1 cm maximum diameter; T_2 = tumor 1 to 3 cm maximum diameter; T_3 = tumor more than 3 cm maximum diameter; T_4 = tumor any size, inflammatory carcinoma; N (Regional Lymph Nodes [RLN]): N_0 = no RLN involved; N_1 = ipsilateral RLN involved; N_2 = bilateral RLN involved; a = not fixed; b = fixed; − = histologically negative; + = histologically positive; M (Distant Metastasis): M_0 = no evidence of distant metastasis; M_1 = distant metastasis.

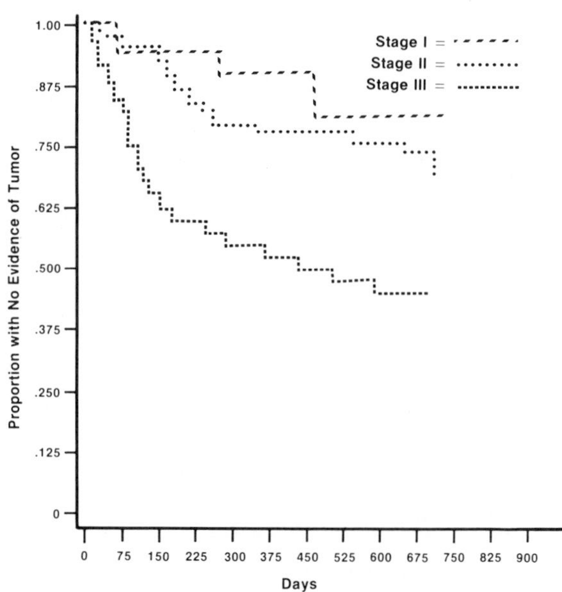

Figure 1. Recurrence (by clinical stage) of mammary tumors in 204 dogs treated with surgical excision. All tumors were diagnosed as adenocarcinomas by using standard, WHO-based histologic criteria. Only animals in stages I, II, and III are included. No significant difference was detected between dogs with stage I and stage II cancers.

years after surgery. The objective of this study was to assess the prognostic significance of the clinical staging (TNM) system. For all malignancies, irrespective of the histologic type, animals presented with stage III tumors (i.e., dogs with primary tumors larger than 3 cm in diameter, with or without lymph node infiltration and fixation) showed a significantly higher risk of disease recurrence within 2 years of surgical excision than did dogs with stage I or stage II tumors (Fig. 1).

Clinical features that do not appear to be of consistent prognostic significance for dogs with mammary gland neoplasia include (1) the location of the primary tumor burden within the mammary chain; (2) whether tumors are located in single or many mammary glands; (3) right-sided versus left-sided mammary chain involvement; and (4) the surgical procedure used to remove each tumor (this includes nodulectomy, simple mastectomy, *en bloc* mastectomy, and complete unilateral mastectomy).

HISTOPATHOLOGY

The development of histopathologic classification systems for canine mammary tumors and the examination of their prognostic significance are among the most controversial topics in veterinary oncology. Morphologically, canine mammary neoplasia is an extremely heterogenous disease. Theilen and Madewell (1979) summarized tumor classification schemes used by various authors and showed that in some systems as many as 22 distinct types of benign and malignant mammary neoplasms have been described. Clearly, the intent of most of these systems was to give the pathologist precise, morphologically descriptive names for as many tumor types as possible. In 1974, the WHO published a classification scheme that, in some form, is used by many veterinary pathologists. The system allows the classification and diagnosis of more than 19 different tumor types. The morphologic basis of this scheme is complex, and it is reviewed elsewhere (Brodey et al., 1983). Table 2 summarizes the various tumor types.

Generally, clinicians evaluating a surgical pathology report of a canine mammary tumor have found it difficult to correlate the WHO histologic diagnosis with a specific prognosis. Some data from mammary tumor studies may be useful, however. Dogs with a diagnosis either of the simple-type or the complex-type of carcinoma appear to have a better prognosis than those given a diagnosis of sarcoma. The latter diagnosis is associated with a recurrence rate of greater than 90 per cent within 2 years of initial surgery, whereas dogs with adenocarcinomas (either simple or complex types) have shown two-year survival rates of about 60 per cent (Misdorp and Hart, 1976; Else and Hannant, 1979). Regarding other WHO types of mammary cancers, Bostock (1975) reported that dogs with carcinomas of the papillary or tubular form have a better overall prognosis than those with solid or anaplastic carcinomas. Papillary and tubular adenocarcinomas are

Table 2. *Different Morphologic Forms of Canine Mammary Tumors**

Benign Mammary Tumors
Benign mixed tumor
Complex adenoma
Fibroadenoma
  Intracanalicular type
  Pericanalicular type
Duct Papilloma
Simple adenoma

Malignant Mammary Tumors
Tubular adenocarcinoma
  Simple and complex types
Papillary adenocarcinoma
  Simple and complex types
Papillary cystic adenocarcinoma
  Simple and complex types
Solid carcinoma
  Simple and complex types
Anaplastic carcinoma
Other carcinomas
  Mucinous, squamous cell, spindle cell
Sarcomas
  Osteosarcoma, fibrosarcoma, and combined forms
Malignant mixed tumor (carcinosarcoma)

*Based on the International Histological Classification of Tumors of Domestic Animals published by the World Health Organization, 1974. Modified from Theilen and Madewell: *Veterinary Cancer Medicine.* Philadelphia: Lea & Febiger, 1979, pp. 192–203.

associated with tumor-related death rates of 21 per cent and 32 per cent, respectively, 2 years after initial surgery. For dogs with solid carcinomas and those with anaplastic carcinomas the tumor-related death rates after 2 years are 53 per cent and 76 per cent, respectively. Few studies have attempted to confirm these findings, however, and more recent reports have disputed their significance.

Dogs with any of the benign forms of mammary neoplasms listed in Table 2 are at minimal risk for tumor recurrence; however, if any normal mammary tissues remain after tumor removal, these animals eventually may develop new primary tumors. In at least one large study (Gilbertson et al., 1983), restrospective comparisons of mammary tumor diagnoses derived by different histologic classification systems revealed that a number of neoplasms previously considered malignant by a WHO-based system were classified as nonmalignant by a newer system. Demonstration that pathologists using various histologic systems may disagree over a feature as fundamental as whether a lesion is benign or malignant is not surprising. In a historical review of more than 5000 dogs whose mammary tumors were removed and submitted for biopsy, slightly less than 50 per cent were given a histologic diagnosis of cancer (Brodey et al., 1983). Traditionally, about 50 per cent of dogs with biopsy-proven malignant mammary tumors suffer recurrence or metastasis after surgical excision; this appears to be true irrespective of the type of surgical procedure used. Thus, although about one half of all canine mammary tumors show a malignant histologic appearance, only about one quarter of the total behave in a malignant fashion subsequent to tumor removal.

To the clinical oncologist, the usefulness of a histologic diagnosis lies in its ability to predict a tumor's biologic behavior. A surgical cure in one half of all dogs with biopsy-proven mammary cancer suggests that the diagnosis of malignancy is offered too liberally. The fault is not with the pathologist who examines the tissues but in the criteria that are used to make the diagnosis. If neither the criteria nor the diagnosis can be shown to have good correlation with prognosis, then the classification system that contains them should be abandoned. Each of the following histologic findings has consistently been correlated with an unfavorable prognosis: evidence of microscopic invasion into tissues past the boundaries of tumor stroma; tumor invasion into lymph nodes, lymph vessels, and blood vessels; features indicative of mammary sarcoma; and features indicative of cellular anaplasia.

In a mammary neoplasm with cellular morphology suggestive of a carcinoma, tumor extension into normal adjacent tissue distinguishes an invasive cancer from a well-circumscribed, also called *in situ,* malignancy. Demonstration of this feature is more likely when at least two or three sections from the tumor are examined. This is particularly important, because many dogs with evidence of invasive cancer also have foci of *in situ* carcinoma elsewhere in the mastectomy specimen (Gilbertson et al., 1983). In addition and not infrequently, a pathologist may interpret carcinoma cells infiltrating into surrounding areas of less malignant-appearing neoplastic tissue as evidence of invasion; in fact, this finding represents carcinoma *in situ.* Clinically, well-circumscribed mammary cancers generally appear as distinct nodules within normal glandular tissue. If the histologic diagnosis is discordant with the clinical impression, this author recommends discussion between clinician and pathologist.

Invasive, also called infiltrative, carcinoma is associated with a significantly higher recurrence rate than noninvasive carcinoma. For this article, recurrence implies postoperative development of either local tumor or regional or distant metastatic lesions. In the studies mentioned, histologically invasive neoplasms had a tumor-related death or a recurrence rate of greater than 70 per cent within 2 years of surgical resection (Fowler et al., 1974; Bostock, 1975; Else and Hannant, 1979; Gilbertson et al., 1983). Except in the study by Else and Hannant (1979), histologically well-circumscribed carcinomas have been associated with less than a 25 per cent rate of tumor-related death or recurrence after 2 years. In the latter report, 40 per cent of dogs with noninfiltrative carcinomas developed, or died from, tumor recurrence within 2 years of diagnosis. Many authors consider these so-called preinvasive malignant mammary proliferations to be precursor lesions of invasive mammary cancer. This concept has been used to justify early mastectomy for the treatment of discrete nodular lesions.

Histologic evidence of tumor invasion into lymph nodes or lymphatic or blood vessels is discussed earlier and appears to represent a poor prognosis. Obviously, submission of adequate tissue specimens and the examination of at least several sections are necessary for evaluation of these features.

The demonstration of highly anaplastic cells is another negative prognostic finding in dogs with mammary carcinomas. Anaplastic tumors are nearly always infiltrative and thus are associated with a recurrence rate similar to that of invasive cancers. All infiltrative carcinomas, however, are not necessarily of the anaplastic form. Because both tumor types are aggressive, it is difficult to determine if anaplastic (invasive) carcinomas correlate with a different prognosis than the invasive nonanaplastic cancers.

The frequency of sarcomas of the canine mammary gland is low, probably accounting for less than 10 per cent of all mammary tumors. Osteosarcoma, compound osteochondrosarcoma (osteochondrosarcoma), and fibrosarcoma are the most commonly reported cell types; often, however, the tumor cells are too poorly differentiated for the tissue origin to be determined. Mammary sarcomas do not often metastasize to regional or distant sites, either before or after surgical removal. Local tumor regrowth is very likely, however, with a recurrence rate approaching 100 per cent. Severe local problems such as ulceration, infection, and difficulties with locomotion may arise in these dogs, and most animals with recurrent mammary sarcomas will die as a result of their disease within 1 or 2 years of initial therapy. In mammary tumor biopsy specimens showing no evidence of sarcomatous lesions, the demonstration of nonmalignant proliferative mesenchymal elements such as bone, cartilage, and hyperplastic myoepithelial cells is usually not associated with an unfavorable prognosis.

As many as 65 per cent of dogs presented for mammary neoplasia show evidence of multiple gland involvement. Examination of all excised tumors frequently reveals both malignant and benign lesions, and several different histologic types may be noted. The likelihood of disease recurrence in dogs with multiple gland involvement is related to the most aggressive lesion found. Additional less-malignant tumors in adjacent tissues do not appear to worsen the prognosis.

SURGICAL THERAPY

Compared with the discussion of histopathologic classification systems, the review of treatment regimens for canine mammary tumors is much less complex. Surgical excision of the neoplasm provides the biopsy specimens necessary for a reliable diagnosis and is the single best method for elimination of all visible disease. At present, the indication for postoperative (adjuvant) therapy is histologic evidence suggesting a high risk of tumor recurrence (i.e., invasive cancer). Forms of adjunctive therapy that may be helpful include the administration of cytotoxic drugs, radiotherapy, and the use of biological response modifiers (immunotherapy).

For most dogs presented with mammary neoplasia the therapeutic objective is to remove all gross evidence of tumor by surgical resection. Exceptions to this include those animals having inflammatory carcinoma or distant metastatic (i.e., stage IV) disease. Among dogs with mammary cancer, the high recurrence rate indicates failure to remove all foci of malignant cells in at least 50 per cent of cases treated with mastectomy. Thus, at the time of initial therapy, at least one half of all dogs with malignant tumors either have cancer cells extending beyond the confines of the resected mammary tissues or have some involvement of regional lymph nodes or more distant sites. Thorough evaluation, including thoracic radiographs, appropriate laboratory analyses, and careful palpation of all mammary glands, peripheral lymph nodes, adjacent soft tissue, and bony structures, is a necessary prerequisite to surgical treatment.

If only local disease is detected, the surgeon has a choice of four procedures: *Nodulectomy* (lumpectomy), the isolated removal of the tumor (or tumors) from within the gland; *simple mastectomy*, the removal of one or more affected glands; *en bloc mastectomy* (modified radical mastectomy), the removal of a group of glands dependent on their lymphatic drainage; and *complete unilateral mastectomy* (radical mastectomy), the removal of all mammary glands ipsilateral to the tumor or tumors, intervening tissues, and regional lymph nodes. The clinical stage and site of involvement as well as the general condition of the dog should dictate which procedure is used.

Nodulectomy has the advantage of being a rapid, low-cost technique for the excision of small, well-circumscribed nodules, such as in dogs with stage I disease. When performed under sedation and local anesthesia, it should result in minimal morbidity to the aged, unhealthy patient. However, because very little of the normal surrounding tissues are removed, it is not possible to evaluate these specimens for histologic evidence of invasiveness or lymph node involvement. If the biopsy subsequently reveals malignancy, then a more aggressive resection, such as a simple or *en bloc* mastectomy, is indicated. Additionally, for dogs with mammary tumors in many glands, *en bloc* or complete unilateral mastectomy may be more practical initially.

The primary disadvantage of simple mastectomy is that, because most canine mammary glands are intimately associated with their fellow ipsilateral glands, isolated removal of a single gland is often more difficult than an *en bloc* resection. Also, unless tumor involves the most posterior (fifth) or the most anterior (first) gland, access to the nearest lymph node is not possible without removal of more than one gland. Review of the regional lymphatics reveals the usefulness of the *en bloc* mastectomy.

The proposed lymphatic drainage of mammary tumors suggests that metastatic cells from glands 1, 2, and 3 generally traverse cranially to the axillary lymph node, whereas cells from glands 4, 5, and, occasionally, gland 3 usually drain caudally to the inguinal node. This scheme was developed from a retrospective necropsy examination of the metastatic pattern of 65 bitches with mammary cancer (Fidler and Brodey, 1967) but has not been confirmed and reported in more recent studies. Nevertheless, the recommended surgical treatment of the majority of canine mammary tumors is the *en bloc* mastectomy technique based on these drainage routes. Tumors in glands 1 or 2 or both are removed by resection of the three most cranial ipsilateral glands and interposing tissue; the axillary node should also be taken if tumor infiltration is suspected. Tumors in glands 4 or 5 or both are removed by resection of the three most caudal ipsilateral glands and intervening tissue; the inguinal lymph node generally adheres to the resected specimen and should be removed, separated, and tagged for histologic examination and clinical staging. Tumors associated with gland 3 should be resected by complete unilateral mastectomy; axillary and inguinal lymph nodes should be left intact or removed as described above. Similarly, this should be the treatment of choice for removal of multiple tumors in both anterior and posterior glands. A less aggressive method for managing tumors in gland 3 is through simple mastectomy.

Theilen and Madewell (1979), this author, and others recommend the *en bloc* mastectomy over complete unilateral mastectomy for most mammary tumors. Certainly, the former technique should be associated with less overall morbidity and expense. Recently, a prospective, randomized trial comparing simple and complete unilateral mastectomy procedures was completed by MacEwen and colleagues (see Harvey and Gilbertson, 1977). Similar to previous retrospective reports, this unpublished study found no significant differences in the rate of tumor-related death or recurrence in dogs presented for mammary carcinoma that were treated with either type of surgery.

Intraoperatively, the surgeon should be prepared for extensive dissection if visible tumor invades into tissues adjacent to the mammary glands. In addition, evidence of dermal infiltration indicates the removal of the overlying skin during the mastectomy procedure. Large surgical wounds may be managed either with or without the placement of subcutaneous drains, rather than by attempts to close the dead space with a large amount of buried absorbable suture (Bright, 1979). Skin closure is best achieved by a continuous subcutaneous pattern followed by apposing-type and, where needed, tension sutures. Aggressive tacking of skin and subcutaneous tissues to deeper structures is seldom necessary.

Monitoring after initial surgical therapy is dependent on the initial clinical stage and histologic diagnosis. Dogs with an increased likelihood for tumor recurrence should be rechecked at least every 1 to 3 months with thoracic radiographs obtained at every other examination visit. In animals with *in situ* carcinoma, rechecks may be scheduled at 3- to 6-month intervals with radiographic evaluation of the chest every 6 months. Benign tumors suggest less aggressive postoperative monitoring, although new primary tumors may still develop.

ADJUVANT THERAPY

Adjuvant therapy offers the most benefit when tumor volume is minimal. The clinician should consider these forms of treatments if the preoperative clinical stage or the histologic diagnosis (or both) suggests an increased risk for tumor recurrence or tumor-related morbidity. Candidates for adjunctive therapy include dogs with any of the following conditions: (1) clinical stage III cancers, prior to surgery, including histologically well-circumscribed malignancies; (2) tumors of any size that show histologic evidence of invasion into adjacent normal tissues, lymphatic structures, or blood vessels; and (3) animals with recurrent or inoperable local cancer or those with distant metastatic (i.e., stage IV) disease. To date, reports regarding the responses to nonsurgical therapy of canine mammary cancer have been anecdotal and poorly controlled. However, some treatments may give hope to clinicians and owners facing the probability of advancing, fatal disease.

Cytotoxic Drug Therapy

Several protocols for mammary carcinoma have been recommended in the veterinary literature (Theilen and Madewell, 1979; Harvey and Gilbertson, 1977). These regimens utilized combinations of cytotoxic agents and caused minimal adverse effects; however, these researchers have not reported significant antitumor effects from these therapies. In women with advanced mammary carcinoma, the use of doxorubicin (Adriamycin, Adria) as a single agent or doxorubicin-containing protocols has resulted in antitumor response rates superior to those reported for other forms of chemotherapy (Forbes, 1982). In a limited number of dogs with metastatic mammary cancer treated with doxorubicin, the author and others have noted objective antitumor responses. Thus, it appears logical to recommend the drug as adjuvant therapy for this disease. Controlled studies in progress should ultimately determine the effectiveness of this protocol. The dosage, treatment intervals, and toxicities of doxorubicin are reviewed in the article entitled Chemotherapeutic Agents Available for Cancer Treatment.

Radiation Therapy

In women with breast cancer, tumor irradiation is reserved for those patients with bulky, nonresectable local disease, those with inflammatory carcinoma, and those with painful bony metastases. Generally the short-term results are good, although most individuals ultimately die from their tumors. The indications for radiotherapy are similar for dogs with mammary cancer. The intent of this form of therapy is not to provide a cure or long-term control but merely to palliate the animal that suffers from advanced disease. The duration of benefit in the limited number of cases reported has been brief, generally less than 2 to 4 months. However, in spite of a grave short-term prognosis, a few pet owners will tolerate the time, expense, and referral required for these treatments. Occasionally, oncologists and radiotherapists are less enthusiastic to administer palliative therapy than the owners are for their pets to receive it. Clinicians attempting to refer animals for such treatments are encouraged to advise the staff of the referral center regarding the expectations of the owners.

Immunotherapy and Hormonal Manipulation

Various forms of immunotherapy have been studied for use against canine mammary tumors. The major rationale for these treatments is that several types of canine mammary tumors generate cellular responses presumed to represent host-versus-tumor reactivity (Else and Hannant, 1979; Gilbertson et al., 1983). Stimulation of the immune system, particularly after tumor removal, may augment these responses and possibly delay recurrence or progression of the tumor.

The most frequently suggested therapeutic agents are classified as nonspecific immunostimulants and include levamisole, *Corynebacterium parvum*, and bacille Calmette-Guérin (BCG). Levamisole and *C. parvum* have been used in several unpublished trials by MacEwen and colleagues and found to offer no significant benefits. In a study referred to elsewhere (Brodey et al., 1983), intravenous therapy with BCG, compared with placebo therapy, resulted in a significantly lower tumor-associated death rate in dogs that had undergone surgical resection of mammary carcinoma. Although the latter report used WHO histologic criteria to classify the tumors, it remains the most positive study regarding the effectiveness of immunotherapy in animals.

Circulating free tumor antigens, antitumor antibodies, and complexes composed of these antigens and antibodies are all thought to inhibit the host's immune response to its tumor. Researchers have proposed that removal of the immune complexes either by plasmapheresis or selective immunoabsorption may improve the immune reaction and possibly result in tumor regression (Matus, 1983). At present, responses to these forms of treatment have been impressive but have not been widely reported and confirmed.

In women, hormonal manipulations are widely accepted in the adjunctive treatment of mammary cancer. The primary indication for these therapies is the presence of estrogen receptors (ER) on the surface of tumor cells; individuals that are ER-positive are more likely to respond favorably to antiestrogen therapy. However, if patients are ER-negative or if the ER status cannot be determined, no hormonal manipulations are recommended. ER determinations in a limited number of canine mammary tumors have revealed that about 60 per cent express the receptors. However, benign tumors appear to be ER-positive more frequently than malignant tumors, and the most histologically aggressive carcinomas are generally ER-negative. Obviously, most clinicians are not routinely able to assay tumors for estrogen receptors. If future studies confirm that tumors with the poorest prognosis also are usually ER-negative, then the various antiestrogen therapies will rarely be indicated.

Ovariectomy performed before the first estrus virtually eliminates the risk of mammary tumor development in dogs. In dogs spayed after the first heat, and up to the age of 2½ years, the risk for tumor development increases. Neutering after 2½ years of age has no sparing effect on the risk of mammary neoplasia. Likewise, many studies have shown no improvement in the rate of tumor recurrence or tumor-associated death in dogs neutered at the time of mammary tumor removal.

General Palliative Therapy

Not infrequently, owners of dogs with advanced mammary cancer request treatments to improve their pet's quality of life. When irradiation and cytotoxic agents have failed or are not acceptable, the clinician may still achieve short-term palliation with basic supportive therapy. Occasionally, surgical debulking or débridement may provide local control of ulcerated, draining masses; however, postoperative wound complications may also result. Hot packs and systemic antibiotics may improve local, secondary bacterial infections. Massages, hot-water soaks, whirlpool treatments, and other forms of physical therapy may help to control limb edema and local discomfort associated with large tumors.

The judicious use of corticosteroids may control tumor-related tissue necrosis and inflammation. These agents also will often improve the appetite and attitude of animals with advanced malignancy. Nutritional support must include an adequate caloric level in a relatively well-balanced and palatable diet. In concert with an increased protein intake, anabolic steroids should help to improve nitrogen utilization. Although it may not occur until very late in the course of a dog's illness, complete anorexia is rarely tolerated by most pet owners.

Pallative management for metastatic disease is primarily symptomatic. Coughing due to pulmonary involvement may be controlled with antitussives. Pleural effusions due to lymphatic obstruction are best treated with intermittent drainage. The use of diuretics in the management of malignant pleural effusion will likely result in dehydration and electrolyte abnormalities before the volume of pleural fluid decreases significantly. Generally, pulmonary metastases must be diffuse before an animal manifests clinical signs of respiratory disease. In addition, metastatic pulmonary nodules from canine mammary cancer may grow at a relatively slow rate, often taking several months to double in size. Thus, euthanasia should not necessarily be recommended when radiographs first demonstrate pulmonary involvement.

References and Supplemental Reading

Bostock, D. E.: The prognosis following the surgical excision of canine mammary neoplasms. Eur. J. Cancer 11:389, 1975.

Bright, R. N.: Mammary neoplasia. Comp. Cont. Ed. Pract. Vet. 1:774, 1979.

Brodey, R. S., Goldschmidt, M. H., and Roszel, J. R.: Canine mammary gland neoplasms. J. Am. Anim. Hosp. Assoc. 19:61, 1983.

Else, R. W., and Hannant, D.: Some epidemiological aspects of mammary neoplasia in the bitch. Vet. Rec. 104:296, 1979.

Fidler, I. J., and Brodey, R. S.: A necropsy study of canine malignant mammary neoplasms. J.A.V.M.A. 151:710, 1967.

Forbes, J. F.: Advanced breast cancer (and quality of life). Clin. Oncol. 1, 917, 1982.

Fowler, E. H., Wilson, G. P., and Koestner, A.: Biologic behavior of canine mammary neoplasms based on a histogenetic classification. Vet. Pathol. 11:212, 1974.

Gilbertson, S. R., Kurzman, I. D., Zachrau, R. E., et al.: Canine mammary epithelial neoplasms: Biologic implications of morphologic characteristics assessed in 232 dogs. Vet. Pathol. 20:127, 1983.

Harvey, H. J., and Gilbertson, S. R.: Canine mammary gland tumors. Vet. Clin. North Am. 7:213, 1977.

Matus, R. E.: Intensive therapeutic plasmapheresis in veterinary medicine. *In* Kirk, R. W. (ed.): *Current Veterinary Therapy VIII*. Philadelphia: W. B. Saunders, 1983, pp. 442–443.

Misdorp, W., and Hart, A. A. M.: Prognostic factors in canine mammary cancer. J. Nat. Cancer Inst. 56:779, 1976.

Susaneck, S. J., Allen, T. P., Hoopes, J., et al.: Inflammatory mammary carcinoma in the dog. J. Am. Anim. Hosp. Assoc. 19:971, 1983.

Theilen, G., and Madewell, B. R.: Tumors of the mammary gland. *In* Theilen, G., and Madewell, B. R. (eds.): *Veterinary Cancer Medicine*. Philadelphia: Lea & Febiger, 1979, pp. 192–203.

Hematology

HEMATOLOGIC CONSEQUENCES OF FELINE LEUKEMIA VIRUS INFECTION

GARY J. KOCIBA, D.V.M.
Columbus, Ohio

Feline leukemia virus (FeLV) infection has been associated with numerous hematologic abnormalities, including anti-proliferative and proliferative disorders. FeLV infects hematopoietic cells and causes a wide variety of hematologic disorders, such as aplasia, immune cell dysfunction, and neoplasia. The changes are inconsistent and do not follow a uniform pathogenetic sequence, thereby leading one to suspect FeLV infection in a diverse group of hematologic disorders. Evaluation of blood or bone marrow specimens for FeLV infection should be an integral part of the diagnostic work-up of cats with hematologic disease. The recent recognition of latent FeLV infection in cats has added support to epidemiologic studies that implicated FeLV in the pathogenesis of some FeLV-negative diseases. The lack of expression of FeLV proteins by blood or bone marrow cells does not exclude the possibility of FeLV-induced disease.

EFFECTS ON LEUKOCYTES

Lymphocytes are among the first cells infected after oronasal exposure to FeLV. Lymphopenia is a relatively consistent change in experimental FeLV infection. The lymphopenia develops coincidentally with the onset of viremia and persists for a variable amount of time. In cats with natural FeLV infection, 25 to 50 per cent of the cats are lymphopenic; the lymphopenia appears to involve B cells as well as T cells. Reactive lymphocytosis occurs in only a few cats with FeLV infection. Neutropenia is a less common manifestation of FeLV viremia but important because it predisposes such cats to secondary infectious diseases. FeLV is the most common cause of neutropenias in cats that are immune to panleukopenia. It is interesting to note that in some cats, granulocytopenic episodes occur in a 10- to 14-day cyclic pattern reminiscent of cyclic hematopoiesis of other species. The bone marrow varies from hypocellular to hypercellular in granulocytopenic cats, with hypercellularity predominating. In some cats with hypercellular bone marrow, the granulocytopenia is secondary to myeloproliferative disease. Difficulty in aspirating bone marrow from neutropenic or anemic cats should not be interpreted as conclusive evidence for aplasia, because frequently "dry taps" are associated with hypercellular marrows or FeLV-associated medullary osteosclerosis.

The hematologic changes of feline panleukopenia (feline infectious enteritis) are not easily distinguished from FeLV-associated neutropenia, although the lymphocyte count may be somewhat lower in cats with panleukopenia and some FeLV-positive cats simultaneously have severe anemia related to erythroid aplasia. The distinction is complicated by the fact that FeLV-pancytopenic cats may have hemorrhagic enteritis that is very similar to that of feline infectious enteritis. Neutrophilia with a mild left shift is present in about one third of cats with FeLV-associated disease.

Although eosinophilia is sometimes observed in FeLV-infected cats, the change does not appear to be specific. In the few cats with hypereosinophilic syndrome that have been positive for FeLV viremia, the viral proteins have not been detected in eosinophilic leukocytes.

IMMUNODEFICIENCY

Immunodeficiency is one of the most frequent and most important effects of FeLV infection. This defect is related to thymic atrophy in young cats, lymphoid atrophy involving T cell-dependent areas and to lesser extent B cell areas, lymphopenia, and T lymphocyte dysfunction. These changes are described in detail in the Immunology section.

No specific therapy for the immunosuppression has been documented to be consistently beneficial, although immune modification by immunosorption of immune complexes or nonspecific stimulation of immunological responses is being evaluated.

CHANGES IN ERYTHROCYTES

Anemia is one of the most common abnormalities associated with FeLV infection. About 70 per cent of cats with naturally occurring anemia are positive for FeLV viremia. The anemia is nonregenerative in most cats. The onset of the anemia is gradual, and clinical signs often do not become apparent until the anemia is very severe. Reticulocytes with coarse clumping pattern are markedly decreased, and punctate reticulocytes usually are also decreased. The erythrocytes have normal morphology in blood films. The erythrocytic indices indicate macrocytic, normochromic or, occasionally, normocytic, normochromic red cells. Erythrocyte macrocytosis and increased anisocytosis occur in many FeLV-infected cats, and these changes are most prominent in those with anemia. Cats that are not anemic or have nonregenerative anemia and have a mean corpuscular volume of greater than 50 fl (μm^3) by electronic measurements (reference range, 37 to 49 fl) have a high probability of being FeLV positive. The mechanism of the macrocytosis is unknown but may be related to persistent macrocytes from a transient, early regenerative response. The anemia and macrocytosis are unresponsive to vitamin B_{12} and folic acid.

The bone marrow of cats with FeLV-induced nonregenerative anemia is usually normocellular or slightly hypocellular. The ratio of myeloid to erythroid cells is increased, owing to erythroid aplasia. There is a paucity of erythroid precursors but normal representation of granulocytic and megakaryocytic cells. Hemosiderin deposits usually are present. Concentration of serum iron is normal. Ferrokinetic studies have confirmed diminished erythropoiesis with decreased plasma iron clearance and decreased incorporation of radio-labeled iron into erythrocytes. Erythropoietin levels are increased. Erythrocyte survival time, determined by chromium-51–labeled red cells, may be normal or decreased.

Occasional cats have hypercellular bone marrow despite the lack of an erythroid regenerative response. The myeloid/erythroid ratio varies but may be decreased with a disproportionate number of immature erythroid precursors and prominent megoblastic changes. These changes generally are unresponsive to vitamin B_{12} and folic acid and are suggestive for preleukemic changes of myeloproliferative diseases but are not conclusive for neoplasia. A few cats with these hematologic changes have recovered coincidentally with reversion from an FeLV-positive to -negative state.

An erythroid regenerative response is observed in about 10 per cent of FeLV-infected, anemic cats. These cats have reticulocytosis and may have nucleated red cells in the circulation and extramedullary hematopoiesis in liver and spleen. Frequently these cats have hemobartonellosis or immune-mediated hemolysis, which probably causes the abrupt onset of anemia in these cats. Cats with FeLV-positive regenerative anemia appear to be susceptible to the spectrum of FeLV-associated diseases, including myeloproliferative disease, lymphosarcoma, and erythroid aplasia.

Treatment of FeLV-associated anemia is symptomatic. The anemia is closely related to the presence of viremia. In cats with regressive infection, the anemia appears to resolve shortly after the cat reverts to FeLV-negative status. Iron therapy is not indicated, as iron stores are adequate and usually are increased in transfused cats. Blood transfusions are effective in prolonging the animal's life, and cats with packed cell volumes less than 10 per cent should receive this therapy. Initial random blood transfusions generally lead to clinical improvement that persists for about 2 weeks. Repeated transfusions from randomly selected feline donors eventually result in shortened erythrocyte survival to less than one week. The prognosis is poor for cats with FeLV-associated anemia because recovery is contingent on clearing of the virus. Some persons advocate the use of prednisone (2 mg/kg PO daily) for treatment of cats with FeLV-associated anemia, but the efficacy of this treatment has not been documented in a controlled study. Anabolic steroids do not seem to be effective. Cats with regenerative anemia should be carefully evaluated for causes of hemolytic anemia, especially *Haemobartonella felis*, immune-mediated hemolysis, and Heinz-body anemia. Specific therapy for these anemias often will lead to improvement but will not remove the predisposition to FeLV-associated diseases.

CHANGES IN PLATELETS

The FeLV infection of megakaryocytes is a consistent finding in FeLV-viremic cats. Bizarrely shaped macroplatelets and transient thrombocytopenia occur in some infected cats. In experimentally infected cats the thrombocytopenia is mild and develops at 2 to 6 weeks after inoculation; generally, it does not persist. Platelet size is variable but the mean platelet volume usually is increased from the reference range of 11 to 18 fl to greater than 30 fl. The macroplatelets are very obvious in cats with severe anemia and their size may overlap with that of feline erythrocytes, leading to erroneous erythrocyte counts. The macrothrombocytosis and nearly normal platelet concentrations are associated with an absolute increase in platelet mass (μl/ml). The total surface area of the macroplatelets is increased, but the estimated surface area of the surface-connected canalicular system is normal. These changes can be explained by increased cytoplasmic growth in megakaryocytes without a proportional increase in membrane demarcation. Decreased platelet half-life has been detected in cats with experimental FeLV infection. The mean platelet half life was 21.5 hours for normal platelets and 11.9 hours for platelets from cats infected with FeLV.

Mild defects in platelet function have been detected in FeLV-infected cats. Prolonged aggregation times have been detected in response to a low concentration of collagen or arachidonic acid but not to adenosine diphosphate. These *in vitro* defects do not manifest themselves in a clinically significant bleeding tendency, and no specific treatment is required.

HEMATOPOIETIC NEOPLASMS

A wide variety of leukemias and lymphosarcoma have been associated with FeLV infection. Myeloproliferative diseases are relatively common in cats, and about 90 per cent of cats so affected are positive for FeLV. The diseases include erythremic myelosis, granulocytic leukemia, erythroleukemia, and megakaryocytic leukemia. It is interesting to note that cats with naturally occurring systemic mastocytosis or eosinophilic leukemia have been negative for FeLV infection.

About 70 per cent of cats with lymphosarcoma have FeLV viremia. The cats with FeLV-negative lymphosarcoma generally are older cats. Epidemiologic studies have demonstrated an association between exposure to FeLV and the development of FeLV-negative lymphosarcoma. Thus, FeLV should be the suspected etiologic agent in most hemolymphatic neoplasms.

References and Supplemental Reading

Cotter, S. M.: Anemia associated with feline leukemia virus infection. J.A.V.M.A. 11:1191, 1979.

Hardy, W. D., Jr., Essex, M., and McClelland, A. J. (eds.): *Feline Leukemia Virus*. New York: Elsevier/North Holland, 1980.

Hardy, W. D., Jr.: Hematopoietic tumors of cats. J. Am. Anim. Hosp. Assoc. 17:921, 1981.

Hardy, W. D., Jr.: Feline leukemia virus non-neoplastic diseases. J. Am. Anim. Hosp. Assoc. 17:941, 1981.

Rojko, J. L., and Olsen, R. G.: The immunobiology of the feline leukemia virus. Vet. Immunol. Immunopathol. 6:107, 1984.

THERAPY FOR DISORDERS OF ERYTHROPOIESIS

DOUGLAS J. WEISS, D.V.M.
St. Paul, Minnesota

Anemia is a sign of disease and not a diagnosis. Development of a rational therapeutic approach to anemia requires definition or diagnosis of the cause of the anemia. Diagnostic techniques include case history, physical examination, complete blood count (CBC), reticulocyte count, clinical chemistry profile, serum iron determination, and bone marrow aspiration and core biopsy.

Disorders of erythropoiesis manifest as a poorly regenerative anemia with or without leukopenia and thrombocytopenia. Based on a CBC, nonregenerative anemias can be divided into refractory anemias (anemia with normal to increased leukocytes and platelet counts), pancytopenia (anemia with leukopenia and thrombocytopenia), and bicytopenia (anemia with leukopenia or thrombocytopenia). Refractory anemias are most often normocytic, but macrocytic and microcytic anemias occur. Normocytic anemias include those caused by primary or secondary failure of erythropoiesis, and can further be differentiated based on the severity of the anemia, serum iron concentration, and bone marrow evaluation. Primary failure of erythropoiesis is characterized by severe anemia, increased serum iron concentration, and severe erythroid hypoplasia or aplasia in bone marrow (Table 1). The only recognized causes of primary normocytic anemia are pure red cell aplasia in the dog and feline leukemia virus (FeLV) infection in the cat (Table 2). Secondary anemias are characterized by mild anemia, low serum iron concentration, and lack of severe erythroid hypoplasia in the bone marrow (Table 1). Further characterization of the cause of secondary anemia involves evaluation for inflammatory, malignant, renal, hepatic, and endocrine diseases (Table 2).

Microcytic anemias occur relatively infrequently except in tropical and subtropical climates, where anemia from hookworm-induced blood loss is common. They are most frequently the result of iron deficiency secondary to chronic blood loss and are characterized by low serum iron concentration and erythroid hyperplasia in the bone marrow (Table 2).

Macrocytic refractory anemias may be either megaloblastic or nonmegaloblastic in type. Megaloblastic anemias result from defective deoxyribonucleic acid (DNA) synthesis. They are characterized by marrow erythroid hyperplasia, maturation arrest, and megaloblastic changes. Nonmegaloblastic macrocytic anemias result from accelerated erythropoiesis or increased surface area of the cell membrane. Such anemias are associated with regenerative anemia, liver disease, splenic disease, and FeLV infection, and they may occur after splenectomy.

Bicytopenia and pancytopenias can be subcategorized as aplastic anemia, marrow stromal disorders, or myelodysplastic disorders based on bone marrow evaluation. In aplastic anemia, proliferation failure at the level of the multipotent hematopoietic stem cell results in a hypocellular bone marrow. Histologically, hematopoietic tissue is replaced by adipose tissue.

Marrow stromal disorders include marrow necrosis and myelofibrosis. Bone marrow necrosis is thought to result from direct toxic marrow damage or marrow ischemia and has been associated with a variety of primary diseases (Table 2). Myelofibrosis has been classified as either primary or secondary. Primary myelofibrosis was thought to be a myeloproliferative disorder, whereas secondary myelofibrosis appeared to be a sequela of marrow stromal injury. Recent evidence, however, suggests that myelofibrosis is always secondary to stromal damage regardless of whether it accompanies myeloproliferative diseases.

Table 1. *Protocol for Differentiation of Primary and Secondary Normocytic, Refractory Anemias in Dogs*

	Hematocrit (gm/dl)	**Serum Iron (μg/ml)**	**Bone Marrow Myeloid/ Erythroid Ratio**
Primary Marrow Failure	5–17	150–400	> 10:1
Secondary Marrow Failure	18–35	30–80	< 10:1

Table 2. *Causes of Nonregenerative Anemias in Dogs and Cats*

Normochromic Normocytic Refractory Anemia
Primary failure of erythropoiesis
- Pure red cell aplasia
- Feline leukemia virus

Secondary failure of erythropoiesis
- Anemia of inflammatory diseases
- Renal disease
- Liver disease
- Hypothyroidism
- Hypoadrenocorticism

Microcytic Hypochromic Refractory Anemia
Iron deficiency anemia

Macrocytic Normochromic Refractory Anemia
Feline myeloproliferative disease
Vitamin B_{12}/folic acid deficiency
Congenital poodle macrocytosis

Aplastic Anemia
Estrogen toxicity
Phenylbutazone toxicity
Chemotherapeutic agents
Ionizing radiation
Benzene toxicity
Organic arsenicals
Feline myeloproliferative disease
Parvovirus enteritis
Ehrlichiosis
Idiopathic

Stromal Disorders of Marrow
Bone marrow necrosis
- Estrogen toxicity
- Parvovirus infection
- Exposure to experimental drugs
- Septicemia
- Ehrlichiosis
- Malignancy
- Disseminated intravascular coagulopathy

Myelofibrosis

Myelodysplastic Syndrome

Myelodysplastic syndromes are a group of related disorders characterized by qualitative defects in hematopoietic stem cells. Clinical features include anemia and leukopenia or thrombocytopenia (or both), hypercellular bone marrow, dysplastic hematopoietic cells, and variable increases in the number of blast cells in peripheral blood and bone marrow. Myelodysplastic syndromes in cats are associated with FeLV infection and may progress to overt leukemia. Myelodysplastic syndromes occur less frequently in dogs.

GENERAL THERAPY

Treatment for disorders of erythropoiesis is primarily supportive and empirical. Recently, however, recognition of the value of immunosuppressive therapy and the development of techniques for bone marrow transplantation have provided new avenues for specific therapy.

Blood Transfusion

Transfusion of whole blood or specific blood components remains the primary supportive therapeutic modality. Blood transfusion is indicated when clinical signs of anemia develop or when the hematocrit is less than 10 per cent. Signs of anemia include anorexia, severe weakness, tachycardia, and orthopnea. Anemia secondary to bone marrow failure often develops slowly, allowing dogs and cats to adapt to the lower hematocrits. Several factors are involved in the adaptation to anemia. Increased concentration of 2,3-diphosphoglycerate in erythrocytes causes the oxygen affinity of hemoglobin to decrease, which thus increases oxygen delivery to body tissues. Cardiac compensation includes increased heart rate, increased stroke volume, and cardiac enlargement. Additionally, oxygenation of vital tissues is enhanced through decreased vascular resistance and decreased plasma volume.

Blood transfusion is not without risk. Side effects include incompatibility of transfused blood cells or plasma, expanded blood volume, iron overload, and sepsis. Hemolytic transfusion reactions are caused by the heterogenicity of antigens (blood groups) on blood cells. Eight erythrocyte groups have been identified in the dog. These are designated DEA 1.1, 1.2, 3, 4, 5, 6, 7, and 8. DEA 1.1 and DEA 1.2 are allelic and therefore cannot be present in the same patient. DEA 1.1 and 1.2 are the most antigenic, but DEA 7 will also produce clinically detectable transfusion reactions. Isolysins to DEA 1.1 and 1.2 do not occur naturally. Sensitization may occur by previous transfusion or when pregnant bitches are sensitized to incompatible fetal blood. Isolysins to DEA 7 have been reported to occur naturally and therefore may be the cause of mild reactions seen with the first transfusion. The remainder of the DEA antigens are either weakly antigenic or are present in greater than 95 per cent of the dog population.

Little information is available on blood groups in cats. Three blood groups (A, B, and AB) have been identified. Group B–positive cats appear to have naturally occurring anti-A antibodies and acute hemolytic transfusion reactions have been reported.

Transfusion reactions can be of several types. Acute hemolytic reactions are caused by administration of blood of groups DEA 1.1 or 1.2 to a sensitized recipient. Rapid intravascular or extravascular destruction of erythrocytes can result in nausea, vomiting, sweating, shivering, pruritis, dyspnea, shock, tachycardia, hypotension, hemoglobinemia, hemoglobinuria, and acute renal failure. In previously unsensitized recipients, destruction occurs 7 to 10 days after transfusion. In acute hemolytic reactions, transfusion should be discontinued and treatment for shock and acute renal failure initiated.

Leukocyte, platelet, and plasma protein incompatibilities can result in one or all of the following: anaphylaxis, vomiting, chills, neurologic signs, and uriticaria. These reactions can be reduced by administration of washed erythrocytes. If whole blood is administered, the severity of plasma reactions can be reduced by pretreatment with antihistamine (diphenhydramine hydrochloride, 4 mg/kg) 20 to 40 minutes prior to transfusion.

Febrile episodes can result from transfusion of incompatible erythrocytes, leukocytes, platelets, or plasma or from transfusion of blood contaminated with bacteria or endotoxins. Febrile reactions can be minimized by proper collection and storage of blood by slowing the rate of blood administration and by administering an antipyretic.

Hospitals treating patients with chronic anemias should maintain suitable donor animals and have facilities for crossmatching blood. Donor dogs must be DEA 1.1-, 1.2-, and 7-negative and, preferably, also negative for 3, 5, and 8. Additionally, dogs should be free of heartworm. Donor cats should be periodically checked for hemobartonellosis and FeLV infection.

Blood can be collected from the jugular vein or femoral artery of the dog and jugular vein of the cat. No more than 20 per cent of blood volume should be collected at 2- to 3-week intervals. Collection containers include commercially available plastic bags or glass bottles containing acid-citrate-dextrose (ACD), citrate-phosphate-dextrose (CPD), or citrate-phosphate-dextrose-adenine (CPDA-1), as the anticoagulant. Plastic bags are preferred because they minimize activation of platelet and clotting factors. Blood can be stored in ACD and CPD for up to 3 weeks at 4°C and in CPDA-1 for up to 35 days.

Blood should be delivered through a commercially available blood administration set, and a blood filter should be used to minimize transfusion of microemboli. The volume of blood to be transfused can be determined from the formulas in Figure 1.

Volume overload is a major concern when one is attempting to correct chronic refractory anemias. Packed RBCs are preferred over whole blood, and the rate of administration should not exceed 10 ml/kg/hr. Clinical signs of vascular overload include uriticaria, pulmonary edema, and vomiting.

Anabolic Steroids

Administration of androgenic compounds to dogs results in increased hematocrit, reticulocytosis, and

DOG:

Anticoagulated blood vol (ml) =

$$\text{body weight (kg)} \times 90 \times \frac{\text{PCV desired} - \text{PCV of recipient}}{\text{PCV of donor in anticoagulant}}$$

CAT:

Anticoagulated blood vol (ml) =

$$\text{body weight (kg)} \times 70 \times \frac{\text{PCV desired} - \text{PCV of recipient}}{\text{PCV of donor in anticoagulant}}$$

Figure 1. Calculation of blood replacement volume for dogs and cats.

erythroid hyperplasia of bone marrow. Androgens also stimulate myelopoiesis and thrombopoiesis to a lesser degree. The erythropoietic effects appear to result from increased erythropoietin production and direct stimulatory effect on bone marrow stem cells. Androgens enter multipotent stem cells and are reduced to 17 keto-derivatives. These 17 keto-derivatives enhance differentiation of multipotent stem cells to committed erythroid stem cells through synthesis of new messenger RNA.

Certain congeners of androgenic hormones are more potent stimulators of erythropoiesis. Alkylated compounds (methyltestosterone, fluoxymesterone, oxymetholone, methandrostenolone, stanozolol, ethylestrenol, norethandrolone) are highly potent but must be administered with care because of potential hepatotoxicity. Prolonged treatment (3 to 6 months) may be required before a response is observed.

Lithium

In mice and humans, lithium salts have been shown to enhance granulopoiesis and thereby induce neutrophilia. Lithium may also cause eosinophilia and thrombocytosis, but it inhibits erythropoiesis. Other effects of lithium include reduced bactericidal capacity of neutrophils and decreased responsiveness of lymphocytes. Prolonged administration of lithium to mice and humans may impair the replicative potential of marrow stem cells.

The utility of lithium carbonate in dogs is less clear. Some investigators have found that administration of lithium carbonate (25 mg/kg, b.i.d.) induces neutrophilia and stimulates granulopoiesis, but others were unable to demonstrate either effect. Lithium does appear to be effective in alleviating the severe cyclic leukopenia associated with cyclic hematopoiesis in gray collie dogs.

Cobalt

Cobalt has been shown to induce polycythemia in dogs and cats. It acts indirectly by inducing tissue hypoxia, which stimulates erythropoietin production. Because of numerous side effects, cobalt is contraindicated in the treatment of anemia.

Hematinics

Numerous pharmaceutic mixtures, including vitamins, minerals, and liver extracts, have been used in the treatment of anemia. These compounds are of no value in treating anemia except when there is a concurrent deficiency of one of the ingredients. When a deficiency is present, it is preferable to supplement only the deficient substance. Additionally, hematinics may induce iron overload, resulting in hemachromatosis.

SPECIFIC THERAPIES

Anemia of Inflammatory Diseases

The anemia associated with inflammatory disorders is mild and blood transfusions are usually not necessary. Therapy should be directed toward elimination of the primary disorder whenever possible. Iron therapy is contraindicated since iron is rapidly taken up by the mononuclear phagocyte system, which is already overloaded with iron. Administration of cobalt alleviates the anemia but is associated with many undesirable side effects.

Anemia of Renal Disease

Administration of anabolic steroids to dogs with chronic renal failure has been recommended to stimulate erythropoiesis, promote positive nitrogen balance, and to stimulate appetite. Although controlled clinical studies have not been done, anabolic steroids seem to be useful in stimulating erythropoiesis. Recently their benefit in inducing positive nitrogen balance and promoting appetite has been questioned. Nandrolone decanoate (Deca-Durabolin, Organon) has been administered at a rate of 5 mg/kg (maximum of 200 mg) per week. Additionally, E-series prostaglandins have been shown to stimulate erythropoietin production by the kidney. The clinical usefulness of prostaglandins in renal disease has not been investigated.

Anemia of Endocrine Disorders

Hormonal replacement therapy results in amelioration of the anemia in both hypothyroidism and hypoadrenocorticism.

Pure Red Cell Aplasia (PRCA)

Severe anemia is often present at the time of diagnosis of PRCA, necessitating whole blood or red blood cell transfusions. Because multiple transfusions may be needed, donor dogs should be of groups DEA 1.1-, 1.2-, and 7-negative, and major and minor crossmatches should be done. Since some dogs have circulating antierythrocyte antibodies, a direct Coombs' test is indicated. If positive, transfusions should be avoided. If the anemia is life-threatening, dogs should be treated with glucocorticoids before blood is administered.

Many cases of canine PRCA are immune-mediated and respond to immunosuppressive therapy. Prednisolone therapy should be initiated (2 mg/kg, divided b.i.d.). If no increase in the reticulocyte count occurs within 2 weeks, the dose should be increased (4 mg/kg, b.i.d.). If the reticulocyte count remains low after 4 to 6 weeks, cyclophosphamide therapy (30 to 50 mg/m^2 body surface area, on 4 consecutive days of each week) should be given and prednisolone therapy should be continued. Cyclophosphamide should be discontinued if neutropenia or thrombocytopenia occur. If the hematocrit and reticulocyte count increase, cyclophosphamide should be discontinued and the prednisolone dosage slowly reduced and given on alternate days.

Aplastic Anemia

Although many cases of aplastic anemia are idiopathic, known causes of the disorder should be ruled out (Table 2). Because idiosyncratic drug reactions may initiate aplastic anemia, all drugs given at or near the time of diagnosis should be discontinued.

Despite the cause of aplastic anemia, symptomatic therapy is often needed. Compatible whole blood or red cell transfusions should be given if severe anemia is present. Antibiotic therapy should be given if severe neutropenia or evidence of inflammation is present. Granulocyte transfusions are of little benefit because of the short half-life of transfused neutrophils. Platelet transfusions are beneficial only if severe thrombocytopenia is present.

Controlled studies of the efficacy of anabolic steroids in aplastic anemia have not been done. However, therapeutic trials in humans and individual case reports of dogs indicate that they are beneficial. Oxymetholone (Anadrol, Syntex; 2 mg/kg PO, b.i.d.) and nandrolone decanoate (Deca-Durabolin, 1.0 to 3.0 mg/kg IM, weekly) are preferred. Higher doses of oxymetholone (5 mg/kg, daily) have been given in human cases which did not respond to the lower dosage. Treatment should be continued for 4 to 6 months because clinical response is often delayed. During treatment, concentrations of serum alanine amino transferase and serum alkaline phosphate should be monitored periodically to evaluate possible hepatotoxicity.

The use of immunosuppressive drugs in the treatment of aplastic anemia is controversial. Administration of glucocorticoid, cyclophosphamide, 6-mercaptopurine, and antilymphocyte globulin have resulted in complete remission in some human cases.

Lithium citrate (Lithonate-S, Rowell; 23.5 mg/kg, b.i.d.) was reported to cause rapid improvement in one dog with aplastic anemia secondary to estrogen toxicity.

Iron Deficiency

The treatment of iron deficiency requires correction of the cause (usually chronic blood loss) and administration of iron. Clinical experience suggests that orally administered iron compounds are often poorly absorbed in dogs. Intramuscular iron dextran (Imferon, Merrill-Dow) is preferred. The formula in Figure 2 has been used to calculate the dosage for humans. Because of possible anaphalactic reactions, an initial test dose should be administered. Daily dosage should not exceed 50 mg in large dogs and 25 mg in small ones.

Bone Marrow Necrosis

Bone marrow necrosis occurs secondary to diseases such as malignancy, disseminated intravascular coagulation, intoxication, and bacterial and viral

Milligrams iron to be injected =

(15 − patient's hemoglobin in gm/dl) × body weight in kg × 3

Figure 2. Formula for calculation of iron-replacement dosage for iron-deficiency in humans.

infections. Attempts should be made to identify and treat the primary disorder. Specific therapy for bone marrow necrosis is unavailable at this time.

Myelofibrosis

Chemotherapeutic agents have not been found to be beneficial in treatment of primary myelofibrosis in humans, but anabolic steroids may be of some benefit. Secondary myelofibrosis is often a sequela of bone marrow necrosis; therefore, the underlying cause of the necrosis should be identified and treated. Antifibrotic drugs such as penicillamine and glucocorticoids have not been evaluated in myelofibrosis.

Myelodysplastic Syndromes

Treatment of idiopathic myelodysplastic syndromes in humans is controversial. Treatment protocols include glucocorticoids, anabolic steroids, and chemotherapeutic drugs. In a single canine case report, treatment with cytosine arabinoside, 6-thioguanine, and prednisolone was of only transient benefit.

References and Supplemental Reading

Barr, R. D., and Galbraith, P. R.: Lithium and hematopoiesis. Can. Med. Assoc. J. 128:123, 1983.

Couto, C. G., and Feldman, B. F.: Therapy for abnormal erythropoiesis. J.A.V.M.A. 181:501, 1981.

Couto, C. G., and Kallet, A. J.: Preleukemic syndrome in a dog. J.A.V.M.A. 184:1389, 1984.

Eldor, A., and Hershko, C.: Androgen-responsive aplastic anemia in a dog. J.A.V.M.A. 173:304, 1978.

Finco, D. R., Barsanti, J. A., and Adams, D. D.: Effects of an anabolic steroid on acute uremia in the dog. Am. J. Vet. Res. 145:2285, 1984.

Killingsworth, R.: Use of blood components for feline and canine patients. J.A.V.M.A. 185:1452, 1984.

Maddux, J. M., and Shaw, S. E.: Possible beneficial effect of lithium therapy in a case of estrogen-induced bone marrow hypoplasia in a dog: A case report. J. Am. Anim. Hosp. Assoc. 19:242, 1983.

Tangner, C. H.: Transfusion therapy for the dog and cat. Comp. Cont. Ed. Pract. Vet. 4:521, 1982.

Weiss, D. J., and Armstrong, P. J.: Nonregenerative anemias in the dog. Comp. Cont. Ed. Pract. Vet. 6:452, 1984.

Weiss, D. J., Miller, M. L., Crawford, M. A. et al.: Primary-acquired red cell aplasia: Response to glucocorticoid and cyclophosphamide therapy. J. Am. Anim. Hosp. Assoc. 20:951, 1984.

ESTROGEN-INDUCED BONE MARROW TOXICITY

ERIK TESKE, D.V.M.

Utrecht, The Netherlands

Estrogens are often used in small animal practice for the treatment of perianal gland adenomas, prostatic hyperplasia, urinary incontinence, pseudopregnancy, prolonged anestrus, and for the prevention of conception following mismating.

In addition to their therapeutic effects, estrogens and the synthetic estrogens can have a toxic effect on the bone marrow. Severe bone marrow depression, characterized by a combination of thrombocytopenia, leukopenia, and anemia, may be the ultimate result of giving estrogen. Endogenous estrogen excess, due to testicular tumor, can also be a cause of bone marrow toxicity. In these cases the hyperestrogenism may be seen in association with seminomas and interstitial cell tumors, but it is most frequently associated with Sertoli cell tumors. Also, one case of granulosa cell tumor of the ovary has been recorded in connection with estrogen-induced bone marrow depression.

To date, estrogen-induced bone marrow toxicity has only been reported in dogs. There is no predeliction for breed or sex, but the disease appears to be more common in older dogs.

PATHOGENESIS

The exact mechanism leading to bone marrow depression is not completely understood, but it is clear that estrogens act during the stage of stem cell differentiation and block the utilization of erythropoietin by these pluripotential stem cells, although the erythropoietin secretion is not inhibited. In the meantime, the proliferation and maturation of the other bone marrow cells are stimulated, finally resulting in bone marrow exhaustion.

As a first change in the peripheral blood, a thrombocytopenia is observed approximately 2 weeks after estrogen administration. Because of the enhanced granulopoiesis, hyperleukocytosis with a left shift develops after 16 to 20 days. At the same time anemia gradually becomes apparent. Because of the inhibited differentiation of the stem cells, the granulopoiesis decreases, which results in a leukopenia after 22 to 25 days.

When a sublethal dose of estrogens is administered, numbers of both granulocytes and platelets may increase again after 30 to 40 days. The anemia may persist for a longer period of time, but it eventually returns to normal. An explanation for the fact that estrogen-induced bone marrow toxicity is seen only in dogs has not yet been found. Recent studies have indicated that plasma proteins of dogs bind sex steroids at a much lower affinity for estrogens than they do in humans, and thus dogs have a less efficient inherent mechanism to buffer an exogenous excess of estrogen.

CLINICAL SIGNS

At the time of presentation the patient may be anorexic, depressed, and febrile. Inflammations, including endometritis, have been observed secondary to the leukopenia. The mucous membranes may be pale and have petechiae. Often there are other hemorrhages, such as in the abdomen, the intestinal tract, the urinary bladder, and the vagina. Less characteristic signs include vomiting, dehydration, and respiratory distress. Most patients die as a consequence of the hemorrhagic diathesis. Other causes of death are severe inflammation, endotoxic shock, and disseminated intravascular coagulation.

DIAGNOSIS

Hematologic findings include severe thrombocytopenia; normocytic, normochromic, nonresponsive anemia; and leukocytosis with left shift or leukopenia, depending on the stage of the disorder. Often the leukocytosis is associated with a monocytosis. The alterations in the bone marrow start with a hyperplasia of the myeloid cells, accompanied by a depression of the erythroid and megakaryocytic cells. As the disorder progresses, a myeloid hypoplasia appears. Eventually a complete disappearance of all myeloid and erythroid elements occurs. The megakaryocytes are largely reduced in numbers, and those that remain are often shrunken. The only cells to be seen in a bone marrow aspiration in this stage of the disease may be reticuloendothelial cells (macrophages), plasma cells, and mature lymphocytes. Fat cells may also be present.

The hematologic findings and the bone marrow alterations, combined with the history and clinical signs, are highly suggestive of estrogen-induced bone marrow toxicity.

TREATMENT

The goals of treatment can be divided into three parts. First of all, any possible life-threatening situation should be corrected. Secondly, estrogen administration should be stopped or, in case of testicular or ovarian neoplasms, surgical removal of the tumor carried out as soon as permitted by the patient's condition. The third part of the therapy should consist of stimulating the bone marrow.

Transfusions with fresh whole blood or with platelet-rich plasma are indicated in severe thrombocytopenia. Platelet-rich plasma can be obtained by centrifuging whole blood at 1500 rpm for 5 minutes and separating the platelet-rich plasma from the cells. When the patient is normovolemic, the rate of administration should not exceed 5 ml/kg/hour. Whole-blood transfusions and packed red blood cells are the treatments of choice for acute severe blood loss and normovolemic anemia, respectively. The amount of whole blood needed to restore normovolemia after acute blood loss will be at least 25 ml/kg. Because of the possibility of repeated blood transfusions, it is recommended to use blood donors typed negative for canine erythrocyte antigens CEA-1 and CEA-2. Instead of prevention of infection with broad-spectrum antibiotics, causal agents in patients with severe leukopenia should be cultured when infection does occur. The antibiogram will guide the clinician in selecting appropriate antibiotic treatment.

Androgens and lithium can be used in an attempt to stimulate the hypoplastic bone marrow. Androgens increase the production of plasma erythropoietin and increase the number of erythropoietin-responsive cells. They also facilitate the oxygen transport to the tissues by stimulating production of 2,3-diphosphoglycerate in the erythrocyte, which decreases the oxygen affinity for hemoglobin. In addition to stimulating erythropoiesis, androgens also may have some stimulating effect on granulopoiesis. The androgens can be divided into two groups: nonalkylated androgens and 17α-alkylated derivatives of testosterone (the latter are inactivated at a lower metabolic rate). Because of the alkylated groups, these androgens can also be used for oral administration. Oxymetholone, an alkylated testosterone derivative, is generally accepted as the best drug to use in cases of bone marrow depression, and it should be given orally at 1 to 3 mg/kg daily. It may take some months to achieve considerable improvement of the bone marrow depression. There seems to be a better response in females to androgen administration than in males, which is probably because of a difference in the metabolism of the hormone in the two sexes. The response to androgen therapy is best when the patients have some erythropoietic and myelopoietic activity left in the bone marrow.

Lithium has been successfully used in gray collies with cyclic granulopoiesis. Lithium stimulates the differentiation of the pluripotential stem cells. The mechanism by which this stimulation is achieved is yet unknown. Like oxymetholone, lithium has to be given for months. The dosage of lithium citrate is 12 mg/kg twice daily orally; lithium carbonate is given in 150- to 300-mg doses, twice daily.

There is little scientific support for the use of corticosteroids and vitamin-mineral supplements in the treatment of estrogen-induced bone marrow toxicity, and in the author's view, they should not be used.

PROGNOSIS

Pancytopenia caused by estrogen toxicity has a very guarded prognosis. Most patients die within 1 or 2 months. The more erythropoietic and myelopoietic activity that remains at the start of treatment, the better the ultimate outcome will be.

It has been stated that when thrombocytopenia lasts more than 2 weeks, prognosis is very poor. However, there are some case reports in which complete recovery has occurred after 30 to 40 days of thrombocytopenia.

In addition to a large individual difference in response to estrogens, age is a major factor influencing the prognosis. As stated before, older dogs are more susceptible to estrogen-induced aplastic anemia than are younger dogs.

PREVENTION

Because of the life-threatening complications of estrogen-induced bone marrow toxicity, alternative therapies should be used whenever possible. Adenomas of perianal glands, for example, are best managed by surgical removal. Also, cryosurgery and castration must be considered. Urinary incontinence of the spayed bitch can be successfully treated with ephedrine (0.5 mg/kg, PO, b.i.d.). Phenylpropanolamine, which is an α-adrenergic stimulant, may also be effective. The dosage of phenylpropanolamine ranges from 12.5 to 50 mg three times a day.

Pseudopregnancy alone usually does not require any treatment. However, when it is associated with lactation, one may consider the use of bromocriptine (0.02 mg/kg, PO, b.i.d. for 10 to 12 days). Induction of estrus with estrogens is of no use since it does not stimulate ovulation. Special treatment schedules with PMSG, HCG, and Gn-RH are more successful.

Aside from causing bone marrow toxicity, estrogens may also induce squamous metaplasia of the prostate when they are used for the treatment of prostatic hyperplasia. This makes the prostate more susceptible to infections. Instead of estrogens, antiandrogenic compounds or castration can be recommended for treatment of this disorder. In Europe delmadinone acetate (1 to 3 mg/kg, IM) is often used as an antiandrogen.

In the treatment of mismating, estrogens are the only drugs currently available. In moderate doses estrogens delay the transport of the ova through the oviduct. It is said that estrogens also may have a degenerative effect on the ova. After administration of estrogen, the endometrium of the uterus resembles the late proliferative phase rather than the secretory phase.

With regard to estrogen therapy, the following should be taken into consideration. Studies on the influence of estrogens on the bone marrow of dogs have revealed that aplastic anemia occurs more rapidly and has a more dramatic course in dogs receiving estradiol than in those treated with diethylstilbestrol. In addition, there is a considerable individual variation in the response to estrogen administration. Diethylstilbestrol is rapidly metabolized in the liver. After parenteral administration, estradiol benzoate persists for several days in the body. Estradiol cypionate takes several weeks to disappear completely.

Because of the alternatives and its possible side effects, estrogen is only indicated for treating mismating. When these drugs are used, the clinician should at least warn the owner of the possible toxic side effects. Diethylstilbestrol, given orally at 0.1 to 1.0 mg/day for 5 days, started within 72 hours after mating, would be the best drug to use. At Utrecht, estradiol benzoate is used (0.01 mg/kg, SC, on the third and fifth day after conception). The dosage of estradiol cypionate is the same as that of estradial benzoate (minimum dose is 0.1 mg) and is given only once. These dosages are only directives, since no substantial research has been done to distinguish between therapeutic and toxic doses of estrogens.

References and Supplemental Reading

Castrodale, D., Bierbaum, O., Helwig, E. B., et al.: Comparative studies of the effects of estradiol and stilbestrol upon the blood, liver and bone marrow. Endocrinology 29:363, 1941.

Couto, C. G.: Therapy for abnormal erythropoiesis. J.A.V.M.A. 181:501, 1982.

Maddux, J. M., and Shaw, S. E.: Possible beneficial effect of lithium therapy in a case of estrogen-induced bone marrow hypoplasia in a dog: A case report. J. Am. Anim. Hosp. Assoc. 19:242, 1983.

Schalm, O. W.: Exogenous estrogen toxicity in the dog. Canine Pract. 5:57, 1978.

Shahidi, N. T.: Androgens and erythropoiesis. N. Engl. J. Med. 289:72, 1973.

Sherding, R. G., Wilson, G. P., and Kociba, G. J.: Bone marrow hypoplasia in eight dogs with Sertoli cell tumor. J.A.V.M.A. 178:497, 1981.

Teske, E., and Feldman, B. F.: Hypoplasia of the bone marrow following estrogen therapy. Tijdschr. Diergeneeskd. 109:357, 1984.

INTERPRETATION OF TESTS FOR IMMUNE-MEDIATED BLOOD DISEASES

ROBBERT J. SLAPPENDEL, D.V.M.
Utrecht, The Netherlands

The immune-mediated blood diseases described in the veterinary literature mainly include the immune hemolytic anemias (IHA) and immune-mediated thrombocytopenias (IMT). Immune mechanisms may also play an important role in aplastic anemias and related disorders, especially pure red cell aplasia (PRCA). No specific tests are available to confirm an immunological mechanism of disease in canine or feline aplastic anemias, but in PRCA the probability of such a diagnosis is often supported by the detection of autoantibodies directed against red cells (see below). Immune mechanisms may also destroy leukocytes, but little is known about the occurrence of immune-mediated leukopenia in animals.

This article will deal with interpretation of tests for IHA and IMT.

IMMUNE HEMOLYTIC ANEMIA (IHA)

IHA may be defined as a hemolytic state in which the premature breakdown of red cells is mediated by antibodies. Disorders of this type can be classified as follows (Wells, 1982): (1) autoimmune hemolytic anemia (AIHA), (2) drug-induced IHA, and (3) alloantibody-induced IHA.

Autoimmune Hemolytic Anemia (AIHA)

In AIHA, increased red cell breakdown is brought about by the production of autoantibodies directed against the patient's own red cells. Clinically, AIHA may be "idiopathic" (a disorder of unknown origin) or "symptomatic" (associated, for example, with neoplastic diseases, systemic lupus erythematosus, or infections). High concentrations of serum antibodies to viral antigens in dogs with AIHA suggest that "idiopathic" canine AIHA may often follow viral infections (Slappendel, 1978). In humans, an association of viral disease and transient AIHA is well known.

In an etiological classification, distinction is made between "true" or primary AIHA and secondary AIHA. Primary AIHA is the result of a breakdown in the immunoregulatory mechanisms, which maintain the normal state of self-tolerance. Secondary AIHA, on the other hand, is associated with an immunological response to exogenous insults, such as infections or toxins. In these cases, the production of antibodies directed against "new" red cell antigens is stimulated. These new antigens may result from the binding of exogenous haptens to membrane proteins, from the adherence of antigen-antibody complexes to the cell membrane, or from membrane insult and exposure of previously hidden antigens. Other types of secondary AIHA include infectious agents that share antigenic determinants with membrane proteins and cause a "cross-reacting" antibody response.

AIHA has been described in both dogs and cats. Many case reports and studies on canine AIHA are available (Halliwell, 1978; Slappendel, 1978, 1979;

Werner, 1980; Switzer and Jain, 1981), but data on feline AIHA are scarce and its incidence seems to be low (Werner, 1980). The following will deal mainly with AIHA in the dog.

The autoantibodies in dogs with AIHA are of two types. By far the most common type are the warm antibodies, which will associate with the red cell antigen more quickly at 37°C than at lower temperatures. Cold antibodies are rare. These antibodies typically do not associate with the antigen at 37°C, although they readily do so as a rule at temperatures below 30 to 35°C. Most probably, the antigens involved are "hidden" at body temperature but become exposed on the red cell membrane at lower temperatures, optimally at 4°C.

The antibodies involved in canine AIHA are usually either IgG or, less frequently, IgM. IgA antibodies have also been identified, mostly in association with IgG and IgM antibodies, but they are extremely rare in both humans and dogs. To date, no IgD or IgE antibodies have been implicated in the origin of AIHA.

Little is known about IgG subclasses in canine AIHA. In human patients, IgG1 and IgG3 seem to predominate, although IgG2 and IgG4 autoantibodies have also been described. IgM and the antibody subtypes IgG1, IgG2, and IgG3 are capable of activating complement components; IgA and IgG4 are not.

The complement system consists of many plasma protein components. A subunit of the first component, C1, contains a receptor for the Fc-portion of immunoglobulins. The interaction of IgG or IgM antibodies with antigens alters the conformation of the Fc-portion of the antibody molecule and enables it to react with this C1 subunit. This reaction initiates the complement cascade. Calcium ions are required for this process.

In the case of IgG antibodies, at least two molecules of IgG in close proximity to one another must react with antigen in order to fix complement. With IgM antibodies, two subunits of the same IgM molecule may serve to activate C1. As a result of the activation of C1 components, C4, C2, and then C3 are activated and fixed on the red cell membrane. If more than 1100 molecules of C3 are fixed per cell, the complement components 5 through 9 may also become activated. The C5–9 complex generated in that way produces small holes in the cell membrane. This leads to passage of water into the cell, cell swelling (spherocytosis), and cell rupture (intravascular hemolysis).

More frequently, however, complement activation does not proceed to the generation of the C5–9 complex. In that case, immune lysis may still take place, but it occurs more slowly in the macrophages of the reticuloendothelial system.

Macrophages possess receptors for C3 and for the Fc-portion of IgG molecules that have reacted with antigen. The adherence of antibody-coated red cells to the phagocytic cells is strongly promoted in that way, and this may lead to partial or complete erythrophagocytosis. Erythrophagocytosis is more efficient when both IgG and C3 are attached to the red cell than when only IgG is present. The presence of C3 without antibody is probably insufficient to cause phagocytosis, but sublytic amounts of other components that participate in the later steps of the complement sequence may be more potent in that respect.

LABORATORY DIAGNOSIS

In a dog with signs of hemolytic anemia, a preliminary diagnosis of AIHA can be made after the detection of autoagglutination, spherocytosis, or abnormal osmotic fragility of red cells. The definite diagnosis depends upon the demonstration by a direct antiglobulin test (DAT) of autoantibodies adsorbed to the patient's red cells. In addition, autoantibodies may be detected free in the serum by the indirect antiglobulin test (IAT) or by other techniques.

AUTOAGGLUTINATION. The presence of immunoglobulins on the red cell membrane may in some instances be detected by their ability to effect spontaneous agglutination. Agglutination is brought about by the linkage of red cells by antibodies connecting the antigen sites on one red cell to the antigen sites on another. Normally, the red cell surface is negatively charged, mainly because of sialic acid residues in the membrane, and the force of this charge keeps individual cells apart. For that reason, the distance between the antigen-binding sites on a single antibody molecule can be important with regard to its agglutinating capabilities. For IgG the distance between antigen-binding sites is about 12.5 to 25 nm, and in saline media this is insufficient for linkage of the red cells. IgG antibodies, nevertheless, may bring about the agglutination of erythrocytes in a medium of high dielectric constant, such as albumin, which dissipates the charge between red cells, thereby allowing closer contact. IgM molecules are larger than IgG molecules and the distance between antigen-binding sites, 30 to 50 nm, is great enough to bring about agglutination of red cells, even in saline.

Spontaneous agglutination of red cells in freshly drawn blood usually indicates the presence of warm- or cold-type IgM antibodies. It may also occur, however, in association with warm-type IgG antibodies. In that case, agglutination seems to be brought about by the combination of a high concentration of IgG and a high dielectric constant of the patient's plasma. As a rule, this type of agglutination disappears when phosphate-buffered saline (PBS) is added to the blood and is promoted by the addition of albumin.

Autoagglutination should be distinguished from rouleaux formation. This may be quite difficult, especially in AIHA, when rouleaux formation may be superimposed upon agglutination. Also, massive rouleaux formation of a normal conformation sometimes simulates true agglutination.

Clumping of red cells due to massive rouleaux formation may often be distinguished from true agglutination by observing that the red cells are mostly arranged side by side, as in the normal rouleaux. Moreover, rouleaux formation, unlike agglutination, is not promoted by the addition of albumin to the blood. It has been suggested that, after the addition of three to four volumes of PBS to the preparation, "pseudoagglutination" due to massive rouleaux formation should either disperse completely or transform itself into typical rouleaux. As mentioned before, however, true agglutination in plasma, caused by warm-type IgG antibodies, may also dissolve in PBS.

In our experience, spontaneous red cell agglutination sometimes occurs in dogs without any clinical or hematological sign of hemolytic anemia and in which neither antibodies against red cells nor cell-bound complement can be demonstrated.

SPHEROCYTOSIS. The presence of spherocytes in a blood smear strongly supports a preliminary diagnosis of AIHA. Spherocytes (microspherocytes) are small, swollen, densely stained erythrocytes that have lost the characteristic central pallor caused by the normal biconcave shape. Their presence indicates a prelytic state of red cells that are attacked by the C5–9 complex or have escaped from phagocytic cells after partial digestion of their membranes. Spherocytosis may occur in all types of IHA and also in a few hemolytic conditions associated with toxic or genetic defects of the red cell membrane.

Spherocytosis is difficult to detect in feline blood smears, since the erythrocytes of cats are normally smaller and denser than those of dogs. The disorder can easily be detected, however, by osmotic fragility tests.

OSMOTIC FRAGILITY. When red cells are suspended in hypotonic saline, water is taken up by the cells until osmotic equilibrium is attained. Normal canine red cells can stand a hypotonic saline dilution provided the concentration is higher than 0.54 per cent sodium chloride (NaCl). At lower concentrations, excessive water uptake causes cell lysis. Spherocytes cannot take up as much water as normal red cells can, and they rupture at higher saline concentrations.

Osmotic fragility can easily be tested in daily veterinary practice. To that purpose, a solution equivalent to 0.54 per cent saline is prepared by diluting three volumes of 0.9 per cent NaCl, or preferably PBS, with two volumes of water. Five drops of blood are added to 5 ml of this dilution. The mixture is incubated for 5 minutes, centrifuged, and read. The presence of intact red cells on the bottom of the tube and a clear supernatant indicates that osmotic fragility of red cells is normal. In the case of spherocytosis, free hemoglobin will somewhat stain the supernatant red. A control test with blood of the patient in 0.9 per cent NaCl should be used as a control. Abnormal osmotic fragility can be demonstrated in about 85 per cent of dogs with AIHA.

Osmotic fragility is higher in cats than in dogs. Therefore, a dilution of five volumes of PBS in two volumes of water, which is osmotically equivalent to 0.64 per cent NaCl, should be used to test osmotic fragility in felines.

DIRECT AND INDIRECT ANTIGLOBULIN TEST (DAT AND IAT). In AIHA, the interaction between antigen and antibody almost always results in the fixation of immunoproteins to the cell membrane. These immunoproteins are antibody, the components of complement, or both. Immunoproteins fixed upon the red cell membrane are usually detected by the DAT. In this test, antiserum containing heterologous antibodies against immunoproteins of the species to be tested is combined with thoroughly washed red cells of the patient. If immunoproteins are fixed to the cell membrane, as in AIHA and other types of IHA, the heterologous antibodies will bind to these molecules. Since one heterologous ("reagent") antibody can fix two autoantibody or complement molecules (even two molecules on separate but adjacent red cells), this results in agglutination and thus yields a positive test.

In the IAT, antiglobulin serum reacts with washed donor red cells that have previously been incubated with serum (or plasma) of the patient. A positive test indicates the presence of free antibody in the serum.

The IAT is a very poor test for diagnosing AIHA. Only in less than 40 per cent of DAT-positive dogs is the concentration of free serum antibody high enough to be detected by IAT. The IAT should therefore never replace the DAT, unless for some reason the patient's red cells are absolutely not available for testing. Under no circumstance should the IAT be positive and the DAT negative.

Blood to be used in antiglobulin tests should be collected in EDTA or ACD to bind the calcium in the plasma, which prevents *in vitro* binding of complement to the red cells. Red cells should be washed at least four times in a large volume of buffered saline in order to remove any nonspecifically bound immunoprotein.

Several techniques for performing the antiglobulin test have been proposed (Dacie and Lewis, 1984). The author prefers a tube method in which the red cells can settle spontaneously (i.e., without centrifugation) during incubation for 1 to 2 hours at the desired temperature (see below). A tube method has the advantage over slide or tile methods in that it is more sensitive and fewer red cells are needed. Though spontaneous sedimentation requires more time, it has the advantage over centrifugation in that results can easily be read macroscopically; the method is also less prone to technical and reading errors. The technique is especially beneficial when antiglobulin tests are to be performed in serial dilutions and at various temperatures, because it does not require the use of an expensive multihead centrifuge.

For the interpretation of test results, understanding and knowledge of the quality and specificity of the antisera one uses is mandatory. Antiserum for canine globulin is prepared by immunizing animals, usually rabbits, with whole canine serum or with specific fractions of canine serum. Whole canine serum is used for the preparation of "broad-spectrum" antisera. Broad-spectrum antisera may also be made by mixing various specific antisera. Specific antisera can be made against IgG, IgM, IgA and against C3 and C4.

Broad-spectrum Coombs' sera should contain strong agglutinating potential for both IgG-coated and complement-coated red cells. However, the anti-C activity of commercial canine antisera is often poor. The activity against IgM and IgA is usually insignificant or absent, but this is irrelevant for the demonstration of AIHA. IgM binds complement, which is detected by the antiglobulin serum. IgA coating of red cells is rare and occurs seldom without IgG coating, which is also detected in the antiglobulin test.

Antisera designed for use in antiglobulin reactions should be free of unwanted specificities; this is accomplished by appropriate absorptions performed by the manufacturers. Unwanted specificities, such as reactivity to albumin or transferrin, may cause false-positive reactions. Unfortunately, verification of the specificity may present major problems, since panels of test cells coated with various types of antibodies are not available. One cannot rely upon precipitin reactions as a criterion of monospecificity, as the antiglobulin reaction for detection of serum protein bound to red cells is several orders of magnitude more sensitive than precipitin reactions.

Heterologous antibodies that cross-react with as yet undefined antigenic sites on canine red cells are regularly present in the sera of rabbits and other species used for the production of antiglobulin sera. In order to prevent false-positive reactions, these antibodies should also be absorbed before the antisera are used in antiglobulin tests. It is not known whether antigens to canine blood groups are involved. We routinely absorb newly obtained antiglobulin sera with a pool of red cells containing at least the strongly antigenic and rather easily obtainable canine erythrocyte antigens CEA-1 and CEA-2 and also CEA-1– and CEA-2–negative cells. (Absorption of antisera with a panel of red cells containing among them all known types of blood-group antigens would probably be most adequate, but this is impossible since completely typed canine red cells are currently almost unobtainable).

The cells are washed six times in a large volume of buffered saline and absorptions are carried out overnight at 4°C with an equal volume of the washed packed cells. Subsequently, the serum is tested at 4°C and at 37°C with a panel of washed red cells from at least five arbitrarily selected normal dogs. Following the above procedure, we have always found the results of these control tests to be negative in our trials.

The optimal dilution of antiglobulin serum for agglutination of IgG-sensitized cells may vary from one antiglobulin serum to another. When a prepared antiserum has strong reactivity against cell-bound IgG, a marked prozone is generally observed when tests employ serial dilutions of the antiglobulin reagent. Thus, to insure optimal detection of IgG antibodies upon red cells, it is essential that a commercial antiserum, designed to be used in a single concentration, is supplied at the correct dilution (i.e., within the optimal midzone range). However, the optimal concentration of a serum for agglutinating IgG1-coated red cells may be different from that required for maximal agglutination of cells coated by IgG2, IgG3, or IgG4. Likewise, the optimal concentration of a broad-spectrum antiserum is usually different for detection of IgG antibodies and for complement components. It is the author's conviction that many of the so-called Coombs-negative AIHAs reported in veterinary literature are attributable mainly to this phenomenon. In veterinary laboratories, DAT is usually performed with a single broad-spectrum antiglobulin serum in a single, fixed concentration. Performing DATs with various specific antiglobulin sera in serial dilutions should reduce the number of false-negative tests considerably.

By using specific antisera containing antibodies to a single immunoprotein, it is possible to discriminate which one of the several immunoproteins is fixed to the membrane. With such antisera, one can distinguish four main types of immunoproteins that coat the red cells of patients with AIHA: (1) type I, in which immunoglobulin alone, usually IgG, is present; (2) type II, in which both immunoglobulin (usually IgG, associated or not with IgM) and complement are present; (3) type III, in which only complement components are detectable; and (4) type IV, in which neither complement nor immunoglobulin is detectable on the red cell.

Type I and Type II Reactions. In our experience, the detection of IgG antibodies by DAT is almost always of clinical significance and indicates a latent or overt IHA. This is true even if the number of antibodies, as indicated by titration, appears to be low. Indeed, comparison between patients of the number of antibody molecules per red cell is an unreliable index of the degree of hemolysis. Within the same patient, however, changes in antibody titer are often associated with predictable changes in the hemolytic state. Also, hemolysis is often more severe in patients with type II DAT than in patients with type I reactions. In patients with type II reactions the situation is often more acute and more serious when both IgG and IgM are detected.

Type III Reactions. The clinical significance of a positive DAT is less obvious when it is caused by complement alone coating the red cells. A strongly positive anti-C′–type DAT is usually associated with distinct clinical signs of red cell breakdown, often including intravascular hemolysis. In these cases, warm- or cold-reacting antibodies may have fixed complement onto the cell membrane and then dissociated from it. Dissociation may have occurred during the washing procedures, but may possibly also occur *in vivo*. In rare cases, for instance, in the so-called cold hemagglutinin disease, such dissociated antibodies are indeed detected in the serum (see below).

When a broad-spectrum antiserum with strong anti-C′ activity is used, most positive DATs are due to a weak type III reaction without detectable antibody in the serum. Interpretation of this kind of type III reaction is difficult. The complement may have been fixed upon the red cell by subdetectable amounts of antibody. This could be an indication of AIHA. However, complement can be fixed to the red cell in a number of ways other than by autoantibodies (for example, by circulating immune complexes that contact the erythrocytes by coincidence). Circulating immune complexes may be present in a wide variety of clinical conditions, including various infectious and neoplastic diseases, and as a consequence of the administration of various drugs. Only rarely, however, does this result in the destruction of red cells.

In "cold hemagglutinin disease" a strongly positive type III DAT is usually present. In this condition, the patient's serum contains a high concentration of autoantibodies directed against red cell antigens that are concealed at body temperature but become exposed upon cooling. The antibodies involved are mostly IgM agglutinins, which readily fix complement. Antigen-antibody binding and complement fixation may occur *in vivo* as the blood circulates to portions of the body that are exposed to a cooler ambient temperature. Especially in a cold climate, strong agglutination of the antibody-coated erythrocytes may cause obstruction within the microcirculation. This may result in necrosis of the extremities (toes, nose, ears, and tail). The antibody dissociates again when the red cells reenter the warmer central circulation; however, the complement remains fixed and, depending upon the degree of its activation, this may induce intra- or extravascular hemolysis.

In the laboratory, the presence of cold agglutinins in the blood may be suspected when the blood agglutinates spontaneously at room temperature, whereas the red cells disperse again upon warming to 37°C. The DAT at 37°C should be distinctly positive with anti-C′ sera, but not with anti-IgG or anti-IgM sera. The diagnosis can be confirmed by demonstrating that the serum, when separated from the patient's red cells at 37 to 40°C, strongly agglutinates donor cells at 4°C, even at high serum dilutions.

(The globulin class of the antibody can be established by immunoelectrophoresis of a concentrated eluate of the patient's red cells. The eluate can be prepared by washing the patient's red cells in PBS at 37 to 40°C, once they have been freed of nonspecifically bound immunoproteins by a minimum of three washings with ice-cold PBS and without any rewarming of the cells in between).

Type III reactions are also found in patients with either a subagglutinating amount of cold agglutinins or incomplete IgM or IgG cold antibodies in the serum. Autoagglutination is very weak or absent, even at 4°C. However, separation of the red cells from the serum, centrifugation, washing, and testing are performed at 4°C. Results of a DAT with monospecific anti-IgM or anti-IgG serum are positive. Clinical signs, due to hemolysis, typically develop in winter and may be serious if ambient temperatures are very low. In our experience, detection of this type of antibody is distinctly related to findings of hemolytic anemia. The incidence of positive DAT at 4°C in nonanemic dogs has been reported to be over 50 per cent (Werner and Halliwell, 1982). In a series of 30 nonanemic dogs tested in our hospital with monospecic anti-IgG, anti-IgM, and anti-C′ sera, DAT at 4°C was consistently negative. In order to avoid false-positive reactions, it is mandatory that the antiglobulin serum, before being used, is absorbed with normal red cells in cold conditions.

Type IV Reactions. AIHA associated with negative DAT may be the result of false-negative reactions. This may occur because of a variety of reasons, including improperly prepared or non-species-specific antisera or from failing to wash the red cells adequately prior to exposing them to the antiglobulin reagent. Very little residual serum protein in the suspending medium is needed to neutralize antibodies in the antiglobulin reagent; this renders them unable to agglutinate coated red cells. As noted above, another important cause of a false-negative DAT may be the prozone phenomenon if the tests are performed with improperly diluted antisera.

Even if tests are performed under optimal conditions and with a set of properly prepared potent antisera, DAT may occasionally be negative despite the fact that both clinical findings and laboratory data are strongly suggestive of AIHA. This may have several causes:

1. Clinical and laboratory findings are suggestive of AIHA, but this is not the correct diagnosis.
2. A dog with cold antibodies in the serum, which has not recently been exposed to low ambient temperatures, may have neither antibody nor complement upon the red cells. In that case, the antibody may only be detected if a DAT is performed at 4°C, as described above.
3. Rarely, red cells may be coated by IgA alone. Most antiglobulin sera lack anti-IgA specificity.
4. Occasionally, the amount of antibody bound to the red cells is too small to be detected by conventional antiglobulin tests. Probably more than 500 molecules of antibody per red cell are required before the DAT is positive, but sometimes smaller amounts of antibody are able to cause considerable hemolysis.

It has been suggested that the DAT may easily become negative once a patient with AIHA is treated with corticosteroids. In our experience, and with the DAT technique described above, this is extremely rare. We routinely perform both clinical and hematologic follow-ups on our patients until the DAT becomes negative. In a few patients this took several years, during which they were undergoing treatment with corticosteroids. Once the DAT became negative, relapses occurred in less than 5 per cent of the patients. This may not be the case when other immunosuppressive drugs are used.

ENZYME-TREATED RED CELLS AND LOW IONIC STRENGTH SOLUTION (LISS). When autoantibodies are present both on the patient's red cells and in the serum but in concentrations too low to cause autoagglutination or even a positive DAT and IAT, their presence in the serum may still be demonstrated by the use of a LISS in combination with donor cells previously treated with papain and incubated with serum of the patient. The LISS presumably reduces the electrostatic barrier surrounding the red cells, thus enhancing the antigen-antibody interaction. Pretreatment of the donor cells with papain presumably modifies the membrane in such a way that more antibody-combining sites become exposed.

It has been suggested that this type of agglutination test is more sensitive than the Coombs' test and is at least as consistent in canine AIHA (Feldmann, 1983). Unfortunately, little is known yet about the incidence of false-positive tests. It is well known from human medicine that both the application of LISS techniques and the use of enzymes are very critical in antibody testing and should only be exercised by experienced staff (Dacie and Lewis, 1984).

Alloantibody-Induced IHA

Alloantibody-induced IHA, occurring after repeated transfusions of incompatible blood, has been described in both dogs and cats. It may also occur in puppies after they drink colostrum that harbors alloantibodies as a result of a previous incompatible blood transfusion. In both cases, the diagnosis can be confirmed by a direct cross-match agglutination test or a DAT. If blood of the puppies is not available, a positive crossmatch in which the serum of the bitch agglutinates the red cells of the sire or an IAT in which the red cells of the sire are tested after incubation with the serum of the bitch is very valuable in supporting the diagnosis.

It should be realized that a crossmatch agglutination test or an IAT is not helpful when a compatible canine blood donor is selected if the recipient has never received a transfusion. Dogs, unlike humans, do not have natural alloantibodies and will not develop them until about 8 to 12 days after an incompatible transfusion. At that time, a high concentration of agglutinating or hemolysing alloantibodies (or both) may be detected within the serum of the recipient by a major crossmatch with incompatible donor cells. After several months, the antibody titer decreases again, and incompatible donor red cells are no longer agglutinated or hemolysed *in vitro* by the serum of the recipient. Low titers of alloantibodies may still be detected for a long time, however, by an IAT in which the donor cells are used after incubation with the recipient's serum or plasma.

Problems and diagnostic procedures related to blood transfusions in cats have been described in the article Feline Blood Transfusion Reactions.

Drug-Induced IHA

Drugs may give rise to a hemolytic anemia of immunological origin. This is difficult to distinguish from a true AIHA. It is thought that in most of these cases the antibodies are directed primarily against the drug and that the red cells are destroyed as "innocent bystanders." IHA may also result from drug-induced chemical alteration of the antigens on the red cell membrane, which elicits an antibody response.

In humans, many cases of drug-induced IHA have been reported, but as yet, little is known about the occurrence of this phenomenon in small animals.

Detailed serologic tests are necessary to confirm the diagnosis.

THE IMMUNE-MEDIATED THROMBOCYTOPENIAS (IMT)

The pathogenesis and classification of IMT are very similar to those of IHA. IMT results from increased platelet destruction, primarily by macrophages. Only rarely does destruction occur by complement-mediated lysis or complement-dependent cytotoxicity after sensitization of circulating platelets with antibody. Platelet production in IMT is usually increased but may also be impaired, and this failure is probably also immune-mediated. Antiplatelet antibodies can cross-react with antigens on the megakaryocytic cell membrane.

Alloantibody-induced IMT may occur after incompatible blood transfusions, but this seems to be of little clinical significance in dogs and cats. Thrombocytopenia of the newborn, due to maternal alloantibodies, as has been described in human infants and in piglets, but it has not yet been reported in puppies or kittens.

Drug-induced IMT, well documented in human medicine, has been suspected in several canine cases, but this diagnosis is difficult to confirm.

Autoantibody-induced IMT is referred to as autoimmune thrombocytopenia or autoimmune thrombocytopenic purpura (AITP).

Autoimmune Thrombocytopenia (AITP)

AITP is one of the most common causes of a hemorrhagic diathesis in dogs, but it is rare in the cat (Jain and Switzer, 1981). AITP, like AIHA, may be "symptomatic" (i.e., secondary to a number of diseases, including infections and neoplastic diseases) or "idiopathic." Approximately 15 per cent of patients with idiopathic AIHA suffer from AITP, which may occur before, at the same time, or after the hemolytic anemia.

The antibodies involved are usually IgG molecules that opsonize the platelet. Platelet destruction is subsequently accomplished by the macrophages in the RES, primarily within the spleen and liver.

A correct diagnosis of AITP is important, since thrombocytopenia may occur in association with many other conditions that should be treated in a different way and that may have a quite different prognosis. Actually, the administration of immunosuppressive drugs, the therapy of choice in most cases of AITP, may be contraindicated in some of these conditions.

The definite diagnosis of AITP depends upon the demonstration of antiplatelet antibodies on the thrombocyte or within the patient's serum. A number of methods to demonstrate antiplatelet antibodies have been developed in the last decade. Sophisticated techniques have shown positive results in almost all human patients with AITP (Wells, 1982). Unfortunately, these methods are generally too complex for routine use.

Even less sophisticated methods, used in veterinary medicine, are still rather complex. These methods include the platelet factor 3 (PF-3) immunoinjury test and the direct immunofluorescence (DIF) of megakaryocytes within a bone marrow smear. In the PF-3 immunoinjury test, platelets from a normal dog are incubated with both a normal dog's globulin fraction (control) and the patient's globulin fraction. If antiplatelet antibody is present in the globulin fraction of the test serum, the antibody "injures" the platelet membrane, thereby exposing PF-3 on its surface. PF-3 enhances the intrinsic blood clotting system, which is evaluated in an adapted, standardized determination of activated partial thromboplastin time (APTT). In a positive test, the clotting time should be at least 10 seconds shorter than that of the normal control (Wilkins and Dodds, 1974).

The method may be somewhat simplified by the use of plain serum instead of a dialized globulin fraction. This modification has the disadvantage, however, that the test becomes inaccurate with hemolytic or lipemic plasmas. Positive PF3 tests were obtained in 60 to 70 per cent of thrombopenic dogs in a study in which the first test method was applied (Wilkins and Dodds, 1974), whereas 37 per cent of the animals showed positive reactions with the adapted method in another study (Jain and Switzer, 1981).

The DIF, with fluorescein-conjugated antiserum to canine IgG on ethanol-fixed bone marrow smears, has been proposed as a sensitive method for the detection of antiplatelet antibodies upon the surface of megakaryocytes (Joshi and Jain, 1976). The specificity and sensitivity of the immunofluorescence test are not precisely known. It is also unknown whether antiplatelet antibodies always cross-react with megakaryocytic antigens. In our trials, interpretation of this test was difficult, as the slide was not counterstained and, more importantly, it was not washed free of nonspecifically bound antibodies or of any other free serum protein. The latter results in a high background fluorescence, which makes the reading of weaker reactions very difficult. The problem can be overcome partially by first suspending and washing the marrow aspirate in PBS. After centrifugation, the cell concentrate is resuspended in diluted fluorescein-conjugated antiserum for canine IgG and inspected under the fluorescence microscope.

References and Supplemental Reading

Dacie, J. V., and Lewis, S. M.: *Practical Haematology,* 6th ed. New York: Churchill Livingstone, 1984.

Feldman, B. F.: Use of low ionic strength solution in combination with papain treated red blood cells for the detection of canine erythrocyte autoantibodies. J. Am. Anim. Hosp. Assoc. 18:653, 1982.

Halliwell, R. E. W.: Autoimmune disease in the dog. Adv. Vet. Sci. Comp. Med. 22:221, 1978.

Jain, N. C., and Switzer, J. W.: Autoimmune thrombocytopenia in dogs and cats. Vet. Clin. North Am. (Small Anim. Pract.) 11:421, 1981.

Slappendel, R. J.: Hemolytic anemia in the dog. Ph.D. Thesis, Elinkwijk, Utrecht, 1978.

Slappendel, R. J.: The diagnostic significance of the direct antiglobulin test (DAT) in anemic dogs. Vet. Immunol. Immunopathol. 1:49, 1979.

Slappendel, R. J., Erp, C. L. G. M., van Goudswaard, J., et al.: Cold agglutinin disease in a toy pinscher dog. Tijdschr. Diergeneeskd. 100:445, 1975.

Switzer, J. W., and Jain, N. C.: Autoimmune hemolytic anemia in dogs and cats. Vet. Clin. North Am. (Small Anim. Pract.) 11:405, 1981.

Wells, J. V.: Hematologic diseases. *In* Stites, D. P., Stobo, J. D., Fudenberg, H. H., et al. (eds.): *Basic & Clinical Immunology,* 4th ed. Los Altos, CA: Lange Medical Publications, 1982, pp. 479–91.

Werner, L. L.: Coombs' positive anemias in the dog and cat. Comp. Cont. Ed. Pract. Vet. 2:96, 1980.

Werner, L. L., and Halliwell, R. E. W.: Diseases associated with autoimmunity. *In* Chandler, E. A., Sutton, J. B., and Thompson, D. J. (eds.): *Canine Medicine and Therapeutics,* 2nd ed. Oxford: Blackwell Scientific Publications, 1984, pp. 270–296.

Wilkins, R. J., and Dodds, W. J.: Idiopathic (immunologic) thrombocytopenic purpura. *In* Kirk, R. W. (ed.): *Current Veterinary Therapy V.* Philadelphia, W. B. Saunders, 1974, pp. 365–367.

THROMBOSIS—DIAGNOSIS AND TREATMENT

BERNARD F. FELDMAN, D.V.M.
Davis, California

Thrombosis with or without embolism of either the venous or arterial systems is often an undiagnosed cause of morbidity and mortality in small animals. The pathogenesis of thrombosis and thromboembolic disease is presented here; it is followed by clinical manifestations, an approach to diagnosis, and a discussion of fibrinolytic agents, anticoagulants, and platelet-function inhibitors used in antithrombotic therapy.

PATHOGENESIS

A thrombus is an intravascular deposit composed of fibrin and the formed elements (cells) of blood. The basic factors contributing to thrombosis are (1) damage to the vascular endothelium, (2) changes in blood flow (rheology), and (3) changes in the constituents of the blood. Most of the thrombotic conditions recognized at present in small animals are associated with infectious agents that result in inflammation and damage to the vascular endothelium. Other types of thromboses occur as part of endothelial or platelet perturbation in disease processes (Table 1). Among the infectious diseases associated with increased risk of thrombotic disease are dirofilariasis (caused by *Dirofilaria immitis*), streptococcal and salmonellal infections (often associated with vegatative endocarditis) of small animals including those in laboratories, and thromboembolic phenomena subsequent to volvulus, torsion, and gastric dilatation in the dog. It should be noted that disseminated intravascular coagulation (DIC), a common sequela of many disease processes such as sepsis, is a microvascular thrombotic event.

Diseases associated with thromboembolic phenomena include hyperadrenocorticism (Cushing's disease), diabetis mellitus, nephrotic syndrome, and many types of metastatic neoplasms.

Thrombosis has been associated with indwelling vascular catheters and fragments of hair in dogs. Numerous reports have appeared in the literature concerning aortic embolism at the terminal aorta of cats with cardiomyopathy. These emboli are often associated with atrial emboli, but the cause is, as yet, specifically undetermined. Polyarteritis, a primary necrotizing inflammatory condition involving small- and medium-sized arteries, may be the result of immune complex disease in the dog and cat.

Thrombi undergo constant structural change. Leukocytes are attracted by chemotactic factors released from aggregated platelets and rapidly accumulate around the platelet aggregate. In addition, the aggregated platelets swell and undergo autolysis, so that after 24 hours only fibrin remains. The subsequent fate of the thrombus represents a balance between forces leading to the deposition and removal of thrombotic material. The factors leading to removal include fibrinolysis, embolization of thrombotic material, phagocytosis of fibrin by leu-

Table 1. Conditions Associated with Thrombosis in Small Animals

Agent	Lesion or Process
Parasites	
Dirofilaria immitis	Affects pulmonary artery, right atrium, vena cava
Sepsis	
Bacteria Viruses Fungi	All cause suppurative inflammatory processes, swelling of endothelial cells, exposure of collagen, and platelet adhesion
Miscellaneous	
Neoplasia	Associated with metastasis
Myeloproliferative disorders	Associated with abnormal platelet function
Aortic embolism (cat)	Affects terminal aorta; associated with cardiomyopathy
Indwelling catheters	Predominantly affects jugular vein
Nephrotic syndrome	Causes pulmonary thrombosis
Cushing's disease (hyperadrenocorticism)	Causes pulmonary thrombosis
Diabetes mellitus	Causes renal glomerular microthrombi
Immune complex polyarteritis	Affects small- and medium-sized arteries
Disseminated intravascular coagulation	Always initiated by a primary process
Congestive heart failure	Causes increased venous stasis
Plasma cell dyscrasias	Causes vascular occlusion and hyperviscosity

kocytes, and organization of the thrombus. If deposition occurs, the thrombus may propagate.

Each of the three components of hemostasis—vascular integrity, platelets, and the coagulation protein (factor) cascade—may be the source of unwanted thrombosis. Each of these three components can be modulated or attenuated to minimize or prevent thrombosis. The fourth hemostatic component, clot lysis, is used to treat thrombosis caused by disorders of the first three hemostatic components.

Major disorders of vascular integrity that promote thrombosis are those involving endothelial injury or pathologic conditions. Atherosclerotic involvement (if it occurs at all in small animal medicine), abnormal venous structures (wall injury, valve abnormalities), and circulatory stasis all may predispose the animal to platelet and fibrin deposition. The treatment of thrombosis caused by disorders of vascular integrity thus involves both the removal of the inciting pathologic disorder and attenuation of the remainder of the hemostatic system, or either of these procedures. Thus, alterations in platelet function (see Salicylate Toxicity) or in the effectiveness of the coagulation cascade may be necessary.

Thrombocytosis, high numbers of circulating platelets (especially associated with myeloproliferative disorders), and many severe inflammatory disorders including solid tumor formation may induce thrombosis. Hemodilution and prevention of circulatory stasis is usually sufficient to minimize problems in this area of hemostasis.

Disorders of the coagulation cascade are numerous and common. The loss of localizing mechanisms may predispose the patient to fibrin formation and thus thrombosis. These could include failure of normal blood flow in circulatory shock, hepatic dysfunction causing inadequate removal of activated coagulation proteins, or lack of activated factor neutralization by acquired deficiency of the normal inhibitor of the coagulation cascade, antithrombin III (AT III). A reduction of coagulation proteins to minimize or prevent thrombosis can be produced with coumarin derivatives. This, along with reestablishment of normal circulatory flow with fluid therapy and fresh plasma (to restore AT III concentrations), is utilized in therapy.

CLINICAL MANIFESTATIONS AND APPROACH

The signs of venous obstruction are consequences of both venous obstruction and local distention (Table 2); the reactive inflammatory response causes pain, tenderness, erythema, and warmth. The clinical manifestations of pulmonary embolism revolve around the single consistent feature of this problem—dyspnea. The mechanism of dyspnea in pulmonary embolism is not completely understood. Possible contributing factors include hypoxemia, splinting of the chest wall caused by pleuritic chest pain, congestive atelectasis, pulmonary infarction, and regional pulmonary edema. Hemoptysis is a relatively infrequent feature of pulmonary embolism. Its presence suggests that pulmonary infarction or congestive atelectasis has occurred and has produced pulmonary hemorrhage. Massive embolism may be associated with syncope.

Detection of venous thrombosis (Table 3) requires sophisticated technologies not usually available and often costly to the veterinary clinician. These in-

Table 2. Factors Involved in the Propagation of Venous Thrombi

Enhancing Factors
Stasis of blood
Increased blood viscosity
Hypercoagulability
Inhibitory Factors
Rapid blood flow
Adequate hydration
Normal hemostatic and fibrinolytic mechanisms
Increased Clinical Risk
Decreased antithrombin III concentration—nephrotic syndrome
Increased coagulation proteins—Cushing's disease
Invasion of endothelial cells—neoplasia

Table 3. *Tests That May Detect Hypercoagulability*

Tests Based on Thrombin Activation
Detection of fibrin(ogen) degradation products
Shortening of thrombin clotting time (TT)
Shortening of the activated partial thromboplastin time (APTT)
Shortening of the prothrombin time (PT)
Decrease in fibrinogen concentration
Tests of Natural Inhibitor Concentration
Antithrombin III—reduced
Protein C—reduced
Less Specific Tests
Platelet adhesiveness—increased
Blood viscosity—increased

clude contrast venography and ultrasound flow detection. Both are available at many veterinary institutions. Clinicians who suspect the presence of venous thrombosis should consult with their veterinary radiologist and hematologist. Blood tests that may provide information on hypercoagulability include increased fibrin (and fibrinogen) degradation products (FDPs, FSPs), shortening of the test times for routine coagulograms (activated partial thromboplastin time, APTT; prothrombin time, PT), decreased concentration of AT III, shortening of the thrombin clotting time (TT), increased platelet adhesiveness, and increased blood viscosity. An awareness of processes that lead to thromboembolic disease (see above) will serve to increase the index of suspicion.

The signs of acute arterial occlusion can be acute pain or chronic intermittent pain, and, in cases frustrating to the clinician, some patients are asymptomatic. Peripheral arterial embolism is usually found in patients with underlying cardiac disease, including arrhythmia or valvular heart disease. A more chronic onset of peripheral arterial thrombosis is associated with limb coldness and paraesthesia. Progression of arterial insufficiency leads to ischemia of distal tissues, ulceration, and possibly gangrene.

Visceral arterial embolism or thrombosis may lead to intestinal or renal infarction and usually results in abdominal pain. Acute mesenteric arterial occlusion produces the triad of sudden abdominal pain, vomiting, and bowel evacuation. Melena usually occurs later. Findings of the abdominal examination are often unimpressive and often show minimal or no tenderness or guarding. Initially, hyperactive bowel sounds may be heard. Later these become hypoactive and then cease.

Acute renal arterial occlusion is usually manifest by sudden flank pain and hematuria. The signs of chronic intestinal ischemia are postprandial abdominal pain, and the resulting food restriction leads to weight loss. As these signs are similar to many acute abdominal problems such as pancreatitis, screening tests must be used to rule out the more common processes. The same laboratory techniques discussed under venous thrombosis may be helpful in the diagnosis of arterial thrombosis as well. In addition, arteriography, perfusion lung scanning, and pulmonary angiography are techniques used to investigate thromboembolic disease of arterial origin.

THERAPY

Two major therapeutic approaches are used in treating thromboembolic disorders: administration of anticoagulants as a preventive measure and administration of thrombolytic drugs as a means of cure. Anticoagulants include heparin for short-term treatment, coumarin derivatives such as warfarin for long-term therapy, and aspirin and dextran as adjunctive antiplatelet therapy.

Heparin

After the subcutaneous injection of 10 to 40 units/kg of either sodium or calcium heparin, sensitive assay techniques can demonstrate the presence of small concentrations of heparin in the plasma of most small animal patients. The amount of heparin revealed peaks about 4 hours after injection and disappears at 8 hours. There is considerable patient variation that is not related to body weight. The peak concentration is influenced by the type of heparin (higher values are achieved with the sodium rather than the calcium salt) and the average molecular weight of heparin (MW 3000 to 37,000; higher values result from heparins of lower molecular weight). Subcutaneous injections of either calcium or sodium heparin every 8 hours will result in fluctuating concentrations of heparin in most patients. Heparin complexes with and activates the serine protease inhibitor AT III. This accelerates the neutralization of all serine proteases among the coagulation proteins, especially activated Factor X and thrombin (IIa). Dosage is varied at 8-hour intervals until the APTT is prolonged from two to two-and-one-half times the preheparin baseline APTT. Complications are hemorrhage (greater with larger doses), hypersensitivity reactions, and modest thrombocytopenia if heparin is used for more than one week. In the event of hemorrhage, heparin activity may be immediately neutralized by protamine sulfate. Heparin cannot dissolve thrombi, but a thrombus may become smaller, because additional thrombus formation is limited and natural fibrinolytic enzyme activity directed against the thrombus will reduce its size. Heparin should never be administered intramuscularly because of the risk of hematoma formation. Because of this, patients receiving heparin therapy should never receive intra-

Table 4. Drugs That Affect Coumarin Derivatives

Drugs That Increase the Effect
Antibiotics (penicillin, cephalosporins, sulfonamides, tetracycline)
Anti-inflammatory analgesics (aspirin, indomethacin, phenylbutazone)
Anabolic steroids
Tranquilizing agents
Thyroxine
Drugs That Decrease the Effect
Barbiturates
Phenytoin
Spironolactone
Griseofulvin

muscular injections. Heparin therapy should *never* be abruptly stopped but should be gradually tapered through 48 hours to prevent rebound hypercoagulability.

Oral Anticoagulant Therapy

The oral anticoagulants consist of two classes of compounds, the coumarins and the indanediones, exemplified by warfarin and phenindione, respectively. This discussion will focus on warfarin, as the indanediones are exceptionally potent drugs. These agents interfere with the action of vitamin K in the hepatic activation of Factors II, VII, IX, and X and of the inhibitor of Factors V and VIII, protein C. Reduction in activity of plasma Factor VII is the main effect in the first several days after induction of therapy. The reduction in other factors quickly follows. The oral anticoagulants render blood hypocoagulable and prevent formation of a thrombus or its further extension. The optimal duration of therapy is wholly dependent upon the initiating problem. We have used this form of therapy for as long as 6 months. It is usually not worthwhile to give oral anticoagulants for less than 6 weeks, as it often takes 2 to 3 weeks to stabilize the patient on the correct dose of the drug (Table 4). The usual dosage is 1 to 5 mg/kg daily. However, individual patient variability is quite large. Coumarin therapy may be abruptly stopped, since no rebound hypercoagulability has occurred either clinically or in laboratory tests.

Aspirin therapy has been discussed in a later article (Salicylate Toxicity) and will not be discussed here other than to note that it is a potent inhibitor of platelet function. Although aspirin is metabolized in less than 1 hour, it irreversibly inhibits platelet cyclo-oxygenase, resulting in failure of the platelet to synthesize prostaglandins G_2 and H_2 and thromboxane A_2. The result is that all platelets circulating before aspirin is metabolized will be rendered nonfunctional. The effect of a single pharmacological dose of aspirin may last up to 10 days. The other nonsteroidal anti-inflammmatory agents (phenylbutazone, indomethacin) have a similar but shorter-lived effect.

Dextran

Dextran has also been used to inhibit platelet function. The effects of dextran are related to dose and are more pronounced with the compounds of higher molecular weight; they reach maximum effect 4 to 8 hours after infusion, suggesting a time-consuming reaction either with the platelets themselves or with plasma proteins.

Thrombolytic Therapy

The major thrombolytic drugs are streptokinase and urokinase, both of which activate plasminogen. Both drugs are expensive, but urokinase is exceptionally so. The following comments on thrombolytic therapy are made with the caveat that clinicians are strongly urged to consult with a veterinary hematologist before embarking on this form of therapy. Dosage will not be discussed.

Streptokinase forms a complex with plasminogen that cleaves additional plasminogen precursors to form plasmin, a potent fibrinolytic enzyme. Administration of streptokinase produces a systemic lytic state defined by several characteristics: depletion of plasminogen; presence of free plasmin in plasma; decrease in α-2-antiplasmin because of its binding to newly formed plasmin; decrease in fibrinogen concentrations; increase in degradation products of fibrin and fibrinogen; and prolonged thrombin clotting time resulting from these circulating degradation products and hypofibrinogenemia.

Although the achievement of a systemic lytic state appears necessary for dissolving a pathologic clot, it increases the risk of uncontrolled bleeding. The change in the plasma coagulation proteins does not in itself cause a bleeding problem. The threat lies in the dissolution of a hemorrhagic plug or the prevention of platelet-plug formation.

Streptokinase is *contraindicated* in patients that cannot tolerate a systemic lytic state without bleeding problems. Grounds for exclusion include a recent (10-day history) of thoracic or abdominal surgery or current gastrointestinal or genitourinary bleeding. Bleeding tendencies or hemostatic abnormalities may be indentified by laboratory tests of bleeding time, platelet count, APTT, PT, TT, or increased fibrin (or fibrinogen) degradation products. The thrombin clotting time is the easiest monitor of fibrinolysis. In many veterinary institutions, plasminogen can be assayed. Marder and Bell reviewed nine studies that compared the effectiveness of heparin and streptokinase. Venography showed, after 5 days of therapy, substantial improvement in 45 per cent of human patients treated with streptokinase but only 5 per cent of the patients treated with heparin.

References and Supplemental Reading

Barrowcliffe, T. W., Johnson, E. A., and Thomas, D.: Antithrombin III and heparin. Br. Med. Bull. 34:143, 1978.

Burns, M. G., Kelly, A. B., Hornof, W. J., et al.: Pulmonary artery thrombosis in three dogs with hyperadrenocorticism. J.A.V.M.A. 178:388, 1981.

Duxbury, B. McD.: Therapeutic control of anticoagulant treatment. Br. Med. J. 284:702, 1982.

Fincell, T. J., and Hill, B. L.: A review of primary cardiomyopathy in the cat. Iowa State Univ. Vet. 45:118, 1983.

Green, R. A., and Kabel, A. L.: Hypercoagulable state in three dogs with nephrotic syndrome: Role of acquired antithrombin III deficiency. J.A.V.M.A. 181:914, 1982.

Hargis, A. M., Stephens, L. C., Benjamin, S. A., et al.: Relationship of hypothyroidism to diabetes mellitus, renal amyloidosis and thrombosis in purebred beagles. Am. J. Vet. Res. 42:1077, 1981.

Hirsh, J., and Brain, E. A.: *Hemostasis and Thrombosis: A Conceptual Approach*, 2nd ed. New York: Churchill Livingstone, 1983.

Keith, J. C., Jr., Rawlings, C. A., and Schaub, R. G.: Pulmonary thromboembolism during therapy of dirofilariasis with thiacetarsamide: Modification with aspirin or prednisolone. Am. J. Vet. Res. 44:1278, 1983.

Loeliger, E. A.: The optimal therapeutic range in oral anticoagulation: History and proposal. Thromb. Haemost. 42:1141, 1979.

Marder, V. J., and Bell, W. R.: Fibrinolytic therapy. *In* Coleman, R. W., Hirsh, J., Marder, V. J., et al. (eds.): *Hemostasis and Thrombosis*. Philadelphia: J.B. Lippincott, 1982, p. 1937.

Sharma, V. R. K., Cella, G., Parisi, A. F., et al.: Thrombolytic therapy. N. Engl. J. Med. 306:1268, 1982.

Statland, B. E., and Ito, R. K.: Thrombolytic therapy: Minimizing the risks. Diag. Med. 7:25, 1984.

ELECTRONIC SIZING OF ERYTHROCYTES AND INTERPRETATION OF THE MEAN CORPUSCULAR VOLUME

M. G. WEISER, D.V.M.

Fort Collins, Colorado

The following information is intended to update the veterinary practitioner's perspective on the mean corpuscular volume (MCV) value, with emphasis on the impact of advances in hematologic instrumentation occurring over the last 20 years. Although the techniques discussed are currently not practical for use in most in-house veterinary hospital laboratories, they are being increasingly utilized by commercial and research laboratories serving veterinarians.

Years ago, it was determined that changes in erythrocyte size during certain disease states were useful in diagnosing human and animal anemias. These size changes, expressed as MCV values, are the basis for the well-known morphologic classification of anemias: microcytic (decreased MCV), normocytic, and macrocytic (increased MCV). Traditional interpretations of MCV values include such disorders as microcytosis which, in the dog, indicates iron deficiency and, more importantly, suggests chronic external blood loss as the cause. Microcytosis is not observed in adult cats. Normocytic anemia is usually due to one of the many causes of bone marrow's failure to produce erythrocytes at the proper rate. Macrocytosis is observed in all species in association with marked erythrocytic regeneration occurring in response to either hemolysis or severe hemorrhage. With maximal stimulation of erythroid marrow, individual erythrocytes at about twice normal volume may be produced. When a minimum of 10 to 20 per cent of the circulating cells are produced under these conditions, the MCV may become increased above normal. Macrocytosis established by maximal regeneration may persist for as long as several weeks after either the cessation of marrow output or the return of erythropoiesis to normal. Macrocytosis, with MCV values in the range of 80 to 100 fl (μm^3) is occasionally observed in normal poodles.

These correlations between MCV and processes affecting erythrocyte size were regarded as useful in early approaches to hematologic disease; however, as more specific diagnostic tests were developed, the MCV value became a less valuable diagnostic tool. In recent years, with the development of automated instrumentation that measures MCV directly, this value has regained popularity in human hematology (Bessman et al., 1983; Fishleder and Hoffman, 1984). This is due to improvements in its reproducibility and new associated measurements such as indices of anisocytosis and the erythrocyte volume-distribution histogram (Fig. 1). These new measurements are becoming routine in human hematologic profiling but to date have received little attention in veterinary hematology.

REVIEW OF TECHNIQUES

The traditional method of determining the MCV value is to calculate it from an erythrocyte count and a value for packed cell volume, determined by the microhematocrit method. The following formula is then used (Schalm, et al., 1975):

$$\frac{\text{PCV} \times 10}{\text{RBC}}$$

There are several disadvantages to this method of determining the MCV:

1. The variation in these primary measurements in the clinical laboratory is at best ±1 unit for the microhematocrit determination and ±5 per cent for the erythrocyte count. Under relatively ideal conditions for these manual methods, the calculated MCV will vary ±4 fl. This variation is about half the reference range in both dogs and cats. The imprecision results in a wider reference range than is necessary, particularly at the upper end of normal.
2. Erythrocytes produced under conditions of iron deficiency, and probably other conditions as well, are less deformable than normal and do not pack completely during microhematocrit centrifugation. The falsely high PCV value due to increased trapped plasma tends to overestimate the calculated MCV value and mask the microcytosis that accompanies iron deficiency.
3. Large platelets may get counted as erythrocytes on electronic cell counters and result in underestimation of the MCV. In anemic cats with large numbers of platelets, this factor may mask an increased MCV associated with recent or ongoing erythrocytic regeneration. The volume of feline platelets is two to four times greater than that of canine platelets.
4. The hypertonicity of excess EDTA causes considerable erythrocyte shrinkage when blood tubes are not filled completely. As much as a 20 per cent decrease in MCV may be observed when less than 0.5 ml of blood is placed in a 2-ml EDTA tube.

In this author's opinion the calculated MCV is not a useful procedure, especially in the veterinary hospital. The effort to count erythrocytes and then calculate the MCV is not worth the interpretive value gained. The imprecision of the procedure and the number of potential sources of error is such that the calculated MCV detects only relatively severe changes in mean cell size and is therefore not sensitive in detecting disease associated with alteration of erythrocyte size.

Modern multi-channel blood cell counters were introduced 20 years ago and have since undergone considerable technologic advances and refinement.

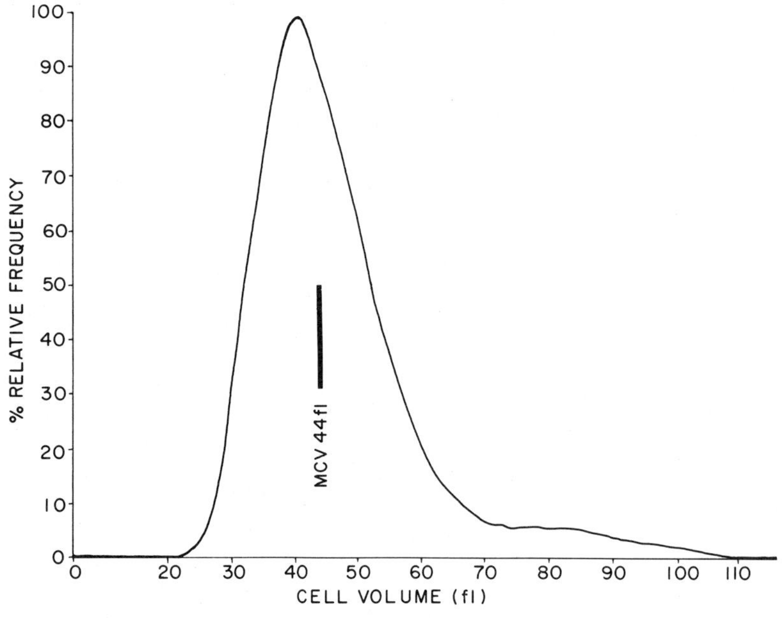

Figure 1. Histogram of a representative volume distribution of feline erythrocytes. The MCV is indicated by the vertical bar. Increased anisocytosis would be shown by widening of the curve. Microcytosis would shift the curve to the left and macrocytosis would shift the curve to the right.

Today these are used by virtually all commercial and human hospital laboratories serving veterinarians.* These counters determine MCV directly and then compute the hematocrit value from the MCV and the erythrocyte count. As each erythrocyte is counted, its volume is detected by a change in electrical current proportional to the volume of electrolyte fluid or diluent displaced by the cell. (For a more detailed explanation, see Weiser, 1981, or Nelson, 1979.) The instrument then derives the MCV by determining the mean of all the individual cell volumes. One of the advantages of this technique is that the sources of error mentioned previously in calculated MCV are not encountered. This determination is quite reproducible; expected day-to-day variation is ±1 or 2 fl. The reference range for MCV is smaller, especially at the upper end of normal. Although the reference range should be determined by each laboratory, experience with several counting systems indicates that a reference range of 37 to 49 fl for cats and 60 to 72 fl for dogs may be used for interpretation of electronic MCV values (Weiser, 1982).

Some advanced cell counters determine an erythrocyte volume-distribution histogram as the cells are counted. A particle size analyzer assigns each erythrocyte in the sample to a narrow size window in a histogram (Fig. 1). The system's computer can analyze the histogram and provide an automated measurement of anisocytosis, the RDW value (red cell distribution width). This value is a coefficient of variation of erythrocyte volumes. In conjunction with the MCV value, an abnormal RDW value can alert the laboratory worker to search for specific erythrocyte defects during the blood film examination. Additionally, inspection of the histogram allows recognition of abnormal erythrocyte subpopulations. Erythrocyte size changes and subpopulation abnormalities are often detectable before the MCV deviates from the normal range. In short, these sensitive new measurements provide an automated method for detection of erythron abnormalities.

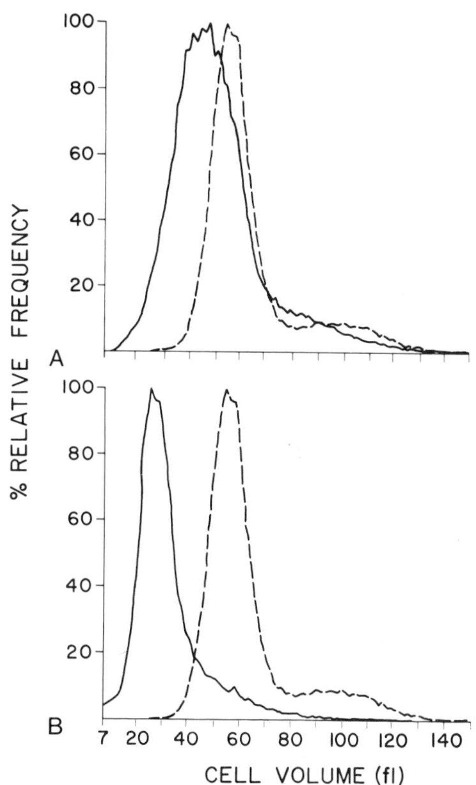

Figure 2. Examples of histograms from dogs with iron deficiency anemia (solid line) and a normal dog (broken line). In *A*, there is increased anisocytosis due to an erythrocyte population consisting of both normocytes and microcytes. In *B*, there has been complete blood repopulation with microcytes. (Reproduced, with permission, from Weiser and O'Grady: Vet. Pathol. 20:230, 1983.)

USE OF NEW HEMATOLOGIC TECHNIQUES IN VETERINARY MEDICINE

Since a high laboratory volume is required to support the expense of this equipment, it is unlikely to be directly used by the veterinarian to diagnose hematologic disease. Rather, it is envisioned that the technician will specialize in using this and other laboratory methods to enhance the quality of data and interpretations available to veterinarians. How are these new technological advances potentially used by laboratories?

1. With electronic MCV values and histograms, disturbances of erythrocyte production that result in altered cell size are more readily detected. For example, a large number of microcytic erythrocytes must be produced before the mean cell size becomes decreased below normal. However, a deviation of the left tail of the histogram toward microcytosis may reveal early iron deficiency in the presence of a normal MCV.

2. By examination of the relative size of erythrocyte subpopulation on the histogram, interpretations can be made about the chronicity or severity of a process (Figs. 2 and 3).

3. Routine use of an erythrocyte histogram along with the MCV value alerts the laboratory technician to search for specific defects on the blood film. For example, a widened histogram with a low or low-normal MCV should increase the suspicion that hypochromic erythrocytes may be present. This defect is frequently missed because it is usually

*Note: In veterinary laboratories these instruments are modified for counting animal cells. However. the unmodified instruments in human laboratories do not accurately count small erythrocytes of some species. In this setting, analysis of canine blood can be considered accurate, but errors will occur in analysis of feline blood. Therefore, laboratories without modified instruments should analyze feline blood by other techniques.

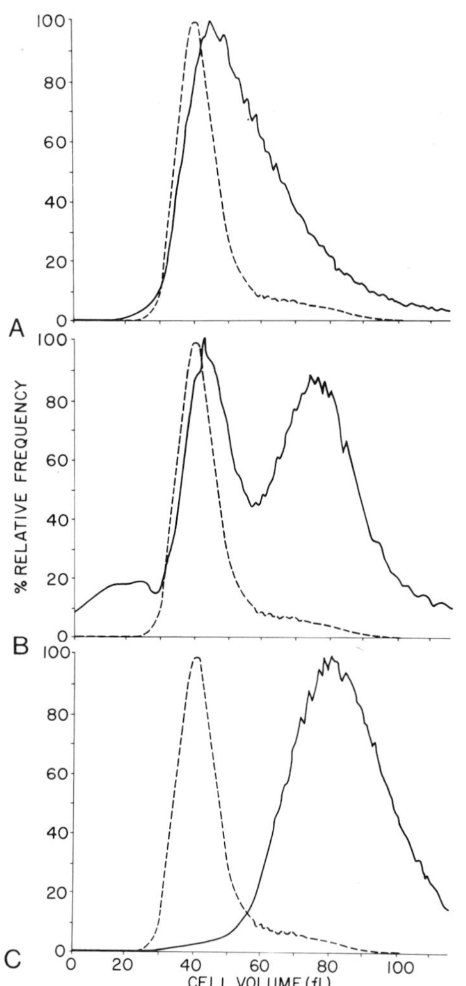

Figure 3. Examples of erythrocyte histograms from cats with feline leukemia virus infection (solid line) and a normal cat (broken line). In *A*, there is increased anisocytosis due to modest production of macrocytes. In *B*, there is a normal subpopulation and a markedly macrocytic subpopulation. In *C*, there has been complete blood repopulation with macrocytic erythrocytes. (Reproduced, with permission, from Weiser and Kociba: Vet. Pathol. 20:687, 1983.)

subtle and the observer does not suspect its presence. Conversely, the presence of questionable defects on the blood film, such as hypochromic cells, may be supported or refuted by features in the MCV and histogram.

4. Inspection of the histogram provides visual confirmation that the cell population has behaved properly with respect to the instrument's counting threshold. This helps ensure counting accuracy for samples having microcytic erythrocytes that may fall below the threshold.

Relatively new observations on MCV interpretation in animals has resulted from routine use of electronically determined MCV and histograms. Microcytosis has been observed in 4- to 7-week-old kittens in association with transient iron deficiency (Weiser and Kociba, 1983a). Kittens rapidly repopulate the blood with normocytic cells after intake of solid food. Microcytosis has been observed in about 75 per cent of dogs with portosystemic shunts; the cause is uncertain at this time (Griffiths et al., 1981). Cats with feline leukemia virus (FeLV) infection have a high incidence of macrocytosis, even those with nonregenerative anemia (Weiser and Kociba, 1983b). This is thought to reflect varying degrees of accelerated erythrocytic regeneration, which establishes macrocytosis, and is then followed by erythroid or total marrow failure attributable to the FeLV infection (see Fig. 3). When observed by the veterinarian, the cat usually has nonregenerative anemia with macrocytosis. Macrocytosis in the cat with either a normal PCV or with reticulocytosis should be interpreted as reflecting current or recent regeneration. However, macrocytosis accompanying nonregenerative anemia has a high probability of being associated with FeLV infection.

References and Supplemental Reading

Bessman, D. J. Gilmer, P. R., and Gardner, F. H.: Improved classification of anemias by MCV and RDW. Am. J. Clin. Pathol. 80:322, 1983.

Fishleder, A. J., and Hoffman, G. C.: Automated hematology: Counts and indices. Lab. Manage. 22:21, 1984.

Griffiths, G. L., Lumsden, J. H., and Valli, V. E. O.: Hematologic and biochemical changes in dogs with portosystemic shunts. J. Am. Anim. Hosp. Assoc. 17:705, 1981.

Nelson, D. A.: Basic methodology. *In* Henry, J. B. (ed.): *Todd-Sanford-Davidsohn Clinical Diagnosis and Management by Laboratory Methods.* 16th ed. Philadelphia: W. B. Saunders, 1979, p. 878.

Schalm, O. W., Jain, N. C., and Carroll, E. J.: *Veterinary Hematology*, 3rd ed. Philadelphia: Lea & Febiger, 1975, p. 66.

Weiser, M. G.: Hematologic techniques. Vet. Clin. North Am. 11:195, 1981.

Weiser, M. G.: Erythrocyte volume distribution analysis in healthy dogs, cats, horses, and dairy cows. Am. J. Vet. Res. 43:163, 1982.

Weiser, M. G., and Kociba, G. J.: Sequential changes in erythrocyte volume distribution and microcytosis associated with iron deficiency in kittens. Vet. Pathol. 20:1, 1983a.

Weiser, M. G., and Kociba, G. J.: Erythrocyte macrocytosis in feline leukemia virus associated anemia. Vet. Pathol. 20:687, 1983b.

Weiser, M. G., and O'Grady, M.: Erythrocyte volume distribution analysis and hematologic changes in dogs with iron deficiency. Vet. Pathol. 20:230, 1983.

PROTEINS INDUCED BY VITAMIN K ABSENCE OR ANTAGONISTS ("PIVKA")

MICHAEL E. MOUNT, D.V.M.
Davis, California

The abbreviation PIVKA is unfamiliar to most veterinarians. Once it is understood, however, the veterinarian will undoubtedly desire to apply a test to determine PIVKA's presence, particularly in relation to anticoagulant poisonings.

Anticoagulant therapy in humans for thrombotic diseases was found to require close monitoring in order to maintain a stable hypocoagulation status with the aim of preventing recurrences of thrombosis. In 1959, the thrombotest (referred to as the "PIVKA test" in our laboratory) was introduced in Europe as a new method for controlling anticoagulant therapy (Owren, 1959). It was a modification and simplification of Owren's prothrombin and proconvertin test (PPT). The PPT was a sensitive indicator of decreased concentrations of Factor II, Factor VII, and Factor X. Clinical application of the thrombotest in humans led to the term PIVKA, which stands for "Proteins Induced by Vitamin K Absence or Antagonists" (Hemker and Muller, 1968). The discovery of "abnormal" coagulation proteins in blood of individuals under anticoagulant therapy supported the existence of PIVKA. The sensitivity of the thrombotest to anticoagulant therapy was attributed to these "abnormal" proteins, which act as inhibitors to this test's reagent.

Immunologic studies verified the nature of the PIVKA and showed that these were nonfunctional precursor forms of vitamin K–dependent Factors II, VII, IX, and X—referred to as PIVKA-II, PIVKA-VII, PIVKA-IX, PIVKA-X, respectively (Hemker and Muller, 1968). These nonfunctional proteins (PIVKA) differ from the functional coagulation proteins only by the lack of modification of the glutamic acid residues that are carboxylated in the functional protein moieties (Gaudernack and Prydz, 1975). The functional coagulation proteins are zymogens capable of being activated to participate in the coagulation cascade, which results in a fibrin clot.

Vitamin K is necessary for the alteration of nonfunctional proteins to functional zymogens. During exposure to anticoagulants, the body's stores of vitamin K are so depleted that a relative absence of vitamin K results in not only a depletion of functional coagulation vitamin K–dependent factors but also in a build-up of PIVKA. Hence, when the thrombotest is performed, it recognizes the occurrence of both events.

Vitamin K–dependent coagulation factors are produced in the liver. Precursor coagulation proteins (nonfunctional forms) are synthesized and stored in the liver microsomal system (Liebman et al., 1982). These precursor coagulation proteins in the liver will be referred to as acarboxy-coagulation proteins. When a relative to absolute vitamin K deficiency occurs, these proteins accumulate and spill over into the circulation; where they are referred to as the PIVKA. In healthy individuals, PIVKA are not present in the circulation. The half-life of circulating PIVKA is similar to or less than that of the functional coagulation proteins. The circulating PIVKA are nonfunctional and not able to be carboxylated to form functional coagulation proteins. However, the acarboxy-coagulation proteins are rapidly converted to functional coagulation proteins after administration of vitamin K.

METHODOLOGY

The original thrombotest reagent contained crude cephalin, thromboplastin from brain, adsorbed bovine plasma, and calcium chloride mixed in proportions so that the assay was sensitive to deficiencies in either the intrinsic or extrinsic pathways used for monitoring anticoagulant-treated patients (Owren, 1959). At that time, PIVKA were not known.

The reagent is produced by Nyegaard and Company, Oslo, Norway. It is distributed in the United States by Accurate Chemical and Scientific Corporation (Westbury, New York). It can be used with capillary blood, citrated capillary blood, venous blood, and citrated plasma; the method depends on equipment available to the laboratory. When a fibrometer is employed, the reagent is reconstituted in a solution of 3.2 mmol/L of calcium chloride and mixed with citrated plasma (this method requires only 30 μl of plasma and 250 μl of reagent). The

Table 1. Conditions Resulting in Vitamin K Absence or Antagonism

Internal Medical Conditions
Malabsorption
Biliary obstruction or fistulae
Intestinal sterilization
Chemically Induced Conditions
Ingestion of anticoagulant rodenticide
Use or overdose of therapeutic anticoagulant

plasma and reagent interact, and the time is measured for the clot to form. The presence of heparin will prolong the thrombotest assay (Owren, 1959).

In humans, the results are expressed as an activity index in which 100 per cent is equivalent to normal activity. Elevation in the thrombotest time results in a lower index percentage. The calculation is given as follows:

$$\frac{\text{Normal thrombotest time in seconds}}{\text{Patient thrombotest time in seconds}} \times 100 = \text{Activity Index as per cent}$$

The data in this text are expressed simply as time in seconds (sec) to complete the thrombotest assay.

APPLICATIONS FOR THE THROMBOTEST

Studies in our laboratory have been performed only in the dog. Normal reference values for the dogs (n = 16) ranged from 16.2 to 19.0 sec with a mean of 17.6 sec and standard deviation (SD) of 0.87 sec. Thrombotest times observed in a normal dog over a 50-day period (n = 30 observations) ranged from 16.4 to 20.9 sec with a mean of 17.5 sec and SD of 0.89 sec.

A decrease in vitamin K–dependent coagulation factors affects the thrombotest assay. The thrombotest is extremely sensitive to plasma concentrations of Factor X (Malia et al., 1980). When only a decrease in factors occurs (without PIVKA formation), as in a congenital factor deficiency or parenchymal hepatic disease, thromboplastins (such as those used in the one-stage prothrombin time assay [OSPT]) are more sensitive indicators of factor deficiency than the thrombotest; this has been demonstrated for Factors II, VII, IX, and X (Soulier, 1964).

Any medical condition producing an absolute to relative vitamin K deficiency would also produce an elevation in the results of the thrombotest assay. This increase is due not only to a decrease in coagulation factors but also to an elevation of circulating PIVKA. Disease conditions that produce a vitamin K deficiency are listed in Table 1 and result in elevation of the PIVKA. Parenchymal liver disease itself does not produce an elevation in PIVKA (Liebman et al., 1982). A clinical study of human patients with liver disease identified PIVKA-positive and PIVKA-negative groups by using the Thrombotest (Malia et al., 1980). Only the PIVKA-positive group demonstrated a response to vitamin K therapy, as evidenced by a dramatic increase in activities of Factors II, VII, and X. There are other assays capable of measuring PIVKA that are more precise (but more involved technically) than the thrombotest (Bertina et al., 1980). They enable a more definitive differentiation of parenchymal liver disease from one of the conditions listed in Table 1 or from such a concomitant disease occurring with parenchymal liver disease.

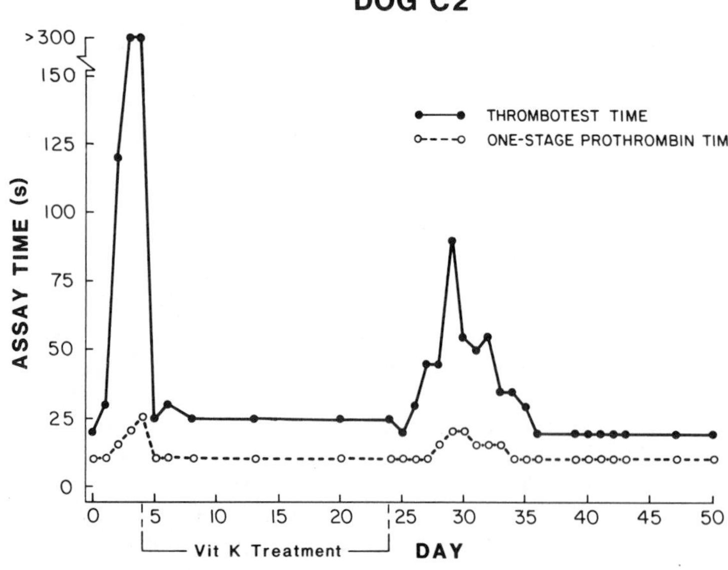

Figure 1. Monitoring of coagulation in a dog that received 2.5 mg diphacinone/kg body weight divided over three days (days 0 to 3) with follow-up therapy of vitamin K_1 at 2.5 mg/kg for 21 days (days 4 to 24). The graph compares the degree of response between one-stage prothrombin time (OSPT) and the thrombotest (PIVKA test). Diphacinone is an indanedione anticoagulant used as a rodenticide. It has a prolonged toxic effect, as indicated by elevation of coagulation time (25 to 35 days).

The most marked increase of PIVKA in veterinary practice is that observed in animals poisoned with anticoagulants. A thrombotest time of 18 sec in a healthy dog would increase to greater than 300 sec when the animal is exposed to an anticoagulant; OSPT would change from a normal activity of 7 sec to a corresponding 25 to 30 sec. Figure 1 illustrates the similarity of response between the thrombotest and OSPT to anticoagulant exposure. The extreme sensitivity of the thrombotest is appreciated by the marked increase in time of assay. This dramatic change may prove helpful to clinicians trying to differentiate causes of anemia. Marked elevation in the thrombotest time would be sufficient evidence to highly suspect anticoagulant poisoning and to initiate vitamin K therapy. Further studies need to be done to evaluate changes in the thrombotest assay in disseminated intravascular coagulopathy (DIC). Elevation of the thrombotest assay times was observed in some forms of low-grade DIC in humans (Slaastad and Godal, 1972). The exact causes were speculative.

SUMMARY

The thrombotest (PIVKA test) is exceptionally sensitive to vitamin K absence or antagonism. In veterinary medicine, anticoagulant poisoning is a disease state in which application of this test offers significant diagnostic information.

References and Supplemental Reading

Bertina, R. M., Van Der Marel-Van Nieuwkoop, W., Dubbeldam, J., et al.: New method for the rapid detection of vitamin K deficiency. Clin. Chim. Acta 105:93, 1980.

Gaudernack, G., and Prydz, H.: Studies on PIVKA-X. Thromb. Diath. Haemorrh. 34:455, 1975.

Hemker, H. C., and Muller, A. D.: Kinetic aspects of the interaction of blood clotting enzymes: VI. Localization of the site of blood-coagulation inhibition by the protein induced by vitamin K absence (PIVKA). Thromb. Diath. Haemorrh. 20:78, 1968.

Liebman, H. A., Furie, B. C., and Furie, B.: Hepatic vitmain K-dependent carboxylation of blood-clotting proteins. Hepatology 2:488, 1982.

Malia, R. G., Preston, F. E., and Holdsworth, C. D.: Clinical responses to vitamin K_1. *In* Suttie, J. W. (ed.): *Vitamin K Metabolism and Vitamin K–Dependent Proteins.* Baltimore: University Park Press, 1980, pp. 342–347.

Owren, P. A.: Thrombotest: A new method for controlling anticoagulant therapy. Lancet 2:754, 1959.

Slaastad, R. A., and Godal, H. C.: Discrepancy between Thrombotest and Normotest—An indicator of disseminated intravascular coagulation (DIC). Scand. J. Haematol. 9:411, 1972.

Soulier, J. P.: Sensitivity of various thromboplastin reagents for the control of anticoagulant therapy. Thromb. Diath. Haemorrh. 13 (suppl.) 363, 1964.

FELINE BLOOD TRANSFUSION REACTIONS

LAURIE A. AUER, B.V.Sc.,
and KEVIN BELL, B.V.Sc.
Brisbane, Australia

The first indication of an incompatible blood transfusion reaction in the cat will probably be the cessation of respiration. If the animal is anesthetized, this may be the only sign of a severe anaphylactoid reaction. Unfortunately, the adverse reactions to introduced blood may negate the beneficial effects of transfusions, which include improved oxygen-carrying capacity and tissue perfusion and the replenishment of blood factors. The feline AB blood group system has been shown to be responsible for blood transfusion reactions in cats receiving incompatible blood for the first time. Severe anaphylactoid reactions characterized by hypotension, cessation of respiration, and cardiac arrhythmias have been observed in approximately 60 per cent of cats in blood group B that receive 1 ml of 50 per cent saline suspension of group A erythrocytes (Auer and Bell, 1983). Incompatibility reactions must be distinguished from other causes of adverse reactions associated with general collection, storage, and procedural practices. These are documented in Table 1 and, for the most part, are preventable.

BLOOD GROUPS OF CATS

There are three blood groups in the feline AB blood group system: A, B, and AB. They are unrelated to the human AB blood group antigens but resemble them in that antibodies, designated anti-

***Table 1.** Transfusion Reactions*

Adverse Reactions	Cause	Precautionary Steps
Citrate toxicity	Large amounts of citrate used as anticoagulant; citrate binds calcium ion, producing a hypocalcemia	Use the correct proportions of ACD to donor blood
Hyperkalemia	Stored (aged) blood has a higher percentage of hemolyzed red cells; the high intracellular potassium ion is released to the plasma and, if transfused, may cause heart failure and possibly death	Check the blood (especially if more than 1 week old) for evidence of hemolysis; cat blood stored in ACD at 4°C generally keeps very well, but cat blood stored in heparin keeps very poorly and pronounced hemolysis is evident after 1 week
Febrile reactions	Bacterial pyrogens	Collect aseptically from healthy donors
Circulatory overload	May result from too-rapid infusion rate; chronically anemic cats have normal blood volumes and increased venous returns due to low viscosity; a sudden increase in venous return may precipitate heart failure	Administer the blood very slowly in cats with chronic anemia or impaired kidneys and control of blood volume (e.g. oliguric cats); look for signs of circulatory overload such as moist rales or distension of veins; the hind-leg veins may be used as a manometer by raising the legs and observing if the veins collapse
Cardiac arrest	Transfusing cold (stored) blood	Warm to 37°C
Pulmonary microembolism	Transfusion of microaggregates formed in stored blood	Filter blood more than 5 days old
Incompatibility Reactions		
Shock	Destruction of donor red blood cells by IV hemolysis; complement is activated with release of anaphylotoxins, which cause release of vasoactive compounds from mast cells, basophils, and other cells	Determine blood type of the donor and recipient cats for the AB blood group system; transfuse only AB-compatible blood; perform crossmatch to detect any other red cell incompatibilities between donor and recipient
Jaundice	Destruction of red blood cells both intra- and extravascularly	Same as above
Disseminated intravascular coagulation	Has not been recorded in cats but there is a possibility of its occurring because of activation of clotting pathways; this leads to the utilization of clotting factors and a resultant tendency for bleeding	Same as above
Renal damage	Has not been recorded in cats but does occur in humans and therefore the possibility of its occurring after adverse reactions in cats should be considered	Same as above
Fever	Either destruction of red blood cells or sensitivity to transfused leukocytes and platelets or both conditions	Same as above

A and anti-B, occur naturally in plasma without any known prior stimuli. It is the binding of these antibodies to the corresponding introduced red cell antigens that initiates a complement-mediated hypersensitivity reaction (Fig. 1) (Brzica, 1982).

The incidences of the A and B antigens appear to vary topographically. A survey of 1895 cats in the Brisbane area of Australia found 73.3 per cent to be group A, 26.3 per cent group B, and 0.4 per cent group AB (Auer and Bell, 1981). This compares with incidences of 85 per cent group A and 15 per cent group B in France (Eyquem *et al.*, 1962), 97 per cent group A and 3 per cent group B in England (Holmes, 1953), and 90.3 per cent group A and 9.7 per cent group B in Japan (Ikemoto *et al.*, 1981). The Australian study demonstrated that 35 per cent of cats in group A possessed circulating anti-B but usually in low titers (less than 2), whereas cats in group AB contained neither anti-A nor anti-B. In contrast, group B cats invariably contained anti-A, and 70 per cent of these cats had agglutination titers greater than 8. Hemolytic titers of greater than 512 were common. Therefore, cats in group B are at greater risk of suffering severe incompatibility reactions. Anti-A is both a strong agglutinin and strong hemolysin. The agglutinating properties of anti-A allow easy detection of incompatibility by a slide agglutination crossmatch.

REACTIONS DUE TO AB BLOOD GROUP INCOMPATIBILITY—CLINICAL PICTURE

Either an immediate or delayed reaction may occur when incompatible blood is transfused into a cat. The severity of the immediate reaction will vary with the titer of circulating isoantibodies and available complement in the recipient and the amount of introduced incompatible erythrocytes. In cats with high titers of isoantibodies, the most severe reactions will occur with as little as 1 ml of introduced red cells. Because of the dilution effect

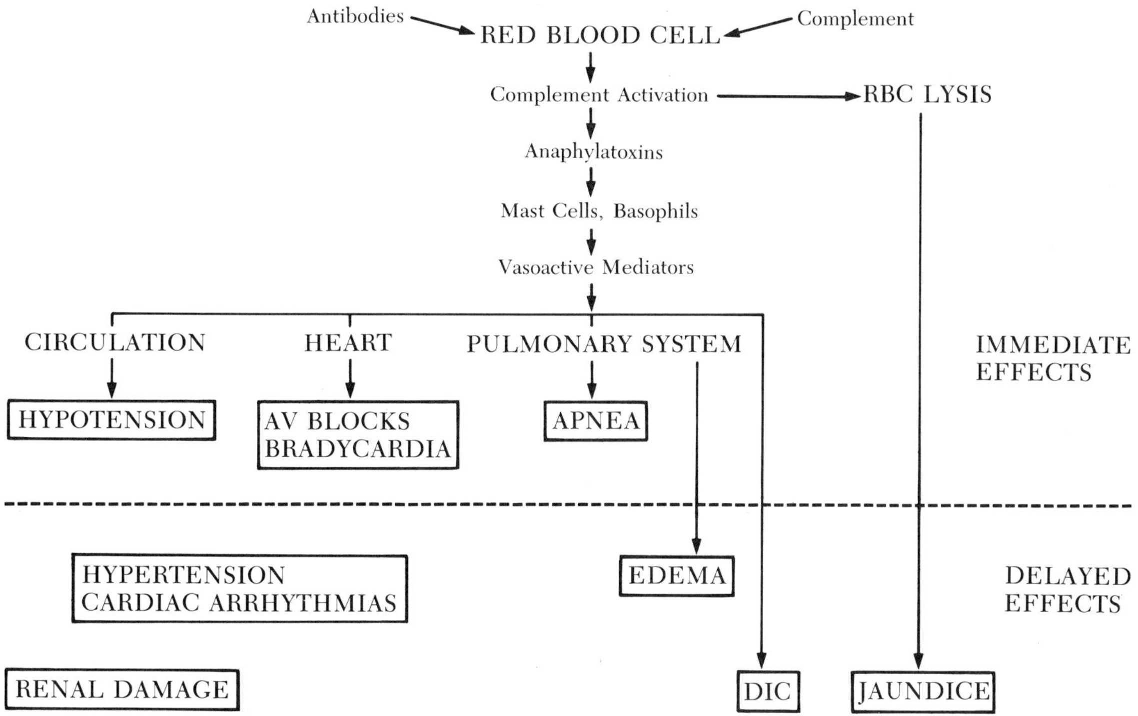

Figure 1. Proposed pathogenesis of an incompatible transfusion reaction illustrating possible serious pathological sequelae of the reaction. Clinical signs are boxed.

of donor blood as it is transfused, high antibody titers in the donor blood are less important as a cause of incompatibility reactions unless large volumes are transfused. Even if no immediate reaction occurs, it is undesirable to transfuse incompatible blood and run the risk of sensitizing the cat to future transfusions. The immune response to foreign red cell antigens also is likely to produce specific antibodies within 10 days; these will shorten the life of the introduced erythrocytes, thereby imposing a burden on the reticuloendothelial system and negating the beneficial effects of the transfusion.

A severe immediate transfusion reaction may be divided into two phases (Auer and Bell, 1983). Phase 1 occurs 30 seconds to 2 minutes after the introduction of the incompatible cells. Severe hypotension occurs simultaneously with bradycardia (approximately half the normal rate) and cessation of respiration. The usual respiratory pattern is a cessation of respiration for 15 to 20 seconds, followed by one or two brief gasps and a further cessation for up to 1 minute. There is sometimes complete absence of electrical activity of the heart for periods up to 18 seconds. Complete atrioventricular block has also been observed. Figure 2*A* illustrates the blood pressure, respiration, and electrocardiogram (ECG) changes of a typical Phase 1 reaction. The clinical signs of such a reaction are a change in body posture from lateral to sternal recumbency, extension of the limbs, opisthotonos, occasionally a distressed meow, and sometimes emesis or defecation (or both). Humans have reported a severe, constricting pain in the chest. Variations of the above reaction occur. In less severe reactions, the hypotension will not be as great and the respiratory and heart rates may increase. The signs associated with Phase 1 are believed to be caused by vasoactive substances released from mast cells and basophils by anaphylatoxins, the products of complement activation (Fig. 1).

The transfusion reaction closely resembles histamine shock with its pulmonary vasoconstriction, peripheral vasodilation, and increased capillary permeability (Rocha e Silva, 1978). However, in contrast to the usual tachycardia produced by histamine, the bradycardia suggests interaction with other mediators including bradykinin, serotonin, prostaglandins, and oxygen-free radicals. A cat is considered to remain in Phase 1 until it no longer shows signs of hypotension. In cats that recover from this phase, the duration of Phase 1 has been observed to vary from 35 seconds to 5 minutes. Although most healthy experimental cats recovered from Phase 1, the clinical situation in which cats are already in shock is potentially more dangerous.

Hematologic measurements taken during Phase

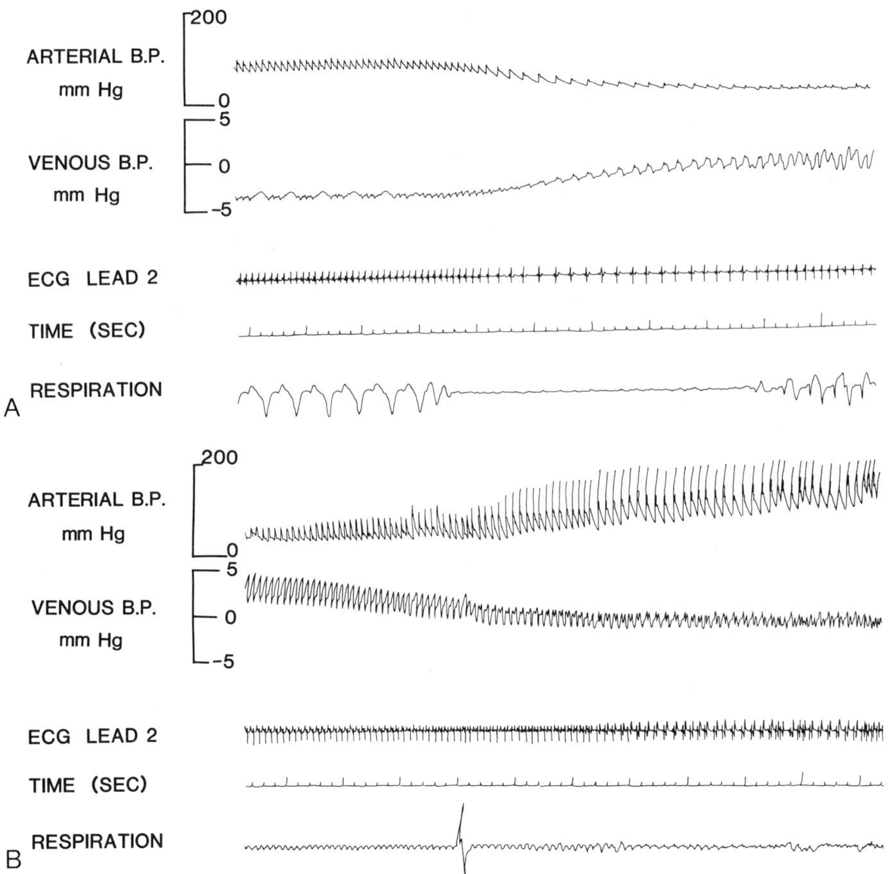

Figure 2. Grass multichannel recordings of a severe, incompatible blood transfusion reaction. *A*, hypotension and apnea of Phase 1, occurring within 2 minutes of the injection of 1 ml of incompatible erythrocytes. *B*, hypertensive compensatory phase commencing 5 minutes after the beginning of Phase 1. (From Auer and Bell: Res. Vet. Sci. 35:145, 1983.)

1 show a hemoconcentration that disappears by 30 minutes. A leukopenia, evident at 2 minutes, persists for at least 2 hours and may be followed later by a leukocytosis. Postmortem examinations often reveal lung congestion and pulmonary edema.

Phase 2 (Figure 2*B*) is a period characterized by markedly elevated arterial blood and pulse pressures (possibly an ischemic response of the central nervous system; values reach 225/125 mm Hg) and increased respiratory and heart rates (probably reflex responses to the hypoxia and hypotension of Phase 1). Heart arrhythmias, most commonly ventricular bigeminy, are prominent in many cats during this phase. Within 30 minutes, most cats stabilize to pretransfusion blood pressures.

Little information is available on the long-term effects of incompatible transfusion reactions. Extrapolation from human reactions would indicate four possible complications. These are disseminated intravascular coagulation, jaundice, fever, and renal damage.

THERAPY

Treatment of a blood transfusion reaction is based on a symptomatic approach extrapolated from other conditions (e.g., anaphylaxis) and other species. Because of the variability of reactions, therapy must be applied according to the presenting problem and with careful appraisal of the stage and degree of the reaction. Therapy will include removing the cause of the reaction, ensuring adequate ventilation and tissue perfusion pressures, and maintaining cardiac function. It is important to assess signs accurately, as treatments that are appropriate for Phase 1 (e.g., epinephrine) may be contraindicated in Phase 2. Over the succeeding few hours and days, the patient must be closely monitored, particularly for coagulopathies, fever, and adequate renal output.

The first action to be taken after an incompatible transfusion reaction is the cessation of the transfusion. Specific therapy must then be instigated; the cardiovascular collapse and apnea receive first priority. Figure 1 outlines the major clinical signs requiring attention during a severe transfusion reaction. As there has been little investigation into the therapy of the feline reaction to an incompatible transfusion, the recommended dose rates of the drugs have been derived from the treatment of anaphylaxis or identical clinical conditions that have been reported in cats by various workers. It may be necessary to change these recommendations when specific clinical and therapeutic data for the transfusion reaction have been accumulated and evaluated.

Hypotension and Apnea

In all transfusion reactions observed by Auer and Bell (1983), the cessation of respiration occurred concurrently with a severe hypotension (mean arterial blood pressure less than 50 mm Hg). Hypotension may be confirmed by a weak or absent pulse and slow, weak, or nonexistent cardiac contractions (by chest wall palpation). If this is the situation, cardiopulmonary resuscitation must be commenced immediately.

External cardiac massage at the rate of at least one compression per second and artificial respiration (if the cat is not breathing) should be initiated (Haskins, 1982; Atwell, 1984). An endotracheal tube must be inserted with minimal disturbance, as lack of continuity of the cardiac massage will allow diastolic and mean blood pressures to fall. Positive pressure ventilation should be given every five cardiac compressions, and oxygen (40 to 60 per cent) will help prevent hypoxia.

If spontaneous recovery of cardiac function has not occurred within 60 to 90 seconds, drug and fluid therapies are indicated. Epinephrine (6 to 10 μg/kg intracardiac [IC] or 20 to 30 μg/kg IV) will increase diastolic pressure and stimulate the heart. If there is no response, this dose may be repeated in 3 minutes. Calcium chloride (0.05 to 0.1 ml/kg of 10 per cent solution IV or IC) will also stimulate the heart. Alternatively, epinephrine may be administered intratracheally to effect rapid absorption and the relief of any bronchospasm. Aminophylline (6 to 10 mg/kg IV or IM, repeated every 6 hours as required) may also be used in the treatment of the bronchospasm.

If possible, colloid fluids should be administered to maintain the intravascular osmotic pressure decreased by the loss of plasma proteins to the extravascular spaces through increased capillary permeability. Initially, the rate of administration may be rapid, but it should be decreased as the reaction proceeds and reassessed according to central venous pressures and cardiac function. Alternatively, compatible blood (preferably an exchange transfusion) may be given if there is danger of hemolytic anemia from the administration of large volumes of incompatible blood.

Bradycardia and Atrioventricular Block

Atropine sulfate (10 to 40 μg/kg IV) may be used to correct a persistent bradycardia or heart block. However, atropine may predispose the patient to sympathetically induced arrhythmias. Other therapy should be employed as needed (Tilley, 1979).

Pulmonary Edema

Pulmonary edema due to the toxic effects of complement activation and granulocyte accumulation in the pulmonary vasculature may occur during the succeeding hours. Effective oxygenation of the "wet lung" syndrome is difficult. Positive pressure oxygen ventilation and high doses of corticosteroids (methylprednisolone, 30 mg/kg, repeated every 6 hours) can be given. The corticosteroids help reduce the defect in permeability of the pulmonary microvasculature. Human experience has shown that they must be given early and not as a heroic last-therapeutic stand. Other drugs that may be of benefit are furosemide (2 to 3 mg/kg IV or IM) and antifoaming agents such as ethyl alcohol (35 to 40 per cent solution, nebulized) to reduce surface tension and improve airway patency. Aminophylline may also be used for bronchodilation (Bonagura, 1977).

Hypertension and Cardiac Arrhythmias

If the cat enters the hypertensive phase of Phase 2, fluid administration must be stopped or adjusted to avoid overloading the circulatory system. If monitoring of central venous pressure (CVP) is not done, a guide to CVP is the collapse of leg veins when the hind leg is raised above the level of the heart. Cardiac arrhythmias may occur at this stage as the heart becomes hyperexcitable from the combined effects of hypoxia, circulating catecholamines, and increased sympathetic activity. An ECG monitor is necessary to diagnose the type of arrhythmia and its severity. The most common arrhythmia is ventricular bigeminy, which usually does not require treatment. More serious arrhythmias should be treated as they arise (Tilley and Weitz, 1977).

Disseminated Intravascular Coagulation

A hemorrhagic diathesis from disseminated intravascular coagulation (DIC) is a dangerous complication of reactions to transfusions of incompatible blood. It is probably triggered by intravascular hemolysis of the transfused red blood cells (releasing thromboplastic substances) and by activation of Factor XIIa of the coagulation process by antigen-antibody complexes. Dodds (1978) details the treatment of this condition. Severe cases may benefit from fluid therapy, blood transfusions, and the use of heparin, but for the last to be effective, it must be started early in the course of the reaction. Dosage recommendations vary, but a reasonable starting dose is 200 units/kg with additional doses required to keep the clotting time of whole blood at levels one-and-one-half to two times above normal. Heparin therapy requires laboratory testing and is not without risk. Extrapolation from human experience indicates that prophylactic treatment with anticoagulant drugs should not be initiated in cats unless a volume greater than 5 per cent of the recipient's blood volume has been transfused.

Hypoxia and Cerebral Edema

Hypoxia and cerebral edema may result from cardiovascular collapse. This is manifested by blindness, persistent coma, or both conditions. Diuretics should be given and repeated every 3 to 4 hours. Ventilation is to be even and controlled to prevent further hypoxia. Mannitol is the diuretic of choice, but it causes poor renal perfusion. Diuretics such as furosemide (Lasix, Hoechst-Roussel; 2 to 3 mg/kg IV) and ethacrynic acid (Edecrin, Merck, Sharp & Dohme) are thought to increase renal cortical blood flow as well as urine flow, but they may be less efficacious in their actions when compared with mannitol.

Renal Damage

Renal damage may be a serious sequela of a transfusion reaction. In humans, the therapy of the reaction to an incompatible blood transfusion is primarily directed toward prevention of renal cortical hypoperfusion (Brzica, 1982). The use of epinephrine in the hypotensive phase may predispose the patient to renal damage because of the drug's vasoconstrictive effects and the subsequent decrease in renal blood flow. Renal damage in humans is unlikely if a volume less than 5 per cent of the recipient's blood volume has been transfused. Renal damage is believed to result from the deposition of antigen-antibody complexes in the kidney and release of toxic mediators, from increased intravascular coagulation, and from renal stasis. If a period of oliguria follows a transfusion reaction, renal damage must be suspected (Mollison, 1983; Cowgill, 1980).

Allergic Reactions

Allergic reactions caused by the presence of foreign proteins in the transfused blood may be treated with corticosteroids. In humans, these are usually mild reactions characterized by urticaria.

Table 2. *The Crossmatch*

1. Collect small samples of donor and recipient blood in heparin or EDTA containers. Separate the plasma and red blood cells (RBC) either by centrifuging for 10 minutes (3000 rpm) or by allowing samples to stand for 30 minutes or longer.
2. Set up the following: (a) donor plasma, (b) recipient plasma, (c) donor 4% RBC suspension (0.2 ml of packed red cells and 4.8 mls 0.9% saline) and (d) recipient 4% RBC suspension.
3. Set up four slides with the following tests:
   Slide 1: 1 drop donor plasma and 1 drop donor RBC suspension (donor control—should not react).
   Slide 2: 1 drop recipient plasma and 1 drop recipient RBC suspension (recipient control—should not react).
   Slide 3: 1 drop donor plasma and 1 drop recipient RBC suspension (minor crossmatch).
   Slide 4: 1 drop recipient plasma and 1 drop donor RBC suspension (major crossmatch).
4. Gently rock the slides from side to side.
5. Look for agglutination reactions on slides 3 and 4, which in the cat will occur within 5 to 15 min at room temperature (22°C). If there is any doubt about the reactions, compare with the control slides 1 and 2. Only anti-A and group A cells will produce a strong agglutination, as anti-B is generally too weak an agglutinin to result in a reaction that is visible to the naked eye. Therefore, a group-B recipient will show a positive reaction on slide 4 with a group-A donor but no reaction on slide 3. The reaction patterns are reversed for A-recipient and B-donor cats (i.e., slide 3 positive and 4 negative). The AB type is so rare (0.4%) that its reactions have not been considered in the crossmatch. Blood typing is a ready alternative to the crossmatch and allows the detection and subsequent maintenance of both A and B donor cats.

CONVALESCENCE

If the cat survives the initial phases of the transfusion reaction, if should be closely monitored over the next few days for signs of delayed reactions. Because of the lack of available information and the potentially serious nature of these reactions, hospital care is indicated and the prognosis should be guarded until there are no signs of renal damage or coagulopathies.

PREVENTION—THE CROSSMATCH

Although the administration of antihistamines is sometimes recommended for both prevention and treatment of transfusion reactions, these agents are considered to be less effective than corticosteroids. Work by the authors indicated that histamine may play a protective role in the recovery from Phase 1 by stimulating H_2 receptors and cardiac contractility. Until this is clarified, it is advisable not to employ the antihistamines.

Once a transfusion reaction occurs, there is little that can be done except symptomatic treatment. Fortunately, the reaction is easily prevented. The strong agglutinating properties of anti-A at room temperature allows easy detection of incompatibility. If the titer of antibodies is too weak to cause visible agglutination, occurrence of a major transfusion reaction is unlikely. However, there is always the danger of the cat mounting a secondary immune response and destroying the introduced erythrocytes. For this reason, it is actually preferable to determine blood type as well as perform a crossmatch. The technique of blood typing has been described by Auer and Bell (1981). Reasonably potent anti-A sera may be obtained from most cats in group B, and their sera can be stored for years at −20°C without loss of potency. The crossmatch will nearly always detect incompatibilities in the AB blood group system of cats. However, it must be remembered that the crossmatch will not detect incompatibilities involving incomplete antibodies. Delayed transfusion reactions, although unlikely, may still occur despite these precautions. Table 2 outlines the procedure for the crossmatch.

CONCLUSION

Little is known about the pathophysiology of the incompatible transfusion reaction in cats. More information is required about the role of the mediators and their possible antagonistic effects. There is still no effective treatment that can reverse the severe hypotension of Phase 1, and almost nothing is known of the long-term effects of the feline transfusion reaction. However, prevention of the transfusion reaction by blood typing or crossmatching allows the veterinarian to avoid the serious consequences of the severe transfusion reaction.

References and Supplemental Reading

Atwell, R. B.: Clinical pharmacology of the cardiovascular system. *In Clinical Pharmacology and Therapeutics*. Sydney: The Post Graduate Committee in Veterinary Science, University of Sydney, Proceedings No. 71, 1984, pp. 253–289.

Auer, L., and Bell, K.: The AB blood group system of cats. Anim. Blood Groups Biochem. Genet. 12:287, 1981.

Auer, L., and Bell, K.: Transfusion reactions in cats due to AB blood group incompatibility. Res. Vet. Sci. 35:145, 1983.

Bonagura, J. D.: Feline cardiovascular emergencies. Vet. Clin. North Am. 7:385, 1977.

Brzica, S. M.: Complications of transfusion. Int. Anaesthesiol. Clin. 20:171, 1982.

Cowgill, L. D.: Management of oliguric and anuric renal failure. *In* Kirk, R. M. (ed.): *Current Veterinary Therapy VII*. Philadelphia: W. B. Saunders, 1980, pp. 1087–1090.

Dodds, W. J.: Management and therapy of bleeding disorders. Small Animal Veterinary Medicine Update Series. Vol. 2, No. 20. Santa Barbara, CA: American Veterinary Publications, 1978.

Eyquem, A., Podliachouk, L., and Milot, P.: Blood groups in chimpanzees, horses, sheep, pigs and other mammals. Ann. N. Y. Acad. Sci. 97:320, 1962.

Haskins, S. C.: Cardiopulmonary resuscitation. Comp. Cont. Ed. Pract. Vet. 4:170, 1982.

Holmes, R.: The occurrence of blood groups in cats. J. Exp. Biol. 30:350, 1953.

Ikemoto, S., Sakuria, Y., and Fukui, M.: Individual difference within the cat blood group detected by isohaemagglutinin. Jpn. J. Vet. Sci. 43:433, 1981.

Mollison, P. L.: Haemolytic transfusion reactions—Treatment of threatened or established renal failure. *In Blood Transfusion in Clinical Medicine*. Oxford: Blackwell Scientific Publications, 1983, pp. 648–649.

Rocha e Silva, M.: Histamine: Its chemistry, metabolism and physiological and pharmacological actions. *In* Eichler, O., and Farrah, A. (eds.): *Handbook of Experimental Pharmacology*. Berlin: Springer-Verlag, 1978, pp. 283–293.

Tilley, L. P.: *Essentials of Feline Electrocardiography*. St. Louis, MO: C. V. Mosby, 1979, pp. 236–239.

Tilley, L. P., and Weitz, J.: Pharmacologic and other forms of medical therapy in feline cardiac disease. Vet. Clin. North Am. 7:415, 1977.

DISORDERS OF IRON METABOLISM

EDWARD A. MAHAFFEY, D.V.M.

Athens, Georgia

Abnormalities in iron metabolism are among the most common causes of anemia in both animals and humans. These abnormalities occur in a variety of disease processes involving all body systems. In developing red blood cells in the marrow, the effect of these pathologic processes is to limit the availability of iron. The diseases can be divided into two general categories: (1) absolute deficiency, in which the total body iron stores are depleted, and (2) relative deficiency, in which the amount of stored iron in the body is adequate for normal hematopoiesis but the iron is unavailable to the developing red cells.

IRON DEFICIENCY

Occurrence

Iron deficiency can result from either inadequate dietary intake or excessive iron loss. Inadequate intake is unlikely to occur in adult dogs or cats fed any commercial diet intended for the species. In contrast, newborn animals have very little stored iron. Milk is quite low in iron content, and nursing puppies and kittens are therefore more likely to develop iron deficiency anemia. A recent publication has documented that the drop in hematocrit that occurs in kittens between 2 and 5 weeks of age is accompanied by low serum iron concentration and the appearance of a population of microcytic red cells in the circulation. The decrease in hematocrit can be prevented by prophylactic iron therapy. Thus, the lower range of hematocrit values for kittens listed in some tables of normal values may reflect mild iron deficiency anemia in those animals.

Three basic concepts are central to a discussion of iron deficiency anemia in adult dogs and cats:

1. Iron deficiency in the adult animal results from excessive iron loss rather than inadequate intake.
2. Iron loss can almost always be equated with blood loss; the one exception is the rare case of intestinal malabsorption in which dietary iron is lost by not being absorbed through the intestinal mucosa.
3. For blood loss to result in iron deficiency anemia, it must be prolonged. A single episode of massive blood loss in an otherwise normal animal obviously will cause anemia, but the normal body stores of iron should be sufficient for synthesis of new hemoglobin during the regenerative response.

The usual causes of iron deficiency anemia in adults include gastrointestinal parasites (especially hookworms) and external parasites such as fleas and ticks. The frequency of severe parasitic infestation in puppies and kittens and the marginal iron status of animals of that age renders them even more vulnerable to iron deficiency. Other causes of iron deficiency include gastrointestinal ulcers and neoplasms, transitional cell carcinomas, and diseases resulting in thrombocytopenia. Veterinarians should also be aware that iron deficiency anemia has occurred in dogs that have been used excessively as blood donors.

Laboratory Findings

Anemia may vary in severity from very mild to life-threatening. Regeneration is usually evident early in the progression of iron deficiency and is detected as polychromasia, anisocytosis, and reticulocytosis, whereas in advanced cases the anemia may be classified as nonregenerative. Hypochromia is usually detected on examination of blood smears; microcytosis is observed less commonly. Other common abnormalities in blood smears of iron-deficient animals include poikilocytosis, leptocytosis, red cell fragmentation, and thrombocytosis.

Erythrocyte indices are among the more useful laboratory tests in detecting iron deficiency, but their determination is practical and accurate only when an electronic cell counter is available. Although hypochromia is detected more often on blood smears than is microcytosis, the mean corpuscular volume (MCV) is more consistently decreased in iron-deficient dogs than is the mean corpuscular hemoglobin concentration (MCHC). This finding is in contrast to some reports of iron deficiency in humans in which the MCHC was the more sensitive indicator.

The serum chemical tests that commonly have been used to evaluate iron status include measurement of serum iron concentration and total iron binding capacity (TIBC). The latter is a measure of both free and iron-bound transferrin. Some laboratories report serum iron and unbound or labile iron binding capacity; the relationship between those measurements and the TIBC is:

TIBC = Serum iron +
Unbound or labile iron binding capacity

Iron deficiency in persons and in some animal species is characterized by decreased serum iron concentration and increased TIBC. In dogs, serum iron decreases during iron deficiency; however, there is no consistent change in TIBC. Iron deficiency anemia in cats is less well characterized. Serum iron decreases, and limited data indicate that there may be modest increases in TIBC.

Therapy

Treatment of iron deficiency anemia must include identification and correction of the cause of anemia, which in most cases means identification of the site and reason for blood loss. Iron replacement therapy has two goals: (1) replacement of iron needed for hemoglobin synthesis to correct the anemia and (2) replacement of storage iron. An important aspect of iron metabolism is that iron deficiency anemia does not develop until the body's iron stores have been depleted. When replacement therapy is begun, iron will first be used by the hematopoietic tissue for synthesis of hemoglobin. Only when the immediate demand for iron for erythropoiesis is satisfied will significant quantities be deposited in fixed macrophages that serve as storage reservoirs of iron. If iron supplementation is stopped as soon as the packed cell volume returns to the normal range, the animal probably remains in a state of iron depletion and is vulnerable to recurrence of anemia.

The packed cell volume of an iron-deficient dog typically returns to normal within approximately 6 to 8 weeks after iron therapy is begun; however, the MCV of some treated dogs may not return to within normal limits for 6 months or longer. Thus, it is prudent to administer supplemental iron therapy for a total of approximately 9 months. Because absorption of iron from the gastrointestinal tract is regulated according to the body's need, iron overload is unlikely to occur with normal supplemental dosages. Iron should be administered orally as ferrous sulfate. A daily dosage of 100 to 300 mg for dogs and 50 to 100 mg for cats should be adequate. The dosage should be reduced by one half after the hematocrit returns to the normal range. Dietary iron supplements can be irritating to the gastrointestinal tract. For that reason, parenteral iron therapy should be considered when the cause of iron deficiency is gastrointestinal blood loss, especially if the site of bleeding is in the stomach or upper small intestine. Parenteral therapy is also necessary when iron deficiency results from malabsorption. A daily dosage of 10 mg/kg of iron dextran injected intramuscularly in divided doses has been recommended for both dogs and cats. Iron dextran is quite irritating and occasionally has been associated with anaphylactic reactions in humans. For those reasons, parenteral iron therapy should be administered only if it is specifically indicated.

The recent evidence strongly indicating that kittens between 5 and 7 weeks of age have hematologic manifestations of iron deficiency raises the question of whether supplemental iron should be given routinely to nursing animals. In the experimental studies, hematologic abnormalities did not develop in kittens supplemented with parenteral iron therapy. There is a considerable body of evidence indicating a relationship between iron and infection. Some bacteria require iron for growth, and limited evidence suggests that animals supplemented with iron may be more vulnerable to bacterial infection. Because it has not been proven that nursing kittens with mild iron deficiency suffer any adverse effects other than the transient hematologic abnormalities, it is premature to recommend routine iron supplementation of nursing animals.

ANEMIA OF INFLAMMATORY DISEASE

Inclusion of the anemia of inflammatory disease in this discussion is relevant because abnormalities in iron metabolism are central in the pathogenesis of the anemia. Also, the hematologic features of the anemia associated with inflammatory disease are sometimes similar to those of iron deficiency anemia.

Occurrence

Anemia of inflammatory disease is probably the most common type of anemia encountered in veterinary medicine. It occurs in both infectious and noninfectious inflammatory diseases and has also been called the *anemia of infection* and the *anemia of chronic disease.* Similar mechanisms are responsible in part for the anemia that accompanies many forms of neoplasia. Because this type of anemia can develop within two weeks after the onset of inflammation, especially in cats, the term *anemia of chronic disease* is not entirely appropriate for this entity as it exists in veterinary medicine.

The pathogenesis of the anemia of inflammatory disease is complex and is not entirely understood. Factors considered most important in the development of anemia are disturbances in iron metabolism, slightly shortened life span of red cells, and an inadequate erythropoietin response for the degree of anemia. Of those factors, the abnormalities in iron metabolism have received the most attention in recent years. The most important flaw in iron metabolism in animals with inflammatory disease is the sequestration of iron in macrophages so that it is unavailable for hematopoiesis. One researcher characterized the anemia as "iron starvation in the face of plenty." Recent work implicates interleukin 1, an inflammatory mediator produced by activated macrophages, as the cause of iron sequestration. Release of iron from hepatocytes and intestinal epithelial cells is also impaired in animals with inflammatory disease.

Laboratory Findings

Anemia varies from mild to moderately severe, but it is often overshadowed by other abnormalities associated with the causative disease process. The PCV of affected dogs seldom drops below 20 per cent, whereas that of affected cats may drop as low as approximately 15 per cent. The anemia is consistently nonregenerative; however, mild reticulocytosis, inappropriately low for the degree of anemia, may occur. Red cell indices usually reveal that the anemia is normocytic and normochromic, although microcytosis and hypochromia are occasionally found.

Serum iron concentrations of animals with experimental inflammatory disease decrease within hours after the onset of inflammation and remain low until inflammation subsides. The TIBC may be normal or decreased. Because the TIBC of dogs with iron deficiency anemia does not increase consistently (as it does in humans), the TIBC is a less valuable marker in dogs for distinguishing iron deficiency anemia from the anemia of inflammatory disease.

The storage of iron in bone marrow in dogs with

the anemia of inflammatory disease is typically abundant; demonstration of iron in bone marrow aspirates requires special staining techniques. That procedure is occasionally used to distinguish the hypoferremia of the anemia of inflammatory disease from that of iron deficiency anemia. In the latter disorder, little or no stainable iron is found. Another technique that is gaining favor in the assessment of iron stores in humans is measurement of serum ferritin. In persons with the anemia of inflammatory disease, the serum ferritin concentration is abnormally high, whereas in those with iron deficiency anemia, the serum ferritin concentration is decreased. Limited research suggests that measurement of ferritin may be similarly useful in assessing iron stores of domestic animals. Ferritin is measured by immunoassay techniques, and species-specific antisera for ferritins of domestic animals are not yet commercially available.

Therapy

There is no specific therapy for the anemia of inflammatory disease. The anemia is not severe enough to justify transfusion, and iron therapy is not beneficial. Gastrointestinal iron absorption is decreased, and even parenteral iron therapy has resulted in only transient increases in serum iron concentration with no lessening of the severity of anemia. Therapeutic efforts should be concentrated instead on treating the underlying cause of anemia, the inflammatory disease.

References and Supplemental Reading

Feldman, B. F.: Hypoproliferative anemias and anemias caused by ineffective erythropoiesis. Vet. Clin. North Am. 11:277, 1981.

Harvey, J. W., French, T. W., and Meyer, D. J.: Chronic iron deficiency anemia in dogs. J. Am. Anim. Hosp. Assoc. 18:946, 1982.

Lee, G. R.: The anemia of chronic disease. Sem. Hematol. 20:61, 1983.

Perman, V., and Schall, W. D.: Diseases of red blood cells. *In* Ettinger, S. J. (ed.): *Textbook of Veterinary Internal Medicine*, 2nd ed. Philadelphia: W. B. Saunders, 1983, pp. 1938–2000.

Weiser, M. G., and Kociba, G. J.: Sequential changes in erythrocyte volume distribution and microcytosis associated with iron deficiency in kittens. Vet. Pathol. 20:1, 1983.

Weiss, D. J., and Krehbiel, J. D.: Studies of the pathogenesis of anemia of inflammation: Erythrocyte survival. Am. J. Vet. Res. 44:1830, 1983.

SALICYLATE TOXICITY

PREM HANDAGAMA, B.V.Sc.

San Francisco, California

Salicylates are salts or esters of salicylic acid. Over-the-counter drug preparations containing salicylates are widely used. Aside from their use as analgesics, salicylic acid and salicylates are also used for many other purposes: as cold medicines, antifungals, shampoos, and wart removers. Salicylates are often found in preparations in which they are least expected (Table 1). Because of the free availability of salicylate preparations for self-medication, they are commonly found in one form or another in most homes. People often use aspirin or other salicylate preparations to medicate their pets, and salicylate poisoning may occur because of overdosing. Ingestion of sugar-coated or flavored children's aspirin preparations by animals is another way by which aspirin poisoning can occur. Although at therapeutic concentrations aspirin has some adverse side effects, salicylates have a definite place in the treatment of small animals. A thorough understanding of their pharmacology and effects on different species is required, however.

PHARMACOLOGY

Absorption of salicylates occurs in the stomach and proximal small intestine. Factors such as gastric emptying time, stomach content, rate of tablet disintegration, and solubility influence the rate of salicylate absorption. As a result, there is considerable individual variation in the rate of absorption of salicylate preparations. Prolonged periods of increased concentrations of salicylates in the blood are obtained with slowly absorbed preparations.

After absorption, salicylates are distributed throughout body fluids. In plasma, salicylates are bound to serum albumin. Hypoalbuminemia can cause lower concentrations of serum salicylate.

The principal site of salicylate metabolism is the

Table 1. *Some Commonly Used Medicinal Preparations Containing Salicylates*

Pain Relievers
Anacin (Whitehall)
Bufferin (Bristol-Myers)
Excedrin (Bristol-Myers)
Ecotrin (Menley & James)
Doan's Pills (Jeffrey Martin)
Momentum (Whitehall)
Ben-Gay (Leeming)
Anti-inflammatory Agents
Di-Gesic (Central)
Ascriptin (Rorer)
Verin (Verex)
Cold Medicines
4-way Cold Tabs (Bristol-Myers)
Bayer Children's Cold Tablets (Glenbrook)
Triaminic (Dorsey)
Coricidin "D" Decongestant Tablets (Schering)
Alka-Seltzer Plus (Miles)
Antidiarrheals
Pepto-Bismol (Procter & Gamble)
Wart Removers (Keratolytics)
Salactic Film (Pedinol)
Verrusol (C & M Pharmaceutical)
Antiseborrheic Medications
Sebucare (Westwood)
Sebulex (Westwood)

liver. Salicylates are metabolized by conjugation with glucuronic acid. Glucuronyl transferase, the enzyme responsible for this reaction, is present in the hepatic microsomal system of mammals. Cats and neonates of most species have low concentrations of glucuronyl transferase. This is thought to be the reason for the inability of these individuals to metabolize salicylates rapidly, and this inability functionally prolongs the metabolic half-life of the compound.

Aspirin is largely excreted by the kidney through a combination of glomerular filtration and proximal tubular secretion. Excretion is influenced by the rate of urine flow and the pH of urine.

EFFECTS ON BLOOD

At therapeutic doses, aspirin has no significant effect on total counts of white blood cells. Aspirin has often been associated with anemia. Although gastrointestinal bleeding is an important side effect of aspirin ingestion, it is not certain if this is the complete cause of anemia. Aspirin-induced bone marrow depression causing neutropenia, thrombocytopenia, and anemia may occur after prolonged use. Serious gastrointestinal hemorrhage following aspirin ingestion occurs only in those animals which, when the hemostatic mechanism is considered, are not clinically normal. The ingestion of aspirin prolongs the bleeding time in healthy animals to a small but significant degree. This is because aspirin is a potent inhibitor of platelet aggregation. However, in the presence of a hemostatic defect such as von Willebrand's disease (vWD), a disease in which platelet adherence is impaired, the combined defect of poor adherence and poor aggregation due to aspirin could lead to serious hemorrhage. In cases of elective surgery, owners should be advised against the use of aspirin for a period of at least 1 week before the procedure. Animals with vWD or aged animals suffering from renal or liver disease may have marginally normal hemostatic systems. After aspirin ingestion these patients may also have excessive bleeding during such minor surgery as tooth extraction.

After vascular trauma, platelets adhere to exposed endothelial connective tissue and subsequently undergo a release reaction. In addition to the release reaction by platelets, arachidonates undergo prostaglandin conversion. The prostaglandins together with released adenosine diphosphate (ADP) can then induce changes in platelet morphology by transforming discs to pseudopodal spheres. Platelets that undergo these changes are able to stick to each other and to platelets that are already adhering to the vessel wall. As the platelet mass enlarges, reactions leading to the formation of thrombin occur. This also induces changes in platelet shape, causes release of more ADP, and activates prostaglandin synthesis from arachidonate. The principal arachidonate product formed in the platelet is thromboxane A_2 (TXA_2), a highly potent platelet-aggregating agent and a substance that causes vasoconstriction. The principal prostaglandin in endothelial cells is prostacyclin or PGI_2, a potent inhibitor of platelet aggregation and a substance that causes vasodilatation.

The anti-inflammatory and antiplatelet properties of aspirin are due mainly to its effect upon arachidonate metabolism. Aspirin inhibits platelet function by acetylating and hence irreversibly inactivating the enzyme cyclo-oxygenase. This effect occurs with small doses, and, despite the short half-life of aspirin, affected platelets are permanently impaired and are unable to aggregate. A single dose of aspirin will increase the bleeding time for as long as 7 days.

Platelets, unlike endothelial cells, are unable to regenerate new enzymes after inactivation by aspirin. Endothelial cells can rapidly regenerate inactivated enzymes. As a result, the synthesis of arachidonate (i.e., PGI_2), in endothelial cells is less susceptible than that of platelets to aspirin inhibition. Doses of aspirin used clinically are not usually high enough to inhibit endothelial PGI_2 synthesis. This antiplatelet effect of aspirin has been utilized in clinical situations in which thrombus formation is a potential secondary complication.

Although there is evidence for the antithrombotic effect of aspirin in the prevention of peripheral ischemia due to thrombocytosis and consequent spontaneous platelet aggregation, further studies are needed to determine the ideal dose of aspirin that will selectively inactivate platelet cyclo-oxygenase without affecting PGI_2 in the vessel walls.

At very high concentrations, aspirin has been shown to possess fibrinolytic activity as measured by the euglobulin lysis test (ELT).

DOSAGE

DOGS. The biological half-life of aspirin in dogs has been shown to be dose-dependent. A dose of 0.4 grains/kg (25 mg/kg) body weight given at 8-hour intervals will maintain the serum salicylate concentration within the desired therapeutic range. It has been suggested that the upper limit for aspirin dosage in dogs would be 50 mg/kg once every 8 to 12 hours. In puppies, the plasma half-life of salicylate is prolonged owing to insufficient amounts of hepatic glucuronyl transferase. Puppies also seem to have difficulty excreting free salicylate, and they lack the ability to form metabolites such as salicylurate.

The recommended dose for relief of pain in the dog is 0.15 grains/kg (10 mg/kg) orally at 8-hour intervals.

Doses of aspirin as low as 0.05 grains (3 mg/kg) inhibit platelet TXA_2 without affecting endothelial PGI_2. This selective inhibition of platelet TXA_2 is responsible for the antiplatelet or antiaggregating effect of aspirin.

CATS. Because of a lack of glucuronyl transferase, cats are unable to conjugate aspirin with glucuronic acid. Thus, the half-life of aspirin in cats is extremely long. It may range from 20 to 25 hours, depending on dosage and factors such as diet and urinary pH. Toxicity often results from doses that have been extrapolated from other species. Aspirin toxicity also occurs when cats are not dosed according to weight. An oral daily dose of 0.4 grains/kg (25 mg/kg) of aspirin is sufficient to obtain a therapeutic blood concentration of aspirin without toxicity. However, the therapeutic dose of aspirin recommended for cats is much lower (10 mg/kg orally every 24 hours).

SIDE EFFECTS OF ASPIRIN THERAPY

Poisoning from ingestion of aspirin and, to a lesser extent, other salicylates is a problem confined to the following clinical situations: (1) ingestion of sugar-coated or flavored children's aspirin and (2) therapeutic intoxication due to incorrect dosing (this is especially true in the cat).

Toxicity

Derivatives of salicylic acid produce the toxic syndrome known as salicylism. Toxic effects are manifest at plasma concentrations in excess of 30 mg/dl. Young animals, for the reasons previously stated, are more susceptible than adults to toxic effects of salicylates. The major toxic signs arise first from central nervous system (CNS) stimulation and secondarily from terminal CNS depression. Central excitation is manifested by hyperpnea, confusion, bizarre behavior or mania, and convulsions. Death is usually due to respiratory failure or cardiovascular collapse.

Hypoglycemia has been reported in some animals with experimental salicylate poisoning, and the administration of glucose has been shown to significantly improve survival. Toxic hepatosis is seen in some animals with excessive doses of salicylates. Less commonly, hemorrhage and renal disturbances may be seen in acute salicylism. A bleeding tendency may be manifested by hematemesis, melena, or petechiae. This may be due, in part, to the induction of hypoprothrombinemia and to the ability of aspirin and other salicylates to inhibit platelet aggregation. Salicylates are gastric irritants. In the worst possible case, fatal peritonitis due to perforation of the gastrointestinal tract could occur. In addition to these dose-dependent effects, signs of drug idiosyncrasy or hypersensitivity may also occur.

Most of these toxic effects are caused by severe disturbance in acid-base balance. A number of factors contribute to salicylate-induced acid-base imbalance, but the chief cause is prolonged hyperventilation and respiratory alkalosis due to CNS stimulation. The respiratory alkalosis may be compounded with metabolic alkalosis when vomiting occurs. One caution: acidosis may occur in some patients.

The clinical signs of chronic salicylate ingestion include vomiting, anorexia, weight loss, anemia, and depression. Some animals with chronic salicylism may develop bone marrow depression, toxic hepatitis, and nephropathy.

In pregnant animals salicylates should be used with caution, as they have been shown to cause reproductive anomalies, fetal resorption, and stillbirths in laboratory animals.

Treatment of Aspirin Toxicosis

Therapy for salicylism is symptomatic and supportive. The major goal is to correct the acid-base imbalance and accelerate excretion of salicylates. Normal renal function should be maintained by correcting dehydration and shock. Salicylate excretion is rapid in alkaline urine.

1. If the patient is presented within 1 hour of aspirin ingestion, emetics are indicated. Apomorphine at a dose rate of 0.04 mg/kg IV or 0.08 mg/kg

IM is an effective emetic in dogs. Syrup of ipecac, 1 to 2 ml/kg orally, may also be used.

2. A slurry of activated charcoal at 2 to 8 gm/kg in a concentration of 1 gm charcoal in 5 to 10 ml water may be administered orally to delay absorption (Note: syrup of ipecac will reduce the adsorptive action of charcoal).

3. Gastric lavage with sodium bicarbonate solution (3 to 5 per cent) may be helpful. The mild alkali delays salicylate absorption.

4. Obtain a blood sample for evaluation of the patient's acid-base status. An analysis of the plasma salicylate concentration may be made at this time to establish the diagnosis.

5. In the presence of established acidosis, sodium bicarbonate therapy (1 to 4 mEq/kg IV every 15 min) is essential.

6. Dehydration is corrected with intravenous administration of lactated Ringer's solution or 5 per cent glucose solution (40 to 50 ml/kg daily as a continuous drip). The glucose may also serve to remedy any concurrent hypoglycemia.

7. Renal function should be supported by correcting dehydration and incipient shock. An alkaline urine may be maintained by administration of sodium bicarbonate if necessary. The administration of diuretics such as furosemide (5 mg/kg IV every 6 to 8 hours) or mannitol (1.0 to 2.0 gm/kg/hr IV) is useful.

8. Sedatives such as phenobarbital (2 to 4 mg/kg) or diazepam (2.5 to 5.0 mg to cats, 2.5 to 20 mg to dogs IV or orally) may be required to control convulsions.

9. The presence of hemorrhagic tendencies due to hypoprothrombinemia may require large doses of vitamin K_1 (2.5 mg/kg divided b.i.d. or t.i.d.) given orally or subcutaneously. Ascorbic acid (25 mg several times daily) has also been shown to be useful when hypoprothrombinemia is present.

10. Although peritoneal dialysis and exchange transfusions have proved useful in salicylate poisoning, alkaline diuretic therapy is usually sufficient.

References and Supplemental Reading

Rainsford, K. D.: *Aspirin and the Salicylates.* Stoneham, MA: Butterworth, 1984.

Taylor, L. A., and Crawford, L. M.: Aspirin-induced gastrointestinal lesions in dogs. J.A.V.M.A. 152:617, 1968.

Yeary, R. A., and Brant, R. J.: Aspirin dosages for the dog. J.A.V.M.A. 167:63, 1975.

Yeary, R. A., and Swanson, W.: Aspirin dosages for the cat. J.A.V.M.A. 163:1177, 1973.

Section 6

DERMATOLOGIC DISEASES

DANNY W. SCOTT, D.V.M.
Consulting Editor

***Additional Pertinent Information Found in* Current Veterinary Therapy VIII:**

Fadok, V. A.: Necrotizing Skin Diseases, p. 473.
Griffin, C. E.: Differential Diagnosis of Nasal Diseases, p. 480.
Miller, W. H., Jr.: The Pruritic Dog, p. 499.
Scott, D. W.: Autoimmune Dermatoses, p. 467.
Scott, D. W.: Chrysotherapy (Gold Therapy), p. 448.
Scott, D. W.: Panniculitis, p. 471.

***Additional Pertinent Information Found in* Current Veterinary Therapy VII:**

Kunkle, G. A.: Zinc-Responsive Dermatoses in Dogs, p. 472.
Scott, D. W.: Canine Pododermatitis, p. 467.
Scott, D. W.: The Differential Diagnosis of Facial Dermatitis, p. 436.

CUTANEOUS MYCOBACTERIOSIS

STEPHEN D. WHITE, D.V.M.
North Grafton, Massachusetts

Mycobacteria are uncommon pathogens in skin diseases of dogs and cats. Three categories of cutaneous mycobacteriosis may be recognized: feline leprosy, cutaneous atypical mycobacteriosis, and cutaneous tuberculosis.

FELINE LEPROSY

Feline leprosy is the name given to a granulomatous skin disease associated with the presence of acid-fast bacilli. The causative organism is thought to be *Mycobacterium lepraemurium,* the agent of rat (murine) leprosy, although not all investigators agree on this point.

The mode of transmission is not known but is thought to be through bites of infected rats. The disease has been encountered in Australia, New Zealand, North America, and Europe. Feline leprosy has not been documented in dogs. Young cats (less than 3 years of age) may be more susceptible, although any age, breed, or sex may be affected.

Lesions are cutaneous nodules, single or multiple, ulcerated or nonulcerated, which may occur in most areas of the skin but most commonly are seen on the head and limbs. These nodules are generally not painful, and systemic signs are usually lacking. Regional lymphadenopathy may be present. The differential diagnoses include other cutaneous mycobacterioses, neoplasia, deep bacterial or fungal infections, foreign body granuloma, and pansteatitis.

Histopathologic examination of the nodules reveals two patterns: (1) epithelioid (tuberculoid) granulomas with areas of caseation necrosis and (2) sheets of macrophages with multinucleated giant cells. Acid-fast stains (Ziehl-Neelson, Fite's) usually demonstrate prominent numbers of mycobacteria. In the granulomas, the bacilli are seen in the areas of caseation necrosis. In the sheets of macrophages, the organisms are found stacked parallel in many of the histiocytes, similar to those of human lepromatous leprosy. Infiltration of nerve bundles with inflammatory cells may be seen. Impression smears of freshly excised tissues will often demonstrate acid-fast bacilli when appropriately stained.

M. lepraemurium is very difficult to grow *in vitro.* A medium termed the *Ogawa egg yolk medium* has been successful (Pattyn and Portaels, 1980). The organism appears as small colonies in 3 to 8 weeks. In animal inoculation studies, *M. lepraemurium* does not kill guinea pigs, and rats and mice develop local and lymph node lesions, usually with demonstrable mycobacteria. Diagnosis of feline leprosy is primarily based on the presence of acid-fast organisms histologically, no evidence of growth on tuberculosis (or other common) culture media, and no usual animal inoculation response pattern of tuberculosis.

Therapy has generally been limited to excisional surgery. This becomes difficult in the cat with multiple lesions but may prove effective in those animals with single or few nodules. Use of antimycobacterial drugs in cats is poorly understood: Efficacy, dosages, and toxicities need further research.* Spontaneous remission does occur, but its incidence is not known.

Although the public health significance of feline leprosy has not been thoroughly investigated, there is at present no evidence that the disease is transmissible to human beings. However, because the causative agent does appear capable of interspecies transmission, some caution is warranted in the handling of suspect animals, tissues, and cultures.

CUTANEOUS ATYPICAL MYCOBACTERIOSIS

Those mycobacteria that do not cause tuberculosis or leprosy (feline, murine, or human) have been categorized as the atypical (opportunistic, anonymous) mycobacteria. These organisms are thought to be ubiquitous in the environment. The atypical mycobacteria have been divided into four groups on the basis of physical and laboratory characteristics. Groups I through III are considered "slow growers," whose initial appearance on culture media

---

*Editor's Note: Dapsone has been frequently used for the treatment of feline leprosy in Australia. Although much remains to be documented about dosage (efficacy and safety) and frequency of remissions induced, present recommendations in Australia suggest a daily dapsone dosage of 1 mg/kg. Hemolytic anemia and neurotoxicity are possible side effects of dapsone administration. Dapsone is *not* approved for use in cats in the United States.

is measured in terms of weeks or months. In Group IV, the "fast growers," growth will usually be seen within 7 days of media inoculation. Almost all reported cases of cutaneous atypical mycobacteriosis in dogs and cats have been caused by Group IV organisms. These include *Mycobacterium fortuitum, M. chelonei, M. phlei,* and *M. smegmatis.*

Cutaneous atypical mycobacteriosis has been described in North America, Australia, and Great Britain, and in both dogs and cats. As there are fewer than 20 cases in the veterinary literature, it is difficult to determine any age, breed, or sex predilection. Lesions are draining tracts, often associated with subcutaneous nodules. These areas are generally nonpainful or cause only mild discomfort when palpated. There may be a predilection for the abdomen and inguinal areas. Systemic signs are usually absent. The mode of transmission is not completely understood, but the organisms are thought to gain entry through wounds. Several of the reported cases have had a prior history of trauma to the affected areas. Differential diagnoses are as for feline leprosy.

Diagnosis is based on histopathologic testing and culture. Histopathologic signs generally are pyogranulomatous inflammation, often with areas of caseation necrosis. In contrast to the case in feline leprosy, the atypical mycobacteria may be difficult to see with acid-fast stains. It has been theorized that some aspect of tissue-fixing affects the organisms' uptake of acid-fast stain. Both a rapid Ziehl-Neelson stain (White et al., 1983) and a method of snap-freezing the formalin-fixed tissues with subsequent acid-fast staining (Gross and Connelly, 1983) have been successful in some cases. Because of this difficulty in fixed preparations, impression smears of biopsy material (before placement in formalin) should also be submitted for acid-fast staining. The Group IV mycobacteria can usually be grown on blood agar or Löwenstein-Jensen media. However, the clinician should notify the diagnostic laboratory of the possibility of a mycobacterium as an etiologic agent.

Treatment for cutaneous atypical mycobacteriosis is not well developed. Surgical excision is occasionally curative but does not seem to be as effective as in feline leprosy. Dehiscence of the incision site and recurrence of the nodules and draining tracts is not infrequent. Medical therapy has not been consistently effective. *In vitro* susceptibility to various antibiotics and antimycobacterial drugs is not reflected by *in vivo* success rates. The reported effectiveness of any therapeutic regimen, surgical or medical, must be suspect, in as much as spontaneous remission occurs in both human and feline cutaneous atypical mycobacteriosis.

The author's current recommendations in otherwise healthy animals with cutaneous atypical mycobacteriosis are to keep the affected area clean and to inform the owners of the difficulty of therapy as well as the possibility of spontaneous remission. If the animal has systemic signs (anorexia, fever) or if the original lesion enlarges or new lesions occur, antibiotic therapy may be initiated based on culture and sensitivity testing. As discussed above with feline leprosy, antimycobacterial drugs should be used with caution because of the lack of definitive knowledge of doses and toxicities in dogs and cats. Surgical excision may be attempted in small lesions, but the owners should be warned of dehiscence and recurrence.

CUTANEOUS TUBERCULOSIS

Tuberculosis in dogs and cats has decreased with the decreased incidence of the disease in humans and cattle. The causative agent is either *Mycobacterium bovis* or *M. tuberculosis.* The latter may be contracted from a human case via airborne infection; the former is usually ingested in infected milk. Dogs are more likely to have *M. tuberculosis;* cats, *M. bovis.* The disease is worldwide in distribution.

Although the lesions are usually in the intestinal or respiratory tract, cutaneous tuberculosis may occur either by hematogenous spread or infected skin wounds. Lesions may be nodules, ulcers, abscesses, or plaques, single or multiple, cutaneous or subcutaneous. These may occur more often on the head and limbs. In contrast to those with feline leprosy and cutaneous atypical mycobacteriosis, tubercular animals often have systemic signs: weight loss, anorexia, fever, or lymphadenopathy. Differential diagnosis is as for feline leprosy.

Diagnosis is by culture and animal inoculation tests. Tuberculosis bacilli generally take 6 to 8 weeks to grow in special media and about as long to cause death in inoculated guinea pigs. Use of intradermal tuberculin as a diagnostic tool is unreliable in dogs and of no value in cats. Histopathologic signs are not diagnostic but include a pyogranulomatous response with variable caseation necrosis and occasional to many bacilli seen on acid-fast stains.

Therapy of confirmed cases of tuberculosis in dogs and cats (or any nonhuman species) is not advised because of the public health hazard they represent. The animal should be euthanized and public health authorities informed.

SUMMARY

Cutaneous mycobacteriosis should be suspected in the dog or cat that presents with nodular skin disease with or without draining tracts. Biopsy samples should be taken for impression smears, culture, and histopathologic and sensitivity tests.

The impression smears and histopathologic samples should be stained and examined for acid-fast organisms, and animal inoculation tests should be performed if tuberculosis is suspected. Therapy is dependent on which mycobacterium is the causative agent and should proceed as outlined above. Although ostensibly rare, the cutaneous mycobacterioses may have been overlooked as differential diagnoses in the past, and with greater awareness of these conditions, many more cases may be reported.

References and Supplemental Readings

Gross, T. L., and Connelly, M. R.: Nontuberculous mycobacterial skin infections in two dogs. Vet. Pathol. 20:117, 1983.

Kunkle, G. A., Gulbas, N. K., Fadok, V., et al.: Rapidly growing mycobacteria as a cause of cutaneous granulomas: Report of five cases. J. Am. Anim. Hosp. Assoc. 19:513, 1983.

McIntosh, D. W.: Feline Leprosy: A review of forty-four cases from western Canada. Can. Vet. J. 23:291, 1982.

Pattyn, S. R., and Portaels, F. G.: *In vitro* cultivation and classification of *Mycobacterium lepraemurium*. Int. J. Lepr. 48:7, 1980.

Parodi, A., Fontaine, M., Brion, A., et al.: Mycobacterioses in the domestic carnivore. Present-day epidemiology of tuberculosis in the cat and dog. J. Small Anim. Pract. 6:307, 1965.

White, S. D., Ihrke, P. J., Stannard, A. A., et al.: Cutaneous atypical mycobacteriosis in cats. J.A.V.M.A. 182:1218, 1983.

Wilkinson, G. T.: *Diseases of Cats*. Vade Mecum No. 3. Sydney: University of Sydney Post-Graduate Foundation in Veterinary Science, 1984, p. 19.

CANINE DEMODICOSIS

KENNETH W. KWOCHKA, D.V.M.

Madison, Wisconsin

Canine demodicosis is an inflammatory, parasitic skin disease in which a larger than normal number of the follicular mite *Demodex canis* inhabit the skin. The initial proliferation of the mites may be due to a genetic or immunologic disorder. In spite of the multiplicity of agents that have been used to treat chronic generalized demodicosis, it remains the most difficult and frustrating non-neoplastic dermatologic condition of the dog.

THE PARASITE

In very small numbers, the *D. canis* mite is a normal inhabitant of the skin of most dogs. When disease is present, the mites populate the skin by the thousands. They reside in hair follicles and occasionally in sebaceous glands and apocrine sweat glands. The life cycle is estimated to be between 20 and 35 days and is spent entirely on the host.

TRANSMISSION

Transmission of mites in all dogs occurs by direct contact during the first 2 to 3 days after birth while the pup is nursing. *In utero* transmission has not been demonstrated. This is substantiated by studies in which pups delivered by cesarean section and raised away from the dam did not harbor mites.

Demodectic mange is not considered to be a contagious disease, since no experimental data have ever demonstrated contagion of *Demodex* mites by themselves to older healthy animals. Attempts to transmit the disease by feeding dogs mites, by injecting mites intraperitoneally or intratracheally, by placing diseased animals in direct contact with neonatal healthy animals, or by directly applying mites to the skin of healthy dogs have failed. Furthermore, mites rapidly die by desiccation on the skin surface at 20°C with a relative humidity of 40 per cent.

PATHOGENESIS

The pathogenesis of this disease is still not completely understood. Since the parasite is found in the normal skin of almost all dogs, the reason for the proliferation of mites and development of clinical disease in certain individuals must be questioned. A number of predisposing factors have been suggested, including age, length of hair, inadequate diet, rapid growth, stress, accidents, boarding, estrus, nursing puppies, hunting or work, heartworms, nervousness, abnormally high or low environmental temperature, serum protein abnormalities, Factor VII deficiency, vaccinations, surgery, parturition, endoparasitism, poor condition, debilitating diseases, and inherited or genetic factors. Although most of these are hard to evaluate, some warrant careful consideration when a dog is presented with generalized demodicosis. The author has examined several bitches that developed generalized demodicosis during or shortly after each estrus or whelping. The disease could be cleared with minimal topical therapy until the subsequent estrus or pregnancy. Neutering was completely curative. The author has also treated two dogs with concurrent heartworm disease that had not completely responded to topical therapy for their generalized demodicosis after more than 1 year. Following therapy and resolution of the heartworm disease, the demodicosis spontaneously resolved without any further topical therapy. Finally, one other dog developed generalized demodicosis each time hookworm ova were found in the stool. Anthelmintic treatment of the hookworms alone resulted in spontaneous regression of the demodicosis until subsequent hookworm infestations.

There is strong evidence of a hereditary predisposition for generalized demodicosis. The disease is most common in certain breeds of purebred dogs and within certain lines of these breeds. It often occurs in littermates or related dogs, and a single bitch may produce multiple litters affected with demodicosis. Culling of affected dams and sires has radically reduced the incidence of generalized demodicosis from individual breeding kennels.

An abnormal immune response that allows mites to proliferate out of control on the skin is still the most accepted explanation for the development of the disease. Neutrophil morphology and function and humoral immunity appear to be normal. Scott and colleagues (1974, 1976, 1979) have hypothesized that generalized demodicosis is the manifestation of a hereditary, specific T-cell defect for *D. canis* in which the mite is allowed to multiply to large numbers and induce a humoral substance that causes generalized T-cell suppression.

In vitro lymphocyte blastogenesis studies conducted by Scott and colleagues (1974, 1976) on dogs with generalized demodicosis demonstrated severely depressed T-cell responses. This T-cell suppression appears to be the result of a serum immunosuppressive factor. Suppressed lymphocytes from dogs with chronic demodicosis respond normally to *in vitro* lymphocyte blastogenesis using phytohemagglutinin, concanavilin A, and pokeweed mitogen when cultured in normal dog serum. Conversely, normal dog lymphocytes have depressed blastogenesis responses when cultured in serum from dogs with generalized demodicosis. As mites are eradicated, measurable T-cell suppression disappears. Thus, any measurable immunosuppression is a result of the disease and large numbers of mites rather than a cause of it. This is further supported by the fact that dogs with localized demodicosis and early generalized demodicosis have normal *in vitro* lymphocyte blastogenesis responses and no serum immunosuppressive factor.

The concept of a serum immunosuppressive factor causing T-cell suppression with large populations of mites has recently been challenged. Barta and colleagues (1983) studied lymphocyte function in dogs with uncomplicated demodicosis, with demodicosis complicated with pyoderma, and with pyoderma alone. There was a good correlation between extent of pyoderma (primary or secondary to demodicosis) and degree of suppression of lymphocyte blastogenesis caused by serum. None of three dogs with uncomplicated demodicosis had detectable suppression of blastogenesis by their serum. The authors suggested that the appearance of suppressive factors in the serum is a consequence of pyoderma and not mites. Further work in this area must include correlating mite numbers per unit area with degree of suppression, since it is possible that any suppression due to the mites may be related to absolute numbers. Work is also needed to prove or disprove the suspected hereditary T-cell defect that allows the mites to multiply initially. Cutaneous ecology should also be studied, since local factors may play a role in the growth and reproduction of demodectic mange mites. Most importantly, in order for practitioners to be able to adequately counsel breeders, studies are badly needed to determine the genetic transmission of the disease.

Although generalized demodicosis is primarily a disease of young dogs, it will occasionally occur spontaneously in older dogs. In these cases, a thorough drug history should be taken to determine if any immunosuppressive drugs have been administered recently, and the presence of any underlying immunosuppressive diseases such as neoplastic disorders or Cushing's syndrome should be investigated. Underlying diseases are often hard to demonstrate at the time the demodicosis is diagnosed, but they will sometimes appear 6 to 12 months later.

CLINICAL SIGNS

The disease is most commonly encountered in purebred dogs younger than 1 year and is manifested in two major clinical forms.

The localized form is characterized by one or more discrete, small focal areas of alopecia with varying degrees of scaling, erythema, follicular plugging, and hyperpigmentation. Pruritus and secondary pyoderma are uncommon. The lesions are usually confined to the head, neck, and forelimbs, although any area of the body may be involved. This form may occur in any breed and in either sex.

Generalized demodicosis occurs primarily in purebred dogs younger than 1½ years. Approximately 10 per cent of localized cases of demodicosis may rapidly or gradually progress to generalized disease. There is usually generalized patchy or diffuse alopecia, erythema, edema, seborrhea, crusting, follicular plugging, lichenification, and a secondary pyoderma. The pyoderma may be either mild and superficial or severe and deep, with furunculosis and cellulitis. Pruritus and a generalized peripheral lymphadenopathy are usually present. Those cases with deep pyoderma may show signs of septicemia and may be febrile, anorexic, lethargic, and severely debilitated. This can be a life-threatening situation demanding immediate aggressive topical and systemic therapy. Generalized demodicosis occasionally occurs in a squamous form without a pyoderma. Demodectic otitis externa has also been reported, as has demodectic pododermatitis. Forms of demodicosis with foot involvement are often difficult to treat successfully.

DIAGNOSIS

Demodicosis is best diagnosed by demonstrating the mites on deep skin scrapings. All pyodermas and seborrheas should be scraped to rule out demodicosis as an underlying cause. Hair should be clipped in the area to be scraped and the skin squeezed gently to help extrude the mites from the hair follicles. A drop of mineral oil should be placed at the site to facilitate picking up material (dry debris is hard to pick up), and the area should be scraped with a No. 10 surgical blade until capillary bleeding is observed. The material should be transferred to another drop of oil on a slide and examined under low-power magnification.

An occasional adult mite may be found on scrapings from normal dogs and does not confirm a diagnosis of demodicosis. If one or two mites are found, scrapings should be repeated. Finding a large number of live adult mites or immature forms and eggs is necessary to confirm the diagnosis.

In very chronic cases, mites may not be demonstrated by skin scraping, since excessive thickening and scarring of the skin may occur and may not allow deep enough penetration. In these rare situations, a biopsy should confirm the diagnosis—mites are found within follicles or within the dermis if follicles have ruptured.

THERAPY

Localized and generalized demodicosis should be considered as two distinct disease entities that require different modes of therapy. In both forms, however, the following are some common considerations:

1. *No corticosteroids!* These drugs are completely contraindicated in any formulation, including topicals, and at any dosage. Corticosteroids may suppress the immune system of an already compromised animal. Localized cases of demodicosis can progress to the generalized form as a result of steroid administration. The pruritus usually associated with generalized disease complicated by a pyoderma will dramatically decrease with antibiotics and topical miticide therapy.

2. If a secondary pyoderma is present, it must be treated based on the severity and depth of infection. A superficial pyoderma limited in distribution can normally be controlled using topical therapy with benzoyl peroxide (Pyoben, Allerderm; OxyDex, DVM) or chlorhexidine (Nolvasan, Fort Dodge) shampoos. Povidone-iodine (Betadine, Purdue Frederick) baths are also effective but can be more irritating than the above products so are not routinely recommended by the author in mild superficial infections.

A generalized superficial pyoderma requires systemic antibiotics in addition to topical therapy. If the infection has not previously been treated, the antibiotic may be chosen empirically since a coagulase-positive *Staphylococcus* is usually isolated. Commonly used antibiotics in this situation include erythromycin (10 to 15 mg/kg PO t.i.d.), chloramphenicol (20 to 50 mg/kg PO t.i.d.) and lincomycin (Lincocin, Upjohn; 20 mg/kg PO b.i.d.). If better assurance of clinical efficacy is desired or if the initial antibiotic fails to give good response within 7 to 10 days, then an aerobic bacterial culture and susceptibility test should be performed. Antibiotic treatment needs to be continued a minimum of 3 to 4 weeks or 1 week after all clinical lesions have resolved.

With deep pyoderma, culture and susceptibility tests are mandatory, followed by an appropriate antibiotic administered for a minimum of 4 to 6 weeks. Even if the antibiotic is expensive, it should be used at the recommended dosage for an adequate period of time to decrease the possibility of poor clinical response, frequent relapses, and the development of antibiotic resistance. Aggressive topical therapy should be instituted by clipping the entire coat followed by warm dilute chlorhexidine (Nolvasan, Fort Dodge) or povidone-iodine (Betadine, Purdue Frederick) solution compresses, whole-body soakings, or whirlpool baths every 12 hours until ulcerated lesions are clean and healed. Heavy sedation or general anesthesia may be necessary for clipping, since ulcerated deep pyoderma lesions are painful.

Topical miticide therapy is started along with treatment of the pyoderma, with two exceptions. If a deep pyoderma is present, no topical parasiticidal agents are used until the erosions and ulcers are healed to minimize the possibility of systemic absorption and toxicity. Also, parasiticidal dippings are never administered to dogs under or recovering from general anesthesia because of possible drug interactions and toxicity.

3. It is important that all dogs that are presented with demodicosis be maintained on a good diet, checked and treated for gastrointestinal parasites, and examined for *Dirofilaria immitis* microfilariae and placed on preventive medication (if appropriate for location and season); all vaccinations should also be current and any concurrent diseases should be treated immediately.

Dogs with localized demodicosis have no demonstrated immunologic deficit, and more than 90 per cent will show a spontaneous cure and disappearance of lesions in 3 to 8 weeks. Thus, the prognosis is excellent, recurrence is extremely rare, and no limitations are placed on breeding. The 10 per cent that are destined to become generalized will do so whether or not therapy is instituted. If the client understands this, then no treatment is necessary. However, if the owner cannot understand this concept, then topical therapy for the localized lesions is indicated. One per cent rotenone ointment (Goodwinol, Goodwinol Products Corp.) or benzoyl peroxide gel (OxyDex Gel, DVM; Pyoben Gel, Allerderm) may be helpful when applied once a day and rubbed well into the individual lesions. The topical acaricidal products will usually cause more alopecia and erythema, making the lesions look worse prior to improvement. The author has seen dogs excoriate "quiet" lesions and create severe pyotraumatic dermatitis after application of rotenone. Conjunctivitis and corneal edema have also been observed after accidental application of rotenone into the eye during the treatment of periocular lesions.

Amitraz (Mitaban, Upjohn), which will be discussed extensively in relation to generalized demodicosis, has apparently been tested and proved safe and efficacious for localized demodicosis. The manufacturer is currently investigating licensure of the product for this use. *Demodex* mites are capable of developing resistance to insecticidal agents. One must question the rationale of using the only product licensed by the Food and Drug Administration (FDA) for generalized demodicosis in every localized case, because 90 per cent will cure themselves, and there is the possible risk of developing resistant mite populations on individual animals.

Before any therapy is instituted for a dog with generalized demodicosis, the veterinarian should spend sufficient time with the owner and explain possible pathomechanisms of the disease, prognosis, and treatment plan including time, effort, and cost involved. The dog's temperament must be such to allow handling for bathing, clipping, and administration of oral medication when antibiotics are needed. There is more reason for optimism in dogs younger than 1 year since as many as 50 per cent may show spontaneous cure; but the prognosis must be worse for old dogs, especially when a treatable underlying disease cannot be found. Other indicators of a more guarded prognosis include a deep pyoderma with isolation of gram-negative organisms such as species of *Pseudomonas*, a severe demodectic pododermatitis, and the presence of the disease in certain breeds, including Old English sheepdogs (the author has never cured one), Scottish terriers, cocker spaniels, Afghan hounds, collies, Doberman pinschers, poodles, and German shepherds. Although amitraz has made treatment and control of clinical lesions easier than older therapies, the client should still be aware that a lifetime of therapy may be necessary for control in those cases that cannot be completely cured. Thus, although clinical control can usually be achieved, generalized demodicosis still carries a guarded prognosis for complete and long-term cure.

A thorough physical examination, complete blood count, serum biochemistry panel, and urinalysis are performed on any dog with generalized demodicosis regardless of age. Although in most cases the abnormalities will be consistent with chronic disease and infection, owners will occasionally spend a great deal of time, effort, and money on unsuccessful therapy only to find that their dog has a nontreatable underlying disease (such as congenital hepatic and renal anomalies in juvenile cases).

Although many products have been claimed as cures for generalized demodicosis (Scott, 1979), most have no scientific basis for their reported efficacy. In order for a drug to be considered effective, the clinical trials should report complete population information, including the dog's age and the form of the disease being treated (localized or generalized). The duration of follow-up before proclaiming complete cures should be a minimum of 1 year with negative skin scrapings and no clinical lesions. Currently, the two most widely used modes of therapy are amitraz (Mitaban, Upjohn) and a topical ronnel (Ectoral Emulsifiable Concentrate, Pitman-Moore) in propylene glycol solution. There are vast differences of opinion among veterinary dermatologists as to which of these products is more effective.

Amitraz, still a fairly new drug, was marketed in August of 1982. It is classified as a monoamine oxidase inhibitor, but the mechanism of its acaricidal action is not known. The product has made treatment of generalized demodicosis much easier than ronnel with propylene glycol, and it is the only drug approved for this use by the FDA. Initial clinical trials conducted or coordinated by the manufacturer reported cure rates ranging from 86 per cent to more than 99 per cent (Folz, 1983). Close

*Table 1. Cure and Toxicity Rates for 18 Dogs Treated for Generalized Demodicosis with Amitraz**

Amitraz Treatment Group (Concentration and Frequency)	Number of Dogs in Group	Rate of Cure	Rate of Toxicity
0.03% (6 ml/gal, every 2 weeks)	5	20% (1 of 5)	40% (2 of 5)
0.03% (6 ml/gal, weekly)	4	75% (3 of 4)	50% (2 of 4)
0.06% (12 ml/gal, every 2 weeks)	4	25% (1 of 4)	50% (2 of 4)
0.06% (12 ml/gal, weekly)	5	80% (4 of 5)	40% (2 of 5)
Totals	18	50% (9 of 18)	44% (8 of 18)

*Reprinted with permission from Kwochka et al.: Comp. Cont. Ed. Pract. Vet. 7:8, 1985.

scrutiny of these trials raised a number of questions as to whether cases were actually cured or just clinically improved but still harboring mites, which would eventually multiply and cause clinical disease when dippings were discontinued. The most important factors frequently overlooked were the length of the follow-up period after cessation of dippings and the number and results of deep skin scrapings at these visits.

A clinical study (Kwochka et al., 1985) was devised using only naturally occurring cases of generalized demodicosis, well-defined population measurements and criteria for end-point cures, and, most importantly, long-term follow-ups with examination and skin scrapings. This trial tested the efficacy and toxicity of amitraz (BAAM, Upjohn) used at two different concentrations and two different frequencies of application (Table 1). Eighteen dogs with an average age of 2.8 years and average disease duration of 11.4 months were treated. The entire coat was clipped on all of the dogs prior to the first dipping, and all dippings were preceded by a 2.5 per cent benzoyl peroxide shampoo (OxyDex, DVM). The follicular flushing activity of benzoyl peroxide may be beneficial in opening affected hair follicles to allow better penetration of the dip. The 19.8 per cent w/w concentrate solution of amitraz was added to warm water to give suspensions of the compound at the two different concentrations (Table 1). The freshly prepared dipping solution was continually saturated over the entire body with a sponge for 10 minutes, and the dog was then allowed to air dry or was blown dry without rinsing. All four feet of each dog were immersed in small bowls of the solution during the 10-minute dipping procedure. The owners were told not to bathe their dogs or let them get wet between dippings. At least six skin scrapings were performed every 2 weeks, and dippings were continued until three consecutive sets of scrapings were negative (no mites, larvae, nymphs, or eggs) at 2-week intervals or for a period of 20 weeks. The dogs were examined and scraped monthly after the last dipping. Cures for this study were designated as those animals with no clinical signs of disease and negative scrapings 6 months after the last dip.

Clinical improvement was evident in all of the dogs, but the overall cure rate was 9 of 18, or 50 per cent (Table 1). The average number of treatments per patient in the nine cured cases was 9.1. Seventy-eight per cent (7 of 9) of the patients treated weekly (regardless of the concentration of amitraz used) were cured, whereas only 22 per cent (2 of 9) of the dogs treated every 2 weeks were cured. There was no significant difference between the cure rates in the groups treated with 0.06 per cent amitraz (56 per cent, 5 of 9) versus those at 0.03 per cent amitraz (44 per cent, 4 of 9). Of the 50 per cent (9 of 18) that were therapeutic failures, six cases never achieved complete regression of lesions or negative scrapings. Three cases (17 per cent) experienced temporary clinical remission and had negative scrapings but later relapsed and had new lesions and viable mites at 4, 5, and 6 months. Switching five of these cases to the FDA-approved amitraz product (Mitaban, Upjohn) did not result in additional cures after 9 to 12 months of treatment. An evaluation of the approved product (White and Stannard, 1983) that has been performed with adequate experimental design and 3-year follow-ups on all animals reported long-term relapses and a cure rate of 53 per cent (18 of 34), similar to our results.

These results suggest that amitraz does not have high efficacy for long-term cures but that better cure rates may be achieved when twice the recommended frequency (weekly) of application is used. Increasing the frequency of application did not result in a greater incidence in toxicity (Table 1). However, the FDA approves current use of amitraz only at 0.025 per cent every 2 weeks. More cases will need to be evaluated before final conclusions can be drawn. In spite of the low cure rate, excellent clinical improvement is seen in most cases and many dogs can be maintained asymptomatic, although still harboring mites, on dippings every 2 to 4 weeks. The author has so far kept dogs totally asymptomatic on maintenance programs for as long as 2 years. It is imperative that these dogs be neutered so that they are not shown or used for breeding and thus perpetuate the disease.

Other advantages of using amitraz include its ease of application in the aqueous form every 2 weeks, owner convenience (since it is approved for application at home), relatively low cost, and low reported toxicity. Drying and flaking of the skin are minor problems encountered on occasion and are easily controlled by adding 1 to 2 capfuls of a bath oil rinse to the dipping solution (Alpha Keri Bath

Oil, Westwood; Humelac, Allerderm). Eight per cent of patients treated will show transient sedation, and 3 per cent will suffer transient pruritus. Other less frequently encountered abnormalities include cutaneous edema and erythema, anorexia, appetite stimulation, bloat, polyuria, polydipsia, ataxia, convulsions, vomiting, diarrhea, personality changes, hypothermia, urinary incontinence, and death. Although many formulations of amitraz are available, only the FDA-approved product (Mitaban, Upjohn) should now be used for legal reasons and because it has been formulated with a very low level of impurities, making it safer for topical use on dogs.

Ronnel still offers the greatest chance for long-term complete cures, with 90 to 92 per cent efficacy in well-controlled studies with long-term follow-ups (Baker et al., 1976; Scott, 1979). The drug was not available for about 2 years but has recently been reintroduced to the market (Ectoral Emulsifiable Concentrate, 33 per cent ronnel, Pitman-Moore). A 4 per cent solution is made by combining 180 ml of the concentrate with 1000 ml of propylene glycol, a good bacteriostatic agent that serves as an excellent vehicle for spreading the ronnel. The solution is stable for approximately 1 month. Water can be used in place of propylene glycol if the patient develops a contact sensitivity, but the aqueous solution is not stable and should be used immediately. The treatment should be instituted only after healing of any deep pyoderma and total clipping of the coat. The solution is shaken well, applied, and massaged into the skin of one third of the body each day on a rotating basis. The solution is allowed to dry without rinsing. Even normal-appearing areas should be thoroughly covered, since spot treatment is not effective. Plastic or rubber gloves must be worn, and dippings should be performed outside or in a well-ventilated area. Ophthalmic ointment should be used to protect the dog's eyes.

As with amitraz, response to therapy should be monitored by skin scrapings. Ideally, live adult mites, dead adults, larvae, and eggs should be counted from several representative skin scrapings prior to therapy to serve as a basis for comparison at follow-up visits. In a busy practice, all of these counts may not be possible, but a rough idea of the ratios of live to dead mites and mature to immature forms should be noted. A favorable response to therapy is indicated by a decrease in live and immature forms. Scrapings are begun 4 weeks after the start of therapy and performed every 2 weeks. Treatment should be continued 3 to 4 weeks after negative (no mites) scrapings and discontinued only after a final set of scrapings at that time. A minimum of 10 scrapings are performed at the final visit, with special attention to previously affected areas, any new clinical lesions, the face, and the feet. Reevaluation with scrapings should be performed every 3 months for 1 year before a case is considered fully cured. Frequent evaluation can often prevent the development of severe clinical lesions in relapsing cases by finding mites and reinstituting therapy prior to extensive hair loss or secondary pyoderma.

Ronnel is a potent organophosphate that is harsh, messy, malodorous, and potentially toxic. Erythema and scaling of the skin, moderate weight loss, and mild salivation are expected side effects, which are reversible on cessation of therapy. Signs of organophosphate toxicity occasionally occur; they include anorexia, excessive salivation, lacrimation, depression, bradycardia, vomiting, diarrhea, muscle fasciculations, and seizures. Therapy should be discontinued, the dog washed to remove any remaining solution, and treatment instituted with atropine and pralidoxime chloride (2-PAM, protopam chloride). After the dog recovers, an alternate miticide should be sought or the frequency of application reduced to one third of the body every other day. Hepatotoxicity has been reported rarely, and usually in dogs on additional drugs. This may lead to speculation about reactions to combination therapy. Oral parasiticidal agents such as ronnel tablets (Ectoral, Pitman-Moore) or cythioate (Proban, American Cyanamid) are not effective modes of therapy and may increase the possibility of organophosphate toxicity.

The practitioner faces a dilemma when deciding which of the two products to use: (1) the FDA-approved amitraz (Mitaban, Upjohn) product, which gives excellent clinical improvement, is fairly inexpensive, is easy to use on a weekly or biweekly basis in an aqueous form, and has low reported toxicity but a low long-term cure rate with frequent relapses, or (2) the non-FDA-approved ronnel (Ectoral Emulsifiable Concentrate, Pitman-Moore) solution, which is time-consuming, messy, potentially hazardous, and more expensive, but is also clinically very effective and has long-term cure rates of 90 to 92 per cent. The decision should be made on an individual basis, and the owner should be fully informed of the two options available and the benefits and drawbacks of each product.

In most cases, the author has found that owners will elect a trial course of amitraz prior to other therapy. Owner compliance with the treatment protocol is of paramount importance in managing a case of generalized demodicosis. It is much easier for a client to spend 30 minutes a week as opposed to 30 minutes a day administering the dippings. The author currently uses amitraz (Mitaban, Upjohn) *weekly* at the manufacturer's recommended concentration (0.025 per cent: 1 vial = 10.6 ml/2 gallons of water) and following the protocol used in the clinical trial (Kwochka et al., 1985) reported earlier in this section. If after 20 weeks there is not complete clearance of the lesions and negative scrapings or if an initially controlled case relapses, the chance of a complete cure with amitraz is small. The owner is then given the option of switching to ronnel in an attempt to achieve a complete cure or switching to a maintenance program using amitraz to control the mites in low enough numbers to keep the dog asymptomatic. The necessary frequency of dippings on a maintenance program will depend on the individual case, but it is generally no longer than every 3 to 4 weeks. These animals should be scraped periodically, as a low number of cases may eventually cure over a long period of time. These cases should also be monitored for relapse while on a long-term maintenance program, since resistant mite populations may develop. The client must be aware of the financial burden of such an indefinite program. If ronnel has been used first and has not resulted in negative scrapings after 4 to 5 months, then amitraz can be tried.

If during initial therapy or maintenance therapy the number of mites or percentage of immature forms dramatically increases, mite resistance may be occurring, and therapeutic disaster is impending. If the treatment protocol has been followed and no concurrent debilitating disease has developed, then a switch to the alternate miticide or doubling the concentration of the product being used (4 per cent to 8 per cent for ronnel and 0.025 per cent to 0.05 per cent for amitraz) would be indicated. If this is not effective, the alternative is a 3 per cent aqueous trichlorfon solution (Neguvon, Haver-Lockhart) applied according to the same protocol as for ronnel or as a whole-body dip every 4 days. If all of these products fail to control the disease, then euthanasia should be considered.

Immunostimulation with drugs such as levamisole or thiabendazole does not alter the course of the disease. Studies are currently being conducted to assess the efficacy of the avermectin compounds for generalized demodicosis.

PROPHYLAXIS

Because of the strong hereditary predisposition for generalized demodicosis, the owner should be strongly advised that the dog should never be used for breeding and that the mating that produced the affected dog should not be repeated. The American Academy of Veterinary Dermatology has passed a resolution that all dogs with generalized demodicosis be neutered. Ideally, all littermates and the sire and dam should be removed from the breeding program, but it is hard to convince a breeder with valuable show dogs to adopt this controversial program since nothing specific is known about how the disease is transmitted genetically.

When to perform the ovariohysterectomy or castration is also an important question. Many dermatologists will recommend not subjecting the patient to anesthesia and elective surgery until well after the disease is cured and therapy is discontinued. The rationale for this is that stress may exacerbate the disease. However, there is also concern that a relapse may occur if the surgery is performed after therapy has been stopped, or that if a bitch comes into estrus during therapy or shortly after therapy the disease may exacerbate. With ronnel, neutering is delayed until at least 6 months after discontinuation of therapy. Estrus can be successfully controlled with mibolerone (Cheque Drops, Upjohn) until the ovariohysterectomy is performed. Since amitraz is used only weekly or biweekly, patients may be successfully neutered while still being treated. The current protocol used by the author is to get the clinical disease well controlled and the mite counts low, skip a week of dipping if on a weekly program (or operate during the nontreatment week if biweekly), during that week perform the surgery (screen with a complete blood count and biochemistry profile), and then continue with dipping the following week. Thus far, no exacerbation of clinical signs, sudden increase in mite counts, or toxicity has been encountered when this protocol is followed.

References and Supplemental Reading

Baker, B. B., Stannard, A. A., Yaskulski, S. G., et al.: Evaluation of topical application of ronnel solution for generalized demodicosis in dogs. J.A.V.M.A. 168:1105, 1976.

Barta, O., Waltman, C., Oyekan, P. P., et al.: Lymphocyte transformation suppression caused by pyoderma—failure to demonstrate it in uncomplicated demodectic mange. Comp. Immunol. Microbiol. Infect. Dis. 6:9, 1983.

Folz, S. D.: Demodicosis (*Demodex canis*). Comp. Cont. Ed. Pract. Vet. 5:116, 1983.

Kwochka, K. W., Kunkle, G. A., and Foil, C. O.: The efficacy of amitraz for generalized demodicosis in dogs: A study of two concentrations and frequencies of application. Comp. Cont. Ed. Pract. Vet. 7:8, 1985.

Miller, W. H.: Canine demodicosis. Comp. Cont. Ed. Pract. Vet. 2:334, 1980.

Muller, G. H., Kirk, R. W., and Scott, D. W.: *Small Animal Dermatology*, 3rd ed. Philadelphia: W. B. Saunders, 1983.

Scott, D. W., Farrow, B. H., and Schultz, R. D.: Studies on the therapeutic and immunologic aspects of generalized demodectic mange in the dog. J.A.A.H.A. 10:233, 1974.

Scott, D. W., Schultz, R. D., and Baker, E.: Further studies on the therapeutic and immunologic aspects of generalized demodectic mange in the dog. J.A.A.H.A. 12:203, 1976.

Scott, D. W.: Canine demodicosis. Vet. Clin. North Am. 9:79, 1979.

White, S. D., and Stannard, A. A.: Canine demodicosis. *In* Kirk, R. W. (ed.): *Current Veterinary Therapy VIII*. Philadelphia: W. B. Saunders, 1983, pp. 484–487.

DIFFERENTIAL DIAGNOSIS OF FELINE MILIARY DERMATITIS

KENNETH W. KWOCHKA, D.V.M.
Madison, Wisconsin

The skin has a limited number of ways in which to react. Thus, a variety of dermatologic and other medical diseases can be manifested by the same or similar clinical cutaneous abnormalities. In veterinary dermatology, there is no better example of this than the feline miliary dermatitis (eczema) complex. Numerous extensive reviews of feline miliary dermatitis have been written in recent years (Willemse, 1980; Scott, 1980; Reedy, 1980; Kunkle, 1982; Ihrke et al., 1983; Muller et al., 1983). All authors agree that the disease complex represents a similar cutaneous reaction pattern to any of a variety of different causes. Thus, before a diagnosis of idiopathic miliary dermatitis is made, a careful search should be undertaken to arrive at a specific diagnosis followed by institution of appropriate therapy.

The disease complex must be carefully explained to owners so that they will understand the necessity of an exhaustive diagnostic workup. In order to successfully define an underlying cause for the condition, the veterinarian must be interested in the case, willing to spend adequate time (often with several office visits needed), and able to formulate a logical step-by-step plan to rule in or rule out the various causes. If, after all of this has been accomplished and a specific cause is still not found, a diagnosis of idiopathic miliary dermatitis is justified.

CLINICAL HISTORY

A carefully taken dermatologic history is invaluable in helping to define a cause for miliary dermatitis. At the very least, the history will indicate which differentials should first be pursued by using specific diagnostic tests. Any history of contagion to other pets or family members would point toward diseases such as flea infestation, pediculosis, dermatophytosis, notoedric mange, cheyletiellosis, otodectic mange, and fur mites (*Lynxacarus radovsky*). Seasonality of the clinical signs would raise suspicion about flea infestation or flea allergy dermatitis, pediculosis, atopy, or trombiculiasis (chiggers). Concurrent gastrointestinal disease may be indicative of food allergy dermatitis or intestinal parasitism. A lack of response to glucocorticoids would suggest food allergy, dermatophytosis, pediculosis, bacterial folliculitis, a drug eruption, feline demodicosis, or idiopathic disease.

Another important indicator in the history is the presence or absence of pruritus. This may be difficult to document in the cat, since true scratching is uncommon. Clues such as alopecia with coarse broken hairs and hyperpigmentation must be carefully evaluated. Pruritic cats will often lick, chew, and groom excessively but in many cases not in the presence of the owners. Irritability, personality change, and twitching of the skin may also be caused by pruritus. True pruritus would be more indicative of allergic or parasitic causes, although it may occur in severe chronic miliary dermatitis due to any cause.

Other helpful historic information includes whether the condition developed acutely (ectoparasites) with no previous skin disease or if it has been chronic, with gradual progression over a longer period of time (allergies).

CLINICAL SIGNS

Any breed, age, or sex of cat may be affected with miliary dermatitis. Initially, there is an erythematous papular reaction covered by small crusts (papulocrustous dermatitis). These lesions may not be obvious visually but detected only by stroking the cat. They usually begin over the dorsum, especially the neck, head, and base of the tail, but may become generalized. Pruritus is variable, but in some cases the self-inflicted trauma may be so intense as to cause extensive hair loss, a severe moist dermatitis, and large, raised plaques. Other signs may include peripheral lymphadenopathy, hyperesthesia, and personality changes ranging from aggression to timidity.

DIFFERENTIAL DIAGNOSIS

The various causes of miliary dermatitis have commonly been grouped into four main categories: allergies, parasites, infectious agents, and miscellaneous causes, including idiopathic disease. These divisions still offer the best classification system for discussing the disorder. A designation of idiopathic disease is given to those cases for which an underlying cause cannot be found after a complete diagnostic investigation.

Allergies

Flea allergy is the most common form of allergic dermatitis in cats and is the most common cause of miliary dermatitis. In parts of the country where fleas are a serious problem, they may account for greater than 90 per cent of the cases of miliary dermatitis (Ihrke et al., 1983). There is no age, breed, or sex predilection, and clinical signs may be seasonal or nonseasonal depending on the section of the country and infestation of the internal environment. The most common areas of the body with miliary dermatitis lesions include the lumbosacral area, medial and posterior thighs, ventral abdomen, head, and neck. In severe chronic cases, there may be generalized involvement.

The diagnosis is made by history, clinical lesions, finding fleas or flea debris, and response to therapy. The failure to find fleas or flea excrement on the cat does not rule out flea allergy dermatitis. Cats may remove such evidence by their fastidious grooming habits, and fleas spend the vast majority of their time off the cat and in the environment. Unfortunately, in an allergic animal, a single flea bite may perpetuate pruritus and dermatitis for several days. Immediate or delayed hypersensitivity reactions to intradermally administered flea antigen may be helpful in making the diagnosis, especially when fleas are not easily found. The author has been pleased with the specificity of a 1:1000 weight/volume aqueous flea antigen extract (Flea Extract 1:1000, Greer) for diagnostic purposes.

The best treatment for a flea-allergic cat is strict topical flea control on the animal, on all contact animals, and, most importantly, in the environment. It is important to eradicate all the fleas and continue therapy as needed to prevent reinfestation. Simply lowering the numbers of fleas is not enough to keep an allergic cat asymptomatic. It is beyond the scope of this article to review all available pesticides. The reader is referred to other references (Bledsoe et al., 1982; MacDonald, 1983; Halliwell, 1983), including the article on parasiticide therapy in this section. The use of the systemic insecticide cythioate (Proban, American Cyanamid) and the potent topical organophosphate fenthion (Spotton, Cutter) in cats is discussed in two references (Halliwell, 1983; Scott, 1984).

Corticosteroids may be necessary to control the pruritus and dermatitis until the flea infestation is brought under control. They may be needed indefinitely in outdoor or indoor-outdoor cats with continual flea exposure from the external environment. Prednisone or prednisolone is used at 1 to 2 mg/kg PO every 12 hours for the first 5 days, followed by a gradual decrease to arrive at an alternate-day maintenance dose, which will keep the patient comfortable (usually 1 to 2 mg/kg PO every other evening). Methylprednisolone acetate (Depo-Medrol, Upjohn) is an effective, injectable glucocorticoid for cats. It is used at a dosage of 5 mg/kg SC and will keep the patient comfortable for 3 to 6 weeks, by which time the fleas should be eradicated. For long-term use, injections should not be given more frequently than every 2 months.

A recent double-blind study (Kunkle and Milcarsky, 1985) evaluated the efficacy of hyposensitization for flea allergy in cats. There was no statistically significant difference in response between the control and treated groups. Only 3 of 17 cats treated with antigen showed improvement in pruritus and dermatitis.

Food allergy is an uncommon disorder in cats but should be considered as a possible cause in any presentation of miliary dermatitis, especially when there is severe pruritus with progression of the miliary lesions to an ulcerative crusting dermatitis of the head and neck. There are no age, breed, or sex predilections. The condition is nonseasonal, and concurrent gastrointestinal signs are rare. The cat may be allergic to any component of the diet, and in most cases the offending food has been fed for 2 years or more.

The diagnosis is made by favorable response to an elimination diet administered over a 3-week period. The diet should consist of foods to which the cat has not been previously exposed. Simply changing commercial foods is not satisfactory, since they usually contain common additives, preservatives, and protein sources. The author has found the most acceptable elimination diet for owner compliance and palatability for the cat to be an additive- and preservative-free strained lamb baby food and rice (not quick-cooking) diet and fresh water. Clinical improvement should be seen within 21 days, and the diagnosis can be further documented by exacerbation of signs within 72 hours after reinstitution of the original diet. If the cat is intensely pruritic, an Elizabethan collar or glucocorticoids (prednisolone or prednisone, 2 mg/kg PO once daily) may be needed for the first 7 to 10 days of the diet to break the itch-scratch-itch cycle. If the affected cat is part of a multiple-cat household, feeding all of the cats the elimination diet or segregating the patient may be necessary to ensure against exposure to other foods.

Therapy consists of avoidance of the offending agent in the diet, but the exact allergen is rarely determined. One new item may be added to the elimination diet every 5 days to create a tolerable balanced diet. Vitamin, mineral, and fatty acid supplementation is important in diets that cannot be balanced. Taurine may be supplemented by adding ½ teaspoon of clam juice to the diet daily. A nutritionally complete homemade diet that may be useful in food-allergic cats has been formulated (Morris, 1977). Experimenting with home-cooked meals is not practical for most busy pet owners. Chicken-based commercial foods may prove useful in some cases. The commercial lamb-based food (Prescription Diet d/d, Hill's) is nutritionally complete for cats, but palatability may be a problem. The addition of one or two boiled eggs per can may improve palatability. During the past 2 years, the author has seen three cats that exhibited signs of food allergy dermatitis while on semimoist packet cat foods. Changing to any brand or flavor of dry or canned food resulted in clearing of lesions. These cats may be allergic to an additive or preservative used in the special processing of these foods. In general, dietary allergies are poorly controlled with glucocorticoids and antihistamines.

Allergic inhalant dermatitis (atopy) should be considered as a possible cause of miliary dermatitis with pruritus, especially if it is seasonal and if there has been a lack of response to flea control and a food-elimination diet. Flea allergy dermatitis and atopy may occur concurrently, as in dogs.

The diagnosis of atopy is made by positive intradermal allergy testing with the same antigens, dilutions, and injection techniques as for dogs. Injections are administered to the lateral thorax with the cat restrained in lateral or sternal recumbency or with the aid of a cat bag. Ketamine hydrochloride (Ketaset, Bristol; 10 mg/kg IM) is effective chemical restraint for the fractious animal. Reactions are read 15 minutes after injection. Evaluation is more difficult in cats than in dogs, since wheals tend to be smaller, flatter, less circumscribed, minimally erythematous, and quick to fade away. Transillumination with a penlight in a dark room and digital palpation will often aid interpretation of reactions.

Therapy consists of avoidance of the allergen (rarely possible), glucocorticoids, or hyposensitization. Reedy (1982) reported a good response to hyposensitization in five of seven cats with miliary dermatitis by using alum-precipitated extracts and a dosage schedule as used in dogs. Prednisone, prednisolone, or methylprednisolone acetate used as described for control of flea allergy dermatitis is also an effective means of control.

Drug eruptions (allergies) may cause a variety of cutaneous and mucocutaneous eruptions. There are few well-documented reports, but miliary dermatitis lesions have been seen with sulfisoxazole and penicillin. Virtually any drug being administered should be considered as a potential cause of the dermatitis. Skin biopsies may be suggestive of a drug allergy (usually not diagnostic) and may help rule out other causes. If miliary dermatitis is the only manifestation of the drug allergy, then discontinuation and avoidance of the drug and chemically related compounds should be curative within 1 to 2 weeks without the need for additional therapy. On rare occasions, reactions may last for several weeks. If the cutaneous reaction is severe, topical symptomatic therapy, glucocorticoids, and evaluation of hematologic, hepatic, and renal status are indicated. More severe concurrent signs (urticaria, angioedema, anaphylaxis) will require glucocorticoids, antihistamines, and epinephrine.

Intestinal parasites (roundworms, tapeworms, hookworms, coccidia) may cause an allergic dermatitis with a pruritic miliary dermatitis. Concurrent gastrointestinal signs would be supportive of this consideration but would also be consistent with food allergy. Any cat presented with miliary dermatitis should have at least one direct fecal smear and one fecal flotation test performed. Use of an appropriate anthelmintic eliminates the parasite and consequently the dermatitis.

If pruritic miliary dermatitis lesions appear in relatively hairless areas such as the ventral abdomen, medial thighs, axillae, perineum, ventral tail, chin, and pinnae, then an allergic contact or irritant contact dermatitis should be considered. True allergic contact dermatitis appears to be a rare, naturally occurring clinical disease. Substances associated with contact dermatitis include neomycin (topical), dichlorvos (flea collars), plants and grasses, carpeting, cleansers, iodine, plastic or rubber compounds that are used to make some pet food dishes, and antioxidants (litter boxes). In true allergic conditions, the offending substance has usually been present in the environment for months to years and only one animal in a multiple-cat household will be affected. A contact irritant dermatitis is caused by a newly introduced substance, and all animals that contact it would be expected to be involved to varying degrees.

The diagnosis is based on the distribution of lesions, supportive biopsy findings, and provocative exposure. Patch testing is impractical in all but the most cooperative of cats and owners. In cases of allergic or irritant contact dermatitis, removal of the offending substance and avoidance of further contact is the preferred therapy. If the offending compound cannot be isolated and identified, glucocorticoids may be useful at the previously described dosages.

Parasites

Excellent photomicrographs of the ectoparasites to be discussed in this section have been presented by Muller and colleagues (1983). These will greatly aid identification of the parasites on skin scrapings.

Species of *Cheyletiella* mites (usually *Cheyletiella blakei* in cats) may infest cats and cause variable clinical signs including a focal or generalized miliary dermatitis with or without pruritus. The mites are surface dwellers, and the entire life cycle is spent on the cat. They are highly contagious, and direct or indirect transmission may occur, including mite attachment to fleas, flies, and lice. It appears that the mites may not be strongly species specific, and other animals and humans in the environment may be affected with a papular pruritic dermatosis. Mites may live off the host in the environment for as long as 2 weeks.

Demonstration of mites to confirm the diagnosis can be very difficult. Examination of scales with a magnifying lens may reveal the moving white mites (walking dandruff). Crusts and scales may be collected from the skin surface and hair by superficial skin scrapings with mineral oil, combing with a very fine-toothed flea comb, or by touching the sticky side of a piece of clear cellophane tape to multiple lesions. Collected material can then be examined microscopically for the eight-legged saddle-shaped body with the characteristic hooked, pinching mouthparts. Occasionally, mites or eggs may be found in fecal flotation samples even when they cannot be demonstrated from cutaneous lesions. Even when all of the above techniques are performed, mites may be overlooked in a significant percentage of cases. A high degree of suspicion warrants a course of appropriate therapy.

The mites are susceptible to most insecticides, but the infestation may be difficult to eradicate unless all animals in the environment are treated as well as the environment itself. Parasiticidal agents such as carbamate powders, pyrethrin or carbaryl shampoos, or 2 per cent lime sulfur dips should be used weekly for a minimum of 4 weeks. The environment should be thoroughly cleaned, vacuumed, and fogged or sprayed with products used for flea control twice at a 2-week interval.

Notoedres cati is a sarcoptid mite that is highly contagious by direct contact and may cause a pruritic miliary dermatitis. It occurs infrequently in the United States, with the exception of several endemic urban areas. The head and neck of the host are most commonly affected, and the pruritus may be so severe that early miliary dermatitis lesions quickly progress to large, thick crusts with excoriation and lichenification. In chronic cases, the forelimbs and perianal area may also be involved. The diagnosis is made by clinical findings (food allergy is the major differential) and skin scrapings. The mites are easily found with superficial scrapings and are similar in appearance to canine sarcoptic mange mites.

A 2 per cent lime sulfur solution applied as a whole-body dip weekly for 4 weeks to all animals in the environment should be effective therapy. Environmental treatment other than washing the cat's bedding and thorough vacuum cleaning is usually not necessary, since the mite does not persist for long off the host. Amitraz used as a single whole-body aqueous dip at a concentration of 0.025 per cent is apparently also effective but is not licensed for use in cats and is toxic even at comparatively low dosage levels.

Otodectic mange (*Otodectes cynotis*) is the most common cause of otitis externa in cats. Owing to the secondary pruritus of the ear canals and ectopic infestations of the mites, a pruritic miliary dermatitis may appear on the head, neck, rump, paws, and perineum. The diagnosis is made by finding the thick, brown-black, dry, crusty exudate in the ear canals; the mites are found on direct otoscopic examination or from ear swabs placed in mineral oil and examined microscopically. Therapy consists of thorough cleaning of the ear canals with a ceruminolytic agent followed by application of an appropriate parasiticide. The author has had best results with a thiabendazole-dexamethasone-neomycin preparation (Tresaderm, Merck, Sharp & Dohme) applied five drops to each ear canal on alternate days for 1 month. A combination of one part rotenone in oil (Canex, Pitman-Moore) diluted with three parts mineral oil and applied twice weekly to the ear canals for 2 weeks beyond clinical cure is also effective but is messy to use and more irritating. To facilitate complete eradication, the entire body should also be treated weekly for 4 weeks with flea powders, sprays, shampoos, or dips. All animals in the environment, whether symptomatic or not, should be treated, since the mite is not host specific and is highly contagious. In chronic recurrent cases, the environment should also be treated with flea preparations, since the mites have been reported to live in the premises for months.

Feline demodicosis is a rare disease, but more cases have been reported recently. There is evidence that two species of *Demodex* mites may inhabit the skin of cats: one found superficially in the stratum corneum, causing mild erythema, alopecia, and pruritus; the other (*D. cati*) in the pilosebaceous apparatus, resulting in alopecia and folliculitis with a clinical presentation possibly mimicking miliary dermatitis. Localized and generalized cases may occur, as well as a demodectic otitis externa. Generalized cases should be evaluated medically for diseases that can cause immunosuppression, such as feline leukemia virus (FeLV) and diabetes mellitus. Deep skin scrapings should confirm the diagnosis. The morphology should be studied to determine if the surface-feeding mite (broad, blunted abdomen) or follicular mite (*D. cati*, elongated) is present. Because of its more superficial location, the former may prove easier to kill and thus carry a better prognosis. Too few cases have been reported to recommend any one best treatment program. Localized cases are usually self-limiting, but a 1 per cent rotenone ointment (Goodwinol, Goodwinol Products Corp.) applied daily until lesions are resolved has been recommended. Excellent results for the generalized form have been reported with topical lime sulfur dips, carbaryl shampoos, rotenone, and organophosphates.

Pediculosis (*Felicola subrostratus*) is rare in the United States but may occasionally present as a variably pruritic miliary dermatitis in neglected debilitated animals in a filthy environment, especially in the winter. Lice are species specific, contagious, but not able to survive off the host for more than a few hours and thus are not of public health significance. The diagnosis is easily made by macroscopic or microscopic examination of hairs for louse eggs (nits) attached to the shafts. Lice are susceptible to most insecticides, and pyrethrin or carbamate powders or shampoos or 2 per cent lime sulfur dips are effective when used on all cats weekly for 4 weeks. A single cleaning and vacuuming of the environment should be sufficient.

The cat fur mite (*Lynxacarus radovsky*) has been reported as a cause of miliary dermatitis and seborrhea sicca in cats. The mites normally attach themselves to the hair shafts and are demonstrated by direct microscopic examination of hairs or superficial skin scrapings. Other diagnostic techniques as listed for cheyletiellosis may also be helpful. Therapy consists of 0.5 per cent malathion or 2 per cent lime sulfur dips or 5 per cent carbaryl powder administered weekly for 3 to 4 weeks.

The small larval form of the harvest mite or chigger (*Eutrombicula alfreddugesi, Bryobia praetiosa, Walchia americana*) may rarely cause pruritic or nonpruritic miliary dermatitis lesions on the head, ears, and paws of outdoor cats. Transmission occurs by contact with the larvae from areas of heavy vegetation, where the adults parasitize grasses, shrubs, and other arthropods. History would contribute to the diagnosis, since the disease is seasonal, occurring in the late summer and fall. The larvae are rarely seen as small (0.2 to 0.4 mm) red, orange, or yellow dots in the center of papules. Scrapings are helpful. Usually the larvae fall off within several days, and the condition gradually resolves without a specific diagnosis being made. Pyrethrin or carbamate powders or shampoos or 2 per cent lime sulfur dips are effective when used as a single application, as long as reinfestation is prevented.

Infectious Agents

Dermatophytosis due primarily to *Microsporum canis* but also to *M. gypseum* and *Trichophyton mentagrophytes* can cause clinical signs of feline miliary dermatitis. A complete discussion of this disease is beyond the scope of this chapter, and the reader is referred to several excellent review articles on the subject (Reedy, 1980; Scott, 1980; O'Neill, 1982a, b; Ihrke et al., 1983; Muller et al., 1983).

True bacterial folliculitis is rare in cats. When it occurs, the chin region is most commonly involved secondary to the follicular plugging of feline acne. Occasionally, a generalized folliculitis may occur, resulting in lesions mimicking miliary dermatitis. Diagnosis of this condition must be confirmed by skin biopsy. Skin scrapings and fungal cultures will rule out other follicular diseases such as demodicosis and dermatophytosis. Bacterial organisms isolated from feline folliculitis include beta-hemolytic streptococci, coagulase-positive staphylococci, and *Pasteurella multocida*. Treatment consists of benzoyl peroxide (OxyDex, DVM; Pyoben, Allerderm) or chlorhexidine (Nolvasan, Fort Dodge) shampoos and systemic antibiotics (penicillin, amoxicillin, ampicillin, cephalexin, hetacillin) for at least 2 weeks, and 1 week beyond complete resolution of clinical lesions.

A pilot study was conducted to define the potential role of bacteria in the development or progression of miliary dermatitis. Quantitative studies showed that the skin (two sites) of four normal cats had a mean of 71 organisms/cm^2. From one lesion-free sample site (sample site matched with normal cats) on four cats with miliary dermatitis, there were 1548 organisms/cm^2 (mean), and from the sites with miliary dermatitis, 1,046,579 organisms/cm^2 (mean).

All of the organisms isolated from the normal and abnormal cats are listed in Table 1. In the normal cats, the organisms most frequently cultured were nonpathogenic species of *Bacillus* and *Micrococcus*. Coagulase-positive staphylococci were cultured from only one of eight sites on the normal cats and constituted only 31 per cent of the microflora present from that site. Pathogenic coagulase-positive staphylococci were present on 50 per cent of the lesion areas cultured and made up 99.5 per cent of the microflora when present. *Staphylococcus epidermidis* was present on 75 per cent of the lesion areas and made up 59 per cent of the flora.

Very low numbers of usually nonpathogenic organisms were found on the normal cat skin. The numbers were lower than the 329 organisms/cm^2 found on normal dogs (Ihrke et al., 1978) and may partially explain the low incidence of bacterial folliculitis seen in the cat. In the four cases studied, a definitive cause of the miliary dermatitis could not be found, and a true bacterial folliculitis was not demonstrated. However, significantly larger numbers of organisms were cultured per square centimeter, and pathogenic staphylococci were present on 50 per cent of the sites. Two of the four cats were completely cured of the miliary dermatitis lesions after 2 weeks on liquid cephalexin (Keflex, Dista; 22 mg/kg PO b.i.d.), and one cat was determined to be 50 per cent improved based on degree of pruritus and decrease in number of lesions. Many

Table 1. Incidence and Composition of Microflora

	Normal Cats (n = 8 Sites)		Cats With Miliary Dermatitis (n = 4)			
			Lateral Thorax		Lesion Areas	
Microbial Groups	*% Incidence*	*% of Flora**	*% Incidence*	*% of Flora**	*% Incidence*	*% of Flora**
Coagulase-positive staphylococci	13	31	0	0	50	99.50
Staphylococcus epidermidis	38	25	50	63	75	59.00
Bacillus spp.	88	41	50	63	25	0.10
Micrococcus spp.	75	28	0	0	25	25.00
Corynebacterium spp.	38	20	0	0	0	0.00
Alpha-hemolytic streptococci	25	51	0	0	0	0.00
Gram-negative rods	38	19	0	0	0	0.00
Gram-positive branching rods	25	6	25	50	0	0.00

*When present

This work was completed by the author and by Susan E. Anderson, D.V.M., while she was a senior student at the University of Florida College of Veterinary Medicine.

more cases need to be evaluated to determine if the coagulase-positive staphylococci represent true secondary pathogens, such as in canine seborrhea, or simply harmless colonizers. The bacteria may not be a primary cause of the development of miliary dermatitis but could be significant enough to warrant appropriate antibiotic therapy as part of the total treatment regimen, especially in cats that are nonresponsive to or intolerant of steroids or megestrol acetate.

Miscellaneous and Idiopathic Causes

Although experimental biotin deficiency has resulted in symptoms of miliary dermatitis, this is not a concern for cats on well-balanced commercial diets. Animals on home-cooked diets should be supplemented with vitamins, minerals, fatty acids, and taurine. Malassimilation or hepatic disease may manifest cutaneous signs associated with nutritional deficiencies or imbalances, but other more serious systemic signs would also be expected.

The early vesicopustular lesions associated with pemphigus foliaceus may mimic miliary dermatitis. However, by the time the cat is presented for examination, the condition has usually progressed to a diffuse crusting dermatitis with severe hyperkeratosis and footpad involvement. Hormonal abnormalities do not have a well-documented relationship to feline miliary dermatitis and thus are not considered in the list of differentials.

DIAGNOSTIC PLAN

The task of formulating a logical diagnostic plan seems at first difficult because of the many possible causes. With appropriate alterations based on the individual animal's clinical history, response to previous therapy, and distribution of lesions, the author has found the following problem-solving approach effective in eliminating within two or three office visits virtually all of the potential causes discussed in this chapter.

At the initial visit, a complete history is taken. If the diet is not complete and balanced, appropriate alterations are made. Any medications that are not absolutely essential for the animal's health are withdrawn. A thorough physical examination is performed, with a diligent search for ectoparasites on the skin surface, coat, and external ear canals (otoscopic examination). Skin scrapings, Wood's light examination, potassium hydroxide (KOH) preps of hairs for fungi, a dermatophyte culture, a fecal smear and flotation test, and ear swabs for cytologic testing and direct examination in mineral oil (if indicated) are performed. If excessive scaling is also present, cellophane tape preps and combings are used to search further for *Cheyletiella* organisms. If fleas or flea debris is seen or if pruritus and history make ectoparasites a strong consideration, then a topical and environmental flea control program is prescribed for 4 weeks, with re-evaluation at that time.

If there is no positive response after 1 month on the parasiticidal treatment program and if the fungal culture is negative, then biopsies are taken, intradermal allergy testing performed, a complete blood count (CBC) evaluated, and another fecal sample submitted. If allergy testing and fecal examination are negative, then a 3-week food-elimination diet is instituted.

A high eosinophil count on the CBC would be most indicative of a parasitic problem and would warrant further investigation for ectoparasites and endoparasites. In rare instances, the author has encountered a peripheral eosinophilia with allergic causes and idiopathic miliary dermatitis.

In most cases, the histopathologic findings are nondiagnostic but help eliminate many possible causes. Large numbers of eosinophils suggest a parasitic cause. Folliculitis and perifolliculitis are indicative of a bacterial disease, dermatophytosis, and demodicosis.

If all of the above procedures fail to establish a

diagnosis, the author may still try a 2- to 3-week course of systemic antibiotics to determine the importance of the bacteria as secondary pathogens. Confinement in a totally different environment for 2 to 3 weeks may be useful to rule out an undefined inhalant or contact allergy as the cause.

This prolonged course of investigation requires a very patient and dedicated owner. However, if no underlying cause has been found, owners should be satisfied with the diagnosis of idiopathic miliary dermatitis, knowing that all diagnostic possibilities have been exhausted.

Treatment of Idiopathic Disease

Megestrol acetate (Ovaban, Schering; Megace, Mead Johnson) has been the most effective drug for achieving clinical remission and long-term control in idiopathic feline miliary dermatitis. Clinical remission is achieved with an oral dose of 2.5 to 5 mg per cat once every other day, followed by weekly maintenance doses. Lifetime maintenance therapy is usually needed. *Megestrol acetate is not licensed for use in cats,* and alarming clinical and experimental side effects are being reported with greater frequency. Some of the reported abnormalities are so serious that the author will only use progestational compounds in severe cases of miliary dermatitis when other drugs (glucocorticoids, antibiotics, antihistamines) have failed to produce adequate control. All potential side effects are fully explained to the owner, frequent rechecks are scheduled during therapy, and the drug is never used more often than once a week at a 2.5-mg total dose.* Progestational compounds are extensively reviewed by Kunkle elsewhere in this section.

Glucocorticoids do not usually control idiopathic miliary dermatitis as well as does megestrol acetate. However, corticosteroids are usually well tolerated in cats and are, therefore, used first. Methylprednisolone acetate (Depo-Medrol, Upjohn) is given SC at a dosage of 5 mg/kg. If a favorable response is noted, the same dosage is repeated twice more at 2- to 3-week intervals. In some cases, long-term maintenance may be achieved with an injection every 8 weeks, but the drug should not be administered any more often than this.

Prednisone or prednisolone may also be tried at 1 to 2 mg/kg PO every 12 hours for 5 to 7 days, followed by a gradual decrease in dosage to an alternate-day maintenance level of 1 to 2 mg/kg. Unfortunately, keeping cats with this disease asymptomatic on alternate-day prednisone or prednisolone therapy is rare. Usually, daily doses of 1 to 2 mg/kg are needed to maintain remission. Miller (1984) switched some cats from 10 mg of prednisone or prednisolone per day to 4 mg of methylprednisolone (Medrol, Upjohn) per day and still maintained remission of miliary dermatitis lesions. This minimized the undesirable side effects of polydipsia, polyuria, and polyphagia. However, the tablet size (1 mg) of the veterinary product makes administration difficult, and the human formulation (4 mg) is expensive.

Dexamethasone is another alternative for treatment. This drug is efficacious in some cases when used at 1 mg total dose PO once a day for 7 days, followed by maintenance therapy at 1 mg twice a week. In cases in which neither glucocorticoids nor progestational compounds at "safe" dosages are controlling the condition, a combination of the two drugs may prove beneficial.

Another drug worthy of consideration is the antihistamine chlorpheniramine, used at 2 mg total dose PO every 12 hours. Chlorpheniramine used with glucocorticoids should also be considered in treatment of refractory cases.

**Editor's Note:* Signing of owner release forms is strongly advised before this drug is used.

References and Supplemental Reading

Bledsoe, W., Fadok, V. A., and Bledsoe, M. E.: Current therapy and new developments in indoor flea control. J. Am. Anim. Hosp. Assoc. 18:415, 1982.

Halliwell, R. E. W.: Flea allergy dermatitis. *In* Kirk, R. W. (ed.): *Current Veterinary Therapy VIII.* Philadelphia: W. B. Saunders, 1983, pp. 496–499.

Ihrke, P. J., Schwartzman, R. M., McGinley, K., et al.: Microbiology of normal and seborrheic canine skin. Am. J. Vet. Res. 39:1487, 1978.

Ihrke, P. J., Reinke, S. I., Rosser, E. J., Jr., et al.: The skin. *In* Pratt, P. W. (ed.): *Feline Medicine,* 1st ed. Santa Barbara, CA: American Veterinary Publications, Inc., 1983, pp. 555–602.

Kunkle, G. A.: Feline miliary dermatitis. Carnation Research Digest 18:1, Spring, 1982.

Kunkle, G. A., and Milcarsky, J.: Double-blind flea hyposensitization trial in cats. J.A.V.M.A. 186:677, 1985.

MacDonald, J. M.: Ectoparasites. *In* Kirk, R. W. (ed.): *Current Veterinary Therapy VIII.* Philadelphia: W. B. Saunders, 1983, pp. 488–495.

Miller, W.: Personal communication, 1984.

Morris, M. L., Jr.: Index of dietetic management. *In* Kirk, R. W. (ed.): *Current Veterinary Therapy VI.* Philadelphia: W. B. Saunders, 1977, pp. 59–73.

Muller, G. H., Kirk, R. W., and Scott, D. W.: *Small Animal Dermatology,* 3rd ed. Philadelphia: W. B. Saunders, 1983.

O'Neill, C. S.: Feline dermatophytosis (Part I). Carnation Research Digest 18:1, Fall, 1982a.

O'Neill, C. S.: Feline dermatophytosis (Part II). Carnation Research Digest 18:6, Winter, 1982b.

Reedy, L. M.: Feline miliary dermatitis with emphasis on dermatomycosis. Comp. Cont. Ed. Small Anim. Pract. 2:833, 1980.

Reedy, L. M.: Results of allergy testing and hyposensitization in selected feline skin diseases. J. Am. Anim. Hosp. Assoc. 18:618, 1982.

Scott, D. W.: Feline dermatology 1900–1978: A monograph. J. Am. Anim. Hosp. Assoc. 16:409, 1980.

Scott, D. W.: Feline dermatology 1979–1982: Introspective retrospections. J. Am. Anim. Hosp. Assoc. 20:537, 1984.

Willemse, T.: Crusting dermatoses in cats. *In* Kirk, R. W. (ed.): *Current Veterinary Therapy VII.* Philadelphia: W. B. Saunders, 1980, pp. 469–472.

DIFFERENTIAL DIAGNOSIS OF SYMMETRIC ALOPECIA IN THE CAT

KEITH L. THODAY, B. VET. MED.
Edinburgh, Scotland

Alopecia may be simply defined as total or partial loss of hair. Although alopecia may be classified according to a number of criteria such as degree (complete or partial) or duration (permanent or transient), the most useful diagnostic feature is the distribution of hair loss. Thus, alopecia may be generalized, regional, or localized, and each of these aspects may either be symmetric or asymmetric.

Alopecia accompanies many feline skin diseases irrespective of origin. Those that cause pruritus usually result in macroscopic skin changes and asymmetric hair loss and will not be dealt with here. It is the aim of this article to discuss those conditions that result in symmetric alopecia and are accompanied by little or no pruritus and minimal skin reaction (Table 1). Cats are far less frequently presented to veterinarians than dogs with a symmetric pattern of hair loss, largely because the associated endocrine disturbances appear to occur less commonly or are, perhaps, less well recognized.

Hair replacement in cats occurs in a mosaic pattern, and adjacent follicles are at different stages of hair growth. The process appears to be governed mainly by the photoperiod and, to a much lesser degree, by temperature. Thus, where day length tends to be reasonably constant (e.g., in the tropics) or in the artificial light of the home, a small amount of hair loss is constant but waves of shedding are not common. In outdoor cats in colder environments, excessive physiologic shedding may result in transient coat thinning.

INVESTIGATING ALOPECIA

As with all cases of dermatologic disorders, investigation into bilaterally symmetric feline alopecia should begin with a thorough history and physical examination, comprehensive details of which are beyond the scope of this article. However, certain

The investigations into thyroid function discussed in this article were supported by grants from the British Small Animal Veterinary Association Clinical Studies Trust Fund.

Table 1. *The Differential Diagnosis of Symmetric Alopecia in the Cat According to Distribution of Hair Loss*

	Regional		**Localized**		
Generalized	***Perineum, Genital Area, Hind Legs, Ventrum, Lateral Abdomen, Distal Forelegs***	***Pinnae***	***Temporal Region***	***Mandible***	***Miscellaneous***
Alopecia universalis Hypotrichosis	Feline endocrine alopecia Flea infestation	Scar tissue: Feline solar dermatitis Frostbite	Preauricular partial alopecia	Acne	Stud tail Linear granuloma
Telogen defluxion	Telogen defluxion				Collar frictional alopecia
Systemic disease	Psychogenic alopecia and dermatitis				
Dermatophytosis	Dermatophytosis	Dermatophytosis	Dermatophytosis		
Demodicosis	Demodicosis	Demodicosis	Demodicosis	Demodicosis	
Hyperadrenocorticism	Diabetes mellitus Estrus	Experimentally produced hypothyroidism			

observations are of particular importance. Initially, the clinician must determine the degree of alopecia in relation to normal individual variations. The regional density of hair varies between animals, particularly in the preauricular, axillary, abdominal, and inguinal areas. The history that the owner gives is helpful in deciding whether a thin coat in these regions is clinically significant.

It is important to note the degree of hair loss and whether hairs appear to have been epilated or are broken. The stage of hair growth should be assessed by gently plucking hairs in affected and nonaffected areas. Generally, telogen (resting) hairs epilate much more easily than those in anagen (active growth). Epilated hairs should be examined microscopically after mounting in mineral oil. Hair that has been bitten has a straight or slightly angled end to the shaft. Telogen hairs show a club root with no root sheaths and a keratinized sac, whereas those in anagen show a larger, expanded, moist, glistening root, which is often pigmented and is surrounded by a root sheath. At present, the assessment of telogen-anagen ratios by microscopic examination of 100 to 200 hairs as suggested by some authors is of minimal value in practice.

A large number of laboratory and other diagnostic tests may need to be carried out in cases of feline alopecia, depending on the suspected cause, but it is essential to check for ectoparasites and dermatophytes in every case. Fleas or their feces may be seen on macroscopic examination or by brushing the coat onto a light-colored surface after spraying with a suitable "invisible" parasiticide. Feces can be simply distinguished from pieces of grit by the reddish-brown halo of blood that forms around them when placed on moist cotton or filter paper. Although deep skin scrapings should always be taken, *Demodex* species on cats occur more superficially than their canine counterparts; mites are confined to the surface keratin or the hair follicle infundibulae.

Dermatophytosis is confirmed by a combination of examination with ultraviolet light (Wood's lamp), direct microscopy, and fungal culture. At the author's clinic, approximately 60 per cent of cases of *Microsporum canis* fluoresce under ultraviolet light. A positive result is apple-green fluorescence of infected hairs. When present, such hairs should always be selected for further investigations. They should be plucked with epilation forceps, and scales and crusts removed with a blunt scalpel blade. In mild cases with minimal changes, a useful alternative is the MacKenzie brush technique. The coat should be brushed with a toothbrush sterilized for 30 minutes in 0.1 per cent chlorhexidine solution; accumulated material for direct microscopic examination is transferred by shaking it onto a slide, and material for culture is removed by shaking or gently pushing the bristles into the medium. Dermatophyte test medium is useful to practitioners, but because the typical colony pigmentation, a useful diagnostic feature, is masked by the medium's color indicator, it should always be used in conjunction with plain Sabouraud agar.

In addition to the tests mentioned, skin biopsy may be of great value in differentiating the causes of symmetric alopecia and will be discussed further as it applies to individual conditions.

GENERALIZED ALOPECIA

ALOPECIA UNIVERSALIS (SPHINX CAT, CANADIAN HAIRLESS CAT). Alopecia universalis is a rare, hereditary, congenital disorder that is bred for selectively by some cat fanciers; the "breeds" are termed *sphinx cats* or *Canadian hairless cats.* Affected animals show a complete absence of primary hairs, and secondary hairs are present only in certain areas, notably the face, tip of the tail, scrotum, and over the back. The skin is oily, has a rancid smell, and may be traumatized by the tongue barbs while grooming. Lipid material may build up under the nail folds.

Antiseborrheic baths such as 1 per cent selenium sulfide (Seleen, CEVA, Abbott) as necessary help to control the oiliness and odor, but nail-fold lipid deposits are best removed manually.

HYPOTRICHOSIS. Hereditary hypotrichosis with an autosomal recessive mode of inheritance has been recorded in Siamese cats. At birth, affected kittens have thin hair, which is lost within 2 weeks. By 10 weeks of age, there is some hair regrowth, but severe hair loss occurs again when these kittens are 6 months old.

The author has seen an adult female Devon rex cat that had bilaterally symmetric trunk hypotrichosis. When it mated with an unrelated Devon rex, five kittens born to it were similarly affected; but when crossed with a Burmese, all progeny had normal coats. The mode of inheritance was not determined (Thoday, 1981b). Hypotrichosis has also been reported in a Mexican breed of cat. No treatment is available for the condition.

TELOGEN DEFLUXION (TELOGEN EFFLUVIUM, TELOGEN DEFLUVIUM). The terms *telogen defluxion, telogen effluvium,* and *telogen defluvium* are used synonymously to denote a state in which the anagen phase of the hair cycle is shortened, resulting in large numbers of hairs entering the resting phase synchronously. Telogen defluxion occurs at times of physiologic stress such as gestation or lactation, in numerous disease states, and with certain drug treatments. Affected hairs are easily epilated both by friction and by normal grooming. The resulting alopecia may be generalized or localized and, particularly when due to environmental friction, tends to be bilaterally symmetric. Specific treatment for telogen defluxion is not required.

SYSTEMIC DISEASE. Diffuse hair loss, mainly affecting the trunk, may be associated with a number of systemic diseases, notably end-stage kidney disease and chronic hepatic conditions. Seborrhea sicca and mild pruritus may also occur. Treatment is directed toward relieving the underlying disease.

DERMATOPHYTOSIS. The physical signs of dermatophytosis in cats are variable and depend on breed, individual susceptibility, and the causal organism. Although many species of dermatophytes have been isolated from cats, in the United Kingdom, 98 per cent of cases are caused by the zoophilic fungus *M. canis*. This is also reported to be the most common isolate in the United States. Cats are probably the natural hosts of this organism. Although the whole myriad of changes associated with feline dermatophytosis may be seen, infection may result in few signs despite widespread involvement. Thus, an asymptomatic carrier state and widespread, diffuse alopecia with small numbers of fractured hairs and mild hyperplasia of the stratum corneum may be the only indications of infection. *Trichophyton mentagrophytes* has zoophilic and anthropophilic forms. The zoophilic form commonly infects rodents, which in turn become potential sources of infection for cats. *T. mentagrophytes* tends to produce a more severe, inflammatory skin reaction than does *M. canis*. *Microsporum gypseum* is a geophilic dermatophyte reported to cause approximately 1 per cent of all cases of dermatophytosis in cats in the United States. Thick, well-circumscribed, tightly adherent, gray crusts are described as typical lesions, but the author has never isolated this organism from a case of feline dermatophytosis in the United Kingdom.

Feline *M. canis* infection may be a self-limiting disease, but, irrespective of other therapy, all cases should have total body clips. The fungistatic antibiotic griseofulvin should be used in all chronic or severe cases at a dose of 80 to 130 mg/kg once daily. This dose is in excess of that recommended by the manufacturers but is more appropriate in the absence of specific metabolism tests in cats (Scott, 1980). A fatty meal enhances the drug's absorption and 2.5 to 5 ml of corn oil is effective and readily taken by cats. Topical treatment is of less value in cats than in humans. Captan and lime sulfur, reportedly very effective in the United States, are not available in the United Kingdom. If necessary, the author uses povidone-iodine washes at weekly intervals. Animals should be reclipped after 1 month and treatment continued until signs of infection have disappeared and cultures are negative.

DEMODICOSIS. Demodicosis, due to infestation by the mite *Demodex cati* and also to a recently described but as yet unnamed species, is a rare but increasingly recognized disease. Pathogenesis is assumed to be similar to that in dogs, and cases in adult cats have been associated with serious systemic disease (leukemia virus infection, diabetes mellitus). Regional symmetric alopecia with minimal skin changes has been described (see below), but the disease can be generalized.

Because so few cases of feline demodicosis have been described, treatment is currently empiric. Presumably because of the often superficial location of feline demodicids, successful therapy has been reported with such simple regimens as weekly pyrethrin-carbamate shampoos and weekly malathion or lime-sulfur dips. In generalized demodicosis in dogs in the United Kingdom, a combination of total body clips, 0.75 per cent rotenone in surgical spirit (Cooper Demodectic Mange Dressing [Concentrate], Wellcome*) applied to one third of the body daily with gauze or cotton swabs, and weekly baths in 1 per cent selenium sulfide has been found to be very successful and warrants a trial in cats. Any underlying accompanying immunosuppressive disease should be identified and treated when possible.

HYPERADRENOCORTICISM (CUSHING'S DISEASE, CUSHING'S SYNDROME). Naturally occurring hyperadrenocorticism is very rare in cats, but cases have been reported to be caused by bilateral adrenocortical hyperplasia (pituitary not examined) and unilateral adrenocortical adenoma. Clinical signs have included polyuria, polydipsia, polyphagia, lethargy, and a pendulous abdomen. The skin may be thin, hypotonic, easily torn, scaly, and hyperpigmented. Varying degrees of hair loss may occur, and in one case this progressed to generalized, bilaterally symmetric alopecia sparing only the head and distal extremities.

Iatrogenic hyperadrenocorticism resulting from long-term glucocorticoid administration has been seen by the author. The systemic signs described above were present, but there were no skin changes. Scott (1984) mentioned three cases associated with megestrol acetate therapy. Cases have also been produced experimentally, albeit with some difficulty, but bilaterally symmetric alopecia was not a feature.

Treatment of the naturally occurring disease by unilateral adrenalectomy has been successful. Medical therapy using *o,p'*-DDD (mitotane; Lysodren, Calbiochem) could pose problems, as cats do not tolerate most chlorinated hydrocarbons.

Differential Diagnosis

In general, the differential diagnosis of the generalized bilaterally symmetric alopecias poses few problems. It is based on history, physical examination, Wood's light examination, microscopic exami-

*This product is not available in the United States.

nation of hair samples and skin scrapings, fungal culture, complete blood count, standard biochemical tests including plasma cortisol responses to stimulation with adrenocorticotropic hormone (ACTH) or its synthetic analogue tetracosactrin (Cortrosyn, Organon) and to suppression with dexamethasone, and skin biopsy.

Alopecia universalis and hypotrichosis are present at or shortly after birth. In alopecia universalis, the remaining hairs lack a properly formed bulb and are easily epilated. On histologic examination, the epidermis is thickened, sebaceous and apocrine glands open directly to the skin surface, and the dermis is normal. In hypotrichosis, hair follicles are small and reduced in number, and many are in telogen with or without hair. In both telogen defluxion and alopecia due to systemic disease, the history is suggestive of the cause and, in this type of alopecia, standard laboratory tests confirm the diagnosis.

Dermatophytosis and demodicosis are diagnosed as discussed previously. In demodicosis, if mites are in hair follicles, histologic examination demonstrates varying degrees of folliculitis and perifolliculitis. If they are in the epidermis, there is a mild superficial perivascular dermatitis, and mites are found in the surface keratin. Reported laboratory abnormalities in naturally occurring and iatrogenic hyperadrenocorticism include leukocytosis, neutrophilia, lymphopenia, eosinopenia, hyperglycemia, elevated alanine aminotransferase and aspartate aminotranferase, hypercholesterolemia, and glucosuria. Response to stimulation with ACTH supported the diagnosis in two naturally occurring cases (excessive response) but was variable in iatrogenic cases (reduced to normal response). A dexamethasone suppression test was diagnostic in one naturally occurring case (minimal response). Histologic examination of affected skin has revealed orthokeratotic hyperkeratosis, epidermal atrophy, follicular keratosis and atrophy, sebaceous atrophy, dermal thinning and atrophy, and telangiectasis of dermal and subcuticular blood vessels.

REGIONAL ALOPECIA

The Perineum, Genital Area, Hind Legs, Ventrum, Lateral Abdomen, and Distal Forelegs

Alopecia with this distribution is commonly encountered in cats and is often diagnosed as feline endocrine alopecia (FEA), but a number of causes are recognized. The author has carried out a study of 51 cats referred to him with a tentative diagnosis of FEA. After a detailed history and physical examination, all animals were subjected to serum cholesterol, total serum thyroxine (T_4) and triiodothyronine (T_3) estimations, skin scrapings for ectoparasites and dermatophytes, fungal culture, fecal examination for ectoparasites, and (in 41 animals) a complete blood count. The final diagnoses are given in Table 2. Cases of pediculosis and mastocytosis did not show this precise distribution of alopecia and should be disregarded. Other disorders that may have similar presenting signs not represented in this study include demodicosis, diabetes mellitus, and alopecia arising during estrus.

***Table 2.** Final Diagnosis in 51* Cats Referred as Suspected Cases of Feline Endocrine Alopecia*

Diagnosis	Number of Cases
Feline endocrine alopecia	26
Flea infestation	9
Probable flea infestation (fleas not seen but responded to parasiticidal therapy)	10
Miliary dermatitis with eosinophilia (? fleas—no follow-up)	1
Telogen defluxion	2
Psychogenic alopecia and dermatitis	1
Pediculosis	1
Mastocytosis	1
Undiagnosed (no follow-up)	1

*One cat had telogen defluxion and fleas.

FELINE ENDOCRINE ALOPECIA. FEA remains a disease of unknown cause and is presumed to be due to hormonal deficiency or imbalance, as there is good response to various hormonal therapies. The condition usually affects males and females at varying intervals after neutering. However, because most cats seen at veterinary clinics are neutered, this predisposition may be apparent rather than real. Indeed, Kirk (1980) reported an even distribution between entire and desexed individuals. Scott (1975) stated that 90 per cent of his cases were neutered males, but this has not been the author's experience. Case data are presented in Table 3.

The condition is bilaterally symmetric and usually begins over the perineum, the genital area, the base of the tail, the posterior or medial thighs, or the ventral abdomen. In addition, the forelegs (elbow to carpus) are commonly affected, sometimes early in the condition. In long-standing cases, hair is lost over the ventral two thirds of the lateral abdomen and less commonly the thorax, but the dorsum is always spared. In most cases, the skin is otherwise macroscopically normal and there is no

***Table 3.** Data on 26 Cases of Feline Endocrine Alopecia*

Breed	Domestic short-hair	24
	Persian cross	1
	Burmese cross	1
Sex	Neutered females	15 (57.7%)
	Neutered males	10 (38.5%)
	Entire male	1 (3.8%)
Age at onset	1 year to 11 years	Mean 4.5 years

pruritus, but occasionally there may be areas of erythema and mild to moderate irritation.

A number of reports state that affected animals are not hypothyroid, but only one author has presented data (Scott, 1975). In the present series, a number of physical and laboratory criteria that might indicate possible hypothyroidism were studied. Serum total T_4 and T_3 concentrations were measured by double antibody radioimmunoassays optimized and validated for cat serum as described previously (Thoday et al., 1984). These data are presented in Table 4. Although some results lie outside the normal ranges, in no single case are abnormal values found for a number of criteria.

Further investigations were carried out into the thyroid status of six cats with FEA by using the thyrotropin (TSH) stimulation test. For this test, a blood sample was taken between 9 and 10 AM, 0.5 IU/kg TSH (Thytropar, Armour) was administered IV, and a second sample was taken 6 hours later. Serum total T_4 and T_3 values were determined, and the results were compared with those obtained from 16 healthy animals using the Mann-Whitney U Test. For T_4, FEA cats had significantly lower values than the healthy cats for the post-TSH concentration ($p < 0.01$) and the absolute increase at 6 hours ($p < 0.05$), but the ratio of post-TSH T_4 concentration to pre-TSH T_4 concentration, a commonly used index of TSH stimulation in dogs, was not significantly different. For T_3, none of these values was significantly different between the two groups. These results suggest that some cats with FEA may have low functional thyroid reserve, but the results need to be substantiated by a larger number of observations.

FEA will respond variably to a number of therapeutic regimens. In the study described, all cases were treated with liothyronine sodium (T_3, Tertroxin, Glaxo) at an initial dose of 20 μg/cat twice daily; this dose was increased by 10 μg twice daily every third day to a maximum of 50 μg twice daily. In 19 cases (73 per cent), there was total hair regrowth within 12 weeks. The response to therapy was markedly reduced with lower dosages. No cat showed signs of thyrotoxicosis, although one developed a systolic cardiac murmur, which resolved completely when therapy was discontinued. Four cases (15 per cent) showed partial hair regrowth, and three cases (12 per cent) did not improve. Thus, the regimen is highly effective and safer than other possible treatments. These include the progestogen megestrol acetate (Ovaban, Schering; Megace, Mead Johnson Pharmaceutical) at a dose of 5 mg every second to third day and oral, depot-injectable or implanted testosterone. With all regimens, a low maintenance dosage (e.g., 30 μg T_3 b.i.d. or 2.5 mg megestrol acetate once or twice weekly) or intermittent higher dosages as described above may be required to maintain normality. Progestational compounds are not approved for use in cats in the United States.

FLEA INFESTATION AND PROBABLE FLEA INFESTATION. Flea infestation without observable pruritus may result in symmetric alopecia and must be carefully ruled out as the cause of FEA. In this study, nine cats with a tentative diagnosis of FEA were found to have fleas or their feces on examination and responded within 6 weeks to weekly sprays with a combination of dichlorvos and fenitrothion (Nuvan Top, Ciba-Geigy) and environmental flea control. In addition, 10 cats without macroscopic evidence of flea infestation responded fully to the same therapy. Of these, nine had high normal (greater than 1.1 × 10^9/L) or elevated (greater than 1.5 × 10^9/L) circulating eosinophil counts. As all were negative for ectoparasites on skin scrapings and for endoparasites on fecal examination and as neither dichlorvos nor fenitrothion has known stimulatory action on hair growth, it was concluded that their dermatoses were associated with flea infesta-

Table 4. *Comparison of Various Criteria of Thyroid Function for Healthy Cats and Cats with Feline Endocrine Alopecia*

Measurement	Normal Range	Range in FEA Cases	Possible Response in Hypothyroidism
Heart rate (per minute)	160–240	144–218	↓
Temperature (°C)	38–39	37.4–39.5	↓
T_4 (nmol/L)	8.5–46.2	7.3–59.8	↓
T_3 (nmol/L)	0.13–1.27	0.16–1.13	↓
Cholesterol (mmol/L)	2.10–6.65	2.49–9.65	↑
Red blood cells (× 10^{12}/L)	5.5–10.0	7.8–10.0	↓
Packed cell volume (L/L)	0.24–0.45	0.34–0.48	↓
Erythrocyte sedimentation rate (mm/hour)	4–13	0–24	↑
Reticulocytes (%)	0.2–1.6	0–13	↓

Normal hematologic and biochemical values from the Clinical Laboratory, Department of Veterinary Medicine, University of Edinburgh, Royal (Dick) School of Veterinary Studies.

Normal T_4 and T_3 values from Thoday et al.: J. Small Anim. Pract. 25:457, 1984.

tion. One animal had miliary dermatitis with eosinophilia. This was diagnosed as probable flea infestation but was lost to follow-up.

TELOGEN DEFLUXION. There were two cases of telogen defluxion, both occurring postpartum.

PSYCHOGENIC ALOPECIA AND DERMATITIS. Psychogenic alopecia with dermatitis is a condition attributed to stress and characterized by excessive licking or hair pulling. "High-strung" breeds such as the Siamese, Abyssinian, and Burmese are most commonly affected. In the author's experience, this condition is uncommon. Details in many reports suggest that the primary or initiating cause was a pruritic or painful lesion such as infected ears or impacted anal sacs, which would make a diagnosis of psychogenic alopecia and dermatitis unlikely. However, occasional cases have been seen in which stress appears to have precipitated the condition. Such stressful events include effects on an animal in a multicat household, disturbances of an excessive pair bond between animal and owner, moving to a new home, or the arrival of a new baby.

The site is usually an area that the cat can lick easily, such as the dorsal lumbar area, tail, medial thighs, and ventral abdomen. Lesions may consist of partial alopecia with or without single or multiple well-demarcated areas of erythema, moist erosions, or ulcerations. In Siamese cats, in which coat color is temperature-dependent, hair may regrow a darker color. In the series described, one animal was shown to have psychogenic alopecia and dermatitis.

Treatment should be directed at determining and, when possible, removing the cause of the anxiety. Oral diazepam (Valium, Roche) at a dose of 1 to 2 mg per cat twice daily is usually effective in controlling the condition. Rarely, oral phenobarbital (2.2 to 6.6 mg/kg b.i.d.), alone or in combination with diazepam, or megestrol acetate (up to 5 mg every second day) may be required. In each case, the drug dosage should be tapered to the minimum when the precipitating cause cannot be identified or removed.

OTHER CONDITIONS. A number of other conditions, not represented in the author's study, may present with lesions similar to FEA.

Dermatophytosis. Dermatophytosis may be localized to the perineum, genital area, hind legs, ventrum, lateral abdomen, and distal forelegs.

Demodicosis. Scott (1984) has reported that feline demodicosis may present with a distribution and appearance identical to FEA. The clinical signs are mild and may consist simply of alopecia with or without broken hairs.

Diabetes Mellitus. Diabetes mellitus that developed during therapy with megestrol acetate is reported to have resulted in ventral midline alopecia in two cats. Both showed accompanying mild seborrhea sicca, and one had bilateral pinnal alopecia.

Table 5. *Data Comparing the Absolute Eosinophil Counts in 41 Cats Referred with a Tentative Diagnosis of Feline Endocrine Alopecia*

Final Diagnosis	Eosinophil Count (× 10^9/L) Median and Range
Feline endocrine alopecia (n = 17)	0.568 (0.127–1.700)
Nonfeline endocrine alopecia (n = 24)	1.365 (0.180–14.196)

Normal range = 0–1.500 × 10^9/L; Mean* = 0.650 × 10^9/L

*From Schalm, O. W., Jain, N. C., and Carroll, E. J.: Veterinary Haematology, 3rd ed. Philadelphia: Lea & Febiger, 1975, p. 109.

Note: For conversion, × 10^9/L = × 10^6/ml

Estrus. Blakemore (cited in Kirk, 1980) reported that cats in estrus tend to shed easily, particularly in the groin. It is likely that this is merely a manifestation of telogen defluxion.

Differential Diagnosis

Differential diagnosis is based on history, physical examination, Wood's lamp examination, microscopic examination of hair samples and skin scrapings, fungal culture, a complete blood count, standard biochemical tests, and the histologic examination of skin biopsies. It is possible that radioimmunoassay of T_4 and T_3 before and after TSH stimulation may be helpful in the future.

Psychogenic alopecia differs from both FEA and telogen defluxion in that the remaining hairs in affected areas do not epilate easily, reflecting the anagen rather than telogen phase, and hairs appear broken when examined macro- and microscopically. Skin biopsy in psychogenic alopecia again shows hairs in anagen, whereas in FEA and telogen defluxion, most follicles are in telogen and lack hairs.

Although there is yet no specific diagnostic test for FEA, in many cases it may be differentiated from clinically similar conditions by a total eosinophil count. Data comparing the total eosinophil counts of 17 cases of FEA with those of 24 cases referred originally as FEA but with alternative final diagnosis are presented in Table 5. The predictive value of the absolute eosinophil count in differentiating FEA from clinically similar conditions is shown in Table 6. Results suggest that this single laboratory test should be carried out routinely on all animals presented with this distribution of alopecia and that in the absence of a definitive alternative diagnosis, all cases warrant a 3- to 6-week trial with a suitable parasiticide to rule out flea infestation prior to therapy for FEA. This is of particular diagnostic importance, as flea-induced lesions may respond to progestogen therapy without attempts at flea control, suggesting incorrectly that the problem is of endocrine origin.

***Table 6.** Predictive Value of the Absolute Eosinophil Count in Differentiating Feline Endocrine Alopecia from Clinically Similar Conditions (From a Study of 41 Cases)*

Absolute Eosinophil Count (× 10^9/L)	Cases		
	FEA	*Non-FEA*	*Total*
> 1.500	1	11	12
< 1.500	16	13	29
Total	17	24	41

Conclusions: Assuming that the prevalence of FEA and clinically similar non-FEA conditions in this study is the same as in the general population,

1. A raised count (>1.500 × 10^9/L) has a 92 per cent predictive value in ruling out FEA.
2. A normal count (<1.500 × 10^9/L) has a 55 per cent predictive value in indicating FEA.

LOCALIZED ALOPECIA

THE PINNAE

SCAR TISSUE. Both ultraviolet radiation and cold may result in bilaterally symmetric alopecia due to scarring.

Feline Solar Dermatitis (Actinic Dermatitis). Feline solar dermatitis is a chronic inflammation of the pinnae and, less commonly, the eyelids and nasal skin of white or partially white cats. Blue-eyed white cats appear to be most commonly affected. Solar dermatitis results from repeated sunburn and damage by ultraviolet light of 3000-nm wavelength and thus is most common in sunny climates. A recent study failed to demonstrate a relationship between the condition and erythropoietic protoporphyria (Irving et al., 1982). Early cases may be seen in young cats, and lesions tend to increase in severity each year. In the acute phase, there is hyperemia, scaling, crusting, and pain, and hair follicles are damaged or destroyed. Initially, lesions heal during the winter months, but, if cases are presented at this stage, the skin is thin and shiny with bilaterally symmetric alopecia. Subsequently, the cartilage may be damaged, causing the pinnae to curl at the edges.

Standard treatments cannot reverse the existing changes and must be directed at preventing progression. Affected animals should be kept out of sunlight from 10 AM to 4 PM and the ears protected with a sunscreen containing para-aminobenzoic acid. Once early lesions have developed, amputation of the poorly protected ends of the pinnae is the most reliable form of treatment and is cosmetically quite acceptable. Recently, an oral combination of β-carotene and canthaxanthin (25 mg active carotenoids) was effective in treating the early stages of the condition and preventing recurrence on reexposure to sunlight (Irving et al., 1982).

Frostbite. Frostbite is a relatively rare condition in cats; however, in extreme conditions or where animals have moved to a cold climate without time to acclimatize, the tips of the ears and the tail (areas where hair covering is sparse and blood supply may be compromised) are at risk.

In the acute phase, the affected tissue is cool, pale, and hypoesthetic but becomes reddened and painful as it thaws. Recovered tissue may show variable degrees of alopecia and scarring and tends to be more susceptible to further cold damage. Amputation of affected areas may be considered to prevent recurrence.

DERMATOPHYTOSIS. Dermatophytosis localized to the pinnae may be encountered.

DEMODICOSIS. Demodicosis, initially localized to the pinnae, may occur.

EXPERIMENTALLY PRODUCED HYPOTHYROIDISM. Although there are numerous anecdotal reports of naturally occurring feline hypothyroidism, the author is aware of only two cases in which the diagnosis has been substantiated by thyroid hormone assays. Martin and Capen (1983) presented photographic evidence of an obese cat that failed to groom itself and in which the serum total T_4 and T_3 concentrations were markedly reduced. No further details were given. Arnold and colleagues (1984) reported a case of primary goitrous hypothyroidism and dwarfism in a 14-week-old kitten; this they attributed to a congenital defect in thyroid hormone biosynthesis. The cat showed numerous abnormalities including dullness, stunted growth, and an enlarged head with shortening of the forehead. Hair was present all over the body but consisted mainly of undercoat with primary hairs scattered throughout. The body temperature was normal, but there was a marked bradycardia. Radiographic investigation revealed almost complete absence of ossification centers of the long bones; there was a mild anemia, and serum total T_4 was undetectable before and after 3 days of TSH stimulation.

The author has never recognized naturally occurring feline hypothyroidism but has produced it experimentally by IV administration of 3 microcuries of ^{131}I to each of two cats. Thyroid ablation was confirmed by the demonstration of subnormal concentrations of total T_4 and T_3 and failure to show any increase in these hormones after TSH stimulation. In a 2½-year follow-up, the cats have shown variable lethargy and appetite, no increase in weight, shortening and broadening of the muzzle, normal heart rate, and a consistently low body temperature. There is a marked, nonpruritic seborrhea sicca, and the hair over the dorsum is matted because of failure to groom. Most of the hair has remained in anagen, hair removed by clipping in multiple sites has regrown, and there is no bilaterally symmetric alopecia with the exception of the pinnae. Both animals have hair loss over the lateral and medial distal halves of the pinnae, and the skin is covered with a thin, brownish-black crust, which can be removed with difficulty to leave shiny but dry epidermis. In the author's experience, such macroscopic changes are unique to hypothyroidism.

DIABETES MELLITUS. Bilateral pinnal alopecia, together with ventral midline alopecia and mild seborrhea sicca, has been reported in a cat that developed diabetes mellitus during therapy with megestrol acetate. After the progestogen was withdrawn and 8 months of insulin therapy was administered, both the diabetes mellitus and the skin condition resolved.

Differential Diagnosis

The diagnosis of bilaterally symmetric pinnal alopecia is based on history, physical examination, Wood's lamp examination, skin scrapings for ectoparasites and dermatophytes, fungal culture, routine biochemical tests, and biopsy. It is possible that cases of naturally occurring feline hypothyroidism are overlooked because they have been assumed to be similar clinically to the human or canine conditions. If experimentally produced and naturally occurring hypothyroidism are similar, then cats presenting as described above should have their serum total T_4 and T_3 concentrations measured, to be followed if necessary by a TSH stimulation test. Histologically, full-thickness pinna biopsies from the hypothyroid animals showed orthokeratotic hyperkeratosis, acanthosis, collagen fibers that were swollen and fragmented and had fewer nuclei, and increased dermal mucin (myxedema).

THE TEMPORAL REGION

PREAURICULAR PARTIAL ALOPECIA. Clinicians are frequently presented with cats that have only a thin covering of hair over the temporal region, between the eye and the ear. This preauricular partial alopecia is normal for these animals, and no treatment is warranted or effective.

DERMATOPHYTOSIS. Dermatophytosis may be localized to this region (see above).

DEMODICOSIS. Feline *Demodex* mites are more common on the head, and lesions as described previously may be localized to the temporal area.

Differential Diagnosis

Differential diagnosis of temporal alopecia is by Wood's lamp examination, skin scrapings for ectoparasites and dermatophytes, fungal culture, and by biopsy if necessary.

THE MANDIBLE

ACNE. Feline acne is a poorly understood condition with no breed, sex, or age predisposition. Suggested causes (for which little firm evidence appears to exist) include genetic predisposition, incorrect eating habits, or failure to clean the area. Acne is probably linked with abnormal function of the sebaceous glands in an area where their density is high.

Patients are presented with comedo formation on the chin and perilabial area, sometimes extending as far as the lip commissures. Mild, diffuse, symmetric alopecia is common. In most cases, there is no pruritus or pain, and the condition may remain static. Occasionally there may be secondary infection with edema, pustules, furuncles, and accompanying pain and self-inflicted trauma.

In most cases of feline acne, no treatment is required, although comedones may be expressed manually. In more severe cases, 50 to 100 per cent ethyl alcohol as a lipid solvent or keratolytic preparations (e.g. sulfur, selenium sulfide, benzoyl peroxide) can be helpful, but therapy may have to be continued indefinitely. In infected cases, the area should be clipped, the lesions evacuated, and systemic antibacterial agents administered.

In humans, the severity of acne is directly related to the rate of excretion of sebum and, if this result is causal, it follows that inhibition of sebum excretion rate should improve acne. While acknowledging the differences between human and feline acne, the author recently has used the vitamin A acid isotretinoin (Roaccutane, Roche) in one severe feline case and knows of its use in one other. At a dose of 5 mg once daily, a marked clinical improvement occurred by 12 weeks, and the dose was subsequently reduced to 5 mg every second day. Isotretinoin acts directly on the metabolism of the sebaceous cell, and, in humans, there are major differences in the components of sebaceous lipid after treatment. Unwanted effects of the drug in humans include desquamation, dryness of the lips, conjunctivitis, dose-related and reversible increases in serum cholesterol and triglyceride, and changes in indices of liver function. Isotretinoin is teratogenic in humans. No unwanted effects were seen in these cats, but the drug is not licensed for veterinary use in the United Kingdom or the United States.

DEMODICOSIS. Demodicosis occurring over the chin may closely resemble feline acnè, with bilaterally symmetric, sharply demarcated lesions of alopecia, scale, erythema, and sometimes hyperpigmentation.

Differential Diagnosis

The differential diagnosis of mandibular alopecia is by history, physical examination, skin scrapings, and biopsy. Histologic examination of feline acne reveals, in the early stages, follicular keratosis, plugging, and dilatation, and subsequently perifolliculitis, folliculitis, and furunculosis.

MISCELLANEOUS CONDITIONS

STUD TAIL. The dorsal surface of the tail of the cat, the so-called supracaudal organ, bears large numbers of sebaceous and apocrine glands. Stud tail is characterized by overproduction of secretions by these glands, resulting in the accumulation of a yellowish-gray, oily material, matting of hair, and variable degrees of alopecia. The condition is more common in entire males (hence its popular name) but also occurs in females and neuters. The cause is unknown, but it has been suggested that it is due to failure to groom in confined animals.

The lesions of stud tail are pathognomonic. Treatment, if required, is as for noninfected acne. The author has not used isotretinoin in this disorder. The effects of allowing the cat a greater degree of freedom should be evaluated. (See also article on progestagens, page 603.)

LINEAR GRANULOMA. Linear granuloma has been arbitrarily classified as a part of the eosinophilic granuloma complex, although whether these conditions are truly related is still uncertain. The cause of linear granuloma is unknown. The condition may occur at any site but is found most commonly over the posterior hind legs or as oral nodules. Skin lesions are well demarcated, raised and firm, yellow or yellowish-pink, and show varying degrees of alopecia. They are seen most commonly in young animals (6 months to 5 years) and are usually otherwise asymptomatic.

Diagnosis is based on history, physical examination, routine hematologic examination (a circulating eosinophilia usually occurs in the oral form), and examination of skin biopsies. Histologically, there is tissue eosinophilia in approximately 50 per cent of cases, together with granulomatous inflammation with marked collagen degeneration.

As linear granulomas are often asymptomatic, treatment may not be required and a gradual spontaneous regression may occur. Systemic glucocorticoids (e.g., 0.5 mg/kg prednisolone b.i.d. initially and reducing) are usually effective in producing a prompt and complete resolution.

COLLAR FRICTIONAL ALOPECIA. Alopecia as a result of simple friction between coat and collar is not uncommon in cats. The lesion and its causal relationship are striking. When the collar is moved, there is a well-demarcated area of often total alopecia in a complete circle and the skin is smooth and shiny. There is no inflammatory response, thereby simply differentiating the condition from flea collar dermatitis, which in the author's experience is extremely rare.

The lesion of collar frictional alopecia is pathognomonic for the condition. Removing the collar results in resolution.

References and Supplemental Reading

Arnold, U., Opitz M., Grosser, I., et al.: Goitrous hypothyroidism and dwarfism in a kitten. J. Am. Anim. Hosp. Assoc. 20:753, 1984.

Irving, R. A., Day, R. S. and Eales, L.: Porphyrin values and treatment of feline solar dermatitis. Am. J. Vet. Res. 43:2067, 1982.

Kirk, R. W.: Feline alopecias. In Kirk, R. W. (ed.): *Current Veterinary Therapy VII*. Philadelphia: W. B. Saunders, 1980, pp. 490–493.

Martin, S. L., and Capen, C. C.: The endocrine system. *In* Pratt, P. W. (ed.): *Feline Medicine*. Santa Barbara, CA: American Veterinary Publications, 1983, pp. 321–362.

Scott, D. W.: Thyroid function in feline endocrine alopecia. J. Am. Anim. Hosp. Assoc. 11:798, 1975.

Scott, D. W.: Feline dermatology 1900–1978: A monograph. J. Am. Anim. Hosp. Assoc. 16:331, 1980.

Scott, D. W.: Feline dermatology 1979–1982: Introspective retrospections. J. Am. Anim. Hosp. Assoc. 20:537, 1984.

Thoday, K. L.: Investigative techniques in small animal clinical dermatology. Br. Vet. J. 137:133, 1981a.

Thoday, K. L.: Skin diseases of the cat. In Pract. 3(6):22, 1981b.

Thoday, K. L., Seth, J., and Elton, R. A.: Radioimmunoassay of serum total thyroxine and triiodothyronine in healthy cats: Assay methodology and effects of age, sex, breed, heredity and environment. J. Small Anim. Pract. 25:457, 1984.

DIFFERENTIAL DIAGNOSIS OF STERILE PUSTULAR DERMATOSES IN THE DOG

DANNY W. SCOTT, D.V.M.
Ithaca, New York

Sterile pustular dermatoses are rare in dogs. These dermatoses account for about 1 per cent of all canine dermatoses seen at the New York State College of Veterinary Medicine. However, due to their pustular nature, these sterile dermatoses are usually misdiagnosed as infectious dermatoses. In addition, some of these sterile dermatoses can be very pruritic, resulting in their being mistaken for allergic or parasitic disorders.

The major sterile pustular dermatoses of dogs include pemphigus foliaceus, pemphigus erythematosus, subcorneal pustular dermatosis, linear IgA dermatosis, and sterile eosinophilic pustulosis (Table 1). In addition, sterile pustules may be occasionally seen in dogs with demodicosis and dermatophytosis. These last two dermatoses have been exhaustively described (Muller et al., 1983) and will not be discussed here.

The keys to initially recognizing the sterile pustular dermatoses are (1) a thorough medical history, (2) a careful physical examination, (3) microscopic examination of direct smears from intact pustules and recent erosions, and (4) careful culturing of intact pustules. These dermatoses (except for sterile eosinophilic pustulosis) often have a waxing and waning course. Thus, the clinician can be misled as to the efficacy of a prescribed treatment regimen. In addition, most of the dermatoses (except for sterile eosinophilic pustulosis) usually show little or no improvement with standard topical, systemic antimicrobial, and systemic glucocorticoid (at anti-inflammatory doses; e.g., 1 mg/kg prednisolone or prednisone per day) treatment protocols.

Pustules are often quite transient skin lesions in dogs, lasting only 2 to 6 hours. Thus, the clinician is often confronted with only the "footprints" of pustules: annular (circular) erosions with peripheral epidermal collarettes. If the finding of intact pustules becomes necessary for accurate diagnosis, patients may have to be hospitalized and examined

Table 1. *Key Laboratory Findings in Canine Sterile Pustular Dermatoses*

Diagnosis	Direct Smear	Skin Biopsy	Direct Immunofluorescence Testing	Other
Pemphigus foliaceus	Neutrophils and/or eosinophils; numerous acanthocytes	Intragranular or subcorneal pustule; marked acantholysis; granular "clingons"; follicular involvement	IgG ± C3 in intercellular spaces of epidermis	
Pemphigus erythematosus	Neutrophils and/or eosinophils; numerous acanthocytes	Intergranular or subcorneal pustule; marked acantholysis; granular "clingons"; follicular involvement	IgG ± C3 in intercellular spaces of epidermis and at basement membrane zone	Positive antinuclear antibody
Subcorneal pustular dermatosis	Neutrophils	Subcorneal pustule	Negative	
Linear IgA dermatosis	Neutrophils	Subcorneal pustule	IgA at basement membrane zone	
Sterile eosinophilic pustulosis	Eosinophils	Intraepidermal eosinophilic pustule; eosinophilic folliculitis	Negative	Eosinophilia (hemogram)

frequently until intact lesions can be found for direct smears, culture, and biopsy.

Microscopic examination of direct smears from intact pustules offers rapid, simple, inexpensive information on possible cause. Smears are usually stained with new methylene blue or Diff-Quik (Harleco). The pustules of bacterial infection are characterized by degenerate neutrophils, some or many of which contain intracellular bacteria.

Skin biopsies are very helpful for determining the nature of sterile pustules. Intact pustules are essential, and early, smaller lesions are more useful than older, larger ones. Biopsies are usually taken with disposable biopsy punches or with a scalpel. Ideally, intact pustules are preserved in both 10 per cent neutral buffered formalin (routine histopathologic examination) and Michel's fixative (direct immunofluorescence testing).

PEMPHIGUS FOLIACEUS

Pemphigus foliaceus is an autoimmune dermatosis of unknown cause. The disease is characterized immunologically by the presence of an autoantibody ("pemphigus antibody") against the glycocalyx of keratinocytes. The proposed pathomechanism of primary skin lesion formation in pemphigus includes (1) the binding of pemphigus antibody at the glycocalyx of keratinocytes, which results in an inhibition of cellular protein and ribonucleic acid synthesis, and (2) resultant activation and release of a keratinocyte proteolytic enzyme ("pemphigus acantholytic factor"), which diffuses into the extracellular space and hydrolyzes the glycocalyx. The resultant loss of intercellular cohesion leads to acantholysis and vesicle formation within the epidermis.

In general, no age, breed, or sex predilections have been reported for canine pemphigus foliaceus. A recent report from California suggests that bearded collies, Akitas, Newfoundlands, and schipperkes may be predisposed to the condition in that region of the United States. Pemphigus foliaceus is characterized by a pustular or vesiculobullous dermatitis. Mucocutaneous orientation may be encountered, but involvement of the oral cavity is very rare. The primary skin lesions are transient, so presenting signs usually consist of erythema, oozing, crusts, scales, alopecia, and annular erosions bordered by epidermal collarettes. Nikolsky's sign may be present.

Pemphigus foliaceus usually begins on the face and ears; commonly involves the feet, footpads (villous hyperkeratosis, or "hard pad"), and groin; and may become multifocal or generalized. The disease usually develops gradually over a period of weeks to months, although acute and generalized cases may occur. Pruritus and pain are variable, and peripheral lymphadenopathy with or without secondary pyoderma may be encountered. Severely affected animals may be anorectic, depressed, or febrile.

Results of routine laboratory examinations (hemogram, serum chemistries, urinalysis, serum protein electrophoresis) are nondiagnostic, often revealing mild to moderate leukocytosis and neutrophilia, mild nonregenerative anemia, mild hypoalbuminemia, and mild to moderate elevations of $alpha_2$, beta, and gamma globulins.

Microscopic examination of direct smears from intact pustules or vesicles or from recent erosions often reveals numerous acantholytic keratinocytes. Occasional solitary acanthocytes may be seen in *any* suppurative dermatosis, but when present in clusters or large numbers in several microscopic fields they are strongly indicative of pemphigus. In pemphigus foliaceus, either neutrophils or eosinophils may be the dominant inflammatory cell type found in direct smears. Neutrophils are usually nondegenerate, and intracellular bacteria are not seen.

Skin biopsies from dogs with pemphigus foliaceus are characterized by intragranular or subcorneal acantholysis, with resultant cleft and pustule or vesicle formation. Within the pustule or vesicle, cells from the stratum granulosum may be seen attached to the overlying stratum corneum (granular "cling-ons"). Either neutrophils or eosinophils may predominate within the pustule or vesicle. These histopathologic changes often involve hair follicles, as well. In addition, a lichenoid band of inflammatory cells may be seen in the superficial dermis.

Direct immunofluorescence testing usually reveals the diffuse intercellular deposition of immunoglobulin (usually IgG), and occasionally complement, within the epidermis. Results of indirect immunofluorescence testing are usually negative.

PEMPHIGUS ERYTHEMATOSUS

Pemphigus erythematosus is an autoimmune dermatosis of unknown cause. The proposed pathomechanism of primary skin lesion formation is basically as described above for pemphigus foliaceus. In addition, ultraviolet light is known to exacerbate canine pemphigus erythematosus.

No age, breed, or sex predilections have been reported for canine pemphigus erythematosus. However, collies appear to be predisposed to the condition in the author's case material. Pemphigus erythematosus is characterized by a pustular or vesiculobullous dermatitis of the face and ears. As the primary skin lesions are transient, presenting lesions usually consist of erythema, oozing, crusts, scales, alopecia, and annular erosions bordered by epidermal collarettes. Nikolsky's sign may be present. Pruritus and pain are variable, and affected animals are usually otherwise healthy. The nose frequently becomes depigmented, whereupon photodermatitis becomes an aggravating factor. If the nasal region is primarily involved, the dogs are usually worse in sunny weather and may be misdiagnosed as having nasal solar dermatitis ("collie nose").

Results of routine laboratory examinations are usually within normal limits. Findings in direct smears and skin biopsies are as described above for pemphigus foliaceus.

Direct immunofluorescence testing usually reveals the diffuse intercellular deposition of immunoglobulin (usually IgG), and occasionally complement, within the epidermis. In addition, immunoglobulin with or without complement is usually deposited at the basement membrane zone of skin lesions. Most dogs also have a positive antinuclear antibody test. Results of indirect immunofluorescence testing are usually negative.

SUBCORNEAL PUSTULAR DERMATOSIS

Subcorneal pustular dermatosis is an idiopathic sterile pustular dermatosis. There is no apparent age or sex predilection. Although many breeds have been reported to be affected, miniature schnauzers have accounted for 38 per cent of the cases.

Affected dogs usually present with a multifocal to generalized pustular dermatitis. The head and trunk are particularly affected, but involvement of the feet is rare. The pustules are nonfollicular and often greenish yellow. Because the pustules are often very transient, presenting lesions usually consist of annular areas of alopecia, erosion, scaling, crusting, and epidermal collarettes. Pruritus varies from extreme to nonexistent. Severely affected dogs may be anorectic, depressed, or febrile.

Results of routine laboratory examinations are usually within normal limits. Occasionally, mild to moderate leukocytosis, neutrophilia, nonregenerative anemia, and hypoalbuminemia may be seen. Microscopic examination of direct smears from intact pustules reveals numerous nondegenerate neutrophils, occasional acantholytic keratinocytes, and no intracellular microorganisms.

Skin biopsies are characterized by subcorneal pustular dermatitis, with neutrophils predominating. Acantholysis is usually minimal but occasionally marked. Hair follicles are rarely involved, and granular cling-ons are not seen.

The result of direct and indirect immunofluorescence testing are negative.

LINEAR IgA DERMATOSIS

Linear IgA dermatosis is an idiopathic, sterile, superficial pustular dermatosis. There is no apparent age or sex predilection. All cases documented, to date, have occurred in dachshunds.

Clinically, linear IgA dermatosis is characterized by a multifocal to generalized pustular dermatitis. The trunk is involved initially. The pustules are both follicular and nonfollicular and transient in nature. Presenting lesions usually consist of annular areas of alopecia, erosion, crusting, scaling, hyperpigmentation, and epidermal collarettes. Pruritus is mild to absent. Affected dogs are otherwise healthy.

Results of routine laboratory examinations are usually within normal limits. Mild to moderate leukocytosis and neutrophilia may occur. Microscopic examination of direct smears from intact pustules reveals numerous nondegenerate neutrophils, occasional acantholytic keratinocytes, and no intracellular microorganisms. Skin biopsy findings are as described above for subcorneal pustular dermatosis.

Direct immunofluorescence testing reveals the deposition of IgA at the basement membrane zone. Results of indirect immunofluorescence testing are negative.

STERILE EOSINOPHILIC PUSTULOSIS

Sterile eosinophilic pustulosis is an idiopathic sterile pustular dermatosis. No age, breed, or sex predilections have yet been recognized.

Affected dogs usually present with an acute onset of multifocal to generalized pustular dermatitis. The trunk is particularly affected, and the pustules are both follicular and nonfollicular in origin. Secondary lesions include annular areas of erosion, crusting, oozing, scaling, alopecia, and epidermal collarettes. Pruritus is usually intense. Some dogs may develop peripheral lymphadenopathy, pyrexia, depression, and anorexia.

Results of routine laboratory examinations usually reveal mild to moderate leukocytosis, neutrophilia, and eosinophilia (1.8 to 5.0 $\times$ 10^3/ml). Microscopic examination of lymph node aspirates from dogs with peripheral lymphadenopathy reveals lymphoid hyperplasia and numerous eosinophils.

Microscopic examination of direct smears from intact pustules reveals numerous eosinophils, nondegenerate neutrophils, occasional acanthocytes, and no intracellular microorganisms. Skin biopsies are characterized by intraepidermal eosinophilic pustules and eosinophilic folliculitis.

The results of direct and indirect immunofluorescence testing are negative.

CONCLUSION

The sterile pustular dermatoses of dogs are rare. However, because of their similarity to infectious, parasitic, and allergic dermatoses, they are frequently misdiagnosed. Direct smears should *always* be included in the laboratory workup of dermatologic cases. Cytologic findings that suggest a sterile pustular process may then be corroborated by culture. The exact nature of the sterile pustular dermatosis may be determined by biopsy, immunopathology, and response to treatment. Therapeutic approaches to these dermatoses may be gleaned from the references.

References and Supplemental Reading

Baker, K. P.: Subcorneal pustular dermatosis seen in dogs. Vet. Rec. 106:420, 1980.

Ihrke, P. J., Stannard, A. A., Ardans, A. A., et al.: Pemphigus foliaceus in dogs: A review of 37 cases. J.A.V.M.A. 186:59, 1985.

McKeever, P. J., and Dahl, M. V.: A disease in dogs resembling human subcorneal pustular dermatosis. J.A.V.M.A. 170:704, 1977.

Muller, G. H., Kirk, R. M., Scott, D. W.: *Small Animal Dermatology*, 3rd ed. Philadelphia: W. B. Saunders, 1983.

Scott, D. W., Miller, W. H., and Lewis, R. M.: Pemphigus erythematosus in the dog and cat. J. Am. Anim. Hosp. Assoc. 16:815, 1980.

Scott, D. W., Manning, T. O., and Smith, C. A.: Linear IgA dermatoses in the dog: Bullous pemphigoid, discoid lupus erythematosus, and a subcorneal pustular dermatitis. Cornell Vet. 72:394, 1982.

Scott, D. W.: Pemphigus in domestic animals. Clin. Dermatol. 1:141, 1983.

Scott, D. W., Walton, D. K., and Smith, C. A.: Unusual findings in canine pemphigus erythematosus and discoid lupus erythematosus. J. Am. Anim. Hosp. Assoc. 20:579, 1984.

Scott, D. W.: Sterile eosinophilic pustulosis in the dog. J. Am. Anim. Hosp. Assoc. 20:585, 1984.

Seiler, R. J., Scott, D. W., and Lewis, R. M.: Comparative immunodermatology. *Immunopathology of the Skin III*. New York: John Wiley & Sons, in press.

PSYCHODERMATOSES

DONNA K. WALTON, D.V.M.

Ithaca, New York

Psychodermatoses are those skin conditions that are self-induced without an existing pathologic cause. Although the lesions are frequently initiated by some pathologic condition, such as ectoparasites or trauma, they are perpetuated by the animal in the nature of a habit.

ACRAL LICK DERMATITIS

Acral lick dermatitis is the most common psychodermatosis of dogs. It is most frequently seen in large or giant breeds of dogs, although any breed may be affected. During the past 10 years, 230 cases of acral lick dermatitis were seen at the New York State College of Veterinary Medicine (NYSCVM). German shepherds, Doberman pinschers, Irish setters, Labrador retrievers, golden retrievers, Great Danes, and St. Bernards made up 47 per cent of these cases but composed only 23.6 per cent of the hospital population. The condition was more common in males than females (ratio of 2:1). There was no age predilection.

Boredom is thought to be the major cause of acral lick dermatitis, and the classic case is an anxious, hyperactive dog who is kenneled or left alone for most of the day. The dog develops an urge to constantly lick the cranial aspect of a distal extremity. Repeated licking produces alopecia, followed by erosion of the epidermis and exposure of the sensory nerves. This causes the dog to continue to lick, resulting in epidermal ulceration and hyperplasia and dermal fibrosis. Clinically, a firm, thickened, ulcerated plaque is produced, which may be surrounded by a hyperpigmented halo.

The lesion may occur on any part of the body but is most frequently present on the cranial carpal or metacarpal area, followed in frequency by the cranial tarsal or metatarsal area. The carpus is thought to be the preferred site because of its accessibility. It has also been suggested that the distal extremities of the dog may have a lower pain or pruritic threshold. Lesions are usually unilateral and solitary. When bilateral lesions are present, the prognosis is poorer. If the lesion is located over a joint, the chronic irritation may result in arthritis or ankylosis of the joint in severe cases.

The diagnosis is often based on history and clinical examination. Other conditions that should be considered in the differential diagnosis include bacterial furunculosis, fungal kerion, foreign body granuloma, trauma, pressure point granuloma, other mycotic granulomas, and neoplasia, particularly mastocytoma and histiocytoma.

Histopathologic examination of a skin biopsy will support the diagnosis with the findings of irregular hyperplasia and ulceration of the epidermis. There is dermal fibrosis along with vertical streaking of collagen in the dermal papillae. A fairly consistent finding is moderate numbers of plasma cells surrounding the apocrine glands. Sebaceous gland hyperplasia is usually prominent. Skin biopsies are most helpful in ruling out many of the similar-appearing dermatoses, along with other diagnostic tests such as skin scrapings, fungal cultures, and impression smears.

Acral lick dermatitis can be a very frustrating disease to treat. Numerous therapies have been proposed, and many are successful, but unless the dog's urgency to lick is removed, one can anticipate failure. Reported therapies have included mechanical restraint (bandages and collars), foul-tasting topical agents, topical steroids, intralesional steroids, intralesional orgotein (Palosein, Diagnostic Data), perilesional cobra venom, acupuncture, radiation therapy, cryosurgery, and surgical excision.

Currently, most cases seen at the NYSCVM are treated initially with the topical application of a mixture of 8 ml of Synotic (Diamond Laboratories) and 3 ml of Banamine (Schering). A few drops of this combination, which becomes warm on mixing, are applied twice daily until the lesion is healed. Owners are instructed to wear gloves while rubbing the medication into the lesion, as Synotic contains dimethyl sulfoxide in addition to a fluorinated corticosteroid. This therapy has been successful in a high percentage of cases. In addition, it is quite safe, inexpensive, and easy to administer.

A thorough history is taken in an attempt to determine the factor that initiated the psychogenic condition. If possible, this factor is removed or corrected. Common recommendations include increased exercise or interaction with household members. The addition of toys, rawhide bones, or a playmate may be helpful. If the initiating cause cannot be determined or cannot be changed, the likelihood of recurrence must be clearly explained to the owner. It is in these cases and in cases of severe bilateral lick dermatitis, particularly in Doberman pinschers and Great Danes, that the use of behavior-modifying drugs is often necessary.

If the inciting cause is predictable, as in the case of fear of fireworks, tranquilizers given prior to the stress may be helpful. In other cases, phenobarbital or progestogen therapy may be required. Phenobarbital is administered at 2.2 to 6.6 mg/kg twice daily. This has a sedative effect and can be used for long or short periods of time.

Progestogens may be helpful because of their calming effect. A repository progesterone (Depo-Provera, Upjohn) given by injection at 20 mg/kg every 3 weeks has been successful in some cases. Megestrol acetate (Megace, Mead Johnson; Ovaban, Schering) given PO at 1 mg/kg once daily and then tapered to a maintenance level tends to be quite successful. However, cost is a factor, and the drug should not be used in intact females. In addition, owners should be informed of the possibility that these drugs may eliminate one behavioral abnormality but produce another.

The prognosis for acral lick dermatitis must be guarded, particularly in severe cases, unless the initiating cause can be identified and corrected. Even then, the animal's psychologic urge to lick must be stopped, an accomplishment that can prove to be difficult.

FELINE PSYCHOGENIC ALOPECIA AND DERMATITIS

Feline psychogenic alopecia and dermatitis are conditions that are the result of chronic chewing and licking by the cat in the absence of a pathologic cause. The conditions may occur in cats of any age or sex but are most frequently seen in the more "high-strung" breeds such as the Siamese, Burmese, Himalayan, and Abyssinian.

In the alopecic form, single or multiple lesions may be present. The most commonly affected areas are the middle of the back, the perineal or genital area, the medial thighs, and the ventral abdomen. The distribution of hair loss may be identical to that of feline endocrine alopecia. Since the hair loss of feline psychogenic alopecia is self-induced, one can differentiate these conditions by examining the affected hairs, which are broken and split in psychogenic alopecia because of the trauma of the cat's teeth and tongue. Dermatophytosis and demodicosis should also be considered in the differential diagnosis, and fungal cultures and skin scrapings are indicated.

In the dermatitic form of this feline psychodermatosis, there is usually a solitary lesion located on an extremity or the abdomen or flank. The major differential diagnosis is indolent (eosinophilic) ulcer or eosinophilic plaque. The latter two conditions should be steroid responsive, whereas the psychogenic condition usually is not.

Therapy must be directed toward identifying the underlying cause. Cats are very perceptive and may be influenced by minor changes in their human and animal companions. They are subject to territory-induced neurosis, and the appearance of a new roaming cat in the neighborhood is frequently stressful. Therapy may include limiting the cat's access to windows from which the intruder is visible. If the underlying cause cannot be determined or corrected, medical therapy may be desired. The alopecic form is frequently not treated in order not to subject the cat to chronic medical therapy. Instead, it may be considered a bad but acceptable habit.

The dermatitic form usually requires medical intervention. Because of the cat's nature, mechanical means of restraint are usually unsuccessful. Foul-tasting agents and topical remedies are rapidly removed by the cat. Sedatives such as diazepam (Valium, Roche; 1.0 to 2.0 mg b.i.d.) and phenobarbital (8 to 16 mg b.i.d.) may be successful in some cases. In other cases, the use of progestational compounds may be necessary. Megestrol acetate (Ovaban) is given at 2.5 to 5.0 mg every other day initially and then tapered to the lowest maintenance dosage possible, given weekly as needed. The side effects of progestational compounds in the cat must be seriously weighed against the severity of the cat's self-induced lesions prior to their chronic use. Megestrol acetate is not approved for use in cats. Alternatively, medroxyprogesterone acetate (Depo-Provera) has been administered by SC or IM injection at 75 to 150 mg per cat. Injections may be repeated as needed, but never more frequently than every 2 to 3 months. This product is not approved for use in cats.

MISCELLANEOUS PSYCHODERMATOSES

There are several other less common psychodermatoses recognized in dogs and cats. Flank sucking is almost exclusively limited to Doberman pinschers. Affected dogs will literally suckle one flank. The area is chronically moist and erythematous, but dermatitis is not usually a significant factor. Several causes including trichuriasis (whipworm infestation) and psychomotor epilepsy have been proposed but not substantiated. Therapy is usually not necessary, as the skin is not damaged. A canine behaviorist should be consulted for help in modifying the habit.

Tail chasing or biting may be seen in young, long-tailed dogs. Again, dermatitis is not usually a significant problem. Young dogs may outgrow the condition; however, if the condition persists, medical therapy is not very rewarding. It has been reported that a small number of bull terriers responded to the injection of 70 per cent ethanol into the first caudal space. This supposedly leaves the motor nerve supply intact but anesthetizes the tail. Tail amputation is not successful, as the patients chase their phantom tail.

Anal licking, a condition most common in poodles, is an almost impossible psychodermatosis to correct. The perianal area will become thickened, hyperpigmented, and lichenified. Anal gland problems have been suggested as an underlying cause; however, anal sac removal does not usually remedy the situation.

SUMMARY

In summary, as our canine and feline companions are forced to adapt to our lifestyles, the occurrence of psychodermatoses should be expected. Various medical therapies may be used in an attempt to correct or control these conditions. However, unless the underlying psychologic causes are identified and corrected, chronic medication along with recurrences and failures must be anticipated.

References and Supplemental Reading

Bullock, J. E.: Acupuncture treatment of canine lick granuloma. Calif. Vet. 32:14, 1978.

Doering, G. G., and Jensen, H. E.: *Clinical Dermatology of Small Animals*. St. Louis: C. V. Mosby, 1973, pp. 125–138.

Krahwinkel, D. J.: Cryosurgical treatment of skin diseases. Vet. Clin. North Am. 10:787, 1980.

Muller, G. H., Kirk, R. W., and Scott, D. W.: *Small Animal Dermatology III*. Philadelphia: W. B. Saunders, 1983, pp. 625–635.

Neibert, H. C.: Orgotein treatment of canine lick granuloma. Mod. Vet. Pract. 56:529, 1975.

Pemberton, P. L.: Canine and feline behavioral control—progestin therapy. *In* Kirk, R. W. (ed.): *Current Veterinary Therapy VIII*. Philadelphia: W. B. Saunders, 1983, pp. 62–71.

Reid, J. S.: Acropruritic granuloma. *In* Kirk, R. W. (ed.): *Current Veterinary Therapy V*. Philadelphia: W. B. Saunders, 1974, pp. 441–443.

Roberts, I. M.: Acral pruritic granuloma. In Kirk, R. W. (ed.): *Current Veterinary Therapy III*. Philadelphia: W. B. Saunders, 1968, pp. 289–290.

Scott, D. W.: Feline dermatology 1900–1978: A monograph. J. Am. Anim. Hosp. Assoc. 16:414, 1980.

Scott, D. W., and Walton, D. K.: Clinical evaluation of a topical treatment for canine acral lick dermatitis. J. Am. Anim. Hosp. Assoc. 20:565, 1984.

ANTIFUNGAL AGENTS IN DERMATOLOGY

CAROL S. FOIL, D.V.M.
Baton Rouge, Louisiana

Medical mycologists often classify the diseases that they study into superficial, subcutaneous, and deep mycoses.

The superficial mycoses that affect small animals are dermatophytosis and surface infections with the yeasts *Candida albicans* and *Malassezia (Pityrosporum)*. These infections are confined to the skin, including the external ear, or mucous membranes and may be treated by either topical or systemic antifungal agents.

Subcutaneous mycoses that are important in small animals include sporotrichosis, pythiosis (phycomycosis), and a variety of opportunistic infections by saprophytes including aspergillosis, phaeohyphomycosis, and mycetomas (Fadok, 1980). With the exception of sporotrichosis, these fungal infections are relatively or completely resistant to chemotherapeutic control. When surgical excision is possible, surgery is the treatment of choice for solitary subcutaneous lesions. If chemotherapy is necessary, sensitivity testing of the isolates is indicated. To date, no chemotherapy has been found to be effective in treating infection with *Pythium*.

The systemic mycoses that commonly have dermatologic lesions are blastomycosis and cryptococcosis. These are treated systemically as discussed in the following sections.

TOPICAL THERAPY

Topical antifungal therapy is useful only in the superficial mycoses. In some form, topical treatment is always indicated in the management of dermatophytosis of dogs and cats. In ringworm infections, scale, crust, exudate, and infected hairs are removed by topical therapy, thus reducing the potential for spread of the infection. In infection of glabrous skin or sparsely haired areas, topical therapy may be used alone to effect a mycologic cure. Also, in extremely inflammatory and secondarily infected lesions, topical treatment with low-potency corticosteroids in combination with antimicrobial agents may hasten resolution of clinical disease.

In the rare case of superficial cutaneous candidiasis or in otic or cutaneous infections with *Malassezia*, topical therapy alone will likely suffice. For candidiasis, the treatments of choice are nystatin-containing compounds. In cases in which *Malassezia* organisms are associated with otitis externa, polyhydroxidine (Xenodine, Xenovet), cuprimyxin (Unitop, Hoffman-LaRoche), and miconazole in combination with low-potency steroids are all effective agents. In many cases, astringent and acidic flushing agents or ceruminolytic compounds with or without topical corticosteroids will resolve *Malassezia*-associated otitis without specific antimycotic therapy.

Topical agents useful in dermatophytosis may be divided into three general categories: keratolytics, antiseptics, and fungicidal antibiotics. Keratolytics include lime sulfur solution (which is also antiseptic), selenium disulfide shampoos, and undecylenic acid and tolnaftate, which are available in cream formulation. Although keratolytic agents may be useful in infections of glabrous skin, they are not effective in the follicular infections of dogs and cats. Tolnaftate cream in particular is widely marketed to veterinarians (Tinavet, Schering); it has been shown to be ineffective in small-animal dermatophytosis (Blakemore, 1974).

Antiseptic preparations include a wide variety of agents that are marketed or available to veterinarians as solutions, incorporated into shampoos, or in cream formulations. These include povidone-iodine in shampoos or solutions (Betadine shampoo, Betadine solution, Purdue Frederick); polyalkyleneglycol-iodine in shampoo (Weladol Shampoo, Pitman-Moore); lime sulfur used as a 2 per cent rinse (Lym Dyp, DVM); technical captan as a rinse (Orthocide, Ortho Chemical); haloprogin-iodinated phenol as a 1 per cent cream or solution (Halotex, Westwood); chlorhexidine as a 2 per cent solution, a 7 per cent ointment, or in a shampoo (Nolvasan solution, Nolvasan ointment, Nolvasan shampoo, Fort Dodge Laboratories); sodium hypochlorite as a 0.5 per cent

(1:20) solution; and cuprimyxin as a cream (Unitop, Hoffman-LaRoche).

For the most part, disinfectant agents are useful mostly as dip solutions or shampoos for treatment of the body as a whole or for extensive lesions. Some, particularly the iodine-containing preparations and lime sulfur, can be drying and irritating. With the exception of povidone-iodine, haloprogin, and cuprimyxin, the commonly used antiseptics are less likely to produce a mycologic cure in follicular dermatophytosis than are ointments containing antimycotic antibiotics (Pascoe, 1984). Therefore, antiseptic preparations should be used as adjunctive therapy to systemic treatment. Products for topical therapy recommended for use in conjunction with systemic therapy in dermatophytosis are listed in Table 1.

Antifungal antibiotics that are useful topically in dermatophytosis include the imidazole derivatives—thiabendazole, clotrimazole, miconazole, and ketoconazole. Of these, thiabendazole is available in a lotion in combination with an antibacterial agent and a corticosteroid (Tresaderm, MSD Ag Vet). This preparation may be used for singular, highly inflamed ringworm lesions on healthy adult dogs. Clotrimazole (Veltrim, Haver-Lockhart) and miconazole (Conofite, Pitman-Moore) are marketed to veterinarians as antifungal agents in cream or lotion form. They are highly effective and are the treatment of choice for localized ringworm lesions in both dogs and cats with or without systemic therapy. Either may occasionally produce an irritant dermatitis. The use of these agents is described in Table 1. All lesions to be treated with these preparations should be clipped widely and cleaned prior to commencing therapy. Both ketoconazole (Cauenbergh et al., 1983) and griseofulvin in dimethyl sulfoxide (Valient and Frost, 1984) have been found to be effective topically in experimental dermatophytosis in guinea pigs. Neither antibiotic is marketed as a topical agent at present, however.

SYSTEMIC ANTIFUNGAL AGENTS

The ideal systemic antifungal agent should have a wide therapeutic index, a broad spectrum of antifungal activity, high efficacy, low toxicity, broad tissue distribution, and oral dosage form (Levine, 1982). Until the development of ketoconazole, the systemic antifungals available in medical and veterinary mycology were very far from this ideal. Most of the other agents described in this article have the disadvantage of a low therapeutic index. In part, this derives from the relative similarity of fungal and mammalian cell systems, at least in comparison with the diversity of structure between animal and bacterial cells. Another difficulty in achieving progress in antifungal chemotherapy has been the relative rarity and great diverisity of the mycotic infections. With the exception of dermatophytosis, these are "orphan diseases," which present great difficulties for development of profitable new therapeutic modalities.

Although ketoconazole's availability in oral form and its low toxicity are great advantages, it has disadvantages as well. It lacks high efficacy and it does not penetrate well into bone and the central nervous system (CNS). As a result, we still must rely on many of the traditional antifungal agents, discussed below, in the treatment of several specific diseases.

Iodides

Sodium and potassium iodide have been used as systemic antifungal agents probably since antiquity. Until the 1940s, these were the only agents available. Their mechanism of action *in vivo* is unknown, although the iodides have been observed to enhance resolution of noninfectious granulomas and to cause an intracellular accumulation of peroxide. The solutions have no efficacy against fungal organisms *in vitro*. Thus, their efficacy has no relationship to the topical use of other iodine-based chemicals. The iodides are readily absorbed when given orally, are widely distributed in the body, and are excreted mainly in the urine.

The spectrum of action of the iodides and indications for use are limited to lymphocutaneous sporotrichosis and occasionally to other subcutaneous opportunistic fungal infections such as basidiobolomycosis.

Table 1. *Products Recommended for Topical Therapy in Dermatophytosis of Dogs and Cats*

Product	Brand Name	Administration	Comments
Povidone-iodine	Betadine solution (Purdue-Frederick)	1:4 in water once daily	Irritating, sensitizing
Chlorhexidine	Nolvasan solution	2% solution daily	
	Nolvasan shampoo (Fort Dodge)	Bathe every 5 days	
Lime-sulfur	Lym Dyp (DVM)	2% solution every 5 to 7 days	Odorous, not for white animals
Captan	Orthocide spray (Ortho Chemical)	2% (2 tbsp/gal)	
Miconazole	Conofite cream, lotion (Pitman-Moore)	Apply b.i.d.	For localized lesions
Clotrimazole	Veltrim (Haver-Lockhart)	Apply b.i.d.	For localized lesions
	Lotrimin (Schering)		

The iodides are provided in saturated (20 per cent) solutions. Dogs are given 1 ml/5 kg on a daily basis for 6 weeks. The dose for cats is 0.5 ml/5 kg/day (Fadok, 1980).

Iodinism can be severe, and anorexia, nausea, salivation, lacrimation, and sneezing are commonly observed. In humans, cutaneous eruptions are seen. Seborrhea sicca may develop in small animals. These signs may necessitate dose reduction or even cessation of therapy.

Griseofulvin

Griseofulvin, a fungistatic antibiotic discovered in 1939, is derived from *Penicillium griseofulvum.* It interferes with renewal of cell walls in actively growing chitinous fungi by binding to ribonucleic acid (RNA), inhibiting protein synthesis, and interfering with microtubule formation. Unfortunately, the spectrum of activity is limited to dermatophytes; the basis for this limitation is unknown. Resistance of dermatophyte isolates to griseofulvin has been documented for some anthropophilic dermatophytes, but treatment failures in veterinary medicine are more likely to be caused by erratic absorption and other pharmacokinetic features of the drug.

Like many antifungal agents, griseofulvin has a very low solubility in water, and gastrointestinal absorption is variable and incomplete. Absorption is enhanced by administration with a fat-containing meal or by formulations using polyethylene glycol (PEG). Particle size (micronization) also greatly affects oral absorption. Divided dosage regimens provide higher absorption levels. Little is known about tissue distribution, but earlier reports about delayed deposition in the skin and hair and of persistence there after cessation of therapy appear incorrect. Levels of griseofulvin in the skin depend on continued administration, and pulse-dosing for preventive purposes probably does not make sense. Griseofulvin metabolites are excreted in both urine and bile. Drugs such as phenobarbital, which enhance liver microsomal functions, will enhance the metabolism of griseofulvin.

Indications for the use of griseofulvin in dermatophyte infections are not well defined experimentally. Some guidelines are given in Table 2.

Dosage and administration of griseofulvin are also controversial. Tablets of either microsize (Fulvicin-U/F, Schering) or ultramicrosize in PEG (Gris-PEG, Dorsey) should be used. A microsize formulation is available as a pediatric suspension (Grifulvin V, Ortho Pharmaceutical, 125 mg/5 ml). The dose for microsize griseofulvin for dogs and cats is 20 to 50 mg/kg in divided doses with fat. The dose for ultramicrosize in PEG is 5 to 10 mg/kg.

A major problem with griseofulvin is its teratogenicity, and its use is absolutely contraindicated in pregnant animals. Otherwise, toxicity in humans and in dogs has been limited and consists mainly of gastrointestinal disturbance. This problem is encountered mainly at higher doses and can be controlled in most cases with divided dosages. Other side effects include various dermatologic eruptions, including photosensitivity, hepatotoxicity, and neutropenia. The latter problem appears to be more prominent with ultramicrosize formulations in PEG when the dose has not been adjusted downward. Recently a series of seven cases of intoxication in cats was reported; the signs included anorexia, lethargy, vomiting and diarrhea, pyrexia, icterus, neurotoxicity, angioedema, and neutropenia (Helton, 1984). In cats in particular, care must be taken to adjust dosages if PEG formulations are to be administered.

5-Flucytosine

5-Flucytosine (Ancobon, Roche) is a fluorinated pyrimidine that is an antimetabolite. Fungi that possess the enzyme cytosine deaminase convert 5-flucytosine (5-FC) to 5-fluorouracil. The compound becomes incorporated into fungal RNA, inhibiting its function. The drug also inhibits deoxyribonucleic acid (DNA) synthesis.

As opposed to other antifungal compounds, 5-FC is well absorbed orally. Distribution within the body is not fully studied, but there is good passage into the cerebrospinal fluid (CSF) (60 to 80 per cent of serum levels). Excretion is through the urinary systems, and impaired renal function necessitates dose reduction.

The spectrum of susceptible yeasts is fairly limited and for practical purposes includes only species of *Candida, Cryptococcus,* and *Cladosporium.* Some other opportunistic saprophytic fungal infections may be caused by susceptible isolates. Even among *Cryptococcus* isolates, considerable variation of *in vitro* mean inhibitory concentration (MIC) measurements are encountered. In addition, emergence of resistance during the course of therapy is a frequent problem.

Because of the problem of resistance, the use of 5-FC is in practice limited to combination therapy with amphotericin B in feline cryptococcosis. The drug is particularly useful in CNS infections with this organism. In addition, some cases of subcutaneous and systemic chromoblastomycosis may respond to 5-FC.

The drug is available in 250- and 500-mg capsules. The dose for dogs and cats is 100 to 200 mg/kg divided three or four times daily. For cats, recompounding of capsules is often necessary.

In humans, bone marrow toxicities occur when serum levels exceed 100 μg/ml. Thus, leukopenia and thrombocytopenia may occur if serum levels

Table 2. *Treatment Recommendations for Various Forms of Small Animal Dermatophytosis*

Dermatophyte Species	Lesion Type	Patient Characteristics	Treatment
Microsporum gypseum	Localized	Dog or cat	Topical, anti-inflammatory
M. gypseum	Multifocal	Dog or cat	Topical, griseofulvin
Microsporum canis	Localized	Dog	Topical
M. canis	Localized	Young, short-haired cat	Topical
M. canis	Any form	Long-haired cat	Topical, griseofulvin
M. canis	Generalized	Dog or cat	Topical, griseofulvin
Trichophyton mentagrophytes	Any form	Dog or cat	Topical, griseofulvin
Any species	Onychomycosis	Dog or cat	Long-term griseofulvin; remove nails; ketoconazole
Any species	Any lesion	Immunocompromised host	Griseofulvin

are not monitored during conditions of renal impairment. There may be some *in vivo* conversion of 5-FC to 5-FU (Diasio et al., 1978). Neurologic signs have been seen with the latter drug in dogs and cats (Harvey et al., 1977). The author has seen aberrant behavior and seizures in a cat with *Cryptococcus* infection during 5-FC therapy. This cat had no CNS infection on postmortem examination.

Amphotericin B

Amphotericin B (Fungizone, Squibb) is a polyene macrolide antibiotic isolated from *Streptomyces nodosus.* The drug is water insoluble and is unstable when suspended in water at 37°C. Instability in the fluid phase makes it difficult to perform *in vitro* sensitivity testing with amphotericin B.

Amphotericin B binds irreversibly to membrane sterols and has a higher affinity for the ergosterol of fungal cells than for cholesterol. Membrane binding impairs membrane uptake mechanisms and causes leakage of cellular constituents. The drug has been reported to be fungistatic at low doses and fungicidal at higher doses. In addition, amphotericin B possesses some poorly defined immunoadjuvant properties.

Amphotericin B is lyophilized in combination with deoxycholate and buffer. It forms an unstable colloid in dextrose solutions. Minimal fungicidal concentration (MFC) and MIC are readily achieved for most fungi by IV administration. The drug is strongly bound to lipoproteins in plasma, but other facets of compartmentalization are poorly understood. The serum half-life is short, but the elimination half-life is extremely prolonged; the drug is excreted in the urine for as long as 60 days after administration. The details of metabolism are not known. The inactivated drug is excreted in urine. As there is poor distribution to the CNS, intrathecal administration may be performed when CNS involvement is present.

Amphotericin B has an extremely broad spectrum. It is the drug of choice in life-threatening systemic mycoses. In declining order of susceptibility are species of *Blastomyces, Histoplasma, Cryptococcus, Candida, Sporotrichum,* and *Coccidioides.* Many saprophytic fungi are susceptible. Resistant strains are infrequent, but more reports are documenting resistance. The aspergilli are most frequently resistant, and susceptibility of the zygomycetes is highly variable. Species of *Pythium* are probably resistant.

Most of the dosage regimens and the recommended total treatment doses have been developed empirically (Table 3). Most regimens call for administration of doses of 0.25 to 1.0 mg/kg two or three times weekly. The drug is administered IV after reconstitution in sterile water and dilution in 5 per cent dextrose solutions (D5W). (Dextrose solutions with pH below 4 should be buffered. Add 1 ml

Table 3. *Guidelines for Systemic Chemotherapy of Selected Mycoses*

Mycosis	Drug(s) of Choice	Dosage and Administration
Microsporum canis infection	Griseofulvin (microsize)	20–50 mg/kg divided b.i.d., 4–6 wk
	Griseofulvin in PEG	5–10 mg/kg daily, 4–6 wk
Trichophyton infection	Griseofulvin (microsize)	20–50 mg/kg divided b.i.d. until culture neg.
	Griseofulvin in PEG	5–10 mg/kg daily until culture neg.
Sporotrichosis	Na or K iodide (20%)	Dogs: 1 ml/5 kg daily, 6 wk Cats: 0.5 ml/5 kg daily, 6 wk
Blastomycosis	Amphotericin B and ketoconazole	0.5 mg/kg 3 times weekly to total dose 6 mg/kg 10–20 mg/kg divided, 3–6 months 30 mg/kg for CNS, bone, eye
Cryptococcosis	Amphotericin B and ketoconazole	0.25–0.5 mg/kg 3 times weekly to 4 mg/kg total dose 5–10 mg/kg divided, 3–6 months
CNS cryptococcosis	Amphotericin B and 5-flucytosine	0.5 mg/kg 3 times weekly to total dose 4 mg/kg 100–200 mg/kg/day divided t.i.d.

potassium phosphate for injection USP per 250 ml D5W.) The reconstituted drug may be stored at refrigerator temperatures for 1 week.

In humans, the final dilution in D5W is recommended to be no greater than 10 mg/100 ml. In veterinary practice, this concentration is often exceeded, and many clinicians can successfully administer the calculated dosage in a bolus of 50 to 100 ml of D5W, given over a 5- to 10-minute period. In such cases, a test dose should always be administered prior to bolus administration. If acute adverse reactions are observed (vomiting, shivering, fever, collapse), a more dilute suspension should be prepared and administered over 1 to 6 hours. The package insert advises to protect the dilute suspension of amphotericin B from light, but this is not necessary except in extremely prolonged administration protocols.

Renal toxicity is the major limitation to the use of amphotericin B. A decrease in glomerular filtration rate (GFR) occurs in virtually every patient that receives amphotericin B. The pathophysiology of this change is not entirely understood. The drug is a renal tubular toxin as well. Both hypokalemia and renal tubular acidosis are common problems in humans but are not commonly observed in dogs and cats. It is important to monitor blood urea nitrogen (BUN) during therapy. Most recommend a temporary suspension of therapy when the BUN exceeds 40 to 50 mg/dl. On the other hand, preexisting renal disease is not a contraindication for the use of amphotericin B. A decreased GFR does not limit drug metabolism.

There are two techniques reported (Said et al., 1980) for trying to reduce the renal toxicity of amphotericin B. The first included the administration of 12.5 gm (or 0.5 to 1 gm/kg) of mannitol in conjunction with slow administration of amphotericin B in D5W. This prevents the rise of BUN in normal dogs given amphotericin B (Said et al., 1980). The author has found it a useful technique in canine patients. Unfortunately, this technique doubles the cost of amphotericin B administration. It has recently been reported both experimentally and clinically that sodium loading of patients prior to amphotericin B administration decreases the renal toxicity, especially in patients with a negative sodium imbalance (Gerkins and Branch, 1980; Heidemann et al., 1983). Clinically, the author has used 0.9 per cent sodium chloride administration at the rate of 5 ml/kg given in two portions, before and after amphotericin B administration. This technique was found helpful in averting overt renal insufficiency in the patients in which the author has seen it used.

Acute adverse reactions may occur during and immediately consequent to IV administration of amphotericin B. In humans, this includes cardiotoxicity, fever, nausea, cramping, leukopenia, and thrombocytopenia. Fever and nausea have been reported in dogs. Other toxicities include anorexia, anemia, and phlebitis. The author has found phlebitis to be a common problem, especially when amphotericin B is administered more than once through the same indwelling catheter. The drug is reported to be safe to use in the second and third trimesters of pregnancy.

Imidazoles

Ketoconazole (Nizoral, Janssen) is the only benzimidazole derivative with any usefulness in the systemic treatment of mycoses in dogs and cats. Other antifungal imidazoles include clotrimazole and econazole, which are too toxic for systemic use. Miconazole is available as an intravenous antifungal agent of broad spectrum, but the vehicle causes a high rate of acute adverse reactions in dogs. It has largely been replaced by ketoconazole for all its indications.

The imidazoles are fungistatic through the inhibition of synthesis of ergosterol, the important sterol of fungal cell membranes. They are very broad-spectrum drugs. Ketoconazole is labeled for human use for candidiasis, coccidioidomycosis, histoplasmosis, chromomycosis, and paracoccidioidomycosis. In addition, it receives wide use in cases of chronic dermatophytosis due to *Trichophyton* infection. *In vitro* activity against *Blastomyces dermatitidis* is variable. *In vitro* and clinical activity against *Sporothrix schenkii* is limited. *In vitro* activity against zygomycetes and other saprophytes is highly variable, and sensitivity testing is indicated in diseases caused by these fungi.

The indications in veterinary medicine are based on clinical experience and anecdotal reports. They have been used for chronic to subacute coccidioidomycosis, canine blastomycosis after therapy with amphotericin B to prevent relapse, nasal and cutaneous cryptococcosis, postsurgically in nasal aspergillosis (sensitivity testing is recommended), chronic to subacute histoplasmosis following amphotericin B therapy, and possibly for chronic onychomycosis caused by *Trichophyton* species. As there are some reports of *Microsporum canis* isolates being resistant to ketoconazole, it is not the drug of choice in this infection.

The drug is rapidly and well absorbed after oral administration in humans. However, 15 to 55 per cent of unchanged drug is excreted in the feces of dogs (Dunbar, 1983b). This is likely due to the fact that oral absorption depends on acidic stomach contents, and stomach acidity is variable in dogs and cats. The drug is extensively metabolized, mostly in the liver. It is well distributed in the dog, although CSF, bladder, bone, and skin concentrations are lowest (Dunbar, 1983a).

The drug is available as 200-mg tablets. The recommended daily dose is 5 to 30 mg/kg given in one or two daily doses (Dunbar, 1983a). The higher doses should be given in infections involving skin, bone, bladder, or CNS (and probably placenta and eye infections). The drug should be given with an acidic or acid-producing meal (after canned food, with or without added tomato juice). Administration should be continued for 3 to 6 months, despite apparent clinical cure, to prevent relapse.

One of the major side effects in animals is anorexia, especially at higher dosages. This may be alleviated to some extent by administering divided doses. Successful administration on an every-other-day basis has been reported in a cat with histoplasmosis (Noxon et al., 1982). Other toxicities are rare and include, in humans, hepatotoxicity and inhibition of testosterone synthesis with gynecomastia and decreased libido. The drug has been used in pregnancy in laboratory animals but is not labeled for this use in humans.

Fungal Vaccines

Vaccines are used widely in northern and central Europe to control epidemic ringworm in cattle, and there has been some interest in development of a vaccine for cattery dermatophytosis. Successful treatment of *M. canis* dermatophytosis in a cat has been reported in Washington (Mosher, et al., 1977). A vaccine for *M. canis* is reportedly marketed in that state for use in cats, but the product has not been approved for interstate marketing, nor have there been any further descriptions of its use in the literature. If such a vaccine becomes available, it could be of great benefit in the control of ringworm in catteries housing long-haired cats.

References and Supplemental Reading

Blakemore, J. C.: Dermatomycosis. *In* Kirk, R. W. (ed.): *Current Veterinary Therapy V.* Philadelphia: W. B. Saunders, 1974, p. 422.

Cauenbergh, G. F. M. I., Degreef, H., and Verhoeve, L. S. G. C.: Topical ketoconazole in dermatology: A pharmacological and clinical review. Mykosen 27:395, 1983.

Chester, D. K.: Superficial fungal infection of the skin. Comp. Cont. Ed. 1:910, 1979.

Diasio, R. B., Lakings, D. E., and Bennett, J. E.: Evidence for conversion of 5-fluorocytosine to 5-fluorouracil in humans: Possible factor in 5-fluorocytosine clinical toxicity. Antimicrob. Agents Chemother. 14:903, 1978.

Dunbar, M.: Ketoconazole: Serum half-life, oral absorption, and tissue distribution in the dog. Presented to Am. Acad. Vet. Dermatol., 1983a.

Dunbar, M.: personal communication 1983b.

Fadok, V. A.: Dermatologic manifestations of the subcutaneous and deep mycoses. Comp. Cont. Ed. Pract. Vet. 2:506, 1980.

Gedek, B., Brutzel, K., Gerlach, R., et al.: The role of *Pityrosporum pachydermatis* in otitis externa of dogs: Evaluation of a treatment with miconazole. Vet. Rec. 17:138, 1979.

Gerkins, J. F., and Branch, R. A.: The influence of sodium status and furosemide on canine acute amphotericin B nephrotoxicity. J. Pharmacol. Exp. Ther. 214:306, 1980.

Green, C. E., O'Neal, K. G., and Barsanti, J. A.: Antimicrobial chemotherapy. *In* Green, C. E. (ed.): *Clinical Microbiology and Infectious Diseases of the Dog and Cat.* Philadelphia: W. B. Saunders, 1984, pp. 144.

Harvey, H. J., MacEwen, E. G., Hayes, A. A., et al.: Neurotoxicosis associated with the use of 5-fluorouracil in five dogs and one cat. J.A.V.M.A. 171:277, 1977.

Heideman, H. Th., Gerkins, J. F., Spickard, W. A., et al.: Amphotericin B nephrotoxicity in humans decreased by salt repletion. Am. J. Med. 75:476, 1983.

Helton, K. A.: Griseofulvin toxicity in cats. Reported to Am. Acad. Vet. Dermatol., 1984.

Jungerman, P. F., and Schwartzman, R. M.: *Veterinary Medical Mycology.* Philadelphia: Lea & Febiger, 1972.

Kirk, R. W.: Dermatophyte infections. *In* Kirk, R. W. (ed.): *Current Veterinary Therapy VI.* Philadelphia: W. B. Saunders, 1977, p. 558.

Levine, H. B.: *Ketoconazole in the Management of Fungal Disease.* New York: ADIS Press, 1982.

Medoff, G., and Kobayashi, G.: Strategies in the treatment of systemic fungal infections. N. Engl. J. Med. 302:145, 1980.

Mosher, C. L., Langendoen, K., and Stoddard, P.: Treatment of ringworm *(Microsporum canis)* with inactivated fungal vaccine. V.M./S.A.C. Aug.: 1343, 1977.

Muller, G. H., Kirk, R. W., and Scott, D. W.: *Small Animal Dermatology*, 3rd ed. Philadelphia: W. B. Saunders, 1983.

Noxon, J. O., Digilio, K., and Schmidt, D. A.: Disseminated histoplasmosis in a cat: Successful treatment with ketoconazole. J.A.V.M.A. 181:817, 1982.

Pascoe, R. R.: Experimental medication of equine ringworm due to *Trichophyton equinum* var. *Autotrophicum.* Aust. Vet. J. 61:231, 1984.

Post, K., and Saunders, J. R.: Topical treatment of experimental ringworm in guinea pigs with griseofulvin in dimethylsulfoxide. Can. Vet. J. 20:45, 1979.

Said, R., Marin, P., Anicama, H., et al.: Effect of mannitol on acute amphotericin B nephrotoxicity. Res. Exp. Med. 177:85, 1980.

Valient, M. E., and Frost, B. M.: An experimental model for evaluation of antifungal agents in a *Trichophyton mentagrophytes* infection of guinea pigs. Chemotherapy 30:54, 1984.

ANTIBACTERIAL THERAPY IN DERMATOLOGY

PETER J. IHRKE, V.M.D.
Davis, California

Antibacterial agents are among the most commonly prescribed medications in small animal practice. However, despite their frequency of use, errors in selection, misuse, and poorly integrated therapeutic plans are common. Most antibiotics or other antibacterial agents used in the treatment of skin diseases in small animal practice are used for canine pyodermas. Antibacterial therapy is not commonly needed for the treatment of feline skin diseases but when indicated is highly specialized. Consequently, this article will stress the use of antibacterial therapy in the treatment of canine skin diseases.

A review of canine pyodermas would be repetitive, since little new clinically useful information has become available in the past several years. Consequently, the reader is referred to a number of recent, exhaustive review articles and book chapters. Pertinent information that has become available since the publication of *Current Veterinary Therapy VIII* will be reviewed. The emphasis of this chapter will be complete case management, including when and how to use systemic, topical, and adjunctive therapy.

OVERVIEW OF PYODERMAS

Pyodermas may be defined as pyogenic, or pus-producing, bacterial infections of the skin. The diversity within this group of diseases is enormous. Visible frank pustules are not always present, since the thinness of canine skin coupled with the frequency of self-trauma leads to the destruction of intact pustules, leaving crusted papules. Further, pustules may be microscopic and identified only by biopsy. Although pyodermas are the most common cause of pustules in dogs, pustules also may be seen with diseases as divergent as demodicosis, dermatophytosis, and pemphigus foliaceus. The scope of canine pyodermas is reviewed in Table 1.

Table 1. *Classification of Canine Pyodermas*

Surface pyodermas
Acute moist dermatitis, pyotraumatic dermatitis
Skin fold dermatitides (intertrigo)
Superficial pyodermas
Impetigo
Superficial folliculitis
Pruritic superficial pyodermas
Deep pyodermas
Deep folliculitis and furunculosis
Cellulitis

Little is known with respect to predisposing and prognostic factors in pyodermas. Poor grooming (especially in long-haired dogs), seborrhea, inflammation associated with any skin disease, pruritus due to any cause, endocrine abnormalities such as Cushing's disease and hypothyroidism, and lack of immunologic competence are all thought to be factors predisposing to the development of pyodermas. Once a pyoderma has been initiated, coexisting disease, pruritus, immunologic competence, inappropriate immunologic response, and initial therapy may all influence prognosis. A failure to recognize predisposing factors and the lack of identification of coexisting disease are the most common reasons for therapeutic failure if proper therapy has been used.

UPDATE ON PYODERMAS

Coagulase-positive staphylococci are the causative agents in most canine pyodermas. Until recently, *Staphylococcus aureus* was thought to be responsible. However, new data indicate that *S. intermedius* is the most common pathogenic staphylococcus encountered in dogs. This information may explain the apparent lack of transmissibility of staphylococcus between dogs and humans.

Work recently completed by Reinke and colleagues at the University of California indicates that acute moist dermatitis (pyotraumatic dermatitis, or "hot spots") should be regrouped as both surface and deep pyodermas. Certain hot spots (including some facial lesions in breeds such as golden retrievers) were histologically documented to be deep folliculitis and furunculosis and required aggressive systemic antibiotic therapy.

DIAGNOSIS OF PYODERMAS

If intact pustules or draining fistulous tracts are present, impression smears stained with a rapid stain such as Diff-Quik (Harleco) are the easiest and potentially most beneficial and rapid diagnostic tests for the documentation of bacterial involvement. Since staphylococci are the primary canine cutaneous pathogens, the presence of both extracellular and intracellular cocci in a smear is supportive of a diagnosis of pyoderma. Bacterial culture, identification, and antibiotic sensitivity testing probably are overused in superficial pyodermas and underused in deep pyodermas. In many circumstances, impression smears are sufficient and empirical therapy is indicated.

Skin biopsy is an often neglected valuable procedure in the diagnosis of pyodermas. As clinicians increase their frequency of taking biopsy specimens in perplexing dermatologic cases, they will note an increased frequency of diagnosed pyodermas, both primary and secondary. Multiple, representative samples should be submitted to either a veterinary dermatologist or a pathologist with a specific interest in dermatology.

When either lack of response to proper therapy or recurrence of a pyoderma suggests that the immune response of a dog may be defective, there currently is no easy, accurate test available to determine immunocompetence. Gross information as to immunocompetence may be derived from a complete blood count and serum electrophoresis. One would expect an absolute neutrophilia in an immunologically competent dog with an ongoing or recurrent pyoderma. Concomitantly, the absolute lymphocyte count should be at least 1000 to 1500/ml of blood for a dog to mount a reasonable cell-mediated response. A broad-based elevation in the beta and gamma region in serum electrophoresis should be noted but is probably less important than indications of T-cell response. *In vitro* lymphocyte blastogenesis and bactericidal assays are available currently, primarily as research tools.

OVERVIEW OF ANTIBACTERIAL THERAPY

In general, systemic antibiotics are not needed in the treatment of most *surface pyodermas.* Superficial bacterial overgrowth certainly contributes to the inflammatory process, but most cases of acute moist dermatitis, "hot spot," pyotraumatic dermatitis, or skin fold dermatitis (intertrigo) will respond to either topical therapy or anti-inflammatory drugs. Acute moist dermatitis without deep bacterial involvement usually responds to gentle cleansing, clipping, topical corticosteroids, and brief (5 to 7 days) systemic corticosteroid therapy at conventional anti-inflammatory dosages (prednisolone or prednisone 1 mg/kg/day). Skin fold dermatitis usually will respond palliatively to topical preparations such as benzoyl peroxide shampoos or gels. Surgical ablation of the underlying anatomic defect is curative. Impetigo, a superficial nonfollicular pyoderma seen primarily in young dogs, may require only topical therapy for successful management. Although canine acne currently is viewed as a disorder of follicular keratinization, secondary folliculitis and furunculosis are common. Benzoyl peroxide shampoos or gels are palliative before puberty, and systemic antibiotic therapy may not be necessary. All other varieties of pyoderma usually require management with systemic antibiotics.

Table 2. *Systemic Dosage Levels of Antibiotics Useful in the Management of Canine Pyodermas*

Generic Name	Route of Administration	Suggested Dosage Level/Kg Body Weight
Erythromycin	PO	10 to 15 mg every 8 hr
Lincomycin	PO	22 mg every 12 hr
Oxacillin	PO	22 mg every 8 hr
Chloramphenicol	PO, IV	50 mg every 8 hr
Trimethoprim-sulfadiazine	PO	30 mg every 12 hr
Cephalexin	PO	22 mg every 12 hr
Gentamicin	SC	1 mg every 8 hr

Key: IV = intravenously; PO = orally; SC = subcutaneously.

Systemic antibiotic therapy is required for the successful management of most *superficial and deep pyodermas.* Although product choice and regimens may vary between clinicians, all other forms of antibacterial therapy should be viewed as adjunctive or ancillary.

Topical therapy may be quite beneficial and will encourage healing, aid débridement, and decrease pruritus or pain. However, shampoos, soaks, or whirlpools should be used in conjunction with systemic antibiotic therapy.

Adjunctive immunomodulatory therapy is controversial in the management of pyodermas. Although killed bacterial products or immune-modulating drugs such as levamisole may be beneficial in certain dogs, they should not be viewed as substitutes for systemic antibiotic therapy.

SYSTEMIC ANTIBIOTIC THERAPY

Antibiotics chosen for the management of canine pyodermas should have a known spectrum of activity against *S. intermedius* (Table 2). Since pyodermas frequently require long-term therapy, narrow-spectrum agents may cause less alteration in gastrointestinal flora. However, the author has seen few problems associated with long-term use of broad-spectrum antibiotics. There is little evidence that bactericidal agents are more effective than bacteriostatic agents if host defense mechanisms are not impaired. If immunosuppression is confirmed or suspected, a bactericidal antibiotic should be selected.

The choice of an antibiotic may be based on empirical considerations or on a bacterial culture and sensitivity test. Empirical therapy is justified initially in the management of most superficial and some deep pyodermas. Empirical therapy also should be used in deep pyodermas while awaiting the results of bacterial culture. Any antibiotic chosen empirically should have a known spectrum of activity against *S. intermedius*. Ideally, the antibiotic should not be inactivated by β-lactamase (pencillinase), since coagulase-positive staphylococci frequently develop the ability to elaborate this enzyme. Erythromycin, lincomycin, and β-lactamase-resistant penicillins such as oxacillin are narrow-spectrum antibiotics that have proved useful empirically.

Erythromycin is a bacteriostatic macrolide antibiotic that inhibits bacterial ribosomal protein synthesis. It is an excellent, inexpensive antibiotic for the treatment of pyodermas. Cross-resistance frequently occurs with lincomycin. The erythromycin base and stearate used in veterinary medicine have a very low toxicity. Vomiting is the only common side effect in dogs. Careful adherence to recommended dosage regimens decreases the occurrence of gastrointestinal upset. Erythromycin may be given to dogs with impaired renal function since it is metabolized and excreted by the liver.

Lincomycin is a macrolide-like antibiotic with a similar mode of action. Although lincomycin is more expensive than erythromycin, it may be given only twice daily and has a much lesser frequency of side effects. Consequently, lincomycin is an excellent antibiotic for dermatologic use. As mentioned previously, cross-resistance with erythromycin is common. If erythromycin proves ineffective, lincomycin should not be chosen as an alternative.

Beta-lactamase-resistant penicillins are excellent bactericidal antibiotics that inhibit bacterial cell wall synthesis. Oxacillin, nafcillin, cloxacillin, and dicloxacillin are all members of this group. In canine pyodermas, staphylococcal resistance to oxacillin is quite rare. Preliminary observations indicate that dicloxacillin may be less effective than oxacillin in dogs. Since food interferes with absorption, this group of antibiotics must be administered at least 1 hour before or after feeding. In general, β-lactamase-resistant penicillins are more expensive than most other orally administered antibiotics except the cephalosporins.

Broad-spectrum antibiotics that have proved useful in empirical therapy include chloramphenicol, the trimethoprim-potentiated sulfonamides (Tribrissen, Burroughs Wellcome), and cephalosporins such as cephalexin. Chloramphenicol is a bacteriostatic antibiotic that inhibits bacterial ribosomal protein synthesis. It has broad-spectrum activity directed against staphylococci and many gram-negative bacteria, with the exception of *Pseudomonas*. Chloramphenicol commonly is used empirically since it is inexpensive and few side effects are seen. Since chloramphenicol causes a reversible depression of liver microsomal enzymes, the effects of liver-detoxified drugs such as barbiturates may be prolonged. Chloramphenicol may be given to dogs with renal disease since it is inactivated by the liver.

Trimethoprim-potentiated sulfonamides such as Tribrissen inhibit sequential steps in bacterial metabolism and are effective against many strains of staphylococci and some gram-negative rods. Tribrissen has been used extensively for canine pyodermas. Keratoconjunctivitis sicca is the most commonly reported side effect, and recent work by Werner and Bright (1983) documents a polysystemic drug-induced immune hypersensitivity disorder in Doberman pinschers. Until more information is available, the author does not recommend Tribrissen for Doberman pinschers.

Cephalosporins are bactericidal antibiotics that attack bacterial cell walls by interfering with polypeptide cross-linkages. They are active against *S. intermedius* as well as many secondary cutaneous pathogens such as *Proteus mirabilis* and some species of *Pseudomonas*. Cephalexin (Keflex, Elanco) has been used extensively in veterinary dermatology. Cefadroxil (Ultracef/Tabs, Bristol), a newly marketed cephalosporin, may also prove useful. Unfortunately, abuse of cephalosporins has led to increased bacterial resistance. Consequently, although cephalosporins are excellent drugs for the management of pyodermas, they should be reserved for severe mixed-bacteria infections or life-threatening disease.

Erythromycin, lincomycin, oxacillin, chloramphenicol, and Tribrissen are the preferred antibiotics for empirical therapy in the treatment of canine pyodermas. Penicillin, ampicillin, amoxicillin, tetracycline, and non-trimethoprim-potentiated sulfa drugs are inappropriate for empirical therapy, since staphylococci isolated from canine pyodermas are sensitive to these antibiotics in fewer than 20 per cent of cultures. Empirical selection is justified if the history, physical findings, and a smear of pustular contents indicate the likelihood of an uncomplicated superficial pyoderma caused by staphylococcus. Empirical therapy with cephalosporin antibiotics is justified only while awaiting bacterial culture in severe, deep, life-threatening pyodermas, since resistance to these potentially lifesaving antibiotics is increasing. On rare occasions, especially in dogs with generalized demodicosis and mixed gram-positive and gram-negative sepsis, the empirical combined use of a β-lactamase-resistant penicillin such as oxacillin and an aminoglycoside such as gentamicin is justified. In general, aminoglycosides (gentamicin, tobramycin, amikacin) have little use in dermatology. Parenteral administration is required, and frequent monitoring is necessary to avoid toxicity. Drug cost, monitoring, hospitalization, nephrotoxicosis, and ototoxicosis limit the use of aminoglycosides.

Bacterial culture and sensitivity testing should be performed when empirical therapy has not been effective. In addition, culture is advisable if infections are deep, chronic, or caused by more than one species of bacteria. If cultures are performed, antibiotics should be chosen not only based on sensitivity testing but also on proven efficacy. In general, antibiotics that are good empirical choices also are employed when culture indicates the likelihood of efficacy.

If a staphylococcus is not isolated as the primary pathogen, reculture should be performed. In mixed infections, if all of the isolates are not sensitive to one antibiotic or if they are sensitive only to an aminoglycoside or cephalosporin, an antibiotic effective against the staphylococcus should be chosen. Since staphylococci create an environment favorable for the replication of other bacteria, usually the elimination of the staphylococci is sufficient to cure a pyoderma.

Improper dosage of systemic antibiotics is a common reason for treatment failure in canine pyodermas. Consequently, all dogs receiving systemic antibiotics should be weighed accurately. Dosage errors occur most commonly with very large or very small dogs.

Systemic antibiotics must be administered for long enough to ensure cure rather than transient remission. Once initiated, antibiotic therapy always should be maintained for a minimum of 10 days. Superficial pyodermas usually require at least 3 weeks of therapy, and antibiotics should be administered for 5 days beyond apparent cure. The duration of required antibiotic therapy for deep pyodermas is highly variable, but antibiotics probably should be administered for at least 2 weeks beyond apparent clinical cure. Therapy lasting 8 to 12 weeks is not uncommon. Owners anxious to discontinue expensive therapy after initial improvement and remission frequently are unwittingly responsible for relapses. The veterinarian should be responsible for the decision to discontinue therapy.

TOPICAL THERAPY

Topical therapy is an important adjunct in the management of canine pyodermas. In general, topical therapy may be employed to decrease pain and pruritus, aid in débridement, and encourage drainage, re-epithelialization, and healing. More subtly, topical therapy may be beneficial in improving the patient's attitude and in maintaining the support of the owner if discouragement is associated with odor or exudation. After apparent cure, shampoos may be beneficial in preventing or delaying the recurrence of pyodermas.

In the management of superficial pyodermas, twice-weekly shampoos aid in the removal of crusts and exudates, thereby speeding recovery. After recovery, the long-term weekly use of antibacterial or antiseborrheic shampoos may discourage exacerbations in dogs susceptible to recurrent pyodermas.

Deep pyodermas require more aggressive topical therapy. Long-haired dogs should be clipped as closely as possible to encourage drainage, discourage matting, and to ensure the successful use of shampoos, whirlpools, or soaks. Initially, in severely exudative deep pyodermas, shampoos and whirlpools may be necessary before clipping can be accomplished. Occasionally, sedation may be indicated. After hair removal, daily antibacterial shampoo and daily or twice-daily whirlpools or soaks may be invaluable during the first 1 to 2 weeks of therapy. After initial hospitalization, shampoos, soaks, or even whirlpools may be continued at home by the conscientious owner. As in the management of superficial pyodermas, after cure, weekly shampoos may prevent recurrences.

Antibacterial shampoos are the most commonly employed effective topical therapy for canine pyodermas. Shampoos remove crusts and scales, discourage matting, and diminish pain and pruritus. Currently, benzoyl peroxide is considered to be the most effective antibacterial agent in shampoos.* Benzoyl peroxide penetrates unchanged through the stratum corneum and follicular orifice and is converted metabolically to benzoic acid within both the epidermis and dermis. In addition to the direct antibacterial action of benzoic acid, benzoyl peroxide–containing products also have a beneficial follicular-flushing effect. The benzoyl peroxide molecule is unstable, and special procedures are required in production and packaging. The author has seen considerable variation in efficacy and the propensity for the development of irritation reactions among the many products marketed. Oxydex (DVM) and Pyoben (Allerderm) are the only brand names currently recommended. Because of the aforementioned problems, the purchase of generic products

**Editor's Note:* Nolvasan shampoo (Fort Dodge) is an emollient product containing chlorhexidine. It is particularly useful in the dog with pyoderma superimposed on a dry skin and coat (seborrhea sicca). Benzoyl peroxide–containing shampoos exacerbate pre-existing dry skin and coat.

and bulk buying with repackaging should be discouraged.

Warm water and contact time are the most important factors in soaks or whirlpools. Dogs should be submerged up to their neck, preferably in whirlpool-agitated water, for a minimum of 10 to 15 minutes daily. The most beneficial agents to add to water in soaks and whirlpools are povidone-iodine (Betadine, Purdue Frederick) or chlorhexidine (Nolvasan, Fort Dodge). Iodine complexed with polyvinylpyrrolidone (povidone-iodine) is less irritating to skin and mucous membranes and is slowly released to the tissues. Further, povidone-iodine is more resistant to inactivation by pus, blood, serum, or necrotic debris. Chlorhexidine is a synthetic, broad-spectrum, biguanide antibacterial agent. Eight ounces or more of a whirlpool concentrate of either product are added to a 20- to 30-gallon tub. Whirlpools remain the least used but most beneficial method of topical therapy in the management of pyodermas.

Topical antibacterial agents in cream, gel, or ointment bases have very limited applicability in the management of pyodermas. The use of benzoyl peroxide products (Oxydex Gel, DVM; Pyoben Gel, Allerderm) in the management of skin fold dermatitides and canine acne is an exception. Because of their messiness, surface area considerations, cost, and the desire of the dog to lick the medication off the skin, topical products containing antibiotics or a combination of antibiotics and corticosteroids should be reserved primarily for otic infections.

ADJUNCTIVE THERAPY

Adjunctive immunomodulatory therapy may be attempted in the treatment of canine pyodermas in patients with a history of response to long-term antibiotic therapy followed by relapse after cessation of therapy. In addition, immunomodulatory therapy may be considered in patients with either confirmed or suspected defects in their ability to cope with bacterial infection. No double-blind studies have evaluated the efficacy of immunomodulatory or immunostimulatory agents in the management of canine pyodermas. In most circumstances, clinicians use such agents in conjunction with antibiotic and topical therapy. Consequently, evaluation has been highly empirical. Claims of efficacy for various products have ranged from zero to as high as 80 per cent. Currently, the author can only recommend two products, Staphage Lysate (Delmont) and levamisole (Levasole, Pitman Moore).

Staphage Lysate is a human product made by lysing cultures of serologic type I and III *S. aureus* with a polyvalent staphylococcus bacteriophage. The ultrafiltrated lysate contains antigenic fractions of *S. aureus* plus active bacteriophage. Clinical benefits may be associated either with stimulation of antibacterial antibody formation or more likely with a beneficial effect on T-cell reactivity to staphylococci. The author uses Staphage Lysate primarily in patients with antibiotic-responsive or partially responsive recurrent pyodermas. This therapy may be most beneficial in patients with pruritic superficial pyodermas. Current protocol at the University of California involves SC administration of 1 ml of Staphage Lysate weekly. If efficacy is noted, long-term therapy is continued. Therapy is discontinued when the clinician or the owner becomes disillusioned with lack of efficacy. Somewhat unscientifically, the author has the clinical impression that Staphage Lysate therapy is beneficial in approximately 20 per cent of patients. No satisfactory method has been determined to delineate in advance which dogs will respond. Kunkle (1985) at the University of Florida has seen quivering and vomiting for as long as 12 hours after injection as an occasional side effect. Antihistamines were not beneficial in eliminating these side effects.

Levamisole is a chemically simple agent with certain immunomodulatory properties. It may restore T lymphocyte and phagocyte function in compromised hosts. Dosage is critical, since higher or lower than optimal dosages may produce immunosuppressive rather than immunostimulatory effects. Somewhat empirically, clinicians have been using 2.2 mg/kg PO every other day in dogs. Although occasional apparent efficacy has been noted, the author believes that levamisole has been effective in fewer than 10 per cent of his patients.

No other immunomodulatory drugs currently are recommended as being even occasionally efficacious.

FACTORS COMPLICATING MANAGEMENT

Treatment failures with properly chosen therapy or disease recurrence usually are associated with the lack of recognition of both intrinsic and extrinsic factors complicating management.

Most dosages of antibiotics recommended for the treatment of pyodermas are largely empirical. Little information is available on dosage required to maintain adequate antibiotic concentrations in the skin. The skin is perfused by only about 4 per cent of cardiac blood output, as compared with 33 per cent for muscle. In one study (Marshall, 1980), subcutaneous tissue received 60 per cent and the dermoepidermal junction received 40 per cent of peak serum concentrations of a synthetic penicillin. In deep pyodermas, sequestered foci of infection further impede antibiotic penetration. Foreign body–type granulomatous response to dermal keratin debris from disrupted hair follicles may prevent the elimination of infection. In addition, many antibiotics are partially inactivated by purulent debris. Penicillins are less effective when obstructed drainage routes, necrotic tissue, or abscesses create conditions that are no longer favorable for bacterial replication, since penicillins are lethal only to bacteria that are rapidly multiplying and synthesizing cell walls. Consequently, higher dosages of systemic antibiotics may be warranted in the management of chronic, deep pyodermas.

Diagnosed or undiagnosed concomitant diseases may hinder management. Pruritus either associated with a pyoderma or associated with another disease is a common complicating factor. The clinician and owner must ascertain if pruritus is still present when a recurrent pyoderma has been abolished. If antibiotic therapy completely eliminates pruritus, then it must be assumed that the pruritus is caused by the pyoderma. In these circumstances, long-term antibiotic therapy and Staphage Lysate may be beneficial. If pruritus is not eliminated by the resolution of the pyoderma, then underlying diseases such as flea allergy, atopy, food allergy, seborrhea, and contact dermatitis must be investigated. If the search for an underlying pruritic disease is not successful, recurrence of the pyoderma is likely.

With or without pruritus, other factors such as demodicosis, seborrhea, hypothyroidism, steroid abuse, or an immunoincompetent host may complicate management. External factors such as owner compliance, vomiting of drug, and drug inactivation by food also must be considered.

ASSESSMENT OF ANTIBIOTIC THERAPY

All dogs receiving systemic antibiotics for the management of pyodermas should be re-examined 7 to 10 days after therapy is initiated. If substantial improvement is not noted, the clinician should re-evaluate the choice and dosage of antibiotic. All potential factors complicating management should be reviewed. If no errors are delineated, then the clinician should consider the basis for diagnosis of pyoderma, since therapeutic failure may be due to misdiagnosis.

References and Supplemental Reading

Ihrke, P. J.: The managment of canine pyodermas. *In* Kirk, R. W., (ed.): *Current Veterinary Therapy VIII*. Philadelphia: W. B. Saunders, 1983, pp. 505–517.

Ihrke, P. J.: Therapeutic strategies involving antimicrobial treatment of the skin in small animals. J.A.V.M.A. 185:1165, 1984.

Ihrke, P. J., Sousa, C. A., and Reinke, S. I.: Diagnostic Techniques in Dermatology. Proc. 51st Meet. Am. Anim. Hosp. Assoc. 1984, pp. 85–88.

Kunkle, G.: Personal Communication, 1985.

Marshall, A. B.: Antibiotic therapy of small animal dermatitis. Br. Vet. Dermatol. Newsletter 2:45, 1980.

Miller, W. H.: The pruritic dog. *In* Kirk, R. W. (ed.): *Current Veterinary Therapy VIII*. Philadelphia: W. B. Saunders, 1983, pp. 499–505.

Muller, G. H., Kirk, R. W., and Scott, D. W.: *Small Animal Dermatology*, 3rd ed. Philadelphia: W. B. Saunders, 1983, pp. 146–149, 158–165, 197–239.

Werner, L. L., and Bright, J. M.: Drug-induced immune hypersensitivity disorders in two dogs treated with trimethoprim sulfadiazine. J. Am. Anim. Hosp. Assoc. 19:783, 1983.

PARASITICIDE THERAPY IN SMALL ANIMAL DERMATOLOGY

J. M. MacDONALD, D.V.M.,
Auburn, Alabama

and T. A. MILLER, D.V.M.
Elwood, Kansas

Parasite-related diseases represent a large portion of small animal dermatology. Regional influences account for some variation of the intensity because of climatic conditions or seasonal changes. Millions of dollars are spent annually by the pet-owning public to fight the adversities of ectoparasites. The market seems flooded with an array of products, and still more are in the formative stage. Sound advice to the pet owner and realistic management of parasitic disease have become increasingly enigmatic for the veterinarian. The era of environmental awareness and increasing concern for human health risks puts further pressure on the veterinarian. What are the characteristics of the ideal parasiticide? It should have desirable efficacy (acute and prolonged), low or no toxicity, no residual environmental accumulation, and minimal ecologic interference. It should be relatively inexpensive, convenient to administer or use, well tolerated by the animal, and aesthetically acceptable to the pet owner. Competitively, manufacturers strive to meet all these expectations. What can veterinarians who dispense products for the control of ectoparasites on companion animals expect from these products? What will they read on the label, and what will it mean? Who determines what may or must appear on the label, and what are the criteria for such determinations?

Most ectoparasiticides and all products for environmental insect control are regulated by the Environmental Protection Agency (EPA). The few products that are administered orally or that are systemically absorbed after dermal application (e.g., cythioate, amitraz, fenthion) are regulated by the Food and Drug Administration (FDA). Products for application to companion animals and the home environment alone are of minor interest to the developers of the new insecticides, since limited potential sales of such products could not justify the cost of obtaining initial registration. Thus, the registration of companion animal formulations is usually obtained last, after efficacy data on crop pests. Extrapolations from efficacy on crop pests to that on pests of companion animals (fleas, ticks, mites) are made freely. Registration of new companion animal ectoparasiticides is often made in the absence of controlled efficacy data on the target insect and with little safety data on the target host (dog, cat, or horse).

Although at this time there is no enforced requirement for efficacy data by the EPA for registration of every companion animal formulation, some companies may conduct such evaluations to generate label efficacy claims. These are usually performed in the following order:

1. Laboratory studies are conducted with the target fleas or ticks in a cage or dish, where they are dusted or wetted with the product to determine immediate efficacy.
2. Residual activity is measured by spraying or wetting a surface with the product to observe efficacy days, weeks, or months after treatment. From these data, manufacturers freely extrapolate claims of residual efficacy under practical conditions on the coat of companion animals and environmental surfaces.
3. Controlled efficacy data are rarely generated on the target parasite with respect to a specific host under practical conditions of experimental or natural infestation and reinfestation. Although efficacy data to support label claims are required by the EPA, few companies subject their formulations to tests outlined in the third category above. Consequently, the veterinarian or consumer may well adopt the attitude of *caveat emptor*.

Registration of some ectoparasiticide products classed as pharmaceuticals and regulated by the FDA require a much larger dossier of supporting data on efficacy and safety. The requirements for FDA registration of new pharmaceuticals are stringent. When treating single animals, it is often difficult for the veterinarian to assess product efficacy accurately and quickly. Pet owners are notorious for misunderstanding and failing to follow instructions. Treatment of a single dog in its home environment cannot be part of an acceptable protocol for scientifically measuring efficacy and residual activity against fleas and ticks. In the absence of published data, veterinarians must use their own judgment from repeated observations. Thus, veterinarians are faced with accepting manufacturers' claims based on limited data or relying on their own observations, which are not controlled. Skepticism about manufacturers' claims of residual activity is justified, unless such claims are well supported.

Assessing product safety is difficult for veterinarians. Caution and warning labels on pesticide products registered by the EPA are designed to protect the user and to warn the veterinarian. When first trying a new product with new active ingredients, be very cautious and monitor safety carefully. Prescribing and dispensing parasiticides is a professional and legal responsibility. Liability is too often taken lightly or ignored completely. Extralabel use of products and improper repackaging procedures constitute most infractions.

REPACKAGING PARASITICIDES

EPA regulations on use, repackaging, or mixing parasiticides are both specific and enforceable. Veterinarians' lack of familiarity with these products leaves them vulnerable to legal assault. Veterinarians can dispense nonrestricted-use pesticides as long as the intended use is consistent with the product's original label specifications.

Repackaging labels must contain the following information on each container:

1. The common or trade names of the product.
2. The names of active ingredients as listed on the original label, with their concentrations.
3. The EPA product registration number.
4. Directions for the prescribed use.
5. A statement of antidote.
6. Directions for the disposal of the pesticide and package.
7. Child hazard warning.
8. Human safety precautionary statements.

SYSTEMS OF PARASITICIDAL APPLICATION

Sprays (Prediluted)

Sprays are the most widely sold ectoparasite control products dispensed by veterinarians (Table 1). Formulations for applying them to small animals and premises differ in many respects. Most animal formulations can be applied to carpets, furnishings, or the pet's bedding, but environmental sprays often contain substances with specific contraindications to application on animals. It is wasteful to apply animal-targeted products, which are usually higher priced, to flooring and furnishings. They often contain repellents, grooming aids, coat conditioners (lanolin, aloe), humectants, and fragrances that are unnecessary and undesirable.

Spray products are prediluted, ready to use, and packaged in 8-, 12-, 16-, 32-, 64-, and 128-oz containers with sprayers controlled by fingertip pumps, triggers, or remote triggers (for gallon bottles). Some products are also packaged in pressurized aerosol containers. Application from pressurized aerosol containers has considerable user appeal, but the noise is resented by pets. Per-unit cost of insecticide in pressurized aerosol packages is about twice that of products marketed in trigger- or pump-sprayer packages, so sales of pressurized products are less.

Trigger sprayers have a history of mechanical problems with defective and leaky pumps. The physical effort and "finger fatigue" resulting from attempts to spray more than 8 to 12 ounces at a time are real drawbacks of manual sprayers. This may be tolerated when applying the product to a small pet, which only requires 2 to 5 ml per pound body weight for good coat cover. The same system used to apply 1 gallon per 1600 to 2000 ft^2 of flooring is a herculean task. This is an additional reason why the pet owner readily treats the pet but does a poor job of environmental control. Prediluted spray products for indoor surface application may be purchased in refill containers and applied by compressed air sprayers. Sprayers should be washed well after use, since seals and pistons may be damaged by prolonged exposure to the organic solvents.

Children and pets should be kept off treated surfaces until the spray dries. There is justified concern about spraying the carpet on which the baby crawls with cholinesterase-depressing insecticides. Residual sprays based on pyrethrins, especially those containing stabilized (Adams) and microencapsulated (3M) pyrethrins, are preferred.

Ready-to-use spray products comprise two classes depending on the liquid diluent (water or isopropanol). Water-based products are cheaper. Alcohol accounts for as much as 50 per cent of the cost in alcohol-based sprays. Water-based products do not penetrate greasy coats and fabrics as rapidly and thoroughly as do alcohol-based products, and the surface does not dry as quickly. Alcohol-based products have a potential flammability risk, their odor may be resented by the animal, and they may irritate inflamed or abraded skin. They dry out the coat, and the solvent redistributes the natural fats and oils. Alcohol-based products may damage wood finished with paints or varnishes, and some plastics. The insecticide solution in alcohol-based products is transported very rapidly through the insect cuticle to produce an immediate effect. In contrast, most insecticides are insoluble in water-based products. They are in an emulsion that does not penetrate the insect but depends on the development of the insecticide's vapor pressure following the drying of the water vehicle.

Most spray products for animals contain synergized pyrethrin for immediate action (as long as 24 hours), although a few contain pyrethroids instead. Some sprays may contain organophosphates or carbamates, either alone or in conjunction with synergized pyrethrins. Many sprays also contain a repellent. Two new patented products contain microencapsulated (3M) or stabilized (Adams) synergized pyrethrins. These products have claims of both immediate and residual efficacy without the use of organophosphates, carbamates, or chlorinated hydrocarbons. It is expected that sprays containing the more stable pyrethroids, particularly permethrin, used alone or in combination with synergized pyrethrin, will predominate in the marketplace within the next few years.

When spraying the pet, care should be taken not to spray the product into its eyes, mouth, or nose. The entire body surface including the legs and tail should be sprayed systematically. Spray may be applied on a cotton swab or with the fingers to areas around the face. All animal sprays, and especially those with flammable bases, should be applied in areas of adequate ventilation. Care should be taken not to expose alcohol-based sprays or recently sprayed animals to open flames. The pet should also be prevented (as much as possible) from licking the wet coat. Alcohol-based sprays dry quickly. Use of water-based products may be accompanied by blow drying the coat to accelerate the drying process. If nursing puppies or kittens are treated, they should not be sprayed completely; rather, small amounts of spray can be applied with a swab or dabbed onto their backs. Ventilation of the nest after treatment of nursing animals is important, especially with alcohol-based sprays. Recommendations and contraindications vary with each product depending on the active ingredient. Give pregnant, sick, convalescent or young animals particular considerations. Read labels and follow instructions closely.

Table 1. *Insecticide Sprays (% w/w)*

Manufacturer*	Product Name	Carbaryl	Propoxur	Malathion	Chlorpyrifos	Methoxychlor	Pyrethrins	Allethrin	Tetramethrin	D-Phenothrin	Resmethrin	Phenothrin	PBO	MGK 264†	MGK 11†	MGK 326†	D-Limonene	Butox. PPG	Linalool
AD	Flea-Off Mist						0.15						1.5	0.5	0.5				
AD	14 Day Residual Mist						0.10						0.37	0.61	0.2	0.2			
AD	Caniderm Mist						0.20						0.75	2.0	0.5				
AD	Feliderm Mist						0.20						0.75	2.0	0.5				
AL	Duo-Cide Spray								0.05	0.1									
AV	Super Veta Flea & Tick Spray							0.15						1.5					
BC	FLT Spray & Aerosol	1.0						0.06						0.6					5.0
BE	Mycodex Mist	2.5						0.06						0.6					
BE	Mycodex Mist Plus	2.5						0.06						0.6					5.0
BE	Mycodex Flea & Tick Spray		0.25																
BE	Mycodex Aqua Spray						0.20						2.0	0.5					
BV	Para Pyrethrin Mist						0.15						1.5	0.33	0.2				
BV	Paramist W.B.						0.15						1.5	0.33					
BV	Para M-1 Press Spray			0.5			0.06						0.48		0.24				
BV	Para S-1 Aerosol	0.5				0.5	0.06						0.48		0.24				
BV	Sendran F+T Spray		0.25																
CA	Aqua-Methrin								0.05			0.1							
CA	DFT Spray	2.5																5.0	
CA	DFT Spray Plus	2.5					0.06						0.6					5.0	
CA	Parid-X Spray						0.18						1.8					10.0	
CA	Parid-X Spray + Carbaryl	1.0					0.18						1.8					10.0	
CA	Parid Press. Spray	2.5																5.0	
CA	Sectrol Spray						0.11						0.22	0.37					

CA	Supra Quick Mist					0.1			0.2	0.33	0.5				
CO	Flair	0.5		0.5		0.06			0.48		0.14		5.0		
CO	Mistaway Xtra					0.15			1.5	0.5	0.5				
DV	Durakyl Spray							0.40							
DV	Durakyl Aerosol						0.15	0.20							
EL	Flyte Spray	0.5				0.15			1.0						
EV	Liqui-Ban				0.22										
EV	Liquidate	0.5				0.05			0.5		0.2				
EV	Liqua-Sect					0.1			0.2	0.33					
EV	Sect-A-Chlor				0.22										
EV	Sect-A-Cide	0.5				0.05			0.1	0.16					
EV	Sect-A-Spray	0.5				0.05			0.5		0.2				
HI	Flea & Tick Spray											5.0			
HI	Flea Pet Spray								0.5					0.93	
NO	Heathcliff's Flea & Tick Spray					0.06			0.12	0.20					
NO	Marmaduke Flea & Tick Spray			0.22											
PF	Clinicare Pet Spray	0.5				0.05			0.1	0.24					
PM	Paladin Spray			0.5		0.06			0.48		0.24				
PM	Pestisol-R Spray		0.5			0.15			1.5	0.5	0.5				
PM	Sprecto Spray	0.5				0.05			0.1	0.4	0.2				
SO	Disrodan Flea/Tick Mist					0.15			1.5	0.33	0.2				
TA	Controller Flea-Kill Mist					0.15			1.5	0.5	0.5				
TA	Controller Flea-Kill Aerosol					0.15			1.5	0.5	0.5				
TA	Controller Flea & Tick Mist					0.15			1.5						
TA	Controller Derm. Mist					0.15			1.5						
TA	Controller Feline Mist					0.15			1.5						
TA	Controller Puppy & Kitten Mist					0.15			1.5						
VK	Pet Spray					0.05			0.1	0.17					
VK	Flea & Tick Pump Spray Mist					0.15			1.5	0.33	0.2				

*See Table 7 for key to manufacturers.
†McLaughlin, Gormley, King Co.

Emulsifiable Concentrates

This group includes dips for animal application and concentrates for yard and kennel sprays. These are usually sold in 4-, 8-, or 16-oz containers for dilution with water.

Dips

Because of their ingredients dips are generally assumed to have some residual activity (Table 2). They are often applied to a pet after shampoos. By action of their detergents or surfactants, most shampoos will kill many of the existing flea population even though they do not contain an insecticide. If an animal is not dried between rinsing off the shampoo and application of the dip, poor results may be achieved because of the dilution factor of the wet coat.

Dips usually contain more toxic insecticides and are stable for a variable amount of time after dilution. This may be as little as 24 hours. Consult labels before use. Discard diluted dips if contaminated with debris, hair, or urine. When discarding any pesticide, follow the label cautions about the risks of environmental contamination. Apply dips at a frequency that is consistent with label restrictions. To obtain maximum efficacy, do not rinse the animal after application of the dip.

Yard and Kennel Sprays

This group contains emulsifiable concentrates containing a residual insecticide (organophosphate or carbamate). Occasionally, such products also contain synergized pyrethrin for its immediate knockdown effect. Since these products are used mostly outdoors, they tend to contain some of the more stable and hence toxic residual insecticides. They also frequently leave stronger odors following application. They must not be applied to animals. These products can be applied by a hose-end sprayer or by compressed air or other power spraying equipment. They should be applied (within reason) anywhere the pet visits and the parasite may be found. Particular attention should be paid to the kennel and doghouse, including the inside walls, ceiling, outside walls, and roof. If the dog has excavated under its house in a dirt run, that area should also be treated. If the pet roams free in the yard, particular attention should be paid to favorite resting places (e.g., crawl space, patio, porch, and favorite shady area under a tree or bush). As with all pesticides, observe directions, cautions, and contraindications. Emulsifiable concentrates are the most concentrated, toxic, and potentially dangerous pesticide formulations available to veterinarians and pet owners.

Shampoos

The main purpose of a shampoo is to clean the coat and skin. The emulsifiers, detergents, and surfactants in shampoos will kill a high proportion of fleas. Insecticidal shampoos are usually formulated with synergized pyrethrin or nonresidual pyrethroids for immediate kill, but they have no residual efficacy. The rationale for this formulation is the common practice of following a shampoo with a residual dip. A few shampoos contain a residual insecticide such as a chlorinated hydrocarbon (lindane) or carbamate (carbaryl), presumably to eliminate the need for subsequent dipping. Shampoos containing cholinesterase-depressing materials should not be followed by the application of a residual dip containing the same class of compound.

Dusts

At one time, dusts were more popular for the control of ectoparasites of companion animals, but they have now been largely replaced by sprays (Table 3). This change can be attributed to a number of reasons. Sprays produce a more rapid and immediate effect. Even dusts that have synergized pyrethrin do not produce the quick kill that one achieves with sprays. Sprays are also easier to apply, especially to the underside of the animal and to areas of thin hair. Sprays do not leave a visible deposit in the coat and on the applicator and surrounding areas, as dusts do.

Dusts are considered to be primarily residual products to send home with the client for continued application to the pet. They are also labeled and recommended for environmental treatment (carpeting, furniture, and vacuum bags) and may be more effective than sprays or foggers for delivering the insecticide to the deepest areas of the carpet, where flea larvae live. Vacuuming will remove the insecticide-coated dust particles and therefore shorten the residual activity. There are few contraindications for dusts, even when they contain some of the more toxic actives. Dusting is one of the safest methods of insect control.

Foggers

Foggers are concentrated insecticide products in pressurized containers designed for total release as a fine aerosol. They are labeled for indoor treatment to control insects (including fleas) and arachnids

Table 2. *Insecticide Dips (% w/w)*

Manufacturer*	Product Name	Carbaryl	Propoxur	Malathion	Dioxathion	Chlorpyrifos	Phosmet	Supona	Rabon†	Lindane	Pyrethrins	Allethrin	Permethrine	Rotenone	Cube Extract	PBO	Amitraz	D-Limonene	Ronnel‡
AD	Flea-Off Dip			53															
BE	Mycodex Dip	8.5																	
BC	Permectrin II												10						
BV	Pro-Kill										0.8			1.1	2.2				
BV	Sendran Flea & Tick Dip		8																
CA	Ban-Guard					3.8													
CO	Dermaton II							12.3											
CO	Conav				27.5														
CO	Expar Dip												3.2						
CO	Kil-A-Mite			15					2										
DV	Durakyl Dip										0.8			1.1	2.2				
HD	Ectocide			57															
HI	VIP Dip II			32															
HI	VIP Flea & Tick Dip																	78	
NO	Norden Flea & Tick Dip					3.8													
PM	Ectoral Emuls. Conc.																		33
PM	Sprecto-D						11.6												
SO	Dirodan Sponge-on							50											
TA	Controller Dog Flea & Tick Dip					4.85													
TA	Controller Cat Flea & Tick Dip											2.95			11.84				
TA	Dermacide Dip			57															
UP	Mitaban																19.9		
VK	Paramite Dip						11.6												

*See Table 7 for key to manufacturers.
†Shell Chemical Co.
‡Dow Chemical

***Table 3.** Insecticide Powders (% w/w)*

Manufacturer*	Product Name	Carbaryl	Chlorfenvinphos	Rabon†	Phosmet‡	Pyrethrins	Rotenone	Cube Extract	PBO	Silica Gel
AD	Flea Off Dust II	12.5				0.1			1.0	10.0
BC	FLT Dust	5.0				0.1			1.0	
BE	Mycodex Powder	5.0								
BV	Para Powder	5.0								
CA	TF7 Powder	5.0								
CO	Dermaton Dust		0.5							
CO	Flea Powder for Cats	3.0								
HI	VIP Tick & Flea Powder	5.0				0.1			0.5	
PM	Diryl Powder	5.0				0.1			1.0	
RI	Ritters Powder	12.0								
SQ	Dirodan Powder			3.0						
TA	Controller Flea & Tick Dust	5.0								
TA	Controller Flea & Tick Dust Plus	5.0				0.01	0.12	0.14	0.1	
VK	Flea & Tick Powder	5.0								
VK	Paramite Powder				5.0					

*See Table 7 for key to manufacturers.
†Shell Chemical Co.
‡Stouffer Chemical Co.

(ticks and mites). Almost all contain one or more residual organophosphate insecticides, the most common being DDVP (Table 4). Some also contain a carbamate, and a few have a synergized pyrethrin or pyrethroids. One brand of fogger (Vet-Kem) contains methoprene (Precor, Zoecon Corp.), an insect growth regulator, in addition to a synergized pyrethrin and an organophosphate (see Table 4).

The convenience of foggers and their availability in supermarkets, lawn and garden shops, pet supply houses, and hardware stores accounts for their popularity. The reputation of fogger efficacy, however, suffers severely from misuse and misrepresentation of label instructions. Six-ounce foggers claim to be able to treat 5000 cubic feet. Few homes with a 7-ft ceiling have rooms with 700 square feet of unobstructed and continuous floor space. Since the droplet size is large, much of the product falls like a fountain within a circle about 15 to 20 ft in diameter around the point of discharge. Corners of rooms and flooring under furniture are not treated, and little of the product flows into closets or through doorways into adjacent rooms. The droplets dry on the surface of the floor covering without penetrating to the location of the flea larvae. Nevertheless, a good residual on the carpet surface will kill many of the larval fleas as they climb through the carpet fibers to pupate at the surface. Adequate treatment requires discharge of one fogger in almost every room, without reference to volume or floor space. Even then, little pesticide reaches sheltered floor surfaces (under beds, sofas, tables, chairs). It is essential to combine fogging with spray application to these sheltered areas, especially those frequently occupied by the pets.

A recent development is the mini-fogger. This device contains a fourfold concentrate (1.5 oz) of active ingredients in a small can with special valving and pressure. The resulting aerosol is much finer. Proponents claim the droplets remain suspended in the air longer, travel farther, pass through open doorways into adjacent rooms more readily, and are deposited more uniformly on sheltered surfaces. Several mini-foggers should be used per house and be strategically placed to obtain maximum coverage of all living areas. Even so, it is beneficial to spray surface areas frequented and favored by the pet, since the flooring and furnishings in those areas have the largest population of developing fleas. Most environments need treatment at regular intervals. If no previous treatment has been applied or if the infestation is significant, repeat treatments at intervals of 2 weeks for at least three treatments before assuming a maintenance schedule.

Systemics

Systemics are insecticide and acaricide products that are distributed by the animal's circulatory system. They act on the ectoparasite when it feeds on the animal's blood or tissue fluids. Systemics may be administered orally, by injection, or by dermal application (with rapid absorption and circulatory dissemination). Cythioate is the only systemic currently registered for use in companion animals.

Two available systemics are not labeled for use on companion animals or for ectoparasite control. Fenthion has been applied to the skin and is approved for use in cattle to control grubs (see page 588). Ivermectin is administered orally to horses and parenterally to cattle and is claimed to control some ectoparasites in addition to helminths. Phosmet applied dermally in a concentrated form is absorbed systemically and has insecticidal activity in cattle. It is also registered in a less concentrated form as a dip for companion animals.

Prescribing or selling these products for small animal use when they are only registered or approved for other species can result in serious malpractice and liability claims against the veterinarian. Note that the labeling of all registered pesticides states, "It is a violation of Federal Law to use this product in a manner inconsistent with its labeling." *That is the law.*

FORMULATIONS AND ACTIVE INGREDIENTS OF PARASITICIDES

Botanicals

PYRETHRIN. Pyrethrin is an extract of the pyrethrum or chrysanthemum flower. It has a very low mammalian toxicity. The commercial product contains six major chemicals with related insecticidal activity, hence the use of the plural, "pyrethrins." The most active are pyrethrins I and II. Pyrethrin II is noted for its very fast knockdown effect on flying insects and flushing action on fleas, and pyrethrin I contributes the major killing component of the extract's activity. Pyrethrins need synergizing to achieve maximum kill of insects. They are never used without synergists. Pyrethrins act on the insect's central nervous system, but there is no evidence yet of a specific enzyme inhibition, as with organophosphates and carbamates. The action is believed to be on excitable cell membranes, causing extended depolarization by maintenance of the sodium ion flow through membrane molecular structures. Pyrethrins are very rapidly degraded by ultraviolet light after application (4 hours or less). Prolongation of the activity to weeks may be accomplished by microencapsulation or stabilization techniques.

Pyrethrin is the most common insecticide in animal sprays and is also included in most shampoos and dusts for animal application. It is also incorporated into foggers and environmental sprays for an immediate insecticide effect. These contain other active ingredients such as organophosphates, carbamates, or synthetic pyrethroids for residual activity. Pyrethrin produces much more rapid action in organic solvent bases (e.g., alcohol) than in water-based emulsion products, in which it is virtually insoluble. There is no evidence of development of resistance in fleas or ticks of companion animals. It is used in the range of 0.05 to 0.20 per cent in ready-to-apply products and 0.2 to 2.0 per cent in concentrated products such as dips or foggers. The pyrethrin-to-synergist ratio is usually about 1:10.

Synergized pyrethrin is available in almost every category of product, including sprays for animals and premises, shampoos, dusts, dips, foggers, mini-foggers, yard and kennel spray concentrates, and wipe-on lotions (Tables 1–4). None of the insecticidal collars contains either pyrethrin or pyrethroids. Stabilized or microencapsulated pyrethrin is used in animal and premises sprays, mini-foggers, and dips. A comparison of pyrethrins and pyrethroids is presented in Table 5.

ROTENONE. Rotenone is an extract from the root of the derris plant. It contains two active ingredients, rotenone (1 part) and cube extracts (2 parts). It is more toxic than pyrethrin but is still considered relatively safe to mammals. It is very toxic to fish and swine. Rotenone is used in combination with synergized pyrethrin, lindane, or carbaryl in occasional dips, dusts, and spot treatment lotions, but its use is uncommon (Table 6). Its action is by paralysis of the insect's cardiovascular and respiratory systems. It does not require synergizing and is usually incorporated in ready-to-apply products at the level of 0.12 per cent (with 0.24 per cent cube extract) and in concentrated products at the level of 1.1 per cent (with 2.2 per cent cube extract).

D-LIMONENE. The insecticidal action of extracts of citrus peel has been known and used for a long time. There is some question of its efficacy compared with that of pyrethrin, rotenone, pyrethroids, and other synthetics. There is one report of severe toxicity to cats from an unregistered citrus extract product. It is used at relatively high levels (5 per cent in shampoos and sprays and 78 per cent in dips), compared with those of other active agents.

Synthetic Pyrethroids

These insecticides are synthesized chemicals modeled on the chrysanthemate molecule of natural pyrethrins, with various substitutions and modifications. The relative risk-benefit ratio of pyrethroids is compared with that of other insecticides in Table 8. A few pyrethroids are presently used in ectoparasiticides or premises sprays and foggers (Table 4). These include D-*trans*-allethrin, resemethrin, tetramethrin, and D-phenothrin. The residual activity of

Text continued on page 583

Table 4. Premise Sprays and Foggers (% w/w)

Manufacturer*	Product Name	Propoxur	Chlorpyrifos	D-Phenothrin	Malathion	Dichlorvos	Ronnel†	Ciodrin	Rabon‡	Pyrethrins	Permethrin	Allethrin	Resmethrin	Tetramethrin	Fenvalerate	PBO	MGK 264§	Methoprene
AD	Anti-Crawl	1.0				0.5												
AD	Surface Spray		0.5									0.5				1.5	0.4	
AD	Anti-Crawl Spray	1.0								0.05						0.1	0.17	
AV	Durafog									0.15						1.5		
AV	Duracide R Spray												6.0					
BE	Mycodex Mini Fogger			0.8								1.29						
BE	Mycodex Room & Carpet Spray		0.5							0.025						0.05	0.084	
BC	Overtime										10							
BV	Para Ban Fogger	1.0				0.5												
BV	Parapremise		0.5										0.1					
CA	Sectrol									0.11						0.22	0.37	
CA	Perm-Fog													0.2	0.4			
CO	Fogger 147	1.0				0.5												
CO	Fogger 5/10	1.0				0.5				0.4						0.8	1.55	
EV	Perm-A-Chlor		0.5															
EV	Sect-A-Cide	0.5								0.05						0.1	0.16	
EV	Sect-A-Fog	1.0				0.5												
NO	Marmaduke Fog	1.0								0.05						0.1	0.16	
PM	Sprecto-CF Fogger		0.05									0.05						
PM	Sprecto F Fogger			0.20								0.32					2.5	

SO	Yard & Kennel Spray Concentrate			5.3		23						
SO	Dirodan Fogger	1.0		0.47								
TA	Controller House & Carpet Spray		0.5									
TA	Controller Indoor Fogger	1.0		0.47								
TA	Yard & Kennel Spray		6.7									
TA	Room Fogger with Dursban		1.0				0.05			0.1	0.16	
VK	Yard & Kennel Spray		6.7									
VK	Siphotrol Premise Spray						0.2			1.0	1.0	0.03
VK	Siphotrol Plus	0.22					0.05			0.1	0.16	
VK	Siphotrol Plus Fogger							0.5				0.15
VK	Vet-Fog Fogger	1.0		0.47								
VK	Siphotrol 10 Fogger											0.15
VK	Siphotrol Plus II Fogger		0.225				0.05			0.1	0.165	0.014
HI	VIP Flea & Tick Fog-ger								0.5	1.0	1.0	
HI	VIP Hookworm (Flea & Tick) Concentrate			4.5	4.8							

*See Table 7 for key to manufacturers.
†Dow Chemical
‡Shell Chemical Co.
§McLaughlin, Gormley, King Co.

Table 5. Pyrethrins and Pyrethroids

Active	Mammalian Oral LD_{50} (gm/kg)	Insect Kill Efficacy (Rel. to Pyrethrum)	Knockdown (Rel. to Pyrethrum)	Synergist Improves Kill	Knockdown Agent Needed	Residual Activity (Days)	Stability (Rel. to Pyrethrum)	Product Uses
Pyrethrins	0.2–>5	1	Good	Yes	No	Hours	1	Sa, Sp, So, Dt, Dp, Fg, Mf, Yk, W
Stabilized pyrethrins	>5	1	Good	Yes	No	14–20	>30	Sa, Sp, Dp, Mf, W
D-*trans*-allethrin	0.5–2.4	4	Fair	Yes	No	Hours	1	Sa, Sp, So, Mf, W
Tetramethrin	2–>5	2	Good	Yes	No	Hours	1	Sa
D-Phenothrin	>5	1	Good	Yes	No	1–4	5–10	Sa, So, Mf
Resmethrin	0.7–>5	3–6	Poor	No	Yes	Hours	1	Sa, Sp, So
Fenvalerate	0.45	?	Fair	No	Yes	14–21	>30	None yet; Yk probable
Permethrin	4–>20	3–6	None	No	Yes	≥28	>40	Sp, Dp
Cypermethrin	0.1–>1	7–13	?	No	Yes	≥28	>40	Not registered
Deltamethrin	0.03–0.06	125–200	None	No	Yes	≥40	>60	Not registered

Key: Sa = animal spray, Sp = premises spray, So = shampoo, Dt = dust, Dp = dip, Fg = fogger, Mf = mini-fogger, Yk = yard and kennel spray concentrate, W = wipe, spot, or dab on.

Mammalian LD_{50} (rat-oral) varies with different solvents, techniques, and reports. Insect killing and knockdown relative to pyrethrins is *not* based on flea or tick data (none published) but on dipterous flies (houseflies, mosquitoes).

Table 6. Insecticide Spot Treatments (% w/w)

Manufacturer*	Product Name	Benzyl Benzoate	Fenthion	Lindane†	Pyrethrins	Rotenone	Cube Extract	PBO	MGK 264‡	MGK 11‡	MGK 326‡	Butox. PPG
AD	Earmite Lotion				0.15			1.5	0.5	0.5	0.5	
BC	Mange Lotion	19		0.1		0.12	0.24					
BV	Pro Spot		5.6									
CA	Mangex	30										
CA	Otomite				0.05			0.5				
CA	Pet-Guard Gel				0.1			1.0				10.0
CA	Supra Wick Roll-On				0.1			0.2	0.33	0.5		
FD	Demodek II	30										
HI	VIP Ointment				0.15			1.0				10.0
PM	Canex Solution					0.12	0.2					
TA	Controller Rep. Oint.				0.18			0.36	0.6	0.5		
TA	Demolene			0.10		0.12	0.24					
TA	Mange Lotion	20		0.25		0.05	1.0					

*See Table 7 for key to manufacturers.

†Recent EPA-mandated label revisions require the remaining lindane-containing products to carry label claims only for mites on dogs.

‡McLaughlin, Gormley, King Co.

Table 7. List of Manufacturers

Code	Manufacturer
AD	Adams Veterinary Research Laboratories, Inc. P.O. Box 971039 Miami, FL 33197
AL	Allerderm, Inc. Hurst, TX 76053
AV	A. V. Labs Miami, FL 33135
BC	Bio-Ceutic Laboratories P.O. Box 999 St. Joseph, MO 64502
BE	Beecham Laboratories 501 Fifth St. Bristol, TN 37620
BV	Bayvet Division Miles Laboratories Box 390 Shawnee, KS 66201
CA	Carson Chemicals, Inc. New Castle, IN 47362
CO	Coopers Animal Health Inc. 520 West 21st St. P.O. Box 167 Kansas City, MO 64141
DV	Dermatologics for Veterinary Medicine, Inc. Miami, FL 33172
EL	Elanco Products Co. 740 South Alabama St. Indianapolis, IN 46285
EV	EVSCO Pharmaceutical Corp. Buena, NJ 08310
FD	Fort Dodge Laboratories, Inc. 800 Fifth St. N.W. Fort Dodge, IA 50501
HD	Hart-Delta, Inc. 5055 Choctaw Dr. Baton Rouge, LA 70805
HI	Hill's Pet Chemicals, Inc. 7781 N.W. 73rd Ct. Miami, FL 33143
NO	Norden Laboratories P.O. Box 80809 Lincoln, NE 68501
PF	Pfizer, Inc. 235 East 42nd St. New York, NY 10017
PM	Pitman-Moore, Inc. P.O. Box 344 Washington Crossing, NJ 08560
SO	Solvay Veterinary, Inc. P.O. Box 7348 Princeton, NJ 08540
TA	TechAmerica Group, Inc. Animal Health Division P.O. Box 338 Elwood, KS 66024
UP	The Upjohn Company 7000 Portage Rd. Kalamazoo, MI 49001
VK	Vet-Kem (A Division of Zoecon Corp.) P.O. Box 340231 12200 Denton Dr. Dallas, TX 75234

these products, in general, is comparable to that of pyrethrin. Like natural pyrethrin, most produce a quick kill. Many benefit also from the inclusion of the synergists that are used with pyrethrin to improve their killing ability.

Mammalian toxicity and safety are variable. Some of the less stable pyrethroids have lower toxicities than pyrethrin (e.g., D-phenothrin, resemethrin, tetramethrin), whereas others are more toxic (D-*trans*-allethrin, cypermethrin, deltamethrin). Some pyrethroids have undesirable side effects. Resmethrin, for example, degrades in ultraviolet light, leaving a heavy odor of stale urine. A bronzing of the human skin may occur with excessive use of some concentrated pyrethroids as a result of photosensitization after exposure to ultraviolet light. Fenvalerate and permethrin tend to be absorbed to synthetic fibers, such as nylon carpet, and either lose their residual activity altogether or are released at sublethal levels. This enhances the development of insecticide resistance. The potential for this development is greater with synthetic monomolecular structures of pyrethroids, especially those with low vapor pressure and more stable molecules that persist in the insect's microenvironment for prolonged periods of time.

The second-generation pyrethroids are less expensive than natural pyrethrin, since they are man-

Table 8. Benefit-Risk Ratio of Insecticide Classes

Class	Mammalian Toxicity (mg/kg)	Insect Toxicity (mg/kg)	Relative Benefit Value
Carbamates	45	2.8	16
Organophosphates	67	2.0	33
Organochlorine	230	2.6	91
Pyrethroid	2000	0.45	4500

Figures are derived by relating the safety factor in mammals (usually rat oral LD_{50}) to the toxicity of that insecticide class to insects (usually contact LD_{50} in flies).

From Elliot, M.: Synthetic Pyrethroids, American Chemical Symposium, No. 42, 1977, p. 2.

ufactured in the United States and pyrethrins are produced in Africa or South America. Their lower cost makes them desirable as insecticides, although they are generally not more effective. Many are marginally safer than pyrethrin, partially because they occur in much purer forms and are not dissolved in the deodorized kerosene solvent used for pyrethrin concentrates. The small difference in safety between pyrethrin and pyrethroids is irrelevant, since pyrethrins already have such a high safety index. This difference should not be a determining factor in final insecticide selection.

Synthetic pyrethroids represent a rapidly evolving and changing aspect of pest control. The changes are so rapid that most publications are outdated by the time of printing. This is particularly true of the third-generation pyrethroids, permethrin and fenvalerate. The synthetic pyrethroids D-*trans*-allethrin, tetramethrin, D-phenothrin, and resmethrin have recently appeared in a number of products. Absence of synergists from some of these formulations may account for the problems in effective insect killing. Only a few of these products will achieve better residual activity than synergized pyrethrin products. Residual claims should be viewed with suspicion unless accompanied by supporting data. All are water based, so immediate flushing of fleas will be inferior to that obtained with alcohol-based sprays.

At this time, the only third-generation, stable synthetic pyrethroid available for use with companion animals is permethrin. Formulations containing permethrin and fenvalerate have been registered with the EPA but are not yet available. Cypermethrin and deltamethrin insecticides have not been registered with the EPA but are being evaluated for agricultural use. It will be several years before companion animal products containing these pyrethroids appear in the United States. However, both are widely used overseas. Because of their high insecticidal activity, only concentrations as low as 0.001 per cent of active insecticide will be needed.

Synergists

In insects, synergists inhibit enzymes that are responsible for oxidative and hydrolytic degradation of pyrethrins and some pyrethroids. Use of synergists extends the period of knockdown and increases the efficacy of killing. A combination of synergists with appropriate pyrethroids or pyrethrin allows conservation of the more expensive active ingredient by producing the same level of efficacy with lower concentrations. Synergists are far less toxic than the active ingredient and therefore are not a reflection of the potential toxicity described on the label.

PIPERONYL BUTOXIDE (PBO). Piperonyl butoxide is a synergist invariably used with pyrethrin, either alone or with *n*-octyl bicycloheptene dicarboxamide. These two agents provide the lethal action to synergize the knockdown and flushing activity of pyrethrin and some of the less stable pyrethroids (D-*trans*-allethrin or D-phenothrin). Efficacy information on PBO was developed primarily on flying insects rather than crawling insects such as fleas. The action of the stable pyrethroids (resmethrin, permethrin, fenvalerate) is not significantly improved by synergists.

PBO is incorporated in ready-to-apply products such as dusts, shampoos, and sprays in the concentration range of 0.1 to 2.0 per cent. It is also included in foggers as a synergist to pyrethrin in the range of 1.0 to 4.0 per cent. Comparable concentrations are found in the concentrated form of dips requiring dilution before use.

There is some evidence that PBO may be toxic to cats. A low incidence of chronic neurologic side effects (tremors, incoordination, lethargy) has been observed with sprays containing levels of PBO equal to or greater than 1.5 per cent.

N-OCTYL BICYCLOHEPTENE DICARBOXIMIDE (MGK 264, McLaughlin, Gormley, King Co.). This synergist may be substituted for PBO and is alleged to have better synergist activity on insects that crawl than on those that fly. It is used with pyrethrin and some of the second-generation pyrethroids, and often in combination with other synergists. MGK 264 has rarely been used as the only synergist. The ratio of pyrethrin or pyrethroid to synergist is usually 1:10, and the synergist may be entirely PBO or a mixture of PBO and MGK 264. In products labeled for cats, the level of PBO may be reduced and a major portion of the synergist activity provided by MGK 264. The objective is to reduce the low risks of side effects associated with PBO. MGK 264 is manufactured in concentrated products for dilution prior to use (including mini-foggers) at levels of up to 7.0 per cent and in ready-to-apply products such as sprays, dips, and shampoos at 0.1 to 2.0 per cent.

Repellents

Repellents are chemicals that cause insects to move away. Many insecticides have repellency. Pyrethrum extract is a potent repellent but is conventionally regarded as an insecticide since it also kills insects. Repellents may be toxic to insects, but usually they are inefficient insecticides. Most repellents are relatively stable compared with pyrethrin.

Many synthetic and some natural compounds are used as repellents. Cost often determines the products in which they are used. Most of those used for application to humans repel mosquitos, gnats, midges, and other insects but are too expensive or have to be used at too high levels to be included in products for companion animals. Very few repellents are approved for application to food animals. This is the reason for label warnings on most equine fly repellents against application to food animals.

Repellents are added to many pesticides for application to companion animals. They contribute to the initial flushing effect and repel biting insects (flies, mosquitoes, and gnats). Since they are more stable than pyrethrin and some pyrethroids, there is some extension of apparent product efficacy since they repel new fleas and ticks longer than active ingredients without the repellent. Most products contain only one repellent, although some contain two or three. Those with three repellents are usually for application to horses, and repellency rather than insecticide activity is the primary objective.

MGK 11 (McLaughlin, Gormley, King Co.). The chemical name of this product is 2,3,4,5-bis (2-butenylene)tetrahydro-2-furaldehyde. It is used in concentrations of 0.1 to 0.5 per cent in sprays, dips, and shampoos. It is the most common repellent used for small animals.

MGK 326 (McLaughlin, Gormley, King Co.). This chemical is di-*n*-propyl isocinchomeronate and is registered for use on both small animals and food animals. Toxicity is less than half that of MGK 11. MGK 326 is not used as the only repellent but is applied in combination with others in sprays, dips, and shampoos.

There is a shortage of technical data on the relative efficacies of these two repellents, especially against fleas and ticks. The choice and concentration of a repellent in a specific product is determined arbitrarily, based more on competitive marketing strategy than on valid scientific data. There are little or no published data comparing the effects of various repellents with each other or even the effect of insecticides with or without repellents.

BUTOXYPOLYPROPYLENE GLYCOL (Butox. PPG). This product is used principally as a fly repellent for application to horses. Only rarely is it used for application to companion animals. The level in equine products is between 5 and 50 per cent. In addition to repelling flies, it has cosmetic value in producing a shine to the coat that is considered desirable in the show ring. Products containing high levels of this repellent may cause dermal irritation if the hair is covered by a harness or collar while still wet.

Chlorinated Hydrocarbons

Ten to 20 years ago, chlorinated hydrocarbons or organochlorines were the insecticides of choice for animals and the environment. The immediate and residual activities were good, and mammalian toxicities were low (except for sensitive animals such as cats and young animals). Because of the stability of chlorinated hydrocarbons, the subsequent accumulation and concentration in the wildlife food chain nearly caused the extermination of some predatory birds. Consequently, this group of insecticides generally has been banned for use.

Only two organochlorines are still available for limited use today. These are γ-benzene hexachloride (γ-BHC, or lindane) and methoxychlor. Considerable effort is being made also to remove these from the marketplace.

The mode of action of organochlorines is similar to that of pyrethrin and the pyrethroids, which block nerve transmissions, induce paralysis of the insect, and produce death.

LINDANE. At the time of this writing, lindane is still available in a few dips and wipe-on lotions. Its only claim for survival in the marketplace is as a treatment for scabies. However, there are other products that make claims against scabies mites. These include carbaryl, phosmet, DDVP, malathion, and propoxur.

METHOXYCHLOR. Methoxychlor is restricted to fly repellent products for horses. These products usually also contain synergized pyrethrin and one or more repellents.

Petroleum Distillate

Petroleum distillate, or deodorized kerosene, is listed on many labels as an active ingredient. In most products, it is present because it is the solvent for pyrethrin and synthetic pyrethroids. Manufacturers have the option, under these circumstances, of including petroleum distillate in the list of active ingredients or in the list of inert ingredients.

Petroleum distillate has some insecticidal activity and was used for this purpose before the development of modern synthetics. As more potent synthetic insecticides became available, this practice was discontinued. Petroleum distillate is still added to some sprays for premises since it volatilizes more rapidly than water and costs about the same as isopropanol.

Insect Growth Regulators

Insect growth hormones (juvenoids, or insect growth regulators [IGR]) are natural chemicals in insects that control various stages of the insect's metabolism, morphogenesis, and reproduction. They are important in reproduction, organ maturation and development, and the development and growth of the larvae. Juvenoids are important as initiators, stimulators, or maintainers of certain functions and are essential for normal development. Methoprene is a chemical with structural and biochemical activities that mimic those of natural juvenile hormone. It has achieved practical use in controlling normal development.

Maturation and pupation of flea larvae is accompanied by and dependent on the absence of the natural juvenile hormone that is essential for earlier larval growth. The provision of a high level of synthetic IGR in the larvae's environment prevents proper maturation and pupation and causes death of the larvae. Application of synthetic IGR in spray or fogger to the indoor environment is designed to interrupt this last stage of flea development and hence prevent the emergence of new fleas. Since the time of action is late in the development of free-living fleas, beneficial effects cannot be expected until 1 to 4 weeks after application. This period depends on the environmental temperature and the rate of larval development. Although initially products introduced contained only a synthetic IGR, new products include synergized pyrethrin for immediate kill of newly emerged fleas and an organophosphate (chlorpyrifos) to provide extended activity. Unfortunately, like those in all indoor sprays and foggers, the active chemicals tend to remain on the carpet surface. It is difficult to deliver the active ingredients to the flea larvae deep in the carpet and furnishings without soaking the materials to an objectionable level. Methoprene is light sensitive, as is pyrethrin, and will not persist outdoors or in bright locations. Its residual activity will be diminished under natural conditions, and it may fail to provide the same activity obtained in the laboratory. Synthetic IGRs are more acceptable in that they pollute the environment less than pesticides such as organophosphates and carbamates, which have undesirable toxicity. However, as with all indoor environmental flea control products, the delivery system rather than the efficacy of the active ingredient presents the greatest problem.

Carbamates and Organophosphates

Both carbamates and organophosphates have been used extensively as insecticides for many years. Both groups exert their toxicity by interfering with the enzyme activity of acetylcholinesterase (AChE). Normally, after transmission of neurogenic impulse across the synapse by means of acetylcholine (ACh), there is binding of AChE, which results in acetylation and ultimate splitting and deactivation of the ACh. Organophosphorous compounds have some structural similarity to the natural substrate, ACh. The final interaction with the enzyme AChE results in its phosphorylation. This phosphorylation is reversible but slow. Carbamates have an effect on the enzyme system by competing with ACh for the active site on the AChE molecule, a process referred to as the carbamylating reaction. Carbamates act to block the enzyme rather than to change it. Hydrolysis of carbamylated cholinesterase reverses the blockage, releasing the AChE for further activity. The final outcome with either organophosphates or carbamates is the depression of available AChE and the accumulation of ACh, resulting in continued neurostimulation.

The intoxication of mammals with carbamates or organophosphates results in neurologic signs resulting from the increased accumulation of ACh. The effects on postganglionic parasympathetics produce miosis, lacrimation, vomiting, diarrhea, salivation, pollakiuria, dyspnea, bradycardia, and hypotension. Behavioral changes may be observed, as well as alteration of memory and learning ability. Abnormal motor activity such as muscle twitching, weakness, paralysis, or seizure activity may be seen. Chronic organophosphate intoxication can result in degeneration of peripheral nerves and long axons in the spinal cord.

Atropine administered parenterally is the preferred treatment for carbamate or organophosphate intoxication. 2-pyridine aldoxime (2-PAM), or pralidoxime chloride (Protopam, Ayerst), contains an oxime hydroxyl group that has greater affinity for positively charged portions of the phosphorylated AChE than the hydroxyl group of water, thereby more rapidly hydrolyzing the enzyme to return it to its natural state. It is of interest that 2-PAM is essentially ineffective in the treatment of carbamate intoxication. Repeated therapy is usually necessary since the duration of activity is short.

Carbamate and organophosphate pesticides must be used with caution and should not be used in combination with other AChE-inhibiting drugs or insecticides. Reputation of certain breed intolerances (such as, perhaps, greyhound) should be respected. Consideration of concurrent medication (anesthetics) or disease (heartworms) should be taken into account when these products are used.

CARBAMATES

CARBARYL. Carbaryl is a member of the aryl methyl carbamates. It has wide application as a pesticide on crops and animals. It is most commonly known by its brand name, Sevin (Union Carbide). Carbaryl is a crystalline solid with minimal solubility in water but soluble in most nonpolar organic solvents. The mammalian toxicity of carbaryl is low (a relatively high oral LD_{50}) compared with other carbamates.

Sevin dust has been used for many years as an insecticide. It is prepared in concentrations of 2 to 10 per cent and is used primarily as a premises treatment. Carbaryl has an alleged reputation for regional ineffectiveness, particularly in the southeastern United States, where an assumed resistance phenomenon has developed in fleas. Preparations for use on the animal include sprays, powders, shampoos, and collars (Tables 1 to 3). Carbaryl is frequently combined with other active agents such as synergized pyrethrins, repellents, or organophosphates. Label claims suggest efficacy against fleas, lice, and ticks for use in both dogs and cats. Carbaryl should not be used on puppies or kittens less than 4 weeks old or on pregnant or lactating animals. Concentrations range from 0.5 to 8 per cent. Usefulness of carbaryl is limited to certain geographic regions; the major disadvantage is the acquired resistance of fleas and ticks. The major advantage of carbaryl is its low toxicity.

BENDIOCARB. Bendiocarb (Ficam, Fisons, B.F.C. Chemicals) is a wettable powder, popular with pest control operators as a premises spray. Its main advantages are its lack of odor, good flea-killing capability, residual efficacy, and low soiling. Bendiocarb has been available only through licensed professional exterminators, although recently there are reports of its being sold in retail stores.

PROPOXUR. Propoxur (Baygon, Bayer; Sendran, Bayvet Division Miles Laboratories) is a natural solid that is nearly insoluble in water but quite soluble in polar organic solvents such as alcohol. Propoxur has a reputation for quick knockdown and residual activity. Propoxur is used most frequently in combination with other active ingredients but may be the only insecticide in some cases (Sendran Flea Collar). It is used in pet shampoos, aerosols, and flea and tick collars approved for dogs and cats. Manufacturers' claims that extended insecticidal activity has been accomplished by the addition of propoxur may have little clinical evaluation to support them. "For extended activity" is a dimensionless phrase, since it is relative. Propoxur, like other carbamates and organophosphates, suppresses AChE activity and must be used with caution.

ORGANOPHOSPHATES

Organophosphate insecticides were developed as a spin-off of production activities of toxic nerve gases during World War II. Since their early beginnings, these compounds have been modified to reduce mammalian toxicity while enhancing insecticidal potency. The outcome is a rather lengthy list of compounds representing some of the most popular pesticides in use today. The mechanism of action has been discussed previously. Keep in mind that each causes AChE depression and, if used concurrently with one another or with other AChE-depressing agents (carbamates), the cumulative effect may have an unfortunate and perhaps fatal outcome. Many pet owners are not aware of this potential problem and are often uninformed of the classification of other products currently in use. The veterinarian's responsibility to inform the owner of the nature of products used cannot be overemphasized. Owners may not realize that use of the malathion bought at the lawn and garden store may potentiate the phosmet dip that the veterinarian dispensed. Client information pamphlets are helpful.

CHLORFENVINPHOS (SUPONA, SHELL). This organophosphate is most familiar to veterinarians as the active ingredient of Dermaton Dip (Coopers Animal Health). It is present in a concentration of 24.5 per cent, which is diluted for use to a 0.1 per cent solution (4 ml/L).

Its use is primarily for flea and tick control. It is an unreliable scabicide and should be avoided for treatment of that disease. Manufacturers' claims of residual activity against fleas are inflated. Dermaton is also used as a premises spray for yards, kennels, and runs. This product is not approved for use on cats. Chlorfenvinphos persists in the soil for a protracted period of time, offering residual environmental insecticide activity.

CHLORPYRIFOS. Chlorpyrifos (Dursban, Dow) is a popular environmental pesticide for the control of a wide spectrum of insects. It is extensively used by professional exterminators. Chlorpyrifos has good efficacy against fleas and is commonly used for that purpose in the Southeast. It is also included in several products to be used on dogs, including sprays and dips (Tables 1 and 2). It is not approved for use on cats and should be avoided on dogs in contact with other forms of organophosphates or carbamates.

CYTHIOATE. Cythioate is the only approved and registered systemic insecticide for small animals. Because it is a systemic, it was subjected to toxicity studies under the direction of the FDA rather than the EPA. Cythioate is administered PO to dogs at 3.3 mg/kg every third day according to insert instructions. Although not approved for cats, it has been used at a dosage of 1.5 to 3.0 mg/kg. The product is available as a 1.6 per cent liquid and in 30-mg tablets (Proban, Bayvet).

This product is probably the single largest-selling veterinary insecticide at the time of this writing. Client acceptance is based primarily on convenience, and it has been heavily promoted to the pet owner. Client pressure has enhanced veterinary use of this product.

Efficacy reports are variable, depending on multiple factors, the first being the accuracy of the observation. Many owners state that *their* pet does not have fleas or a flea problem, despite the identification of a significant flea burden at the time of veterinary examination. Accurate appraisal of flea infestation by owners is at best speculative. Another factor influencing cythioate efficacy is the amount of environmental control. In those situations in which rigorous environment treatment schedules are adhered to, there is an obvious enhancement (as would be expected with many products). There is a definite individual variation of the intensity of parasitism among dogs. Product efficacy therefore can be more of an expression of host appeal than true parasiticidal potency. Because cythioate is a systemic parasiticide, there is no repellent activity or immediate insecticidal effect. Obtaining a blood meal by the insect is a prerequisite to insecticide efficacy and implies that the parasite will have the opportunity to feed. Another prerequisite for effective insecticidal activity is the appropriate blood level of the drug. Cythioate blood levels are maintained for only 6 to 12 hours following medication. Therefore, the interval between treatments is long enough for blood levels to fall below effective limits. Increased frequency of therapy can result in toxicosis. Concurrent use of external organophosphate products can potentiate the toxicity of cythioate. It is essential before placing an animal on systemic organophosphates to be aware of coexisting therapy (systemic or external) and the health status of the animal (hepatopathy, heartworms). The use of cythioate has limited value for dogs with flea allergy, since the insecticidal effect occurs after a blood meal and, therefore, after the deposition of the antigen in the skin. Owners are frequently given a false sense of security when treating their flea-allergic animal with cythioate. Owners who assume that there cannot be a flea-related problem if their dog is taking the pill often require strong persuasion to convince them to the contrary.

DIAZINON. Diazinon (Geigy) is a popular organophosphate used for application to premises. It is minimally soluble in water but quite soluble in most organic solvents. Desirable characteristics include minimal resistance by most insects and a long residual effect. It is produced in several different forms, including a powder, liquid, and microencapsulation. It is readily available in most lawn and garden stores. Separate preparations for outside and inside application are available.

DICHLORVOS (VAPONA, SHELL; DDVP). Dichlorvos was once more popular than it is today. It has rather quick knockdown insectidal action but little residual efficacy. Use of this insecticide in small animals is in the form of flea collars or tags.

DIOXATHION. Dioxathion (Delnav, Nor Am Co.) is an insecticide with limited application in small animals. It is used in sprays, dips, pour-ons, and back rubbers for large animals. It is recognized for long residual insecticidal and acaricidal activity. Insects may be killed by ingestion of or physical contact with the insecticide. Dioxathion decomposes rapidly in an alkaline medium and is not heat stable. It is formulated as a spray or dip for use in dogs. Application may be repeated every 7 days. A 0.5 per cent dioxathion solution is used for spraying the premises.

FENTHION. Fenthion is a very potent organophosphate formerly approved only for large animal use and now approved for canine use as well (Pro-Spot, Bayvet). It is an oily liquid with an offensive pungent odor. It is extremely stable and therefore tends to persist for long periods. It is primarily used as a pour-on for the control of *Hypoderma* grubs in cattle. Use of fenthion in dogs has been for flea control, although there have been some anecdotal reports of its use in demodicosis. Dosage in dogs has been rather empiric and varies from 20 to 33 mg/kg. The dosage recommended by the manufacturer is 4 to 8 mg/kg. According to unpublished research, dogs will become intoxicated following a dosage of 90 mg/kg administered every 2 weeks for three treatments. A predictable lethal dose is 270 mg/kg as a single treatment. Despite the seemingly large difference between therapeutic dose and intoxicating dose, this drug has been responsible for more unintentional intoxications than any other parasiticide currently available. It is only conjectural whether this represents a poorly calculated dose, inappropriate application, individual sensitivity to the drug, or the potential intoxicating properties of fenthion. The important point is that this drug has potential dangers to animals *and* to humans in contact with the drug or treated animals.

Enthusiasm for fenthion is based on the convenience of a weekly or biweekly treatment. Efficacy of fenthion is probably overrated, although it definitely has good insecticidal effect on fleas. Unfortunately, it does not provide the total flea control necessary for the treatment of flea-allergic animals. The risk-benefit ratio must be considered strongly before selecting this drug. Because of the systemic absorption, sick animals or those with subclinical hepatopathies have a high risk of side effects. Because preparations of synergized pyrethrins or pyrethroids are effective and lack toxicities and insecticide buildup, there is little indication for the use of fenthion in its current form.

MALATHION. Malathion is a popular organophosphate for use as both a treatment for premises and as a dip for dogs and cats. It is safe for general use. Malathion is formulated with other insecticides because of its compatibility and low toxicity. As a premises treatment, malathion is also prepared in granular form. It is highly effective in flea control.

PHOSMET. Phosmet (Stouffer) is a popular organophosphate primarily used for small animal therapy. It is the principal active ingredient in Paramite (Vet-Kem) dip. Phosmet may be used on cats but should never be used on either cats or dogs younger than 8 weeks. Treatment should not be repeated more frequently than every 7 days. It is recognized as a scabicide with good efficacy.*

RONNEL. Ronnel (Dow Chemical abroad) is an

**Editor's Note:* Phosmet, along with oher organophosphate products, is frequently ineffective for the treatment of canine scabies in the Northeast.

organophosphate with low mammalian toxicity. It is used primarily on dogs but occasionally as a spray for premises. Ronnel is a potent insecticide and acaricide. It is effective as a scabicide and has been used as a 4 per cent solution in propylene glycol for the treatment of demodicosis. Ronnel was not commercially available as an approved small animal product for a period of time but has recently been placed back on the market as Ectoral (Pitman-Moore).

Formamidines

The formamidines are a group of newly formulated acaricidal compounds whose mechanism of action is inhibition of monoamine oxidase. They are effective against organisms that have developed resistance to organophosphates and carbamates. Amitraz is the formamidine used most in veterinary dermatology. It is used primarily as a demodecide, although it is an effective scabicide. (Refer to the article on Canine Demodicosis for further information on the use of amitraz.) This product is very unstable and deteriorates rapidly by oxidation and exposure to ultraviolet light. When it is applied as a 0.025 per cent solution, it may produce transient sedation, depression of rectal temperature, elevation of blood glucose, and seizures. Acute death has been observed following treatment with amitraz, but a confirmed cause-and-effect relationship has not been established. Amitraz is *not* an organophosphate; therefore, conventional treatment of organophosphate intoxication is of no value.

Miscellaneous Insecticides

BENZYL BENZOATE. Benzyl benzoate is an effective agent against most ectoparasites but is outdated by more contemporary agents. It is primarily used for spot treatment as an acaricide and frequently is combined with other active ingredients.

SULFUR. One of the oldest acaricidal drugs, sulfur is still recognized as a reliable scabicide. The formulation is usually a concentrated lime sulfur orchard spray, which is diluted to a 2 per cent solution. Scalding of the skin has been observed when the product was inappropriately applied full strength. It can be safely used on dogs and cats as well as on most other mammals. Sulfur is also used in shampoos and dusts. Sulfur-containing oral preparations sold in pet stores are of little benefit in controlling fleas.

IVERMECTIN. Ivermectin is a synthetically modified derivative of a group of agents called avermectins. It is noted for anthelmintic activity against nematodes and microfilariae. It is effective as a miticide, particularly against *Sarcoptes scabiei* and *Otodectes cynotis* but has minimal effect against *Demodex canis*. *This product is not currently licensed in the United States for use in dogs.* However, experimental oral therapy appears to be effective at a dose rate of 200 μg/kg. A single oral dose has been shown to completely cure cases of canine scabies. Proper licensure and approval should be obtained before use in small animals.

PRINCIPLES OF PARASITICIDAL THERAPY IN DERMATOLOGY

The usefulness and reputation of any parasiticidal formulation is directly related to its application. Too frequently, a product may gain the notoriety of having poor efficacy when in fact it is doing what is expected of it but the source of the parasite has not been addressed. We often hear, "I wish they would invent something that would kill fleas." There are many products that are nearly 100 per cent effective as insecticides against fleas. There are few, however, that have a residual killing or repellent effect. The recognition of a persistent flea burden is interpreted as a lack of insecticidal potency rather than the reinfestation of the animal. Success can only be derived from consideration of all factors related to the treatment program. The successful management of ectoparasitic diseases requires knowledge of (1) life cycle of the parasite, (2) habitat of the parasite, (3) asymptomatic carrier state, (4) contagiousness of the parasite to humans and other animals, and (5) recognized activity of the parasiticide.

Life Cycle of the Parasite

The first concern for rational therapy is to *know* the parasite. Awareness of the life cycle is a prerequisite to the successful treatment. Most parasiticides are directed against a specific stage of the life cycle (usually the adult stage) and have virtually no effect on the other developmental periods. As a rule of thumb, the treatment of obligate parasites requires the use of an adulticide at an appropriate interval (weekly) for the length of the life cycle plus 1 week. Parasites that have more complex life cycles in which the parasitism is interrupted by periodic molts in the environment require modification of the treatment protocol. The use of combined active ingredients merits further consideration. The addition of methoprene as a flea larvacide in combination with an adulticide will affect the life cycle. The interval of environmental treatment will require alteration from the conventional procedures. In situations in which the life cycle of the parasite is ongoing, as with fleas in the warmer climates, treatment requires a more persistent and regular approach.

Habitat of the Parasite

Eradication of the parasite requires knowledge of its habitat. Obligate parasites pose one set of treatment plans, whereas a parasite that has widespread environmental territory requires an entirely different approach. Unfortunately, these factors are frequently overlooked. Most "failures" of flea control programs relate to ignoring the environment rather than to total ineffectiveness of the product. Proper preparation of the animal may entail removing all the hair and then providing an adequate contact time for penetration of the active ingredient. The treatment of *Pelodera strongyloides* points out the necessity for environmental treatment. As a free-living nematode, the source of the parasite (e.g., moist straw) is the primary treatment consideration. Treating the animal is really not necessary since the disease is self-limiting *if* the source is removed.

Asymptomatic Carrier State

Concern for this aspect of treatment is often overlooked. Animals that are in contact with the parasite but not demonstrating clinical signs cause treatment problems. Most cases are relatively clear-cut, although controversies exist regarding the asymptomatic carrier state of specific parasites. The variation of symptoms among parasitized animals is most representative of the host reactivity to that parasite rather than to parasite load or a unique pathogenicity. The asymptomatic carrier state is best exemplified by flea infestation. Some dogs may harbor thousands of fleas and have minimal pruritus (or dermatitis), whereas others with hypersensitivity show intense skin lesions but few fleas. Cats can be asymptomatic flea carriers. Overlooking the family cat, whose environmental boundaries are frequently unrestricted, will bring failure to the best flea control program.

Highly contagious diseases may be overlooked in the absence of "total family" involvement. Canine scabies is an example of a highly contagious disease that is usually associated with all animals on the premises. However, cases can be found that demonstrate positive skin scraping and yet are asymptomatic carriers. All animals in contact with parasites need to be treated despite the lack of clinical signs.

Recognized Activity of the Parasiticide

The variations of parasiticide formulations pose a further concern in treatment. Range of potencies, concentrations, systems of application, and efficacy are all factors to be considered. It is helpful to determine whether a product has good insecticidal or acaricidal properties, or both. A product that may show excellent acaricidal efficacy may have poor insecticidal activity or the reverse. This is not always described accurately by the manufacturer. Actual use is the best testimonial to the efficacy of a product. There may be a regional influence on the reputation for efficacy. One insecticide may be favored in some geographic areas but viewed as useless in other regions. It is advisable to use a product with recognized efficacy for the parasite but to consider regional variations.

There are numerous home remedies that gain local popularity. Most have no scientific basis for efficacy, and many show no more than a placebo effect when subjected to stringently controlled studies. Thiamine, brewer's yeast, and colloidal sulfur are examples. Parasite appetite for the host is variable, too. One dog may attract only few fleas, but another in the same household may carry a severe flea burden. Only a controlled study with an acceptable number of treated and untreated dogs can determine true insecticide efficacy.

Contagiousness to Humans or Other Animals

Diseases with public health implications attract attention from the aspect of treatment urgency. The "decontamination" process should be expedited to remove the source of infestation even though the treatment will not directly affect the persons involved. Referral to a physician or dermatologist is indicated for treatment of affected humans.

Treatment of contagious parasitic disease is most troublesome in large kennels or catteries. Treatment must be based on regimentation requiring the treatment of all animals. Selective animal treatment is futile. For best results, one must obtain total adherence to a complete treatment program. Convincing owners and managers of the need to comply with this principle may be difficult when many dogs need to be treated. Success of a treatment program is only as good as owner compliance. There is no substitute for good client education, and time-consuming discussions can be replaced by descriptive information pamphlets. The excuse that time constraints prohibit good client education is ill founded. The success of any parasite control program relies on it.

References and Supplemental Reading

Casida, J. E. (ed.): *Pyrethrum: The Natural Insecticide.* New York: Academic Press, 1973.

Coats, J. R. (ed.): *Insecticide Mode of Action.* New York: Academic Press, 1982.

Elliott, M. (ed.): *Synthetic Pyrethroids: A Symposium Sponsored by the Division of Pesticide Chemistry at the 172nd Meeting of the American Chemical Society, San Francisco, CA., Aug. 30–31, 1976.* Washington, D.C.: American Chemical Society, 1977.

Georgi, J. R.: *Parasitology for Veterinarians*, 4th ed. Philadelphia: W. B. Saunders, 1985.

MacDonald, J. M.: Ectoparasites. *In* Kirk, R. W. (ed.): *Current Veterinary Therapy VIII.* Philadelphia: W. B. Saunders, 1983, pp. 488–495.

Wilkinson, C. F. (ed.): *Insecticide Biochemistry and Physiology.* New York; Plenum Press, 1976.

NUTRITIONAL THERAPY IN VETERINARY DERMATOLOGY

VALERIE A. FADOK, D.V.M.
Gainesville, Florida

Nutrition plays an important role in the development and maintenance of normal skin and coat. Testimonial evidence suggests that some dogs and cats eating complete and balanced diets may show improvement in coat and skin condition after fat, vitamin, and mineral supplements are given. Many nutritionists, however, believe that supplementation of complete and balanced diets is neither necessary nor desirable. It is important to remember that nutritional supplements, particularly the fat-soluble vitamins, can cause toxicosis when given in high dosages for a long period of time. Also, the injudicious addition of specific supplements to a diet may cause subtle dietary imbalances. Recently, individual vitamins and minerals have been used to treat specific dermatoses. These dermatoses may not reflect actual dietary deficiencies; therefore, the vitamins and minerals may have pharmacologic effects. This article will review the important nutrients, effects of deficiency and toxicity, and established uses for nutritional therapy in veterinary dermatology.

NUTRITIONAL FACTORS IN SKIN AND COAT MAINTENANCE

Dogs and cats require energy, amino acids, fatty acids, glucose precursors, vitamins, and minerals for growth and maintenance. Experimental diets have revealed the effects of specific nutrient deficiencies. The skin is a highly active metabolic organ; a deficiency in any of the nutrients mentioned above can result in abnormal keratinization of skin and hair, as well as quantitative and qualitative changes in sebaceous and epidermal lipids. Associated clinical signs often include a poor, dry coat and scaly skin. One rarely can differentiate these conditions by physical examination. Specific deficiencies are not common in clinical practice; however, dietary imbalances can occur in pets fed incomplete home-prepared diets or inappropriately supplemented diets. The interaction of nutrients is complex; the use of each nutrient depends on appropriate levels and utilization of the others. A listing of recommended daily allowances for proteins, fats, vitamins, and minerals is available (National Research Council [NRC], 1974, 1978). Quality pet foods labeled "complete and balanced" contain these nutrients in levels greater than those recommended.

Dietary protein and the essential amino acids are important precursors of the structural proteins of developing skin and hairs. Protein is used by the body most efficiently when optimal energy is provided by fats and carbohydrates. Protein and calorie malnutrition results in a sparse, dry, fragile coat with decreased hair diameter and atrophic scaly skin, as the body tries to conserve protein synthesis for more vital structures. Protein and calorie excess in adult dogs results in obesity, and in the growing dog, skeletal abnormalities (Sheffy, 1979a).

Dietary fat provides an important source of energy. The polyunsaturated fatty acids (linoleic, linolenic, and arachidonic acids) are used in the production of cell membranes and prostaglandins. Dogs can convert linoleic to linolenic and arachidonic acids. Cats cannot desaturate linoleic acid and therefore require all three in the diet (NRC, 1978). Dogs and cats fed an experimental fat-deficient diet develop dull, dry coats, alopecia, and scaling skin. This syndrome can be seen occasionally in pets eating diets in which the fats have become rancid as a result of prolonged storage or diets that are prepared at home and not supplemented. Dogs with malabsorptive disorders will also develop signs of fatty acid deficiency. Recommendations for fat supplementation have been published (Muller et al., 1983). Fats of both animal and vegetable origin are suggested. Excess supplementation of fat should be avoided, as it may cause obesity and loose stools.

Both water-soluble and fat-soluble vitamins are important for normal skin growth and metabolism. The B-complex vitamins are important constituents of coenzymes and cofactors in protein, carbohydrate, and fat metabolism. Cats and dogs fed diets deficient in individual B vitamins will develop dry, scaly skin and alopecia. B-complex vitamins commonly are added to commercial pet foods. Supplementation is only necessary in anorectic patients or those eating imbalanced diets. Toxicosis has been created in laboratory animals (including dogs and cats) and in humans with thiamine given by both parenteral and oral routes; signs included central nervous system disturbances and allergic reactions, including anaphylaxis. Apparently, thiamine hydrochloride can induce hypersensitivity in certain individuals; sensitivity has been demonstrated by intradermal testing and passive transfer. Niacin and pyridoxine have also caused toxicoses experimentally (Rechcigl, 1978). B-vitamin toxicoses require dosages more than 1000 times the daily requirement. Hypersensitivity reactions, although rare, could occur from repeated parenteral administration of B-complex vitamins at normal dosages. Vitamin C is not normally required in the diet of dogs or cats, as the liver can synthesize it from glucose. High dosages of vitamin C have been associated with toxic changes in liver, thyroid, and bone and with fetal damage in laboratory rodents. Side effects of large doses of vitamin C in humans are rare but may include intestinal and urinary lithiasis, thrombosis, hemolysis, metabolic acidosis, and development of scurvy after cessation of excess supplements (Rechcigl, 1978). Alterations in uric acid metabolism also occur in humans and may represent a contraindication for megadose use in Dalmatians.

The fat-soluble vitamins A, D, and E are required in the diet of dogs and cats. Vitamin A is an important regulator of metabolism in epithelial and bony tissue and is involved in the production of visual pigment. Unlike dogs, cats cannot convert plant carotenes to vitamin A (retinol); cats require preformed vitamin A in their diet. Vitamin A deficiency results in epidermal and mucosal hyperkeratosis and increased susceptibility of the skin to infection. Marked follicular hyperkeratosis (phrynoderma) occurs in humans (Fine and Moschella, 1985). Vitamin A toxicosis clinically is very similar to deficiency and is characterized by a dry, scaly skin. Other signs include malaise, abdominal discomfort, nausea, vomiting, skeletal hyperostosis, irritability, and icterus. Hypervitaminosis A has occurred in cats fed diets high in liver. The recommended allowances for dogs are 110 IU/kg for adults and twice that for puppies; the allowance for cats is twice that for dogs (NRC, 1974, 1978). The dosage required to produce hypervitaminosis A in dogs is greater than 100 times the recommended daily allowance (NRC, 1974).

Vitamin D is important in the skin because its precursor, 7-dehydrocholesterol, is present in epidermal and sebaceous lipids. This molecule is converted to pre-D_3 by ultraviolet light; it then is transformed to D_3, which enters the circulation by binding with a carrier protein. Canine and feline diets are supplemented with vitamin D, because production in the skin by ultraviolet irradiation is not sufficient to meet their needs. Symptoms of deficiency include rickets and abnormal tooth eruption, as well as abnormalities in calcium and phosphorus metabolism. Hypervitaminosis D results in hypercalcemia, increased bone density, and calcification of soft tissues. The toxic dosage is 500 times the recommended level for growth, which is 22 IU/kg. Adult maintenance dosage is 11 IU/kg (NRC, 1974).

Vitamin E (the tocopherols) and selenium work in concert to protect cell membranes against peroxidation and destruction by oxygen-derived free radicals. Dietary requirements for vitamin E are increased when levels of ingested polyunsaturated fatty acids and sulfur-containing amino acids are increased. Dietary vitamin E and selenium levels are also related, having a sparing effect on each other. Vitamin E plays an important role in the protection of vitamin A and its precursor from oxidation in the gastrointestinal tract and within cells. Vitamin E deficiency causes dermatologic signs similar to those seen with deficiencies of fatty acids: dry scaly skin and alopecia. Inflammation may also be present. Cats fed diets high in polyunsaturated fats (all-fish diets) without concomitant supplementation of vitamin E develop pansteatitis, characterized by painful nodules in the subcutaneous tissue and abdominal fat. Foods that become rancid will be deficient in vitamin E, as the tocopherols are susceptible to oxidation. The recommended daily allowance for vitamin E for adult dogs is 1.1 IU/kg and for puppies 2.2 IU/kg (NRC, 1974). For cats, 4 mg α-tocopherol per day is suggested (Mellentin, 1977). Vitamin E toxicosis has been demonstrated in laboratory animals and humans; clinical signs include muscular weakness and fatigue. In addition, hepatic lipid deposition and teratogenicity have been noted in rats (Rechcigl, 1978).

Minerals are the inorganic nutrients essential for life. They are divided into the major minerals, or macrominerals (calcium, magnesium, potassium, sodium, chlorine, phosphorus, sulfur), and the trace minerals, or microminerals (chromium, copper, iodine, manganese, nickel, silicon, vanadium, cobalt, fluorine, iron, molybdenum, selenium, tin, zinc). These elements are considered essential for animals; however, research about specific canine and feline requirements for trace minerals is scanty. Specific requirements for dogs have been established for iron, copper, iodine, and zinc (Sheffy, 1979b). Guidelines have also been established for manganese and selenium supplementation based on research data accumulated from other species. Trace minerals are involved in growth and regeneration of tissues, as well as for hormone and enzyme production. Each mineral is in delicate equilibrium with the others; imbalances can occur easily. Although absolute deficiencies are rare, relative deficiencies can be created by oversupplementing one or two minerals. Commercial dog and cat foods are supplemented with many of the trace minerals, making the addition of extra supplements unnecessary for most pets.

Mineral interactions of importance to the skin are those between zinc, copper, and calcium, because absorption of these minerals is interrelated. Excess dietary calcium will depress zinc absorption; excess zinc will depress copper absorption. It is known that vegetable fiber and phytin from cereal grains and soybeans depress calcium, zinc, and magnesium absorption.

Zinc plays an important role in maintaining homeostasis in many tissues. It is an important component of many enzyme systems and affects nucleic acid metabolism and immune function. Foods of both plant and animal origin contain zinc, although that in plants is less available for the reasons stated above. Deficiency results in impaired growth and development, decreased utilization of protein, decreased resistance to infection, decreased wound healing, behavioral changes, and dermatologic disease.

Zinc deficiency syndromes are well documented in human and veterinary medicine. A relative zinc deficiency can be noted in puppies and dogs eating diets high in vegetable matter, particularly if calcium supplements are added to the diet. Generic dog foods have been associated with a dermatologic disease comparable to relative zinc deficiency. Affected dogs have dull, scaly coats and erythematous crusted lesions around eyes, muzzle, ears, and pressure points. The footpads may become extremely hyperkeratotic. Zinc deficiency has been created experimentally in cats, resulting in alopecia, crusting, and scaling. Cats require higher levels of zinc if fed a diet high in vegetable protein (NRC, 1978). Good-quality commercial foods have zinc added in levels adequate for most pets.

Relative copper deficiency can cause decreased pigmentation of the skin and hair. Faulty keratinization results in scaly skin and a dull, rough coat.

VITAMIN AND MINERAL THERAPY

Many veterinarians, breeders, and pet owners believe that the coat and skin of some dogs and cats improve when supplements containing vitamins, minerals, and fatty acids are added to the basic diet. Most dogs and cats eat complete and balanced diets; it would seem that addition of extra vitamins and minerals is redundant, and could be harmful, if given in high dosages. Factors such as stress, illness, and medications may affect the dietary requirements of individual patients; however, not enough information is available to enable specific dosage recommendations to be made. The author does not routinely supplement the diet of dermatologic patients unless the animal is not eating a complete and balanced commercial diet.

VITAMIN A AND RETINOIDS

Naturally occurring vitamin A is an alcohol, all-*trans* retinol. It is oxidized in the body to retinal, an aldehyde, and retinoic acid. Retinol is stored in the liver; retinoic acid is not. Each of these compounds has variable metabolic and biologic activities. Retinol and retinoic acid are important in the induction and maintenance of normal growth and differentiation of keratinocytes. Depending on the amount of retinoid added and the cell system used, retinoids may have either stimulatory or inhibitory effects on epidermal growth (Chytil, 1983). The specific roles of these compounds within keratinocytes are under active and enthusiastic investigation at this time.

The efficacy of vitamin A and synthetic retinoids in the treatment of keratinization disorders in humans not caused by a deficiency suggests a pharmacologic as well as physiologic role for these compounds. Vitamin A has also been used in dogs to treat idiopathic seborrhea (Ihrke and Goldschmidt, 1983; Parker et al., 1983). Canine seborrhea is characterized by abnormalities in epidermal cell turnover rate and keratinization and results in clinical signs of increased scaling, with or without excessive oiliness and inflammation. One group of investigators (Ihrke and Goldschmidt, 1983) correlated the histopathologic finding of marked follicular keratosis with response to vitamin A at the approximate daily oral dosage of 1000 IU/kg. Marked improvement was noted in three dogs after 8 weeks of therapy. After 1 to 4 years of daily vitamin A administration, no recurrence of clinical signs or toxicosis was seen. Another group (Parker et al., 1983) reported one case of vitamin A–responsive seborrhea in a Labrador retriever, characterized histologically by marked follicular keratosis, with both orthokeratotic and parakeratotic hyperkeratosis and dyskeratosis. The dog was treated with 50,000 IU vitamin A twice daily for 2 months, then 50,000 IU daily, with marked improvement noted within the first 5 weeks. After 2 years, the dog was clinically normal and had no evidence of toxicosis. This author has had some success with vitamin A in the treatment of idiopathic seborrhea but has been unable to correlate the finding of follicular keratosis with successful response to vitamin A. Because the signs of idiopathic seborrhea are nonspecific and can be seen in association with other diseases, each patient should be evaluated to rule out allergic, parasitic, endocrine, and other causes of seborrhea. Concomitant bacterial infections should be treated specifically. If no underlying diseases can be found, vitamin A therapy can be attempted on a trial basis for 8 weeks. Biopsies showing follicular keratosis may lend support but will not necessarily predict a response to vitamin A. A useful product is Aquasol-A (USV Laboratories), given PO at a dosage of 1000 to 2500 IU/kg daily. This dosage is less than 10 times the toxic dose for dogs. Aquasol A is miscible in water, allowing for increased and more efficient absorption. If successful, daily therapy may be required for the remainder of the dog's life. The dog should be monitored for signs of toxicosis, which include loss of appetite and weight, bone and joint pain, and development of dry, scaly skin.

The mechanism of action of vitamin A in canine seborrhea is not known, but it probably represents a pharmacologic effect rather than a physiologic one. It has been suggested that the effects of excess retinoids on epithelial tissue may result from a combination of their physiologic effects and toxic, lytic effects on cell membranes (Chytil, 1983).

The use of synthetic retinoids in human dermatology has awakened an interest in their possible efficacy in the treatment of veterinary dermatoses. Two compounds have been used extensively in humans: 13-*cis*-retinoic acid (isotretinoin), which is actually a natural metabolite of ingested retinol, and etretinate, an aromatic retinoid (Dicken, 1984). Isotretinoin (Accutane, Hoffman-LaRoche) is approved for use in the United States in humans and is extremely effective in the treatment of cystic acne, in which it reduces inflammation and decreases the size and output of sebaceous glands. Patients treated for 4 months will often remain in remission for as long as 3 to 4 years. Isotretinoin has been used successfully to treat keratinization disorders such as Darier's disease and ichthyosis, as well as precancerous and cancerous epithelial lesions. Treatment of squamous or basal cell carcinoma with isotretinoin results in decrease of tumor size but does not cure the patient (Dicken, 1984). Patients with disorders of keratinization require daily therapy to remain in remission. Side effects of isotretinoin in humans include cheilitis in virtually 100 per cent of patients, and facial erythema, dry skin, pruritus, and conjunctivitis. Laboratory side effects of significance include elevated triglyceride levels in greater than 25 per cent of patients. The severity of these side effects appears to be dose related and rarely causes the patient to discontinue treatment. Of increasing concern is the development of skeletal hyperostosis in patients with disorders of keratinization who are taking isotretinoin at high dosages for long periods of time. Dosages in humans have varied from 0.5 to 4.0 mg/kg divided twice daily. Experiences with this drug in the treatment of cystic acne have shown that lower dosages may be equally effective and have fewer side effects, although numbers of relapses may increase (Dicken, 1984).

Because isotretinoin affects keratinization and sebum production, a study was designed to evaluate the response to isotretinoin of eight dogs with idiopathic seborrhea (Fadok). Response to isotretinoin was compared with that of an identical-appearing placebo. The biopsies from these dogs showed severe follicular keratosis. The dogs were treated for 2 months at a dosage of 3 mg/kg given once daily. Only one showed significant response, but relapse occurred 2 months after withdrawal of the drug. Readministration of isotretinoin resulted in remission of clinical signs. Elevations in triglyceride levels were noted in three dogs given this dosage. Another investigator has used isotretinoin at 1 mg/kg twice daily for 5 months in four seborrheic cocker spaniels with equally discouraging results (Kwochka, 1984). A clinical report describes the efficacy of isotretinoin at a dosage of 0.25 mg/kg twice daily for 1 month in the treatment of one seborrheic cocker spaniel (Bates, 1984). This patient was normal for longer than 6 months, but relapsed. Periodic readministration of the drug has induced remission of clinical signs, but time between relapses has decreased (Bates, 1985). Based on the above experiences, the use of isotretinoin in the treatment of seborrhea would be limited. A relatively low dosage, 0.25 to 0.5 mg/kg twice daily, could be tried after underlying causes for seborrheic skin disease were ruled out. A positive response should be evident within 1 to 2 months. A patient taking the drug should be evaluated periodically by physical examination, complete blood count, and serum chemistries, including triglyceride and cholesterol levels. The potential for the dog to develop skeletal hyperostosis after long-term therapy is not known. Retinoids are teratogenic in laboratory animals and humans and therefore should not be administered to pregnant animals.

Etretinate, a synthetic retinoid approved for use in humans in Europe, has shown improved efficacy over isotretinoin in the treatment of disorders of keratinization, especially psoriasis (Dicken, 1984). Etretinate, unlike isotretinoin, is stored in the liver and therefore has a prolonged elimination time; it may also have more potential for cumulative toxicity. Side effects in humans are similar to those caused by isotretinoin. The skeletal hyperostosis associated with chronic isotretinoin therapy has not been reported in patients taking etretinate for long periods. Like isotretinoin, etretinate is teratogenic. Due to its anti-inflammatory action, etretinate has been used with success in limited numbers of human patients with T-cell lymphoma, cutaneous lupus erythematosus, dermatitis herpetiformis, bullous pemphigoid, and vasculitis (Dicken, 1984). When approved for use in the United States, etretinate would be available to evaluate for the treatment of canine seborrhea.

The potential for the use of retinoids in veterinary oncology has not been explored. The retinoids may be of value in the treatment of canine ichthyosis.

VITAMIN E

Vitamin E has been reported to be efficacious in the treatment of canine discoid lupus erythematosus and epidermolysis bullosa simplex. There are anecdotal reports of efficacy in canine pemphigus foliaceous and acanthosis nigricans. Vitamin E has been used in the treatment of a variety of dermatologic diseases in humans, with the most convincing results seen in epidermolysis bullosa. The mechanism of action may be related to the stabilization of cell and lysosomal membranes against damage induced by peroxides and free radicals. The therapeutic dosage of vitamin E in dogs is 100 to 400 IU D, L-α-tocopherol acetate given PO twice daily. The author's experience with vitamin E alone in the therapy of canine discoid lupus erythematosus has been limited to five cases. Only one had significant remission of clinical signs. One patient showed no further progression of clinical signs while on vitamin E but seemed to get worse after therapy was stopped. Three patients failed to respond to vitamin E at all. In a series of 16 reported cases, seven were shown to respond to vitamin E alone (Scott et al., 1983). Evidence of clinical improvement may not be seen for 30 to 60 days. Evaluating the response to vitamin E may be difficult, as individual response may depend on initial severity of clinical signs and degree of exposure to ultraviolet light, which can cause exacerbation. This disease may wax and wane regardless of therapy.

Trial therapy with vitamin E in patients with mild forms of discoid lupus erythematosus or in those who cannot tolerate corticosteroids can be recommended at the above dosage, as no side effects have been observed. Although not common, side effects associated with megadoses of vitamin E in humans (800 IU/day/adult) have included severe muscular weakness and fatigue. Allergic contact dermatitis has been induced in humans with topical application of vitamin E (Rechcigl, 1978).

OTHER VITAMINS

Vitamin C (ascorbic acid) has been used in humans to treat a variety of diseases characterized by defects in neutrophil function, including chronic granulomatous disease, Chédiak-Higashi syndrome, hyperimmunoglobulinemia E syndrome, and recurrent cutaneous staphylococcal infections (Fine and Moschella, 1985). Defects in neutrophil chemotaxis were associated with lowered leukocyte ascorbate levels. Patients given 1 to 2 gm of ascorbic acid daily showed improvement in neutrophil chemotaxis as well as in clinical signs. One veterinary investigator has attempted to treat canine patients with recurrent staphylococcal infections with no identifiable predisposing causes with oral vitamin C. No improvement was noted (Schultz, 1985). At the current time, there are no indications for the treatment of canine and feline dermatoses with megadoses of vitamin C.

There are sporadic reports in the human literature of the efficacy of high doses of niacin in the treatment of neutrophil-amplified disorders such as dermatitis herpetiformis and a type of neutrophilic vasculitis, erythema elevatum diutinum. Its use apparently is not widespread in human dermatology, and no work in veterinary medicine has shown a use for this or other B-complex vitamins in the treatment of neutrophil-amplified diseases in dogs.

B-complex vitamins in brewer's yeast, and thiamine in particular, have been touted as adjunctive therapy in the management of flea allergy dermatitis because of putative repellent action. It has been shown that neither brewer's yeast nor thiamine is effective in repelling fleas.

MINERALS

Zinc supplements are useful in the treatment of specific dermatoses. A zinc-responsive dermatosis occurs in Siberian huskies and malamutes (Kunkle, 1980) and occasionally in other breeds such as the Great Dane. Affected dogs are fed complete and balanced diets yet develop erythematous, crusted lesions around the eyes, mouth, ears, and pressure points. Hyperkeratosis of footpads may be pronounced. Histopathologic study of skin biopsies shows diffuse parakeratotic hyperkeratosis, which extends into the hair follicles, as well as significant inflammatory infiltrates in the dermis. Lesions may appear in puppies prior to or during puberty. Some dogs develop lesions spontaneously as young adults. Significant lymphadenopathy can accompany these lesions. The lesions are similar to those in humans with acrodermatitis enteropathica, a hereditary disorder characterized by impaired ability to absorb zinc. A similar mechanism of altered absorption has been postulated for these dogs; it has been demonstrated that malamutes have a genetic defect characterized by decreased zinc absorption in the gut (Muller et al., 1983). The oral administration of zinc causes rapid resolution of the skin lesions within 7 to 10 days. Ten mg/kg of zinc sulfate can be given once daily, or divided and given twice a day. Once remission is achieved, the dosage can be lowered to the daily maintenance dose required to keep the dog symptom free. These dogs seem to require zinc supplementation for life. The dosage may need to be increased during times of stress, such as estrus, pregnancy, and lactation. Zinc gluconate could also be used, as long as the same amount of elemental zinc is given. A 220-mg capsule of zinc sulfate contains 55 mg of elemental zinc. A product containing zinc methionine (Zinpro, Zinpro Corp.) has been advocated, as absorption of zinc is increased when it is complexed with amino acids. Each tablet contains 15 mg elemental zinc; the suggested label dosage is one tablet/10 kg. This dosage can be increased if needed. Dosage can be adjusted to maintenance after remission is achieved. The most significant side effects associated with zinc therapy include inappetence, nausea, and vomiting, which can be managed by dividing the daily dosage into two portions and administering the drug with food.

Zinc-responsive dermatitis is also noted in puppies that are vigorously supplemented with calcium or fed inexpensive diets high in vegetable fiber and soybean meal. Lesions are similar to those described above. The footpads can become hyperkeratotic and fissured. These dogs may have significant lymphadenopathy and malaise. They respond to treatment with zinc at the dosages described above. Any dietary imbalances should be corrected and the dog placed on a reputable brand of commercial dog food. Once in remission, zinc supplementation can be discontinued.

Zinc has been suggested for use in the therapy of burns, wound healing, seborrhea, and recurrent pyodermas. No controlled studies have shown that zinc supplementation is efficacious in the treatment of these diseases.

References and Supplemental Reading

Bates, J. R.: Treatment of idiopathic seborrhea in a dog. Mod. Vet. Pract. 65:725, 1984.

Bates, J. R.: Personal communication, Imperial, MO, 1985.

Chytil, E.: Vitamin A and the skin. *In* Goldsmith, L. A. (ed.): *Biochemistry and Physiology of the Skin*, Vol. 2. New York: Oxford University Press, 1983, pp. 1187–1199.

Dicken, C. H.: Retinoids: A review. J. Am. Acad. Dermatol. 11:541–554, 1984.

Fadok, V.: The use of isotretinoin (Accutane) for canine idiopathic seborrhea. Am. J. Vet. Res., submitted for publication.

Fine, J. D. and Moschella, S. L.: Diseases of nutrition and metabolism. *In* Moschella, S. L., and Harley, J. H.: *Dermatology*, 2nd ed. Philadelphia: W. B. Saunders, 1985, pp. 1422–1532.

Ihrke, P. J., and Goldschmidt, M. H.: Vitamin A-responsive dermatosis in the dog. J.A.V.M.A. 182:687, 1983.

Kunkle, G. A.: Zinc-responsive dermatoses in dogs. *In* Kirk, R. W., (ed.): *Current Veterinary Therapy VII*. Philadelphia: W. B. Saunders, 1980, pp. 472–476.

Kwochka, K.: Unpublished data presented at annual American Academy of Veterinary Dermatology meeting, 1984.

Mellentin, R. W.: *Basic Guide to Canine Nutrition*, 4th ed. White Plains, NY: Gaines Professional Services, 1977, pp. 1–98.

Muller, G. H., Kirk, R. W., and Scott, D. W.: *Small Animal Dermatology*, 3rd ed. Philadelphia: W. B. Saunders, 1983, pp. 477–480, 582–586, 657–666.

National Research Council: *Nutrient Requirements of Cats*. Washington, D.C.: National Academy of Sciences, 1978.

National Research Council: *Nutrient Requirements of Dogs*. Washington, D.C.: National Academy of Sciences, 1974.

Parker, W., Yager-Johnson, J. A., and Hardy, M. H.: Vitamin A responsive seborrheic dermatosis in the dog: A case report. J. Am. Anim. Hosp. Assoc. 19:548, 1983.

Rechcigl, M. (ed.): *CRC Handbook Series in Nutrition and Food. Section E: Nutritional Disorders. Vol. 1: Effects of Nutrient Excesses and Toxicities in Animals and Man*. West Palm Beach, FL: CRC Press, 1978.

Schultz, K.: Personal communication, University of Wisconsin, Madison, 1985.

Scott, D. W., Walton, D. K., Manning, T. O., et al.: Canine lupus erythematosus. II. Discoid lupus erythematosus. J. Am. Anim. Hosp. Assoc. 19:481, 1983.

Sheffy, B. E.: Meeting energy-protein needs of dogs. Comp. Cont. Ed. Pract. Vet. 1:345, 1979a.

Sheffy, B. E.: The nutritionally essential mineral elements. Comp. Cont. Ed. Pract. Vet. 1:673, 1979b.

ANTISEBORRHEIC AGENTS IN DERMATOLOGY

WILLIAM H. MILLER, JR., V.M.D.

Philadelphia, Pennsylvania

"Death is the goal of every epidermal cell, and it is achieved in an orderly manner. Like the leaves of autumn, the epidermal cells, having lived their season, eventually dry out and peel off" (Montagna, 1965).

If every epidermal cell behaved in such an orderly fashion, there would be no need for antiseborrheic products—but indeed the need exists. *Seborrhea* is a term used to describe a variety of conditions in which the skin becomes flaky (seborrhea sicca), greasy (seborrhea oleosa), or both. These cutaneous changes can be caused by a wide variety of conditions that result in some alteration in the normal process of keratinization with or without an alteration in function of the sebaceous glands.

THE NORMAL SKIN

The epidermis of an animal is in a balanced state of renewal in which new cells are produced to match the number of cells lost to the environment. Cells move from the basal cell layer (the mitotic zone of the epidermis) to the skin surface (the stratum corneum) approximately every 3 weeks. This transit time is called the epidermal turnover rate. As the cells migrate upward, they undergo a variety of changes, collectively called keratinization. The cells produce keratin, which is a tough fibrous protein, and lipids. By the time a cell reaches the stratum corneum, it is a flat, anuclear, dead piece of keratin that is joined to similar cells. The stratum corneum of the normal dog is approximately 50 cell layers thick. The stratum corneum cells are held together by intercellular bridges, and the intercellular spaces are filled with—among other things—sebaceous lipids, epidermal lipids, and apocrine sweat. As the cells reach the outermost layers of the stratum corneum, the intercellular bonds are lost and the cells are shed into the environment. Most surface cells are not lost individually but in groups called squames. Normally the squame is so small that it is invisible to the unaided eye.

The sebaceous glands are simple alveolar holocrine glands, which for the most part empty into the hair follicles. Sebum, the product of these glands, is primarily composed of sterol and wax esters and coats the hairs and, through grooming, covers the skin surface. Secretion is under hormonal control.

In addition to the protective effect of sweat and sebum, a natural moisturizing factor has been described in humans. Lactic acid, carboxylic acid, and urea are the most important components of this factor, and these agents are humectants (hygroscopic chemicals that help to absorb water). They also impart a certain plasticity to keratin in the absence of water. It is unknown whether or not these compounds are important in dogs.

SEBORRHEIC SKIN

Any process that affects the epidermal turnover rate, process of keratinization, glandular function, or cohesiveness of scales can cause seborrheic signs. (Refer to Ihrke, 1979, for a complete description of the seborrheic skin disease complex.)

The histopathologic findings in seborrheic skin are not specific and can be characterized as a hyperplastic superficial perivascular dermatitis with hyperkeratosis and follicular keratosis. There may also be histopathologic signs of secondary events such as pyoderma or signs of an underlying endocrine disorder.

Pathophysiologic events known to occur in seborrheic skin include an increase in the epidermal turnover rate to as brief a period as 3 days, an alteration in the cutaneous lipid layer so that there is a decrease in the diester waxes and an increase in free fatty acids, and an increase in the number of pathogenic bacteria on the skin. The exact roles that the altered lipid layer and bacterial flora play is unknown, but they can aggravate any pre-existing condition.

ANTISEBORRHEIC THERAPY

Since most seborrheic dogs have some definable underlying disorder that causes the skin changes, the main thrust of therapy is an accurate diagnosis. If an underlying disease can be identified and resolved, the seborrheic changes will become less severe with time and eventually will spontaneously resolve. Antiseborrheic therapy should be used in these animals to hasten this return to normal, but the therapy will only be necessary for a short period of time. In the case of idiopathic or primary seborrhea, the therapy will be lifelong.

Antiseborrheic agents are numerous, and each has some specific advantages and disadvantages. Agents that have application in the treatment of seborrheic dogs are discussed below.

Nutrition

Normal dietary intake of essential fatty acids, protein, trace minerals (especially zinc), and vitamins A, B, and E is necessary to maintain the normal epidermis of the dog. Standard high-quality commercial foods usually meet or exceed all of the dog's nutritional requirements, so nutritional seborrheas, with the exception of essential fatty acid deficiencies, are infrequent. Breed idiosyncrasies and imbalanced diets can produce seborrheas associated with vitamin deficiencies or excesses or trace mineral imbalances (see Nutritional Therapy in Veterinary Dermatology).

Linoleic acid is essential in the diet of all dogs. Dogs also have the requirement for arachidonic acid and linolenic acid, but these can be synthesized from linoleic acid. In essential fatty acid deficiency, the epidermis becomes hyperproliferative, with an alteration in the barrier function and increased transepidermal water loss. Epidermal lipids, produced during keratinization, are markedly depressed with a fatty acid deficiency. Sebaceous lipids appear not to be affected, but some fat-deficient dogs appear to have an initial decrease in sebum production followed by an overcompensatory increase. Correction of the dietary deficiency or topical application of linoleic acid corrects the barrier defect and returns the epidermis to normal.

Water

Water is necessary for maintaining the flexibility and normalcy of the epidermis. The stratum corneum receives its water by external application (humidity) and transpiration or transepidermal water loss. Water can be drying or moisturizing, depending on the method of application.

With decreased environmental humidity, the epidermis dehydrates and dries. Humidity-damaged dry skin has a normal turnover time and the stratum corneum is of normal thickness, but there is a decrease in transepidermal water loss, further drying the skin. The decreased transepidermal water loss is due to an increase in the sebaceous lipids of the stratum corneum. The cracks and fissures of the surface cells allow the lipids to sink to the deeper zones of the stratum corneum, where they are retained as a barrier to water loss rather than shed with cells as they are lost.

Moisturizers, Bath Oils, and Humectants

These agents are intended for rehydration and subsequent softening of the epidermis. For the maximum effect, the skin should be hydrated first and then covered with an occlusive oil such as petrolatum. Obviously this is impractical in dogs. Bath oils are highly dispersible agents that have appropriate emulsifiers to distribute the oil in water. Humectants use components of the natural moisturizing factor, such as carboxylic acid and lactic acid, to rehydrate the skin without oil.

Keratolytic and Keratoplastic Agents

Keratolytic agents are used to remove all or part of the stratum corneum. The agents do not truly lyse cells, but, since most keratolytic agents are irritants, they cause cellular damage that results in ballooning of the cell and subsequent shedding. Aqueous maceration favors desquamation.

Keratoplastic agents alter the normal process of keratinization. The mode of action varies but probably is due to cytostatic effects on the basal cell layer. Most of the antiseborrheic agents are both keratolytic and keratoplastic.

The agents described in the paragraphs that follow are those that are most widely used in antiseborrheic products.

TARS. Crude coal tars are the product of the distillation of bituminous coal in the absence of oxygen. The crude product is composed of thousands of components, so the standardization of a final product can be very difficult. Coal tar solutions of various strengths are used in antiseborrheic products.

Tars are keratolytic, keratoplastic, antipruritic, and vasoconstrictive. Initially, the skin shows a hyperplastic response to the application of a tar because of the irritant nature of these products. After prolonged use, tars produce an atrophogenic (keratoplastic) effect because they cause a suppression of deoxyribonucleic acid (DNA) synthesis in the epidermis.

Tars, depending on the purity, strength, and state of refinement, can be irritating and will leave an unpleasant odor on the animal. Light-colored coats can be stained. Tars are photodynamic compounds, and photosensitization could occur, especially in white animals. Tar preparations have their greatest application in the greasy forms of seborrhea.

SULFUR. Sulfur is keratolytic, keratoplastic, antipruritic, and antibacterial and is a mild follicular flushing agent. The mode of keratolytic action is thought to be an inflammatory process that causes an increased sloughing of cells. The formation of hydrogen sulfide and pentathionic acid is responsible for its keratolytic as well as its antimicrobial activity. The keratolytic activity of sulfur is enhanced when it is incorporated in a nonemulsive or grease base. The keratoplastic effect probably is a cytostatic one similar to that of coal tars.

Sulfur products can be drying, and they can leave their typical odor on the coat. Sulfur is not a very effective degreasing agent and thus finds most of its use in the dry form of seborrhea. Because of their keratolytic and antibacterial effects, sulfur products are very useful when a pyoderma is present, regardless of whether the underlying seborrhea is dry or greasy.

SALICYLIC ACID. Salicylic acid is keratolytic, keratoplastic, mildly antipruritic, and bacteriostatic. The keratolytic effect is thought to be due to the lowering of the pH of the skin, resulting in an increase in the hydration of the keratin and swelling of the cells. Salicylic acid works best in an emulsion type of base. When salicylic acid is combined with sulfur, a synergistic effect occurs and the keratolytic effect is more pronounced.

Salicylic acid is used in combination with other products.

SELENIUM SULFIDE. Selenium sulfide is keratolytic and keratoplastic because it depresses the epidermal cell turnover rate and interferes with hydrogen bond formation in the keratin. It is also a good degreasing agent. Selenium sulfide can be staining and irritating and often is drying.

BENZOYL PEROXIDE. Benzoyl peroxide is keratolytic, antibacterial, degreasing, and antipruritic and is a strong follicular flushing agent. At 5 per cent concentration, the product is very irritating. Benzoyl peroxides are very useful in the greasy form of seborrhea, especially if there is a secondary bacterial component.

MISCELLANEOUS AGENTS. Alpha-hydroxyacids, which include lactic acid, have been shown to affect keratinization through a nonkeratolytic mechanism. Propylene glycol, fatty acids, and resorcinol also have keratolytic affects.

Hormones

Many seborrheic dogs have underlying endocrine disorders that cause their skin lesions. In these cases, appropriate hormonal therapy corrects the disease and resolves the seborrheic lesions. Hormones do have effects on the epidermis and sebaceous glands and may be useful in the treatment of nonhormonally induced seborrheas.

CORTICOSTEROIDS. Glucocorticoid steroids are agents with complex anti-inflammatory and immunosuppressive effects. In the skin, corticosteroids are profoundly atrophic because of their effect on protein catabolism, their ability to suppress DNA synthesis and therefore inhibit epidermal cell renewal, and their suppression of sebaceous gland function. Additionally, the normal process of keratinization is altered as a result of the stabilization of intracellular lysosomes.

In addition to their effects on the skin, glucocorticoid steroids, either through topical or systemic application, have many serious side effects that include iatrogenic hyperadrenocorticism, increased susceptibility to infection (especially of the skin and urinary tract), diabetes mellitus, gastric ulceration, and pancreatitis. Typically, the effects and side effects of steroids depend on the dose and its duration, but some individuals are much more sensitive than others.

ESTROGENS. At physiologic levels, estrogens are thought to stimulate epidermal mitosis and maintain normal keratinization. At therapeutic levels, estrogens have an atrophic effect on the epidermis and decrease sebum production. Bone marrow suppression (especially of the red cell series) and hepatic changes can occur as side effects of their use.

ANDROGENS. Androgens increase epidermal mitotic activity, thereby increasing cell turnover time and epidermal thickness. They also increase the size of sebaceous glands and sebum production. Aggression (both behavioral and sexual) increased lacrimation, and hepatic changes can occur with the use of androgens.

PROGESTATIONAL COMPOUNDS. At reasonable pharmacologic doses, progestational compounds have very little effect on the skin. In women, topical application can decrease sebum production. Progestational compounds bind androgen receptors and inhibit the enzyme 5-α-reductase, which converts testosterone to dihydrotestosterone, the active substance. Because of these effects, progestational compounds can act as antiandrogenic agents.

Retinoic Acids

Vitamin A is necessary to maintain the normal keratinization of the epidermis. Dietary insufficiencies or excesses of vitamin A can cause various seborrheic conditions. The retinoic acids, derivatives of vitamin A, were developed to treat disorders of keratinization without the toxic side effects of natural vitamin A.

Retinoic acids are available in both oral and topical forms. Topical retinoic acid can be irritating. It causes an increase in epidermal turnover time and reduces the cohesiveness of keratinocytes. Isotretinoin (13-*cis*-retinoic acid) is the commonly used oral retinoid, and in humans it causes sebaceous gland atrophy, alteration of keratinization of the pilosebaceous canal, and a reduction in the cutaneous response to inflammation.

APPROACH TO ANTISEBORRHEIC THERAPY

Every clinician has a favorite approach to the treatment of seborrheic animals and uses the agents that seem most effective. So many agents are available that it is best to know just a few and use these to the exclusion of all others unless their cost, elegance, or efficacy becomes questionable.

Every generalized seborrheic case should be suspect as a fatty acid deficiency and treated as such. In mice, topical application of essential fatty acids has proved to be just as effective in the correction of the epidermal changes as dietary supplementation. In light of this, the author prefers the application of either sesame oil rinse (Veterinary Dermatology Products [VDP]) or HY-LYT*efa (Dermatologics for Veterinary Medicine [DVM]) over dietary addition of fatty acids. In the purest approach, these agents should be used alone; the animal should not be bathed for 4 to 6 weeks, and then its condition should be re-evaluated. If improvement is not seen, fatty acid deficiency is unlikely. If the problem is resolved, topical therapy can be continued or the diet can be modified if that approach is more convenient for the owner. Initially the oils are applied once daily as a rinse or a spray, and then the frequency is decreased as needed. Good grooming by brushing or cloth wiping is essential to clean the skin and hair and prevent excessive oil buildup.

Most cases of generalized seborrhea will require bathing to clean and medicate the skin. A shampoo should be used twice weekly initially until the skin is normal, and then the frequency should be decreased to the lowest acceptable level. This decrease in frequency is especially important when tar-based shampoos are used. The owner should lather the dog well and let the shampoo contact the skin for at least 10 minutes to allow for any keratoplastic effects. Gentle massage of the skin helps lift the dead scales and improves the efficiency of the bathing.

The choice of shampoos depends on the dryness or greasiness of the condition and the individual owner and clinician. For seborrhea sicca, the author prefers sulfur-based products (Sebbafon, Winthrop; SebaLyt, DVM), Nolvasan (Fort Dodge), or Allergroom (Allerderm). Nolvasan is a chlorhexidine-containing emollient shampoo that is especially useful for seborrhea sicca complicated by superficial pyoderma. Allergroom is a hypoallergenic emollient shampoo. Usually the owner is given samples of each and allowed to select the preferred product. Depending on the severity of the condition, bathing may be the only therapy necessary. In those dogs with residual flaking after the bath or with recurrence of flaking before the next bath, bath oils or humectants are used. Bath-oil rinses are applied after the skin is hydrated by bathing. If the agents are used at times other than after bathing, water should be applied to the skin first by misting. Plant mister bottles are an excellent way to moisturize the skin and apply bath oils or humectants. Sesame oil rinse, HY-LYT*efa and Humilac (Allerderm) are all acceptable. Because of its humectants and lactic acid, Humilac tends to have more residual activity and therefore requires less frequent application.

In the greasy seborrheas, benzoyl peroxides, coal tars, and selenium sulfide all can be used. Benzoyl peroxides (OxyDex, DVM; Pyoben, Allerderm) should be used under careful supervision since they can be irritating and cause flaking if used too long. Normally these products are used until the greasiness disappears, and then a different shampoo is used as a replacement or alternately with the benzoyl peroxide.

Most tar shampoos actually are a combination of tars, sulfur, and salicylic acid in various strengths (Lytar, DVM; Allerseb T, Allerderm; Mycodex Tar and Sulfur, Beecham), but some are pure tar shampoos (Pragmatar, Norden; Clear Tar, VDP). These products can be used in either the dry or the greasy form but often can make seborrhea sicca worse because they are too drying. The author uses these products infrequently because of their side effects, and then only in greasy seborrheas. The shampoo can be used as the sole agent, as a replacement, or as an alternate for benzoyl peroxide. If these shampoos are used appropriately, the coat should retain a small amount of oil, so bath oils are unnecessary.

Selenium sulfide is fairly effective in greasy seborrheas, but it can be staining and irritating, especially the veterinary formulation. The human product, Selsun Blue (Abbott), is more elegant, less irritating, and can be purchased without a prescription in pharmacies.

Apart from bathing, the only treatments that find much use in seborrheic therapy are corticosteroid applications. Retinoic acids have not been used extensively, and the reports on their efficacy are conflicting. Further studies need to be completed before their use is recommended. Sex hormone therapy usually is very unrewarding unless an underlying imbalance in these hormones is the cause of the seborrhea. In most seborrheic dogs, the sebaceous glands appear normal histopathologically. If on biopsy the glands appear hypertrophied, sex hormone therapy may be of some value. Estrogens or progestational compounds, because of their antiandrogenic effects, would be the drugs of choice. A response should be seen within 2 weeks, and if none is noted the therapy should be discontinued. Androgens, although they stimulate sebaceous gland secretion, usually are of no benefit in treating seborrhea sicca, and they can cause formation of comedones.

Corticosteroids have no place in the long-term treatment of seborrhea sicca, since they tend to cause dryness of the skin. A short course of therapy during the initiation of antiseborrheic therapy will not be harmful. In seborrhea oleosa or seborrheic dermatitis, pruritus is frequent because of the inflammation in the skin and the free fatty acids on the skin surface. Bathing may lessen the pruritus. Often the pruritus is due to a secondary bacterial infection, in which case appropriate antibiotic therapy decreases the itching. However, if bathing and antibiotic therapy fail to lessen the itching, corticosteroids will be necessary. Topical corticosteroids are most appropriate when the itching is localized. Initially a potent fluorinated steroid in an ointment base (Valisone, Schering) should be used. Ointments occlude the skin surface and hydrate the epidermis, hastening their antiseborrheic effects, but they are greasy and messy. Creams are not as effective but are more acceptable to the client, so they have received wide use. The drug should be applied three to four times daily until the desired effect is achieved. At this point, a less potent agent such as hydrocortisone (1 or 2.5 per cent) should be used to keep the condition in remission.

Often, topical application of a steroid is inappropriate because of the widespread nature of the problem. Systemic drugs are then indicated, but only short-acting oral drugs (prednisone, prednisolone, methylprednisolone) should be used. Judicious use of topical steroids can lessen the amount of oral drug needed. If the animal's pruritus is constant despite bathing and other appropriate therapy, alternate-day steroid therapy can be used, but the owner should be warned of the systemic side effects and that the animal's response to the drug probably will lessen with time. Additionally, if the steroids must be discontinued (for whatever reason), the skin condition will worsen significantly and be much more troublesome to control.

Through careful selection of antiseborrheic agents, most seborrheic dogs can be adequately maintained. After the regimen is determined, it should be continued for as long as it works. Most seborrheic dogs experience a flare in their condition at changes of the season. Dry dogs are worse in the winter and greasy dogs are worse in the summer. If the animal's condition exacerbates, the frequency of bathing is increased until the skin adjusts to the new environmental conditions. If the skin does not respond to the increased effort, a new shampoo should be selected, since some resistance may have developed. If resistance (tachyphylaxis) occurs, the new shampoo should be effective.

References and Supplemental Reading

Austin, V. H.: A clinical approach to abnormal keratinization diseases of the dog. Comp. Cont. Ed. Pract. Vet. 5:890, 1983.

Chesterman, K. W.: An evaluation of O-T-C dandruff and seborrhea products. J. Am. Pharm. Assoc. NS12:578, 1972.

Halliwell, R. E. W.: Seborrhea in the Dog. Comp. Cont. Ed. Pract. Vet. 1:227, 1979.

Ihrke, P. J.: Canine seborrheic disease complex. Vet. Clin. North Am. 9:93, 1979.

Maibach, H. I., and Lowe, N. J.: *Models in Dermatology*. Vol. 1. Basel: Karger, 1985.

Mandy, S. H., and Kramer, K. J.: Moisturizers, bath oils, and dry skin. Dermatology 2:43, 1979.

Montagna, W.: The skin. Sci. Am. 212:56, 1965.

Muller, G. H., Kirk, R. W., and Scott, D. W.: *Small Animal Dermatology*, 3rd ed. Philadelphia: W. B. Saunders, 1983.

Scott, D. W.: Topical Cutaneous Medicine, or Now What Should I Try. Proc. Am. Anim. Hosp. Assoc. 45:89, 1979.

PROGESTAGENS IN DERMATOLOGY

GAIL A. KUNKLE, D.V.M.

Gainesville, Florida

In recent years, progestational compounds have proved to be both advantageous and deleterious for the treatment of skin disorders of small animals. These drugs have been dispensed repeatedly by veterinarians to give rapid symptomatic relief of several feline and a few canine dermatoses. Progestagens can without doubt be therapeutically beneficial, and in a few cases they have given owners an alternative to euthanasia of the pet. However, when therapy is so effective at relieving signs, the veterinarian's search for a cause of a skin disorder becomes less diligently pursued and an actual diagnosis may be ignored. Thus, the widespread use of these drugs has impeded the accumulation of knowledge regarding causes of these dermatoses and especially has hindered progress in feline dermatology.

PROGESTATIONAL COMPOUNDS

The progestagens are synthetic steroid substances that possess physiologic activity similar to progesterone. They suppress release of gonadotropins. Their effects on androgen and estrogen activity reportedly differ in species, change with dosage, and vary in different target organs. They suppress adrenocortical secretion, presumably through suppressing release of adrenocorticotropic hormone (ACTH). The pharmacologic properties that usually suggest their use in dermatology are (1) their effects on behavioral centers in the hypothalamus and limbic systems and (2) their little-understood anti-inflammatory activity in the cat.

MEGESTROL ACETATE. Megestrol acetate (Ovaban, Schering; Megace, Mead Johnson) is a potent synthetic oral progestagen originally marketed for veterinary use in suppression of canine estrus and treatment of pseudopregnancy. Although it is widely used in Europe for this purpose, its primary use in the United States is in the treatment of feline dermatoses.

The drug is supplied in a palatable tablet of either 5 mg or 20 mg. Since cats find this tablet especially tasty, proper precautions should be taken to prevent them from ingesting large quantities. Although recommended dosages vary, the most commonly used regimen for cats is 2.5 to 5.0 mg daily or on alternate days initially, with a declining dosage to follow after remission of symptoms (1 to 3 weeks). When withdrawal of the drug results in recurrence of lesions, long-term maintenance therapy of 2.5 to 5.0 mg once or twice weekly may be necessary for control. Dogs are usually treated with 2 to 4 mg/kg daily for behavior-related dermatoses.

Megestrol acetate is *not* approved by the Food and Drug Administration for use in cats.

INJECTABLE PROGESTATIONAL COMPOUNDS. Medroxyprogesterone acetate (MPA) (Depo-Provera, Upjohn) is an injectable repository progestagen. Upjohn also markets an oral form of this drug, but it is not used in veterinary medicine. Repository progesterone (in oil) is periodically marketed for veterinary use by various veterinary suppliers. Side effects with progestational compounds can be serious, and injectable products are preferred only in patients in which oral medication presents a significant problem. Recommended dosages of the injectable products vary widely, and cats generally receive 50 to 100 mg and dogs 20 mg/kg. Administration of these injectable products may be repeated in 3 to 6 months if needed. Behavior-related dermatoses may require higher levels or more frequent administration because of variations in individual response to the drug. The solubility of injectable progestagens in tissue and subsequent metabolism may also vary from pet to pet, so effects of these products may be extended for many months in some animals.

Most often, injectable and oral progestagens can be used interchangeably, as they have common effects. However, it is reported that occasionally one product will cause a more dramatic clinical response in the same cat than in another.

Feline Uses

EOSINOPHILIC GRANULOMA COMPLEX (EGC). Progestational compounds have been used successfully in the treatment of all three forms of EGC. They are most useful in the treatment and management of oral lip ulcers and the oral collagenolytic granulomas, both of which may become refractory to corticosteroids. The cause of these forms is unknown at this time.

The eosinophilic plaque form of EGC deserves further investigation in individual cases. This clinical entity may occur with generalized pruritus, and in those cases the cause of the pruritus should be investigated. Flea allergy, food allergy, or atopy should be considered. Occasionally, a mechanical or chemical irritant may result in a clinical lesion compatible with a diagnosis of eosinophilic plaque. Removing the inciting cause may eliminate the need for specific symptomatic therapy.

MILIARY DERMATITIS. Miliary dermatitis represents a complex of diseases that result in a local or generalized crusting dermatosis. All cases of this clinical entity deserve diagnostic investigation. Flea allergy, food allergy, inhalant allergy, ectoparasitism, dermatophytosis, and bacterial folliculitis are among some of the causes responsible for the clinical symptoms of miliary dermatitis. A thorough history, skin scrapings, fungal cultures, and allergy testing are indicated in many cases. When it is impossible to pinpoint the underlying cause, glucocorticoid therapy is usually effective. Therefore, a diagnosis of miliary dermatitis does not usually warrant therapy with progestagens.

SELF-INDUCED HAIR LOSS. There are two groups of cats that will lick and pull hair, often in a symmetric pattern from the trunk and extremities. In the first group, or the majority of cases, these cats cause no excoriations or obvious lesions on the skin itself. Some of these cats have true pruritus, which results in their increased grooming activity. Why these cats do not excoriate themselves is unclear. The second group of cats have no apparent pruritus and pull hair or excessively lick for behavior-related reasons (psychogenic alopecia). Most cases of pattern hair loss in which the hairs are broken or stubby should first be investigated for underlying causes of pruritus. Hair loss occurring *only* on body regions easily accessible to a cat in a reclining or sitting position (such as the inside and outside of the front legs, the abdomen, and the lateral thighs) may suggest that the cat is overzealously grooming for behavioral reasons.

Cats in the group with pruritus-induced hair loss benefit most from treatment for the specific cause of the pruritus. Cats with psychogenic-induced hair loss may benefit from megestrol acetate or behavioral modification. Mechanical barriers such as an Elizabethan collar may be adjunctive to breaking a habit of excessive licking. Sometimes cats may have a combination of both problems—a temporary pruritic condition may have initiated licking and a subsequent bad habit developed but did not regress when the source of the itch was removed.

Cases of self-induced hair loss in cats are often more disconcerting to the pet's owner than they are troublesome to the pet. Although progestagens may be effective in managing these cases, the risks of side effects should always be considered. These agents are best used temporarily and as adjunctive therapy.

ENDOCRINE ALOPECIA (FEA). The author believes this to be a very rare condition of castrated male cats in which symmetric alopecia occurs in the groin and caudal thighs. A mechanical barrier such as an Elizabethan collar should not result in improvement of the coat in true cases of FEA, since the hair is falling out and not being pulled out. Reportedly, cats with FEA have an easily epilated coat, although this can be difficult to assess clinically. Affected cats respond best to sex hormone supplementation. Although some clinicians have reported success with progestagen treatment, these drugs rarely seem indicated in this disease.

FELINE HYPERESTHESIA. This rare feline condition is one that can cause frustration, present a dilemma to the cat's owner and veterinarian, and cause apparently intense pain to the cat itself. In this syndrome, cats show heightened sensitivity in the thoracolumbar region. Simply touching the skin of this area may induce severe muscle spasms and yowling to almost seizurelike proportions. Neurologic examinations and necropsies of these cases have shown no specific pathologic mechanism for this hyperesthesia. This condition should be differentiated from steatitis (with subcutaneous ceroid deposits) resulting from vitamin E deficiency. Cats with signs of hyperesthesia may respond to phenobarbital, diazepam, and in some cases progestational compounds. Euthanasia may eventually be necessary if the severity of symptoms increases.

STUD TAIL. Progestational compounds can be used to control a local seborrheic disorder of sexually active male cats known as stud tail. This is generally an unaesthetic condition but one that causes little other problem. Veterinarians should remember, however, that progestational compounds may suppress spermatogenesis and thus are best avoided in males intended for breeding.

OTHER DISORDERS. In cats, progestational compounds exhibit potent anti-inflammatory effects by unknown mechanisms. There are rare instances when potent anti-inflammatory properties may be required to treat cases in which glucocorticoid therapy is not totally effective.

The exact effects of progestational compounds on the immune system of cats are unknown. Some dermatologists have found megestrol acetate to be occasionally beneficial in treating feline autoimmune skin disease in cases refractory to high doses of corticosteroids. Other immunosuppressive chemotherapeutic agents such as azathioprine and gold salts should be considered as options when megestrol acetate treatment is proposed in the management of autoimmune skin disease.

Canine Uses

BEHAVIOR- OR PSYCHOGENIC-RELATED DERMATOSES. Progestational compounds have been used with mixed results in the treatment of dermatoses caused by or complicated by abnormal behavior. It is often difficult for a veterinarian presented with a long-standing skin problem to assess the true cause and to ascertain how much of the dermatosis was initiated by the dog's behavior. However, there is little doubt that factors such as boredom, positive reinforcement from the owner, insecurity, and failure of adaptation to environmental change may significantly contribute to some skin diseases.

The classic "boredom dermatosis" is acral lick dermatitis, once presumed to be due primarily to self-trauma by the dog. We now find that many of these cases respond dramatically to extended courses of systemic antibiotics, suggesting that there is an infectious cause. In other cases of lick granuloma, symptomatic treatment with topical or intralesional anti-inflammatory compounds may be efficacious. In still others, behavior seems to play a primary role, and the dog may initiate a new lesion overnight. Progestagen therapy alone is not commonly effective in the medical management of these patients, but in cases unresponsive to antibiotics, progestagens may be a helpful adjunct when used with mechanical barriers (Elizabethan collar or bandages) for interruption of the lick cycle. They also may be advantageous when initiating behavior modification. These drugs are not useful for long-term management of canine acral lick dermatitis.

Flank sucking, an undesirable habit of some Doberman pinschers, and foot chewing in toy poodles are sometimes unexplained by known disease entities. These traits may subsequently be attributed to inappropriate behavior. However, therapy with drugs, including progestagens, is usually unrewarding.

SEBORRHEA. When megestrol acetate was first sold in this country, it was hoped that through its indirect antiandrogen effects it would be useful in the treatment of seborrhea. However, it has *not* been efficacious in therapy of this clinical complex.

HORMONAL ALOPECIA. Very rarely, spayed female dogs will present with symmetric alopecia that cannot be attributed to hypothyroidism, hypoestrogenism, hyperadrenocorticism, or hyposomatotropism. These dogs may show regrowth of hair when supplemented with megestrol acetate at 1 to 2 mg/kg/daily. Therapy may later be tapered significantly for maintenance of a normal coat. The risk of potential side effects should always be considered, especially in long-term maintenance therapy.

Side Effects

FELINE. There are four major side effects that the clinician should consider seriously before instituting the use of a progestagen in cats. Any of these can ultimately result in death of the pet. There has been no positive relationship shown between these side effects and dose or duration of therapy.

1. The most serious of these is the *adrenocortical suppression,* which occurs in all cats given progestagens. In one study, significant impairment of adrenocortical function was noted after 2 weeks of megestrol acetate (2.5 mg/cat) on alternate days. Others have noted suppression of adrenocortical function in cats given megestrol acetate only once weekly (2.5 or 5.0 mg). These effects are rather rapid in onset, but the adrenal is slow to recover. Some cats given small weekly maintenance doses for long periods have taken 12 weeks or longer to regain their adrenal function after cessation of megestrol acetate. This delayed recovery is a probable reflection of the long half-life of progestational compounds in cats. Since these compounds seem to have mild glucocorticoid effects in cats, this fact coupled with the long half-life probably helps to prevent acute crises when the drug is suddenly withdrawn. However, when surgery or some other definitive stress is predicted for a cat that has just discontinued megestrol acetate, short-term supplementation with oral glucocorticoids might prevent a crisis.

2. *Mammary changes* have been repeatedly noted in cats given progestational compounds. The most common change is fibroadenomatous hyperplasia, or feline mammary hypertrophy. This condition occurs in both intact or neutered male and female cats. Its occurrence does not necessarily correlate with the dose or duration of therapy. It has been seen within a few weeks after institution of standard doses. Microscopically there is proliferation of mammary duct epithelium and stroma. Cases may spontaneously regress over weeks once the progestagen is discontinued. In other cases, the mammary tissues may be painful, ulcerated, and draining, necessitating surgical resection.

Mammary neoplasias have also been linked to progestational therapy in cats. Mammary tumors in cats are usually malignant and carry a poor prognosis. Since one cannot clinically distinguish neoplasia from hypertrophy, mammary masses in cats always should be pursued diagnostically through biopsy or cytologic examination.

Clinicians should flag the records of feline patients that are receiving megestrol acetate, so that they are reminded to palpate the mammary glands whenever the cat visits the office.

3. *Diabetes mellitus* is a rather serious side effect that occurs in some cats given megestrol acetate. Its appearance does not seem to be related to dose or duration, and it has occurred as early as 2 weeks after institution of therapy. In many cases, insulin therapy is needed; some of these cats will require decreasing amounts of insulin over the next weeks to months, and in most of these cases the diabetes is transient. In a few cases, however, cats have required lifelong management of their diabetes in spite of discontinuation of megestrol acetate. In a few cases, cats have been refractory to insulin and death has occurred.

4. *Pyometra,* especially stump pyometras, can be serious sequelae to megestrol acetate therapy. If any significant area of the uterus is left during ovariohysterectomy, the cat is predisposed to pyometra if megestrol acetate is prescribed.

The statistical incidence of these side effects is not reported and is unlikely to be in the near future. Large prospective investigations with clinical patients would be necessary. Although many practitioners use these drugs routinely and report no obvious complications, evidence continues to accumulate regarding the side effects listed above.

Some clinicians have suggested that side effects may be compounded by the concurrent use of glucocorticoids. Certainly the pathophysiologic mechanisms that result in adrenocortical suppression and diabetes mellitus would suggest that simultaneous glucocorticoid therapy might complicate problems. Thus, combination therapy should be restricted to very refractory cases.

CANINE. In dogs and other species in which values have been measured, circulating levels of growth hormone may increase with the use of progestagens. Acromegaly has been known to occur in a few dogs given these drugs.

General Effects

In both dogs and cats, personality changes often are noted with the use of progestagens. These effects vary widely in different pets, but those most frequently noted include increased affection or friendliness, calmness or tranquility, and lethargy. Occasionally a "people-oriented" pet may become more reserved and withdrawn. The actions of these drugs on the hypothalamus and limbic system not only result in these mentioned side effects but also are responsible for their therapeutic use in behavior problems. Other effects include polydipsia, which is not usually noted by the owner, and polyphagia, which may be marked in many individuals. Weight gain is a common result of therapy with this drug in cats and dogs unless dietary intake is restricted.*

Injections of progestagens may cause local alopecia, atrophy, and depigmentation. These changes are usually temporary but may be permanent. This side effect usually can be avoided by giving injections intramuscularly and not subcutaneously.

Because progestational compounds suppress spermatogenesis, their use should be restricted to male dogs and cats not intended as breeding animals.

**Editor's Note*: Iatrogenic Cushing's syndrome has also been noted in dogs and cats treated with megestrol acetate.

Pyometra has been documented in females after the use of the long-acting progesterone compounds. Although the oral form of megestrol acetate has been marketed as a "birth control" drug, manufacturers recommend limited use in estrus postponement to avoid uterine changes. Mammary changes including hypertrophy and neoplasia have also been repeatedly reported.

WHEN TO USE THESE DRUGS

Veterinarians should try to answer the following questions honestly when they reach for a progestational compound:

1. Have you investigated the cause of this dermatosis?
2. Have you attempted to treat the specific cause when it is known?
3. Have other drugs with fewer potential side effects been considered or used?
4. Is the owner well informed regarding the possible side effects?
5. Is the drug approved for use in the species you are treating and, if not, has the owner been so informed?
6. Do the symptoms warrant the use of the drug?

References and Supplemental Reading

Chastain, C. B., Graham, C. L. and Nichols, C. E.: Adrenocortical suppression in cats given megestrol acetate. Am. J. Vet. Res. 42:2029, 1981.

Eigenmann, J. E., and Venker-van Haagen, A. J.: Progestagen-induced and spontaneous canine acromegaly due to reversible growth hormone overproduction: Clinical picture and pathogenesis. J. Am. Anim. Hosp. Assoc. 17:813, 1981.

Elling, H., and Ungemach, F. R.: Progesterone receptors in feline mammary cancer cytosol. J. Cancer Res. Clin. Oncol. 100:325, 1981.

Gosselin, Y., Chalifoux, A., and Papageorges, M.: The use of megestrol acetate in some feline dermatological problems. Can. Vet. J. 22:382, 1981.

Hayden, D. W., Johnston, S. D., Kiang, D. T., et al.: Feline mammary hypertrophy/fibroadenoma complex: Clinical and hormonal aspects. Am. J. Vet. Res. 42:1699, 1981.

Kunkle, G. A.: Vet. Clin. North Am. [Small Anim. Pract.] 14:1065, 1984.

Ogilvie, G. K.: Feline mammary neoplasia. Comp. Cont. Ed. Pract. Vet. 5:384, 1983.

Pemberton, P. L.: Canine and feline behavior control: Progestin therapy. *In* Kirk, R. W. (ed.): *Current Veterinary Therapy VII*. Philadelphia: W. B. Saunders, 1983, pp. 62–71.

Scott, D. W.: Feline dermatology 1900–1978: A monograph. J. Am. Anim. Hosp. Assoc. 16:331, 1980.

FELINE POXVIRUS INFECTION

L. R. THOMSETT, F.R.C.V.S.
London, England

Since the mid-1970s, several cases of poxvirus infection have been reported in domestic and exotic felines in Europe. Based on these initial observations, it is thought that the prevalence of clinical disease in cats is low. However, because of the similarity of the viruses isolated from cats to cowpox virus and the susceptibility of cows and humans to infection with cowpox virus, much interest has been generated in the feline disease.

The precise identity of the poxvirus isolated from cats is currently controversial. Cowpox virus is a member of the *Orthopoxvirus* genus, as are smallpox and vaccinia viruses. All orthopoxviruses have similar morphology and share common antigens, so that differentiation between isolates of these viruses is not always readily achieved or clear. Initial descriptions of the poxvirus isolated from cats concluded, on the basis of morphologic and cross-neutralization studies, that the isolates were cowpox virus. However, a recent study involving transmission of the virus isolated from a cat to cattle concluded that the virus was unlikely to be cowpox virus. These investigators suggested that the feline virus be called after the host of origin (e.g., catpox virus or feline poxvirus).

Feline poxvirus infection has been recorded in cats from 2 months to 12 years of age, with no apparent predilections for breed or sex. The most common presenting sign is the development of multiple, circular, 5- to 10-mm diameter skin lesions, which include crusted papules, plaques, nodules, and crateriform ulcers. Pruritus is variable, and the lesions occur most commonly on the face, limbs, paws, and dorsal lumbar area. Initial skin lesions may develop at the site of a reported bite wound. Systemic signs may or may not be present and include some combination of anorexia, lethargy, pyrexia, vomiting, diarrhea, conjunctivitis, dyspnea, and jaundice.

The differential diagnosis includes bacterial and fungal infections, the eosinophilic granuloma complex, and neoplasia (especially mast cell tumor and lymphosarcoma). Definitive diagnosis is made by skin biopsy, serologic testing, and virus isolation. Dermatohistopathologic findings include hyperplasia, ballooning degeneration, reticular degeneration, microvesicle formation, and necrosis of affected epidermis and the outer root sheath of the hair follicle. Eosinophilic intracytoplasmic inclusion bodies are found within keratinocytes. Serum samples and fresh biopsy or scab material in viral transport medium are submitted to an appropriate diagnostic laboratory for serologic examination and viral isolation (hemorrhagic pocks are produced on the chorioallantoic membranes of hen eggs), respectively.

Therapy is symptomatic. Most cats recover spontaneously within 1 to 2 months. Glucocorticoids are contraindicated.

The epizootiology of feline poxvirus infection is poorly understood. It is hypothesized that cats become infected accidentally and that the virus reservoir is some yet unidentified small wild mammal.

References and Supplemental Reading

Baxby, D., Ashton, D. G., Jones, D., et al.: Cowpox virus infection in unusual hosts. Vet. Rec. 104:175, 1979.

Baxby, D., and Gaskell, R. M.: Cowpox in cats. Vet. Rec. 111:132, 1982.

Gaskell, R. M., Gaskell, C. J., and Evans, R. J.: Natural and experimental poxvirus infection in the domestic cat. Vet. Rec. 112:164, 1983.

Hoare, C. M., Gruffy, D. D., and Jones, T. J.: Cowpox in cats. Vet. Rec. 114:22, 1984.

Martin, W. B., Scott, F. M. M., and Lauder, I. M.: Poxvirus infection of cats. Vet. Rec. 115:36, 1984.

Martland, M. F., Fowler, S., and Poulten, G. J.: Poxvirus infection of a domestic cat. Vet. Rec. 112:171, 1983.

Schönbauer, M., Schönbauer-Länele, A., and Kölbl, S.: Pockeninfektion bei einer Hauskatze. Zentralbl. Veterinarmed. [B] 29:434, 1982.

Thomsett, L. R., Baxby, D., and Denham, E. M. H.: Cowpox in the domestic cat. Vet. Rec. 108:567, 1978.

Webster, J., and Jeffries, A. R.: Cowpox. Vet. Rec. 114:151, 1984.

SULFONES AND SULFONAMIDES IN CANINE DERMATOLOGY

DANNY W. SCOTT, D.V.M.

Ithaca, New York

Sulfones first attracted attention because of their chemical relationship to the sulfonamides, and they were first used extensively in the 1940s for the treatment of leprosy in humans. The sulfonamides were the first truly effective chemotherapeutic agents to be employed in medical practice for the prevention and cure of nontreponemal bacterial infections in humans. However, the sulfonamides are now of very limited use as antibacterial agents, having been replaced by a succession of newer, more effective, and less toxic agents. More recently, the sulfones and certain sulfonamides have been employed by dermatologists and rheumatologists for the treatment of a variety of disorders. Most of these disorders are characterized by being noninfectious, presumably immune mediated, and associated with tissue neutrophilia.

MECHANISM OF ACTION

The antimicrobial activity of these drugs is based on a competition with para-aminobenzoic acid for incorporation into folic acid in susceptible bacteria. However, this does not explain their efficacy in the predominantly noninfectious disorders for which they are currently used.

Sulfones have potent anti-inflammatory actions in many animal models of inflammation. They inhibit formation of edema (irritant and foreign body reactions) and Arthus reactions but have no demonstrable inhibitory effects on histamine, serotonin, bradykinin, prostaglandins, immune-complex formation, cell-mediated immunity, or humoral immunity. The antipyretic and analgesic properties of the sulfones are comparable to those of phenylbutazone. They have also been shown to suppress the release of β-glucuronidase from phagocytosing macrophages.

The current theory on the mechanism of action of these drugs in the disorders for which they are prescribed centers around an effect the drugs have on the neutrophil. These drugs have been shown to inhibit the neutrophil's cytotoxicity system, which is mediated by myeloperoxidase, hydrogen peroxide, and halides. When the neutrophil phagocytizes bacteria or immune complexes, hydrogen peroxide and myeloperoxidase are released into surrounding tissues to catalyze the formation of free iodine from sodium iodide. When this reaction is dampened by sulfones, inflammation is markedly decreased. These drugs do not appear to have any effect on neutrophil chemotaxis, random motility, or phagocytosis *in vitro*. Significantly, despite this effect on neutrophils, there is no apparent increased susceptibility to bacterial infections in patients receiving these drugs.

METABOLISM

The metabolism and distribution of these drugs have been studied in humans and laboratory animals but *not* in dogs. Most orally administered sulfones are metabolized to the parent compound, dapsone. Absorption of dapsone from the gastrointestinal tract is slow and nearly complete; about 85 per cent of a given dose is absorbed. Peak serum levels occur in 2 to 6 hours. With continued administration, serum levels reach a plateau in 8 to 10 days.

There is considerable retention of sulfones in the body. After repeated doses of dapsone, trace amounts can be detected in the blood for more than a month after the last dose. The long half-life and persistence within the body are associated with high levels of protein binding and enterohepatic recycling. The sulfones are retained to varying degrees in skin, muscle, liver, and kidneys. About 80 to 90 per cent of an administered dapsone dose is excreted in the urine, and about 10 per cent is recoverable from the bile.

Of the sulfonamides, only sulfapyridine and sulfasalazine have been found to be effective. Sulfasalazine is presumed to work by being broken down to sulfapyridine by colonic bacteria.

CLINICAL USE

The sulfones and sulfonamides have been used to manage an amazing array of diseases in humans (Table 1). In dogs, these agents have been used successfully to treat subcorneal pustular dermatosis, cutaneous vasculitis, linear IgA dermatosis, pemphigus foliaceus, and pemphigus erythematosus. The reader is referred to the supplemental reading list (especially Muller et al., 1983) for discussions of these diseases. Only dapsone (Avlosulfon, Ayerst) and sulfasalazine (Azulfidine, Pharmacia) have been used in dogs. In humans, dapsone is usually the drug of choice as it is more effective and usually better tolerated.

Table 1. *Human Diseases That May Respond Favorably to Sulfones and Sulfonamides*

Dermatitis herpetiformis
Subcorneal pustular dermatosis
Pemphigus
Pemphigoid
Discoid lupus erythematosus
Systemic lupus erythematosus
Relapsing polychondritis
Rheumatoid arthritis
Herpes gestationis
Vasculitis
Erythema elevatum diutinum
Sterile nodular panniculitis
Acute febrile neutrophilic dermatosis (Sweet's syndrome)
Pustular psoriasis
Acropustulosis of infancy
Granuloma faciale
Alopecia mucinosa
Cystic acne
Benign familial pemphigus (Hailey-Hailey disease)
Epidermolysis bullosa acquisita
Linear IgA dermatosis
Pyoderma gangrenosum
Pyoderma vegetans
Leprosy
Actinomycotic mycetoma
Brown recluse spider bites (loxoscelism)

Because metabolic studies with these drugs have not been conducted on dogs, currently recommended regimens for the use of dapsone and sulfasalazine are totally empirical. Initially, dapsone or sulfasalazine is given orally at a dosage of 1 mg/kg or 20 mg/kg, respectively, three times daily. A good clinical response should be seen within 1 to 4 weeks. Dapsone should *not* be continued at these "induction" doses for longer than 4 weeks, as the likelihood of toxicity becomes greater.

After remission is achieved, "maintenance" doses of the drugs are sought. The drugs are first given twice daily for 2 weeks, then once daily. Occasionally, the drugs can be given *every other* day and still secure clinical remission. In most instances, owing to the nature of the diseases being treated, therapy must be continued for long periods of time if not for life.

The author has found dapsone to be most useful in the management of subcorneal pustular dermatosis and cutaneous leukocytoclastic vasculitis, although not every case is completely controlled. The few dogs that do not totally respond are markedly improved and are satisfactory pets as far as their owners are concerned. The response of dogs having pemphigus foliaceus, pemphigus erythematosus, and linear IgA dermatosis is much more unpredictable. About 50 per cent of the cases in which the drug has been used have shown a beneficial response. In dogs with pemphigus, dapsone has had a marked steroid-sparing effect but has not been effective for total control by itself.

Interestingly, the author has seen two dogs with subcorneal pustular dermatosis become apparently refractory to the effects of dapsone after long periods of drug-induced remission. These dogs were then satisfactorily managed with sulfasalazine.

Table 2. Side Effects of Sulfones and Sulfonamides in Humans

Hemolysis
Methemoglobinemia
Dermatitis
Nausea
Vomiting
Headache
Dizziness
Fatigue
Anorexia
Shortness of breath
Nervousness
Hepatotoxicity (hepatitis; cholestatic jaundice)
Nephrotoxicity
Neuropathy (motor)
Lymphadenopathy
Psychosis
Leukopenia
Agranulocytosis

SIDE EFFECTS

In humans, the side effects attributable to these drugs are legion (Table 2). The least serious but most bothersome side effects are nausea, vomiting, headache, weakness, dizziness, fatigue, anorexia, shortness of breath, and nervousness. These are dose related and occur in 20 to 38 per cent of the patients. Hemolysis is common but is severe *only* in patients who lack glucose-6-phosphate dehydrogenase. Heinz body formation may be seen. Cutaneous eruptions develop in about 10 per cent of the patients taking these drugs and include morbilliform eruptions, erythema multiforme, erythema nodosum, toxic epidermal necrolysis, and exfoliative erythroderma. Hepatotoxicity, leukopenia, and agranulocytosis are rare (0.1 to 5 per cent of the patients) and not related to dose (idiosyncratic).

In dogs, side effects associated with dapsone administration have included mild anemia (normocytic, normochromic), mild neutropenia, severe thrombocytopenia, mild to moderate asymptomatic elevations of liver enzymes, vomiting, diarrhea, clinical hepatotoxicity, and generalized erythematous maculopapular dermatitis. Mild asymptomatic anemia, neutropenia, and elevated levels of liver enzymes are commonly encountered during induction therapy and do not usually necessitate stopping treatment. These measures return to normal as maintenance doses are achieved. Vomiting and diarrhea are usually avoided by giving the drug with food. Clinical hepatotoxicity, severe thrombocytopenia, and cutaneous eruptions are rare. The most common side effect associated with sulfasalazine is keratoconjunctivitis sicca, which is usually irreversible. As this effect is relatively mild and easily managed with artificial tears, sulfasalazine treatment is not usually stopped.

In rodents, chronic toxicity studies with sulfones have indicated that the drugs are carcinogenic. There is no information to suggest that a similar phenomenon occurs in humans or dogs.

All side effects usually respond rapidly and completely to stopping the causative drugs. In humans, vitamin E is believed to partially or totally correct hemolysis, and glucocorticoids are thought to benefit patients with leukopenia or agranulocytosis. Activated charcoal is recommended for cases of acute toxicosis. As concerns interactions with other drugs, caution is indicated during the concurrent use of other oxidant agents (enhanced erythrocyte toxicity). In humans, patients who react adversely to one of the sulfone or sulfonamide drugs may take another with no difficulty. However, the incidence of cross-reactivity is estimated to be 20 per cent.

Because of the potential side effects associated with sulfones and sulfonamides, it is recommended that a hemogram, urinalysis, and blood urea nitrogen and alanine amino transferase levels be checked every 1 to 2 weeks during induction therapy. During maintenance therapy, the same values should be checked every 1 to 3 months. Dogs receiving sulfasalazine should also have their tear production closely monitored so that artificial tear therapy can be instituted if needed.

References and Supplemental Reading

Baker, K. P.: Subcorneal pustular dermatosis seen in dogs. Vet. Rec. 106:420, 1980.

Barranco, V. P.: Inhibition of lysosomal enzymes by dapsone. Arch. Dermatol. 110:563, 1974.

Barranco, V. P.: Dapsone—other indications. Int. J. Dermatol. 21:513, 1982.

Berstein, J. E., and Lorincz, A. L.: Sulfonamides and sulfones in dermatologic therapy. Int. J. Dermatol. 20:81, 1981.

Coburn, P. R., and Shuster, S.: Dapsone and discoid lupus erythematosus. Br. J. Dermatol. 106:105, 1982.

Elonen, E., Neuvonen, P. J., and Halmekoski, J.: Acute dapsone intoxication: A case with prolonged symptoms. Clin. Toxicol. 14:79, 1979.

Fadok, V. A., and Barrie, J.: Sulfasalazine responsive vasculitis in the dog: A case report. J. Am. Anim. Hosp. Assoc. 20:161, 1984.

Goodman, L. S., and Gilman, A.: *The Pharmacological Basis of Therapeutics*. New York: MacMillan, 1975.

Jablonska, S., and Chorzelski, T.: When and how to use sulfones in bullous diseases. Int. J. Dermatol. 20:103, 1981.

Katz, S. I.: Sulfones and sulfapyridine. J. Am. Acad. Dermatol. 3:80, 1980.

Katz, S. I.: Bullous systemic LE: Response to dapsone. J. Am. Acad. Dermatol. 8:738, 1983.

King, L. E., and Rees, R. S.: Dapsone treatment of a brown recluse bite. J.A.M.A. 250:648, 1983.

Lang, P. G.: Sulfones and sulfonamides in dermatology today. J. Am. Acad. Dermatol. 1:479, 1979.

Lees, G. E., McKeever, P. J., and Ruth, G. R.: Fatal thrombocytopenic hemorrhagic diathesis associated with dapsone administration to a dog. J.A.V.M.A. 175:49, 1979.

Lewis, A. J., Gemmell, D. K., and Stimson, W. H.: The anti-inflammatory profile of dapsone in animal models of inflammation. Agents Actions 8:578, 1978.

Mackel, S. E.: Treatment of vasculitis. Med. Clin. North Am. 66:941, 1982.

Manning, T. O., and Scott, D. W.: Cutaneous vasculitis in a dog. J. Am. Anim. Hosp. Assoc. 16:61, 1980.

McKeever, P. J., and Dahl, M. V.: A disease in dogs resembling human subcorneal pustular dermatosis. J.A.V.M.A. 170:704, 1977.

Morgan, R. V., and Bachrach, A.: Keratoconjunctivitis sicca associated with sulfonamide therapy in dogs. J.A.V.M.A. 180:432, 1982.

Muller, G. H., Kirk, R. M., and Scott, D. W.: *Small Animal Dermatology III*. Philadelphia, W.B. Saunders, 1983.

Piamphongsant, T.: Dapsone for the treatment of vesiculo-bullous and pustular diseases. Int. J. Dermatol. 21:512, 1982.

Ruzicka, T., and Goerz, G.: Dapsone in the treatment of lupus erythematosus. Br. J. Dermatol. 104:53, 1981.

Scott, D. W., Manning, T. O., and Smith, C. A.: Linear IgA dermatoses in the dog: Bullous pemphigoid, discoid lupus erythematosus, and a subcorneal pustular dermatitis. Cornell Vet. 72:394, 1982.

Stendahl, O., Molin, L., and Dahlgren, C.: The inhibition of cytotoxicity by dapsone. J. Clin. Invest. 62:214, 1978.

CANINE EPIDERMOTROPIC LYMPHOMA

(Mycosis Fungoides and Pagetoid Reticulosis)

DONNA K. WALTON, D.V.M.

Ithaca, New York

Mycosis fungoides is a type of lymphoma that has clinical and histologic characteristics distinguishing it from other cutaneous lymphosarcomas, either primary or secondary. This condition has been well documented in humans. In the past 15 years, mycosis fungoides has been described in several dogs and, recently, in one cat.

Alibert, a French dermatologist, originally described the disease in humans in 1806 and named it mycosis fungoides in 1832 because he thought the cutaneous tumors produced in the late stage of the disease resembled mushrooms. By 1872, most authors believed that mycosis fungoides was a form of cutaneous lymphoma. More recently, the disease has been grouped with several malignant skin diseases under the heading of cutaneous T-cell lymphomas. There currently is much controversy concerning the genesis of human mycosis fungoides. It has been suggested that chronic stimulation of Langerhans' cells and T-lymphocytes by persistent environmental antigens may result in a reactive inflammatory process that eventually becomes malignant.

HUMAN MYCOSIS FUNGOIDES

Clinically, the classic, progressive behavior of mycosis fungoides in humans may be divided into three stages. The premycotic, or eczematous, stage is characterized by localized patches of erythema and scale. Pruritus is variable. During the plaque stage, firm, raised papules coalesce to form smooth, solid plaques that are erythematous and may be scaly. These may or may not be pruritic. It is during the third, or tumor, stage that the malignant nature of this disease becomes obvious. Tumors are usually firm, sessile, and may be brightly erythematous. They appear to be painless and are rarely pruritic. They may regress spontaneously or enlarge, ulcerate, and become secondarily infected. The premycotic and plaque stages may be present for prolonged periods of time before the disease advances to the tumor stage. Mycosis fungoides is ultimately fatal, with metastasis to lymph nodes and internal organs.

In addition to the classic, progressive appearance of mycosis fungoides in human beings, several clinical variations have been recognized. The d'emblée form begins in the tumorous stage without clinical evidence of the premycotic or plaque stages. This form appears to progress more rapidly to its fatal outcome. Erythroderma may be present during any of the stages. When it is generalized, pruritic, and the most prominent feature, it has been termed "l'homme rouge" (red man) or erythrodermic mycosis fungoides. The Sézary syndrome was originally described in patients that showed circulating atypical mononuclear cells (mycosis cells) in their peripheral circulation in addition to the presence of cutaneous signs. Although this syndrome has been referred to as the leukemic form, the bone marrow appears to be unaffected. Pagetoid reticulosis (localized epidermotropic reticulosis, or Woringer-Kolopp disease) appears clinically to be a localized form of mycosis fungoides. Controversy abounds as to whether the prominent cells in this variant are histiocytes or stimulated T-lymphocytes (as in other forms of mycosis fungoides).

Mycosis fungoides appears to affect all races equally. Males are affected more frequently than females (2:1), and the disease is most commonly diagnosed in patients 40 to 60 years of age.

CANINE MYCOSIS FUNGOIDES

A disease resembling mycosis fungoides was first described in dogs by Kelly and colleagues in 1972. Since that time, at least 23 canine cases have been added to the veterinary literature. The comparison of these canine cases with human mycosis fungoides has been based on clinical and histologic similarities. Histologically, mycosis fungoides is an epidermotropic disease, meaning that the abnormal lymphocytes appear to be attracted to the epidermis and the epithelium of the outer root sheath of the hair follicle.

Although T-cell proliferation is the documented abnormality in humans, this has not been proved in published cases in dogs. One reason for this is that canine T cells lack classic T-cell markers. There are anecdotal reports in which most lymphocytes in these epidermotropic lymphomas have been shown *not* to be B cells. This suggests that they may be T cells. Further studies in this area are currently in progress. Electron microscopy may also be helpful in distinguishing between B and T cells. A case of feline mycosis fungoides with documented T-cell proliferation has recently been reported. In this instance, T-lymphocytes were identified by the guinea pig erythrocyte rosetting technique and by determination of surface feline thymocyte antigen.

Since 1975, 26 cases of canine mycosis fungoides have been evaluated at the New York State College of Veterinary Medicine (NYSCVM) (Table 1). The age of these dogs at the time of diagnosis ranged from 5 to 16 years. The majority of the dogs were between 10 and 13 years of age. Males and females were equally represented, and neutering did not appear to have any effect on disease incidence. When these 26 cases are added to those already in the literature, some breeds appear to be overrepresented. Breeds in which three or more cases have been seen include mixed-breed dogs (7), poodles (6), cocker spaniels (4), boxers (3), golden retrievers (3), Labrador retrievers (3), and Scottish terriers (3). Two cases have been recognized in Irish setters, bulldogs, and Shetland sheepdogs. Breed predilection is difficult to determine from these data, as these cases are from different hospitals in various parts of the country. There are no data to evaluate the frequency with which these breeds are seen at these various hospitals, and thus the relative risk of mycosis fungoides in these breeds cannot be determined.

Clinical Signs

At presentation, a dog with mycosis fungoides may exhibit any of several cutaneous signs. Some cases are presented with a tentative diagnosis of seborrhea or atopy. These dogs may demonstrate generalized erythema, scale or crust formation, and multifocal or generalized alopecia. Pruritus is frequently a complaint, and it may be poorly responsive to systemic glucocorticoid therapy. Ten of the 26 dogs in this study presented in this manner. These signs were the most common in previously reported cases; they were reported either singularly or together in 18 cases.

Ulceration, with a predilection for the oral cavity, mucocutaneous junctions, and sometimes the ventral abdomen, is another frequent presenting feature. This occurred in 14 of the dogs evaluated at the NYSCVM. Interestingly, in three of these cases (Cases 2, 4, and 9), the ulcerative lesions were limited to the oral cavity and were the only lesions evident. Because of the distribution of ulcerative lesions in the oral cavity, at the mucocutaneous junctions, and on the ventral abdomen, dogs with this condition are frequently suspected of having autoimmune skin disease—specifically, pemphigus vulgaris, systemic lupus erythematosus, or bullous pemphigoid. These diseases may have the identical clinical appearance, and without histopathologic and immunofluorescent testing, the definitive diagnosis cannot be determined.

In seven cases evaluated at the NYSCVM, the presenting complaint was a single cutaneous mass (cases 20 through 26). In five of these cases, the mass was located at the mucocutaneous junction of the lip. Most of these individual tumors were either ulcerated or depigmented.

Dogs with mycosis fungoides commonly have peripheral lymphadenopathy either at diagnosis or at some later time during the disease progression. This may be due to tumor invasion of the lymph node but is more often a result of inflammatory skin disease (dermatopathic lymphadenopathy).

Based on the cases of mycosis fungoides in the literature and those in this study, it does not appear that canine cases can be easily separated into the stages that are recognized in humans. Clinical variations in dogs are best represented by generalized erythema or scaling; ulceration, with a predilection for the mucocutaneous junctions; and focal, ulcerative tumor formation. Too few cases have been followed for extended periods of time to determine if these clinical variations actually represent progressive stages of the disease in the dog. The fact that these signs (erythema, ulceration, and tumors) may be seen simultaneously in the same dog just adds confusion to any attempt to stage this disease.

***Table 1.** Cases of Mycosis Fungoides Evaluated at the New York State College of Veterinary Medicine (NYSCVM)*

Case No.	Breed	Sex	Age at Diagnosis (Years)	Duration Prior to Diagnosis (Months)	Follow-Up
1	Welsh corgi	M	12	5	E
2	Mix	M	9	6	UK
3	Irish setter	M	11	ND	UK
4	Mix	F	10	3	E—7 months
5	Pug	F	5	3	E—13 months
6	Golden retriever	FS	11	2	E—2 months
7	Labrador retriever	FS	14	3	E—2 months
8	Gordon setter	M	11	8	E—8 months
9	Scottish terrier	M	12	10	D—1 months
10	Border collie	M	13	ND	UK
11	Mix	MC	12	2.5	UK
12	Basenji	F	10	ND	E—1.5 months
13	Weimaraner	MC	13	14	D—3 months
14	Yorkshire terrier	F	8	2	UK
15	Scottish terrier	FS	12	12	D—1 month
16	Beagle	F	13	3	UK
17	West Highland white terrier	F	UK	3	UK
18	Boxer	M	6	24	UK
19	Labrador retriever	M	16	4	E—9 months
20	Belgian sheepdog	M	10	ND	Recurrence E—6 months
21	Shetland sheepdog	FS	8	0.5	No recurrence—23 months
22	Boxer	M	11	0.5	Recurrence E—10 months
23	Cocker spaniel	FS	13	ND	No recurrence—10 months
24	Mix	FS	5	1	No recurrence—28 months
25	Mix	F	11	ND	Recurrence E—15 months
26	Golden retriever	MC	14	1	UK

Key: E = euthanatized, D = died, ND = not determined, UK = unknown.

Perhaps mycosis fungoides should join other dermatologic conditions (i.e., hypothyroidism and systemic lupus erythematosus) as being thought of as a "great impersonator."

Diagnosis

The diagnosis of canine mycosis fungoides is based on both historic and physical examination findings and results of histopathologic tests of the skin. Occasionally, hematologic studies or examination of lymph nodes will reveal the presence of large mononuclear cells (12 to 20 μm) with a highly convoluted nucleus. These cells are commonly referred to as mycosis cells. Their occurrence suggests the diagnosis of mycosis fungoides; however, microscopic examination of skin biopsies must be performed to confirm the diagnosis. In general, laboratory tests (hemogram, serum biochemistry evaluation, immunofluorescence tests, and so forth) may be helpful to rule out other disease entities but do little to establish the diagnosis of mycosis fungoides.

Definitive diagnosis is based on the microscopic examination of skin or mucosal biopsies. Multiple biopsies should be taken from a variety of early and late lesions. Biopsies from the margins of a lesion may be helpful; however, large amounts of normal-appearing skin should not be submitted because, in the preparation of sections for examination, lesions may be missed in the plane of sectioning. In this regard, biopsies taken from a central area of ulceration may be nondiagnostic, in that the epidermis with its pathognomonic changes may be absent. Preparation of the skin for biopsies should be minimal (gentle clipping and a *light* alcohol swab), as even mild trauma with a gauze sponge may remove the affected epidermis and its changes that are necessary for definitive diagnosis.

Skin biopsies in 10 per cent formalin and the findings of historic and physical examinations should be submitted to a veterinary dermatohistopathologist. If this is not possible, samples should be submitted to a veterinary pathologist with an interest in dermatology. The microscopic changes seen in mycosis fungoides are frequently subtle, especially in early cases, and unless one is familiar with these changes, they may be overlooked.

Examination of skin sections under scanning power reveals a lichenoid pattern (a band of mononuclear cells "hugging" the epidermis). It is this pattern that separates epidermotropic lymphoma from the B-cell lymphomas located in the middle to deep dermis or subcutaneously. This lichenoid pattern is not diagnostic of mycosis fungoides and may be seen with other canine dermatoses such as systemic or discoid lupus erythematosus, bullous pemphigoid, pemphigus erythematosus, a Vogt-Koyanagi-Harada–type of syndrome, and drug eruptions.

On closer examination, the lichenoid cellular infiltrate of mycosis fungoides is composed of neutrophils, small mononuclear and plasma cells, and large atypical mononuclear cells. These cells have a large, irregular nucleus that is folded and grooved. There is abundant eosinophilic cytoplasm. Pautrier microabscesses are collections of two to ten of these pleomorphic, atypical mononuclear cells (mycosis cells) within the epidermis. In later lesions, these cells may become more monomorphous. The occurrence of Pautrier microabscesses appears to be pathognomonic for mycosis fungoides. The lichenoid cellular infiltrate and Pautrier microabscesses may affect the outer root sheath of the hair follicle and the secretory epithelium of apocrine sweat glands in the same manner.

Treatment

Several therapeutic regimens have been described in both case reports and review articles in the veterinary literature. The most commonly discussed treatment involves the use of topical nitrogen mustard (mechlorethamine hydrochloride; Mustargen, Merck, Sharp & Dohme). In 50 ml of water, 10 mg is dissolved and applied to the clipped skin surface two to three times a week initially. As the lesions regress, the drug is applied when needed for maintenance. A major disadvantage of this treatment regimen is a high incidence of contact sensitivity in persons exposed to this drug. A recent report suggests that nitrogen mustard may be less irritating to humans if used with an ointment base. Regardless, strong, specific precautions to decrease owner contact must be stressed if this method of therapy is elected.

Topical nitrogen mustard has been used alone and also in combination with oral prednisolone and cancer chemotherapy. Clinical improvement appears to be greatest when these regimens are used together. There is a report from the University of Pennsylvania of one dog treated with topical nitrogen mustard and oral prednisolone; its lesions resolved, and the dog remained in clinical remission for 2½ years before dying of an unrelated cause. The success in this case appears to be the exception. In several cases, clinical improvement has been seen; however, nitrogen mustard therapy has not appeared to prolong the survival time, which ranged from 1 to 7 months.

Chemotherapy with various combinations of prednisolone, chlorambucil, vincristine, cyclophosphamide, and methotrexate has also resulted in clinical improvement for 1 to 5 months in some cases. Reported unsuccessful treatments have included oral nitrogen mustard and intravenous doxorubicin hydrochloride (Adriamycin, Adria).

A recent report describes a treatment protocol using oral prednisolone along with a placental lysate (Scott's A510, Scott Biologicals) given intradermally, 0.1 ml once daily. In the case discussed, clinical remission was maintained for 25 months before the dog was euthanized for an unrelated cause. This placental lysate, which was developed for its antineoplastic effects, is currently licensed for use in canine arthritis in California.

In one documented case of feline mycosis fungoides, tumor excision was followed by intravenous and intralesional administration of fibronectin. Fibronectin is a glycoprotein dimer that can be isolated from heparinized plasma. The antineoplastic properties of fibronectin appear to be related to its ability to attract macrophages and monocytes to areas of tissue injury where fibrin and denatured collagen are present. In this feline case, there was a 75 per cent reduction in tumor load and no evidence of systemic involvement 7 months after diagnosis. The use of fibronectin in cases of canine mycosis fungoides has not been reported.

With the exception of total excision of localized tumors, treatment aimed specifically at mycosis fungoides has not been used in those cases evaluated at the NYSCVM. The reasons for this have been twofold. First, the use of topical nitrogen mustard, which has generally been the treatment of choice in humans and dogs, does present significant dangers to the pet owner because of its strong contact-sensitizing activity. This, combined with the fact that treatment with nitrogen mustard or any other chemotherapeutic regimen seldom appears to affect survival time in humans, encouraged us to compare survival times in our untreated dogs with those reported in the literature for treated dogs.

Although no specific anticancer treatment is given at the NYSCVM, measures are taken in an attempt to keep the animal as comfortable as possible until the inevitable systemic signs become evident. These measures include the use of anti-inflammatory doses of prednisolone to decrease pruritus and inflammation. Antiseborrheic and antibacterial shampoos are also used to minimize discomfort and reduce seborrheic changes and secondary bacterial infections.

Prognosis

The prognosis in cases of generalized canine mycosis fungoides is poor. Since the dogs in the NYSCVM study were not given specific anticancer therapy, the natural progression of the disease may be evaluated to some extent. The average duration of clinical signs prior to diagnosis was 6.5 months. When follow-up information was available, the average time from diagnosis until euthanasia, or occasionally natural death, was 4.5 months. The longest duration following diagnosis was in Case 5, in which the dog was euthanatized 13 months after diagnosis, when the disease had progressed to oral ulceration and generalized erythema with pruritus and pain. No cutaneous nodules were evident at this time. The duration from onset of clinical signs to diagnosis and from diagnosis to natural death or euthanasia in the dogs evaluated at the NYSCVM is very similar to that in previously reported cases. In those publications in which it was available, the average time from onset to diagnosis was 7 months and the duration following diagnosis was 3.5 months.

In cases in which a focal tumor is diagnosed as mycosis fungoides, the prognosis is somewhat more optimistic. Follow-up information was available for six such cases seen at the NYSCVM. Three were euthanatized in 6 to 15 months (average 10 months) after the recurrence and spread of cutaneous nodules. The other three were normal and had no recurrence after 10, 23, and 28 months.

Mycosis fungoides is ultimately a fatal disease, and present treatments appear to do little to affect the disease progression. However, treatment in some cases may reduce the animal's discomfort.

Only one animal from this study (Case 15) was examined postmortem. In this case, there was no gross evidence of tumor invasion of internal organs. In previous reports, the disease has been shown to be capable of metastasizing to the lymph nodes, liver, spleen, kidneys, lungs, and tonsils. In many instances, there has been no evidence of extracutaneous involvement, except for the occasional spread to lymph nodes.

This is somewhat similar to the progression of mycosis fungoides in humans. In various studies, the duration from the onset of clinical signs to histologic diagnosis may range from 5 to 10 years. Average survival time following diagnosis is approximately 5 years. Survival time in humans is most affected by the stage of disease at diagnosis and the person's occupation. Male industrial workers tend to have a shortened survival time, perhaps because of chronic antigenic exposure. The presence of multiple cutaneous tumors, ulcerative lesions, or enlarged lymph nodes worsens the prognosis. When all of these are present at diagnosis, only 50 per cent of affected individuals survive for 1 year. If hepatomegaly or splenomegaly is also evident, the average survival time is shortened to 3 months.

Although it was previously thought that mycosis fungoides remained localized to the skin until the late stages of the disease, when it could rapidly and widely disseminate, there is new evidence in humans to suggest that systemic spread may occur early in the course of the disease. There may not be clinical evidence of extracutaneous involvement, but various sophisticated laboratory techniques (cytogenic studies, electron microscopy) may suggest its presence. This may help to explain the apparent lack of effect of topical therapy on disease progression.

PAGETOID RETICULOSIS

Pagetoid reticulosis is an epidermotropic lymphoproliferative disease that may be a variant of mycosis fungoides. Clinically, in humans it usually presents as a localized cutaneous tumor, frequently erythematous and scaly, with a predilection for the distal extremities. There is debate as to the genesis of the abnormal mononuclear cells found in this disease (either reactive or neoplastic T-lymphocytes or histiocytes). Pagetoid reticulosis differs histologically from mycosis fungoides. The most prominent difference is that pagetoid reticulosis tends to spare the subepidermal areas and limits itself to epidermal invasion of abnormal mononuclear cells. These atypical mononuclear cells tend to be monomorphous, whereas those in mycosis fungoides are polymorphous. Pautrier microabscesses may be evident, or the infiltrate may be more diffuse within the epidermis. The course of pagetoid reticulosis also differs from that of mycosis fungoides. It appears to be a relatively benign disease in humans, and surgical excision or radiation therapy may be curative. Recurrence has been encountered, but visceral involvement has not been reported.

Pagetoid reticulosis has previously been reported in dogs. Johnson and colleagues discussed the case of a 9-year-old female Scottish terrier with ulcers, vesicles, and plaques affecting the oral mucosa, nasal epithelium, and footpads. Histologically, the lesions in this case were identical to those in pagetoid reticulosis. The dog was euthanatized, and on necropsy examination, no extracutaneous lesions were identified.

Since 1975, four cases of canine pagetoid reticulosis have been evaluated at the NYSCVM (Table 2). In these cases, the clinical appearance resembled mycosis fungoides, pemphigus vulgaris, systemic lupus erythematosus, and bullous pemphigoid. Oral or facial ulceration or both were present along with generalized seborrhea and erythema. Brightly erythematous tumors developed in Case 4.

The disease in these four dogs resembled pagetoid reticulosis on histologic examination, in that atypical mononuclear cells were limited to the epidermis and outer root sheath of the hair follicle. In original biopsies, the dermis was spared. In Case 4, which was followed to euthanasia and postmortem examination, the atypical mononuclear cells diffusely affected the epidermis and dermis in later stages of the disease. The cells remained monomorphous. In this instance, the disease spread to the liver, spleen, lungs, and multiple lymph nodes.

Table 2. *Cases of Pagetoid Reticulosis Evaluated at the NYSCVM*

Case No.	Breed	Sex	Age at Diagnosis (Years)	Duration Prior to Diagnosis (Months)	Follow-Up
1	Mix	FS	12.5	ND	UK
2	Poodle	F	12	6	UK
3	Mix	M	11	3	D—5 days
4	Golden retriever	FS	12	4	E—5 months

Key: E = euthanatized, D = died, ND = not determined, UK = unknown.

Canine pagetoid reticulosis, unlike its human counterpart, appears and behaves clinically very much like mycosis fungoides. Although its histologic appearance differs from mycosis fungoides, it does share many similarities. Perhaps it is a variant of mycosis fungoides with more precise epidermotropism and cellular monomorphism.

SUMMARY

Canine epidermotropic lymphoma (mycosis fungoides and pagetoid reticulosis) is clinically an uncommon disease. When it presents as a pruritic, erythrodermic, and seborrheic disorder, it may frequently be misdiagnosed as seborrhea or atopy. In other cases, especially those with ulcerative lesions, autoimmune skin disease is the major differential diagnosis. Various treatments have been suggested, but none appears to influence the survival time or the fatal nature of the disease. Treatment is aimed at improving the comfort of the animal. Based on a limited number of canine cases, the prognosis is poor, and suspected survival time ranges up to several months.

Further studies are needed with recently described treatment regimens. Additional studies are also needed to confirm that canine mycosis fungoides is indeed a T-cell neoplasia, as is the case in humans.

References and Supplemental Reading

Ackerman, L.: Oral T cell-like lymphoma in a dog. J. Am. Anim. Hosp. Assoc. 20:955, 1984.

Bender, W. M.: Nontraditional treatment of mycosis fungoides in a dog. J.A.V.M.A. 185:900, 1984.

Brown, N. O., Nesbitt, G. H., Patnaik, A. K., et al.: Cutaneous lymphosarcoma in the dog: A disease with variable clinical and histologic manifestations. J. Am. Anim. Hosp. Assoc. 16:565, 1980.

Caciolo, P. L., Hayes, A. A., Patnaik, A. K., et al.: A case of mycosis fungoides in a cat and literature review. J. Am. Anim. Hosp. Assoc. 19:505, 1983.

Halliwell, R. E. W., Gorman, N. T., Calderwood, M., et al.: A case of canine mycosis fungoides. Dermatol. Reports 1:1, 1982.

Johnson, J. A., and Patterson, J. M.: Canine epidermotropic lymphoproliferative disease resembling pagetoid reticulosis in man. Vet. Pathol. 18:487, 1981.

Kelly, D. F., Halliwell, R. E. W., and Schwartzman, R. M.: Generalized cutaneous eruption in a dog with histological similarity to human mycosis fungoides. Br. J. Dermatol. 86:164, 1972.

McKeever, P. J., Grindem, C. B., Stevens, J. B., et al.: Canine cutaneous lymphoma. J.A.V.M.A. 180:531, 1982.

Miller, W. H., Jr.: Canine cutaneous lymphomas. *Current Veterinary Therapy VII. In* Kirk, R. W. (ed.) Philadelphia: W. B. Saunders, 1980, pp. 493–495.

Muller, G. H., Kirk, R. W., and Scott, D. W.: *Small Animal Dermatology III.* Philadelphia: W. B. Saunders, 1983.

Shadduck, J. A., Reedy, L., Lawton, G., et al.: A canine cutaneous lymphoproliferative disease resembling mycosis fungoides in man. Vet. Pathol. 15:716, 1978.

Thrall, M. A., Macy, D. W., Snyder, S. P., et al.: Cutaneous lymphosarcoma and leukemia in a dog resembling Sézary syndrome in man. Vet. Pathol. 21:182, 1984.

Wall, A. E.: Cutaneous lymphosarcoma in a Shetland collie. Vet. Rec. 95:150, 1974.

Zenoble, R. D., and George, J. W.: Mycosis fungoides-like disease in a dog. J. Am. Anim. Hosp. Assoc. 16:203, 1980.

Section 7

OPHTHALMOLOGIC DISEASES

THOMAS J. KERN, D.V.M.,
and RONALD C. RIIS, D.V.M.
Consulting Editors

***Additional Pertinent Information Found in* Current Veterinary Therapy VIII:**

Betts, D. M.: Diseases of the Orbit, p. 577.
Kern, T. J.: Ocular Emergencies, p. 531.

***Additional Pertinent Information Found in* Current Veterinary Therapy VII:**

Martin, C. L.: The Ophthalmic Examination and Anamnesis, p. 505.
Peiffer, R. L., Jr.: Ophthalmic Disorders of Proven or Suspected Genetic Etiology in the Dog and Cat, p. 587.
Scagliotti, R. H.: Neuro-ophthalmology, p. 510.

CLINICAL ASPECTS OF OPHTHALMOLOGY IN CAGED BIRDS

LORRAINE G. KARPINSKI, V.M.D.,
and SUSAN L. CLUBB, D.V.M.
Miami, Florida

Unlike birds of prey, which seem primarily to have traumatic ocular problems (Murphy et al., 1982), caged birds seem to have infectious ocular problems. Although not all etiologic agents of these diseases are known, some description, management, and treatment can be suggested.

ANATOMY

When treating ocular problems in birds, it is important to keep in mind some of the anatomic differences between birds and mammals. The shape of the avian eye varies from species to species. The anatomic structures absent in mammals are the striated musculature of the iris and the ciliary body, the scleral ossicles, and the pecten.

The musculature of the iris and ciliary body in birds is striated rather than smooth; therefore, dilatation for ophthalmoscopy or for therapeutic benefit cannot be achieved by application of parasympatholytic drugs (e.g., atropine, tropicamide). Agents that paralyze skeletal muscles must be used. Bellhorn (1981) suggested the topical use of a 3 mg/ml solution of a dry crystalline preparation of D-tubocurarine in 0.025 per cent benzalkonium chloride. Commercially prepared aqueous solutions of tubocurarine do not readily pass through the corneal layers.

The anterior sclera of birds contains 11 to 15 sclerotic plates. These help give shape to the globe and provide support for the ciliary body. They are clinically important when enucleation of the eye is indicated.

Birds have a true anangiotic (avascular) retina, but they do possess a pecten, a heavily pigmented, highly vascular, pleated structure extending from the optic disc into the vitreous. Ultrastructurally, the pecten capillaries resemble those of organs with secretory function, such as the ciliary body of mammals, and the pecten may produce intraocular fluid.

EXAMINATION

Chemical restraint may be necessary for complete ocular examination. Ketamine in combination with a topical ophthalmic anesthetic is sufficient for most procedures. Ketamine does not cause consistent pupillary dilatation in birds. Therefore, topical muscle-paralyzing agents may be necessary for examination of the posterior pole.

In a laterally recumbent bird under ketamine anesthesia, the anterior chamber of the lower eye may collapse. The eye returns to a normal appearance within a few minutes after repositioning. Recovery areas should be padded to prevent periocular bruising, which may occur as a result of head tossing.

Iris color should be noted since in many species it may be an indication of age or sex. Fledgling macaws (*Ara* spp.) have brown irises, which fade to gray within the first year. Between 1 and 3 years, the irises appear white and turn yellow as the bird matures. Young Amazon parrots (*Amazona* spp.) have brown irises, which become red-orange as they age. Iris color in African gray parrots (*Psittacus erithacus*) changes from brown through gray to white. Many species of cockatoos (*Cacatua* spp.) show sexual dimorphism in iris color. Adult males have dark brown to black irises and adult females have red irises. The young of both sexes have brown irises.

GENERAL EYE PROBLEMS IN BIRDS

Most ocular disorders diagnosed in mammals are recognized in birds. Management is similar to that of mammals; however, treatment frequency may need to be decreased to minimize stress.

Dermoids, birth defects of the cornea, occur sporadically. One case of unilateral dermoid was observed in a cockatiel. The dermoid contained a single filoplume lash.

Uveitis, with lowered intraocular pressure, a cloudy cornea, hyperemic iris, and aqueous flare, is seen unilaterally or bilaterally and may be a reflection of some systemic disease (e.g., salmonellosis or avian pox). Hypopyon, which is an accumulation of thick cellular material in the anterior chamber, may result. Adhesions of the inflamed iris to the lens or cornea, known as synechiae, are common sequelae. Uveitis in birds is treated with topical corticosteroids. Dexamethasone and 1 per cent prednisolone in ointment or drop form are the drugs of choice.

Corneal damage may occur from an abrasion, an infectious process, or a laceration. Corneal ulcers in birds are treated with topical antibiotics. Cycloplegics, commonly used in mammals, are of no therapeutic value. Acetylcysteine (Mucomyst 10 per cent, Mead Johnson Pharmaceutical) should be used topically in conjunction with antibiotics in the treatment of deep corneal ulcers. This collagenase inhibitor can be applied as a drop or, with less stress, as an ocular spray every few hours. Many corneal ulcers will result in relatively permanent but clinically insignificant corneal crystals. Severe corneal lacerations should be repaired surgically.

Trauma may result in hyphema, usually originating from the iris or ciliary body. Topical corticosteroids are indicated to minimize any uveitis as this clears.

Cataracts are seen sporadically, especially in older birds, but also as a result of injury or previous intraocular inflammation. When it is indicated, cataracts may be removed surgically. Phacoemulsification, when available, allows lens removal through a small incision and leaves minimal lens debris.

Primary neoplasia of the eye and adnexa is rare in birds. Orbital sarcoma, glioma of the optic nerve, lipogranuloma of the eyelid, and trichoepithelioma of the eyelid have been reported.

SPECIFIC EYE DISEASES AFFECTING BIRDS

Avian Pox

Avian poxvirus infections occur in a wide variety of species of birds. Newly imported parrots from South and Central America are often infected with pox. In most cases, the disease has run its course by the time the bird reaches the pet owner. However, many cases may leave residual scars or chronic ophthalmic problems for which veterinary care may be sought.

The eye lesions of parrot pox are most often seen 10 to 14 days after infection and are usually the first lesions observed. Lesions may be unilateral or bilateral. The first signs observed are mild blepharitis and a serous ocular discharge. The lids swell and paste together. Caseous white masses and fluids collect under the lids. The cornea becomes edematous and ulcerated. These ulcers may become chronic and may perforate. At 12 to 18 days after infection, dry crusty scabs form around the margins of the lids and may completely seal the lids shut. These scabs progressively become leathery in texture and subsequently dry and fall off. Clinical illness lasts 2 to 6 weeks.

Many of the birds that do recover will suffer residual effects. Distorted lids, loss of periocular pigmentation and filoplume lashes, subepithelial corneal crystals, and chronic corneal ulcers are common. Chronic tearing may occur as a result of damage to the lacrimal drainage apparatus. In some cases, the eye may be lost as a consequence of perforated ulcers or panophthalmitis.

Treatment is aimed at secondary bacterial and fungal infections and providing supportive care. Vitamin A supplementation has been clinically effective in decreasing severity of the infection if given prior to the onset of lesions or in the very early stages of the disease. Intramuscular administration of 10,000 to 25,000 IU of vitamin A per 300 gm body weight once weekly is recommended. After the appearance of eye lesions, the vitamin A is much less effective. Systemic antibiotic therapy is often necessary.

Treat eye lesions routinely with a baby shampoo wash followed by merbromin solution rinse and the application of chloramphenicol ophthalmic ointment. Use gauze or cotton swabs to gently clean early eye lesions with dilute baby shampoo (Johnson's Baby Shampoo, Johnson & Johnson). Daily cleaning and opening the lids in the early stages of disease often decreases the formation of disfiguring scabs. The merbromin eyewash is prepared by adding 1 oz of 2 per cent merbromin (Mercurochrome; Hynson, Westcott, & Dunning) to 4 oz of eyewash solution. After formation of the scabs, the eye can be treated by gently lifting the lateral side of the scab, just enough to medicate the eye. Scabs should not be removed because of the potential damage this would cause to the lids. Far less damage will occur if the scabs are allowed to drop off naturally. The most common secondary bacterial invaders are *Escherichia coli, Pseudomonas,* and *Proteus.* Fungal infections (candidiasis and aspergillosis) often occur in the eye secondary to pox.

Eye lesions due to avian pox infections may also be seen in canaries, birds of prey, pigeons, and gallinaceous birds. Treatment of pigeon pox lesions is similar to that of pox in parrots. In canaries, individual treatment may be impractical because of their size and the very high mortality rate. Antibiotic preparations sprayed into the eyes may be helpful. Pox infections in birds of prey in the United States are usually self-limiting and cause relatively little damage. Topical treatment of the lesions, however, may be helpful.

Cockatiel Conjunctivitis

Cockatiels (*Nymphicus hollandicus*), especially the white or albino mutations, are very often afflicted with a conjunctivitis of unknown cause. It has often been speculated that this syndrome is caused by *Mycoplasma;* however, this has not been confirmed despite repeated isolation attempts.

The condition begins with mild blepharitis and serous ocular discharge. The conjunctiva becomes inflamed and begins to swell at the medial canthus. The conjunctival vessels become engorged, and the conjunctiva protrudes from under the lids. If the condition is allowed to progress, the tissue will become infiltrated. This conjunctivitis is often associated with upper and lower respiratory tract infections. Nasal discharge, plugged nares, sneezing, coughing, and dyspnea may be observed.

The eye lesions are easily treated and respond to a variety of antibiotic ophthalmic preparations with or without corticosteroids. Recurrence, however, is common. Systemic therapy with chlortetracycline (CTC) in feed appears to be the most effective treatment. The easiest and most readily accepted form of medicated feed is CTC-impregnated millet (Keet Life, Hartz Mountain). The treatment period should be approximately 30 days. This diet is not balanced, but nutritional deficiencies are unlikely to develop during this time. Vitamins can be added to water, but calcium should not be supplemented as it inhibits absorption of CTC. Medicated parrot pellets provide more balanced nutrition but are rejected by approximately 5 per cent of cockatiels. A mixture of impregnated millet and pellets provides a good alternative. As supplemental therapy, eye lesions can be sprayed with tylosin (Tylan Powder, Elanco) mixed 1:10 with water. Birds can easily be treated several times daily with minimal stress. Surgical removal of the infiltrated conjunctiva in chronic cases has not been rewarding.

There is some evidence that this disease may be transmitted to offspring, so infected birds should not be used as breeders.

Lovebird Eye Disease

This disease of unknown cause has been observed only in lovebirds (*Agapornis* spp.) and is more severe in mutation lovebirds than in the wild types. It is most often observed in peach-faced mutations (*Agapornis roseicollis*). Other species are affected but to a lesser degree. This is a severe and highly fatal systemic disease that has a concurrent ocular manifestation. The first signs of the disease are depression, blepharitis, and a slight serous ocular discharge. As the disease progresses, the lids become hyperemic and swollen and the ocular discharge becomes more severe. Weight loss and severe depression ensue. If kept in a flock, an affected bird is often assaulted by cage mates. Medical management has been unrewarding. Death usually occurs within a few days after the appearance of lesions.

Renal adenovirus has been demonstrated by electron microscopy in some affected birds, but its direct association with this syndrome has not been proved.

The disease does seem to be stress related, and birds will often develop symptoms 1 to 2 weeks after a stress such as shipping. The only measure that has been helpful in the management of the disease is placing the birds in a nonstressful environment and using no treatment. This syndrome has been observed only in birds bred in captivity. Birds from affected flocks should not be used as breeders.

Mynah Eye Disease

Three distinct eye problems have been observed in mynahs (*Gracula* spp.). They may be unrelated or may be different stages of the same disease.

Corneal scratches may occur during shipping. Mynahs move around excessively in shipping crates and tend to scratch their corneas. In one study, 96 of 100 birds examined after shipping were affected. In most cases, the cornea will regrow epithelium within 24 to 48 hours without treatment.

Keratitis is usually observed within a week after shipping. Lesions include corneal irregularities and loss of corneal transparency, ranging in severity from mild corneal edema to complete corneal opacity. Most cases regress spontaneously within weeks, but some may persist several months. Therapy does not seem to affect the course of the disease. Scarring of the cornea may result in severe cases.

Chronic keratoconjunctivitis is a sequela to the keratitis syndrome. A large mass of infiltrated conjunctiva can be found under the lower lid. In order to see this tissue, the lid must be everted. The entire cornea is often ulcerated. Vascularization of the cornea may occur with chronicity. Surgical removal of the redundant conjunctival tissue and topical antibiotic therapy may result in at least temporary resolution of the ulcers. Systemic aspergillosis is found in many chronically affected birds.

Rhinitis and Sinusitis

Upper respiratory inflammation is often accompanied by conjunctivitis and ocular discharge. Although the initiating cause may be chlamydial, viral, mycoplasmal, fungal, or bacterial, other factors are also important in the initiation of upper respiratory tract disease, including hypovitaminosis A, chills, irritating fumes, or a dusty environment.

Many cases respond favorably to treatment with vitamin A, alone or in conjunction with systemic and topical antimicrobials. Some chronic cases may result in the accumulation of caseous material under the eyelids and in the sinuses. In most cases, alleviation of the sinusitis or rhinitis will relieve the ocular problems.

Chronic Conjunctivitis in Amazon Parrots

Chronic conjunctivitis may be associated with upper respiratory tract infections in Amazon parrots. Conjunctival tissue may become edematous, inflamed, and infiltrated. Topical corticosteroids or surgical removal of excessive conjunctival tissue may be helpful. Chronic or intermittent corneal ulcers may accompany this chronic conjunctivitis.

Periorbital Abscesses

A possible sequela to chronic upper respiratory tract disease is periorbital abscess. This is most often seen in cockatiels and may occur above or below the orbit. Abscesses are much less likely to occur in sinusitis cases that are treated with antibiotics in the early stages. They are much more common in the pet bird whose owner fails to notice the symptoms of sinusitis for a period of time. Surgical removal of caseous material and the use of systemic antibiotics are indicated. Caseous masses above the eye that are not too large may be successfully removed through the conjunctiva, resulting in faster healing and less lid distortion.

Lacrimal Sac Abscesses

Lacrimal sac abscesses are often confused with periorbital abscesses. The cause is unknown; however, they usually accompany or follow sinusitis in psittacine birds. They are presented as swellings anteroventral to the medial canthus. The swelling is usually movable and hard. If pushed toward the eye, caseous material can usually be seen in the lacrimal punctum, which is usually enlarged. In mild cases, the material may be removed simply by expressing it gently out of the lacrimal punctum. In more severe cases, cannulation of the punctum may be required to break up the caseous material so that it may be flushed out or removed in pieces with a pair of fine ophthalmic forceps. Daily flushing with rather large volumes (2 to 10 ml) of saline may be required to remove the caseous material. Appropriate antibiotics may be included in the saline flush. In severe cases, some distortion of the lids, with or without chronic epiphora, may occur. Surgical removal is not recommended except in the most severe cases because of the potential for spread of the infection and excessive scarring of periorbital tissues.

Sunken Eyes and Sinuses in Macaws

A peculiar sinusitis that has been observed in macaws (*Ara* spp.) results in sinking of the eyes into the orbit. In very severe cases, the eye may recede far into the orbit and move ventrally so that the pupil is bisected by the ventral rim of the orbit. It is often accompanied by collapse of the tissues over the sinuses.

A copious, thick, mucoid to mucopurulent material is contained within the sinuses and may be discharged from the nostril. A mucoid discharge may also collect under the lids and drain from the eye. Caseous material may form in the choanal cleft. Culture of sinus aspirates usually reveals *E. coli*, *Klebsiella*, or *Pseudomonas*. Combined infections are common. In one yellow-collared macaw (*Ara auricollis*), a pure culture of *Haemophilus* was obtained on necropsy.

Despite the shocking appearance of this disorder, it responds well to therapy. These birds are routinely treated with carbenicillin (100 mg/kg IV or IM b.i.d. or t.i.d.) and gentamicin (10 mg/kg IM b.i.d. or t.i.d.) or amikacin (40 mg/kg IM once daily or b.i.d.). The sinuses must be flushed daily with large volumes (10 to 30 ml in each nostril) of saline mixed with the appropriate antibiotic. The sinuses are flushed by inserting the end of a syringe into the nostril and gently pushing the solution through the sinuses and out the choana. The bird can be held on its side or upright. In some cases, fluids may emerge from the nasolacrimal duct into the eye. Topical antibiotic ophthalmic preparations are helpful in the treatment of accompanying conjunctivitis. Recovery is usually complete after 2 weeks of vigorous treatment.

Scarlet (*Ara macao*) and green-winged macaws (*Ara chloroptera*) are most often affected and respond well to treatment. The condition in miniature macaws, especially yellow-collared macaws, is more likely to become chronic. A similar condition, observed in Amazons and cockatoos with chronic sinusitis, is usually not responsive to therapy and may be unrelated.

Punctate Keratitis in Amazon Parrots

A mild transient punctate keratitis has been observed in Amazon parrots imported from Central America. The first signs are mild blepharospasm and serous ocular discharge. The lesions are most often bilateral.

Initial lesions appear as slight irregularities of the medial cornea. In approximately half of the cases, the lesions will progress over the entire surface. In many cases, this will resolve spontaneously within a week. Transient superficial staining with fluorescein may be observed at this time. There may be concomitant anterior uveitis, evidenced by aqueous flare, iritis, and fibrin deposits in the anterior chamber. Anterior or posterior synechiae may result. Fewer than 5 per cent of these birds will develop a deep corneal ulcer. As the disease progresses, some birds will develop sinusitis.

Most cases will regress spontaneously within 1 to 2 weeks. Treatment of the superficial eye lesions has been attempted with a variety of topical antibacterial, antiviral, and chemical preparations. No treated group has shown a significant improvement over untreated controls.

A more chronic form occurs in Amazon parrots from northern South America. These birds have less intraocular involvement, but the percentage of long-term corneal defects is higher.

Treatment is recommended for cases that develop a mucoid or mucopurulent nasal discharge, deeply staining corneal ulcers, or uveitis. Therapy in sinusitis should be aimed at secondary invaders and the provision of adequate levels of vitamin A. Uveitis should be treated with a topical antibiotic-corticosteroid ophthalmic preparation. Systemic antibiotics may be indicated. Mild residual blepharospasm may be evident for several weeks to months.

Hereditary Cataracts in Canaries

Slatter and colleagues (1983) reported hereditary cataracts in a breeding group of Yorkshire and Norwich canaries (*Serinus canarius*) in which excellent long-term pedigrees were available. The birds were presented with gradual onset of a "crash landing" syndrome followed eventually by refusal to move from the perch. Mature bilateral cataracts were observed in all of the six birds examined. After studying the pedigree of the Yorkshire canaries, which included seven generations over 15 years, they hypothesized that the syndrome was produced by a fully penetrant recessive allele at an autosomal locus.

Ocular Parasitic Diseases

Knemidokoptic mites (*Knemidokoptes pilae*) cause lesions (scaly face) of the cere and periorbital area in budgerigars (*Melopsittacus undulatus*) and occasionally other species. Historically, the condition has been treated with a variety of topical acaricides. Application of these compounds around the eyes often leads to irritation, and repeated application for a number of weeks is required. An infestation can now be very effectively treated with a single IM dose of ivermectin (Ivomec, Merck Sharp & Dohme). Ivomec is diluted 1:8 with propylene glycol and administered at the rate of 0.1 ml/kg (200 μg/kg) SC or PO (0.01 to 0.02 ml for a budgerigar). Very extensive or severe infections may require a second dose.

Oxyspirura mansoni is a small, slender nematode that may be found behind the nictitating membrane or in the conjunctival sac and lacrimal duct. It commonly occurs in cockatoos and has been reported in domestic poultry, mynahs, house sparrows, and doves.

Following instillation of a topical anesthetic, worms can be found by lifting the nictitating membrane. In heavy infestations, the eyelids may appear swollen or distended and the bird may scratch at the eye.

Light infestations result in little or no discomfort to the bird, and treatment is not warranted. Worms can be removed manually, but many will escape into the lacrimal duct. Worms will die after treatment with ivermectin, but frequent washing of the eye is required to remove the decaying worms.

An unidentified nematode was observed in the anterior chamber of a blue-and-gold macaw (*Ara ararauna*). Surgical removal was successful.

SURGICAL PROCEDURES

Suturing the external eyelids is an easy and effective alternative to third eyelid or conjunctival flaps in birds. Use a small cutting needle with a small diameter and nonabsorbable suture material to place a single horizontal mattress suture in the lids. Third eyelid flaps are not recommended because of the intrinsic muscular control of the nictitating membrane.

Enucleation in birds is a disfiguring procedure because of the relatively large volume of the globe. A transconjunctival approach is used, and care must be taken to minimize traction and trauma to the optic nerve, which is short and is close to the optic chiasm. Excessive trauma in the posterior pole of one orbit may affect the other optic nerve, resulting in blindness.

Evisceration of the ocular contents is preferable. The cornea is removed, and the intraocular contents are teased free and removed. The conjunctiva is closed over the globe with small-diameter absorbable sutures. The eyelid borders are trimmed close to their margins and then sutured edge to edge with fine-diameter nonabsorbable suture.

Removal of exuberant granulation tissue from the conjunctiva in mynahs can be done with the bird under ketamine or inhalation anesthesia together with a topical anesthetic. The base of the tissue to be removed is carefully crushed with Allis tissue forceps and cut with small scissors along the indicated line. Bleeding is minimal, and suturing is not required.

A lacrimal sac abscess sometimes requires surgical drainage, although repeated flushing may be adequate. Birds have an upper and a lower nasolacrimal punctum. Topical anesthesia is required for flushing. A nasolacrimal cannula may be used. Alternatively, the plastic portion of a feline indwelling IV catheter (Sherwood Industries) is used. It is pliable and blunt enough to reach the deep recesses of the expanded sac and to disrupt the inspissated material. Sterile saline with or without an appropriate antibiotic is used as the flushing solution. In cases that cannot be flushed and in periorbital abscesses, surgical removal of the material is indicated.

References and Supplemental Reading

Bellhorn, R. W.: Laboratory animal ophthalmology. In Gelatt, K. N. (ed.): *Veterinary Ophthalmology*. Philadelphia: Lea & Febiger, 1981.

Clubb, S. L.: Therapeutics in avian medicine: Flock vs. individual bird treatment regimens. Vet. Clin. North Am. [Small Anim. Pract.] 14: 345, 1984.

Murphy, C. J.: Raptor ophthalmology. Proc. Ann. Meet. Assoc. Avian Vet. 1984, pp. 43–58.

Murphy, C. J., Kern, T. J., McKeever, K., et al.: Ocular lesions in free-living raptors. J.A.V.M.A. 181:1302, 1982.

Slatter, D. H., Bradley, J. S., Vale, B., et al.: Hereditary cataracts in canaries. J.A.V.M.A. 183:872, 1983.

OPHTHALMIC DISEASES OF REPTILES

NICHOLAS J. MILLICHAMP, B.VET. MED.,
College Station, Texas

and ELLIOTT R. JACOBSON, D.V.M.
Gainesville, Florida

Diseases of the eyes of reptiles are frequently seen in veterinary practice. Although the approach to treatment is similar to that in mammals, anatomic differences in the reptile eye cause conditions unique to reptiles. This is further complicated by the predisposition of reptiles to certain systemic diseases that are rarely encountered in mammals.

CLINICAL ANATOMY

The anatomy of the lizard eye is the most typical of the reptile pattern. The eyelids are well developed, and the lower lid is the more movable. Most species have third eyelids. In some families the lower lid is modified to form a transparent window to enable vision with the lids closed, and geckos have fused lids that form a transparent spectacle. The globe has hyaline cartilage in the anterior sclera, forming a ring of approximately 14 scleral ossicles behind the corneoscleral limbus and adjacent to the ciliary body.

Chelonian (turtle) eyes are similar to those of lizards. The orbital (harderian and lacrimal) glands are very large in most chelonians, a fact of some significance in vitamin A deficiency. The nasolacrimal duct is absent, and tears are lost by spillage onto the face and evaporation.

Crocodilians have well-developed eyelids with a tarsal plate in the upper lid. The strength of closure of the eyelids and the presence of a third eyelid make examination of the eye particularly difficult in these animals.

The iridal muscle is striated in reptiles and is largely under voluntary control. Conventional mydriatic agents (parasympatholytics) are therefore ineffective in reptiles. Lizard, chelonian, and crocodilian eyes submitted for histolopathologic examination require decalcification prior to routine processing.

The eyes of all snakes are covered anteriorly by a transparent spectacle, formed embryologically by the fusion of the eyelids. This structure appears impervious to topical medications, thus making treatment of the globe difficult. In all reptiles with a spectacle, microsilicone injections have shown this structure to be highly vascular. This is significant when differentiating normal vascular patterns from inflammatory neovascularization in the spectacle or cornea.

The spectacle is periodically replaced along with the rest of the skin during molting cycles. The frequency of ecdysis depends on the nutritional state and rate of growth of the animal, its age, environmental conditions, and systemic or dermatologic disease. The molting cycle begins with dulling of the skin, especially well seen in normally iridescent species. A cloudy appearance develops in the spectacle, which becomes an opaque bluish color over the course of a few days. These color changes are due to (1) thickening of the skin as the new epidermis is produced and (2) breakdown of the inner layers of the old epidermis to leave a fluid lubricating layer between the old and new tissue. Gradually, the cloudy appearance is lost, and the spectacle becomes transparent again just before the snake molts.

Snakes have a harderian gland but no lacrimal gland. Tears are secreted into the space between the spectacle and the cornea (subspectacular space) and drain to the roof of the mouth or base of the duct of the vomeronasal organ through the nasolacrimal duct.

OCULAR EXAMINATION

In most reptiles seen in clinical practice, the small size of the eye makes it desirable to use some form of magnification to perform an ocular examination. Although this is best accomplished with a slit-lamp biomicroscope, the +25 or +40 diopter lenses of a direct ophthalmoscope are adequate in most instances.

Mydriasis can be achieved by examining the eye under general anesthesia, which relaxes the striated iridal sphincter muscle. Alternatively, the fundus can be viewed with a dim light through a small pupil with the direct ophthalmoscope. In larger species (varanid lizards and crocodilians), the pupil can be dilated by intracameral injection of curare. In adult alligators, 0.05 to 0.1 ml of D-tubocurarine (Squibb, 20 units/ml) can be injected into the anterior chamber with a 27- or 30-gauge needle, which is advanced under the conjunctiva and through the corneoscleral limbus after topical ophthalmic anesthetic is applied to the cornea. It may be necessary to paralyze the orbicularis oculi muscle to prevent blepharospasm with 2 per cent lidocaine (Carter-Glogan Labs) injected subcutaneously dorsal and lateral to the eye to temporarily block the palpebral nerve branches. Mydriasis may persist from 30 minutes to several hours.

PERIOCULAR SKIN INFECTIONS

The periocular scales may be involved in various skin diseases, including herpesvirus infections in young marine turtles and poxvirus infections in juvenile caimans. Fungal infections of the skin may involve the spectacle and periocular scales and can be severe enough in some instances to progress to fungal endophthalmitis. Biopsy and culture from lesions may reveal various agents including species of *Penicillium*, *Geotrichum*, *Fusarium*, and *Trichoderma*.

Soaking the animal in chlorhexidine (0.26 ml/L of water) for 1 to 2 hours, especially when it is shedding, may be effective in the early stages of some infections. Culture of fungal organisms and application of more specific antifungal agents (including tolnaftate, miconazole, and nystatin) may be attempted.

Periorbital infections may occur with various bacterial species, including *Pseudomonas* and *Escherichia coli*. The signs include swelling of eyelids due to granuloma formation or exophthalmos and palpebral edema due to retrobulbar abscessation and cellulitis. Abscesses should be lanced, curetted, cultured, and treated with systemic and topical antibacterial agents. Due to the inspissated nature of the pus encountered in reptile abscesses, effective drainage is difficult. Early therapy with appropriate antibiotics is necessary to avoid septicemia. Autogenous bacterins have proved valuable in treating recurrent *Pseudomonas* infections.

RETAINED SPECTACLES

Spectacle retention is associated with inadequate nutrition, poor environmental conditions, or systemic disease. Over several molts, a thick layer of old spectacles accumulates, putting pressure on the cornea beneath. These may be removed after dampening the scales with artificial tears to render them more pliable. Fine forceps and magnification are required to ensure that only the dead outer layers are removed. If the new spectacle is removed accidentally, exposure keratitis will result and the eye may be lost. To avoid this, it is better not to remove tightly adherent spectacles but rather to wait until the next molt. In the intervening period, treat any skin disease, correct the cage humidity, and ensure that the animal is well hydrated. Tightly adherent spectacles can be loosened by soaking the snake in water or using the mucolytic agent acetylcysteine (Mucomyst, Mead Johnson Pharmaceuticals) applied topically to the retained spectacle.

Abscessation of the subspectacle space occurs in snakes and those lizard species with spectacles. It may occur unilaterally or bilaterally. Infection can reach this site either from penetrating injuries to the spectacle, by ascent through the nasolacrimal duct from the mouth (e.g., in cases of ulcerative stomatitis), or possibly as hematogenous extension of systemic disease. These infections often are seen as a ballooning of the spectacle, with or without palpebral edema (the latter a more consistent finding in lizards), and a white or yellow exudate beneath the spectacle.

The globe is often not involved in the early stage of subspectacle abscessation. Initial therapy requires providing a drainage route for the pus (since the nasolacrimal duct frequently becomes blocked), coupled with culture and appropriate antibacterial therapy. Under general anesthesia, a 30-degree wedge can be excised from the ventral quadrant of the spectacle, enabling cultures to be taken and topical antibiotics to be instilled. Inspissated pus should be flushed from the subspectacle space. Species of *Pseudomonas* are often cultured from the abscesses in snakes, and therapy with topical gentamicin solution or ointment and systemic gentamicin (Schering, 2.5 mg/kg IM every 72 hours) may effect a cure.

The nasolacrimal duct can also be congenitally absent or become blocked by pressure from adjacent tissue (granulomas or neoplasia) or by fibrosis (burn injuries to the roof of the mouth). In these cases, the spectacle is distended by an accumulation of clear tears. Wedge excision of the spectacle will relieve the distension, although the drainage site heals over a period of time. Another approach is to create a new drainage route between the subspectacle space and the mouth (conjunctivoralostomy). With the animal under general anesthesia and after a wedge of the spectacle is removed, a curved 22-gauge or 18-gauge needle (depending on the size of the reptile) is passed into the subspectacle space and through its ventral aspect, passing between the maxillary and palatine bones to reach the roof of the mouth. A 2-0 nylon suture or 0.0025-inch outer diameter Silastic tubing is then passed through the needle. The needle is retracted, and the nylon or Silastic tubing is sutured in place to create a passage between the subspectacle space and the mouth. The tube is left in place for 4 to 8 weeks while antibiotic therapy is maintained. Patency of the duct can be assessed by injecting 10 per cent sodium fluorescein beneath the spectacle with a 30-gauge needle and observing the roof of the mouth with a cobalt blue light source.

Bacterial conjunctivitis appears to be rare in reptiles, although it may occur in association with upper respiratory tract infection. Bacteria isolated include *Aeromonas liquefaciens* and species of *Pseudomonas* in lizards and *Pasteurella* in chelonians. Topical applications of broad-spectrum antibiotics are effective, provided underlying systemic diseases can be controlled. Chelonians are often seen with excessive tearing and blepharedema after hibernation. This usually resolves within a few days, once the animals begin feeding. The periocular region should be cleaned with moist cotton.

Corneal ulcers may occur occasionally and can be diagnosed by fluorescein staining of the ulcerated area. Application of a broad-spectrum antibiotic ophthalmic solution is effective therapy in most cases.

Uveitis with hypopyon may occur secondary to systemic bacterial infection and in rare cases of lymphoreticular neoplasia. Other signs include corneal opacification and vascularization of the cornea and iris. Bacteria that may be isolated systemically include species of *Klebsiella*, *Aeromonas*, and *Pseudomonas*. Diagnosis of the underlying cause is often not made until necropsy, although bacterial culture from blood samples and tracheal aspirates may be revealing in reptiles with bacteremia or respiratory infections. Therapy with broad-spectrum antibiotics systemically is the most likely means of resolving such cases of uveitis.

Panophthalmitis may result from penetrating injuries, extension of subspectacle infection, or hematogenous spread of systemic bacterial infections. The only means of therapy is enucleation and use of broad-spectrum antibiotics.

NUTRITIONAL DISEASE

Vitamin A deficiency in aquatic chelonians causes squamous metaplasia of the orbital glands and their ducts. Desquamated material blocks the ducts, and the glands increase in size, resulting in orbital and eyelid edema and secondary conjunctivitis and blepharitis. Occasionally there is secondary bacterial infection. The condition may be confused with infectious conjunctivitis. It develops most often in young, rapidly growing turtles fed a diet of skeletal muscle meat and dried insects. In the early stages, the eyes remain open and the animal may still be induced to eat, enabling a change of diet and supplementation with cod-liver oil. Commercial trout pellets are a good balanced diet for young turtles and should be fed routinely to aquatic turtles. As the edema worsens in untreated animals, the eyelids become tightly closed, and the animal refuses to enter water to eat. If untreated, animals so affected eventually will die. Squamous metaplasia of the renal, pancreatic, gastrointestinal, and respiratory epithelium contributes to the animal's demise in untreated cases. In the later stages, it is necessary to give vitamin A parenterally to effect a cure. Hatchlings and very small juvenile turtles may receive a dose of 1000 to 5000 IU of vitamin A, depending on size, at weekly intervals for at least three treatments or until the eyelid edema subsides. Topical applications of antibiotics may be required in cases complicated by bacterial infection.

NEOPLASIA

Fibromas, papillomas, and fibropapillomas occur in adult green sea turtles and involve the eyelids and other areas of the integument. Neoplasia involving the eye in reptiles is otherwise rarely reported.

MISCELLANEOUS

Congenital abnormalities seen in reptiles include cyclopia and microphthalmos. These frequently occur with skeletal abnormalities.

Cataracts may be unilateral or bilateral, congenital or acquired. No surgical therapy has been reported, nor is it justified. Posterior segment abnormalities are rarely reported and are difficult to diagnose and treat. Retinal degeneration may be seen as a sporadic finding in most of the reptile genera.

References and Supplemental Reading

Frye, F. L.: *Biomedical and Surgical Aspects of Captive Reptile Husbandry.* Edwardsville, KS: Veterinary Medicine Publishing Co., 1981, p. 228.

Millichamp, N. J., Jacobson, E. R., and Wolf, E. D.: Diseases of the eye and ocular adnexa in reptiles. J.A.V.M.A. 183:1205, 1983.

Walls, G. L.: *The Vertebrate Eye and Its Adaptive Radiation.* Bloomfield Hills, MI: Cranbrook Institute of Science, 1942, p. 607.

DISORDERS OF THE EYELIDS AND CONJUNCTIVA

MARK P. NASISSE, D.V.M.

Raleigh, North Carolina

Diseases of the eyelids and conjunctiva are probably the most frequently treated ophthalmic disorders in small animal practice. In addition to being common, the diseases of these structures are of a considerable variety. Congenital, inflammatory, and neoplastic disorders all occur with frequency and with clinical signs varied enough to make diagnosis a challenge for even the experienced ophthalmologist. The significance of eyelid and conjunctival diseases is further emphasized by their ability to adversely affect the nearby globe, frequently leading to loss of vision.

DISEASES OF THE EYELIDS

Disorders of Abnormal Structure and Function

Among the diseases most likely to cause vision-threatening corneal damage are the structural and functional defects of the eyelids. Although these may be secondary to some primary insult such as trauma and cicatrix formation, most of these disorders are present congenitally. Dogs and cats are occasionally born with incomplete development of the eyelid, leaving a residual notch-like defect (coloboma) at the lid margin or in some cases a complete lack of the eyelid (agenesis). Although far more commonly a corneal problem, dermoids occasionally occur on the eyelids and interfere with eyelid function. These problems are uncommon, have no specific breed predilection, and are easily corrected surgically in all but the most severe cases.

The eyelids of puppies and kittens are normally closed at birth and remain so for the first 10 to 14 days of life (physiologic ankyloblepharon). If the eyelids do not open spontaneously, the ankyloblepharon may become pathologic, contributing to formation of bacterial and viral conjunctival infections. The problem is treated by splitting the palpebral fissure with the blade of a small scissor. Ankyloblepharon associated with conjunctival infection is more fully discussed with diseases of the conjunctiva.

Entropion

Entropion is an inward rolling of the eyelid margin that occurs most commonly as the result of a congenital weakness of the supporting collagenous layer of the eyelid. Although any breed may be affected, the chow chow, Chinese shar-pei, English bulldog, and the sporting breeds (setters and retrievers) are predisposed. Cats are affected less commonly, but the problem is sometimes seen in the Persian breed.

The potential corneal irritation by contact with eyelid cilia gives entropion its significance as a threat to vision. The clinical signs are extremely varied, depending on the duration, severity, and stiffness of the offending cilia. In mild cases, only blepharospasm and epiphora are evident. Chronic cases are characterized by corneal neovascularization, pigmentation, and eventual scarring. If the severity of the irritation exceeds the ability of the cornea to respond with the production of protective scar tissue, corneal ulceration and perforation may occur.

Any chronically painful ocular disease can cause blepharospasm accompanied by secondary entropion. Initially, the entropion is spastic and reversible, but it can become permanent if the cause of the pain goes uncorrected.

Regardless of the cause, the treatment of choice for entropion is surgical correction. The modified Hotz-Celsus procedure (Bistner, 1977) is universally applicable and can be modified for the specific area of the lid involved. If lateral canthal laxity is present, as typically found in the St. Bernard, the modified Hotz-Celsus procedure using a V-shaped incision corresponding to the lateral canthus is effective. A more sophisticated procedure involves repositioning the lateral portion of the orbicularis muscle (Wyman, 1971). If the entropion is associated with an abnormally small palpebral fissure, as is commonly found in the chow chow, the modified Hotz-Celsus procedure is combined with permanent lateral canthotomy. Entropion in the chow chow is also frequently aggravated by redundant facial skin, which may require concurrent excision. Entropion involving only the medial canthus in brachycephalic breeds is most easily corrected with permanent medial canthus closure (Jensen, 1979).

However, it is not the surgical procedure but the preoperative considerations that are the most challenging part of entropion correction. It is advisable to correct the congenital forms of entropion only after the animal has matured sufficiently to allow maximal spontaneous correction by the changing skull and facial features. Puppies with severe entropion may be temporarily managed with a temporary tarsorrhaphy placed as early as 2 weeks of age. In certain breeds, especially the shar-pei, permanent correction may not be necessary. If the animal reaches 6 months of age with a persistent problem, surgical correction can be performed with less likelihood of overcorrection.

Prior to correcting any case of entropion, it is important to determine the extent to which secondary blepharospasm is contributing to the problem. The instillation of a topical anesthetic before surgery will alleviate the entropion due to pain-associated blepharospasm, making accurate estimation of the anatomic component possible.

Ectropion

Ectropion, an outward deviation of the eyelid margin, may develop after trauma (cicatricial ectropion) but most commonly occurs as a developmental defect in spaniels (English springer and cocker), setters, hounds, and the giant breeds. Clinical signs develop as a result of the eyelid's inability to properly protect the cornea and maintain and distribute the tear film. Unlike the case in entropion, the potential for vision-threatening complications is low. Chronic ectropion is usually associated with only conjunctival hyperemia and persistent ocular discharge, which are easily controlled with periodic irrigation or application of an antibiotic-corticosteroid ophthalmic ointment. As a result, surgical correction is only indicated when the ectropion is severe or cosmetically unacceptable. The modified Kuhnt-Szymanowski procedure (Bistner et al., 1977; Munger and Carter, 1984) provides excellent cosmetic results and may be combined with the modified Hotz-Celsus procedure in those cases in which the central lower lid is ectropic but the lid is entropic at the medial and lateral extremities (e.g., St. Bernards, Newfoundlands, Great Pyrenees). Cicatricial ectropion is effectively corrected with the Y-V procedure.

Trichiasis

Trichiasis is the abnormal projection toward the eye of cilia or facial hairs that originate from a normally placed follicle. Any canine breed may be affected, but the problem is most common in the brachycephalic breeds, in which an excessive nasal skin fold puts cilia in close proximity to the cornea. In cats, the Persian and Himalayan breeds occasionally have such problems.

This abnormality becomes significant if the hairs contact the cornea in sufficient numbers to produce irritation. The long-term result is corneal ulceration, scarring, or both. A less significant manifestation of trichiasis is the epiphora seen in miniature and toy poodles. Cilia projecting from follicles in, or adjacent to, the medial canthus contact the tear film and through capillary action contribute to the tear overflow.

Treatment for trichiasis must be tailored to the patient's needs and coexisting problems. In show dogs and cats, relief of minor trichiasis is easily accomplished with daily application of a nonirritating lubricant (petrolatum) to keep the cilia away from the eye. In severe cases, surgical intervention is necessary either by excision of skin folds or by permanently narrowing the medial portion of the palpebral fissure. Closure of the medial canthus (Jensen, 1979) easily and effectively corrects the problem with little alteration in the cosmetic appearance of the animal.

Distichiasis

Probably the most common of the eyelash disorders, distichiasis is the presence of cilia that originate from an abnormal follicle, usually the orifice of the meibomian glands. The disease is seen frequently in the American cocker spaniel, toy and miniature poodle, Shih Tzu, and golden retriever and sporadically in other canine breeds. Cats are rarely affected.

Distichiasis is not always a clinically significant problem, depending on the number and structure of the abnormal cilia. Dogs with fine and soft cilia, as those typically seen in the cocker spaniel, usually require no treatment. Clinical signs develop when the cilia, even if few in number, are coarse and stiff; corneal contact is extremely irritating and rapidly results in ulceration.

A multitude of procedures have been advocated for the treatment of distichiasis, including manual epilation, electrolysis, surgical excision of isolated follicles, resecting the cilia-bearing tarsoconjunctiva with lid-splitting techniques, and cryosurgery. All these procedures suffer from inherent inadequacies. Cilia that are epilated rapidly regrow. Due to the small follicle size, electrolysis is both tedious and difficult to perform, and recurrences are common. Accurate surgical excision of the abnormal cilia and follicle is extremely difficult and can result in eyelid disfiguration that, if accompanied by regrowth of the cilia, leaves a complication even more serious and difficult to correct than the original problem. Cryosurgery offers the most practical, effective, and safe method of correcting distichiasis (Wheeler and Severin, 1984). Under general anesthesia, the lid is everted and immobilized with a chalazion forceps. A cryoprobe (activated by either nitrous oxide or liquid nitrogen) is pressed to the conjunctiva over the follicle to be destroyed. The freeze is continued until the ice ball extends to the lid margin. A double freeze-thaw cycle reduces the rate of recurrence. The abnormal cilia will fall out, usually within 1 month. Severe temporary swelling of the eyelids occurs but can be minimized by pretreatment with flunixin meglumine, 0.5 mg/kg intravenously (Banamine, Schering). Depigmentation of the lid margin also occurs but is temporary, and pigmentation returns in several months. Cryosurgery offers the distinct advantage of allowing retreatment of any cilia regrowth without the fear of causing permanent lid disfiguration.

Ectopic Cilia

Although they are the least common eyelash disorder, ectopic cilia are more likely to cause serious corneal ulceration than either trichiasis or distichiasis. Ectopic cilia are those cilia emerging from a misplaced follicle. Most cases represent a congenital malformation and are therefore clinically apparent early in life. Ectopic cilia also occur in older animals, the follicle misplacement apparently occurring secondary to trauma or deviation of cilia growth by a glandular inflammatory process. In either case, ectopic cilia tend to be few in number and usually emerge from the palpebral conjunctiva several millimeters from the eyelid margin.

Ectopic cilia, because they project directly toward the globe, are nearly always associated with corneal ulceration. They are small and sparse, so diagnosis depends on a careful and deliberate examination of the conjunctiva with the aid of good magnification. Treatment is easily effected by sharp excision of the misplaced follicle.

Abnormalities of Palpebral Fissure Size: The Exophthalmos-Lagophthalmos Syndrome

One of the most underdiagnosed and important problems in clinical ophthalmology is what might best be termed the exophthalmos-lagophthalmos syndrome. In all brachycephalic breeds of dogs, particularly the Pekingese, Lhaso Apso, and Shih Tzu, two anatomic abnormalities occur as the result of the compact facial and skull configuration. The palpebral fissure is invariably too large, and the orbit is excessively shallow. As a result, the eye protrudes (exophthalmos) and the eyelids incompletely cover the eye during reflex blinking (lagophthalmos). The eye is not adequately protected, and the lids incompletely distribute the tear film. This combination of abnormalities is responsible for a large proportion of the corneal ulcers seen in these breeds of dogs.

This problem is easily misdiagnosed, as deliberate evaluation of blinking effectiveness is necessary to establish the presence of this functional abnormality. In many cases, the owner will notice that the eyelids remain partially open as the animal sleeps. During examination, blinking must be observed for both frequency (normal is four to five times per minute) and completeness. If blinking is infrequent or the lids fail to cover the globe completely, the problem is likely to be significant. Lagophthalmos is further implicated as the cause of the problem when corneal ulceration or pigmentation is found in the central cornea, where exposure is maximized.

Correction of both lagophthalmos and excessive palpebral fissure size is easily accomplished with a permanent partial tarsorrhaphy. This is effective not only in protecting the cornea but also reduces the risk of traumatic proptosis. The author's preference is the pocket flap technique originally described by Jensen. Performing the surgery at the medial canthus also protects the cornea from trichiasis if excessive nasal skin folds are present.

Inflammatory Diseases

HORDEOLUM

A hordeolum is a staphylococcal infection of either the marginal eyelid glands (external hordeolum) or the tarsal (meibomian) glands (internal hordeolum). It occurs primarily in young dogs. The conjunctiva becomes inflamed, and small white accumulations of inflammatory cells may be seen subconjunctivally at the base of the meibomian glands. Hot compresses combined with a broad-spectrum antibiotic ointment (Neosporin, Burroughs Wellcome) applied three to four times daily are curative. Larger areas of abscessation may be gently expressed under topical anesthesia with a cotton-tipped swab.

CHALAZION

If the excretory ducts of the meibomian glands become obstructed, retained lipid secretions incite a granulomatous inflammatory response termed a chalazion. Chalazions commonly occur after inflammation of the gland or in conjunction with tumors that obstruct the duct system. Chalazions are nonpainful white swellings that are easily recognized when the lid margin is everted. Treatment is surgical curettage of the retained secretion through a small conjunctival incision. If the chalazion is big enough to cause distention of the eyelid skin, incision and curettage through the skin side of the eyelid may be easier. A broad-spectrum antibiotic ointment should be applied postoperatively three or four times daily.

STAPHYLOCOCCAL BLEPHARITIS

Pathogenic staphylococci (*Staphylococcus intermedius* and *S. epidermidis*) are capable of infecting the eyelids of dogs and causing blepharitis. There is hyperemia and swelling of the lid margin, which may be accompanied by purulent ocular discharge and conjunctivitis. Bacterial infection of the tarsal (meibomian) glands may occur at the same time. Acute infections respond well to a 2- to 3-week course of appropriate systemic and topical antibiotics. If the blepharitis is chronic, associated with generalized pyoderma, or secondary to seborrhea, the response to therapy is slow and frequently incomplete.

Staphylococcal blepharitis also occurs in a chronic form thought to represent a hypersensitivity to the bacterial cell wall antigen. The blepharitis is recurrent, with eyelid edema and a mucopurulent ocular discharge. Long-term antibiotic therapy is necessary. Staphylococcal bacterins are nonspecific stimulators of the immune system, and both commercial (Staphage Lysate, Delmont; Staphoid A-B, JenSal) and autogenous bacterins have been recommended.

MYCOTIC BLEPHARITIS

Blepharitis can be caused by the common small animal dermatophytes, *Microsporum canis*, *M. gypseum*, and *Trichophyton mentagrophytes*. The infected area is usually alopecic, with scales and varying degrees of inflammation. When the eyelid margin is involved, there is concurrent conjunctivitis and mucopurulent ocular discharge. Although potassium hydroxide preparations of perilesional hair may reveal spores, culture is necessary for a definitive diagnosis.

Mycotic blepharitis can be treated topically with the common dermatologic preparations of miconazole (Conofite, Pitman-Moore), thiabendazole (Tresaderm, Merck Sharp & Dohme), and haloprogin (Halotex, Westwood). Treatment should be preceded with an application of ophthalmic ointment (Lacrilube, Allergan) to prevent corneal irritation. When more extensive lesions are present, systemic therapy with griseofulvin (Fulvicin, Schering; Grifungal, Pitman-Moore) at a dose of 90 to 130 mg/kg daily for 6 weeks is more reliable.

PARASITIC BLEPHARITIS

Local or generalized dermatologic mite infestations can involve the eyelids. In dogs, demodicosis frequently occurs on the eyelids and characteristically produces a circular area of alopecia. Generalized demodicosis also affects the eyelids, but the clinical significance is negligible in light of the generalized lesions. Therapy for eyelid demodicosis differs from demodicosis in other body areas only by the necessity to consider the health of the cornea and conjunctiva when applying potentially irritating therapeutic agents. Although localized demodicosis is usually self-limiting, the eyelid lesions may be treated with dermatologic creams (Goodwinol, Goodwinol; Canex, Pitman-Moore) after the application to the eye of a bland ophthalmic ointment. The current drug of choice for treating generalized demodicosis is amitraz (Mitaban, Upjohn), and information concerning its use can be found elsewhere in this text. Cats also suffer from demodicosis but far less commonly.

Sarcoptic mange also involves the eyelids but is easily resolved along with the generalized infestation with application of lindane (KIL-A-MITE, Burroughs Wellcome) or lime sulfur dips. After protective ophthalmic ointment is applied to the eyes, the dip can be safely and thoroughly applied to the eyelids with a soaked cotton ball.

ALLERGIC BLEPHARITIS

Allergic blepharitis is most likely to occur as a component of atopic dermatitis (allergic inhalant dermatitis). In addition to axillary and inguinal pruritus, the face and eyelids may be involved. Affected dogs frequently paw at or rub the face and eyelids on the carpet, leaving the eyelids swollen and inflamed. Alternate-day systemic corticosteroid therapy is effective; however, skin testing and hyposensitization may provide more permanent relief.

Blepharitis also develops in a small percentage of patients after chronic administration of certain ophthalmic medications. This is a local hypersensitivity reaction to either the drug or the preservative used in its preparation. Neomycin is most often involved. The skin below the medial canthus becomes hyperemic, swollen, and eventually excoriated, and secondary bacterial infection causes a purulent discharge. Withdrawal of therapy causes a rapid resolution of the clinical signs. An antibiotic-corticosteroid ophthalmic preparation applied three to four times daily will reduce the inflammation and speed recovery.

AUTOIMMUNE BLEPHARITIS

Although it is uncommon for autoimmune diseases to spare the rest of the skin in preference for the eyelids, the lesions may be more noticeable on the face and eyelids, especially early in the course of disease. Pemphigus and systemic lupus erythematosus are the two most likely considerations. Pemphigus vulgaris affects the mucocutaneous junction of the eyelids, producing erosions and ulcerations. Pemphigus foliaceus and erythematosus may appear on the face and eyelids as a vesicobullous or pustular lesion. Early in the course of lupus erythematosus, the eyelids may appear swollen and eventually progress to the more typical vesicobullous and ulcerative lesions. The reader is referred to other sources for details concerning diagnosis and treatment of the autoimmune skin diseases (Muller et al., 1983).

IDIOPATHIC BLEPHARITIS

A bilateral blepharitis confined to the medial canthus occurs without an identifiable cause in the German shepherds, long-haired Dachshund, and toy and miniature poodles. The eyelid skin of the medial canthus becomes inflamed and ulcerated, and the condition responds to topical antibiotic-corticosteroid preparations. Although the cause is speculative, infiltration of the affected skin with lymphocytes and plasma cells and the occasional concurrent presence of chronic superficial keratitis suggest this to be an immune-mediated phenomenon.

Neoplastic Diseases

Tumors of the eyelids are very common in small animals, especially dogs. Although dogs and cats can exhibit the same neoplasms, significant differences exist in the relative prevalence of the different tumors and their behavior. In general, feline eyelid tumors are likely to be malignant, and squamous cell carcinoma is the most common. This tumor appears as an ulcerative lesion anywhere on the lid margin and has a predilection for white cats. Cats are also predisposed to eyelid fibromas and fibrosarcomas; the latter may be associated with feline leukemia virus infection. Other less common feline eyelid tumors include neurofibroma, neurofibrosarcoma, mast cell, and sebaceous gland tumors (adenoma and adenocarcinoma).

Eyelid tumors of dogs are usually benign. Adenomas of the sebaceous (meibomian) glands are most common, have a characteristic pedunculated appearance, and can usually be seen arising from the meibomian glands if the lid is everted. Melanomas are also common, are usually located at the lid margin, and are also generally benign. Other canine eyelid tumors include papilloma, sebaceous gland adenocarcinoma, malignant melanoma, mast cell tumors, histiocytoma, and squamous cell and basal cell carcinoma.

Most eyelid tumors are easily removed by surgical excision. Full-thickness V-resection safely allows removal of tumors involving as much as one third of the eyelid margin. Following removal of larger tumors, the defect can be closed with sliding grafts, bucket handle, or lip-to-lid flaps (Gwin, 1980; Pavletic et al., 1982). If available, cryosurgery is also an effective method of treating many eyelid tumors. For feline squamous cell carcinomas, when determining the margins of the tumor is usually difficult, excision is unpredictable. In these cases, either cryosurgery, hyperthermia, or implantation of radioactive seeds (iridium) may be necessary. Histopathologic evaluation of all eyelid tumors is advisable, but it is especially important in cats and in dogs with invasive or recurrent lesions.

DISEASES OF THE CONJUNCTIVA

The conjunctiva lines both the globe (bulbar conjunctiva) and the eyelids (palpebral conjunctiva) and functions as (1) a protective covering to the eye and its adnexa, (2) a source of the mucus component of the tear film, and (3) the first line of defense against potentially invading organisms. The conjunctiva responds with a variety of reactions to a diverse group of local and systemic diseases. Because the conjunctiva has a strategic location and is highly visible, changes occurring in it are frequently the first clinical signs of disease noticed.

Response of the Conjunctiva to Disease

INFLAMMATION VERSUS HYPEREMIA

It is tempting to refer to the reddened conjunctiva as inflamed. In the strictest sense, however, a diagnosis of conjunctivitis is justified only when the traditional criteria for inflammation are satisfied. The vessels of the conjunctiva frequently become engorged with blood in the absence of true inflammation. Common examples are glaucoma, uveitis, and disturbances in systemic circulation. The term *hyperemia* is more appropriate in these situations and avoids attributing unjustified significance to the conjunctival reaction. Accurately distinguishing conjunctival hyperemia from inflammation is not only important in the diagnosis of ocular disease but is crucial if therapy is to be appropriately directed.

CONJUNCTIVAL HEMORRHAGE

The conjunctiva is richly perfused with capillaries that easily rupture when traumatized. Because of its visibility, conjunctival hemorrhage usually looks more severe than it is and spontaneously resolves without specific therapy in several days. A topical antibiotic may be applied prophylactically three or four times daily. The primary significance of conjunctival hemorrhage is that it alerts the clinician that other more serious ocular damage may be present. Conjunctival hemorrhage that occurs spontaneously or fails to resorb quickly indicates the potential presence of a systemic bleeding disorder.

CHEMOSIS

Edema causes the conjunctiva to appear puffy and paler than normal. It occurs in the early phase of local allergic conditions, as part of a generalized hypersensitivity reaction, early in the course of feline chlamydial infection, and in response to irritating stimuli. Chemosis responds dramatically to corticosteroid administration but will resolve without complication after correction of its underlying cause. Topical hyperosmotic agents (e.g., 5 per cent sodium chloride [Muro 128, Muro]) are also effective symptomatic therapy.

FOLLICLE FORMATION

Small follicles of proliferated lymphoid cells are normally present on the bulbar surface of the nictitating membrane but can appear on any of the conjunctival surfaces under pathologic conditions. Follicle formation has been specifically attributed to chlamydial conjunctivitis in cats; however, they may appear after chronic conjunctivitis of any cause. In most situations, follicle formation suggests chronic antigenic stimulation. Follicles are, in themselves, insignificant and may persist long after the cause has disappeared.

Structural Defects

Structural defects of the conjunctiva are rare. Symblepharon is an adhesion of the conjunctiva either to itself or to the eyelids or cornea. Symblepharon may be a congenital lesion or may occur secondary to either inflammation, trauma, or surgery. Correction is surgical but is necessary only in unusually severe cases.

Canine Conjunctivitis

Conjunctivitis has traditionally been considered to be the most common of all ophthalmic disorders. However, very few animals have gone blind or lost vision as the result of conjunctival inflammation alone. All too often, because of the high frequency of conjunctival inflammation, a diagnosis of conjunctivitis is hastily assigned to other more serious ocular diseases such as glaucoma, keratoconjunctivitis sicca, and uveitis. An appreciation of conjunctival diseases is important not only because they are common but also because recognizing and correcting potentially vision-threatening diseases often depends on first distinguishing them from conjunctivitis.

BACTERIAL

An almost unlimited variety of bacteria are routinely recovered from the canine conjunctival sac, implying that they are not by themselves pathogenic. The normal host defense mechanisms must be impaired to allow the organism to proliferate. The usual causes are trauma or irritation (most commonly from eyelash disorders), inadequate tear production, or exposure to irritating stimuli such as inappropriately applied dips and shampoos. Bacterial conjunctivitis frequently accompanies chronic pyoderma, seborrheic dermatitis, and otitis externa. The foremost consideration in treating bacterial conjunctivitis is to identify and correct the primary cause. Once this is accomplished, the disease responds rapidly to broad-spectrum ophthalmic antibiotic solutions or ointments applied four times daily. An excellent choice is the combination of neomycin-bacitracin-polymyxin (Neosporin, Burroughs Wellcome; Trioptic-P, Beecham). This drug is bactericidal, inexpensive, and available under numerous trade names as both ointments and solutions. It has a spectrum of activity that is effective in the vast majority of cases. There is little justification for treating routine conjunctivitis with the more expensive aminoglycoside antibiotics unless indicated by culture and sensitivity results. When conjunctivitis fails to respond as expected, the clinician should look for another diagnosis and not a different drug.

Opinions vary as to the necessity of concurrent corticosteroid administration in the treatment of bacterial conjunctivitis. In the author's opinion, they are rarely indicated; if the diagnosis and choice of antibiotic are correct, resolution of the problem is rapid without the nonspecific suppression of clinical signs afforded by corticosteroids. It is important for the clinician to know that when the conjunctivitis appears improved, it is because the bacteria are eliminated and not simply because the signs are distorted.

VIRAL

The only common viral cause of canine conjunctivitis is canine distemper. In addition to showing the upper respiratory signs of coughing and nasal discharge, acutely infected dogs usually have conjunctivitis that is serous in character, rapidly becoming purulent as secondary bacteria become involved. The disease is complicated by decreased tear production. Treatment is nonspecific and consists of application of a broad-spectrum antibiotic ointment or solution three to four times daily and artificial tears as needed. Irrigating excess exudate from the eye prior to therapy is also helpful.

Feline Conjunctivitis

Conjunctivitis in cats differs from that in dogs by having a greater number of infectious causes and a greater variety of clinical signs. In addition, feline conjunctival pathogens tend to be more selective in the clinical signs they produce. Cats do suffer from bacterial conjunctivitis; however, because of both the lower incidence of adnexal diseases that predispose the conjunctiva to irritation and the lower numbers of resident flora, feline conjunctivitis is likely to be caused by either chlamydia, mycoplasma, or the feline herpesvirus (Nasisse et al., 1984).

CHLAMYDIA

The causative agent of feline chlamydial conjunctivitis is *Chlamydia psittaci.* The organism is primarily a conjunctival pathogen but does affect, to a lesser extent, the nasal mucosa. Clinical signs are serous conjunctivitis, chemosis, blepharospasm, and sometimes conjunctival follicle formation. The disease typically starts unilaterally, affecting the second eye 1 week later. With chronicity, the discharge becomes mucopurulent to purulent. Sneezing and nasal discharge are inconsistent findings. The clinical course may range from 3 to 6 weeks.

A presumptive diagnosis is based on a history of unilateral progressing to bilateral conjunctivitis in conjunction with suggestive clinical signs. Conjunctival scrapings stained with Giemsa or similar stain (Diff Quik, Harleco) may reveal intracytoplasmic inclusion bodies that focus in the plane of the epithelial cell nucleus. The best method of diagnosis is by fluorescent antibody testing of conjunctival scrapings. The treatment of choice is tetracycline ophthalmic ointment (Terramycin, Pfizer; Achromycin, Lederle) applied four times daily. Although the response to therapy is usually good, a carrier state and recurrent infections can occur. Systemic tetracycline therapy may be beneficial in these instances.

MYCOPLASMA

Mycoplasma conjunctivitis can be caused by *Mycoplasma felis* and *M. gatae.* Unlike chlamydial pathogens in chlamydial conjunctivitis, mycoplasma is probably not a significant pathogen unless the animal's defense mechanisms have been weakened by some form of stress. The disease is usually bilateral, with chemosis and serous to mucoid ocular discharge. A characteristic finding attributed to mycoplasma infection is the formation of a conjunctival pseudomembrane. The clinical course is approximately 1 month.

The clinical signs may be suggestive but are rarely diagnostic. Cytologic examination of the conjunctiva reveals a predominantly polymorphonuclear reaction. Intracytoplasmic inclusions that focus at the level of the cell membrane may be seen but are an inconsistent finding. Culture offers the only means of definitive diagnosis but is rarely necessary. Response to topical tetracycline ophthalmic ointment applied four times daily is good.

FELINE HERPESVIRUS

The feline herpesvirus (rhinotracheitis virus) is capable of producing a variety of ocular lesions in addition to upper respiratory tract infection. The most common clinical syndrome is the acute conjunctivitis that accompanies the upper respiratory tract infection. The conjunctivitis is usually bilateral and is characterized by conjunctival hyperemia, blepharospasm, and ocular discharge that begins as serous in nature but progresses to mucopurulent as the infection persists. Sneezing and nasal discharge are accompanying features. This acute form of the disease is most common in young cats and kittens, and the conjunctivitis resolves with symptomatic antibiotic therapy when the viral infection has run its 2- to 3-week course.

Feline herpesvirus infection may also occur as a chronic ocular condition without the upper respiratory tract involvement. This is more common in older cats, and the clinical signs range from conjunctivitis to superficial or deep keratitis. Occasionally, early in the course, the virus causes corneal ulcers that are linear and branching (dendritic) in appearance. This is the only sign considered pathognomonic for ocular herpesvirus infection. These branching ulcers may enlarge and coalesce to form suggestive geographic ulceration. In a small percentage of cases, stromal keratitis develops that is characterized by a combination of edema, vascularization, and cellular infiltration. In chronic cases, a decrease in tear production may also be noticed.

In acute infection, when upper respiratory involvement is present, history and clinical signs are usually enough to make a tentative diagnosis. Laboratory diagnosis is necessary in chronic cases. Cytologic study of the conjunctiva is an unreliable method of diagnosis, as the cellular reaction is variable and the presence of diagnostic inclusion bodies is rare. Virus culture is effective but impractical in most clinical settings. Fluorescent antibody testing of conjunctival scrapings is inexpensive, reliable, and practical, as samples for testing are easily obtained and may be mailed to the laboratory.

Treatment of chronic ocular herpesvirus infection is difficult at best. Three topical antiviral drugs exist in ophthalmic form: idoxuridine (Stoxil, SmithKline Beckman; Dendrid, Alcon), adenine arabinoside (Vira-A, Parke-Davis), and trifluridine (Viroptic, Burroughs Wellcome). Unfortunately, clinical response to their use is unpredictable and frequently disappointing. The major indication for their use is keratitis. Antiviral ointments should be used five times daily. Solutions require instillation every 1 to 2 hours for the first day and five times daily thereafter. Corticosteroids are contraindicated in most infections because they inhibit host defense mechanisms and perpetuate the infection. However, they are used as a last resort to suppress corneal scarring in cases of chronic stromal keratitis.

The prognosis for cats with ocular herpesvirus infection is dependent on the form of the disease. Acute upper respiratory infection, although followed with an estimated carrier rate of 80 per cent, usually resolves without serious consequence. If the conjunctivitis becomes chronic or the cornea is involved, the prognosis is guarded, as in all likelihood the problem is not the virus but an inadequate immune response to it on the part of the animal.

MISCELLANEOUS

Feline reovirus and feline calicivirus infection can cause conjunctivitis in cats, but the infection is mild and of lesser significance than with the previously described pathogens.

MIXED INFECTIONS

Much of the difficulty in differentiating the types of feline conjunctivitis based solely on clinical signs stems from the frequent occurrence of more than one pathogen. Infection of the conjunctiva with any of the previously described organisms predisposes to secondary infection with another.

Neonatal Conjunctivitis

Conjunctivitis that occurs in either cats or dogs within the first few weeks of life is termed neonatal conjunctivitis. The cause is usually bacterial in dogs but in cats may be caused by any of the previously described pathogens. The clinical signs are identical to other forms of conjunctivitis except that infection may occur before the eyelids open. Retained exudate will give the closed eyelids a distended appearance. Treatment is drainage of the retained exudate by splitting the palpebral fissure with the blade of a small scissor, followed with topical antibiotics four times daily until resolved.

Allergic Conjunctivitis

In dogs, allergic conjunctivitis is caused most commonly by the same factors responsible for allergic blepharitis. Certain topical medications, vaccine reaction, and atopic skin disease are common causes. Cats are affected less commonly, but by the same causes. Allergic conjunctivitis responds dramatically to topically applied corticosteroid ophthalmic preparations, provided any systemic reaction is treated concurrently.

Neoplastic Diseases

Conjunctival tumors occur rarely. Hemangiomas appear occasionally and are typically small, distinctly vascular in appearance, and easy to excise. Papillomas and melanomas can also occur on the conjunctiva. Most other tumors affecting the conjunctiva are extensions of tumors originating in one of the adjoining structures. Examples are the scleral pseudotumors (fibrous histiocytoma, nodular granulomatous episclerokeratitis), and limbal melanomas.

DISEASES OF THE THIRD EYELID

Eversion or Inversion of the Cartilage

A congenital weakness of the cartilage of the third eyelid may allow inversion or eversion of the third eyelid margin. The condition usually occurs in dogs in the first few years of life. The folded nictitating membrane appears protruded from the medial canthus and may mimic a prolapse of the gland. Surgical excision of the folded portion of the cartilage allows the membrane to return to a normal position.

Idiopathic Protrusion in Cats

In cats, the nictitating membrane will occasionally protrude from the medial canthus with no apparent cause. The condition is bilateral and is associated with no other ophthalmic abnormalities. However, the third eyelid is sometimes protruded enough to obstruct vision. Systemic examination likewise reveals no abnormalities. A diagnosis of idiopathic protrusion is made when other causes of nictitans protrusion are ruled out; protrusion also occurs in Horner's syndrome, when ocular pain causes retraction of the globe, or if loss of orbital fat or dehydration results in enophthalmos.

Idiopathic nictitans protrusion spontaneously resolves in 4 to 8 weeks. If the protruding third eyelid is particularly troublesome, symptomatic relief can be gained by applying 1 per cent epinephrine ophthalmic solution once or twice daily.

Plasma Cell Infiltration

In German shepherds, the third eyelid occasionally becomes thickened and irregular as the result of infiltration with plasma cells. The condition is bilateral and may or may not be associated with superficial keratitis (pannus). Like pannus, the condition responds to therapy with topical corticosteroid ophthalmic ointments or solutions, and its cause is presumed to be immunologic in origin.

Neoplasia

Neoplasms of the third eyelid are rare in small animals. In cats, fibrosarcoma has been described, and squamous cell carcinomas sometimes involve the third eyelid. If the third eyelid appears diffusely swollen, lymphosarcoma is a consideration. In dogs, hemangiomas of the nictitans occur infrequently. Suspicious lesions of the third eyelid should be carefully studied by biopsy, as the *only* indication for complete removal of the nictitating membrane is extensive involvement by a malignant neoplasm.

Prolapse of the Gland

Prolapse of the gland of the third eyelid ("cherry eye") occurs commonly in dogs. The cause is either a weakness of the third eyelid's T-shaped cartilage, a weakness of the fibrous tissue anchoring the gland, or both. The traditional treatment by gland excision is undesirable, as inadequate tear production can result. Techniques to surgically anchor the prolapsed gland in its proper position have been described and include suturing the gland to the periorbital fascia, suturing the gland to one of the extraocular muscles, suturing the gland to the sclera, and anchoring the gland to the base of the third eyelid. All these procedures are effective; different techniques work better for different surgeons. It is most important to appreciate that the

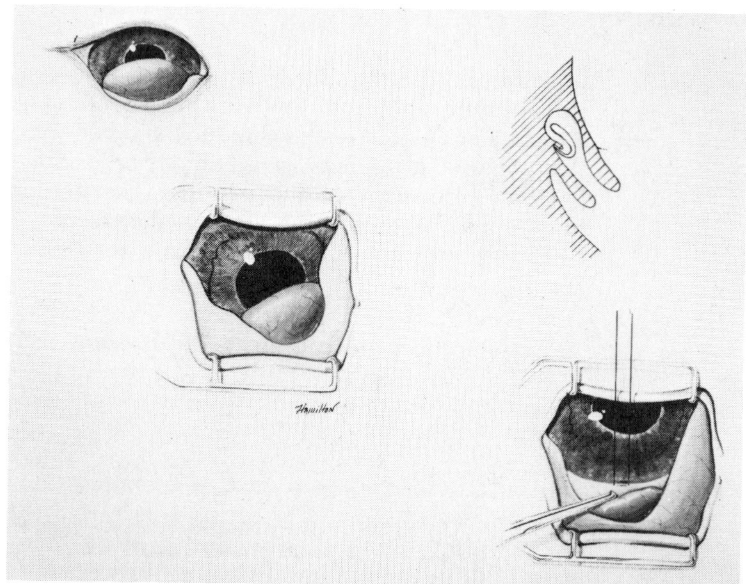

Figure 1. The typical prolapse of the nictitans gland causes the "cherry eye" appearance in the upper left. For maximum exposure, place a lid speculum and a 4–0 silk stay suture in the limbus at the 6 o'clock or ventral position. Position the globe upward as far as possible to expose the fornix between the nictitans and the bulbar conjunctiva. (Courtesy of R. C. Riis, Cornell University.)

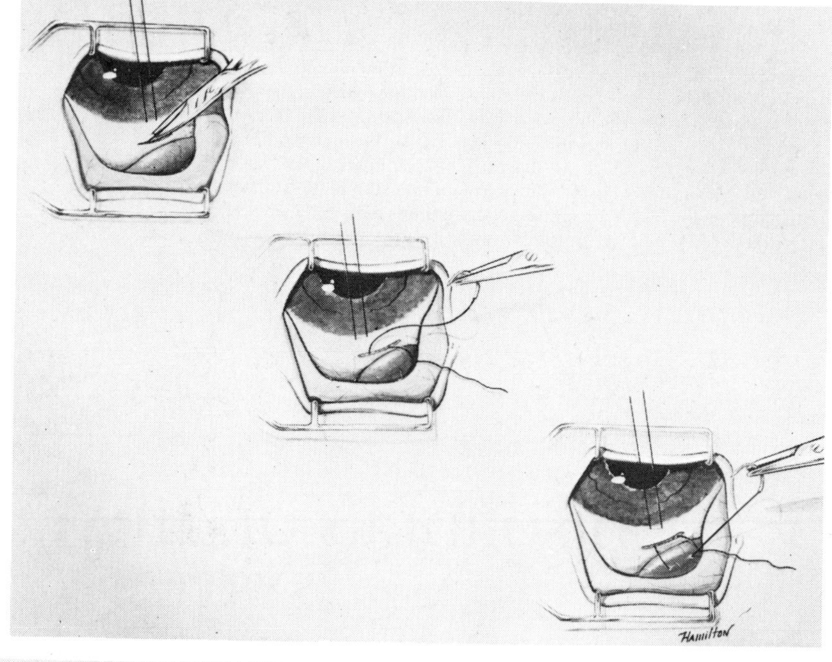

Figure 2. The upper left shows the ventrally exposed fornix being superficially incised to expose underlying bulbar fascia and sclera. The center exposure depicts anchoring a 5–0 Vicryl suture into the sclera with a mattress pattern. If this suture is correctly anchored, the globe can be moved in any direction with the suture. The mattress pattern is continued into the dorsal portion of the prolapsed gland, as shown in the lower right. This portion of the pattern has to be fairly deep but not necessarily into the cartilage. (Courtesy of R. C. Riis, Cornell University.)

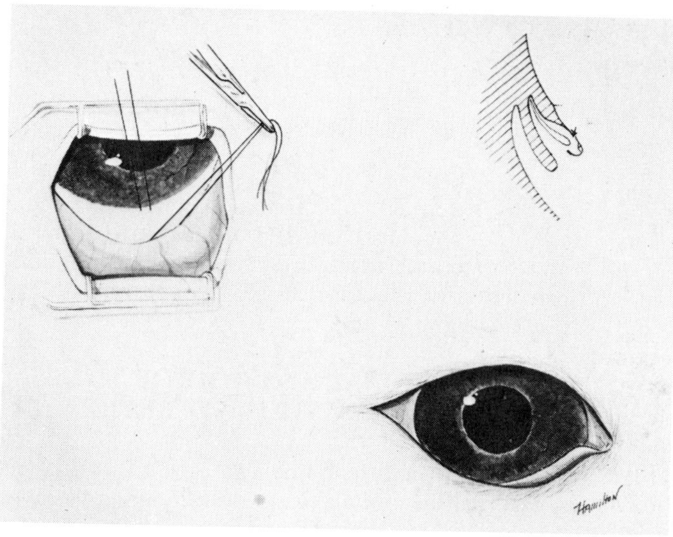

Figure 3. The upper left drawing shows the repositioning of the gland when the suture is tied. The conjunctival incision and the reaction incited by the dissolving Vicryl suture should stimulate an adhesion. The proper placement will account for immediate cosmesis as well as time for the adhesions to form. Once the stay suture is removed, the downward globe rotation will take the gland to its normal position, as shown in the right upper (side) and lower views. (Courtesy of R. C. Riis, Cornell University.)

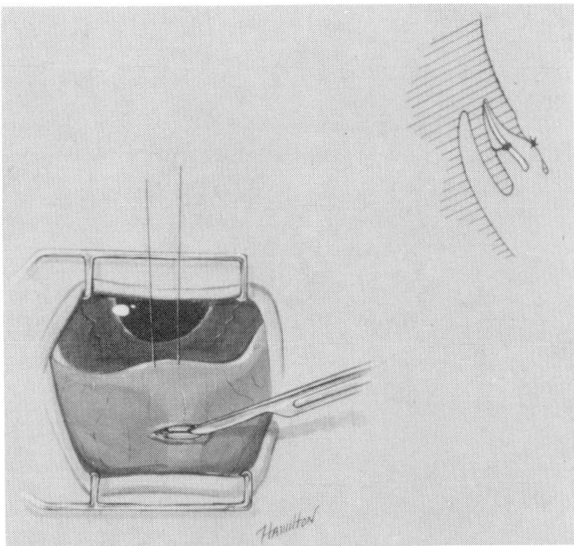

Figure 4. If the prolapsed gland is of long standing or in an older animal, the cartilage of the nictitans will be permanently deformed. In these cases, to make the "tack-down" successful, include an extra step to incise the base of the cartilage. Expose the anterior surface of the nictitans by placing a 4–0 silk traction suture in the margin and pull dorsally. Incise through anterior conjunctiva and cartilage as shown. The conjunctiva does not have to be sutured. Postoperative treatment should be topical broad-spectrum antibiotic ointment three times daily for 2 weeks. (Courtesy of R. C. Riis. Cornell University.)

prolapsed gland is actually flipped over and not simply protruding from the palpebral fissure (Figs. 1 to 4). For any of these techniques to be effective, the prolapsed gland must be accurately repositioned prior to placement of the sutures. The author's preference is to suture the gland to the sclera with 5–0 Vicryl with a small swaged cutting needle.

References and Supplemental Reading

Bistner, S. I., Aguirre, G., and Batik, G.: *Atlas of Veterinary Ophthalmic Surgery*. Philadelphia: W. B. Saunders, 1977.

Gwin, R. M.: Selected blepharoplastic procedures of the canine eyelid. Comp. Cont. Ed. Pract. Vet. 2:267, 1980.

Jensen, H. E.: Canthus closure. Comp. Cont. Ed. Pract. Vet. 1:735, 1979.

Muller, G. H., Kirk, R. W., and Scott, D. W.: Small Animal Dermatology, 3rd ed. Philadelphia: W. B. Saunders, 1983.

Munger, R. J., and Carter, J. D.: A further modification of the Kuhnt-Szymanowski procedure for correction of atonic ectropion in dogs. J. Am. Anim. Hosp. Assoc. 20:651, 1984.

Nasisse, M. P., Cook, C. S., Peiffer, R. L., et al.: *Feline Infectious Conjunctivitis*. (Schering Continuing Education Series.) Princeton: Veterinary Learning Systems, 1984.

Pavletic, M. M., Nafe, L. A., and Confer, A. W.: Mucocutaneous subdermal plexus flap from the lip for lower eyelid restoration in the dog. J.A.V.M.A. 180:921, 1982.

Wheeler, C. A., and Severin, G. A.: Cryosurgical epilation for the treatment of distichiasis in the dog and cat. J. Am. Anim. Hosp. Assoc. 20:877, 1984.

Wyman, M.: Lateral canthoplasty. J. Am. Anim. Hosp. Assoc. 7:196, 1971.

DISORDERS OF THE LACRIMAL SYSTEM

THOMAS J. KERN, D.V.M.
Ithaca, New York

The presence and importance of the precorneal tear film are most evident when its normal functions become impaired. Both secretory and excretory lacrimal dysfunctions in dogs and cats may cause clinical signs that demand accurate diagnosis and appropriate therapy. Disorders of lacrimal secretion are most simply classified as states of tear deficiency or tear excess. Tear deficiency results from lacrimal secretory failure or impaired access of normally formed tears to the conjunctival sac through the lacrimal ductules. Excessive lacrimation is stimulated by external ocular irritation, intraocular pain, and photophobia. Disorders of tear excretion involve congenital or acquired structural or functional obstruction of the nasolacrimal excretory pathways at one or more sites.

FUNCTIONAL ANATOMY OF THE LACRIMAL SYSTEM: SECRETION

The precorneal tear film comprises three layers: an external oil monolayer, a middle aqueous layer, and an inner mucin layer. The extremely thin outer layer of lipids is secreted by the meibomian glands of the eyelid margin. It retards evaporation and maintains surface tension necessary for normal tear distribution and breakup. The innermost glycoprotein or mucin layer produced by conjunctival goblet cells binds the aqueous middle layer of the tear film to the hydrophobic corneal epithelial cell membranes.

The middle aqueous layer of the tear film, accounting for more than 98 per cent of tear volume, is produced by the main orbital lacrimal gland and the gland of the nictitans. Both are mixed mucoserous, compound tubuloacinar glands with parasympathetic innervation. The presence and importance of accessory conjunctival lacrimal glands in the dog and cat are uncertain. The lacrimal gland lies in a fold of periorbital fascia, superotemporal and closely apposed to the globe, beneath the orbital ligament. The nictitans gland lies on the inner surface of the third eyelid at the base of the T-shaped cartilage of the nictitans. Ten to 20 lacrimal ductules transmit tears from the glands to the conjunctival sac. In dogs, approximately 70 per cent of tear volume is produced by the orbital lacrimal gland and 30 per cent by the gland of the nictitans. In normal dogs, either gland alone is credited with maintaining adequate tear secretion in the other gland's absence (Gelatt and Gwin, 1981). Similar quantitative data for the cat's lacrimal gland secretion is unavailable.

Vital functions of the tear film include the following: nourishment of the cornea and conjunctiva, ocular surface lubrication, mechanical cleansing of the cornea and conjunctival sac, immunologic defense of the ocular surface through secretory immunoglobulins and lysozyme, and formation of the major refracting surface in visual image formation.

LACRIMAL SECRETORY DISORDERS

Excessive Lacrimation

Even when the normal nasolacrimal system is functionally patent, increased lacrimation may overwhelm it and result in tear overflow, or epiphora. Both external ocular and intraocular discomfort cause reflex excessive lacrimation (Table 1). Eyelid deformities, congenital anomalies, conjunctivitis, ulcerative keratitis, glaucoma, uveitis, and ocular foreign bodies must all be ruled out. Therapy is targeted toward correction of the underlying disorder.

Keratoconjunctivitis Sicca

Keratoconjunctivitis sicca (KCS) may be defined as the progressive inflammatory and degenerative changes of the cornea and conjunctiva caused by deficient tear secretion. Almost by definition, KCS results from a quantitatively reduced aqueous tear component, though functional deficiencies of the meibomian glands (producing an abnormal oily layer) or conjunctival goblet cells (resulting in deficient ocular surface mucin) may also cause corneal and conjunctival dryness and reduced surface wettability. In animals, discrimination of aqueous-deficient from oil- and mucin-deficient dry eye syndromes is difficult.

Table 1. Causes of Lacrimal Hypersecretion

External ocular irritation	
Eyelids	Blepharitis Distichiasis/ectopic cilia Trichiasis Entropion Prominent nasal folds Lagophthalmos Nictitans gland prolapse
Conjunctiva	Conjunctivitis
Cornea	Ulcerative keratitis
Intraocular discomfort	
Uveitis	
Glaucoma	
Photophobia	Secondary to mydriasis or uveitis

Although its initial presentation is frequently unilateral, KCS in most instances eventually involves both eyes. KCS occurs sporadically in individual dogs and cats of most breeds as well as in mixed-breed animals. In a statistical review of KCS occurrence in dogs and cats, certain breeds of both species are overrepresented (Tables 2 and 3). No sex predilection was evident. KCS was most frequently diagnosed in dogs and cats 7 years of age and older (Table 4). The number of KCS diagnoses per 1000 admissions was notably higher in dogs than in cats.

CAUSES

Although several causes of KCS in dogs are known or postulated, documentation of the specific cause in individual cases is difficult. Congenital anomalies, infectious agents, and toxic, neurologic, inflammatory, immune-mediated, and iatrogenic factors may all be associated.

Congenital alacrima occurs rarely, often only unilaterally, as severe xerosis, most commonly in toy breeds of dogs.

Canine distemper virus, by virtue of its epitheliotropism, may cause both acute lacrimal adenitis and acute conjunctivitis with primary or secondary (often transient) KCS. Chronic KCS may result if lacrimal gland destruction has been extensive or if conjunctival cicatrization occludes the lacrimal ductules.

Several drugs may produce transient and even

Table 2. *KCS Diagnosis by Breed—Dogs**

Breed	Diagnoses/1000 Admissions This Breed × 10^3
Bulldog	321.2
Lhasa apso	167.0
West Highland white terrier	133.0
Sealyham terrier	128.6
Pug	97.0
Bloodhound	77.4
Pekingese	77.1
Shih Tzu	74.6
Cocker spaniel	70.1
Kerry blue terrier	69.3
Bull terrier	63.3
Boston terrier	53.7
Yorkshire terrier	47.7
Miniature poodle	35.3
Dachshund	30.3
Miniature schnauzer	30.3
Chow chow	2.51
Golden retriever	2.34
Old English sheepdog	2.22
Great Dane	2.21
Labrador retriever	2.19
Alaskan malamute	2.08
Doberman pinscher	2.08
Afghan hound	0.73
Dalmatian	0.67

*Based on retrospective analysis of 491,917 canine patient records in the Veterinary Medical Data Program, Inc., a consortium of 20 veterinary college referral teaching hospitals.

permanent KCS in some dogs. Sulfasalazine (Azulfidine, Pharmacia) sulfadiazine (alone and with trimethoprim [Tribrissen, Burroughs Wellcome]), atropine, phenazopyridine (Azo Gantrisin, Roche), and sulfisoxazole have been implicated (Morgan and Bachrach, 1982; Kaswan et al., 1983). Recovery of normal tear secretion is possible but unpredictable if drug administration is discontinued.

Aqueous secretory cells in the lacrimal glands require cholinergic innervation to function, whereas mucus-secreting cells are autonomous. Some animals with facial nerve palsy or peripheral denervation of the parasympathetic lacrimal nerve develop KCS.

Chronic conjunctivitis, especially with conjunctival ulceration, occasionally scars the lacrimal ductules and prevents tear access to the conjunctival sac, causing chronic KCS. Acute conjunctival inflammation may transiently cause secondary KCS by a similar, although reversible, mechanism. Postinflammatory KCS may be the most frequent dry eye syndrome in cats.

Table 3. *KCS Diagnosis by Breed—Cats**

Breed	KCS Diagnosis/1000 Admissions This Breed × 10^3
Burmese	41.2
Abyssinian	26.7
Himalayan	19.6
Persian	2.6
Mixed-breed (including domestic long-hair)	2.2
American domestic short-hair	1.5

*Based on a retrospective analysis of records of 202,374 feline patients in the Veterinary Medical Data Program, Inc., a consortium of 20 veterinary college referral teaching hospitals.

Table 4. *Age at KCS Diagnosis**

Age (Years)	No. of KCS Diagnoses/1000 Admissions × (10^3)	
	Dogs	***Cats***
1	1.5	0.8
1–2	5.2	1.4
2–4	13.1	3.4
4–7	35.6	5.2
7–10	64.5	9.6
10–15	74.1	8.0
15+	41.4	15.9

*Based on a retrospective analysis of records of 491,921 canine and 202,385 feline patients in the Veterinary Medical Data Program, Inc., a consortium of 20 veterinary college referral teaching hospitals.

Immune-mediated lacrimal gland destruction has been postulated to occur in dogs (Kaswan et al., 1984). Biopsies of lacrimal and nictitans glands from a large series of dogs with KCS showed multifocal mononuclear cell infiltration with variable fibrosis, atrophy, fatty infiltration, and ductular dilatation. In this series, 90 per cent of the dogs had elevated $beta_2$ or gamma globulins.

Dryness of the oral and nasal mucosa does occur in some dogs, suggesting multiple gland involvement. Xerostomia is a contraindication for parotid duct transposition. KCS may occur in animals with other known or suspected immunologic dysfunctions, such as systemic lupus erythematosus, rheumatoid arthritis, autoimmune hemolytic anemia, chronic active hepatitis, and certain endocrinopathies (hypothyroidism, hypoadrenocorticism, hyperadrenocorticism, diabetes mellitus).

In certain breeds at risk for KCS (e.g., American cockers, English bulldogs), surgical excision of a prolapsed gland of the nictitans may promote or accelerate KCS development. In these dogs, the main lacrimal gland may not sustain adequate tear production for unknown reasons.

Hypovitaminosis A is an unlikely cause of canine or feline KCS. Seborrhea and demodicosis have been empirically associated with canine KCS, though the relationships are unclear.

DIAGNOSIS

Clinical Signs

The severity of clinical signs is proportional to the relative degree of dryness and its duration. The hallmark of KCS at all stages is the presence of mucoid or mucopurulent ocular discharge. Mucin produced by conjunctival goblet cells is not properly admixed with and dispersed by aqueous tears; it accumulates as mucus threads, which entrap debris and bacteria. In addition, blepharospasm, subtle to severe corneal epithelial and stromal ulceration, and conjunctivitis are prominent. When corneal ulceration occurs, secondary reflex uveitis develops with attendant miosis and aqueous flare.

Superficial corneal neovascularization progresses if KCS persists undiagnosed or is inadequately treated. Corneal melanosis frequently develops in dogs, as melanocytes colonize the basal epithelial layers. Partial, then complete, blindness ensues.

Secondary bacterial conjunctivitis is present in most untreated cases of KCS. Even with specific prolonged therapy, tear-deficient animals develop recurrent bouts of bacterial conjunctivitis that require treatment. Chronic dacryocystitis frequently accompanies chronic KCS. Blepharitis due to chronic conjunctivitis or self-trauma commonly develops.

Animals with lagophthalmos or conformational exophthalmos, already on the verge of exposure keratopathy, may show clinical signs in early KCS when ocular surface dryness is still minimal.

Confirmation

Ideally, the Schirmer's tear test (STT) (CooperVision) should be part of every complete ocular examination. Most importantly, every animal presented with mucoid or mucopurulent ocular discharge must have this test performed *prior to the instillation of any diagnostic eye drops!* Large mucus strands may be removed from the eye first *without* irrigation. The STT strip tip is creased and inserted over the lower lid into the conjunctival sac and is left for 1 minute. Normal canine STT values are 20 mm wetting/minute (± 5 mm SD). Normal feline values are 17 mm wetting/minute (± 6 mm SD). As performed, the STT in animals measures the sum of basal and reflex tear secretion. In the presence of typical clinical signs, values less than 10 mm/minute are indicative of KCS. More severe clinical signs are usually evident with STT values less than or equal to 5 mm/minute. Animals with dry eyes presumably secondary to conjunctival inflammation and possible obstruction of the lacrimal ductules may exhibit STT values in the range of 5 to 15 mm/minute. The significance of low STT values in the absence of clinical signs is unknown; idiopathic corneal and conjunctival hypesthesia may be considered.

Conjunctival culture collection should be performed immediately prior to or following STT if the clinician anticipates it will be needed. Here again, bacteriostatic agents in diagnostic eye drops will negate the results if collection is performed after their instillation. Exfoliative conjunctival cytologic specimens, collected with Kimura spatula, scalpel blade butt, or cotton swab, should be obtained from all eyes with mucoid discharge. Slides stained with new methylene blue, Wright's, Giemsa, or Diff-Quik (Harleco) stains should be carefully examined for representative cell population (neutrophils, lymphocytes), intracellular bacteria (in neutrophils, epithelial cells), and fungi (very uncommon in small animals).

Fluorescein dye staining of the ocular surface should be performed to identify corneal ulceration. Examination under cobalt-blue–filtered light will reveal even minor dye retention.

The use of 0.5 per cent rose bengal dye has been promoted for the specific diagnosis of KCS. Rose bengal, a very irritating dye that stains devitalized corneal and conjunctival epithelial cells, is minimally retained by the normal ocular surface. Its retention is enhanced in many conditions in which the ocular surface is damaged (e.g., exposure keratitis, recurrent corneal erosions, KCS). Therefore, rose bengal dye retention is *not* pathognomonic for KCS! Because of the test's subjective interpretation, potential for irritation, and lack of specificity, the author does not recommend its routine use.

TREATMENT

When clinical signs and ocular examination results confirm or strongly suggest KCS, the clinician should attempt to estimate the likelihood that the condition is primary (i.e., due solely to lacrimal secretory failure) or secondary (i.e., possibly due to lacrimal ductular obstruction by conjunctival inflammation from another ocular condition). In either instance, specific KCS therapeutic objectives must dictate the treatment plan. For secondary KCS, additional therapy for the inciting ocular disorder should be considered and added when appropriate.

The objectives of KCS treatment include the following:

1. Dryness relief by
   a. Tear replacement
   b. Tear stimulation
2. Bacterial infection resolution by
   a. Antibiotic application
   b. Ocular discharge control
3. Resolution of corneal complications
4. Conjunctivitis reduction

Medical therapy of KCS should be recommended for a minimum of 1 month to assess the following:

1. Whether tear deficiency is transient or likely to be permanent
2. The feasibility of effective treatment by the owner

In truth, successful medical therapy of KCS and its

sequelae is difficult for most owners to accomplish over the long term.

For tear replacement, a regimen combining solutions and ointment is usually most practical and effective. Artificial tear solutions may contain the following:

1. Agents that increase surface tension and decrease evaporation (e.g., 0.2 to 1.0 per cent methylcellulose and derivatives, 1 to 3 per cent polyvinyl alcohol)
2. Agents that increase the solution's affinity for the corneal surface and prolong tear film break-up time (e.g., polyvinylpyrrolidone)
3. Preservatives (thimerosal, benzalkonium chloride, chlorobutanol, disodium edetate).

The solutions' major limitation is short duration of action (½ to 2 hours) (Havener, 1983). To be effective, they must be instilled as often as possible, at least four times daily. The selection of an artificial tear preparation that is effective in individual instances is, at best, a trial-and-error process. All preparations have some drawbacks; for example, the numerous commercial products containing benzalkonium chloride probably will disrupt the remaining outer oily layer of the dry eye's tear film. Hypotonic tear preparations (e.g., Hypotears, CooperVision) may be more soothing than isotonic or hypertonic products. Useful preparations for initial tear replacement therapy in dogs and cats include Adsorbotear (Alcon), Adapt (Alcon), Liquifilm Tears (Allergan), Tears Naturale (Alcon), and Hypotears (CooperVision). Alternatively, slow-release hydropropylmethylcellulose inserts (LacriSerts, Merck, Sharp & Dohme) may be used one or twice daily.

Ophthalmic ointments containing sterile petrolatum ointment with lanolin (LacriLube, Allergan; DuraTears, Alcon), or without (Ophthalmic Base Ointment, Pharmafair) should be used at bedtime and at intervals (e.g., t.i.d., q.i.d.) during which solution instillation is not possible.

Stimulation of tear production from residual functional lacrimal tissue is often possible. Oral administration of one or two drops of 2 per cent ophthalmic pilocarpine twice daily for a 25-pound dog may increase STT values to a beneficial level. Maximal effect is gained 45 to 60 minutes after administration and maintained for only a few hours or less. STT improvement with pilocarpine should be documented before prescription for long-term therapy to spare the owner and animal useless treatment. Dosage can be increased in increments of one drop twice daily until STT values increase or toxic signs are noted. If vomiting, diarrhea, ptyalism, bradycardia, or anorexia develops, the dose should be reduced, a lower concentration (0.5 to 1.0 per cent) substituted, or the medication discontinued entirely. *Oral pilocarpine administration is contraindicated in animals with compensated or medically controlled congestive heart failure, pancreatitis, or chronic diarrhea.* Pilocarpine therapy is most effective for animals with measurable, although marginal, tear secretion, and its efficacy will diminish as tear secretion by the lacrimal glands progressively fails.

For most animals, the optimal frequency of tear replacement or stimulation has been achieved when ocular discharge accumulation between treatments is consistently minimal.

Bacterial keratoconjunctivitis, whether suspected or documented by conjunctival cytologic examination or culture, should be treated with topical antibiotics for prolonged (14 to 21 days) but not indefinite periods. Chronic antibiotic therapy promotes overgrowth of resistant bacterial strains. For the recurrent episodes of bacterial keratoconjunctivitis to which animals with KCS are prone, bacterial culture and sensitivity testing are frequently more expedient and economical than indiscriminate broad-spectrum antibiotic treatment. Ocular discharge control is imperative for both the animal's comfort as well as infection treatment and prevention. In most instances, regular cleansing with eyewash prior to treatment is recommended. For extremely tenacious or voluminous discharges, instillation of 5 to 10 per cent acetylcysteine (quarter- to half-strength 20 per cent Mucomyst, Mead Johnson) several times daily for a few days will help to control the mucus component. Acetylcysteine requires refrigeration and has a shelf life after opening of only 4 days.

Most animals with chronic KCS eventually require *intermittent, judicious* treatment with topical corticosteroids to control corneal neovascularization and discourage corneal melanosis. This can be safely accomplished if the treatment intervals are *short* (b.i.d. to q.i.d. for 7 to 14 days), if therapy is begun *only* after corneal ulceration has been ruled out by *fluorescein dye application*, and if *follow-up evaluation* is conducted at the end of the treatment period.

When corneal ulceration complicates KCS, topical antibiotic therapy and 1 per cent atropine (to abolish ciliary muscle spasm and cause mydriasis) are indicated for use until epithelialization is complete. Corticosteroids are always *contraindicated* while ulceration or untreated infection is present.

If medical therapy for KCS is assessed to be unsuccessful or impractical after a minimum of 1 month's trial, surgical parotid duct transposition (PDT) may be considered for the dog or cat. Surgical results will be unsatisfactory in animals with concurrent xerostomia or lagophthalmos. PDT is not a panacea for KCS management; its sequelae include chronic facial wetness and moist dermatitis, mineral precipitation on the cornea and eyelids, idiopathic ocular irritation, and delayed corneal wound healing. Nonetheless, for selected owners and animals, PDT can be a manageable alternative to medical therapy. Superficial keratectomy, if contemplated, should be performed *prior* to PDT; if performed following PDT, permanent stromal opacification may result.

PROGNOSIS

The prognosis for KCS resolution with therapy generally seems directly related to the STT values at first diagnosis; that is, animals with consistently low (0 to 5 mm/minute) STT values seem most likely to have or develop chronic KCS and its sequelae. Some animals, especially those whose dry eye syndromes are secondary to other conjunctival disease, completely recover. Routine use of the STT in complete ocular examination will identify many of these unsuspected transient KCS cases.

Owners should be apprised early of the potential necessity for chronic therapy. With diligent treatment by the owner and regular follow-up by the veterinarian, many animals can be maintained comfortably with useful vision for many months or years. With poor or no treatment, KCS rapidly causes chronic painful blindness.

PREVENTION

Dogs that have undergone partial or complete nictitans gland (NG) removal for gland hypertrophy and prolapse ("cherry eye") (and, perhaps, cats, in which the condition is far less frequent) may be at increased risk for KCS development. Breeds of particular concern are English bulldogs and American cocker spaniels. In normal dogs, removal of either the main orbital lacrimal gland or the NG does not produce KCS. In dogs with marginally low tear secretion, compromise of either gland's function may precipitate KCS or accelerate its onset.

The alternative to NG excision for prolapse is surgical replacement of the gland. At least three surgical techniques have been described and illustrated. The prolapsed gland may be sutured to the fibrous orbital rim near the medial canthus (Kaswan and Martin, 1983), the ventromedial equatorial sclera (see Disorders of the Eyelids and Conjunctiva), or the ventral epibulbar fascia (Blogg, 1980). Long-term follow-up of dogs undergoing surgical NG replacement will be necessary to determine its efficacy and benefit.

Dogs receiving lacrimotoxic drugs should undergo periodic ocular examination and STT during treatment to identify incipient KCS while it may still be reversible.

FUNCTIONAL ANATOMY OF THE LACRIMAL SYSTEM: EXCRETION

The tear film appears invisible on the cornea and conjunctiva except for a concave outer surface, or meniscus, at the upper and lower eyelid margins. Here the outer oil layer prevents tear spillage onto the lids. Tears do not flow over the eye by gravity; rather, a thin film is spread over the cornea and conjunctiva by blinking and ocular movements. Between blinks, about 20 per cent of the aqueous tear volume evaporates, causing increased osmolarity and admixture of the outer oily and inner mucin layer. This admixture encourages tear film breakup before and during blinking as well as the subsequent resurfacing of the eye with new layers of tear film components.

During blinking, the lateral canthus closes before the medial canthus, propelling the tear film toward the nasolacrimal puncta. Tears are drawn to the medial canthus into a lacrimal lake and then into the puncta by capillary action, facilitated by a passive lacrimal pump mechanism activated by blinking. The lower punctum is normally present about 5 mm from the medial canthus, in the palpebral conjunctiva on the bulbar side of the eyelid mucocutaneous junction. The upper punctum is similarly located on the upper lid. Normal function of the lower punctum appears more critical to tear drainage. Each punctum drains into a short canaliculus, and the two canaliculi join in a rudimentary lacrimal sac encased within the lacrimal bone. The nasolacrimal duct exits the sac, passes rostrally through the lacrimal canal of the lacrimal and maxillary bones, continues deep to the nasal mucosa, and opens onto the ventrolateral floor of the nasal vestibule (Pollock, 1979). Many dogs have an accessory opening of the duct into the nasal cavity at the level of the canine tooth root.

LACRIMAL EXCRETORY DISORDERS

Clinical Signs

Epiphora, or abnormal tear flow down the face, is the most consistent clinical finding in both lacrimal hypersecretion and functional excretory obstruction. Causes of lacrimal hypersecretion are numerous and must be ruled out by complete ocular examination before epiphora assessment can proceed (Table 1).

Lacrimal drainage dysfunction may be congenital or acquired, structural or functional (Table 5).

Diagnostic Evaluation of Epiphora

Functional nasolacrimal excretory patency can be demonstrated by the primary fluorescein dye test, in which the precorneal tear film stained with fluorescein is tracked to its exit from the nasolacri-

***Table 5.** Causes of Lacrimal Excretory Dysfunction*

Congenital
Structural
Imperforate puncta
Nasolacrimal duct atresia
Functional
Punctal malposition (e.g., due to ectropion, entropion)
Conformational exophthalmos/lagophthalmos
Facial hair wick: medial entropion, aberrant medial canthal dermis, trichiasis
Conformational lacrimal lake impairment
Acquired
Structural
Punctal stenosis: postinflammatory, postneoplastic
Nasolacrimal duct obstruction
Dacryocystitis
Foreign body
Nasal mass: inflammatory, neoplastic
Punctal malposition: posttraumatic, cicatricial
Functional
Facial nerve palsy
Buphthalmos
Pathologic exophthalmos: orbital neoplasia or inflammation

mal duct in the anterior nasal vestibule. If dye appears at the external nares in 5 to 7 minutes (a positive test), the excretory system's functional patency is confirmed. In this instance, orthograde nasolacrimal flushing with saline or eyewash is superfluous. If dye is absent from the external nares (a negative test), three conditions must be ruled out: (1) functional drainage abnormality (e.g., lagophthalmos, punctal malposition, facial nerve palsy), (2) physical obstruction, and (3) anomalous nasolacrimal duct opening into the posterior nasal or oral cavities (occasionally noted in brachycephalic dogs and cats). Following a negative primary fluorescein dye test, nasolacrimal flushing through one punctum is necessary to rule out and sometimes to relieve nasolacrimal duct obstruction. If irrigation does not demonstrate or establish patency, duct cannulation with 0 to 2–0 monofilament nylon or prolene may be attempted to relieve or bypass an obstruction. If successful, cannulation can be maintained for 7 to 14 days by suturing the thread to the facial skin proximally near the medial canthus and distally near the external nares. If the system is freely patent on irrigation, functional drainage abnormality and anomalous nasolacrimal duct exit must be ruled out by inspection.

DACRYOCYSTITIS

Dacryocystitis, inflammation of the lacrimal sac that usually extends to the canaliculi and nasolacrimal duct, may be primary or secondary, infectious or sterile. Primary dacryocystitis may be promoted by a foreign body (most commonly, a weed seed) or lacrimal sac injury. Secondary dacryocystitis may accompany chronic KCS or primary bacterial conjunctivitis, or it may ensue following acquired nasolacrimal duct obstruction. Most dacryocystitis, whether primary or secondary, probably involves bacterial infection during at least part of its course.

The clinical signs of primary dacryocystitis may be either dramatically evident or subtle and nonspecific. Subcutaneous medial canthal swelling may be visible; the animal may show discomfort as the swelling is massaged, and exudate may be expressed through the puncta into the conjunctival sac. More commonly, persistent mucopurulent discharge is centered at the medial canthus and conjunctivitis is absent.

The clinical signs of secondary dacryocystitis are often overshadowed by those of the inciting conjunctivitis or nasolacrimal duct obstruction. In both primary and secondary dacryocystitis, epiphora is often attendant to the nasolacrimal obstruction caused by lacrimal sac inflammation.

Initial diagnostic evaluation of suspected dacryocystitis should include exfoliative cytologic examination, Gram stain, and bacterial culture collection (if indicated) of expressed exudate prior to instillation of any diagnostic eye drops. Thorough nasolacrimal irrigation with saline or eyewash solution should then be performed to (1) remove exudate, (2) flush out a foreign body, if present, and (3) relieve primary or secondary nasolacrimal duct obstruction. For persistent and recurrent dacryocystitis, dacryocystorhinography using 50 to 90 per cent sodium diatrizoate (Hypaque, Winthrop) or 40 per cent iodized poppy seed oil (40 per cent Lipiodol, Fongera) is indicated in an attempt to identify a foreign body or characterize nasolacrimal duct obstruction.

The objectives of dacryocystitis therapy include (1) relief of obstruction; (2) foreign body removal, if present; (3) elimination of infection; and (4) reduction of inflammation. Topical aqueous antibiotic therapy, specified by culture and sensitivity results when available, should be administered frequently for 14 to 21 days. Periodic nasaolacrimal irrigation with saline, eyewash, or an antibiotic-fortified solution of either during this treatment interval is useful to maintain patency. Topical aqueous corticosteroids may be added judiciously, if deemed necessary, after the apparent or proven infection appears controlled. Indwelling catheterization of the nasolacrimal duct with 0 to 2–0 monofilament suture or polyethylene tubing can be maintained during treatment if obstruction recurs.

LACRIMAL EXCRETORY DYSFUNCTION: SURGICAL THERAPY

In many instances, correction of tear excretory dysfunction is optional. Indications for surgical therapy include recurrent moist facial dermatitis and an owner's insistence on cosmetic correction. Specific surgical therapy must be tailored to the individual patient after thorough ocular and adnexal examination confirms the correctable cause. In actual practice, animals presented for evaluation of epiphora often have several conformational abnormalities that must be identified and assessed.

Congenitally imperforate puncta and acquired cicatricial punctal stenosis can often be corrected by careful incision with a No. 11 Bard-Parker scalpel blade over the punctum after topical anesthesia. This minor surgery should be immediately preceded by nasolacrimal irrigation to tent the overlying conjunctiva and to determine patency of the nasolacrimal duct. To discourage closure during healing, topical antibiotic-corticosteroid drops or ointments should be used for 7 to 14 days.

Correction of congenitally imperforate nasolacrimal ducts and acquired duct obstruction that cannot be relieved by vigorous irrigation or suture cannulation may require rather extensive surgery. This is rarely indicated because of the relatively minor sequelae of untreated epiphora. Conjunctivorhinostomy, the establishment of a fistula between the lacrimal lake at the medial canthus and the upper nasal passages through the lacrimal bone, has been successfully performed on selected animals. Conjunctivorhinostomy has also been reported in the dog (Gelatt and Gwin, 1981). In both procedures, a silicone or polyethylene cannula must be sutured in place and left for several weeks to encourage permanent fistulization.

Punctal malposition due to conformational exophthalmos, entropion, ectropion, or eyelid scarring is frequently difficult to correct well enough for perfect physiologic function. Anatomically perfect surgical correction of eyelid conformation abnormalities may be partially effective, however, in this regard.

Epiphora associated with an inadequate lacrimal lake at the medial canthus occurs frequently in dogs with tight eyelid conformation or exophthalmos. Excision of the NG to encourage pooling of tears near the puncta or to reduce tear volume should be condemned, since KCS may develop as a long-term sequela.

Epiphora secondary to facial hair wicking is associated with medial or lateral entropion, trichiasis, or aberrant medial canthal dermis. Specific surgical correction of the entropion, trimming of excessively long facial hair, or excision of aberrant medial canthal skin may improve the clinical signs of tearing.

Animals with epiphora due to conformational exophthalmos, lagophthalmos, or facial nerve palsy may benefit from permanent partial lateral canthorrhaphy to shorten the palpebral fissure and to improve their blinking effectiveness.

FACIAL TEAR STAINING: MEDICAL THERAPY

Oral tetracycline has been used with variable success in an intermittent or continuous regimen to control staining of facial hair due to epiphora. Administered at 5 to 10 mg/kg/day (Gelatt and Gwin, 1981) or 50 mg/dog/day (Kaswan and Martin, 1983), tetracycline does not decrease tear flow but may bind to or alter chromatic compounds that stain light-colored hair. Lacrimotoxic drugs should *not* be administered to resolve epiphora. Their effects are unpredictable and potentially irreversible.

LACRIMAL SYSTEM NEOPLASIA

Neoplasms of the lacrimal and nictitans glands, although rare, do occur in dogs and cats. Adenomas and adenocarcinomas have been reported. Clinical signs referable to an orbital disorder are usually evident before KCS sequelae are notable. Surgical excision is the usual treatment, and the prognosis is guarded.

The lacrimal excretory system may be secondarily obstructed by maxillary sinus or nasal cavity neoplasms. Epithelial and connective tissue tumors predominate. Prognosis even with radical surgery is poor.

References and Supplemental Reading

Blogg, J. R.: Diseases of the eyelids. *In* Blogg, J. R. (ed.): *The Eye in Veterinary Practice—Extraocular Disease*, 1st ed. Philadelphia: W. B. Saunders, 1980, pp. 341–344.

Gelatt, K. N., and Gwin, R. M.: Canine lacrimal and nasolacrimal systems. *Veterinary Ophthalmology*. Gelatt, K. N. (ed.). Philadelphia: Lea & Febiger, 1981, pp. 309–329.

Havener, W. H.: Wetting agents. *Ocular Pharmacology*, 5th ed. St. Louis: C. V. Mosby, 1983.

Kaswan, R. L., and Martin, C. L.: Diseases of the lacrimal apparatus. *In* Kirk, R. W. (ed.): *Current Veterinary Therapy VIII*. Philadelphia: W. B. Saunders, 1983, pp. 549–554.

Kaswan, R. L., Martin, C. L., and Chapman, W. L.: Keratoconjunctivitis sicca: Histopathologic study of the nictitating membrane and lacrimal glands from 28 canine cases. Am. J. Vet. Res. 45:112, 1984.

Morgan, R. W., and Bachrach, A.: Keratoconjunctivitis sicca associated with sulfonamide therapy in dogs. J.A.V.M.A. 180:432, 1982.

Pollock, R. V. H.: The eye. *In* Evans, H. E., and Christensen, G. C. (ed.): *Miller's Anatomy of the Dog*, 2nd ed. Philadelphia: W. B. Saunders, 1979, pp. 1073–1127.

DISEASES OF THE CORNEA

DARIEN L. NELSON, D.V.M.,
Garden Grove, California

and ALAN D. MACMILLAN, D.V.M.
San Diego, California

CORNEAL ANATOMY AND PHYSIOLOGY

The proper diagnosis and treatment of corneal disease are dependent on a basic understanding of the anatomy and physiology of the cornea.

The cornea is the clear anterior portion of the eyeball. The functions of the cornea are to (1) provide a fibrous tunic to maintain the shape of the globe and protect the intraocular structures, (2) provide a powerful refracting surface, and (3) maintain transparency to allow the passage of light through its medium.

From anterior to posterior, the cornea is composed of four distinctive layers: the epithelium with its underlying basement membrane, the substantia propria (or stroma), Descemet's membrane, and the endothelium.

The corneal epithelium consists of approximately five to seven layers composed of outer squamous epithelium, wing cells, basal cells, and a thick underlying basement membrane.

The substantia propria present beneath the epithelium represents about 90 per cent of the corneal thickness. The stroma is composed of lamellae (parallel bundles of collagen fibers), fibroblasts (keratocytes), and ground substance.

Descemet's membrane, or the posterior limiting membrane, lies between the stroma and the endothelium. This membrane is an exaggerated basal lamina produced throughout life by the endothelium.

The corneal endothelium is the innermost layer and consists of a single layer of cells.

The cornea is a relatively thin structure. In dogs and cats, the central cornea varies in thickness from approximately 0.6 to 1.0 mm. The peripheral cornea is thinner (about 0.4 to 0.6 mm).

The transparency of the cornea is necessary for normal vision. This transparency is due to the cornea's state of relative dehydration, avascularity, lack of pigmentation, and the normal arrangement of stromal collagen fibrils. Corneal dehydration is dependent on the integrity of the epithelium and endothelium, which provide a physical barrier against the influx of tears and aqueous humor. The corneal endothelial cell-pumping mechanism, which results in the removal of excessive interstitial water, is also an important factor in maintaining corneal dehydration.

In order for the cornea to remain healthy, the eyelids, the tear film, aqueous humor, and intraocular pressure must be normal. Oxygen and necessary nutritive requirements are provided to the avascular cornea by the limbal vessels, the tear film, and the aqueous humor.

SIGNS OF CORNEAL DISEASE

Signs of ocular pain and irritation such as blepharospasm, epiphora, enophthalmos, prolapse of the nictitans, eye rubbing, and conjunctival hyperemia may or may not occur, depending on the type of corneal disease present.

The cornea is a highly sensitive structure. Pain is most likely to occur with loss of epithelium. Ocular pain due to corneal disease is usually relieved following application of topical anesthesia. Pain due to anterior uveitis or glaucoma is not relieved by topical anesthesia, and this procedure may therefore be helpful in diagnosing corneal disease.

A change in corneal transparency may be due to neovascularization, edema, cellular infiltration, pigmentation, calcium or lipid deposition, or loss of the normal arrangement of collagen fibrils.

Corneal neovascularization may involve large branching vessels that occur in the superficial corneal stroma and are most often associated with primary corneal disease. Smaller straight vessels that are located within the deeper stroma usually indicate intraocular disease such as anterior uveitis.

Corneal edema is a nonspecific pathologic state that may be due to primary corneal disease or may be secondary to intraocular disease such as glaucoma, uveitis, or anterior lens luxation. Corneal edema results from either loss of epithelial integrity or endothelial disease. Chronic or severe edema may result in bullous keratopathy, in which fluid accumulates in vesicles or bullae between the layers of epithelium. Corneal ulceration may occur following rupture of these vesicles.

Superficial corneal pigmentation may occur as a congenital defect or may occur spontaneously but usually develops following chronic keratitis. Deep corneal pigmentation is usually due to uveal adhesions (e.g., persistent pupillary membranes, anterior synechiae) but may occur without any known cause.

CONGENITAL ABNORMALITIES

Microcornea (abnormally small cornea) is most often associated with microphthalmia and is most common in certain breeds (Australian shepherds, collies, miniature schnauzers). It is usually associated with other congenital ocular malformations. Macrocornea (enlarged cornea) is rare; however, it may be associated with buphthalmia due to congenital glaucoma.

Persistent pupillary membranes (PPMs) consist of persisting embryonic tissues that arise from the anterior surface of the iris. The pupillary membrane is a sheet of mesoderm carrying anastomosing blood vessels during embryologic development. Atrophy of this membrane begins during fetal life and should be complete by 4 to 8 weeks of age in the dog and cat. Corneal opacification occurs as a result of an adhesion from the persistent membrane to the endothelium. Descemet's membrane may also be abnormal. The severity of opacification depends on the extent and number of adhesions. Medical treatment will not resolve the opacification but may be indicated if the cornea is secondarily inflamed. PPMs occur more commonly in certain breeds of dogs, including the basenji, chow chow, Doberman pinscher, and golden retriever. Dogs of other breeds, mixed-breed dogs, and cats are occasionally affected.

Dermoids are skinlike masses usually containing hair; they occur on the eyelids, conjunctiva, or cornea. If the anomaly is present on the cornea, it usually is associated with varying amounts of blepharospasm and mucopurulent discharge. A superficial keratectomy is required to remove the abnormal tissue. Topical antibiotics are recommended immediately postoperatively, but topical corticosteroids may be used after re-epithelialization.

KERATITIS

Superficial Ulcerative Keratitis

Superficial ulcerative keratitis may be caused by trauma, foreign bodies, eyelid abnormalities (e.g., entropion, distichiasis, ectopic cilia), infectious diseases, tear film abnormalities, or exposure due to lagophthalmos.

Clinical signs include blepharospasm, mucoid ocular discharge, epiphora, conjunctival hyperemia, enophthalmos with prolapse of the nictitans, and rubbing at the eye. Corneal edema and neovascularization may also be present.

The cause of the ulcer should be determined, if possible. The lid surfaces, nictitating membrane, and the globe should be examined with a good light source and magnification for abnormalities or foreign bodies. A Schirmer's tear test should be performed if poor tear production is suspected.

Bacterial cultures and sensitivity tests are usually not indicated, since primary bacterial or fungal involvement as a cause of superficial ulceration is rare. A wide-spectrum antibiotic such as chloramphenicol or a combination of neomycin-bacitracin and polymixin B is usually adequate in preventing secondary bacterial infection.

Fluorescein staining is a useful diagnostic procedure. Fluorescein dye in solution will not penetrate an intact epithelial layer; however, it will be absorbed by the hydrophilic stromal layer and the inter-epithelial cell cement substance. Therefore, a positive dye test indicates partial or full-thickness loss of the epithelial layer. Descemet's membrane also does not stain, and this should be considered when a deep corneal ulcer is evaluated.

Proper instillation of the dye is important to avoid false-positive or false-negative results. The edge of the dye strip should be touched to the palpebral or bulbar conjunctiva. If a normal tear volume is present, the dye will be distributed across the corneal surface by the tear film after blinking. If the tear volume is low, instillation of artificial tears may be necessary. A Schirmer's tear test should be performed before artificial tears are instilled. False-positive test results may occur if the fluorescein strip is touched directly to the cornea. Topical anesthetics can be toxic to the epithelium, and can also cause false-positive results.

Re-epithelialization of an uncomplicated superficial corneal ulcer should be complete within 3 to 4 days. Should this not occur, a complication is present. The complication should be identified and resolved. Simply altering the antibiotic treatment is not recommended, since primary infection rarely is a complicating factor. A tendency to rub the affected eye is usually present, since pain is often associated with this type of ulceration. Rubbing can prevent healing. The use of a properly fitting Elizabethan or Buster Brown collar will eliminate this complication. Lid position should be evaluated. Primary entropion as the initiating cause can be differentiated from secondary spastic entropion due to pain through the use of topical anesthetics. Spastic entropion will be relieved by topical anesthesia; primary anatomic entropion will persist.

Ectopic cilia that penetrate through the palpebral conjunctival surface of either the upper or lower eyelid are a common cause of refractory ulcerations but may be difficult to find. The eyelids are everted, and a bright light source and high magnification are used to see the cilia. Surgical excision of the cilia and related follicles is then indicated.

Chronic superficial ulcers due to the presence of abnormal epithelium surrounding the ulcer have been previously described as boxer, dendritic, indolent, and refractory ulcers or erosions. A buildup of necrotic abnormal epithelium surrounding the ulcer prevents healing by interfering with epithelial mitosis and migration. The pathogenesis leading to development of the abnormal epithelial tissue is not well understood. Causative factors probably involve mechanical trauma, entrapped debris under the epithelial edges, degeneration or lack of a basement membrane, and primary epithelial dystrophy. Reepithelialization cannot occur unless the abnormal epithelium is removed either by superficial keratectomy or chemical cautery (e.g., 2 per cent tincture of iodine). In many cases, this can be done in the examination room and under topical anesthesia. Physical débridement can be done with a cotton swab or fine forceps. A chemical cauterant can then be applied to the affected area with a cotton swab. General anesthesia and a more extensive keratectomy may be necessary in other cases. A nictitating membrane flap may also be used as a protective bandage. Rubbing the eye should be prevented by utilization of a restraint collar. A topical broad-spectrum antibiotic should be instilled four to six times daily to prevent secondary infection. A topical cycloplegic-mydriatic (e.g., 1 per cent atropine) instilled three times daily may help relieve pain. Subepithelial edema may be reduced with the addition of a hyperosmotic ophthalmic solution or ointment (e.g., sodium chloride 2 or 5 per cent, Muro 128, Muro). Corticosteroids are contraindicated because they retard epithelial replication, an effect that may prevent or delay healing.

Deep Corneal Ulcers

Ulceration with extension into the corneal stroma can result in corneal perforation and loss of vision. Proper management of a deep corneal ulcer is dependent on the identification and resolution of any complicating factors.

Primary bacterial infection may be more likely in a deep rather than superficial corneal ulceration. Some of the more common organisms involved include *Staphylococcus, Streptococcus, Proteus, Escherichia coli,* and *Pseudomonas.*

Collagenase-associated ulcers have a "melting" or "mushy" appearance. Corneal epithelial cells, fibroblasts, and leukocytes as well as some bacteria (especially *Pseudomonas*) can produce a collagenase that causes rapid corneal breakdown and can lead to perforation. Vigorous therapy with proper antibiotics and an anticollagenase agent are recommended. Cultures and sensitivity should be taken, followed by immediate instillation of a broad-spectrum antibiotic (e.g., gentamicin, chloramphenicol, or tobramycin) every hour until culture results are available.* An anticollagenase agent such as 10 or 20 per cent acetylcysteine (Mucomyst, Mead Johnson) is commercially available. Concentrations between 5 and 10 per cent of this drug are recommended in order to ensure comfort and efficacy. The commercially available 20 per cent solution can be mixed with a selected antibiotic solution at a ratio of 1:1. Acetylcysteine solutions must be kept refrigerated. The patient should be treated with this mixture every hour until there is evidence of response. The dosage may then be reduced to every 3 to 4 hours. Topical 1 per cent atropine should be given three times daily, particularly if there is severe pain, often due to concurrent anterior uveitis. Systemic antibiotics as well as systemic corticosteroids may be occasionally recommended in the face of associated anterior uveitis. A restraint collar should be applied. A bulbar conjunctival flap is placed if there is inadequate response to medication or danger of perforation.

Deep stromal ulcers and descemetocoeles are common in the brachycephalic and exophthalmic breeds. The cause of this type of ulcer is usually unknown; however, it is thought to be related to trauma or exposure. The ulcers are usually oval to round and have steep margins. The surrounding cornea is often uninvolved, and there is typically no associated neovascularization. If a descemetocoele is present, the base of the ulcer will appear clear and glassy and will not retain fluorescein dye, although the walls of the corneal pit do stain. A descemetocoele should be considered an ophthalmic emergency, since rupture can easily occur.

Most of these ulcers are nonhealing and require surgical intervention. A nictitating membrane flap alone is generally not beneficial. Either a partial bulbar conjunctival flap pulled across the affected area and sutured directly to the cornea or a complete 360-degree conjunctival flap will help to promote healing by directly adhering to and filling in the ulcerative defect and by providing a direct source of blood supply to the area.

Another method of surgical therapy, which we prefer, is a free conjunctival graft. A plug of conjunctival tissue is harvested from the palpebral conjunctiva of the lower eyelid. This graft is then

**Editor's Note:* Subconjunctival antibiotics (e.g., 5 mg gentamicin) may also be given once daily until corneal collagenolysis stops.

placed into the defect and the margins sutured directly to the surrounding cornea. Most grafts remain viable and grow into the defect. Postoperatively, the animals are treated with topical antibiotics and a topical mydriatic-cycloplegic four to six times daily. They are sent home wearing a restraint collar. Topical treatment is usually altered in about 4 to 6 weeks to include topical corticosteroids to reduce the associated inflammation.

Corneal Perforations

Corneal perforation can occur as a direct result of trauma or subsequent to rupture of a deep corneal ulceration.

Rupture of the cornea will result in loss of aqueous and collapse of the globe. The iris may or may not prolapse depending on the extent of the corneal defect. Damage to the lens and retinal detachment can also occur.

These events lead to iridal inflammation with leakage of fibrin and cells from the iridal vessels into the anterior chamber. If the corneal defect is small, it may become plugged with fibrin and the anterior chamber may re-form. However, aqueous leakage will probably continue. The iris itself may plug the corneal defect, forming an anterior synechia. The amount of iris protruding through the defect is variable.

Surgical correction is indicated in all of these cases. The prolapsed portion of iris should be excised if it is necrotic or cannot be easily reintroduced into the anterior chamber. Necrotic corneal tissue should also be conservatively excised. Anterior synechiae can be broken down by gentle pressure with a cyclodialysis spatula. The anterior chamber should be flushed with a balanced salt solution. The corneal defect should be closed directly if possible. If the defect is too large, a bulbar conjunctival flap, a conjunctival graft, or a corneal scleral transposition can be performed. The anterior chamber is then re-formed with air or a balanced salt solution. A nictitating membrane flap may also be sutured in place for additional protection. Postoperative treatment should include a restraint collar; topical antibiotics and a mydriatic-cycloplegic four to six times daily; and systemic antibiotics, all administered for 2 to 4 weeks.

Mycotic Ulcerations

Fungal ulcers are rare in dogs and cats. Fungal contamination should be considered in trauma-induced ulceration that is not responsive to antibiotic therapy, in the immune-deficient patient, or following long-term use of topical corticosteroids.

Although many species of fungi can infect the cornea, *Aspergillus* and *Candida* are the most common in dogs and cats. Diagnosis is tentatively based on microscopic observations of fungal elements following corneal scrapings and confirmed by fungal culture.

Treatment of keratomycosis may be complicated because of the limited availability of antifungal medications. Nonophthalmic drugs such as nystatin (Mycostatin, Squibb) and amphotericin B (Fungizone, Squibb) have had limited use. Since they are nonophthalmic drugs, they can be irritating. A new ophthalmic preparation, natamycin (Natacyn, Alcon), is now commercially available. It has a wide spectrum but is relatively expensive.

Feline Herpetic Keratitis

Herpesvirus can affect both the conjunctiva and cornea in cats. It is most common in young kittens and is often associated with active rhinotracheitis. Respiratory infection may be severe and complicated by oral ulceration. Unilateral or bilateral keratoconjunctivitis without systemic disease caused by herpesvirus can also occur in older cats.

Cats with herpes keratitis commonly are presented with a seromucoid discharge, conjunctival hyperemia, chemosis, superficial corneal neovascularization, and corneal ulcerations. The viral ulcerations may have a typical pattern and have been described as punctate, dendritic, or geographic. The ulcers are generally superficial, involving only the epithelium and outer stroma. Multiple punctate areas may stain with fluorescein dye, or there may be a branching or dendritic pattern, or large, irregular ulcers may be visible.

Clinical diagnosis is generally made on the typical appearance of the ulceration. A few commercial diagnostic laboratories are able to perform indirect fluorescent antibody tests on conjunctival or corneal scrapings; however, these tests are not readily available.

Antiviral medications include idoxuridine (Herplex, Allergan; Stoxil, Smith, Kline & French), cytosine or adenosine arabinoside (Vira-A, Parke-Davis), and trifluridine (Viroptic, Burroughs-Wellcome). Frequent topical application (every few hours) is generally recommended.

Nonulcerative Keratitis

Corneal inflammation can occur as a result of direct external irritation or secondary to other ocular disorders. Initiating causes to consider include lid abnormalities, low tear production, corneal ulcers, primary infections, anterior uveitis, and glaucoma. Resolution of secondary keratitis is dependent on identification and proper treatment of the primary ocular disease.

Primary corneal inflammation is a specific disease entity unrelated to other ocular diseases. The most common form of primary superficial keratitis known to occur in dogs has been termed degenerative pannus. It occurs most frequently in the German shepherd; however, it can occur in greyhounds, mixed breeds, and others.

Although the cause is unknown, the chronicity may be due to a cellular hypersensitivity against some certain protein. A familial predisposition is also a consideration. The age of onset in the German shepherd is usually between 3 and 5 years. The initial clinical signs involve a superficial subepithelial fibrovascular ingrowth into the cornea from the inferior temporal perilimbal quadrant. This is a bilateral disorder, and clinical signs are usually similar in both eyes. The nictitating membrane may also be affected, appearing red, thickened, and inflamed. Multiple central corneal punctate subepithelial opacities may develop in eyes with pannus. If left untreated, the vascular ingrowth progresses across the cornea followed by melanin depositions. Untreated dogs can suffer severe loss of vision.

The condition will be chronic, and the owner should be made aware that treatment is limited to controlling the disease and is not curative. Corticosteroids are considered the treatment of choice. Frequent topical application of a potent corticosteroid (e.g., 1 per cent prednisolone acetate or 0.1 per cent dexamethasone) is usually all that is required to bring the condition under control. Initially we recommend treatment six times daily. If the neovascularization has receded at the time of re-examination a few weeks later, the frequency of application is reduced to three times daily for another 3 to 4 weeks. Once the vascular ingrowth has completely receded, a maintenance dosage is established. Each dog will differ; however, most can be maintained on as infrequent a treatment schedule as once daily or once every other day. If the disease is recognized early and the owners are diligent with treatment, the prognosis for vision is good. Should a case be presented with extensive corneal pigmentation and vision loss, a superficial keratectomy is recommended to restore vision. Once the active inflammation is controlled medically, the keratectomy is performed. We generally make a nicitating membrane flap for protection. The dog is sent home with a restraint collar and topical antibiotics and a mydriatic-cycloplegic to be applied four to six times daily. The animal is re-evaluated in 1 week. The flap is removed and the cornea examined for fluorescein dye retention. Usually a week is sufficient time for complete re-epithelialization, and fluorescein dye stain is negative. Topical corticosteroid therapy is then resumed to reduce the inflammation and avoid repigmentation.

Pigmentary Keratitis

Pigmentary keratitis occurs frequently in pugs and other exophthalmic breeds. The corneal pigmentation typically involves the medial aspect of the cornea and is usually caused by irritation from a medial canthal entropion as well as from the nasal folds. A surgical medial canthal closure resolves the entropion, prevents the nasal fold from contacting the cornea, and narrows the palpebral fissure. Blepharoplasty helps protect the globe from injury by reducing lagophthalmos and exposure keratitis.

Interstitial Keratitis

Interstitial keratitis involves inflammation of the deeper corneal layers. Severe corneal edema and deep limbal vascularization are usually present. This type of inflammation is most frequently associated with intraocular inflammation. Efforts should be made to define the cause of the keratitis as well as to identify and properly treat any intraocular disease (anterior uveitis, glaucoma, anterior lens luxation).

Keratoconjunctivitis Sicca–Associated Keratitis

Corneal disease related to low tear production can involve corneal neovascularization, edema, pigmentation, and ulceration, depending on the severity and chronicity. However, it should be emphasized that all patients presented with excessive mucoid discharge and conjunctival and corneal inflammation should be evaluated with a Schirmer's tear test for adequate tear production. (Keratoconjunctivitis sicca is discussed in depth in the article entitled Disorders of the Lacrimal System.)

Feline Proliferative Keratitis (Eosinophilic Keratitis)

A unilateral or bilateral proliferative granulomatous keratitis can occur in cats. This disease is characterized by superficial neovascularization and infiltration of inflammatory cells into the cornea, usually beginning at the temporal limbus. In severe cases, the cornea may be thickened and raised, with white plaque-like formations. Fluorescein dye may be retained if the epithelial layer is disrupted. The cause of this inflammatory disease is unknown. Histologically, the influx of inflammatory cells can include eosinophils, plasma cells, histiocytes, lymphocytes, and giant cells. The cases that reveal a large number of eosinophils may be related to the eosinophilic granuloma complex known to occur in cats.

Treatment with topical or systemic corticosteroids

will help control the disease. Alternatively, megestrol acetate (Schering) will usually cause regression of the inflammatory lesions within 2 to 3 weeks. A dosage of 0.5 mg/kg daily until a response is noted and then a maintainance dose of 1.25 mg two to three times weekly may be required to prevent recurrence.

FELINE CORNEAL SEQUESTRUM

This corneal disorder is seen only in cats. It is primarily a disease of Persian, Siamese, and related breeds, although other types of cats may occasionally be affected. It is usually unilateral but occasionally affects both eyes. The cause is unknown, and the sequestrum has been observed to form in at least two apparently different circumstances.

The first involves nontraumatized corneas. Close examination with a biomicroscope initially reveals a light brown discoloration within the superficial stroma. At this stage, there are no visible associated signs of corneal inflammation. The sequestrum then increases in area and becomes darker so that it is visible to the unaided eye. It may eventually extend into the deeper stroma, and it usually extends to involve the epithelium, when it appears as a superficial brown or black plaque at the corneal surface. Even at this stage, there is often no associated visible corneal inflammatory response unless the epithelium is disrupted.

The second apparent route of sequestrum formation occurs within corneas with obvious inflammation. In these instances, the cornea is chronically inflamed (e.g., corneal ulcer due to entropion irritating the cornea) and the sequestrum forms within the site of the corneal disorder. A marked inflammatory keratitis with vascular ingrowth and corneal edema is usually associated with this type of sequestrum.

It is our opinion, based on watching several innocuous-appearing sequestra present some months later as markedly inflamed corneas, that almost all corneas with sequestra will benefit from early surgical removal by lamellar keratectomy. Even in the early cases showing little discomfort or tearing, surgery will result in clearer, healthier corneas than those that do not have surgery or have it later. To wait and watch only permits the sequestrum to extend to deeper stroma and eventually become a large plaque. In all cats, except those with high anesthetic risk, it is preferable to operate rather than hope the plaque will spontaneously slough and result in a clear, noninflamed cornea.

A lamellar keratectomy to remove a sequestrum should employ proper ophthalmic surgical instrumentation and magnification. Simply scraping the cornea is not a proper technique. As stated above, early surgery before the sequestrum involves the deeper stroma should result in complete excision. Following the keratectomy, we suture in place a nictitating membrane flap, and the eye is treated with topical antibiotics and a mydriatic-cycloplegic four to six times daily for 10 to 14 days. At that time, the nictitating membrane flap is lowered, and if epithelialization is complete, topical corticosteroids are used to treat any residual keratitis. Often there is no obvious keratitis and thus no need for further therapy.

Owners should be advised that sequestra may recur, sometimes many years later and sometimes in the other eye.

Proliferative Keratoconjunctivitis (Fibrous Histiocytoma)

An inflammatory disease known to occur most frequently in the collie has been termed proliferative keratoconjunctivitis, fibrous histiocytoma, nodular episcleritis, or nodular fasciitis. The disorder is characterized by the presence of bilateral pink, fleshy, raised, corneal masses that begin at the temporal limbus and may progress across the central cornea. The nictitating membrane may also be thickened with nodular lesions. Chronic cases can result in opacification of the cornea. The cause is unknown, although there appears to be a familial basis. (This condition is discussed further in the article entitled Tumors of the Eye and Adnexa.)

CORNEAL DYSTROPHY

Corneal dystrophies, which occur most often in dogs and are only rarely observed in cats, are usually bilateral within the central cornea and are symmetric in both eyes, although one eye may be more extensively involved than the other. They are usually slowly progressive, and the corneal opacity may become quite obvious over a period of many years. Fortunately, corneal dystrophies rarely cause blindness. Corneal dystrophies are not known to be associated with any systemic disease. The appearance of each corneal dystrophy varies with the area of the cornea that is primarily involved; however, the appearance of a dystrophy is usually quite characteristic for each affected breed. Corneal dystrophies should be considered inherited, although to date, none of the described corneal dystrophies in dogs and cats have a clearly defined mode of inheritance. Affected animals should not be bred.

Typical examples of canine dystrophies are described below, based on the primary area of corneal involvement.

Epithelial Layer Dystrophies

The types of corneal dystrophies in Shetland sheepdogs and boxers (and occasionally others), although affecting initially the epithelium and sharing certain other features, are by no means identical. Treatments, however, are similar. When ulceration is present, use of topical antibiotics and protection of the cornea are indicated. When the ulcerations have healed and there is residual keratitis, topical corticosteroids are indicated. The periods of quiescence when the cornea is smooth and uninflamed are periods of no treatment.

Signs of corneal epithelial dystrophy vary depending on the stage of the disease. In general, affected corneas exhibit a focal deterioration of the epithelial layers in one or multiple areas, resulting in erosion and ulceration. Epithelial healing is usually slower than normal and often will take many weeks. Affected corneas usually exhibit an associated inflammatory response of edema and corneal vascularization in varying degrees, depending primarily on the chronicity of the episode. Ulceration recurs following varying periods during which the cornea is apparently normal.

Therapy varies with the stage of the disease. The diseased margins of the ulcerations should be débrided (using a cotton swab or if necessary a lamellar keratectomy with a chemical cauterant) to hasten healing. The patient should be made comfortable by using soft contact bandage lenses or third eyelid flaps with topical antibiotic drops and atropine for its cycloplegic effect. A restraint collar is recommended.

Stromal Layer Dystrophies

The Siberian husky and Samoyed breeds exhibit a dystrophy that affects the corneal stroma. The usual age of onset of subtle clinical signs is between 6 and 24 months. The corneal opacities slowly increase in size and area and are usually obvious by 2 to 4 years of age. This dystrophy seldom causes visual impairment, but a few cases of older dogs (over 9 years) with opaque central corneas and blindness have been reported. Clinically affected dogs exhibit a corneal opacity that is shaped like a football or doughnut within the central cornea. At magnifications provided by a slit-lamp biomicroscope, the opacities are seen as crystalline deposits within the deep corneal stroma or an indistinct "haze," which can be located at any level of the stroma. Histochemically, the opacities contain neutral fats, phospholipids, and cholesterol. Electron microscopy reveals the crystals to be similar to cholesterol. Serum lipid levels have been normal in several affected dogs.

Of perhaps most importance to clinicians, stromal corneal dystrophies in any breed are usually unassociated with ocular inflammation; thus, there is no treatment. If secondary corneal inflammation is observed, then appropriate topical medication is indicated.

Endothelial Layer Dystrophy

In our referral practice, the most frequently encountered breed with this corneal dystrophy is the Boston terrier. Chihuahuas are also often affected. We examine several new cases yearly, almost all referred for glaucoma. This dystrophy is also observed infrequently in other breeds of dogs (including mixed breeds) and rarely in cats.

Although the initiating factors of this dystrophy are unclear, it is known that endothelial cell dysfunction and cell loss allow the aqueous to enter the stroma, causing lamellar separation and stromal thickening. The stromal edema may subsequently cause formation of epithelial bullae (fluid-filled clefts), which may in turn cause ulceration.

In our practice, affected dogs are usually presented at 6 to 8 years of age with corneal clouding that, if bilateral, is usually asymmetric. At this time there are usually no signs of inflammation or discomfort. As the dystrophy progresses (most do progress slowly), a larger area of the cornea will become cloudy and there may be signs of discomfort and inflammation—all probably due to bulla formation with subsequent ulceration. It is the combination of corneal edema with ocular inflammation and discomfort that makes this disorder clinically appear similar to glaucoma.

Medical therapy of the disorder is generally unrewarding. Hypertonic sodium chloride solutions or ointments (Adsorbonac, Alcon; Muro 128, Muro) may be useful in controlling the epithelial edema and bulla formation. This may require long-term, frequent medication to be effective. When corneal ulcerations are present, topical antibiotics should be used to help prevent secondary infection. Topical corticosteroids are of doubtful value in treating the dystrophy; however, they may be used to control the secondary ocular inflammation.

Surgical therapy to correct the primary problem consists of full-thickness corneal transplants, which are both infrequently performed and infrequently successful. Corneal ulcerations that do not respond to medical therapy require appropriate surgical measures (discussed earlier under Keratitis).

CORNEAL DEGENERATIONS

Corneal degenerations usually involve opacification due to lipid or calcium deposition. Unlike a dystrophy, the degenerative change is nonfamilial and may be associated with inflammatory reactions and secondary ulceration. The condition may be a primary degeneration or associated with other ocular abnormalities or systemic disease. Primary corneal degenerations usually occur in older dogs. Lipid or calcium keratopathy can develop subsequent to systemic diseases associated with hypercholesteremia, hyperlipemia, and hypercalcemia.

Treatment may or may not be indicated, depending on the existence of an underlying systemic disease, the extent of opacification, and the presence of any associated inflammation or ulceration. Should an underlying systemic disease be present, it should be identified and treated accordingly. Topical medical treatment will not alter the opacifications; however, topical corticosteroids and antibiotics are used to control corneal inflammation and ulcerations, respectively. The likelihood that a superficial keratectomy will be beneficial is debatable. If the opacification is extensive and vision is compromised, a keratectomy could be indicated to remove the outer affected corneal layers. However, the lipid deposition may recur. A keratectomy is indicated if a nonhealing ulcer is associated with degenerative changes in the superficial layers of the cornea. Excision of the abnormal tissue should help promote healing. A nictitating membrane or conjunctival flap may be indicated, depending on the severity. Postoperative treatment with topical and systemic antibiotics is recommended.

EPITHELIAL INCLUSION CYSTS

Epithelial inclusion cysts occur in the dog as isolated, benign, raised corneal masses that involve the epithelial layers. The surrounding stroma may be inflamed. Usually the cause is unknown but is suspected to be traumatic. Superficial keratectomy is generally successful in resolving the problem without recurrence.

DISORDERS OF THE ANTERIOR UVEA

C. SUE WEST, D.V.M.,
and KATHLEEN P. BARRIE, D.V.M.
Tampa, Florida

The uveal tract is a highly vascularized and pigmented structure whose main function is to provide nutrition to other parts of the eye. This vascular tunic is composed of the iris and ciliary body (anterior uvea) and choroid (posterior uvea). The corneoscleral shell surrounds it externally, and the retina lines its posterior aspect internally. Although this chapter will discuss the anatomy and diseases of the anterior uvea, it must be remembered that many of the conditions described also involve the choroid.

ANATOMY

The diaphragmlike iris is the most anterior part of the uveal tract. It separates the aqueous-filled anterior and posterior chambers and is supported posteriorly by the anterior lens surface. The iris consists of a network of connective tissue, muscle, blood vessels, and nerves. The iris vascular stroma is of mesodermal origin, and the anterior three fourths provides nutrition to the anterior segment by diffusion into the aqueous. The iris blood vessels in dogs are much less rigid than in humans and as a result are more prone to hemorrhage and inflammatory changes. The basilar artery, which forms an incomplete ring in the dog, may be found in either the iris root or ciliary body. These anatomic variations are important considerations in iridal surgery.

The iris muscles and posterior pigmented epithelium are neuroectodermal in origin. The iris sphincter and dilator muscles control pupil size, regulating the amount of light reaching the retina. These muscles are innervated by the autonomic nervous system. The sphincter muscle, which circles the iris at the pupillary zone, controls pupillary constriction. This constriction is mediated by the parasympathetic branches of the oculomotor nerve (cranial nerve III). Dilation is mediated through the cervical sympathetic trunks to the thin, wide, peripheral dilator pupillae muscle. The posterior pigmented epithelium consists of two layers and is located directly behind the dilator muscle. It lines the back surface of the iris, and an extension forms the pigmented ruff of the pupil.

The color of the iris can vary from dark brown to blue to white in dogs and blue to green to yellow in cats. This is dependent on the number of melanocytes in the stroma and the thickness of the anterior limiting membrane of the iris. The dog's iris color may vary from monochromia to heterochromia. The cat's iris is usually one color. The canine pupil is round, whereas the feline pupil is a vertical slit when constricted and round when dilated.

The ciliary body is located posterior to the iris and anterior to the choroid. The base of the iris and the anterior ciliary body join with the corneoscleral shell in the area adjacent to the limbus to form the iridocorneal angle. The ciliary body can be divided into the *pars plicata* and the *pars plana*. The junction of the ciliary body with the choroid and the retina is termed the *ora ciliaris retinae* (ora serrata). The 70 to 80 ciliary processes in the pars plicata form accordionlike folds through which the lens supensory ligaments (zonules of Zinn) pass. The ciliary body is covered by two layers of epithelial cells. The innermost nonpigmented epithelium of the pars plicata is the site of aqueous humor production and extends posteriorly over the pars plana to join the neuroretina. The underlying pigmented epithelium is contiguous with the posterior pigmented epithelium of the iris and the retinal pigmented epithelium. The smooth muscle fibers of the ciliary muscles (longitudinal, oblique, and circular) are poorly developed in domestic animals; the longitudinal muscle has some effect on aqueous outflow. Because of this poor muscular development, accommodation in dogs and cats is limited.

EXAMINATION

Examination of the anterior uvea should be performed in a darkened environment. The direct ophthalmoscope or a penlight may be used as the light source, with appropriate magnification (a head loupe of 4× or greater magnification). The best diagnostic tool for examining the iris and ciliary body is the biomicroscope. It provides stereopsis, variable magnification, and variable light intensity and beam size and allows optical dissection of the anterior half of the globe.

The anterior chamber should be observed for depth and clarity, flare, hypopyon, or hyphema. The iris surface should be relatively smooth; a rough appearance indicates iritis. Changes in color may indicate inflammation or neoplasia. Surface hemorrhage and pigment changes should be observed. Variation in iris thickness may indicate the presence of tumors, cysts, or atrophy. The pupillary light response (PLR) demonstrates sphincter and dilator muscle function. Pupils should be equal in size and respond readily to light. Normal PLR should be equal in both eyes with a consensual response present in the opposite eye. A miotic pupil may indicate iritis, Horner's syndrome, or other neurologic disorders. A dilated, nonresponsive pupil may be the result of iris atrophy, fear, glaucoma, the use of mydriatic agents, or neurologic disease. Absence of PLR should not be used as the sole determinant of retinal function! An eye with a normal retina may have no light response because of iris atrophy. Light sensitivity may be easily determined by using a bright light source and watching for a blink or squint response. In any case, a complete retinal examination must be performed before a diagnosis is made. Subtle differences in direct and consensual light responses will be detected as the observer gains experience.

Examination of the ciliary body is limited, since most of it is obscured by the iris. Use of the indirect ophthalmoscope and mydriatic agents allows partial visualization of the pars plana. The presence of ciliary cysts and tumors can be detected with this method. The iridocorneal angle is observed with the use of a gonioscopic lens and the indirect ophthalmoscope or biomicroscope. In most animals, these techniques can be used without anesthetic, or in the case of gonioscopy, with the use of a topical anesthetic agent such as 0.5 per cent proparacaine hydrochloride (Ophthaine drops, Squibb).

CONGENITAL AND DEVELOPMENTAL ANOMALIES

Many congenital defects of the anterior uvea have been reported in dogs and cats, but few have clinical significance. The potential genetic implications should be considered when breeding stock is selected.

Persistent Pupillary Membranes

During development of the eye, the pupil is closed with a thin membrane, the tunica vasculosa lentis. The pupil is formed by absorption of the membrane during the last trimester of gestation and the first few weeks postpartum. If there is incomplete atrophy of the fetal vascular arcades and the mesodermal tissue, persistent pupillary membranes (PPMs) result. These strands arise from the collarette region of the iris and may extend from the iris to the cornea, lens, or other portions of the iris, crossing over the pupil in some cases. They do not affect pupil response but may cause some distortion. They may be pigmented or nonpigmented. Strands attached to the cornea may cause endothelial opacities. Focal capsular cataracts may be observed in dogs with lenticular attachments of the PPMs. Although PPMs are commonly seen in many breeds, genetic significance has not been determined except in the basenji. In most cases, vision is not affected and no treatment is necessary. Many of the strands disappear with age.

Heterochromia Iridis

Heterochromia can be a normal finding due to variation in pigmentation of a part or all of the iris. The color change may involve one or both eyes and may be partial or complete. Hypopigmentation with concurrent hypoplasia of the iris can be related to coat color. The merling gene in a variety of dog breeds (collies, Shetland sheepdogs, Great Danes) causes hypopigmentation of the iris and fundus. Multiple ocular anomalies may be associated with heterochromia in some breeds (homozygous merled Australian shepherds). Subalbinotic animals and true albinos will lack pigmentation of the iris. Waardenburg's syndrome (white coat, blue eyes, and deafness) has been described in cats and dogs. Bluesmoke Persian cats with Chédiak-Higashi syndrome exhibit photophobia, iris hypopigmentation, and hypoplasia. These animals also have cataracts and chorioretinal hypopigmentation associated with the syndrome. Partial albinism is observed in Siamese cats; these animals may also have iris and chorioretinal hypopigmentation, iris hypoplasia, photophobia, strabismus, and nystagmus.

Aniridia and Colobomas of the Anterior Uvea

Aniridia or total absence of the iris is rare in dogs and cats. Usually, rudimentary iris structures are present. When a portion of the iris fails to develop and a defect results, the condition is called iris coloboma. Iris colobomas may occur alone or in association with a coloboma of the ciliary body and choroid. Typical colobomas occur in the region of the embryonic cleft (6 o'clock position) and are the result of abnormal closure of the embryonic cleft. Atypical colobomas are those occurring in regions other than the 6 o'clock position. The condition can be unilateral or bilateral. The exposed iris pigmented epithelium in eyes with partial iridal colobomas may be mistaken for melanomas. Full-thickness colobomas (pseudopolycoria) can be various sizes and shapes that will change with mydriasis. When colobomas are present, increased amounts of light reach the retina, causing some animals to exhibit increased sensitivity to light.

Polycoria

Polycoria is the presence of more than one functional pupil. This is a rare condition, and in most cases, the defect is truly a coloboma.

Dyscoria and Corectopia

Dyscoria is an abnormally shaped pupil not associated with a coloboma. Corectopia is displacement of the pupil. These congenital defects may be associated with other ocular abnormalities, and a complete intraocular examination should be performed.

Primary Iris Atrophy

Primary iris atrophy results in multiple holes in the iris stroma without involving the sphincter muscle, mimicking polycoria. Senile iris atrophy is differentiated by its location at the pupillary margin, giving the pupil a ragged appearance and a poor pupillary light response.

Anterior Uveal Cysts

Formation of cysts from the pigmented epithelium of the iris or the epithelium of the ciliary body can be congenital or acquired. Cysts can be fixed or free floating within the anterior and posterior chambers. The cysts may be found unilaterally or bilaterally and may be singular or multiple in number. Clinically, the cysts are a dark color but can be transilluminated. Sudden movement of the head will often cause the cyst to rise up into the anterior chamber. The ability of the pigmented mass to be transilluminated differentiates the cyst from an iris tumor. When the cysts are very large, fine-needle 30-gauge) aspiration or laser phototherapy can be performed, but in most cases no treatment is necessary.

ATROPHIES AND DEGENERATIONS

Senile Iris Atrophy

This condition occurs in adult animals that were normal when they were young. It is frequently encountered in toy and miniature poodles, miniature schnauzers, and Chihuahuas. The atrophy involves the sphincter region of the iris. This gives the pupillary margin a scalloped appearance and can produce a slow or incomplete pupillary reflex. The degeneration can become more severe, affecting the bulk of the iris. Multiple holes can develop, resembling polycoria. Dogs with iris atrophy may exhibit photophobia.

Iridal and Ciliary Cysts

Iris and ciliary cysts may be seen in the older animal. They are histologically the same as those described under congenital anomalies. They are usually black, spherical, and free floating. They must be distinguished from intraocular tumors. A cause has not been ascertained in the dog, although in humans iris cysts are associated with chronic inflammation and the use of topical miotic agents (2 per cent pilocarpine hydrochloride).

Ectropion Uveae

Ectropion uveae is seen in dogs and cats. Eversion of the pigmented epithelium is usually a sequela to uveitis. True ectropion involves eversion of the sphincter muscle, stroma, and pigmented epithelium secondary to shrinkage of the anterior surface of the iris. The dark brown appearance of the pigmented epithelium around the pupil is a striking finding when seen in the cat. Proliferation of the pigmented epithelium onto the anterior surface of the iris without muscle or stromal involvement gives a similar appearance.

UVEITIS

Anterior uveitis is inflammation of the iris and ciliary body. Anterior uveitis (iridocyclitis) can be classified as (1) exogenous: trauma to the globe or infective agents, (2) endogenous: nongranulomatous (viral, bacterial) or granulomatous, (3) hypersensitive, or (4) idiopathic.

The cause of uveitis is often difficult to determine. A thorough physical examination with appropriate laboratory tests should be performed prior to implementing intensive therapy. Unfortunately, a specific cause is seldom identified. Therefore, the clinician should try to catalog each patient according to ocular and systemic signs. This will help rule out many of the known offending diseases.

Once a complete history is taken and physical and ocular examinations are completed, the clinician may need to perform hematologic tests (complete blood count, serum chemistries). If indicated, serologic tests for systemic mycoses and immune-mediated, parasitic, or viral (feline leukemia virus [FeLV], feline infectious peritonitis [FIP]) diseases can be implemented.

The greatest success in demonstrating a causative agent is by fine-needle aspiration of ocular fluids. This can severely damage the eye and is used only if a specific group or individual agent is suspected. To obtain aqueous, a 25- to 30-gauge needle is inserted into the paralimbal conjunctiva of the anesthetized animal. The needle is directed into the anterior chamber and kept parallel to the iris. A small amount (0.1 to 0.2 ml) of aqueous is slowly removed. As the needle is withdrawn, the tract should seal itself. Complications of this procedure include iris hemorrhage, increased inflammation, and continuous leakage of aqueous.

Vitreal aspiration is also performed in the anesthetized animal. A 20-gauge needle is inserted into the globe posterior to the equator. Aspiration of vitreous may be difficult and requires constant pressure on the syringe. A variable amount of fluid can be removed. As the needle is withdrawn, a hemostat or fine forceps may be needed to prevent leakage of intraocular fluid. Because complications with this technique are severe (ciliary body hemorrhage, retinal detachment, or retinal hemorrhage), it is not recommended for use in eyes that function and is used only as a last resort.

The initial inflammatory response to local cellular injury is hyperemia of iridal vessels and edema, allowing release of mediators of inflammation (prostaglandins, fibrinogen, antibodies). Prostaglandins released from damaged tissues further increase capillary permeability, altering the blood-aqueous barrier. This produces mild smooth muscle contraction leading to miosis. With breakdown of the blood-aqueous barrier, inflammatory cells invade the anterior chamber and uveal tissue. This stimulates release of chemoattractant substances such as platelet products, endotoxins, and other exudates. Therefore, the primary inflammatory response causes a more severe secondary response and thus a vicious cycle. Antiprostaglandin therapy is the current area of interest in ocular therapeutics.

The pathophysiologic result of anterior uveitis is centered around ocular immunology. It is believed that the uvea functions as a regional lymph node. Sensitized lymphocytes can accumulate in the uvea and become immunologically competent. Antibodies can be produced locally and be involved in cell-mediated response. All four classic types of the immune response have been demonstrated within the eye: (1) immediate, (2) cytotoxic, (3) immune complexes, and (4) cell mediated.

Signs of Uveitis

The signs of anterior uveitis are varied (Table 1). They can be unilateral or bilateral, depending on the inciting agent. Close examination of the anterior chamber will reveal a loss of clarity to the aqueous. This is due to an increase in protein and inflammatory cells (flare). Cellular and proteinaceous debris may adhere to the posterior cornea (keratic

Table 1. Signs of Acute and Chronic Anterior Uveitis

Acute	Chronic
Painful	Infrequently painful
Ocular hypotony	Phthisis bulbi
Corneal edema	Bullous keratopathy
Hypopyon, fibrin, hyphema	Fibropupillary membranes
Swollen iris, vessel engorgement	Hyperpigmentation to synechiation of the iris
Aqueous flare	Aqueous flare
Debris on the anterior lens capsule	Secondary cataract
Conjunctival congestion	Secondary glaucoma

precipitates), anterior lens capsule, and the iris. On examination of the limbus, circumcorneal vascular injection extending into the corneal stroma may produce a brush border effect. Corneal edema is diffuse and may cause subtle to severe opacification. Along with fibrin and accumulation of inflammatory cells (hypopyon), hemorrhage into the aqueous (hyphema) may be found. The animal may exhibit mild to severe photophobia, enophthalmos, epiphora, and blepharospasm. Along with miosis, the iris may be swollen and have engorged vessels.

The more chronic signs of anterior uveitis are influenced by the cause and duration of the inflammation. Posterior synechia (adherence of the iris to the anterior lens capsule) is the most frequent finding. Hyperpigmentation of the iris and pigmented cells on the anterior lens capsule or posterior cornea may be found. If the posterior synechiae involve the entire pupil, an iris bombé with secondary glaucoma will develop. Anterior synechia (adherence of the iris to the cornea) will cause pathologic changes in the cornea. Secondary glaucoma may develop acutely as a result of obstruction of the iridocorneal angle with inflammatory debris or from extensive peripheral anterior synechiae. Peripheral anterior synechia will produce glaucoma because it results in the collapse of the iridocorneal angle. Corneal endothelial death from chronic uveitis will produce persistent corneal edema and may lead to a bullous keratopathy. Fibropupillary membranes can extend across the iris or involve the posterior cornea. Secondary cataracts can develop from altered lens metabolism. Finally, severe chronic anterior uveitis may produce irreversible damage to the ciliary body, resulting in ocular hypotony and phthisis.

Treatment

The objectives of treatment of anterior uveitis are to suppress inflammation and thereby decrease secondary disease, relieve pain by producing iridocycloplegia, and eliminate noxious agents.

Anti-inflammatory agents are the most important aspect of uveitis therapy. Corticosteroids can be administered topically, subconjunctivally, and systemically. One or all three routes may be used. Corticosteroids reduce the amount of exudate, increase cellular membrane integrity, inhibit release of lysozymes, and decrease circulating lymphocytes.

Topical medication will allow immediate drug levels into the anterior chamber. The more potent topical corticosteroids are dexamethasone and prednisolone acetate. Oral prednisolone (2 mg/kg) can be given concurrently with topical corticosteroids. Intravenous corticosteriods can be given in more severe disease. Subconjunctival injection is used in those cases that cannot be treated routinely or in chronic cases in which parenteral administration is difficult or contraindicated. Nearly all injectable corticosteroids can be used subconjunctivally. The short-acting agents are prednisolone and hydrocortisone. The intermediate-acting drugs are triamcinolone and dexamethasone. Those drugs that last longer than 10 days are Depo-Medrol (Upjohn) and betamethasone.

Antiprostaglandin therapy is a promising method of uveitis treatment. Presently, aspirin is the most commonly used agent, given at a dose of 10 mg/kg orally. Phenylbutazone can be administered orally, 20 mg/kg. Flunixin meglumine (Banamine, Schering), although not approved for use in small animals, has been used with caution at 0.50 to 1.00 mg/kg intravenously. Antiprostaglandins can cause systemic side effects such as bleeding, vomiting, diarrhea, and renal dysfunction. New antiprostaglandins for topical and sytemic use are presently being investigated and will be available in the near future.

Antimicrobial agents are used in uveitis therapy against specific organisms or supportively. Penetration of most antibiotics occurs in the inflamed uvea as a result of the breakdown of the blood-aqueous barrier. Antimicrobial drugs are administered topically or systemically.

Various mydriatics are used to induce mydriasis and cycloplegia. These drugs will help to minimize formation of posterior synechiae and relieve pain. In the most complicated uveitis cases, they must be administered with caution because of the chance of producing secondary glaucoma. Topical 1 per cent atropine, 10 per cent phenylephrine, and 0.25 per cent scopolamine can effectively be used alone or together.

INFECTIOUS AGENTS

Refer also to Section 12 for additional information on infectious agents.

INFECTIOUS CANINE HEPATITIS. Canine adenovirus type 1 (CAV) is the infectious agent of canine hepatitis. The virus replicates in reticuloendothelial cells, parenchymal cells, and vascular endothelium. The disease can be fatal in young dogs, whereas it may be subclinical in adult animals. The ocular signs may be observed in 20 per cent of the dogs recovering from the disease. These dogs develop anterior uveitis and corneal edema.

The incidence of the disease has been reduced because of widespread vaccination programs. The original vaccine available was a modified live CAV-1 strain. Anterior uveitis identical to the natural disease occurred with certain strains of CAV-1. The attentuated CAV-2 vaccine has greatly reduced the occurrence of the "vaccinated disease."

The pathologic changes produced by the virus are due to an Arthus reaction; virus replicates in the anterior uvea and corneal endothelium, followed by an antigen-antibody reaction, forming soluble immune complexes that evoke inflammation. Thus the endothelium, owing to lack of regeneration, is permanently lost. The result is chronic corneal edema, often referred to as "blue eye."

Treatment is aimed at minimizing the immune reaction. Topical and systemic corticosteroids can be administered. Mydriatics may also be beneficial.

LEPTOSPIROSIS. *Leptospira icterohaemorrhagiae* can produce anterior uveitis due to direct infection by the leptospira organism. Topical treatment is directed at reducing the inflammatory response. Systemically administered streptomycin is also indicated.

SEPTICEMIA/BACTEREMIA. Generalized systemic septicemias can produce ocular disease including anterior and posterior uveitis and panuveitis. Whenever the animal is debilitated by a septic disease, the clinician should evaluate the eyes.

SYSTEMIC MYCOSES. Blastomycosis is frequently encountered in dogs and cats. Panuveitis or endophthalmitis may be found alone or with systemic disease. The more common ocular signs are granulomatous chorioretinitis followed by retinal detachment, optic neuritis, and anterior uveitis. Aspiration of subretinal fluid will frequently identify the thin-walled budding cell. *Blastomyces dermatitidis* is a 7 to 10μm, budding yeast.

Cryptococcus neoformans has been observed in cats and dogs. The organism is a saprophyte found in soil and in pigeon droppings. *Cryptococcus* has a predilection for the brain and meninges. Ocular findings are mainly associated with granulomatous chorioretinitis with secondary retinal detachment, although anterior uveitis with hyphema may be found. Aspiration of the vitreous or subretinal fluid may find round or oval organisms with a thick mucinous capsule 4 to 7μm in diameter.

Coccidioidomycosis (valley fever), caused by *Coccidioides immitis*, is a common fungal infection in the southwestern United States. The arthrospores are found in the dust and are acquired by inhalation. The ocular signs are characterized by a granulomatous panuveitis and keratitis. Aspiration of the vitreous may yield a small yeast cell (2 to 5μm), found most commonly within the cytoplasm of macrophages. In tissue, a thick-walled spherule (20 to 50μm) filled with endospores can be found.

Geotrichum candidum is a rare mycotic disease encountered in domestic animals. Ocular disease has been described in dogs. A severe panophthalmitis with secondary retinal detachment is seen. The oval, yeastlike cell may form pseudohyphae and can be identified in tissue sections.

Histoplasma capsulatum can produce granulomatous panuveitis in dogs and, rarely, in cats. It is endemic in the central Mississippi and Ohio River valleys. Ophthalmic examination may reveal fluffy exudates in the retina, exudative retinal detachment, thickened iris, and aqueous flare. The organism occurs in reticuloendothelial cells as a thin-walled yeastlike organism (2 to 4μm) with a spherical, basophilic body surrounded by an unstained zone.

Protothecosis is caused by colorless algae found throughout nature. The disease has been reported in dogs, cats, wild animals, fish, and humans. In dogs, 50 per cent of those infected showed ocular disease, a granulomatous chorioretinitis with secondary retinal detachment.

Aspiration of the fluid from the posterior or anterior segment, depending on the ocular disease, may reveal mycotic organisms. Ten to 20 per cent potassium hydroxide (KOH) and Parker ink or india ink will outline the walled organisms of *Blastomyces*, *Cryptococcus*, and *Coccidioides*. Biopsies of other organs or lymph node aspirates can be stained with periodic acid–Schiff (PAS) or other hematologic stains to reveal the fungus. Histoplasmosis is rarely diagnosed by direct smears. (Refer to the article entitled Contemporary Ocular Therapeutics for treatment suggestions.)

PARASITIC UVEITIS

Toxoplasmosis

Toxoplasmosis is a widely disseminated disease found in humans and animals. The cat is the definitive host of *Toxoplasma gondii*, a small intracellular protozoan. The disease is thought to occur by ingestion of sporozoites in feces, insects, or infected muscle or by transfer across the placenta. Ocular lesions in dogs are most frequently chorioretinitis and optic neuritis; less common are anterior uveitis and extraocular muscle or orbital disease. Cats showing ocular signs usually are systemically infected with *Toxoplasma* organisms. Chorioretinitis and a granulomatous anterior uveitis are found, although anterior segment disease is more frequently seen. Diagnosis of toxoplasmosis is usually made by running serial titers, fecal examinations, and identification of organisms in ocular tissue.

Leishmaniasis

Leishmania donovani, a protozoan found in southern Europe, Asia, Africa, and South America, has been reported in dogs in the United States originating from these areas. Although severe keratitis and conjunctivitis are the most common ocular findings, anterior uveitis can be noted.

Ehrlichiosis

Tropical canine pancytopenia is caused by *Ehrlichia canis,* a rickettsial organism. In association with the systemic manifestations of severe anemia, extraocular and intraocular hemorrhage can be found. Systemic tetracyclines are indicated.

Ocular Filariasis

Immature canine heartworm, *Dirofilaria immitis,* can be found in aberrant locations such as the anterior chamber or vitreous. Diagnosis is made by observing the worm in the anterior chamber. Mild anterior uveitis occurs. Treatment is surgical removal of the worm. The animal is placed under general anesthesia. A limbal incision is made to allow small forceps to enter the anterior chamber and remove the worm. The incision is closed with one or two 8–0 absorbable sutures. Postoperative therapy for anterior uveitis is indicated.

FELINE UVEITIS

A significant number of cats that develop a unilateral or bilateral anterior uveitis are positive for feline leukemia, infectious peritonitis, or toxoplasmosis.

Feline infectious peritonitis (FIP) is caused by a coronavirus. It is a multisystemic, immune-mediated, necrotizing vasculitis. Ocular signs develop in 25 per cent or more in the noneffusive form of the disease. Affected cats may present with pyogranulomatous anterior uveitis, iritis, and aqueous flare with hemorrhagic precipitates. The posterior segment may show chorioretinitis, retinal hemorrhage, and retinal detachment.

FeLV is an oncornavirus causing panuveitis or discrete ocular neoplasms. Anterior uveitis, either unilateral or bilateral, is the most common ocular finding. Iritis, aqueous flare with hypopyon, and, more chronically, pigmentary changes in the iris are seen. Posterior segment disease, including chorioretinitis and retinal detachment, are encountered in the later stages. Corticosteroids aid in reducing some of the ocular signs.

LENS-INDUCED UVEITIS

Lens-induced uveitis is the result of cataract formation. The breakdown of the lens capsule allows lens protein, normally isolated from the body, to be exposed. The immune system reacts to this protein as foreign, producing a hypersensitivity reaction. In dogs, this phenomenon may go unrecognized until secondary problems such as glaucoma develop. Treatment with topical corticosteroids and cycloplegics is necessary.

HYPHEMA

Hyphema is associated with many systemic disorders. Bleeding disorders, whether inherited or acquired, can produce hemorrhage within the ocular tissues. Blunt trauma to the head can produce hyphema. Foreign body penetration of the globe can produce intraocular hemorrhage. Hyphema is common with primary and metastatic intraocular tumors. If there is hemorrhage in an older animal, the clinician should consider a diagnosis of intraocular tumor. Congenital anomalies such as collie eye anomaly and retinal dysplasia in Bedlington terriers can cause chronic hyphema. Chronic glaucoma may also produce chronic hyphema.

Treatment of hyphema is dependent on the cause. Control of the iridocyclitis is of primary concern. Use of topical antibiotic-corticosteroid ophthalmic solutions every four hours is indicated. The use of mydriatics may be helpful, although one must monitor intraocular pressure carefully.

HYPERLIPIDEMIA

Lipid-laden aqueous has been reported in dogs and cats. It is associated with tremendous elevation of lipoproteins in the serum. It is thought that anterior uveitis allows the breakdown of the normal blood-aqueous barrier to the large fat molecules, allowing lipids to enter the aqueous. Treatment with topical corticosteroids and mydriatics is indicated. Eliminating the intake of dietary fats is necessary, as well as pursuing the cause of the lipemia. (Note: Uveal neoplasms are discussed in the article Tumors of the Eye and Adnexa.)

References and Supplemental Reading

Bergsma, D. R., and Brown, K. S.: White fur, blue eyes and deafness in the domestic cat. J. Heredity 62:171, 1971.

Collier, L. L., Bryan, G. M., and Prieur, D. J.: Ocular manifestations of the Chediak-Higashi syndrome in four species of animals. J.A.V.M.A. 175:587, 1979.

Gelatt, K. N., and McGill, L. D.: Clinical characteristic of microphthalmia with colobomas of the Australian shepherd dog. J.A.V.M.A. 162:393, 1973.

Gwin, R. M., Wyman, M., Lim, D. J., et al., Multiple ocular defects associated with partial albinism and deafness in the dog. J. Amer. Anim. Hosp. Assoc. 17:401, 1981.

Keller, W. F., The canine anterior uvea. *In* Gelatt, K. N. (ed.): *Veterinary Ophthalmology*. Philadelphia: Lea & Febiger, 1981, pp. 375–389.

Schlaegel, Jr., T. F., Pathogenesis of Uveitis. *In* Duane, T. (ed.): *Clinical Ophthalmology*. Vol. 4. New York: Harper & Row, 1980, Chapter 40, pp. 1–6.

Shimada, K.: The immune system in the eye and allergic uveitis. Jpn. J. Immunol. 23:469, 1979.

Sonntag, H. G.: Essentials of microbiology in uveitis. *In* Krause-Mackin, E., and O'Connor, G. R. (eds.): *Uveitis, Pathophysiology and Therapy*. New York: Thieme-Stratton, 1983, p. 31.

Theodore, F. H., Bloomfield, S. E., and Mondino, B.: Pathology of the Immune Responses. *In Clinical Allergy and Immunology of the Eye*. Baltimore, Maryland: Williams & Wilkins, 1983, pp. 18–27.

Yanoff, M., and Fine, B. S.: Uvea. *In* Duane, T. D., and Jaeger, E. H. (eds.): *Biomedical Foundations of Ophthalmology*. Vol. 3. New York: Harper & Row, 1983, Chapter 11, pp. 1–17.

CANINE AND FELINE GLAUCOMAS

DENNIS E. BROOKS, D.V.M.

Gainesville, Florida

AQUEOUS HUMOR DYNAMICS AND INTRAOCULAR PRESSURE

Aqueous humor is an optically transparent fluid that fills the anterior and posterior chambers of the eye. It provides nutrition and removes waste products from the avascular intraocular structures.

Aqueous humor is produced in the ciliary body by active secretion and ultrafiltration of plasma. The enzyme carbonic anhydrase participates in the energy-dependent secretory phase of aqueous production. Most of the aqueous humor flows from the posterior chamber, through the pupil, to the anterior chamber, and exits at the iridocorneal angle into the intrascleral venous plexus. A small percentage of the outflow in dogs and cats (uveoscleral or nonconventional) also exits through the iris, ciliary body, choroid, and sclera. The balance between formation and drainage of aqueous humor maintains intraocular pressure (IOP) within a normal range of 15 to 25 mm Hg. All ocular structures are subjected to this pressure, which stabilizes the shape of the globe and preserves the precise optical relationships of the various refractive components of the eye.

By definition, glaucoma is increased IOP with associated visual deficits. In most cases in dogs and cats, glaucoma is caused by obstruction or stenosis of the aqueous humor outflow pathways. Obstruction of venous blood flow from the eye or head may also be associated with elevation of IOP in rare cases. It remains a challenge to the veterinarian to detect the early subtle disturbances of glaucoma and to effectively treat this condition. Delayed or inadequate therapy can lead to irreversible blindness and a painful, cosmetically unacceptable eye.

PATHOLOGIC EFFECTS OF GLAUCOMA

All ocular tissues are eventually affected by the elevated IOP. The presence, individually or as a group, of a "red eye," corneal edema, mydriasis, blepharospasm, blindness, and buphthalmos can be explained by the increased IOP.

Glaucoma produces tension in the corneoscleral coat, resulting in stretching and disruption of the corneal and scleral collagen lamellae. If the IOP cannot be reduced, an overall increase in the size of the globe may result (buphthalmos). This change may occur more rapidly in young dogs and cats.

Ruptures of the cornea's inner limiting (Descemet's) membrane may accompany the elevated corneal tension and buphthalmos to produce multiple, linear corneal striae. Persistent corneal endothelial damage can result in corneal edema.

Buphthalmos causes increased tension on the lens zonules. Zonular disinsertion results in lens subluxation or luxation. It may not always be possible in dogs and cats to ascertain whether the presence of a luxated lens caused glaucoma and buphthalmos or whether the luxated lens is a secondary result of a previously existing glaucoma.

Pupillary light reflexes may be normal, slow, or absent in early glaucoma, depending on the functional status of the iris sphincter muscle, retina, and

Table 1. Goniomorphology in Canine Primary Glaucoma

Breed	Morphology
Afghan	Goniodysgenesis
American cocker spaniel	Narrow; goniodysgenesis
Basset hound	Open to narrow; goniodysgenesis (congenital). Anterior uveitis may be concurrent.
Beagle	Open
Bedlington terrier	Narrow to closed
Brittany spaniel	Narrow to closed
Dachshund	Narrow to closed
Dalmatian	Narrow to closed
English cocker spaniel	Open; narrow
English springer spaniel	Narrow to closed
Fox terriers (smooth- and wire-haired)	Narrow to closed
Great Dane	Goniodysgenesis
Malamute	Narrow to closed
Norwegian elkhound	Open; narrow to closed
Saluki	Goniodysgenesis
Samoyed	Goniodysgenesis; narrow to closed
Sealyham terrier	Narrow to closed
Siberian husky	Narrow; goniodysgenesis
Toy and miniature poodles	Open; narrow

optic nerve. Acute elevation of IOP (greater than 45 mm Hg) causes paralysis of the iris sphincter and dilator muscles. Retinal atrophy is clinically manifested in advanced glaucoma by tapetal hyperreflectivity and retinal vessel attenuation.

Prolonged or recurrent elevations of IOP lead to degeneration of the optic nerve, with excavation or cupping of the optic nerve head. Cupping occurs as a result of a progressive posterior movement of the scleral lamina cribrosa and a decrease in the thickness of the rim of the optic nerve head due to axonal and glial degeneration. Axonal degeneration of the optic nerve probably results from the blockade of axoplasmic transport by mechanical compression of axons at the lamina cribrosa and local tissue ischemia caused by vascular insufficiency.

TYPES OF GLAUCOMA

Glaucoma is divided into primary (including congenital) and secondary categories. The iridocorneal angle may be open, narrow, or closed in either type. Abnormal development of the iridocorneal angle (goniodysgenesis) has been noted in some breeds (Table 1). Evaluation of the iridocorneal angle is performed with gonioscopy in the dog but may be performed with focal illumination in the cat.

Primary glaucoma in dogs is a breed-related, hereditary condition. Predisposition to primary open-angle glaucoma in the Persian and Siamese cat breeds has also been noted, but in the author's experience, domestic short-hairs are more often affected. In both dogs and cats, affected animals may present with only one eye involved, but the risk is very high for development of glaucoma in the other eye.

Secondary glaucoma is more commonly encountered than primary glaucoma in dogs and cats. The elevated IOP results from other disease processes within the eye. The glaucoma may be open or closed angle, and in some instances is associated with pupillary block. The condition tends to be unilateral without an inherited basis.

Obstruction of an open iridocorneal angle can occur with red blood cells from hyphema; inflammatory debris and cells from uveitis, intraocular infection, or trauma; and neoplastic cells from intraocular tumors. Cats, in particular, presented with unilateral glaucoma and anterior uveitis or hyphema should be carefully examined for intraocular or systemic neoplasia, systemic viral infection (feline leukemia virus [FeLV], feline infectious peritonitis [FIP]), toxoplasmosis, and systemic mycosis.

Leakage of lens proteins into the aqueous humor from mature or hypermature cataracts may be associated with severe uveitis. Iridocorneal angle obstruction by lens proteins, inflammatory debris, large lens particles, and macrophages is possible. The organization of inflammatory exudate in the iridocorneal angle can result in peripheral anterior synechiae and can further aggravate the already compromised drainage angle.

Secondary closed-angle glaucoma is caused by anterior movement of the peripheral iris into the drainage angle. Age-related lens growth, lens intumescence during rapid cataract formation, anterior lens luxation, and iris and ciliary body tumors can cause angle narrowing or closure.

Several breeds of terriers appear predisposed to lens luxation with or without glaucoma. The condition may be associated with inflammation and pupillary block. The specific cause in many breeds is not known. This condition occurs in Jack Russell, Sealyham, Welsh, Manchester, Boston, Cairn, Tibetan, smooth- or wire-haired, and toy fox terriers, as well as several non-terrier breeds (e.g., Norwegian elkhound, Brittany spaniel). In most non-terrier canine breeds and cats, lens luxation is most often the end result of zonular disinsertion in a buphthalmic globe and can exacerbate glaucoma already present.

CLINICAL SIGNS OF ACUTE AND CHRONIC GLAUCOMA

The presentation of a patient with a painful, red eye requires that glaucoma be ruled out among the possible diagnoses of conjunctivitis, uveitis, or keratitis. Pain manifested as depression, anorexia, rubbing at the eye, and squinting is common. Congestion of episcleral vessels, diffuse corneal edema, a fixed and dilated pupil, and blindness will occur as the IOP increases. The onset of clinical signs in cats is often insidious, as cats are less likely to demonstrate the acute intense corneal edema and episcleral congestion exhibited in dogs.

Signs of chronic glaucoma are dramatic. They include combinations of the early signs with buphthalmos, lagophthalmos, exposure keratitis, luxated lens, corneal striae, optic nerve atrophy with cupping, and retinal atrophy.

TONOMETRY

IOP must be accurately measured to diagnose glaucoma. The normal canine and feline IOP is 15 to 25 mm Hg. An IOP greater than 30 mm Hg is considered pathologic and diagnostic for this condition. It is possible to crudely evaluate IOP digitally if the IOP is very high or low, but this is not satisfactory to evaluate clinical response to therapy. The Schiotz's indentation tonometer allows the practitioner to diagnose and evaluate treatment in small animals with glaucoma. Practice improves technique and reliability. The tonometer is held vertically and placed on the center of the cornea after the application of topical anesthesia. Several tonometer values are averaged and used to convert the scale readings on a conversion table to mm Hg IOP. Schiotz's tonometric values may be artifactually low in the presence of corneal edema and high in the presence of an anteriorly luxated lens. The Schiotz's tonometer must not be used if ocular perforation is suspected or within 1 month after intraocular surgery.

TREATMENT

The objectives of therapy are to maintain vision and eliminate pain by (1) increasing aqueous outflow, (2) decreasing aqueous production, and (3) preventing or delaying glaucoma in the other eye. Primary glaucoma may be more difficult to control than secondary glaucoma because it is eventually bilateral, and blindness is a possible sequela despite therapy. The author nevertheless recommends prophylactic therapy for the unaffected eye in animals afflicted with unilateral primary glaucoma. In secondary glaucoma, the inciting cause is identified and either removed or suppressed. Topical corticosteroids may be indicated to diminish inflammation when nonseptic anterior uveitis is also present.

Medical therapy and cyclocryotherapy are the treatments of choice in animals with a history of acute primary or secondary glaucoma. Treatment should be instituted to reduce the IOP as soon as possible to alleviate pain and preserve vision. Animals presented with a history and clinical signs of chronic glaucoma should be considered for medical and surgical therapy. Tonometry is recommended to effectively manage therapy, as the iridocorneal angle gradually closes in most types of glaucoma and the initially effective treatment becomes inadequate at a later time.

Table 2. *Pharmacologic Agents for Medical Treatment of Glaucoma*

Carbonic-anhydrase inhibitors (oral)
Acetazolamide (Diamox, Lederle): 10 to 25 mg/kg divided 2 to 3 times daily
Dichlorphenamide (Daranide, Merck, Sharp & Dohme): 10 to 15 mg/kg divided 2 to 3 times daily
Methazolamide (Neptazane, Lederle): 5 mg/kg divided 2 to 3 times daily
Parasympathomimetics (topical)
1 to 2 per cent pilocarpine every 6 hours
0.125 to 0.25 per cent demecarium bromide (Humorsol, Merck, Sharp & Dohme): 1 to 2 times per day
0.125 to 0.25 per cent echothiophate iodide (Phospholine Iodide, Ayerst): 1 to 2 times per day
Sympathomimetics (topical)
1 to 2 per cent epinephrine (P_2E_1, Person and Covey): 2 to 3 times per day (may be combined with 2 per cent pilocarpine)
0.1 to 0.5 per cent dipivalyl epinephrine (Propine, Allergan): 2 to 3 times per day
Beta-adrenergic antagonists (topical)
0.50 per cent timolol maleate (Timoptic, Merck, Sharp & Dohme): 2 to 3 times per day
Hyperosmotics
20 per cent mannitol: 1 to 2 gm/kg IV; repeat in 6 hours if necessary
50 per cent glycerol: 1 to 2 ml/kg PO; repeat in 8 hours if necessary

Medical Therapy

Multiple drug therapy to decrease IOP by reducing production of aqueous humor and diminishing the resistance to aqueous humor outflow is the most effective approach (Table 2).

Carbonic-anhydrase inhibitors reduce ciliary-body production of aqueous humor independent of diuresis. These drugs can cause metabolic acidosis, and the dosage should be carefully adjusted to minimize side effects, which include panting, nausea, and vomiting. Non-carbonic anhydrase–inhibiting diuretics do *not* significantly reduce IOP!

Topical parasympathomimetic drugs act primarily to cause ciliary muscle contraction, increasing the outflow of aqueous humor. This action is independent of their effect on the iris sphincter muscle. Parasympathomimetics are contraindicated in glaucoma associated with anterior uveitis. They should be used with caution in glaucoma associated with anterior lens luxations.

Topical sympathomimetic drugs reduce IOP by decreasing production of aqueous humor and increasing outflow. These drugs are most effective in reducing IOP when combined with parasympathomimetics.

Topical β-adrenergic antagonists decrease production of aqueous humor, but the specific mechanism of action is not known. The ocular hypotensive effects are additive to those of carbonic-anhydrase inhibitors, parasympathomimetics, and sympathomimetics.

Oral and intravenous hyperosmotic agents lower IOP rapidly by osmotically reducing the volume of the vitreous. They are used in the emergency treatment of acute glaucoma but are ineffective or impractical for long-term or maintenance therapy. Less benefit may occur in the inflamed eye because of the disruption of the blood-aqueous barrier.

Mannitol (1 to 2 gm/kg) is administered intravenously over a 15- to 20-minute period. Glycerol (50 per cent, 1 to 2 ml/kg) is administered orally. It is readily absorbed from the gastrointestinal tract but may produce emesis. The osmotic effect of oral glycerol is more variable and less rapid than that of intravenous mannitol, but oral glycerol may be more convenient in that it can be safely administered by the owner in an emergency to mitigate an acute attack of glaucoma prior to the patient's presentation to a veterinarian. Water should be withheld for 30 to 60 minutes after administration of hyperosmotic agents.

The author prefers the carbonic-anhydrase inhibitors, dichlorphenamide or methazolamide, in combination with topical pilocarpine (2 per cent) or pilocarpine (2 per cent) with epinephrine (1 per cent), for the initial maintenance therapy in most types of glaucoma. Changes in therapy may be necessary as the disease progresses. More potent longer-acting parasympathomimetics or β-adrenergic antagonists can then be used. Mannitol therapy is added to this regimen in cases of acute glaucoma. In situations in which parasympathomimetics are ineffective or contraindicated, β-adrenergic antagonists may be effective in lowering IOP.

Surgical Therapy

Surgery should be considered when the IOP cannot be controlled medically, especially when vision is still present. Anteriorly luxated lenses should be removed in functioning eyes to relieve pupillary block and prevent corneal damage due to the lens touching the corneal endothelium.

Surgical procedures may be thought of as divided into those that increase aqueous humor outflow and those that decrease aqueous humor production. The combined iridencleisis-cyclodialysis filtering procedure is preferred by the author to increase aqueous humor outflow. Details of the surgical technique may be found in the supplemental readings.

Cyclocryotherapy has been found to be effective in decreasing production of aqueous humor by the selective transcleral freezing with nitrous oxide of the ciliary body. This may require repeated applications for optimal IOP control.

Enucleation or evisceration with prosthetic silicone implants is indicated when vision is lost in uncontrolled primary glaucoma and in selected instances of secondary glaucoma when the cause is documented. The source of pain is removed, and no further medication is necessary. The cosmetic appearance of the prosthetic implant is usually preferred to that of enucleation. Prosthetic implants should not be used when glaucoma is or may be associated with intraocular infection or neoplasia.

References and Supplemental Reading

Brightman, A. H., Magrane, W. G., Huff, R. W., et al.: Intraocular prosthesis in the dog. J. Am. Anim. Hosp. Assoc. 13:481, 1977.

Gelatt, K. N.: The canine glaucomas. *In* Gelatt, K. N. (ed.): *Textbook of Veterinary Ophthalmology.* Philadelphia: Lea & Febiger, 1981, pp. 390–435.

Meredith, R. E., and Gelatt, K. N.: Cryotherapy in veterinary ophthalmology. Vet. Clin. North Am. 10:837, 1980.

Moses, R. A.: Intraocular pressure. *In* Moses, R. A. (ed.): *Adler's Physiology of the Eye,* 7th ed. St. Louis: C. V. Mosby, 1981, pp. 227–254.

Peiffer, R. L.: Feline ophthalmology. *In* Gelatt, K. N. (ed.): *Textbook of Veterinary Ophthalmology.* Philadelphia: Lea & Febiger, 1981, pp. 521–568.

Sears, M. L.: The aqueous. *In* Moses, R. A. (ed.): *Adler's Physiology of the Eye,* 7th ed. St. Louis: C. V. Mosby, 1981, pp. 204–226.

DISEASES OF THE LENS AND VITREOUS

FRANS C. STADES, D.V.M.
Utrecht, The Netherlands

The lens is a uniquely biconvex intraocular organ capable of changing its refractive index by accommodation. It is a part of the refractive system of the eye, which functions to focus light rays on the retina. The lens is enclosed in an elastic capsule suspended from the ciliary body by very fine, zonular fibers, which attach radially at the equator. After fetal development, the lens loses its blood supply and becomes an isolated tissue, nourished solely through its capsule by the surrounding aqueous and vitreous humor. Waste products are removed by the same media. Metabolic dysfunction of the lens, either primary or secondary (i.e., from irradiation or from metabolic, toxic, nutritional, electrical, or mechanical insults) may result in opacities of the lens contents or its capsule. This is called a cataract.

The vitreous is a transparent structure that fills the globe behind the lens. It serves as a highly elastic hydrogel, keeping the retina in place against the choroid. The hyaloid-vessel system that penetrates the vitreous regresses a few weeks after birth; like the lens, the vitreous has no blood supply. Both the lens and vitreous lack nervous innervation.

To understand the pathologic changes of the lens and vitreous, and for correct diagnoses of the subsequent entities, appreciation of the main features of their ontogenesis, anatomy, physiology, and clinical examination is essential.

ONTOGENESIS

The vitreous originates essentially from both neuroderm and surface ectoderm, whereas the lens derives solely from surface ectoderm. When the primary optic vesicle protrudes from the forebrain and approaches the surface ectoderm, it induces the surface ectoderm to thicken, forming the lens placode. The placode invaginates, separating from the surface ectoderm and forming the lens vesicle at about day 19 post coitum (p.c.). At this stage, the lens has the shape of a spherical cone. The cellular material of the primitive vitreous (PV) fills the space in the optic cup, extending from the primitive retina to the lens vesicle. At this same time, the PV is penetrated by the hyaloid artery (HA), which extends to the posterior pole of the lens and divides into a capillary network that surrounds the lens. This is called the tunica vasculosa lentis (TVL). This network extends to the anterior surface of the lens and returns to anastomose with the annular vessel around the optic cup (the site of future iris development). Small, vascular loops arise from the annular ring vessel and extend to the anterior pole of the lens, forming the pupillary membrane (PM). At about day 45 p.c., the HA-TVL-PM system surrounds the rapidly growing lens, which is gradually assuming its mature lenticular form. From this point on, the vascular system begins regression. The posterior part of the HA-TVL system disappears approximately 2 to 3 weeks after birth. Anteriorly, the PM vanishes by 3 to 4 weeks after birth. Remaining parts of the HA-TVL-PM system that are still present 8 weeks after birth will not undergo further regression and will persist throughout life. At 6 to 8 weeks after birth, in puppies and kittens, a short remnant of the hyaloid artery is seen as a very small, white, spiral-shaped strand on the posterior pole of the lens (Mittendorf's dot). This is located just beneath and in between the ventral suture lines of the lens. This strand can only be seen with the use of a slit-lamp biomicroscope (15 to 20 power).

In the primitive lens itself, the epithelial cells at the posterior pole start to elongate, forming the primary fibers. Degeneration of their nuclei follows, and they migrate toward the center of the lens. These cells remain throughout life as the embryonic nucleus. Cells at the equatorial region of the lens proliferate and form secondary fibers. This is a continual process throughout life. The anterior tips of the elongating fibers lie under the lens epithelium, and the posterior ends lie directly under the posterior capsule. Where the fibers meet under the anterior epithelium, a Y- or X-shaped suture-line pattern is formed. Since the fibers are oriented with their anterior ends nearest to the anterior pole and their posterior ends farthest from the posterior pole, the posterior suture-lines form an inverted shape of the anterior pattern (⅄ or X). These fibers constitute the fetal nucleus. This structure is distinctly visible (by slit-lamp biomicroscope) directly under the capsule at 3 to 4 weeks after birth, in the still hazy infantile lens.

The lens capsule is primarily derived from the basement membrane of the lens epithelium, but some of it comes from the TVL–endothelial cell membrane material. Its formation starts at the posterior pole of the lens during the time when the TVL is surrounding the lens.

The zonular fibers seem to be produced by the endothelial cells of the TVL and by debris that surrounds the TVL, located in the vicinity of the equator. This process begins at the time when regression of the TVL starts. The zonular fibers were formerly incorrectly called "tertiary vitreous."

ANATOMY, PHYSIOLOGY, AND BIOCHEMISTRY

The anterior capsule of the lens lies directly behind the iris, in the posterior chamber. It is through the posterior chamber that the aqueous continuously flows, from the ciliary body toward the anterior chamber. The lens is thereby freshly bathed with aqueous. The lens enlarges as it ages, and there is more contact between the anterior lens capsule and the back of the iris. This forces the iris forward, following the convex shape of the lens and narrowing the anterior chamber angle. The lens usually measures 9 to 14 mm in diameter and is approximately 7 mm thick. It is usually somewhat larger than the diameter of the total dilated pupil. The lens is surrounded by a highly transparent capsule, which is approximately 50 μm thick anteriorly and 5 μm posteriorly. Although it contains no elastic fibers, the anterior capsule can resist relatively high tension forces, as long as it is not sharply perforated. The posterior capsule, however, is very delicate and should only be handled with great care.

The lens capsule, with its contents, is suspended by the zonular fibers. These fibers consist of numerous small, collagenous fibrils, which attach to the capsule at the equatorial region of the lens. On the other end, they insert into the depressions both in between and at the bases of the ciliary processes.

The lens consists of approximately 65 per cent water and 35 per cent proteins. The remaining material is composed of small amounts of minerals, sugars, and lipids.

The physiologic state of the lens proteins is an important factor in maintaining its transparency. Lens proteins are isolated from the rest of the body by the lens capsule at about the time when the HA-TVL network is surrounding the primitive lens fibers. This is most probably before the immune system becomes competent. Hence, animals may produce antibodies to their own lens proteins. This is clinically illustrated by a phacoanaphylactic reaction following either lens trauma or an extracapsular lens extraction. Additional complications arise if, at a later date, it becomes necessary to operate on the other eye. This is one reason favoring bilateral extracapsular lens extraction done in one procedure.

Since the lens has no blood supply, all nutrients and waste products must be exchanged through the capsule and into the aqueous. The main energy requirement of the lens is for growth of the fibers and maintenance of transparency. In order to remain transparent, the lens cannot contain high concentrations of pigmented respiratory enzymes.

Glucose is used as the main source of energy. Because of the very limited amount of oxygen in the aqueous, most of the glucose metabolism in the lens occurs through (1) the anaerobic Embden-Meyerhof pathway in addition to (2) the pentose shunt, (3) the breakdown of sorbitol and fructose, and (4) the Krebs cycle (mainly for the epithelial cells).

The vitreous is a large, highly elastic hydrogel, filling the globe behind the lens and keeping the retina smooth against the choroid. Because of its very low cellular content, there is a poor understanding of its anatomy and physiology. About 1 per cent of the vitreous consists of a meshwork of polygonal fibrils, which enclose single vitreous cells. The remaining 99 per cent is water. The fibril meshwork consists of highly polymerized hyaluronic acid and collagen, which allows for a high viscosity. Demarcation of the boundaries of the vitreous onto surrounding structures results from the condensations of fibrils, which are not true membranes. These condensations, as well as the colloid structure, guarantee the constant percentage of water within the aqueous that is necessary for a constant volume. This also prevents the invasion into the vitreous of cells, from either the aqueous or retinal capillaries, that could potentially disturb the visual axis.

Age Changes

Growth continues in the equatorial region of the lens throughout the life of the animal. This forms the adult nucleus, with the cortex around it. The suture lines in these layers have the shape of a Y anteriorly and a ⅄ posteriorly. Because of the continuous addition of fibers, the cortex thickens. Centrally the nuclei become more sclerotic, particularly because of the decrease in the percentage of soluble proteins. At 5 to 6 years of age, in both dogs and cats, there is a gradual but distinct loss of transparency in the center of the lens. This is referred to as nuclear sclerosis or, incorrectly, senile cataract.

Although this loss of transparency, which is especially visible in direct light, may be alarming to the owner or even the practitioner, it does not significantly affect the vision of the animal. Both indirect and, to a lesser extent, direct ophthalmoscopic examination of the retina remain possible. This is true even with 15- to 20-year-old animals.

Shortly after birth, the vitreous is still somewhat hazy but gradually clears. Demarcation structures of condensed vitreous fibrils around the regressed HA-TVL system (canalis hyaloideus and space of Erggelet) are rarely distinctly visible with routine slit-lamp biomicroscopy (10 to 20 power). Improved visual access to the vitreous is achieved with the use of a special fundus contact lens placed on the cornea. During aging, some condensation of vitreous material is expected. This is visible in the slit-lamp microscope beam as fine, white, cotton-wool-like strands. At an advanced age, the vitreous gradually dehydrates, resulting in decreased colloid stability, liquefaction, and the formation of fluid-filled cavities. This can be appreciated during both the slit-lamp microscopic and direct ophthalmoscopic examination and also, less commonly, during a hand slit-lamp, penlight, or direct ophthalmoscopic examination. This change is seen as a floating or streaming activity of the vitreous behind the lens; it follows the movements of the globe.

EXAMINATION OF LENS AND VITREOUS

A thorough examination of the lens requires a widely dilated pupil. Before mydriasis is induced, pupillary responses should be evaluated. Dilation should never be performed in cases of either primary or secondary glaucoma as it will increase the intraocular pressure significantly. Fifteen minutes prior to examination, apply a short-acting topical mydriatic such as 1.0 per cent tropicamide. In puppies and kittens, 1 drop of 0.5 to 1.0 per cent atropine is advised to induce sufficient mydriasis. This should be done at least 30 minutes prior to examination. The owner should be warned of possible secondary reactions, such as foamy salivation or vomiting directly following application.

Slit-lamp biomicroscopy is the most informative method of examination of lens and vitreous. If it is not available, examination with a penlight, flashlight, direct ophthalmoscope (including a slit-beam), or even an indirect ophthalmoscope may be very informative. The biomicroscopic appearance of the normal lens is produced by the difference in optical densities of the different media. Inspection should begin anteriorly with the dark aqueous. It follows the convex anterior capsule and epithelium into the deeper zones of discontinuity, which mark the subsequent layers of the nuclei. It concludes at the concave posterior capsule. Behind the posterior capsule, the light beam is lost in the dark vitreous. For inspection of the peripheral and posterior vitreous, special fundus contact lenses (Lovac fundus contact lenses, Medical Workshop, Groningen; H ruby or fundus lenses, West Coast Optical Instruments) with or without mirrors, respectively, are necessary. The zones of discontinuity are best seen with a thin slit-beam. Moreover, the observer must move the slit-beam focus (or the head of the animal) from front to back, left to right, and to the equatorial area. The direction of inspection must also move from left to right.

Other techniques used for this are wide-beam illumination and retroillumination. In the latter, a direct ophthalmoscope is used with a high-plus lens held about 10 cm from the eye. The light beam should point slightly upward onto the tapetum lucidum. If the technique is performed correctly, opacities are silhouetted against the fundus reflection. Indirect ophthalmoscopy is especially useful in cases of advanced cataracts because it permits inspection of the fundus, even through a very small transparent pinhole within the cataract. When funduscopy is no longer possible, the cataract is referred to as mature.

Transillumination through the sclera is of some value in ruling out large retrolental tumors. However, ultrasonography is far more selective for detection of tumors, detachments, hemorrhages, and foreign bodies in the retrolental space. Electroretinography is very useful in cases of mature cataracts to rule out retinal abnormalities, such as progressive retinal atrophy. It is advisable to document changes in lens shape, position, or transparency (or any other abnormalities found). This is useful for current records and for the later evaluation of progression of changes.

CONGENITAL AND DEVELOPMENTAL ANOMALIES

Aphakia

Aphakia, or absence of the lens, is a rare anomaly. In this abnormality, no sign of development of the lens is present. In general, this is part of a group of other severe ocular developmental disturbances, such as microphthalmia, microcornea, and a totally dysplastic globe. In a dysplastic globe, there may be a cyst or vesicle in the orbit, underneath the skin; it may occur with or without a lid fissure and contains parts of retina and uvea but no lens.

Coloboma

A coloboma of the lens is characterized by an equatorial notching. The zonular fibers are either deficient or absent in this area. Often there are other anomalies associated with it, or it is part of a syndrome of developmental errors, such as persistent hyperplastic TVL and PV (PHTVL/PHPV). The missing fibers cause unequal tension on the equator. The underlying cause for the defect may be a developmental error of the TVL in that area or a decreased or aberrant lens fiber activity.

Spherophakia and Microphakia

These conditions are both due to abnormal lens shapes; the lens may be either spherical or too small when examined in cross section. The central part may have a "normal" size, but the periphery is volume deficient. This causes a central bulging and a flattening in the periphery. In cases in which the lens diameter is too small, elongated ciliary processes may be present. Here, in general, normal lens metabolism is or has been deficient and results in either congenital or juvenile cataracts. Microphakia and spherophakia are often seen as part of other syndromes, such as PHTVL/PHPV.

Lenticonus (Globus)

Lenticonus, or globus, is defined as a cone- or globe-shaped bulge of the lens. It occurs most commonly in a central and posterior position and less frequently in the anterior part of the lens. A posterior conus may reach as far back as halfway to the retina. The capsule in this area may show dysplastic or degenerative changes, such as irregularity, dissolution, complete disappearance, or capsular rents. This directly or at a later time influences lens metabolism and thus results in a cataract. In most cases, the cataract will start in the dysplastic area of the capsule and later progress to a mature cataract. For this reason, a posterior conus usually can only be appreciated prior to development of a central anterior cataract and therefore is seen only in young dogs. Lenticonus is often associated with other anomalies or as part of syndromes such as PHTVL/PHPV. It is important to appreciate posterior lenticonus clinically before lens extraction is considered, because it may require a deep vitrectomy, which is a serious operative risk. In Doberman pinschers, posterior lenticonus is an inherited anomaly, as part of PHTVL/PHPV.

Persistent Hyaloid Artery

Larger parts of the obliterated hyaloid vessel that persist (without any other anomalies found, as in PHTVL/PHPV) are referred to as persistent hyaloid artery (PHA). This is a misleading term, as these remnants do not contain any blood. The small, off-white point of attachment to the posterior capsule is called Mittendorf's dot. The PHA is usually seen as a white thread, variable in length and up to 0.5 mm in diameter. It may move with the eye movements. Less frequently, it is seen as a complete thread extending from the lens to the center of the optic disk. Very rarely, other strands that do not follow the former hyaloid canal are found. These are presumably remnants of the vasa hyaloidea propria. In the case of a singular PHA, vision will not be influenced. PHA is usually an incidental finding during ophthalmic examination.

Persistent Hyperplastic Tunica Vasculosa Lentis and Primary Vitreous (PHTVL/PHPV)

PHTVL/PHPV refers to a group of dysplastic developmental anomalies that occur in the area between the HA, TVL, and the posterior part of the lens. In both animals and humans, it is a rare anomaly. Doberman pinschers are the exception, in which it occurs as an inherited disease. In the isolated cases found in different breeds, it may be either unilateral or bilateral. In Dobermans, the severe grades are always bilateral. PHTVL/PHPV seems to originate from a (hereditary) disharmony in the ontogenesis of the posterior capsule of the lens and the TVL. This is followed by a failure of the HA-TVL system to regress.

Clinically, in puppies as young as 4 weeks, severe grades of PHTVL/PHPV are recognized as leukocoria (white pupil) because of a whitish sheet behind the pupil. PHTVL/PHPV in Dobermans is characterized by bilateral (or less frequently, unilateral) retrolental pigmented fibrovascular tissue dots on the posterior capsule of the lens (grade 1). These dots can only be diagnosed with the use of a slit-lamp microscope (15 to 20 power).

The severe cases are characterized by a bilateral, retrolental, more or less pigmented, fibrovascular plaque located in the center of the posterior capsule of the lens. These are grade 2 cases, and they contain grade 1 dots in the periphery of the posterior capsule. The fibrovascular plaque of grade 2 can be associated with distinct persistent or patent parts of the HA-TVL system (grade 3). Sometimes a hyaloid vein may even be found. A posterior lenticonus is ranked as grade 4, and combinations of grades 2, 3, and 4 are classified as grade 5. Other associated anomalies such as microphakia, lens coloboma, retro- or intralental pigmentation, calcium or blood deposits, and elongated ciliary processes can also be found (grade 6). All severe grades (2 to 6) are accompanied by progressive cataracts, which start posteriorly and gradually involve the entire lens. In cases with a thin plaque (grade 2), cataracts generally progress slowly. A mature cataract results at about 5 to 6 years of age. In cases with heavy plaques or severe deformities of the posterior capsule (grades 4 to 6), dogs will be blind before they are 1 or 2 years old. All severe grades may be associated with persistent strings of the anterior TVL or persistent (epi)pupillary membranes. These are important signs of PHTVL/PHPV, in the event that inspection of the posterior lens is obscured by a cataract. Some eyes are found to be microphthalmic. Fundus abnormalities are limited to Bergmeister's papillae, and, infrequently, rosette-like areas (folds) of retinal dysplasia may also be present.

If the cataract is only in the central vision axis, therapy consists of one drop of 0.5 per cent atropine into the eye each morning. In cases of mature cataracts, only lens extraction may restore vision. There is a tendency to develop retropupillary membranes after extracapsular lens extraction. Therefore, in severe cases of PHTVL/PHPV, intracapsular extraction with anterior vitrectomy and cutting of the hyaloid artery appears to be the most promising technique. However, tearing of the zonular fibers is difficult. Complications such as hemorrhage from the transected HA and direct or subsequent retinal detachment (by traction bands) are to be expected. Because it is necessary to operate deep within the eye in cases of PHTVL/PHPV, addition of a muscle relaxant during anesthesia (see later discussion of lens extraction) is even more essential than it is in normal cataract surgery.

Although several severe cases of PHTVL/PHPV in Dobermans have been reported from all over Europe and the United States, the main source seems to be in the Netherlands (more than 250 severe cases during the past decade). A possible explanation may be that a few unrecognized carriers (or dogs in grades 2 to 6) were by chance used as breeding stock, just after World War II, to rebuild what is now a relatively large Dutch Doberman population.

PHTVL/PHPV in Dobermans has proved to be a hereditary defect. It is most likely an autosomal incomplete dominant trait, with variation in the expression. It is assumed that the heterozygous dogs for the mutant gene may be phenotypically free or show only grade 1 aberrations. Because therapy is relatively difficult, elimination of this disorder should rely on litter examinations and subsequent breeding programs.

CATARACT

Any opacity in the lens or its capsule is called a cataract. In animals with cataracts, it is important to know the age of onset, the location and type involved, and the degree of maturation and progression. It is also advisable to investigate initial signs of the cause of the cataract and to determine what therapy is possible.

Formation

Cataract formation is generally caused by reduced oxygen intake and a subsequent increase in water content. This causes swelling (intumescent cataract) of the lens, followed by dehydration.

In diabetes mellitus, concentration of glucose increases in the aqueous and subsequently in the lens. The excess glucose is diverted to the sorbitol pathway, resulting in accumulation of polyhydric alcohols. Because of the insolubility of these compounds, increased osmolarity results, causing the lens to hydrate and swell. The resulting loss of transparency is probably due to secondary cell membrane disruption, as well. Interruption of the ion pump in the cell membrane and a decreased percentage of soluble proteins are other causes for the loss of transparency, which may result in cataract. Early signs of cataract are vacuolization of the active cells of the lens (mainly equatorial region) and cyst formation in the intercellular spaces.

Attempts to retard cataract formation have not been successful. Moreover, those therapies that require intraocular administration may result in serious eye damage due to development of post-traumatic uveitis.

Congenital Cataract

Congenital cataracts are opacities present when the eyes first open, or within 8 weeks of age (an arbitrary cutoff point). Small, white, dense opacities in or near the suture lines (e.g., a Mittendorf's dot) or in the embryonic or fetal nucleus or at attachment points of associated anomalies (e.g., persistent pupillary membranes) are generally congenital. These cataracts are mostly nonprogressive or very slowly progressive and will not interfere with vision. In the case of a nuclear cataract having a diameter equal to that of the pupil diameter in daytime, 0.5 per cent atropine applied to the eye each morning may be helpful in restoring some vision. These cataracts are suspected to be hereditary entities in the Bouvier, German shepherd, and golden retriever.

Another type of cataract is suspected to be hereditary in such breeds as the beagle, Bouvier, Boston terrier, cavalier King Charles spaniel, German shepherd, golden and Labrador retrievers, Old English sheepdog, and West Highland white terrier. This is a characteristically larger dense cataract in the posterior pole. If gray cloudy areas or vacuoles are present, progression is most likely. Other causative factors that may contribute to cataract formation are irradiation, drugs, metabolic disease, infections, and malnutrition during gestation. However, when no distinct cause can be found (along with the fact that considerable inbreeding is common in many relatively rare breeds), hereditary factors should always be suspected when a bilateral cataract is present. For these reasons, examination of the littermates and both parents is important. When possible, a later backbreeding of the affected animal with a parent or another affected animal is highly informative to the breeder, if a genetic link is suspected. Otherwise, in cataracts of suspected hereditary origin, further breeding of the affected animal or its direct relatives should be avoided.

Although therapy (i.e., lens extraction) in very young animals is possible, the postoperative complication rate is markedly higher than it is in adults. Young animals are more active and untrained, and after the operation the patient is still missing its normal lens function. The owner should be well aware of these higher risks and later handicaps before deciding whether or not to keep or buy the animal.

Developmental Cataract

Cataracts that present after the first 8 weeks of life are called juvenile cataracts. Their cause and morphology follow the same pattern as for congenital cataracts. Other inherited diseases (e.g., progressive retinal atrophy [PRA], retinal dysplasia, or diabetes mellitus) are important contributory factors in the elderly animal. The term *senile cataract* may be used for small extra opacifications, which exceed normal lens sclerosis in old animals. These progress so slowly that, in general, there is no significant deterioration of vision.

Juvenile cataracts in young animals generally have a soft, fluffy appearance. In elderly animals, the nuclear area dehydrates progressively. The lens becomes a hard, breakable core, which shows suture-line bursts and is found in a soft, sticky cortex. When vision no longer exists and inspection of the fundus is no longer possible, the cataract is then referred to as mature. Later, the cortex may liquefy (hypermature). In the end stage, the cortex becomes glistening and milky, containing a small shrunken core with or without a wrinkled capsule (Morgagnian cataract). In some cases, the liquefied contents escape through the capsule, resulting in cataract resorption, which restores partial vision. On the other hand, the cortical material in the anterior chamber may cause a phacoanaphylactic reaction, resulting in uveitis and secondary glaucoma and requiring specific treatment.

The time course for maturation of a cataract is difficult to predict except in cases of diabetes mellitus, in which the cataract generally becomes mature within a few months. Until now, the only therapy has been lens extraction.

Pupillary responses are unreliable criteria for ruling out diseases such as PRA. This means that, in cases of bilateral mature cataracts, electroretinography (ERG) is the only way of diagnosing such underlying retinal dysfunctions. For these reasons, the patient should be sent directly to the cataract surgeon for evaluation of the deeper parts of the eye before the cataracts are mature or bilateral. In case of bilateral, mature cataracts, the patient should have an ERG prior to cataract surgery.

Indications and Contraindications for Cataract Surgery

Besides the ophthalmologic or overall physical health status of the patient, the animal's temperament and the owner's motivation are equally important when considering cataract surgery. These should be evaluated with the owner to estimate the operation risk and probable success rate. However, the primary indication for surgery is the degree to which the animal is handicapped. Many owners want to have their pet operated on even when, after evaluation, the animal appears to function successfully in its particular environment. In the owner's opinion, losing sight is a tragic occurrence; but realistically, the pet is losing one of its minor sense organs.

Preoperative Management

Prior to surgery, the owner should train the patient to accept wearing a protective collar (which is necessary postoperatively) as well as to tolerate topical and oral medication. Preoperative mydriasis (1 to 2 days before surgery) is achieved by using topical 1 per cent atropine, twice daily. One hour before surgery, 10 per cent phenylephrine may be helpful to induce mydriasis. Suppression of inflammatory reactions during and after surgery can be achieved with topical 0.1 per cent dexamethasone four times daily. This should be started 2 days before surgery. Also, one drop of topical anesthetic (oxybuprocaine 0.4 per cent)* given both 5 and 10 minutes preoperatively and 1 per cent indomethacin* both 1 and 3 hours preoperatively may aid in diminishing miosis. The latter medication also helps to control uveal exudation during intraocular surgery.

Anesthesia and Preparations for Intraocular Surgery

Two different methods of anesthesia are available to prevent exophthalmos and rotation of the globe during surgery, both of which are normally induced

*These preparations are unavailable in the United States.

with most forms of anesthesia. One method is halothane–nitrous oxide anesthesia with artificial respiration. Five minutes prior to actual surgery, a muscle relaxant such as pancuronium bromide (Pavulon, Organon) 0.05 to 0.1 mg/kg IV is given. This method allows for correct positioning of the globe during surgery.

One disadvantage of this method is the necessity of artificial respiration. It is good practice always to antagonize the muscle relaxant with 0.5 mg atropine IV followed a few minutes later with 0.5 mg per 10 ml neostigmine methylsulfate (Prostigmin, Roche) solution IV, given to effect.

The positioning of the patient and the head is important. The patient should lie with its head resting on the end of a table that is elevated about 5 degrees. The head should be positioned so the iris is in a plane that is more or less parallel to the floor. This is best effected by the use of a special vacuum cushion (Vapac, Howmedica). In this way, the vitreous, even when opened, will not tend to prolapse into the anterior chamber. Prolapse may occur when a cataractous posterior capsule is removed or an intracapsular lens extraction is to be performed. Also, in cases of lens luxation with glaucoma, these methods for anesthesia (the tilted table and the cushion) prevent the need for use of osmotic diuretics such as mannitol.

Because of the much larger cornea and deeper anterior chamber of animals (in comparison with humans) combined with the difficulty required to place the limbal plane into a horizontal position, the use of an operating microscope in animals has a more limited advantage. However, a 5- to 10-power magnifying loupe or microscope is indispensable for intraocular surgery.

Lens Extraction

The easiest approach to opening the eye is through a 160-degree dorsolateral limbal incision. This lessens the trauma, prevents hemorrhage, and is quick as well. Moreover, the prevention of postoperative astigmatism using a conjunctival flap method is less important in animals than it is in humans.

The most commonly used method for lens extraction in small animals is the extracapsular procedure. With this method, the posterior segment is not opened and ciliary hemorrhage is therefore prevented. However, postoperative lens-induced uveitis due to the liberated lens proteins is a disadvantage. Intracapsular lens extraction, the tearing of the zonular fibers, is difficult, and zonulysis by α-chymotrypsin (1:5000 to 1:7000) induces postoperative uveitis. In extracapsular extraction, disruption of the anterior capsule, with a still-closed anterior chamber (using a bent 0.5-mm cannula, as performed in humans), has no main advantage in animals because of the strength of the anterior capsule. Instead, anterior capsule removal can be accomplished by using two 0.2-mm toothed forceps; one serves for fixation while the other is used for rotating and tearing. The cortex and nucleus are then removed by loop and strabismus hook or flushing. Flushing is done with lactated Ringer's solution or, preferably, a specially balanced salt solution. The flushing is alternated with mild suction to remove remaining cortical fibers in both the equatorial area and against the posterior capsule. This is most important in preventing synechia and lens-induced postoperative uveitis. Twelve to 15 interrupted sutures using 8–0 silk or nylon are necessary for a good watertight and "barking-resistant" closure of the cornea. The sutures are removed 9 to 12 days postoperatively. Following the surgery, two 10-mg deposits of long-acting prednisolone are injected subconjunctivally.

Intraocular and intracorneal lens implants ranging from 14 to 33 diopters have been used in dogs after extra- and intracapsular procedures. They are well tolerated by the dog's eye. However, they introduce additional postoperative complications such as uveitis, secondary glaucoma, corneal edema, and iris atrophy, particularly after intracapsular procedures. Moreover, the estimation of the exact diopter strength in animals is difficult. For this reason, there is no real advantage of a lens prosthesis over an aphakic eye.

Discission and aspiration or phacofragmentation methods are limited in the lens to soft contents, which are generally only found in young animals. Rotoextractors are not efficient in removing the hard nucleus found in older animals or the plaques found in PHTVL/PHPV.

When possible, lens extraction should be performed bilaterally. This serves to restore optimal visual capacity, as well as to prevent the phacoanaphylactic reactions that occur when a second eye is operated on at a later time.

Postoperative Treatment and Complications

It is most important to have a cooperative and quiet (nonbarking) dog, especially during the first postoperative week. Should tranquilization become necessary, acepromazine is the most helpful. The patient should wear a protective collar for 2 weeks following surgery and should be kept on the leash for 3 to 4 weeks. Additional postoperative treatment consists of neomycin-polymyxin B eye drops four times daily for 2 weeks, topical 1 per cent atropine four times daily for 4 weeks, and 0.1 per cent dexamethasone for 4 to 6 weeks.

The most frequent postoperative complication is anterior uveitis. This may further result in synechia, deformed pupils, or complete occlusion of the pupil, in which case the dog becomes blind again. Secondary glaucoma may develop but is rare. However, the owner should be warned of this possibility before surgery, because it results in a return to blindness as well as pain for the patient and sometimes causes the loss of the eye.

LENS LUXATION

Luxation of the lens is the most common eye anomaly in many of the smaller breeds of terriers. However, it is infrequent in other breeds and rare in cats. Subluxation refers to a rupture of a region of the zonular fibers resulting in a minor displacement of the lens. In complete luxation, all fibers are disrupted, and the lens generally displaces in a ventral direction, leaving an aphakic crescent in the dorsal part. Luxations in young animals with gel-like vitreous generally go toward the anterior chamber. In cases of a liquefied vitreous, as found in many older patients, luxations occur more easily posterior and ventrally toward the vitreous space. In the predisposed breeds, such as the Welsh, Sealyham, fox, Tibetan, and German hunting terriers, the luxation occurs bilaterally, or the second eye follows the first luxation within a few months. The possible causes in hereditary luxations include a decreased number of zonular fibers and inflammatory reactions of the fibers, causing degenerative changes. The extra stress that the fibers endure in the highly active (barking) terriers may be another contributing factor inducing the rupture of already deficient fibers.

Therapy

Therapy consists of immediate initiation of glaucoma therapy. (See the article entitled Canine and Feline Glaucomas.) In anterior luxations (but also eventually in those that are posterior), glaucoma subsequently develops. The best therapy consists of intracapsular cryoprobe lens extraction. After the anterior chamber is opened, the lens is carefully attached with the cryoprobe (be careful not to touch the corneal endothelium or iris), twisted once around, and cut away from the vitreous with scissors. Prolapsed vitreous in the anterior chamber is picked up with a cellulose sponge and cut in front of the pupil. The cornea is closed by its presuture, and a large air bubble is placed in the anterior chamber, preventing further vitreous prolapse. It is important to keep this air bubble as large as possible during corneal suturing. After closure, a small, flattened irrigation cannula is inserted between sutures at the highest point of the wound. The cannula is then rotated 90 degrees. This allows the air to escape, and flushing solution can then be inserted. In cases of chronic anterior luxation, the capsule of the lens may be attached to the corneal endothelium. For this procedure, the capsule should be opened and transected as far as possible from the corneal adhesion. Extraction by force of the adhered capsule will cause severe endothelial damage and result in irreversible corneal edema.

Postoperative treatment is the same as for cataract extraction, with the exception of the use of atropine. Instead of atropine, topical 1 per cent pilocarpine is administered three times daily for prevention of vitreous prolapse.

OTHER VITREAL ABNORMALITIES

Vitreous Floaters

A floater, or musca volantis (gliding fly), is a small opacity in the vitreous; its shadow may stimulate the retina. Floaters may consist of small condensations of vitreous fibrils, of larger cholesterol crystals, or of small groups of white or red blood cells or pigment. Humans see them most readily against bright light. They usually move in the same direction as ocular movements. They are commonly found on routine examinations of elderly dogs. In rare cases, history reveals abnormal "flycatcher" or "mouse-trapper" reactions observed by the owner. These are sometimes only induced after illumination with a flashlight.

These cases should not be dismissed as insignificant. Careful inspection of the vitreous and the periphery by the use of a fundus contact lens, when possible, is indicated. In cases of a unilateral floater, the abnormal eye should be blindfolded with tape to see if the abnormal behavior stops. Sometimes the behavior of the dog is so disturbing to the owners that the problem must be solved by permanent tarsorrhaphy or even enucleation. Although vitrectomy would be indicated (when available), vitreous hemorrhages from the perforation through the ora serrata are more likely to occur in animals. When the floater consists of blood or exudate (generally darker and less circumscript), the origin of the floater in the retina or uvea should be found and treated when possible.

Asteroid Hyalosis

In asteroid hyalosis, several very small, somewhat pigmented dots are uni- or bilaterally scattered throughout the vitreous. They may move with eye movements but return to their place once the eye is still. They may be pigmented remnants of the hyaloid vessel system or degenerative calcium-lipid spheres in elderly dogs. They do not interfere with vision and do not require treatment.

Synchysis Scintillans

In synchysis scintillans, numerous cholesterol crystals with the appearance of sugar granules are settled at the lowest part of the vitreous space. The vitreous is generally liquefied and, when the eyes are moved, the crystals whirl through the vitreous like a snowstorm behind the lens. This abnormality may be found unilaterally or bilaterally in older dogs. It seldom interferes with vision, and therapy has not been described.

Injury to the Lens and Vitreous

Blunt trauma may cause contusions of the globe. Lesions may include subconjunctival hemorrhage, edema, ruptures of the sclera and cornea, hyphema, uveitis, indentation cataract, lens luxation, vitreous hemorrhage, retinal detachment, or glaucoma. Cataracts may develop many weeks after the injury. Secondary hemorrhage may develop 2 to 3 days after the injury. Therapy includes topical 1 per cent tropicamide, antibiotic-corticosteroid eye drops, and glaucoma therapy to lower intraocular pressure. The patient should be kept as quiet as possible.

Blunt trauma resulting in rupture of the globe with prolapse of the lens or vitreous material will generally cause panophthalmitis or glaucoma and result in subsequent blindness and possibly loss of the eye. Thorough questioning of the owner is necessary to determine if vitreous gel or lens material has prolapsed. This is an important criterion in determining the prognosis.

Penetrating trauma may be due to a cat nail, thorn, air rifle bullet, or shotgun pellet that penetrates the eye at high velocity. Prolapse of the lens contents or vitreous may occur at the entry or exit site of the foreign body. The penetration tunnel will be marked by synechiae, traction bands, and hemorrhage. X-ray examination of the skull may reveal the penetrating foreign body. Vitreous surgery currently used in humans is still an open field in veterinary ophthalmology.

Vitreous Hemorrhage

Hemorrhage in the vitreous, not originating from trauma, may vary from floaters to total filling of the vitreous cavity with blood. There is loss of fundus detail, and the fundus reflection is either red or totally absent. Hemorrhage is often due to rupture of a retinal vessel or is uveal in origin. It may also be complicated by retinal detachment. The origin may be hereditary in the collie eye anomaly or in congenital retinal detachment (dysplasia).

Other cases of vitreous hemorrhage usually originate from very serious ocular disease (e.g., chorioretinitis, retinal detachment) or may be due to systemic diseases (e.g., feline infectious peritonitis or leukemia or other malignancies in other species).

Vitreous Inflammation (Infection)

Vitreous inflammation has a wide spectrum of manifestations. It can be seen as various-sized clots of exudate, abscesses, or endophthalmitis formation. These inflammations are generally due to the same serious ocular or systemic diseases mentioned above. In rare cases, when therapy is successful, floaters, traction bands, or larger scars remain and affect vision. Retinal detachment due to traction bands may develop following the initial disease.

RETINAL DETACHMENT AND TUMORS

In cases of retinal vessel movement or if tissue is visible directly behind the lens, most often there is total retinal detachment. In some rare cases, a tumor filling the vitreous space may be accompanied by retinal detachment.

References and Supplemental Reading

Aguirre, G. D., Rubin, L. F., and Bistner, S. I.: Development of the canine eye. Am. J. Vet. Res. 33:2399, 1972.

Barnett, K. C.: Hereditary cataract in the dog. J. Small Anim. Pract. 19:109, 1978.

Bistner, S. I., Aguirre, G. D., and Batik, G.: *Atlas of Veterinary Ophthalmic Surgery*. Philadelphia: W. B. Saunders, 1977.

Davson, H.: *Physiology of the Eye*, 4th ed. New York: Churchill-Livingstone, 1980.

Gwin, R. M., and Gelatt, K. N.: The lens. *In* Gelatt, K. N. (ed.): *Veterinary Ophthalmology*. Philadelphia: Lea & Febiger, 1981, pp. 435–447.

Gwin, R. M., Warren, J. K., Samuelson, D. A., et al.: Effects of phacoemulsification and extracapsular lens removal on corneal thickness and endothelial cell density in the dog. Invest. Ophthalmol. Vis. Sci. 24:227, 1983.

Jaffe, N. S.: Cataract Surgery and Its Complications. St. Louis: C. V. Mosby, 1976.

Luntz, M. H.: Clinical types of cataract. *In* Duane, T. D., and Jeager, E. A. (eds.): *Clinical Ophthalmology*. New York: Harper & Row, 1982.

Martin, C. L.: Zonular defects in the dog. A clinical and scanning electron microscope study. J. Am. Anim. Hosp. Assoc. 14:571, 1978.

Playter, R. F.: The development and maturation of a cataract. J. Am. Anim. Hosp. Assoc. 13:317, 1977.

Pollet, L.: Refraction of normal and aphacic canine eyes. J. Am. Anim. Hosp. Assoc. 18:323, 1982.

Rathbun, W. B.: Biochemistry of the lens and cataractogenesis. Current concepts. Vet. Clin. North Am. [Small Anim. Pract.] 10:377, 1980.

Stades, F. C.: Persistent hyperplastic tunica vasculosa lentis and persistent hyperplastic primary vitreous (PHTVL/PHPV) in 90 closely related Doberman pinschers. Clinical aspects. J. Am. Anim. Hosp. Assoc. 16:739, 1980.

Yakely, W. L.: A study of heritability of cataracts in the American cocker spaniel. J.A.V.M.A. 172:814, 1978.

DISEASES OF THE RETINA AND OPTIC NERVE

NITA L. IRBY, D.V.M.
Kennett Square, Pennsylvania

The retina is a highly complex, specialized neuroectodermal tissue that lines the inner part of the eye from the ora ciliaris retina and ciliary body posteriorly. It is bounded anteriorly by the vitreous body. Externally, the retina lies against and is nourished, in part, by the choroid. A single layer of low cuboidal epithelial cells, the retinal pigment epithelium (RPE), is the outermost layer of the retina, adjacent to the choroid. This layer is then closely applied to a nine-layered sheet of sensory and glial tissue. The retina is a normally transparent layer, except where it overlies pigmented epithelium. The neural retina is firmly bound to the RPE at the ora serrata anteriorly and is firmly attached at the optic nerve posteriorly. Between these points, the retina is easily separated from the adjacent RPE. The blood supply to the inner two thirds is through the short posterior ciliary arteries. The retina is composed mostly of rods, but an area of increased cone density, the area centralis, occurs 3 to 4 mm dorsolaterally to the optic nerve. The retina is very susceptible to many insults and lacks regenerative potential.

The optic nerve is formed by coalescence of the ganglion cell axons and is composed of bulbar, retrobulbar or orbital, and intracranial portions. The optic disc, or bulbar portion of the optic nerve, is the only portion visible with an ophthalmoscope. The size, apparent position in relation to the tapetum, and degree of myelination of the optic disc vary greatly in the dog.

CONGENITAL DEFECTS

Retinal dysplasia is characterized histologically by disorganized, folded retina composed of immature neural elements with primary involvement of the outer retinal layers; it may be focal, multifocal, or diffuse. Ophthalmoscopically, the folds may appear as linear or round, gray elevations in the nontapetal fundus, or gray, hyperreflective scars associated with pigment disturbances in the tapetal fundus. Retinal dysplasia may be a focal lesion or associated with microphthalmia and other congenital ocular anomalies. Prenatal infections (canine herpesvirus and adenovirus, feline leukemia, and panleukopenia), irradiation, nutritional deficiencies, and trauma may produce dysplastic lesions in immature retinas but are difficult to prove. The cause may also be genetic (as in the Bedlington terrier, Australian shepherd, Sealyham terrier, Labrador retriever, beagle, American cocker spaniel, English springer spaniel, and collie), and affected individuals should be removed from breeding programs. Folds present in mildly affected individuals may disappear with age. In Labrador retrievers, the retinal dysplasia may be associated with skeletal chondrodysplasia.

Collie eye anomaly (CEA), or collie scleral ectasia syndrome, is an autosomal recessive disease that affects approximately 90 per cent of the collies in the United States. The primary lesion in CEA is choroidal hypoplasia, which appears as a pale, depigmented area, temporal to the optic disc, with exposure of a decreased number of underlying choroidal vessels. Surrounding RPE may also lack pigment. The lesion may vary in size from less than one disc diameter to three to four times larger than the disc. Small lesions present in puppies at 6 weeks of age may become pigmented by 1 year of age. Known to breeders as "go-normals," these animals are nonetheless affected and should be removed from breeding programs even though the overlying retina is normal.

A second defect, present in approximately 25 per cent of CEA cases, is an excavation of the posterior sclera or optic nerve and is known as a scleral ectasia or coloboma, respectively. The defects may be large or small in diameter or depth, and their size does not change with age. The defect may be lined with choroid or normal to dysplastic retina.

A third component of CEA, retinal detachments, is present in approximately 7 per cent of affected dogs. The majority of detachments occur within the first year and may be accompanied by severe intraocular hemorrhage. Early detachments are often evident adjacent to extensive colobomas. Tortuous primary retinal vessels may also be seen in CEA-affected individuals, but their significance is unknown.

A disease clinically similar to CEA occurs in a low percentage of shetland sheepdogs and Australian sheepdogs, but the pattern of inheritance has not been determined. Some German shepherds may exhibit the same spectrum of anomalies seen in CEA.

Optic nerve hypoplasia may be seen alone or with other ocular defects. It appears sporadically in many breeds but may be inherited in the beagle, poodle, and other breeds. Ophthalmoscopically, the optic disc is small and pale, and retinal veins may be dilated and tortuous. Pupillary light reflexes and vision are variable, depending on the degree of hypoplasia. Visual deficits are often not noticed in animals affected unilaterally.

Optic nerve colobomas are most commonly seen as part of CEA but may be seen in other breeds. The defect results from a failure of closure of the fetal fissure and may involve the entire optic nerve head. The affected area appears out of focus, and retinal vessels may appear to arch over the margins and disappear into large defects. Vision acuity in affected individuals is variable.

PROGRESSIVE RETINAL ATROPHY

The term *progressive retinal atrophy* (PRA) describes a group of hereditary retinal diseases, present in many different breeds of dogs, with similar clinical signs and ophthalmoscopic features but with unique physiologic and biochemical differences. The disease is common in the toy and miniature poodle, Irish setter, miniature schnauzer, English and American cocker spaniel, Norwegian elkhound, collie, Samoyed, Gordon setter, golden retriever, and Tibetan terrier breeds. An autosomal recessive transmission has been documented in the miniature poodle, Irish setter, collie, and Norwegian elkhound and is likely in other breeds. There is no sex predisposition. The age of onset of disease is determined by the pathogenesis of the disease and varies among breeds, from 6 months in the Irish setter and collie to middle age in the poodle and miniature schnauzer. The disease may be detected much earlier (by 6 weeks in the Irish setter and 9 to 12 weeks in the miniature poodle) with electroretinography (ERG). PRA may be subclassified, depending on the developmental abnormality present, into rod–cone dysplasia (early-onset PRA), rod dysplasia with cone degeneration (usually 1 to 3 years of age), and rod–cone degeneration (older animals).

The clinical signs of PRA are similar, regardless of the breed affected. Defective night vision (nyctalopia) is the first clinical sign but is often not detected or considered significant by many owners. As the disease progresses, day vision is progressively impaired. Central vision may persist for some time, because some owners report "sudden blindness" in their pets that have advanced disease, ophthalmoscopically. Owners are often unaware of visual problems until the dog is taken out of its home environment, probably because the slow onset of the disease allows the dog to accommodate. The resting pupil position and pupillary light reflex are often normal until late in the disease; therefore, pupillary light reflexes are a very poor indicator of retinal function. Cataracts often develop in eyes of dogs affected with PRA, thus necessitating ERG prior to cataract surgery in suspect breeds if the fundus cannot be seen.

Ophthalmoscopically, affected individuals first exhibit a gray, granular appearance of the peripheral tapetal retina when viewed with low-intensity illumination, with slight attenuation of the secondary retinal arterioles. The gray appearance is not due to pigmentary changes but results from diffraction of reflected light through the disorganized retina. Under bright-intensity light, the granular areas may appear hyperreflective. Early lesions are difficult to detect in the nontapetal portion of the fundus. As retinal disorganization and thinning progress centrally, the tapetum becomes increasingly hyperreflective, with centripetal attenuation of the retinal vessels. The end-stage lesions are uniform retinal thinning (with resultant increased reflectivity of the tapetum), severe vascular attenuation, and optic nerve atrophy. The nontapetal fundus becomes more lightly pigmented as a result of loss of retinal pigment epithelial cells; occasional hyperpigmented foci may be seen, however.

As stated above, an ERG is very beneficial in the diagnosis of PRA. Affected animals may be detected at early ages and eliminated from breeding stock, or animals of known status may be kept for test-breeding purposes. Suspect animals of any age can be confirmed with an ERG. Importantly, PRA can be diagnosed even in the presence of complete, mature cataracts, thus eliminating affected animals from surgery. There is no known treatment for PRA; the incidence of the disease can be controlled by careful breeding of unaffected individuals.

Central progressive retinal atrophy (CPRA) is rarely encountered in the United States but is common in Great Britain and Europe. It is most often noted in the Labrador, golden, and Chesapeake Bay retrievers, border collies, briards, Shetland sheepdogs, and English springer spaniels. CPRA usually appears between 2 and 6 years of age. It is a disease primarily involving the RPE, with secondary photoreceptor degeneration. Early in the disease there are hypertrophy and hyperplasia of RPE cells in the area centralis. Later, light brown lipofuscin-like granules accumulate in the hypertrophied RPE cells, and retinal degeneration follows. In every stage of the disease, the pathologic findings are more severe in the central portions of the retina.

The clinical presentation of patients affected with CPRA corresponds to the pathologic findings. Observant owners report visual acuity that is poor in bright light but improves in dimly lit situations, distant vision that is superior to near vision, and the ability to see moving objects better than still ones. The appearance through the ophthalmoscope also corresponds to the pathologic findings, and lesions are evident before decreased visual acuity is noted. The earliest changes noted are small, brown pigment clumps in the area centralis, with eventual involvement of the entire retina. Even in late stages of the disease, the lesions are most obvious clinically in the tapetal fundus. End-stage disease shows loss of pigmentation, loss of retinal vessels, and atrophy of the optic disc. The pattern of inheritance of the disease is unclear, and expression of the disease may be modified by environmental factors. An experimentally produced disease similar to CPRA ophthalmoscopically and histologically in beagles fed vitamin E–deficient rations has been reported. There is no treatment documented at the present time; however, until the retinal degeneration becomes advanced, visual acuity may be improved by dilating the pupils.

Retinal atrophy also occurs in cats, but not as frequently as in dogs. Feline central retinal degeneration, secondary to taurine deficiency, may be a slowly progressive disease. The earliest lesion is a granular appearance of the area centralis; this progresses to a larger, elliptical area of hyperreflectivity. Later, similar lesions may be seen nasal to the optic disc. Affected animals at this stage have normal vision clinically, but ERG will show reduced cone function. If taurine deficiency is prolonged, diffuse retinal atrophy may result. Cats are unable to synthesize taurine and must receive it in their diet. Meats, milk, and fish are all excellent sources of this amino acid.

An autosomal recessive PRA has been described in large numbers of Abyssinian cats in Sweden. The ophthalmoscopic changes in the Abyssinian cat are similar to those described above for dogs, except that 2- to 3-year-old affected individuals showed a complete change in color of the tapetum. The entire tapetum appeared gray, and the periphery was a darker gray. The earliest lesions were seen in cats 1 to 2 years of age. A progressive retinal atrophy has been described in Persian cats; rod–cone dysplasia has been described in a family of domestic shorthair cats.

Hemeralopia (day blindness) is much less common and has been reported only in the Alaskan malamute and miniature poodle. It is an autosomal recessive trait in the malamute. The dogs appear blind in daylight but have good vision at low light intensity and are ophthalmoscopically normal. ERGs recorded with bright light intensity, with flickers of 25 Hz or greater, can confirm the diagnosis. Diagnosis can also be made by histopathologic examination of affected retinas.

INFLAMMATORY DISEASES

Retinitis may occur unilaterally or bilaterally, in any age or breed or sex. The retina may be affected primarily, but, because of the close association of the retina and the choroid, it is often difficult to differentiate retinitis from choroiditis. Both of these tissues and adjacent vitreous may be inflamed simultaneously. Active retinal inflammation is characterized by perivascular or subretinal exudates, edema, cellular infiltrates, granulomas, or retinal detachments. Affected areas have fuzzy margins and are raised. Against the tapetal background, affected areas appear dull and dark, but the same lesion against a dark area of the fundus appears grayish white. Perivascular sheaths or "cuffs" and hemorrhages are seen variably. Resolution of active disease may lead to retinal degeneration, necrosis, and eventual atrophy with focal to multifocal areas of increased tapetal reflectivity. Retinal atrophy is evidenced in the nontapetal fundus as light brown areas. In either portion of the fundus, lesions may be associated with hyperpigmented clumps that result from proliferating, hyperplastic pigment epithelial cells. Retinal vessels associated with lesions may be attenuated.

There are many causes of retinochoroiditis and chorioretinitis in small animals, many with identical clinical appearances. *Toxoplasma gondii* is a common cause of retinochoroiditis in dogs and cats. Viral causes include canine distemper, feline infectious peritonitis (FIP), and the feline leukemia virus. A granulomatous chorioretinitis, as well as anterior uveitis, is often present in systemic mycotic diseases such as blastomycosis, histoplasmosis, cryptococcosis, and coccidioidomycosis, and in ocular disease due to the colorless algae *Prototheca*. Diagnosis of many of these diseases is facilitated by complete physical and neurologic evaluations, since they are usually multisystemic. Repeated serologic examination, aqueous or vitreous paracentesis, and spinal fluid paracentesis are helpful. If a specific cause can be found, treatment should be directed accordingly. The use of systemic corticosteroids is controversial in many of these diseases but may be indicated if blindness is imminent. Topical and subconjunctival corticosteroids penetrate minimally to the retina and choroid. Focal retinitis of unknown cause should not be treated.

Papillitis is defined as inflammation of the optic nerve head. *Optic neuritis* is a nonspecific term denoting inflammation anywhere along the nerve or tract. Numerous diseases should be considered in the differential diagnosis of optic neuritis, including canine distemper, cryptococcosis, toxoplasmosis, feline infectious peritonitis, lymphosarcoma, trauma, reticulosis, orbital neoplasia or abscess, and possibly an extension of disease from adjacent sinuses.

The optic disc may or may not be involved in

cases of optic neuritis. The typical historic finding in cases of bilateral optic neuritis is sudden, complete blindness. Astute owners may notice visual deficits prior to complete blindness. On examination, the animals often have widely opened, staring eyes with dilated, unresponsive pupils if the disease is bilateral. Unilateral cases may have normal resting pupil positions in room light. Careful testing will show an afferent pupil deficit (no direct or consensual response) when the affected eye is stimulated. If the optic disc is involved in the inflammatory process, it will appear large, swollen, and hyperemic and will have fuzzy borders. Hemorrhages may or may not be present. The peripapillary retina is often detached secondarily to the "pull" of the protruding disc or from subretinal exudates. Cases of retrobulbar optic neuritis, tentatively diagnosed when no disc abnormalities are evident, must be differentiated from sudden acquired retinal degeneration (SARD) via ERG (see page 673). In the author's experience, SARD is much more common than optic neuritis of any cause. This recently recognized syndrome may explain many of the cases of presumed optic neuritis seen in the past that did not respond to therapy, even when appropriate therapy was instituted rapidly.

The presence of other neurologic deficits would give further support to a diagnosis of optic neuritis, and careful cranial and peripheral nerve examinations should be performed. Other diagnostic procedures should include a cerebrospinal fluid paracentesis with opening pressure, total and differential cell counts, protein, and possibly culture, serologic, or fluorescent antibody determinations. Regardless of the cause, restoration of vision requires the immediate administration of local and systemic corticosteroids at immunosuppressive levels (2 mg/kg) to reduce inflammation and prevent demyelination of the optic nerve. Judicious corticosteroid use is indicated in suspected infectious cases. Additional initial therapy must be based on initial laboratory findings and clinical impressions. Generally, cases treated within 2 weeks from onset of disease have the best chance for restoration of vision following institution of therapy. These cases will usually have improvement in vision within 24 to 48 hours. Corticosteroids should be withdrawn very slowly, and the owner should monitor visual acuity (ability to catch toys, treats) and pupillary light reflexes daily. Recurrences are common. Systemic broad-spectrum antibiotics are recommended during immunosuppression.

VASCULAR DISEASES

Retinal hemorrhages may result from trauma, bleeding disorders, blood parasites, hyperviscosity syndromes, retinal inflammation, neoplasia, and congenital retinal or vascular anomalies (CEA, preretinal arterial loops). Retinal hemorrhages in cats occur with severe anemia, feline infectious peritonitis, and lymphoreticular diseases. Another common cause of focal to extensive retinal hemorrhage (with associated preretinal and subretinal exudates, retinal edema, and occasional destruction of the tapetum) is systemic hypertension secondary to renal disease, hyperadrenocorticism, or hypothyroidism. Primary hypertension has not yet been reported in dogs or cats. The retinal hemorrhages encountered with secondary hypertension may occur in any layer and often extend into the vitreous. Choroidal hemorrhages or infarcts may also occur and may explain the tapetal color changes seen in some cases.

As with inflammatory retinal diseases, patients with retinal hemorrhages require careful systemic and laboratory evaluation, including clotting profiles. A direct arterial blood pressure measurement to rule out hypertension should be performed in all cases of retinal hemorrhage with no apparent cause.

There is no specific treatment for retinal hemorrhages, but the inciting cause, if known, should be resolved as quickly as possible. Small hemorrhages often resolve without consequence, whereas large hemorrhages into the vitreous may result in immediate or delayed retinal detachment (vitreous traction bands). Many cases will have unilateral involvement initially, but, untreated, bilateral involvement is likely. Treatment of canine hypertension has been attempted with several antihypertensive drugs, but results to date are not encouraging, most likely because of poor control of the primary disease.

RETINAL DETACHMENT

Retinal detachment is a misnomer for what is actually a retinal separation. The separation occurs between the RPE and photoreceptor layers of the retina. A true retinal detachment would detach the RPE from adjacent choroid. Retinal detachments can be categorized into three basic groups: (1) those caused by subretinal exudates, tumors, or hemorrhage, which push the retina inward; (2) those that occur when the retina is pulled forward (vitreal traction bands secondary to vitreal inflammatory lesions or loss of the vitreous body); and (3) those occurring secondary to retinal tears, holes, or cysts. The cause should be pursued, but bear in mind that some retinal detachments reattach with tranquilization (rest), diurectics, corticosteroids, and time.

MISCELLANEOUS DISEASES

Peripheral cystoid retinal degeneration occurs in older dogs and is characterized by cyst formation within the peripheral sensory retina. One or many cysts may be present. The lesions can be best visualized with maximum mydriasis and indirect ophthalmoscopy. Visualization may be enhanced with scleral depression. The lesions are interesting to examine but have little clinical significance.

Sudden acquired retinal degeneration (SARD), also known as silent retina syndrome or metabolic toxic retinopathy, is a recently described syndrome causing sudden, apparently total, and permanent blindness in otherwise generally healthy animals. Affected animals examined soon after the onset of the disease appear normal ophthalmoscopically. The hallmark of the disease is a completely extinguished electroretinogram. The clinical presentation is identical to retrobulbar optic neuritis, and an ERG is mandatory for diagnosis. The disease is encountered equally in mixed-breed and purebred dogs, and it is therefore unlikely to be inherited. Affected dogs range in age from 6 to 14 years, may be of either sex, and are often obese. The incidence is more common in winter months. Dogs examined several months after onset of the disease show typical, nonspecific retinal degeneration, progressing to complete atrophy within approximately 1 year. No consistent hematologic or biochemical abnormalities have been found in affected dogs. Morphologic examination of tissue from affected dogs shows a rapid, widespread loss of structural integrity affecting rods and cones equally. The remainder of the retina degenerates slowly. The cause of this syndrome is unknown, in spite of multiple diagnostic efforts. The disease should be distinguished from retrobulbar optic neuritis, which, depending on the cause, will often respond to treatment. SARD-affected dogs have remained healthy for years after diagnosis, but they never regain sight.

Papilledema is defined as a noninflammatory swelling of the optic nerve head causing it to bulge into the vitreous. In primates, papilledema results from increased intracranial pressure, but this phenomenon rarely occurs in dogs and cats, perhaps due to anatomic differences. The condition must be differentiated from pseudopapilledema or excess myelination of the optic disc. Papilledema has been described in canine distemper, canine hypertension, optic nerve or orbital tumors, and low intraocular pressure. Papilledema may not result in loss of vision, in contrast to papillitis.

References and Supplemental Reading

Acland, G. M., Irby, N., Aguirre, G. D., et al.: Sudden acquired retinal degeneration in the dog: Clinical and morphological characterization of the "silent retina" syndrome. Trans. 15th Ann. Sci. Prog. Am. Col. Vet. Ophthalmol. Atlanta, November, 1984.

Aguirre, G. D.: Hereditary retinal diseases in small animals. Vet. Clin. North Am. 3:515, 1973.

Aguirre, G. D.: Retinal degeneration associated with the feeding of dog foods to cats. J.A.V.M.A. 172:791, 1978.

Aguirre, G. D., and Laties, A.: Pigment epithelial dystrophy in the dog. Exp. Eye Res. 23:247, 1976.

Bellhorn, R. W., Aguirre, G. D., and Bellhorn, M. B.: Feline central retinal degeneration. Inves. Ophthalmol. Vis. Sci. 13:608, 1974.

Irby, N.: Silent retina syndrome, an etiology of acute blindness in the dog. American College of Veterinary Ophthalmology, Lake Tahoe, 1982.

Narfstrom, K.: Progressive retinal atrophy in the Abyssinian cat. Svensk. Vet. 33:147, 1981.

Narfstrom, K.: Hereditary progressive retinal atrophy in the Abyssinian cat. J. Hered. 74:273, 1983.

Riis, R. C., Sheffy, B. E., Lowe, E., et al.: Vitamin E deficiency retinopathy in dogs. Am. J. Vet. Res. 42:74, 1981.

West-Hyde, L., and Buyukmichi, N.: Photoreceptor degeneration in a family of cats. J.A.V.M.A. 181:243, 1982.

Wolf, D., Vainisi, S. J., and Santos-Anderson, R.: Rod cone dysplasia in the collie. J.A.V.M.A. 173:1331, 1978.

OCULAR INFECTIOUS DISEASES

LOUIS J. LARATTA, D.V.M.
Ithaca, New York

The eyes can be involved in infectious diseases from direct environmental exposure, from hematogenous dispersion, or from migration of infectious agents from adjacent tissues. Infections localized to the eyelids, conjunctiva, and cornea are commonly seen in small animal practice. Predisposing factors such as conformational and functional eyelid abnormalities and precorneal tear film abnormalities may lower the normal resistance of the ocular and adnexal surfaces. These factors should be minimized or corrected when treating the infectious disease. Traumatic eye injuries are often complicated by opportunistic pathogens. Common bacterial organisms identified in surface infections usually repre-

Text continued on page 678

Table 1. *Infectious Bacterial Diseases Localized to Ocular and Adnexal Surfaces*

Ocular Signs or Lesions	Diagnostic Features	Objectives of Therapy	Therapy*
***Staphylococcus* or *Streptococcus* spp.**			
Conjunctivitis	Thick, mucopurulent ocular discharge, phagocytized bacteria on cytologic examination of conjunctiva, isolation of organism by culture	Control infection	Topical, broad-spectrum antibiotics (e.g., neomycin-polymyxin B–bacitracin, gentamicin) t.i.d-q.i.d.
Ulcerative keratitis	Yellow to white corneal infiltrates adjacent to ulcerated area	Control infection and preserve pupillary aperture/cycloplegia	Topical atropine sulfate 1% once or twice daily (to effect)
Blepharitis (*Staph.*)	Severe eyelid hyperemia and swelling	Control infection	Systemic broad-spectrum antibiotics (e.g., oxacillin [22 mg/kg PO t.i.d.], amoxicillin trihydrate/clavualanate potassium [13.75 mg/kg PO b.i.d.])
		If chronic, immunostimulation	Homologous *Staphylococcus* bacterin injection
***Pseudomonas* spp.**			
Conjunctivitis	History of previous topical or systemic glucocorticoid therapy or corneal trauma	Control infection	Intensive topical broad-spectrum antibiotic solutions (e.g., gentamicin, tobramycin) (every 1–2h), with or without subjconjunctival or systemic antibiotics
Ulcerative keratitis or collagenase-mediated stromal "melting"	Rapidly progressive corneal liquefaction, degeneration, and perforation	Control infection and arrest collagenase activity ("melting")	Topical acetylcysteine 10% solution, one drop every 1–2 hours (to effect) or topical disodium edetate solution every 1–2 hours (to effect) (may be irritating)
		Preserve pupillary aperture/cycloplegia	Topical atropine sulfate 1% solution q.i.d.

*Refer to Table 6 for trade names and manufacturers.

Table 2. *Systemic Infectious Viral Diseases*

Ocular Signs or Lesions	Objectives of Therapy	Therapy*	Systemic Signs or Lesions	Diagnostic Features
Infectious Canine Hepatitis				
Corneal stromal edema (diffuse)	If active, decrease uveal inflammation	Topical glucocorticoids (e.g., dexamethasone 0.5–1.0%) t.i.d.–q.i.d.	History of recent (2–3 weeks) vaccination or unvaccinated, fever, tonsillitis, pharyngitis, coughing, peripheral lymphadenopathy, hepatomegaly, petechiae, ecchymoses	Leukopenia (lymphopenia and neutropenia), thyrombocytopenia, increased liver enzymes, bilirubinuria, proteinuria
Anterior uveitis	Preserve pupillary aperture/cycloplegia	Topical atropine sulfate 1% once or twice daily		
Secondary glaucoma (especially Afghan, basset hound, American cocker spaniel, Siberian husky, Samoyed)	Decrease aqueous production	Carbonic anydrase inhibitors (e.g., dichlorphenamide PO 2–10 mg/kg, once daily to t.i.d. initially) Topical timolol maleate 0.5% one drop once or twice daily		
	Facilitate aqueous outflow	Discontinue cycloplegics Supportive systemic therapy		
Canine Distemper Virus				
Keratoconjunctivitis sicca (lacrimal adenitis)	Tear replacement	Topical artificial tear solutions every 2–3 hours Topical ophthalmic lubricant t.i.d.–q.i.d.	Depression, fever, nasal discharge, coughing, dyspnea, anorexia, vomiting, diarrhea, dehydration, seizures, paresis, paralysis, blindness	Clinical signs, lymphopenia, positive fluorescent antibody test (FA) on epithelial cells (e.g., conjunctival), with or without distemper intracellular inclusions in erythrocytes, lymphocytes

Table continued on opposite page

Table 2. *Systemic Infectious Viral Diseases* Continued

Ocular Signs or Lesions	Objectives of Therapy	Therapy*	Systemic Signs or Lesions	Diagnostic Features
Keratoconjunctivitis sicca (*continued*)	Increase tear production	Oral 2% pilocarpine 1–4 drops once or twice daily		
Ulcerative keratitis	Control or prevent secondary bacterial infection	Topical broad-spectrum antibiotics (e.g., neomycin-bacitracin–polymyxin B ointment) t.i.d.–q.i.d.		
	Preserve pupillary aperture/cycloplegia	Topical atropine sulfate 1% once or twice daily		
Optic neuritis or chorioretinitis	If no systemic signs, decrease uveal inflammation	For optic neuritis: oral prednisolone 2 mg/kg once daily for 5 days then 1 mg/kg for 5 days, then decrease to alternate-day therapy and half dosage		
	Prevent secondary infection	Systemic broad-spectrum antibiotics (e.g., ampicillin 20 mg/kg PO t.i.d.)		
		Supportive systemic therapy		
Feline Leukemia Complex				
Anterior uveitis: including keratic precipitates, hypotony, aqueous flare, hypopyon, posterior synechiae, granulomatous iris infiltration	Decrease uveal inflammation	Topical antibiotic-glucocorticoids (e.g., neomycin-polymyxin B–dexamethasone ointment)	Effusive form: fever, anorexia, lethargy, icterus, dyspnea, abdominal distention	Pale, yellow to amber pleural fibrinous fluid, high protein content, supportive serologic testing
	Preserve pupillary aperture/cycloplegia	Topical atropine sulfate 1% ointment once or twice daily	Noneffusive form: fever, malaise, mesenteric lymphadenopathy, pneumonia, vasculitis, paresis, paralysis, seizures	Pyogranulomatous lesions: supportive serologic testing
Secondary glaucoma	Decrease aqueous production	Carbonic anhydrase inhibitors (e.g., dichlorphenamide PO 2–10 mg/kg once daily to t.i.d. initially		
		Topical timolol maleate 0.5% one drop once or twice daily		
	Facilitate aqueous outflow	Discontinue cycloplegics		
		Supportive systemic therapy		
Feline Viral Rhinotracheitis (Herpes)				
Corneal ulceration or keratitis	Inhibit virus replication	Topical idoxuridine or vidarabine 4–6 times/day	Depression, sneezing, oculonasal discharge, coughing, oral ulcers	Clinical signs and positive FA of conjunctival or nasal epithelial cells
Conjunctivitis	Prevent or control secondary infection	Topical oxytetracycline or chloramphenicol t.i.d.–q.i.d.		
Blepharospasm	Preserve pupillary aperture/cycloplegia	Topical atropine sulfate b.i.d.–t.i.d.		
Chemosis	Reduce chemosis	Topical 5% NaCl (hyperosmotic) ointment b.i.d.–t.i.d.		
Feline Calicivirus Disease				
Conjunctivitis	Prevent or control secondary infection	Topical oxytetracycline or chloramphenicol t.i.d.–q.i.d.	Depression, fever, sneezing, oculonasal discharge, coughing, oral ulcers	Clinical signs and positive FA of conjunctival or nasal epithelial cells
Blepharospasm	Preserve pupillary aperture/cycloplegia	Topical atropine sulfate b.i.d.–t.i.d.		
Chemosis	Reduce chemosis	Topical 5% NaCl (hyperosmotic) ointment b.i.d.–t.i.d.		

*Refer to Table 6 for trade names and manufacturers.

Table 3. Miscellaneous Systemic Infectious Disease

Ocular Signs or Lesions	Objectives of Therapy	Therapy*	Systemic Signs or Lesions	Diagnostic Features
Chlamydia psittaci (felis)				
Conjunctivitis	Control infection	Topical oxytetracycline or chloramphenicol ointment t.i.d.–q.i.d. (2–3 weeks duration)	Occasional fever, oculonasal discharge	Occasional conjunctival intracytoplasmic inclusions (if early); relapses occur
Blepharospasm Chemosis	Reduce chemosis	Topical 5% NaCl (hyperosmotic) ointment b.i.d.–t.i.d.		
Mycoplasma felis				
Conjunctivitis, with or without pseudomembrane formation	Control infection	Topical oxytetracycline or chloramphenicol ointment t.i.d.–q.i.d. (2–3 weeks duration)	Occasional oculonasal discharge	Occasional conjunctival cell membrane organisms
Blepharospasm Chemosis	Reduce chemosis	Topical 5% NaCl (hyperosmotic) ointment b.i.d.–t.i.d.		
Rickettsia				
Ehrlichia canis				
Hyphema Uveitis	Decrease uveal inflammation	Topical antibiotic/glucocorticoid (e.g., neomycin-polymyxin B-dexamethasone) ointment t.i.d.–q.i.d.	Fever, anorexia, dyspnea, lymphadenopathy; if chronic, depression, weight loss, epistaxis, petechiae	Clinical signs: acute: monocytic morula inclusions, increased liver enzymes, increased globulins; chronic: pancytopenia, serologic testing
Subconjunctival hemorrhage	Preserve pupillary aperture/cycloplegia	Topical atropine sulfate 1% b.i.d.–t.i.d. (to effect)		
	Control infection	Systemic tetracycline therapy Supportive systemic therapy		
***Haemobartonella* spp.**				
Retinal hemorrhages (secondary to anemia)	Control infection	Systemic tetracycline, with or without systemic glucocorticoid therapy Supportive systemic therapy	Depression, weakness, anorexia, weight loss, pale mucous membranes	Regenerative anemia, parasites on erythrocytes
Protozoan (Toxoplasma gondii)				
Anterior uveitis Chorioretinitis Optic neuritis	Decrease uveal inflammation	Topical antibiotic/glucocorcoticoid (e.g., neomycin-polymyxin B–dexamethasone) ointment t.i.d.–q.i.d.	May or may not show multifocal CNS abnormalities, fever, dyspnea, myositis, hepatitis, lymphadenopathy	Fecal oocysts (feline), supportive serologic testing
Myositis (extraocular muscle)	Preserve pupillary aperture/cycloplegia	Topical atropine sulfate 1% b.i.d.–t.i.d. (to effect)		
	Control infection	Systemic trimethoprim/sulfadiazine and folic acid supplementation		

*Refer to Table 6 for trade names and manufacturers.

Table 4. Systemic Bacterial Infectious Diseases

Ocular Signs or Lesions	Objectives of Therapy	Therapy*	Systemic Signs or Lesions	Diagnostic Features
Brucella canis				
Anterior uveitis (including hypotony, aqueous flare, hypopyon)	Decrease uveal inflammation	Topical antibiotic-glucocorticoid ointment (e.g., neomycin-polymyxin B–dexamethasone) ointment t.i.d.–q.i.d.	Epididymitis, prostatitis, abortions, diskospondylitis, glomerulonephritis, meningoencephalitis	Serologic tests, blood culture
	Preserve pupillary aperture/cycloplegia	Topical atropine sulfate 1% once or twice daily (to effect)		
	Control infection (difficult)	Systemic oxytetracycline or minocycline		
***Leptospira* spp.**				
Anterior uveitis (including hypotony, aqueous flare, hypopyon)	Decrease uveal inflammation	Topical antibiotic-glucocorticoid ointment (e.g., neomycin-polymyxin b–dexamethasone) ointment t.i.d.–q.i.d.	Fever, myalgia, anorexia, vomiting, dehydration, petechiae, ecchymoses, icterus	Renal impairment, increased serum liver enzymes, thrombocytopenia, serologic testing, leptospiruria
	Preserve pupillary aperture/cycloplegia	Topical atropine sulfate 1% once or twice daily (to effect)		
	Control infection	Systemic penicillin		
Other				
Bacteremias (e.g., *Staphylococcus* spp., *Streptococcus* spp., *Escherichia coli*)				
Endophthalmitis	Control infection	Subconjunctival, intracameral, parenteral broad-spectrum antibiotics	Variable depending on organs involved including fever, tachycardia, cardiac arrhythmias, cardiac murmurs	Leukocytosis with left shift, monocytosis, anemia, hematuria, pyuria, bacteriuria, blood culture
Secondary glaucoma	Decrease aqueous production	Carbonic anhydrase inhibitors, (e.g., dichlorphenamide PO 2–10 mg/kg once or twice daily initially)		
		Topical timolol maleate 0.5% one drop once or twice daily		
	Facilitate aqueous outflow	Discontinue cycloplegics		

*Refer to Table 6 for trade names and manufacturers.

Table 5. *Systemic Mycotic Infectious Diseases*

Ocular Signs or Lesions	Objectives of Therapy	Therapy*	Systemic Signs or Lesions	Diagnostic Features
Cryptococcus neoformans *Blastomyces dermatitidis* *Coccidioides immitis* *Histoplasma capsulatum*				
Granulomatous uveitis (including aqueous flare, chorioretinitis, retinal detachment, optic neuritis)	Control infection (difficult)	Systemic amphotericin B with or without ketoconazole	Cough, dyspnea, nasal discharge, fever, draining skin lesions, localized peripheral lymphadenopathy, lameness, gastrointestinal disturbances *(Histoplasma)*, CNS disturbances *(Cryptococcus)*	Geographic location, leukocytosis, monocytosis, organism identified by biopsy, cytology, or culture, serologic testing
	Decrease aqueous production	Carbonic anhydrase inhibitors (e.g., dichlorphenamide PO 2–10 mg/kg once or twice daily initially Topical timolol maleate 0.5% one drop once or twice daily		
	Facilitate aqueous outflow	Discontinue cycloplegics		

*Refer to Table 6 for trade names and manufacturers.

sent the overgrowth of a particular organism present as part of the normal flora. Table 1 lists common organisms involved in surface infections, outlines therapeutic objectives, and suggests therapy. Many systemic infectious diseases involve the ocular tissues. However, the chief complaint may or may not relate to an ocular problem. A thorough ophthalmic examination can provide valuable diagnostic clues to an undiagnosed systemic disease. Tables 2 through 6 list documented ocular signs and lesions associated with systemic infectious diseases and offer guidelines for approaching ocular therapy in such cases. The importance of specific systemic therapy, if available, and supportive care for patients with these diseases listed cannot be overemphasized.

Table 6. *Veterinary Ophthalmic Agents**

Generic Name	Trade Name	Manufacturer
Acetylcysteine 10% solution	Mucomyst	Mead Johnson
Amoxicillin trihydrate and clavualanate potassium	Clavamox	Beecham
Artificial tears	Tears Naturale	Alcon
Atropine	Atropine sulfate 1%	Pharmfair
Chloramphenicol	Chloromycetin	Parke-Davis
Dexamethasone	Maxidex, Maxitrol	Alcon
Dichlorphenamide	Daranide	Merck Sharp & Dohme
Disodium edetate solution	Endrate	Abbott
Gentamicin	Gentocin	Schering
Idoxuridine	Stoxil	SmithKline Beckman
Neomycin, polymyxin B, and bacitracin	Neosporin	Burroughs Wellcome
Oxacillin	Bactocill	Beecham
Oxytetracycline	Terramycin	Pfizer
Pilocarpine	Pilocar	CooperVision
Sodium chloride (NaCl) 5%	Muro 128	Muro
Timolol maleate	Timoptic	Merck Sharp & Dohme
Tobramycin	Tobrex	Alcon
Vidarabine	Vira-A	Parke-Davis

*See also page 684, Contemporary Ocular Therapeutics.

References and Supplemental Reading

Barlough, J. E.: Serodiagnostic aids and management practice for feline retrovirus and coronavirus infections. Vet. Clin. North Am. 14:955, 1984.

Bistner, S., and Shaw, D.: Intraocular inflammation. *In* Kirk, R. W. (ed.): *Current Veterinary Therapy VIII.* Philadelphia: W. B. Saunders, 1983, pp. 582–589.

Ford, R. B.: Infectious respiratory disease. Vet. Clin. North Am. 14:985, 1984.

Gaskin, J. M.: Microbiology of the canine and feline eye. Vet. Clin. North Am. 10:303, 1980.

Green, C. E.: *Clinical Microbiology of Infectious Diseases of the Dog and Cat.* Philadelphia: W. B. Saunders, 1984.

Martin, C. L.: The eye and systemic disease. *In* Kirk, R. W. (ed.): *Current Veterinary Therapy VII.* Philadelphia: W. B. Saunders, 1980, pp. 593–600.

Peiffer, R. L., Jr.: Ocular manifestations of systemic disease. *Textbook of Veterinary Ophthalmology.* Gelatt, K. N. (ed.). Philadelphia: Lea & Febiger, 1981, pp. 699–723.

TUMORS OF THE EYE AND ADNEXA

RONALD C. RIIS, D.V.M.
Ithaca, New York

ADNEXAL TUMORS

Ocular tumors may be associated with the adnexal structures, extraocular tissue, or intraocular tissue or may involve several of these tissues. Each of these three general areas have tissue characteristics for tumor predilection types. When the wide variety of types of tissues around the eye are taken into consideration, almost any type of tumor may be found. However, some are more common than others.

Eyelid tumors are among the most commonly encountered. Fortunately most are benign sebaceous gland adenomas arising from the meibomian glands. Inflammatory involvement of these glands may be the precursor to their enlargement. It has been estimated that 44 to 60 per cent of the lid tumors in dogs are sebaceous gland tumors. Other epithelial tumors such as papillomas, squamous cell carcinomas, and basal cell carcinomas are less common. In general, lid tumors are not highly malignant but may be locally invasive and disfiguring and may impair normal lid function. Most of these tumors are amenable to a variety of therapies, but the smaller the tumor the easier it is to treat.

Surgical excisional biopsy is recommended for most lid tumors. Tumors as large as 1 cm^2 can be removed by a wedge or pentagonal excision, but if more than one fourth to one third of the eyelid is excised, blepharoplastic procedures using sliding skin grafts and tarsoconjunctival grafts should be performed. Cryotherapy, thermotherapy, immunotherapy, and radiotherapy are alternate methods of treatment.

Debulking lid tumors prior to additional therapy is a wise idea to obtain adequate samples for histologic confirmation and to minimize the tissue mass that has to be destroyed by thermotherapy, cryotherapy, immunotherapy, chemotherapy, or radiation therapy.

Conjunctival tumors are almost always some form of epithelial proliferation. These vary from epithelial hypertrophic plaques to papillomas to carcinomas. The depth and breadth of their involvement is extremely variable. Fortunately, they are also treatable by means other than surgery.

A pseudotumor caused by repository corticosteroids given subconjunctivally may be confused with nodular episcleritis, focal scleritis, granulomatous sclerouveitis, or a focal tumor. They are distinctly yellow and mobile. Pseudotumors have been noted to occur after the eye is treated for other conditions by an injection. They may have to be surgically removed if they appear to cause an inflammatory reaction.

Fibrous histiocytomas (FH) are inflammatory in cellular morphology but proliferate significantly from the eyelid and conjunctival surfaces. These tumors can be very invasive; however, they usually respond to a combination of therapies (see Chemotherapy). Several rare experiences with this tumor suggest that it has the ability to alter its characteristics and become neoplastic (i.e., change into a fibrosarcoma, possibly stimulated by steroid therapy).

FH are noted more frequently in the collie, but other breeds also have been affected. Nodular fasciitis (NF) is similar histologically, also involving the fascia of the episclera, nictitans, and subcutaneous tissues of the eyelids. The author believes that NF and FH are the same tumor, both sensitive to similar therapy as discussed later.

Conjunctival nevi and primary epibulbar melanomas should be monitored for size enlargement over extended periods rather than subjected to hasty surgical excision. They should be removed when their growth is documented or when they become invasive. They are benign, however.

Plasmomas and hemangiomas are similar benign tumors that appear red to pink and nodular. They are variably responsive to topical steroids, but some require more radical therapy.

Other conjunctival tumors usually arise from deeper orbital structures and manifest as a swelling, which either displaces the globe or impairs extraocular muscle function. These are orbital tumors that can be primary from tissues surrounding the globe or from cavities adjacent to the orbit. Since this area contains a wide variety of tissues, almost any type of tumor may develop. With the exclusion of cystic structures from the primary lacrimal gland, accessory lacrimal gland, or zygomatic salivary glands, all other masses within the extraocular category are usually neoplastic.

Radiographic evaluations of the skull and orbit aid in deciding the course of therapy. During anesthesia for radiographs, a biopsy of the tumor or fluid aspiration for cytologic testing and composition is recommended. For swellings ventral to the globe, sialograms of the zygomatic tissues can be informative. Other special techniques may give added information, but the patient's welfare should be seriously considered before performing positive contrast orbitograms, negative contrast (air) orbitograms, computed tomography, angiograms or venograms, or thecograms.

Meningiomas are the most frequent primary extraocular or orbital neoplasms that invade the globe.

A recent report (Kern, 1985) of orbital tumors in small animals indicated that the majority were malignant.

GLOBE TUMORS

Intraocular tumors may be neoplastic or benign tissue. These tumors may be noted on the iris surface, protruding into the pupil space from the ciliary area, displacing the lens, or emerging through the sclera.

Generally, intraocular tumors are identified as either pigmented or nonpigmented and can be primary or metastatic.

Malignant melanomas are the most common intraocular uveal neoplasms. They are usually pigmented and most frequently involve the iris and ciliary body. With clinical signs of persistent iridocyclitis, hyphema, glaucoma, and pain, always rule out the possibility of an intraocular neoplasm.

The most common primary, nonpigmented anterior uveal tumors are the adenomas and adenocarcinomas. They are usually noted at the iris base, bulging through the iridocorneal angle, or as a mass arising behind the iris into the pupil. Neuroectodermal neoplasms or embryonic medulloepitheliomas are also nonpigmented but are less common.

If a nonpigmented intraocular tumor of the anterior uvea can be precisely localized by the use of gonioscopy, direct and indirect ophthalmoscopy, or transillumination and ultrasonography, surgical removal by iridectomy or cyclectomy may be possible. For those tumors that cannot be localized, enucleation or exenteration is recommended.

Adenocarcinomas are invasive as well as proliferative. Adenocarcinomas are more likely to cause intraocular complications. These include glaucoma, lens displacement, and retinal detachment. Primary adenocarcinomas of the uveal tract are known for their pulmonary and liver metastases.

The secondary intraocular tumors occur by extension from the orbit, conjunctiva, or cornea and enter the globe through the optic nerve or cornea or by hematogenous spread. The sclera is most resistant to external invasion. Depending on the tumor cell morphology and characteristics, penetrance into the globe is variable. Hematogenous metastasis to the eye from other organs should always be ruled out when a primary site away from the eye is noted. It is believed that in cases of generalized neoplasia, intraocular metastasis is fairly common in animals.

Metastasizing or secondary intraocular tumors are frequent enough to warrant an ocular evaluation in each case in which neoplasia is diagnosed. Lymphosarcoma, adenocarcinoma, hemangiosarcoma, giant cell sarcoma, fibrosarcoma, and transmissible venereal tumor may affect the uvea secondarily. If uveitis or hyphema does not respond to uveitis therapy and if the cause remains unclear, the patient should be thoroughly re-evaluated for a primary neoplasm that has secondarily metastasized to the ocular uveal tissue. The evaluations should always include chest radiographs. Metastatic intraocular carcinomas may originate from the breast, lung, gastrointestinal tract, ovary, uterus, kidney, liver, pancreas, testicle, thyroid, prostate, salivary glands, and skin glands. Remember that in cats, feline lymphosarcoma-leukemia complex is the most frequent intraocular neoplasm, but it may involve any or all ophthalmic structures.

Intraocular extensions from the optic nerve are seen with meningiomas, astrocytomas, gliomas, gangliogliomas, and reticulosis. These cases may appear clinically as an optic neuritis (e.g., blindness with a dilated, unresponsive pupil).

Contagious venereal tumor (CVT) in dogs is the only naturally transmissible neoplasm known to infect small animals. Histologically, this tumor is characteristically a round cell sarcoma, appearing extraocularly with the ability to penetrate the sclera and invade uveal tissue.

RETICULOSIS

Reticulosis or chronic granulomatous encephalitis, a common cause of optic neuropathy, is a proliferation of reticulohistiocytic or mononuclear cells thought to originate from the adventitial layers of blood vessels in the central nervous system (CNS). Blindness caused by reticulosis may be reversed by giving systemic corticosteroids. A diagnostic plan should include a cerebrospinal fluid (CSF) tap. A relatively low nucleated cell count made up of mononuclear cells (10 to 100 cells/μl) and a moderately elevated total protein (30 to 100 mg/dl) rule out infectious causes, and intense steroid therapy can be initiated without fear of unwanted complications. The following plan of prednisone or prednisolone therapy should be effective:

2 mg/kg/day for 1 week, then
1 mg/kg/day for 1 week, then
0.5 mg/kg/day for 1 week, then
0.5 mg/kg/every other day for 1 week, then
0.25 mg/kg/every other day for 1 week, then
0.25 mg/kg/every third day for 1 week.

During the first 2 weeks, the patient should be given chloramphenicol 20 to 25 mg/kg orally to cover the immunosuppressed state. In addition to oral medication, retrobulbar steroids (6 mg/eye prednisolone acetate) or flunixin meglumine (12 to 15 mg/eye) has been used. If vision returns with this therapy, it usually does so in the first 2 weeks. If vision is lost again while the steroids are being reduced, return to the previous level and maintain at that dose for 2 weeks. The prognosis is guarded.

Other useful diagnostic aids may include ocular ultrasonography and brain scans. They are especially helpful in the evaluation of the eye structures if hyphema is present or if the cornea or the lens is opaque. Ultrasonography is excellent to display the presence of a retinal detachment, tumor, foreign body, or lens displacements. Brain scans using technetium^{99m} citrate have been beneficial, as increased uptake in the area of the optic nerves or within the CNS signifies proliferating or inflammatory cell invasion.

SURGICAL THERAPY OF SUPERFICIAL TUMORS

In dogs, lid margin extirpation techniques are usually curative for small tumors. Conjunctivocorneal tumors should be removed by superficial keratectomy and conjunctival dissection. Care should be taken to limit surgical manipulation of tumors that etiologically stem from virus. Suspicious tumors in this category are papillomas, venereal tumors, and fibrosarcomas. Cryosurgery destroys such tumors *in situ*, minimizing virus seeding and providing acceptable cosmetic results. Avoid cryosurgery of the cornea. Electrosurgery or electrocautery of lid tumors is not successful and, therefore, not recommended. In addition, scarring resulting in lid deformity is a likely sequela. The excision of a tumor with sharp dissection or electroscalpel and proper suturing of the healthy margins is recommended.

CRYOSURGICAL TREATMENT OF NEOPLASIA

The success of cryotherapy of benign or neoplastic tumors is dependent on the relative rate of freezing and thawing rather than on the lowest temperature achieved during the procedure. Some tissues are less sensitive to cryosurgery than others.

Keep in mind the following guidelines:

1. The more rapid the rate of freezing, the greater the cellular death.
2. The slower the rate of thawing, the greater the cellular death.
3. A double or triple freeze-thaw cycle may ensure maximal cellular death.
4. The rate at which the cells are frozen and thawed is more important than the final temperature.

A typical tumor is frozen 1 minute at $-80°C$, allowed to thaw, and refrozen.*

THERMOTHERAPY

Exposing the tumor cells to noncoagulating temperatures between 41 and 50°C potentiates the efficacy of chemotherapy, immunotherapy, and radiotherapy. It also destroys the malignant cells because of their increased sensitivity to higher temperature. Several thermotherapy units are available (Hyperthermia Unit, Los Alamos Scientific Laboratories, Los Alamos, New Mexico; RL/22A Thermoprobe LCF Device, Hach Chemical Company, Loveland, Colorado).

The thermotherapy routine for sensitive tumors (carcinomas, FH) of the lids and conjunctiva is simple. After topical or general anesthesia, clean the area with a surgical preparation solution. Protect the cornea with a corneoscleral contact or fitted Styrofoam cover. Calibrate the probe at $50 \pm 1°C$ for 30 seconds and apply the probe in overlapping sites, including normal tissue at the margins of the lesion. After thermotherapy, medicate the site with topical antibiotics for 2 weeks.

BETA RADIATION THERAPY

For carcinomas of the cornea, beta ray therapy has been quite successful following debulking of the tumor by keratectomy to a healthy level of normal cornea. One report recommends a surface dose of 25,000 rep.† from a 50 to 55 megacurie ^{90}Sr applicator in one dose, whereas another suggests 8000 to 10,000 rads per site using another source (Strontium Applicator #SIA-20, Amersham Company, Arlington Heights, Illinois).

CHEMOTHERAPY

FH tumors are sometimes responsive to topical, intralesional, subconjunctival, or systemic corticosteroids or combinations of these. If the tumors proliferate despite steroids or continually return, consider the use of an immunosuppressive agent (Imuran) along with local treatment of antibiotic corticosteroids (Maxitrol, Alcon).

Azathioprine (Imuran, Burroughs Wellcome) has been a valuable adjunct treatment. Dogs are administered 2 mg/kg daily for 2 weeks, re-evaluated, and

*A cryosurgery system that has worked well is manufactured by Frigitronics of Connecticut, Shelton, Connecticut.

†Roentgen-equivalent-physical.

Table 1. *Epithelial Tumors and Tumorlike Lesions of the Eyelids, Conjunctiva, and Cornea*

A. Sebaceous gland tumors
B. Papilloma
C. Squamous cell carcinoma
D. Basal cell tumor
E. Epidermal plaque
F. Dermoid
G. Epidermoid cysts

then reduced to 1 mg/kg on alternate days for 2 weeks and then 1 mg/kg once weekly for 1 month. Both liver enzymes and total white cell counts should be monitored during the use of this drug. Discontinue using it if complications are noted.

IMMUNOTHERAPY

Some of the epithelial and mesenchymal tumors of the eye may respond to immunostimulation (Tables 1 [B,C] and 2 [A]). Therapy with mycobacterial cell wall fractions have been shown to possess antitumor activity. Two commercially available preparations are Regressin (Ragland Research) and Ribigen (Ribi Immunochem Research). These preparations must be injected into the tumor as well as into the adjacent tissue. Since the reaction to be expected is inflammation, use only topical antibiotics for several weeks. The injection may have to be repeated. The author has found this therapy ineffective against fibrous histiocytomas (FH) and would not recommend it for large intraocular tumors for fear of inciting a destructive uveitis. Immunotherapy of anterior uveal neoplasms with immunoregulin (Immunovet) shows promise.

Table 2. *Mesenchymal Tumors*

A. Extraocular
  Tumors of fibrous tissue
    Fibroma
    Fibrosarcoma
    Round cell sarcoid (CVT)
  Tumors of muscle
    Rhabdomyosarcoma
  Tumors of blood vessels
    Hemangioma
    Hemangiosarcoma
  Lymphosarcoma
  Mesenchymal tumors of peripheral nerves
    Perineural fibroblastoma
    Neurofibrosarcoma
  Mast cell tumor
  Canine histiocytoma and fibrous histiocytoma
B. Optic nerve and nerve sheath
  Meningioma
  Reticulosis
C. Uveal tract
  Hemangioma
  Leiomyoma

Table 3. *Neuroectodermal Tumors*

Iridociliary epithelium
  Adenoma
  Adenocarcinoma
Other
  Astrocytoma
  Medulloepithelioma

UVEAL MELANOMAS

Primary intraocular malignant melanomas are always respected, but they are feared most when they appear in the ciliary body or posterior pole of the globe. Once these tumors invade the ciliary body and choroid, it is likely they have spread to other organ sites. The diagnostic studies used in evaluating intraocular melanomas are many. Fluorescein angiography is useful in differentiating choroidal melanomas (mottled hyperfluorescence) from subretinal hematomas (nonfluorescent). Melanomas become progressively more hyperfluorescent in the late phases of circulation of dye and in melanomas with necrosis. Dye leakage into the aqueous or vitreous may indicate the relative neoplastic character of the tumor. Fluorescein is given as an IV bolus 10 to 20 mg/kg (Fluorescite 10 per cent Injection, Alcon).

Ultrasonography is useful in estimating the size, shape, and location of the tumor. The characteristic beta-scan features of a choroidal melanoma, although rare in animals, include acoustic hollowness (internal sonolucency), choroidal excavation, and orbital shadowing. Beta scan is especially informative if the tumor has caused retinal detachment, bleeding into the vitreous, and even extrascleral extension.

The management of uveal melanomas includes the following alternatives: observation, photocoagulation, radiotherapy, surgical resection, enucleation, or exenteration.

Observation

There is very good evidence that many melanomas are dormant or slowly growing tumors that rarely cause visual or systemic problems. Simple observation is recommended for small- to medium-

Table 4. *Melanogenic Tumors*

Eyelids and Conjunctiva
  Benign melanoma (nevus)
  Malignant melanoma
Uveal tract
  Benign melanoma
  Malignant melanoma
    Epithelioid cell type
    Spindle cell type
    Mixed cell type

sized iris and ciliary body melanomas that have caused no symptoms and appear clinically dormant. Precise measurements, photographs, ultrasonography, and fluorescein studies (if available) every 3 to 6 months are indicated.

Photocoagulation

This option is currently used in humans. Moderately intense xenon or argon laser energy to the tissues surrounding the tumor destroys the tumor's blood supply. After several photocoagulation sessions, the tumor itself is photocoagulated. This alternative is applicable to small posterior uveal melanomas.

Radiotherapy

This could include many types of treatment, but only episcleral cobalt plaques sutured over the base of the tumor are currently used to treat choroidal melanomas in humans. Indications for this treatment in a functioning eye have included medium to large melanomas with evidence of growth causing complicating symptoms. After a delivery of about 10,000 rads, the cobalt plaque is removed. Most melanomas in humans treated in this way have shown good tumor regression. External beam irradiation may be used for metastatic tumors to the choroid. Techniques may vary, but a lateral portal is often used to deliver 2000 to 4000 rads to the eye.

Surgery

Surgical resection has been used in animals with primary conjunctival-scleral melanomas and iris base melanomas. Defects left by the resection have been repaired with donor scleral grafts, homografts, or a sliding Tenon's fascial patch. Melanoma confined to the iris may be excised by a sector iridectomy with little complication, but those melanomas requiring iridocyclectomy may have complications such as subluxation of the lens, vitreous hemorrhage, or retinal detachment.

All too often, enucleation or exenteration was the treatment immediately recommended for eyes with melanomas. The trend now is more conservative. It might be well for us to classify animal melanomas into five categories, as for humans: (1) nonsuspicious nevus, (2) suspicious nevus, (3) small melanoma, (4) medium-sized melanoma, and (5) large melanoma. A nonsuspicious nevus is any flat lesion with benign characteristics. A suspicious nevus is between 3 × 3 mm and 5 × 5 mm in diameter and as much as 2 mm thick. A small melanoma is from 5 × 5 × 2 mm up to 10 × 10 × 3 mm. A medium-sized melanoma is 10 × 10 × 3 mm to 15 × 15 × 5 mm. A large melanoma is more than 15 × 15 × 5 mm. Although the indications for a specific method of treatment depend on a number of complex factors, the final treatment selected depends partly on the size of the lesion.

When should an eye be enucleated if a melanoma is diagnosed or suspected? Most veterinarians are uncertain how to handle a malignant melanoma. The majority practice immediate enucleation because this procedure requires no further consideration. The security provided by removing the tumor completely is most comforting. Consider the following factors:

1. Malignant melanomas usually grow slowly; therefore, quick decisions are usually not necessary when tumors are discovered.
2. There is agreement that the larger the tumor the worse the prognosis.

Malignant melanomas follow these principles more than other tumors. The most prognostic characteristic of a melanoma is the cell type. Prior to knowing the cell type, the rate of growth accounting for its size is extremely prognostic. If one waits long enough, enucleation will become mandatory in all malignant melanomas because pain, glaucoma, and blindness force the surgery. Unfortunately, by then the tumors are so large that the prognosis after enucleation is very poor. The main debate is whether enucleation for malignant melanoma improves the prognosis at all. It has been suggested that in humans enucleation may enhance the dissemination of tumor cells. Improved enucleation techniques are therefore encouraged. These techniques include periocular infiltration with 1 to 5 ml xylocaine in combination with epinephrine to constrict the orbital vasculature. Alternatively, use the "no touch" technique, which freezes the blood supply to the tumor before enucleation. Bear in mind that cardiac complications (fibrillations) may occur with the use of epinephrine and halothane anesthesia. It is good technique to avoid any manipulation of the tumor or adjacent ocular structures while performing the enucleation.

Enucleation in dogs and cats should be considered in the following instances:

1. After observation, an increase in size above 10 × 10 × 2 mm is documented.
2. The tumor character prevents preserving the globe.
3. The tumor has caused an obvious decrease in visual ability.
4. The patient is young (less than 5 years).
5. The tumor is located within 2 disc diameters around the optic nerve head.
6. The tumor is diffusely growing.

Several of the above conditions are usually noted, but the greater the number, the more seriously enucleation should be considered. We almost never enucleate for small melanomas but encourage enucleation if the eye becomes blind or secondary glaucoma develops.

Exenteration of the orbital contents is not performed for tumors confined to the intraocular structures. If clinical evidence of extrascleral extension is present, excise a limited amount of orbital tissue, conserving enough periorbital fascia to close the orbit. Following both enucleation and exenterations, silicone ball implants have been placed into the orbits to aid the cosmetic appearance.

OPTIC NERVE AND CNS TUMORS

When a tentative diagnosis of bilateral disease of the optic nerves or optic chiasm is made, skull radiographs usually appear normal. A vascular contrast study of the orbits and a cavernous sinus venogram comparing the filling characteristics of the ophthalmic vein and orbital plexus may be rewarding. By injecting contrast material into the angularis oculi vein on each side while temporarily occluding the jugulars, one can demonstrate by contrast flow a filling deficit in the vascular area of the orbital plexus or base of the brain. Because the cannulation or injection of the facial or angularis oculi vein is difficult, a cutdown for visualization is recommended.

Brain tumors in dogs may first be suspected by a visual deficit or abnormal eye characteristics. A recent report (Turrel et al., 1984) of successful treatment with external beam megavoltage radiation is encouraging. X-ray computed tomography was used to localize and assess the treatment response. Radiation doses of 3000 to 3600 rads were given in five or six sessions over 14 to 19 days. Complete tumor regression as determined by tomographic scans, improved clinical signs, and reduction in medications were documented in all irradiated dogs. The 1-year survival rate for these dogs was 100 per cent. The majority of these tumors originated from CNS tissue.

References and Supplemental Reading

Gwin, R. M., Gelatt, K. N., and Williams, L. W.: Ophthalmic neoplasms in the dog. J. Am. Anim. Hosp. Assoc. 18:853, 1982.

Kern, T. J.: Orbital neoplasia in 23 dogs. J.A.V.M.A. 186:489, 1985.

Kircher, H., Garner, F. M., and Robinson, R. F.: Tumors of the eye and adnexa. Bull. WHO 50:135, 1974.

Latimer, C. A., Wyman, M., Szymanski, C., et al.: Azathioprine in the management of fibrous histiocytoma in 2 dogs. J. Am. Anim. Hosp. Assoc. 19:155, 1983.

Martin, C. L.: Canine epibulbar melanomas and their management. J. Am. Anim. Hosp. Assoc. 17:83, 1981.

Turrel, J. M., Fike, J. R., LeConteur, R. A., et al.: Radiotherapy of brain tumors in dogs. J.A.V.M.A. 184:82, 1984.

Vandevelde, M.: Primary reticulosis of the central nervous system. Symposium on advances in veterinary neurology. Vet. Clin. North Am. 10:57, 1980.

Williams, L. W., Gelatt, K. N., and Gwin, R. M.: Ophthalmic neoplasms in the cat. J. Am. Anim. Hosp. Assoc. 17:999, 1981.

CONTEMPORARY OCULAR THERAPEUTICS

MILTON WYMAN, D.V.M.
Columbus, Ohio

The therapeutic effect of any medication depends on an accurate diagnosis, an appropriate drug selection, and an effective route of administration. This is especially true as it relates to ocular disease. All clinicians have their "pet cures" and swear by all that is holy that they work time after time. Many times these "remedies" are not evaluated by a controlled study, but we recognize that clinical improvement is demonstrable. The author would like to register doubt about this type of drug evaluation and suggest that the patient may have responded without any medication. In other words, be critical of the effectiveness of a treatment regime if it is evaluated solely by clinical impression. The nature of the disease, the drug selected, and its route and method of administration are the three primary considerations in effective ocular disease control.

There is a lack of unanimity regarding the most efficacious route of administration of ocular medication. The author describes those medications currently available, with emphasis on those methods that have been used and advocated and some that may be available in the future.

Topical application is an effective and practical method. It is useful in conjunctival, corneal, and anterior segment diseases. The therapeutic concentration is dependent on differential solubility, drug concentration, vehicle, contact time, frequency of application, and bioavailability. One can clearly see that many of these factors are interdependent; therefore, some discussion is prudent.

The cornea is the major barrier to intraocular penetration of topically applied drugs. The corneal layers (epithelium, stroma, Descemet's membrane, and endothelium) approximate a fat-water-fat sandwich. Thus, penetration into the anterior segment is best achieved by agents that are soluble in both water and fat. We also must determine if penetration is necessary. For example, corneal pannus, as observed in German shepherds, does not require penetration into the anterior segment but requires higher concentrations in the superficial structures. Therefore, a drug that will remain on the surface for a long time and that is predominately lipid soluble should be selected.

Another important aspect is bioavailability. Similar agents are supplied by different pharmaceutical companies. Some of them are inexpensive, but the active agents may be "vehicle bound" so that they are not available. Be aware that the cheaper drugs are not necessarily the best buy.

Contact time is dependent on vehicle, degree of inflammation, and tear flow. *Aqueous solutions* flow very rapidly from the surface via the nasolacrimal drainage apparatus. This is clearly demonstrated in cats after placing a drop of atropine on the cornea. They taste the bitter alkaloid that was transmitted through the nasolacrimal drainage apparatus to the nose and into the mouth, and profuse salivation is stimulated. The rapidity of this phenomenon staggers the imagination, but it demonstrates that solutions are rapidly removed from the corneal surface. Solutions are useful, but they must be applied more frequently in order to reach adequate therapeutic concentrations. The clinician should also recognize that dacryocystitis is best treated with appropriate solutions applied to the corneal surface, since they are removed by this route.

In contrast to solutions, viscid vehicles such as the *ophthalmic ointments* remain on the surface longer and provide greater contact time. These agents have historically been considered more irritating, resulting in retarded healing. Recent evaluation of vehicles demonstrates that if solutions are placed on the eye so that drug concentration equals that obtained with ointments, there is no difference in rate of healing between the two. Because of this and the convenience of less frequent medication to obtain therapeutic levels, ointments are extremely useful for topical medication, and they are the author's choice.

The failure of therapeutic response is often due to inadequate frequency of medication. It is the author's belief that part of our job as veterinarians is to educate our clients and encourage them to become members of the treatment team for their pets. They must be educated to follow instructions to medicate the eyes as often as instructed. The veterinarian should decide the necessary frequency, instruct clients on the method of treatment, and make them partially responsible for the response. Clients should also be advised to return with their medication when the patient is re-evaluated. It is not unusual to prescribe ointments every 4 hours for 1 week, and have them return with three quarters of a ⅛-oz tube left after 6 days of medication. Realizing that compliance is a problem, the clinician should try to place the responsibility of the therapeutic response on the clients' shoulders. In conjunction with this, the veterinarian may offer to hospitalize the pet, at considerable cost, and medicate the animal for the client. Those who accept this service observe marked improvement, which makes them realize that frequency is an important part of therapy and, had they complied, it would have been more economical for them. Compliance can be stimulated by showing photos of effective response, thereby educating the client.

The degree and severity of inflammation also affect contact time. Vascular dilation may increase drug uptake into the general circulation. This may decrease contact time, requiring more frequent application in order to establish local therapeutic concentrations. Systemic absorption does occur and must be taken into consideration when treating frequently with a potent drug such as 1 per cent atropine sulfate. Indiscriminate use may result in systemic atropinization, particularly in small patients.

Increased lacrimation also contributes to contact time. Normally, the animal's reflex tearing is five times greater than in humans. When a normally lacrimating eye is irritated, tear flow is copious. Therefore, one drop of an aqueous solution on the corneal surface is rapidly diluted as well as quickly removed. In contrast, a hyposecretor will not establish the same dilution; however, the agent may dry and not be adequately distributed across the eye. These characteristics must be identified and proper steps should be taken to correct them (e.g., increasing frequency of medication or selecting an ointment vehicle in lieu of a solution).

Subconjunctival injection is a method of providing a greater concentration to superficial structures and better absorption for drugs that are poorly absorbed. It is important to understand that it is not a panacea and should be used with caution and reservation. Subconjunctival injections used in humans are performed two or three times per day, in addition to frequent topical medication, and the patient is usually hospitalized. Single injections are unlikely to provide better levels than frequent topical applications of a good ophthalmic ointment vehicle. Subconjunctival injection may predispose to granulomas as well as cause patient discomfort or other more serious injury to the globe.

Parenteral and *oral routes* are most applicable to the posterior uvea, retina, or vitreous. Topical medications do not reach therapeutic levels in these regions. Therapeutic levels also are best accomplished in the lids and orbit by the parenteral or oral routes. The author is convinced that, if antibiotics or other drugs are necessary for blepharitis, topical application is not as efficacious as the systemic route.

Retrobulbar medication is most often used in food-producing animals, particularly for regional anesthesia. The author believes that retrobulbar injection has very limited use in small animals and, when used, is for diagnostic purposes such as immobilization of the globe for electroretinography (ERG) or contrast radiography. Some authors recommend retrobulbar injections of steroids and other agents as a part of the therapy for traumatic proptosis. The author is adamantly opposed to even the smallest retrobulbar injection, which will further compromise an already compromised periorbital space. Systemic medication will provide therapeutic levels without adding to space-occupying debris.

Intraocular injections are limited to last-resort efforts to save the globe or for intentional destruction of the eye. Intraocular mycosis or bacterial infections have been medicated by this route. Sight is often lost, but the globe may be saved for cosmetic purposes. Absolute glaucoma has also been managed by intraocular injection of an aminoglycoside, which destroys the ciliary body secretory structure, resulting in phthisis bulbi. The practitioner should not consider this approach in a sighted eye that could possibly be salvaged.

Prolonged release devices such as hydrophilic lenses and permeable membrane devices (Ocusert, Alza) provide slow, constant release of drugs for several hours. This is the basis for effective ocular drug concentrations. The technical problem of developing conformation to corneal curvature (allowing adequate retention and patient comfort) is the weak link in this route. However, for their future potential as a delivery system and as a protective bandage, these devices show great promise.

AUTONOMIC DRUGS

Although this is a very important group of drugs in human ophthalmology, many of these agents have not been thoroughly investigated for use in veterinary ophthalmology. There are, however, several drugs that are effective, useful, and important in veterinary ocular therapeutics.

Adrenergic Agents

These drugs produce mydriasis, cycloplegia, vasoconstriction, and alterations in intraocular pressure. Sympathomimetic drugs produce mydriasis but not cycloplegia. Of greatest importance among this group is epinephrine, which is vasoconstrictive and reduces intraocular pressure. It is generally thought that pressure reduction results from decreased aqueous production due to a beta-stimulating sympathetic effect on the secretory mechanism. In addition, epinephrine improves the facility of outflow. This is not an immediate reaction but often takes several weeks to months to demonstrate in humans.

A pro-drug, dipivalyl epinephrine, does not become activated until it passes through the cornea. This allows a much lower concentration of the active agent, thus producing less ocular irritation. It has the same hypotensive effect as epinephrine without the topical vasoconstrictive effect.

Phenylephrine 10 per cent and 2.5 per cent are direct-acting sympathomimetic agents that can be used as mydriatics and for symptomatic treatment of Horner's syndrome.

Anticholinergic Agents

This group of drugs is extremely valuable in veterinary ocular therapeutics, particularly in the management of iridocyclitis. The most commonly used agent is *atropine sulfate*, which blocks the response to acetylcholine in smooth muscles and secretory glands innervated by postganglionic cholinergic nerves. Atropine is both a mydriatic and a potent cycloplegic. The mydriasis is enhanced by sympathomimetic drugs, but cycloplegia is not, since sympathomimetics have insignificant cycloplegic action. Normal heavily pigmented eyes will take longer to dilate but remain dilated for many days once dilation occurs.

Atropine sulfate is biphasically soluble and easily and quickly passes through the conjunctiva and cornea. The practitioner must remember that other agents (prostaglandins) have a direct effect on smooth muscles and may compromise the mydriatic effect of atropine or other mydriatic agents. Atropine relieves pain due to ciliary muscle spasms and minimizes predisposition to posterior synechiae by dilating the pupil. Dilation results in a decrease in iridal surface adjacent to the anterior lens capsule, which in turn decreases the potential for complete posterior synechiae and iris bombé. Another beneficial effect of atropine is the restoration of normal vascular permeability of the inflamed eye. This action decreases cells and protein (flare) in the anterior chamber by an unidentified or indirect mechanism.

*Table 1. Cholinergic Action**

Direct
- Acetycholine: Not routinely used in veterinary ophthalmology.
- Methacholine: No longer commercially available.
- Carbachol: Not routinely used in veterinary ophthalmology.
- Pilocarpine: Most commonly used cholinergic agent.

Indirect (anticholinesterases)

Reversible
- Physostigmine: Not routinely used in veterinary ophthalmology.
- Neostigmine: Not routinely used in veterinary ophthalmology.
- Edrophonium: Tensilon test for myasthenia gravis.

Irreversible
- Isoflurophate (diisopropylflurophosphate, DFP)
- Echothiophate
- Demecarium

*Modified from Havener, W. H.: Ocular Pharmacology. 5th ed. St. Louis: C. V. Mosby, 1983.

Scopolamine is more potent than atropine on a weight-for-weight basis. Its duration of action is shorter than atropine; however, it produces more adverse reactions than atropine in humans. It is available as a combination drug with phenylephrine (Muro #2, Muro) and is used for preoperative mydriasis as well as iridocyclitis. The author does not recommend its use in combination with atropine.

Tropicamide has excellent biphasic solubility, which helps explain its very rapid onset of action and short duration. It is less potent as a cycloplegic but adequate as a mydriatic for ophthalmoscopic examination in animals. It is not pigment dependent, unlike atropine or the less frequently used homatropine. It is extremely safe as a mydriatic for ophthalmoscopy, and, because it has a rapid onset and short duration, it is the drug of choice for this purpose at the 1 per cent concentration (Mydriacyl, Alcon). Homatropine has less cycloplegic effect as compared with atropine but may substitute for atropine if a patient is intolerant to atropine. It is available as a 1 to 5 per cent solution.

Cyclopentolate, in contrast to atropine, produces mydriasis and cycloplegia of equal duration. Atropine produces longer mydriasis than cycloplegia. Cyclopentolate has more adverse clinical effects in animals than do any of the other agents in this group. The worst clinical reaction is severe chemosis and conjunctival hyperemia. This is usually transient, but, because of the high incidence of this adverse effect and the limited benefits derived from the drug, the author does not recommend its use in veterinary ophthalmology.

Cholinergic Agonists

This group of drugs (Table 1) produces responses similar to those of acetylcholine. The group has also been called parasympathomimetic because reactions mimic the parasympathetic autonomic nervous system. Clinically, these drugs are useful in management of glaucoma, as diagnostic agents for pupillary abnormalities, and as lacrimomimetics. The agents are classified according to their direct or indirect actions.

Pilocarpine is the most widely used cholinergic agent in veterinary medicine. It is a direct-acting cholinergic agent used in glaucoma therapy and as a lacrimomimetic. Pilocarpine also affects the cardiovascular system, exocrine glands, and smooth muscle. The effect on the cardiovascular system is usually a fall in blood pressure.

Pilocarpine also increases salivation, sweating, lacrimation, and gastric secretions. Its effect on smooth muscle is contraction, which increases tone and motility in the gut, ureters, urinary bladder, gallbladder, biliary ducts, and bronchiolar musculature. The eye is affected by pupillary constriction and contraction of the ciliary musculature, which most probably is responsible for increased aqueous outflow and reduced intraocular pressure. There is also evidence that prolonged therapy decreases aqueous production.

Pilocarpine is most often used in the management of glaucoma. Its efficacy is directly related to the early recognition of the disease. Chronic, absolute glaucoma will not respond well to any agent; therefore, early recognition, client education, and frequent (once every 3 to 6 months after regulation) re-evaluation of the intraocular pressures are mandates for effective control. One must always remember that there is no cure for glaucoma, only control.

Pilocarpine is available in 0.025 to 10 per cent solutions; however, the author prefers 1 or 2 per cent concentrations. Concentrations over 4 per cent are extremely irritating and have no clinical advantage. In addition to the solutions, a sustained release membrane-bound drug is available for use in humans. This insert (Ocusert, Alza) has been proved extremely toxic in the author's clinical and investigational experience because dogs secrete five times or more tears than do humans. This elutes the agent more rapidly, resulting in a faster absorption (via the drainage apparatus as well as conjunctival vessels). Secondly, losing the insert with subsequent ingestion by the patient (two out of six animals tested) also occurs.

Pilocarpine is also commercially available in combination with 1 per cent epinephrine bitartrate in 1, 2, 3, 4, and 6 per cent concentrations. This combination has been helpful in control of early onset glaucoma.

The frequency of administration should be two to four times daily. It has been demonstrated that 4 times per day is more effective in humans. Often the client complains that the animal is worse with medication. The most frequent complaint from the

Table 2. Formula for Modified Severins' Solution

Mucomyst 20 (Mead Johnson)	6 ml
Pilocarpine 1 or 2%	6 ml (Modified Severins' #1 or #2, respectively)*
Adapt (Alcon)	6 ml
Gentamicin for injection (100 mg/ml)	2 ml
	20 ml

*Severins' #1 solution contains pilocarpine 1%; #2 contains pilocarpine 2%.

owner is a "red eye and squinting," particularly seen with early occult glaucoma. Indeed, in a normal eye, pilocarpine will produce every clinical characteristic of Horner's syndrome. (It can be used to demonstrate Horner's to students.) This implies that pilocarpine stimulation results in an overpowering of the sympathetic innervation to the eye. The author is of the opinion that client education is most important and neglecting this results in noncompliance. The irritative reactions are usually transient (about 3 to 4 days), and thereafter the patient becomes more tolerant to the drug. The higher the concentration, the greater the reaction. Although it has been reported that animals become sensitized to pilocarpine, resulting in irritation associated with prolonged treatment, this may be the exception to the rule once the patient has become tolerant to the drug.

Pilocarpine has also been used as a lacrimomimetic. It is advisable to administer it orally in the food once or twice daily. Because of its systemic absorption and potential toxicity, the author advocates topical administration using a modified Severins' solution (Table 2). This is less toxic and more efficacious if some lacrimation is present. Absolute sicca will not respond to pilocarpine stimulation and, indeed, the clinical disease may be worsened by the irritation caused by the medication. Modification of Severins' solution is described in Table 2. The frequency of medication can be hourly and adjusted according to response. The mixture should be refrigerated; however, the drug is more irritating when it is cold than when it is at room temperature. A daily supply can be kept in a small medicine dropper vial stored at room temperature.

Demecarium results from linking two molecules of neostigmine. This increases its potency and duration. It is available in 0.125 or 0.25 per cent solutions. It is used as a substitute for the shorter-acting pilocarpine if resistance or irritation occurs. The author does not recommend it except as a last resort because it has no advantage over pilocarpine.

Organophosphates

Isoflurophate (DFP) is an irreversible anticholinesterase. It produces intense miosis and ciliary body musculature contraction and is of long duration. It is available as an 0.025 per cent ointment. Because of its relative toxicity, the author does not recommend this drug for use in veterinary ophthalmology.

Echothiophate is also an irreversible anticholinesterase agent. It is available in 0.03, 0.06, 0.125, and 0.25 per cent concentrations. Like DFP, this drug is extremely potent, and the author does not use it.

LOCAL ANESTHETICS

Injectable anesthetics (Table 3) are used more often for facial, retrobulbar, or tissue infiltration in large animals than in small animals. Some surgeons use this method of anesthesia in aged or debilitated small animals in which general anesthesia may be detrimental.

Topical anesthetics (Table 4) should be limited to diagnostic or minor surgical procedures. *They should not be used for therapeutic purposes.* The drug of choice is proparacaine hydrochloride 0.5 per cent. The method of application is important. In order to effectively anesthetize the cornea or conjunctiva, one or two drops should be placed on the eye; after 2 to 5 minutes the procedure is repeated. Corneal sensitivity should be determined prior to performing the intended technique.

Indications for topical anesthesia include tonometry, suture removal, corneal débridement, cytologic tests, simple biopsies, lacrimal irrigation, eversion of the lids, and subconjunctival injections.

Contraindications for topical anesthesia include routine treatment, use prior to obtaining a culture specimen or prior to performing a Schirmer's tear test, and use in conjunction with sodium fluorescein for staining ocular tissues.

ANTI-INFLAMMATORY DRUGS

Steroidal Anti-inflammatory Agents

Corticosteroids are the most frequently used drugs to control ocular inflammation. The ocular effects of corticosteroids include decreased cellular and fibrinous exudation and tissue infiltration, retarded epithelial and endothelial regeneration, inhibited fibroblastic and collagen-forming activity, reduced capillary permeability, suppressed migration of leukocytes to the site of injury, inhibited release of hydrolytic enzyme from leukocytes, and decreased postinflammatory vascularization and scarring. These effects result from unknown mechanisms. The cause of the inflammatory lesion is not eliminated by corticosteroid therapy, even though the inflammatory response is inhibited.

Table 3. Injectable Local Anesthetics

Generic Name	Proprietary Name	Dosage Form*	Onset of Action	Duration of Action
Procaine hydrochloride	Novocaine	1, 2, and 10% solution	7–8 min	30–45 min (60 min with epinephrine)
Lidocaine hydrochloride	Xylocaine	0.5, 1, 1.5, 2, and 4% solution	4–6 min	40–60 min (120 min with epinephrine)
Mepivacaine hydrochloride	Carbocaine	1, 1.5, 2, and 3% solution	3–5 min	120 min
Bupivacaine hydrochloride	Marcaine	0.25, 0.5, and 0.75% solution	5–11 min	480–720 min with epinephrine
Etidocaine hydrochloride	Duranest	0.5, 1, and 1.5% solution	4–6 min	300–600 min

*Some concentrations are commercially available with epinephrine. Hyaluronidase may be added to increase diffusion of the anesthetic.

From Bartlett, J. D., and Jaanus, S. D.: *Clinical Ocular Pharmacology*. Boston: Butterworths, 1984, p. 136.

The route of administration and dosage is often a point of controversy. It is the author's belief that the nature, extent, and location of the inflammation are important criteria for establishing the route, drug, and dosage. For superficial corneal and conjunctival lesions, topical medication is the choice, in contrast to a posterior segment lesion, which would require systemic administration. An antibiotic corticosteroid combination, preferably an ointment (Tables 5 and 6), is also recommended.

Subconjunctival (sub-Tenon's capsule) injections should be used only as a last resort. The repositol drug methylprednisolone acetate (Depo-Medrol, Upjohn) has been used to provide prolonged steroid levels. Some investigators suggest that 2 to 4 weeks of constant corticosteroid therapy is possible by this method. The author has observed many ocular granulomas and corneal ruptures following subconjunctival corticosteroid administration. Subconjunctival corticosteroids may be used only if a greater anti-inflammatory effect is needed beyond that obtained with topical or systemic administration.

Corticosteroids should not be used indiscriminately. They can potentiate infection (particularly mycosis) and collagenase activity, as well as decrease epithelial sliding and mitosis. Corticosteroids should not be used in ulcerative keratitis, particularly those in which keratomalacia is evident.

Nonsteroidal Anti-inflammatory Agents

Prostaglandins are mediators of certain aspects of the inflammatory process. Prostaglandins are liberated at the inflammatory site in addition to the slow-reacting substances of anaphylaxis released locally, such as histamine, bradykinin, 5-hydroxytryptamine, and several other chemotactic agents.

The prostaglandins are very potent. They increase vascular permeability, may be chemotactic, and act directly on smooth muscle, resulting in severe contraction. The prostaglandins are grouped according to the arrangement of their ketone and hydroxyl groups. These are E, F, A, B, C, and D. Prostaglandins E and F have demonstrated a role in ocular inflammation. PGE_1, PGE_2, and PGF_2 have been isolated from plasmoid or secondary aqueous in humans and some animals. The ocular response to prostaglandin release in rabbits has been well documented: miosis, injection of conjunctival vessels, flare, increased intraocular pressure, and pain. Recent work has demonstrated that the elevated pressure is transient and probably the result of increased aqueous production secondary to a breakdown of the blood-aqueous barrier and decreased pressure.

Aspirin is still a very effective antiprostaglandin and can be used in dogs and cats. Aspirin can be administered prior to elective intraocular surgery

Table 4. Topical Anesthetics

Generic Name	Proprietary Name (Manufacturer)	Dosage Form
Cocaine hydrochloride	(Schedule II—controlled substance)	1–4% solution, prepared from the bulk powder
Tetracaine hydrochloride	Pontocaine (Breon)	0.5% solution 0.5% ointment
Piperocaine hydrochloride	M-Z* (Smith, Miller, Patch)	0.75% solution, in combination with 0.25% zinc sulfate and 0.125% phenylephrine
Benoxinate hydrochloride	Fluress (Barnes-Hind)	0.4% solution, in combination with 0.25% sodium fluorescein
Proparacaine hydrochloride	Ophthaine (Squibb); Ophthetic (Allergan); Alcaine (Alcon)	0.5% solution

*No longer commercially available.

From Bartlett, J. D., and Jaanus, S. D.: *Clinical Ocular Pharmacology*. Boston: Butterworths, 1984, p. 137.

Table 5. *Antibiotic-Corticosteroid Combinations: Ointments*

Generic Name	Trade Name	Manufacturer
Neomycin sulfate, polymyxin B sulfate, and dexamethasone	Maxitrol AK-Trol	Alcon Akorn
Neomycin sulfate and hydrocortisone acetate	Neo-Cortef 0.5% Neo-Cortef Blephamide (0.2%)	Upjohn Allergan
Neomycin sulfate, ZN bacitracin, polymyxin B sulfate, and hydrocortisone	Cortisporin AK-Sporin HC	Burroughs Wellcome Akron
Neomycin sulfate and prednisolone acetate	Neodelta-Cortef 0.5% and 0.25%	Upjohn
Neomycin sulfate and prednisolone phosphate	Neo-Hydeltrasol	Merck, Sharp & Dohme
Neomycin sulfate and methylprednisolone	Neo-Medrol	Upjohn
Chloramphenicol, polymyxin B sulfate, and hydrocortisone acetate	Ophthocort	Parke-Davis
Chloramphenicol and prednisolone	Chloroptic-P S.O.P.	Allergan
Sulfacetamide sodium and prednisolone sulfate	Cetapred AK Cide Metimyd Blephamide	Alcon Akorn Schering Allergan
Sulfacetamide sodium, prednisolone acetate, and phenylephrine hydrochloride	Vasocidin	CooperVision

From Wyman, M.: *Manual of Small Animal Ophthalmology.* New York: Churchill Livingstone, in press.

to minimize postoperative inflammation. The recommended dose for dogs is 25 to 35 mg/kg daily and for cats 15 mg/kg every third day. However, the author recommends 1 grain/10 kg two or three times daily for dogs and cats.

Flunixin meglumine (Banamine, Schering) is also a very potent and effective antiprostaglandin. It has not been approved for use in small animals. The author recommends 0.250 mg/kg IV once daily for no more than 5 days at a time. The manufacturer provides the drug in concentrations of 50 mg/ml. By withdrawing 0.1 ml in a TB syringe and diluting it with 0.9 ml of water for injection, one can administer an accurate amount without fear of overdosing the small patient. This drug is also used preoperatively, administered IV 30 minutes prior to anticipated surgery. Although the drug has been recommended for IM injection, it is extremely irritating.

Other agents will be forthcoming, and some practitioners use phenylbutazone in small animals; however, the author does not.

ANTIBIOTIC DRUGS

Tables 5 through 8 list various antibiotics used in ophthalmology. The effective management of ocular infections is based on the following guidelines:

1. Establish an accurate diagnosis.
2. Select the appropriate drug for the causative organism (Table 9).
3. Select the appropriate route of administration.
4. Re-evaluate critically for response.
5. Institute supplemental physical therapy when necessary (e.g., warm compresses).
6. Evaluate for adverse drug reaction.
7. Avoid combinations of antibiotics *not* commercially available.

The practitioner should select an effective agent against the causative organism. The most accurate method is to isolate the organism, identify it, and determine sensitivity to available agents by culture and sensitivity techniques. This is certainly necessary for serious stromal keratopathies, nonresponsive oculopathies, or ocular lesions that are progressing during therapy. For simple lesions that experience and knowledge identify as infections, broad-spectrum antibiotics or combinations are usefully employed without specific identification.

Table 6. *Antibiotic-Corticosteroid Combinations: Solutions*

Generic Name	Trade Name	Source
Neomycin sulfate, polymyxin B sulfate, and dexamethasone 0.1%	Maxitrol AK-Trol	Alcon Akorn
Neomycin sulfate and hydrocortisone acetate	Neo-Cortef 1.5%	Upjohn
Neomycin sulfate, polymyxin B sulfate, and hydrocortisone	Cortisporin	Burroughs Wellcome
Neomycin sulfate and prednisolone	Neo-Delta-Cortef AK-Neo-Cort	Upjohn Akorn
Neomycin sulfate and prednisolone phosphate	Neo-Hydeltrasol	Merck, Sharp & Dohme
Neomycin sulfate and dexamethasone phosphate	NeoDECADRON	Merck, Sharp & Dohme
Chloramphenical and hydrocortisone acetate	Chloromycetin Hydrocortisone	Parke-Davis
Oxytetracycline hydrochloride and hydrocortisone acetate	Terra-Cortril	Pfizer
Sulfacetamide sodium 10% and prednisolone acetate	Isopto Cetapred AK-Cide Blephamide Metimyd Suspension	Alcon Akorn Allergan Schering

From Wyman, M.: *Manual of Small Animal Ophthalmology.* New York: Churchill Livingstone, in press.

Table 7. Individual Topical Antibiotics

Individual Agent	Manufacturers	Available Vehicles
Chloramphenicol	Alcon, Akorn, Allergan, Parke-Davis	0.5% solutions and 1% ointments
Colisitin sulfate (polymyxin E)	Professional Pharmacol.	0.012% solution
Gentamicin*	Schering and Allergan	0.3% solution 0.3% solution
Sulfa		
Sulfacetamide Na	Alcon, Allergan	10, 15, 30% solution
Sulfisoxazole diolamine	Schering, Cooper, and Roche	10% ointment 4% solution 4% ointment
Tetracycline	Lederle	1% solution 1% ointment
Tobramycin†	Alcon	0.3% solution 0.3% ointment
Bacitracin	Lilly and Upjohn	500 units/gm ointment
Chlortetracycline	Lederle	1% ointment
Erythromycin	Dista	0.5% ointment
Neomycin	Upjohn	0.35% ointment

*Preferable drugs for *Pseudomonas*.
†Excellent for *Pseudomonas* but expensive.
From Wyman, M.: *Manual of Small Animal Ophthalmology*. New York: Churchill Livingstone, in press.

The practitioner should administer the antibiotic by the route that will provide the greatest therapeutic level to the diseased part. For most conjunctival and corneal infections, topical therapy is effective and simple. It can be accomplished by the client and is relatively inexpensive. The anterior segment can also be medicated topically. In addition, systemic or subconjunctival injections may be indicated. Subconjunctival administration is used as a last resort or for those specific antibiotics that do not penetrate the eye. Treat inflammatory diseases of the lids systemically and with warm compresses. This produces vasodilation, which increases local immune factors assisting in controlling the infection.

Table 8. Combination Topical Antibiotics

Combination of Agents	Manufacturers	Available Vehicles
Neomycin sulfate and polymyxin B sulfate	Alcon and Allergan	Solution and ointments
Neomycin sulfate,* polymyxin B sulfate, and gramicidin	Burroughs Wellcome, Dow, and Pharmafair	Solution
Neomycin sulfate,* polymyxin B sulfate, and bacitracin	Upjohn, Dow, Allergan, and Burroughs Wellcome	Ointment
Oxytetracycline hydrochloride and polymyxin B	Pfizer	Ointment

*Preferable drug for spectrum without culture sensitivity.
From Wyman, M.: *Manual of Small Animal Ophthalmology*. New York: Churchill Livingstone, in press.

Re-evaluating the response to therapy is also important. The patient should be seen initially every 2 to 3 days, depending on the type of lesion present. Those infections involving the cornea or anterior segment in particular should be critically evaluated early in order to adjust the therapy if necessary. This method will also provide for evaluation of the possible adverse reaction that is relatively rare but must always be considered.

Clients should also be informed of any possible reaction to expect when medicating the patient's eyes. Client compliance is a very important part of effective therapy, and clients who are aware of the expected response will be more likely to follow instructions.

The veterinarian should also remember that combinations of broad-spectrum antibiotics (e.g., chloramphenicol and gentamicin) may be antagonistic to each other. Therefore, it is prudent to avoid using combinations not commercially available.

ANTIBACTERIAL DRUGS

These drugs can be divided into groups according to their action on the parts of the organism or its metabolism. Many drugs will demonstrate multiple action sites; however, their predominant action is to affect the cell wall, the cell membrane, protein synthesis, or intermediary metabolism (Table 10). Antibacterial drug concentrations and dosages for topical and subconjunctival routes are also listed in Table 11.

Ocular penetration is also variable and is dependent on biphasic solubility, plasma protein binding, particulate size, and peak serum concentration. These measurements, however, are primarily related to the normal intact eye. In the inflamed eye, the corneal epithelial, blood-aqueous or blood-vitreous barriers are disrupted, providing an avenue for drug penetration not possible in a normal eye.

ANTIVIRAL AGENTS

The development of antiviral agents has been much slower than that of antibacterial agents. This is primarily because of the host-parasite relationship associated with viral replication. Since viral propagation relies on the cell mechanism of the host, the antiviral agent must act intracellularly and specifically for the virion rather than the host cell. This has been accomplished by developing drugs that have a greater toxicity for the viral particle than for the host cell. Another mechanism inhibits specific and unique viral enzyme systems that are not present in the host cell (e.g., acyclovir for herpes simplex). Most of the available antiviral agents today inhibit the synthesis of DNA by competing for

Table 9. *Susceptibility of Common Ocular Pathogens to Antibiotics**

Organism	Ampicillin	Chloramphenicol	Bacitracin	Carbenicillin	Cephalosporin	Gentamicin	Tobramycin	Methicillin	Nafcillin	Neomycin	Colistin	Polymyxin B	Penicillin G	Vancomycin	Tetracycline	Sulfonamides	Kanomycin	Erythromycin
Gram-positive cocci																		
Staphylococcus (Penicillin–S)	S	S	S	S	S	S	S	S	S	S	R	R	S	S	S	V	V	S
Staphylococcus (Penicillin–R)	R	S	S	R	S	S	S	S	S	V	R	R	R	S	V	V	V	S
Streptococcus spp. (B)	S	S	S	S	S	V	R	S	S	R	R	R	S	S	R	V	R	S
Gram-positive rods																		
Corynebacterium spp.	S	S	S	S	S	S	S	S	S	S	S	S	S	S	S	S	S	S
Gram-negative rods																		
Pseudomonas spp.	R	V	R	S	R	S	S	R	R	R	S	S	R	R	R	R	R	R
E. Coli	V	V	R	S	V	S	S	R	R	V	S	S	R	R	V	V	V	R
Proteus spp.	S	V	R	S	V	S	S	R	R	V	R	R	R	R	R	R	V	R
Haemophilus spp.	V	S	R	S	V	S	S	R	R	S	S	S	V	R	S	R	R	V
Enterobacter	R	V	R	R	R	S	S	R	R	S	V	V	R	R	R	R	R	R
Moraxella	S	S	R	S	S	S	S	S	S	S	S	S	S	S	S	S	S	S
Chlamydia	R	S	R	R	R	V	V	R	R	R	R	R	R	R	S	S	V	R
Mycoplasma spp.	R	S	R	R	R	R	S	S	R	S	R	R	R	R	S	R	V	S

*Information compiled from Dr. Joseph Kowalski's data

Sensitivity studies: S = 85% of the organisms tested were susceptible; V = > 50% and < 85% of the organisms were susceptible; and R = < 50% of the organisms tested were susceptible.

From Wyman, M.: *Manual of Small Animal Ophthalmology*. New York: Churchill Livingstone, in press.

purine and pyrimidine bases, the building blocks for DNA and RNA synthesis.

The available ocular antiviral agents are only effective against herpesviruses. They are only available for topical use. It is the author's opinion that in cat corneal herpetic ulcers or conjunctivitis, antivirals not only are therapeutically helpful but contribute to a diagnosis if healing occurs subsequent to treatment. Table 12 lists the commercially available antiviral agents.

Table 10. *Sites of Action for Antibacterial Agents*

Affects Cell Wall	Affects Protein Synthesis
Penicillins	Aminoglycoides
Penicillin G	Streptomycin
Penicillin V	Neomycin
Phenethicillin	Kanamycin
Methicillin	Gentamycin
Nafcillin	Tobramycin
Oxacillin	Amikacin
Cloxacillin	Chloramphenicol
Ampicillin	Erythromycin
Amoxicillin	
Carbenicillin	
Carbenicillin indanyl	
Ticarcillin	
Cephalosporins and cephamycins	
Bacitracin	

Affects Cell Membrane	Affects Intermediary Metabolism
Polymyxin B	Sulfonamides
Polymyxin E (colistin)	Sodium sulfacetamide
Gramicidin	

Table 11. *Concentrations and Dosages of Principal Antibiotics*

Antibiotics	Topical	Subconjunctival
Ampicillin	. . . .	50–250 mg
Bacitracin	10,000 units/ml	10,000 units
Carbenicillin*	4.0 mg/ml	100 mg
Cephaloridine	. . . .	100 mg
Cephalothin	. . . .	50–100 mg
Chloramphenicol	5 mg/ml	500–100 mg
Clindamycin	. . . .	15–40 mg
Colistin	5–10 mg/ml	15–37.5 mg
Erythromycin	. . . .	100 mg
Gentamicin*	8–15 mg/ml	20–40 mg
Lincomycin	. . . .	150 mg
Methicillin	. . . .	150–200 mg
Neomycin	5–8 mg/ml	250–500 ug
Penicillin G	100,000 units/ml	0.5–1.0 million units
Polymyxin B	16,250 units/ml	10 mg
Streptomycin*	. . . .	50–100 mg
Tobramycin	3 mg/ml	. . . .
Vancomycin	50 ml/ml	25 mg

*Incompatible mixture for IV administration.

Revised from Henkind, P., Walsh, J. B., and Berger, A. W. (eds.): Copyright© *PDR for Ophthalmology 1983*. Published by Medical Economics Company Inc., Oradell, NJ 07649.

Table 12. Antiviral Agents

USP or NF Name	Dosage
5-Iodo-2 deoxyuridine (IDU) (Herplex, Allergan) (Stoxil, SmithKline Beckman)	Ointment 0.5%: 5 times/day; solution 0.1%: every 2 hours for 5–7 days
Adenine arabinoside (ARaA) (Vira-A, Parke-Davis)	Ointment 3%: 5 times/day for 5–7 days

Note: Antivirals are compatible with antibiotic preparations.

ANTIFUNGAL AGENTS

Systemic mycosis with secondary ocular involvement is the most frequent ocular mycosis observed in small animals. The horse is the animal in which keratomycosis is most commonly observed. The practitioner's index of suspicion should be raised in severe nonresponsive corneal disease in any domestic animal. The corneal lesions are usually due to saprophytic fungi in debilitated or immunosuppressed patients or those that have received prolonged topical antibacterial and corticosteroid treatment. The available drugs are few and expensive and sometimes not available in an ophthalmic form. It is imperative that specific identification and sensitivity tests be performed to aid in selection of a therapeutic agent. The sensitivity tests are not routinely performed in laboratories, which makes it difficult to complete the necessary evaluations. (The diagnostic laboratory at the New York State College of Veterinary Medicine, Cornell University, performs antifungal sensitivity tests.)

The antifungal agents can be divided into broad classifications.

Polyene antibiotics include the following:

1. Nystatin (very toxic, mainly used topically)
2. Amphotericin B (systemic, subcutaneous, topical)
3. Natamycin (topical solution, very expensive)

Pyrimides such as flucytosine (5-fluourocytosine) are administered orally.

Imidazoles include the following:

1. Miconazole (systemic, topical)
2. Ketoconazole (systemic, topical)
3. Clotrimazole (topical)
4. Econazole (topical)
5. Thiabendazole (systemic)

Table 13 lists some antifungal agents used in ophthalmology.

ANTIENZYME AGENTS

Corneal lysis as a result of enzyme digestion is a common clinical occurrence. It is rapid and devastating to the cornea. Certain bacteria *(Pseudomonas)* secrete proteases that cause lysis of the corneal matrix. This releases other necrotoxins and stimulates leukotaxis. In a complex fashion, polymorphonuclear neutrophils, keratocytes, and necrotic epithelium liberate collagenase, resulting in further lysis. The liberation of collagenase, once initiated, can continue after the initial infection has been brought under control. It is prudent to incorporate an anticollagenase agent in the presence of signs of corneal melting (keratomalacia).

Agents that have been used include *N*-acetylcysteine 10 and 20 per cent (Mucomyst 10 and 20 per cent, Mead Johnson), disodium edetate (EDTA), and dimethylcysteine. The author recommends mixing equal parts of Mucomyst 20 with Adapt (Alcon) and treating every 4 hours. The frequency should be adjusted as necessary.

Chelators of zinc ions have also been used successfully. Disodium EDTA (Endrate, Abbott) can be used by withdrawing 0.4 ml of Adapt from a 15 ml vial and replacing it with 0.4 ml of Endrate. This solution can be used every 4 hours and adjusted as necessary. Dimethylcysteine (penicillamine [Cuprimine, Merck, Sharp & Dohme]) capsules can be made into a 0.15 M solution applied every 4 hours, and adjusted as necessary. One of the most potent anticollagenase agents available is the α-2-macroglobulins in whole fresh blood. This can be obtained from the patient if necessary (by venipuncture) and dropped on the eye until more appropriate drugs are available.

CAUTERANTS

These agents have long been used in ophthalmology. Their indiscriminate use is dangerous. The action of most of these agents provides a method of superficial chemical keratectomies. These agents can be used to sterilize septic lesions, remove superficial necrotizing corneal epithelium and stroma, and seal small corneal leaks. Some of the agents have some anticollagenase effect, which is poorly documented (e.g., iodine). Specific agents include trichloracetic acid crystals, liquid phenol, and iodine preparations. The author limits use to the iodine agents, which include 7 per cent tincture, 2½ per cent tincture, Lugol's solution, and Xenodine (Squibb). The cornea or the animal should be anesthetized. The area should be stained to identify the extent of the lesion and then dried with a sterile cotton applicator before the cauterant is applied. A cotton applicator is dipped into the solution, and the excess is removed by rolling on the back of a sterile glove. The lesion is swabbed, and all excess is thoroughly irrigated away with a collyrium.

Table 13. *Antifungal Agents*

USP or NF Name	Dosage	Spectrum	Toxicity
1. Amphotericin B (Topical solution) (Subconjunctival injection)	2.5–10 mg/ml of diluent (distilled water or 5% dextrose solution) 750 μg/ml of diluent (as above) every other day		
2. Amphotericin B (Intravenous)	0.15–1.0 mg/kg IV 3 times weekly for 2–4 months utilizing a preparation of 0.1 mg amphotericin B/ml solution obtained by diluting 50 mg of powder in 10 ml sterile water and then diluting final concentration 0.1 mg/dl in 5% dexrose solution	*Blastomyces* *Candida* *Coccidioides* *Histoplasma*	Fever, nausea, vomiting, renal impairment, hematuria, albuminuria, increased BUN, bone marrow depression, thrombophlebitis at site of injection
3. Amphotericin B (Intravitreal)	5–10 μg		
4. Nystain (Topical)	Ointment 100,000 units/gm	*Aspergillus* *Candida*	
5. Flucytosine	(a) PO: 200 mg/kg body weight/day ÷ t.i.d. (b) Topical: 1% solution	*Candida* *Cryptococcus*	Diarrhea, nausea, bone marrow suppression
6. Natamycin (Topical suspension)	5% Suspension	*Candida* *Aspergillus* *Cephalosporium* *Fusarium* *Penicillium*	
7. Miconazole and Econazole	Topical, 1% solution in arachis oil	*Candida* *Aspergillus*	Phlebitis, GI disturbance, enhances Coumadin effect, ocular irritant
8. Ketoconazole	(a) Dog: 10–20 mg/kg in a single daily dose or divided b.i.d. (b) Cat: 10–20 mg/kg b.i.d. every other day or 50 mg/kg once daily	*Blastomyces* *Cryptococcus* *Histoplasma*	

Revised from Henkind, P., Walsh, J. B., and Berger, A. W. (eds.): *PDR for Ophthalmology 1983*. Oradell, NJ: Medical Economics, 1982, p. 6.

INHIBITORS OF AQUEOUS SECRETION

Carbonic-anhydrase inhibitors are used in the medical management of glaucoma. They block the combination of carbon dioxide plus water to form carbonic acid and vice versa. The bicarbonate ion is reduced, resulting in decreased aqueous production. The exact mechanism is difficult to explain because of the low bicarbonate ion concentration in aqueous; however, production is decreased 50 to 60 per cent. A reasonable explanation may be the relative regional acidosis due to increased hydrogen ion concentration that occurs in the epithelium of the ciliary processes. Although these agents are diuretics, they are not used as such. This was demonstrated when bilateral nephrectomized rabbits treated with a carbonic-anhydrase inhibitor had decreased intraocular pressures. It is mundane, but imperative, to state again that *these agents are not used as diuretics* and that *the most effective diuretics* (e.g., furosemide [Lasix, Hoechst-Roussel]) *cannot be used for glaucoma therapy.*

Agents and dosages are as follows:

1. Acetazolamide (Diamox, Lederle): 10 to 30 mg/kg divided t.i.d.
2. Methazolamide (Neptazane, Lederle): 4 to 8 mg/kg divided t.i.d.
3. Dichlorphenamide (Oratrol, Alcon; Daranide, Merck, Sharp & Dohme): 2 to 5 mg/kg divided t.i.d. (the author's preference).

These agents often produce signs of metabolic acidosis, although dichlorphenamide causes the fewest complications. (Other agents that affect aqueous production have previously been described under Autonomic Agents.)

Table 14. Artificial Tear Solutions

Product and Ingredients	Product and Ingredients	Product and Ingredients
Adapettes (Alcon)	Isopto Tears (Alcon)	Methulose (Softcon)
Adsorbobase*	Hydroxypropyl methylcellulose	Methylcellulose 0.25%
Thimerosal 0.002%	0.5%	Buffered solution
Disodium edetate 0.05%	Benzalkonium chloride 0.01%	Benzalkonium chloride 0.004%
Adapt (Alcon)	Lacril (Allergan)	Tearisol (CooperVision)
Adsorbobase*	Hydroxypropyl methylcellulose	Hydroxypropyl methylcellulose
Hydroxyethyl cellulose 0.55%	Polysorbate 80, gelatin A, buffered	0.5%
Thimerosal 0.002%	isotonic solution	Benzalkonium chloride 0.01%
Disodium edetate 0.05%	Chlorobutanol 0.5%	Edetate disodium
Adsorbotear (Alcon)	Liquifilm Forte (Allergan)	Buffered isotonic solution
Adsorbobase*	Polyvinyl alcohol 3%	Tears Naturale (Alcon)
Hydroxyethyl cellulose	Thimerosal 0.002%	Duasorb polymeric system with
Buffered isotonic solution	Edetate disodium	dextran
Thimerosal 0.002%	Liquifilm Tears (Allergan)	Benzalkonium chloride 0.01%
Disodium edetate 0.05%	Polyvinyl alcohol 1.4%	Edetate disodium 0.05%
Hypotears (CooperVision)	Chlorobutanol 0.5%	Visculose (Softcon)
Lipiden polymeric system	Lyteers (Barnes-Hind)	Methylcellulose 0.5 or 1.0%
Benzalkonium chloride 0.01%	Hydroxyethyl cellulose 0.2%	Buffered solution
Edetate diusodium 0.03%	Buffered isotonic solution	Benzalkonium chloride 0.004%
Nonionic tonicity adjusters	Benzalkonium chloride 0.01%	
Sterile hypotonic solution	Disodium edetate 0.05%	

*Adsorbobase = polyvinylpyrrolidone-soluble polymers (PVP) 1.67% with water.
Revised from Henkind, P., Walsh, J. B., and Berger, A. W. (eds.): *PDR for Ophthalmology 1983*. Oradell, NJ: Medical Economics, 1982, p. 12.

OSMOTIC AGENTS

Parenteral drugs are used in glaucoma management to reduce intraocular pressure rapidly and safely in an emergency. The reduction in pressure results from osmotic tension applied to the contents of the eye, mainly the vitreous. The eye is surrounded by a vascular network, the uvea. Osmotic agents cannot penetrate the normal blood-ocular barrier, so a gradient of osmotic tension results. The vitreous, which is about 99 per cent water, becomes smaller. This results in a rapid lowering of the pressure and a posterior displacement of the lens iris diaphragm, which also provides a wider drainage angle. The author has demonstrated this phenomenon with ocular ultrasonography before and after mannitol administration. The method of administration should include withholding water for 2 to 4 hours after delivery. Specific agents available for intravenous or oral administration include mannitol 15 to 20 per cent, 1 to 2 gm/kg slow push IV; and glycerol, 1 to 2 gm/kg PO (causes emesis in many instances).

Topical hyperosmotic ointments are used for symptomatic treatment of an overhydrated (edematous) cornea. They are not curative but are effectively used for endothelial dystrophic keratopathy, which results in corneal edema. The frequency of medication varies with the severity of the lesion. The author prefers the ointment form.

Specific topical osmotic agents include the following: sodium chloride solutions 2 to 5 per cent (Adsorbonac, Alcon; Muro 128, Muro) and sodium chloride ointments 5 per cent (5 per cent Muro 128, Muro).

STAINS (DYES)

These are used as diagnostic aids. They may be used to identify lesions of the corneal or conjunctival epithelium, patency of the nasolacrimal drainage apparatus, and integrity of the retinal vasculature; as a study of aqueous dynamics; and, in humans, for applanation tonometry.

Specific Agents

Fluorescein sodium-impregnated strips are sterile and disposable. (The available solutions are dangerous since they support the growth of *Pseudomonas* and are easily contaminated.) The involved eye is irrigated, and a drop of sterile collyrium is placed on the end of the strip. This is placed on the dorsal bulbar conjunctiva, carefully avoiding the corneal surface. This is important, particularly in cats, because the strip may remove the mucin portion of precorneal film, causing a false-positive dye retention. Because of the water solubility of the dye and the pH at which this agent fluoresces, epithelial defects will appear green. This can be accentuated by using an ultraviolet light source (Wood's light), which enhances fluorescence.

Observing the external nares for the presence of the dye can identify the patency of the nasolacrimal drainage apparatus. Variations in the nasolacrimal duct may cause a false-negative dye passage, and irrigation may be necessary to more definitely identify an obstruction or patency.

Intravenous fluorescein is available in sterile form. This is used to identify abnormalities within the posterior segment by fluorescein angiography. It requires special filters and techniques that are beyond the scope of this article to discuss.

Rose bengal is a vital dye that stains necrotic or dying cells and mucus brilliant red. It is used in human medicine primarily as an adjunct for early detection of keratoconjunctivitis sicca (KCS). It is nonspecific, irritating, and will stain clothing and other objects. It does not add any additional information to a good ocular workup and essentially is not necessary as a diagnostic tool in veterinary ophthalmology.

TEAR REPLACEMENT AGENTS

Decreased tear production is extremely common (see Keratoconjunctivitis Sicca). There are many commercially available tear replacement agents. One of the most important criteria is contact time, and the practitioner should keep this in mind when designing a regimen for a patient with keratoconjunctivitis sicca. Other factors include (1) the degree of lacrimal deficiency, (2) the presence of other associated or concomitant oculopathies, (3) owner compliance, and (4) the age of the patient.

Polyvinylpyrrolidone (Adapt or Adsorbotear, Alcon) is the author's preference. It is similar to bovine mucin and is compatible with most ophthalmic medications, as well as being an excellent surface wetting agent. This characteristic provides longer contact time.

Other available solutions include polyvinyl alcohol, methylcellulose, and ethylene glycol polymers (similar to polyvinylpyrrolidone). These are found as vehicles for many of the ophthalmic drugs. Table 14 lists tear replacement agents.

Oily or ointment bases contain refined petrolatum, lanolin, and peanut oil. These are sophisticated agents that provide prolonged contact without adverse side effects and little competition with fat-soluble agents, increasing the bioavailability of the drugs carried by them. Some ointment agents used to supplement tears include Lacri-Lube S.O.P. (Allergan), AKWA Tears ointment (Akorn), Duratears (Alcon), Murocel (Muro), Duolube (Muro), and Ophthalmic Base (Pharmafair).

Section 8

DISEASES OF CAGED AND EXOTIC PETS

MURRAY E. FOWLER, D.V.M.
Consulting Editor

Additional Pertinent Information Found in **Current Veterinary Therapy VIII:**

Brooks, D. L.: Rabbit Gastrointestinal Disorders, p. 654.
Bush, M.: External Fixation to Repair Long Bone Fractures in Larger Birds, p. 630.
Clark, J. D.: Rabbit Pasteurellosis, p. 669.
Emanuelson, S.: Avian Trichomoniasis, p. 619.
Ensley, P.: Parasitic Diseases of Cage Birds, p. 641.
Fowler, M. E.: Disinfectant and Insecticide Usage Around Birds and Reptiles, p. 606.
Galvin, C.: The Feather Picking Bird, p. 646.
Jacobson, E. R.: Parasitic Diseases of Reptiles, p. 599.
Kennedy-Stoskopf, S.: Avian Pox in Caged Birds, p. 633.
Mainster, M. E.: Scaly Face in Budgerigars, p. 626.
Mehren, K. G.: Gout, p. 635.
Meier, J. E.: Salmonellosis and Other Bacterial Enteritides in Birds, p. 637.
Phillips, L. G., Jr.: Total Parenteral Nutrition in Exotic Animals, p. 657.
Redig, P. T.: Aspergillosis, p. 611.
Sawyer, B. A.: Bumblefoot in Raptors, p. 614.

> Notice: The blood levels of lead in psittacine birds that are given on page 618 of *Current Veterinary Therapy VIII* are incorrect. See page 713 of this edition, the article Lead Poisoning in Psittacine Birds, for detailed information.

OROPHARYNGEAL DISEASES IN CAGED BIRDS*

KEVEN FLAMMER, D.V.M.
Raleigh, North Carolina

Oropharyngeal diseases are common in caged birds, and inspection of the oral cavity should be a routine part of the physical examination. The beak of most avian species can be opened manually, but a speculum is required for psittacine birds. Parrot beaks can be opened with a forceps or with gauze strips looped around the upper and lower beaks.

The anatomy of the avian oropharynx differs from that of mammals. The floor of the mouth is occupied by the tongue and glottis (Fig. 1). The glottis is located within the oral cavity, just caudal to the base of the tongue. The morphology of the tongue varies, depending on the feeding habits of the bird. Most birds (e.g., passerines, pigeons, poultry, and raptors) have a narrow, pointed, heavily keratinized tongue. The tongue in psittacine birds is used primarily for manipulating food and is rounded and fleshy. A slit in the roof of the mouth, the choana, forms the opening of the nasal passageway. In most birds this passageway communicates with the external nares and the periorbital sinuses. Its edges are lined by a number of small papillae. Salivary glands are located in numerous locations in both the roof and floor of the oral cavity.

Disease-related changes in the oropharynx include depigmentation, blunting or swelling of the choanal papillae, and the presence of exudates, plaques, and abcesses. Microscopic examination of an impression smear of material from the lesion will

*Note: FDA approval has not been obtained for use of any drug in nondomestic avian species.

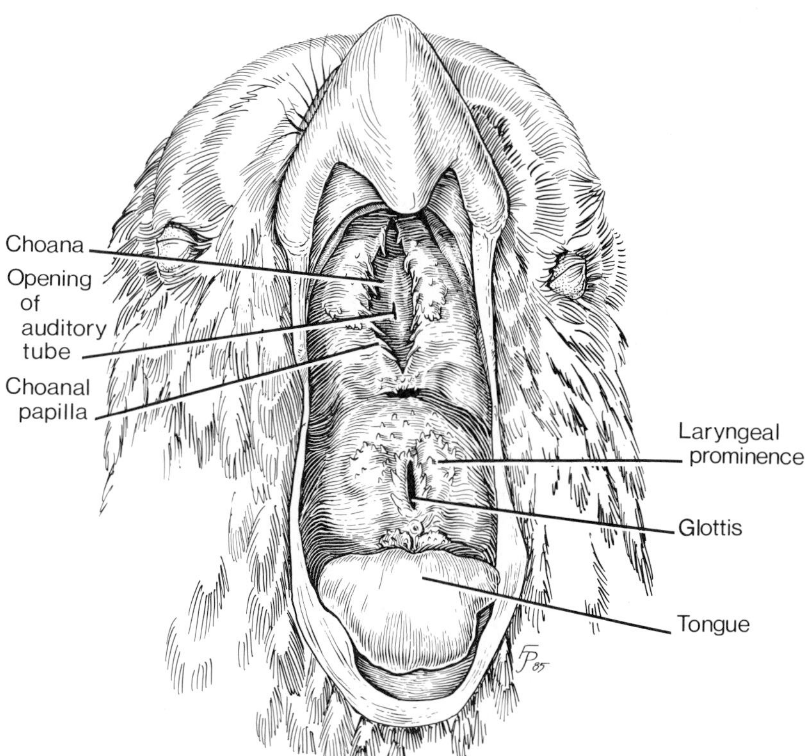

Figure 1. Anatomy of the avian oropharynx.

frequently reveal the causative agent. Caution must be used when the presence of bacteria and fungi is found, since these opportunists may secondarily invade lesions caused by another agent. Recovery of a microbial pathogen does not necessarily rule out other causes. Biopsy and histopathlogic tests may be necessary for a definitive diagnosis.

VITAMIN A DEFICIENCY

Vitamin A deficiency is most commonly diagnosed in psittacine birds, particularly Amazon, pionus, and eclectus parrots. Vitamin A deficiency causes changes in epithelial tissue, leading to increased keratinization and squamous metaplasia.

Deficient birds are prone to ocular, sinus, and respiratory infections. Early clinical signs include swelling and depigmentation of the choanal papillae. Later, increased keratinization of mucous membranes and the degeneration of mucosal glands results in the formation of abscesses, which frequently become secondarily infected with opportunistic bacteria and yeast. These abscesses first appear as small, rounded swellings that may eventually become large and confluent. Abscesses are most easily identified on the roof of the mouth, and they are filled with a watery or cheesy white pus. This exudate is easily removed without causing damage to the underlying tissue. In contrast, plaques of primarily microbial or viral origin form a pseudomembrane that adheres to the underlying mucosa and leaves a raw, hemorrhagic surface when forcibly removed.

A definitive diagnosis of vitamin A deficiency is difficult to make. Examination of biopsy material from the oropharyngeal glands may reveal characteristic changes of squamous metaplasia of epithelial cells. Assays for vitamin A in liver tissue are available but require a larger tissue sample than can be obtained from a living bird. Most often, a presumptive diagnosis is made from the dietary history, clinical signs, and response to therapy.

Therapy consists of supplementing vitamin A, treating oral abscesses, and controlling secondary infections. Initially, a single intramuscular injection of vitamin A (10,000 to 20,000 IU/kg) should be given, since epithelial changes caused by the deficiency may reduce absorption of orally administered vitamin in the intestines. Once stabilized, the patient should be fed a balanced diet and should receive a vitamin A supplement in the form of an avian multivitamin mix added to the drinking water or a suitable food vehicle (e.g., cooked mash). Natural sources of vitamin A include carrots, spinach, and dried red peppers. Small oral abscesses will often resolve with vitamin A therapy alone. Large abscesses should be carefully lanced and the abscess material removed and cultured. A small amount of antibiotic ointment placed into the incision will help control hemorrhage and microbial infections. Infected lesions can be treated with appropriate antibiotics, selected on the basis of culture and sensitivity of organisms recovered from the surgical site.

AVIAN POXVIRUS

Avian poxvirus infection is most often encountered in canaries, pigeons, and psittacine birds. Among the psittacines, recently imported Amazon parrots (especially blue-fronted), pionus parrots, lovebirds, and Australian parakeets are most frequently affected.

Pox lesions are manifested in two main forms, which may appear concurrently. In the dry or cutaneous form, crusts and proliferative wartlike nodules appear on the unfeathered portions of the body, especially in areas surrounding the eyes and beak. In the wet, or diphtheritic form, the earliest lesions are swelling, erosion, and depigmentation of the choanal papillae. Later, white, slightly raised plaques form on the mucous membranes of the oral cavity, esophagus, crop, sinuses, and trachea. These plaques may join to form large diphtheritic pseudomembranes that tightly adhere to the mucosa. If the pseudomembrane is forcibly removed, it will leave a raw, hemorrhagic, eroded surface.

A presumptive diagnosis can be made from the history and clinical signs. A definitive diagnosis is made by taking a biopsy of the lesion and culturing the virus or identifying the characteristic intracytoplasmic inclusions (Bollinger's bodies) in epithelial cells. Secondary infections by bacteria and yeast are common.

There is no specific treatment for poxvirus, but supportive care (e.g., warmth, force-feeding, and fluid maintenance) and control of secondary infections will reduce mortality. No vaccine is commercially available.

BACTERIA

Gram-negative organisms (e.g., *Escherichia coli*, *Klebsiella*, and *Pseudomonas*) and species of *Staphylococcus* are frequently isolated as secondary invaders but may also cause primary oral lesions. Most of the primary bacterial lesions the author has identified are discrete, rounded, slightly raised, yellowish plaques. These plaques are firmly attached and will leave a small, hemorrhagic hole if forcibly removed. Primary bacterial disease may also mimic early signs of pox or vitamin A deficiency. One species of *Staphylococcus* was responsible for an outbreak of oropharyngeal disease in a mixed collection of Amazon parrots. Lesions started as a slight swelling and depigmentation of the choanal papillae and progressed to erosion of the edges of the choanal slit. The birds were fed a supplemented diet, so vitamin A deficiency was ruled unlikely. The collection was successfully treated with ampicillin (150 mg/kg orally twice daily for 7 days).

Bacterial infections are identified by examining cultures and gram-stained impression smears of the lesion. Topical therapy with antibiotic ointments is occasionally successful, but more often systemic treatment is required. The proper antibiotic should be selected on the basis of susceptibility testing since the resistance of oral isolates is difficult to predict.

CANDIDA

Candida albicans frequently causes oropharyngeal disease in young and nestling birds. The mouth, crop, esophagus, and distal alimentary tract may be involved. Early infection with *Candida* causes a white, velvety, exudate (resembling a Turkish towel) that covers the mucosal surface and can be scraped away without causing hemorrhage. More chronic lesions, and those in more keratinized regions of the mouth (such as the tongue and commissures of the beak), cause firm, brownish plaques that adhere more tenaciously to the underlying mucosa.

Candida organisms are gram-positive, budding, and oval shaped. In most cases they can be demonstrated on an impression smear of the lesion. The fungi can also be cultured on blood agar or Sabouraud dextrose-agar plates.

Several drugs are available for treating candidiasis. Nystatin is the primary drug of choice, but it must come in contact with the lesions since it is not absorbed from the gut. Oral suspensions (300,000 IU/kg) can be given directly into the mouth or through a crop tube twice daily for 7 to 10 days. Flocks of birds can be treated by adding a nystatin premix (Myco 20, Squibb) to a cooked mash or other food vehicle at the rate of 5 gm of Myco 20 per pound of food. Oral lesions can also be treated topically with a plasticized cream containing amphotericin B (Fungizone Cream, Squibb) or with a topical cream containing miconazole (1% Conofite, Pitman-Moore). Ketoconazole (Nizoral, Janssen; 10 to 15 mg/kg orally twice daily for 10 to 14 days) or flucytosine (Ancobon, Roche; 250 mg/kg orally twice daily for 7 to 10 days) can be used for *Candida* infections that are refractory to nystatin treatment. Chlorhexidine (Nolvasan, Fort Dodge) has activity against *Candida* and can be added to the drinking water at the rate of 10 ml/gallon for 10 days. This dose may reduce the severity of a mild outbreak but should not be relied upon as the sole means of treatment.

TRICHOMONAS

Trichomoniasis is caused by the protozoan parasite *Trichomonas gallinae* and is frequently encountered in gallinaceous birds, pigeons, and raptors. Among the pet birds, canaries and finches are most often infected and may exhibit a significant mortality rate. In most cases parasitic invasion is limited to the oral cavity, crop, and esophagus, but in young pigeons and poultry the disease can spread systemically and affect multiple organ systems. In the mouth, *Trichomonas* causes small, white, sticky plaques that *rapidly become confluent*, yellowish-brown, cheesy masses. This exudate can be removed without causing damage to the underlying mucosa. In severe cases accumulation of this cheesy material can interfere with swallowing and closure of the beak. Other signs include depression, weight loss, and the inability to eat or drink.

Trichomoniasis is easily diagnosed by microscopically examining a warm saline wet mount of material collected by swabbing or scraping a lesion. *Trichomonas gallinae* is flagellated, pear-shaped, and moves with a characteristic spiral motion.

Most infected birds respond quickly to treatment with dimetridazole (Emtryl, Salsbury). Flocks of larger psittacine birds, pigeons, and raptors can be treated by adding 1 level teaspoon of Emtryl per gallon of drinking water for 5 days. Toxicity has been reported at this dose in finches, budgerigars, cockatiels, and very young pigeons, so small and young birds should be treated with smaller amounts. The author has safely and effectively used ¾ tsp/gallon drinking water for 4 days in cockatiels and finches. Birds that are reluctant to eat or drink can be tube-fed with dimetridazole (50 mg/kg once or twice daily) until they are drinking on their own.

Signs of dimetridazole toxicity include depression, refusal to eat, ataxia, staggering, and death. In finches depression may be the only outward sign, followed by death within 12 to 24 hours. If abnormal signs are exhibited, treatment should be stopped immediately. General supportive care is also important in reducing mortality rates.

CAPILLARIA

Capillaria worms most commonly infect the alimentary tract distal to the mouth, but they are occasionally responsible for oral lesions as well. Petrak (1982) reported caseous, yellow, diphtheritic membrane lesions in the mouth of wild blue jays. The presence of capillarid eggs in scrapings of the necrotic debris confirmed the diagnosis. *Capillaria* infestation is difficult to eradicate, and repeated treatment may be necessary. Oral administration of levamisole, either as a single bolus through a crop tube (15 to 30 mg/kg), or by adding 2.25 mg/gallon drinking water for 4 to 5 days, is sometimes successful. Use of ivermectin (0.20 mg/kg intramuscularly) has also shown promising results. Treatment with either drug should be repeated in 10 to 14 days. Strict clean-up of the aviary to remove old droppings that may harbor *Capillaria* eggs is necessary to prevent post-treatment reinfection. Housing the birds in suspended cages with wire bottoms that allow droppings to pass out of the cage will also reduce the incidence of reinfection.

OTHER CAUSES OF OROPHARYNGEAL DISEASES

Trauma to the oral cavity can cause injuries that may become secondarily infected by yeast and bacteria. In baby birds hand-fed by catheter-tipped syringes, the syringe tip will occasionally cause oral abrasions. Psittacine birds are fond of chewing and may eat objects that can cause splinters or chemical burns in the mouth. In birds suffering respiratory distress, both the glottis and the choanal slit should be examined in order to make sure that a seed or other piece of debris is not plugging the opening of either orifice.

SUMMARY OF THE DIAGNOSTIC APPROACH TO OROPHARYNGEAL LESIONS

1. Examine the bird for associated clinical signs.
2. Examine and characterize the lesion.
3. Culture the lesion.
4. Swab the lesion and prepare:
   A. A direct saline wet mount to check for *Capillaria* eggs and *Trichomonas*.
   B. A gram-stained smear to examine for microorganisms.
5. If these tests do not yield a suitable diagnosis, or if pox virus is suspected, submit a biopsy of the lesion.

References and Supplemental Reading

Campbell, T. W.: Diagnostic cytology in avian medicine. Vet. Clin. North Am. 14:317, 1984.

Clubb, S. L.: Therapeutics in avian medicine. Vet. Clin. North Am. 14:345, 1984.

Emanuelson, S.: Avian trichomoniasis. *In* Kirk, R. W. (ed.): *Current Veterinary Therapy VIII*. Philadelphia: W. B. Saunders, 1983. pp. 619–621.

Kennedy-Stoskopf, S.: Avian pox in caged birds. *In* Kirk, R. W. (ed.): *Current Veterinary Therapy VIII*. Philadelphia: W. B. Saunders, 1983, pp. 633–635.

Petrak, M. L. (ed.): *Diseases of Cage and Aviary Birds*, 2nd ed. Philadelphia: Lea & Febiger, 1982.

Pitts, C.: Hypovitaminosis A in psittacines. *In* Kirk R. W. (ed.): *Current Veterinary Therapy VIII*. Philadelphia: W. B. Saunders, 1983, pp. 622–625.

ENDOCRINOLOGY OF BIRDS

ROBERT D. ZENOBLE, D.V.M.,
and ROBERT J. KEMPPAINEN, D.V.M.

Auburn, Alabama

Endocrine testing in dogs and cats is well established in veterinary medicine, and many practicing veterinarians are routinely diagnosing and treating endocrinopathies in animals. This interest in clinical endocrinology has been extended to the care of avian patients. Established testing protocols and hormone values for normal pet birds have only recently become available for avian practitioners (Lothrop et al., 1985; Rosskopf et al., 1982; Walsh et al., 1985; Zenoble et al., 1985). Most of the earlier published data on hormone levels in pet birds were based on measurements of hormones important in mammals. In certain instances, such as in thyroid and pancreatic endocrine function, the avian and mammalian species are similar. However, the physiology of the adrenal glands of birds is substantially different from that of mammals. The endocrine systems of domestic fowl have been studied and offer a base from which caged-bird endocrinology can be examined. In all studies published, domestic fowl and psittacine birds are similar.

ENDOCRINOLOGY OF THE ADRENAL GLAND

Birds have paired adrenal glands located anterior and medial to the anterior pole of the kidneys and immediately posterior to the lungs. They are light yellow to orange in color and are triangular or oval in shape. In contrast to those of mammals, avian adrenal glands have no defined cortex or medulla. Islets of medullary cells are diffusely spread throughout the cortical tissue. The avian adrenal cortex is not grossly divided into distinct functional regions; however, the area of mineralocorticoid production is in the subcapsular zone and the area of glucocorticoid production is predominantly the inner zone.

In the species of birds studied (chicken, turkey, pigeon, sparrow, and duck), corticosterone is the major glucocorticoid, and cortisol is very low in concentration. Aldosterone is the principal mineralocorticoid. Plasma corticosterone levels show a circadian rhythm under light-dark cycles that is altered if the bird is kept in continuous light. The concentration of plasma corticosterone varies according to season, sexual activity, and molting cycle. Stresses, such as cold temperature, surgical procedures, or handling, cause an increase in plasma corticosterone levels. Endogenous release of ACTH stimulates synthesis and release of corticosterone but not aldosterone. The exogenous administration of ACTH will cause corticosterone to be released and hence can be used to measure adrenal gland capacity and function.

The resting level of corticosterone can be influenced by numerous factors; therefore, the ACTH stimulation test is used to evaluate the capacity of the gland under maximal activation. Blood samples are taken from the patient prior to and approximately 1.5 hours after ACTH is administered. ACTH as cosyntropin (Cortrosyn, Organon) is administered intramuscularly, 0.125 mg per bird.

Levels of cortisol and corticosterone before and after ACTH administration in several psittacine species and one species of raptor are shown in Table 1. Corticosterone concentration was markedly increased after ACTH administration but cortisol did not rise significantly. Comparison of the various species shows some differences, but this variation does not reduce the clinical value of the test. Several birds were given saline injections instead of ACTH to determine the effects of capture and endogenous ACTH release. A rise in corticosterone occasionally occurred after saline administration; however, the responses were significantly less than those seen after administration of exogenous ACTH.

There are case reports describing adrenal insufficiency in pet birds, but cortisol and not corticosterone was the glucocorticoid measured. Conclusions from these case reports must be considered invalid until they are reconfirmed by measuring the appropriate glucocorticoid. The adrenal glands of birds that die of bacterial septicemia occasionally show histopathologic lesions, but one should not interpret that as adrenal insufficiency. Ideally, practitioners wishing to evaluate adrenal function in birds should test healthy, matched individuals and submit these samples to the laboratory for comparison. Adrenal insufficiency should be suspected when no increase in corticosterone is seen after ACTH administration. An empirical regime for replacement therapy for adrenal insufficiency has been suggested by Rosskopf: dexamethasone (2 mg/ml), 0.1 to 0.2 ml, and fluorocortisone acetate (0.1 mg), ¼ to 1 tablet per 4 ounces of drinking water.

Treatment with glucocorticoids for prolonged periods would likely result in secondary adrenal gland atrophy and a reduced response to ACTH stimulation. Spontaneous hyperadrenocorticism (Cushing's disease) should show an exaggerated response to exogenous ACTH administration.

ENDOCRINOLOGY OF THE THYROID GLAND

In the dog, thyroid-stimulating hormone (TSH, or thyrotropin) stimulates the thyroid gland to synthesize and release thyroxine (T_4) and a small amount of triiodothyronine (T_3). Measurements of resting, unstimulated concentrations of T_4 and T_3 do not always definitely identify animals with deficient glandular function. Administering TSH and measuring the change in concentration of circulating T_4 more accurately evaluates the functional capacity of the thyroid gland. Resting levels of T_4 and, particularly, T_3 are influenced by non-thyroid associated factors such as stress, disease, and surgery. These factors do not inhibit the response of the thyroid to TSH in the dog, and the same is presumably true in birds.

The thyroid glands in avian species are paired organs, oval in shape and dark red in color. They are located on either side of the trachea, cranial to the syrinx and just exterior to the thoracic cavity. The size of the thyroid gland and its secretory activity is influenced by numerous factors such as age, sex, diet, species, and season.

Synthesis of thyroid hormones in birds is similar to that in mammals. Iodine is concentrated in the thyroid gland and thyroid proteins are iodinated to form thyroglobulin, which contains monoiodotyrosine, diiodotyrosine, triiodothyronine, and thyroxine. Both triiodothyronine and thyroxine are found in the plasma of birds. In blood, they are bound to plasma proteins such as thyroxine-binding globulin and albumin. Synthesis and release of the thyroid hormones are governed by their concentration in circulation and pituitary release of TSH. The thyroid-pituitary feedback mechanism is similar to that found in mammals. The secretion of TSH and the circulating levels of thyroid hormones are influ-

Table 1. *Influence of ACTH (Cosyntropin) on Plasma Corticosterone and Cortisol*

	Pre-ACTH		Post-ACTH	
Species	*Corticosterone* (μg/dl)	*Cortisol* (μg/dl)	*Corticosterone* (μg/dl)	*Cortisol* (μg/dl)
Red-lored Amazon (*Amazona autumnalis*)				
n = 10	1.01	0.223	4.75	0.234
n = 4 (Saline injection)			1.83	0.36
Blue-fronted Amazon (*Amazona aestiva*)				
n = 10	2.04	≤0.16	10.4	0.253
n = 4 (Saline injection)			1.76	≤0.16
African gray parrot (*Psittacus erithacus*)				
n = 10	2.24	≤0.16	4.75	≤0.16
n = 4 (Saline injection)			1.68	≤0.16
Bald eagle (*Haliaeetus leucocephalus*)				
n = 10	6.64	≤0.16	12.1	≤0.16
n = 2 (Saline injection)			7.0	≤0.18

Note: ≤0.16 = lowest detectable amount of cortisol

enced by season of the year, photoperiod, gonadal activity, and molt cycle.

Thyroid hormones have potent metabolic effects in all body tissues. Thyroidectomy in domestic poultry results in stunted growth in young birds, decreased feather growth, decreased gonadal weight and function, and lowered egg production. Experimental hyperthyroidism in domestic poultry results in an increase in metabolic processes, which results in weight loss.

Goiter has been documented in caged birds; it occurs when dietary iodine is inadequate. Iodine is essential for the biosynthesis of thyroid hormones, and iodine deficiency causes lowered levels of circulating T_3 and T_4 because of decreased production. Decreased concentrations of thyroid hormone result in an increased release of thyrotropin (TSH) from the pituitary because of a negative feedback system. Constant stimulation of the thyroid gland by thyrotropin causes hyperplasia and glandular enlargement. Metabolically, these birds have hypothyroidism even though they show glandular hyperplasia. The clinical manifestation of goiter is related to the physical expansion of the thyroid and not to low levels of hormone production. Thyroid enlargement can impinge on the trachea, causing dyspnea and a squeaking or clicking noise with respiration. Goiter is most often found in parakeets, but it can potentially occur in any bird on an iodine-deficient diet. Diagnosis is often based on characteristic respiratory signs and history of an iodine-deficient diet. Therapy is dietary replacement of iodine and a balanced diet.

Hypothyroidism has been documented in caged birds, but the bases of the diagnoses have been measurement of resting concentrations of thyroid hormone and response to thyroid hormone replacement. It is known that dogs may have low resting concentrations of thyroid hormone without actually having hypothyroidism. A firm diagnosis of hypothyroidism cannot be established simply because a clinical sign is altered or corrected after administration of thyroid hormones. A more secure diagnosis of hypothyroidism is made after a lack of response is demonstrated to exogenous TSH administration.

The TSH stimulation test for the assessment of thyroid gland function in birds is similar to that in dogs. Blood is collected prior to and about 6 hours after intramuscular administration of TSH, (Dermathycin, Jen-Sal; 1 unit per bird). The resting levels of T_4 and T_3 were low in most birds tested by our laboratory, but they dramatically increased after TSH administration (Table 2). Poststimulation levels of T_4 were high enough to be accurately measured; however, many birds had resting levels below the sensitivity limit of the hormone assay.

Hormone values determined by standards prepared in canine plasma were different from those prepared in avian plasma (Table 2). The type of radioimmunoassay can influence the range of values, and it is therefore necessary to determine if the laboratory has tested the species in question and has established a range of normal values when it is employed to determine hormonal concentrations in birds. If not, control samples may be submitted from matched, healthy birds to assist in proper assessment of potentially diseased patients (Table 2).

ENDOCRINOLOGY OF THE PANCREAS

The pancreas releases several hormones, of which insulin is the most important to the host. Diabetes mellitus has been diagnosed in caged birds and has been successfully managed with insulin injections. Hyperglycemia and glucosuria are seen in diabetic birds in response to insulinopenia and carbohydrate intolerance. Direct measurement of serum insulin is not needed for the diagnosis of diabetes mellitus.

Table 2. Plasma T_4 and T_3 Concentrations in Birds Before and After TSH Administration

Species	Pre-TSH T_4 (μg/dl) Assay 1*	Pre-TSH T_4 (μg/dl) Assay 2†	Pre-TSH T_3 (ng/dl) Assay 1*	Pre-TSH T_3 (ng/dl) Assay 2†	Post-TSH T_4 (μg/dl) Assay 1*	Post-TSH T_4 (μg/dl) Assay 2†	Post-TSH T_3 (ng/dl) Assay 1*	Post-TSH T_3 (ng/dl) Assay 2†
Red-lored Amazon (*A. autumnalis*) n = 14	≤0.15	0.43	105	156	1.92	6.11	111	137
Blue-fronted Amazon (*A. aestiva*) n = 12	≤0.15	≤0.15	160	107	2.24	7.64	244	260
African gray parrot (*P. erithacus*) n = 12	≤0.15	≤0.15	179	175	0.97	1.79	182	184

*Samples determined against standards in canine plasma
†Samples determined against standards in avian plasma

The insulin molecules among many species of animals, including birds, are similar. We have measured circulating plasma levels of insulin and glucose randomly in 10 Amazon parrots. The means were 9.1 μU/ml (SD 3.2 μU/ml) for insulin and 310 mg/dl (SD 45 mg/dl) for glucose. No special modification of the assay was made for this procedure.

Endocrine function has been extensively studied in domestic fowl and various other species of birds. In all instances, results in the nondomesticated birds were very similar to those in domestic fowl. The endocrine function of psittacine birds has been minimally studied, and when data for psittacines are unavailable, the domestic fowl should be used as a model.

References and Suggested Reading

Epple, A., and Stetson, M. H. (eds.): *Avian Endocrinology*. New York: Academic Press, 1980.

Jones, I. C., and Henderson, I. W. (eds.): *General, Comparative and Clinical Endocrinology of the Adrenal Cortex*. New York: Academic Press, 1976.

Lothrop, C. D., Jr., Loomis, M. R., and Olsen, J. H.: Thyrotropin stimulation test for evaluation of thyroid function in psittacine birds. J.A.V.M.A. 186:47, 1985.

Rosskopf, W. J., Woerpel, R. W., Rosskopf, G., et al.: Normal thyroid values for common pet birds. V.M./S.A.C. 77:409, 1982.

Skurkie, P. H. (ed.): *Avian Physiology*. New York: Springer-Verlag, 1975.

Walsh, M. T., Bildegreen, R. A., Clubb, S. L., et al.: Effect of exogenous ACTH on serum corticosterone and cortisol concentrations in the moluccan cockatoo (*Cacatus moluccensis*). Am. J. Vet. Res. 46:1584, 1985.

Zenoble, R. D., Kemppainen, R. J., Young, D. W., et al.: Endocrine responses of healthy parrots to ACTH and thyroid/stimulating hormone. J.A.V.M.A., in press.

EMERGING VIRAL DISEASES OF PSITTACINE BIRDS

LINDA J. LOWENSTINE, D.V.M.
Davis, California

With the increased popularity of exotic psittacines in the avicultural and pet trade has come awareness of viruses that affect these birds. Much of the recent information and cataloging of viruses has come both from investigators in Europe and through the quarantine and testing procedures employed by the departments of agriculture (USDA) in the United States and Britain. In addition, several of the large private quarantine or avicultural facilities now employ full-time veterinarians, and many of our veterinary schools have initiated programs in exotic avian medicine.

For the practioner, and even for the academician, this is a confusing era in psittacine medicine. New viruses are often described without an account of the clinicopathologic entities associated with them. New clinical syndromes that are of probable, but not proven, viral cause are also being identified. In addition, much recent knowledge has not yet been presented in standard texts and is found only in the proceedings or abstracts of meetings or made known through conversations between people actively involved in the field. All of this is indicative of an exciting and rapidly evolving discipline. It is the purpose of this article to acquaint the practitioner with some of the emerging disease entities associated with viruses in psittacine birds.

USDA QUARANTINE PROCEDURES AND ISOLATION OF VIRUSES FROM PSITTACINES

The USDA requires that all birds presented for importation into the United States be held in either a USDA-operated or a privately owned, USDA-approved quarantine facility for 30 days. During this time, tissue samples are taken from birds that die and cloacal swabs are taken from living birds. These samples are cultured in embryonated chicken eggs. Embryo-lethal viruses are tested for hemagglutinating activity, and positive viruses are examined serologically to identify Newcastle disease viruses, influenza viruses, and other paramyxoviruses. Election microscopy is also employed for morphologic classification. Non-Newcastle hemagglutinating and nonhemagglutinating embryo-lethal viruses are inoculated into 4- to 6-week-old chickens and turkeys to determine pathogenicity. Isolation of viruses virulent to domestic poultry results in shipments of exotic birds being refused entry into the United States. Entry is allowed to lots of birds from which mesogenic or lentogenic Newcastle disease virus, paramyxovirus or other hemagglutinating viruses, or viruses that are nonhemaggluting and embryo-lethal but not virulent for poultry are isolated. This last category includes psittacine herpesviruses, poxviruses, and adenoviruses, in order of frequency of isolation. In addition, the testing procedure will not detect many of the less virulent (non-embryo-lethal) avian viruses, such as some adenoviruses, some strains of influenza viruses, and infectious laryngotracheitis virus, among others.

The importance of these regulations for the practitioner is that birds that are infected or have been exposed to a variety of viruses gain access to the pet, zoo, and avicultural trade. These viruses pose no threat to the domestic poultry industry but can be significant causes of morbidity and mortality in psittacine birds themselves. Complicating matters further is the fact that, in spite of attempts to prevent unquarantined exotic birds from entering the United States, smuggled birds, especially from Latin America, suffering from velogenic Newcastle disease or other viral maladies may be presented for veterinary attention. "New viruses" are also being recognized in domestically reared psittacine birds; perhaps these organisms emerge from latency in the face of other disease conditions or management-related stresses. Intercurrent infections (e.g., reovirus and adenovirus, or pox and adenovirus) have also been recognized both in recent imports and in domestically reared birds.

DISEASES OF PROVEN OR PROBABLE VIRAL CAUSE

Table 1 lists viruses that have been isolated from psittacine birds, the species from which they are reported, and clinical signs or postmortem findings. It must be realized that Koch's postulates have not always been rigorously fulfilled and that the isolation of virus from moribund or defunct birds is often the sole criterion for deciding the viral cause of these conditions. In Table 2 diseases are listed that have even more nebulous proof of viral origin. In these conditions the assumption is based on identification of viral particles by transmission election microscopy (TEM) or by the presence of lesions that are reminiscent of those seen that are of proven viral cause in other species (e.g., myelo- and lymphoproliferative disorders in chickens and cats).

From the practical standpoint of differential diagnosis in the clinical setting, these entities will be presented in more detail according to their major clinical signs.

Diseases With Cutaneous or Mucocutaneous Lesions

Poxviruses in many species are notorious for producing both proliferative and necrotizing cutaneous lesions. In psittacine birds the warty excrescences of dry pox occur less frequently than in some other orders of birds, although this may differ with the strain of virus and species of bird. Conjunctivitis (especially in blue-fronted Amazons) and necrotizing oropharyngitis leading to depigmentation are most commonly seen. Nasal and tracheobronchial lesions have also been reported, as well as systemic disease associated with myocardial and hepatic necrosis. Demonstration of the cytoplasmic inclusions in diphtheritic lesions or in scabs is pathognomonic. The highly contagious psittacine poxviruses can be fairly readily cultured on the chorioallantoic membrane of chick eggs, although several passages may be required. Latent infections with fecal shedding have been suspected by researchers in Europe.

Proliferative, but rarely necrotizing, oropharyngeal and cloacal lesions have been reported in Amazons and macaws. These papillomatous lesions are thought to be infectious because they may occur in several birds in the same household or aviary. Attempts to demonstrate virus by TEM, culture, and immunohistochemical methods have proved unsuccessful to date. Diagnosis is based on histo-

Table 1. *Viruses Isolated from Psittacine Birds*

Type of Virus	Species Affected	Syndromes Seen
DNA Viruses		
Poxviruses	Amazons, macaws, *Pinous* parrots, many species	Conjunctivitis, wet pox; rarely, dry pox; fatal systemic disease
Herpesviruses	Amazons, many species of both Old and New World psittacines, cockatoos, budgies	Fatal hepatitis/splenitis; systemic disease; tracheitis; proliferative bronchitis; proliferative foot lesions; feather deformities
Papovaviruses	Budgerigars, many other species	Systemic disease; morbidity and mortality in nestlings
Papillomaviruses	African gray parrot	Facial warts
Adenoviruses	Budgerigars, lovebirds	Hepatitis; pancreatitis, inapparent infections
RNA Viruses		
Reoviruses	Variety of species	Inapparent infection; hepatosplenitis; fatal systemic disease
Paramyxoviruses PMV-1 (Newcastle disease)	Budgies, Amazons, conures, lovebirds, "parrots," other psittacines	Neurologic signs, especially tremors, ataxia, and paralysis; conjunctivitis; diarrhea; fatal systemic disease
PMV-2 Yucaipa virus	African gray parrots, parrots	Catarrhal pneumonia; emaciation; fatal systemic disease
PMV-3	Lovebirds, conures, Amazons, cockatiels, budgies, macaws, *Neophema* spp.	Neurologic signs (torticollis, tremors); diarrhea; inapparent infections
PMV-5 Kunitachi virus	Budgerigars	Diarrhea; dyspnea; hepatic and renal necroses with syncytial cells
unclassified paramyxoviruses	Budgerigars, lories	Diarrhea with gastrointestinal edema and hemorrhage; splenomegaly
Influenza viruses (Type A)		
H3N8	Psittacines (not specified)	Enteritis; air sacculitis; emaciation
H7N2	Parakeets	Fatal infection
H4N1	Parakeets, parrots, cockatoos	Fatal infection

pathologic findings. Recurrence after surgical removal has been seen in some cases. In addition, there has been a suspected association with cholangiocarcinomas in three cases.

Cutaneous wartlike lesions have been seen on the face of an African gray parrot and on the feet and legs of cockatoos and macaws. In the cockatoos and macaws, particles similar to herpesvirus were demonstrated by TEM but immunohistochemistry examination for papillomavirus antigens was negative. The lesions in cockatoos were papillary and quite horny, whereas those in macaws were flatter, more plaquelike, and depigmented. They were often present at the time of importation, and they frequently recurred after surgical removal. They may persist for many years but are of low infectivity and little clinical consequence. Diagnosis is based on histopathologic results; attempts to isolate the virus in embryonated chicken eggs has failed. Its relationship to other psittacine herpesvirus infections is unclear. In the African gray, particles similar to those of papillomavirus were seen on TEM, and genus-specific papillomavirus antigens were demonstrated by immunohistochemistry.

A far more significant and more widely reported syndrome associated with papovavirus infection is

Table 2. *Psittacine Diseases of Suspected Viral Cause*

Disease	Species Affected	Syndrome	Suspected Agent
Beak and feather disease, keratodysgenesis, naked cockatoo disease	Cockatoos, lovebirds, others	Feather deformity and loss; beak deformity; susceptibility to opportunistic pathogens	Parvo-like virus, densovirus, or picornavirus (seen on TEM)
Macaw wasting disease, infiltrative splanchnic neuropathy	Macaws, conures, others	Proventricular dilatation; encephalitis and ganglioneuritis	Unknown—probably an RNA virus
Mucosal papillomas	Amazons, macaws, others	Cloacal, oropharyngeal, or tracheal papillomas	Papovavirus (papillomaviruses)
Lymphoproliferative and myeloproliferative disorders	Red shining parrot, conures, budgies	Lymphosarcoma; infiltrative leukemias	Retrovirus
Cutaneous papillomas of feet and legs	Cockatoos, macaws	Warts and depigmented plaques on shanks and toes	Herpesvirus (seen on TEM)
Lymphoplasmacytic meningoencephalitis	*Pionus* spp.	Torticollis; high morbidity, moderate mortality; survival possible if bird is eating	Unclassified hemagglutinating virus (paramyxo-like particles seen on TEM)

the so-called budgie fledgling disease. This is a systemic disease causing morbidity and mortality in young birds of a variety of psittacine species. The most apparent manifestation is failure of feather growth and development that is due to infection of the follicular epithelium. Hepatic and renal necroses and involvement of other organs are also seen. Diagnosis is based on histopathologic demonstration of karyomegaly associated with clear to basophilic inclusion bodies. The basophilic inclusions can be confused with those seen in adenovirus infections, which may also cause hepatic or renal necrosis (though no cutaneous abnormalities) in budgies and lovebirds. The diagnosis should therefore be confirmed by TEM or by virus isolation. Psittacine papovaviruses have been isolated in chicken eggs, but sometimes they prove to be more particular and require psittacine eggs or primary budgerigar fibroblast cultures for growth. This disease is contagious and adult birds may be inapparent carriers.

Yet another disease condition with cutaneous manifestations is "cockatoo beak and feather disease." This syndrome goes by a variety of names, including "psittacine beak and feather disease" or "dyskeratogenesis." Although most often seen in white cockatoos of the genus *Cacatua*, this entity has also been reported in other psittacine birds, especially lovebirds. In this condition, feather follicles are active but new feathers fail to emerge from the sheaths. In some cases the sheaths split in an irregular fashion, giving the emerging feather a beaded appearance. Pulp hemorrhage is seen, and when feathers do emerge from their sheaths, the callamus or shaft appears weakened and the feathers break off or split. The feather tracts of the sides and flanks are usually the first to be affected, but any or all of the tracts, including those on the wings, crest, and tail, may be damaged.

In addition, beak deformities may occur with initial overgrowth of the upper and lower horny covering (ramphotheca) and the subsequent separation of ramphotheca or oral mucosa from the underlying bone. This ulceration or separation is usually first apparent on the palate of the upper mandible just at the junction between the palate and the hook of the beak.

Affected birds are usually young and may be recently imported or captively bred and reared. The disease does occur in sulfur-crested cockatoos in the wild and probably occurs in other species as well. It is thought to be fairly contagious, although the rate of transmission is uncertain. Adult birds without feather abnormalities have been found to have successive clutches with affected young, and therefore an inapparent carrier state probably exists. Some affected birds may survive for several years with feathering abnormalities alone. The usual course is more rapid, especially once beak lesions occur. An apparent increased susceptibility to opportunistic pathogens leads to death usually within 6 months to a year after diagnosis.

Tentative diagnosis may be based on the clinical appearance of the bird and the elimination of nutritional problems and the more rare endocrine abnormalities or ectoparasites as causes. Diagnosis is confirmed by histopathologic tests. The finding of the triad of individually necrotic cells in pulp and follicular epithelium, large cells with basophilic cytoplasmic granules in pulp and epithelium, and inflammation of the feather pulp is virtually pathognomonic. Electron microscopy reveals paracrystalline arrays of tiny viral particles in the nuclei of individually necrotic epithelial cells and in cytoplasmic granules of the large basophilic "botryoid cells." These particles are morphologically compatible with parvoviruses and the inclusions stain positively for DNA with Feulgen stain. There is some debate, however, as to their exact morphologic classification. Virus cultivation to date has been unsuccessful.

An additional condition associated with feathering abnormalities has been reported in budgerigars in Europe. Herpesvirus particles have been demonstrated and isolated from feathers of dead-in-the-shell and "feather-duster" chicks. This entity has not been reported in the United States. Diagnosis would rely on histopathologic and TEM results.

Diseases with Central Nervous System Signs

Several of the paramyxoviruses (PMVs) have been associated with neurologic signs. The differential must always include Newcastle disease virus (NDV), since this is a reportable disease. Differentiation relies on culture and histopathologic testing. Histopathologic findings alone are not always definitive, since both NDV and PMV-3 infections produce similar lesions, including multifocal gliosis with neuronophagia, mild lymphocytic perivascular cuffing, and vascular endothelial swelling or hyperplasia. Clinical signs are not a reliable method of differentiation but may serve to increase an index of suspicion of NDV if limb paralysis is present. In PMV-3 infection in species of *Neophema*, torticollis or stargazing is a prominent feature. If the birds do not die during the acute phase of the disease and if the torticollis is not severe enough to prevent eating, the birds will survive with the persistent neurologic deficit.

Similar torticollis has been observed in a group of *Pionus* parrots from a lot with high morbidity and mortality. Pox was present in several birds as well. A nonclassified hemagglutinating virus was isolated from cloacal swabs in quarantine. Many of the birds were left with residual torticollis, circling, and intention tremors, which worsened when they were excited. At the time of euthanasia, all birds had a severe lymphoplasmacytic meningomyeloencephalitis and choroiditis. At that time, several weeks after the original isolation of the virus, no viruses were cultured from nervous tissue or other organs.

It is not clear whether inapparent carrier states exist with paramyxovirus infection. Prevention by vaccination, primarily for Newcastle disease, is being investigated in Europe.

Another recently described syndrome in psittacine birds that has been associated with neurologic lesions is the "macaw wasting disease," also called "proventricular dilatation syndrome" and "infiltrative splanchnic neuropathy." This syndrome, most often described in young blue-and-gold macaws, has also been seen in other species, including conures. Presumptive diagnosis is based on finding atony of crop and proventriculus, atrophy of the gizzard musculature, and progressive, relentless weight loss. Consistent necropsy findings have included mild nonsuppurative encephalitis and visceral ganglioneuritis. A viral cause is strongly suspected but not substantiated. The mode of transmission or degree of infectivity are, as yet, unknown.

Diseases with Systemic or Visceral Involvement

Hepatitis is among the most common postmortem diagnoses in psittacine birds. The best described of the psittacine viral diseases is herpesvirus hepatosplenitis or Pacheco's disease. This disease, first described in the 1930s, made its re-emergence in this country in the late 1970s. There is a high degree of morbidity and mortality; the clinical signs of bright yellow-green diarrhea and ruffled feathers precede death by only a day or two. Definitive diagnosis relies on histopathologic results coupled with TEM or virus isolation. The virus is easily cultured. Syncytial cells and intranuclear inclusions are key histologic findings.

Although the usual case of Pacheco's disease produces an acute infection, herpesvirus-associated diseases that are less fulminating and show widespread systemic involvement (including the respiratory tract, esophagus, intestines, pancreas, and kidneys) have been noted in recent years. Whether this is due to a difference in host or virus is uncertain. Classic Pacheco's is highly contagious, whereas this less acute form may not be. Latent carriers, in both forms, are strongly suspected (e.g., Nanday and Patagonian conures), and there are instances in which isolated birds have died from disseminated herpesvirus infection without recent exposure to other birds.

Another newly described viral disease presenting with signs and lesions similar to Pacheco's disease is psittacine reovirus infection. Reoviruses were first isolated from shipments of birds that showed no increase in mortality and the reoviruses were initially considered to be nonpathogenic. However, recent outbreaks of clinical disease and mortality have been associated with isolation of reoviruses from diseased birds and demonstration of viral particles by TEM in the lesions. Enteritis, splenomegaly, and hepatomegaly are accompanied by acute hepatic necrosis. The lesions might be confused with those of Pacheco's disease, except that no syncytia or intranuclear inclusions are present.

Infection with paramyxovirus-5, reported in budgies, has similar clinical signs and portmortem lesions, including the formation of syncytial cells. In addition, disseminated adenovirus infection in lovebirds may also present with hepatic necrosis, pancreatitis, and renal tubular necrosis. Histopathologic tests in these cases reveal large intranuclear inclusion bodies but no syncytial cells. Thus, some of the recently described viral isolates have signs and lesions overlapping those of each other and of Pacheco's disease. Little is known about the infectivity or pathogenesis of reoviruses, PMV-5, or adenoviruses in psittacine birds. Inapparent carriers and latent infections are suspected in both reovirus and adenovirus infections of lovebirds.

Respiratory involvement may accompany systemic infections in diseases such as Newcastle disease, PMV-2 infection, or influenza. Primary respiratory involvement has been described in Amazon parrots suffering from severe tracheitis. The virus isolated in Germany is somewhat similar, but not identical, to infectious laryngotracheitis virus (a herpesvirus) of chickens, and it is quite distinct from Pacheco's agent. It is infectious but not necessarily lethal. In some cases the fibrinous tracheitis leads to a persistence of respiratory rales for many months. Diagnosis relies on demonstrating the virus in lesions by TEM or culture of the virus from pharynx or trachea.

Proliferative bronchitis, associated by TEM with herpesvirus particles in nuclear inclusions found in syncytia and individual cells, has been described in species of *Neophema* in this country. Dyspnea was the dominant clinical sign. Attempts at virus isolation have failed. Thus, the relationship between this entity, "*Amazona* tracheitis," and Pacheco's disease remains unclear.

Enteritis with clinical signs of diarrhea is also more commonly seen in conjunction with systemic disease than it is as a primary entity. This is especially true of the paramyxovirus infections. Viral diarrhea should be suspected when hemmorrhages and edema are seen in the intestinal wall. Virus isolation from spleen and from intestinal swabs should be attempted.

SUMMARY

From reading this chapter, it should become apparent to the practitioner that our knowledge of viral diseases in psittacine birds is rudimentary at best. Much confusion exists because of overlapping clinical, gross, and histopathologic signs. Electron microscopy and virus cultivation are necessary diagnostic adjuncts that are not always available. In addition, the fastidious nature of some of these viruses has frustrated isolation attempts, and the value of the species affected has often precluded fulfilling Koch's postulates. Nonetheless, progress is being made. It is an exciting era in avian medicine and one in which every clinician can participate. The accumulation of good clinical and pathologic data will help to better define and to someday prevent or treat these emerging viral diseases of psittacine birds.

References and Supplemental Reading

Bernier, G., Morin, M., and Marsolais, G.: A generalized inclusion body disease in the budgerigar. Avian Dis. 25:1083, 1981.

Gerach, H.: Virus Diseases in Pet Birds. Proc. Ann. Meet. Assoc. Avian Vet., San Diego, 1983, pp. 87–109.

Graham, D. L.: An update on selected pet bird virus infections. Proc. 1984 Assoc. Avian Vet., International Conference on Avian Medicine, Toronto, 1984, pp. 267–280.

Pass, D. A., and Perry, R. A.: The pathology of psittacine beak and feather disease. Aust. Vet. J. 61:69, 1984.

Lowenstine, L. J.: Diseases of psittacines differing morphologically from Pacheco's disease but associated with herpesvirus-like particles. Proc. 31st West. Poultry Dis. Conf. 1984, pp. 141–142.

Senne, D. A., Pearson, J. E., Miller, L. D., et al.: Virus isolations from pet birds submitted for importation into the United States. Avian Dis. 27:731, 1983.

COCKATOO BEAK AND FEATHER DISEASE SYNDROME

ELLIOTT R. JACOBSON, D.V.M.
Gainesville, Florida

HISTORICAL PERSPECTIVE

A syndrome of feather loss and malformation, often associated with beak necrosis, has been seen in a variety of psittacine species and has been termed *psittacine beak and feather disease syndrome* (Perry, 1981). In Australia, this syndrome has been observed predominantly in sulphur-crested cockatoos (*Cacatua galerita*), but it also has been identified in other Australian white cockatoos including the galah (*Eolophus roseicapillus*), little corella (*C. sanguinea*), and Major Mitchell cockatoo (*C. leadbeateri*). This syndrome has not been noted in species of black cockatoos. In a series of flocks studied in the wild in Australia over a four-year period, approximately 10 to 20 per cent of the sulphur-crested cockatoos manifested gross signs of the syndrome. Other psittacines that are reported to show a similar feather or beak dysplasia (or both) are lovebirds (*Agapornis* spp.) and budgerigars (*Melopsittacus undulatus*).

In the United States, a similar syndrome has been seen in both cockatoos recently imported from Indonesia and in captively bred and reared cockatoos. These species of cockatoo include lesser sulphur-crested (*C. sulphurea*), Moluccan (*C. moluccensis*), triton (*C. g. triton*), umbrella (*C. alba*), citron (*C. s. citrino-cristata*), Goffin (*C. goffini*), and red-vented (*C. haematuropygia*). In cockatoos imported by a large business in southern Florida, less than 1 per cent of cockatoos were noted to be affected.

Since information on the pathologic characteristics of this disease has only recently been reported in cockatoos and since no histopathologic studies have been reported for other species of psittacines, the syndrome will be termed *cockatoo beak and feather disease syndrome* (CBFDS), and this article will deal exclusively with the disease in cockatoos.

CBFDS has been noted for many years, and numerous causes, including endocrine disturbances, nutritional problems, infectious agents, toxicologic principles, and behavioral abnormalities, have been proposed. Although there has been some suggestion that CBFDS may be caused by an adrenal insufficiency, in a group of cockatoos with BFDS, both thyroxine and corticosterone levels were found within the normal range after TSH and ACTH stimulation, respectively. Thus it appears that CBFDS is not due to a primary disease of the thyroid or adrenal cortex.

GROSS FEATURES

In two recent reports (Pass and Perry, 1984; McOrist, 1984), the gross and histopathologic features of CBFDS in captive and wild sulphur-crested cockatoos were described. The author's own experiences with CBFDS in Indonesian cockatoos is similar to the descriptions given in these reports. The syndrome, although most commonly seen in cockatoos less than one year of age, has been diagnosed in older birds. Often, early in the onset of the disease, when only a few feathers are affected, the disorder can go unrecognized. The disease is generally chronic and progressive, and increasingly more feather tracts become involved over time (Fig. 1). The reason for a particular feather tract manifesting lesions appears to depend on the stage of the molt cycle of individual tracts. In affected birds, with time, as more and more feathers are replaced, more and more abnormal feathers are noted. The feather loss appears symmetrical. Newly emerging feathers from affected follicles may fail to exsheath. Feathers that do exsheath often have fragmented barbs and barbules. Feather sheaths may be clubbed and show constrictions. Some feathers completely fail to develop, and what remains is a featherless papilla. The primary wing feathers appear to be the last to become severely affected.

A corresponding hyperkeratosis with elongation of toenails and the upper beak commonly occurs, particularly in sulphur and lesser sulphur-crested cockatoos. The beak often will develop fissures in the distal end and will slowly undergo a progressive necrosis (Fig. 2) with involvement of the underlying bones. Secondary gram-negative bacteria and opportunistic fungi became established in these lesions and can commonly be isolated.

PATHOLOGIC FINDINGS

Histologic examination of affected feathers reveals necrosis of the cells within the epidermal collar (see Lucas and Stettenheim, 1972) and epidermal hyperplasia. Hyperkeratosis of the feather sheath results in the constriction and clubbing of the feathers seen at gross examination. Similar changes are seen within the epithelium giving rise to the beak.

Within affected growing feathers, the feather pulp shows diffuse infiltrates of inflammatory cells, including heterophils and small mononuclear cells; multinucleated giant cells are seen in areas of hemorrhage. Scattered throughout the pulp and epidermis, often in large numbers, are large macrophages containing variously sized inclusions that appear basophilic or magenta-colored when stained with hematoxylin and eosin (H & E; Fig. 3). Electron microscopy reveals that these inclusions consist of crystalline arrays of viral particles measuring approximately 20 to 22 nm. Also seen are mononuclear cells containing smaller basophilic granules (with H & E) of uniform size; these cells are also seen in developing feathers of clinically healthy cockatoos and appear to be morphologically similar to basophils.

In two lesser sulphur-crested cockatoos examined at necropsy, eosinophilic intranuclear inclusions were seen within hepatocytes. In a previous report (Rosskopff et al., 1981), similar inclusions seen in the liver were thought to represent herpesvirus inclusions. In the author's experience these inclusions represent an intranuclear metabolite, probably accumulating secondary to the primary disorder.

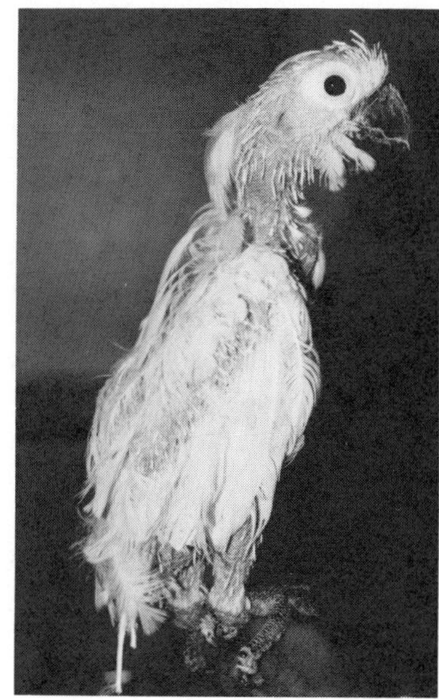

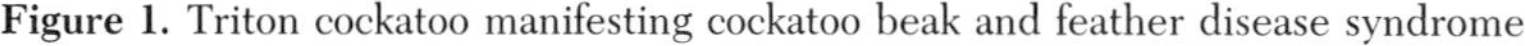

Figure 1. Triton cockatoo manifesting cockatoo beak and feather disease syndrome

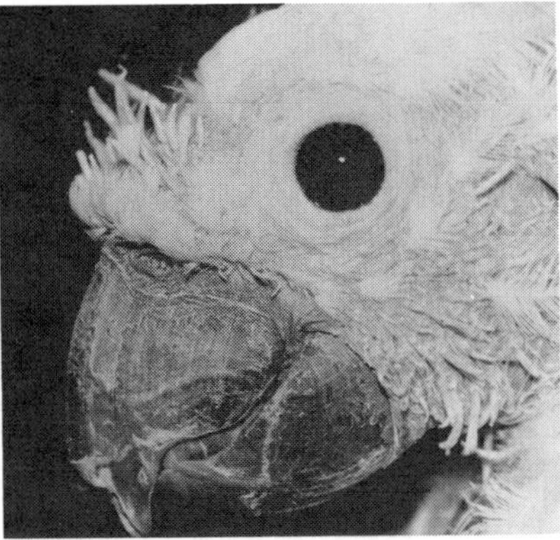

Figure 2. Lesser sulphur-crested cockatoo with necrosis of the distal end of the upper beak.

Unfortunately, the agent seen in CBFDS has not been isolated, and ultimate identification will depend on isolation in tissue culture. Additionally, since Koch's postulates need to be fulfilled to establish a causative relationship, the connection between the virus and the syndrome can only be speculated. Still, the consistent presence of this agent in cockatoos in Australia and in examined birds in the United States and its absence from a series of clinically healthy birds examined by the author makes "guilt by association" very convincing. Because of this limited information, clinically healthy cockatoos should not be exposed to affected cockatoos.

DIAGNOSIS AND TREATMENT

Cockatoo beak and feather disease syndrome is easily diagnosed in suspected birds by either biopsy and histologic evaluation of affected recently emerging feathers or by examination of a Wright-Giemsa–stained cytologic preparation of pulp from an affected feather. When biopsies are taken, a recently emerging feather should be taken along with its follicle. A minimum of six feathers per bird should be evaluated, and ideally several feather tracts should be sampled. Birds are easily anesthetized with ketamine given intravenously, and skin samples of full thickness should be taken circumferentially around an affected, newly emerging feather. Mature feathers are relatively acellular and have limited value in arriving at a diagnosis. The biopsy should be fixed in either neutral buffered 10 per cent formalin or Trump's solution (McDowell and Trump, 1976). In the author's opinion, demonstration in the pulp and epidermis of macrophages containing inclusions and the presence of gross signs of the disease are diagnostic.

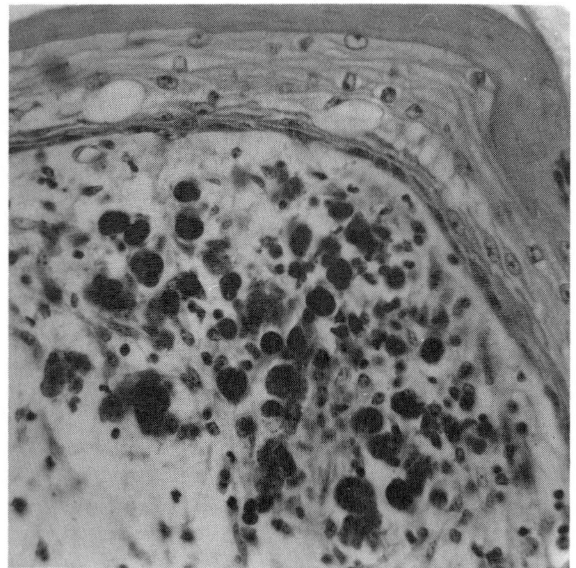

Figure 3. Photomicrograph of an affected feather at biopsy. Note numerous macrophages containing inclusion bodies within the distal end of the pulp.

Unfortunately, there are no chemotherapeutic agents that have been found effective in controlling this disease. Secondary bacterial and mycotic invaders can be controlled with appropriate antibiotics and antifungal drugs. There are no studies demonstrating the effectiveness of antiviral drugs or immunopotentiating drugs such as ImmunoRegulin (ImmunoVet). Birds showing involvement of a significant number of contour feathers easily become hypothermic and need to be kept warm. With time, many of these birds appear to become severely immunocompromised and die of secondary bacterial infections.

The client owning a cockatoo with CBFDS should be made aware that the disease is slowly progressive and the outcome is always fatal. However, birds may survive for several years. Again, affected birds should be kept separate from healthy birds. Many clients desire to keep these birds, even though the bird may be severely affected and quite unattractive. Clients should be encouraged to have their cockatoo euthanized when the bird's quality of life has deteriorated to the point where there is obvious suffering.

References and Supplemental Reading

Lucas, A. M., and Stettenheim, P. R.: Avian anatomy. Integument. Parts I and II. Agriculture Handbook 362. Washington, D. C.: U.S. Department of Agriculture, U.S. Government Printing Office, 1972.

McDowell, E. M., and Trump, B. F.: Historical fixatives suitable for diagnostic light and electron microscopy. Arch. Pathol. Lab. Med. 100:405, 1976.

McOrist, S., Black, D. G., Pass, D. A., et al.: Beak and feather dystrophy in wild sulphur-crested cockatoos (*Cacatua galerita*). J. Wildl. Dis. 20:120, 1984.

Pass, D. A., and Perry, R. A.: The pathology of psittacine beak and feather disease. Aust. Vet. J. 61:69, 1984.

Perry, R. A.: A psittacine combined beak and feather disease syndrome. *In* Hungerford, T. G. (ed.): Proceedings No. 55 of Courses for Veterinarians. Cage and Aviary Birds. Sydney, Australia: The Post-Graduate Committee in Veterinary Science, 1981, pp. 81–87.

Rosskopff, W. J., Woerpel, R. W., Howard, E. B., et al.: Chronic endocrine disorder associated with inclusion body hepatitis in a sulphur-crested cockatoo. J.A.V.M.A. 179:1273, 1981.

LEAD POISONING IN PSITTACINE BIRDS

SCOTT E. McDONALD, D.V.M.

Westchester, Illinois

Lead poisoning is a common toxicologic problem encountered in many species of wild birds and has been well documented in free-living waterfowl that ingest spent lead shot. It is estimated that lead poisoning kills as many as two million ducks and geese annually, which is 2 to 3 per cent of the fall population of all species of waterfowl. The disease is not uncommon in caged birds, particularly pet psittacines that are allowed to fly free throughout the house. The inquisitive, yet destructive, nature of these birds attracts them to many household objects, which they may grasp with their beak and manipulate in their mouth. Sources of lead that psittacines may pick at and ingest include lead-based paint, lead shot, bullets, solder, fishing sinkers, bird toys (containing lead weights), linoleum, putty, ceramics, curtain weights, and foil from the top of wine bottles.

CLINICAL SIGNS

Lead is a systemic, heavy-metal poison that adversely affects all body systems to which it is distributed, especially the nervous, digestive, and hematopoietic systems. It operates at the molecular level by inhibiting the activities of enzymes that are required by all cells.

Lead poisoning in birds produces clinical signs that are often vague; they consist of nonspecific gastrointestinal, renal, and neurologic dysfunction. In pet birds, the onset of disease is often acute, and the usual history is of a normal, healthy bird that suddenly becomes ill. Clinical signs observed in psittacine birds have included lethargy, depression, weakness, anorexia, regurgitation, polyuria (hemoglobinuria in some species), diarrhea, ataxia, head-tilt, blindness, circling, and convulsions. Birds may present with only mild depression or they may be critically ill with seizures and at a point near death. Two key symptoms that should always arouse the clinician's suspicion of lead poisoning in free-flying psittacine birds are hemoglobinuria and abnormalities of the central nervous system (CNS).

Birds with lead poisoning usually do not show signs of illness until several days after ingestion of lead. However, once symptoms develop, the course of the disease may be rapid, leading to death within 48 hours.

The severity of disease is dependent upon the amount of lead ingested over a period of time, the size of the particles, and the factors affecting absorption of lead in the gut, such as the type and amount of abrasive material present in the gizzard. In one study involving ducks, it was found that fewer birds died in a group fed oyster-shell grit than did those fed quartz grit or no grit at all (Longcore et al., 1974). Apparently the more abrasive oyster-shell grit hastens the mechanical degradation and subsequent passage of lead particles through the gut. Grit is frequently not fed to larger parrots, which may prolong the retention of lead particles in the ventriculus and therefore increase absorption and thus the severity of toxicity. Ingestion of many small fragments of lead is more likely to induce acute toxicity than one or two large pieces. This is due to a larger surface area from which lead can be eroded and absorbed. However, large pieces do not tend to move out of the ventriculus as quickly as small fragments, and as small amounts of lead

Notice: Lead levels for blood of psittacine birds given on page 618 of *Current Veterinary Therapy VIII* are incorrect. They are superseded by values given in this article.

continue to be absorbed daily, the course of disease becomes chronic and potentially more severe.

In a study to evaluate the clinical signs and hematologic and biochemical measurements of lead poisoning in psittacine birds, 30 6- to 8-month-old clinically healthy cockatiels (*Nymphicus hollandicus*) were separated into three groups of ten (McDonald and Lowenstine, 1983). The birds in the first group (Group A) were force-fed three pieces of No. 12 lead shot, whereas those in the second group (Group B) were given one piece of No. 12 lead shot. This shot was approximately 1 mm in diameter, and each piece weighed between 9 and 10 mg. The third control group (Group C) did not receive lead shot. Birds were examined daily for clinical signs of lead poisoning. Blood samples were taken before administration of shot and then 1, 2, 4, 8, 15, 20, and 28 days later.

Clinical signs indicative of lead toxicosis were not observed in birds of Group A or B until the fourth day. The number of sick birds was highest and the clinical signs most severe between days 6 and 12. Greenish-black diarrhea and mild polyuria were the most common and sometimes only symptoms seen. It occurred in all 10 birds of Group A and in seven birds of Group B by day 12. Generalized weakness, characterized by lethargy, ruffled feathers, partial or complete anorexia, and weight loss was the next most prevalent sign; it was seen in nine birds of Group A but in only four from Group B. Inability to fly, ataxia, and seizures were seen less often, but when present, death was usually imminent. Five of 10 birds in Group A died of suspected lead poisoning between the sixth and twelfth days, whereas only two birds from Group B died during this same period.

The greenish-black diarrhea seen in nearly all affected cockatiels was the result of increased quantities of biliverdin, which was excreted in the bile because of the hemolytic effect of lead. Anemia was a significant laboratory finding in all lead-dosed birds. Polyuria, a common finding in larger psittacines (Woerpel and Rosskopf, 1982), was not a significant symptom in these birds. Polyuria may be a clinical manifestation of the renal tubular necrosis induced by lead intoxication.

Hemoglobinuria, which has previously been reported only in Amazon species (Woerpel and Rosskopf, 1982), was not observed in cockatiels. It is associated with intravascular hemolysis. The abnormally watery droppings may be slightly tinged pink, or, if urates are still prominent, the color and consistency may resemble that of tomato soup (Galvin, 1983). Hemoglobinuria is commonly misdiagnosed as bloody diarrhea.

Lead encephalopathies are the result of diffuse and perivascular edema, increase of cerebrospinal fluid, and necrosis of individual nerve cells scattered throughout the CNS (Smith and Jones, 1972). Lead may also act directly at the neuronal level by inducing changes in basic metabolism in the brain (Bull et al., 1975). Lead-induced demyelination is thought to be the cause of peripheral neuropathies (Hunter and Haigh, 1978). Peripheral nerve damage may account in part for the muscular weakness that is commonly associated with lead poisoning.

RADIOGRAPHIC FINDINGS

Radiographs should be taken of birds with a history and clinical signs suggestive of lead poisoning in order to reveal lead particles in the gastrointestinal tract. Substances containing lead are radiopaque; the heavy metal densities are easily discernible from oyster-shell or quartz grit, small stones, or pieces of bone. Lead particles are usually seen within the ventriculus but they may also be detected in the crop or proventriculus if recently ingested or in the intestines or cloaca if they are being eliminated. The presence of metallic particles indicates but does not confirm the disease. In addition, one cannot always eliminate the possibility of lead poisoning based on negative findings from a radiograph, since the lead particles may have been recently broken down or eliminated. Intoxication is most reliably confirmed by the determination of lead concentration in the blood. The presence of lead shot in muscle or subcutaneous tissues is not thought to be a major health hazard as it is not readily absorbed from these sites.

In the cockatiel study, whole-body radiographs were taken of all birds prior to shot administration, 24 hours later, and then at weekly intervals (in Groups A and B) to detect when lead shot had been completely eroded and absorbed or eliminated. In only one bird was the correct number of shot not present in the ventriculus at 24 hours; this bird was redosed. Rapid elimination of shot was uncommon; 88 per cent of all pellets were still visible on the eighth day. During this time, all pieces of shot were severely eroded by the action of the gizzard and grit and presumably absorbed. Only 11 per cent remained at two weeks, and by day 20, all pellets were totally eroded or eliminated. In one bird a radiograph taken at 2 weeks showed an eroded pellet that was present within the intestines; thus indicates that lead particles can pass out of the ventriculus prior to their complete degradation.

LABORATORY FINDINGS

Lead causes profound alterations in hemoglobin synthesis (Fig. 1). It inhibits heme synthetase, the enzyme responsible for incorporation of iron in protoporphyrin IX (PP) to form heme (Schalm et

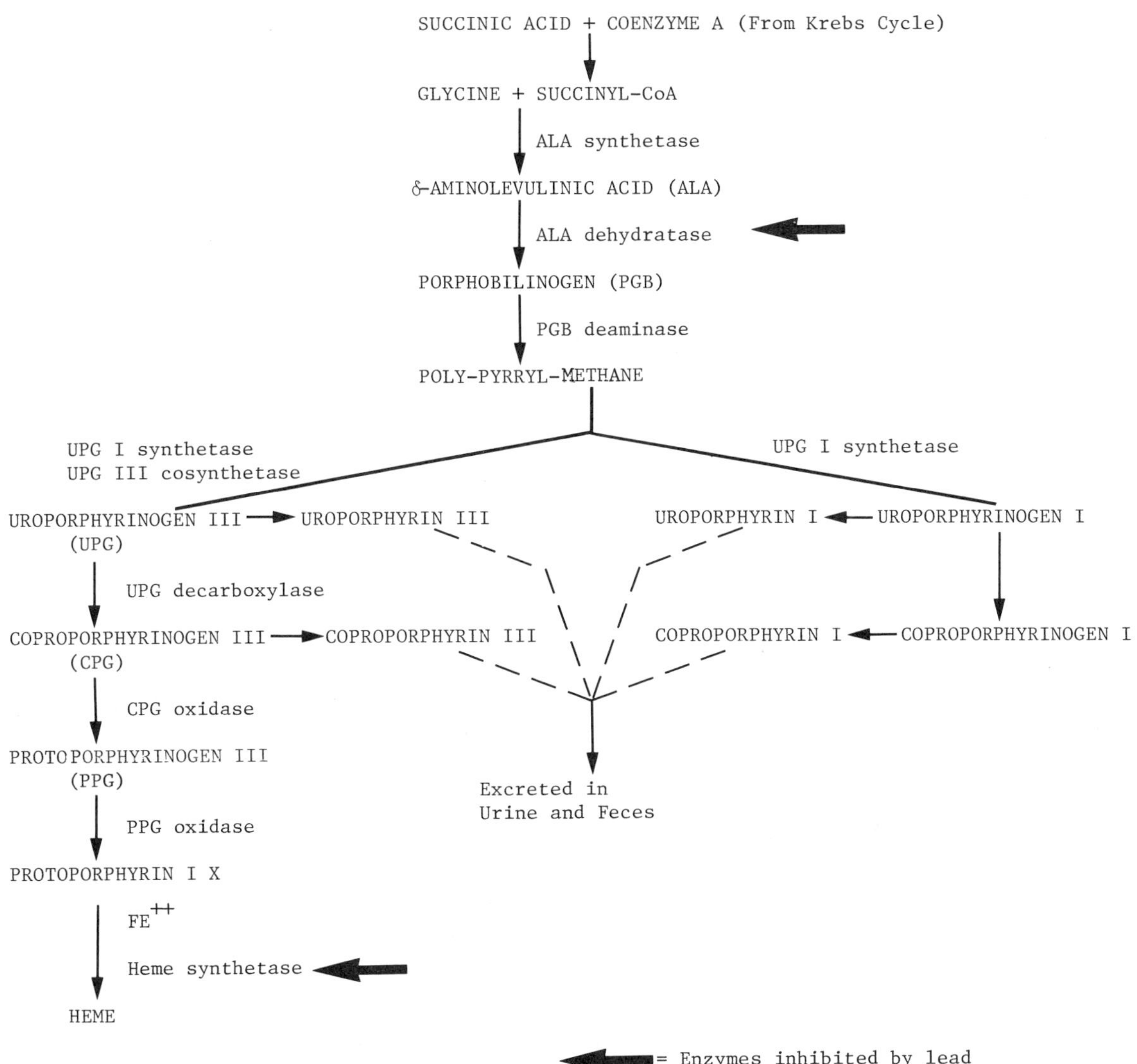

Figure 1. Schematic representation of the steps involved in biogenesis of heme. (From Schalm et al.: *Veterinary Hematology.* Philadelphia: Lea & Febiger, 1975.)

al., 1975). As a result, PP accumulates in erythrocytes.

Hematologic findings in birds with lead poisoning are not as characteristic or consistent as they are in mammals. A hypochromic, regenerative anemia is the primary finding in birds. Basophilic stippling, which is a consistent finding in dogs, has rarely been reported in birds. In lead-dosed cockatiels, hematocrit and hemoglobin concentrations were significantly decreased from predose values and control birds by the second day after lead ingestion and remained low through day 28.

The definitive diagnosis of lead poisoning is based on the direct measurement of lead levels in the blood or in the tissues of the liver or kidneys. In humans, blood concentrations of 40 to 60 μg/dl indicates exposure to lead, whereas levels of 80 to 100 μg/dl constitute an emergency situation (Berkow et al., 1977). In dogs, values of 40 to 50 μg/dl are abnormally high, and findings of 60 μg/dl or more are virtually diagnostic of lead poisoning (Kowalczyk, 1980). The significance of blood lead levels in birds is more variable than in mammals and may be the result of several factors, such as species resistance to lead, the chronic nature of the poisoning, and the bird's diet, environment and physical condition. In sandhill cranes (Kennedy et al., 1977) and in an eastern turkey vulture (Janssen et al., 1979), diagnosis was confirmed on the basis of blood lead concentrations ranging from 146 to 376 μg/dl. A diagnosis was also made in a sick Cuban whistling tree duck that had a blood lead level of 163 μg/dl, compared with 32 μg/dl found in an apparently healthy cagemate (Janssen et al., 1979). In studies involving mallard ducks and bald eagles, levels as high as 500 μg/dl were reported; death occurred in some birds but not in others (Roscoe et al., 1979; Hoffman et al., 1981). Chickens reportedly show no signs of disease with blood lead concentrations as high as 800 μg/dl (Peckham, 1978).

In cockatiels, blood lead levels were less than those reported elsewhere. Values ranging from 44 to 129 μg/dl were measured in these birds 1 to 2 days before death, and gastrointestinal signs were present in birds with levels as low as 23 μg/dl. The highest blood lead concentration measured in predosed or control cockatiels was 14 μg/dl. Blood lead levels in all treated birds exceeded 28 μg/dl 24 hours after receiving shot. Peak concentrations were seen in 80 per cent of the birds on day 4 (range, 45 to 129 μg/dl).

The diagnosis of lead poisoning in five Amazon parrots was based on the presence of metallic densities in their ventriculi and their response to therapy (Rosskopf, 1984). Three of these birds had blood lead levels between 77 and 166 μg/dl before treatment. The other two birds had blood lead levels of 29 and 54 μg/dl after calcium ethylenediaminetetraacetate (CaEDTA) therapy had commenced. Five other Amazon parrots were evaluated for lead poisoning as a result of CNS abnormalities. None of these birds had metallic densities in their digestive tracts and all had blood lead levels ranging from less than 5 to 13 μg/dl. Several of these birds were treated with CaEDTA with no response, and the others were ultimately diagnosed as having some other disease.

In mallard ducks, tissue concentrations of lead ranging from 6 to 20 ppm in the liver or kidney indicates acute exposure to lead (Longcore et al., 1974). With the exception of one bird (liver lead level of 2 ppm), lead levels in the liver of cockatiels that died were consistent with these values (six birds; range, 7.6 to 17.5 ppm).

The measurement of some of the metabolites (or their associated enzymes) resulting from the interference by lead with heme synthesis is also of diagnostic value. The measurement of PP is a simple diagnostic test useful in screening waterfowl for lead poisoning. In mallards, lead concentrations greater than 40 μg/dl are considered indicative of ingestion of at least one pellet of No. 4 lead shot two days to one month before testing (Roscoe et al., 1979). A value of 234 μg/dl was reported in an eastern turkey vulture that contained lead material in its ventriculus (Janssen et al., 1979).

In cockatiels, predose values were similar to those found in mallards, but in some birds the levels were as high as 90 μg/dl. The mean PP concentration was 34 μg/dl (range, 5 to 90 μg/dl), and 86 per cent of these values were below 60 μg/dl. On the first day after lead dosing, the mean PP concentration rose to 200 μg/dl. The levels continued to rise, reaching maximum mean values of over 1100 μg/dl on day 15 before decreasing precipitously. No significant difference was detected between PP concentration in birds that received three pellets of lead shot versus those that received only one at any interval.

In humans, aminolevulinic acid dehydrase (ALAD) activity is an accurate and sensitive indicator of the amount of circulating lead, and it is partly inhibited by low lead levels that do not cause any other measurable biochemical effects (Hernberg et al., 1970. The sensitivity of this enzyme to lead has been demonstrated in a number of avian species. Retention of lead shot for a minimum of 24 hours has resulted in inhibition of ALAD activity for 4 weeks (Hoffman et al., 1981). In ducks, blood samples with less than 50 ALAD units were regarded as abnormal and were shown consistently to contain elevated lead residues greater than 20 μg/dl (Dieter, 1977).

In cockatiels, the mean value for ALAD enzyme units measured in undosed controls was 175. Erythrocytic ALAD activity was depressed by 85 per cent in birds of Group A and by 70 per cent in birds of Group B, compared with predose values or with undosed controls analyzed concurrently. Depression occurred within 24 hours of lead shot ingestion and remained consistently low for 28 days, at which time sampling was discontinued.

Normal values for blood lead concentration, PP, and ALAD were determined in clinically healthy cockatiels. Blood lead concentrations in excess of 20 μg/dl, PP measurements greater than 240 μg/dl, and ALAD units less than 86 were highly significant ($p < 0.01$) and indicative of lead exposure. Clinical signs increased in severity as blood lead concentrations increased above 40 μg/dl, PP levels exceeded 500 μg/dl, and ALAD units decreased below 50.

Blood lead levels, PP values, and ALAD units can all be determined in as little as 50 μl of whole blood for each measurement. This allows one to safely sample birds as small as parakeets with the extraction of no more than enough blood to fill one or two heparinized microhematocrit tubes. Practitioners should contact a human clinical laboratory, especially one that deals with pediatric samples in which microtechniques are commonly used, for processing these toxicologic tests. Most veterinary reference laboratories still use laboratory techniques in which several milliliters of whole blood are required to determine blood lead concentrations. Veterinary laboratories are also unlikely to run samples for PP and ALAD, since these tests are rarely requested. It should be noted that because PP is not bound to zinc in birds, as it is in humans, adjustments must be made to the spectrofluorometer from which these measurements are determined. If the proper instrument alterations are not made, the laboratory will automatically test for zinc PP and obtain a result that is invalid in avian species. The instrument adjustments are described in the veterinary literature (Roscoe et al., 1979).

Psittacine birds dying of lead poisoning often reveal no remarkable gross pathologic lesions. Retrieving from the intestinal tract metallic particles that could be analyzed for lead is potentially rewarding. In waterfowl that have died of lead toxicosis, lesions reported have included emaciation with severe muscle atrophy; atrophic liver, kidneys, and intestines; enlarged gallbladder filled with bile; and proventricular and esophageal impaction (Wobeser, 1981). These signs are very nonspecific and are similar to those of starvation. Waterfowl usually die of chronic lead poisoning, whereas in psittacines the disease is more acute in nature. Therefore, even these lesions may rarely be encountered.

A detailed description of the histopathologic signs of lead poisoning in birds (Canada geese) has been well documented (Cook and Trainer, 1966). The primary lesions are found in the liver and kidneys. The findings in psittacine birds are consistent with what has been reported.

In the livers of seven cockatiels that died of lead toxicosis, Kupffer cells were greatly swollen. These cells, as well as hepatocytes, contained pigment that varied from finely granular in shape and golden brown in color to coarse and nearly black. All pigment was positive for trivalent iron when stained with Prussian Blue. Lead causes the formation of hemosiderin because of the excessive destruction of erythrocytes. Kidney lesions consisted of renal tubular necrosis characterized by tubular dilation, flattening and necrosis of tubular epithelial cells, and the accumulation of brightly eosinophilic concretions (iron pigments). Both proximal and distal tubules were affected. Small, granular, acid-fast inclusions, characteristic of lead poisoning in mammals and some other birds, were seen in epithelial cells of the proximal tubules of only one bird.

TREATMENT

If the history, clinical signs, and radiographic findings suggest lead poisoning, treatment should commence immediately. One should not wait for the determination of blood lead levels or the results of other biochemical tests before chelation therapy is started. Even if the patient does not have lead poisoning, the therapy will not harm the bird. This clinical approach is also justified in situations in which economics dictate a conservative work-up. Blood collected for toxicologic tests should always be done before the onset of chelation therapy, but in a severely debilitated patient, the stress of this procedure may be prohibitive. Chelation therapy should always take precedence over blood collection.

The purpose of therapy in lead poisoning is (1) to remove lead from the blood and body tissues as rapidly as possible and (2) to remove lead, if still present, from the gastrointestinal tract, particularly the ventriculus, so that further absorption is prevented. Supportive therapy is indicated as needed.

Lead that is absorbed is effectively removed by using a chelating agent. These agents combine with lead to form nontoxic complexes that are rapidly removed from the blood by the kidneys. The drug of choice is CaEDTA, which is supplied as calcium disodium edetate injection (Havidote, Haver-Lockhart; Calcium Versenate, Riker Laboratories). The dosage for either agent is the same, and this author gives 35 to 40 mg/kg twice daily for 5 days. The drug is not diluted and is given intramuscularly. In humans, renal damage has occurred from excessive doses of CaEDTA, but this has not been reported in birds. Nonetheless, treatment should not continue for more than 5 consecutive days. As demonstrated in cockatiels, lead particles may take up to several weeks or longer to be completely eroded or eliminated. In such cases, a second 5-day regimen of CaEDTA therapy is instituted after a 5- to 7-day waiting period. Therapy is indicated in this manner until no lead particles are visible on serial radiographs. This author has not had to subject a bird to more than two treatment regimens before all lead particles were removed. However, in most of these cases lead fragments were minuscule (less than 1 mm in diameter). Surgical intervention may be necessary if larger fragments are ingested.

Response to chelation therapy is dramatic. Often the bird is asymptomatic within 48 to 72 hours, especially if CNS involvement is negligible. The prognosis is more guarded when neurologic signs are present, but even some of these birds can make apparently complete recoveries. Permanent mental deficiencies and recurrent seizures are a common sequelae of lead poisoning in children (Kowalczyk, 1980), but this author is unaware of such occurrences in pet birds. Seizures in psittacine birds may be controlled with diazepam (Valium, Hoffman-LaRoche) given at a rate of 0.5 to 1 mg/kg, intramuscularly, two to three times daily as needed.

In addition to CaEDTA, supportive care is indicated for critically ill birds. Antibiotics are used to prevent secondary infection, corticosteroids are given to help alleviate shock, and fluids are administered to combat dehydration due to fluid loss of decreased intake. Birds that are completely or partially anorectic are force-fed daily, and they are placed in a warm environment (85°F) to minimize stress.

To enhance the movement of small lead fragments (less than 1 mm) from the ventriculus, warm, liquefied peanut butter is mixed with mineral oil in a

2:1 ratio and administered through a stomach tube. The purgative action of these substances will often eliminate lead particles within a period of several days. Birds the size of cockatiels receive 1 ml of this formula daily, Amazon parrots 10 ml, and macaws as much as 20 ml.

Oral administration of magnesium sulfate at a dosage of 0.5 to 1.0 gm/kg has also been advocated as a cathartic and as an aid in reducing lead absorption by causing the formation of insoluble lead precipitates (Galvin, 1983). A 5 per cent solution in the drinking water can be given to asymptomatic patients who have lead particles that would take up to several weeks to be broken down and eliminated.

Ventriculotomy has been successfully performed in psittacine birds that have ingested unusually large pieces of lead that would not pass (Woerpel and Rosskopf, 1982). However, the potential risk of this procedure is considered high, and it should not be performed unless absolutely necessary. Prior stabilization of the patient with chelation therapy is critical to the success of the surgery.

Surgical removal of lead fragments from the crop is much less risky and may be indicated to prevent additional particles from moving farther down the digestive tract, especially in a bird that already harbors lead fragments in its ventriculus and exhibits signs of plumbism. In such patients, the surgery can be performed by using only physical restraint, thus avoiding the added risks of general anesthesia.

The author has successfully removed lead shot from the gizzard of a red-tailed hawk by using a noninvasive suction technique. With the bird lightly sedated, an appropriately sized suction tube was passed down the esophagus, through the proventriculus, and into the gizzard. Seen with a fluoroscope, the tip of the tube was directed toward the shot, which was removed by aspiration. This procedure would be difficult to perform in psittacine birds because of their smaller size and the presence of a pendulous crop, which impedes the passage of a stomach tube. However, it is conceivable that a suction tube could be successfully passed into the gizzard by a cropotomy procedure and that lead particles could be aspirated out, especially in the larger psittacine species.

References and Supplemental Reading

Berkow, R. (ed.): *The Merck Manual.* Rahway, N. J.: Merck and Co., 1977, p. 1070.

Bull, R. J., Staneszek, P. M., O'Neill, J. J., et al.: Specificity of the effects of lead on brain energy metabolism for substrates donating a cytoplasmic reducing equivalent. Environ. Health Perspec. 12:89, 1975.

Cook, R. S., and Trainer, D. O.: Lead toxicity in Canada geese. J. Wildl. Manage. 30:1, 1966.

Dieter, M. P.: Use of the ALAD blood enzyme bioassay to monitor lead contamination in the canvasback duck population. Proc. Symp. Environmental Pollutants, University of Connecticut, Storrs, 1977.

Galvin, C.: Acute hemorrhagic syndrome of birds. *In* Kirk, R. W. (ed.): *Current Veterinary Therapy VIII.* Philadelphia: W.B. Saunders, 1983, pp. 617–619.

Hernberg, S., Nikkanen, J., Mellin, G., et al.: δ-aminolevulinic acid dehydrase as a measure of lead exposure. Arch. Environ. Health 21:140, 1970.

Hoffman, D. J., Pattee, O. H., Weimeyer, S. N., et al.: Effects of lead shot on ALAD activity, hemoglobin concentration, and serum chemistry in bald eagles. J. Wildl. Dis. 17:423, 1981.

Hunter, B., and Haigh, J. C.: Demyelinating peripheral neuropathy in a guinea hen associated with subacute lead intoxication. Avian Dis. 22:344, 1978.

Janssen, D. L., Robinson, P. T., and Ensley, P. K.: Lead toxicosis in three captive avian species. Proc. Am. Assoc. Zoo Vet., 1979, pp. 40–42.

Kennedy, S., Crisler, J. P., Smith, E., et al.: Lead poisoning in sandhill cranes. J.A.V.M.A. 171:955, 1977.

Kowalczyk, D. F.: Lead poisoning. *In* Kirk, R. W. (ed.): *Current Veterinary Therapy VII.* Philadelphia: W.B. Saunders, 1980, pp. 136–141.

Longcore, J. R., Locke, L. N., Bagley, G. E., et al.: Significance of lead residue in mallard tissues. USDI Fish and Wildlife Service, Special Scientific Report. Wildlife 182:1, 1974.

McDonald, S. E., and Lowenstine, L. J.: Lead toxicosis in psittacine birds. Proc. 25th Ann. Int. Symp. Zoo and Wild Anim. Med. Vienna, 1983.

Peckham, M. C.: Poisons and toxins. *In* Hofstad, M. S. (ed.): *Diseases of Poultry.* Ames, Iowa: Iowa State University Press, 1978, pp. 909–913.

Roscoe, D. E., Nielson, S. W., Alamola, A., et al.: A simple quantitative test for erythrocytic protoporphyrin in lead-poisoned ducks. J. Wildl. Dis. 15:127, 1979.

Rosskopf, W. J.: Personal communication, 1984.

Schalm, O. W., Jain, N. C., and Carroll, E. J.: *Veterinary Hematology.* Philadelphia: Lea & Febiger, 1975, pp. 377–379.

Smith, H. A., Jones, T. C., and Hunt R. D.: *Veterinary Pathology.* Philadelphia: Lea & Febiger, 1972, pp. 956–961.

Wobeser, G. A.: *Diseases of Wild Waterfowl.* New York: Plenum Press, 1981, pp. 151–159.

Woerpel, R. W., and Rosskopf, W. J.: Heavy-metal intoxication in caged birds I-II. Comp. Cont. Ed. Pract. Vet. 4:9, 10, 1982.

REHABILITATION OF OIL-CONTAMINATED BIRDS

F. JOSHUA DEIN, V.M.D.,
and LYNNE S. FRINK, M.A.
Wilmington, Delaware

Oil has long been demonstrated to have a negative impact on waterbirds, both as a result of contamination from chronic oil pollution and from major oil-spill incidents on waterways around the world (Michael, 1977). It has been estimated that one million birds die annually in the European North Atlantic as a result of oil pollution; the extent of worldwide mortality is not known (Croxall, 1979). A major concern is that species most commonly affected are those that are not prolific breeders and whose populations are not easily monitored in the wild; such species include alcids (e.g., murres, auklets), gannets, and loons.

Historically, salvage responses to major spills have been terrible failures, and bird mortality has exceeded 80 per cent. Organizations in the United States and abroad have directed time and energies to solving the problems associated with rehabilitation of oiled birds. Since its organization in 1976, Tri-State Bird Rescue and Research (TSBRR) has been involved in both responses to and research on oil spills and with this experience has decreased mortality rates to an average of 15 per cent.

The presence of oil in the environment can affect birds in many different ways. These effects can been categorized as environmental, behavioral, external, and internal; a collection of review articles and an extensive bibliography describing them are available (Barnes and Rosie, 1983, Light and Lanier, 1978).

The environmental effects involve the microorganisms, invertebrates, and fish, which are part of the waterbirds' food web. Studies have shown that oil can cause behavioral and reproductive changes in these food sources, resulting in a decrease in available food (Percy, 1977).

Oil-induced behavioral changes in birds can result in such serious problems as altered courtship rituals and variations in nesting and nestling behavior. These changes can have significant adverse effects on successful reproduction and on survival of offspring. Some of the most disastrous of the internal effects of oil are on the reproductive system. Delays in laying time, decreases in the numbers of eggs laid, decrease in eggshell thickness and hatching success, embryonic death, teratogenicity, and degeneration of ovarian follicles have all been reported in experimental birds. Post-hatching effects such as decreased rates of growth and feather development and delays in initiation of thermoregulatory ability have also been described.

Other physiologic and pathologic consequences of ingested oil are also significant. Alteration of normal endocrine and osmoregulatory functions resulting from oil ingestion have been intensively studied. Direct toxic effects on the gastrointestinal tract, pancreas, and liver have all been documented. These effects generally cause loss of digestive and absorptive efficiency with subsequent loss of fitness. Oil-aspiration pneumonia is common in victims of oil spills. Visceral gout due to kidney damage as a direct toxic effect of oil or due to dehydration is a common postmortem finding. Ingested oil has been shown to cause Heinz-body anemia in experimental situations. Related research has also shown a decrease in red cell mass as a result of oil ingestion.

The external effects of oil are the most noticeable and the most immediately debilitating. They are also the ones most readily counteracted. Oil destroys the waterproofing and insulating properties of plumage, and the bird may suffer from hypothermia and have difficulty swimming or flying. If food is scarce or foraging behavior is hampered, there may be a negative energy balance, resulting in decreased body condition. Irritation of eyes and obstruction of ears, nares, and mouth are frequently seen.

It is important to note that each of these effects may not cause death in itself but may decrease the bird's ability to pursue normal activities necessary for survival. Stressful conditions and loss of fitness provide ample opportunity for secondary infections, especially aspergillosis. An additional concern is the potential for latent carriers to begin shedding disease organisms, which may lead to epornitics both in the wild and in the rehabilitation center.

REHABILITATION OF OILED BIRDS

Rehabilitation of oiled birds can be divided into four major steps: (1) stabilizing the bird, (2) removing the oil from the feathers, (3) removing the cleaning agent from the feathers, and (4) restoring feather structure.

Stabilizing the Bird

Routine physical examination of oiled birds should include noting the extent and distribution of oil on the body, the attitude of the bird on arrival, its weight, and its cloacal temperature. Oil should be removed from the nares and mouth with swabs, and eyes should be flushed with ophthalmic irrigation. Hematocrit and total protein should be determined. Birds should be tube-fed a warm electrolyte and elemental nutrient solution (e.g., ProSobee [Mead Johnson] diluted with multielectrolyte solution) at 10 to 30 ml/kg and Pepto-Bismol (Norwich) at 1 to 3 ml/kg. This process should be repeated every eight hours until the bird has been cleaned and allowed access to food and water. The bird should be kept warm in an environment free from external stressors. Oil ingestion through feather preening can be discouraged by wrapping the bird loosely in a disposable diaper. The diaper should be changed regularly to avoid cloacal impaction and soiling of the feathers with fecal matter. Cleaning should not begin unless the bird is alert, is responsive to its surroundings, and has a normal cloacal temperature (greater than 101°F). Although prophylactic use of many medications has been suggested, there is no evidence that they are efficacious (Lauer et al., 1982).

Removing Oil From the Feathers

The most important requirements for cleaning are large amounts of water (103 to 104° F) and an effective cleaning agent. Eighty to 100 gallons of water delivered over 15 to 30 minutes are needed for cleaning one bird the size of a goose (4 to 7 kg). Numerous cleaning agents have been tested in rehabilitation of oiled birds; most have proven to be too dangerous, toxic, irritating, ineffective in removing oil, or difficult to rinse out (Williams, 1978). TSBRR currently uses Lux Liquid Amber industrial detergent (Lever Brothers), or Dawn dishwashing detergent (Procter & Gamble). Cleaning should be undertaken in an area that is warm, quiet, and free from drafts.

For the cleaning process a single bird is placed in a 10-gallon tub containing a 4– to 15–per cent concentration of detergent in water at a temperature of 103 to 104°F. One person ladles the detergent solution over the bird's body and wings while another strokes in the direction of feather growth. It is important that the feathers not be scrubbed, since this will disrupt the delicate feather structure and delay the return to a waterproof condition. The bird's head should be restrained; ophthalmic solution should be used frequently to flush any detergent that may come in contact with the eyes.

The bird should be removed from the tub when the water is dirty and lightly rinsed under a warm-water spray. The entire washing process is immediately repeated in a fresh tub of detergent solution. The bird may require three or more washings; weathered or heavy oils are particularly difficult to remove. Tarry residue can often be softened with a small amount of warm mineral oil prior to the detergent washing, although mineral oil itself is a feather contaminant and must be completely washed out.

Removing the Cleaning Agent from the Feathers

The rinsing process is crucial to the successful cleaning of oiled birds; any detergent residue will prevent waterproofing. This is carried out through a combination of rinses under a forced spray of warm water (103 to 104°F) and moving the bird through one or more tubs of clean water. Special attention should be given to the vent, breast, and underwings. The bird is not acceptably well rinsed until the water beads off the feathers in small, sparkling droplets. The bird's feathers are then gently blotted with clean, dry towels. When all necessary materials are assembled in advance, the entire cleaning process should take 20 to 40 minutes.

Restoring Feather Structure

After rinsing, the bird is placed in a holding pen until it dries. The pen should be lined with sheets, curtained to limit human intrusion, and provided with heat lamps positioned to allow the bird to find a comfortable ambient temperature. Diving birds should be provided with foam padding under the sheeting to prevent breast trauma. When the bird is dry, food and water should be offered and the bird observed to determine if it is eating. Twenty-four hours after cleaning, the bird is allowed free access to water for swimming. The water can be slightly warm for the first swim; later it is kept at room temperature. We use pens that measure 4 ft by 8 ft and that have sloped ramps, which allow the birds to enter and leave the water at will (Fig. 1). The pens are curtained and have heat lamps on one side. Pools should have constant surface overflow drainage to remove debris and residues from the water. Birds usually take to the water readily; when they experience any lack of waterproofing, they leave the water to preen. This continual swimming

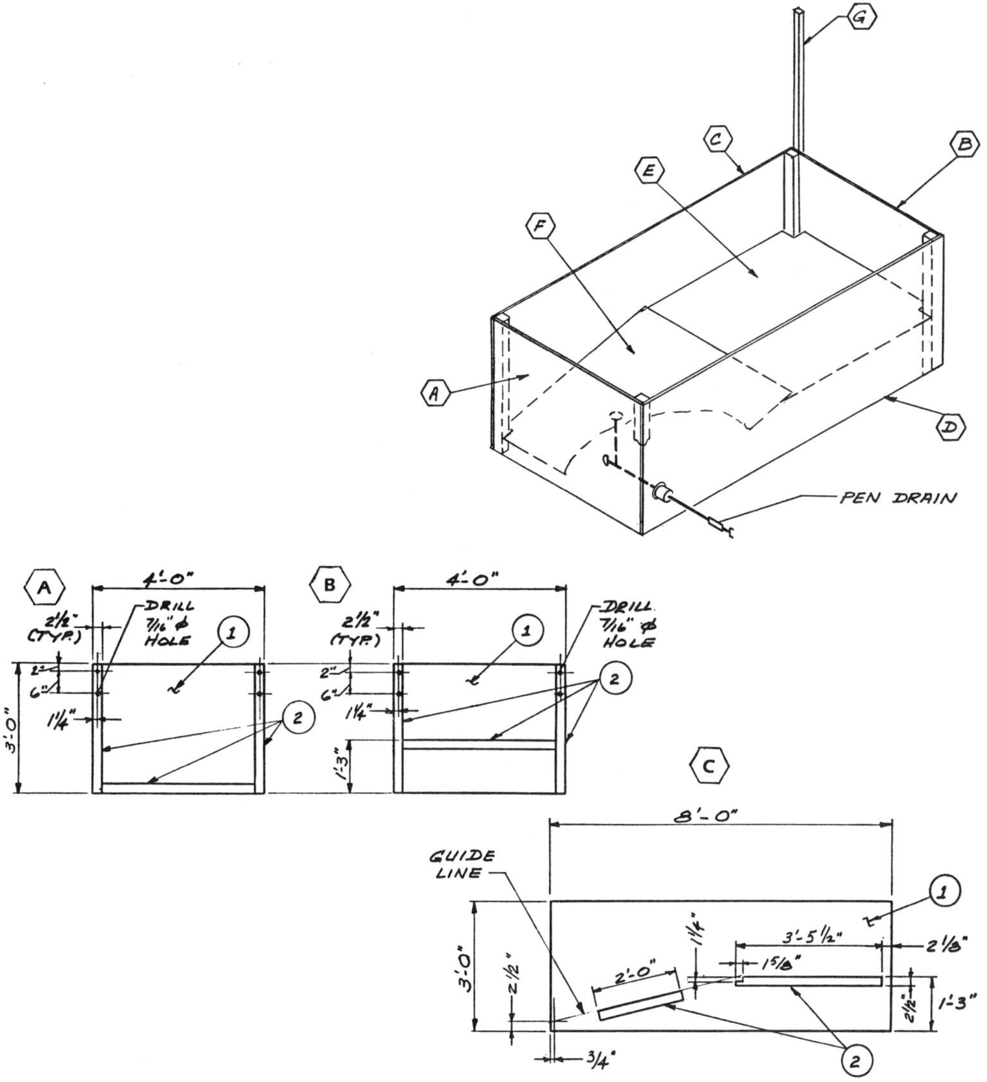

Figure 1. Oiled birds undergoing rehabilitation need free access to a pool. The "puddle pen" can be easily constructed from plywood, double-headed 8-penny nails, and bulkhead fittings if continual drainage is desired. (The bulkhead fittings and gasket should be installed first; then the PVC piping is fitted by force.) Two sheets of 6-mil polyethylene (8 ft × 12 ft) are stapled to the inside of the pen. Clean indoor-outdoor carpeting or sheets should be laid over the elevated, dry area of the pen (section *E*), and the excess should trail onto ramp *F* and be secured there to provide footing for the birds. The pool should be filled to the edge of *E*. Sheeting or drapes are hung from posts *G* in order to screen the area and prevent dabbling ducks and geese from jumping out of the pen. Diving ducks cannot take flight from these pools.

and preening is required for restoring the waterproof feather structure. This restoration does not require, but is further enhanced by, the reapplication to the feathers of oil from the uropygeal gland during preening. Birds that are adequately waterproofed will be able to remain in the water for 15 to 90 minutes, depending on the species, with feathers that still appear dry. The outer contour feathers of diving birds may become wet, but the down feathers remain dry. Waterproofed birds must be acclimated for release by gradual exposure to prevalent external temperatures. This can be accomplished by lowering the temperatures of the indoor holding area or by placing the bird outside for a longer period of time each day. In very cold climates this may take 3 or more days.

A bird slated for release should be of average weight for its species and sex. It should be adequately muscled so that it can forage normally in the wild. Birds should be free from any obvious signs of disease and should be released early in the day in suitable habitat. Those that are to be returned to a marine environment should be fed normal saline (0.9 per cent) for 2 to 3 days prior to release to allow the nasal salt gland to resume normal functioning.

The ease with which the rehabilitation of oiled birds is carried out varies according to species.

Mallard ducks, for example, can be easily treated in only a few days. Ocean birds (e.g., loons), however, are more difficult to house, feed, and waterproof, and they are more susceptible to land-based diseases. Oiled raptors, woodpeckers, and passerine (perching) species have been treated by using the above methods; the basic techniques are altered slightly in each case to conform to the special needs of the species (Jones, 1984).

SPECIAL CONSIDERATIONS FOR LARGE NUMBERS OF BIRDS

A major oil-spill crisis involving many birds requires special preparation and procedures. Since the rehabilitation of a large number of birds requires many people working long hours over a number of days, it is essential to train and organize the participants to perform in an efficient manner. Volunteers can be divided into four major groups:

The *facility management* group controls access to the cleaning center, sets up the work areas, maintains records, and is responsible for volunteer scheduling and welfare. The *medical treatment* group conducts physical examinations and performs treatments and, if necessary, triage. The *cleaning group* is responsible for cleaning, rinsing, and drying the birds. The *rehabilitation group* provides long-term rehabilitative care, including the feeding, swimming, and maintenance of the washed birds.

Group leaders should train members in their responsibilities within the overall organizational structure. This training should ideally take place prior to a spill, but it must occur before rehabilitation begins. Written instructions and posted flow charts are very valuable in transmission of information. Admittance to the facility must be controlled, and only trained workers and qualified personnel should be allowed into bird holding areas.

During a major spill, each bird should be banded at admittance, and individual records should be maintained for each step of the rehabilitation process. Statistical analysis of previous efforts indicate that there is a correlation between mortality and body weight and temperature (Lauer et al., 1982). Treated diving ducks with a body weight or temperature at or above average for their species achieved a 100 per cent release rate. Survival was reduced when either temperature or weight fell below these limits (66 per cent and 75 per cent, respectively), and the poorest chance for survival occurred when both measurements were low (38 per cent). Triage should be performed accordingly when an overwhelming number of birds are involved.

CONCLUSION

In most cases, oiled birds can be successfully rehabilitated with the above procedures. As experience with oiled birds is gained, the entire process can be carried out quickly and the bird can be released after a relatively short stay in captivity. Problems arise most frequently when one of the aforementioned steps is altered in some small way (e.g., by using the wrong detergent, too little water, water that is not warm enough, or insufficient rinsing). Every effort must be made to avoid any dogmatic adherence to the unsuccessful outdated cleaning methods (e.g., plucking, cornmeal, kitty litter, turpentine, and so forth). Properly handled birds can be returned to the wild with minimal or no lasting adverse effects.

References and Supplemental Reading

Barnes, S. A., and Rosie, D. G. (eds.): *The Effects of Oil on Birds: Physiological Research, Clinical Applications, and Rehabilitation*. Wilmington, DE: Tri-State Bird Rescue and Research, 1983.

Croxall, J.: Birds and oil pollution. *In* Cooper, J. E., and Eley, J. T. (eds.): *First Aid and Care of Wild Birds*. North Pomfret, VT: David and Charles, 1979, pp. 174–191.

Dolensek, E. P., and Bell, J.: *Help! A Step by Step Manual for the Care and Treatment of Oil-Damaged Birds*. New York: New York Zoological Society, 1977.

Harris, J. M.: Management of oil-soaked birds. *In* Kirk, R. W. (ed.): *Current Veterinary Therapy VII*. Philadelphia: W. B. Saunders, 1980, pp. 687–91.

Jones, B.: Handling small numbers of oiled birds. *In* Beaver, P. (ed.): *Wildlife Rehabilitation. Vol. 2*. New York: National Wildlife Rehabilitators Association, 1984, pp 121–127.

Lauer, D. M., Dein, F. J., and Frink, J. A.: Rehabilitation of ruddy ducks *(Oxyura jamaicensis)* contaminated with oil. J.A.V.M.A. 181:398, 1982.

Light, M., and Lanier, J. J.: *Biological Effects of Oil Pollution—A Comprehensive Bibliography With Abstracts*. Washington, DC: U.S. Department of Transportation, 1978.

Michael, A. D.: The effects of petroleum hydrocarbons on marine populations and communities. *In* Wolfe, D. A. (ed.): *Fate and Effects of Petroleum Hydrocarbons in Marine Ecosystems and Organisms*. New York: Pergamon Press, 1977, pp. 129–137.

Percy, J. A., and Mullin, T. C.: Effects of crude oil on the locomotory activity of arctic marine invertebrates. Marine Pollution Bulletin 8:35, 1977.

Williams, A. S.: *Saving oiled seabirds*. Washington, DC: American Petroleum Institute, 1978.

AVIAN GIARDIASIS

KAREN E. ROERTGEN, D.V.M.
Sacramento, California

Infection of exotic birds with the protozoan parasite *Giardia* can manifest itself in a number of ways; the range is from asymptomatic carriers to birds that show the classic symptoms mimicking those found in other species of animals suffering from the disease giardiasis. General symptoms in all animals include a loose, watery stool; malabsorption disorders; flatulence; steatorrhea; weight loss; and a deterioration of the quality of the skin, hair, or feathers. The diagnosis of giardiasis in domestic animals has increased rapidly in the past few years, and the disease was first described in pet birds in the 1970s. At this time it is considered to be an emerging zoonosis.

LIFE CYCLE

The protozoan parasite *Giardia* is an inhabitant of the upper small intestine. It is a member of the same order as the *Hexamita* organisms, which cause catarrhal enteritis in turkeys and the more severe ulcerative enteritis of pigeons. The parasite occurs in two forms, the motile trophozoite and the nonmotile cyst. The trophozoite is a somewhat pear-shaped creature; when viewed on the side it is crescentic in shape. It has two nuclei, which impart a characteristic facial appearance. The movement of the trophozoite is best described as a "falling leaf" motion. This form is 10 to 20 μm long and 5 to 15 μm wide; cysts are approximately two-thirds the size of trophozoites.

The life cycle is a direct one. The trophozoites attach to the intestinal mucosa by means of a ventral sucking disc. They divide by binary fission. Nuclear division occurs in the lower intestine, and the mature cyst with four nuclei is discharged with the feces. Cysts become infective in 1 to 7 days. The prepatent period in birds is 4 to 8 days.

Endosymbiotic bacteria of the protozoan may play an important part in the varying pathogenicity, metabolism, host specificity, and antigenic surface characteristics of the parasite. All of the endosymbionts found so far have been gram-negative organisms.

PATHOGENESIS

Giardial infections are, as mentioned before, very similar in all species of animals. The disease can range in severity from acute to subacute to chronic. It should be noted that the majority of infections in most species are asymptomatic. The clinical severity of the infection also has no relation to the infective dose.

Significant associations or predispositions to clinical giardiasis have been reported in humans with achlorhydria, hypogammaglobulinemia, previous antibiotic therapy, and decreased secretory IgA levels (Hartong, 1979). Malabsorption disorders associated with the disease have also been studied more extensively in human medicine, and one report cited 60 per cent of patients with steatorrhea and others with deficiencies of folic acid (40 per cent), vitamin B_{12} (50 per cent), fat-soluble vitamins (50 per cent) and general disaccharidases (80 per cent). Hypocarotenemia and abnormal absorption tests for D-xylose were also common (Hartong, 1979).

Factors involved in the cause of the syndrome include one or all of the following: (1) blanketing of the mucosal surface by *Giardia*, which decreases its absorptive and digestive capability, (2) release of substances that decrease function of the microvilli and activity of enzymes, (3) direct irritation of the mucosa, causing excessive mucus secretion, (4) bacterial overgrowth, and (5) bile salt abnormalities secondary to bacterial deconjugation.

Histologic changes in cases of giardiasis are the exception and not the rule. When present, they usually consist of villus atrophy, decreased height of the columnar epithelium, and possibly infiltration of the lamina propria with lymphocytic cells. The exact role of the immune response in the disease is uncertain, but both aspects of the response (humoral and cell-mediated) appear to be involved. Histologic changes are seen more commonly in immunodeficient patients, and synergism between *Giardia* and enterobacteria has been theorized to play a part in such cases.

EPIDEMIOLOGY

Giardia lamblia is the most commonly encountered intestinal parasite in humans in the United States and Great Britain. Its prevalence is from 2 to 20 per cent worldwide and 8 per cent in the United States. Studies of prevalence in parakeets have indicated a rate of 65 to 70 per cent. Immature animals tend to have higher rates of infection. The organism is passed on by the fecal-oral route or by the ingestion of contaminated food or water. Cysts will remain viable for up to 3 months. The disease was first seen in birds in Texas, where large-scale breeders of parakeets began experiencing epidemics of a "wasting syndrome." The nestlings especially were affected; they showed up to 90 per cent mortality and the survivors showed 50 per cent morbidity. The outbreaks were usually related to the recent introduction of new birds. Desquamation of the crop and erosions of the gizzard were found at necropsy. In some of these cases, budgie nestling virus was also thought to be involved. Simultaneous outbreaks of giardiasis and chlamydiosis have been reported, and improper disinfection procedures and lack of chemotherapy might have promoted the number of subclinical carriers of both diseases.

THE SYNDROME IN BIRDS

When seen in clinical practice, parakeets harboring *Giardia* have usually come from an environment with many other birds and questionable sanitation. They are usually less than a year of age. (Budgies with giardiasis don't live long!) Cockatiels with the disease have shown a greater age 171stribution and may come from relatively isolated surroundings. Additionally, a larger percentage of them are either asymptomatic or subclinical carriers.

"Classic" avian giardiasis is more often seen in parakeets. They are emaciated and are unable to maintain their weight in spite of a voracious appetite. Young birds are often presented for crop stasis or stunted growth. The droppings are light-colored, large, and either loose or pasty.

Cockatiels often present with more diverse signs. Their feathers may be greasy or oily, and the owner's complaint is often that of a feather problem or pruritus. The droppings may or may not be normal in appearance, and the parasite may be discovered only by a routine fecal examination.

Not all feather problems in such birds can be attributed to *Giardia;* however, the documented malabsorption that occurs with this disease could significantly affect the nutritional status of the bird enough to cause abnormalities in molting, regrowth, and weatherproofing of the feathers. Another factor to be remembered is the high degree of association between giardiasis and other compounding illnesses.

DIAGNOSIS

Giardia cysts are shed inconsistently; therefore, the larger the number of samples tested, the better the chance of diagnosis. (Ten to 50 per cent of humans with multiple negative results on fecal examination react positively to one of the other more invasive tests.) Medications such as kaolin, antacids, oily laxatives, and antibiotics decrease the chance of obtaining a positive result on a fecal exam. If the feces is fresh, it may be possible to detect motile trophozoites as well as cysts.

A direct smear of the droppings, mixed with saline, is often used to aid in diagnosis. The cysts can be seen better after a drop of Lugol's iodine is added, but this will destroy the motility of any trophozoites. Cysts can be seen at 400× magnification; trophozoites usually require higher power in order to be discernible.

Fecal samples can also be preserved with PVA (polyvinyl alcohol) and thus collected over a long period of time by the owner. A sample thus preserved can later be stained with trichrome, as described in *The Manual of Clinical Microbiology,* by Lennette. Many suspicious cases have been proved to be infected in this manner. This technique is also of benefit for follow-ups on post-treatment checks of aviaries.

TREATMENT

Whenever a bird is found to be shedding *Giardia,* it, and all other birds in the aviary, should be treated. The infected bird is a reservoir for other birds, and it is capable of shedding the cysts for months or years. The owner should be warned of possible toxicity to nestlings and younger birds. If not visibly affected, they should be removed from the treatment group. Emphasis should be placed first on cleaning and disinfecting the premises and then on treating the birds. Post-treatment cleaning and disinfecting should also receive high priority. New birds should show negative results on serial fecal examinations before they are admitted to a treated group, and no group of birds should be considered successfully treated until multiple fecal exams, collected at least one month after cessation of treatment, show negative results. It may be necessary to treat the group 3 to 4 times in order to control the situation, and in some instances eradication of the parasite may be achieved only by repopulation of the aviary with specific-pathogen free (SPF) birds. Periodic monitoring of representative fecal exams from each group is advocated for all aviaries. Installing suspended cages, changing to a more easily sanitized cage floor, or preventing access to the cage floor with wire mesh can minimize recontamination. Containers of water and food should be positioned so as to minimize their potential as fecal reservoirs. Two drugs are currently used to control giardiasis in caged birds. Dimetridazole (Emtryl, Salsbury Laboratories) has been used in a solution of 0.02 to 0.04 per cent* in the drinking water for 5 days, followed by a withdrawal period of 5 days and a second course of treatment for another 5 days. The dose should be halved on hot days or when used on breeding birds in order to avoid the toxicity problems associated with increased water consumption. Signs of toxicity are head pressing, convulsions, and ataxia. The second drug in use is ipronidazole (Ipropran, Hoffman-LaRoche). It is also administered in the drinking water, at a dosage of 0.5 gm/gallon for one week.

Besides the problems with potential toxicity of these drugs, there seems to be an association with a large number of post-treatment bacterial and fungal infections of the alimentary tract. Whether they were pre-existing and subclinical or iatrogenic is uncertain. Certainly bacterial overgrowth is known to occur in giardiasis in other animals. There is another side to these secondary infections, however, and that is the spectrum of activity of the nitroimidazoles used to treat the disease. Some of the drugs in this family are used to treat anaerobic infections in humans. It is possible that Emtryl and Ipropran may have similar effects and may be affecting the intestinal flora of the bird in other ways, paving the way for opportunistic pathogens. In any case, owners should be forewarned of the possible side effects so that they realize the importance of post-treatment rechecks. It is a good idea to prepare and stain the droppings of the treated bird in order to check for inordinate numbers of gram-negative bacteria or yeast.

*Note: An approximately 0.03 per cent solution is made by dissolving ¼ tsp. powder in 2 quarts of water.

As mentioned before, routine chlorination of the drinking water, which is effective in controlling coliforms, is ineffective against *Giardia* cysts. They remain viable in cold, clear water for up to 3 months, and neither iodine solutions nor chlorination will kill them. The least expensive way of killing the cysts seems to be boiling the water, particularly in areas in which they are highly endemic.

Because of the potential for cross-species transmission, the need for treatment and strict sanitation should be emphasized to the owner. Once they understand the basic aspects of the parasite's life cycle, owners are more willing to put effort into preventative management, which, in the end, is the only way to ensure success in treating this avian problem.

References and Supplemental Reading

Davies, R. B., and Hilber, C. P.: Animal reservoirs and cross-species transmission of *Giardia*. *In* Jakubowski, W., and Hoff, J. C. (eds.): *Waterborne Transmission of Giardiasis*. Cincinnati, OH: United States Environmental Protection Agency (EPA–600/9–79–0001), 1979, pp. 104–125.

Hartong, W. A., Gourley, W. K., and Arvanitakis, C.: Giardiasis: Clinical spectrum and functional-structural abnormalities of the small intestinal mucosa. Gastroenterology 77:1, 1979.

Lennette, E., Spaulding, E., and Truant, J.: *Manual of Clinical Microbiology*, 2nd ed. Washington, DC: American Society for Microbiology, 1978.

Panigrahy, B., Elissalde, G., Grumbles, L. C., et al.: Giardia infections in parakeets. Avian Dis. 22:815, 1978.

Scholtens, R. E., New, J. C., and Johnson, S.: The nature and treatment of giardiasis in parakeets. J.A.V.M.A. 180:170, 1982.

Wolfe, M. S.: Giardiasis. J.A.M.A. 233:1362, 1975.

Yamashita, T., Hirai, K., Shimakura, S., et al.: Recent occurrence of chlamydiosis and giardiasis in budgerigars in Japan. Jpn. J. Vet. Sci. 43:963, 1981.

CYTOLOGY IN AVIAN DIAGNOSTICS

TERRY W. CAMPBELL, D.V.M.

Manhattan, Kansas

Cytodiagnosis can be a valuable diagnostic tool for the avian veterinarian. It is a simple, rapid, inexpensive diagnostic procedure that can be performed in the veterinary clinic. Cytologic specimens are easily obtained and cause little tissue injury since only a small sample is required. Examination of the cellular response in a lesion often provides an excellent evaluation of the nature of the disease process involved. The veterinarian can determine whether the primary response is inflammatory or neoplastic or whether tissue hyperplasia has occurred; occasionally, the cause of the disorder can be identified.

Diagnostic cytology has a few limitations that the

veterinarian should recognize. Cytologic interpretations may differ from those obtained from histologic examination of the same lesion. Cytologic inspection does not provide information concerning cellular architecture, lesion size, or invasiveness of a malignant lesion. Also, the predominant cellular response may not represent the primary lesion. An example would be an ulcerated neoplastic lesion that reveals evidence only of the secondary inflammation when examined cytologically. Occasionally, one is unable to characterize the cellular response in a cytologic sample and must rely on histologic interpretations. However, cytodiagnosis can often provide a strong presumptive diagnosis that will complement the histologic evaluation. Armed with a presumptive diagnosis obtained from cytodiagnosis, the veterinarian can begin therapy while waiting for histologic or other supportive laboratory results.

SAMPLING PROCEDURES

The method of fine-needle aspiration biopsy is commonly used for obtaining cytologic samples. The sample is aspirated into a needle bore, deposited onto a glass microscope slide, and smeared by using a "squash prep" method. Contact smears are also commonly used. These are made by pressing on a slide removed masses or exposed lesions. Tissues that exfoliate poorly require scraping of the cut surface with a scalpel blade to improve the cellular distribution of the sample. Fluid samples are obtained by aspiration or a cotton swab. Smears from fluids are made with the conventional two-slide wedge, coverslip, or "squash prep" method (especially for thick fluids or if particles of solid tissue are present). Fluids in cells may require concentration techniques, such as sediment smears (centrifugation at 1800 rpm for 10 min) and cytocentrifuge smears (Cytospin, Shandon Southern Instruments).

Blood can be collected by several methods: jugular venipuncture, cutaneous ulnar (wing vein) venipuncture, medial metatarsal venipuncture, toenail clip method, cardiac puncture, or occipital venous sinus puncture (Campbell and Dein, 1984; Vuillaume, 1983). Blood smears are made in the same manner as mammalian blood smears; however, the coverslip method appears to cause less cellular smudging. Sites for bone marrow aspiration biopsy include the sternum and the proximal tibiotarsus. Jamshidi (Kormed) bone marrow biopsy/aspiration needles (20 or 22 gauge) or disposable modified Illinois sternal/iliac bone marrow aspiration needles (adult or pediatric sizes) can be used. Indications for bone marrow evaluation include leukopenia, nonregenerative anemia, thrombocytopenia, abnormal cells in the peripheral blood, and a leukocytosis due to a leukemia. Crop aspiration is indicated in cases of vomiting, regurgitation, delayed crop emptying, and other crop disorders. The procedure requires a mouth speculum; sterile, soft plastic or rubber tube; and syringe. The tube should be gently passed into the crop for aspiration. Aspirate from the upper respiratory sinus should be obtained from birds with sinusitis. When the bird's head is held firmly, a sinus aspirate can be obtained by inserting a needle with syringe attached directly into the sinus. The needle is inserted at the commissure of the mouth, directed to a point midway between the eye and the nares, and passed under the zygomatic bone and parallel to the side of the head (Campbell, 1984). A misdirected needle may puncture the ocular orbit and globe or a muscle mass. A tracheal aspirate is obtained by passing a sterile, soft plastic or rubber tube through the glottis, into the trachea, and ending near the syrinx at the thoracic inlet. Sterile saline (1.0 to 3.0 ml/kg body weight) is infused into the trachea and immediately reaspirated back into the syringe. This procedure usually requires a general anesthetic. Large birds can be intubated with a sterile endotracheal tube, which decreases contamination from the oral cavity. The sample usually requires concentration procedures for proper evaluation. A swab sample from an air sac can be obtained during an otoscope laparotomy, laparoscopy, or exploratory surgical laparotomy. Abdominocentesis is indicated whenever ascites, peritonitis, hemoperitoneum, or other abdominal effusions are suspected. A needle is inserted into the abdominal cavity at the ventral midline immediately distal to the point of the sternum (keel) and directed to the right to avoid the gizzard.

STAINING

Stains used in veterinary cytodiagnosis include Papanicolaou's stain, Sano method or its modifications, new methylene blue, hematoxylin-eosin, Romanovsky's stains (i.e., Giemsa and Wright's stains), and "stat" stains such as Diff-Quik (Harleco), a rapid, modified Wright-Giemsa stain (Clark, 1981; Lillie, 1977). Special stains include Gram's stain for bacteria, acid-fast stain for tubercle bacilli, Giménez and Macchiavello's stains for chlamydia, and Sudan stains for fat (Clark, 1981; Lillie, 1977). The cell descriptions used in this text are based on Wright's stain or the Diff-Quik stain, which are commonly used by practicing veterinarians.

GENERAL PRINCIPLES OF CYTODIAGNOSTIC INTERPRETATIONS

The cytologic appearances of many cells obtained from avian tissues and fluids are similar to those described for mammals. Rebar (1978) and Perman and colleagues (1979) have provided two handbooks on veterinary cytology to assist the practitioner in the evaluation of specimens. These handbooks would also be beneficial to the avian veterinarian. Cells obtained in cytologic samples are classified into one of the four major cytologic tissue groups: hemic, epithelial-glandular, connective, or nervous tissue (Perman et al., 1979). Details of these groups can be found in the references, where illustrations enhance the descriptions (Campbell, 1984; Campbell and Dein, 1984; Perman et al., 1979). Also, the predominant cellular response can be classified into one of three major cytodiagnostic groups: inflammation, hyperplasia, or neoplasia (Perman et al., 1979; Rebar, 1978).

MAJOR CYTODIAGNOSTIC GROUPS

Inflammation

Inflammatory cells include heterophils, eosinophils, basophils, lymphocytes, plasma cells, and macrophages. Plasma cells are round to oval lymphocytes with an abundant, deeply basophilic cytoplasm. The round nucleus is eccentrically located and contains coarse hyperchromatic chromatin. Plasma cells have prominent Golgi complexes. Macrophages are large, irregular cells that have abundant, granulated blue cytoplasm, which often contains phagocytic vacuoles and foreign material. Inflammatory lesions are classified as acute, chronic-active, or chronic, based on their cytologic response (Rebar, 1978). Acute inflammation shows a predominance of heterophils (greater than 70 per cent of the inflammatory cells). Heterophils become degenerate when exposed to a toxic environment (i.e., overwhelming bacterial infections). Degenerative features include increased cytoplasmic basophilia, vacuolization, degranulation, and nuclear karyolysis or karyorrhexis. Karyolysis is represented cytologically by a swollen nucleus with poorly defined pink, homogeneous chromatin. Karyorrhexis is nuclear fragmentation. Nuclear pyknosis indicates a slow aging of the cell in a nontoxic environment and is represented by a small, dense, deeply basophilic nucleus. Chronic-active inflammation also shows a predominance of heterophils (50 to 70 per cent of the inflammatory cells), but a mixture of other cell types are also present (i.e., lymphocytes, plasma cells, and macrophages). The heterophils are usually nondegenerate. Chronic inflammation shows a predominance of mononuclear cells (greater than 50 per cent of the inflammatory cells) such as lymphocytes and macrophages. Granulomatous reactions, a type of chronic inflammation, are represented by macrophages and multinucleated giant cells. The macrophages often coalesce into netlike sheets. If heterophils are mixed among the macrophages, the term *pyogranulomatous reaction* is used. Causative agents, such as foreign bodies, fungi, and tubercle bacilli are noted for establishing chronic inflammatory lesions. Background material of inflammatory lesions often shows an increased granular precipitation and protein aggregation.

Tissue Hyperplasia

Hyperplastic tissue reveals a uniform population of normal-appearing cells when examined cytologically. The cells may show signs of immaturity (e.g., cytoplasmic basophilia). Tissue hyperplasia often results from tissue injury. Epithelial or fibrous proliferation surrounding areas of chronic inflammation is an example of tissue hyperplasia.

Neoplasms

The general cellular features of neoplasms include a population of cells that appear related (cells with a common origin) but exhibit various degrees of pleomorphism. This feature differentiates neoplasia from hyperplasia. Certain types of neoplasms tend to exfoliate well and occur in clumps or sheets (e.g., carcinomas), whereas others exfoliate poorly and occur as single cells (e.g., sarcomas). Nuclear features of neoplasms include nuclear enlargement, a variation in size and shape (suggesting rapid or abnormal mitosis), variable nuclear-cytoplasmic ratio, nucleolar variations (variable sizes, shapes, number, and staining quality), multinucleation (uneven numbers suggest asynchronous cell divisions), irregularity of the chromatin and nuclear membrane, and abnormal mitotic figures (Perman, 1979; Campbell, 1984). Cytoplasmic features of neoplasms include a small cytoplasmic volume (may be normal in some cells, such as lymphocytes), variable cytoplasmic borders, cytoplasmic basophilia (indicates a high concentration of RNA and rate of metabolism), large vacuoles, and inclusions (e.g., pigment granules, phagocytosis of other cells, and nuclear fragments) (Rebar, 1978; Campbell, 1984). Neoplasms can be classified as carcinomas, sarcomas, or discrete cell neoplasms (Rebar, 1978). Carcinomas have large round to oval cells with epithelial cell features; they exfoliate in sheets or clumps and have distinct cytoplasmic borders. Adenomas and adenocarcinomas have large cytoplasmic secretory vacuoles and tend to form multinucleated giant cells. Cells from sarcomas resemble connective tissue cells and exfoliate poorly. These cells are often elongated or spindle-shaped with indistinct cytoplasmic borders. They frequently have large nuclei (occasionally multinucleated) with distinct nucleoli. Discrete cell neoplasms are derived from cells that have no normal cellular interactions. Lymphoid leukosis (lymphosarcoma) is an example of a discrete cell neoplasm found in birds. This neoplasm is represented by a marked number of immature lymphocytes (i.e., lymphoblasts and prolymphocytes) with frequent mitotic figures and many pale-blue cytoplasmic fragments in the background. Other cytologic features that are suggestive of a neoplasm include the appearance of peripheral blood in a body cavity in a bird with no history of trauma; this is the result of spontaneous hemorrhage due to an ulcerated neoplasm. Hemangiosarcomas often have such a pattern. The presence of foreign cells (ectopic cells) in the tissue is suggestive of a metastatic neoplasm.

CYTOLOGIC FEATURES OF BODY FLUIDS AND TISSUES

Body Fluids and Abdominal Effusions

Normal abdominal effusions have a low volume and cellularity. They contain an occasional macrophage and mesothelial cell. Normal mesothelial cells adhering to serosal surfaces vary in size and shape and appear flat. They occur singly or in clusters. Nuclei are centrally located and the cytoplasm has a homogeneous appearance. Mesothelial cells become reactive when they are exposed to long-standing abdominal effusions or when serous membranes are irritated. Reactive mesothelial cells are round to oval and often show multinucleation, mitotic figures, cytoplasmic vacuolization, and scalloped cytoplasmic margins. They appear larger and more basophilic than normal mesothelial cells. Reactive mesothelial cells become transformed into phagocytic cells that resemble macrophages. Transformed mesothelial cells appear in long-standing transudative fluids or exudates.

Abdominal transudates result from hypoproteinemia, cardiac insufficiency, and hepatic cirrhosis (Campbell, 1984). These transudates are characterized by a low cellularity, specific gravity less than 1.020, total protein less than 3.0 gm/dl, and color that ranges from clear to pale yellow. The cellular content of transudates reveals primarily mononuclear cells (macrophages and mesothelial cells) on a clear background. Transudates become modified with hydrostatic pressure changes or if they are allowed to stand for long periods of time. Modified transudates show an increase in cellular and protein content and in heterophils and reactive or transformed mesothelial cells.

Exudative effusions are caused by infectious agents, irritating chemicals, and neoplastic effusions. They are characterized by a high cellularity (predominantly inflammatory cells), specific gravity of 1.020 or greater, total protein greater than 3.0 gm/dl, and thick granular background. Exudates vary in color, are often viscous, frequently clot, and often have a foul odor. Chronic exudates often contain many lymphocytes and plasma cells.

Hemorrhagic effusions are indicated by a predominance of peripheral blood in the fluid. Acute hemorrhagic effusions resemble peripheral blood. Thrombocytes indicate active hemorrhage or peripheral blood contamination of the sample. Chronic or resolving hemorrhagic effusions show varying degrees of erythrophagocytosis (e.g., macrophages containing intact or fragmented erythrocytes and iron pigment).

Malignant effusions have exudative features but contain neoplastic cells. Occasionally, they are accompanied by hemorrhagic effusion.

Upper Alimentary Tract (Buccal Cavity, Esophagus, Crop)

The buccal cavity is lined with cornified squamous epithelium and the esophagus and crop (ingluvies) are lined with noncornified stratified squamous epithelium (Banks, 1974). Cytologic study of normal tissue reveals many squamous epithelial cells with varying degrees of cornification. Young squamous cells are round to oval with abundant blue cytoplasm and central vesicular nuclei. The mature squamous cell is larger, is polygonal in shape (with angular or folded margins), and has a small condensed nucleus. Many extracellular bacteria are present in cytologic samples from the upper alimentary tract. They show a wide variation in morphology and are often associated with squamous epithelial cells. *Alysiella filiformis* is a normal inhabitant of the avian upper alimentary tract and is often associated with squamous cells (Campbell, 1984). It occurs as pairs of cells arranged in unbranched, ribbonlike filaments. Normal samples also show a moderate amount of debris and foreign material (e.g., plant fibers and crystals).

Inflammatory lesions of the upper alimentary tract (stomatitis, esophagitis, and ingluvitis) show a variable number of squamous epithelial cells and amount of background debris. There are numerous inflammatory cells. Bacterial phagocytosis indicates a septic lesion. Parabasalar cells indicate an ulcerative lesion or traumatic exfoliation. These cells are round epithelial cells with scant, deeply basophilic cytoplasm and large central nuclei. Fibroblasts are associated with chronic ulcerative lesions.

Candidiasis is indicated by a large number of oval, thin-walled budding yeast cells (3 to 6 μm in diameter) that stain a dark blue with Wright's stain. There is usually a marked amount of background debris, but few inflammatory cells are present unless mucosal ulceration has occurred. The presence of *Candida* pseudohyphae (or true mycelium) and blastospores indicate mucosal invasion, possible systemic involvement, and a poor prognosis. Trichomoniasis is best identified on a wet mount smear, which reveals the motile, piriform, flagellate protozoa. Trichomonads are identified by their undulating membranes and anterior flagellae. Acute septic inflammatory lesions show a predominance of heterophils that may be degenerate and contain phagocytized bacteria. Bacteria represented by one morphological type should be viewed with suspicion.

Hypovitaminosis A causes hyperkeratosis of squamous epithelium and squamous metaplasia of nonsquamous epithelium. Lesions due to hypovitaminosis A show a large number of cornified squamous epithelial cells with little background debris and no evidence of inflammation.

Cloaca and Vent

The cloaca is the common orifice of the digestive, urinary, and reproductive tracts. It is lined by simple columnar epithelium and lymphatic nodules (Banks, 1974). The vent is the external opening to the cloaca and is lined with cornified stratified squamous epithelium (Banks, 1974). The normal cytologic appearance of this area shows a variable number of columnar epithelial and cornified or noncornified squamous cells. There is usually a large number of extracellular bacteria, represented by a wide variety of morphological types and a moderate amount of background debris. Inflammation involving this area shows many inflammatory cells. Parabasalar cells suggest ulcerative lesions. Granulomatous cellular reactions and neoplasms can also be found in this area.

Upper Respiratory Tract

The nasal and infraorbital sinuses are lined by nonkeratinizing stratified squamous epithelium (Banks, 1974). The trachea and primary bronchi are lined by pseudostratified ciliated columnar epithelium with goblet cells, and the syrinx is lined with bistratified squamous or columnar epithelium (Banks, 1974). Normally, samples from the upper respiratory sinuses are poor in cells and show little background debris. There is an occasional squamous cell and a few extracellular bacteria. Material from the normal trachea and bronchi also has few cells and contains a variable number of ciliated columnar respiratory epithelial cells. These cells are shed singly or in clusters, vary in size and shape, and have an abundant granular basophilic cytoplasm. They have an eccentric, round to oval nucleus on the narrow pole of the cell and prominent eosinophilic cilia at the opposite, wider pole. Normal tracheal and bronchial cytologic samples also contain goblet cells, which secrete mucin. These cells resemble ciliated respiratory epithelial cells but lack cilia, often have an indistinct cytoplasmic margin, and have prominent eosinophilic cytoplasmic granulation. An occasional heterophil, eosinophil, lymphocyte, macrophage, or mesothelial cell can be found in samples from this area.

Cytologic characteristics of sinusitis include an increased number of inflammatory cells and background debris. Bacterial phagocytosis indicates a septic sinusitis. Chlamydial organisms are identified as small, basophilic, coccoid, intracytoplasmic inclusions within macrophages and epithelial cells. Special staining with Giménez or Macchiavello's stains will aid in the detection of *Chlamydia*. The chlamydial elementary bodies (200 to 300 μm) stain red with both stains, whereas the larger, initial bodies (900 to 1000 μm) stain red with Giménez stain and blue with Macchiavello's stain. Chronic sinusitis lesions show an increased number of lymphocytes and plasma cells.

Tracheobronchitis is indicated by an increased number of inflammatory cells and amount of background debris. The epithelial cells may show degenerative changes such as loss of cilia, karyorrhexis, and cytoplasmic vacuolization. An increase in mucin is represented by a thick purple background when stained with Wright's stain. Hypersensitivity reactions (i.e., allergies) are indicated by an increased number of eosinophils and goblet cells.

Lower Respiratory Tract (Lungs and Air Sacs)

The lung air capillaries and air sacs are lined by simple squamous epithelium (Banks, 1974). Normal lung imprints obtained at necropsy show a marked amount of peripheral blood due to the great vascularity of the tissue. Lung imprints often show an alveolarlike pattern. Imprints or swabs of air sacs, obtained during necropsy or exploratory laparotomy, normally yield poorly cellular samples with occasional noncornified squamous cells. Inflammatory lesions (pneumonia and air sacculitis) reveal large numbers of inflammatory cells with an increased amount of background debris. Bacterial involvement is indicated by phagocytized bacteria. Mycotic lesions show fungal elements (i.e., hyphae and spores). Aspergillosis is indicated by branching septate hyphae, spores, and conidiophores. Mycotic lesions have chronic inflammatory cellular patterns with formation of multinucleated giant cells. Chlamydiosis of the air sacs reveals a marked number of mononuclear inflammatory cells (primarily macrophages), degenerate cells, and cytoplasmic chlamydial inclusions.

Skin and Subcutis

The skin is composed of keratinized, stratified, squamous epithelium, and exfoliation produces primarily cornified, squamous epithelial cells (Banks, 1974). Bacterial skin infections show a large number of inflammatory cells (primarily heterophils) and phagocytized bacteria. Nonpathogenic surface bacteria are extracellular. Fungal involvement reveals fungal elements and a granulation reaction. Hyperkeratosis is primarily indicated cytologically by cornified squamous epithelial cells on a clear background. Knemidokoptic mange is best detected by demonstrating the mites on a wet mount by using mineral oil from a skin scraping. Pox lesions reveal a marked number of inflammatory cells. Pox is diagnosed by the identification of swollen epithelial cells with large cytoplasmic vacuoles that push the nucleus to one edge of the cell. The vacuoles (Bollinger bodies) contain small, pale, eosinophilic inclusions (Borrel bodies) when stained with Wright's stain. Xanthomatosis of the skin is indicated by many macrophages, multinucleated giant cells, and cholesterol crystals, which are translucent crystals of varied geometric shapes that often dissolve in Wright's stain. Subcutaneous lipomas demonstrate numerous background droplets of fat (best seen with new methylene blue or Sudan stains) and adipose cells, are round with foamy cytoplasm that contain large secretory (fat) vacuoles, and have a nucleus located at the cell's edge. Subcutaneous lymphoid neoplasms (e.g., lymphoid leukosis and Marek's disease) contain numerous immature lymphocytes. Feather cysts (feathers growing within their follicle) reveal a variable number of erythrocytes and inflammatory cells along with erythrophagocytosis, marked amount of background debris, and feather fragments. Numerous fibroblasts may be seen in chronic lesions.

Conjunctiva and Cornea

Normal conjunctival and corneal samples show a few cells on a clear background. The cells are predominately noncornified epithelial cells, and they occur singly or in sheets. They have a lightly basophilic cytoplasm and round to oval vesicular nuclei. Inflammatory lesions (conjunctivitis and keratitis) are indicated by a large number of inflammatory cells and degenerate epithelial cells. Chronic lesions show keratinization of the epithelial cells and conjunctival goblet cells. Conjunctival goblet cells are large cells with abundant, foamy cytoplasm that contains large secretory vacuoles; the cells have an eccentric nucleus. Chlamydial or mycoplasmal inclusions may be present and are best detected by using special stains.

Synovial Fluid

Normal avian joints contain very little fluid; however, a diseased joint that is distended with fluid may provide enough sample for cytologic evaluation. Normal synovial fluid contains few cells and has a thick, coarsely granular background (mucin). The predominant cells are mononuclear leukocytes. Septic arthritis is indicated by a large number of inflammatory cells (primarily heterophils) and phagocytized bacteria. Traumatic arthritis shows a variable number of erythrocytes and leukocytes; an increased number of macrophages, showing erythrophagocytosis, appear as the lesion becomes chronic. Degenerative joint disease is marked by an increased cellularity (primarily mononuclear cells) and decreased background granulation (poor mucin content). Articular gout produces a large number of inflammatory cells and urate crystals. These crystals are amorphous or needlelike birefringent crystals under polarized light. The fluid produced by articular gout appears dense, white, or yellow, and it is cloudy on gross examination.

Liver

Antemortem liver samples can be obtained for cytologic study by aspiration or excisional biopsy. Normal liver tissue provides highly cellular imprints and reveals a thick background with many cell fragments and free nuclei. There is usually a marked amount of peripheral blood. Hepatocytes occur singly, in sheets, or clustered. They are round to oval and show abundant basophilic cytoplasm and coarse granulation. The hepatocyte nuclei are eccentric in location, contain coarse chromatin, and have a single prominent nucleolus. Occasionally, binucleated cells and mitotic figures are seen. Hepatic samples also contain spindle-shaped stromal cells, lymphocytes, plasma cells, and macrophages (often containing iron pigment). The lymphoid aggregates found in hepatic preparations are composed primarily of small, mature lymphocytes. Abnormal findings include degenerate hepatocytes (suggesting postmortem autolysis or hepatocellular necrosis), swollen hepatocytes (enlarged, vacuolated hepatocytes are seen with hepatic lipidosis), increased number of inflammatory cells, a large number of plasma cells (reactive lymphoid response), and cells with neoplastic features from primary or ectopic neoplasms.

Spleen

Splenic samples are obtained at necropsy or by excisional biopsy. Normal splenic tissue shows a marked amount of peripheral blood and a heavy background of cellular debris. There are many free nuclei. Macrophages with varying degrees of erythrophagocytosis are common. Lymphoid components are predominantly small, mature lymphocytes but there is also an increased number of plasma cells with reactivity (e.g., systemic chlamydiosis or other antigens). Splenic stromal cells have indistinct cytoplasmic margins with a variable amount of pale blue cytoplasm. The nucleus is eccentric and round to oval; it contains coarse chromatin. Abnormal findings include schizont stages of blood parasites, chlamydial inclusions, marked erythrophagocytosis (seen with hemolytic anemias), fungal elements, and an increased number of inflammatory cells.

References and Supplemental Reading

Banks, W. J.: *Histology and Comparative Organology: A Text-Atlas.* Baltimore: The Williams & Wilkins Co., 1974.

Campbell, T. W.: Diagnostic cytology in avian medicine. Vet. Clin. North Am. [Small Anim. Pract.] 14:317, 1984.

Campbell, T. W., and Dein, F. J.: Avian hematology, the basics. Vet. Clin. North Am. [Small Anim. Pract.] 14:223, 1984.

Clark, G. (ed.): *Staining Procedures.* Baltimore: The Williams & Wilkins Company, 1981.

Lillie, R. D. (ed.): *H. J. Conn's Biological Stains.* Baltimore: The Williams & Wilkins Company, 1977.

Perman, V., Alsaker, R. D., and Riis, R. C.: *Cytology of the Dog and Cat.* South Bend, IN: American Animal Hospital Association, 1979.

Rebar, A. H.: *Handbook of Veterinary Cytology.* St. Louis, MO: Ralston Purina Company, 1978.

Rebar, A. H., and Boon, G. D.: Diagnostic cytology in small animal practice. Proc. Am. Anim. Hosp. Assoc. 1980, p. 131.

Vuillaume, A.: A new technique for taking blood samples from ducks and geese. Avian Pathol. 12:389, 1983.

INTERPRETATION OF SEROLOGIC TEST RESULTS FOR CHLAMYDIOSIS

JAMES E. GRIMES, PH.D.

College Station, Texas

The diagnosis of *Chlamydia psittaci* infection in avian species depends upon isolation of the agent or serologic testing. Isolation of chlamydia is more costly and requires considerable time; and because the organism is intermittently shed in feces, the results of isolation attempts may be misleading. Therefore, serologic testing can be of value because it can be done more rapidly. However, interpretation of the results may require careful evaluation of the disease signs, duration of the illness, and the development of antibody during an infection.

Because of the importation of psittacine birds for the pet trade during the past several years, the need for diagnosing or ruling out chlamydiosis has become an important consideration. From 1978 to 1984, 3,485 single sera have been tested by direct complement fixation in the author's laboratory with an antigen produced from cell culture–grown chlamydiae. The titers of these sera have been published (Grimes, 1985b). These titers ranged from 8 to over 256, and the vast majority were almost equally distributed between 8, 16, and 32. About 57 per cent were negative (values lower than 8) for antibody activity. Some paired serum samples and other sets of specimens, consisting of feces or cloacal swabs and serum, have been tested. Results of these tests will be used as a basis for interpreting serologic tests for chlamydiosis.

The signs of chlamydiosis may be any or all of the following: conjunctivitis with lacrimation, sinusitis with nasal discharge, dyspnea, anorexia, diarrhea, and emaciation. Because of the variability in the occurrence of signs, it may sometimes be necessary to rule out a chlamydial infection by laboratory tests. The forms of chlamydiosis in psittacines can vary from acute to chronic. The chronic form may be manifested as (1) a completely asymptomatic carrier; (2) a low-grade, chronic infection with intermittent periods of illness and remission; or (3) a continuously ill bird.

Test results in which there is no detectable antibody activity against chlamydial antigen may indicate that (1) the bird has not had any previous experience with chlamydia; (2) the illness is chlamydiosis in the acute stage and there has been insufficient time for antibody production to reach a detectable level; or (3) the bird is anergic and thus will not respond to antigenic stimulus by producing immunoglobulins. With such varied results, the veterinarian must make a clinical diagnosis based upon the disease signs present and treat the bird accordingly.

To confirm a clinical diagnosis, a second serum should be submitted about 3 weeks after the first to determine if there is a change in antibody titer. (Results in this laboratory indicate that the usual interval of 2 weeks apparently is not always sufficient to detect a significant—fourfold or greater—rise in chlamydial antibody titer in psittacine birds). Examples of significant rises in titer are shown in Table 1 (first five pairs).

Because an untreated bird might die before the second serum sample is taken, the veterinarian should initiate treatment. Remember, however, that correct antibiotic treatment, which diminishes the antigenic stimulation, may delay or completely suppress development of detectable antibody levels.

The alternative to serologic testing, culturing of feces for *Chlamydia*, has drawbacks related to cost, time, and lack of sensitivity. Isolation attempts should be considered, but culturing samples from birds recently treated with chlamydiastatic antibiotics should not be considered.

The results of tests done by the author on 147 sets of specimens (serum and feces or cloacal swabs) from individual birds are shown in Figure 1. These results indicate that there is a positive correlation between the isolation of *Chlamydia* and the height of the antibody titer. It is obvious that there is a broad "gray area" for those trying to confirm whether or not a bird is infected with *Chlamydia* on the basis of a single antibody titer. Birds that have no demonstrable antibody activity, or titers of 8, 16, 32, and possibly even 64 may pose some problem in the determination of a definitive diagnosis. Give careful consideration to the signs presented. The laboratory tests are only an aid to the final interpretation and diagnosis. Any bird, with or without detectable antibody, should be considered to be infected when there are classic signs of chlamydiosis. Even a relatively high titer, 64 or 128, could be residual from a very recent infection. We have found that antibody titers increase rapidly but decrease very slowly. Examples of titer decreases are shown in Table 1 (last five pairs), and the results of tests showing titer decreases in nine pairs of sera have been published (Grimes, 1984).

The possibility that stable titers are indicative of constant low-level or intermittent antigenic stimulation from a chronic infection should be considered. Isolation attempts should be made in order to explain the meaning of stable titers.

Although this is not correct in every instance, we have found a titer that is greater than or equal to 64 to be an indicator of probable current infection. Isolation attempts indicate that almost 30 per cent of birds with a titer of 64 are infected at the time such a measurement is taken (Fig. 1). However, it is not possible for the serologist to make the diagnosis; that must be done by the veterinarian, who can evaluate the history and the clinical signs and judge the meaning of a given titer. The author states on laboratory reports that a titer greater than or equal to 64 indicates that the bird is probably infected. A titer of 8, 16, or 32 is currently interpreted to mean that the bird is possibly infected, and a notation is made that submission of a second serum for detection of any titer change is indicated if signs of chlamydiosis are present. A titer lower than 8 is reported as negative. However, titers within this range are now footnoted to indicate that a second specimen should be submitted in 3 weeks if signs of chlamydial infection are present.

The test results on paired sera in Table 1 show increases or decreases in titer to be highly variable. This variation may depend on such things as (1) the ability of the individual bird to respond, (2) the titer of the first specimen, (3) the interval between

***Table 1.** Examples of Increase or Decrease in Chlamydial Antibody Titer by Direct Complement Fixation Tests on Paired Sera From Psittacine Birds*

Bird Tested	Titer of Serum *No. 1*	*No. 2*	Amount of Change	Approx. No. Days Between Sera
Double yellow-headed Amazon	< 8*	64†	≥ 16-fold	41
Yellow-naped Amazon	< 8	≥ 256	≥ 32-fold	32
Blue-fronted Amazon	8	64‡	8-fold	43
Blue-fronted Amazon	16	≥ 256	≥ 16-fold	41
Double yellow-headed Amazon	64	≥ 256§	≥ 4-fold	25
Cockatoo	64	16	4-fold	32
Green-winged macaw	64	16	4-fold	281
Scarlet macaw	256	64	4-fold	86
Yellow-naped Amazon	≥256	32	≥ 8-fold	51
Double yellow-headed Amazon	≥256	64	≥ 4-fold	69

*A cloacal swab submitted with the serum was culture-negative for chlamydiae.
†A cloacal swab submitted with the serum was culture-positive for chlamydiae.
‡A third serum submitted 61 days after the second had a titer of 128.
§A third serum submitted 165 days after the second had a titer of 32.

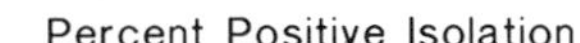

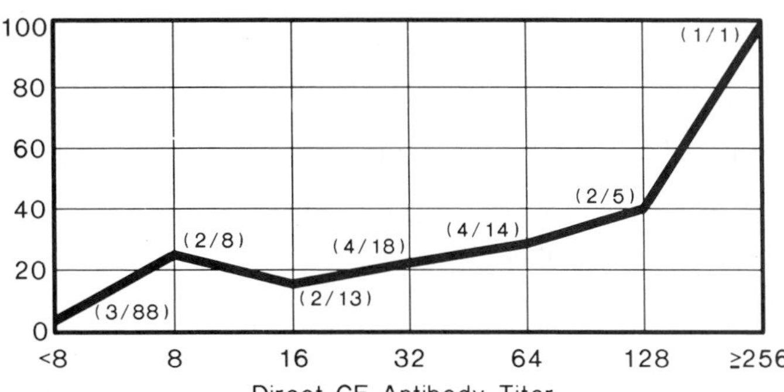

Figure 1. Correlation of serologic titer and attempts at isolation of *Chlamydia*.

collection of the two sera, (4) the severity of the infection, and (5) any treatment with chlortetracycline or other chlamydiastatic antibiotics. Other things that may influence the development of antibody are the "strain" of *C. psittaci*, its pathogenicity, and the species of bird; however, these aspects have perhaps not been studied sufficiently. There is no reliable, simple method to differentiate between isolates. In this laboratory, it has been shown that the infectivity for cell cultures of various isolates of avian *C. psittaci* is highly variable (Winsor and Grimes, unpublished data). It is not known, however, if this characteristic has any effect on pathogenicity for the bird or the elicitation of antibody.

We have determined that the larger psittacine birds, macaws, cockatoos, Amazon parrots, and African gray parrots can be tested by direct complement fixation. Many smaller birds (e.g., cockatiels) also respond to produce complement-fixing antibodies. However, results of direct complement fixation tests on sera from some smaller species, especially lovebirds, budgerigars, and young African grays, apparently are not reliable.

In conclusion, the final interpretation of serologic tests for chlamydial antibody activity must be done by the veterinary clinician after consideration of the history and the signs of disease. The interpretation of chlamydial antibody titers is not always clear-cut. Tests may need to be done on additional specimens, particularly on properly spaced sets of serum and feces.

References and Supplemental Reading

Grimes, J. E.: Direct complement fixation and isolation attempts for detecting *Chlamydia psittaci* infection of psittacine birds. Avian Dis. 29:873, 1985.

Grimes, J. E.: Enigmatic psittacine chlamydiosis: Results of serologic testing and isolation attempts, 1978–1983, and considerations for the future. J.A.V.M.A. 186:1075, 1985b.

Grimes, J. E.: Serological and microbiological detection of *Chlamydia psittaci* infections in psittacine birds. Avian/Exotic Pract. 1:6, 1984.

Grimes, J. E., and Panigrahy, B.: Potential increase of chlamydiosis (psittacosis) in pet bird owners in Texas. Tex. Med. 74:74, 1978.

McDonald, S. E., and Bayer, E. V.: Psittacosis in pet birds. Calif. Vet. 35:6, 1981.

Mohan, R.: Epidemiologic and laboratory observations of *Chlamydia psittaci* infection in pet birds. J.A.V.M.A. 184:1372, 1984.

AN UPDATE ON ANTIBIOTIC THERAPY IN BIRDS

MICHAEL R. LOOMIS, D.V.M.
Asheboro, North Carolina

Rational antibiotic therapy in birds is in its infancy. However, the same sound medical expertise governing the use of antibiotics in any other field of medicine should also affect the use of antibiotics in birds. Antimicrobial therapy must be individualized on the basis of the clinical situation, microbiologic information, and pharmacologic considerations.

THE CLINICAL SITUATION

The clinical situation defines if, when, and how antibiotic therapy is delivered to birds. Not all moribund birds required antibiotic therapy. Every attempt should be made to document the presence of a disease that is treatable by antibiotics before such therapy is initiated.

Several laboratory and clinical techniques are available to identify avian disease conditions in which antibiotic therapy is appropriate. Culture and sensitivity testing lie at the heart of most of these techniques.

A complete blood count can reveal a bacterial infection. Birds respond to bacterial infections with a leukocytosis that is primarily a heterophilia. Follow-up counts of white blood cells can be used to monitor the efficacy of antibiotic treatment (Dein, 1982). Normal hematologic values are available for many species of birds.

Clinical judgment must be relied upon in many cases in which no tangible evidence exists for the presence of a bacterial pathogen. Response to treatment in some instances may be the only indication that a bacterial pathogen was present. This may be of academic significance if a therapeutic success was achieved; however, it should be kept in mind that antibiotic treatment of an untreatable disease (e.g., a virus) is an underlying cause of treatment failure (i.e., the bird dies).

The manner in which the bird is housed can dictate the treatment method. Although it may be relatively easy to treat an individually housed bird with a parenteral antibiotic several times a day, it may be logistically impossible to treat a flock with the same disease in this manner. It may be necessary to treat flocks by using antibiotics in water or in food. Neither of these methods is ideal. Adequate levels of chlortetracycline have been maintained in parrots by using pelletized food containing the antibiotic (Landgraf et al., 1981). Dosage regulation in food is generally more accurate than in water if the bird can be converted to a medicated food. A balance must be struck between the ideal treatment regimen and a regimen in which compliance can be met in order to reach the therapeutic goal.

The condition of the patient may define when treatment should begin. The practitioner may not wish to subjugate an extremely ill bird to the stress of a diagnostic work-up prior to the initiation of antibiotic therapy. In such a situation, supportive care, including fluid and oxygen therapy and treatment for hypothermia and shock, coupled with administration of a broad-spectrum antibiotic may be given before a diagnostic work-up is begun. Nebulization therapy can be considered. Therapeutic levels of tylosin have been reached in lungs and air sacs by means of nebulization (Locke and Bush, 1984). The continuation of antibiotic therapy should be contingent upon a diagnostic work-up.

MICROBIOLOGIC INFORMATION

Culture and sensitivity testing provide the bulk of the microbiologic information. Easily accessible portals for culture collection are the crop and cloaca for suspected gastrointestinal infections, the choana for suspected upper respiratory infections, and the cloaca for some suspected urogenital infections. The normal flora of these orifices can vary with the species and, to a certain extent, within a species; they must be considered when culture results are interpreted.

Other sources of culture include needle aspirates of the infraorbital sinus and of visible or palpable masses. Biopsies for culture, impression smears, and histopathologic tests can be taken by laparoscopy from liver, kidneys, spleen, lungs, and air sacs. Blood cultures can also be taken. The results of blood cultures are more reliable in larger birds, owing to the larger blood samples available for culture.

The Gram stain is an extremely useful technique in avian medicine. If the normal flora of an orifice is known, a Gram stain may indicate the presence of a potential pathogen before the results of a culture test are received. By monitoring the sensitivity of isolates over time, one can begin to see patterns. These patterns, coupled with Gram staining results, can lead to an educated guess of the pathogen and an appropriate antibiotic to use prior to the receipt of culture results.

Once culture results are available, treatment should conform to culture and sensitivity findings.

It is important to monitor the response of the infective agent to the drug. Not doing so is a second cause of treatment failure. The emergence of resistant organisms or L-forms, or the existence of mixed infections may be detected by follow-up microbiologic evaluations.

PHARMACOLOGIC CONSIDERATIONS

Probably the most serious underlying cause of treatment failure is the use of an inadequate dosage regimen, which can result from the use of an inadequate dosage rate, an inadequate dosage interval, an inadequate duration of treatment, or any combination of these conditions. Dosage rates and intervals for use of several antibiotics (based on pharmacokinetics) in various species of birds are given in Table 1.

Due to the large number of species of birds kept in captivity and the proliferation of new antibiotics, there will never be a comprehensive formulary for

Table 1. Guidelines for Antibiotic Regimens in Birds

Antibiotic	Species	Route*	Dose Rate (mg/kg)	Dose Interval (hours)	Minimum Plasma Concentration Maintained (mg/ml)†	Half-Life (hours)	Reference
Pencillin G	Domestic turkey	IM	100 mg procaine and 100 mg benzathine	48	0.1	3	Hirsh et al., 1978
Ampicillin trihydrate	Pigeon	IM	25	8		1.28	Bush et al., 1979
	Emu	IM	15–20	12		1.67	Bush et al., 1979
	Gallinule	IM	25	8		1.0	Bush et al., 1979
	Hawks	IM	15	12		2.65	Bush et al., 1979
	Cranes	IM	15–20	12		1.55	Bush et al., 1979
Ampicillin	Amazon parrot	PO	150–200	8–12	1.3–5.8		Ensley and Janssen, 1981
	Amazon parrot	IM	100	4	0.65		Ensley and Janssen, 1981
	Pigeon	IM	150	2	2	0.45	Dorrestein et al., 1984
	Pigeon	PO	150	6	2	1.04	Dorrestein et al., 1984
Amoxycillin	Pigeon	IM	150	4	2	0.57	Dorrestein et al., 1984
	Pigeon	PO	150	6	2	1.07	Dorrestein et al., 1984
Cephalothin	Eastern bobwhite quail	IM	100	6	Less than 2	0.3	Bush et al., 1981
	Pigeon	IM	100	6	Less than 2	0.7	Bush et al., 1981
	Rosy-billed duck	IM	100	6	Less than 2	0.6	Bush et al., 1981
	Sandhill crane	IM	100	6	Less than 2	0.9	Bush et al., 1981
	Emu	IM	100	6	Less than 2	0.9	Bush et al., 1981
Cephalexin	Eastern bobwhite quail	PO	35	6	Less than 2	1.5	Bush et al., 1981
	Pigeon	PO	50	6	5	1.0	Bush et al., 1981
	Rosy-billed duck	PO	25	6	Less than 2	0.6	Bush et al., 1981
	Sandhill crane	PO	25	6	Less than 2	0.9	Bush et al., 1981
	Emu	PO	35	6	3	2.1	Bush et al., 1981
Gentamicin	Greater sandhill crane	IM	5	8	3	2.73	Custer et al., 1979
	Ring-necked pheasant	IM	5	8	Less than 2	1.25	Custer et al., 1979
	Japanese quail	IM	10	6	Less than 2	0.7	Custer et al., 1979
	Domestic chicken (1 day old)‡	IV	0.2 mg		0.2 at 24 hours	4.4	Spreat and Bickford, 1977
	Domestic chicken (1 day old)‡	SC	0.2 mg		0.2 at 24 hours	4.4	Spreat and Bickford, 1977
Chloramphenicol	Domestic chicken	IM	50	12	1.2 ± 0.6	2.56	Clark et al., 1982
	Domestic turkey	IM	50	12	0.31 ± 0.2	1.86	Clark et al., 1982
	Ruddy shelduck	IM	50	12	0.2 ± 0.2	1.58	Clark et al., 1982
	Muscovy duck	IM	50	12	0.1 ± 0.0	1.31	Clark et al., 1982
	Egyptian goose	IM	50	12	0.3 ± 0.2	1.46	Clark et al., 1982
	Budgerigar	IM	50	12	0.7 ± 0.4	2.09	Clark et al., 1982
	Red-shouldered hawk	IM	50	12	1.6 ± 0.7	2.35	Clark et al., 1982
	Golden eagle	IM	50	12	2.7 ± 1.2	2.67	Clark et al., 1982
	Red-tailed hawk	IM	50	12	0.7 ± 0.2	2.68	Clark et al., 1982
	Cooper's hawk	IM	50	12	3.0 ± 0.9	3.03	Clark et al., 1982
	Broad-tailed hawk	IM	50	12	1.2 ± 0.2	2.02	Clark et al., 1982
	Barred owl	IM	50	12	1.2 ± 0.2	1.97	Clark et al., 1982
	Macaw	IM	50	6	1.0 ± 1.1	0.66	Clark et al., 1982
	Sun conure	IM	50	6			Clark et al., 1982
	Nanday conure	IM	50	6			Clark et al., 1982
	Bald eagle	IM	50	24	1.5	4.80	Clark et al., 1982
	Peafowl	IM	50	24	1.5	4.72	Dein et al., 1979
	Spot-billed duck	IV or IM	22	3	5		Dein et al., 1979
	Spot-billed duck	IV or IM	92	6	5		Dein et al., 1979
	Spot-billed duck	IV or IM	213	8	5		Dein et al., 1979

Table continued on opposite page

Table 1. Guidelines for Antibiotic Regimens in Birds Continued

Antibiotic	Species	Route*	Dose Rate (mg/kg)	Dose Interval (hours)	Minimum Plasma Concentration Maintained (mg/ml)†	Half-Life (hours)	Reference
Oxytetracycline (long-acting)	Ring-necked pheasant	IV	45	8	5	2.5	Teare, in press
	Ring-necked pheasant	IM	60	24	5	14.9	Teare, in press
	Great horned owl	IM	20	24	5	26.4	Teare, in press
	Amazon parrot	IM	80	24	5	16.0	Teare, in press
Chlortetracycline	Pigeon	PO	95	6	1	2.25	Dorrestein et al., 1984
	Pigeon	PO	190	8	1	2.25	Dorrestein et al., 1984
Chlortetracycline (fed with grit)	Pigeon	PO	30	6	1	5.0	Dorrestein et al., 1984
	Pigeon	PO	95	12	1	5.0	Dorrestein et al., 1984
Doxycycline	Pigeon	IM	10	6	1	4.43	Dorrestein et al., 1984
	Pigeon	PO	7.5	6	1	5.12	Dorrestein et al., 1984
	Pigeon	PO	25	12	1	5.12	Dorrestein et al., 1984
	Pigeon	PO	150	24	1	5.12	Dorrestein et al., 1984
Doxycycline (fed with grit)	Pigeon	PO	3	6	1	9.81	Dorrestein et al., 1984
	Pigeon	PO	7.5	12	1	9.81	Dorrestein et al., 1984
	Pigeon	PO	25	24	1	9.81	Dorrestein et al., 1984
Tylosin	Bobwhite quail	IM	25	6	1	1.2	Locke et al., 1982
	Pigeon	IM	25	6	1	1.2	Locke et al., 1982
	Greater sandhill crane	IM	15	8	1	1.2	Locke et al., 1982
	Emu	IM	25	8	1	4.7	Locke et al., 1982
Trimethoprim	Pigeon	PO	10	6	1	3.2	Dorrestein et al., 1984
Trimethoprim/sulfatroxazole	Pigeon	PO	10/50	12	0.25/1		Dorrestein et al., 1984
Trimethoprim/sulfamethoxazole	Pigeon	PO	10/50	12	0.02/9		Dorrestein et al., 1984
Flumequine	Pigeon	IM	30	8	1	1.69	Dorrestein et al., 1984
	Pigeon	PO	25–30	8–12	1	1.57	Dorrestein et al., 1984

*Key: IM = intramuscular; IV = intravenous; PO = oral; SC = subcutaneous.
†Some of these determinations were made on a single injection of the antibiotic. With multiple doses, levels may be higher.
‡Values are for a total single dose of 0.2 mg per chick.

birds based on pharmacokinetics. Table 1 can be used only as a broad guideline to determining the appropriate dosage regimen for birds. One must use a table such as this with the understanding that there will be treatment failures.

Ideally, the minimum inhibitory concentration (MIC) of an antibiotic for a given organism should be known in order to formulate a dosage regimen. Plasma concentrations of the antibiotic also should be followed during the course of the treatment to ensure that the MIC is met and toxic concentrations of the antibiotic are not achieved. These procedures are impractical in most veterinary clinics.

Although plasma concentrations of an antibiotic are an indication of effective treatment dosages, the concentration of the antibiotic at the target tissue should also be considered. For example, tylosin levels can be higher in kidneys, liver, and lungs than they are in plasma (Locke et al., 1982).

Over-reliance on antibiotics is a third underlying cause of treatment failure. It may be necessary to use antibiotic therapy in conjunction with other treatment methods. Since bird pus inspissates, it may not be possible to resolve an abscess with antibiotics alone because of the difficulty of achieving appropriate antibiotic levels at the site of infection. Surgical removal of the inspissated pus in addition to antibiotic treatment may lead to a more acceptable treatment outcome. One should also be on the lookout for underlying metabolic, neoplastic, toxic, parasitic, or viral diseases that may be the primary insult leading to a secondary bacterial infection.

It should be kept in mind that a patient cannot be rendered bacteriologically sterile with antibiotics; therefore, the host immune mechanism must be operative to cure an infection.

Finally, one should strive to minimize the appearance of resistant organisms. This may be done by using suitable dosage regimens, beginning treatment early, continuing treatment long enough to eradicate the pathogens, avoiding the use of antibiotics for minor infections, and as mentioned earlier, monitoring the progress of treatment with microbiologic methods.

References and Suggested Readings

Bush, M., Locke, D., Neal, L. A., et al.: Pharmacokinetics of cephalothin and cephalexin in selected avian species. Am. J. Vet. Res. 42:1014, 1981.

Bush, M., Locke, D., Neal, L. A., et al.: Gentamicin tissue concentrations in various avian species following recommended dosage therapy. Am. J. Vet. Res. 42:2114, 1981.

Bush, M., Neal, L. A., and Custer, R. S.: Preliminary pharmacokinetic studies of selected antibiotics in birds. Proc. Am. Assoc. Zoo Vet. 1979, pp. 45–47.

Clark, C. H., Thomas, J. E., Milton, J. L., et al.: Plasma concentrations of chloramphenicol in birds. Am. J. Vet. Res. 43:1249, 1982.

Clubb, S. L.: Therapeutics in avian medicine. Vet. Clin. North Am. [Small Anim. Pract.] 14:345, 1984.

Custer, R. S., Bush, M., and Carpenter, J. W.: Pharmacokinetics of gentamicin in blood plasma of quail, pheasants, and cranes. Am. J. Vet. Res. 40:892, 1979.

Dein, F. J., Monard, D. F., and Koalczyk, D. F.: Pharmacokinetics of chloramphenicol in Chinese spot-billed ducks. Proc. Am. Assoc. Zoo Vet. 1979, pp. 48–50.

Dein, F. J.: Avian clinical hematology. Ann. Proc. Assoc. Avian Vet. 1982, pp. 5–29.

Dorrestein, G. M., van Gogh, H., Rinzema, J. D., et al.: A preliminary report of pharmacokinetics and pharmacotherapy in racing pigeons. Ann. Proc. Assoc. Avian Vet. 1984, pp. 9–23.

Ensley, P. K., and Janssen, D. L.: A preliminary study comparing the pharmacokinetics of ampicillin given orally and intramuscularly to psittacines: Amazon parrots and blue-naped parrots. J. Zoo Anim. Med. 12:42, 1981.

Fudge, A. M.: Avian antimicrobial therapy. Ann. Proc. Assoc. Avian Vet. 1983, pp. 162–183.

Hirsh, D. C., Knox, S. J., Conzelman, G. M., et al.: Pharmacokinetics of penicillin G in the turkey. Am. J. Vet. Res. 39:1219, 1978.

Kollias, G. V.: Use of antibiotics in birds: A review with clinical emphasis. Ann. Proc. Am. Anim. Hosp. Assoc. 1982, pp. 9–12.

Landgraf, W. W., Ross, P. F., Cassidy, D. R., et al.: Concentration of chlortetracycline in the blood of yellow-crowned Amazon parrots fed medicated pelleted feeds. Avian Dis. 21:14, 1981.

Locke, D., Bush, M., and Carpenter, J. W.: Pharmacokinetics and tissue concentrations of tylosin in selected avian species. Am. J. Vet. Res. 43:1807, 1982.

Locke, D., and Bush, M.: Tylosin aerosol therapy in quail and pigeons. J. Zoo Anim. Med. 15:62, 1984.

Spreat, S. R., and Bickford, S. M.: Pharmacodynamics of gentamicin in day-old chicks. W. Poult. Dis. Conf. 26:101, 1977.

Teare, J. A.: Pharmacokinetics of a long-acting oxytetracycline preparation in three species of birds. Am. J. Vet. Res., in press.

PLANT POISONING IN PET BIRDS AND REPTILES

MURRAY E. FOWLER, D.V.M.
Davis, California

Veterinarians are frequently consulted by clients about suspected ingestion of ornamental plants by household pets. Numerous lists are circulated that list plants that are purportedly dangerous. Many of these lists have been copied from other lists and perpetuate misinformation. One should not assume that birds or reptiles are susceptible to the same plants as humans or any other mammal. Many lists continue to include plants that are known to produce only allergic dermatitis or rhinitis in humans. It is totally inappropriate to consider such plants as hazardous to birds or reptiles.

There is little question that birds and reptiles are susceptible to plant poisoning. However, veterinarians should understand the interactions between toxic substances found in plants and the animals that consume them. Additionally, the marked differences in the anatomy and physiology of birds and reptiles, as contrasted with mammals, make it unwise to extrapolate information about poisoning from mammals to other classes or vice versa.

WHY POISONOUS PLANTS?

Herbivorous animals (insects, fish, amphibians, reptiles, birds, and mammals) coevolved with the plants in their native environments (Fowler, 1983). Successful plants developed methods to prevent total predation. These included harsh outer coats, thorns, spines, and chemical compounds (secondary plant compounds, SPC) that make the plant unpalatable or lethal to a predator. During the evolutionary process animals countered by avoiding the plant; by minimizing the risk through eating a small amount of each of many different plants, thus diluting potentially poisonous substances; by developing chemical or microbial means of degrading poisonous substances in the gastrointestinal tract; and, finally, by developing general and specific detoxification mechanisms (Fowler, 1983).

A seesaw of the development of more potent toxic agents by the plant and better detoxification methods by the animal kept a balance. Death caused by poisonous plants was rare. Many of the protective behaviors were learned by animals from parents, siblings, or social interactions. Specific detoxification methods were genetically controlled and had to be periodically primed by exposure to low levels of the toxic agent. Over 8600 species of birds and 4000 species of reptiles have evolved in habitats with hundreds of thousands of species of plants. It is ridiculous to assume that all species are equally susceptible to every poisonous plant.

Mankind has not only moved animals to new environments, exposing them to plants for which they may not have developed protective mechanisms against SPCs, but plants have been moved all over the world by the ornamental horticulture trade. Finally, animals have been provided with feeds that were not included in their pristine diets. Birds and reptiles raised in captivity have not been afforded the opportunity to learn avoidance or dilution behaviors, nor have any species been able to keep degrading or detoxification mechanisms primed and ready to deal with SPC ingestion.

It has been estimated that over 40 per cent of plants contain secondary SPCs that may be a deterrent or actually poisonous to herbivorous animals (Fowler, 1983). Considering the hundreds of thousands of plant species world wide, it is not possible to make a complete list of plants that are (or are not) poisonous for any species of bird or reptile.

UNIQUE BIOLOGY OF BIRDS AND REPTILES

There are marked differences between mammalian species in their response to ingestion of poisonous plants. Although it has not been proved, there is ample reason to assume that birds have those same species differences. There are also wide differences between mammals and birds. One basic difference is in the anatomy and function of the kidney. Glomerular filtration is less important and tubular filtration is more important in birds than in mammals. Both birds and reptiles possess a renal portal circulation (RPC), but in birds it is only partially functional (Feldman and Kruckenberg, 1975).

The significance of an RPC is that blood from the caudal areas of the body, including a section of the mesenteric circulation, may pass through the kidney before returning to the heart. In birds, the RPC may be functional or not, depending on the physiologic state of the bird and a variety of unknown factors. Apparently, a sphincter on the vein can either direct blood into the kidney or divert it directly to the liver in the hepatic portal system. Blood from the RPC is not carried to the glomeruli but bathes the renal tubules. Any toxin that could be excreted by the kidney tubule would be removed before it reaches the systemic circulation. Conversely, nephrotoxic substances may thus reach the kidneys in higher concentration and cause more severe damage. The facts are that little is known about the function of detoxification mechanisms in birds and reptiles.

Many species of birds are migratory and others move to new habitats when food becomes scarce. Migratory birds may have had a broader evolutionary exposure to secondary plant compounds. This does not mean, however, that captive migratory birds of the same species are capable of dealing with such SPCs. The microsomal enzyme systems for detoxification may be genetically programmed, but unless the systems have been primed and periodically stimulated with small doses, the systems may not be able to mount a protective response.

Some, but not necessarily all, birds and reptiles are capable of emesis. Emesis may be induced by action directly on the central nervous system. Cardioactive glycosides and apomorphine act in this manner. Other toxins (rhododendrons, veratrums) cause emesis by local irritation of the epithelium of the pharynx, esophagus, or stomach. Any plant that causes emesis in a bird or reptile capable of it is less likely to cause poisoning in that species.

Such interactions have interesting and profound ecologic implications. The monarch butterfly and its caterpillar are rarely preyed upon by birds. The deduction of the reason for this was one of the first examples of the importance of SPCs in the ecologic scheme. Monarch caterpillars feed exclusively on milkweeds, species of *Asclepias*. Other caterpillars are killed by the cardioactive glycosides found in this plant. The monarch larvae actually sequester the glycoside, which passes through the chrysalis stage on into the mature butterfly (Fowler, 1983).

If a bird is unwise enough to gulp down a monarch, the glycoside will cause emesis in the bird. Any experienced bird will avoid both the green and yellow caterpillar and the red and brown butterfly. To go one step further, other species of moths and butterflies have developed similar color patterns in order to mimic the monarch and profit from the avoidance pattern.

PLANT IDENTITY

There are three questions for which it is always difficult to obtain factual answers when a client calls or arrives at the clinic on an emergency: (1) Did the bird or lizard actually eat the plant? (2) How much did the pet consume? and (3) What is the identity of the plant?

Ornamental plant identification is not easy. Clients may have their own common names for plants, which makes it difficult to look up the proper name. It is surprising how many people do not know the names of plants they have purchased to decorate their home. No busy practitioner can know all the native and introduced ornamental plants, but the client may be requested to quickly take a suspected plant to a nursery for identification. Ask for a scientific name, because the use of common names is hopeless. Other sources of help in plant identification include the curator of a local college herbarium, landscape horticulturists and architects, botanical museum curators, and garden clubs. Agricultural plants may be identified by agricultural commissioners, county and state agricultural agents, or botanists in the state department of agriculture. Native wild plants can be identified by many nature buffs or through some of the previously mentioned resources (Crockett, 1971–1975; Graff, 1980; *Sunset Western Garden Book*, 1968).

The more difficult problem is the identification of plant segments removed from the crop or stomach of the animal by aspiration or vomiting, or at necropsy. Seeds are valuable, because they are commonly used to identify plants taxonomically. Thus there are keys available and individuals with the skills necessary to make the identification. Leaf segments are another matter. Pharmacognosy (the science of plant use in pharmacology) provides detailed microscopic identification of plants used in the pharmaceutical industry. This is not a readily available source, and many plants are not included in the list of those so identified.

A few plants have structures such as unique patterns of leaf veins that will allow quick identification. More commonly it is necessary to collect as much of the plant material as possible and take it or send it to a professional botanist. Even then it may be extremely difficult to make a precise identification. Leaf structure is rarely used in taxonomic keys. Herbariums are the most fruitful resource because they at least have preserved specimens for comparison. Small particles of plant or seed material should be placed in a vial of 50 per cent isopropyl alcohol to prevent destructive drying or decomposition. Larger plant segments should be refrigerated if material can arrive at the identifier within a few days. Otherwise the material should be dried by pressing it flat between sheets of newspaper or a large magazine.

PLANT POISONING IN SPECIFIC ANIMALS

Birds

There are few documented cases of plant poisoning in caged birds (Table 1). Table 2 lists the plant species that have been reported as poisonous to gallinaceous birds (chickens, turkeys, quail, pheasants) and anseriforms (ducks, geese, and swans). Table 3 lists plants containing toxic agents similar to those that are known to affect birds.

Plant poisoning must be a rarity in birds. There is a National Animal Poison Control Center housed within the College of Veterinary Medicine at the University of Illinois. In the quarterly progress report for 1984 are listed all the calls received about plant poisoning during a three-month period. Over 270 calls were received for all species, including 24 for birds and none for reptiles. Three of those calls were for information only. Ten were simple exposures with no report of clinical signs. In six cases the toxicologists felt that there was no connection between the illness and the suspected plant toxicity. In only three cases was true toxicity suspected, and in only one case was a diagnosis of toxicity justified. Granted, not everyone knows that this fine facility is available for helping veterinarians and bird owners, but if these results are indicative of overall action, plant poisoning is of minimal concern with most household birds.

In the only documented experimental trial of plant poisoning in psittacine birds, the investigator conducted feeding trials and forced feeding experiments with five household plants—oleander (*Nerium oleander*), lily of the valley (*Convallaria majalis*), rhododendron (*Rhododendron indicum*), philodendron (*Philodrendron scandens*), and poinsettia (*Euphorbia pulcherrima*)—to budgerigars (*Melopsittacus undulatus*) (Hoffmann, 1980).

The author's conclusions were that none of these plants constitute a major hazard for the budgerigar. The rhododendron and philodendron were readily consumed, but large quantities (2 to 10 gm/kg) of force-fed material were required to produce clinical signs (Hoffmann, 1980).

Both oleander and lily of the valley contain digitalislike glycosides. In mammals, the lethal dose of oleander leaf is 100 mg/kg. In the budgie, 20 to 100 times more oleander was required to cause death. Since the resistance in the budgie seemed to be so high, the investigator conducted a trial with a purified glycoside, digoxin. The dose of digoxin necessary to induce mild clinical signs of toxicity

Table 1. *Reported Plant Poisoning in Caged Birds*

Scientific Name	Common Name	Species*	Clinical Signs	Pathologic Effects	Plant Parts Involved	Toxic agent	Reference
Aspergillus flavus	Mycotoxin (aflatoxin)	Budgerigar (C), red-headed parrot (C)	Peracute death	Acute catarrhal gastritis and enteritis, hepatic necrosis, renal necrosis	Moldy millet	Mycotoxin	Cuturić et al., 1964
Convallaria majalis	Lily of the valley	Budgerigar (E)	Weakness, apathy, diarrhea, emesis		Leaves	Cardioactive glycoside	Hoffmann, 1980
Daubentonia punicea, Sesbania punicea	Purple sesbane, purple rattlebox	Pigeons (C and E)	Vomiting; green, watery droppings; weakness; emaciation (12 seeds sufficient for effect)	Green staining of gizzard, duodenitis, splenomegaly, and nephromegaly; histonecrotic enteritis, cloudy swelling of hepatocytes	Seeds		Emmel, 1943
Euphorbia pulcherrima	Poinsettia	Budgerigar (E)	Minimal signs; small quantities of red-colored feces (from red bracts); some diarrhea		Bracts, red leaves	Resin	Hoffmann, 1980; Petrak, 1982
Lantana camara	Lantana	Unknown	Weakness, diarrhea	Gastroenteritis, hepatic necrosis	Green fruits	Hepatotoxin	Petrak, 1982
Nerium oleander	Oleander	Budgerigar (E)	Apathy, diarrhea, weakness, tetanic spasm, salivation, emesis, ataxia, death	Gastritis, enteritis, hemorrhage in subcutis, heart fully filled with blood	Leaves	Cardioactive glycoside	Hoffmann, 1980
Philodendrom scandens	Philodendron	Budgerigar (E)	Severe choking, emesis of mucus and plant material, diarrhea	Hyperemia of mucous membranes of crop, stomach, and intestine; mucus in ingesta, pasty vent	Leaves	Proteins cause histamine reaction	Hoffmann, 1980; Petrak, 1982
Rhododendron simsii (indicum)	Rhododendron	Budgerigar (E)	Weakness, apathy, choking, emesis, pasty vent		Leaves	Andromedotoxin	Hoffmann, 1980
Solanum pseudocapsicum	Jerusalem cherry	Unknown	Diarrhea	Gastroenteritis	Fruits	Solanine-alkaloidal glycoside	Petrak, 1982
Taxus baccata	Yew	Pheasants (C)	Death; no other signs	Gastritis, duodenitis, hyperemia of liver	Needles	Alkaloid-taxine	Petrak, 1982

*Key: C = clinical report; E = experimental report.

Table 2. *List of Plants with Documented Clinical or Experimental Poisoning in Poultry and Waterfowl*

Scientific Name	Common Name	Affected Birds
Abrus precatorius	Precatory bean	Fowl
Acacia decurrens	Wattle	Poultry
Aesculus glabra	Ohio buckeye	Chick
Agrostemma githago	Corncockle	Chicken
Ammi majus	Bishops weed	Chicken, turkey, goose
Arctium minus	Burdock	Pheasant
Argemone mexicana	Mexican poppy	Chicken
Asclepias spp.	Milkweed, cotton bush	Chicken
Astragalus emoryanus	Locoweed, milk vetch	Chicken
Brassica rapa	Rape	Chicken
Cassia occidentalis	Coffee senna	Chicken
Cestrum diurnum	Jasmine, jessamine	Chicken
Claviceps purpurea	Ergot	Chicken, goose
Conium maculatum	Poison hemlock	Chicken
Coriandrum sativum	Coriander	Chicken
Crotalaria goreensis	Rattlebox, Crotalaria	Chicken
C. retusa		Chicken
C. spectabilis		
Cymopterus watsonii	Parsley	Duckling
C. longipes		
Datura stramonium	Jimson weed, thornapple	Chick
Gelsemium semperivirens	Yellow jasmine	Chick, poult
Glottidium vesicarium	Glottidium	Chicken
Gypsophila vaccaria		Poultry
Heliotropium spp.	Heliotrope	Chicken
Klanchoe spp.	Felt plant, maternity plant, air plant, panda plant	Chick, duck
Karwinskia humboldtiana	Coyotillo	Chicken
Lathyrus spp.	Sweet pea	Poultry
Lupinus albus	Lupine	Chicken
Melia azedarach	White cedar, China berry	Chicken
Microcystis aeruginosa	Blue-green algae	Poultry, waterfowl
Nerium oleander	Oleander	Chicken, goose
Nicotiana tobacum	Tobacco	Chicken
Phaseolus vulgaris	Navy bean	Quail
Phytolacca americana	Pokeweed	Turkey
Quercus incana	Oak	Poultry
Ricinus communis	Castor bean	Duck
Robinia pseudoacacia	Black locust	Chicken
Sesbania drumundii	Coffee bean, rattlebush rattlebox, coffeeweed	Poultry, chicken
Solanum malocoxylon	Nightshade	Chick
Solanum spp.	Nightshade	Chicken, duck
Sterculia foetida	Australian flame tree, flame tree	Chick
Theobroma cacao	Cacao	Chicken
Trichodesma incanum	Camel bush	Fowl
Trisetum flavescens	Grass	Chick
Vicia spp.	Hairy and Common vetch	Chick
Xanthium spp.	Cocklebur	Chicken
Zygadenus spp.	Death camus	Chicken

was 2.2 mg/kg. In humans, the digitalization dose of digoxin is approximately 0.017 mg/kg (Hoffmann, 1980).

Unfortunately, at the conclusion of this important piece of work the author perpetuated folly by listing a lot of plants causing poisoning in humans and domestic animals.

In every list of potential poisonous plants for birds, authors have perpetuated the idea that numerous *Prunus* species (apricot, almond, peach, nectarine, cherry, choke cherry, and laurels) and many other species containing cyanogenic glycosides are a hazard to birds. The facts are that cyanide poisoning by ingestion of plants containing cyanogenic glycosides has not been documented in poultry, waterfowl, or pet birds, though it is true that birds are susceptible to the cyanide ion if it is freed from the glycoside moiety. Cyanide poisoning is rare in other animals with simple stomachs, such as swine and horses. Perhaps the enzymatic degradation of the glycoside to free cyanide ion is more rapid in the ruminant or detoxification mechanisms are more effective in simple-stomached animals.

Many ornamental plants produce brightly colored berries and fruits, and birds are attracted to them. Both in the free-living state and in captivity, birds utilize berries and fruits extensively for food. Birds also play a vital part in the dispersal of plants by transporting seeds that traverse the digestive tract to other locations in the environment. Some seeds

Table 3. *Additional Plants That Should be Considered Potentially Poisonous to Birds**

Cardioactive glycosides	
Thevitia peruviana	Yellow oleander
Digitalis purpurea	Purple foxglove
Araceae Plants Producing Stomatitis (Philodendrons)	
Alocasia antiquorum	Elephant ear, alocasia
Caladium spp.	Caladium
Calla palustris	Wild calla, water arum
Dieffenbachia spp.	Dumbcane
Epiprenum (Scindapsus) spp.	Malanga, elephant ear, devil's ivy, variegated philodendron
Monstera spp.	Cut-leaf philodendron, Mexican breadfruit, mother-in-law plant, Swiss-cheese plant
Philodendron spp.	Philodendrons
Symplocarpus foetidus	Skunk cabbage
Xanthosoma spp.	Malanga
Zantedeschia aethiopica	Calla lily, arum lily
Ericaceae (Heaths) Containing Andromedotoxin (Rhododendrons)	
Kalmia spp.	Mountain laurel
Leucothoe spp.	Black laurel, Leucothoe
Pieres spp.	Andromeda
Rhododendron spp.	Azaleas, rhododendrons

*Based on the plant's content of toxic agents known to be poisonous to caged birds, poultry, or waterfowl.

actually require a pregermination sojourn through a digestive tract.

Berries have frequently been implicated as a source of poisoning. Some berries are indeed dangerous, especially in the immature or unripe stage. A common shrub often thought to be poisonous is the pyracantha or firethorn (*Pyracantha* sp.). The berries are not poisonous intrinsically. However, they may be a hazard, since the mature fruits will start to macerate and ferment. Because the berries are high in carbohydrates, the fermentation process yields alcohol. Migratory fruit-eating birds, such as the cedar waxwing (*Bombycilla cedrorum),* are frequently seen exhibiting the same type of neural signs shown by inebriated humans. And just as in humans, trauma may bring about demise or injury from flying into plate-glass windows, doors, or other similar objects.

Plants containing pyrrolizidine alkaloids are a significant hazard to mammals, but no poisonings have been reported in caged birds. In one experimental trial with quail, the author concluded that quail were highly resistant to the oral effects of pyrrolizidine alkaloids (Buckmaster et al., 1977). Species of *Crotalaria* contain these alkaloids, and poisoning in chickens (although not the classic hepatocytomegaly) has been reported.

Mushrooms and toadstools are also listed as dangerous for birds, yet no cases have been reported to justify inclusion of fungi (except ergot) as hazards for birds. A potential poison-plant hazard is mycotoxicosis associated with the ingestion of poorly stored seeds and grains. Aflatoxicosis has been documented in galliforms (turkeys and chickens), anseriforms (ducks and geese), and budgerigars.

Reptiles

Only one documented case of plant poisoning in reptiles has been reported (Holt et al., 1979), and that is circumstantial, based on a stomach filled with the flowers of buttercups (*Ranunculus* sp.). Either plant poisoning is rare or is not being recognized as a cause of disease in herbivorous reptiles.

A mimeographed publication has been circulated by a group of dedicated turtle and tortoise conservationists, TEAM (Turtle and Tortoise Education Adoption Media). A series of line drawings of approximately 80 species of poisonous plants was published over a two-year period. This anonymous author is to be congratulated for making an effort to educate owners of chelonian of the hazards of poisonous plants. Unfortunately, the material was taken directly from publications on human plant poisoning. The clinical signs described are those of human poisoning and may have no relevance to poisoning in the turtle or tortoise.

CONCLUSIONS

Plants may contain no toxic chemicals but still be toxic as a result of spraying with pesticides or fertilizers that may be hazardous to a herbivorous pet. Herbicides containing arsenic are frequently applied to lawns for weed control. Labels on these products specify the length of time that animals should be kept off the lawn. These directions must be closely followed to prevent unnecessary exposure.

Herbivorous and omnivorous birds and reptiles may ingest plants as a normal consequence of feeding. Carnivorous species may consume plant material through ingestion of prey species. Birds and reptiles that would not ordinarily consume herbaceous material may do so as a result of boredom or lack of proper food.

The author is not so naive as to assume that only those plants listed are poisonous to birds and reptiles. However, to list plant after plant without justification is unwise.

If a bird or reptile becomes ill after ingestion of a plant, the clinician should use symptomatic and general nursing therapy since there are no antidotes for the vast majority of plant poisons. Rapid evacuation of the gastrointestinal tract by mineral oil is warranted. Activated charcoal is indicated as well.

Because of space considerations in this volume, a list of references on plant poisoning in poultry and waterfowl is not provided here. The author will supply it to interested readers.

References and Supplemental Reading

Buckmaster, G. W., Cheeke, P. R., Arscott, G. H., et al.: Response of Japanese quail to dietary and injected pyrrolizidine (*Senecio*) alkaloid. J. Anim. Sci. 45:1322, 1977.

Crockett, J. U.: *Time-Life Encyclopedia of Gardening.* (15 volumes on different types of ornamentals such as evergreens, trees, and vines.) Alexandria, VA: Time-Life Publications, 1971–1975.

Cuturić, S., Herceq, M., and Huber, I.: Aflatoxicosis in undulated parrots (budgerigars). Verh. Int. Symp. Erkrank. Zoo. 11:129, 1964.

Emmel, M. W.: *Daubentonia punicea* poisoning in pigeons. J.A.V.M.A. 102:294, 1943.

Feldman, B. F., and Kruckenberg, S. M.: Clinical toxicities of domestic and wild caged birds. Vet. Clin. North Am. 5:653, 1975.

Fowler, M. E.: Toxicities in exotic and zoo animals. Vet. Clin. North Am. 5:685, 1975.

Fowler, M. E.: *Plant Poisoning in Small Companion Animals.* St. Louis: Ralston Purina, 1981.

Fowler, M. E.: Plant poisoning in free-living wild animals: A review. J. Wildl. Dis. 19:34, 1983.

Graff, A. B.: *Exotica Series* 3, 10th ed. E. Rutherford, NJ: Roehrs, 1980.

Hoffmann, H.: Die Wirkung toxischer pflanzeninholtsstoffe auf den Wellensittich im appetenzversuch und nach Zwangsverabreichung. Ein Beitrag zur Gefahrdung von Stubenvogeln durch Zierpflanzen. (The effect of toxic plant constituents on the budgerigar in appetite experiments and after forced feedings. Contribution on the risk to cage bird from ornamental plants.) Inaugural Dissertation, Tierarztliche Hochschule, Hannover, 1980.

Holt, P. E., Cooper, J. E., and Needham, J. R.: Diseases of tortoises: A review of seventy cases. J. Small Anim. Pract. 20:269, 1979.

Jordan, W. J.: Yew (*Taxus baccata*) poisoning in pheasants (*Phasianus colchicus*). Tijdschr. Diergeneeskd. 89(Suppl.1):187, 1964.

Oehme, F. W., and Davis, J. W.: Plants poisonous to free-living or caged mammals and birds. *In* Hoff, G. L., and Davis, J. W. (eds.): *Noninfectious Diseases of Wildlife.* Ames, IA: Iowa State University Press, 1982, pp. 8–23.

Petrak, M. L.: Poisoning and other casualties. *In* Petrak, M. L. (ed.): *Diseases of Cage and Aviary Birds,* 2nd ed. Philadelphia: Lea & Febiger, 1982, p. 646.

Sunset Western Garden Book. Menlo Park, CA: Lane Magazine and Book, 1968.

THE USE OF IVERMECTIN IN BIRDS, REPTILES, AND SMALL MAMMALS

JAMES G. SIKARSKIE, D.V.M.
East Lansing, Michigan

The avermectins are a group of antiparasitic drugs produced by the actinomycete *Streptomyces avermitilis.* They have broad-spectrum efficacy against a variety of nematode and arthropod parasites. Ivermectin is presently marketed in the United States in injectable form for cattle (Ivomec, Merck & Co.) and as an oral paste for horses (Eqvalan, Merck & Co.; Zimectrin, Farnum).

Although not completely understood, at least part of the mechanism of action is stimulation of the inhibitory neurotransmitter γ-aminobutyric acid (GABA) from presynaptic nerve terminals and the potentiation of GABA binding at postsynaptic receptors. The susceptible parasite becomes paralyzed and is dislodged or dies. A variety of nematodes, insects, and arachnids are susceptible to this method of action, but cestodes and trematodes are not affected because they do not use GABA in neurotransmission.

Gamma-aminobutyric acid is not found in the mammalian peripheral nervous system but is present in the central nervous system. At routine dosages, ivermectin does not cross the blood-brain barrier and is considered safe for use in mammals. In theory there could be a risk when it is used in animals with disorders of the central nervous system. Presumably the drug works in a similar manner in birds and reptiles, although there seems to be more variation in dose among reptilian species than in birds and mammals. Fatal toxicity has been reported in dogs, usually collies and similar types; it is apparently caused by ivermectin's crossing the blood-brain barrier.

There also have been some allergic reactions and deaths in dogs treated with injectable ivermectin containing polysorbate 80 as a stabilizer. This formulation has been removed from the market and is no longer available. The present injectable formu-

Editor's Note: This drug, like many others used in exotic and nondomestic species, has been used by the author in an extra-label manner. Report of this trial use must be interpreted carefully by clinicians proposing similar use. The use of ivermectin is not approved by the Food and Drug Administration, and signed, informed owner consent should always be obtained.

lation Ivomec (for cattle) contains propylene glycol as a carrier, which probably will cause fewer local or allergic reactions.

Ivermectin in propylene glycol is not soluble in water or saline, and this complicates the dilution procedure often necessary in the treatment of small exotic species. In our clinic, one part Ivomec is diluted in nine parts propylene glycol, resulting in a solution of 1 mg/ml. This solution is administered subcutaneously at 100 μg/lb or approximately 0.1 ml/lb body weight. If sterile diluent is not readily available commercially, the propylene glycol used to treat ketotic cattle can be placed in a vented bottle and autoclaved in a gravity cycle unit at 250°F for 10 minutes. The solvent can also be passed through a Millipore filter and stored in a sterile vial until needed. It is recommended that the diluted product be used the same day, since no information is available on the stability of the product after dilution. Caution should be exercised in disposing unused drug, as it can contaminate ground water or run-off and kill a variety of marine life. Ivermectin is sensitive to ultraviolet light, and reasonable precautions for disposal should suffice; the drug should be stored in the dark to prolong its shelf life. There is also some evidence that ivermectin can increase the effect of diazepam. This tranquilizer should therefore be given cautiously if ivermectin has been recently administered (Williams and Yarbrough, 1979).

The use of ivermectin is certainly not without risk, and it is important that the risks and benefits are explained to the client. Good relationships between the doctor, client, and patient are essential whenever a veterinarian is using a drug in an "extra-label" manner, which is the usual case in nondomestic animal medicine. Special owner consent forms should be completed.

Most parasitic conditions are not immediately life-threatening, but any parasite is a potential problem for all animals. This is especially true for confined nondomestic species for which diet, environment, vaccination schedule, and other "routine" health maintenance considerations are not specifically known to the same degree as they are for domestic species. Drug treatments always carry a risk of side effects and of the stress resulting from the therapeutic procedure. Ivermectin is a new treatment that has a great potential for use in nondomestic animals because of its margin of safety, broad spectrum of activity, lack of resistant parasites, ease of administration, and residual duration of effect. The safety of ivermectin and its efficacy against a variety of parasites in domestic species has been reviewed (Campbell, 1981; Campbell and Benz, 1984), and new information on its use is regularly published.

IVERMECTIN IN BIRDS

Ivermectin is a useful product for treating avian parasites. It must be diluted for accurate dosages in patients weighing less than 1 pound. The standard dose of 200 μg/kg or approximately 100 μg/lb has been used at our clinic. The author has treated a variety of raptors and other wild species such as ring-billed gulls, ravens, whistling and mute swans, Canada geese, and turkeys. One great horned owl and one red-tailed hawk were treated with ivermectin delivered at 200 μg/lb. The owl was anorectic for 2 days, but this may have been the result of its caging. A number of other raptors were treated with ivermectin (100 μg/lb) with no observed side effects. Treated birds included nine great horned owls, two barred owls, two snowy owls, two common barn-owls, two American kestrels, nine red-tailed hawks, and two broad-winged hawks. Treatment was successful for ascarids and *Capillarida* in raptors and for scaly-leg mites (*Knemidocoptes*) in a variety of pet birds and poultry. Chickens with a severe infestation of scaly-leg mites were successfully treated with 1 mg/lb or 10 times the regular dose of ivermectin without any adverse effects. It is also reported to be effective against air sac mites (*Sternostoma*), oxyspirurids, and stomach worms (*Tetrameres*). The author has not experienced, nor are there any published accounts of, side effects or complications in any species of birds at the dose of 200 μg/kg body weight. The author prefers injecting the drug subcutaneously and has not had any problems at the injection site even when standard unsterilized propylene glycol was used as the diluent. Propylene glycol can cause muscle irritation if administered intramuscularly, so it is recommended that the oral or subcutaneous route be used.

IVERMECTIN IN REPTILES

Ivermectin should be used with caution in reptiles. There have been unpublished reports of mortality associated with its use in young alligators, and there are published reports of paralysis and fatalities in turtles and tortoises treated with this drug (Teare and Bush, 1983). Doses as low as 25 μg/kg caused paresis in leopard tortoises, but this dose once a week is considered a safe starting point for treatment of chelonian species in which the advantage of an injectable anthelmintic is obvious. Ivermectin at a dose of 200 μg/kg has also been used safely in a variety of snakes including pythons, corn snakes, rat snakes, and garter snakes (Lawrence, 1984).

Ivermectin has been used to treat nematodes as well as ticks and mites. There have not been many reported or published experiences regarding the use of ivermectin in reptiles, and the veterinarian should be cautious, especially when treating turtles and tortoises. Special owner consent forms should be completed.

IVERMECTIN IN SMALL MAMMALS

Ivermectin is a useful product in small mammals. The equine paste formulation can be used for many species. This product is supplied in a 1.87 per cent paste, which provides 18.7 mg/ml. There are approximately 6 ml in a single-dose syringe. The marks on the plunger are adequate for dosing a large animal, but the product is softer than most equine pastes and can easily be transferred to a 10-ml syringe and measured exactly to at least 0.2 ml. This paste can be mixed in the food of a variety of animals. The bovine injectable product Ivomec, which is a 1 per cent solution, can also be given orally and, as pointed out earlier, can easily be diluted with propylene glycol for accurate treatment of small species.

The injectable ivermectin is especially useful in the treatment of small carnivores and rodents because the risk of being bitten during attempts at oral dosage is avoided. The following small mammals (two each) were treated with ivermectin (100 μg/lb) with no observable side effects: striped skunk, European ferret, river otter, badger, raccoon, coatimundi, arctic fox, rabbit, and guinea pig. Treatment was administered by a subcutaneous injection made through a fabric net. A net can be purchased (as a smelt or landing net) or homemade with a wooden handle, electrical conduit for the hoop, and a nylon laundry bag for the net. Injection through a net is a common technique for vaccinating intractable patients, and another injection would take care of a variety of internal and external parasites. So far there is no evidence that ivermectin affects the immune response of animals to common vaccines.

Ivermectin is useful for treating wildlife. As an oral preparation, it has been used to treat free-ranging wolves in Alaska for lice. It has been used in bighorn sheep for scabies and in moose to treat winter ticks. At Michigan State University, ivermectin in a single 100 μg/lb subcutaneous dose was used to treat notoedric mange in fox squirrels. The residual effect apparently killed any eggs that hatched later, as hair growth in the squirrels started quickly after treatment and was complete in 3 to 4 weeks. The author has used ivermectin in raccoons for treatment of *Baylisascaris procyonis*. A single treatment probably kills immature roundworms and certainly results in passage of dead adults for 4 to 5 days after treatment.

The author has not seen nor knows of any reported side effects of ivermectin delivered subcutaneously at 200 μg/kg to nondomestic species of mammals for a variety of parasites. It has been used successfully to treat primates with *Pneumonyssus* lung mites, which are normally difficult to eradicate.

CONCLUSIONS

Ivermectin is a good antiparasitic agent for birds and mammals and is useful in some reptiles such as snakes, but it can cause toxicity in others, especially turtles and tortoises. Its efficacy, when delivered either orally or parenterally, and its margin of safety, broad spectrum, and lack of resistant parasites will cause an increase in its use in nondomestic animals. It is likely that with the increased use of ivermectin, parasites will develop resistance to the drug within a few years. Ivermectin is not related to any current drugs, so the best plan may be to rotate its use with that of other successful treatments, especially in confinement situations, in order to prolong the usefulness of ivermectin as a successful therapeutic treatment for a variety of internal and external parasites.

It appears that some individuals or some species are more sensitive to the drug than others; this is now being discovered with its increased use in dogs and reptiles. As with any drug, one should look at alternative treatments and select the one with the best benefits and least known risks.

References and Supplemental Reading

Bowen, J. M.: The avermectin complex: A new horizon in anthelmintic therapy. V.M./S.A.C. 76:165, 1981.

Campbell, W. C.: An introduction to the avermectins. N.Z. Vet. J. 29:174, 1981.

Campbell, W. C., and Benz, G. W.: Ivermectin: A review of efficacy and safety. J. Vet. Pharmacol. Ther. 7:1, 1984.

Egerton, J. R., Ostlind, D. A., Blair, L. S., et al.: Avermectins, new family of potent anthelmintic agents: Efficacy of the B_{1a} component. Antimicrob. Agents Chemother. 15:372, 1979.

Lawrence, K.: Ivermectin as an ectoparasiticide in snakes. Vet. Rec. 115:441, 1984.

Teare, J. A., and Bush, M.: Toxicity and efficacy of ivermectin in chelonians. J.A.V.M.A. 183:1195, 1983.

Williams, M., and Yarbrough, G. G.: Enhancement of in vitro binding and some of the pharmacological properties of diazepam by a novel anthelmintic agent, avermectin B_{1a}. Eur. J. Pharmacol. 56:272, 1979.

DEALING WITH THE EGG-BOUND BIRD

RICHARD R. NYE, D.V.M.
Des Plaines, Illinois

Egg-binding is a condition caused by the obstruction of the oviduct by a developing egg. The material present in the oviduct can be in the form of a developing or fully formed egg, concretions of egg material, degenerating egg material, or excessive secretion of the uterine mucosa.

The reproductive tract of the female bird consists of a developed left ovary and left oviduct. The right ovary and oviduct degenerate, but occasionally, remnants may be present. According to Petrak, the oviduct may be divided into five anatomical segments. The most cranial segment is the infundibulum, which is a flattened funnel that receives the egg. The egg is passed by muscular contractions to the magnum, a thick-walled, glandular area that secretes the albumen. The isthmus, the next section, is a thin-walled area and secretes shell membranes. The final glandular area is a very muscular dilated region known as the shell gland or uterus. This is where the shell is applied; it is also the area of the oviduct most commonly obstructed. The final segment of the oviduct is the vagina, which has a well-developed, muscular sphincter that expels the egg into the cloaca.

The exact cause of egg-binding is unknown, but it has been speculated by several observers to be due to atony or spasms of the oviduct. These oviduct changes can be caused by age, obesity, poor nutrition, stress from chilling, overbreeding or breeding out of season, specific calcium deficiency, or salpingitis.

The bird is presented to the clinic with different degrees of distress depending on the location of the obstructing material and the length of time the bird has been trying to pass the egg.

Many birds, especially parakeets, will present with the egg intact in the distal oviduct, which will be prolapsed through the cloacal opening. There will be a thin mucous membrane over the egg and, depending on the length of time of exposure of the oviduct tissue, it may be hemorrhagic or dry and necrotic. Instead of sitting on the floor of the cage and straining, the bird may be perched upright, exhibiting only a small amount of dyspnea. Some of the hemorrhage and necrosis can be the result of self-mutilation.

The diagnosis of the problem when the egg and the oviduct have prolapsed through the cloacal opening is easy. This condition requires prompt action so that a minimal amount of oviduct tissue becomes dried and necrotic or even secondarily infected. In this case an incision in the oviduct over the egg is made, and the oviduct mucosa is gently separated from the eggshell. It is important to remove all of the shell and yolk material from the oviduct and to remove as much necrotic uterine tissue as possible to allow healthy tissue to be sutured prior to replacement through the cloaca. Suturing may be done with 5–0 or 6–0 absorbable suture material.

If the remaining tissue is unable to be sutured and a deficit must be left in the uterine wall, the possibility of an egg or egg material passing into the abdominal cavity exists. If the bird is a chronic egg layer, surgical removal of the oviduct should be considered. In either case, the bird should be given systemic antibiotics.

If the egg has passed into the cloaca, a bit of lubrication placed in the cloaca and digital pressure on the cranial pole of the egg will aid in its passage.

Another common location of the egg is the distal portion of the oviduct or uterus. The bird strains but is unable to pass the egg through the uterocloacal orifice. This bird will usually be fluffed and dyspneic, and tends to seek a corner on the floor of the cage, where it remains quiet and depressed.

The best initial therapy is to administer calcium gluconate (1 per cent solution, 0.01 to 0.02 ml/gm body weight) intramuscularly, provide moist heat (80 to 85°F) such as in an incubator, and allow the bird 24 hours to pass the egg itself. It is also good to take an abdominal x-ray to eliminate the possibility of complication from a second egg.

If the egg lodged in the distal oviduct does not pass within 24 hours after initial therapy, lubrication can be accomplished by using surgical lubricant infused through an open-end 5-French plastic urinary catheter. Dilation of the cloacal sphincter allows a view of the uterocloacal orifice, where the oviduct enters the cloaca on the left lateral wall. The eggshell may be visible through the orifice.

If lubrication and digital pressure fail to dislodge the egg, an 18-gauge needle can be inserted into the egg and the contents aspirated. Digital pressure externally on the abdominal wall can then crush the egg (the shell pieces usually remain attached to the shell membrane), and with a small forceps the shell and membrane can be gently extracted from the oviduct; care should be taken not to traumatize the oviduct mucosa. A follow-up radiograph should be taken to ensure removal of all shell fragments. The presence of large fragments could possibly lead to penetration of the oviduct wall and subsequent peritonitis. A catheter containing a warm solution of saline and povidone-iodine can be reinserted into the uterocloacal orifice and the oviduct gently flushed.

If the bird is presented when the distal oviduct and egg have passed into the cloaca, the diagnosis of egg-binding is made by abdominal palpation. Prior to any attempt at removal it is always wise to take a radiograph of the abdomen, since occasionally a second egg may be present but not palpable, and the bird could be presented again within 24 hours in a critical condition.

The treatment for this condition can be handled in a simple way without anesthesia or by a laparotomy incision.

The simple method involves dilation of the cloacal sphincter by using a forceps or an otoscope cone to reveal the obstructing egg within the oviduct in the cloaca. An incision can be made in the oviduct wall with a No. 11 blade or a fine-wire electrosurgery needle. Proceed as before and use an 18-gauge needle to aspirate the egg contents. Compress the shell exteriorly and use rat-tooth forceps or Allis tissue forceps to remove the shell and membrane through the incision. The oviduct can be flushed with a solution of saline and povidone-iodine through a 5-French plastic urinary catheter. In this case no attempt is made to suture the oviduct wall. The bird is placed on systemic antibiotics to help prevent peritonitis.

If on examination or radiographs a second egg is present or if the cloacal sphincter cannot be dilated sufficiently to show the prolapse, a laparotomy is indicated.

The last location at which the egg or egg material can be causing obstruction is the mid-body of the oviduct. (These birds are not commonly presented to the veterinarian unless the owner notices the subtle changes in the bird's demeanor.) These birds will frequently be perching, may be ruffled, and may be unsteady on the perch. They may sit with feet apart and may appear to be straining to defecate. They are usually lethargic, depressed, and anorexic. In many parrots for which the sex is undetermined, the early signs of sexual activity or reproduction (e.g., increased dropping size, behavioral changes) can be confused with signs of egg-binding, so the birds will not be presented until they are in a more advanced stage of the condition.

The author has seen a case of egg-binding in which the abdomen of an African gray parrot was distended and fluctuant but radiographs revealed no abnormal calcified densities, only the presence of an amorphous soft tissue density just cranial to the pelvic inlet. Because of the weakened, depressed condition of the bird and a history of recent laying, exploratory surgery was performed to reveal an egg that was bound by a slightly calcified, roughened membrane in the distal oviduct. There were no observable problems with the ovary and no evidence of egg peritonitis. Removal of the egg and therapy, including intramuscular calcium gluconate and subcutaneous fluids, reversed the condition in 24 to 36 hours, and no further problems ensued.

If a laparotomy is indicated, use the technique described by Harrison (1984). Make an incision from side to side about 1 cm below the sternal border. Enter the abdomen on the left side. The swollen oviduct is immediately evident. An incision should be made in the oviduct in an area of decreased vascularity over the egg or egg material. After the oviduct is opened, the intact egg or yolk material should be gently removed so as not to contaminate the abdominal cavity or traumatize the oviduct mucosa. If the bird has had repeated incidents of egg-binding, it may be advisable to remove the oviduct to prevent ovulation and further egg laying. The oviduct is sutured with 5–0 or 6–0 absorbable suture in a continuous pattern. The abdominal musculature is closed in a continuous pattern with 4–0 or 5–0 absorbable suture, and the skin is closed with absorbable sutures in a continuous pattern.

After all of these procedures, it is important to keep the bird on an appropriate systemic antibiotic for 5 to 7 days to help prevent peritonitis. The clinician should also attempt to evaluate possible causes in each individual case of egg-binding so that the client can be advised regarding changes in diet (i.e., supplements of vitamins or minerals), medications to be used or tried, and the prognosis regarding recurrence.

References and Supplemental Reading

Harrison, G. J.: New Aspects of Avian Surgery. Vet. Clin. North Am. 14(2):363, 1984.

Petrak, M. L.: *Diseases of Cage and Aviary Birds.* Philadelphia: Lea & Febiger, 1982, pp. 462–464.

Steiner, C. V., and Davis, R. B.: *Caged Bird Medicine.* Ames, IA: Iowa State University Press, 1981, pp. 111–112, 141.

Stunkard, J. A., Russell, R. J., and Johnson, D. K.: *A Guide to Diagnosis, Treatment, and Husbandry of Caged Birds.* Edwardsville, KS: Veterinary Medicine Publishing, 1980, pp. 6–7, 26–27.

Wallach, J. D., and Boever, W. J.: *Diseases of Exotic Animals.* Philadelphia: W.B. Saunders, 1983, pp. 961–962.

CRYPTOSPORIDIOSIS IN REPTILES

DON GILLESPIE, D.V.M.
Santa Barbara, California

Cryptosporidium is a coccidian parasite related to *Eimeria, Isospora, Sarcocystis,* and *Toxoplasma.* Its life cycle resembles that of other intestinal coccidians, and an infective oocyst containing four sporozoites is passed from the affected host. Infections have been reported from many species of wild and domestic mammals and birds as well as from humans, suggesting a broad host range similar to that of *Toxoplasma.* Two consistent factors of clinical disease from mammalian studies appear to be age and immune status of the host. Very young and immune-deficient animals appear to be at higher risk. The studies also suggest inapparent infection as the usual outcome in immunocompetent animals.

Cryptosporidium has been noted in reptiles such as lizards and snakes since 1925, but clinical problems have only been reported in snakes. The author's experience in both zoological and private practice has been mostly with rat snakes (corn snakes, *Elaphe guttata*; trans-Pecos rat snakes, *Elaphe subocularis*) and various rattlesnakes (*Crotalus* species), but reports of infection in boa constrictors (*Constrictor constrictor*), Gaboon vipers (*Bitis gabonica*), red-bellied snakes (*Pseudechis porphyriacus*), and other species suggest susceptibility in all snakes.

Cryptosporidiosis has not been as extensively studied in reptiles as it has been in other animals, and the life cycle is unknown. Whereas human and calf isolates have been successfully transmitted to other birds and mammals, reptile isolates did not induce infection in mice. This may suggest adaptation of the parasite to poikilothermic animals, but more studies in this area are needed. Infection in reptiles is usually detected as a clinical rather than a subclinical problem.

CLINICAL SIGNS

Cryptosporidium usually inhabits the microvillus border of the intestines and colon, resulting in villous atrophy and subsequent watery diarrhea in mammals. Postprandial regurgitation 2 to 3 days after eating, which is due to gastric hypertrophy, has been the consistent clinical sign in snakes. Regurgitation may not be constant, and the snake may act normal otherwise. Often a firm mid-body swelling may be palpated, and weight loss is present in chronic cases. A history of recent collection or importation is often discerned, suggesting that stress and altered immune status may play a role in development of the clinical disease.

Cryptosporidiosis is only one cause of regurgitation, and others that must be ruled out include management practices (temperature, water availability, and handling), internal abscesses, neoplasias, parasitism, and bacterial or viral gastroenteritis.

DIAGNOSIS

After ruling out management-related causes for regurgitation, direct and sucrose-flotation fecal exams may demonstrate characteristic oocysts. Bacterial culture may be indicated if secondary infections are suspected. Ultrasound may confirm extragastrointestinal masses (neoplasias or internal abscesses), and contrast radiography may be used to confirm gastric involvement. Because of the risk of inspissation of barium in the gastrointestinal tract, direct exam by stomach washings with normal saline or the use of laparotomy or endoscopy and biopsy are preferred approaches. Mucus on regurgitated meals has also yielded *Cryptosporidium* oocysts. Even if other pathologic conditions are found, persistent regurgitators should be evaluated thoroughly before cryptosporidiosis is ruled out.

Biopsy samples may be studied using hematoxylin-eosin, toluidine blue, Giemsa, and Masson trichrome stains. Pathologic changes include edema and thickening of the gastric mucosa and accentuation of the longitudinal rugae. Microscopically, these changes are noted along with atrophy of granular cells. Cystic changes in gastric glands and focal mucosal necrosis are present. All developmental forms may be present lining the microvillar surfaces.

Direct or flotation fecal samples, mucus smears, or stomach washings may be stained with Giemsa to reveal blue oocysts 2.6 to 6 μm diameter, often with four or five fixed red granules. Yeasts will appear similar but often have amorphous masses of red granules. Differentiation by modified Ziehl-Neelsen staining reveals that *Cryptosporidium* oocysts are acid fast whereas yeasts are not. Also, iodine will stain fecal matter and yeasts while oocysts remain colorless. For fecal flotations, immediate examination of a saturated sucrose solution is preferred; saturated sucrose is superior to other commonly used solutions.

TREATMENT AND CONTROL

Over 50 different compounds have been evaluated and failed to prevent or modify cryptosporidiosis consistently in humans and other mammals. Clinical experience with various anticoccidial drugs in reptiles has been uniformly disappointing. Animals with confirmed cases may live months to years, depending on the degree of involvement and supportive measures such as liquid tube feeding. Generally the prognosis is grave, and euthanasia is the best alternative unless valuable specimens are involved.

Control measures would include complete isolation of infected specimens, caging, and handling equipment. Other specimens in the collection should also be tested for the presence of *Cryptosporidium*. Recent evidence suggests use of 5 per cent ammonia or 10 per cent formalin as the only reliable disinfectants used to control oocysts in the environment.

In light of an associated outbreak in immunocompetent humans of cryptosporidiosis from infected calves as well as cross-transmission between many species, reptilian cryptosporidiosis must be considered a potential zoonosis. Immune-deficient persons must be considered at risk when handling infected snakes, equipment, or housing.

References and Supplemental Reading

Angus, K. W., Hutchison, G., Campbell, I., et al.: Prophylactic effects of anticoccidial drugs in experimental murine cryptosporidiosis. Vet. Rec. 114:166, 1984.

Brownstein, D. G., Strandberg, J. D., Montali, R. J., et al.: Cryptosporidium in snakes with hypertrophic gastritis. Vet. Pathol. 14:606, 1977.

Campbell, I., Tzipori, A. S., Hutchison, G., et al.: Effect of disinfectants on survival of *Cryptosporidium* oocysts. Vet. Rec. 111:414, 1982.

Current, W. L., Reese, N. C., Ernst, J. V., et al.: Human cryptosporidiosis in immunocompetent and immunodeficient persons: Studies of an outbreak and experimental transmission. N. Engl. J. Med. 308:1252, 1983.

Jacobson, E. R.: Parasitic diseases of reptiles. *In* Kirk, R. W. (ed.): *Current Veterinary Therapy VIII*. Philadelphia: W.B. Saunders, 1983, pp. 599–606.

Kirkpatrick, C. E., and Farrell, J. P.: Cryptosporidiosis. Comp. Cont. Ed. Pract. Vet. 6:154, 1984.

McKenzie, R. A., Green, P. E., Hartley, W. J., et al.: *Cryptosporidium* in a red-bellied snake (*Pseudechis porphyriacus*). Aust. Vet. 54:365, 1978.

Tzipori, S. R., Campbell, I., and Angus, K. W.: The therapeutic effect of 16 antimicrobial agents on *Cryptosporidium* infection in mice. Aust. J. Exp. Biol. Med. Sci. 60:187, 1982.

REGURGITATION IN SNAKES

THOMAS J. BURKE, D.V.M.

Urbana, Illinois

All snakes apparently possess the ability to regurgitate, although in well-kept specimens this is an uncommon clinical symptom. Physiologic emesis such as occurs in some birds and carnivorous mammals does not appear to occur in snakes. Vomiting should be regarded therefore as a sign that the patient is ill or that there is a serious error in its management by the owner. Snakes are poikilothermic and thus are dependent on environmental temperature and their innate strategies for temperature gathering (e.g., basking) and avoidance in the maintenance of proper digestive function. Vomiting appears to be an active process in snakes. The author has never witnessed passive regurgitation in any snake.

The vomitus usually contains undigested or partially digested food. In severe cases of infectious gastroenteritis the vomitus may contain dark blood and mucus. Mucus alone has been seen as an agonal sign. The owner may mistake the appearance of blood or mucus in the cage as an abnormal stool, and unless the patient has been observed vomiting one may be misled by an incorrect history. Helpful clues are that vomitus usually has a lower pH than stool and urates are not deposited with the material in question. With time the pH will rise, presumably as a result of bacterial fermentation. The amount of blood present may also buffer the gastric acid in the vomitus.

There are many causes of vomiting, but they can be placed in three general categories for the purpose of differential diagnosis: (1) inflammation (gastroenteritis), (2) obstruction, and (3) poor husbandry. When dealing with "pet" snakes, the author has found the third category to be the most common cause of regurgitation.

Gastritis may be caused by a variety of infectious agents, including metazoan and protozoan parasites (especially amoeba) and bacteria (usually gram-negative bacilli). Parasitic and bacterial infections generally produce other signs of illness, particularly anorexia, decreased activity, and diarrhea. The voluntary ingestion of noxious chemicals is not known to occur in snakes.

Obstruction of the gastrointestinal tract is usually the result of external pressure from other organs that are pathologically enlarged as a result of neoplastic, metabolic, or inflammatory disease. Voluntary ingestion of foreign bodies is far less common than with other reptiles and, when found, seems to be associated with small pieces of cage substrate ingested with prey.

When the snake is maintained at suboptimal temperature, digestion does not occur and prey may act as a foreign body. Some degree of bacterial fermentation does take place. The time interval between ingestion and vomiting is variable but is usually in the range of 3 to 5 days. The vomitus contains recognizable prey and usually a quantity of mucus. Radiographs taken before vomiting will show delayed decalcification of the prey's skeleton (highly visible beyond 50 hours).

Excessive handling of snakes within the first 24 to 36 hours after eating frequently causes vomiting. Owners should be cautioned to avoid handling their snakes for 2 days after feeding.

Metabolic causes of gastritis common in mammals, such as uremia and hepatic failure, have not been documented as causes of regurgitation in snakes, although it may be seen as an agonal sign in any disease.

The clinical approach to a snake presented for regurgitation is fairly straightforward and should always include a detailed history, especially concerning management and husbandry. If the owner is unable to provide details about temperatures in the patient's immediate environment, they should be instructed to use a room thermometer to determine the temperature in several places in the cage. The most common cause of vomiting seen by the author is poor temperature management. The second is excessive handling of the snake after it has eaten. The patient should be maintained in a cage large enough to provide a temperature gradient from its optimal digestive temperature to one several degrees cooler. Some means of allowing the snake to bask in order to warm up is ideal. Arboreal species should also have the ability to climb to various points below the heat source and also to do the same in a nonbasking area to cool themselves. Subterranean heat sources are not sufficient alone but may be used as supplemental heat sources. Supplemental heat should be available to the snake *24 hours a day*. For this reason, the overhead heat source should be a red heat bulb or some other device that does not emit white light. Rapid daily temperature changes such as those produced by turning off the heat lamp at night are far more stressful on poikilothermic than on homeothermic animals.

A complete physical examination should be performed with special attention given to abdominal palpation to detect intra-abdominal masses. If one is assured that husbandry is adequate and the results of the physical examination are normal, then ancillary diagnostic aids are employed. These include fecal flotation and direct microscopic examination for parasite ova or protozoa, Gram stain of the vomitus in order to look for an overabundance of gram-negative bacteria, and radiographic examination. Barium contrast studies are indicated if none of the above provide a possible diagnosis. Gastroscopy may be employed by using flexible fiberoptic instruments if the patient can tolerate the chemical restraint necessary for the procedure.

Treatment obviously depends upon the diagnosis. The reader is referred to other articles in this volume for the treatment of various parasites. Therapy for bacterial gastritis depends upon the result of culture and sensitivity testing. While this is pending, the author usually begins treatment with parenteral gentamicin (2.5 mg/kg IM every 72 hours) and oral neomycin (15 mg/kg b.i.d.) with concomitant administration of live *Lactobacillus*. If dehydration is evident, the patient is given warm lactated Ringer's solution at the rate of 10 to 25 ml/kg via intracoelomic injection. The patient should be maintained at 78 to 85°F during treatment.

Intraluminal foreign bodies, including undigested prey, are treated with lubricant laxatives (given orally) and several daily 15-minute swims in tepid water. If results are not obtained within 72 hours, gastrotomy is recommended.

Extraluminal obstruction should be approached by exploratory coeliotomy; either the obstruction should be extirpated or a biopsy should be taken for study.

SHELL DISEASE IN TURTLES AND TORTOISES

WALTER J. ROSSKOPF, JR., D.V.M.
Hawthorne, California

Veterinarians involved in the treatment of chelonian species are frequently presented with patients manifesting signs of shell disease. These cases may be primary in nature or secondary to systemic disease conditions.

NORMAL ANATOMY

Structural details of the shell are diagrammed in Figures 1 through 3. The shell encloses the body so completely that only the head, limbs, and tail protrude. There is a wide range of species variation in structural anatomy among the various chelonian families, considering that some are strictly terrestrial, some are amphibious, and some are entirely aquatic. Some species have soft shells and others have shells with moveable parts or hinges.

The shell consists of an inner bony capsule, a layer of vascularized "skin," and an outer covering of large, horny plates in most turtles and tortoises. This outer covering varies from soft skin in the soft-shelled turtles to a leatherlike covering in some marine species. The dorsal shell, the carapace, is distinguished from the ventral part, or plastron.

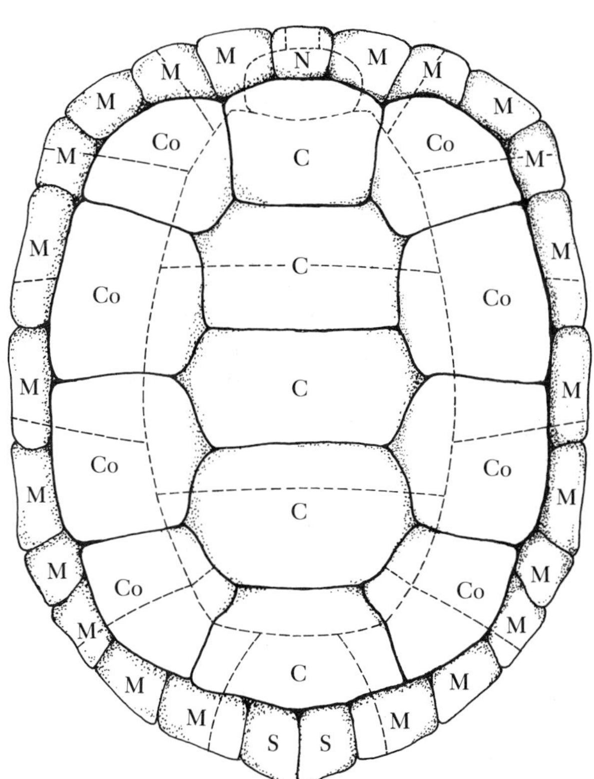

Figure 1. Scute terminology of the carapace. *C*, centrals; *Co*, costals; *M*, marginals; *N*, nuchal; *S*, supracaudals.

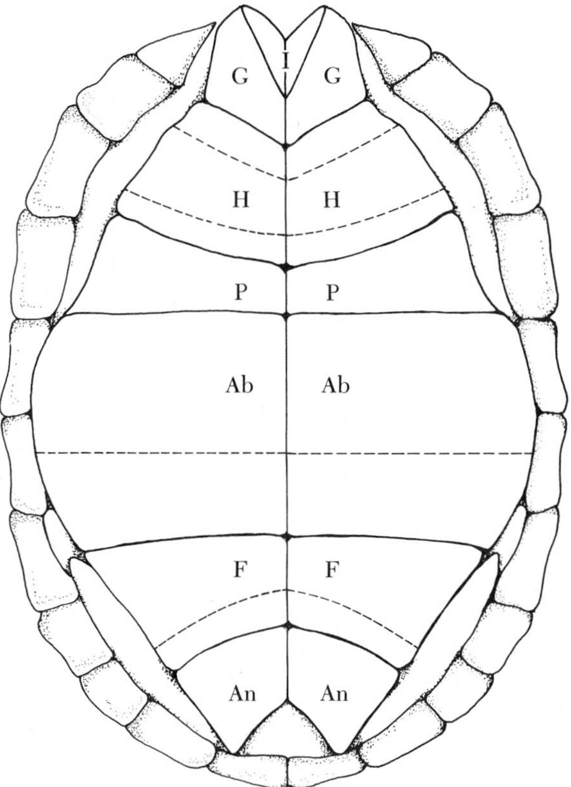

Figure 2. Scute terminology of the plastron. *Ab*, abdominal; *An*, anal; *F*, femoral; *G*, gular; *H*, humeral; *I*, intergular; *P*, pectoral.

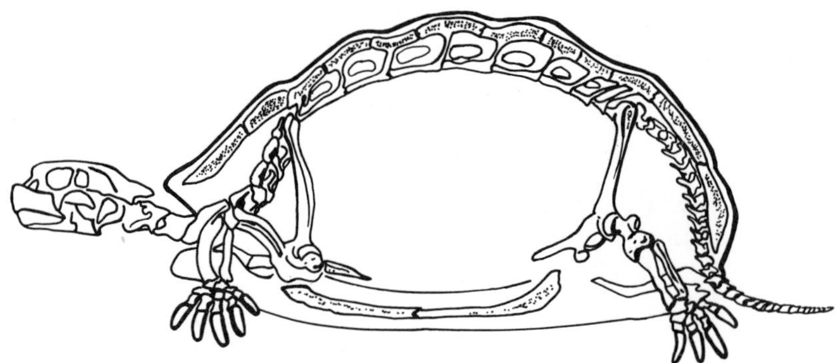

Figure 3. Skeleton and shell structure of a tortoise.

The two are joined at the side by the "bridge." The carapace and plastron are each composed of a number of elements, usually paired in a regular, symmetric pattern.

Many aquatic turtles, and some terrestrial species as well, have evolved single or double transverse hinges in the plastron where elastic cartilaginous tissue is interposed between two adjacent plate pairs. In this way the plastron, usually quite rigid, is divided into movable anterior and posterior sections that the animal can fold upward to close the apertures between the top and bottom of the shell. In such turtles, the bridge joining carapace and plastron has lost its rigidity and become more flexible by the inclusion of cartilage and bands of connective tissue. An identical mechanism, found in the carapace of the hinged tortoise, allows the posterior part to snap down like the visor of a helmet to protect the rear quarters.

The shape of the pancake, or Tornier's, tortoise (*Malacochersus tornieri*) is quite different from that of all other testudinids. Its shell appears flat as a board, is barely ossified, and is so soft that it yields under pressure. When these tortoises were first discovered, this condition was thought to be a malformation similar to that caused by rickets. This species, when disturbed, will wedge itself in rocky crevices. It can anchor itself with its legs and wedge the flexible shell against the walls of its hiding place so tightly that one can hardly pull it out by hand.

DEFORMITIES

A wide variety of deformities of the carapace or plastron may be seen. These may be due to (1) congenital anomalies, (2) healed injuries, (3) healed lesions of disease, and (4) vitamin, mineral, and other dietary imbalances.

Congenital lesions seen by the author have included missing sections of scutes and accompanying bone, unusual asymmetric scute and bone patterns, and extra scutes and sections of bone. One hatchling desert tortoise had an anomaly (missing nuchal bone plate) that appeared similar to an anomaly in the Galapagos tortoise that was selected for on Hood Island. One wonders if this characteristic could have been selected for in time in our desert if this animal had been allowed to live in the wild and had prospered.

Large, granulated filling defects are frequently encountered in desert tortoises from injuries occurring in the wild. Animals that have survived massive burns are frequently encountered with patterns of scar tissue on the shell. Healed wounds from the gnawing of predatory mammals are often seen.

Pitting of the carapace and plastron from old, healed lesions of osteomyelitis (shell rot) is common in water turtles. The scar tissue will be made up of granulation tissue with no evidence of active infection.

Evidence of calcium deficiency and other mineral, vitamin, and dietary imbalances are seen in most captive water turtles that are not caught when mature. A malformed shell is often the result of a calcium-deficient (i.e., all-meat) diet during the turtle's formative years. As the hobbyist learns how to properly feed his charges (i.e., give a balanced ration such as dry dog or cat food or trout chow), these animals return to good health. However, they remain "marked for life" with a humped, small, upcurved or otherwise deformed shell from the scar tissue that formed in an attempt to strengthen the bone when calcium was not available in adequate amounts or in proper balance with other vitamins and nutrients (fibrous osteodystrophy). Many clients who see a normal adult red-eared slider for the first time (over 8 inches in length with a perfectly smooth shell) are, needless to say, shocked.

Shell deformities may also occur from apparent overuse of various nutrient materials. The difficulty in providing a normal diet to the various chelonian species kept as pets has resulted in a wide variety of suggested diets with dietary vitamin and mineral additives included. Most veterinarians and zoologists treating chelonians have found that feeding excess protein and often insufficient minerals to captive exotic tortoises will result in incredibly rapid growth, producing large specimens with mounded shell bone plates. As a result, most captively raised tortoises can be differentiated from their wild counterparts. Zoos have experimented for years with diets to avoid this unnatural look in their captively hatched tortoises. The answer to this problem is difficult because of the wide variety of species present, their individually different requirements, and the usual inability in providing exactly what these animals eat in the wild. Commercial pelleted foods that are being studied show promise. In the future, pelleted rations will be developed for many of the species kept in captivity.

TRAUMATIC INJURIES

Clinicians are frequently presented with turtles and tortoises suffering from traumatic injuries to the shell. Prognosis depends on the extent of the injury, the amount of blood lost, the previous health status of the individual, and the degree of internal involvement (i.e., lungs, kidneys, liver, spinal column). Causes of traumatic injury include automobiles and lawnmowers (most frequently in the spring, when animals wake from hibernation and begin to wander and when the first grass is cut), dog attacks, bites (in soft-shelled species from fighting among themselves), sharp aquarium rocks, bruising, and shell cracks from falls, paint and chemicals, and burns. Disease arising from improper housing will be discussed later.

The two most frequently seen causes of shell injury are automobiles and dog attacks. The clinician must first, of course, stop the bleeding and treat for shock. *Involved repair of shell injuries should not be attempted until the patient is stable.* If the shell is badly cracked and the viscera are exposed, a decision must be made as to whether there is a reasonable enough chance of saving the patient to warrant treatment. It is amazing what degree of injury a chelonian patient can sustain and still survive, but some injuries are obviously beyond our present capabilities, especially if large areas of shell are missing or if intestinal rupture with major peritoneal contamination has occurred.

If an injury is severe, the usual procedure of this author is to stop the bleeding by using standard techniques without anesthesia (hemostats and tying, cautery, Gel Foam [Upjohn], or pressure), approximate the shell edges, apply an antibacterial cream to external cracks, and bandage with a plastic coated gauze pad and a flexible adhesive bandage. Plastic wrapping works well to prevent pneumoperitoneum and can be placed over the gauze pads. The animal is then given a shock dose of dexamethasone (0.45 to 0.91 mg/kg IM into the axillary area [because of the renal portal system]), an antibiotic (see treatment section) is injected subcutaneously into the axillary area, and the patient is placed on a warm heating pad (low setting). A blood sample is taken by nail-clipping technique to establish baseline values for monitoring the case (see Table 1 for suggested normal values for some species). The clinician should expect to see signs of stress in the hemogram in most cases. If blood pressure is low (chelonians in stress will have less blood in their extremities), often only slides can be obtained. Initial packed cell volume (PCV) values will be higher than equilibrated values taken later. If fluid therapy is desired, subcutaneous or intraperitoneal fluids (the latter if shell damage is not extensive) may be given (the author prefers normal saline). Transfusions can be given in some cases through the jugular vein or cutdown axillary vein (in some species). The author has given desert tortoise blood to desert tortoises and other species with no apparent reactions on first transfusion. Extensive blood loss may result in thrombocytopenia and spontaneous bleeding in desert tortoises. (One theory is that desert tortoises convert thrombocytes to red cells in time of need.) Response of the bone marrow can be rapid but usually takes weeks to replace lost blood.

After the patient is stabilized and organ function has been examined by serum chemistry readings in severe injuries, shell repair can be undertaken. In simple cases, the shells of tortoises and land turtles are simply pieced together, and antibacterial cream is applied after the area is first cleansed with washes

Table 1. *Suggested Blood Values for Some Chelonian Species**

	Desert Tortoise	Box Turtle	Red-Eared Slider
WBC (× $10^3/mm^3$)	3–8	5–11	6–13
Neutrophils (%)	0–3	0–1	0–1
Heterophils (%)†	35–60	30–60	20–60
Lymphocytes (%)	25–50	25–60	15–40
Monocytes (%)	0–4	0–2	0–1
Eosinophils (%)	0–4	0–10	0–15
Basophils (%)†	2–15	2–10	5–40
PCV (%)	23–37	25–40	25–40
Thrombocytes	Present	Present	Present
Polychromasia	Slight	Slight	Slight
Anisocytosis	Slight	Slight	Slight
Blood parasites	Occasionally *Plasmodium*	Occasional	Common
SGOT (IU)	10–105	15–200	50–250
Total protein (gm/dl)	2.5–5.0	2.5–6.0	2.5–6.0
Glucose (mg/dl)‡	35–150	50–180	35–180
Uric acid (mg/dl)	2.2–7.2	0.2–7.1	1.0–5.0
BUN (mg/dl)	< 1–30	10–90	10–110

*Based on author's data.

†Stress may elevate heterophils in certain species (e.g., desert tortoises and box turtles) and basophils in other species (e.g., water turtles).

‡Stress and excitement may increase glucose values. Inanition or hibernation may decrease glucose values.

of povidone-iodine solution (PI). The area is then bandaged for stabilization. Most minor cracks will granulate and stabilize in 2 to 3 weeks. If extra stabilization is desired, one to three surgical steel wire sutures may be applied by using a hobby drill, and then the cream and bandages can be applied.

If extensive damage has occurred, fiberglass and quick-setting acrylic resin is used. Many brands are acceptable. The author prefers to let the wounds granulate 1 to 3 weeks before this is done to allow more thorough cleansing of the injured areas and to prevent leakage of acrylic into the body cavity. Standard bandages and wires may be used to stabilize the injury prior to the application of acrylic resin. In order to avoid chronic abcessation, care must be taken not to trap dirt, detritus, or other contaminated material under the acrylic. The author much prefers wire, antibacterial cream, and changeable bandages to acrylic resin for that reason. Acrylic resin is preferred for use after abdominal surgery. In young, growing animals (most land tortoises theoretically grow for life but after maturity growth is minimal), the acrylic patch will eventually need routing and removal. Antibacterial cream, used in human burn patients, is always used over the wounds prior to repair. Silvadene cream (Marion Laboratories) is effective against gram-negative contaminants common in chelonians, and it is especially effective against the ubiquitous *Pseudomonas* organisms. The author has seen very few wound infections when using Silvadene, which is much preferred over the nitrofurantoin (Furacin, Norwich-Eaton) and PI (Betadine, Purdue Frederick) creams in vogue in veterinary medicine. Silvadene is also advantageous in that it is water soluble.

A common injury seen in large land tortoises is a crack between the pectoral and abdominal scutes. This injury results from a fall and creates a box-turtle-like hinge effect, which will interfere with the tortoise's walking and normal functioning. Acrylic resin is used to stabilize the area in smaller animals, but more sturdy material such as aluminum rods or splinting material may be necessary to reinforce the repair in large tortoises. Care must be taken not to make the repair too heavy or cumbersome or the tortoise will not be able to ambulate normally.

In water turtles, extra care is needed in severe shell injuries, as dehydration can quickly become a problem if the animals are kept out of water. Also, water turtles cannot eat out of water. As a result, the author prefers to use acrylic resins with these animals as a means of returning them to their environments faster. Daily intraperitoneal injections of lactated Ringer's may be necessary if extensive, out-of-water recovery time is necessary.

Repair of dog-bite injuries depends, of course, on the extent of the injury. Minor injuries are first cleansed with PI scrub. The animal is soaked in PI solution. (A rule of thumb is to make the soaking solution tea-colored.) Antibacterial cream and bandages are then used as necessary, and dressings are changed daily at first. Eventually, wounds are allowed to granulate, and PI soaks are continued with bandage changes made less frequently. Water turtles are often soaked daily in PI and are allowed to eat in a clean feeding tank and kept dry for extended periods or until acrylic repair is attempted.

Clients must be warned of the danger of infestation with fly larvae (myiasis). Any chelonian wound seems to attract flies, and turtles and tortoises neglected for more than 12 to 24 hours may be discovered teeming with maggots. If this occurs, careful PI and peroxide soaking and hand removal of these creatures must be instigated. Maggots must breathe air, and they usually quickly surface from submerged wounds, although several days may be necessary to expose all of them. The author avoids the use of ether because of its high volatility and associated pain.

Antibiotic therapy is of paramount importance in any chelonian shell injury because of the presence of numerous symbiotic gram-negative organisms found on the skin and shell (e.g., *Pseudomonas, Proteus*). See treatment section for a full discussion of available antibiotics.

Paint injuries were formerly common when water turtles were painted with designs for the tourist trade. This, of course, resulted in toxic reactions and shell deformities if the animal was fortunate enough to survive. Usually, these turtles would die from the usual dietary and husbandry practices at the time. Today, we are occasionally presented with land tortoises that have been painted by unknowledgable people for "esthetic" purposes or for identification. One desert tortoise the author saw was painted completely yellow for a purported satanic rite! Affected animals are bathed with a mild soap in an attempt to loosen the paint. Mineral-oil baths, alternated with detergent, will help. In general, the author tries to handle these cases in the same manner as for oil-soaked birds. Never allow clients to sandpaper the shell, for obvious reasons. Paint thinner is dangerous but can be judiciously used in land tortoises if followed by an immediate, thorough bath. Never use any product such as paint thinner on a water turtle. Use an eye ointment in the eyes before the animal is bathed.

All types of burns are handled in the same manner as human burns. Antibiotics, proper supportive care, and antibacterial cream are routinely used by the author for such cases.

For all animals with shell injury, the use of the clinical laboratory will aid the clinician in handling the patient. As with other species, infection and internal complications can be diagnosed and monitored by the interpretation of blood slides and blood chemistry values.

SYSTEMIC CONDITIONS THAT AFFECT THE SHELL

Dietary Deficiencies

As previously mentioned, deficiencies of proteins, minerals, vitamins, and other nutrients will affect the shell's growth and appearance. Calcium deficiency disease (nutritional hyperparathyroidism) is most common. In herbivorous tortoises (e.g., desert tortoises) that are fed improperly balanced rations, the results can be devastating. Most commonly, in southern California, the clinician is presented with a young desert tortoise hatchling fed mainly human salad ingredients such as iceberg lettuce, tomatoes, melons, and so forth. Unsuspecting clients often do not realize that these products contain mainly water and have little nutrient value. Work by Fowler has shown that the nutrient makeup of many naturally occurring desert forage and edible plants consumed by desert tortoises is high in protein and minerals. Clients must be encouraged to feed foods such as natural grasses, alfalfa hay, alfalfa sprouts, clover, guinea pig chow, rabbit chow, dandelion, and high-protein supplements such as low-fat dry dog food (moistened) instead of the usual "tortoise foods." The usual salad ingredient can be used in moderation to supply water and serve as a vehicle for vitamin and calcium powders. A stubborn hatchling can often be acclimated to eating a more nutritious diet by offering it a "burrito" in which some food it has grown accustomed to (to such as lettuce) wraps more nutritious food inside.

Diets deficient in minerals will lead to softening of the shell in herbivorous tortoises (often one can see through the shell and observe internal organs) and weakening of the animal's condition until disease takes over. Treatment of these pitiful cases may require addition of calcium, injections of B-complex and other vitamins, administration of antibiotics, and force-feeding. Many of these animals are damaged beyond repair. Those recovering will be deformed for life.

Deficiency problems in carnivorous water turtles usually arise from eating all-meat diets such as beef heart, hamburger, smelt, and shrimp. A change to dry cat food, dry dog food, trout chow, or live food (guppies, goldfish) will arrest the deformity if it is not too late (e.g., the heart muscle may be flabby), but the turtle will remain stunted or deformed (in one case, the turtle grew but the shell stopped growing). Injectable vitamins, calcium, and antibiotics are often necessary.

In omnivorous chelonians such as box turtles fed mainly vegetation or fruit by unknowledgable clients, dry or semimoist dog food will help arrest the animal's deficiency problems. The author much prefers prepared animal foods to natural diets because of the clean nature of dog food, its availability, and known successes with its use. Live food such as mealworms and crickets are usually not balanced nutritionally unless they are raised in calcium-vitamin powder; in addition, this type of food may not be available and can be contaminated. For omnivorous species such as box turtles, a diet of one-half dog food and one-half fruit and vegetation seems to work well. There are many other regimens, of course, and success stories abound for many lay feeding regimens for various species.

Generalized Infections

The shell and associated skin may reflect the general health of the turtle or tortoise. This is especially true of water turtles and less true of land animals. The author has seen many land tortoises that are dying of kidney or liver failure but that have beautiful shells. In water turtles, on the other hand, the shell may begin to crack or peel unnaturally as an internal disease advances. Clinicians should realize that scutes will be shed in young turtles as they grow, but the scutes should look healthy and clean. Very fine air bubbles can be seen under the scutes of young desert tortoises that are healthy (cause unknown). This can represent shell rot in its early stages in water turtles, however.

Shell Problems Associated With Special Environmental Requirements

Some chelonian species have specific environmental requirements associated with shell health. A classic case is the diamond-back terrapin (*Malaclemys terrapin*). These turtles live in the brackish coastal waters of the eastern United States. If they spend too much time in fresh water, they develop skin and shell ulcerations and eventually die. Their food in the wild consists mainly of hard-shelled mollusks. The excess salt they consume is excreted by means of special glands at the eye. Hobbyists usually add a teaspoonful of sea salt to each gallon of aquarium water for diamond-back terrapins.

Neoplasia

The author has seen several rare cases of shell neoplasia, resulting in abnormal swellings. Despite the incredibly long life span of many of these turtles and tortoises, this condition is very uncommon. One swelling associated with the posterior carapace in a desert tortoise was classified as a chondroma. Shell abcesses tend to invade the inside of the body (with minimal external swelling) in chelonians, in the author's experience.

INFECTIOUS DISEASES

There are many infectious organisms that may be associated with shell disease. Minor infections may involve the skin and subcutaneous tissue. As the infection spreads, the underlying bone becomes involved, resulting in osteomyelitis or "shell rot." Once osteomyelitis occurs, the organisms may invade the blood and initiate systemic disease. For this reason, the author prefers to treat most shell disease systemically. Infectious agents may be opportunistic pathogens that invade a weakened animal or enter through damaged skin. Other agents are more pervasive.

Most shell infections in turtles and tortoises result from poor husbandry practices. Poor feeding methods and inadequate diets lead to a weakened animal. Abrasive aquarium rocks result in shell and skin injuries. Overcrowding leads to fighting and its resulting injuries. Poor cleanliness results in a buildup of pathogenic bacteria in the water that may enter the subcutaneous tissue under loose scutes and eventually invade the bone.

Algal Shell Disease

The shells of aquatic turtles are frequently covered with algae. Such growth is thought to be symbiotic, providing camouflage for the turtle in its native habitat. In captive situations, the algae may penetrate the shell, resulting in erosion of the underlying bone, secondary infection, and internal disease.

Algal shell disease is often complicated by unsanitary conditions leading to a buildup of bacterial pathogens. Prevention of disease by adequate sanitation and periodic cleaning of the turtle's shell if algae begins to appear is of paramount importance. PI solution is most often used to clean the shell. The use of a Vita-Lite (Duro-Test) provides adequate lighting without encouraging plant growth in the aquatic environment. In the author's experience, turtles that spend large amounts of time basking out of the aquatic environment (e.g., *Pseudemys* or *Chrysemys* species) have less trouble with algae than turtles that spend most of their time submerged (musk turtles or snapping turtles).

If skin penetration of algal growth has occurred, treatment with systemic antibiotics and PI solution should be instituted (see therapy section).

Bacterial Shell Disease

Most cases of shell disease are caused by bacterial pathogens. Again, many of these diseases are precipitated by environmental problems such as abrasive rocks, overcrowding, inadequate sanitation, and poor diet. The reader is referred to *Current Veterinary Therapy VII* for a discussion of environmental considerations for water turtles.

There are two specific bacterial pathogens that cause chelonian shell disease. *Ulcerative shell disease* (infectious shell rot, spot disease, or shell rust) is a contagious, chronic condition characterized by blotchy darkening, loosening, and shedding of the keratinized shell plates of the plastron and carapace. It is caused by a gram-negative bacillus, *Beneckea chitinovora*. The condition has been described in several species of freshwater turtles. Affected shell plates slough, leaving raw ulcers and a brownish-yellow pseudomembrane from which the organism can be cultured. The disease is spread directly through unsanitary conditions and shell lesions or indirectly through intermediate hosts. The intermediate hosts include crayfish, lobsters, crabs, and other crustaceans that frequently harbor *B. chitinovora*. Because of this, *water turtles should not be fed or housed with crustaceans.*

The other specific bacterial pathogen, *Citrobacter freundii*, results in *septicemic cutaneous ulcerative disease* of turtles, or SCUD. *Citrobacter freundii* is a gram-negative rod frequently found in soil and water and in the intestinal tract of various animals. Turtles are thought to become infected through skin abrasions while in contaminated water. Clinical signs in turtles include lethargy, reduced muscle tone, paralysis of limbs, loss of claws or digits, and cutaneous vasodilation, hemorrage, and ulceration. Hemolysis and multiple foci of necrosis are found in internal organs. The disease is transmissable to frogs, which also develop superficial ulcers and fatal septicemia.

Because of the occurrence of these bacterial pathogens, it is always good to back medical treatment with a Gram stain and culture and sensitivity testing.

Other causes of bacterial shell disease are numerous. A wide variety of gram-negative and gram-positive pathogens may invade the shell if poor sanitation, poor health, injury, or a combination of these conditions predisposes the animal to infection. The author has seen shell disease result from such gram-negatives organisms as *Pseudomonas, Aeromonas, Proteus, Serratia, Klebsiella, Escherichia coli,* and many others. Mycobacterial infections have been seen. Common gram-positive organisms such as *Staphylococcus aureus* and α-hemolytic *Streptococcus* have been isolated from shell lesions in turtles and tortoises. In many cases, multiple organisms have been isolated in shell disease. In the author's opinion, most of these are opportunistic pathogens, usually normal inhabitants of the skin, digestive tract, or soil, which gain a foothold if conditions are conducive to their growth (e.g., filth, poor diet, abrasions, or injury).

Fungal Shell Disease

A wide variety of fungal organisms have been isolated from the shell lesions of sick turtles and tortoises. They include *Fusarium solanae,* species of *Aspergillus, Penicillium, Mucor,* and many others.

Parasitic Shell Disease

Parasitic diseases of the shell are rare in turtles and tortoises seen in practice. Leeches may be found under the edges of the shell in newly caught water turtles. Ticks will occasionally be found under the shell margins of desert tortoises. One report has been made of a tick with its mouthparts imbedded in the carapace of an African tortoise. Barnacles may be found on the shells of sea turtles.

The most commonly seen disease associated with parasites of turtles and tortoises is myiasis, caused by maggot infestation. Flies will lay eggs on any chelonian wound, and the eggs may hatch in 12 to 24 hours. These flesh-eating maggots will quickly invade the body of the animal and will produce incredible damage. The author once saw a Galapagos tortoise die from maggot-induced pneumonia as a result of one small bullet hole in the carapace. Turtles and tortoises with shell injuries must be kept away from flies. If fly larvae are present, they must be soaked out with peroxide and PI baths before damage becomes irreparable.

Viral Shell Disease

Little is known about viral diseases in turtles and tortoises. Many diseases will be discovered to be of viral origin as further work is done. The only virus so far described in association with shell disease in turtles and tortoises is gray patch disease of green sea turtles (*Chelonia mydas*). This disease is caused by a herpesvirus and is characterized by cutaneous infection in animals 2 to 3 months old. Epidermal cells contain basophilic intranuclear inclusion bodies.

DIAGNOSIS OF SYSTEMIC DISEASE

The clinician, when presented with a case of shell disease, must first evaluate the patient. A physical exam is performed and a history is taken. Does the animal appear normal in stature and appearance? Is the diet and husbandry adequate? Are other animals involved? Are signs of other disease evident (i.e., upper respiratory disease, swollen eyes, or soft shell)? When did the lesions first appear? How rapidly are they spreading? Is the patient's appetite normal, diminished, or nonexistent?

After the patient's general condition is evaluated, a decision is made as to the necessity of obtaining blood samples or cultures. Economic constraints may be placed on the veterinarian and limit diagnostic procedures.

In the individual valued pet, the author prefers to collect a blood sample. Samples are taken by nail clipping or venipuncture (axillary or jugular). Coverslip slides are made for all turtles, tortoises, and water turtles to avoid crushing and damaging the blood cells. A microhematocrit tube is used to obtain blood for a PCV and, in many cases, a blood chemistry evaluation.

A swab of the shell lesion for Gram staining and possible culture and sensitivity testing is usually taken. This is especially important if systemic involvement is suspected.

THERAPY

Therapy often includes daily PI soaks after débridement of shell lesions. A typical regimen may be to soak a tortoise in tea-colored PI solution for 1 hour, two times daily. A water turtle may be kept out of water for most of the day except during meals. At those times, a PI-soaked gauze pad may be used to keep the lesions wet and Silvadene cream or other antibiotic may be applied afterwards. Intraperitoneal fluid therapy may be necessary if a water turtle is to be kept dry for long periods of time. In cases of minor shell involvement, the turtle may be kept out of water for only a limited period several times a day, during which PI solution is painted on the shell.

Careful attention to cleanliness is of paramount importance in the treatment of shell disease, especially in water turtles that may swim in contaminated water. Frequent water changes must be made. The turtle is best treated in an isolation tank unless the clinician feels that the disease in noncontagious during therapy or that the animal is more likely to recover if living with others (some gregarious animals will not eat away from the group).

The choice of a systemic antibiotic must be made for all but the most superficial disease. Treatment regimens are found in Table 2. The author's antibiotics of choice include gentamicin, carbenicillin (except in desert tortoises, in which it frequently causes peeling skin reactions), a gentamicin-carbenicillin combination, piperacillin, ticarcillin, cefotaxime, tobramycin, and amikacin. The use of a penicillin derivative (carbenicillin, piperacillin,

Table 2. *Antibiotics and Antimicrobial Drugs Used in Turtles and Tortoises*

Type of Drug (Generic Name)	Brand Name and Manufacturer (Strength)	Dosage	Length of Treatment
Aminoglycosides			
Amikacin*	Amikin, Bristol (250 mg/ml)	10 mg/kg daily, water turtles; every other day, land turtles and tortoises	7–10 days
Gentamicin*	Gentocin, Schering (50 mg/ml)	5–10 mg/kg daily, water turtles; every other day, land turtles and tortoises	7–10 days
Tobramycin*	Nebcin (Dista, Eli Lily) (10 mg/ml)	10 mg/kg daily, water turtles; every other day, land turtles and tortoises	7–10 days
Penicillin Derivatives			
Ampicillin	Polyflex, Bristol (100 mg/ml)	20 mg/kg daily	1–2 weeks
Carbenicillin†¶	Geopen, Roerig (100–200 mg/ml)	50–100 mg/kg daily	1–2 weeks
Piperacillin†	Pipracil, Lederle (100–200 mg/ml)	50–100 mg/kg daily	1–2 weeks
Ticarcillin†	Ticar, Beecham (100–200 mg/ml)	50–100 mg/kg daily	1–2 weeks
Cephalosporins			
Cefotaxime‡	Claforan, Hoechst Roussel (200 mg/ml)	20–40 mg/kg daily	1–2 weeks
Other Antibiotics			
Chloramphenicol	Chloromycetin, Parke-Davis (100 mg/ml)	20 mg/kg b.i.d.	1–3 weeks
Antifungals			
Ketoconizole	Nizoral, Janssen (250 mg/tablet)	25 mg/kg daily, orally	2–4 weeks
Amphotericin B§	Fungizone, Squibb (10 mg/ml)	1 mg/kg daily, intraperitoneally	2–4 weeks

*Advisable to begin therapy with 20 ml/kg fluid injection; hydration is essential with aminoglycosides—monitor uric acid levels when possible.

†100 mg/kg used in animals under 3 lbs.

‡40 mg/kg used in animals under 3 lbs.

§Dilute at least tenfold in lactated Ringer's solution; monitor with serum chemistries when possible.

¶Frequently associated with peeling skin reactions in desert tortoises and therefore should not be used in that species.

ampicillin, ticarcillin) or a cephalosporin (e.g., cefotaxime) in addition to an aminoglycoside (amikacin, tobramycin, gentamicin) has a potentiating effect on both drugs, and as a result, combination therapy is very efficacious in cases of shell disease. Ampicillin is rarely useful for most chelonian infections, despite earlier successes by the author, since it has a limited gram-negative spectrum. (It is only occasionally effective against *E. coli* and other gram-negative organisms.) Chloramphenicol is bacteriostatic and less desirable as a result, although it is preferred by many investigators. The author's studies have shown 50 per cent efficacy *in vitro* with chloramphenicol. Tetracycline is virtually worthless in chelonian infections, in the author's experience. Antibiotics are usually given subcutaneously or intramuscularly in the axillary region (due to the renal portal system).

For fungal infections, the author has used Tinactin cream (Schering) for localized infections and amphotericin B and ketoconizole for systemic or deeper infections. Localized yeast infections respond to nystatin cream. Ketoconizole is used if systemic yeasts are suspected.

Therapy for shell infections may involve surgical débridement of wounds and removal of sequestered bone in deep osteomyelitis. Thorough treatment is required, or walled-off abscesses may develop and result in chronically draining tracts or septicemic deaths. A progressively increasing monocyte count is usually associated with abscessation in chelonians. The author knows of one case in which a leopard tortoise died of acute septicemia 4 years after a walled-off shell lesion occurred. The *Proteus* organism originated from a slow-growing cyst that had been followed radiographically for 4 years. The lesion eventually burst, showering the tortoise's body with bacterial emboli. In water turtles, removal of dying or damaged scutes may be necessary to properly curette lesions. Damaged scutes may trap contaminated water, and removal is indicated if water or air bubbles are evident under them. If thorough surgical débridement is necessary, the author prefers ketamine as an anesthetic (20–40 mg/kg). Ketamine may be followed by intubation and administration of halothane or isoflurane. If respiratory depression occurs with ketamine, positive pressure oxygenation and fluid therapy are effective to remove the anesthetic from the system, as the contractile ability of the chelonian heart keeps it beating. (The heart of a euthanized chelonian will often beat for hours after death.)

References and Supplemental Reading

The inclusion of extensive lists of references is discouraged in *Current Veterinary Therapy*. The author will provide a list of 36 references to those who wish to delve more deeply into the subject.

DENTAL PROBLEMS IN RABBITS AND RODENTS

PAMELA H. EISELE, D.V.M.
Davis, California

Dental problems are fairly common in rabbits and rodents. Affected animals may be presented with a number of clinical signs, including a gradual decrease in food intake that may progress until eating stops completely, drooling with resultant wetting of the skin and fur around the mouth and under the chin ("slobbers"), swelling under the jaw, weight loss, and obviously maloccluded and overgrown teeth.

MALOCCLUSION

The most frequently seen dental problems are usually those associated with malocclusion. The incisors of rabbits and rodents have open roots and grow continuously throughout the life of the animal. In the rabbit, this can amount to more than 2 mm of growth each week. Additionally, the cheek teeth of rabbits and of some of the rodent species such as the guinea pig and chinchilla are also open-rooted and continuously growing. Normal wear is required to keep this type of tooth from becoming overgrown. Consequently, any factor preventing normal occlusion and wear can lead to overgrown teeth. Such factors include inherited malocclusions, malocclusions secondary to dietary imbalances, malocclusions secondary to jaw trauma and malalignment or to breakage or loss of an opposing tooth, and inadequate roughage in the diet.

Malocclusion in the Rabbit

Malocclusion in the rabbit is usually a primary problem of malaligned incisors and, secondarily, their overgrowth. Eventually, this may lead to inadequate wear of the cheek teeth so that they become overgrown as well. The affected rabbit may be presented for slowly decreasing food intake or may be off feed totally. It may appear hungry when food is placed in front of it, yet is unable to prehend or chew the food properly. Other presenting signs include weight loss, dehydration, and excessive salivation and drooling.

Differential diagnoses to be ruled out include water deprivation or inability to use the water source, unpalatable feed, gastric trichobezoars or hairballs, and some systemic diseases. A number of these can be eliminated from consideration by a good history of the course of the disease and a description of the animal's home environment and care.

A diagnosis can be made upon careful examination of the animal's teeth and oral cavity. The rabbit should be properly restrained in a cat or rabbit restrainer or wrapped in a towel so that it cannot break its back if it jumps during the examination. The incisors can be easily examined by retracting the animal's lips. The occlusion of the cheek teeth, however, is most easily evaluated by radiography or by examination of the back of the oral cavity with the animal under light general anesthesia. This can be facilitated by using an oral speculum or strips of gauze to hold the animal's mouth open. An otoscope or small laryngoscope blade offers a suitable light source for the examination. The mouth should be examined for broken or missing teeth and ulcerations in addition to maloccluded teeth.

Adequate anesthesia for the oral examination can be attained with the combination of xylazine (Rompun, Haver-Lockhart) 2 to 5 mg/kg and ketamine (Vetalar, Parke-Davis) 35 to 50 mg/kg given intramuscularly. The rabbit should be carefully re-

---

Note: No anesthetics are approved for use in these species but the drugs and doses referred to in this article are widely used and accepted.

strained so that it does not injure its back when the injections are made. It should be sufficiently relaxed for examination within 5 to 10 minutes after the drugs are given. An alternate technique employs the use of an inhalant anesthetic administered in oxygen with the rabbit in an anesthetic chamber. Halothane at 2 to 4 per cent can be used for induction until the rabbit relaxes adequately for the examination. The animal should be carefully observed during the induction period so that it does not become too deeply anesthetized. Halothane at 0.5 to 1.5 per cent can be used to maintain the rabbit under anesthesia for longer periods of time if necessary. Although many rabbits have high levels of atropinesterase, atropine sulfate at 0.05 to 0.1 mg/kg subcutaneously can be given as a preanesthetic to help reduce oral secretions in those animals that are sensitive to its effects. As these drugs do not have established withdrawal times in rabbits, they should not be used in rabbits intended for use as food.

The dentition of rabbits differs from that of the rodents in that there are two rows of upper incisors (Table 1). The first pair of upper incisors are the large front teeth. Directly behind them are the tiny peglike secondary incisors. The large single pair of lower incisors should occlude behind the primary upper incisors with the small secondary ones.

Although both maxillary and mandibular prognathism are seen in rabbits, the latter seems to be more common. In animals with this condition, the maxilla is shortened in relation to the mandible. This appears to be an inherited trait, and animals with this defect should not be used as breeding stock. Mandibular prognathism will first manifest itself as an edge-to-edge bite of the lower incisors with the primary upper incisors when the animal is three weeks of age or older. As the discrepancy between the lengths of the mandible and maxilla increases, the lower incisors will completely miss occluding with the primary upper incisors and will grow out in a large arc in front of the animal. Matted hair may accumulate around the base of these teeth and should be removed. The upper primary incisors grow in a smaller arc than the lower ones, and they curl within the mouth or alongside of it. They can pierce the roof of the mouth or the buccal lining, causing tissue trauma, pain, and excessive salivation.

Treatment consists of clipping the incisors with small animal nail trimmers (Resco, TECLA) or wire cutters in such a way as to provide the animal with an occlusion that is as close to normal as possible. It is essential to restrain the rabbit properly during the teeth trimming process (see description for the initial oral exam). If adequate restraint cannot be achieved in this manner, light general anesthesia as described above can be used for the procedure. Care should be taken to hold the trimmer steady as the sliding blade is moved so that the teeth are not snapped off or split. The eyes of attending personnel should be protected from flying tooth fragments. Rough tooth edges can be smoothed with a dental abrasive or file. Occasionally, occlusion approaches normal after the overgrown teeth are trimmed, but usually the teeth need to be trimmed throughout the rest of the animal's life at intervals that vary with the individual rabbit.

In the rabbit, overgrowth of the cheek teeth is much less common than incisor overgrowth. It may be a primary problem or secondary to incisor overgrowth and the associated inability to close the mouth and chew properly. Normal cheek teeth occlude on a level plane. Overgrown cheek teeth occlude unevenly. The lower teeth usually form sharp points on the lingual side, whereas the upper teeth form points on the buccal side. This can be detected with radiographs and by physical examination of the oral cavity, as described above. These overgrown teeth can be trimmed back to a more normal shape with a bone forceps and rongeurs and filed smooth with the animal under general anesthesia. As for overgrown incisors, this procedure may need to be repeated at intervals throughout the animal's life.

Some rabbits will be reluctant to eat for several days after tooth trimming. These animals can be offered soft food such as fresh, washed greens during this period to encourage them to eat.

Malocclusion in the Guinea Pig

Malocclusion in the guinea pig contrasts with that in the rabbit in that it is usually a primary problem

Table 1. *Dental Formulas for Rodents and Rabbits**

Species	Incisors	Canines	Premolars	Molars	Open-rooted Cheek Teeth
Chinchilla	1/1	0/0	1/1	3/3	Yes
Guinea pig	1/1	0/0	1/1	3/3	Yes
Hamster	1/1	0/0	0/0	3/3	No
Mouse	1/1	0/0	0/0	3/3	No
Rat	1/1	0/0	0/0	3/3	No
Rabbit	2/1	0/0	3/2	3/3	Yes

*Key: Number of upper teeth/number of lower teeth.

causing overgrowth of the cheek teeth, with or without secondary overgrowth of the incisors. The most anterior cheek teeth are often the most severely affected. As in the rabbit, the maxillary teeth overgrow on the buccal side, whereas the mandibular teeth overgrow lingually. The sharp tooth edges may injure the oral mucosa and the lower cheek teeth may overgrow until they have formed an arch entrapping the tongue and causing ulceration of its surface. Affected animals become emaciated as their ability to feed becomes impaired, and they may drool excessively because of oral irritation or inability to swallow normally (due to entrapment of the tongue). Food particles and hair may accumulate around the base of the overgrown teeth and gingivitis may develop.

Diagnosis is made, as in the rabbit, by physical examination of the oral cavity with the animal under light anesthesia and by radiography. If possible, the guinea pig should be fasted for 6 hours prior to anesthetic induction so that the mouth will be emptied of food. If this cannot be done, the oral cavity may have to be cleaned out before the cheek teeth can be evaluated. Ketamine (25 to 35 mg/kg) and xylazine (2 to 5 mg/kg) can be given intramuscularly to achieve adequate anesthesia for examination of the mouth.

Temporary correction of the condition may be attempted by trimming the affected teeth as for the rabbit and providing appropriate supportive care. This may include fluid therapy and vitamin C supplementation. The guinea pig has an absolute requirement for this vitamin and may have a deficiency if it has been unable to eat for some time. If a dietary imbalance is implicated as a cause of tooth malformation, it should be identified and corrected.

The causes of cheek teeth malocclusion and overgrowth in the guinea pig are not well defined. Genetic factors may be of importance, since an increased incidence of malocclusion has been seen in some strains and has been eliminated by removing affected animals and their close relatives from the breeding stock. Nutritional factors may also affect the development of teeth and bones. Fluorosis has been associated with deficient tooth development, resulting in both overgrowth and excessive wear of the cheek teeth in guinea pigs. Fluorosis can be differentiated from inherited malocclusion in a number of ways. In cases of fluorosis, animals of all ages are affected and one dental arcade will be overgrown although the opposing arcade will be worn down. The syndrome is also associated with an increased incidence of abortions and stillbirths. Inherited malocclusions generally cause problems in younger animals, in which both upper and lower arcades are overgrown. Other dietary factors, such as imbalances in calcium and phosphorus, may also cause dental malformations. Prevention of malocclusion in guinea pigs may be aided by feeding a properly formulated guinea pig food and by breeding only those animals with normal teeth.

Malocclusion in Other Rodents

Overgrown teeth can also cause problems in other species of rodents, both domestic and wild. In general, diagnosis and treatment are similar to those described for the rabbit and guinea pig.

Incisor overgrowth is seen in rats fed powdered diets. Treatment is to trim the teeth and change to a harder diet if possible. Overgrowth can also occur when opposing teeth are lost or broken, in which case the overgrown tooth is trimmed periodically until the broken tooth grows back in.

Chinchillas and other rodents with open-rooted cheek teeth are susceptible to the overgrowth of these teeth as seen in the guinea pig. In some cases this can be detected by palpating the prominent root projections on the sides of the mandible.

MISCELLANEOUS DENTAL PROBLEMS

Rabbits and rodents occasionally suffer from dental disease not related to malocclusion. They may develop abscesses associated with the teeth, mandible, and surrounding soft tissues. These present as swellings around the face and jaw and may be further delineated radiographically. Treatment by drainage of the abscess and removal of the affected tooth has been only rarely reported and has not been associated with good clinical results. Removal of an open-rooted tooth should not be undertaken lightly, since the root may comprise 80 per cent of the total length of the tooth and extraction creates a malocclusion with the opposing tooth.

Rats and hamsters are susceptible to the development of experimental dental caries. When kept as pets, these animals should not be fed table scraps but should be maintained on a nutritionally balanced rodent diet.

Rodents in laboratory animal facilities may be maintained on water acidified with hydrochloric acid as part of a preventive disease program. This can cause demineralization of the teeth, leading to the excessive erosion of the occlusal surfaces of the molars that is sometimes seen in these animals.

CONCLUSIONS

It is important to consider dental disease in the differential diagnosis when presented with a rabbit or rodent with apparent anorexia and weight loss, with or without ptyalism. Without a timely diagnosis and correction of the conditions described, these animals may die from inanition. The occurrence of major dental problems in rabbits and rodents may be minimized by offering a complete, balanced animal food appropriate for the particular species and by removing animals with heritable dental defects from the breeding stock.

References and Supplemental Reading

Clark, J. O.: Biology and diseases of other rodents. *In* Fox, J. G., Cohen, B. J., and Loew, F. M. (eds.): *Laboratory Animal Medicine*. New York: Academic Press, 1984, pp. 196–197.

Harkness, J. E., and Wagner, J. E.: *The Biology and Medicine of Rabbits and Rodents*. Philadelphia: Lea & Febiger, 1983, pp. 129–130.

Kraus, A. L., Weisbroth, S. H., Flatt, R. E., et al.: Biology and diseases of rabbits. *In* Fox, J. G., Cohen, B. J., and Loew, F. M. (eds.): *Laboratory Animal Medicine*. New York: Academic Press, 1984, p. 234.

Lindsey, J. R., and Fox, R. R.: Inherited diseases and variations. *In* Weisbroth, S. H., Flatt, R. E., and Kraus, A. L. (eds.): *The Biology of the Laboratory Rabbit*. New York: Academic Press, 1974, pp. 383–385.

Rest, J. R., Richards, T., and Ball, S. E.: Malocclusion in inbred strain-2 weanling guinea pigs. Lab. Anim. 16:84, 1982.

Sedgwick, C. J.: Anesthesia for rabbits and rodents. *In* Kirk, R. W. (ed.): *Current Veterinary Therapy VII*. Philadelphia: W. B. Saunders, 1980, pp. 706–710.

Wagner, J. E.: Miscellaneous disease conditions of guinea pigs. *In* Wagner, J. E., and Manning, P. J. (eds.): *The Biology of the Guinea Pig*. New York: Academic Press, 1976, p. 228.

Williams, C. S. F.: *Practical Guide to Laboratory Animals*. St. Louis: C. V. Mosby, 1976, p. 165.

ESTROGEN-INDUCED PANCYTOPENIA IN THE FEMALE EUROPEAN FERRET

THERESA PARROTT, D.V.M.,
and JOHN PARROTT, D.V.M.
Pembroke Park, Florida

The European ferret's small size and ease of maintenance have increased its popularity as a domestic pet. Ferrets kept as companion animals are often maintained as solitary pets.

Female ferrets are induced ovulators. Estrus is indicated by pronounced vulvar swelling. Those females that are not bred or stimulated to ovulate can remain in estrus for a period of time exceeding one year. It has been reported that long periods of high levels of estrogen in the blood can produce bone marrow suppression with pancytopenia. A history of prolonged estrus, together with clinical and laboratory findings, facilitate diagnosis of the disease.

CLINICAL PRESENTATION

A history consistent with the pancytopenic syndrome is that of acute lethargy and anorexia after being "in heat" for 2 or more months. Many times, owners do not relate the presence of vulvar swelling with the onset of estrus. The age of affected ferrets will range from 8 months (the time of sexual maturity) to 7 years. Although most females are maintained as isolated pets, several have had a history of recent (less than 12 months) separation from a male.

On examination, pale mucous membranes may be observed. Ecchymotic or petechial hemorrhages may be evident within the oral mucosa and subcutis. Auscultation frequently reveals a systolic murmur with a weak and rapid femoral pulse. Respiration may be labored, and rectal temperature is usually subnormal. Stools are often dark with a mucoid consistency. Partial or complete alopecia may be evident. Weight loss is a constant finding (Table 1). Hematologic values are always altered (Table 2).

Table 1. Normal Biological Data for Ferrets

Adult Weight (average)	
Male	1360 gm
Female	680 gm
Adult Length	
Male	450–510 cm
Female	350–425 cm
Rectal Temperature	38.8° C
Respiration Rate	33–36/min
Heart Rate	216–242/min

Table 2. *Blood Values for Ferrets*

	Normal Animals	Pancytopenic Animals
PCV (%)	35.0–51.0	4.0–17.0
Total protein (gm/dl)	5.8–7.4	5.5–12.0
Platelets/μl	78,000–500,000	33,000–420,000
WBC/μl	9,000–13,000	2,000–6,900
Segmented cells (%)	65	18–53
Band cells (%)	—	0–7
Lymphocytes (%)	35	33–87
Eosinophils (%)	0	0–7
Monocytes (%)	0	0–1
RBC × 10^6/μl	9.98	1.2–3.0

TREATMENT

Frequently an animal is presented as a critical care emergency. Treatment for hypothermia and dehydration are first and foremost. A small animal incubator is ideal for a rapid increase in environmental temperature, but if an incubator is not available, heating pads or thermal water units can be used.

An intravenous catheter is used whenever possible. In anemic animals, development of hematomas is common. Catheter placement sites in order of ease of access are lateral saphenous, cephalic, and jugular veins. Hematomas, body structure (short limbs and neck), and an anemic condition often require the use of cut-down techniques. Once a catheter is placed, a warmed lactated Ringer's solution is started at a slow drip. Intravenous prednisolone sodium succinate (Solu-Delta Cortef, Upjohn; 7 to 35 mgs) can be given to help counteract shock. If tranquilization is needed for catheter insertion and fluid administration, ketamine hydrochloride (Ketaset, Bristol Laboratories) can be given at a dosage of 10 to 30 mg/kg intramuscularly or subcutaneously.

Blood is collected for a packed cell volume (PCV), total protein, and complete blood count (CBC). If the PCV is less than 10 per cent (as in most cases presented), a ferret blood donor is found. A male ferret is used whenever possible, as the body size of the male (twice that of the female) will allow for a larger volume of whole blood to be collected for transfusion. The donor animal is anesthesized with ketamine hydrochloride (20 to 40 mg/kg). The jugular vein is the site of choice for blood collection. The ventral neck is clipped and surgically prepared. A 20-gauge needle is used on a heparin-coated, 20- or 30-ml syringe. The amount of blood to be collected for transfusion is calculated by using the formula in Table 3.

Transfusion is best done immediately after blood is collected. Blood should be transfused at the rate of 0.25 to 0.5 ml/min. An increase of 4 to 10 per cent is desired in the post-transfusion PCV. The intravenous catheter should be maintained while the ferret is recovering and stabilizing from the presenting crisis. Antibiotics are started to guard against opportunistic bacterial pathogens.

The problem of elevated blood estrogen levels over the long term with bone marrow suppression must be taken into account and corrected. Current therapies for estrus termination include surgery, the use of human chorionic gonadotropin (HCG), or both treatments. Results with the latter are not predictable. Of the ferrets treated with the recommended dose of 50 to 100 IU intramuscularly of HCG, over 65 per cent remained in estrus. Signs of estrus remission may take up to 30 days to occur. An increased incidence of hair loss is also noted after use of injectable HCG. Hair loss does not coincide with ovulation; on the contrary, the animal will often remain in estrus.

Surgery (ovariohysterectomy) is the authors' treatment of choice. Once the hematocrit of the transfused animal has reached 11 per cent or greater and its vital signs are stable, the ferret is reevaluated for surgery. Once a decision is made to proceed with surgery, the objective is to minimize the time required for anesthesia and surgery.

The ferret is anesthesized with ketamine hydrochloride at a dose of 20 to 40 mg/kg and prepared for surgery. During surgery, the patient is maintained on methoxyflurane (Metofane, Pitman-Moore) and oxygen. A ventral midline approach is used and care is taken to expose sufficient uterine tissue to allow ligature of the uterine body just anterior to the cervix. Speed with minimal tissue trauma is most desired.

During postsurgical recovery, it is important to monitor the patient's temperature. Fatalities due to hypothermia from extended surgical procedures are common in this species.

After surgery, the ferret's PCV may drop 3 to 7 per cent over 24 to 48 hours. If the decrease in hematocrit is greater than 7 per cent or vital signs deteriorate, another transfusion may be indicated. Using the same donor for serial transfusions has posed no problem in past experiences. If available, a new donor should be used for any additional transfusions.

Postsurgical anorexia may require forced feeding of a high-calorie, vitamin-mineral supplement. Zu/Preem monkey chow (Hill's Pet Products) with either BVMO (Burns-Biotec) or Nutrical (Evsco) is ideal. Feeding may be done by syringe or gastric tube. Feedings of 10 to 25 ml, three to four times

Table 3. *Calculations for Volume of Blood to be Transfused*

(A) Total blood volume = 75 ml/kg × recipient's weight
(B) RBC (mass) = (A) × PCV of recipient
(C) RBC (desired mass) = (A) × PCV desired
(D) RBC (required) = (C) − (B)
(E) Blood volume (required) = (D) ÷ PCV of the donor

daily are continued until the patient begins to eat. Antibiotics are continued for up to 10 days after surgery. Steroids are not recommended. For 10 to 14 days after surgery, blood samples are taken every 48 to 72 hours. If the animal is discharged, the owners are instructed to bring the patient back at least once a week for continued monitoring of the blood. If the ferret's PCV begins to decline, the patient is placed on an intravenous drip. A high percentage of these animals will need repeated transfusions of whole blood once a decline in PCV is observed. As many as 18 transfusions have been accomplished in the same patient with success. Time between transfusions has been as little as 3 days to as long as 4 weeks. Rejuvenation of the bone marrow is correlated with the length of estrus and the peripheral blood values of the presenting patient.

If the patient recovers from surgery, the prognosis for full recovery is greatly increased, even when serial blood transfusions are necessary. The survival rate of the pancytopenic animal will vary with the animal's age, the duration of estrus prior to treatment, and the degree of bone marrow suppression. Ferrets that present with secondary bacterial infections or renal impairment (or both) warrant a less favorable prognosis. Most fatalities occur within the first 48 hours after presentation and directly after surgery. Bone marrow aspirates on these ferrets are not routinely performed, but an aspirate may help the clinician develop a clearer picture of the response anticipated with medical treatment or surgery.

PREVENTION

It is recommended that the owners of female ferrets have their pets spayed as soon as maturity is reached and estrus is observed.

References and Supplemental Reading

Bernard, S. L., Leathers, C. W., Brobst, D. F., et al.: Estrogen-induced bone marrow depression in ferrets. Am. J. Vet. Res. 44:657, 1983.

Kociba, G. J., and Caputo, C. A.: Aplastic anemia associated with estrus in pet ferrets. J.A.V.M.A. 178:1293, 1981.

Ryland, L. M.: Remission of estrus-associated anemia following ovario-hysterectomy and multiple blood transfusions in a ferret. J.A.V.M.A. 181:820, 1982.

Hammond, J., Jr., and Chesterman, F. C.: *U.F.A.W. Handbook*. Baltimore, MD: Williams & Wilkins, 1982.

Wallach, J. D., and Boever, W. J.: *Diseases of Exotic Animals*. Philadelphia: W. B. Saunders, 1983.

PHYSICAL RESTRAINT AND SEXING TECHNIQUES IN SMALL MAMMALS AND REPTILES

NANCY KOCK, D.V.M.,
and MICHAEL KOCK, B. VET. MED.
Davis, California

FERRETS

Ferrets, like dogs and cats, are members of the order Carnivora, and share some of the characteristics common to these more usual pets. They belong to the family Mustelidae, having long bodies, long tails, and short legs. Their anal glands are well developed, and their secretions may make the adult males, in particular, unacceptable house pets.

Pet ferrets are usually used to handling and, unless agitated, will not bite. Gloves can be used for difficult animals, or they can be grasped around the thorax with a thumb underneath the chin, controlling the mandible (Fig. 1).

Sexing of ferrets is quite easy. The males, or hobs, usually weigh two to three times more than the females, and, like dogs, they have a penis located on the caudal ventral abdomen. Both sexes experience atrophy of the reproductive organs after the breeding season each year and subsequent hypertrophy at the beginning of the next season.

RABBITS

Rabbits belong to the order Lagomorpha; there are over 100 breeds recognized by the American Rabbit Breeders' Association. Pet rabbits, used to

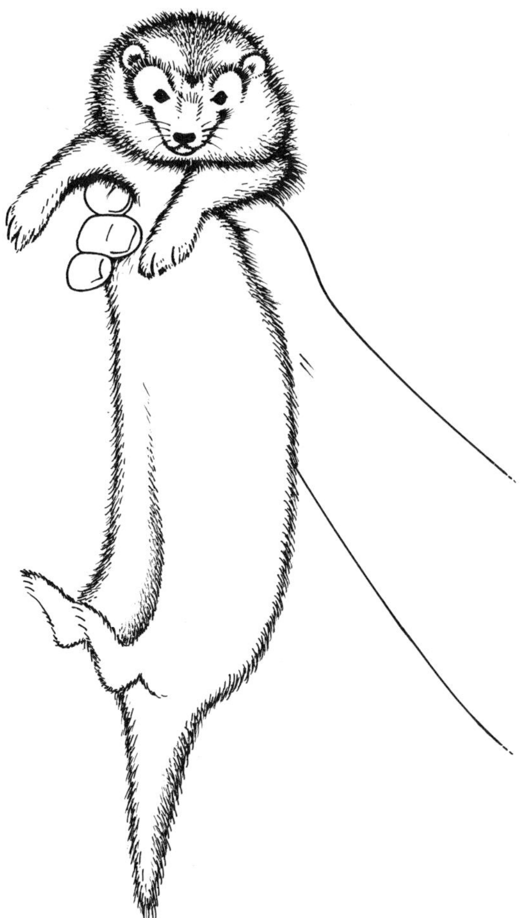

Figure 1. Proper restraint of a ferret.

handling, usually present few problems to veterinarians, but those raised in colonies for meat or fur can be quite difficult to restrain. Care should always be taken to ensure that the hindquarters are well supported when rabbits are carried, for nervous animals often kick with their powerful back legs in escape attempts, which can result in broken backs. The skeleton of the rabbit comprises 7 per cent of its total body weight. This, along with the well-muscled back legs, makes for an unfortunate combination in captive situations, rendering the lumbar spine especially vulnerable to trauma. Even when caged, extremely agitated rabbits have been known to break their own backs.

Rabbits can be firmly grasped by the scruff of the neck and then lifted enough to support the body under the rump with the other hand (Fig. 2). When they are to be carried for distance, they can be held close to the body with the head tucked between the handler's arm and body; again the posterior end is supported with the other hand.

Sexing young rabbits can be done by applying gentle pressure around the genital orifice and everting the genitalia with the thumbs while the animal is held in a cupped hand on its back. The penis will protrude in the male, or buck, equally all the way around. In the female, or doe, the vulva will only protrude anteriorly, and will become a slit at its posterior end. Adult males have obvious

Table 1. *Reproductive Information on Ferrets*

Lifespan	Record: 13 years
Gestation	41 days
Litter size	5 to 15; average, 8
Weaning	6 weeks
Breeding	March through August in the Northern Hemisphere
Sexual characteristics	Male: 1350–2700 gm body weight; penis present on ventral abdomen Female: 450–900 gm body weight

Table 2. *Reproductive Information on Rabbits*

Lifespan	5–10 years
Gestation	30–32 days
Litter size	Average, 8; depends on breed
Weaning	6–8 weeks
Breeding	Year-round, with decreases in production during the fall and winter
Sexual characteristics	Male: Eversion of penis: adults have hairless inguinal pouches Female: Slitlike vulva

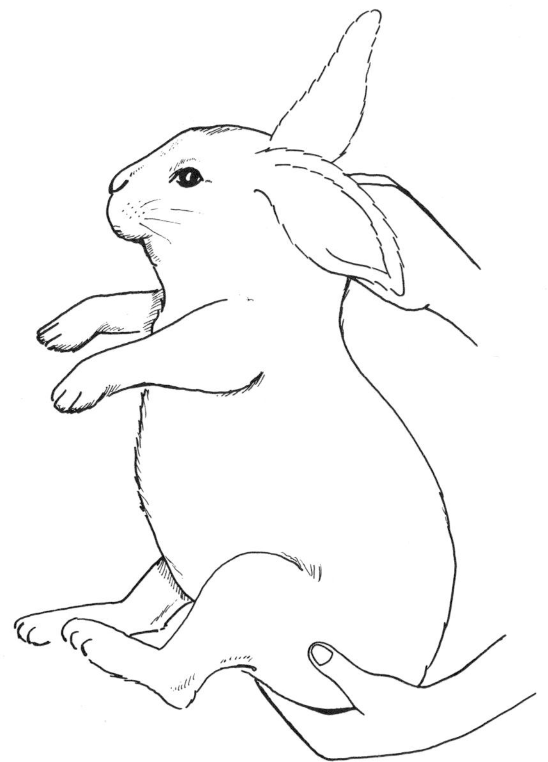

Figure 2. Proper restraint of a rabbit.

hairless inguinal pouches, even though the testicles may not be visible; they can be drawn up into the abdomen through the open inguinal ring. Again, with proper restraint, the penis can be extruded if the sex of the animal is in question.

RODENTS

Rats, mice, and gerbils can all be restrained similarly. By grasping the base of the tail with one hand and elevating the rear legs (preferably on a rough surface so the animal will attempt to hold with its forelegs), the handler can lift the rear legs, forming an angle of about 45 degrees from the table (Fig. 3). The scruff of the neck can be grasped with the other hand (see Fig. 7). Care should be taken so that the animal does not turn and bite. Gerbils usually do not bite but may have seizures with handling. These are quite common, have a genetic basis, and are not life-threatening. Rats and mice, however, very often try to bite when restrained, and with large rats an alternative hold may be preferred. They can be grasped in a manner similar to holding a ferret, with the fingers around the thorax and the thumb underneath the chin (Fig. 1).

Rats, mice, and gerbils can all be successfully sexed by comparing the anogenital distances between males and females (Fig. 4). The males consistently have longer distances. In gerbils this distance in the male is approximately 10 mm and only 5 mm in the female. In rats and mice it is usually twice as long in males as it is in females.

Guinea pigs rarely bite but may get excited in a veterinary clinic and run off the end of the examining table. They can easily be handled but seem to resent being grasped by the scruff of the neck. Instead, they can be grasped around the thorax and lifted. Care should be taken to support the rear quarters, especially of larger or pregnant animals (Fig. 5).

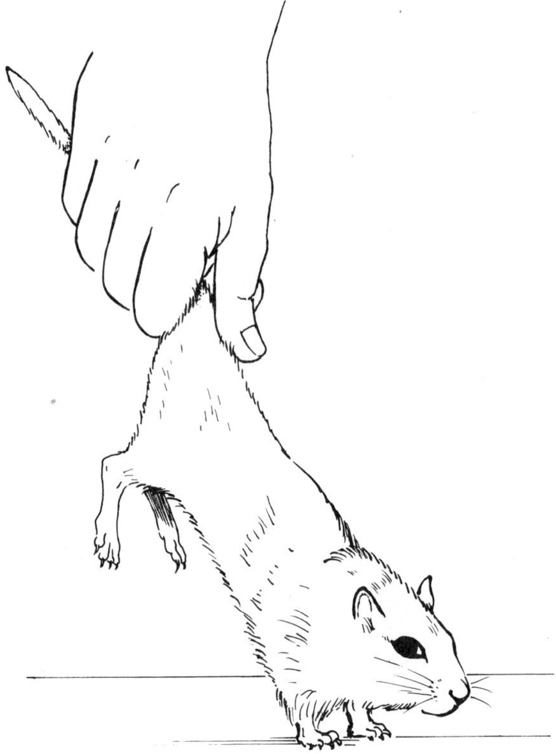

Figure 3. When restraint of a mouse, gerbil, or rat is attempted, the base of the animal's tail should be grasped and its hind quarters lifted off the table. The scruff of the neck can then be more easily grasped for full restraint (see Fig. 7).

Sexing guinea pigs is not as straightforward as in other rodents, as there is no significant difference between the anogenital distances of males and females. The genital opening of the female is a Y-shaped fold of skin, whereas that of the male is a slit (Fig. 6). Testes can usually be palpated in adult males, and in even the youngest males the penis can be extruded with gentle digital pressure around the genital orifice.

Table 3. *Reproductive Information on Rodents*

	Lifespan	Gestation	Litter Size	Sexual Characteristics
Chinchilla	Up to 16 years	105–115 days	Average, 2	Anogenital distance is twice as long in males; females have a large cone-shaped genital papilla; females are usually larger
Guinea pig	6–8 years	59–72 days (depends on litter size)	2 to 6	Female genital opening is Y-shaped; male opening is a slit; penis can be extruded in the male
Hamster	2–3 years	16 days	5 to 10	Female is often larger; male has large testicles that make the tail appear rounded; female's tail is more pointed
Gerbil	2–4 years	22–26 days	4 to 5	Anogenital distance is longer in males
Mouse	1–2 years	20 days*	5 to 10	
Rat	2–3 years	22 days*	Average, 9	

*Longer gestations occur when females conceive on the postpartum estrus, which results in delayed implantation.

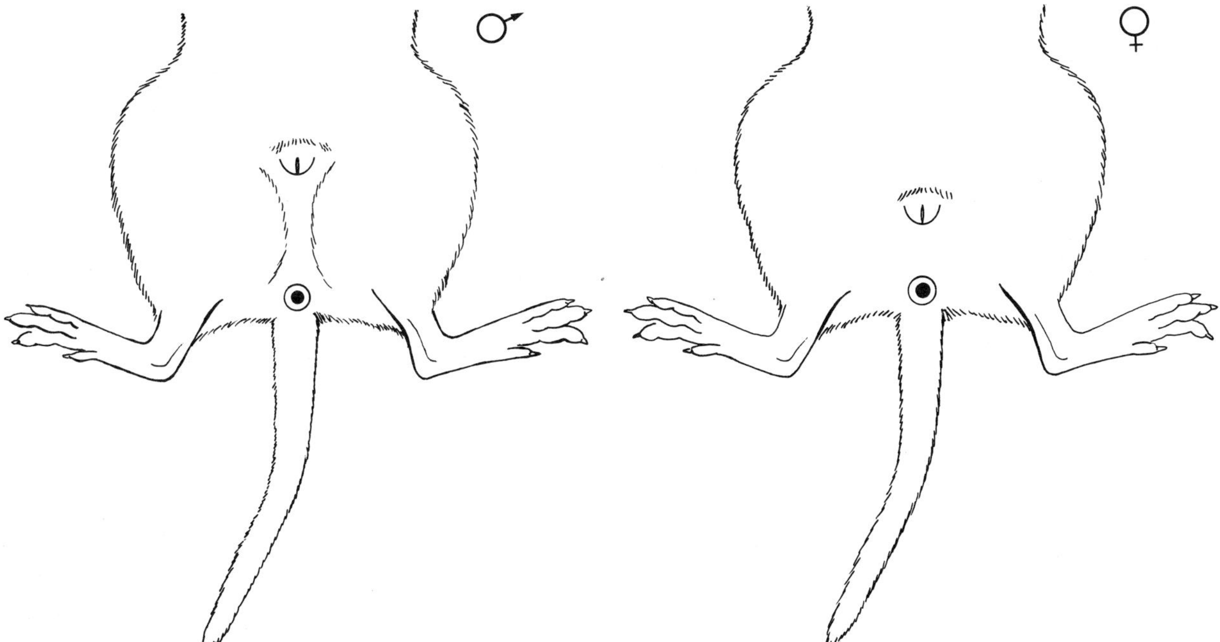

Figure 4. The anogenital distance can be used as a reliable measure for sexing mice, rats, gerbils, hamsters, and chinchillas. The distance in the male is generally twice that in the female.

Hamsters can be difficult to restrain and will bite, especially if disturbed while sleeping. They have an abundance of loose skin around the scruff of the neck. If this skin is not gathered into the handler's hand sufficiently, the animal can still turn and bite even while being held by the scruff (Fig. 7).

Sexing hamsters is again based upon a longer anogenital distance in the male. One can also compare the perineal margins of hamsters placed in dorsal recumbency. The males have more rounded margins, owing to the presence of the scrotal sacs, whereas those of the females are more pointed and the tails are more prominent (Fig. 8). Females, in general, also tend to be larger.

Chinchillas rarely bite but may urinate when excited. They can be grasped in the same way as the guinea pig and restrained (Fig. 5), or they can be lifted by the tail and onto the opposite forearm of the handler (Fig. 9).

Table 4. *Sexual Characteristics of Snakes*

Male	Female
Paired hemipenes	
Tail is evenly tapered from cloaca to tip	Tail narrows abruptly at cloaca and remains so to tip.
Large spurs occur on either side of the cloaca of the boa constrictor	Spurs, if present, are smaller
Probe may be inserted into paracloacal sinus to a depth of 7 to 12 scales	Probe may be inserted into paracloacal sinus to a depth of only 3 to 5 scales

Sexing chinchillas can be challenging, for the females have a large cone-shaped urogenital papilla that resembles a penis. The vagina is closed except during estrus and is therefore not conspicuous. Testicles cannot be palpated in the males as they are inguinal, not scrotal. The most reliable method

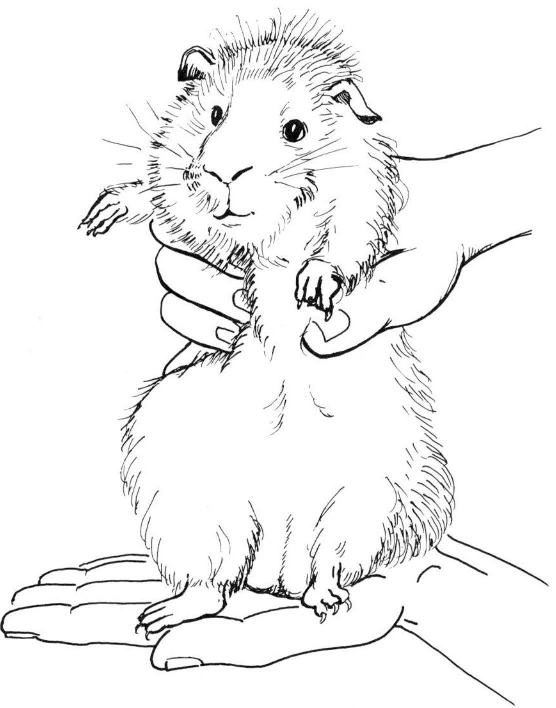

Figure 5. Proper restraint of a guinea pig.

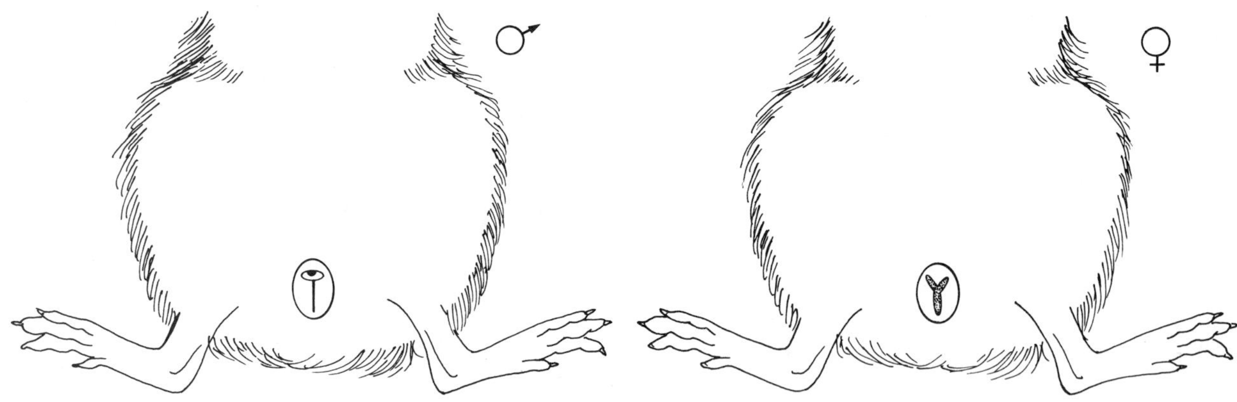

Figure 6. The anogenital distance is not a reliable marker for sexing guinea pigs. In the female the genitalia appear as a Y-shaped fold, whereas in the male they form a slit. Gentle digital pressure around the male genitalia is usually successful in everting the penis.

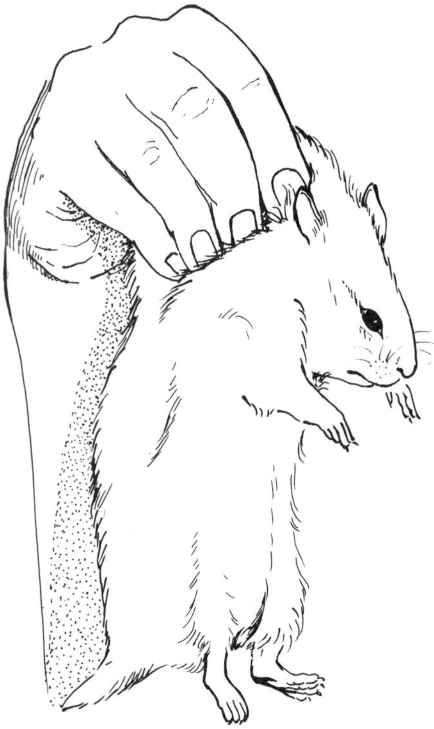

Figure 7. Proper restraint of rats, mice, and hamsters. When hamsters are restrained, it is important to gather the abundant amount of skin in the region of the scruff to avoid being bitten.

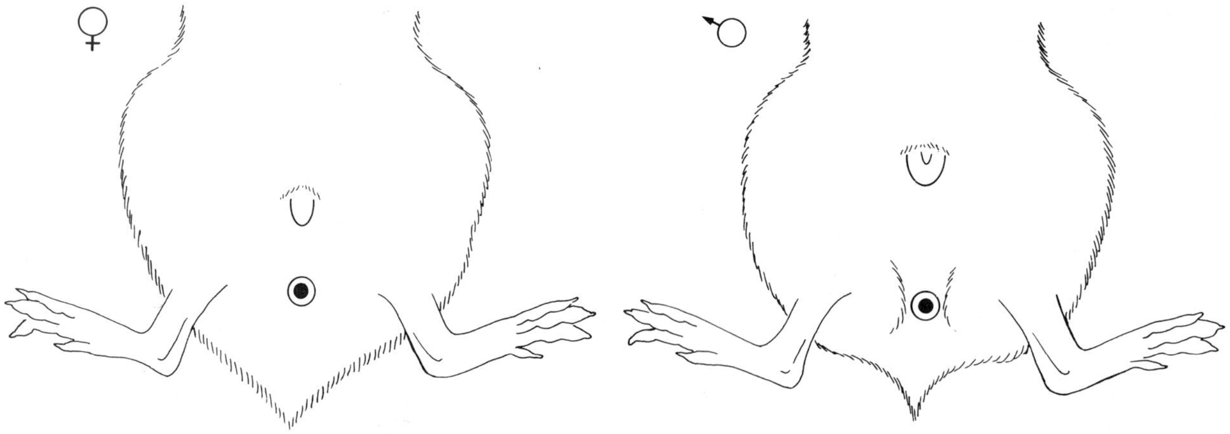

Figure 8. In hamsters the anogenital distance in the male is usually twice that in the female. The scrotal sac in the male gives a rounded appearance to the perineal region; in the female it is more pointed.

Table 5. Sexual Characteristics of Lizards

Male	Female
Often more highly colored, especially during breeding season	
Often body size is larger	Body size is smaller
Femoral glands are present on caudoventral aspect of thigh (green iguana).	If present, femoral glands are less prominent
Some species have dimorphism (male Jackson chameleon has three rostral horns)	

for sexing these animals is by comparing the anogenital distance, which is usually twice as long in males as it is in females.

REPTILES

Reptiles require careful and specialized handling techniques. These animals can be dangerous; they vary from extremely venomous snakes to large constrictors and from snapping turtles to long-clawed lizards. A knowledge of basic handling techniques should be refined by all practitioners who expect to encounter these varied creatures of the animal world.

When sexing these animals it is important to be aware that the ovaries and testes are internal organs. It is often difficult to distinguish their sex by superficial examination, but the evaluation of certain characteristics will help the practitioner in determining the sex of these animals.

SNAKES

Handling constrictor snakes usually requires two people, depending on the size of the snake. It is essential to maintain a firm grip behind the head while supporting the snake's body (Fig. 10*A*). Venomous snakes should be handled by using a snake noose around the base of the neck or by transferring the snake into a clear plastic tube (Fig. 10*B*). Once its head is in the tube, the snake can be coaxed forward until one half of the snake is in the tube; the handler holds the tube and snake with the same hand. It is important to ensure that the tube is small enough in diameter to prevent the snake from turning around. If necessary, general anesthesia may be attempted by using ketamine hydrochloride at 50 to 100 mg/kg intramuscularly. The ambient temperature should be maintained relatively constant, between 75 to 85° F, throughout the procedure and during recovery.

Sexing of snakes is best accomplished by inserting a probe into the paracloacal sinuses. A blunt-ended metal probe (40 to 60 mm long and 1 to 2 mm in diameter) can be gently manipulated into the paracloacal sinuses (Fig. 11). The insertion is continued caudally, and in the male snake the probe can be inserted at least two to three times the depth achieved in the female. In the male, this depth represents the inverted hemipenes, and in the female, these sinuses are short and nonfunctional.

LIZARDS

When handling lizards, one should not attempt to grasp them by the tail. They should be grasped with two hands; one holds the animal firmly behind the head with the fingers controlling the front legs, and the other holds the lizard similarly around the abdomen with the fingers controlling the hind legs. This will prevent the lizard from biting, using its claws to scratch the handler, and whipping its tail. Gloves can be used when larger species are handled.

Sexing of lizards is often difficult, and laparoscopy has been utilized in some species.

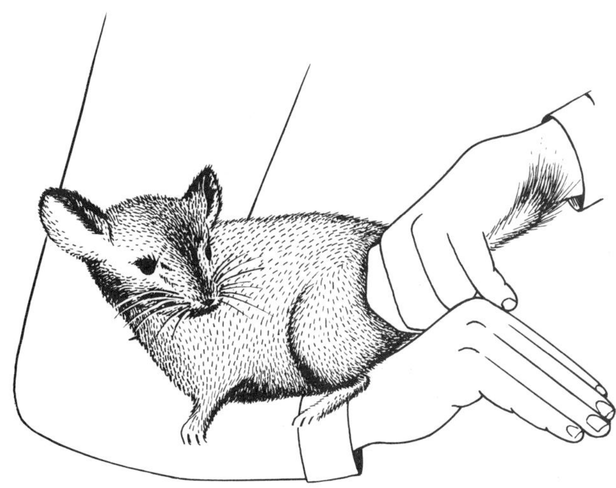

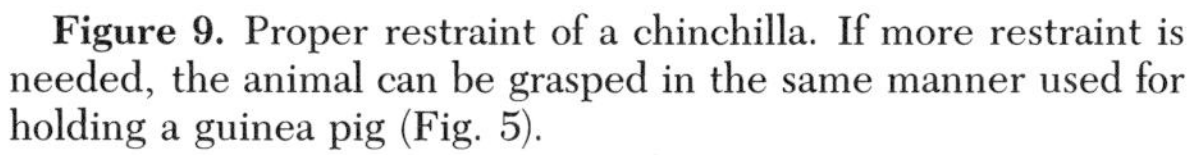

Figure 9. Proper restraint of a chinchilla. If more restraint is needed, the animal can be grasped in the same manner used for holding a guinea pig (Fig. 5).

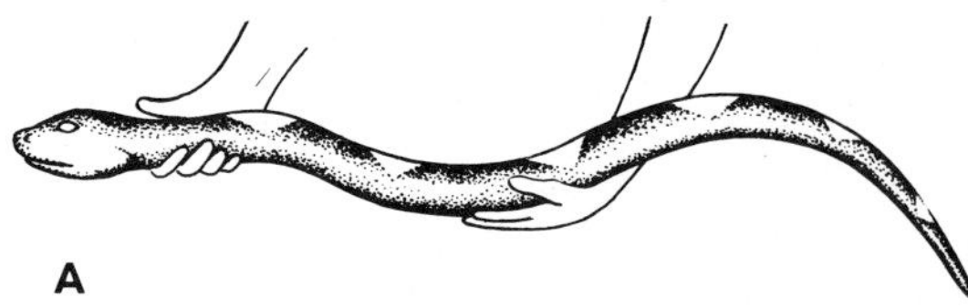

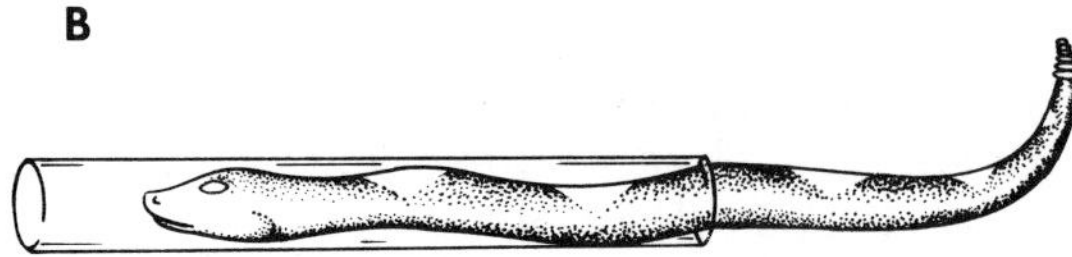

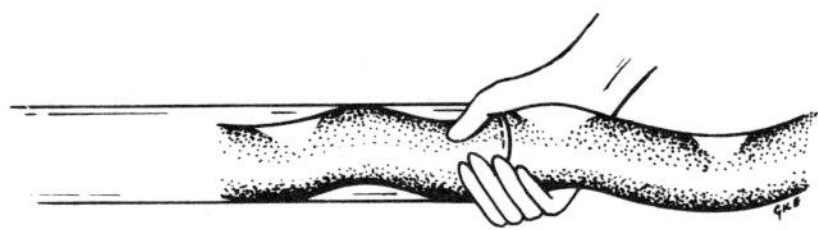

Figure 10. *A*, Proper restraint for a constrictor snake. *B*, A venomous snake should first be restrained with a snake noose or transferred to a clear plastic tube. One hand should be used to hold both the body of the snake and the tube.

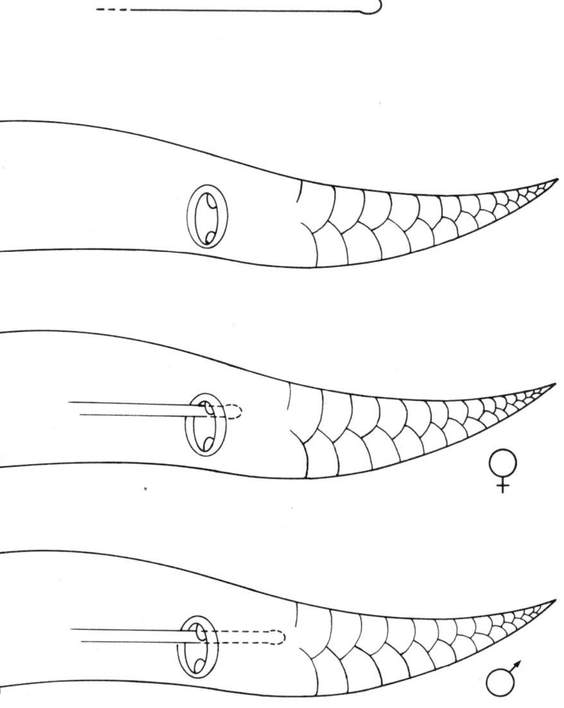

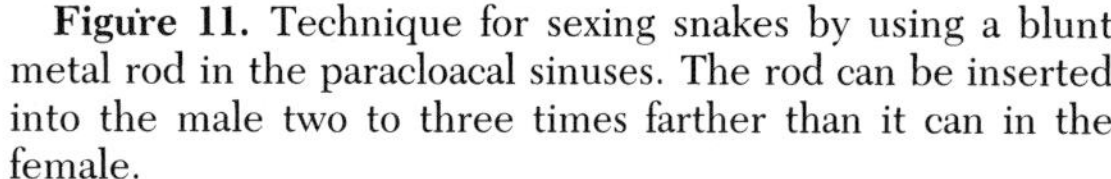

Figure 11. Technique for sexing snakes by using a blunt metal rod in the paracloacal sinuses. The rod can be inserted into the male two to three times farther than it can in the female.

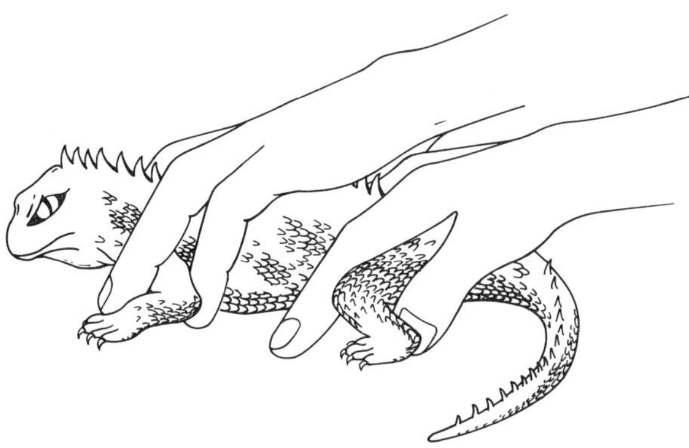

Figure 12. Proper restraint of a lizard. Both hands are used to grasp the lizard; one restrains the head and front legs, and the other holds the rear legs and tail.

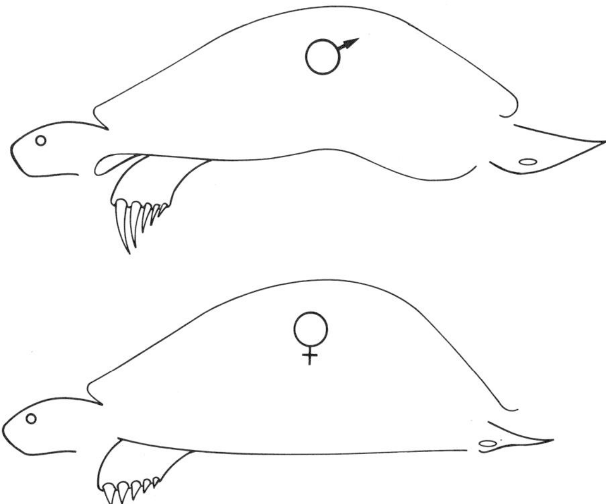

Figure 13. Schematic drawing of the prominent anatomical features in male and female turtles and tortoises. These differences are summarized in Table 6. The difference in the plastron pertains to tortoises only.

TURTLES AND TORTOISES

Turtles and tortoises can be handled by holding the plastron and carapace with two hands and rolling the animal into ventral or sternal recumbency.

***Table 6.** Sexual Characteristics of Tortoises and Turtles*

Male	Female
Tortoises have concave plastrons (Fig. 13), and the anterior gular projection of plastron may be well developed and scooplike in shape	Relatively flat plastron
Male box tortoises have red irises	Irises are brown
In both tortoises and turtles the tail length is longer, broader, and less tapered	Tails are narrower, shorter, and more tapered
In tortoises and turtles the cloacal opening is more posterior	
In turtles the claws are longer, especially on the front legs	

Turtles tend to be more aggressive than tortoises, and more care needs to be taken to avoid being bitten. Snapping turtles in particular can be dangerous to handlers, and small specimens can be manipulated by the tail.

The sexing techniques for turtles and tortoises are summarized in Table 6 and Figure 13.

References and Supplemental Reading

Fowler, M. E.: *Restraint and Handling of Wild and Domestic Animals.* Ames, IA: Iowa State University Press, 1978.

Fowler, M. E. (ed.): *Zoo and Wild Animal Medicine,* 1st ed. Philadelphia: W.B. Saunders, 1978.

Frye, F. L.: *Biomedical and Surgical Aspects of Captive Reptile Husbandry.* Edwardsville, KS: Veterinary Medical Publishing, 1981.

Harkness, J., and Wagner, J.: *The Biology and Medicine of Rabbits and Rodents.* Philadelphia: Lea & Febiger, 1978.

Marcus, L. C.: *Veterinary Biology and Medicine of Captive Amphibians and Reptiles.* Philadelphia: Lea & Febiger, 1981.

Williams, C.: *Practical Guide to Laboratory Animals.* St. Louis: C.V. Mosby, 1976.

PREVENTIVE MEDICAL CARE FOR THE PET FERRET

R. WAYNE RANDOLPH, V.M.D.
Flemington, New Jersey

The domestic ferret (*Mustela putorius furo*) is a fun-loving, gregarious member of the family Mustelidae that has become increasingly popular as a household pet. For some time it has been commonly employed as an important laboratory animal. In some states the keeping of ferrets is prohibited, whereas in others there are laws regulating the possession of these animals. It is prudent to review state statutes before obtaining such a pet.

Female ferrets (called jills) are seasonally polyestrus and induced ovulators. Males (called hobs) are not sexually active year-round, but vary in their sexual activity according to the photoperiod. The domestic ferret exists only in captivity and is not a wild animal. Two color varieties are recognized: the fitch ferret is buff with a black mask, tail, and limbs; the albino ferret is white with pink eyes.

This article describes some medical, surgical, and husbandry practices that will help to keep the ferret both well and a good pet.

VACCINATIONS

Canine Distemper

Ferrets are highly susceptible to canine distemper; virtually 100 per cent of positive cases die. Protection against this disease is afforded by vaccination with a modified live virus of chicken embryo origin. Vaccines developed from ferret cell cultures are to be rigidly avoided, as incomplete attenuation can lead to clinical disease with canine distemper. A killed virus vaccine of high antigenicity, developed by new techniques, might be preferred over the modified live virus product, but it is not currently available.

First vaccination is administered at 6 to 10 weeks of age or at first presentation, which, in clinical practice, tends to be about 10 to 14 weeks of age (Table 1). A second dose is administered 3 to 4 weeks later; yearly boosters are given thereafter.

Panleukopenia

To date panleukopenia has not been reported to occur in the ferret. For this reason most clinicians choose not to vaccinate against this disease.

Another group, however, chooses to vaccinate against this disease for the following reasons: (1) it seems phylogenetically peculiar that the ferret is the only mustelid unsusceptible to panleukopenia, and (2) vaccination against panleukopenia may provide immunity against infection with parvovirus (if this disease occurs in the ferret). For those opting to vaccinate, a killed vaccine of feline cell origin is used according to the same regimen as for canine distemper vaccination (Table 1).

Rabies

Although rare, rabies has been reported to occur in the ferret. The use of rabies vaccine in ferrets

***Table 1.** Schedule for Vaccination and Examination of Ferrets*

Age	Procedure
6 to 10 weeks (or first presentation)	First CDV* First PV† (optional) Fecal exam Physical exam Husbandry consultation
10 to 14 weeks (3 to 4 weeks after first presentation)	Second CDV Second PV (optional) Physical exam Husbandry review
4½ to 6 months	Spaying or castration Descenting Rabies vaccine‡ (optional) Fecal exam
15 months (1 year after second CDV)	CDV (annual) PV (annual, optional) Rabies vaccine (annual; optional) Fecal exam Physical exam

*Canine distemper vaccine; modified live virus of chicken embryo cell origin; administered subcutaneously

†Panleukopenia vaccine; killed virus of feline cell origin; delivered subcutaneously

‡Killed vaccine of murine origin; delivered intramuscularly

remains controversial because labeling does not support its use in this species. When used, only a killed virus product should be selected, preferably of murine origin. Under no circumstance should a live virus product be used. Vaccinations are at 3 to 6 months of age and yearly thereafter.

PARASITES

Dirofilariasis

Dirofilariasis has been reported to occur both naturally and experimentally in the ferret. Microfilaremia is uncommon, as is the case in other abnormal hosts infected with *Dirofilaria immitis*. Ferrets infected with *D. immitis* may present in respiratory distress secondary to congestive heart failure.

The scope of this problem is not fully appreciated at present. In enzootic areas of *D. immitis*, it seems reasonable to consider the use of a prophylactic medication. Diethylcarbamazine at the standard canine dosage (2.5 mg/0.45 kg) might be employed in these enzootic areas.

Ear Mites

Infestation with ear mites (*Otodectes cynotis*) is a particularly common malady of ferrets, especially kits obtained from a commercial source. Diagnosis is straightforward; brown, waxy debris is observed in the opening of the external ear canal. The veterinarian should confirm the presence of mites with an otoscope or examine some waxy debris microscopically. Head shaking and ear scratching are *uncommon* signs of ear mite infestation in the ferret.

Commercial feline preparations for ear mites can be employed safely. Treatment, however, must be diligent. Treatment failure is common and typically occurs for the following reasons: (1) the patient squirms and resists treatment, (2) the small diameter of the ear canal precludes easy application of the preparation along the canal's length, and (3) the ferret's body is not treated. Good client instruction will help to circumvent these problems. The whole body of the ferret should be treated with an appropriate flea product. A combination of thiabendazole, dexamethasone, and neomycin (Tresaderm, Merck, Sharp & Dohme) has proved a successful ear mite preparation.

Fleas

Fleas (*Ctenocephalides* spp.) can present a problem, especially when ferrets are housed with dogs and cats. The veterinarian should check regularly for these parasites as one would on a dog or cat.

Table 2. *Ferret Anesthetic Regimen*

Drug	Dosage	Route of Administration
Acepromazine	0.2–0.5 mg/kg	Intramuscular, subcutaneous
Ketamine*	20–35 mg/kg	Intramuscular
Halothane	To effect, if needed	Face mask

*Administered with or shortly after the acepromazine

Moderate scratching is normal in the ferret and does not by itself constitute a diagnosis of flea infestation. Those flea products safe for use on cats may be used on the ferret.

The wearing of a prescription, feline flea collar can be an effective prophylactic measure. One standard cat collar will yield three ferret collars. A cat flea collar can be cut into thirds, one of these pieces is held around the ferret's neck, and the ends are sewn together with needle and thread. Most but not all ferrets will leave these collars on.

SURGERY

Two prophylactic procedures, neutering and descenting, are commonly practiced in the pet ferret. Hobs are castrated in order to decrease aggression, inappropriate urination, and body odor. Jills are spayed to avoid pregnancy, false pregnancy, and pancytopenia during estrus and to reduce body odor. Both genders are descented to help alleviate body odor.

Ferrets are robust anesthetic and surgical patients. Multiple anesthetic regimens have been described. The one depicted in Table 2 has proved safe, easy, and efficacious. Acepromazine and ketamine are administered together; halothane delivered by face mask is used only if needed. To curb loss of body heat, a heating pad is always employed. Leg restraints are easily fashioned from ½-inch surgical adhesive tape.

Ferrets usually reach sexual maturity in the first spring after their birth; hence, they become sexually active at different ages. Neutering is safely performed at 5 months of age but may be performed either earlier or later.

In order to be spayed, jills are placed in dorsal recumbency and, after a ventral midline incision is made, standard canine and feline procedure is followed. Castration of hobs is performed according to closed, standard canine procedure. Small sutures should be made with material of sizes 3–0 and 4–0.

Descenting, or surgical removal of the paired musk-producing glands lateral to the anus, is always performed *after* the neutering operation to preserve the sterility of the instruments. Many procedures have been described, but the author prefers the closed technique as used for standard excision of canine anal sacs. The veterinarian should not attempt to inject the glands with contrast material as the duct openings are too small.

HOUSING

Appropriate and adequate housing is necessary to promote good health and to avoid husbandry problems. Although outdoor housing is acceptable, most owners prefer to house their pets indoors.

Within the home a cage is required. How much time the pet is held in this cage remains a personal decision on the part of the owner; however, most ferrets are caged at least during the night. Such a cage ought to be constructed of impermeable material to avoid the absorption and retention of odors. Ideal materials include plastic, fiberglass, and metal mesh; a sliding bottom tray for cleaning is helpful. A small bed for sleeping is kept within the cage; it can be a small box, towel, or blanket. Without a bed a ferret will sleep in its litter.

Ferrets are easily trained to use a litter box and one box should be maintained in the cage and at least one other within the home. Any small plastic container will do. The bottom of the litter box must be weighted to avoid spillage, and the box should always be placed in a corner.

In order to maintain a ferret's safety, the owner's home must be "ferret-proofed." These small mustelids can easily crawl through an aperture 2 inches in diameter, so attention should be given to the bottom of appliances (stove, refrigerator, washer), spaces around plumbing and pipes, and openings into the walls. Without this attention, ferrets will be lost.

DIET

Nutritional requirements have not been determined for this carnivore. Experience, however, has shown they do well on a diet of high-quality, commercial cat food. Dry or canned food may be fed, and table scraps can be added in small amounts. The author prefers to feed a diet of dry food only, because it aids in preventing the buildup of dental calculus and the development of subsequent periodontal disease.

Young ferrets (6 months of age and younger) are given free access to food. Adults are fed twice daily to avert obesity, which can occur in later life. The owner should be aware that these creatures tend to relocate and cache their food, which can present a particular problem with canned food and table scraps.

Water must be always available. If a water bowl is used, it should have a weighted bottom to prevent spillage by these active, messy eaters. The hanging water bottle of the rabbit or hamster type, which is less messy, is preferred.

Bones of all types are avoided to prevent gastrointestinal blockage. A dry, brittle hair coat with dry, scaly skin, occurring especially during the cold months, may necessitate the addition of small amounts of saturated and unsaturated fatty acids to the diet. Commercial preparations (e.g., Nutriderm, Norden) are useful for this purpose.

CARE

When a ferret is chosen, one should obtain a young kit (aged 5 to 6 weeks), preferably from a breeder who selects for good temperament. Ferrets get along well with dogs, cats, birds, and other animals, providing they have become accustomed to these other animals. Households with ferrets tend to keep more than one; two is probably the ideal minimum.

Claws may be trimmed by using either a human or animal nail trimmer. A thin, lightweight pet collar (cut-down cat collar) with an identification tag and bell is useful. The attached bell aids in locating the ferret. Most but not all ferrets will tolerate these collars.

Ferrets are susceptible to infection with a number of strains of human influenza virus. The disease is nonfatal, and the treatment is symptomatic. It might be wise not to handle pet ferrets when human family members suffer with this problem.

If keeping a pet ferret can be said to have one drawback, it is the animal's body odor. Three sources contribute to this odor: (1) the gonads, (2) the paired scent glands adjacent to the anus, and (3) sebaceous glands in the skin. Odor from the first two sources is eliminated surgically, whereas bathing helps to dissipate odor emanating from the skin. Ferrets are bathed easily and as needed (up to 1 to 2 times per week). A mild baby shampoo should be selected; dandruff and herbal shampoos should be avoided.

References and Supplemental Reading

Ryland, L. M., and Gorham, J. R.: The ferret and its diseases. J.A.V.M.A 173:1154, 1978.

Ryland, L. M., Bernard, S. L., and Gorham, J. R.: A clinical guide to the pet ferret. Comp. Cont. Ed. Pract. Vet. 5:25, 1983.

Wallach, J. D., and Boever, W. J.: *Diseases of Exotic Animals.* Philadelphia: W. B. Saunders, 1983, pp. 495–533.

Williams, C. S. F.: *Practical Guide to Laboratory Animals.* St. Louis: C. V. Mosby, 1976, pp. 65–71.

Winsted, W.: *Ferrets.* Neptune City, NJ: T.F.H. Publications, 1981.

CARE AND FEEDING OF ORPHAN MAMMALS AND BIRDS

RICHARD H. EVANS, D.V.M.
Brighton, Illinois

In the last 10 years in North America, there has been a tremendous proliferation of organizations devoted to rehabilitating and releasing back to the wild orphaned or injured wild mammals and birds. Two national organizations, the Wildlife Rehabilitation Council and the National Wildlife Rehabilitators Association, have been chartered to promote the dissemination of knowledge on rehabilitation through an annual convention or symposium and a multitude of publications. With this proliferation of rehabilitation centers has come a desperate need for experienced, competent veterinary assistance. One of the chief drawbacks many veterinarians have in rendering assistance to rehabilitators is a lack of knowledge on formulating and administering artificial diets.

The objective of this article is to describe diets and feeding techniques that have been used successfully in rearing wild animals. It is hoped that such knowledge will help make the clinician more confident and competent in caring for them.

The veterinarian should also be cognizant that possession of wild animals for reasons other than emergency medical treatment without appropriate state or federal permits is illegal. Most birds are protected under the Migratory Bird Act. Fur-bearing mammals usually are protected under state regulations. Marine mammals are strictly controlled by both state and federal laws. In fact, since the latter species are rather difficult to rear without considerable experience, they are not dealt with in this article; they should be referred to the nearest licensed marine mammal rehabilitation center. These centers can be contacted through the state department of conservation, fish and wildlife, or natural resources.

MAMMALS

Initial Patient Evaluation

Upon receiving an orphaned mammal, the veterinarian's first act should be to determine what species it is and its age. Aging methods and other biological data are detailed in *Wild Mammals of North America* (Chapman and Feldhamer, 1982). A physical examination, as complete as the animal will allow, should be conducted, since the animal must be healthy, normothermic (see Table 1 for normal body temperature) and in positive hydration status before feeding can commence. Since small, unfurred neonatal animals are not able to thermoregulate but have a tremendous surface area for heat loss, they readily become hypothermic after as little as 45 to 60 minutes of exposure to ambient temperatures. Hypothermia may result in impairment of sucking reflex, gastrointestinal motility, and digestion. A variety of devices are available for rewarming; they include heating pads, hot-water bottles, and heat lamps. In our experience, none are as effective in raising body core temperature as a warm-water bath and massage and immediate drying under a heat lamp or hair dryer. Hydration status should be assessed by standard methods for neonates. A balanced electrolyte replacement fluid should be given orally or subcutaneously unless dehydration is severe, in which case the intravenous route can be used. Remember that neonates have two to three times the fluid requirements of adults. A highly successful regimen has been to give 40 to 50 ml of Normosol-R (Abbott) per kg of body weight in divided doses every 12 to 24 hours until rehydration is complete.

Diets

The professional and lay literature contains a vast array of milk replacer formulas for small sucklings. Many formulas have nothing more to recommend them than a statement that they have been used successfully to rear a wild orphaned mammal. Data on growth rate and physical and behavioral development that could be compared to that reported in the biologic and zoologic literature are lacking. As a result, we do not know whether the diet was truly

Text continued on page 778

Table 1. Diets for Suckling Mammals

Species	Body Temperature (°F)	Suckling Diet	Feeding Interval	Weaning Age (weeks)	Weaning Diet
Opossum	90–99	Esbilac (Borden) and/or Multimilk (Borden)*	6 to 8 times daily	13–15	Mink pellets (National, Milk Specialites Co.) dog or cat food
Armadillo	84–98	Esbilac and/or Multimilk*	3 to 5 times daily	8–12	Cat or Kitten Chow (Ralston Purina); Mink pellets; dog or cat food
Nutria	97–100	Esbilac and/or Multimilk*	3 to 5 times daily	6–8	Rabbit or rodent pellets (Ralston Purina)
Beaver	98–100	Esbilac and/or Multimilk*	4 to 8 times daily	6–9 (begins as early as 1 month)	Rodents or rabbit pellets; selected shrubs, twigs, branches
Woodchuck and other marmots	99–100	Esbilac and/or Multimilk*	3 to 5 times daily	6–8	Rodent or rabbit diets
Ground squirrels	98–99	Esbilac and/or Multimilk*	3 to 5 times daily	6–7	Rodent diets
Tree squirrels (gray, red, fox, flying)	98–102	Esbilac and/or Multimilk*	3 to 6 times daily	6–8	Rodent pellets
Muskrat	98–101	Esbilac and/or Multimilk*	3 to 6 times daily	5–8	Rodent or rabbit pellets
Jack rabbit	101–103	KMR (Borden)	1 to 3 times daily	4	Rabbit pellets
Cottontail rabbit	100–103	Esbilac and/or Multimilk*	1 to 3 times daily	3–4	Rabbit pellets; fresh grass clippings
Badger	99–101	Esbilac and/or Multimilk*	3 to 5 times daily	10–12	Dog or cat food with supplemental rodents
Bobcat	100–103	KMR	3 to 5 times daily	7–8	Mink Chow (Ralston Purina); Kitten Chow
Coyote	100–103	Esbilac and/or Multimilk*	3 to 5 times daily	5–7	Puppy Chow (Ralston Purina)
Raccoon	100–103	KMR	3 to 5 times daily	13–16	Puppy Chow; Mink Chow
Red fox; gray fox	100–102	Esbilac and/or Multimilk*	3 to 5 times daily	7–8	Puppy Chow; supplement 10% with ground whole rodents
River otter	99–102	KMR	3 to 5 times daily	12–13	Mink Chow; supplement 10% with ground whole rodents
Skunk	101–102	KMR	3 to 5 times daily	8	Mink Chow; Kitten or Puppy Chow; grubs and insects
Wolf	100–102	Esbilac and/or Multimilk*	3 to 5 times daily	8–12	Mink Chow; Kitten or Puppy Chow; grubs and insects

Table continued on opposite page

Table 1. *Diets for Suckling Mammals* Continued

Species	Body Temperature (°F)	Suckling Diet	Feeding Interval	Weaning Age (weeks)	Weaning Diet
Mink	99–102	KMR; Esbilac and/ or Multimilk*	3 to 5 times daily	4–6	Mink Chow; Kitten or Puppy Chow; grubs and insects; supplement 10% with ground whole rodents
Weasels	100–103	KMR; Esbilac and/ or Multimilk*	3 to 6 times daily	3–5	Mink Chow; Kitten or Puppy Chow; grubs and insects; supplement 10% with ground whole rodents
White-tailed deer and other cervids	98–101	Doe Milk Replacer (Foremost McKesson); Lamb Milk Replacer; evaporated milk (undiluted liquid)	Days 1 and 2: 50–60 ml bovine colostrum every 3 hours Days 3 and 4: 85 ml bovine colostrum every 4 hours (if colostrum not available, use milk replacer) Days 5 and 7: Slow concentration method (i.e., 50% colostrum and 50% milk replacer to 100% milk replacer); 100–200 ml 4 times daily Days 8 to 20: 250–350 ml milk replacer 3 times daily (should have access to parasite-free soil at this age) Days 21 to 34: 850 ml, 2 times daily Days 35 to 70: 100 ml, 2 times daily	10–13	Browse, alfalfa hay, and complete wild ruminant diet
Peccary	99–102	SPFLac (Borden); Esbilac and/or Multimilk*	4 to 6 times daily	10–12	Pig starter and grower

*Multimilk is a new, multipurpose milk replacer containing 53% fat and 34.5% protein with only trace amounts of carbohydrates. It has the same vitamin and mineral content as Esbilac. This product is meant to be used either alone as a high-fat and high-protein milk replacer or to alter fat, protein, and carbohydrate levels of Esbilac or KMR. Multimilk replaces whipping cream, eggs, and other substances that have been used to alter the concentrations of Esbilac or KMR.

adequate. The information presented in Table 1 on artificial milk replacers, feeding amounts, and intervals includes only those methods that have successfully supported an adequate growth rate and physical and behavioral development (to the extent that such facts are known).

When feeding wild animals the diets listed in Table 1, the clinician should insist that a minimum data base, including periodic physical examinations, be kept on each animal or in the case of litters, a representative sample. The correlation of this data base with the results of physical examinations will enable growth problems or diseases to be diagnosed early in their development and for rigorous therapeutic measures to be instituted before the problems become life-threatening. Such therapies are especially important in cases of diarrhea, because even a moderate fluid loss in neonates may result in death within 48 hours. During the first few weeks of life, the animal should be weighed every 48 to 72 hours, preferably in the morning, when its digestive tract is empty. During the later suckling period, weights can be obtained at weekly intervals. Weights should be plotted in graph form for ease in determining the animal's growth rate. Patterns of defecation and urination, including stool color and consistency, should be recorded. Milk feces appear golden-brown to brown in color and are about the consistency of peanut butter. Physical and behavioral development (e.g., eye opening, tooth eruption, pelage development, vocalization, locomotion, and sibling interaction) should be described. Physical exams should be conducted at weekly intervals. Particular attention should be paid to the respiratory and digestive systems, since aspiration pneumonia as well as nutritional and infectious enteropathies are the most common complications of hand rearing.

Methods of Feeding

To institute feeding, the desired formula is warmed to the animal's body temperature and diluted to a 30 per cent concentration with tap water. This mixture is offered for the first few feedings. The formula can then be diluted to 50 per cent for a few more feedings, after which full-concentration formula is offered within a minimum of 24 to 48 hours. This slow elevation of formula concentration allows the microbial flora, especially in mammals with ceca, to adapt to the new diet. Initial full-concentration feeding will usually result in loose stools and diarrhea in short order. Diet acceptance and stool quality should be constantly monitored, for the vast majority of maladaptive nutritional enteropathies will occur at this time. Usually a normally colored but slightly to moderately loose stool can be expected until about 72 to 96 hours after the institution of feeding. If loose stools continue beyond this period or diarrhea develops, the animal is not adapting to its new diet and therapy is in order (see below).

The clinician should always bear in mind that the term *milk replacer* is somewhat of a misnomer because this type of formula generally does not entirely support a growth rate equal to that of mother's milk. Furthermore, there is some evidence that special requirements for amino or fatty acids in some wild species may not be met by commercial milk replacers for dogs and cats. Every attempt should be made to wean the animal onto a solid diet as soon as possible. Tree squirrels are able to begin eating semisolid or solid food when their incisors are developing, at 3 to 5 weeks, whereas raccoons and related species begin eating these foods around 6 to 7 weeks. Lagomorphs will begin eating grass as early as 10 days of age. Growth rate charts will show the typical biphasic mammalian pattern—a plateau during this weaning period and another rise when weaning is complete.

The techniques of bottle feeding are quite simple and not unlike those for human neonates. However, constant vigilance is necessary to avoid problems such as aspiration pneumonia. With a commercial human or animal nursing bottle (Pet Nurser, Borden) and an appropriately sized nipple (premature infant or Borden's Pet Nurser Nipple), the neonate is allowed to suckle from a "natural position." A properly suckling neonate should have to perform some degree of work to obtain milk; it should not flow freely from the bottle. The nipple orifice may have to be altered to facilitate the correct flow of milk. Hoofed stock are fed standing or in sternal recumbency with a sheep's or lamb's nipple. Neonatal procyonids, canids, mustelids, rodents, and lagomorphs are best fed in the sitting position (rear legs only) with the forefeet elevated to at least the level of the stomach; this position facilitates gravity flow of milk to the stomach. In rodents such as tree squirrels, a regular-tipped, 1- to 3-ml syringe allows better control over milk delivery. Opossums pose special problems because the semipermanent mouth-to-nipple attachment in the pouch does not require as good a suckling reflex as is needed by eutherian mammals. As a result, very often opossums (especially those weighing less than 50 grams) must be fed by intubation.

In many instances, getting the neonate to accept the nipple may be a frustrating experience. Rodents usually take the nipples readily; however, lagomorphs are notorious for resisting attempts to get them to suckle. Deer do not like any manipulation of their heads during feeding, but placing a hand behind and on the back of the head of young carnivores seems to help. Covering the eyes of young raccoons assists their concentration on suckling. Many times it may be necessary to use one hand to hold the mouth and lips closed around the nipple to facilitate suckling (especially in deer and raccoons). Great care should be exercised in this manipulation; avoid obstructing the trachea or nose as well as touching the eyes.

In certain species, especially tree squirrels and very young raccoons, the suckling reflex may be so vigorous that the animal may aspirate some milk into its upper respiratory system. Milk bubbling from the nose is evidence of aspiration. In these instances, the bottle should be removed immediately and the nostrils cleared by suction. Feeding may be resumed, but the bottle may have to be withdrawn at intervals to slow down the animal's suckling pace. If the problem persists, excessive milk flow may be the cause and a nipple with a smaller orifice should be selected. The use of regular-tipped syringes instead of nursing bottles (as described earlier) allows a slower and much more controllable milk delivery.

Do not allow the animal to suckle freely until it decides it has had enough. Since artificial milk replacers are usually highly palatable, overeating and subsequent diarrhea become common sequelae to this practice. (The author has not-so-fond memories from "back in the early days" of a score or more of bloated, semicomatose, diarrheic, crying raccoon kits, the result of overfeeding.) A proper volume of milk per feeding can be determined by considering the animal's daily caloric needs, the caloric density of the formula, and the animal's comfortable stomach capacity. At the author's center, feeding charts are being developed in which the standard metabolic rate is used to establish daily caloric needs. Feeding intervals are calculated by equating these needs with a comfortable stomach capacity, which in most small animals (excepting lagomorphs) appears to be approximately 40 to 60 ml per kg of body weight. Table 2 is an example of such a chart. This has been used successfully for several years on raccoons. In general, carnivores and rodents consume 20 to 30 per cent of their body weight daily in milk. The opossum and armadillo consume about 20 per cent per day, whereas hoofed stock consume about 10 per cent of their body weight daily. Table 2 and daily milk consumption values are general guidelines; not all individuals adhere to them. Periodic weighing will allow the clinician to assess whether a particular volume of milk is supporting a good growth rate. Sometimes individuals grow poorly on the amounts shown here but will show adequate growth after a 20 per cent rise in daily volume. Remember that energy is the most important regulator of growth at these ages.

Since most small mammals do not defecate or urinate without maternal stimulation until the middle of the suckling period, it is necessary after each meal to stimulate the animal by patting (not rubbing) its rectum and genitals with a cottonball or gauze pad soaked in warm water. Yellow stains on the pad are indications of urination. The armadillo and white-tailed deer appear to be the exceptions to this rule; they will urinate and defecate on their own at a very early age, usually 1 to 2 weeks. Failure to elicit defecation is not uncommon during the first 1 to 3 days of feeding; as artificial milk replacers approach 100 per cent digestability, it takes several feedings to form sufficient feces to produce a bowel movement. During rectogenital stimulation, the genitals, especially the penis in tree squirrels, should be examined to ensure that they have not been mutilated. Occasionally siblings of these species will suckle on any handy appendage between feedings, and some quite severe mutilations can occur.

When the neonate appears to be eating semisolid or solid food and has developed cheek teeth, weaning can begin by slowly limiting milk intake and watching for an increase in consumption of solid foods. When the animal is eating sufficient amounts of solid food, the stools will be tubular and brown in color and composed of fine granules.

Although selection and delivery of an appropriate milk replacer is of paramount importance in rearing orphan wild mammals, success obviously cannot be achieved without proper environment and housing. It is beyond the scope of this article to describe all of the environmental factors that need to be controlled and the types of housing that are needed. However, a few brief comments are in order.

A photoperiod close to that occurring in the wild, proper humidity (especially important with the opossum, which lives in a humid pouch), and an ambient temperature correlated to the animal's age-dependent thermoneutral zone are necessary. Usually 85°F is adequate for the first week of life in all but marsupials, which should be kept at a temperature ranging from 90 to 95°F and a relative humidity of 65 to 70 per cent. The ambient temperature should be that which maintains a normal body temperature (see Table 1).

Water and feed bowls for weaning animals should be inedible and not easily overturned (e.g., small fire-glazed crockery pots). Cage furniture such as "jungle gym" arrangements of tree branches and logs will help develop the finely tuned motor skills characteristic of rodents, raccoons, and similar species. Pits made from filling a plastic litter pan with washed and baked sand is ideal for burrowing carnivores and rodents. A nest box should always be supplied for carnivores, lagomorphs, large rodents (especially nocturnal varieties) and opossums. One half of a plastic dog-carrying crate makes an excellent secluded home. Small rodents, especially

Table 2. Daily Feeding Chart for Suckling Raccoons

Body Weight				Daily Energy Requirement*	Recommended Amount per Feeding‡	Amount Fed at Various Intervals§			
oz	*lb*	*gm*	*kg*			3×	4×	5×	6×
2.82	0.17	75	0.08	21 (22)†	4.0			4.4	3.7
3.53	0.22	100	0.10	25 (26)	5.0			5.2	4.3
4.59	0.28	125	0.13	30 (32)	6.5			6.4	5.3
5.29	0.33	150	0.15	34 (36)	7.5			7.2	6.0
6.35	0.39	175	0.18	39 (41)	9.0		10.25	8.2	6.8
7.05	0.44	200	0.20	42 (44)	10.0		11.00	8.8	7.3
7.41	0.46	210	0.21	43 (46)	10.5		11.50	9.2	7.7
7.76	0.49	220	0.22	45 (47)	11.0		11.75	9.4	
8.11	0.51	230	0.23	47 (49	11.5		12.25	9.8	
8.46	0.53	240	0.24	48 (51)	12.0		12.75	10.2	
8.82	0.55	250	0.25	50 (52)	12.5		13.00	10.4	
9.88	0.61	275	0.28	54 (57)	14.0		14.25	11.4	
10.58	0.66	300	0.30	57 (60)	15.0	20.0	15.00	12.0	
11.64	0.72	325	0.33	61 (64)	16.5	21.3	16.00	12.8	
13.40	0.83	375	0.38	68 (71)	19.0	23.6	17.75	14.2	
14.11	0.88	400	0.40	70 (74)	20.0	24.6	18.50	14.8	
17.64	1.10	500	0.50	83 (88)	25.0	29.3	22.00	17.6	
21.16	1.32	600	0.60	96 (101)	30.0	33.6	25.30	20.2	
				Beginning Weaning Process					
24.69	1.54	700	0.70	107 (113)	35.0	37.6	28.30	22.6	
28.22	1.76	800	0.80	118 (125)	40.0	41.7	31.30	25.0	
31.74	1.98	900	0.90	129 (136)	45.0	45.3	34.00		
35.27	2.20	1000	1.00	140 (147)	50.0	49.0	36.75		
38.80	2.43	1100	1.10	150 (158)	55.0	52.7	39.50		
42.32	2.65	1200	1.20	161 (170)	60.0	56.7	42.50		
45.85	2.87	1300	1.30	171 (180)	65.0	60.0	45.00		
49.38	3.12	1400	1.40	181 (190)	70.0	63.0	47.50		

*Daily energy requirement = 2.5 ($70 \times BW^{0.75}$), in kcal.

†Value in parenthesis is amount of KMR (Borden) in milliliters that is equivalent to the daily energy requirement.

‡Recommended amount per feeding = maximum of 50 ml/kg body weight.

§Amounts fed at various intervals, determined by dividing recommended amount per feeding into the amount of KMR needed to fulfill daily energy requirement.

the nocturnal species such as the flying squirrel, are best housed in plywood nest boxes (not plastic, which is frequently eaten).

Problems of Hand Raising

A brief discussion of the most common maladies encountered in suckling mammals is necessary here, but readers are referred to standard veterinary medical texts for more in-depth coverage.

Without a doubt the most common problems a clinician will encounter are (1) runting, (2) aspiration pneumonia, (3) enteropathies, and (4) infectious diseases.

True runting must be differentiated from pseudorunting. In the latter case, a depression in the growth rate is caused by inadequate energy intake; this is rather easily resolved by increasing the daily caloric intake. Work at the author's center has revealed two types of runting. In the first type, the growth curve has a normal configuration but is shifted in time (i.e., growth is retarded until late in the suckling period or just after weaning). Opossums, especially when received weighing less than 50 grams, seem inordinately prone to this phenomenon. Cases of the second type of runting show a growth curve that is not only shifted but also markedly depressed. With a little time and patience, cases of the first type usually become robust, healthy juveniles, whereas those of the second type seldom recover and usually die of malnutrition and starvation regardless of the kind of supportive therapy they receive. The key to resolving runting in "type 1" cases is to limit the daily caloric intake to the apparent rather than the real age-dependent caloric requirements and to raise the caloric intake slowly as weight gain is noted.

Aspiration pneumonia is a very common sequela to bottle feeding in suckling rodents, lagomorphs, and, to a lesser extent, carnivores. Overfilling the stomach by gavage, overfeeding from free access to food and subsequent passive regurgitation, and overzealous suckling usually precipitate this problem. Unfortunately, the relative inactivity of most suckling mammals usually prevents development of dyspnea until the condition is well advanced or even terminal. Mild cases, however, will frequently resolve spontaneously but usually result in some degree of pulmonary tissue loss. Aspiration pneumonia is most successfully treated by preventing it in the manner described above.

By far, nutritional enteropathies are the most common problem the clinician will confront. Diarrhea, malnutrition or starvation, and poor physical development are hallmark signs. Most cases are the result of either overfeeding or too-rapid initiation of artificial milk replacers in recently orphaned animals. In either event, an imbalance in bacterial flora and the proliferation of enterotoxigenic aerobic (e.g., *Escherichia coli, Enterobacter*) or anaerobic (e.g., *Clostridium* spp., *Bacteroides fragilis*) bacteria occurs and perpetuates the osmotic diarrhea caused by overfeeding. Enteric virus (rotavirus) and protozoan parasites such as *Girardia* or *Cryptosporidium* are also common secondary invaders. Treatment usually involves immediate cessation of milk feeding, rapid and aggressive rehydration (either orally or intravenously, depending on the severity of the problem), and reinstitution of feeding when diarrhea has subsided. Treatment can be a no-win fight between (1) resting the bowel and starving the animal to death and (2) reinstituting feeding, which results in exacerbation of the problem. Usually, when diagnosis is early and the above treatment regimen is initiated, the problem will resolve in 48 to 96 hours.

Generally, neonatal mammals suffer from few infectious diseases other than those occurring secondary to nutritional abuse. Viral diseases such as canine distemper, feline panleukopenia, and canine parvovirus, however, are especially dangerous and highly lethal problems in canids, procyonids, mustelids, and felids. The clinician should give careful thought to expending large amounts of time, effort, and funds on treating such diseases, which are commonly associated with high mortality. Furthermore, such animals constitute a grave risk to the organization's orphan mammal population. A variety of bacterial diseases, such as pneumonia caused by *Pseudomonas*, respiratory disease caused by *Klebsiella*, and generalized or enteric salmonellosis, are seen but generally secondary to nutritional abuse, unsanitary rearing conditions, or runting syndromes. Helminth parasites cause important disorders predominantly in carnivores, especially procyonids and mustelids, in which the roundworm of the genus *Baylisascaris* can result in sometimes severe enteritis. Eggs of this parasite are not usually detectable in animals under 8 weeks old, as the prepatent period averages about 60 days. The same parasite can readily produce cerebrospinal nematodiasis, especially in rodents.

BIRDS

Initial Patient Evaluation

As noted in the section on mammals, species identification and an initial physical examination are absolute necessities in the treatment of incoming orphaned birds. Hypothermia and dehydration should be corrected immediately. Warm-water baths with massage work rather well in naked nestling birds, but wetting a feathered bird is not advised. Feather structure can be damaged in attempts to dry the bird. An incubator is an excellent means of elevating the body temperature of a feathered bird. Heating pads are less effective, since they tend to distribute heat unevenly. Remember that hypothermia can result in gastrointestinal hypomotility and maldigestion. Identification of nestling birds, particularly passerines, has been extremely difficult if not impossible in the past. However, with the advent of new field guides on nestlings, the job is easier (Harrison, C., 1978). Categorization of size, bill structure (especially bill commissure and phalanges), and down pattern usually enable at least an identification of family. It is also helpful to have the nest the bird came in, since species may be determined with the aid of field guides to nest structures (Harrison, H., 1975).

Once the bird is normothermic, rehydrated, and judged to be free from diseases or other abnormalities, it can be placed in an appropriately sized artificial nest and fed.

Diets

Table 3 lists appropriate diets for most species of common birds. It is, however, incomplete, because at present there is not sufficient data on many of the lesser known species to warrant dietary recommendations.

As previously stated, there are many diets other than those listed that have been used to raise avian species. However, as in the case of mammals, data supporting their effectiveness are not available. The diets in Table 3 have, for the most part, been evaluated in controlled experiments. In the songbird section (Passeriformes, Piciformes, and Apodiformes) recommended diets are the result of recent experiments by a noted New England rehabilitation center specializing in these species. Their experiments have produced excellent growth and development in birds fed according to the methods described below. Readers should note that these methods are very similar to those that occur in the wild. The addition of live insects has been shown to promote the early development of foraging behavior. Songbird species can be nested in facial tissue or paper towels in plastic fruit baskets on a heating pad or in an incubator, where the temperature should be between 80 and 90°F when they are naked nestlings, 80 to 85°F when they are covered with down, and 70 to 80°F when they are feathered.

Pigeons and doves are rather easy to raise. A

Table 3. Diets for Nestling Birds

Species	Diet
Passeriformes, Piciformes, Apodiformes	
Ground insectivores: robins, thrushes, towhees	1 cup Purina Hi-Pro Dog Food softened in water (or Hills' p/d dog food), ½ cup mynah bird food or turkey pellelts, two soft-boiled eggs, ⅓ cup cooked Roman Meal cereal, 1 tsp. dark loam, 1 tsp. dolomite vitamin and mineral mix, berries; this mixture is mixed 1:1 with earthworms
Aerial insectivores; swallows, kingbirds, phoebes, swifts, wrens	1 cup of high-protein pablum, ¼ cup cooked Roman Meal cereal, 1 cup of dried insect mix (fish food) and one soft-boiled egg; this mixture is mixed 1:1 with live insects
Insectivorous omnivores: blackbirds, orioles, thrashers, mockingbirds, warblers, tanagers	Same as for ground insectivores, except cooked Roman Meal cereal is increased to ⅔ cup and insects or worms can be used
Omnivores: jays, shrikes, crows, grackles	Same as for insectivorous omnivores, but lean hamburger is added (not more than 10% of diet)
Granivores: finches, chickadees, juncos	Same as for insectivorous omnivores; at day 10, 20% of diet is seeds
Frugivores: waxwings, woodpeckers, flickers	Same as for insectivorous omnivores, but 20% of diet is berries
Columbiformes	
Pigeons, doves	Same as for granivores, or mix equal amounts of chicken starter and wild bird seed made to a slurry with water
Caprimulgiformes	
Nighthawks, whip-poor-will	Same as diet for aerial insectivorous passeriformes
Ciconiiformes	
Herons, egrets, bitterns	Minced or ground skinned, whole rodents for the first 10 to 14 days, after which chopped rodents of sufficiently small size can be fed; fresh or recently thawed fish at a rate of 30 to 60% of body weight daily; may need to supplement with vitamins (i.e., vitamin E, thiamine)
Gruiformes	
Coots, gallinules, rails	Commercial poultry, gamebird, or waterfowl diets with supplements of insects, minced rodents, and aquatic vegetables
Cranes	A mixture of commercial poultry diet and ground rodents or a commercial crane diet (Ziegler Brothers), given freely with water
Galliformes	
Pheasant, quail, grouse, turkey	Commercial gamebird, turkey, or chicken starter and growing ration; supplement with insects; allow grit
Anseriformes	
Duck, geese	Commercial duck, gamebird, or turkey starter and grower; supplement with fresh aquatic vegetables; all should have access to grit
Charadriiformes	
Gulls, terns, plovers, sandpipers	These species are omnivores and do well on a mixture of dog food, ground or minced rodents, insects, and fish
Falconiformes and Strigiformes	
Hawks, owls	Ground or minced, skinned, and beheaded *adult* rodents or plucked day-old cockerels or quail rolled in bone meal (for falcons) for the first 2 to 10 days; thereafter, fur and feathers can be fed in moderation with chopped whole animals until the bird is forming pellets well; then allow free access to food

foster hen can be obtained from a local pigeon breeder; she can do a much better job than you can. Although pigeon milk has yet to be duplicated, the diets listed in Table 3 have been used with very good success.

Nighthawks are intriguing aerial insectivores. They can be raised successfully but require an intensive amount of work and prolonged force feeding. When these birds are force fed, care should be taken with the mandible, since it has a mid-shaft hinge and can be fractured easily.

Readers may find it unusual that no mention is made here of feeding fish to birds of the heron family. Work at the author's center with a large number of these species has shown that in order to maintain or increase the weights of these birds, 30 to 60 per cent of a bird's body weight in food must be consumed daily. In certain portions of the country (especially its interior), fish are expensive and hard to obtain in an appropriate size and quantity. Our experiments have shown an equal, if not better, growth and development with decidedly fewer procurement problems when ground or chopped rodents are used for food. The birds readily accept this diet, since most consume mice and other small rodents in the wild. If fish are offered, they should be fresh or recently thawed. Avoid using fish that have been frozen for an excessively long period of time (months). Vitamin supplements such as vitamin E and thiamin should be given periodically because of the rapid breakdown of these micronutrients in the carcasses of fish, especially smelt and herring. When the bird is eating on its own, the food should be placed in a small pool or bucket of water so that the bird can mimic adult foraging behavior.

Common species of Galliformes and Anseriformes, except wood ducks, are seldom difficult to raise. Because the wood duck is an aquatic insectivore, it must be fed in this manner. However, despite some rather ingenious methods by rehabilitators to mimic the natural feeding behavior of wood ducks, they still remain extremely difficult to raise in captivity.

In the order Gruiformes, the rails and gallinules are typically fussy eaters. Frequently they will put themselves into the throes of starvation while they decide to eat what has been prepared for them. Constant monitoring of their body weight may reveal that supplemental force feeding is necessary.

Birds of prey are not very difficult birds to raise, provided they are fed proper diets. There is usually sufficient yolk in the newborn to sustain them for 8 to 12 hours after hatching. For the first 2 days only muscle meat should be fed, but the crop should not be filled to capacity. At day 3, skinned whole, ground, or minced adult rodents are fed until the crop is about three-quarters full. Whole adult rodents should not be withheld from these birds for more than 3 days, since raptors are very susceptible to the development of metabolic bone disease in as short a time as 5 to 10 days.

Methods of Feeding

The actual hand feeding of baby birds is not difficult but can be tedious and very time-consuming. Those who undertake it must be willing to spend their waking hours stuffing food into seemingly bottomless pits. Forceps or toothpicks can be used to deliver small bits of food. As an alternative, a 1- to 3-ml syringe with the needle adaptor removed makes a good food delivery system. One should refrain if possible, from prying open the bird's mouth to feed it (see the section on force feeding for further details). Instead, the food-begging reflex can be elicited by tapping the bill (the yellow or orange phalanges at the base of the bill in passerines) or feathers around the bill; this stimulates the bird to gape for food. Frequently, only sight or sound around the nest will stimulate the begging reflex. Thus, a tap at the side of the nest can elicit begging. Some who work in rehabilitation are even able to mimic the calls made by mother birds to elicit food begging. The feeder should be consistent in the type of stimulus used to elicit begging. Jumping around confuses the bird into not responding at all. The bird should not be allowed simply to eat until it stops begging for food, as this reflex is not precisely attuned to gastrointestinal filling. Such factors as sibling competition may foster begging well beyond the point at which the bird is full.

The amount to feed an orphan bird at one session and the number of times a day to feed it are dictated by the fullness of the crop and the rate of growth and development of the species. Growth is best monitored by frequent weighings and observations on physical development, particularly plumage. For very young songbirds the following feeding regimen utilizing the diets in Table 3 has been developed. This regimen is very similar to that occurring in the wild and results in a crop that is usually always one-half to three-quarters full.

1. Days 0 to 4: feed every 10 to 15 minutes from 6:00 AM to 10:00 PM.
2. Days 4 to 10: feed every 15 to 20 minutes from 6:00 AM to 10:00 PM.
3. Days 10 to 14: feed every 45 to 60 minutes from 6:30 AM to 9:30 PM.
4. Day 15 and onward: feed every 60 to 90 minutes from 7:00 AM to 9:00 PM.

Under no circumstances should birds be fed so that their crops are packed full at each feeding. This can result in crop atony or impaction. Many small meals a day are far better than one or two "gut-busters." After each bit of food is given, a liberal amount of water should follow to ease passage of the food through the esophagus and help supply daily water needs. Once a meal is completed, the bill and surrounding skin should be cleaned of pieces of food that can dry and become a source of irritation and infection.

Every attempt should be made to promote self-feeding as early as possible. This usually requires efforts to get the bird to recognize his feed within a container such as a small bowl. Gently submerging the bird's beak into the feed or playing with the feed in an attempt to entice the bird to eat it can be successful in promoting self-feeding. Once the bird is feeding itself, one must be extremely vigilant to make sure that it is taking in sufficient feed and not merely playing with its food.

As in the case of mammals, frequent physical examinations, serial weighings, and analysis of physical and behavioral development should be undertaken to ensure that the bird is progressing as expected. Reliance on body conformation as discerned by palpation can frequently be misleading as feathers can hide a multitude of problems. Readers should consult the list of suggested readings for information on specific species.

Once the bird's flight feathers have grown, it is said to be in the fledgling stage, at which time it begins to learn to fly. Appropriately sized and constructed avaries are required at this time. For most passerines, a cage measuring 6 × 6 × 6 feet is adequate, whereas Great Horned Owls require a minimum size of 40 × 10 × 10 feet. Hawks and owls can be given flight experience by common falconry techniques. Cages should be constructed so that birds do not injure their feathers. Readers can consult the previously mentioned national rehabilitation organizations for minimum standards on cages for various species.

Problems of Hand Raising

Some words of caution are in order concerning the hand raising of orphan birds. Early in the bird's life it undergoes a process called imprinting, during which it learns what species of animal it is. This process is a conglomeration of innate responses to several stimuli such as sight and sound. If the parent on which this bird is imprinting is not of its own species (such as occurs with cross-fostering, when a bird is raised by a similar species or even a human), it will imprint on that species. Incorrectly imprinted birds are usually very aggressive hunters and strong fliers but may not necessarily be tame. Abnormal behavior is commonly seen during the breeding season in incorrectly imprinted birds. Those that imprint on a human will frequently select a human for breeding and end up by being killed by an irate citizen.

To overcome these problems, a foster parent program should be utilized. This program uses an unreleasable adult of the species in question that serves as either a true foster parent and actually raises the orphan or is only a role model for the orphan while it is hand fed. Alternatively, hand puppets or photographs can be used to mimic adults, but they are no substitute for foster parenting. In addition, these programs are an excellent productive use of unreleasable adults. Passerines have added problems, since these species must learn a particular song to complete their breeding cycle. In some cases the song is taught to the young by the adult. This task can be carried out by foster parents or records of the adult song.

FORCE FEEDING SMALL MAMMALS AND BIRDS

In some instances, neonatal birds and small mammals will refuse to eat on their own and must be nourished forcibly. Great care and forethought should be given to force feeding any animal. First, problems of management should be ruled out (e.g., a problem with the size, consistency, taste, or amount of diet fed or a housing and environment arrangement that produces stress and prevents the animal from feeding). Certain groups of birds, especially waders such as herons, egrets, rales, coots, and gallinules, will often simply not eat if other species (including humans) are within the range of sight or hearing. These birds are very secretive by nature and easily become emotionally upset when gawked at while feeding. Conversely, the author has found that some species such as ducks, geese, and ospreys will frequently eat if they are put in a situation of conspecific competition for food. With small nocturnal rodents and lagomorphs, the same type of fright and stress reactions occur, not uncommonly resulting in acute death. Certain species have particular, often peculiar, eating habits or requirements, thus requiring a thorough understanding of the animal's natural history.

To make sure that no injury, disease, or other anomaly prevents feeding, the clinician should conduct a thorough physical examination that concentrates on the digestive system. Immediate steps should be taken to resolve any problems by appropriate medical or surgical therapies.

If, after all enticements, the patient still will not eat, force feeding must be started. If too long a period passes before this decision is made, the animal may begin the procedure in the throes of starvation. Nestling passerines, for example, can succumb to starvation in 1 to 3 days, whereas young carnivores may die in about a week. The clinician should also be aware that without food, neonates have no source of water. Dehydration is far more life-threatening at this age than starvation.

There are several types of force feeding that can be used in these cases. The method that accomplishes feeding quickly and with the least amount of stress to the animal should be employed. In decreasing order of stress placed on the animal and of frustration by the feeder, these methods are (1) oral force feeding, (2) pharyngeal or upper esophageal bolus intubation feeding, and (3) gavage, or intubation of the stomach or crop. Obviously, the third method is the most appropriate in terms of speed of feeding and reduced stress.

For oral force feeding, the animal's jaw or bill is opened (technique is described later) and small pieces of food are placed deep into the pharynx, behind the glottis. This will usually stimulate swallowing. A small amount of water should be placed into the mouth to facilitate swallowing and esophageal passage of food.

To deliver a pharyngeal or upper esophageal bolus, a short length of plastic or metal tubing of large diameter (i.e., 1 to 10 ml syringe with its needle adapter end removed) is used. The animal is properly restrained with its head and neck nearly vertical, the tube is passed swiftly over the tongue to the upper pharynx, and the bolus is deposited. This procedure should be done swiftly so that breathing is not restricted too long. This is the normal method for feeding in raptors that swallow

Table 4. *Feeding Tube Sizes*

Weight of Animal	French Size
Less than 50 gm	3–5
50–100 gm	5–10
100–500 gm	10–14
500–1000 gm	15–18
1 kg–2 kg	18–20
2 kg–5 kg	20–24
5 kg–10 kg	28–30
10 kg–20 kg	32–34*

*Human adult gastric lavage kit (No. 8881-750015, Monoject, Sherwood Medical Industries).

their prey whole. Again, sufficient water should be given to allow smooth passage of the bolus.

Gavage should not be used routinely as a method of feeding simply because it is quicker. Impairment of a suckling reflex, disorders of digestive function, regurgitation, and gastrointestinal atrophy from rapid gastric distention can result with chronic use of gavage. Gavage should never be performed if there is a possibility of impaired gastrointestinal motility. Any animal given xylazine may have varying degrees of compromised gastrointestinal motility for several hours after recovery. Birds suffering from lead poisoning frequently show atony of the upper gastrointestinal tract.

The procedure for gavage feeding is actually quite simple in theory but in practice requires considerable skill. One must first select an appropriately sized feeding tube. Gavage tubes come in a variety of types and consistencies; medical-grade polyvinyl or polypropylene, semirigid to soft, and flexible varieties are sufficient for most small mammals and birds (Monoject, Sherwood Company). For hoofed stock such as white-tailed deer fawns, the author has found that human gastric gavage kits that contain 140-ml syringe and 3 feet of clear polyvinyl tubing are the perfect choice (Monoject, Sherwood Company). All gavage tubes should have rounded or blunted atraumatic ends. The tube's rigidity may be altered by heat or cold. Polyvinyl tubes usually are soft and pliable at body temperature but become more rigid at lower temperatures. It is not necessary to sterilize the tubes before each use, but they should be thoroughly cleaned inside and out with an all-purpose disinfectant. Cold or heat sterilization will tend to cause degenerative changes in these tubes over time.

Table 4 lists sizes of tubes that are appropriate for an animal's body weight. In general, as large and as flexible a tube as possible should be selected. A tube about the size of the trachea will greatly reduce problems with tracheal intubation, tube coiling or folding, pharyngeal or esophageal puncture, and delivery of food with thick consistencies. Alternatively, rigid, ball-tipped steel tubes can be used for rodents and other small carnivores. However, these tubes require considerable skill in use and are frequently of insufficient length.

Before a syringe filled with milk is attached to the tube, the tube should be cut or marked to denote the length that should be inserted to reach either the stomach or crop. Measuring the distance from the tip of the nose or beak to the manubrium of the sternum as the animal is stretched, usually on its back, will guarantee placement of the tube in the stomach. This distance should not be measured when the animal is in a contorted position, because an artificially shortened distance will be obtained. To determine the distance to the crop, the distance from the nose or break to the caudal extent of the thoracic inlet should be measured.

Once an appropriately sized tube has been selected, a syringe is filled with 2 to 5 ml more diet than is required and is attached to the tube. For diets other than liquids, a Luer-tip syringe will fit most tubes. Gouging out the tip in the center of the Luer mounting with one blade of a pair of scissors will produce a greater orifice. If only regular-tip syringes are available, the first few inches of most tubes should be removed for a proper fit, since this area of the tube is usually several diameters wider than the tube size. Do not try to use small-bore tubes to deliver thick diets, as the excessive pressure needed to pass the food can lead to filling the stomach with a bolus or worse, detachment of the tube from the syringe and spraying of the diet over both operator and facilities. The tube should be well lubricated with a water-soluble jelly before it is used.

Gavage should not be performed by only one operater; those working alone have a good chance of hurting both the patient and themselves. One person should hold or restrain the animal while the tube is passed by another. In birds, the mouth can usually be opened by grasping the beak and prying apart the bills very carefully. A hemostat, toothpick, or similar device can also be inserted into the commissure of the bill. Slow, deliberate pressure on the bills will fatigue the jaw muscles. The bills of wading birds such as herons and egrets are usually razor-sharp or serrated and should be handled with care; they can inflict deep wounds on fingers or can impale an eye with lightning speed and accuracy.

Caution should also be used with small nestling birds (such as passerines) that have pliable, uncalcified bills and with nighthawks, which have hinged mandibles. Excessive pressure on these species can cause irreparable damage to their bills. Be wary of raptorial birds that can exert tremendous pressures with their beaks (e.g., a mature bald eagle can severely injure a finger).

To avoid many of these problems, the bird can be grasped from behind with thumb and index finger on either side of its head at the base of the skull. The index and middle fingers can then be inserted between the fleshy base of the bill and the bills pried apart. As an alternative method, a variety of specula may be used to open the mouth (e.g., canine tooth specula or dowl rods with holes drilled in their centers through which the tube can be passed).

Intubation of birds is made rather easy since the glottis is located at the base of the tongue and can be easily avoided by passing the tube over the tongue, along the roof of the mouth, and down into the esophagus.

To prevent gravity backflow, the bird should be held in an upright position with the head well above the stomach during intubation and for a short time after withdrawal of the tube. When the tube passes into the stomach, resistance will be felt at the crop and the gastric entrance. Slow back-and-forth manipulations may be necessary to move the tube below these areas. After the food is dispensed, the tube is withdrawn in a slow, steady manner while negative pressure is applied to prevent any residual food dripping from the tube into the glottis.

The anatomic placement of the glottis in mammals makes intubation more difficult than it is in birds. The animal is placed in a horizontal position and its head is elevated by a hand that is held under the jaw but does not restrict the trachea; a tube can then be passed blindly over the tongue and into the glottis. Contact with the glottis will stimulate the gag reflex, and the animal will swallow. Immediately after this response, the tube can be slid into the esophagus. Check to make sure that the tube is in the esophagus by palpation or external observation. Additionally, suction on the tube at this point will not draw back air if the tube is in the esophagus. Once the operator is assured that the tube is in the esophagus, the tube can be passed to the desired length. Usually, but not always, the gag reflex may be triggered if the tube is placed in the trachea. In another method, mouth specula (e.g., wood blocks, dowel rods, or saw retractors) can be used to open the mouth and, usually, the glottis.

For hoofed stock such as fawns of the white-tailed deer, appropriate intubation techniques for bovine or equine animals can be used. Restraint by an experienced person is necessary so that the operator can avoid having to handle the patient.

One of the most common problems in young rodents, opossums, and lagomorphs is pharyngeal perforation. The tube eventually becomes placed subcutaneously over the shoulder, and a tremendous inflammatory lesion results from instillation of diet in this area. Since these species usually have thin skin and little fur, the tube can be readily seen as it transverses the cervical subcutus.

After the diet is delivered into the stomach of a mammal, the tube is withdrawn in the same manner as for birds.

Another useful technique for carnivores and birds (especially raptors) is pharyngostomy or exteriorization of the esophagus and the cranial cervical area, which allows ease of intubation. This technique is especially useful for animals with fractured jaws. An appropriate surgical text can be consulted for the proper procedure.

In orphaned suckling mammals, an appropriate milk-replacer diet (Table 1) should be used for force feeding. Otherwise healthy weaned or adult mammals and nestling or fledged adult birds (i.e., those possessing normal gastrointestinal function and not suffering from starvation) can be fed their normal diets by grinding it and mixing it with sufficient water to obtain a slurry that will pass through the gavage tube. The amount of water used must be enough to supply the animal's daily maintenance needs: 50 ml/kg body weight.

For animals suffering moderate to severe starvation, the group of appropriate diets under consideration should not include the normal diet, which requires significant loss of energy merely to digest it. Elemental diets containing amino acids, fatty acids, glucose, and vitamins and minerals should be used to promote a rapid return to positive nutritional balance.

The author has had some rather amazing success by using a complete and balanced human tube-feeding diet (Isocal, Mead Johnson) on a variety of species. This diet is given on the basis of daily caloric requirements (in kcal), which can be calculated from the animal's body weight (BW) as follows:

Nonpasserine adult birds and mammals: 70 to 90 $\times$ $BW^{0.75}$

Nonpasserine juvenile birds and mammals: 2 to 3 (70 to 90 $\times$ $BW^{0.75}$)

Adult passerine birds: 140 $\times$ $BW^{0.75}$

Young passerine birds: 2 to 3 (140 $\times$ $BW^{0.75}$)

Thus, a bird requiring 40 kcal of energy a day is fed 40 ml of Isocal (1 kcal/ml) over a 24-hour period. Other more concentrated elemental diets that are hypertonic should be avoided, as they may lead to such osmotic disorders as diarrhea. In adult raptors, hypertonic elemental diets will usually cause sloughing of the superficial keratin layer of the ventriculus after two feedings. This is no cause for alarm, since the lining is rapidly regenerated. It is important to note that fecal volume will be dramatically reduced with these diets because of their very high digestability.

Although the author has kept many species (goshawks, crows, herons, small carnivores) alive and in positive nutritional balance for up to 4 weeks on these diets, prolonged feeding is not recommended. Patients should be encouraged to feed themselves as soon as possible.

References and Supplemental Reading

Beaver, P. (ed.): Raising the American robin. *In* Beaver, P. (ed.): *Wildlife Rehabilitation*. Vol. 4. Hauppauge, NY: Suffolk, in press.

Chapman, J. A., and Feldhamer, G. A.: *Wild Mammals of North America*. Baltimore, MD: Johns Hopkins University Press, 1982.

Evans, A., and Evans, R. H.: Raising raccoons for release. *In:* Beaver, P. (ed.): *Wildlife Rehabilitation*. Vol. 3. Hauppauge, NY: Suffolk, 1985, pp. 92–136.

Evans, R. H.: Rearing orphaned North American mammals. Vet. Clin. North Am., in press.

Fowler, M. E.: Care of orphaned wild animals. Vet. Clin. North Am. [Small Anim. Pract.] 9:447, 1979.

Fowler, M. E.: Force-feeding techniques in wild animals. J. Zoo Anim. Med. 12:3, 1981.

Harrison, C.: *A Field Guide to the Nests, Eggs and Nestlings of North American Birds*. Glasgow: William Collins, 1978.

Harrison, H. H.: *A Field Guide to Birds' Nests*. Boston: Houghton Mifflin, 1975.

McKeever, K.: *Care and Rehabilitation of Injured Owls*. Lincoln, Ontario: W. F. Rannie, 1983.

Pekins, P. J., and Mautz, W. W.: A new fawn feeding schedule. Wildl. Soc. Bull. 13:174, 1985.

Readers should also consult Volumes 1, 2, and 3 of *Wildlife Rehabilitation*, the proceedings of the first three annual symposia of the National Wildlife Rehabilitators Association. They can be obtained by writing RR#1, Box 125E, Brighton, IL 62012.

Section 9

NEUROLOGIC AND NEUROMUSCULAR DISORDERS

A. DE LAHUNTA, D.V.M.
Consulting Editor

***Additional Pertinent Information Found in* Current Veterinary Therapy VIII:**

LARYNGEAL PARALYSIS IN DOGS

JOAN A. O'BRIEN, V.M.D.
Philadelphia, Pennsylvania

Paralysis is the most common cause of laryngeal dysfunction in nonbrachycephalic breeds of dogs. Laryngeal paralysis can occur as an acquired or congenital disease. The paralysis may be partial, causing signs only in a working animal, or complete, causing severe, fatal dyspnea.

SIGNS

Signs of disease are similar in both the congenital and acquired forms. Signs in congenital disease may be noticed as early as 6 weeks of age. Severity of signs depends on the mass and number of laryngeal muscles affected. A mildly affected dog may fatigue easily and breathe noisily with exertion during racing, heavy work, or overheating. Voice changes (e.g., hoarseness) may be present but are often not noted. Affected dogs can often cry and howl normally. Severely affected animals exhibit stridor, cyanosis, and dyspnea with mild exertion or excitement. Gagging, regurgitation, and collapse may also occur (see Table 1). Signs are often first noted or become worse in hot weather. In both the acquired and congenital forms of laryngeal paralysis, there may be clinical or electromyographic evidence of polyneuropathy. Temporary megaesophagus, gastroesophageal reflux, hiatal hernia, and esophagitis have been seen radiographically and endoscopically in some of these dogs (see Table 1).

BREED

Congenital familial paralysis has been recognized in the Bouvier des Flandres (Venker-van Haagen et al., 1978), blue-eyed Siberian huskies and blue-eyed cross of husky and racing sled dogs (O'Brien, 1985). It is inherited as an autosomal dominant in the Bouviers. The inheritance pattern is under study in the other dogs.

Acquired paralysis is most common in middle-aged to aged dogs of large and giant breeds (Table 1).

DIAGNOSIS

Diagnosis is based on compatible signs and is confirmed by laryngoscopy, electromyographic findings of denervation potentials, and histologic evidence of denervation atrophy of the laryngeal muscles. Differential diagnosis must include central neural degeneration and multiple peripheral neuropathy as well as primary myositis, malignancy (laryngeal, vagal, or recurrent nerve), trauma, myasthenia gravis, or laryngeal collapse (Table 1). Laryngeal paralysis has also been reported in dogs with hypothyroidism.

THERAPY

Sedation as needed (all doses are at lower end of range and may be adjusted if necessary) with low doses of promazine (Sparine, Wyeth), 2 mg/kg, and prednisolone, 0.5 mg/kg orally (for its anti-inflammatory effect), when combined with avoidance of exertion may give brief, temporary relief from bilateral paralysis and is useful in cases of mild unilateral paralysis. Definitive therapy for bilateral paralysis is surgical enlargement of the glottic opening. This may be done through the mouth by means of vocal cord resection and partial unilateral arytenoidectomy (O'Brien et al., 1973), or by a unilateral lateralization and permanent fixation of the arytenoid cartilage (Venker-van Haagen, et al., 1978). A temporary tracheostomy is performed before either surgical approach. An illustrated and detailed description of both surgical approaches has been presented (Harvey and Venker-van Haagen, 1975). Both methods have been successful and yielded good results when performed by experienced surgeons. The tracheostomy tube usually can be removed within 24 hours postoperatively. Since aspiration pneumonia has been one of the most serious postsurgical complications, all feeding and watering are supervised for the first day or two and may be withheld if vomiting occurs. Slow intravenous or subcutaneous metoclopramide (Reglan, Robins) at 0.05 mg/kg is given 10 to 20 minutes before small feedings to help prevent vomiting. If the regurgitated material has been bloody, cimetidine (Taga-

Table 1. *Results in 29 Dogs with Severe Laryngeal Disease* (*2-Year Study*)

Breed	Sex and Age (Years)	CPK	Thyroid Status	Signs	Methods of Diagnosis and Results	Laryngeal Muscle Biopsy	Treatment	Responses and Follow-Up
Labrador Retrievers:	Male, 11	88	ND	Panting, presented for prostatitis	L: left-sided laryngeal paralysis	ND	None	Treatment for prostatitis; euthanized 1 year later with posterior paresis; no necropsy
	Male, 12	120	TSH normal	Stridor and dyspnea with exertion or excitement; gagging, chronic or acute	L, R, Flu: BLP; temporary megaesophagus	Denervation atrophy	Surgery	Good for 1 year; still alive; no respiratory or gastrointestinal signs except hoarse bark
	Female, 14	220	TSH and T_4 0 to 1.3	Dyspnea and stridor, almost continuous gagging, vomiting, hind leg weakness	L, R, Flu, EMG: BLP; temporary megaesophagus, hiatal hernia, aspiration pneumonia, fibrillations	Denervation atrophy	Surgery; webbed at 6 wks; reoperated	Good; severe CNS signs 8 months later; no thyroid therapy given; euthanized, no necropsy
	Female, 13	100	TSH normal	Panting, heat intolerance, hind end weakness	L, R: BLP	ND	Surgery refused	Good 5 months later
	Female, 13	190	TSH and T_4 0.9 to 1.7	Intermittent stridor, gagging, bloody vomitus, hind leg weakness	L, R, Flu: BLP; hiatal hernia; temporary megaesophagus	ND	Surgery refused; cimetidine and metoclopramide administered; initial thyroid replacement therapy	Fair; still shows stridor but gastrointestinal response good; taken off thyroid medication; TSH repeated 4 months later with normal response; no clinical change; 1.5 year survival; euthanized for posterior paresis, no necropsy
	Male, 12	85	TSH normal	Gagging, dyspnea, bark decreased; bloody, streaked vomit	L, R, Flu: Temporary megaesophagus; hiatal hernia; BLP	Denervation atrophy	Laryngeal surgery	Good; no airway or gastrointestinal disorders; 1 year later still alive
	Male, 11	75	ND	Gagging, voice decreased, intermittent stridor and dyspnea	L, R: Left laryngeal paralysis, right laryngeal paresis	ND	Refused surgery; sedation and steroids administered	Acute respiratory distress and death 4 months later, no necropsy
Irish Setters:	Female, spayed, 11	700	TSH normal	Chronic or acute dyspnea, stridor, gagging, vomiting	L, R, Flu: BLP; hiatal hernia; temporary megaesophagus	ND	Laryngeal surgery; metoclopramide administered	Good, but euthanized 6 months later in renal failure; no necropsy
	Female, 11	ND	ND	Panting, voice decreased, intermittent dyspnea	L: BLP	ND	Laryngeal surgery	OK at 6-week check-up; 2 years later, good
	Male, castrated, 13	258	ND	Dyspnea	L, EMG: BLP; fibrillation	ND	Laryngeal surgery	Good at 3 months; no further follow-up
Newfoundlands:	Male, 9	253	ND	Intermittent dyspnea, clumsy	L, EMG: BLP; multiple sites of fibrillation	Denervation atrophy	Laryngeal surgery	Good airway, but euthanized 6 months later for progression of polyneuropathy
	Male, 10	206	ND	Chronic intermittent dyspnea, gagging, weak hind leg	L, EMG: BLP; multiple sites of fibrillation	Denervation atrophy	Laryngeal surgery	Airway good, but euthanized 5 months later for progression of polyneuropathy
	Female, spayed,	700 2 800	ND	Dyspnea, gagging, vomiting, knuckling of limbs, aspiration pneumonia	L, R, EMG: multiple abnormal muscles; BLP	Myositis	Laryngeal surgery; prednisolone	No measurable response; dysphagia; euthanized; diffuse myositis on necropsy

West Highland White Terriers:	Male, aged	ND	ND	Severe dyspnea	L: BLP with or without collapse	ND	Laryngeal surgery; weight reduction; permanent tracheostomy	OK 6 weeks after surgery
	Female, spayed, 3	ND	ND	Severe intermittent dyspnea, gagging, vomiting, collapse	L: BLP; positive response to edrophonium chloride indicated presence of myasthenia gravis	Normal muscle	Vocal cord resection	Owner elected euthanasia
	Male, 13	ND	ND	Intermittent, severe stridor and dyspnea	L: BLP with or without collapse; EMG: normal	ND	Laryngeal surgery	Euthanized for "growth" at unknown site 1 year later
St. Bernards:	Female, spayed, 11	ND	ND	Severe dyspnea and stridor, acute emergency	L	ND	None	Cardiac arrest occurred before surgery became necessary
	Male, 5	ND	ND	Noisy respiration, panting	L: BLP	ND	Rest; refused surgery	Lost to follow-up
Bull Terrier:	Male, 12	632	TSH and T_4 0.5 to 0.8	Dyspnea, gagging stridor, vomiting	L, R: BLP; aspiration pneumonia; temporary megaesophagus	ND	Laryngeal surgery; initial thyroid replacement therapy	On thyroid medication for 3 months after surgery; when therapy was discontinued, response to TSH test was normal; alive and well 2 years later; no further treatment
Mixed Breeds:	Male, aged	ND	ND	Dyspnea, cyanosis, gagging	L: BLP	Denervation atrophy	Laryngeal surgery	Good, no follow-up
	Male, 8	72	ND	Dyspnea	L, EMG: Multiple muscle abnormalities; BLP		None	Euthanasia, no necropsy
German Shorthair Pointer:	Female, spayed, 3	ND	ND	Chronic noisy breathing; Horner's syndrome, anorexia, dyspnea	L, R: Right-sided laryngeal paralysis, large mediastinal mass	ND	None	Euthanasia; right vagal nerve overgrown by mediastinal mass; lymphosarcoma
Great Dane:	Male, 10	400	T_4 normal	Chronic wheezing, worse with heat and exertion	L: BLP	ND	Laryngeal surgery	Good airway 1 year after surgery; weak posterior limbs
Rottweiler:	Female, 5 months	ND	ND	Clumsy puppy, severe dyspnea, could not see well	L, R, EMG: BLP, proprioceptive dysfunction; cataracts	ND	None	Euthanized; multiple congenital neural abnormalities; cerebellar atrophy, laryngeal muscle degeneration and atrophy
Brittany Spaniel:	Male, 14	83	TSH normal	Panting, stridor with exertion, weak hind limbs	L, R: BLP	ND	Refused surgery; rest, steroids	Overall worsening, died 2 years later of "heat exhaustion"
Standard Poodle:	Male, 12	130	ND	Noisy breathing, howling	L, EMG: BLP	ND	Laryngeal surgery; webbed at 1 month; reoperated	Good until webbing, then good again; lost to follow-up
Miniature Poodle:	Female, 10	ND	ND	Dyspnea, stridor, tracheal trauma	L: BLP; bite wound; severe sepsis	ND	Multiple repairs; severe infection	Died of sepsis 1 month after surgery
Siberian Huskies:	Male, 6 months	ND	ND	Dyspnea from 7 weeks of age	L: BLP	ND	Laryngeal surgery	Good 6 months after surgery
	Female, 7 months	100	T_4 normal	Dyspnea at 12 weeks; fatigue while playing	L, EMB: Fibrillations; BLP, worse on left side		Cage rest	OK at rest 1 year later

Key: BLP = bilateral laryngeal paralysis; CPK = creatine phosphokinase; EMG = electromyography; Flu = fluoroscopic esophagram; L = laryngoscopy; ND = not done; R = radiography; T_4 = thyroxine (µg/dl); TSH = thyroid-stimulating hormone. Laryngeal surgery entailed vocal cord resection (per os) and unilateral partial arytenoidectomy. Samples for TSH test were taken 2 hours after intravenous administration of thyrotropin (5 µg for animals weighing less than 50 lb; 10 µg for larger animals).

T_4 levels of 1 µg/dl and above were accepted as normal for the lab at this time; T_4 levels after administration of TSH were expected to double by 2 hours per sample.

met, SmithKline Beckman) is also given intravenously (0.5 mg/kg) or orally (2 mg/kg every 6 hours). Metoclopramide is continued orally at home until there is no evidence of gagging.

Prognosis for untreated paralysis is dismal since animals may literally be asphyxiated. Unilateral paralysis can progress to severe bilateral disease. The prognosis in terms of airway competence and quality of life after surgery is good. Animals still have noisy breathing, and a muted bark. They also may have some exercise intolerance. Since most have some degree of polyneuropathy, the overall prognosis must be open and should be discussed with the owner before laryngeal surgery. The author has treated aged dogs with acquired laryngeal disease that lived for 4 or more years after surgery before developing severe gait abnormalities, but severe, progressive, incapacitating hind limb weakness has also occurred within 3 months of laryngeal surgery (Table 1). Clinical signs in dogs with congenital laryngeal paralysis usually do not worsen after 6 months of age. The author has seen dogs with clinical and endoscopic evidence of unilateral paralysis or paresis that have compensated by using the more functional side of their larynx and have become highly successful racing dogs. Litter mates of those dogs may be clinically normal but show electromyographic evidence of laryngeal denervation. Thus, selection of nonaffected individuals is difficult if only clinical observations are used. Laryngoscopy and electromyographic studies are recommended for definitive diagnosis.

References and Supplemental Reading

Harvey, H. J., Irby, N. L., and Watrous, B. J.: Laryngeal paralysis in hypothyroid dogs. *In* Kirk, R. W. (ed.): *Current Veterinary Therapy VIII*. Philadelphia: W.B. Saunders, 1983, pp. 694–697.

Harvey, C. E., and Venker-van Haagen, A. J.: Surgical management of pharyngeal and laryngeal airway obstruction in the dog. Vet. Clin. North Am. 5:515, 1975.

O'Brien, J. A.: Hereditary laryngeal paralysis in the racing sled dog (Husky). Proceedings of the Voorjaarsdagen International Congress, Amsterdam, Holland, 1985.

O'Brien, J. A., Harvey, C. E., Kelly, A. E., et al.: Neurogenic atrophy of the laryngeal muscles of the dog. J. Small Anim. Pract. 14:521, 1973.

Venker-van Haagen, A. J., Hartman, W., and Goedegebuure, S. A.: Spontaneous laryngeal paralysis in young Bouviers. J. Am. Anim. Hosp. Assoc. 14:714, 1978.

GOLDEN RETRIEVER MYOPATHY

JOE N. KORNEGAY, D.V.M.
Raleigh, North Carolina

Muscle diseases in dogs may be categorized as either inflammatory or degenerative. The most common inflammatory muscle disease is polymyositis, an apparently immune-mediated disease that causes weakness and muscle pain. Degenerative muscle diseases are either acquired or congenital. The acquired degenerative myopathies usually follow nutritional deficiencies (selenium, vitamin E) or endocrinopathies (hypothyroidism, hyperadrenocorticism). Congenital muscle diseases have been described in Labrador retrievers, chow chows, Irish terriers, and golden retrievers. The golden retriever myopathy remains poorly defined, as only brief descriptions have been included in overviews of canine muscle disease. These cases and three additional dogs studied at the University of Georgia and North Carolina State University are the basis of this report.

CAUSE AND PATHOGENESIS

All affected golden retrievers have been males, suggesting that the disease is acquired as a sex-linked trait. In this way, the golden retriever myopathy resembles Duchenne's muscular dystrophy of humans and a muscle disease identified in Irish terriers. Both Duchenne's muscular dystrophy and the Irish terrier myopathy are linked to the X chromosome; males are affected and females serve as carriers. The clinical and pathologic features that the golden retriever myopathy shares with these two myopathies suggest that these disorders may have a common pathogenesis as well. However, the pathogenesis of these and other congenital muscle diseases remain unclear. Neurogenic, vascular, and membrane hypotheses have been proposed to account for human muscular dystrophies.

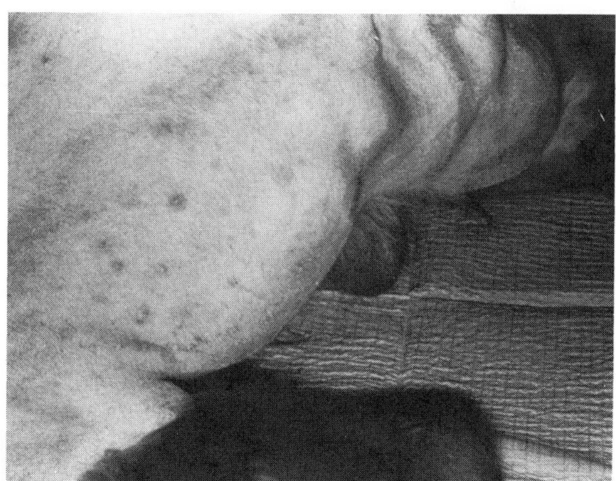

Figure 1. Lateral view of left pelvic limb of adult golden retriever with myopathy. Note the hypertrophy of the semimembranosus and semitendinosus muscles.

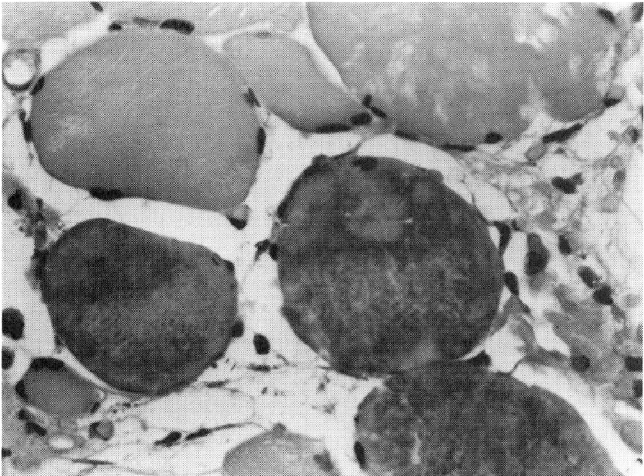

Figure 3. Photomicrograph of transverse section of muscle from golden retriever with myopathy. The three fibers at the bottom are necrotic and mineralized (hematoxylin-eosin × 100).

CLINICAL SIGNS

Initial clinical signs are noted around 6 to 8 weeks of age and include stiffness of gait, thoracic limb abduction, enlargement of the tongue, and simultaneous advancement of the pelvic limbs ("bunny hopping"). Perhaps because of their enlarged tongues, affected dogs have dysphagia and salivate excessively. These clinical signs usually worsen with exercise and gradually progress. As the dogs grow, appendicular muscles may become atrophied or hypertrophied (Fig. 1). The severity and progression of these signs vary: some dogs remain functional for several years, and others require euthanasia before 1 year of age. Some dogs are nearly normal in size and others are stunted.

DIAGNOSIS

Serum muscle enzymes are dramatically increased at 6 to 8 weeks of age and remain elevated in adults with this disorder. Creatine kinase often exceeds 5000 IU/L, and the enzyme concentration increases even more after exercise. Clinically normal females from affected litters may have mildly elevated levels of serum creatine kinase. Accordingly, quantification of creatine kinase may serve to identify carriers.

On electromyographic evaluation, all muscles have bizarre, high-frequency discharges that persist (pseudomyotonia) (Fig. 2). There are no fibrillation potentials, and conduction velocity of motor nerves is normal.

At necropsy of one dog, the tongue, diaphragm, semimembranosus, semitendinosus, biceps femoris, and muscular layers of the esophagus were hypertrophied. Other muscles were either grossly normal or mildly atrophied. Similar histopathologic changes have been seen in all muscles examined. Abnormalities include marked variation in fiber size, numerous hyaline fibers, occasional internal nuclei, and a mild proliferation of endomysium (Fig. 3).

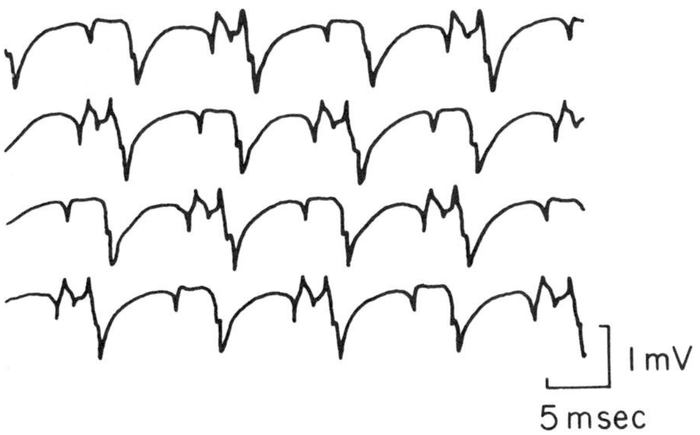

Figure 2. High-frequency discharges recorded from muscle of golden retriever with myopathy.

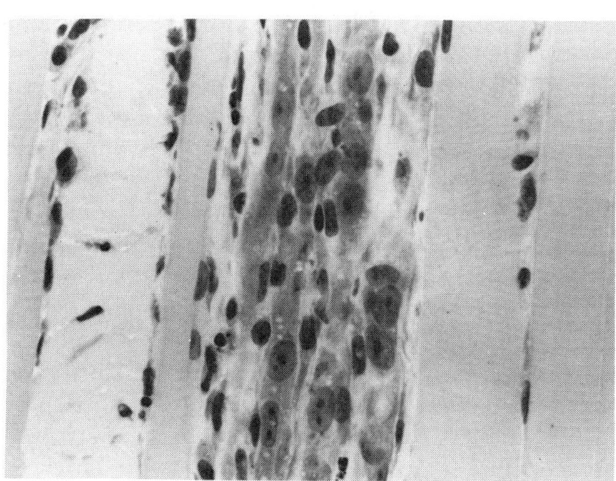

Figure 4. Photomicrograph of longitudinal section of muscle from golden retriever with myopathy. Small basophilic fibers and chains of nuclei with prominent nucleoli at the center of the picture are indicative of regeneration (hematoxylin-eosin × 100).

Severely affected dogs have numerous necrotic fibers that mineralize and are eventually removed by macrophages. Clusters of small basophilic fibers and chains of nuclei with prominent nucleoli also are present (Fig. 4), indicating attempted regeneration. On histochemical evaluation, neither muscle fiber type is selectively affected. However, fiber type grouping has been seen. Electron microscopic changes evident in affected fibers include disruption of myofibrillar organization, dilatation of sarcoplasmic reticulum, increase in glycogen, and both hyperplasia and hypertrophy of mitochondria.

TREATMENT

Little has been done to treat affected golden retrievers. Membrane stabilizing agents such as quinidine, procainamide, and phenytoin have been used with some success in the Irish terrier myopathy and chow chow myotonia, so may have benefit in golden retrievers. However, any improvement probably would be incomplete and only temporary.

References and Supplemental Reading

Cardinet, G. H., and Holliday, T. A.: Neuromuscular diseases of domestic animals: A summary of muscle biopsies from 159 cases. Ann. N.Y. Acad. Sci. 26:290, 1979.

de Lahunta, A.: *Veterinary Neuroanatomy and Clinical Neurology*. Philadelphia: W.B. Saunders, 1983, p. 87.

Wentink, G. H., van der Linde-Sipman, J. S., Meijer, A. E. F. H., et al.: Myopathy with a possible recessive X-linked inheritance in a litter of Irish terriers. Vet. Pathol. 9:328, 1972.

PERIPHERAL VESTIBULAR DISEASE IN SMALL ANIMALS

KENNETH L. SCHUNK, D.V.M.
Grafton, Massachusetts

Disorders of the vestibular system are common in small animals and result in a clinical syndrome characterized by head tilt, ataxia with preservation of strength, and nystagmus. These signs may result from lesions of either the peripheral (membranous labyrinth, vestibular ganglion, and vestibular portion of cranial nerve VIII) or the central (vestibular nuclei and vestibular portion of the cerebellum) vestibular systems. Since most disorders affecting the peripheral vestibular system can be managed more successfully than can diseases involving the central vestibular system, it is important for the clinician to know the differences between them, based on abnormalities found on neurologic examination and the results of diagnostic tests. In addition, the specific cause for the peripheral vestibular dysfunction should be identified, since certain diseases require a specific therapy and may have a different prognosis.

ANATOMY AND PHYSIOLOGY. The vestibular receptors are located within the membranous labyrinth, which is contained in the bony labyrinth of the petrous temporal bone. The bony labyrinth consists of the vestibule, three semicircular canals, and the cochlea, and it contains perilymph, fluid similar in composition to cerebrospinal fluid (CSF). The membranous labyrinth contains endolymph and consists of the saccule and utriculus, three semicircular ducts, and the cochlea duct. The cochlea and cochlear duct are components of the auditory system.

Each part of the membranous labyrinth of the vestibular system contains a specialized receptor that is innervated by the vestibular portion of cranial nerve VIII. At one end of each semicircular duct there is a dilation called the ampulla, which houses the peripheral receptor. The receptor consists of a membranous ridge of connective tissue, termed the *crista*, and neuroepithelial cells covered by a gelatinous material, called the *cupula*. The neuroepithelium consists of supporting cells and hair cells; the hair cells have many stereocilia and a single kinocilium on their luminal surface and function by detecting deflections of the cupula. Because of the orientation of the three semicircular ducts, movement of the head in any plane or angular rotation stimulates the vestibular neurons, which function in dynamic equilibrium. The receptors are not affected by a constant velocity of movement. Each semicircular duct on one side can be paired to a semicircular duct on the opposite side, and movement in one plane stimulates the activity of the neurons of one duct and inhibits their activity in the opposite duct of the synergic pair.

In the utriculus and saccule, the receptors consist of maculae with neuroepithelial cells covered by a gelatinous material, the otolithic membrane. Calcareous crystalline bodies called statoconia are present on this membrane, and their movement in relationship to the stereocilia and kinocilia of the epithelial cells results in stimulation of the vestibular neurons. Gravitational forces affect the position of the statoconia, since the macula in the saccule is oriented in a vertical direction, whereas the macula of the utriculus is in a horizontal position. The maculae are responsible for the sensation of the static position of the head relative to the force of gravity. In addition, linear acceleration or deceleration of the head is detected by the macula of the utriculus; the macula of the saccule is more sensitive to vibrational stimuli.

After originating at the hair cells of the crista ampullaris, macula utriculi, and macula sacculi, the axons of the vestibular portion of cranial nerve VIII enter the cranial cavity via the internal acoustic meatus. Their bipolar cell bodies are located within the petrous temporal bone in the vestibular ganglion. The vestibular neurons enter the rostral medulla at the cerebellomedullary angle. Most of these neurons terminate in the vestibular nuclei in the rostral medulla; the remainder enter the cerebellum to terminate in the fastigial nucleus and flocculonodular lobe.

The vestibulospinal tract originates from the vestibular nuclei and descends in the ipsilateral ventral funiculus and terminates on interneurons in the ventral gray column. The interneurons are facilitory to ipsilateral alpha and gamma motor neurons innervating the extensor muscles and inhibitory to ipsilateral alpha motor neurons to the flexor muscles. Some interneurons cross to the contralateral side and are inhibitory to the alpha and gamma motor neurons to the extensor muscles (de Lahunta, 1983).

The vestibular nuclei send axons rostrally in the medial longitudinal fasciculus and reticular formation to the nuclei of cranial nerves III, IV, and VI. Therefore, changes in head posture will be accompanied by coordinated conjugate eyeball movements.

SIGNS OF VESTIBULAR DISEASE

Unilateral Peripheral Disease

Signs of unilateral peripheral vestibular disease include a head tilt toward the side of the lesion, nystagmus, and asymmetrical ataxia with preservation of strength. The ataxia is characterized by leaning, drifting, and falling toward the side of the lesion. The animal may also circle tightly in the same direction as the head tilt. There may be a curvature of the trunk with the concavity directed to the side of the lesion, and the animal often prefers to lean or walk along a wall on the affected side for support. There is a decrease in extensor tone of the limbs on the affected side and an increase in extensor tone on the opposite side. Infrequently, animals with acute peripheral vestibular lesions will roll to the side of the lesion. The degree of head tilt will vary, and blindfolding the patient will usually make the head tilt more obvious. These signs can be explained by the loss of activity of the vestibulospinal tract ipsilateral to the lesion.

Nystagmus is an involuntary rhythmic oscillation of the eyeballs that usually has a fast and slow phase. The nystagmus should be described by the direction of the fast component. During movement of the head in a normal animal, the eyes move away from the direction the head is turning and then quickly jerk back to that direction. This is known as vestibular nystagmus and occurs in a normal animal when its head is moved in any direction. The fast phase of the nystagmus is toward the direction the head is rotated.

If an animal is rotated, nystagmus occurs during the initial acceleration, and the direction of the fast phase is in the direction of the rotation. Once the velocity of the rotation is constant, nystagmus does not occur. When the rotation of the animal is stopped suddenly, postrotatory nystagmus is present for a short interval, and the direction of the fast component is opposite that of the rotation. Postrotatory nystagmus can be tested clinically in small animals to measure the functional integrity of each peripheral vestibular system. Although the duration of the postrotatory nystagmus is variable, it should be approximately the same when the animal is spun in either direction. The postrotatory nystagmus will be reduced or absent when the patient is rotated in the direction opposite to the side of the lesion.

In animals with unilateral peripheral vestibular disease, horizontal or rotary nystagmus occurs with the fast component away from the side of the lesion. This may be observed when the head is held in its normal position (spontaneous nystagmus) or when the head is fixed in an abnormal position (positional nystagmus). The direction of the nystagmus should not change regardless of the position of the head. In some animals a concomitant eyelid contraction may be observed with the nystagmus.

In most animals with unilateral peripheral disease, the eyeball ipsilateral to the lesion is deviated ventrally. This can best be seen when the head is straightened and the nose is elevated; this is referred to as vestibular strabismus. There is no paralysis of the extraocular muscles, since the eyeball can move in all directions. Vestibular strabismus and abnormal nystagmus result from the dysfunction within the vestibular system and its influence on cranial nerves III, IV, and VI.

Postural reactions such as hopping, placing, and conscious proprioception are normal, except for the righting response. In patients with severe ataxia due to a peripheral vestibular lesion, it is often difficult to evaluate the postural reactions critically, and serial neurologic examinations should be performed.

Vomiting may occur in any vestibular disorder but is more common in animals with acute peripheral vestibular disease. This is due to the central connections from the vestibular nuclei to the vomiting center in the reticular formation of the brain stem.

Bilateral Peripheral Disease

In animals with bilateral peripheral vestibular disease, head tilt and nystagmus are often absent. The animal exhibits a symmetrical ataxia and usually has a crouched gait with a tendency to stagger or fall to either side. This may resemble cerebellar ataxia; however, there is no hypermetria or intention tremor. Head movements consist of wide excursions from side to side and are characteristic of bilateral vestibular dysfunction. Normal vestibular nystagmus and postrotatory nystagmus cannot be elicited. The animal may also be deaf if the auditory system is involved in the disease process.

Central Vestibular Disease

Lesions involving the vestibular nuclei, fastigial nuclei, or the flocculonodular lobes of the cerebellum result in signs that are similar to those seen in peripheral vestibular disorders. These animals usually exhibit, in addition to the vestibular signs, evidence of brain stem or cerebellar dysfunction.

Clinical signs consistent with a lesion of the central vestibular pathways are "central" nystagmus, upper motor neuron paresis and general proprioceptive ataxia (usually ipsilateral to the lesion), cerebellar ataxia, deficits of cranial nerves other than VII, and disturbances to the sensorium. The nystagmus resulting from disorders of the central vestibular system may be in any direction. Vertical nystagmus, nystagmus with the fast phase directed toward the head tilt, or nystagmus that changes directions with different positions of the head indicate a central lesion.

DISEASES OF THE PERIPHERAL VESTIBULAR SYSTEM

Idiopathic Benign Vestibular Disease in Dogs

This disease is the most common cause of unilateral peripheral vestibular disease in geriatric dogs. The mean age of onset is 12.5 years (Schunk and Averill, 1983). The disease is characterized by a peracute onset of unilateral peripheral vestibular signs. The degree of ataxia is usually moderate (the dog is able to stand but stumbles and falls to the affected side) or severe (unable to stand or walk without assistance); rolling is not a common sign. The nystagmus often has a rotary component. Transient nausea and vomiting occur in approximately one third of the cases.

The diagnosis is made by eliminating the other causes of peripheral vestibular dysfunction. The absence of physical abnormalities of the tympanic membrane and the absence of radiographic changes within the tympanic bulla or petrous temporal bone in patients with a peracute onset of unilateral peripheral vestibular signs but without a history of trauma are diagnosed as having idiopathic benign vestibular disease. In patients in which CSF analysis has been performed, the results have been normal. Radiographs of the tympanic bullae and petrous temporal bone and examination of the tympanic membrane under anesthesia are necessary to rule out the diagnosis of otitis media or otitis interna.

Therapy is not recommended; corticosteroids do not alter the clinical recovery of the animal. Since the vomiting is usually not severe and stops within the first 24 to 36 hours, antimotion drugs are usually not administered.

The prognosis for recovery is good to excellent. Spontaneous nystagmus is usually present for the first 3 to 4 days but then disappears. An abnormal positional nystagmus in the same direction as the spontaneous nystagmus can usually be elicited for another few days. Over the first week, the ataxia usually improves to the point where the animal is able to walk without falling but will still lean and drift to the affected side. Over the next 2 weeks the gait continues to improve. The head tilt usually resolves within the first month, but occasionally it will persist indefinitely. After the animal has recovered or compensated for the lesion, the dog may show a transient disturbance of balance if stressed. Recurrent attacks are unusual but may occur on the same or opposite side.

The pathogenesis of this disease is unknown. Cases examined histologically have not revealed any lesions within the labyrinth, vestibular nerve, vestibular ganglion, or CNS. A neuritis of the vestibular portion of cranial nerve VIII and dynamic abnormalities of endolymphatic fluid within the membranous labyrinth are possible causes. Experimentally, labyrinthectomy produces an identical clinical syndrome, from which the animal recovers by compensation that is dependent on central vestibular structures (Carpenter et al., 1959).

Idiopathic Vestibular Neuropathy in Cats

Idiopathic vestibular neuropathy is a common disease in adult cats of any age. The history of a peracute onset of a loss of balance and the neurologic examination findings of unilateral peripheral vestibular dysfunction are almost identical to those found in dogs. This disease may have a higher incidence in the summer and early fall (de Lahunta, 1983). Vomiting is not as common in cats as it is in dogs. The results of all diagnostic tests, including radiographs of the tympanic bullae and petrous temporal bone and physical examination of the tympanic membrane, are within normal limits. Spontaneous recovery is usually complete over a 2- to 3-week period. Occasionally, transient vestibular attacks have been observed in cats that recover to normal in 1 to 3 days. The pathogenesis of this disease is poorly understood. No therapy is recommended, and the prognosis is excellent.

Otitis Interna

Extension of otitis media to otitis interna is the most common cause of inflammatory vestibular disease (Chrisman, 1982). Vestibular signs occur when the middle ear inflammation affects the function of the membranous labyrinth. Most cases of otitis media are caused by bacteria and are secondary to otitis externa, although extension from the pharynx through the auditory tube also occurs. Hematogenous spread of infection to the middle and inner ears appears to be uncommon. The disease occurs at any age. In one study the mean age of onset was 8.5 years with a range of 6 months to 18 years (Schunk and Averill, 1983). Although otitis media and otitis interna may be seen in any breed, cocker spaniels and other long-eared dogs with chronic otitis externa are commonly affected. The rate of onset is variable, and signs appear acutely or insidiously over a period of several weeks.

The vestibular signs are consistent with a unilateral peripheral vestibular lesion. The most significant sign is a head tilt. The ataxia is usually mild or not present at all, and nystagmus may not be seen. In addition to the vestibular signs, an ipsilateral facial paresis or palsy or Horner's syndrome may be observed on neurologic examination; these may be caused by involvement of the facial nerve and sympathetic innervation within the middle ear. Facial weakness is present in over half of the cases of otitis media and interna. Since the facial nerve contains parasympathetic preganglionic neurons that produce secretion of lacrimal glands, facial palsy may be accompanied by decreased tear formation and keratitis sicca. Unilateral deafness may occur, but this is difficult to determine clinically.

Bilateral occurrence of both otitis media and otitis interna is occasionally seen with or without bilateral facial weakness. If the disturbance to the vestibular system is symmetrical, signs of bilateral vestibular disease will be present. However, most cases have asymmetrical vestibular involvement resulting in asymmetrical vestibular signs. Deafness may occur in animals with bilateral otitis media and interna.

The diagnosis of otitis media and interna is based on finding physical or radiographic evidence of non-neoplastic, nontraumatic lesions in the middle or inner ear or both areas. The patient should be anesthetized, and ventrodorsal, oblique lateral, and open-mouth skull radiographs should be taken. Radiographic evidence of otitis media and interna include increased thickness of the bones of the tympanic bullae and bony labyrinth of the petrous temporal bone, with or without increased density within the tympanic bullae. The open-mouth view is the most useful in evaluating changes of the tympanic bullae. Radiographs may appear normal in animals with acute infections. Bilateral radiographic abnormalities are often found in animals with unilateral vestibular signs due to otitis media and interna. Radiographic evidence of bone lysis is not common with this condition, and its presence suggests the possibility of a tumor.

While the patient is under anesthesia, the external ear canal, tympanic membrane, and pharynx should be examined carefully. Most cases of otitis media occur by extension from otitis externa, so if inflammation is present, specimens for culture should be taken from the horizontal ear canal. The tympanic membrane should be identified. If necessary, exudate can be suctioned from the ear canal by using a straight Frazier suction tube. Only low negative pressure should be used in order to avoid damaging the tympanic membrane. The eardrum is normally pearl-gray in color and translucent; the manubrium of the malleus can be seen through the ventral portion of the tympanic membrane, the pars tensa. Most dogs with otitis media and interna have an eardrum that appears abnormal or ruptured.

Myringotomy with a 20-gauge, 3.5-inch spinal needle should be performed in animals with radiographically abnormal petrous temporal bones or diseased tympanic membranes. The needle should be inserted through the edge of the eardrum at the 6 o'clock position, and samples should be obtained for culture and cytologic tests. If exudate is not obtained from the middle ear cavity, 0.25 to 0.5 ml of sterile saline can be instilled and then aspirated and used for testing. This same procedure can be performed when the tympanic membrane is ruptured. It is important to obtain samples for culture, since most cases are caused by a bacterial infection and respond to appropriate long-term antibiotic therapy. The author does not recommend routine flushing of the outer ear canal for otitis externa. This procedure occasionally results in signs of acute otitis interna and even though the tympanic membrane was probably ruptured before the ear canal was flushed, the procedure can result in perforation of the eardrum. The pharynx should be examined carefully, since otitis media may occur by extension from the pharynx through the auditory tube.

Inflammatory polyps are common in cats with otitis media and interna and originate within the middle ear secondary to chronic inflammation. The polyp is often seen deep within the external ear canal, near the level of the tympanic membrane. Occasionally, a polyp may extend down the auditory tube and can be found protruding into the pharynx. It is important to rule out the presence of an inflammatory polyp in cats with otitis media and interna since surgical excision is necessary in these cases.

The treatment of otitis media and interna is dependent on the clinical and radiographic findings. A medical approach is used in most cases unless radiographs reveal a moderate or marked increased density in the tympanic bulla, suggesting the presence of a large quantity of exudate in the middle ear. In the author's experience, most cases of otitis media and interna can be treated successfully with long-term (4 to 6 weeks) systemic antibiotics. If a culture has been performed and sensitivity is known, the appropriate antibiotic is administered. Otherwise, treatment with chloramphenicol (Chloromycetin, Parke-Davis), 25 to 50 mg/kg in dogs and 20 mg/kg in cats, repeated every 8 hours, or cephalexin (Keflex, Dista), 30 mg/kg for both groups, repeated every 8 hours, has been used successfully. Long-term therapy with chloramphenicol should be used with caution in cats because of its propensity to cause anorexia, weight loss, and blood dyscrasias. Long-term therapy with systemic aminoglycosides should be avoided because they may cause degeneration within the vestibular and auditory systems. Systemic corticosteroid therapy is not recommended by the author but has been used initially for a few days to reduce the inflammation within the vestibular system. Topical medications, based on the results of culture and sensitivity tests, are used to treat associated otitis externa. Gentamicin (Gentocin, Schering) has been used in cases with ruptured tympanic membranes; this drug has no known side effects but should be used with caution.

Surgical exploration and drainage is indicated in cases with significant amounts of exudate within the middle ear cavity or in cats suspected of having an inflammatory polyp. The author's procedure of choice is the osteotomy of the ventral bulla. Horner's syndrome has occasionally been observed after surgical removal of an inflammatory polyp.

The prognosis for most cases of otitis media and interna is good if treated properly. Recurrences following withdrawal of antibiotic therapy may occur. The most common residual vestibular symptom after therapy is a head tilt, which may never resolve completely. The prognosis is guarded in cases with osteomyelitis involving the petrous temporal bone. Extension of an inner ear infection to the brain stem is rare; if this occurs despite CSF culture and aggressive systemic antibiotic therapy, the prognosis is grave. Facial nerve paralysis and Horner's syndrome are usually permanent sequelae of otitis media. If keratitis sicca is present owing to facial nerve involvement, the use of artificial tear preparations will be necessary. Reduced auditory function may be permanent but will not be clinically significant unless the infection is bilateral.

Neoplasia

Tumors such as osteosarcomas, fibrosarcomas, and chondrosarcomas, originating in the osseous bullae or bony labyrinth, may involve the peripheral vestibular structures. Carcinomas of the squamous cells and ceruminous glands may spread locally and damage the vestibular apparatus within the inner ear.

In addition to signs referable to vestibular dysfunction, facial weakness or Horner's syndrome is often seen on neurologic examination. These tumors are usually evident on plain radiographs of the skull. The presence of bony lysis on radiographs should strongly suggest the possibility of neoplasia. The diagnosis can be confirmed after a biopsy is taken of the lesion. Since these tumors are locally invasive, total resection is not possible in most cases.

Neurofibrosarcomas and neurofibromas of cranial nerve VIII are rare in the dog and cat. They should be suspected in animals with slowly progressive peripheral vestibular signs that are unresponsive to therapy. Skull radiographs are normal at the onset, but lysis of the petrous temporal bone may be seen later (Chrisman, 1982). These tumors tend to grow along the vestibulocochlear nerve and eventually compress the brain stem, resulting in central vestibular symptoms.

Trauma

Head trauma may result in fractures of the petrous temporal bone or tympanic bulla. Hemorrhage, with or without a ruptured tympanic membrane, may be seen on otoscopic examination of the ear. Serial neurologic examinations should be performed in order to differentiate peripheral from central vestibular trauma. Significant improvement within 72 hours suggests that the lesion is peripheral (Chrisman, 1980). If the disturbance is primarily limited to the peripheral system, the prognosis is better, since compensation will occur if the brain stem and cerebellum are not involved.

Congenital Peripheral Vestibular Disorders

Purebred cats and dogs that develop a head tilt, circling, or rolling from birth to 3 months of age should be suspected of having a congenital vestibular disorder. Unilateral congenital disease has been reported in German shepherd, English cocker spaniel, and Doberman pinscher dogs and in Siamese and Burmese cats (de Lahunta, 1983). Clinical signs of bilateral peripheral vestibular dysfunction and deafness have been reported in beagles (de Lahunta, 1983). Findings of all ancillary tests are normal. The prognosis for animals with unilateral involvement is good, since they are often able to compensate and become acceptable pets. Deafness may accompany the vestibular signs and is usually permanent. A developmental abnormality of the peripheral vestibular system is suspected, but histologic evidence of disease has not been found. No effective therapy is available.

Effects of Toxins

Aminoglycoside antibiotics are known to cause degeneration within the vestibular and auditory systems. Prolonged administration of high doses or use of these drugs in patients with impaired renal function usually produces the degeneration. In cats, streptomycin more commonly affects the vestibular receptors but may also involve the auditory receptors. Dihydrostreptomycin, neomycin, gentamicin, kanamycin, and vancomycin usually affect the auditory system, but the vestibular system is also susceptible. Degeneration within the vestibular structures may result in unilateral or bilateral peripheral vestibular symptoms. Deafness may occur with or without vestibular dysfunction. Any animals receiving these drugs should be monitored for loss of hearing or vestibular signs. If the drug is discontinued immediately, the vestibular symptoms usually improve; however, deafness is often irreversible (Chrisman, 1980). Degenerative changes are observed histologically in the hair cells of the vestibular receptors as well as in the fastigial nuclei and flocculonodular lobes of the cerebellum.

Polyneuropathy

Occasionally, adult dogs have been observed with unilateral or bilateral peripheral vestibular symptoms and facial paresis or paralysis. The results of diagnostic tests, including skull radiographs, examination of the tympanic membrane, and CSF analysis, are normal. The cause of this condition is unknown. In some cases, hypothyroidism has been present, but appropriate thyroid therapy is usually not beneficial. Spontaneous recovery has been reported (de Lahunta, 1983).

References and Supplemental Reading

Carpenter, M. B., Fabrega, H., and Glinsmann, W.: Physiological deficits occurring with lesions of labyrinth and fastigial nucleus. J. Neurophysiol. 22:222, 1959.

Chrisman, C. L.: Vestibular diseases. Vet. Clin. North Am. 10:103, 1980.

Chrisman, C. L.: *Problems in Small Animal Neurology.* Philadelphia: Lea & Febiger, 1982, pp. 250–275.

de Lahunta, A.: *Veterinary Neuroanatomy and Clinical Neurology*, 2nd ed. Philadelphia: W.B. Saunders, 1983, pp. 238–254.

Schunk, K. L., and Averill, D. R., Jr.: Peripheral vestibular syndrome in the dog: A review of 83 cases. J.A.V.M.A. 182:1354, 1983.

GENERALIZED TREMOR SYNDROME

BRIAN R. H. FARROW, B.V.Sc.
Sydney, Australia

Generalized tremor or shaking results from involuntary, repetitive, rhythmic muscle contractions that are of fairly uniform amplitude and frequency and involve the body, head, and limbs. This tremor may be the principal manifestation of a variety of disorders in animals. Conclusive evidence regarding the pathophysiologic basis of generalized tremor is not yet available; however, a number of observations suggest that generalized tremor results from a diffuse disorder of the central nervous system. One such observation is the appearance of a generalized tremor resulting from certain metabolic conditions and intoxications that are known to affect the central nervous system diffusely. In cases of tremor that may be absent at rest and made worse with excitement or exercise, it seems likely that involvement of the cerebellum plays a significant role but is not the sole source of the signs.

Although tremor as a clinical sign has been associated with lesions of hypomyelination, many tremor syndromes occur in which no structural abnormalities can be detected in either nervous or other tissues. This observation, together with the rapid recovery seen in some tremor disorders, suggests that in many cases a reversible biochemical lesion affects neurotransmission and is the pathophysiologic basis of the tremor. Studies using tremorgenic mycotoxins provide support for this notion by indicating their role in influencing neurotransmitter activity (Mantle and Penny, 1981).

Generalized tremor associated with disorders of myelination, both congenital and acquired, have been reviewed by Mayhew and colleagues (1984). The diseases showing hypomyelination tend to be congenital and become manifest as the affected animals begin to walk, whereas those disorders characterized by demyelination tend to develop later in life. Occasionally tremors occur with diffuse, nonsuppurative encephalomyelitis (de Lahunta, 1983) or other encephalopathies such as certain lysosomal storage diseases. Tremor also can often be a manifestation of a number of metabolic conditions and intoxications. These include hypocalcemia, hypoglycemia, azotemia and hyperammonemia, and poisoning with metaldehyde, organophosphate, chlorinated hydrocarbon, fluoroacetate, strychnine, and, occasionally, lead.

IDIOPATHIC GENERALIZED TREMOR (SHAKER DOGS)

Apart from disorders of myelination, metabolic conditions, and intoxications that may cause generalized tremor, a condition is seen in dogs throughout the world in which generalized tremor of unknown cause is the dominant feature. It occurs predominantly in small dogs, and the vast majority of cases have a white coat. Although it has been observed occasionally in other small breeds, such as the beagle, Yorkshire terrier, Australian silky terrier, and miniature pinscher, this condition is seen most frequently in small white dogs, particularly the Maltese terrier and West Highland white terrier.

The onset is usually sudden; first signs generally appear between 9 months and 2 years of age, although occasionally younger and older animals have been seen. Detailed questioning of owners has failed to identify any prior significant illnesses, and they emphasize the suddenness of onset. The tremor is generalized and varies from mild to so severe that the whole animal shakes and normal locomotion is difficult. The tremor is exaggerated by handling, forced locomotion, and excitement, and it diminishes markedly at rest or with relaxation. The dogs are alert and responsive and generally have no other neurologic deficits. Occasional animals are seen with a head tilt, suggesting focal vestibular involvement. Rarely, a shaking dog may convulse, but in general the tremor is the only manifestation of abnormality. Results of routine hematologic and biochemical tests are normal. Cerebrospinal fluid evaluation may show normal values or reveal a mild increase in lymphocytes (more than 5 per microliter). In cases in which euthanasia has been performed and detailed histologic examination of nervous tissues has been undertaken, a very mild, diffuse, nonsuppurative meningoencephalomyelitis may be seen. Lesions consisting of mild lymphocytic perivascular cuffing are most apparent in the cerebellum but are not confined to that structure. The choroid plexus and meninges may also show infiltration by lymphocytes and plasma cells. There are no associated parenchymal lesions evident. In some animals in which euthanasia has been requested because of their disease, there are no visible lesions despite detailed examination. Serologic and viral isolation studies have not revealed a cause.

Treatment

When a specific cause of the generalized tremor can be demonstrated, appropriate specific therapy should be instituted. In cases of unknown cause that occur in young adults of the small breeds (usually white), most dogs respond in a few days to immunosuppressive doses of glucocorticosteroids. Prednisone or prednisolone is given at approximately 3 mg/kg each morning for 5 days and then decreased to alternate mornings for an additional 5 days before a phased withdrawal of medication; this usually results in a dramatic disappearance of clinical signs. Some cases will remain free of clinical signs after the withdrawal of medication, whereas others need to be maintained on low-dose, alternate-day therapy to control clinical signs. Sometimes successfully treated cases will relapse months later and require reinstitution of glucocorticosteroid therapy. If left untreated, the signs may persist for life, although their severity may decrease.

Because the histologic lesions are very mild and often absent, it is unlikely that these changes are the cause of the dramatic clinical signs. Nevertheless, the presence of lymphocytes around blood vessels in the nervous system and in the cerebrospinal fluid of some cases may indicate an underlying immune-mediated disorder. This suggestion is supported by the remarkable response seen to immunosuppressive levels of glucocorticosteroids. The fact that by far the majority of affected dogs are white in color seems more than coincidental, as does the predominance of affected Maltese terriers and West Highland white terriers. As both melanin and the catecholamine neurotransmitters are derived from tyrosine, it is hypothesized (Farrow and de Lahunta, unpublished data) that these dogs are in some way predisposed to develop immunologic reactions that are directed at cells involved in the elaboration and release of certain neurotransmitters. There is a precedent for this general concept: the Vogt-Koyanagi-Harada syndrome, which occurs in both humans and dogs, is the result of an immunologic disease directed against melanin-producing cells (Lubin et al., 1981) and accounts for the vitiligo, poliosis, uveitis, and leptomeningitis that occur. The common denominator in these two diseases may be their involvement with the metabolism of tyrosine and their embryologic origin from neural crest.

References and Supplemental Reading

de Lahunta, A.: *Veterinary Neuroanatomy and Clinical Neurology*, 2nd ed. Philadelphia: W.B. Saunders, 1983, p. 150.

Lubin, J. R., Loewenstein, J. L., and Frederick, A. R.: Vogt-Koyanagi-Harada syndrome with focal neurologic signs. Am. J. Ophthalmol. 91:332, 1981.

Mantle, P. G., and Penny, R. H. C.: Tremorgenic mycotoxins and neurological disorders—A review. *In* Grunsell, G. S. G., and Hill, F. W. G.: *The Veterinary Annual*, 21st Issue. Bristol: Scientechnica, 1981, pp. 51–62.

Mayhew, I. G., Blakemore, W. F., Palmer, A. C., et al.: Tremor syndrome and hypomyelination in lurcher pups. J. Small Anim. Pract. 25:2551, 1984.

FELINE DYSAUTONOMIA

N. J. H. SHARP, B. VET. MED.,
Liverpool, England

and A. S. NASH, B.V.M.S.
Glasgow, Scotland

In late 1981 an apparently new disorder of unknown origin appeared in the feline population of the United Kingdom. Correspondence from Key and Gaskell (1982) first drew attention to the condition with a series of five cases exhibiting clinical signs such as dilated pupils, dry mucous membranes, constipation, and megaesophagus. Nash and others (1982) then related these signs to lesions found in autonomic ganglia. Various names have been ascribed to this condition including the Key-Gaskell syndrome, feline autonomic polyganglionopathy, the dilated pupil syndrome, and, more recently, feline dysautonomia. The last is, we feel, the most appropriate term because it denotes dysfunction of the autonomic nervous system, which is the only consistent factor in the presentation. Since its appearance, feline dysautonomia has become established throughout the United Kingdom as an important cause of both morbidity and mortality. It has also been described in isolated case reports from both Norway and Sweden.

The condition is most frequently encountered in young domestic cats of previous good health and from a wide range of environments. Epidemiological surveys (Rochlitz, 1984; Sharp et al., 1984) have failed to reveal evidence of contagion or a relationship to any factor in management or the environment, although further, more extensive studies are in progress.

CLINICAL SIGNS AND DIAGNOSIS

The time of development for the classic clinical signs is variable and ranges from rare, peracute cases to chronic ones with a more gradual onset of signs over several weeks. Most cats present over a period of 48 hours and may initially seem to be in the early stages of "cat flu" or may show a transient fever with diarrhea.

The most frequently encountered clinical signs include dilated, nonresponsive pupils; regurgitation associated with megaesophagus; constipation; dryness of both nasal and ocular mucous membranes; depression; anorexia; dehydration; and weight loss. The incidence of the main clinical features is shown in Table 1, and these have been extensively reviewed by Rochlitz (1984) and Sharp and colleagues (1984). Prolapse of the nictitating membrane may mask the pupillary signs, and the administration of barium prior to lateral thoracic radiography may be necessary to reveal the extent and severity of the megaesophagus. A valuable diagnostic feature is the marked decrease in tear production as measured by the Schirmer tear test; normal values of more than 10 mm of tears in one minute frequently drop to as low as 2 or even 0 mm in affected cats. Bradycardia with a heart rate of less than 120 beats per minute is seen in some cats, and in some animals this may fall to as low as 90 beats per minute. Results of hematologic and plasma biochemical tests and urinalysis in most cases are within normal limits, although the significance of large numbers of Heinz bodies noted in the red blood cells of some cats is unknown.

Differentials to diagnosis are few, and they occur mainly before the full syndrome is apparent. They include intestinal obstruction and early "cat flu"; in cases presenting with dysuria and retention cystitis, the feline urologic syndrome should be considered.

At present, final diagnosis depends on recognition of the pathognomonic degeneration within autonomic ganglia (Griffiths and Sharp, in press; Sharp et al., 1984).

THERAPY

Most cats will present with varying degrees of dehydration and anorexia, which initial therapy must therefore correct. Further therapy can then be divided into supportive measures and more specific attempts at autonomic stimulation.

Table 1. *Major Clinical Features of Feline Dysautonomia*

Feature	Number of Cases Investigated	Number of Cases Affected	Percent of Cases Affected
Depression and anorexia	40	40	100
Constipation	39	37	95
Dry rhinarium	38	36	95
Reduced tear production	27	25	93
Megaesophagus	37	34	92
Dilated pupils	40	36	90
Regurgitation or vomiting	38	31	82
Prolapsed membrane	35	25	71
Reduced or absent photomotor reflex	30	21	70
Dry oral mucosa	39	27	69
Bradycardia (< 120/min)	37	22	59
Areflexic anus	24	7	29
Fecal incontinence	35	7	20
Urinary incontinence	39	7	18
Paresis or collapse	28	5	18
Proprioceptive deficits	28	4	14

Perhaps one of the most important duties of the clinician is to make the owner fully aware of both the guarded overall prognosis and the likely extended nature of the clinical course, during which time an often considerable degree of nursing at home may be required.

Initial therapy will normally consist of administration of intravenous fluid such as physiologic saline solution to correct the estimated fluid deficit. This is continued at a maintenance dose of 40 to 60 ml/kg body weight per day for several days as required and can be combined with a multivitamin preparation. The feeding of liquified nutrients by hand or by carefully using a syringe should be encouraged, provided it does not induce repeated regurgitation. Alternatively, stomach intubation, in which a urethral catheter is inserted into the nostril, has been described (Rochlitz, 1984) and has been well tolerated, provided that a local anesthetic spray is applied to the nares. Administration of corticosteroids or megestrol acetate has been reported by some workers to stimulate appetite and general demeanor, and it may be continued every other day for several months. Broad-spectrum antibiotic administration for one to two weeks is indicated in debilitated animals to prevent secondary infection of the respiratory and urinary tracts. When regurgitation is frequent, the use of the parenteral route for these drugs may be more reliable.

Constipation can cause considerable distress, and liquid paraffin (mineral oil) at a dose of 2 to 5 ml orally on alternate days may be helpful. A safer alternative is danthron laxative (Dorbanex, Riker Labs) at a dose rate of up to 5 ml of a 5 mg/ml solution orally per day. If conservative laxative therapy is ineffective, then careful use of an enema is indicated. Cases exhibiting urinary retention will require regular manual evacuation of the bladder, which is normally well tolerated.

Parasympathomimetics are often beneficial and can be administered either by tablet, such as bethanechol hydrochloride (2.5 mg daily), or in ophthalmic solutions, such as 0.5 per cent physostigmine or 1 per cent pilocarpine at a dose of one drop in one or both eyes once or twice daily. Each preparation is capable of causing a systemic effect, although this may be more reliable when eye drops are used in cases with severe megaesophagus.

After 1 to 2 weeks of such intensive therapy, a reassessment should be made of the situation in order to determine whether there has been a positive response, with improvement or at least stabilization of the patient. Cases with a particularly poor prognosis and in which early euthanasia should be considered include those with persistent regurgitation, which complicates attempts to maintain an adequate oral intake of fluid. A more optimistic outlook is suggested in cases that maintain adequate hydration and tolerate supplemented feeding or even show an interest in voluntary intake. This should be encouraged by allowing the animal access to fresh water, milk, and aromatic foodstuffs. The transfer of food taken by any method into the stomach may be encouraged by nursing the animal in an upright position for 10 minutes after feeding.

Cases that have stabilized should be returned to the owner with instructions to maintain the oral intake of fluid and food, but they should be examined at first every few days to ensure that progress is maintained. Antibiotic therapy can be stopped, but steroid or progestogen administration should be continued if there has been apparent benefit. Oral delivery of multivitamins and laxatives should be continued as necessary, and the owner should be instructed on how to manually express the bladder if urinary retention is present. Minimal resistance normally occurs during this procedure, so iatrogenic rupture is unlikely. Long-term administration (up to 6 months) of parasympathomimetics has not caused difficulties. Variation exists as to the best dose and preparation, and this will need to be determined by trial and error for each individual case. A regular consultation once or twice a month is indicated to reassess the prognosis and to modify drug therapy as necessary. Gradual withdrawal of drug therapy should be instituted as return to normality occurs.

COMPLICATIONS

These may either occur as a result of attempted treatment or because of the effects of the disorder.

The use of parasympathomimetic drugs should be undertaken with care. They should not be used in combination, and even when used individually they may sometimes result in overdosage manifest by hyperesthesia, muscular fasciculations, abdominal cramp, and diarrhea. Fortunately, these are easily countered with atropine, but this is an undesirable treatment because it temporarily exacerbates the parasympathetic dysfunction. The use of flea collars or products containing organophosphate compounds should also be avoided during treatment.

Liquid paraffin may well increase the risk of inhalation because of its bland taste, so a combination with pilchard oil (a strong fish oil) may help counter this effect and will also serve as a supplement of fat-soluble vitamins. Barium studies will also increase the risk of inhalation, particularly in debilitated animals, and caution should be adopted; the use of barium is preferably restricted to mild or stabilized cases.

Anesthesia with a variety of parenteral and inhalation agents has had fatal consequences in several cases and should be performed with caution.

The condition carries the risk not only of inhalation pneumonia but also of upper respiratory and oropharyngeal infection due to devitalized mucous membranes, and urinary retention predisposes the animal to cystitis.

A complication seen relatively late in the course of the condition has been that of fecal incontinence. Three cats that were otherwise recovering well became socially unacceptable and had to be destroyed.

PROGNOSIS

Twenty to 40 per cent of affected cats are likely to recover, but initial severity does not appear to be particularly useful in assessing the eventual outcome. The cat's general demeanor and its response to treatment are more reliable indicators. The likely time for recovery ranges from 2 to 12 months. In some cases recovery is complete, but in many, residual features, such as dilated pupils, intermittent regurgitation, or a failure to regain full body weight and condition, persist.

References and Supplemental Reading

Griffiths, I. R. G., and Sharp, N. J. H.: Feline dysautonomia (the Key Gaskell Syndrome) An ultrastructural study of autonomic ganglia and nerves. Neuropathol. Appl. Neurobiol. 11:17, 1985.

Key, T., and Gaskell, C. J.: (Correspondence.) Vet. Rec. 110:160, 1982.

Nash, A. S., Griffiths, I. R. G., and Sharp, N. J. H.: (Correspondence.) Vet. Rec. 111:370, 1982.

Rochlitz, I.: Feline dysautonomia (the Key Gaskell or dilated pupil syndrome): A preliminary review. J. Small Anim. Pract. 25:587, 1984.

Sharp, N. J. H., Nash, A. S., and Griffiths, I. R. G.: Feline dysautonomia (the Key Gaskell syndrome): A clinical and pathological study of forty cases. J. Small Anim. Pract. 25:599, 1984.

NEUROAXONAL DYSTROPHY AND LEUKOENCEPHALOMYELOPATHY OF ROTTWEILER DOGS

CHERYL L. CHRISMAN, D.V.M.
Gainesville, Florida

Neuroaxonal dystrophy and leukoencephalomyelopathy are two degenerative disorders of the nervous system of Rottweiler dogs. These conditions currently are considered as distinct entities owing to their differing clinical signs and neurohistologic lesions (Chrisman et al., 1984; Cork et al., 1983; Gamble and Chrisman, 1984).

NEUROAXONAL DYSTROPHY

Pups affected with neuroaxonal dystrophy may appear clumsy, but a neurologic disorder may not be suspected until the gait of the dog is critically evaluated by a breeder, trainer, judge, or veterinarian. By the time a deficit is first suspected, the dog may be 12 to 24 months old. The main neurologic deficit at that time is a symmetrical dysmetria of all four limbs. Most dogs exhibit hypermetria of the thoracic limbs at this stage; however, a few have hypometria. Patellar reflexes are hyperactive with clonus. The other spinal reflexes are normal, and limb strength and conscious proprioception are normal as well. An astute observer may detect a slight intention tremor or mild incoordination of the head and neck in some young affected dogs. Malformation of the cervical vertebrae and distemper myelopathy might produce these signs, so they should be considered in the list of differential diagnoses. Results of complete blood counts, serum chemistry profiles, cervical vertebral column radiographs, cerebrospinal fluid analysis, myelography, electromyography, and electroencephalography are all normal. These findings may not completely rule out the possibility of distemper myelopathy, but, unlike distemper, neuroaxonal dystrophy appears to have a characteristically insidious progression over several years.

By approximately 4 years of age, the menace response (blinking the eyelids to a threatening gesture) may be depressed. Mild head and neck incoordination and a positional nystagmus when the animal is laid on its side or back may be observed. The dysmetria of the limbs worsens, and hypermetria of thoracic and pelvic limbs is commonly seen. Patellar reflexes remain hyperactive with clonus, and a crossed extensor response and positive Babinski response may also be observed. Limb strength and conscious proprioception are still normal. Findings of neurologic diagnostic tests remain normal.

By approximately 5 to 6 years of age, head and neck incoordination and intention tremors are obvious. The menace response remains depressed. Positional as well as spontaneous nystagmus is apparent. Dysmetria of the limbs, most often hypermetria, is moderate to severe and remains symmetrical. No weakness or loss of conscious proprioception is seen. Patellar reflexes remain hyperactive with clonus. Crossed extensor reflexes are present, as are positive Babinski responses. Responses to neurologic diagnostic tests remain normal. Neuroaxonal dystrophy is suspected from the progression of the signs and the normal diagnostic test results. The diagnosis is only confirmed by necropsy. Axonal spheroids are disseminated throughout the gray matter of the nervous system in all structures except the cerebral cortex. The most severe lesions are usually the presence of spheroids in the nucleus of the dorsal spinocerebellar tract and the loss of Purkinje's cells in the vermis and flocculus of the cerebellum, which accounts for the progressive dysmetria and head and neck incoordination as well as the nystagmus. Spheroids are also found in the vestibular and other nuclei of the brain stem; lesions in these areas may account for nystagmus as well as hyperactive spinal cord reflexes.

Currently there is no known treatment for neuroaxonal dystrophy, and all cases studied have been progressive. However, affected dogs may remain acceptable pets for many years because of the slow progression of signs. From preliminary breeding studies, a recessive mode of inheritance with possible variable penetrance is suspected (Cork et al., 1983).

LEUKOENCEPHALOMYELOPATHY

Leukoencephalomyelopathy has been described in two Rottweilers—a four-year-old male and a three-year-old female who had progressive ataxia and weakness of all four limbs for 9 and 7 months, respectively. Neither of these dogs had a prior history of neurologic deficit. These affected dogs had dysmetria, hypermetria, and hyperactive patellar reflexes with clonus, similar to the signs in dogs with neuroaxonal dystrophy. The differentiating neurologic features, however, were the lack of any head involvement, an obvious weakness in all four limbs, and a conscious proprioceptive deficit of the rear limbs.

Complete blood counts, serum chemistry profiles, electromyography, electroencephalography, vertebral column radiography, cerebrospinal fluid analysis, and myelography all showed normal results. The male was treated with corticosteroids for 2 months with no improvement and had continued progression of signs. A diagnosis of leukoencephalomyelopathy was made after necropsy. Demyelinating lesions were found in the spinal cord, brain stem, and deep cerebellar white matter in both dogs. Some axonal spheroids were found in the accessory cuneate nucleus, nucleus gracilis, cuneate nucleus, and the nucleus of the dorsal spinocerebellar tract in the male dog. The most severe lesions in both dogs were demyelination of the dorsal and lateral funiculus of the spinal cord, which accounted for the dysmetria, quadriparesis, and conscious proprioceptive deficits.

Currently no treatment is known for leukoencephalomalacia. The dogs had a common grandsire on their sire's side, and this common grandsire had offspring with neuroaxonal dystrophy. Further studies are needed on the cause of leukoencephalomyelopathy and its relationship to neuroaxonal dystrophy.

References and Supplemental Reading

Chrisman, C. L., Cork, L. C., and Gamble, D. A.: Neuroaxonal dystrophy of Rottweiler dogs. J.A.V.M.A. 184:464, 1984.

Cork, L. C., Troncoso, M. D., Price, D. L., et al.: Canine neuroaxonal dystrophy. J. Neuropathol. Exp. Neurol. 42:286, 1983.

Gamble, D. A., and Chrisman, C. L.: A leukoencephalomyelopathy of Rottweiler dogs. Vet. Pathol. 21:274, 1984.

CANINE WOBBLER SYNDROME

ERIC J. TROTTER, D.V.M.

Ithaca, New York

"Wobbles" was first described in the horse by Dimock and Errington in 1939. A "Wobbler syndrome" in large breeds of dogs, predominantly Great Danes and Doberman pinschers that showed similar signs of cervical myelopathy, was later reported by LaCroix (1970) and de Lahunta (1971). In the 1970s, significant effort was devoted to further description of the vertebral column and spinal cord lesions in the horse and the dog by a number of authors (see references). The various hypotheses of causes and pathogenesis, the assortment of breeds affected, the variances in neurologic dysfunction, and the numerous types of spondylopathic changes responsible for the cervical myelopathy have resulted in many different names for this syndrome. Its names include progressive cervical spinal cord compression, cervical spondylosis, cervical spondylolisthesis, wobblers, caudal cervical subluxation, cervical vertebral instability, Great Dane ataxia, cervical spondylopathy, caudal cervical spondylopathy, caudal cervical malformation-malarticulation, cervical vertebral stenosis, cervical myelopathy, midcervical spondylolisthesis, cervical spondylotic myelopathy, caudal cervical spondylomyelopathy, and, most recently, dynamic compression of the cervical spinal cord. The common denominator in this syndrome is the typical neurologic dysfunction of bilaterally symmetric spastic paraparesis, tetraparesis, and ataxia, which results from any one or more of the various spondylopathies that cause spinal cord compression, contusion, stretching, or ischemia in the caudal cervical region of large dogs. The original name, canine wobbler syndrome, is based on a graphic description of the neurologic signs and does not imply the origin or pathogenesis of the disorder; perhaps it should have been retained.

The spinal cord compression, contusion, stretching, or intermittent ischemia most often results in varying degrees of bilateral, symmetric, spastic paresis and ataxia of the pelvic limbs with an awkward swaying movement of the hindquarters. Although in most instances a thoracic limb deficit is not reported by the owner, careful examination reveals mild thoracic limb dysfunction. Neurologic deficits range from minimal spastic paresis and ataxia to nonambulatory tetraparesis. In most affected dogs, upper motor neuron (UMN) signs predominate, although the lesion, or lesions, are most often located in the caudal cervical segments. Scapular muscle atrophy due to lower motor neuron (LMN) involvement is noted occasionally and reflects the chronic nature of the lesion and neuronal loss from the gray matter of the C_6 and C_7 segments. The onset of neurologic dysfunction is most often insidious, and cervical pain is usually absent. An acute onset and the presence of prominent cervical pain are more typical signs of cervical intervertebral disc protrusion or extrusion than they are of this more chronic cervical spondylotic myelopathy. The signs are usually progressive, although long static periods do occur. These animals have no history of external injury or medical illness.

In ambulatory dogs, the signs are most evident when the animals arise from a recumbent position. The pelvic limb gait is often characterized as awkward and swaying, owing to the long, and often asymmetric, stride. Overextension, wide stance, and crouching in the pelvic limbs are typical. The pelvic limbs frequently cross each other, abduct widely, and, in severe cases, collapse. The dorsal aspects of the claws are often worn because of dragging of the limb on protraction or stepping with the dorsal surface of the paw on the ground. Deficits are greatly exacerbated on turning. Thoracic limb signs, when present, are similar but usually less remarkable. Thoracic limb spasticity is most frequently observed in the Doberman pinscher. The greatest deficits are usually noted with hopping and proprioceptive positioning. Hypertonia and hyperreflexia are frequently observed in both pelvic and thoracic limbs. Some dogs present as nonambulatory tetraparetics that may have a slight amount of hypalgesia. These signs indicate a lesion in the white matter of the cervical spinal cord that predominantly involves ascending proprioceptive tracts (with resultant ataxia) and descending motor tracts (with resultant spastic paresis). The predisposition of these breeds to a variety of musculoskeletal disorders may complicate the neurologic examination of ambulatory patients.

Although reported in other breeds of dogs, this disorder appears to be most common in the Great Dane and Doberman pinscher. Many clinical and pathologic features of this syndrome resemble those observed in horses with this syndrome and in humans with cervical spondylotic myeloradiculopathy. The pathogenesis and origin may be similar. Altered spinal biomechanics (which appears to be the unifying feature of these disorders) result in a variety of spondylopathic changes and subsequent spinal cord compression and ischemia. In humans as well as in older dogs, cervical intervertebral disc degeneration (as opposed to cervical disc protrusion) in this dynamic region of the spine leads to instability, abnormal motion, and abnormal stresses at this and adjacent articulations (MacNab, 1983). As usual, osteoarthrosis ensues. The resultant degenerative changes of the ligamentous and osseous components of the symphyseal (intervertebral disc) and synovial (articular process) joints may cause spinal cord attenuation or neurovascular compromise at one or many locations. The roles of instability in young dogs and of these sequelae resulting in spinal cord compression in older patients are less certain. In some cases, spinal cord compression, contusion, stretching, or ischemia appears to be the direct result of any of a variety of malformations or malarticulations of the osseous or ligamentous structures of the cervical spine at one or more levels. Clinical and experimental evidence suggest a role of genetics as well as nutrition in the development of this disorder (Hedhammer et al., 1974; Conrad, 1973; Selcer and Oliver, 1975).

Congenital or developmental stenosis of the cervical vertebral canal predisposes the dog to cervical myelopathy (Epstein et al., 1979; Hinck and Sachdev, 1966). Minimal encroachment on a relatively "tight" vertebral canal by normally innocuous osseous or ligamentous lesions may, in these individuals, result in significant spinal cord attenuation. Flexion or extension of the cervical spine well within a normal range of motion may, in affected individuals, exacerbate the spinal cord compression, contusion, stretching, displacement, or ischemia. Infolding, or "buckling," of redundant dorsal longitudinal or interarcuate ligaments occurs with extension. Extension may also dramatically increase spinal cord compression in dogs with elongation of the vertebral arches or dorsal laminae of one or more of the caudal cervical vertebrae. Flexion of the cervical spine in the presence of malformation of the craniodorsal aspect of one of the cervical vertebral bodies, even without instability at this articulation, increases spinal cord compression or stretching. Extreme caution must be exercised during neurologic examination or other manipulation of the patient, especially during endotracheal intubation and positioning for myelography, when general anesthesia precludes self protection.

The neurologic dysfunction is caused by attenuation of the spinal cord from one or more spondylopathologic conditions at one or many locations. The attenuation is caused by the deformity of the vertebral canal, which may be confirmed by myelography. Abnormalities that do not directly result in spinal cord compression are nevertheless significant, as they represent "footprints" of disease. These abnormalities have probably resulted from altered spinal biomechanics (i.e., from abnormal stresses on the osseous and ligamentous structures of the caudal cervical spine). These changes, evident on plain radiography, show no evidence of compromise of the subarachnoid space on myelography and may include (1) exostoses, which are most often on the cranioventral aspects of the vertebral bodies; (2) degenerative periarticular osseous changes typical of arthritis; (3) degenerative changes of the associated intervertebral discs; (4) reactive changes on the dorsal spines; (5) degenerative or reactive changes of the ligamentous supporting structures of the ventral aspect of the vertebral column; (6) loss or production of bone at the ventral aspects of these vertebrae; and (7) ankylosis of symphyseal joints.

In many affected dogs multiple abnormalities may be revealed on plain films of the normally extended cervical spine. With myelography, one (most commonly) or multiple sites and types of spinal cord attenuation may be confirmed in the individual patient. There is frequently a discrepancy between the lesions that appear to be most significant on examination of plain films and those that are confirmed with myelography. The bizarre and often extensive secondary bony changes representing the body's response to abnormal forces are not usually indicative of the exact site or sites of spinal cord compression.

Rational medical, surgical, and adjunctive medical therapies of canine wobbler syndrome have evolved from the study of all aspects of this disorder and of related disorders in man. Because of the variety of malformations and malarticulations, their static or dynamic natures, the secondary changes, the existence of multiple-level lesions, and their variable courses, no single therapeutic regime can be logically recommended. The therapy must be that most suited to the successful control of signs or to the correction of the individual's particular spondylopathies. Treatment must be further modified by the surgeon's previous experiences with the various medical and surgical techniques and their associated hazards. Judgment is also influenced by the surgeon's previous experiences with the morbidity, mortality, and postoperative responses, complications, and care inherent in various medical and surgical techniques used in patients of different ages and with different neurologic deficits. In humans, "the management of cervical spondylotic myeloradiculopathy by a variety of approaches has passed through many phases, and initial optimistic results have been tempered by experience with larger groups of patients and improved diagnostic and technical facilities. The variety of procedures now in use provide ample evidence that no one technique will solve all the unique problems presented by this disorder" (Epstein and Janin, 1983). Management of patients with the cervical myelopathy resulting from various spondylopathies of wobbler syndrome has followed an identical trend.

In recent years, numerous studies have been conducted to standardize models of spinal cord injury, to elucidate the pathophysiologic characteristics of acute and chronic spinal cord injuries, and to investigate the efficacy of many therapeutic measures. An extensive pharmacopeia has permitted the prevention, modification, or reversal of many of the postulated biochemical components of the vicious cycle of autodestruction that occurs in acute spinal cord injury. The mechanism of action of many of the pharmaceutical agents has been investigated, although not necessarily agreed upon, at the cellular or molecular level. Controversy still exists regarding the relative efficacy of the various therapeutic regimens, including some of those that were previously almost universally accepted. An in-depth discussion of research into spinal cord injury is beyond the scope of this paper, but some of the more recent conclusions are presented for discussion of this more chronic cervical myelopathy and its operative and nonoperative treatment. The pathophysiologic responses of the spinal cord to compression are, in some ways, similar in both acute and chronic cases. Alteration or minimization of the pathologic changes that result from spinal cord attenuation is the goal of most methods of therapy.

Experimental studies have confirmed the separate but additive effects of compression and ischemia on the canine cervical spinal cord (Hukuda and Wilson, 1972; Gooding et al., 1975). There is general agreement on the effect of reduced blood flow to the spinal cord and the histopathologic result of relative ischemia in both acute and chronic spinal cord compression. Both experimental and clinical evidence suggest that the spinal cord lesions are due more to ischemia induced by compression than to direct neural damage due to spinal cord attenuation.

Most investigations of acute experimental spinal cord trauma report encouraging results with parenteral glucocorticosteroid therapy. Many mechanisms of action have been postulated to explain the beneficial effects of these agents in both acute and chronic spinal cord compression. Although incapable of increasing blood flow to the spinal cord, glucocorticoids, probably through stabilization of parenchymal and vascular biologic membranes, appear to decrease some of the pathologic results of reduced spinal cord perfusion, most notably edema and its progressive deleterious effects. These agents may reduce edema directly by maintaining vascular integrity of spinal cord microcirculation. Simultaneously, they prevent autolysis and demonstrate a myelin-sparing effect through their stabilizing influence on lysosomal membranes, thereby preventing the release of proteolytic enzymes and esterases that result in the hydrolytic destruction of the phospholipids in myelin (Campbell et al., 1974). Other studies relate the beneficial effects of dexamethasone on the maintenance of cellular integrity (as seen in its preservation of the potassium content of the injured spinal cord) rather than on the direct reduction of edema (Lewin et al., 1974).

The extremely rapid (less than 24 hours) and often remarkable improvement seen after the administration of glucocorticoids to many dogs with this cervical myelopathy cannot logically be expected and is not caused by the elimination of further injury and by the "overnight" remyelination of axons that are still intact. However, resolution of ischemia-induced edema from spinal cord attenuation, which is further aggravated by the additive effect of direct neural deformation or compression, may account for the dramatic results.

Improved diagnostic techniques, an expanded but still incomplete understanding of the pathophysiologic results of this disorder, a re-evaluation of the initial cases with particular attention to the occurrence of long-term postoperative complications, and an increased experience with the various modes of operative and nonoperative management of this disorder have resulted in modification of the management of these patients. Nonoperative treatment is now used, at least on a trial basis. Alternate-day administration of oral glucocorticoids is highly satisfactory in many cases. In retrospect, it appears possible that the early encouraging results with surgical intervention were due, at least in part, to the administration of glucocorticoids pre-, intra-, and postoperatively. Some of these patients may have regained functional status in spite of, rather than due to, the surgery. However, glucocorticoids are not the ultimate answer in all cases. Severely, especially chronically, affected animals (with severe or nonambulatory tetraparesis) rarely show a satisfactory response to medication alone. Thus, although the initial enthusiasm for surgery has waned, we have not abandoned surgery but have adopted flexibility in deciding treatment protocols.

At present, dogs with signs of mild to moderate paraparesis, tetraparesis, or ataxia are usually managed by the oral administration of glucocorticoids. After a 48- to 72-hour trial period to determine steroid responsiveness (at an oral dose of 1 to 2 mg/kg of prednisolone twice daily) the loading dose is decreased gradually over a 5-day period to a dosage of 0.5 to 1.0 mg/kg on alternate days. Dogs of the most frequently affected breeds that show a typical history for this disorder, the usual neurologic signs, and a satisfactory response to steroid administration require no further diagnostic workup. The administration of glucocorticoids results in sufficient improvement in many patients to allow return to functional status as a companion animal. Only rarely are signs completely relieved. Even with relatively severe neurologic deficits, some cases respond rapidly and dramatically. Often after a few months, steroid administration may be discontinued without deterioration in neurologic status. In some cases, intermittent exacerbations remain responsive to steroids. Patients have been managed with this regimen for periods as long as 5 years. This may have been the result of the long static periods typical of the disorder, spontaneous resolution due to revascularization, development of collateral circulation, remodeling of the spine with maturity, compensation, or ankylosis.

In nonresponsive patients, diagnostic evaluation is continued, and the most appropriate method of surgical intervention is determined by many factors: neurologic progression, specific myelographic findings at one or several locations, patient age, coexistent disorders, financial implications, and the surgeon's experience with the various techniques. One must also consider the associated risks, advantages, and complication rates of surgical approaches. Even with surgery, the prognosis in nonambulatory patients is poor. Some recover remarkably well, but the majority, although usually nonprogressive postoperatively, do not regain a satisfactory functional status. It is hoped that increased experience will lead to increased success in predicting the reversibility of spinal cord lesions in affected animals.

References and Supplemental Reading

Campbell, J. B., DeCrescito, V., Tomasula, J., et al.: Effects of antifibrinolytic and steroid therapy on the contused spinal cord of cats. J. Neurosurg. 40:726, 1974.

Chambers, J. N., and Betts, C. W.: Caudal cervical spondylopathy in the dog: A review of 20 clinical cases and the literature. J. Am. Anim. Hosp. Assoc. 13:571, 1977.

Chrisman, C. L.: Cervical spondylolisthesis in the canine. Speculum 24:14, 1972.

Chrisman, C. L.: The diagnosis and management of dogs and cats presented with quadriparesis and paraparesis. Proc. Am. Anim. Hosp. Assoc. 48th Ann. Meet. 1981, pp. 245–254.

Conrad, C.: Motion of the canine cervical vertebral column in the median plane. A radiographic method of analysis. M.S. Thesis, Cornell University, Ithaca, NY, 1973.

de Lahunta, A: Cervical spinal cord contusions from spondylolisthesis (A wobbler syndrome in dogs). *In* Kirk, R. W. (ed.): *Current Veterinary Therapy IV*. Philadelphia: W.B. Saunders, 1971, pp. 503–504.

de Lahunta, A.: Progressive cervical spinal cord compression in Great Dane and Doberman pinscher dogs (a wobbler syndrome). *In* Kirk, R. W. (ed.): *Current Veterinary Therapy V*. Philadelphia: W.B. Saunders, 1973, pp. 674–675.

de Lahunta, A.: *Veterinary Neuroanatomy and Clinical Neurology*. Philadelphia: W.B. Saunders, 1977.

Denny, H. R., Gibbs, C., and Gaskell, C. J.: Cervical spondylopathy in the dog: A review of thirty five cases. J. Small Anim. Pract. 18:117, 1977.

Dimock, W. W., and Errington, B. J.: Incoordination of equidae: Wobblers. J.A.V.M.A. 95:261, 1939.
Epstein, J. A., and Janin, Y.: Management of cervical spondylotic myeloradiculopathy by the posterior approach. *In* The Cervical Spine Research Society: *The Cervical Spine*. Philadelphia: J.B. Lippincott, 1983, p. 402.
Epstein, J. A., Carras, R., Hyman, R. A., et al.: Cervical myelopathy caused by developmental stenosis of the spinal canal. J. Neurosurg. 51:362, 1979.
Gage, E. D.: Disc syndrome in the large breed dog. J. Am. Anim. Hosp. Assoc. 5:93, 1969.
Gooding, M. R., Wilson, C. B., and Hoff, J. T.: Experimental cervical myelopathy: Effects of ischemia and compression of the canine cervical spinal cord. J. Neurosurg. 43:9, 1975.
Hedhammer, A., Wu, F. M., Krook, L., et al.: Overnutrition and skeletal disease: An experimental study in growing Great Dane dogs. Cornell Vet. 64:1, 1974.
Hinck, V. C., and Sachdev, N. S.: Developmental stenosis of the cervical spinal canal. Brain 89:27, 1966.
Hoerlein, B. F.: *Canine Neurology*, 2nd ed. Philadelphia: W.B. Saunders, 1971, pp. 267–276.
Hukuda, S., and Wilson, C. B.: Experimental cervical myelopathy: Effects of compression and ischemia on the canine cervical spinal cord. J. Neurosurg. 37:631, 1972.
Hurov, L. I.: Treatment of cervical vertebral instability in the dog. J.A.V.M.A. 175:278, 1979.
LaCroix, F. A.: Diagnosis of orthopedic problems peculiar to the growing dog. V.M./S.A.C. 65:229, 1970.
Lewin, M. G., Hansebout, R. R., and Pappius, H. M.: Chemical characteristics of traumatic spinal cord edema in cats. J. Neurosurg. 40:65, 1974.
MacNab, I.: Symptoms in cervical disc degeneration. *In* The Cervical Spine Research Society: *The Cervical Spine*. Philadelphia: J.B. Lippincott, 1983, p. 388.
Mason, T. A.: Cervical vertebral instability (wobbler syndrome) in the dog. Vet. Rec. 104:142, 1979.
Mayhew, I. G., de Lahunta, A., Whitlock, R. H., et al.: Spinal cord disease in the horse. Cornell Vet. 68:1, 1978.
Olsson, S. E., Stavenborn, M., and Hoppe, F.: Dynamic compression of the cervical spinal cord. A myelographic and pathologic investigation in Great Dane dogs. Acta Vet. Scand. 23:65, 1982.
Parker, A. J., Park, R. D., Cusick, P. K., et al.: Cervical vertebral instability in the dog. J.A.V.M.A. 163:71, 1973.
Parker, A. J., Park, R. D., and Gendreau, C.: Cervical disc prolapse in a Doberman pinscher. J.A.V.M.A. 163:75, 1973.
Parker, A. J., Park, R. D., and Henry, J. D.: Cervical vertebral instability associated with cervical disc disease in two dogs. J.A.V.M.A. 163:1369, 1973.
Raffe, M. R., and Knecht, C. D.: Cervical vertebral malformation: A review of 36 cases. J. Am. Anim. Hosp. Assoc. 16:881, 1980.
Rendano, V. T., and Smith, L. L.: Cervical vertebral malformation-malarticulation (wobbler syndrome)—The value of the ventrodorsal view in defining lateral spinal cord compression in the dog. J. Am. Anim. Hosp. Assoc. 17:627, 1981.
Seim, H. B., and Withrow, S. J.: Pathophysiology and diagnosis of caudal cervical spondylo-myelopathy with emphasis on the Doberman pinscher. J. Am. Anim. Hosp. Assoc. 18:241, 1982.
Selcer, R. R., and Oliver, J. E.: Cervical spondylopathy—Wobbler syndrome in dogs. J. Am. Anim. Hosp. Assoc. 11:175, 1975.
Swaim, S. F.: Ventral decompression of the cervical spinal cord in the dog. J.A.V.M.A. 164:491, 1974.
Trotter, E. J., and de Lahunta, A.: Caudal cervical vertebral malformation-malarticulation. *In* Bojrab, M.J. (ed.): *Pathophysiology in Small Animal Surgery*. Philadelphia: Lea & Febiger, 1981, pp. 761–763.
Trotter, E. J., de Lahunta, A., Geary, J. C., et al.: Caudal cervical vertebral malformation-malarticulation in Great Danes and Doberman pinschers. J.A.V.M.A. 168:917, 1976.
Wagner, P. C., Bagby, G. W., Grant, B. D., et al.: Surgical stabilization of the equine cervical spine. Vet. Surg. 8:7, 1979.
Wright, F., Rest, J. R., and Palmer, A. C.: Ataxia of the Great Dane caused by stenosis of the cervical vertebral canal: Comparison with similar conditions in the basset hound, Doberman pinscher, ridgeback, and the thoroughbred horse. Vet. Rec. 92:1, 1973.
Wright, J. A.: A study of the radiographic anatomy of the cervical spine in the dog. J. Small Anim. Pract. 18:341, 1977.
Wright, J. A.: Congenital and developmental abnormalities of the vertebrae. J. Small Anim. Pract. 20:625, 1979.
Wright, J. A.: The use of sagittal diameter measurement in the diagnosis of cervical spinal stenosis. J. Small Anim. Pract. 20:331, 1979.

DISKOSPONDYLITIS

JOE N. KORNEGAY, D.V.M.
Raleigh, North Carolina

Diskospondylitis is concurrent intervertebral disc infection and vertebral osteomyelitis of contiguous vertebrae. First reported in humans as early as 1887 and in dogs in the 1960s, diskospondylitis (vertebral osteomyelitis) has been diagnosed with increasing frequency in dogs in recent years. The clinical features and treatment of 56 dogs with diskospondylitis evaluated during a 5-year period at the University of Georgia Veterinary Medical Teaching Hospital (GVMTH) are the basis of this chapter.

CASE SIGNALMENT AND CLINICAL FEATURES

Diskospondylitis primarily affects large dogs (Fig. 1), and males outnumber females by approximately 2 to 1. Affected dogs usually are middle-aged (Fig. 2). German shepherds and Great Danes appear to be affected more frequently than other breeds.

Table 1. *Clinical Signs Seen in 56 Dogs with Diskospondylitis*

Clinical Signs	Number of Affected Dogs
Hyperesthesia	42
Paresis or complete paralysis	26
Pyrexia	18
Stilted gait	16
Depression	15
Weight loss	14
Anorexia	10
Lameness	7
Abdominal pain	4

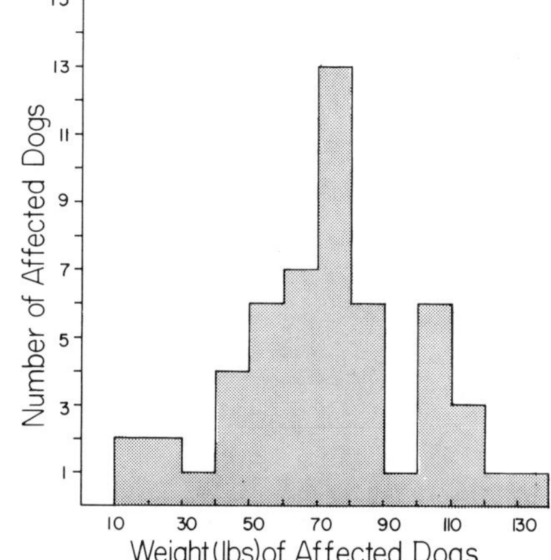

Figure 1. Histogram of weights (in pounds) of 56 dogs with diskospondylitis.

Clinical signs include hyperesthesia, paresis or complete paralysis, stilted gait, depression, weight loss, and pyrexia (Table 1). Both neurologic dysfunction and evidence of systemic disease are usually seen, but each can occur separately.

The midthoracic spine, C_{6-7}, and L_7–S_1 are the most common sites involved (Fig. 3). Involvement of multiple disc spaces is occasionally seen and usually occurs at adjacent disc spaces, suggesting local spread of infection. The thoracic spine is predisposed to involvement of multiple, adjacent disc spaces.

CAUSES AND PATHOGENESIS

Causes of diskospondylitis in dogs include migration of foreign bodies and fungal or bacterial infection. *Staphylococcus aureus* is the most common organism associated with diskospondylitis in dogs. It is frequently isolated by culture of either blood, urine, or bone. *Brucella canis* and species of *Streptococcus* are cultured occasionally from affected dogs. Other bacteria are viewed as contaminants unless isolated from infected bone or multiple blood cultures.

In humans, diskospondylitis generally occurs secondary to hematogenous dissemination of bacteria from infections elsewhere in the body. Subchondral vascular loops in the vertebral epiphyses evidently slow circulation of organisms and allow their colonization in the vertebral body. These bacteria then diffuse through the cartilaginous end plate of the vertebral body to reach the disc and to the adjacent vertebrae through freely communicating venous sinuses. Humans commonly have concurrent infections in the urinary tract, which may serve as the primary site of infection. Concurrent bacteremia and urinary tract infection also are seen occasionally in dogs with diskospondylitis. However, a direct cause-and-effect relationship has not been established in most of these cases. Other potential primary sites of infection identified in affected dogs include bacterial endocarditis, dermatitis, and orchitis due to *B. canis*.

Diskospondylitis can occur secondary to disc surgery in humans and has been diagnosed in several dogs subsequent to disc fenestration. However, the rarity of diskospondylitis in dachshunds suggests that neither disc disease nor disc surgery significantly predisposes dogs to its occurrence. Although trauma has been reported as a possible predisposing factor in dogs with diskospondylitis, a history of trauma rarely has been present in affected dogs

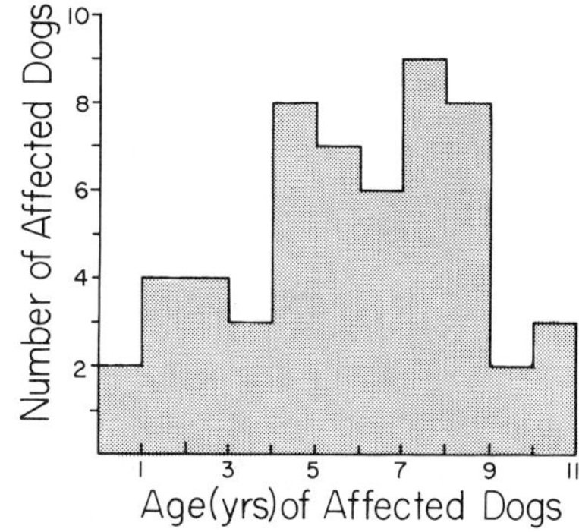

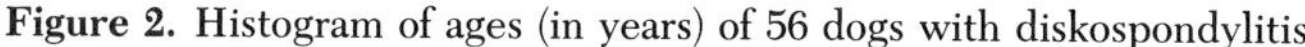
Figure 2. Histogram of ages (in years) of 56 dogs with diskospondylitis.

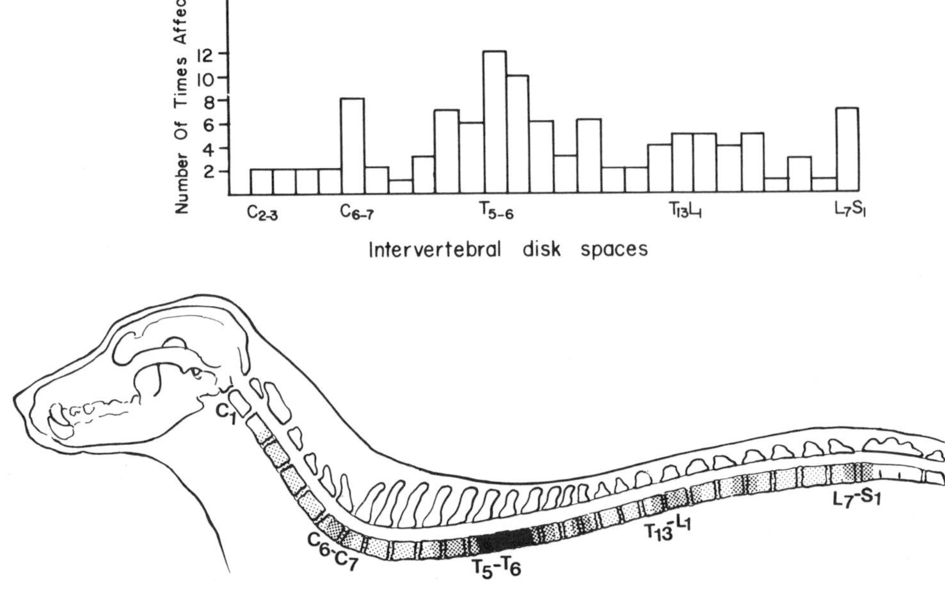

Figure 3. Distribution of lesions in 56 dogs with diskospondylitis.

evaluated by the author. Nevertheless, the prevalence of diskospondylitis in large, male dogs suggests that stresses placed on the spine by increased size and activity may play a role.

Spinal cord compression by new bone and fibrous connective tissue leads to the neurologic deficits seen in dogs with diskospondylitis. Instability and resulting vertebral subluxation occur less frequently. Infection rarely extends to the spinal cord and meninges in dogs with hematogenous infection, but it is relatively common in those with infection subsequent to foreign body migration.

DIAGNOSIS

RADIOLOGY. Diagnosis of diskospondylitis is usually based on the radiographic presence of characteristic lesions of vertebral lysis, sclerosis, and spondylosis (Fig. 4). These lesions may not be seen until 4 to 6 weeks after the onset of infection; thus, dogs may have clinical signs of diskospondylitis and be radiographically normal. Use of radionuclide imaging in these dogs may be helpful in defining the bony lesion. Serologic evaluation for *B. canis* and cultures of blood and urine also may indirectly identify the causative organism in dogs showing no radiographic changes and will allow the initiation of antibiotic therapy.

Diskospondylitis should not be confused with spondylosis deformans, a common, usually benign, vertebral lesion often present in older large dogs. Although spondylosis and sclerosis are features of both spondylosis deformans and diskospondylitis, vertebral lysis is seen only in diskospondylitis (Fig. 4). Vertebral tumors also cause bone lysis but usually do not affect adjacent vertebrae.

CLINICOPATHOLOGY. Consistent abnormalities in blood chemistry are not present in dogs with diskospondylitis. Leukocytosis is present infrequently. Pyuria, bacteriuria, or both are present in about 50 per cent of the cases. The results of cerebrospinal fluid analysis are usually normal, except for a mild elevation of protein levels.

MICROBIOLOGY. Bacterial cultures of blood have been positive in about 75 per cent of dogs with diskospondylitis that were evaluated by the author. *Staphylococcus aureus* is the most common organism identified. *B. canis* and species of *Streptococcus* are isolated occasionally. Other bacteria are considered to be contaminants unless isolated on multiple cultures.

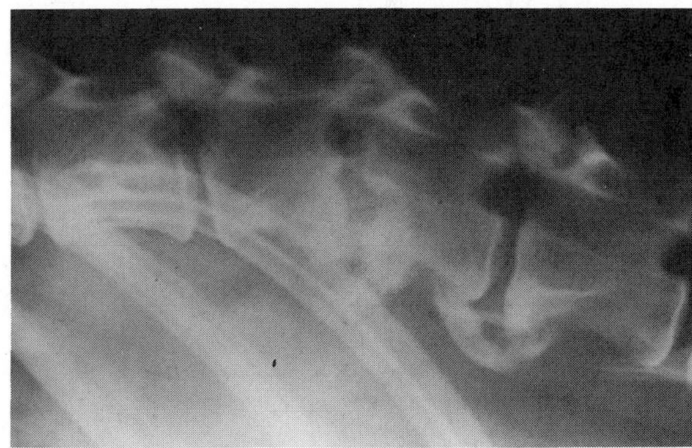

Figure 4. Radiographic demonstration of diskospondylitis at L1–2. Note the lysis of vertebral endplates, sclerosis, and spondylosis. There is also spondylosis at L2–3 but no evidence of lysis.

Cultures of bone are done if treatment includes vertebral curettage. Cultured bacteria from bone show antibiotic sensitivities that are similar, if not identical, to those of bacteria found in the blood. For this reason, bacteria identified on blood cultures are regarded as the causative organisms even though bone cultures may be unavailable or negative.

Urine cultures are positive in only about 25 per cent of dogs with diskospondylitis. Isolated organisms other than *S. aureus* are not viewed as the cause of the vertebral lesion unless they are also cultured from either blood or bone.

The tube agglutination test for *B. canis* is positive in about 10 per cent of dogs with diskospondylitis. Titers from 1:250 to 1:500 are considered indicative of bacteremia; titers between 1:50 and 1:100 suggest exposure with possible progression to bacteremia; a titer of 1:25 may occur because of cross agglutination with another organism. *Brucella canis* is also usually isolated from cultures of blood in seropositive dogs.

TREATMENT

A variety of treatment regimens have been used for dogs with diskospondylitis. A combination of spinal cord decompression, spinal column immobilization, and systemic antibiotic therapy resulted in clinical resolution of diskospondylitis in 28 of 30 dogs in one study. Other dogs have been managed successfully with curettage, drainage, and irrigation of the vertebral lesion. Antibiotic therapy alone also has been used.

Criteria utilized by the author in selecting a therapeutic regimen include (1) degree of neurologic dysfunction, (2) results of *B. canis* titer and blood cultures, (3) multiplicity of lesions, and (4) surgical accessibility of the lesion site.

Dogs with little or no neurologic dysfunction are treated with antibiotics alone. The selection of antibiotic is based on results of serologic tests or blood cultures. If these results are negative, the causative organism is assumed to be *S. aureus* and the antibiotic is chosen accordingly (see Table 2). Dogs that fail to improve clinically within 5 days of the onset of antibiotic therapy are reassessed. Solitary lesions that are readily accessible are curetted and cultured. Dogs with multiple, widely spaced lesions or lesions that are not readily accessible are treated with a different antibiotic.

Dogs with moderate to marked neurologic dysfunction usually have spinal cord compression due to either fibrosis or exostosis. Myelography in these dogs may be helpful in determining the extent and location of the compression. The offending bone or fibrous tissue is removed by either hemilaminectomy or dorsal laminectomy. Although it provides better exposure, a dorsal laminectomy entails removal of the dorsal spinous processes, which may be needed for spinal stabilization. The hemilaminectomy usually provides adequate exposure and preserves the dorsal spines for placement of plates if there is instability. The lesion is curetted, and necrotic bone and disc material are removed. Antibiotic therapy is instituted on the basis of cultures of affected bone and is continued for at least 4 to 6 weeks after surgery. Dogs with acutely progressive clinical signs should be treated parenterally for the first 3 to 5 days.

Table 2 lists results of antibiotic sensitivities of bacteria isolated from either blood or bone of dogs with diskospondylitis that were evaluated at the GVMTH. Table 3 lists antibiotics and the dosages used to treat affected dogs; the preferred antibiotic is listed first. Bactericidal antibiotics such as the cephalosporins and semisynthetic, penicillinase-resistant penicillins are preferred in treating *S. aureus*. Less expensive antibiotics such as chloramphenicol and trimethoprim do not appear to be as effective. Penicillin or ampicillin usually is ineffective. A staged-treatment regimen of tetracycline and streptomycin is used to treat diskospondylitis due to *B. canis* (Table 3), and intact dogs are also neutered. *Streptococcus* is treated with a bactericidal antibiotic that is selected on the basis of results from culture and sensitivity tests of blood or bone samples. Ampicillin or penicillin usually is effective.

Affected dogs should be evaluated clinically and radiographically at 2-week intervals during treatment. In the dog with evidence of clinical or radiographic deterioration, either the lesion is curetted or a different antibiotic is used.

Table 2. *Results of Antibiotic Sensitivities of Bacteria Isolated from Blood or Bone of Dogs with Diskospondylitis*

		Antibiotic and Efficacy Percentage												
Bacterium	**Number of Isolates**	*Ampicillin*	*Cephalothin*	*Chloramphenicol*	*Cloxacillin*	*Erythromycin*	*Gentamicin*	*Lincomycin*	*Penicillin*	*Streptomycin*	*Sulfadimethoxine*	*Tetracycline*	*Trimethoprim*	*Triple sulfa*
Staphylococcus aureus	30	27	97	83	93	77	83	46	20	60	11	57	65	10
Brucella canis	5	100	60	100	20	100	100	20	100	100	0	100	40	0
β-hemolytic streptococcus	2	100	100	100	100	100	0	100	100	0	0	100	100	0

Table 3. Antibiotics and Dosages Recommended for Treatment of Diskospondylitis in Dogs

Bacterium	Antibiotic and Dosage
*Staphylococcus aureus**	Cephradine†: 20 mg/kg t.i.d. orally for 4 to 6 weeks Cloxacillin: 10 mg/kg q.i.d. orally for 4 to 6 weeks
Brucella canis	Tetracycline hydrochloride‡: 20 mg/kg t.i.d. orally for 3 weeks Streptomycin: 20 mg/kg b.i.d. IM for 5 days at onset of tetracycline Skip 3 weeks and repeat this regimen
β-hemolytic streptococcus*	Ampicillin: 20 mg/kg t.i.d. orally for 4 to 6 weeks Penicillin: 40 units/kg q.i.d. orally for 4 to 6 weeks

*The preferred antibiotic is listed first. Dogs with acutely progressive clinical signs should be treated parenterally for 5 days and then orally for at least 4 to 6 weeks.

†A number of cephalosporins are available. Cephradine (Velosef, Squibb) is used because of its availability and expense. Cephalexin (Keflex, Dista) also has been used.

‡Minocycline hydrochloride also has been used and may be more efficacious. However, it also is more expensive.

Blood cultures should be repeated in dogs that deteriorate and in all cases 2 weeks after cessation of antibiotic therapy.

PROGNOSIS

Dogs with little or no neurologic dysfunction usually respond to antibiotic therapy alone or in combination with vertebral curettage. Some dogs deteriorate despite treatment, so owners should be informed of this possibility. The prognosis for dogs with marked neurologic dysfunction is guarded regardless of the treatment regimen. However, some of these dogs respond favorably, so treatment should be encouraged.

Recurrence rarely is a problem in dogs infected with *S. aureus* but is common in dogs with infections of *B. canis*. Owners should be advised of the difficulty encountered in eliminating *B. canis* from the infected animal and should be cautioned as to the potential need for repeated treatment. However, most dogs with diskospondylitis due to *B. canis* infection can be either cured or kept relatively free of clinical signs with periodic treatment.

Diskospondylitis due to *B. canis* does not progress as rapidly as that due to *S. aureus*, and it rarely necessitates spinal cord decompression or spinal immobilization. In contrast, lesions resulting from *S. aureus* often progress rapidly and are likely to require more extensive therapy.

PUBLIC HEALTH SIGNIFICANCE

Human infections with *B. canis* are rare but do occur. They are usually mild and respond to tetracycline therapy. Owners should be advised of this potential public health risk but they should not be overly alarmed.

References and Supplemental Reading

Kornegay, J. N.: Canine diskospondylitis. Comp. Cont. Ed. Pract. Vet. 1:930, 1979.

Kornegay, J. N., and Barber, D. L.: Diskospondylitis in dogs. J.A.V.M.A. 177:337, 1980.

MENINGITIS

WILLIAM R. FENNER, D.V.M.
Columbus, Ohio

Meningitis is an inflammation of the meninges that does not primarily involve the nervous tissue. Because there is such a close and intimate relationship between the brain parenchyma and the meninges, those cases of meningitis that involve both meninges and neural parenchyma are known as meningoencephalitis or, if they involve both the spinal cord and brain, as meningoencephalomyelitis. Inflammations of the meninges may be produced by a variety of causes that include infections (i.e., viral diseases such as canine distemper and feline infectious peritonitis [FIP]); mycotic infections such as cryptococcosis, blastomycosis, or histoplasmosis; rickettsial diseases such as Rocky Mountain spotted fever; and bacterial infections. In addition, there is a variety of unclassified or unknown causes of meningitis such as granulomatous meningoencephalomyelitis, a steroid-responsive suppurative meningitis of young dogs, the meningitis that follows myelography, and that which follows subarachnoid hemorrhage. In infectious cases, ways that the infection may arise include secondary reactions to systemic infection, from trauma to the cranium or spine, from nasal or ear infections, or from migration of foreign bodies. For this reason, careful scrutiny of the entire patient for an underlying cause is indicated.

CLINICAL APPEARANCE

Clinically, inflammatory and infectious diseases of the nervous system may be categorized as progressive diseases that usually have an acute or subacute onset. On general physical examination, many affected animals will be febrile. With the disorders that affect many systems (e.g., FIP, canine distemper, or systemic fungal infections), there may also be other signs of involvement (e.g., diarrhea, ascites, or cough). Many of these diseases will be associated with retinal abnormalities, which can be seen when a careful fundoscopic examination is performed. In animals with meningitis, significant neck and back pain usually occurs. Cases of meningitis are often associated with fever, which may be a result of endogenous pyrogen release or of other factors such as muscle fasciculations. The inflammation of the meninges tends to be generalized. For this reason the clinical signs are usually multifocal. Findings of the neurologic examination are usually normal except for the presence of severe pain and a stiff, stilted gait. This gait has been described as "walking on eggs," since affected animals walk very cautiously, as if on hot coals. Additionally, the animals seen by the author have turned "en bloc" (i.e., they turn their entire body rather than turn their neck or twist their spine). Although the pain is most easily reproduced by manipulation of the neck, most of these animals have back pain as well. Because the pain is so generalized, it is easy to mistakenly assume that the animal has generalized muscle or joint pain, such as would be seen with polymyositis or polyarthritis.

Even though pain is the predominant sign in infectious meningitis, the condition may spread to the adjacent tissues of the central nervous system (CNS) and cause ataxia, weakness, and changes in reflexes. These signs are multifocal and may reflect brain involvement as well as spinal cord infection.

In addition, in some patients, vasculitis may occur secondary to the meningitis, which may result in infarction of CNS parenchyma. If this occurs, signs of CNS dysfunction will be present in addition to the neck and back pain. Finally, in some cases of meningitis, there may be obstruction of flow or absorption of spinal fluid, which will cause secondary hydrocephalus and, subsequently, seizures, behavior changes, or loss of consciousness.

Differentials for meningitis include inflammation of cervical discs, diskospondylitis, vertebral tumors, spinal nerve root tumors, and epidural abscesses. Other causes of pain and fever are polyarthritis (rheumatoid, bacterial, or associated with lupus), polymyositis, bacterial endocarditis, and pyelonephritis.

DIAGNOSTIC EVALUATION

The diagnosis of meningitis or encephalitis in dogs and cats requires that a careful history be taken. Prior evidence of respiratory disease could suggest the presence of canine distemper encephalomyelitis. The physical examination may reveal systemic illness in cats with feline infectious peritonitis, in all species with systemic fungal infections, and in dogs with canine distemper. Cats with cryptococcosis frequently have chronic rhinitis and a mucopurulent nasal discharge. Diagnostic tests would include spinal radiographs as well as cerebrospinal fluid (CSF) taps. These patients should not undergo myelograms until the CSF is shown to be negative, since the contrast agent could exacerbate the meningitis.

When evaluating the CSF tap, the clinician should look for changes in pressure, clarity, color, cytologic characteristics, and protein. The cytologic sample should be examined carefully for microorganisms, and Gram stains should be used if suspicious bodies are seen. In addition, the CSF should be cultured.

In animals with ventriculitis, ependymitis, or meningitis, determination of the cell types after spinal fluid is collected can provide etiologic information. Inflammatory cells may be mononuclear cells (such as lymphocytes and macrophages) or polymorphonuclear leukocytes (neutrophils). A predominantly neutrophilic pleocytosis is generally seen in acute, severe viral infections and in bacterial infections. It is also seen in young dogs in the early stages of an acute, sterile, suppurative, steroid-responsive meningitis. Both bacterial meningitis that has been treated with antibiotics and the steroid-responsive meningitis of dogs in its later stages are predominantly mononuclear. A mixed mononuclear-polymorphonuclear infiltrate is seen in chronic granulomatous diseases, parasitic diseases, and protozoal diseases. A primarily or pure mononuclear infiltrate is most frequently seen in viral infections or chronic and resolving infections of other origins.

CLINICAL CONDITIONS

A nonbacterial suppurative meningitis has been reported in young dogs, especially beagles. These animals are febrile and have severe neck pain. The meningitis is not responsive to antibiotics, but as the disease normally waxes and wanes, initially it may appear that antibiotics are partially effective.

These animals are usually under 18 months of age, although the author has seen this condition in older animals (up to 4 years of age). The initial signs are acute in onset, but because the condition waxes and wanes, it may exist for several months prior to diagnosis. Although highly responsive to steroids, these animals usually do not respond to other anti-inflammatory drugs (e.g., aspirin or phenylbutazone). The underlying pathologic condition in these animals is vasculitis, which may result in spinal cord infarction. If that occurs, signs of CNS dysfunction such as weakness and ataxia may be seen. Cytologic tests of CSF in the early stages of this condition reveal a moderate (20 to 200 white blood cells [WBCs]/μl) or greater neutrophilic pleocytosis. The cells are well preserved, and no organisms are seen. The protein elevations are variable, with values of 50 mg/dl or greater common, although it is unusual for measurements to exceed 500 mg/dl.

Animals with this type of meningitis usually rebound rapidly and completely with immunosuppressive doses of steroids (2 mg/kg of prednisone per day, given for 10 days, then tapered slowly over 1 month). The cultures must be negative before steroid treatment is instituted.

Bacterial meningitis has been reported in dogs. Although an uncommon disease, it is one that should be in the differential diagnosis of an animal that presents with acute neck pain, fever, and nuchal rigidity. Signs of parenchymal involvement of the CNS are not common, although weakness and ataxia may occur with bacterial meningitis. Occasionally, cranial nerve dysfunction is found, especially in animals that develop an abscess at the site of involvement.

The diagnosis of bacterial meningitis is based on the presence of large numbers of WBCs, predominantly polymorphonuclear neutrophil leukocytes (PMNs), in CSF; great amounts of CSF proteins; and organisms either phagocytized by PMNs or free in CSF. The diagnosis is further confirmed by positive bacteriologic culture. Species of *Staphylococcus* and *Pasteurella* are the predominant organisms in bacterial meningitis in the dog; therefore, initial therapy, pending culture results, should be intravenous penicillin or ampicillin unless Gram's staining indicates infection by a gram-negative organism. Definitive treatment is administration of high levels of an antibacterial drug that is known to cross the blood-brain and CSF-brain barriers and to which the organism is susceptible. Such drugs include chloramphenicol, the sulfonamides, trimethoprim, and the cephalosporins. In addition, penicillin and ampicillin usually cross the blood-brain barrier adequately during inflammation. Antibacterial drugs are grouped as bactericidal (those that cause death of bacteria) and bacteriostatic (those that inhibit growth or reproduction of bacteria in order to enhance their removal by the body's immune system).

In general, the bactericidal antibiotics are most effective against rapidly dividing cells. They act by reversal mechanisms, which may include inhibition of cell wall synthesis, leading to osmotic lysis; interference with protein synthesis and subsequent accumulation of toxic metabolic by-products; or direct injury to the cell membrane. Examples of bactericidal antibiotics include penicillin, the cephalosporins, vancomycin, bacitracin, the aminoglycosides, and the polymyxins. Bacteriostatic antibiotics may interfere with protein synthesis by affecting synthesis of one-carbon fragments. Examples of bacteriostatic antibiotics include chloramphenicol, tetracycline, erythromycin, the sulfonamides, and trimethoprim. Initial selection of any of these antibiotics should be based on the results of a Gram's stain of CSF and on knowledge of the relative ability of available drugs to reach the CSF. Most patients will respond well to treatment.

Another cause of meningitis in dogs is granulomatous meningoencephalomyelitis (GME), also called inflammatory reticulosis. This is a disease of unknown pathogenesis that may affect animals at any age, although generally it affects adults. The disease has a predilection for the brain stem and cerebellum; therefore, ataxia, pathologic nystagmus, head tilt, weakness of limbs, and cranial nerve deficits are the most common signs. The signs are asymmetric and reflect a multifocal disease process. Animals with this disorder may have remarkable neck pain from meningitis and may also be persistently febrile. The animals may have optic nerve dysfunction, although many appear normal upon fundic examination. Animals with GME usually do not show any evidence of systemic illness. The signs in GME typically wax and wane, and frequently they are responsive to steroids. The spinal fluid of an affected animal frequently shows a mixed mononuclear-polymorphonuclear pleocytosis that may have very high numbers of white cells. There is often moderate to marked elevations of spinal fluid protein as well; the author has seen protein elevations over 1 gm/dl. The disease carries a guarded to grave prognosis, although steroids may cause temporary remissions.

The most common meningoencephalomyelitis of cats is feline infectious peritonitis. This disease causes a vasculitis and an associated pyogranulomatous inflammation of ependyma and meninges. Affected animals have predominantly cerebellar and vestibular signs, but they show evidence of associated brain stem, spinal cord, and, occasionally, cerebral disorders as well. Animals with FIP frequently will undergo vascular changes in the eyes as well as corneal and retinal changes. They may show evidence of systemic illnesses associated with weight loss, depression, or mild anemias. Occasionally animals will have the pleural and peritoneal effusions that are typical of "wet" FIP; however, the majority with nervous system involvement have the "dry" form of FIP. These animals frequently will have marked elevations of serum globulins and may occasionally have hyperviscosity syndrome, which includes sludging of blood and subsequent vascular accidents. Analysis of spinal fluid from these animals reveals a pyogranulomatous inflammation consisting of a mixture of mononuclear cells and polymorphonuclear leukocytes in the spinal fluid and moderate to marked elevations of spinal fluid protein. Currently, the success of treatment for these disorders is quite poor. In addition, treatment of FIP has limited success. Corticosteroids have been shown to cause temporary remission of signs in FIP. Other immunosuppressive drugs such as melphalan and cyclophosphamide have also been used but have generally shown poor long-term results.

A disease process that affects all species is mycotic meningitis. Fungal infections primarily cause a granulomatous meningitis and ependymitis and produce secondary involvement of the brain parenchyma. Infection with *Cryptococcus neoformans* is the most common. The clinical signs are variable, depending upon the area most greatly affected, and may reflect involvement of any portion of the CNS. Granulomas may affect cranial nerves as they exit the brain stem. Generally, the clinical signs are gradually progressive. The animals frequently have a systemic illness, especially respiratory disease. This and other systemic signs such as bone infections or chronic gastrointestinal disorders may also be seen in animals with fungal infections. Chorioretinitis is frequently seen with all of the fungal infections, and many affected animals have granulomatous disease of the uvea as well. Spinal fluid in these animals will reveal a granulomatous inflammation by the presence of both mononuclear and polymorphonuclear leukocytes and by mild to moderate elevations of protein. Fungal infections may also cause an eosinophilic pleocytosis in spinal fluid. Fungal organisms may be seen in the spinal fluid, especially with cryptococcal infections, and the organisms will be present on smears of nasal exudate or the material drained from fistulas of skin infections. Serologic testing may be beneficial in the diagnosis of this disease.

Treatment of fungal infections of the CNS currently consists of the use of intravenous amphotericin B, either alone or in combination with oral flucytosine, with which it may be synergistic. Both of these drugs poorly penetrate the blood-brain barrier. Of the two, amphotericin B appears the most effective in CNS infections.

Amphotericin B is given in low initial doses (0.22 mg/kg), which are slowly raised with progressive treatments to 0.4 and then to 0.75 mg/kg. Therapy is continued three times weekly at the maximum dose until renal complications arise or a cumulative dose of 7 to 20 mg/kg has been given. Flucytosine is usually given at 37.5 mg/kg four times daily for 6 weeks. Ketoconazole has proved to be an effective treatment for the various systemic fungal infections, and although expensive, it has less severe side effects than amphotericin B. Although not generally believed to cross the blood-brain barrier, ketoconazole has been found by at least one author to be effective in the treatment of CNS infections if used at a dose of 40 mg/kg/day and given in combination with parenteral amphotericin B. The use of intrathecal amphotericin B has been suggested but may not be needed if parenteral amphotericin is combined with either flucytosine or a high dose ketoconazole.

Treatment with a single antimicrobial agent is the method of choice for treatment of CNS infections.

There are certain combinations of antimicrobials that appear to diminish the effectiveness of each other. These include the combinations of chloramphenicol and penicillin and of ampicillin and oxytetracycline. These combinations should specifically be avoided.

In severe infections or in immunosuppressed patients, it is advised that a parenteral route of administration be used. The use of parenteral drugs ensures higher levels of drug in the tissues and removes the variable of intestinal absorption. Some specific drugs, such as the aminoglycosides, are not absorbed from the gastrointestinal tract and must be given parenterally regardless of the severity of the infection. Other drugs, such as amphotericin B, must be given by a specific route because they produce local tissue injury. If the infection is not severe and the indicated drug is well absorbed from the gastrointestinal tract, then oral administration is generally satisfactory. All drug dosages should be based on lean body weight.

Overall, the therapy for meningitis should be geared to the underlying cause. There is no currently effective therapy for a viral infection. The protozoal and fungal disorders may be treated with appropriate antimicrobials; however, success at present appears to be limited. Bacterial diseases should be treated vigorously with antibiotics, and the success rate is higher in these disorders. In the absence of any evidence of infection, and especially if the dog is under 18 months of age, it should be treated with corticosteroids in immunosuppressive doses. These dogs have a generally good long-term prognosis.

References and Supplemental Reading

Braund, K. G.: Encephalitis and meningitis. Vet. Clin. North Am. 10:31, 1980.

Chrisman, C. L.: *Problems in Small Animal Neurology*. Philadelphia: Lea & Febiger, 1982.

de Lahunta, A.: *Veterinary Neuroanatomy and Clinical Neurology*. Philadelphia: W.B. Saunders, 1983.

Fishman, R. A.: *Cerebrospinal Fluid in Diseases of the Nervous System*. Philadelphia: W.B. Saunders, 1982.

Greene, C. E.: Meningitis. *In* Kirk, R. W. (ed.): *Current Veterinary Therapy VIII*. Philadelphia: W.B. Saunders, 1983, pp. 735–738.

Harcourt, R. A.: Polyarthritis in a colony of beagle dogs. Vet. Rec. 102:519, 1978.

Hoff, E. J., and Vandvelde, M.: Necrotizing vasculitis in the central nervous system of two dogs. Vet. Pathol. 18:219, 1981.

Igarashi, M., Gilmartin, R. C., Gerald, B., et al.: Cerebral arteritis and bacterial meningitis. Arch. Neurol. 41:531, 1984.

Joshua, J. O., and Ishmael, J.: Pain syndrome associated with spinal hemorrhage in the dog. Vet. Rec. 83:165, 1968.

Kelly, D. F., Grunsell, C. S., and Kenyon, C. J.: Polyarteritis in the dog. Vet. Rec. 92:363, 1973.

Kornegay, J. N., Lorenz, M. D., and Zenoble, R. D.: Bacterial meningoencephalitis in two dogs. J.A.V.M.A. 173:1334, 1978.

Moore, P. M., and Cupps, T. R.: Neurologic complications of vasculitis. Ann. Neurol. 14:155, 1983.

Oliver, J. E., and Lorenz, M. D.: *Handbook of Veterinary Neurologic Diagnosis*. Philadelphia: W.B. Saunders, 1983.

Russo, E. A., Lees, G. E., and Hall, C. L.: Corticosteroid responsive aseptic suppurative meningitis in three dogs. Southwest. Vet. 35:197, 1983.

THERAPY OF CENTRAL NERVOUS SYSTEM INFECTIONS

MICHAEL D. LORENZ, D.V.M.
Athens, Georgia

Appropriate therapy for an infection of the central nervous system (CNS) is based on the identification of its cause and the selection of an appropriate antimicrobial agent. Drugs effective against an infection in most body systems may not be effective in treating CNS infections because their penetration into the CNS is limited by the blood-brain barrier (BBB).

The combined functions of the CNS capillaries and the choroid plexus form a physiologic barrier to the movement of many drugs from plasma into cerebrospinal fluid or nervous tissue. In capillaries outside the CNS, drugs pass from plasma through clefts between endothelial cells and through fenestrations in the capillary basement membrane. In the CNS, the capillary intercellular clefts are sealed and the capillary basement membrane has no fenestrations. To penetrate the CSF, a drug must penetrate the endothelial cell of the capillary, a basement membrane, and, finally, the processes of glial cells that surround the capillary.

Penetration of an antimicrobial agent into the CNS is largely a function of its endothelial membrane solubility. In general, antimicrobial agents that are highly soluble in lipids, are poorly bound to plasma proteins, and have a low degree of ionization at physiologic pH penetrate the CNS in amounts usually effective to inhibit or destroy the etiologic agent. The degree of penetration may be enhanced with inflammation, since the capillary permeability may be increased. However, as the infection (and associated inflammation) subsides, the drug may be excluded, resulting in a poor therapeutic response.

Table 1. *Achievable Concentrations of Antimicrobial Drugs in CSF and CNS*

	High	Adequate	Inadequate
Microbicidal drugs	Trimethoprim Metronidazole	Penicillin Ampicillin Methicillin Oxacillin Carbenicillin	Cephalosporins Aminoglycosides Polymyxin B
Microbiostatic drugs	Chloramphenicol Sulfonamides	Minocycline Doxycycline Tetracycline Flucytosine	Amphotericin B Ketoconazole Erythromycin Lincomycin

*Table 2. Antimicrobial Drugs Usually Effective in the Treatment of CNS Infection**

Disease or Organism	Drugs Used *Recommended*	*Alternate*
Bacterial meningitis		
Staphylococcus	Ampicillin Amoxicillin	Trimethoprim Chloramphenicol
Streptococcus	Penicillin	Erythromycin
Actinomyces	Ampicillin	Minocycline
Escherichia coli	Ampicillin	Trimethoprim Chloramphenicol
Pseudomonas	Carbenicillin	Chloramphenicol Gentamicin†
Pasteurella	Ampicillin	Trimethoprim
Brucella	Minocycline	
Salmonella	Trimethoprim	Chloramphenicol
Anaerobes	Ampicillin Metronidazole	Amoxicillin Carbenicillin
Acid-fast bacteria		
Atypical	Sulfonamides Trimethoprim	
Mycobacterium	Isoniazid and ethambutol	Rifampin, ethionamide, and cycloserine
Bacterial Abscess	Same as for bacterial meningitis; also treat with surgical drainage	
Fungal Meningoencephalomyelitis		
Histoplasma, Blastomyces, Coccidioides, and *Candida*	Amphotericin B and ketoconazole	
Cryptococcus	Amphotericin B, ketoconazole, and flucytosine	
Aspergillus	Amphotericin B, flucytosine, and thiabendazole	
Sporothrix	Amphotericin B	Sodium iodide
Prototheca	Amphotericin B and minocycline	
Rocky Mountain Spotted Fever		
Meningoencephalitis	Chloramphenicol	Tetracycline

*Data compiled from references
†Intrathecal administration

In general, the three most important questions to answer in selecting antimicrobial therapy are: (1) Will the drug be effective against the suspected infectious agent? (2) Does the drug effectively penetrate the BBB? and (3) Can the drug be safely administered in dosages above those commonly given when the infectious agent causes disease in non-CNS tissues?

ANTIMICROBIAL THERAPY

Antimicrobial agents are grouped by their ability to achieve concentrations in the CNS sufficient to inhibit or kill the microorganism *throughout the period of therapy.* Table 1 lists these drugs relative to achievable concentrations in the cerebrospinal fluid (CSF) and CNS. If at all possible, intravenous therapy should be used to ensure the highest plasma concentration possible and adequate CSF and CNS concentrations. Because phagocytic cells are less effective in the CSF, bactericidal drugs should be used whenever possible for treating bacterial meningitis. Table 2 lists various CNS infections and the most appropriate drugs for treatment.

Bacterial Meningitis

Meningitis in dogs and cats is rare and usually results from infection that extends locally or hematogenously from other areas of the body. Of the various organisms listed in Table 2, *Staphylococcus* is most important in the dog; the usual source of infection is endocarditis, prostatitis, diskospondylitis, or chronic recurrent pyoderma. In the absence of data confirming the type of CNS infection, one should proceed on the assumption that staphylococci are present. Ampicillin, 5 mg/kg intravenously every 6 hours for at least 7 to 10 days, should be given. Chloramphenicol can be substituted for ampicillin only when the organism is known to be sensitive to its action and when treatment with ampicillin has failed.

Although gentamicin penetrates the CNS very poorly, it is acceptable to combine the drug with ampicillin, since it is assumed that the primary focus of infection is not in the CNS. A dosage of 1 to 2 mg/kg subcutaneously every 8 hours is recommended. Proper hydration and renal function must be maintained. Under no conditions should the aminoglycosides be given as the sole antibiotic in bacterial CNS infections.

Gram-negative infections are extremely difficult to treat because the antibiotics most successful against them may not penetrate the CNS. The most effective drugs include high doses of ampicillin, carbenicillin, trimethoprim, or chloramphenicol. With *Pseudomonas* infections resistant to carbenicillin, the administration of intrathecal gentamicin should be considered.

Synergistic antibiotic combinations include penicillin or ampicillin plus an aminoglycoside (such as gentamicin) against enterococci and staphylococci, carbenicillin and gentamicin against *Pseudomonas*, and amphotericin B and flucytosine against *Cryptococcus.* Synergistic activity is compromised when one drug fails to penetrate the CNS. Antagonism occurs between ampicillin and oxytetracycline and between penicillin and chloramphenicol.

MYCOTIC INFECTIONS

The drugs used in the treatment of mycotic infections in the CNS are outlined in Table 2. Mycotic infections in this system have a poor prognosis, since the most effective drugs fail to penetrate the CNS in significant concentrations. In general, amphotericin B (0.4 mg/kg intravenously every 3 days) is recommended for histoplasmosis, blastomycosis, coccidioidosis, and candidiasis. Flucytosine, 0.25 to 0.30 mg/kg/day, is added to the dose of amphotericin B for the treatment of CNS cryptococcosis. Many clinicians may be tempted to treat CNS mycotic infections with ketoconazole alone since it can be given orally and is relatively inexpensive compared with amphotericin B therapy. However, ketoconazole penetrates the CNS poorly even when high doses are given. Therefore, ketoconazole should be viewed as adjunctive therapy with amphotericin B.

The combination therapy outlined above has the potential for several side effects, including renal toxicity, liver toxicity, and bone marrow suppression. Anorexia and vomiting may be observed.

ANTI-INFLAMMATORY THERAPY

Glucocorticoids have been advocated in the treatment of CNS infection to relieve edema and inflammation. Their use is associated with increased morbidity, mortality, and relapses. The doses of glucocorticoids required to control CNS edema suppress host defense mechanisms, and this author cannot therefore support the use of glucocorticoids in CNS infections.

Other anti-inflammatory compounds such as aspirin may be used to help control pain. Codeine may be useful in suppressing pain associated with meningitis.

References and Supplemental Readings

Green, C. E.: Infections of the central nervous system. *In* Greene, C. E. (ed.): *Clinical Microbiology and Infectious Diseases of the Dog and Cat.* Philadelphia: W.B. Saunders, 1984, pp. 284–300.

Lorenz, M. D.: Principles of medical treatment of the nervous system. *In* Oliver, J. E., and Lorenz, M. D. (ed.): *Handbook of Veterinary Neurologic Diagnosis.* Philadelphia: W.B. Saunders, 1983, pp. 122–130.

BRAIN TUMORS IN DOGS AND CATS

RICHARD A. LeCOUTEUR, B.V.Sc.
Fort Collins, Colorado

and JANE M. TURREL, D.V.M.
Davis, California

A dog or cat with a brain neoplasm is considered by most veterinarians to have a guarded to poor prognosis. This conclusion results largely from an inability to localize a brain tumor accurately and, consequently, to provide definitive treatment. With the development of effective localizing techniques such as x-ray computed tomography (CT) and their application in animals, accurate information regarding location, size, and extent of a brain tumor has become available. In turn, treatments of intracranial neoplasms have been developed for use in animals. Radiation therapy, complete excision, or partial surgical resection, either alone or in combination, are now being used in several veterinary institutions to treat canine and feline brain tumors. Results in animals support continued development of these therapeutic modalities. The purpose of this article is to summarize for practicing veterinarians techniques of diagnosis of intracranial tumors in animals and to outline currently available methods of treatment.

INCIDENCE

There is little information in the literature concerning the incidence of brain tumors in animals. The incidence rate (number of cases per 100,000 of the population at risk) of nervous system tumors has been estimated in dogs and cats to be 14.5 and 3.5, respectively.

Brain tumors occur more often in dogs than in other domestic species. Dogs also have the broadest spectrum of tumor types. There is a higher incidence among certain breeds, such as boxers, Boston terriers, and bulldogs. A gender predisposition has not yet been demonstrated. The highest incidence appears to be in dogs between 6 and 11 years of age. Similar information for cats has not been reported.

The incidence of metastatic brain tumors in animals is not known, largely because the central nervous system is not routinely examined at necropsy. It may be expected that the frequency of diagnosis of metastatic tumors will increase. This will occur with improved diagnostic imaging techniques and increased longevity of patients with primary tumors that have been treated with advanced surgical, chemotherapeutic, or radiotherapeutic methods.

CLASSIFICATION

Intracranial neoplasms may be classified as either primary or secondary. Primary neoplasms arise from brain or meningeal stem cells. They rarely metastasize to sites outside the nervous system, although in some cases local spread along cerebrospinal fluid (CSF) pathways may occur. Occasionally, more than one primary brain tumor will occur in an animal (e.g., multiple meningiomas in cats). Secondary tumors comprise either metastases from a primary tumor located outside the nervous system or tumors that affect the brain by local invasion from adjacent non-neural tissues such as bone. Lymphosarcoma of the brain is considered to be a secondary tumor, often occurring late in the course of multicentric lymphosarcoma. Occasionally, it may occur solely as a brain tumor. It can, however, occur in the brain simultaneously with the development of multicentric lymphosarcoma.

Central nervous system tumors in animals are classified according to the same criteria used in the classification of human tumors (Table 1). Despite histologic similarities between human and animal brain tumors, there is a need for a veterinary classification of gliomas, many of which are unclassifiable according to criteria currently used. There are published accounts of predilection sites for various tumor types, but such data are based on low numbers of tumors, and exceptions occur with

Table 1. *Classification of Tumors of the Central Nervous System in Dogs*

Primary Neoplasms	Secondary Neoplasms
Neuroectodermal Tumors	***Metastatic Tumors***
Astrocytoma	Mammary gland adenocarcinoma
Oligodendroglioma	Pulmonary carcinoma
Glioblastoma multiforme	Prostatic carcinoma
Glioma (unclassified)	Salivary gland adenocarcinoma
Ependymoma	Hemangiosarcoma
Choroid plexus tumor	Fibrosarcoma
Spongioblastoma	Malignant melanoma
Medulloblastoma	Lymphosarcoma
Neuroblastoma	
Ganglioneuroma	
Mesodermal Tumors	***Primary Tumors of Surrounding Tissues***
Meningioma	Osteoma
Primary reticulosis	Osteosarcoma
Lipoma	Chondroma
Chordoma	Chondrosarcoma
Angioblastoma	Hemangioma
Sarcoma	Hemangiosarcoma
Ectodermal Tumors	Fibrosarcoma
Craniopharyngioma	Epidermoid cyst
Pituitary adenoma	Multilobular osteoma or chondroma
Cylindromatosis epithelioma	
Olfactory gland adenocarcinoma	
Malformation Tumors	
Epidermoid	
Dermoid	

sufficient frequency to render this information of limited clinical usefulness.

ETIOLOGY

The cause of intracranial neoplasms is unknown. In a few patients an identifiable genetic or environmental factor may be implicated. For example, there is a high incidence of meningiomas reported in cats with mucopolysaccharidosis. Several viruses can produce a variety of brain tumors in experimental animals. The possible role of viral infections in spontaneous brain tumors remains undetermined.

PATHOGENESIS

Brain tumors cause dysfunction by destroying nervous tissue and compressing adjacent anatomic structures. Interference with cerebral circulation, local necrosis and edema formation, or disturbance of the dynamics of CSF flow may result in further nervous system damage. The precise location of a brain tumor may be masked by more generalized secondary effects, which include elevated intracranial pressure (ICP), brain herniation, or hydrocephalus. Increased ICP is often associated with edema and less commonly with hemorrhage or infarction, and it may occur in association with either a rapidly growing tumor or a slowly growing tumor that has

Table 2. *Clinical Signs Commonly Associated with Brain Tumors*

Generalized (Nonfocal)*
Depressed state of consciousness
Behavioral change
Head pressing
Pacing
Papilledema
Localized (Focal)
Signs of Local Brain Dysfunction
Hemiparesis
Circling
Hemisensory abnormalities
Visual field deficits
Cranial nerve deficits
Seizures
Focal or secondary generalized
Specific Neurologic Syndromes
Cerebellomedullary angle
Vestibular
Hypothalamo-hypophyseal
Cerebellar

*Often associated with increased intracranial pressure

reached a large size. Tumors that obstruct CSF flow or result in brain herniation may also result in a rapid and severe rise in ICP.

Primary brain tumors usually grow slowly and result in a chronic clinical progression. Occasionally, clinical abnormalities will be evident only after the compensatory mechanisms of the brain are exhausted. In these instances, a sudden onset of severe neurologic dysfunction may occur in the absence of any premonitory signs. If a tumor erodes or obstructs a blood vessel, causing hemorrhage or infarction, an acute onset of neurologic deficits may ensue. Secondary brain tumors, particularly those that are highly malignant, often demonstrate more acute progression.

CLINICAL SIGNS

The location of a lesion and its rate of progression determine the clinical signs associated with a brain tumor. Localized (focal) abnormalities are seen most frequently and result from direct compression, invasion, or irritation of a region of the brain. Generalized (nonlocalizing) signs result from secondary effects such as elevated ICP.

Clinical signs commonly associated with a brain tumor are summarized in Table 2. It should be remembered, however, that intracranial neoplasia must be considered as a cause for all neurologic syndromes that can be localized in the brain. This is true regardless of rate of progression, signalment of the animal, and location (focal, multifocal, or diffuse) of the lesion in the brain.

DIAGNOSIS

It is possible on the basis of signalment, history, and physical and neurologic examinations to localize a lesion to the brain and, in some cases, to determine laterality or approximate location. A similar neurologic syndrome will result from any one of many different disease processes occurring at a given location. Many degenerative, metabolic, inflammatory, toxic, and vascular diseases may result in clinical signs similar to those seen with a brain tumor. These other causes must be eliminated before the diagnosis of brain tumor is made.

A minimum data base for an animal with a brain lesion should include a complete blood count, serum chemistry analyses, urinalysis, and plain radiographs of the thorax and abdomen. These tests are especially important when a metastatic brain tumor is suspected or when clinical signs of metabolic or endocrine disturbance are present.

Analysis of CSF is an essential ancillary test in the diagnosis of a brain tumor. It not only serves to help rule out inflammatory diseases but also may support a diagnosis of intracranial neoplasm. The results of CSF analysis most often seen with a brain tumor are elevated pressure and increased protein in the presence of a normal cell count. This is a variable finding, however, and it is possible to have normal results on these tests. Tumor cells are rarely seen in CSF.

Electroencephalography (EEG) may be helpful in the diagnosis and localization of a cortical tumor. A focal abnormality may be demonstrated, or confirmation of generalized brain dysfunction may be possible. As with CSF analysis, EEG does not provide a definitive diagnosis but may support the presence of a brain lesion. Another electrophysiologic technique that may provide useful information in the localization of brain stem lesions is the brain stem auditory evoked response (BAER). Reports on its use for the localization of brain stem tumors in animals do not exist at this time.

Radiographs of the skull appear normal in most animals with primary brain tumors. They may demonstrate bone tumors resulting in secondary effects on brain and infrequently show calcification associated with a meningioma.

The diagnostic methods listed above, either alone or in combination, are often useful in determining the presence of an intracranial neoplasm, but they seldom provide specific information regarding its precise location, size, and extent. More advanced techniques have been developed to meet this need. Radiographic techniques that use contrast materials (ventriculography, arteriography, sinus venography, and optic thecography) can help in many instances to confirm the location of a neoplasm within the calvaria. These techniques are limited, however, in their ability to define precise size and extent of a neoplasm and its relationship to adjacent structures. This is also true of nuclear medicine studies (radioisotope brain scans).

The recent application of CT in animals has resulted in renewed interest in the localization and treatment of brain neoplasms. The primary strength of CT is its ability to localize a lesion precisely in three dimensions and to define the size and extent of that lesion. After a lesion is identified, CT provides an accurate means for treatment planning and follow-up. The limited accessibility and high cost of CT systems have restricted their use in veterinary medicine to veterinary institutions that possess the equipment and to those human hospitals that will scan animals.

Another diagnostic technique with capabilities similar to CT is magnetic resonance imaging (MRI), which is now available to several veterinary institutions. The basic strength of MRI will be the identification of specific tissue types based on their chemical characteristics. The diagnostic specificity of MRI may eventually obviate the need for biopsy of lesions prior to treatment.

TREATMENT

The essential goals of brain tumor therapy are: (1) to control elevated ICP and other secondary tumor effects and (2) to eradicate the tumor or to decrease its size.

Control of Secondary Effects

The treatment of intracranial neoplasms has been, for the most part, palliative and noninvasive. Survival times are short (2 to 3 months), as progression of the tumor is inevitable. Therapy is symptomatic and is aimed at reducing elevated ICP and edema, controlling seizures, and providing supportive care. Corticosteroids and anticonvulsants have been widely used for these purposes. Dexamethasone (0.25 to 2 mg/kg repeated every 6 hours) may be administered intravenously in acute episodes of cerebral edema. Prednisolone or prednisone can be given orally on a daily or alternate-day therapy regimen to correct or control chronic secondary effects of a brain tumor. A dose of 0.5 to 1 mg/kg repeated every 12 hours is recommended for several days; then a decreasing dosage plan can be followed over the next week or month, depending on the patient's needs. Phenobarbital (1 to 2 mg/kg repeated every 12 hours) administered orally is the anticonvulsant drug best suited for use in dogs and cats.

Corticosteroids have proved to be of considerable benefit to patients with both primary and metastatic brain tumors. Reduction of edema is the most likely mechanism of action, although there is some evidence for specific antitumor effects. Corticosteroids are also used in conjunction with other treatments, such as surgery or radiation therapy.

Eradication or Reduction in Size

Reduction in the size of a brain neoplasm is the most important consideration for the long-term survival of an animal with a brain tumor. Four treatment methods, used alone or in combination, exist for this purpose: (a) surgery, (b) radiation therapy, (c) chemotherapy with cytotoxic agents, and (d) immunotherapy (or biologic response modification). At this time, only surgery and radiation therapy have been reported for use in dogs and cats with intracranial neoplasms.

SURGERY. Prior to the use of CT, neurosurgical management of brain tumors was largely limited to removal of superficial meningiomas or bony lesions that compressed the brain. Neurosurgical intervention is considered essential in the management of most brain tumors, whether it be complete excision, partial removal (debulking), or biopsy prior to definitive therapy. The development of advanced neurosurgical techniques, such as the infrared carbon-dioxide laser, intraoperative ultrasound, and bipolar coagulators, and the use of advanced neuroanesthetic techniques to manage elevated ICP have increased patient survival significantly.

Complete removal of a brain tumor will be limited by the location and invasiveness of a lesion. Meningiomas are almost always histologically benign and often can be removed completely. Partial removal of brain tumors may give symptomatic relief and will decrease tumor bulk prior to other modes of therapy. Malignant brain tumors rarely can be completely excised. Generally, by the time they are detected, they have invaded deep areas of the brain. In such cases, internal decompression of the tumor may be attempted by removing as much of the tumor as possible prior to the use of radiotherapy. Surgery is rarely indicated when an animal has a metastatic brain tumor. Surgical biopsy of a brain tumor is recommended prior to radiation therapy or other treatment modalities. This biopsy information will ultimately be used to provide data regarding the response to treatment of various tumor types in animals.

RADIATION THERAPY. The aim of radiation therapy is to destroy a neoplasm and at the same time minimize the damage to any normal tissue that must be included in the irradiated volume. Careful treatment planning is required to achieve these objectives. Except for surgically accessible, benign tumors such as meningiomas, radiation therapy is indicated for most primary brain tumors. It is used either alone or after surgical intervention. Radiation therapy is also indicated when a tumor is a metastasis.

External-beam, megavoltage irradiation has been demonstrated to be effective in the treatment of canine brain tumors and is currently utilized for the treatment of brain tumors in cats and dogs at several veterinary institutions. There are variations in the total dose given, the number of fractions, and the time over which it is given. These have been empirically determined. Factors such as tumor type, radioresponsiveness, and anatomic location may determine the treatment dose. At the University of California, Davis, and Colorado State University, Fort Collins, total radiation doses currently used are 4000 or 4800 rads given in 10 to 12 fractions over 22 to 26 days. Results at both institutions are extremely encouraging, and many animals have tumor regression and clinical improvement after radiation therapy. Some dogs and cats experience gradual reversal of symptoms throughout treatment. Many animals improve with surgical resection and decompression prior to radiation therapy.

New techniques are being developed to improve the effectiveness of radiotherapy. For example, superfractionation (with two or more fractions per day) may be utilized. Also, radiation enhancers (sensitizers) such as misonidazole can be employed. These drugs substitute for oxygen in hypoxic areas of brain tumors and may render them more radiosensitive. Brachytherapy, or interstitial radiation therapy, is a method of implanting radioisotopes (e.g., ^{125}I) intratumorally to deliver high radiation doses to relatively hypoxic tumors. Hyperthermia and photoradiation therapy may also be used to potentiate the effects of radiation therapy. These techniques have received little attention in veterinary medicine up to this time.

CHEMOTHERAPY. In humans, chemotherapy is currently being actively investigated for use in combination with other treatments for brain tumors. However, there are several factors that must be considered in their use. The first, unique to the brain, is that the blood-brain barrier may prevent exposure of all or some of the tumor to a chemotherapeutic agent injected parenterally. Second, tumor cell heterogeneity may be such that only certain cells are sensitive to a given agent. Third, a tumor may be sensitive only at doses that are excessively toxic to normal brain or to other organs of the body.

Several chemotherapeutic agents have proved to be at least modestly efficacious in treating malignant gliomas in humans. As single agents, BCNU (a lipid-soluble nitrosourea) and procarbazine (a monoamine oxidase inhibitor) have demonstrated a modest increase in patient survival in randomized clinical studies. Further investigation of chemotherapy for brain tumors in animals seems warranted.

IMMUNOTHERAPY. This mode of therapy has not yet been attempted in animals. It involves the modification of the immune response of a patient so that a tumor may be eliminated immunologically. Current efforts are concentrating on the recognition of specific tumor-associated antigens, which could in turn be used to immunize a patient against the tumor from which the antigens were isolated. Monoclonal antibody–defined, tumor-associated antigens are being explored as targeting carriers of radiation for imaging and therapy and of other cytotoxic agents. This therapy, either alone or as an adjunct to other treatments, may improve survival in the future of patients with brain tumors.

CONCLUSIONS

There have been few reports in the literature concerning therapy of brain tumors in dogs and cats. Most existing reports concern the surgical removal of superficial tumors. Recently, the use of radiation therapy in dogs with intracranial neoplasms was reported. Results of this study were encouraging; survival times of some dogs with brain tumors were greater than one year, and quality of life after therapy was excellent. Currently, radiation therapy for brain tumors, either alone or after surgery, is used at several veterinary institutions. This trend parallels the rapid development and availability of advanced diagnostic modalities such as CT, which allows accurate localization of a tumor and permits monitoring of tumor regression, progression, or recurrence after therapy.

This article has outlined the principles, availability, and potential usefulness of various techniques for the diagnosis and treatment of brain tumors in dogs and cats. Referral of animals with brain tumors to veterinary institutions that possess advanced surgical and radiotherapeutic capabilities should be offered to animal owners. As the number of treated animals increases, diagnostic and therapeutic techniques will be refined and improved. These data will, in turn, provide a basis for rational treatment plans and improved survival of dogs and cats with brain tumors.

References and Supplemental Reading

Braund, K. G.: Neoplasia of the nervous system. Comp. Cont. Ed. Pract. Vet. 6:717, 1984.

Edwards, M. S., Levin, V. A., and Wilson, C. B.: Brain tumor chemotherapy: An evaluation of agents in current use for phase II and III trials. Cancer Treat. Rep. 64:1179, 1980.

Fike, J. R., Cann, C. E., Davis, R. L., et al.: Radiation effects in the canine brain evaluated by quantitative computed tomography. Radiology 144:603, 1982.

Fike, J. R., LeCouteur, R. A., Cann, C. E., et al.: Computerized tomography of brain tumors of the rostral and middle fossas in the dog. Am. J. Vet. Res. 42:275, 1981.

Gutin, P. H., Phillips, T. L., Wara, W. M., et al.: Brachytherapy of recurrent malignant brain tumors with removable high-activity iodine-125 sources. J. Neurosurg. 60:61, 1984.

LeCouteur, R. A., Cann, C. E., and Fike, J. R.: Computed tomography. *In* Gourley, I. G., and Vasseur, P. B. (eds.): *General Small Animal Surgery*. Philadelphia: J.B. Lippincott, 1985, pp. 989–1002.

LeCouteur, R. A., Fike, J. R., Cann, C. E., et al.: Computed tomography of brain tumors in the caudal fossa of the dog. Vet. Radiol. 22:244, 1981.

LeCouteur, R. A., Fike, J. R., Cann, C. E., et al.: X-ray computed tomography of brain tumors in cats. J.A.V.M.A. 183:301, 1983.

Mahaley, M. S., Jr., and Gillespie, G. Y.: Immunotherapy of patients with glioma: Fact, fancy, and future. Prog. Exp. Tumor Res. 28:118, 1984.

Oliver, J. E., and Lorenz, M. D.: *Handbook of Veterinary Neurologic Diagnosis*. Philadelphia: W.B. Saunders, 1983.

Tew, J. M., Feibel, J. H., and Sawaya, R.: Brain tumors: Clinical aspects. Semin. Roentgenol. XIX:115, 1984.

Turrel, J. M., Fike, J. R., LeCouteur, R. A., et al.: Radiotherapy of brain tumors in dogs. J.A.V.M.A. 184:82, 1981.

Walker, R. W., and Posner, J. B.: Central nervous system neoplasms. *In* Appel, S. H. (ed.): *Current Neurology*. Vol. 5. New York: Wiley Medical Publications, 1984.

Wara, W. M., and Sheline, G. E.: Radiation therapy for intracranial tumors. *In* Schneider, R. C., Kahn, E. A., Crosby, E. C., et al. (eds.): *Correlative Neurosurgery*, 3rd ed. Springfield: Charles C Thomas, 1982.

Zaki, F. A.: Spontaneous central nervous system tumors in the dog. Vet. Clin. North Am. 7:153, 1977.

CONGENITAL PORTOSYSTEMIC SHUNTS IN CATS

SHARON A. CENTER, D.V.M.,
WILLIAM E. HORNBUCKLE, D.V.M.,
Ithaca, New York

and THOMAS D. SCAVELLI, D.V.M.
New York, New York

Portosystemic vascular anomalies have been commonly reported in dogs and less commonly in cats. This condition was first recognized in cats in 1980 and is associated with clinical features similar to those occurring in dogs (Vulgamott et al., 1980). Neurologic signs predominate and are typically episodic in occurrence. Recognition of hepatic encephalopathy as the cause of the neurologic impairment is possible on the basis of hepatic function tests. The definitive diagnosis may be substantiated with contrast venography, two-dimensional ultrasonography, surgical exploration, and liver biopsy.

Three major types of portal vein anomalies described in cats include a direct portocaval or portoazygous shunt, a patent ductus venous, and aplasia or hypoplasia of the portal vein with the development of collateral shunting vessels (Carr and Thornburg, 1984; Gandolfi, 1984; Hawe and Mullen, 1984; Levesque et al., 1982; Parker, 1982; Rothuizen et al., 1982; Vulgamott et al., 1980). The patent ductus venosus is an intrahepatic shunt that is more commonly reported in dogs. Most of the portosystemic vascular anomalies in cats are extrahepatic. In the authors' experience, the left gastric vein represents the major collateral communication in 50 per cent of affected cats.

Changes in hepatic morphology of cats with congenital portosystemic shunts include atrophy of the hepatic lobule, centrolobular fatty change, and portal vein hypoplasia or periportal fibrosis. In some cases there are no apparent abnormalities of the portal triads.

FELINE HEPATIC ENCEPHALOPATHY

The syndrome of hepatic encephalopathy may develop owing to insufficiency of the portohepatic circulation or as a direct result of severe hepatocellular dysfunction. Hepatic encephalopathy is infrequently recognized in cats. When acquired, hepatobiliary insufficiency is the cause of hepatic encephalopathy, and the animal usually has such obvious clinicopathologic abnormalities as bilirubinuria or hyperbilirubinemia. Central nervous system disturbances have also been reported in neonatal cats with kernicterus. Hepatobiliary disorders associated with hepatic encephalopathy in cats are listed in Table 1. Although dogs with occult cirrhosis may present primarily with encephalopathic signs, this is an uncommon presentation for cats, which usually die of abnormalities attributable to hepatobiliary dysfunction before neurologic signs of hepatic impairment are recognized.

Multiple factors are considered to interact in the generation of hepatic encephalopathy (Hoyumpa and Schenker, 1982; Sherding, 1981; Tams, 1985;

Table 1. *Liver Diseases Associated with Hepatic Encephalopathy in the Cat*

Portosystemic vascular anomaly
Hepatic lipidosis
Cholangiohepatitis
Cholangitis
Experimentally induced arginine deficiency
Toxic hepatopathy
Hepatic degeneration
Cirrhosis

Vulgamott, 1985; Zieve, 1982). Metabolic imbalances and toxins are thought to be synergistic in the origination and perpetuation of the neurologic abnormalities. The alimentary tract is the major source of many of these substances. Pathogenetic mechanisms by which encephalopathic signs occur include alteration of the blood-brain barrier, disruption of cellular energy metabolism, or abnormal neurotransmission.

A major substance implicated in the pathogenesis of hepatic encephalopathy is ammonia, which is largely derived from the gastrointestinal tract, especially the colon. In addition, peripheral tissue metabolism, particularly of the skeletal muscles, may generate substantial amounts of ammonia. In the gastrointestinal tract endogenous urea, which diffuses into the intestinal lumen, is hydrolyzed by bacterial ureases to ammonia. Ammonia is also generated within the gastrointestinal tract from exogenous dietary amines and from the metabolism of glutamine. In the normal animal, ammonia of enteric origin is absorbed into the portal circulation and transported directly to the liver. Within the liver, the Krebs-Henseleit urea cycle detoxifies ammonia to urea. Approximately 75 per cent of the urea generated in the liver is excreted by glomerular filtration. The remainder diffuses into the intestinal lumen, where it is decomposed to ammonia, is reabsorbed, and subsequently re-enters the urea cycle. Another route of ammonia detoxification is in the kidney, through glutamine synthesis. In the completely hepatectomized animal, the role of the kidney in ammonia detoxification may become more important.

Hyperammonemia as a result of an enzyme deficiency in the urea cycle (e.g., arginosuccinate synthetase) has been reported in dogs. Spontaneous enzyme deficiencies in the urea cycle have not been reported in cats. However, experimentally induced arginine deficiency has resulted in feline hepatic encephalopathy. This amino acid deficiency is inducible in cats because of their dependence on preformed dietary arginine. Since arginine is an essential component of the urea cycle, its absence results in decreased ammonia detoxification.

The importance of hyperammonemia in the generation of hepatic encephalopathy is controversial. Nevertheless, most cats presenting with encephalopathic signs due to portosystemic vascular anomalies have increased blood ammonia values. There appears to be no correlation between the magnitude of ammonia increase and the severity of the neurologic signs in individual cats. The proposed mechanisms of ammonia intoxication include a direct depressant effect on neuronal membranes associated with altered ion transport, interference with mitochondrial metabolism, diminution of excitatory neurotransmitters, decrease in cerebral energy stores, and alteration of the blood-brain barrier.

Other toxins derived from the gastrointestinal tract that are implicated in the generation of hepatic encephalopathy include mercaptans, skatoles, indoles, and short-chain fatty acids. Mercaptans are derived from dietary methionine by bacterial deamination within the gastrointestinal tract. These substances are normally efficiently removed from the portohepatic circulation by the liver and detoxified. Lipotrophic medications containing methionine may precipitate neurologic signs in animals with hepatic insufficiency and thus should be avoided in patients with portosystemic vascular anomalies. Intestinal bacterial deamination of dietary tryptophan results in the formation of skatoles and indoles. Insufficient hepatic metabolism of these substances results in their accumulation and, subsequently, signs of cerebral intoxication. Tryptophan intoxication, characterized by ataxia and visual disturbances, was induced in a dog with a portosystemic circulatory anastomosis. Reduced clearance of short-chain fatty acids in patients with hepatocellular insufficiency appears to intensify the neurologic effects of the cerebral toxins previously discussed.

Abnormal patterns of plasma amino acids, characterized by increased concentrations of aromatic amino acids (phenylalanine, tyrosine, free tryptophan) and decreased concentrations of the branched-chain amino acids, have been described in humans, dogs, and rats displaying signs of encephalopathy. The occurrence of such aberrations is undocumented in cats. Maladjustment of amino acid ratios is purported to result in the accumulation of false neurotransmitters and the decreased synthesis of normal excitatory neurotransmitters.

The inhibitory neurotransmitter gamma aminobutyric acid (GABA) is increased in hepatic insufficiency owing to decreased hepatic metabolism of GABA originating from the intestinal tract. There is some evidence that increased serum concentrations of GABA may pass through an altered blood-brain barrier and bind to synaptic membranes.

Increased serum bile acids have been postulated to augment the neurologic effects of other encephalopathic toxins. The alteration of the blood-brain barrier that has been recognized in experimental animals with portacaval anastomoses may result from increased concentrations of circulating bile acids. An increase in serum bile acid values has been documented in cats with either acquired or congenital hepatic insufficiency. In cats with portosystemic vascular anomalies, postprandial values of serum bile acid are consistently increased more than five times normal.

Since hepatic encephalopathy is a multifactorial neurophysiologic aberration, other metabolic imbalances may influence the expression of the neurologic signs. Hypoglycemia can cause a problem in patients with portosystemic vascular anomalies because of their diminished gluconeogenesis capabilities, abnormal responsiveness to glucagon, and deficient hepatic glycogen stores. Neuroglycopenia may develop in these patients and aggravate the pre-existing neurologic signs. Hypokalemia, alkalemia, and hypoxia may synergistically interact with many of the toxins causing hepatic encephalopathy. Another factor that may contribute to the neurologic signs observed in cats with hepatic insufficiency is thiamine deficiency. This is important because cats may become thiamine-deficient after prolonged periods of inappetence. Cats suffering from hepatic encephalopathy may experience recurrent anorexia.

The histologic lesions of the central nervous system of cats with hepatic encephalopathy due to portosystemic vascular anomalies have been typified by polymicrocavitation and by hypertrophy and proliferation of astrocytes.

HISTORY AND PHYSICAL EXAMINATION

Most cats with portosystemic vascular anomalies demonstrate neurobehavioral signs at a young age. These cats are brought for examination between 2 and 25 months of age and have shown encephalopathic signs for 2 to 10 months prior to presentation. Although central nervous system signs predominate, inappetence, polyphagia, diarrhea, occasional vomiting, polydipsia, and lower urinary tract signs have occurred in some cats. Clinical signs of encephalopathy are episodic and alternate with periods of normalcy. The signs may last for 12 to 48 hours and can occur at a frequency of once per month or up to several times per week. Neurologic manifestations are best characterized as a diffuse, symmetric, central nervous system aberration, and they may include abnormal behavior, depression, agitation, aggression, weakness, ataxia, dementia, head pressing, propulsive circling, mydriasis, blindness, and grand mal seizures..Some cats have neurologic signs that intensify within several hours after eating. Many cats exhibit excessive salivation or drooling and have consequently been treated for upper respiratory disease. In some instances, symptomatic treatment with broad-spectrum antibiotics has ameliorated the recurrent clinical signs. Slow recovery from general anesthesia with substances requiring hepatic biotransformation or excretion has also been observed.

The findings of physical examination are generally unremarkable, with the exception of the abovementioned neurologic signs and a tendency toward small body stature. There appears to be no predilection for a certain breed or sex. In the authors' experience, four of eight cats with documented portosystemic vascular anomalies have had substantial systolic cardiac murmurs. One of these cats had multiple cardiac malformations. Renal enlargement and absence of the spleen have also been observed.

CLINICOPATHOLOGIC EXAMINATIONS

Routine hematologic and biochemical profiles rarely provide evidence of hepatocellular insufficiency in cats with portosystemic vascular anomalies. Hematologic abnormalities identified in some cats have included poikilocytosis and microcytic anemia. Poikilocytosis is recognized as a nonspecific erythrocytic change in cats with any form of liver disease. Microcytosis, sometimes associated with mild anemia, has also been reported as a common hematologic feature in dogs with portosystemic vascular anomalies.

Serum biochemical abnormalities identified during routine screening may include a modest increase in levels of alanine aminotransferase and alkaline phosphatase. Values for urea nitrogen are usually normal but may be slightly decreased. Blood glucose values are usually in the low-normal range. Since normal stressed cats generally have hyperglycemia, the relative hypoglycemia observed in these cases may represent abnormal blood glucose regulation; this condition has been observed in other species with portosystemic vascular anastomoses.

Examination of the urine may reveal the presence of ammonium biurate crystalluria. There appears to be no correlation between the detection of ammonium biurate crystals and the magnitude of hyperammonemia. The formation of ammonium biurate crystals is influenced largely by the urine pH; crystal precipitation occurs more frequently in non-neutral urine. These crystals are inconsistently present in cats with portosystemic vascular anomalies. Cystic calculi of urate composition have been described in one cat with a portovascular anomaly.

The most important tests for the diagnosis of hepatic insufficiency in cats with portosystemic vascular anomalies are measurements of blood ammonia, both fasting and 2-hour postprandial serum bile acids, and the 30-minute percentage retention of sulfobromophthalein (BSP). Measurements of blood ammonia and bile acids are the preferred diagnostic procedures. When given at the recommended dose of 5.0 mg/kg, the plasma clearance of BSP is too rapid to be a sensitive indicator of hepatobiliary function in the cat. Percentages for BSP 30-minute retention in dogs (less than or equal to 5.0 per cent) are not the same as those in cats, which have normal values that are less than or equal to 3.0 per cent (Center et al., 1983). Increased BSP retention in dogs with portosystemic vascular anomalies is an inconsistent finding. Similar observations have been made for cats.

Blood ammonia values provide the only direct evidence of hepatic encephalopathy available to the practitioner. Unfortunately, this analytic procedure is fraught with many inconveniences. The metabolic generation of ammonia in improperly managed whole blood can invalidate the blood ammonia test. Since ammonia is so labile, coordination of clinical testing and laboratory analysis is essential. Animals with portosystemic vascular anomalies inconsistently demonstrate hyperammonemia after meals or a prolonged fast. Hyperammonemia is more consistent in these patients after the oral administration of ammonium chloride. Although some investigators have cautioned that encephalopathic signs may be precipitated by oral dosage of ammonium chloride (0.1 gm/kg), the authors have never seen this sequela in cats with portosystemic vascular anomalies.

Serum bile acids are sensitive and specific indicators of hepatic insufficiency resulting from hepatocellular failure or insufficient hepatoportal circulation. Measurement of serum bile acids has been shown to be more sensitive than BSP testing and equivalent in sensitivity to the ammonia tolerance test in the diagnosis of portosystemic venous anastomosis (Center et al., 1985a). Animals with substantial hepatic insufficiency commonly show increased fasting values for bile acid but may show values within the normal range if the fast is prolonged (over 24 hours). The increase in values for serum bile acid 2 hours after a meal identifies animals with hepatocellular insufficiency. Values for serum bile acid in cats with portosystemic vascular anastomoses are within the normal range or mildly increased after a prolonged fast but are markedly increased 2 hours after a meal. The range of fasting values in four cats was 1.8 to 50.5 μM/L (normal, 1.7 ± 0.3 μM/L), and the mean value 2 hours after a meal in three cats was 80.8 to 124.2 μM/L (normal, 8.3 ± 0.8 μM/L). Since the bile acid test is more convenient for the clinician, laboratory technician, and patient, it is the preferred diagnostic test in the authors' clinic.

RADIOGRAPHIC EXAMINATIONS

Plain abdominal radiographs generally disclose a small hepatic silhouette in cats with portal vein anomalies. Diminished hepatotrophic factors within the portal circulatory system and reduced sinusoidal blood volume are believed to be responsible for the reduction in hepatic size. Decreased abdominal and subcutaneous fat has been seen in some cats. Cardiomegaly has been observed by the authors in four cats that also had cardiac murmurs.

Definitive diagnosis of a portosystemic vascular anomaly is confirmed by contrast portal venography. Reported techniques include transabdominal splenoportography, femoral arterial catheterization for cranial mesenteric or celiac arterioportography, and direct catheterization of a mesenteric or splenic vein. The preferred technique is catheterization of a jejunal-mesenteric vein through a small abdominal incision, performed with the patient under general anesthesia.

A 20- to 18-gauge over-the-needle catheter is aseptically secured into a mesenteric vessel with a size 000 suture. After survey abdominal radiographs are taken, proper catheter placement may be verified by an injection of 2 to 3 ml of contrast medium. Radiographs are taken immediately after the test injection or, if available, fluoroscopy is used to visualize the catheter's location. Contrast material (5 to 10 ml total dose, 1 to 2 ml/kg of aqueous iodine contrast medium containing 25 to 40 per cent iodine) is rapidly injected by hand into the catheter for the definitive study. Radiographs are taken immediately and up to 10 seconds after the injection. If necessary, the contrast study may be repeated up to two times. The jejunal-mesenteric vein used for contrast injection is ligated when the study is completed (V. Rendano and A. Dietze, Cornell University).

The portogram in the normal cat will demonstrate the hepatic portal vessels within several seconds of injection of contrast material. At 10 seconds, contrast material will be present in the caudal vena cava and in the heart. If the cat is abnormal, the shunting vessel will be revealed within several seconds. The caudal vena cava and heart will be illuminated more rapidly than in the normal animal. The radiographic assessment of normal portohepatic venous channels cannot be used to select surgical candidates. Radiographic evidence of liver perfusion is usually absent because of the increased resistance to hepatic perfusion owing to the hypoplastic character of the hepatoportal system and the decreased resistance to blood flow within the shunting vessel. It may be necessary to repeat the radiographic contrast studies after surgery if portovenous atresia or induced portovenous hypertension is suspected.

ULTRASONOGRAPHY

Two-dimensional ultrasonography may be used to verify the existence of a portosystemic shunt. This is a noninvasive procedure that does not require general anesthesia, and it is considered by the authors to be a useful clinical screening test. Nevertheless, contrast portography remains the preferred method of shunt localization for surgical intervention.

MEDICAL TREATMENT

The major objective of medical treatment is to control or minimize the episodic manifestations of hepatic encephalopathy (Hoyumpa and Schenker, 1982; Sherding, 1981; Tams, 1985; Vulgamott, 1985). Dietary management is directed toward the quantitative restriction of foods rich in protein. It is the impression of the authors that cats with portosystemic vascular anomalies do well on several prescription diets (i/d, k/d; Hill's Pet Products) and on diets rich in rice or pasta supplemented with small amounts of cottage cheese. Additionally, a diet formulated for dogs with hepatic insufficiency is highly palatable to some cats and may be useful in the management of this disorder. We have observed the precipitation of encephalopathic signs in three cats with portosystemic shunts that were fed feline c/d prescription diet (Hill's Pet Products). These signs occurred within 2 to 6 hours of food ingestion. An additional dietary consideration is vitamin supplementation (but *no* products containing methionine). Cats undergoing prolonged periods of inappetence should be supplemented with thiamine (vitamin B_1), 50 mg orally twice daily for at least 1 week, and also with other forms of water-soluble vitamins.

Since many of the toxic substances implicated as a cause of the syndrome of hepatic encephalopathy arise within the alimentary canal, the adjustment of enteric organisms and ingesta may modulate the clinical signs. Cleansing colonic enemas consisting of warm isotonic saline or other polyionic fluids help to eliminate toxic substances directly during an encephalopathic crisis.

The oral administration of lactulose, a synthetic disaccharide, is useful in the management and prevention of hepatic encephalopathy. This substance cannot be digested by mammalian enzymes but is fermented in the alimentary canal by enteric organisms. The beneficial attributes of lactulose include the lowering of colonic pH, which results in trapping ammonium ions within the gut; decreased intestinal transit time owing to a cathartic effect; and a protection against enteric endotoxins. The usual dose of lactulose for cats is 0.25 to 1.0 ml orally. The dose is individualized on the basis of stool consistency and is titrated until a semiformed stool is obtained. Unfortunately, cats resent the taste of lactulose, and excessive doses of this drug can induce flatulence, diarrhea, and dehydration.

The oral administration of antibiotics has decreased the encephalopathic signs in several cats with portosystemic vascular anomalies. Neomycin, an aminoglycoside, is the most commonly used antibiotic in the management of hepatic encephalopathy. It exerts its effects by modifying the enteric flora that contribute to the production of cerebral toxins. The dosage recommended for the cat is 10 to 20 mg/kg orally twice daily. Neomycin is reported to act synergistically with lactulose in lowering blood ammonia, and a combination of these drugs is currently recommended for use in humans with hepatic encephalopathy. Lactulose or neomycin used singly or in combination may also be colonically administered in cleansing enemas. In the experience of the authors, the administration of ampicillin or amoxicillin has had therapeutic value in controlling episodes of encephalopathy in some cats. However, the use of nonabsorbable aminoglycoside antibiotics given orally is preferred.

Metronidazole has recently been advocated for the management of hepatic encephalopathy in humans and in dogs. The beneficial effects of this drug result from the selective killing of anaerobic bacterial organisms, which are considered an important source of ammonia production. Although there has been limited experience with this drug in cats, the following dosage has been recommended: 7.5 mg/kg orally three times daily for 2 to 4 weeks or longer, as indicated by response to therapy (Tams, 1985).

Since the regulation of blood glucose may be deficient in patients with portosystemic vascular anomalies, blood sugar should be closely monitored. During and after general anesthesia, prolonged diagnostic procedures, or surgery, intravenous therapy with dextrose-fortified solutions should be administered. Continuous infusions of 2.5 to 5.0 per cent dextrose in water or in balanced electrolyte solutions are recommended.

SURGICAL CORRECTION

Surgical occlusion of the shunting vessel is the preferred therapeutic option (Birchard, 1984; Breznock, 1979; Levesque et al., 1982). If the portal blood flow can be surgically redirected to the liver, affected patients will often be relieved of their encephalopathy. The surgical technique involves partial ligation of the shunt. A celiotomy is performed, the portal vein is isolated, and its course to the liver is identified. If the portal vascular anomaly is not readily apparent, then a through-the-needle catheter (17 to 22 cm) may be passed by way of a mesenteric vein to reveal the major pathway of blood flow to the shunt. Once the shunt is identified, a partial occlusion is then performed by means of a single ligature of monofilament nonabsorbable material (silk or nylon). It is important not to ligate the vessel lumen completely if portal hypertension results from temporary shunt occlusion. Estimation of portal hypertension by observation of the mesenteric vasculature and visceral perfusion is unreliable and potentially dangerous, because hypertension may not be apparent until 12 to 24 hours after surgery. Direct measurement of portal pressure by a manometer (normal canine mesenteric pressure, 8 to 13 cm H_2O) is recommended. The shunt's diameter is gradually decreased by 60 to 80 per cent or until the mesenteric pressure is increased by 10 cm H_2O over the preligation value. In some cases, a series of surgical procedures may be necessary for safe and effective occlusion of the vessel. Reports in dogs recommend occluding the shunt diameter by 70 to 80 per cent during the initial surgery. The mesenteric veins in cats are much smaller than those in dogs, and it is therefore more difficult to quantitate the degree of closure. To avoid excessive shunt occlusion, a 20-gauge plastic catheter can be used to adjust the tautness of the ligature. The catheter is placed parallel to the shunting vessel, the ligature is applied over the shunt and catheter, the first knot is placed, and the catheter is then removed.

Medical management should be sustained for 2 to 4 weeks after the remission of clinical signs. Return to normal diet and activity should be gradual. Improvement following shunt ligation may be monitored by liver function tests.

References and Supplemental Reading

Birchard, S. J.: Surgical management of portosystemic shunts in dogs and cats. Comp. Cont. Ed. Pract. Vet. 6:795, 1984.

Breznock, E. M.: Surgical manipulation of portosystemic shunts in dogs. J.A.V.M.A. 174:819, 1979.

Carr, S. H., and Thornburg, L. P.: Congenital portacaval shunt in two kittens. Feline Pract. 14:43, 1984.

Center, S. A., Baldwin, B. H., de Lahunta, A., et al.: Evaluation of bile acid concentrations for the diagnosis of portosystemic venous anomalies in the dog and cat. J.A.V.M.A. 186:1090, 1985.

Center, S. A., Baldwin, B. H., Erb, H., et al.: Bile acids in the diagnosis of hepatobiliary disease in the dog. J.A.V.M.A. 187:931, 1985.

Center, S. A., Bunch, S. E., Baldwin, B. H., et al.: Comparison of sulfobromophthalein and indocyanine green clearances in the cat. Am. J. Vet. Res. 44:727, 1983.

Gandolfi, R. C.: Hepatoencephalopathy associated with patent ductus venosus in a cat. J.A.V.M.A. 185:301, 1984.

Hawe, R. S., and Mullen, H. S.: An unusual portacaval anomaly as a cause of hepatic encephalopathy in a cat. J. Am. Anim. Hosp. Assoc. 20:987, 1984.

Hoyumpa, A. M., and Schenker, S.: Perspectives in hepatic encephalopathy. J. Lab. Clin. Med. 100:477, 1982.

Levesque, D. C., Oliver, J. E., Cornelius, L. M., et al.: Congenital portacaval shunts in two cats: Diagnosis and surgical correction. J.A.V.M.A. 181:143, 1982.

Parker, A. J.: Differential diagnosis of brain disease—feline behavior. Mod. Vet. Pract. 63:711, 1982.

Rothuizen, J. van den Ingh, T. S.G.A.M., Voorhout, G., et al.: Congenital porto-systemic shunts in 16 dogs and 3 cats. J. Small Anim. Pract. 23:67, 1982.

Sherding, R. G.: Hepatic encephalopathy in the dog. Comp. Cont. Ed. Pract. Vet. 3:55, 1981.

Tams, T. R.: Hepatic encephalopathy. Vet. Clin. North Am. 15:177, 1985.

Vulgamott, J. C., Turnwald, G. H., King, G. K., et al.: Congenital portacaval anomalies in the cat: Two case reports. J. Am. Anim. Hosp. Assoc. 16:915, 1980.

Vulgamott, J. C.: Portosystemic shunts. Vet. Clin. North Am. 15:229, 1985.

Zieve, L.: Hepatic encephalopathy. *In* Schiff, L., and Schiff, E. R. (ed.): *Diseases of the Liver*, 5th ed. Philadelphia: J.B. Lippincott, 1982, pp. 433–459.

HEAD TRAUMA AND NERVOUS SYSTEM INJURY

WILLIAM R. FENNER, D.V.M.

Columbus, Ohio

Traumatic injuries of the head are common in dogs and cats. They are often severe and are frequently frustrating to manage. In a recent review it was found that about 20 per cent of all traumatic injuries in dogs and approximately 35 per cent in cats involved the head. Of the total number of injuries, 10 per cent were severe and 10 per cent life-threatening (Kolata et al., 1974). The bony skull and spinal fluid afford the central nervous system (CNS) considerable protection from injury. For this reason, trauma that causes CNS injury is usually major and clearly identifiable, either historically or on physical examination.

Head injuries may cause neurologic signs by damaging the peripheral nervous system (PNS), the CNS, or both. Although the signs of PNS injury are often permanent, they are rarely life-threatening. CNS injury often is life-threatening but causes fewer long-term deficits. The diagnostic approach to both types of injury is the same, but the therapeutic approach differs.

GOALS OF THERAPY

The principal goals of therapy in head injury are to reduce tissue swelling, decrease intracranial pressure, and maintain vascular perfusion and thus oxygenation. Achieving these goals serves to preserve the greatest amount of functional tissue. Regardless of therapy, a certain amount of neural tissue will be irreparably injured at the time of trauma. The clinician cannot reverse this initial damage but can attempt to prevent its progression (Averill, 1981; Cooper, 1979; Jennett and Teasdale, 1981).

To improve the survival rate in head trauma as well as the quality of survival, the clinician must rapidly classify the location, extent, and severity of the injury. This allows the prompt establishment of appropriate therapy.

PATIENT APPROACH

The history of trauma to the nervous system usually indicates an acute injury. The signs usually reach their maximum severity within hours of the accident, and, if the injury is not fatal, they are followed by a period of stabilization and resolution.

The first step in evaluating the patient is to diagnose and correct life-threatening non-neural injuries. Shock, and its associated hypotension, can cause CNS hypoxia and brain edema. CNS hypoxia may be potentiated by severe pneumothorax or traumatic cardiac arrhythmia if these injuries are not fatal in themselves. When instituting fluid therapy for shock, one should be aware that the blood-brain barrier will not be intact in the patient with CNS disease. In this situation, the massive volumes of fluid required for treatment of shock may aggravate cerebral swelling and attendant neurologic signs. After ensuring an airway, stabilizing cardiac output, and controlling any life-threatening hemorrhage, the veterinarian should begin the neurologic evaluation.

The neurologic history should include not only the trauma but also other major concurrent metabolic or neurologic disease. A patient with preexisting neurologic disease such as epilepsy may display abnormalities not related to the head injury. Animals with severe metabolic diseases such as diabetes will be more difficult to treat if their underlying disease is not recognized.

The neurologic examination should be rapid and complete: the level of consciousness, pupil size and symmetry, eye movements, and spinal reflexes are emphasized. The injury should be localized and classified as either CNS or PNS and as diffuse or focal.

CLASSIFICATION OF INJURY

The neurologic examination is the first step in differentiating a CNS injury from a PNS injury. The CNS above the foramen magnum consists of three parts: cerebrum, cerebellum, and brain stem. Each of these parts serves some separate or unique function, and each has some function in association with other parts of the CNS (Fig. 1). Thus, an injury to any portion of the CNS can cause varying degrees of weakness (paresis) or loss of coordination (ataxia) in one or more limbs. In addition, an injury to either the cerebrum or brain stem can cause increased tone and abnormal (increased) reflexes in the limbs. These reflex changes reflect the loss of upper motor neuronal influence over the limbs.

The changes in the unique (localizing) function in combination with the reflex changes allow the clinician to decide which portion of the CNS is affected. The cerebral functions are those of intellect and vision. The unique signs of cerebral disease include epilepsy and visual, behavioral, and mental changes. Brain stem function can be thought of as controlling the "head" and vegetative body functions. Dysfunction of the brain stem will be seen as paralysis of cranial nerves, loss of balance, loss of consciousness, and cardiac and respiratory abnormalities. The cerebellum serves to coordinate motor movements. Cerebellar injury may cause ataxia of the head and body.

In contrast to CNS injury, which causes limb signs and evidence of brain dysfunction, PNS injuries usually cause signs limited to the areas innervated by the damaged cranial nerve (CN). An exception to this is the vestibular nerve (CN VIII), which is responsible for maintaining balance. Damage to this nerve may cause ataxia, circling, falling, and disorientation. Injury to the peripheral portion of CN VIII is common and is often mistaken for injury to the CNS. The facts that other cranial nerves are not involved, that limb reflexes are normal, and that consciousness is preserved all suggest peripheral nerve injury. A review of the neurologic examination can be found in textbooks of veterinary neurology (de Lahunta, 1983; Hoerlein, 1980; Palmer, 1977).

TREATMENT OF PNS INJURIES

After the injury is localized, therapy can be instituted. In injuries of the PNS that do not involve the vestibular nerve, treatment is usually not required. A careful examination should be performed for skull fractures that may have entrapped or severed a peripheral nerve. If these are found, surgical correction of the fracture may result in return of function to the injured nerve. There may be a concomitant loss of lacrimation in animals with

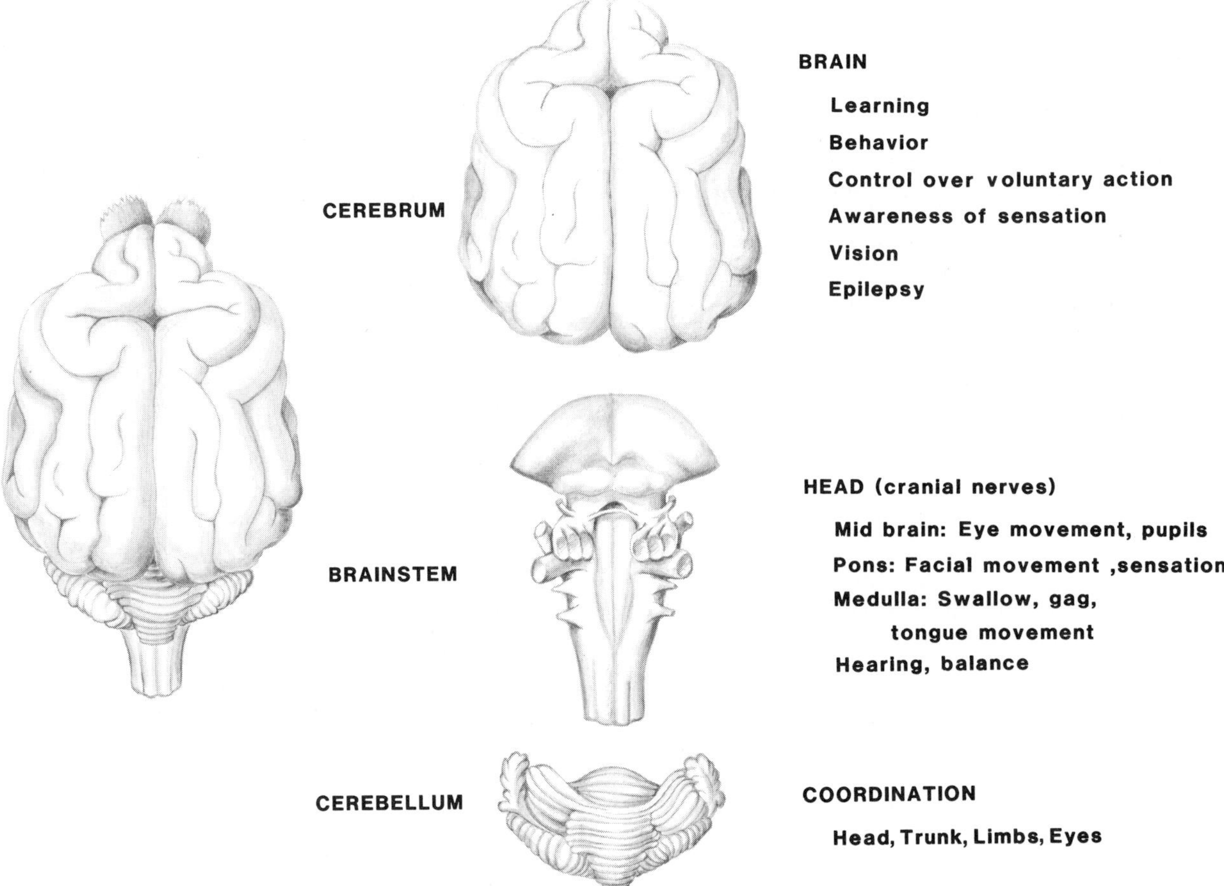

Figure 1. Summary of functions associated with major anatomic levels. (Adapted from Daube: *Medical Neurosciences.* Boston: Little, Brown and Co., 1978.)

facial paralysis. Tear production should be evaluated by a Schirmer tear test. If lacrimation is inadequate, the cornea should be moistened at frequent intervals with artificial tears.

Animals with peripheral vestibular disease may injure themselves further because their disorientation causes them to roll and thrash about violently. These animals may require mild sedation or light restraint to prevent additional injury. If physical restraint is used, body temperature should be monitored frequently, because these animals may become hyperthermic while struggling to free themselves.

Vestibular disorders usually appear worse than they actually are, and the tendency is to overtreat a benign PNS injury rather than perform a critical neurologic examination. Even with total destruction of the inner ear, signs begin to resolve in less than 2 weeks with or without treatment (Baloh and Honrubia, 1980). An otoscopic examination should be performed to detect hemotympanum.

In summary, peripheral nerve injuries are usually complete (total loss of function of the involved nerve), they rarely require treatment, and, with the exception of vestibular injuries, they rarely cause signs beyond focal loss of function.

EVALUATION OF CNS INJURIES

When a patient with CNS injury is evaluated, several steps should be taken rapidly. First, the skull should be palpated for fractures. If skull fractures are present and fragments are depressed into the cranial vault, they may compound the injury. Depressed fractures should be elevated as soon as the animal's condition is stable. Second, a record should be made of the animal's level of consciousness, pupil size and symmetry, pupillary responsiveness, and presence or absence of physiologic nystagmus (doll's eye maneuver). These tests aid in differentiating animals with cerebral and brain stem injury. Brain stem injury carries a grave prognosis. An animal with such an injury is more likely to have permanent sequelae and is least likely to be responsive to therapy.

The level of consciousness may be abnormal in one of two ways (Fig. 2). The animal may have an

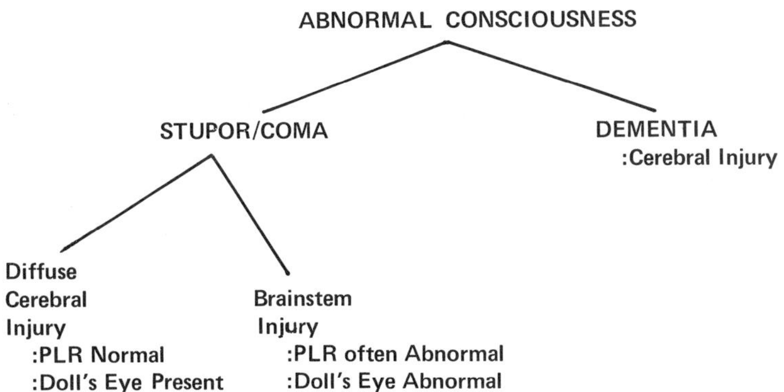

Figure 2. Two ways in which the level of consciousness may be abnormal.

abnormal *content* of consciousness (i.e., it appears to be awake but does not respond properly to its environment). In this case, cerebral injury should be suspected. If the animal has an abnormal *level* of consciousness such as stupor or coma, either generalized cerebral injury or brain stem injury should be suspected. A change in the level of consciousness during the observation period is more significant than the level of any one time. In humans, 50 per cent of head injury patients with coma die. If coma persists beyond six hours, mortality increases. The anatomic site of the lesion causing coma is also important, because 85 to 95 per cent of humans with coma and signs related to brain stem injury will die (Plum and Posner, 1980). The author's experience with dogs parallels the observations in humans that patients with cerebral injuries respond more favorably than those with brain stem injuries.

Abnormal pupil size may be seen with either cerebral or brain stem injury. The animal with cerebral injury will have abnormally small pupils that are responsive to light and will still display physiologic nystagmus (Fig. 3). The animal with brain stem injury may have abnormally large or abnormally small pupils. If the injury is in the midbrain, the pupils will be abnormally large and nonresponsive to light and physiologic nystagmus will be absent. If the injury is in the pons, the pupils will be abnormally small (pinpoint) and poorly responsive or nonresponsive to light and physiologic nystagmus will be absent. Recent reports indicate that certain cerebellar injuries also may cause abnormal pupil size. The animals with cerebral or brain stem injury and abnormal pupil size that the author has seen have also had an abnormal level of consciousness. This would not be expected with cerebellar injury. Therefore, if the animal has abnormal pupil size, normal consciousness, and normal physiologic nystagmus, cerebellar injury (or a peripheral nerve injury) should be suspected.

When evaluating animals with abnormal pupil size, the veterinarian should remember that ocular injury may be responsible. Careful examination of the globe should reveal the injury. Animals may also suffer injury to the optic nerve. If both optic nerves are involved, the pupils will be abnormally large and nonresponsive to light, but normal physiologic nystagmus should be present.

The animal's posture and response to external stimuli should be recorded. Animals with lesions of the rostral brain stem (midbrain) may have spasms of decerebrate posturing, which look very similar to the opisthotonic posture of cerebellar injury. The presence of coma or stupor serves to identify the behavior as decerebrate posturing, as opposed to the opisthotonos of cerebellar disease. Decerebrate posturing is more commonly episodic than constant and is induced by noxious stimuli. It is a poor prognostic sign in an otherwise stable patient.

Examination of the spinal reflexes helps to confirm the presence of a lesion involving the CNS and may show that the animal has spinal as well as intracranial injury. This combination of injuries is rare in the author's experience, but when it does occur the spinal injury is treated. Later, when the patient remains nonambulatory after apparent improvement of the head injury, a complete neurologic examination is performed and the second lesion is localized.

TREATMENT OF INTRACRANIAL INJURY

After the animal's injury to the cerebrum, brain stem, or cerebellum is localized, therapy should be instituted (Fig. 4).

In treating injuries of the CNS, an attempt is made to decrease both the size of any intracranial masses and the metabolic needs of the CNS and to provide oxygen and glucose for the metabolic needs that remain.

As a rule, the author hospitalizes and observes

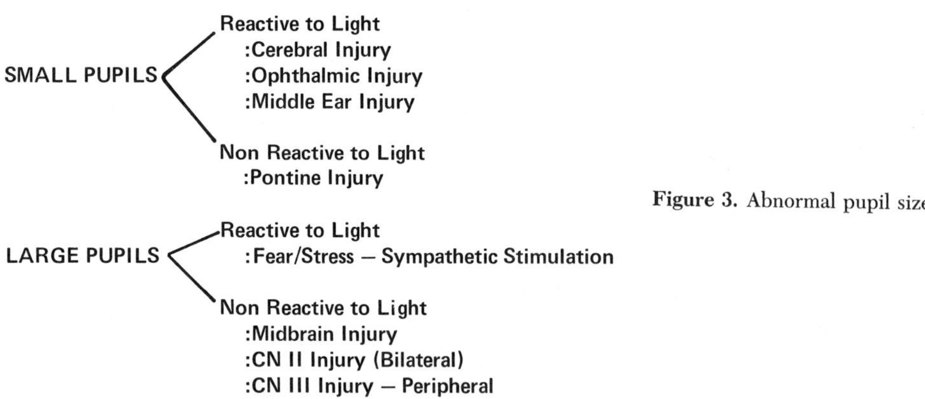

Figure 3. Abnormal pupil size.

for at least 24 hours any traumatized animal with either historic or clinical evidence of neurologic dysfunction. The first line of treatment in intracranial injury is corticosteroids. Although there is no standard dosage for corticosteroids in head trauma, the author uses a dosage of dexamethasone 0.2 mg/kg of body weight given as a bolus, followed by the same amount on a daily basis in two or three divided doses. This dosage is lower than those recommended by others, and dosages as high as 2.0 mg/kg of body weight four times per day for 1 to 3 days have been suggested (Kirk and Bistner, 1985). The author uses the lower dosage in the absence of shock. If the animal is in shock, a dosage of 2.0 mg/kg of body weight is given as the initial bolus.

The animal is then placed in 40 per cent oxygen with its head elevated, and it is observed and evaluated. If necessary, the animal is carefully re-

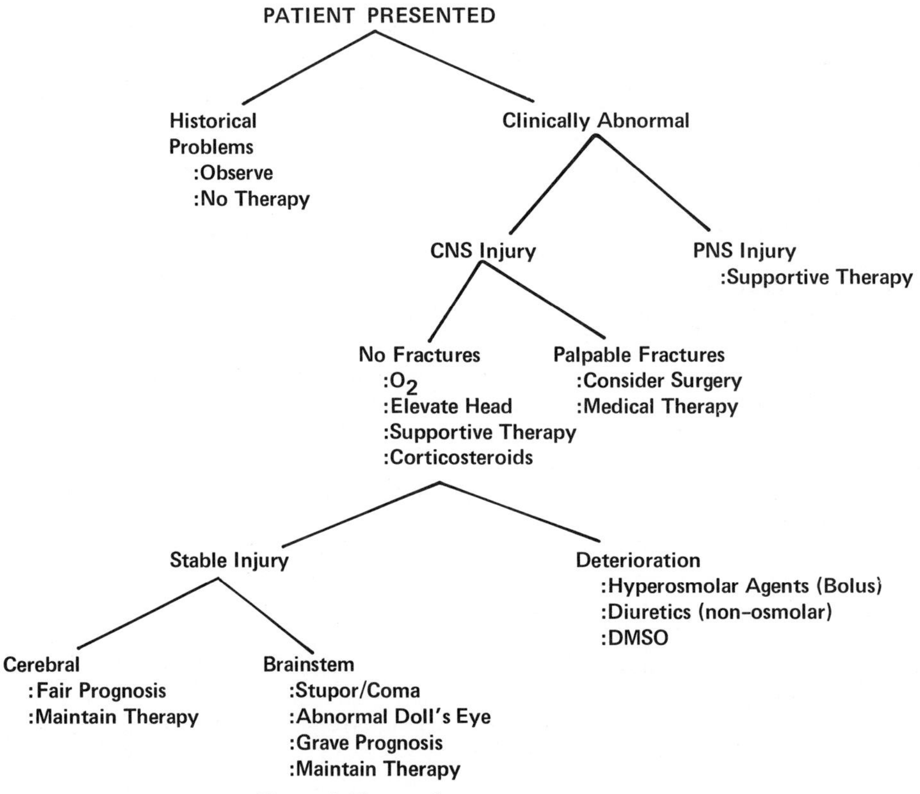

Figure 4. Therapy for intracranial injury.

strained to prevent further self-injury; sedative drugs are avoided. Supportive fluid therapy is provided if warranted by the animal's clinical condition. The head is elevated to improve venous drainage, thereby decreasing the size of the vascular component of intracranial contents. The enriched oxygen atmosphere is used because hypoxia potentiates CNS edema (Jennett and Teasdale, 1981).

Hypercarbia causes vasodilatation and a decrease in cerebral perfusion pressure, which increases edema and intracranial pressure. A decrease in consciousness often causes decreased ventilation. Although maintenance of airways is often difficult in small animals, the high oxygen atmosphere may help prevent hypercarbia.

Although steroids have not been clearly demonstrated to be beneficial experimentally, they are routinely used because of the clinical impression that they are efficacious. Large volumes of fluids are not administered to the animal with head trauma unless shock is present. Fluids are given judiciously to prevent extravasation of excess fluid across an already damaged blood-brain barrier, which may worsen cerebral edema.

Although the use of hyperosmolar agents has been advocated, the author rarely uses them except in animals that are *in extremis* or in those that display rapid deterioration. The animal with intracranial injury may have an altered blood-brain barrier, and hyperosmolar agents can leak across this barrier into the damaged neural parenchyma. Fluid will follow the hyperosmolar agent into the central nervous system rather than be removed from it into the vascular compartment. In addition, there is evidence that hyperosmolar agents are effective only in acute states and should be used only once rather than on a repeated basis (Fishman, 1980; Sklar, 1979).

If the animal has seizures, the author administers diazepam (Valium, Roche) intravenously at 0.25 to 0.50 mg/kg of body weight as needed. If diazepam is ineffective, phenobarbital is used to effect. Oral maintenance therapy with phenytoin (Dilantin, Parke-Davis) 30 mg/kg three times daily is used in animals weighing less than 10 kg. In animals over 10 kg, phenobarbital (1 to 2 mg/kg twice daily) is used for oral therapy. Although phenytoin is less sedative than barbiturates, its short half-life and poor absorption necessitate dosage that is prohibitively costly in animals over 10 kg.

At this point, initial therapy is complete. The patient is re-evaluated on an hourly basis. If the animal shows deterioration despite therapy, hyperosmolar agents may be used. Mannitol is given once only at a minimum dosage of 1.5 gm/kg body weight. Other drugs that may be tried are acetazolamide (Diamox, Lederle) and furosemide (Lasix, Hoechst). Although they act by different mechanisms, both are believed to decrease the production of cerebrospinal fluid and may lower intracranial pressure. Lowering intracranial pressure would facilitate resolution of edema. The use of dimethyl sulfoxide (DMSO) intravenously in conjunction with corticosteroids has been advocated, although the author has not used this drug.

Signs of deterioration include a decline in the level of consciousness, development of bradycardia, loss of physiologic nystagmus, and loss of pupillary responsiveness to light. An animal that is recumbent owing to cerebral or brain stem injury may develop ataxia and other signs of cerebellar disease as it improves and begins to walk. This is an unmasking of a previous injury and not a sign of deterioration.

In the author's experience, exploratory craniotomies in animals with head trauma are rarely required. If there is no objective surgical lesion (e.g., fracture), surgery is not indicated.

The objectives of treatment of intracranial injury are alleviation of brain edema and prevention of deterioration. A certain amount of irreversible injury that is present cannot be treated and may result in sequelae.

The sequelae of head trauma include neurogenic pulmonary edema, permanent neurologic deficits, epilepsy, and internal hydrocephalus. Permanent neurologic deficits may be central or peripheral in nature. Peripheral nerve injuries are usually focal and are rarely debilitating. Sequelae to central nervous system injuries include marked personality changes, visual deficits, circling, weakness in one or more limbs, and other deficits that may make the animal an unacceptable pet. On the initial neurologic examination it is impossible to determine whether an animal will have residual sequelae. The animal with brain-stem injury is more likely to have permanent deficits than is the animal with cerebral injury. Animals with cerebellar injury are likely to recover completely.

The onset of epilepsy may be at the time of head trauma or may be delayed for hours, days, or weeks. In most cases, post-traumatic epilepsy begins within 1 week of injury. Delayed post-traumatic epilepsy is relatively easy to manage and does not usually require special therapy. Hydrocephalus as a sequela to head trauma is a reported phenomenon that the author has rarely seen. It is reported to cause a rapidly progressive decline in the level of consciousness days or weeks after the animal appears to have recovered from head injury. The prognosis in these animals is considered to be grave.

In summary, the treatment of head trauma consists of preventing further injury and administering corticosteroids, enriched oxygen mixtures, and supportive care. The prognosis is largely determined by the site of injury, and animals with PNS injuries tend to have good prognoses. Animals with CNS injuries can be divided into three categories. Animals with cerebellar injuries have a good prognosis, those with cerebral injury have a guarded to fair prognosis, and those with brain stem injuries have a grave prognosis.

References and Supplemental Reading

Averill, D. R.: Brain injury. *In* Bojrab, M. (ed): *Pathophysiology in Small Animal Surgery.* Philadelphia: Lea & Febiger, 1981, pp. 218–219.

Baloh, R. W., and Honrubia, V.: *Clinical Neurophysiology of the Vestibular System, Contemporary Neurology Series.* Vol. 18. Philadelphia: F. A. Davis, 1980.

Cooper, P. R.: The treatment of head injury. *In* Rosenberg, R. (ed.): *The Treatment of Neurological Diseases.* New York: Spectrum Publications, 1979.

de Lahunta, A.: *Veterinary Neuroanatomy and Clinical Neurology,* 2nd ed. Philadelphia: W.B. Saunders, 1983.

Fenner, W. R.: Seizures and head trauma. Vet. Clin. North Am. 11:31, 1981.

Fishman, R. A.: *Cerebrospinal Fluid in Diseases of the Nervous System.* Philadelphia: W.B. Saunders, 1980.

Hoerlein, B. F.: *Canine Neurology,* 3rd ed. Philadelphia: W.B. Saunders, 1978.

Jennett, B., and Teasdale, G.: Management of Head Injuries. Philadelphia: F. A. Davis, 1981.

Kirk, R. W., and Bistner, S: *Handbook of Veterinary Procedures and Emergency Treatment,* 4th ed. Philadelphia: W.B. Saunders, 1985.

Kolata, R. J., Kraut, N. H., and Johnston, D. L.: Patterns of trauma in urban dogs and cats: A study of 1000 cases. J.A.V.M.A. 164:499, 1974.

Palmer, A. C.: *Introduction to Animal Neurology,* London: Blackwell Scientific Publications, 1977.

Plum, F., and Posner, J. B.: *The Diagnosis of Stupor and Coma,* 3rd ed., *Contemporary Neurology Series,* Vol. 19. Philadelphia: F. A. Davis, 1980.

Sklar, F. H.: Treatment of increased intracranial pressure. *In* Rosenberg, R. (ed.): *The Treatment of Neurological Diseases.* New York: Spectrum Publications, 1979.

Snyder, B. D., Lloyd, J. C., Cleeremans, B., et al.: Mannitol pharmacokinetics and serum osmolality in dogs and humans. Ann. Neurol. 14:183, 1983.

ANTICONVULSANT DRUG THERAPY IN COMPANION ANIMALS

SUSAN E. BUNCH, D.V.M.

Raleigh, North Carolina

INTRODUCTION

Incidence of Seizure Disorders

The seizure disorder is a common clinical problem requiring chronic medical management in small animals. Published epidemiologic reports in humans indicate an incidence of 0.5 to 1.0 per cent. The only comparable veterinary data available were collected in one study that showed that seizure disorders made up 1 per cent of all canine illnesses diagnosed at a veterinary teaching hospital. A retrospective evaluation of canine and feline hospital records over a six-year period at the New York State College of Veterinary Medicine (NYSCVM) revealed an incidence of 2.3 per cent of all sick dogs examined and 1 per cent of all sick cats examined, suggesting that seizures are more common in dogs than in cats.

Definitions of Seizures and Seizure Phases

Seizures are the clinical manifestation of a paroxysmal cerebral disorder. They may represent a systemic illness that causes central nervous system (CNS) dysfunction or a primary intracranial disease. In either case, the fundamental event is a disturbance in the excitability of the CNS that results in a focus of excessive neuronal discharge. It is important to note that even normal nervous tissue can be made hyperexcitable under appropriate conditions. If the stimulus is sufficient, the seizure threshold is exceeded, and normal inhibitory mechanisms fail; this abnormal discharge is allowed to spread, resulting in a seizure. When seizures become recurrent and are associated with nonprogressive intracranial disease that may be inherited or acquired, the term *epilepsy* may be used.

The two basic categories of seizures are focal, or partial, and generalized. *Focal seizures* are caused by a localized area of neuronal dysfunction that results in clinical signs compatible with the area of involvement in the brain and are usually acquired. The prototype of focal seizures in humans is the scar left by trauma to the head that remains as an irritable focus. Examples in dogs include psychomotor seizures characterized by marked changes in behavior or hallucinations ("fly biting"). Frequently, seizures may begin as partial seizures and develop into generalized seizures by a process termed *secondary generalization.*

Generalized seizures begin abruptly, are distinguished by the absence of localizing signs, and are usually accompanied by interruptions in consciousness. Generalized seizures may be classified by the presence of violent muscular activity, *grand mal seizures*, or the absence of such activity, *petit mal seizures.* Most seizures observed in small animals are of the grand mal type. Although true petit mal seizures probably occur in small animals, documentation has been difficult because the more common focal motor seizure is frequently misinterpreted as a petit mal seizure.

The mechanisms involved in the initiation, spread, and termination of a seizure discharge are not clearly understood, although considerable advancements in the comprehension of these events have been made in recent years. Currently under investigation are factors such as the role of neurotransmitter metabolism, the contribution of CNS inhibitory substances such as gamma aminobutyric acid, and changes in neuronal cell membrane physiology. The importance of these studies lies not only in clarification of the pathogenesis of seizures but also in the pharmacology of the therapeutic agents selected to control them.

The actual seizure (ictus) is preceded by an aural or *preictal phase* commonly characterized by behavioral changes and autonomic signs that may last minutes to days. The next phase, the *seizure* itself, usually lasts one to two minutes unless *status epilepticus* is developing. Finally, the *postictal phase* may be very short, with immediate return to normalcy, or may last for hours, during which behavioral changes, disorientation, and temporary blindness are typical. The description and duration of the seizure phases may be useful in localizing the excitable focus, especially in partial seizure disorders. They do not, however, provide information as to the exact cause or severity of the seizure disorder nor do they influence the therapeutic approach.

Causes of Seizures

The causes of seizures have been addressed in previous publications and will not be considered in depth here. Intracranial causes include various infections (canine distemper, feline infectious peritonitis, blastomycosis, toxoplasmosis, cryptococcosis), head trauma, developmental abnormalities (hydrocephalus, lissencephaly), lysosomal storage diseases, neoplasia (primary or metastatic), inflammatory conditions (parasitic migration, reticulosis), vascular impairment (feline ischemic encephalopathy), genetic predisposition (German shepherd, beagle, Belgian tervueren, keeshond, collie, and poodle, with Irish setter, Saint Bernard breeds suspected), and idiopathic epilepsy. Systemic illnesses that may have central nervous system sequelae include hypocalcemia, hypoglycemia, cardiopulmonary insufficiency, thiamine deficiency, intoxication (lead, strychnine, organophosphates), uremia, hepatic encephalopathy, hyperlipidemia, hyperviscosity syndrome, and heat stroke.

Diagnosis

The diagnostic approach to a patient presented for evaluation of a seizure disorder consists of a careful analysis of the history of the patient, a physical examination, a neurologic examination, clinical laboratory analyses, and radiography.

HISTORY. The attending veterinarian must rely on the owner's description to differentiate seizures from other episodic syndromes such as syncope, cataplexy, myasthenia gravis, or polymyositis. Once it has been established that a seizure actually occurred, specific attention is given to elements of the history that would contribute to the differential diagnosis. The age of the patient is valuable, since inherited or congenital seizures usually begin at less than three years of age. Geriatric patients with seizures beginning late in life, especially with localizing neurologic signs, are most likely to have a space-occupying lesion in the CNS. Since certain breeds are predisposed to particular CNS diseases, breed information is useful also. Background history should include vaccinations received, illnesses unrelated to the current complaint of seizures such as difficult delivery as a puppy or head trauma, evidence of infectious disease, and information regarding the state of health of littermates, parents, and other animals at home. Information about environmental conditions is essential in determining whether there has been exposure to toxins or contagious agents endemic to specific geographic locations. A detailed account of all phases of the seizure is needed to classify the seizure as focal or generalized and to determine what conditions, if any, might be considered provocative. For example, cats with thiamine deficiency may show seizures with handling. Equally important is knowledge of the interictal period. Patients genetically predisposed to seizures appear healthy between episodes, whereas those with structural lesions of the CNS are likely to have clinical signs of illness between seizures.

PHYSICAL EXAMINATION. A careful physical examination may reveal the presence of systemic infection, cardiac irregularities, respiratory inadequacy, external trauma, or perhaps tumors. Although seizures can accompany advanced renal or hepatic disease, it is unlikely that they will be the sole presenting clinical sign. Ocular examination is also important, since fundic lesions are often associated with various systemic and intracranial disorders.

NEUROLOGIC EXAMINATION. A complete neurologic examination is valid only if performed during the interictal period. All aspects of the nervous system, including spinal reflexes, postural reactions, and cranial nerves, should be evaluated. If interictal neurologic signs are present, then there is structural brain disease. Single mass lesions such as a tumor or infarct produce specific localizing signs. Metabolic diseases may produce diffuse cerebral signs or no interictal signs. Abnormal findings in more than one part of the nervous system suggest multifocal involvement. A normal interictal neurologic examination supports a tentative diagnosis of *idiopathic epilepsy* or an episodic metabolic illness such as hypoglycemia. It is also possible that seizures may be the first sign of intracranial disease not yet associated with neurologic deficits. Regardless of the cause of seizures, serial neurologic examinations are invaluable in assessing the course of illness.

CLINICAL LABORATORY EVALUATION. Ideally, baseline laboratory data should be obtained for all seizure patients before therapy is instituted, not only for diagnostic purposes but to supply a reference point should problems develop in the future. Selection of laboratory tests should be guided by evaluation of information gained from the history and the results of physical and neurologic examinations. Clinical laboratory evaluation may include a hemogram to determine whether *lead intoxication* (large numbers of nucleated red blood cells, basophilic stippling) or *systemic infection* (leukocytosis or leukopenia, depending on the offending organism) is present, a chemistry profile to assess *liver and kidney function*, urinalysis, and, in selected cases, a 30-minute BSP per cent retention test and a determination of plasma ammonia concentration.

Whole blood, obtained after at least a 12-hour fast and preserved in sodium fluoride, is preferred for accurate determination of glucose concentration. *Hypocalcemia* of sufficient magnitude to cause seizures is usually detectable by routine serum analysis. The persistence of conspicuous *lipemia* in a serum sample harvested more than 8 hours postprandially signifies altered lipid metabolism and may be related to metabolic diseases such as diabetes mellitus or may be without an identifiable cause. Idiopathic hyperlipidemia is occasionally associated with seizures in humans and in dogs. *Elevated serum proteins*, especially in the globulin fraction, are frequently seen with feline infectious peritonitis.

Cerebrospinal fluid (CSF) should be evaluated when empirical anticonvulsant therapy has not been successful, when abnormalities are detected in the neurologic examination, or when neoplasia, meningeal infection, encephalitis, or other intracranial disease is suspected. A complete evaluation of the CSF includes measurement of opening pressure and protein and cytologic examination. Culture and sensitivity tests are performed when there are more than 5 white blood cells per microliter or when the predominant cell is the polymorphonuclear cell. Antibody titers to canine distemper, feline infectious peritonitis, and toxoplasmosis may indicate active infection. Additional analyses may be performed in selected cases but are not considered routine (glucose concentration, enzyme activities, Pándy's test).

RADIOGRAPHY. Radiographs of the skull generally are helpful only in cases of head trauma or intracranial neoplasia. Fractures or superficial tumors that may be treated surgically are rarely identified. Most patients with seizure disorders have normal survey radiographs of the skull. Contrast procedures using a positive or negative medium may outline the dilated ventricles of hydrocephalus. Angiography may reveal abnormal vascular patterns in neoplasms, hematomas, and infarctions, but it is not used routinely. Survey thoracic radiographs may occasionally disclose evidence of primary or metastatic neoplasia that may be related to CNS neoplasia.

For selected cases and usually only at referral institutions where specialized equipment is available, electroencephalography, scintigraphy, and computed tomography may confirm a working diagnosis. Each procedure is relatively safe and noninvasive.

This introduction represents only an overview of the information available on seizure disorders in companion animals. Thorough reports of the pathophysiology, description, and diagnosis of seizures have been published previously, and readers are encouraged to consult the references listed at the end of this article.

CHRONIC MEDICAL THERAPY OF SEIZURE DISORDERS

Indications for Therapy

If specifically treatable intra- or extracranial diseases have been ruled out during the diagnostic evaluation, one must assume that a nonprogressive seizure disorder exists. The remaining discussion will pertain only to canine and feline patients with a seizure disorder of this type.

The many factors influencing the decision to begin therapy can be placed in two groups: patient factors and client factors. Patient factors are as follows.

SEIZURE FREQUENCY. It is not necessary to begin anticonvulsant therapy in a young patient that has experienced only one seizure. Rather, a pattern of repetitive seizures must exist before a long-term commitment to therapy is made. Patients with seizures that occur more than once monthly or patients that have clusters of seizures are candidates for extended therapy.

CHARACTER OF THE VARIOUS SEIZURE PHASES. If the seizures are particularly objectionable, such as psychomotor seizures during which the patient becomes vicious, or if the pre- and postictal phases are characterized by intolerable changes in excretory habits, then control of the episodes must be attempted.

Perhaps more important than the patient factors are the client factors. The owners must be informed of all the ramifications of seizure disorders and continued anticonvulsant therapy. Frequently, owners interpret anticonvulsant therapy as curative. The definition of successful management of most veterinary patients is a reduction in the severity, frequency, and, possibly, duration of seizures. Although most patients will improve with drug therapy, 20 to 30 per cent will never be controlled despite intensive medical treatment. Each patient must be treated individually, and many medication changes may be required to reach optimal control. If high dosages of drugs are required, the risk of developing drug-induced complications increases and must be weighed against the benefits of therapy. The veterinarian must explain to the client that once therapy has begun, the prescribed dosage schedule must be followed *exactly*, usually for the life of the patient. The client must understand that the drugs most commonly used must be given two to three times every day, regardless of the inconvenience. Moreover, the cost of the drugs can be considerable. Polydipsia, polyuria, and sometimes polyphagia and weight gain are expected side effects of all the commonly used anticonvulsant drugs. With barbiturate derivatives, personality changes are common. These considerations must be made clear to the owner before therapy, so that maximal owner compliance can be achieved.

Primary Anticonvulsant Drugs

In keeping with the goal of anticonvulsant therapy, the perfect drug should control seizures without toxic effects. Many drugs are available to treat the large variety of seizure disorders that occur in humans. Because a vast majority of seizures seen in companion animals are of the generalized, grand mal type, the drugs found efficacious for these seizures in humans are the most commonly used anticonvulsant drugs in animals. The recommended dose ranges for dogs and cats and the desirable serum concentrations are listed in Table 1.

PHENOBARBITAL

Phenobarbital (Luminal, Winthrop) was the first barbiturate derivative approved for anticonvulsant use in humans. It has been found effective for generalized grand mal seizures as well as simple partial seizures. It acts by raising the threshold of electrical excitability and shortening the duration of afterdischarges in the motor cortex. Thus, the overall effect is to suppress the spontaneous electrical discharges and, to a limited extent, prevent their spread to other areas of the brain. It is interesting to note that phenobarbital is the most effective of the primary anticonvulsants in delaying the progressive intensification of seizure activity known as "kindling." Experimental evidence suggests that repeated application of certain drugs or an electrical stimulus to the cerebral cortex induces changes in excitability that facilitate the development of recurrent seizures. This implies that the probability of establishing repetitive seizures increases with each episode. It is not known with certainty whether "kindling" occurs in spontaneous seizure disorders; however, human patients seem to be more effectively controlled when anticonvulsant therapy is started early.

Biotransformation of phenobarbital to inactive metabolites that are excreted in the urine takes place in the microsomal enzyme fraction of the liver. The elimination half-life has been found to be 36 to 46 hours in the dog; data are not available for the cat. With continued oral administration of phenobarbital, effective steady-state serum and tissue concentrations are achieved only after 7 days. As a result, there is a lag period during which there is limited anticonvulsant efficacy. To expedite therapeutic effect, the recommended dosages of 5 to 16 mg/kg/day for the dog and 2.2 to 4.4 mg/kg/day for the cat divided twice or three times daily may be doubled for the first 4 days. Unfortunately, the anticipated side effects of sedation, ataxia, polydipsia, and polyuria may be especially marked during the loading period, making this practice undesirable. These side effects generally diminish with time even during continued administration.

Despite the long-standing availability of phenobarbital, little is known about its metabolic effects. Although it is a controlled substance, it is a safe, inexpensive, effective anticonvulsant for dogs and is *the* drug of choice in cats. The author does not believe that the controlled drug classification of phenobarbital should discourage its use as the first drug chosen for a seizure-control regimen.

PRIMIDONE

Primidone (Mylepsin, Fort Dodge) is a desoxybarbiturate that is metabolized by the microsomal

Table 1. *Drugs, Dosages (Canine and Feline), and Therapeutic Serum Concentrations (Canine) of Anticonvulsant Drugs*

Drug	Dose Range Dog	Dose Range Cat	Therapeutic Serum Concentration (μg/ml)
Phenobarbital	5–16 mg/kg/day divided b.i.d. or t.i.d.	2.2–4.4 mg/kg/day divided b.i.d. or t.i.d.	15–45
Primidone*	15–80 mg/kg/day divided b.i.d.	—	15–45 (phenobarbital metabolite)
Phenytoin†	20–35 mg/kg t.i.d.	2–3 mg/kg/day; 20 mg/kg/week	10–20§
Carbamazepine‡	4–8 mg/kg b.i.d.	—	5–10§
Valproic acid‡	75–200 mg/kg t.i.d.	—	50–100§
Diazepam	5–15 mg t.i.d.	2.5–5.0 mg t.i.d.	—

*Not approved for use in cats.
†Neither approved nor recommended for use in cats (see text).
‡Not approved for use in dogs or cats.
§Serum concentrations considered therapeutic in humans.

enzyme fraction of the liver to phenobarbital and phenylethylmalonamide (PEMA). All three components have inherent anticonvulsant activity and contribute to the efficacy of the drug. With repeated dosing, the phenobarbital fraction accumulates and the remaining fractions do not. It is likely that phenobarbital is responsible for most of the anticonvulsant activity of primidone. Like phenobarbital, primidone generally causes polydipsia, polyuria, and polyphagia and may cause personality changes in certain patients.

Primidone is approved for use only in dogs. It is not a controlled substance but is five to ten times more expensive than phenobarbital at beginning recommended dosages (15 mg/kg divided twice daily).

PHENYTOIN

Of the three primary anticonvulsant drugs traditionally used in veterinary medicine, phenytoin (Dilantin, Parke-Davis) has received the most attention recently because of several interesting experimental studies. In humans, phenytoin is degraded to parahydroxy metabolites and has a half-life of 22 hours. By contrast, in dogs phenytoin is rapidly transformed to primarily a metahydroxy metabolite and has a half-life of 4 hours. The biotransformational reactions take place in the microsomal enzyme fraction of the liver in both species. Phenytoin stimulates its own degradation in the dog, a process that occurs in humans only at high dosages. It is possible that the metahydroxylation step in dogs occurs more rapidly than the parahydroxylation step in humans, which may also contribute to the difference in phenytoin half-life in the two species. Since brain concentrations of phenytoin are directly related to serum levels, phenytoin is of questionable efficacy as an anticonvulsant because serum levels cannot be maintained. To achieve and sustain effective blood levels of phenytoin in the dog based on human therapeutic ranges, 60 to 105 mg/kg/day must be given, which is greater than the starting dosage of 4 to 8 mg/kg/day suggested by the Food and Drug Administration. Unfortunately, studies to determine the dose and serum level of phenytoin necessary to protect against chemically or electrically induced seizures have not been done in the dog. Cardiac arrhythmias caused by digitalis intoxication in dogs can be suppressed with phenytoin at a serum concentration of 10 μg/ml. Whether a similar serum concentration would be effective in anticonvulsant therapy is not known. One study in dogs has been reported that correlated successful therapy using 6.6 to 11 mg/kg with serum concentrations of 1.5 to 3.0 μg/ml. Recently, another study of dogs with seizures receiving anticonvulsant drug therapy reported that of 77 dogs given phenytoin, only three were controlled, and two of the three dogs had also concurrently received phenobarbital.

Phenytoin acts by stabilizing neuronal membranes and subduing the spread of electrical activity from the seizure focus. There is a negligible effect on the focus itself. Although phenytoin has been in use for years, many clinicians consider it inadequate. Not until recently, however, were there experimental data to support these observations. Some individuals improve with phenytoin therapy, perhaps because of individual variation in biotransformation of the drug. However, the author cannot recommend it as an effective anticonvulsant drug because of its short half-life and the unreasonable dosages required.

Pharmacokinetic studies of phenytoin in cats have revealed a plasma half-life that varies from 41.5

hours in kittens to a range of 24 to 108 hours in adult cats. Signs of toxicity developed with low daily doses of phenytoin and were associated with high plasma concentrations. Because of these findings, phenytoin is considered unsuitable as an anticonvulsant drug for cats unless it is given at 2 to 3 mg/kg/day or 20 mg/kg/week and suspended as soon as sedation, ataxia, or anorexia is noticed.

Miscellaneous Primary Anticonvulsant Drugs

PARAMETHADIONE

The main indication for use of paramethadione (Paradione, Abbott) in humans is petit mal seizures. The drug has also been found effective against experimentally induced seizures in dogs. For this reason, a preliminary study was designed in 1975 using canine seizure patients uncontrolled with conventional therapy and canine seizure patients not receiving drugs. Sixty-five per cent of the previously uncontrolled patients improved, and the response in the new patients was similar to that achieved with traditional anticonvulsants (70 per cent improvement). Paramethadione has not been stringently studied in dogs and cannot be recommended until more information is available.

CARBAMAZEPINE

Although carbamazepine (Tegretol, Geigy) is the first drug of choice for trigeminal neuralgia in humans, it has been found to be as effective as phenytoin in the treatment of grand mal seizures and psychomotor seizures. Both the parent drug and its main metabolite, carbamazepine-10,11-epoxide, have potent anticonvulsant activity. The half-life of the drug decreases from 35 hours to 10 to 20 hours with repetitive administration. The recommended starting dosage is 100 to 200 mg twice daily, but because there is marked tendency for the drug to stimulate its own degradation, the dosage must be increased to maintain optimal serum concentrations (see Table 1). The most common side effects are bone marrow depression and, occasionally, hepatitis. There is no sedative effect of carbamazepine, as there frequently is with phenobarbital and phenytoin in humans.

Recently, carbamazepine in both liquid and tablet forms has been evaluated in dogs. The liquid was absorbed rapidly, but serum concentrations were variable and declined rapidly (half-life of 1 to 2 hours). As in humans, dogs transform the parent drug to the epoxide metabolite, but serum levels of both compounds decrease considerably with repeated administration. Because of these characteristics carbamazepine has not been found to be suitable for extended anticonvulsant therapy in dogs.

Carbamazepine has not been evaluated in cats.

VALPROIC ACID

Over the past few years since its approval in 1978, valproic acid (VPA) (Depakene, Abbott) has shown considerable promise in the treatment of various types of human epilepsy. Pharmacologic characteristics of the drug in dogs are different from those in humans. The average half-life in dogs is 2.8 hours, and it does not change with prolonged treatment, in contrast to phenytoin. In addition to VPA, two metabolites found in the plasma of dogs have anticonvulsant activity. Moreover, there is less protein binding of VPA in dogs than in humans, which allows greater concentrations of the free, active drug to enter the CNS. These two factors suggest that lower dosages, and thus lower serum levels, might be sufficient to control seizures in dogs. However, because of its short half-life, VPA must be given either at very high dosages or very frequently to maintain a steady serum concentration.

In a recent clinical study of 57 canine seizure patients, VPA (30 to 40 mg/kg/day) was added to the existing therapy of phenytoin and phenobarbital or primidone or was given alone or in combination with phenobarbital. The most improvement was observed in dogs treated with a combination of VPA and phenobarbital. Serum concentrations were not evaluated, so conclusions about adequacy of the dosage cannot be made. On the basis of the canine pharmacology of VPA and the accepted human therapeutic serum ranges (see Table 1), the estimated dosage of VPA alone needed to achieve effective levels is 220 mg/kg three times daily. If the increased serum level of phenobarbital in the presence of VPA observed in humans occurs in dogs, then the improvement observed in the dogs treated at the lower dosage of VPA in the clinical study may be a result of this effect.

A distinct advantage of VPA as an anticonvulsant drug is that the half-life does not decrease with chronic administration. However, until more experimental work with VPA has been done in dogs, we can only speculate on the dosage, serum therapeutic ranges, efficacy, and long-term side effects.

The clinical usefulness of VPA in cats has not been investigated.

Combinations of Drugs

It is preferable to begin therapy with one drug, usually phenobarbital or primidone, and wait for three seizure cycles before the effectiveness of the treatment is assessed. If there has not been any improvement, the veterinarian should increase the dosage and wait. If there still is no improvement, the addition of other drugs should be considered. Doses should always begin at the lower end of the dose range, then be increased when necessary. Some patients cannot be controlled with one drug, and some respond to one drug and not another, even if they are of the same class of drugs and are given in adequate dosages.

The use of combination preparations such as Dilantin with phenobarbital or Mebroin (Winthtrop; 60 mg phenytoin plus 90 mg mephobarbital per tablet) is not advisable. Separate preparations allow each patient to be treated more accurately.

If there is a need to change therapy and a desire to withdraw a drug completely, the veterinarian should NOT make sudden changes. This is especially important when using the barbiturate derivatives, which cause habituation. When these drugs are stopped abruptly, seizures may become more severe and more difficult to control or may progress to *status epilepticus*. For safe withdrawal, the dosage should be reduced by 30 per cent every 7 days. This rule of thumb also applies to patients whose dosages are being reduced to the minimum maintenance level after a period of satisfactory control, usually 6 months to 1 year.

Summary

The two drugs that remain effective for seizures in dogs are phenobarbital and primidone. Recent experimental studies of phenytoin in both dogs and cats have shown it to be unsatisfactory for various pharmacologic reasons. The limited information available on newer drugs, such as carbamazepine and valproic acid, is an insufficient basis on which to make recommendations. Phenobarbital remains the drug of choice for seizure disorders of cats. Single agents are preferable, but combinations of drugs may be necessary.

Secondary or Adjunct Anticonvulsant Drugs

DIAZEPAM

If the preictal phase is sufficiently long and clearly demarcated, diazepam (Valium, Roche) can be used during that time in both dogs and cats to reduce the severity of the coming seizure. The usual starting dose is 2.5 to 15 mg three times daily. As a primary anticonvulsant, diazepam has not been useful because of expense, controlled drug classification, and short half-life. Its primary indication is in the treatment of *status epilepticus*, which will be discussed later.

Complications of Chronic Therapy

Much has been learned in recent years about the many adverse effects of chronic anticonvulsant therapy in humans. The factors that influence the development of these problems are duration of therapy; use of multiple drugs, perhaps at high dosages; and failure to recognize subtle evidence of intoxication.

Similar complications may occur in animals since the same anticonvulsant drugs are used in their treatment. However, animals seem to be remarkably resistant to most of the toxic effects seen in humans. For this reason, only the complications that have been reported or that the author has seen will be discussed. Adverse effects were not recognized in the few cats that underwent long-term anticonvulsant therapy examined at the NYSCVM, so the following discussion pertains only to dogs.

ENZYME INDUCTION

Phenobarbital, primidone, and phenytoin belong to the group of compounds capable of altering the activity of the metabolizing enzymes located in the smooth endoplasmic reticulum of the liver. The biotransformation of both endogenous and exogenous compounds can be accelerated by this process of *enzyme induction*. Substances given concurrently with anticonvulsants will be metabolized more rapidly, resulting in lower serum concentrations of the parent drug. Some drugs, including phenytoin and carbamazepine, given chronically will stimulate their own degradation as well. In addition, endogenous compounds such as cortisol are affected, leading to stimualtion of ACTH and adrenal hypertrophy. Enzyme induction has been implicated in the pathogenesis of such drug-induced complications as folate deficiency and metabolic bone disease in humans.

Membrane-bound enzymes other than drug-metabolizing enzymes can also be induced by the anticonvulsant drugs. The best example is alkaline phosphatase (AP) of hepatic origin. Elevated serum AP activity not related to hepatic injury can be expected within 1 month of anticonvulsant therapy. Because the AP isoenzyme induced by the anticonvulsants is the same as that associated with hepatic injury, it is difficult to distinguish the benign drug-induced effect from a more serious hepatotoxic reaction without the benefit of other tests of liver function.

When more than one anticonvulsant drug is used, drug interactions can be expected. Concurrent administration of phenytoin and a barbiturate derivative in humans results in lower serum concentrations of phenytoin and higher concentrations of phenobarbital than when either is administered alone. This does not appear to be of clinical significance. Similar studies have not been done in dogs, but the successful use of phenytoin-barbiturate combinations is probably attributable to the barbiturate contribution in most cases. In addition, as mentioned before, the metabolism of phenytoin is too rapid to be of long-term benefit, especially in the presence of a barbiturate.

The activity of drug-metabolizing enzymes can be inhibited by certain compounds. For example, administration of chloramphenicol in addition to phenytoin or phenobarbital results in accumulation of the anticonvulsant drug and clinical signs of toxicity (sedation, ataxia, prolonged anesthesia).

FOLATE DEFICIENCY

Megaloblastic anemia caused by folate deficiency is seen in 0.15 to 0.75 per cent of human seizure patients. It is most commonly associated with the administration of phenytoin and can occur at any time after initiation of therapy. Folate concentrations are classically subnormal in the serum, erythrocytes, and CSF. The condition can be reversed with folic acid supplementation, 1 to 2 mg/day. The author has observed megaloblastic anemia, leukopenia, and thrombocytopenia in dogs given phenytoin experimentally. Whether folate deficiency was causative, however, was not determined. Because seizures may be aggravated in some human patients given folic acid for megaloblastic anemia, folic acid must be used cautiously.

GINGIVAL HYPERPLASIA

The most common chronic toxic effect of phenytoin therapy in humans is gingival hyperplasia, occurring in as many as 50 per cent of treated patients. Periodontal disease or other diseases caused by poor oral hygiene aggravate the gingival hyperplasia. The hyperplasia will regress within 6 months if phenytoin is discontinued and secondary infection is controlled. Gingival hyperplasia was reported in a dog receiving twice daily 100 mg of phenytoin for 3 years. The author has not recognized this as a common complication caused by phenytoin in dogs.

HEPATOTOXICITY

Hepatic disease caused by anticonvulsant drug therapy in humans is most commonly associated with phenytoin. Phenytoin hepatotoxicity has been determined to be an idiosyncratic hypersensitivity reaction resulting in lesions varying from mild cholestatic hepatitis to massive hepatic necrosis. In a published review of 23 human cases, 17 (74 per cent) developed signs of hepatotoxicity within 6 weeks of starting therapy and nine (39 per cent) subsequently died.

Published reports of hepatic injury associated with anticonvulsant therapy in dogs are rare. Reports of single cases of toxic reactions caused by primidone and phenytoin suggest that these are idiosyncratic drug reactions. Cirrhosis of the liver was diagnosed at the NYSCVM in five dogs that received primidone alone or in combination with other anticonvulsant drugs for 2 to 3 years. Increased activities of AP and alanine aminotransferase (ALT) and BSP retention may be observed in as many as 50 per cent of seizure patients receiving anticonvulsant therapy. This may represent a tolerable degree of hepatic injury. Severe hepatic disease, however, occurs much less frequently (estimated range 6 to 15 per cent).

Hepatic function should be evaluated before and every 6 months after starting anticonvulsant therapy. Any increase in serum gamma glutamyl transferase activity (GGT) (more than 2 to 4 IU/L), fasting bile acid retention (more than 10 μmol/L), BSP retention (more than 5 per cent at 30 minutes), or ammonia intolerance suggests hepatic dysfunction. When this occurs, the anticonvulsant drug dosages should be reduced to the minimum needed to control seizures. In the presence of liver dysfunction, the metabolism of the primary anticonvulsants may be delayed and toxicity could result if dosages are not decreased. More importantly, the drugs may be the cause of the liver disease, either directly or indirectly.

ACUTE MEDICAL THERAPY—STATUS EPILEPTICUS

Repeated seizures within a short period of time and without recovery constitute *status epilepticus*. The neuronal damage, hyperthermia, acidosis, and possible cardiac arrhythmias that occur during *status epilepticus* may cause death unless the seizures are stopped. Thus, *status epilepticus* is a true medical emergency.

The following diagnostic and therapeutic approach is recommended.

1. If there is not too much muscular activity, an indwelling intravenous catheter should be inserted, not only to administer medications but to draw blood samples for laboratory analysis. *If possible*, a blood sample should be collected for determination of glucose and calcium concentrations.

2. To stop the seizures, diazepam can be given at 5 to 20 mg intravenously, depending on the size of the patient. Slow test boluses of glucose and calcium gluconate may be given first to determine whether hypoglycemia or hypocalcemia is causative.

If not and if one bolus of diazepam is inadequate, the diazepam should be repeated every 10 minutes for three doses.

3. If diazepam is not sufficient, pentobarbital should be given slowly to effect. The onset of action of pentobarbital is faster than that of phenobarbital, although phenobarbital has more anticonvulsant activity.

4. The veterinarian should ensure a patent airway and use an endotracheal tube if necessary. Body temperature, acid-base balance, electrolyte status, fluid balance, and cardiovascular integrity should also be regulated.

5. Once the seizures are controlled, the remaining diagnostic tests may be pursued. No definitive judgments about neurologic status should be made until the patient is fully recovered, which may take days.

6. During recovery, phenobarbital may be given intramuscularly in low doses (0.5 mg/kg three times daily) to provide anticonvulsant effects. When the patient is able to swallow, oral phenobarbital can be given at the usual recommended dosages.

7. Occasional seizure activity during recovery is acceptable. The clinician should not attempt to stop it completely, because oversedation may be dangerous.

SUMMARY OF RECOMMENDATIONS

For chronic therapy of both canine and feline seizure patients, the veterinarian is given the following recommendations:

1. Start with phenobarbital at the low end of the recommended dose range. Measure serum concentrations 8 to 12 hours post dose at 2 weeks after treatment was initiated. If seizures are uncontrolled and serum concentrations are inadequate, increase the dosage of phenobarbital to achieve established therapeutic levels. If seizures continue despite adequate serum concentrations, consider reducing phenobarbital while simultaneously adding primidone (conversion rate: 250 mg primidone will provide serum phenobarbital levels similar to those for 65 mg phenobarbital).

2. Seizures will be controlled in most dogs with phenobarbital or primidone given at dosages guided by serum concentrations of phenobarbital. Occasionally, both barbiturates given in combination will be effective when each drug given singly was not. Seizure control correlates best with serum concentration of phenobarbital rather than with drug dosage.

3. Consider adding phenytoin only if phenobarbital and primidone have not been effective. Other, unapproved, drugs may be tried only with the informed consent of the owner.

4. After satisfactory control of seizures has been reached (reduction in frequency and severity of seizures for two to three seizure cycles), recheck the patient every 6 months to evaluate the drug regimen, the seizure history, hematologic values and, especially, hepatic function. After 6 to 12 months of *satisfactory* control an attempt can be made to gradually reduce the amount of drugs given.

5. Because most seizures in cats examined at the NYSCVM have been caused by organic diseases, there is little information available on prognosis and side effects of long-term therapy in cats with nonprogressive seizure disorders.

6. Euthanasia of the animal must remain as an option for owners who choose not to start or continue a lifelong commitment to a dog with seizures.

References and Supplemental Reading

Bunch, S. E., Baldwin, B. H., Hornbuckle, W. E., et al.: Compromised hepatic function in dogs treated with anticonvulsant drugs. J.A.V.M.A. 184:444, 1984.

Cunningham, J. G., Haidukewych, D., and Jensen, H. A.: Therapeutic serum concentrations of primidone and its metabolites, phenobarbital and phenylethylmalonamide in epileptic dogs. J.A.V.M.A. 182:1091, 1983.

Farnbach, G. C.: Serum concentrations and efficacy of phenytoin, phenobarbital, and primidone in canine epilepsy. J.A.V.M.A. 184:1117, 1984.

Greene, C. E., and Oliver, J. E.: Neurologic examination. *In* Ettinger, S. J. (ed.): *Textbook of Veterinary Internal Medicine*. Vol. 1. Philadelphia: W.B. Saunders, 1983, pp. 419–460.

Holliday, T. A.: Seizure disorders. Vet. Clin. North Am. 10:3, 1980.

Kay, W. J.: Epilepsy in cats. J. Am. Anim. Hosp. Assoc. 11:77, 1975.

Kornegay, J. N.: Feline neurology. Comp. Cont. Ed. Pract. Vet. 3:203, 1981.

Loscher, W.: Plasma levels of valproic acid and its metabolites during continued treatment in dogs. J. Vet. Pharmacol. Therap. 4:111, 1981.

Oliver, J. E.: Seizure disorders in companion animals. Comp. Cont. Ed. Pract. Vet. 2:77, 1980.

Prichard, J. W.: Phenobarbital: Introduction. *In* Glaser, G. H., Penry, J. K., and Woodbury, D. M. (eds.): *Antiepileptic Drugs: Mechanisms of Action*. New York: Raven Press, 1980, pp. 473–491.

Roye, D. B., Serrano, E. E., Hammer, R. H., and Wilder, B. J.: Plasma kinetics of diphenylhydantoin in dogs and cats. Am. J. Vet. Res. 34:947, 1973.

Russo, M. E.: The pathophysiology of epilepsy. Cornell Vet. 71:221, 1981.

Schwartz-Porsche, D., Loscher, W., Frey, H. H.: Treatment of canine epilepsy with primidone. J.A.V.M.A. 181:592, 1982.

Shepherd, D. E., and de Lahunta, A.: Central nervous system disease in the cat. Comp. Cont. Ed. Pract. Vet. 2:306, 1980.

Woodbury, D. M., Penry, J. K., and Schmidt, R. P. (eds.): *Antiepileptic Drugs*. New York: Raven Press, 1972.

Yeary, R. A.: Serum concentrations of primidone and its metabolites, phenylethylmalonamide and phenobarbital, in the dog. Am. J. Vet. Res. 41:1643, 1980.

Section 10

GASTROINTESTINAL DISORDERS

DAVID C. TWEDT, D.V.M.
Consulting Editor

***Additional Pertinent Information Found in* Current Veterinary Therapy VIII:**

Hardy, R. M.: Hepatic Biopsy, p. 813.

Strombeck, D. R., and Feldman, B. F.: Acute Pancreatitis, p. 810.

Strombeck, D. R., Schaeffer, M. C., and Rogers, Q. R.: Dietary Therapy for Dogs with Chronic Hepatic Insufficiency, p. 817.

STOMATITIS

PATRICK J. McKEEVER, D.V.M.
St. Paul, Minnesota

Stomatitis, or inflammation of the oral mucosa, is a common problem faced by the small animal practitioner. Because of the varied causes such as infectious organisms, physical agents, systemic disease, and immunologic disorders, a specific diagnosis requires an extensive and carefully developed diagnostic plan that includes a complete history, physical examination, and laboratory evaluation. Treatment for many types of stomatitis is prolonged, and some disease states responsible for stomatitis cannot be cured but are controlled through continuous use of medications.

Specific diagnosis of infectious conditions by culture is complicated because of the extensive and varied flora of the oral cavity, difficulty in determining which organisms are pathogens, and difficulty in culturing some of the organisms because of their unique nutrient requirements.

PLANT AWN STOMATITIS

ETIOLOGY. Plant awn stomatitis frequently results when a dog tries to chew out or remove plant awns that are embedded in the coat and causing irritation to the skin. The bristles of these awns, especially burdock (*Arctium* sp.), erode and become embedded in the gingiva and tongue. As these awns may pass intact through the digestive tract of horses, they may occasionally cause stomatitis in dogs who play with and chew on horse fecal material.

CLINICAL FINDINGS. Lesions are generally located in the gingiva surrounding the incisors and canine teeth. Gingivitis, small papules or vesicles of the mucosa, and shallow ulcers of the tongue are the only findings in mild cases. In severe cases, multiple papules, nodules, and hyperplasia of the gingiva are observed. Small splinters of plant material are often seen protruding from these papules or nodules. In addition, some affected animals may have extensive erosions of the tongue covered by a thick white-gray pseudomembrane.

DIAGNOSIS. The diagnosis is confirmed by either observing the plant material while examining the animal's mouth, finding plant material in scrapings of papules or necrotic debris, or finding plant material in biopsies of affected tissues.

TREATMENT. No treatment is necessary in mild cases with minimal lesions. Plant material embedded in the mucosa will either slough out or be broken down and absorbed as a result of inflammation. In severe cases, plant bristles seen protruding from tissues and extensive pseudomembranous tissue should be scraped away using a scalpel blade. After they are scraped, affected tissues should be flushed with 1 per cent hydrogen peroxide solution. Finally, and most important, the animal's access to areas contaminated with the offending plant material must be stopped.

NECROTIZING ULCERATIVE STOMATITIS

ETIOLOGY. The cause of necrotizing ulcerative stomatitis is not completely understood. *Staphylococcus aureus,* hemolytic streptococcus, Pseudomonas, and *Pasteurella multocida* have been cultured from infected tissues. Spirochetes (Vincent's stomatitis) and fusiform bacilli have been identified in impression smears of affected tissues. Undoubtedly, there are other aerobic and anaerobic organisms that may cause or contribute to the condition. Other undetermined systemic factors also may play a role in the development of the disease.

CLINICAL FINDINGS. Gingivitis and ulcerations of gingival tissues are the lesions most consistently found. The ulcerations are often covered by a grayish mass of necrotic tissue and other oral debris. Affected tissues bleed easily when touched. Salivary secretions are increased, and halitosis is severe. Lesions are painful. It is difficult for some affected animals to eat, and most resist examination of the mouth. In severe cases, the disease process may affect alveolar bone.

DIAGNOSIS. There are no specific diagnostic procedures that will provide a definitive diagnosis of necrotizing ulcerative stomatitis. A tentative diagnosis is based on clinical findings and culture or observation of one or more of the organisms discussed as causes.

TREATMENT. Specific therapy depends on the organisms cultured and their sensitivities. Most animals respond well to either amoxicillin every 12 hours or ampicillin every 8 hours given at an oral dose of 20 mg/kg for 20 days. An alternative would be clindamycin 5 mg/kg orally every 12 hours for 20 days. Necrotic debris and any plaque on the teeth should also be removed and the ulcerated areas flushed one to three times daily with 1 per cent hydrogen peroxide.

CANDIDAL STOMATITIS

Etiology. *Candida albicans* is the yeast organism responsible for this form of stomatitis. Generalized disease states or a compromised immune system play important roles in reducing host resistance to *C. albicans* in humans. At present, these factors have not been documented as playing important roles in candidal stomatitis in dogs.

Clinical Findings. A white plaque of dead epithelial cells (pseudomembrane) located on the buccal mucosa is the outstanding feature of candidal stomatitis. Often there are small white satellite lesions surrounding the main plaque. Halitosis, if present, is not severe. Excessive salvation is rarely present.

Diagnosis. The diagnosis is confirmed by the culture of candidal organisms from or the identification of yeast organisms in impression smears of pseudomembrane.

Treatment. Systemic treatment of choice would be ketoconazole (Nizoral, Janssen) 10 mg/kg every 8 hours orally until the lesions resolve. In addition, 1 per cent clotrimazole (Lotrimin, Schering) in Orabase (Hoyt) can be compounded by a pharmacist and applied to the lesions three to four times a day. If any conditions exist that may decrease host resistance, they should also be corrected, if possible.

NOCARDIAL STOMATITIS

Etiology. *Nocardia* organisms are the causative agents.

Clinical Findings. Severe halitosis is the hallmark of nocardial stomatitis. In early or mild cases, gingivitis, especially around the gingival sulcus, is the predominant finding. A small amount of exudate is often noted in association with the inflamed tissues. In severe cases, areas of gray necrotic infected tissue are often found in the periodontal areas. This causes the periodontal membrane to recede and the crevicular epithelium to extend downward, thereby creating a periodontal pocket. As these pockets deepen, the teeth become loose as a result of destruction of their supporting structures. If the disease is allowed to progress, teeth may become more loose or fall out. The infection and lesions of necrotic tissue may also appear on the lips, buccal mucosa, and soft palate. In severe cases, infection may also spread to regional lymph nodes and adjacent skin. Excessive salivation is present in a majority of the cases and often contains a purulent exudate. The condition is painful, and all affected animals resist examination of the mouth. Severely affected animals are reluctant to eat.

Diagnosis. The diagnosis is based on clinical findings plus culture of *Nocardia* organisms. Culture of these organisms can be difficult, as the abundant flora of the mouth will often overgrow the *Nocardia*. Therefore, when culture material is submitted, the laboratory should be notified that *Nocardia* is a differential diagnostic consideration. It may also be helpful if impression smears of affected tissue are submitted with the culture.

Treatment. Sulfadiazine is given orally at a dosage of 80 mg/kg every 8 hours until there is resolution of the lesions. Alternatively, ampicillin or amoxicillin 20 to 30 mg/kg may be given orally every 8 or 12 hours, respectively.

Prognosis. Seventy per cent of the cases will respond to therapy within 6 weeks. However, 30 per cent, which generally represent severe cases, do not respond favorably.

STOMATITIS ASSOCIATED WITH PERIODONTAL DISEASE

Stomatitis may result from the extension of infection and plaque accumulation in periodontal disease. Plaque removal by routine dental procedures and antibiotic therapy (ampicillin 20 mg/kg every 8 hours) is accepted therapy. A program of routine brushing of the teeth to prevent plaque buildup should be instituted.

VIRAL STOMATITIS

Erosions and ulcers of the oral mucosa often occur in cats infected with either feline rhinotracheitis (feline herpesvirus) or feline calicivirus (feline picornavirus). Feline calicivirus is more frequently responsible for the development of oral lesions, whereas feline rhinotracheitis virus is more likely to produce severe and extensive general lesions. Infection with either feline panleukopenia or feline leukemia virus may result in stomatitis; however, other organs are typically affected.

STOMATITIS ASSOCIATED WITH POISONS

All heavy metal poisons may cause oral inflammation and ulceration. Thallium, which in the past has been used as a rodenticide, has been responsible for most cases in this group. It is less readily available today, so cases are rare. Oral ulcers occasionally occur in animals that chew on the house plant *Dieffenbachia*.

STOMATITIS ASSOCIATED WITH SYSTEMIC DISEASE

Uremia resulting from renal disease is a common cause of oral ulcerations in dogs. In this condition, ammonia (resulting from bacterial action on urea that diffuses into saliva), dehydration, and bleeding tendencies that occur late in the disease all contribute to the syndrome.

Oral ulcerations are often features of the autoimmune diseases pemphigus vulgaris, bullous pemphigoid, and systemic lupus erythematosus. Lesions of pemphigus vulgaris and bullous pemphigoid first develop as vesicles, which rapidly rupture leaving ulcers. In contrast, only ulcers are found with systemic lupus erythematosus.

Oral ulcerations are a severe recurrent problem in gray collies afflicted with the simple recessive autosomal disease that causes cyclic neutropenia (gray collie syndrome).

References and Supplemental Reading

Cheville, N. F.: The gray collie syndrome. J.A.V.M.A. 1952:620, 1968.

Conroy, J. D.: Immune-mediated diseases of skin and mucous membranes. *In* Ettinger, S. J. (ed.): *Textbook of Internal Medicine*. Vol. 2. Philadelphia: W. B. Saunders, 1983, pp. 2145–2158.

Dietrich, U. B.: Dental care: Prophylaxis and therapy. Canine Pract. 3:44, 1976.

Findlay, G. H.: Superficial fungus infections. *In* Thomas B. Fitzpatrick (ed.): *Dermatology in General Medicine*, 2nd ed. New York: McGraw-Hill, 1971, pp. 1520–1521.

Harvey, C. H., O'Brien, J. A., Rossman, L. E., et al.: Oral, dental, pharyngeal, and salivary gland disorders. *In* Ettinger, S. J. (ed.): *Textbook of Internal Medicine*. Vol. 2. Philadelphia: W. B. Saunders, 1983, pp. 1127–1191.

Kaplan, M. K., and Jeffcoat, M. K.: Acute necrotizing ulcerative gingivitis. Canine Pract. 5:35, 1978.

MEGAESOPHAGUS IN THE DOG

MICHAEL S. LEIB, D.V.M.

Blacksburg, Virginia

Megaesophagus is one of the most common causes of regurgitation in dogs. Usually it is an idiopathic disorder, but it may occur secondary to polysystemic disease (Table 1). As a descriptive term, megaesophagus simply refers to a dilated esophagus from any cause. To avoid confusion, the author prefers not to use the term *megaesophagus* to describe conditions such as vascular ring anomaly, esophageal stricture, and esophageal foreign bodies that may produce esophageal dilation. For the remainder of this discussion, the term *megaesophagus* will refer to a specific syndrome characterized by a dilated hypoperistaltic esophagus.

Table 1. *Rule-Outs for Regurgitation*

Megaesophagus—idiopathic
Megaesophagus—secondary
Myasthenia gravis
Systemic lupus erythematosus
Polyneuropathy
Polymyositis
Hypoadrenocorticism
Vascular ring anomaly
Foreign body
Esophagitis
Stricture
Extraesophageal compression
Motility disorder—segmental
Spirocerca lupi
Tumor
Granuloma or abscess
Diverticula
Gastroesophageal intussusception
Esophageal-pulmonary fistula

In the veterinary literature, *achalasia* has frequently been used as a synonym for *megaesophagus*. Achalasia in humans is characterized by aperistalsis, regurgitation, and a hypertensive lower esophageal sphincter. Achalasia has not been reported in dogs, suggesting that this term should not be used interchangeably with megaesophagus. Hoffer and colleagues (1979) define megaesophagus developing after maturation as acquired achalasia. At the present time, there is no evidence to justify the use of separate terms for adult- and juvenile-onset megaesophagus.

Megaesophagus has been reported infrequently in cats. Because the anatomy and physiology of the feline esophagus differ from those of dogs, megaesophagus in cats probably represents a different pathophysiologic syndrome. Megaesophagus is a component of a recently reported autonomic polyganglionopathy in cats seen in England and termed the *Key-Gaskell syndrome*. Other clinical signs associated with this syndrome include persistent pupillary dilation, decreased lacrimal and nasal secretions, bradycardia, and constipation. The remainder of this article will deal with megaesophagus in dogs.

PHYSIOLOGY AND PATHOPHYSIOLOGY

The canine esophagus is a striated muscular tube that transports food from the pharynx to the stomach. Unlike the small intestine, the esophagus requires a centrally mediated nervous reflex pathway for controlling its motility. Esophageal distension from an intraluminal bolus produces sensory impulses transmitted via the vagus nerves to the medullary swallowing center through the nucleus solitarius. Inhibitory impulses are sent to the respiratory center in the medulla to prevent aspiration of ingesta during swallowing. An abnormality in this region may explain aspiration pneumonia commonly encountered in dogs with megaesophagus. The swallowing center sends impulses to the nucleus ambiguus, which contains the cell bodies of the lower motor neurons that supply the esophagus. Lower motor neurons travel to the esophagus in the vagus nerves. Motor impulses cross the neuromuscular junction to striated muscle fibers, initiating regional muscular contractions. As the food bolus is propelled aborally, sensory information initiates a continuation of the peristaltic reflex arc, causing progressive transport of the bolus.

When a food bolus approaches the aboral esophagus, signals are sent to the lower esophageal sphincter, causing relaxation and opening of the sphincter and allowing food to enter the stomach. Synchronous function of the lower esophageal sphincter requires a normal esophagus orad to the sphincter to relay sensory information. Local esophageal disease or surgical removal of this area results in asynchronous function of the lower esophageal sphincter, failure of the sphincter to open, and retention of esophageal contents. After successful passage of a food bolus through the lower esophageal sphincter, contraction of the sphincter occurs, maintaining a high-pressure zone that prevents gastroesophageal reflux.

Primary esophageal peristalsis is defined as the muscular wave of contraction initiated by a food bolus as it passes through the cricopharyngeal sphincter (upper esophageal sphincter) into the esophagus. If the primary peristaltic wave passes over the bolus, failing to propel it to the stomach, a secondary wave of peristalsis is initiated by esophageal distention. An identical reflex pathway controls both primary and secondary peristalsis.

Any abnormality along the peristaltic reflex pathway may result in esophageal dysfunction and megaesophagus. Megaesophagus may be secondary to an abnormality of the neuromuscular junction, as occurs in myasthenia gravis; an abnormality of striated muscle, associated with polymyositis and systemic lupus erythematosus; and defects in peripheral nerves such as occurs in giant axonal neuropathy.

Although pathophysiology has not been studied in large numbers of dogs with megaesophagus, research has indicated that the lower motor neuron segment of the peristaltic reflex pathway can be normal. All reported resting pressures of the lower esophageal sphincters in dogs with megaesophagus have been normal. Direct nerve stimulation and electromyography of the esophagus have been normal in some dogs with megaesophagus. The location of the lesion in idiopathic megaesophagus is thought to involve either the sensory receptors, afferent vagal fibers, or medullary connections between the tractus solitarius and swallowing center. Pathophysiologic differences between juvenile- and adult-onset forms have not been identified.

HISTORY AND CLINICAL SIGNS

Megaesophagus occurs most commonly in the recently weaned puppy; however, several large case studies have indicated that 30 to 40 per cent of all affected dogs may be older than 1 year at the time of diagnosis. Approximately one third of all cases seen by the author have been older than 5 years. Megaesophagus affects many breeds of dogs. Great Danes, Irish setters, and German shepherds are at increased risk. There does not appear to be a sex predisposition. Megaesophagus has been shown to be hereditary in wire-haired fox terriers and miniature schnauzers. Since it may also be hereditary in other breeds, veterinarians should discourage the breeding of affected dogs or the sire and dam of affected dogs.

The most common clinical sign associated with megaesophagus is regurgitation of food and water. In a young puppy, the owner will commonly describe regurgitation soon after the initiation of solid food. Occasionally, regurgitation of bitch's milk may be noticed by an observant owner. Affected puppies do not grow as rapidly as normal littermates, develop a rough, dry coat, and generally are considered runts of the litter. Megaesophagus may affect single or multiple littermates or, rarely, the entire litter. The frequency and severity of regurgitation vary among affected dogs.

Adult dogs developing megaesophagus usually have a sudden and severe onset of regurgitation and weight loss. If megaesophagus is secondary to a primary neuromuscular disorder, generalized signs of weakness may be evident. In some cases of myasthenia gravis, regurgitation may precede the clinical signs of muscle weakness.

Respiratory disease, secondary to aspiration pneumonia, is very common in megaesophagus. Approximately two thirds of dogs with megaesophagus seen by the author have clinical or radiographic evidence of aspiration pneumonia. Clinical signs include coughing, tachypnea, dyspnea, mucopurulent nasal discharge, and pyrexia. Aspiration pneumonia is a major cause of morbidity and mortality. Approximately 15 per cent of dogs with megaesophagus may present with only a history of respiratory disease and no evidence of regurgitation.

The frequency and severity of clinical signs vary greatly among affected individuals. Dogs with megaesophagus will often show waxing and waning periods of clinical signs without any apparent predisposing factors. Unless severe aspiration pneumonia is present, dogs usually maintain an excellent appetite. Occasionally, megaesophagus may occur as an incidental finding in an asymptomatic dog.

Physical examination often reveals a thin dog in poor condition. Thoracic auscultation may reveal bilateral crackles, most prominent over the cranial ventral lung fields, indicating aspiration pneumonia. Bulging of the cervical region adjacent to the thoracic inlet, secondary to an enlarged esophagus, may be seen on expiration. This may be demonstrated by compressing the thorax with the dog's mouth closed and the nares occluded.

DIAGNOSTIC PLAN

The initial step in evaluation of any case of regurgitation is to distinguish between regurgitation and vomiting. Most owners will report that their dog with megaesophagus vomits. Only with a careful history and physical examination can the veterinary clinician clearly identify the patient's problem as regurgitation and then pursue a diagnostic plan.

Regurgitation is a passive process. Food retained in the esophagus is moved along the path of least resistance to the pharynx by changes in body position, excitement, muscle activity, or other causes of increased intrathoracic pressure. As the food reaches the pharynx, it may initiate a gag reflex and then be expelled from the oral cavity. Regurgitation most commonly occurs soon after eating but may be delayed 12 to 24 hours. The longer the interval between eating and regurgitation, the less the material will appear undigested. The regurgitated food may assume a cylindrical shape and be covered with mucus.

Vomiting is a centrally mediated reflex that consists of hypersalivation, frequent swallowing, and nausea followed by abdominal contractions producing retching and finally the expulsion of gastric and duodenal contents. The presence of bile identifies duodenal contents and indicates vomiting rather than regurgitation. After identifying the animal's problem as regurgitation, the clinician should compile a ranked rule-out list (Table 1) and pursue a thorough and logical diagnostic plan.

Radiography is the most important part of the diagnostic plan. A normal esophagus is usually not visible on survey thoracic radiographs. With megaesophagus, survey radiographs may reveal the presence of an enlarged esophagus containing gas, fluid, or food. An air-filled esophagus may produce a "tracheal stripe," as the esophageal wall silhouettes with the tracheal wall. Often the trachea will be depressed cranial to the heart on the lateral view. Evidence of aspiration pneumonia consisting of peribronchial and alveolar infiltration and pulmonary consolidation is often seen.

If survey radiographs fail to provide a definitive diagnosis, a barium contrast esophagram should be performed. Only 3 to 5 seconds are necessary for transport of a barium bolus through a normal esophagus into the stomach. Liquid barium sulfate alone or mixed with food will outline the dilated hypoperistaltic esophagus. In most cases of megaesophagus, the entire thoracic esophagus is uniformly dilated. The esophagus tapers to a conical shape as it approaches the diaphragmatic hiatus. This tapering of the esophagus does not suggest cardiospasm or achalasia as previously suggested in the literature, but represents normal anatomic relationships. Approximately 40 per cent of cases also have a dilated cervical esophagus. This estimate may be falsely low, because many esophageal radiographic studies do not routinely include cervical radiographs. The degree of esophageal dilation is greater in the thoracic esophagus than in the cervical esophagus, because more area is available for dilation in the thoracic region. A large ventral esophageal sacculation occasionally may be seen cranial to the heart. This condition must be differentiated from a vascular ring anomaly, in which an esophageal constriction at the base of the heart and a normal esophagus aboral to the constriction should be seen.

A variable esophageal motility pattern in dogs with megaesophagus is seen with fluoroscopy. In the author's experience, approximately 70 per cent of affected dogs have no primary or secondary peristaltic contractions. There is considerable difference in the motility pattern of the remaining cases; however, in all affected dogs, esophageal motility is reduced. Often, radiographic studies show that barium is retained in the esophagus and does not pass through the lower esophageal sphincter and enter the stomach even when the x-ray table is tilted. This does not represent achalasia or a hypertensive lower esophageal sphincter, but an asynchronously functioning sphincter. The lower esophageal sphincter will not sequentially open to allow barium to enter the stomach if it does not properly receive sensory information from the esophageal segment orad to the sphincter.

Radiographic findings do not correlate well with clinical signs or prognosis. The author has seen littermates with identical radiographic findings who had vastly different signs. Often, during waxing and waning periods in an affected dog there are no radiographic changes in esophageal motility to explain the changing clinical signs.

In an adult dog, a careful neurologic examination should be performed to rule out neuromuscular disease producing secondary megaesophagus (Table 1). Specific laboratory tests to evaluate polysystemic diseases such as hypoadrenocorticism and systemic lupus erythematosus should be performed if the history and physical examination provide evidence that these primary diseases may exist.

TREATMENT

Although the treatment plan is controversial, most veterinary gastroenterologists recommend medical management for megaesophagus. Two large case studies have indicated that surgical treatment has been associated with higher mortality than medical management and generally produces poor results. The difficulty in adequately evaluating surgery as a treatment for megaesophagus has been compounded by the almost universal addition of medical management to surgical treatment. One author has reported favorable surgical results using a modified Heller's myotomy in a limited number of cases of mature-onset megaesophagus. This surgical procedure reduces lower esophageal sphincter resting tone but still allows the sphincter to maintain enough of a high-pressure zone to prevent gastroesophageal reflux. Surgical treatment does not improve esophageal peristalsis, and medical management must be used to assist in delivery of food to the stomach through a weakened sphincter.

Medical management consists of elevated feedings, allowing gravity to aid movement of food through the esophagus. Dogs can be rapidly trained to eat with their forelegs elevated on a table, step, or feeding rack. They should remain elevated at a 45-degree angle for 10 to 15 minutes after eating. With small dogs, owners can hold the animals upright after eating.

The consistency of food that affected individuals can best tolerate will vary. Most dogs will regurgitate least often if they are fed a gruel of canned food and water. The author starts with a ratio of one can of dog food to one to two cans of water blended together and administered in an amount necessary to supply caloric needs of the animal. Owners should try various food consistencies to determine which works best for their dog. The optimal food consistency may change over time.

Treatment for aspiration pneumonia is often necessary during acute exacerbations. Because many genera of bacteria may be involved, appropriate antibiotic therapy should be based on culture and sensitivity testing of a transtracheal wash. The author has found that many bacterial isolates are sensitive to chloramphenicol. Before the bacterial culture results have been obtained, initial therapy with chloramphenicol, 50 mg/kg every 8 hours, is initiated. Parenteral antibiotics must be used because frequent regurgitation interferes with the absorption of oral medication. The concurrent use of glucocorticoids for the initial treatment of aspiration pneumonia is controversial and is not suggested by the author.

PROGNOSIS

The overall prognosis for megaesophagus remains poor. In two large case studies, approximately 70 per cent of dogs died or were euthanized because of megaesophagus. In the author's experience, most dogs are dead within 18 months of initial diagnosis. The author found that dogs showing signs prior to 1 year of age had a significantly better chance of surviving 12 months after diagnosis than dogs developing signs after 2 years of age. Causes of death and euthanasia include progressive emaciation, aspiration pneumonia, persistent regurgitation, and unwillingness of owners to manage their dogs with special diets or to tolerate persistent clinical signs.

The veterinary literature contains isolated case reports suggesting improvement or cure of dogs with megaesophagus. In many instances, long-term follow-up and radiographic re-evaluation are lacking. In 95 per cent of the author's cases in which follow-up radiographs were performed, there was no improvement of esophageal function. Fewer than 5 per cent of dogs reported in the literature were free of clinical signs when re-evaluated.

Occasional well-documented cases of improvement or cure have been encountered, especially in young puppies. The canine esophagus is not functionally mature at birth but matures during the first 6 months of life. Improvement in young puppies with megaesophagus may represent a static disease process and maturation of esophageal function. If megaesophagus is secondary to polysystemic disease, successful management of the primary condition may lead to improvement or cure of esophageal dysfunction. Although improvement occasionally occurs in young puppies, it rarely occurs in older dogs with idiopathic megaesophagus.

References and Supplemental Reading

Cox, V. S., Wallace, L. J., Anderson, V. E., et al.: Hereditary esophageal dysfunction in the miniature schnauzer dog. Am. J. Vet. Res. 41:326, 1980.

Harvey, C. E., O. Brien, J. A., Durie, V. R., et al.: Megaesophagus in the dog: A clinical survey of 79 cases. J.A.V.M.A. 165:443, 1974.

Hendricks, J. C., Maggio-Price, L., and Dougherty, J. F.: Transient esophageal dysfunction mimicking megaesophagus in three dogs. J.A.V.M.A. 185:90, 1984.

Hoffer, R. E., MacCoy, D. M., Quick, C. B., et al.: Management of acquired achalasia in dogs. J.A.V.M.A. 175:814, 1979.
Leib, M. S.: Megaesophagus in the dog. Part I—Anatomy, Physiology and Pathophysiology. Comp. Cont. Ed. Pract. Vet. 5:825, 1983.
Leib, M. S., and Hall, R. L.: Megaesophagus in the dog. Part II—Clinical aspects. Comp. Cont. Ed. Pract. Vet. 6:11, 1984.
Osborne, C. A., Clifford, D. M., and Jessen, C.: Hereditary esophageal achalasia in dogs. J.A.V.M.A. 151:572, 1967.

CHRONIC GASTRITIS

DAVID C. TWEDT, D.V.M.,
and MICHAEL L. MAGNE, D.V.M.
Fort Collins, Colorado

Chronic gastritis collectively describes a number of clinical entities due to diverse causes. The definition is quite broad and has many different meanings. The clinician frequently uses the term to describe clinical conditions associated with chronic vomiting in which all other causes have been ruled out. With the use of fiberoptic endoscopes, the clinical diagnosis is now strengthened by observation of certain characteristic mucosal abnormalities. Radiologists also have their own set of criteria for the diagnosis based on selected contrast studies. To pathologists, chronic gastritis represents certain characteristic inflammatory changes. All these criteria are presumptive and quite variable. Some dogs, for example, may have histologic changes representing chronic gastritis and no clinical signs related to gastric disease. More often, dogs have signs of chronic intermittent vomiting and never have histologic confirmation of chronic gastritis. A precise definition of chronic gastritis must therefore most correctly be restricted to the dog that has both the clinical signs and characteristic histologic lesions within the gastric mucosa. This precise definition requires a gastric mucosal biopsy. Methods include the use of either suction biopsy capsules or biopsy forceps during endoscopic examination or surgical excision. Chronic gastritis at our institution appears to be of higher incidence than previously thought, and several distinct types of chronic gastritis have been identified in dogs.

ETIOPATHOGENESIS

In most cases of chronic gastritis, the cause is never determined. An understanding of the pathophysiology of mucosal damage together with the knowledge gained in experimental studies in dogs enables one to predict how chronic gastritis may develop.

The normal *gastric mucosal barrier* is generally resistant to the abrasive or toxic effects of ingested foodstuffs and is also impervious to the effects of hydrochloric acid and the digestive enzyme, pepsin. This barrier consists of two parts, the mucous layer lining the surface of the epithelial cells and the mucosal epithelial cell membrane. The mucous coat functions in a minor role, predominantly in lubrication. The gastric epithelial cells are regarded as the most important part of the barrier. The precise anatomic site of the epithelial barrier is believed to be the lipoprotein layer of the plasma membrane. Damage to this barrier may result by disruption of intercellular tight junctions or by direct cytologic damage.

Various physiochemical factors have been shown to cause damage to the gastric mucosal barrier. *Ingested exogenous factors* within the gastric lumen may result in mucosal damage. These include a long list of drugs, various toxins, and many dietary constituents, as well as abrasive or foreign material. *Alteration in blood flow* to the gastric mucosal microcirculation will also potentiate formation of gastric mucosal lesions. Mucosal ischemia results in a decrease in gastric mucosal energy and rapid cellular death. *Endogenous factors* will also bring about mucosal damage. States of excessive gastric acid production or reflux of bile or pancreatic enzymes into the gastric lumen result in damage to the gastric mucosal barrier. Endogenous hormonal imbalances or immune-mediated mechanisms may play a causative role in mucosal damage.

Damage to the gastric mucosal barrier results in a series of pathologic events beginning with the back-diffusion of luminal gastric acid through the damaged mucosa. Local tissue inflammation occurs from direct damage by acid. Damage then extends deeper to the blood vessels and nerves located in the subepithelium. Mast cells present in the submucosa and lamina propria degranulate on contact with acid, releasing histamine, heparin, and kinins. Released histamine stimulates adjacent parietal cells to secrete additional hydrochloric acid. The increased production and further back-diffusion of hydrochloric acid appear to be a key factor in perpetuation of most gastric mucosal lesions.

The stomach is constantly exposed to an infinite number of dietary antigens, chemicals, and microbial agents. Damage to the gastric wall permits the entry of these constituents, which may cause either direct damage or initiate an immune response stimulated by continued irritation. Experimental studies in dogs have demonstrated a variety of immunologic phenomena in association with chronic gastritis and support the hypothesis of this etiopathogenesis. Mucosal damage with the subsequent release of certain gastric antigens causing either cellular or humoral immune response may also play a role in the development of autoimmune-mediated cases of chronic gastritis.

CLASSIFICATION OF CHRONIC GASTRITIS

Chronic gastritis can be classified into three broad categories: those types that are erosive, those that are nonerosive, and those that are quite specific, based on histologic evaluation.

Erosive Gastritis

Animals with erosive gastritis have lesions associated with multiple mucosal erosions or ulcers and variable inflammatory infiltrates. The gastric lesions may be acute or chronic. The causes of erosive gastritis are many and often occur secondary to certain clinical situations or therapies. The presence of blood in the vomitus generally signifies an erosive gastritis and generally dictates aggressive medical management. The reader should refer to the article in *Current Veterinary Therapy VIII* on gastric ulcers (Twedt, 1983) for the diagnosis and therapy of conditions causing gastric mucosal ulceration.

Nonerosive Gastritis

This subclassification is commonly referred to as "chronic gastritis" and is the most common gastritis observed in dogs. The gastric changes are nonspecific and appear to be the result of a final common pathway of inflammation in response to many forms of injury. There are two histologic patterns of nonerosive gastritis: chronic superficial gastritis and chronic atrophic gastritis.

CHRONIC SUPERFICIAL GASTRITIS

Chronic gastritis in dogs is characterized by excessive but variable inflammatory cell infiltrates, particularly lymphocytes and plasma cells, and fibrosis. The inflammatory changes generally affect only the superficial epithelium and adjacent lamina propria. Many of the gastric lesions probably result through repeated exposure to the suspected agent. Once the cause has been removed, the changes appear to be reversible and the prognosis for chronic superficial gastritis is therefore generally good.

CHRONIC ATROPHIC GASTRITIS

This nonerosive gastritis is characterized by a thinner than normal mucosa and a reduction in the size and depth of the gastric glands. The parietal cells are often replaced by mucus-secreting cells, and there is a variable inflammatory component similar to that of chronic superficial gastritis. Available information suggests that gastric atrophy is the end stage of an inflammatory process starting as a superficial gastritis and ultimately progressing to the atrophic form. The time sequence of this progressive lesion is unknown but probably takes months to occur. There is evidence that immunologically mediated mechanisms are responsible for atrophic gastritis, since inflammatory atrophic lesions have been produced experimentally in dogs by immunizing them with their own gastric juices. This experimental model appears quite similar to the naturally occurring disease.

With the loss of gastric glands as well as numbers of parietal cells, gastric acid production should logically be reduced. Dogs with atrophic gastritis evaluated by the authors were found not to be achlorhydric but probably had less than maximal gastric acid output, although total secretory capacity was not measured. Acid reduction from atrophic gastritis in dogs has also been associated with secondary intestinal bacterial overgrowth leading to malabsorption and diarrhea. Plasma gastrin levels may be elevated in dogs with atrophic gastritis because of the loss of negative feedback by gastric acid on gastrin release.

Clinical Findings. Dogs with chronic nonerosive gastritis have vomiting as the salient clinical feature. The vomiting need not be continuous and is usually intermittent, ranging from once daily to only several times a week. The vomitus frequently consists of either mucus and gastric secretions sometimes containing bile or simply undigested food. Vomiting of a meal appears to have no specific relationship to eating. Other less frequent signs associated with chronic gastritis include belching, pica (such as ingestion of grass), polydipsia, anorexia, and weight loss or diarrhea. Rarely, animals may exhibit a "praying position" of relief secondary to gastric pain. Most animals with chronic nonerosive gastritis are in good physical condition.

The diagnosis is based on the clinical signs of

gastric disease and histologic confirmation through a mucosal biopsy. Barium radiographic contrast studies generally fail to distinguish cases of chronic nonerosive gastritis. Secondary motility abnormalities may result, causing delayed gastric emptying of barium or altered gastric contractions on fluoroscopic examination. The endoscopic appearance of the mucosal surface may frequently be normal. Changes observed in some cases of chronic nonerosive gastritis include hyperemia, a patchy and pale mucosal color, or mucosal ulceration. Frequently the mucosa will bleed easily when touched with the endoscope. In atrophic gastritis, submucosal vessels may easily be observed through the thin mucosal surface.

TREATMENT. The primary objective in the management of nonerosive gastritis should be to identify and remove the inciting cause. Failure to do so dictates institution of dietary management or medical therapy. The prognosis is generally good for most cases of chronic nonerosive gastritis.

Most dogs with chronic gastritis tend to tolerate a canned, meat-based diet better than a dry, high-fiber diet. The diet ideally should be bland, low in fat, low in nondigestible fiber, nonallergenic, and should meet the daily caloric requirements. Although there is no conclusive evidence that dietary allergy or sensitivity is the cause of chronic gastritis in dogs, a "semipure" diet without additional additives should be selected. The commercial diet (Intestinal diet, Hill's Pet Products) is adequate for most cases. Commercial "all-natural" diets or home diets such as cottage cheese and rice may also be beneficial. The animal should be fed several small meals daily.

Since back-diffusion of hydrochloric acid is a perpetuating factor in gastric mucosal damage, the administration of agents that block acid production are indicated. Cimetidine (Tagamet, SmithKlein Beckman) is given at the rate of 5 to 10 mg/kg body weight every 6 to 8 hours for a period of 2 to 4 weeks. The use of acid-blocking agents in the management of atrophic gastritis may be questionable in theory, but since most cases are not completely achlorhydric, blocking remaining acid secretion appears to be clinically beneficial.

In suspected immune-mediated gastritis, immunosuppression may be indicated in the therapy and azathioprine (Imuran, Burroughs Wellcome) has been shown in dogs to prevent experimentally produced immune atrophic gastropathy. Corticosteroids may also be useful for both their anti-inflammatory effects and reported action of stimulating regeneration of gastric parietal cell mass. The clinical effectiveness of immunosuppressive therapy for chronic nonerosive gastritis has not yet been determined in dogs.

Specific Types of Gastritis

There are several distinct histologic patterns included in the classification of chronic gastritis. These conditions are quite uncommon, and the causes of each are seldom determined.

CHRONIC HYPERTROPHIC GASTRITIS

This condition is characterized by a macroscopic thickening of the gastric mucosa by large rugal folds. Microscopically, there is typically glandular proliferation and cystic dilatation, foveolar hyperplasia, and various inflammatory cellular infiltrates. Mucosal ulceration may be present. The hypertrophic changes may be either diffuse, involving only the pyloric antral region, or arise as focal mucosal polyps. The cause of this condition or group of histologically similar conditions is speculative. Experimental data and clinical evidence in humans suggest that immune-mediated inflammation, hormonal influence, environmental factors, and genetic predisposition are all important in the pathogenesis.

In dogs, mucosal hypertrophy may result secondary to excessive hormonal trophic factors. Histamine, gastrin, and acetylcholine are known trophic factors that may be responsible. Chronic hypertrophic gastritis has been observed in basenji dogs with renal tubular defects and elevated plasma gastrin levels. The altered renal metabolism of gastrin and subsequent hypergastrinemia may be the cause of these hypertrophic changes. We have observed gastric mucosal hypertrophy and hypergastrinemia in dogs with gastrinomas (Zollinger-Ellison syndrome) and in a dog with primary hypergastrinism due to antral mucosal G-cell hyperplasia. In the latter case, the dog had marked elevations in plasma gastrins. Some dogs with systemic mast cell neoplasia may have mucosal hypertrophy and ulceration due to the action of released histamine by these tumors. Pyloric outflow obstruction secondary to antral and pyloric mucosal hypertrophy has been reported in nervous, small breeds of dogs, suggesting a behavior-related, neuroendocrine cause.

CLINICAL FINDINGS. Dogs with hypertrophic gastritis usually exhibit typical signs similar to those of chronic nonerosive gastritis. Vomiting is almost always a feature. It may be severe and contain both a large volume of gastric acid and blood if associated with increased acid production and mucosal ulceration, or the vomiting may be intermittent for months or years, containing undigested food if resulting from a partial pyloric outflow obstruction. Other signs include anorexia, belching, abdominal pain, melena, polydipsia, diarrhea, and weight loss.

The diagnosis of hypertrophic gastritis is based on clinical signs and histologic confirmation. Barium contrast radiographs often show markedly thickened gastric rugal folds. Sometimes these hypertrophic lesions are localized. Lesions located within the pyloric-antral portion of the stomach may result in delayed gastric emptying and a narrow antral region. Endoscopy confirms the radiographic findings and can identify associated mucosal ulceration or erosions. Biopsies taken through the endoscope or by suction capsules may suggest the diagnosis, but often a diagnosis requires a full-thickness biopsy obtained at laparotomy to demonstrate the characteristic hypertrophic changes.

TREATMENT. The therapy for chronic hypertrophic gastritis can only be supportive if a cause cannot be identified and removed. The prognosis for improvement is therefore quite variable. Dietary recommendations given for chronic nonerosive gastritis should be included in the management. Conditions associated with hypergastrinemia, hyperchlorhydria, or mucosal ulceration should be managed with acid blockers such as cimetidine, (5 to 10 mg/kg every 6 to 8 hours) or ranitidine (Zantac, Glaxo; 0.5 mg/kg every 12 hours). Ranitidine is reported to be six to ten times more potent than cimetidine and should be considered if the desired response is not obtained using cimetidine.

When mucosal hypertrophy acts as a mechanical obstruction blocking pyloric outflow, surgical intervention is required. In such conditions focal mucosal resection and pyloroplasty or possibly more radical procedures such as pyloric and antral resection may be required.

EOSINOPHILIC GASTRITIS AND GRANULOMA

This is a rare condition characterized as a diffuse eosinophilic and fibrous tissue infiltration involving many or all layers of the stomach wall. Less frequently reported are discrete single or multiple granulomatous nodules. Eosinophilic lymphadenitis and vasculitis also occur. The gross lesions may appear as a scirrhous thickening of the gastric wall, often resembling gastric neoplasia.

The cause of the eosinophilic infiltration in the stomach is unknown. Some authors suggest that it is immunologically mediated, perhaps due to an allergic or parasitic cause. Microfilaria were observed in some gastric histologic sections from dogs with diffuse eosinophilic gastritis. Dogs experimentally infected with *Toxocara canis* were found to have focal eosinophilic gastritis, but the lesions rarely contained larva and vasculitis was not found. This latter condition may be similar to the syndrome "eosinophilic gastroenteritis," in which there is either a segmental or diffuse infiltration of eosinophils in the mucosa and submucosa of the stomach or intestine. Although the clinical presentation of the two conditions may be similar, they differ significantly in their pathologic features.

CLINICAL FINDINGS. The clinical features are those of chronic gastritis. Vomiting is attributed to gastric wall involvement or pyloric outflow obstruction. Signs associated with mucosal ulceration may also be present. Some cases of eosinophilic gastritis may show a peripheral eosinophilia, although this is not a consistent finding. Barium contrast studies may reveal thickened mucosal folds, nonspecific narrowing, or nodular filling defects. These findings often have a striking resemblance to gastric neoplasia. Endoscopic findings confirm radiographic changes, and mucosal biopsies reveal evidence of eosinophilic infiltrates.

TREATMENT. Dietary control should be attempted, since a dietary allergy may be a causative factor. Dogs with eosinophilic gastritis placed on controlled nonallergenic diets reportedly showed clinical improvement and resolution of peripheral eosinophilia.

Corticosteroids are also indicated in the management of these cases. Prednisone at 0.5 mg/kg daily should be administered for 1 to 2 weeks, followed by a gradual tapering in the dose to 0.12 mg/kg every other day. The response to corticosteroids is usually favorable; however, some cases may require long-term management.

Other Conditions

Granulomatous gastritis is a condition characterized by the presence of tissue granulomas as the predominant histologic finding. The condition is unusual and may result from infections, allergic conditions, or possibly foreign body migration into the gastric wall. Fibrosing granulomatous gastritis is also reported in dogs with gastric phycomycosis. The lesions in these dogs are associated with diffuse or segmental transmural thickening with granulomatous inflammation. Special fungal stains are required to identify the organism. The prognosis for gastric phycomycosis is generally poor, since no current antifungal agent seems effective against this pathogen. Surgical resection, if possible, appears to offer a more successful outcome. An isolated case of *histiocytic gastritis* with *amyloidosis* in a dog has also been reported. The lesions were isolated to the stomach, and no cause was identified.

References and Supplemental Reading

Breitschwerdt, E. B., Ochoa, R., and Waltman, C.: Multiple endocrine abnormalities in basenji dogs with renal tubular dysfunction. J.A.V.M.A. 182:1348, 1983.

Davenport, H. W.: Prevention and suppression by azathioprine of venom-induced protein-losing gastropathy in dogs. Proc. Nat. Acad. Sci. 73:968, 1976.

Happe, R. P., Van Der Gaag, I., and Wolvekamp, W. T. C.: Pyloric stenosis caused by hypertrophic gastritis in three dogs. J. Small Anim. Pract. 22:7, 1981.

Hayden, D. W., and Fleischman, R. W.: Scirrhous eosinophilic gastritis in dogs with gastric arteritis. Vet. Pathol. 14:441, 1977.

Kipnis, R. M.: Focal cystic hypertrophic gastropathy in a dog. J.A.V.M.A. 173:182, 1978.

Krohn, K. J. E., and Finlayson, D. C.: Interrelations of humoral and cellular immune responses in experimental canine gastritis. Clin. Exp. Immunol. 14:237, 1973.

McLeod, C. G., Linglinios, P. C., and Brown, J. C.: Ulcerative histiocytic gastritis with amyloidosis in a dog. Vet. Pathol. 18:117, 1981.

Miller, R. I.: Gastrointestinal phycomycosis in 63 dogs. J.A.V.M.A. 186:473, 1985.

Skillman, J. J. and Slen, W.: Gastric mucosal barrier. Surg. Annu. 4:213, 1972.

Strombeck, D. R.: *Small Animal Gastroenterology.* Davis, CA: Stonegate Publishing, 1979, pp. 110–124.

Twedt, D. C.: Gastric ulcers. *In* Kirk, R. W. (ed.): *Current Veterinary Therapy VIII.* Philadelphia: W. B. Saunders, 1983, p. 705.

Twedt, D. C., and Wingfield, W. E.: Diseases of the stomach. *In* Ettinger, S. J. (ed.): *Veterinary Internal Medicine*, 2nd ed. Philadelphia: W. B. Saunders, 1983, pp. 1233–1277.

Van Der Gaag, I., Happe, R. P., and Wolvekamp, W. Th. C.: A boxer dog with chronic hypertrophic gastritis resembling Menetrier's disease in man. Vet. Pathol. 13:172, 1976.

Van Kruiningen, H. J.: Giant hypertrophic gastritis of basenji dogs. Vet. Pathol. 14:19, 1977.

Walter, M. C., Goldschmidt, M. H., Stone, E. A., et al.: Chronic hypertrophic pyloric gastropathy as a cause of pyloric obstruction in the dog. J.A.V.M.A. 186:157, 1985.

GASTRIC DILATATION-VOLVULUS

E. CHRISTOPHER ORTON, D.V.M.
Fort Collins, Colorado

Gastric dilatation-volvulus (GDV) initiates a series of metabolic events that if unabated result in death. Few disease syndromes challenge the veterinarian's medical and surgical skills to the extent that GDV does. Much is known regarding the pathophysiology of GDV, and yet determination of the underlying cause of GDV has eluded the veterinary profession. More research must be conducted on the origins of GDV before individual dogs at high risk to develop it can be identified and before reliable advice on prevention of GDV can be given. However, the origin of the disease becomes a secondary concern to the veterinarian presented with a dog succumbing to GDV. Therefore, the emphasis in this chapter will be on the management of GDV once it occurs. Much progress has been made toward development of a logical and consistent approach to the management of dogs with this disorder, although controversy still exists.

INCIDENCE

Giant breeds of dogs including the Great Dane, St. Bernard, and borzoi are the most likely to develop GDV. The German shepherd and Irish setter also frequently present with GDV, more because of their popularity than because of a high incidence within the breed. Dogs are most likely to develop GDV between the ages of 2 and 10 years. Although early studies indicated a greater prevalence of GDV in male dogs, recent studies have shown no sexual predisposition for the disease.

ETIOLOGY

In normal dogs, the pylorus is tightly fixed to the cranial right quadrant of the abdomen by the hepatoduodenal ligament, lesser omentum, and common bile duct. Even though the pylorus in normal dogs can be forced to the left and placed in a volvulus position, it immediately returns to its normal position once released. The stomach of a dog that has experienced GDV, however, can easily be placed in the volvulus position and remains in an abnormal position once released. Thus, a fundamental abnormality associated with GDV is laxity of the hepatoduodenal and hepatogastric ligaments, leading to a high degree of mobility of the stomach within the abdomen.

Dogs experiencing gastric dilatation almost invariably also have gastric volvulus. Once the stomach becomes distended in the volvulus position, gastric emptying becomes difficult because of twisting of the cardia and obstruction of the pylorus by the distended fundus. Conversely, the distended fundus locks the mobile stomach in the volvulus position and does not allow the stomach to return to its normal position. Thus, both gastric dilatation and a predisposition for gastric volvulus must be present to produce the GDV syndrome. Simple gastric dilatation does not produce gastric volvulus in an otherwise normal stomach. Any attempt to explain the cause of GDV must address this fact. It is possible that chronic gastric retention due to delayed gastric emptying results in continuous traction on the gastric ligaments, particularly in deep-chested dogs. Such a mechanism would explain both a tendency toward gastric dilatation and excessive gastric mobility within the abdomen, allowing gastric volvulus.

Aerophagia is the major source of gastric gas and is thought to contribute to gastric dilatation in most cases of GDV. It is unknown at this time whether aerophagia initiates or merely contributes to GDV.

PATHOPHYSIOLOGY

Pathophysiologic alterations associated with GDV can be attributed to (1) gastric wall ischemia and (2) circulatory shock arising from occlusion of the caudal vena cava and portal vein by the distending stomach.

According to Laplace's law, gastric wall tension is directly proportional to both intragastric pressure and gastric radius. Thus, even though intragastric pressures are not markedly elevated in most dogs presenting with GDV (20 to 25 mm Hg), gastric wall tension increases dramatically as a result of the combined effect of a moderate increase in gastric pressure and gastric dilatation. Gastric ischemia occurs when gastric wall tension increases sufficiently to occlude intramural gastric vessels. Additionally, the short gastric and left gastroepiploic arteries may be partially occluded by the gastric malposition.

Necrosis and sloughing of the gastric mucosa result from the combined effect of gastric ischemia and gastric acid. Gastric ischemia compromises the gastric mucosal barrier, which normally protects the gastric mucosa from the digestive effects of gastric acid and pepsin. As GDV becomes prolonged, necrosis extends into the gastric muscular wall, resulting eventually in gastric rupture and peritonitis.

In addition to local gastric injury, GDV induces circulatory shock by occluding the caudal vena cava and portal vein. Occlusion of the caudal great veins reduces venous return to the heart, which in turn dramatically decreases cardiac output and mean arterial pressure.

Shock initiates a series of compensatory neurohumoral mechanisms. Baroreceptors responding to arterial hypotension increase sympathoadrenal activity, resulting in tachycardia, vasoconstriction, and splenic contraction. Atrial stretch receptors detect reduced right atrial filling pressure, which stimulates release of antidiuretic hormone (ADH), a potent vasoconstrictor. Renin, released from the kidney in response to renal hypotension, initiates activation of angiotensin II, also a potent vasoconstrictor. Reduced capillary hydrostatic pressure encourages an interstitial to intravascular fluid shift, thereby aiding venous return.

Although neurohumoral compensatory mechanisms improve arterial pressure, apparently stabilizing the patient, occult compromise of vital organs results from reduced perfusion associated with intense arterial vasoconstriction. As shock becomes prolonged, decompensation results from multiple organ failure.

Under physiologic conditions, the heart normally extracts a large portion of the oxygen carried by arterial blood (i.e., large difference in arteriovenous oxygen tension [PO_2]). Oxygen delivery to the heart is therefore critically dependent on coronary blood flow. Reductions in coronary blood flow associated with shock, coupled with increased myocardial oxygen demands secondary to sympathetic-induced increases in heart rate and contractility, result in myocardial ischemia. Multifocal myocardial necrosis results from prolonged ischemia.

Ischemic injury to endothelial cells initiates a series of microvascular changes. Activation of the complement, bradykinin, coagulation, and fibrinolysin cascades results from endothelial damage and exposure of subendothelial tissues to Factor XII. Aggregation of leukocytes and platelets results in release of histamine, serotonin, prostaglandins, and lysosomal enzymes. The eventual result is increased capillary permeability and microvascular sludging.

Renal manifestations of shock are essentially those of acute renal failure. Oliguria results from a disproportionate decrease in urine production compared with renal blood flow. A diminished ratio of cortical to medullary perfusion is thought to be responsible.

Dogs are particularly vulnerable to splanchnic ischemia. Gastrointestinal hemorrhagic necrosis results in sequestration of fluid within the bowel as well as endotoxemia. Endotoxemia accelerates microvascular alterations by activation of complement through the alternative pathway. Zymogenic and lysosomal enzymes released from the ischemic pancreas combine to produce myocardial depressant factor, which compounds the negative inotropic effect produced by myocardial ischemia.

Acute respiratory failure occurs as a relatively late sequela to shock. Pulmonary microvascular injury results in interstitial pulmonary edema. Eventually, alveolar collapse results in decreased pulmonary compliance, increased airway resistance, increased work of respiration, and hypoxemia secondary to ventilation-perfusion mismatch.

Ultimately, shock reaches a point of irreversibility. That is, despite apparent improvement with therapy, death will result regardless of therapy. The mechanism of irreversibility is unknown but, in dogs, has been linked to endotoxemia secondary to splanchnic ischemia. At present, irreversibility cannot be clinically recognized, leaving the veterinarian no choice but to initiate therapy and hope that shock has not reached an irreversible stage.

MANAGEMENT

Decompression

The most urgent concern on presentation of a dog with GDV is gastric decompression. Gastric decompression immediately improves cardiac output and arterial blood pressure by relieving caudal vena caval and portal venous occlusion. Gastric decompression is accomplished by passing a small flexible orogastric tube. The tube is passed through a padded mouth speculum held firmly in place by the operator. Physical restraint is used, preferably with the dog placed in a sitting position. Chemical restraint is generally avoided because of the shock condition of the patient. A small orogastric tube can be passed into the stomach regardless of gastric volvulus in the majority of cases. If an orogastric tube will not pass, then intragastric pressure should be reduced by gastrocentesis. Gastrocentesis is performed in an aseptically prepared area caudal to the costal arch on the right flank with two to three 20-gauge hypodermic needles. Relief of intragastric pressure by gastrocentesis will then allow passage of an orogastric tube. Once positioned, the orogastric tube is used to remove as much gastric liquid and gas as possible. Removal of solid gastric contents may be aided by gastric lavage with warm water.

In the event that an orogastric tube cannot be passed following gastrocentesis, the patient should be prepared for immediate exploratory celiotomy. Alternatively, a temporary gastrostomy may be performed if the patient is an unsuitable candidate for anesthesia. (See Treatment of Gastric Dilatation and Torsion in the Dog in *Current Veterinary Therapy VI* for details.) However, it should be emphasized that inability to pass an orogastric tube is rare following adequate gastrocentesis.

Shock Therapy

Shock therapy is instituted immediately after gastric decompression. Intravenous administration of crystalloid fluids constitutes the basis of shock therapy. A balanced electrolyte solution such as lactated Ringer's is generally the crystalloid fluid of choice. Sodium chloride (0.8 per cent) solution is indicated in rare instances of metabolic alkalosis produced by gastric fluid sequestration. Rapid initial administration of crystalloid fluids at 90 ml/kg every 30 minutes is indicated if the patient is in shock. Subsequent fluid therapy must be titrated to the patient's condition. If the patient responds to initial fluid administration as indicated by improvement in the quality of pulse and reduction in the pulse rate, then fluid administration may be reduced to maintenance levels (60 ml/kg/24 hours). However, if clinical signs of shock persist, then fluid administration should continue at a high rate until a response is noted. The packed cell volume (PCV) and total protein should be monitored regularly during fluid therapy for shock. Whole blood or plasma should be administered if PCV falls below 20 per cent or total protein falls below 3.5 gm/dl, respectively. Whole blood should be cross-matched prior to administration, as antigen-antibody complexes associated with a transfusion reaction can accelerate microvascular alterations already present.

Although controversial, corticosteroids are indicated particularly if septic shock is suspected. Either prednisolone sodium succinate (10 mg/kg) or dexamethasone sodium phosphate (4 mg/kg) is thought to be effective. Broad-spectrum systemic antibiotics are also indicated, particularly if sepsis is suspected. Intravenous sodium penicillin G (40,000 U/kg) or ampicillin (22 mg/kg) and gentamicin (2.2 mg/kg) is an effective bactericidal combination. A trimethoprim and sulfonamide combination may also be effective.

Correction of acid-base disorders is ideally based on arterial blood gas analysis. Early cases may present with either metabolic alkalosis or metabolic acidosis. Hypoventilation produced by the distended stomach may complicate the acid-base picture by producing respiratory acidosis. Advanced

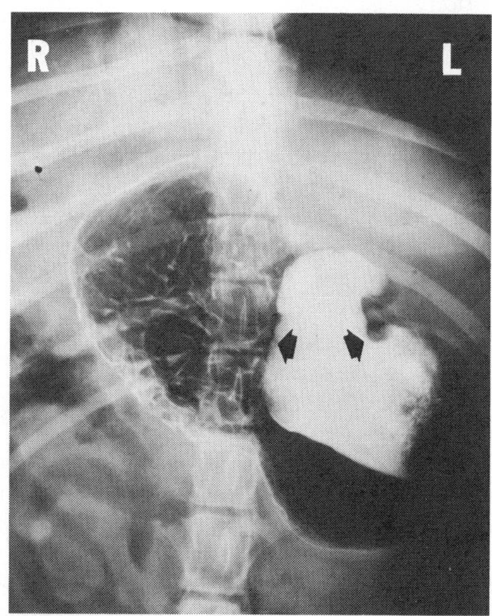

Figure 1. Barium gastrogram of a dog taken after decompression of a gastric dilatation-volvulus. Note that the pylorus (arrows) is located to the left of midline. Any position of the pylorus other than at the far right should be considered abnormal.

cases of GDV invariably show a moderate to severe metabolic acidosis. Bicarbonate therapy is indicated in these cases based on the formula 0.3 × base deficit (mEq/L) × body weight (kg). The calculated bicarbonate dose should be administered by intravenous boluses not larger than 1 mg/kg every 15 minutes. If blood gas analysis is unavailable, then the indiscriminate use of bicarbonate should be avoided because of its potential to cause hyperosmolality, alkalosis, and paradoxical cerebrospinal fluid acidosis. In cases of mild responsive shock, bicarbonate therapy is probably unnecessary. In cases of severe progressive shock, an empirical dose of 1 mg/kg of bicarbonate will likely do more good than harm.

Recent experimental data indicate that nonsteroidal anti-inflammatory drugs such as flunixin meglumine (1.1 mg/kg) administered early in the course of endotoxemia prevent prostaglandin-mediated hypotension. Such data offer hope that microvascular alterations associated with GDV may be improved by flunixin meglumine. However, more data are necessary before a universal recommendation regarding these drugs can be made. Intravenous doses of flunixin meglumine should not be repeated more than twice because of adverse gastrointestinal side effects associated with this drug in the dog.

After gastric decompression and initiation of shock therapy, radiographs may be taken to demonstrate the presence of gastric volvulus. Barium will aid in identifying the position of the pylorus, which is most important in determining the presence of gastric volvulus. Since the stomach may partially derotate after gastric decompression, any pyloric position other than the far right cranial abdominal quadrant must be considered evidence that gastric volvulus existed prior to decompression (Fig. 1). Noncritical evaluation of postdecompression radiographs has contributed to the misconception that gastric dilatation often occurs without gastric volvulus.

Surgery

It is now widely accepted that all dogs experiencing GDV are candidates for exploratory surgery. Controversy arises as to when surgery should be performed. Many clinicians favor a period of stabilization following gastric decompression. It is

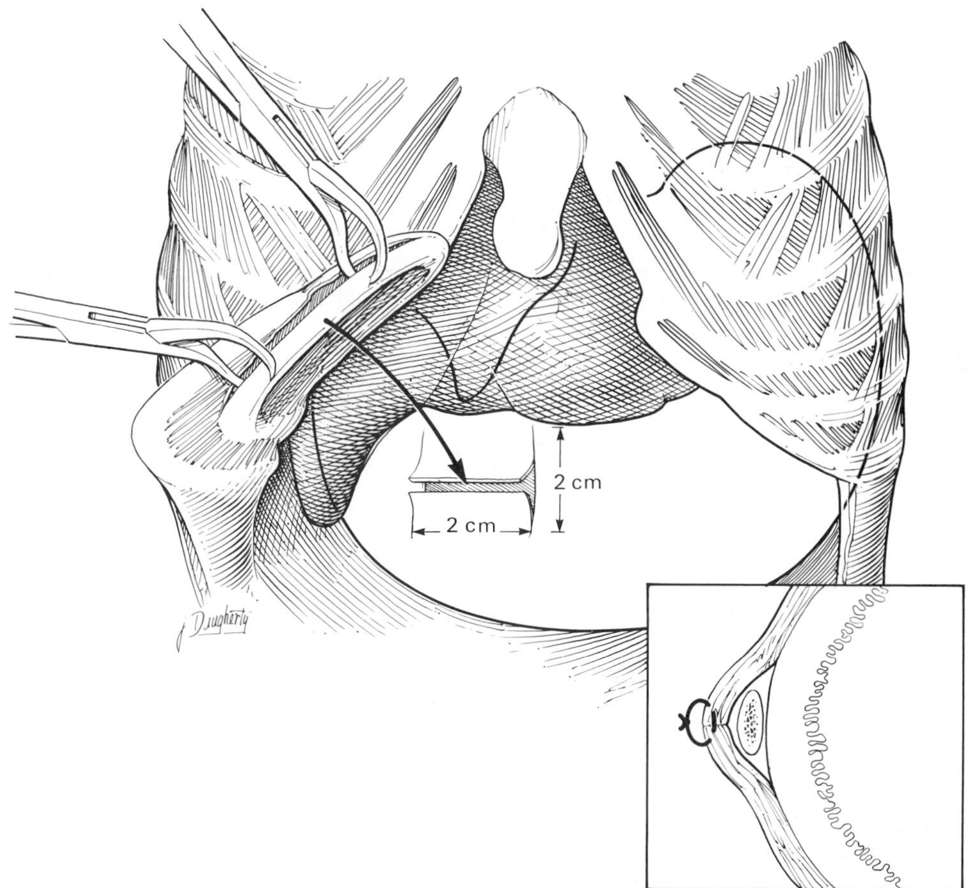

Figure 2. Circumcostal gastropexy. Seromuscular flaps are elevated on the pyloric antrum of the stomach and sutured around rib 11 or 12 (inset) on the right side.

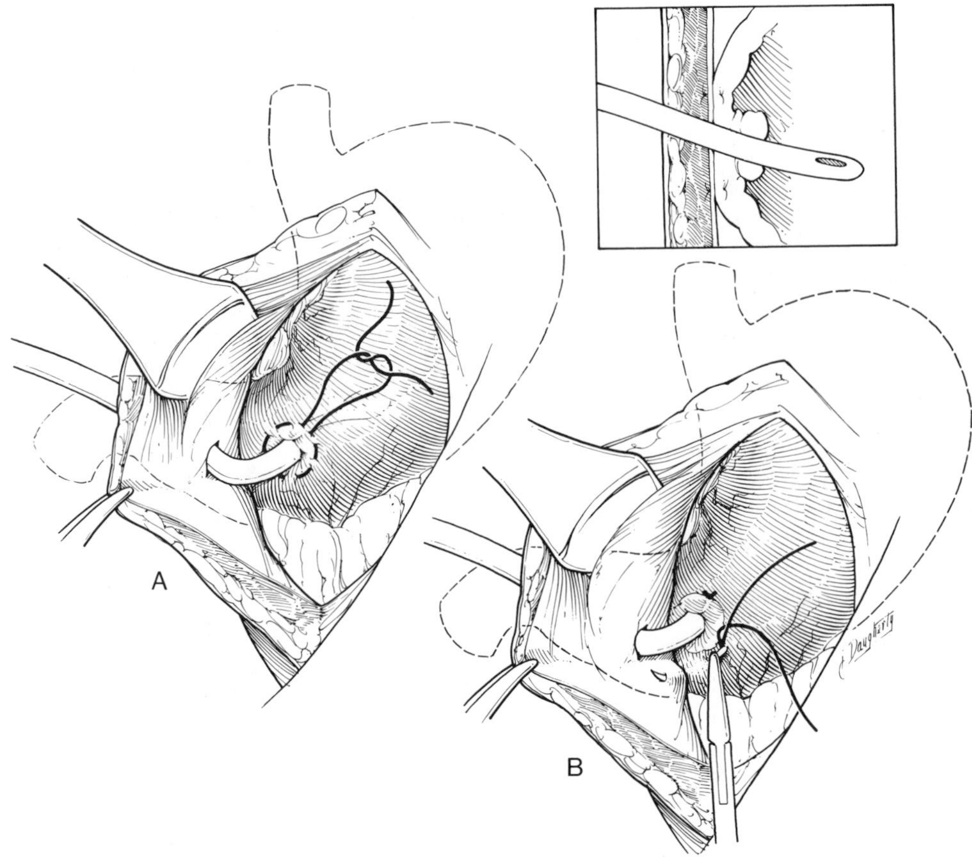

Figure 3. Tube gastrostomy. *A*, The Foley catheter is passed through stab incisions in the right abdominal wall and pyloric antrum of the stomach. *B*, The catheter balloon is inflated (inset) and a gastropexy is performed around the catheter.

thought that once the stomach is decompressed the immediate emergency is over. However, if the gastric muscular wall is necrotic, then the patient will fail to stabilize and is at risk for gastric rupture. The presence of dark hemorrhage in the gastric lavage has been suggested as a barometer of gastric wall necrosis; however, this is not a completely reliable indicator. Since gastric viability cannot be accurately assessed without exploratory surgery, the author favors exploratory surgery approximately 1 hour after gastric decompression and initiation of shock therapy. Additionally, there is currently no evidence that any significant stabilization occurs once effective shock therapy has been administered. In fact, by delaying the surgery, the clinician will likely have to contend with several of the sequelae of shock during the anesthetic period, including ventricular tachyarrhythmias.

Anesthesia must be carefully induced in patients undergoing exploratory surgery for GDV. Thiobarbiturates should be avoided in most cases. Preanesthetic sedation with diazepam or oxymorphone or both followed by mask induction with halothane or isoflurane is a reliable method of induction. Vital signs, electrocardiogram, and blood pressure (direct or indirect) must be monitored during anesthesia and surgery.

Exploratory surgery for GDV has three goals: (1) repositioning of the stomach and spleen, (2) assessment of gastric and splenic viability, and (3) gastropexy. Gastric repositioning is most easily accomplished with the stomach decompressed. Passage of a stomach tube during surgery will allow the surgeon to evacuate the stomach, facilitating repositioning. A surgeon standing on the right side of the patient would reposition the stomach by pulling the pylorus up (toward the incision) and to the right and pushing the fundus down (away from the incision) and to the left. Once the stomach is repositioned, viability of the stomach should be assessed. The surgeon's attention should be directed toward the greater curvature in the areas supplied by the short gastric and left gastroepiploic arteries. Assessment of gastric viability is subjective and is based on color, pulse, and motility of the gastric wall. If gastric wall viability is suspect, then a partial gastrectomy is performed. The spleen must also be carefully assessed for viability. Once repositioned, the spleen should contract somewhat. Thrombosis of the splenic vasculature is indication for splenectomy.

Gastropexy is highly effective in preventing recurrence of GDV and is therefore indicated in all dogs undergoing exploratory surgery for GDV. Circumcostal gastropexy produces an effective long-term gastropexy and is preferred by the author when stomach viability is normal (Fig. 2). Tube gastrostomy also produces a long-term gastropexy and has the added advantage of continuous postoperative decompression (Fig. 3). Tube gastrostomy is preferred for dogs undergoing partial gastrectomy in order to keep the gastrotomy incision completely decompressed during the postoperative period. The tube is left in place at least 5 days postoperatively to ensure adequate adhesion between the stomach and abdominal wall.

POSTOPERATIVE MANAGEMENT

Postoperative management is directed largely toward problems associated with gastric injury and the sequelae to shock. The completeness of postoperative management largely determines the outcome in dogs with GDV. The immediate postoperative period is most critical. Problems that arise during this time and that must be addressed quickly include shock, hypothermia, acidosis, electrolyte imbalance, endotoxemia, septicemia, and hypoventilation.

Fluid therapy is based on the clinical findings. Shock that persists into the postoperative period must be treated vigorously with crystalloid fluids. Whole blood and plasma must be administered to maintain the PCV and total protein above critical levels. Shock doses of corticosteroids may be repeated, particularly if endotoxemia is evident. Systemic antibiotics are generally continued into the postoperative period, particularly if endotoxemia or gastric mucosal compromise is present. Once shock is controlled, intravenous maintenance fluids are indicated until sufficient oral intake is possible, usually 1 to 5 days. Gastric fluid loss during this period should be estimated from the gastrostomy tube and replaced intravenously.

Acid-base balance should be monitored with arterial blood gas analysis when possible. Metabolic acidosis should be corrected with sodium bicarbonate when present. Empirical administration of bicarbonate in the absence of blood gas analysis should be avoided unless moderate to severe progressive shock persists into the postoperative period. Electrolytes should be monitored daily until the patient is eating. A deficit in total body potassium levels is usually present in GDV patients owing to gastrointestinal loss and reduced intake of potassium. Serum potassium levels must be interpreted in light of acid-base abnormalities. Elevations in serum potassium secondary to acidosis may mask a deficit in total body potassium. Potassium chloride should be added to intravenous maintenance fluids until oral intake resumes (Table 1). Intravenous potassium administration should never exceed 0.5 mEq/kg body weight per hour.

Cardiac arrhythmias are a common sequela of GDV. Ventricular tachyarrhythmias including premature ventricular contractions, paroxysmal ventricular tachycardia, and multifocal ventricular tachycardia are most frequently described. Premature atrial depolarization, atrial fibrillation, and sinus bradycardia are also seen. Ventricular tachyarrhythmias are thought to arise from myocardial ischemia secondary to shock and are generally self-limiting in 2 to 4 days. Ventricular tachyarrhythmias should be treated if (1) the origin is multifocal, (2) the rate exceeds 140 bpm, (3) the premature complexes are associated with weak pulse, pulse deficits, or shock, or (4) the complexes demonstrate R on T phenomena. Intravenous lidocaine infusion at 70 to 100 μg/kg/minute is usually an effective method of control. Hypokalemia potentiates ventricular tachyarrhythmias and must be corrected in order for antiarrhythmic therapy to be effective. (See the article on cardiac arrhythmias, page 346, for details regarding therapy.)

Disseminated intravascular coagulation (DIC) is a less common but life-threatening sequela of GDV. Diagnosis of DIC is based on demonstration of several alterations, listed in order of reliability: (1) increased partial thromboplastin time, (2) decreased antithrombin III, (3) increased prothrombin time, (4) decreased platelet count, (5) red blood cell fragments on blood smear, (6) decreased fibrinogen, and (7) increased fibrin degradation products. The treatment of DIC remains controversial. Early low-grade DIC (hypercoagulable phase) may be controlled with low-dose heparin therapy (50 to 100 U/kg SC t.i.d.). Acute florid DIC (consumptive phase) requires the administration of fresh cross-matched whole blood. Continued hemorrhage following whole blood transfusion is indication for

Table 1. *Potassium Chloride Supplementation*

Serum K^+ (mEq/L)	KCl Added to Maintenance Fluids*
>3.5	Add 5 mEq/250 ml
3.0–3.4	Add 7 mEq/250 ml
2.5–2.9	Add 10 mEq/250 ml
<2.4	Add 12 mEq/250 ml

*Administration rate is 60 ml/kg/24 hours.

high-dose heparin therapy (300 to 400 U/kg SC t.i.d.).

References and Supplemental Reading

Fallah, A. M., Lumb, W. V., Nelson, A. W., et al.: Circumcostal gastropexy in the dog: A preliminary study. Vet. Surg. 11:9, 1982.
Muir, W. W.: Acid base and electrolyte disturbances in dogs with gastric dilatation-volvulus. J.A.V.A.M.A. 181:229, 1982.
Muir, W. W.: Gastric dilatation-volvulus in the dog, with emphasis on cardiac arrhythmias. J.A.V.M.A. 180:739, 1982.
Orton, E. C., and Muir, W. W.: Hemodynamics during experimental gastric dilatation-volvulus in dogs. Am. J. Vet. Res. 44:1512, 1983.
Parks, J. L., and Greene, R. W.: Tube gastrostomy for the treatment of gastric volvulus. J. Am. Anim. Hosp. Assoc. 12:168, 1976.
Wingfield, W. E., Betts, C. W., and Rawlings, C. A.: Pathophysiology associated with gastric dilatation-volvulus in the dog. J. Am. Anim. Hosp. Assoc. 12:136, 1976.

THERAPEUTICS OF GASTROINTESTINAL DISEASES*

ROBERT C. DENOVO, JR., D.V.M.
Knoxville, Tennessee

The gastrointestinal tract is a complex and highly integrated system that is easily disrupted by a multitude of diseases. Frequently, the exact cause of disease is undetermined, making specific therapy impossible. Indeed, the emphasis of management of gastrointestinal disease is too often directed toward symptomatic control of vomiting and diarrhea and less attention is paid to the etiology of the illness. Primary efforts in the management of gastrointestinal disorders should always be directed toward localizing disease to a particular portion of the gut and determining a cause. A more rational therapeutic plan can then be formulated.

This article describes the uses of a variety of drugs for the treatment of gastrointestinal disorders. The categories of drugs include antibiotics, antiemetics, antacids, antidiarrheals, absorbents, antisecretories, and corticosteroids. Effective use of these drugs requires knowledge of diseases affecting the gastrointestinal tract, an understanding of the pathophysiology involved, and an understanding of mechanisms of drug actions on the gut.

ANTIMICROBIALS

The proper role of antimicrobial drugs in the treatment of most gastrointestinal diseases remains the subject of controversy. Antibiotics unfortunately continue to be used in the routine management of both acute and chronic gastrointestinal diseases with little regard for potential adverse effects. Primary bacterial infection is not a major cause of gastrointestinal disease in dogs and cats; however, the potential for secondary bacterial invasion is a valid therapeutic concern. When using antimicrobials, one must consider their effects on the normal microflora within the lumen and the microflora adhering to the mucus layer of the wall of the intestinal tract. This resident flora is composed of a stable system of aerobic and anaerobic microbes that are a vital component of the mucosal defense barrier. The flora compete with pathogenic bacteria for receptor sites on epithelial cells. Few bacterial pathogens can successfully compete with the normal flora and colonize the intestinal wall (Simon and Gorback, 1982). Antimicrobials can significantly damage the protective flora and allow invasion of antibiotic-resistant strains of pathogenic bacteria. Consideration must also be given to the increased pool of resistant organisms created through the use of antimicrobial agents. Bacterial plasmids, extrachromosomal units of DNA that contain genetic information for antibiotic resistance, can pass from one bacterium to another. The mechanism of plasmid resistance to one drug can also produce cross-resistance to other antimicrobial agents. Therefore, selection for plasmid-induced resistance by the use of one drug could result in the development of resistance to a number of antibiotics.

Despite the potential deleterious effects of the use of antimicrobials in gastrointestinal disorders,

---

**Editor's Note:* A number of the drugs in this article do *not* have Food and Drug Administration clearance for the veterinary uses described by the author. He has used them carefully for clinical trials with the owners' prior informed consent. Readers are cautioned to use similar discretion until such time as official approval may be granted for their routine use.

there are specific conditions in which their use is justified. Dosages of selected antibiotics are listed in Table 1.

Acute Gastroenteritis

In general, antibiotics should be used only in those patients in which damage to the intestinal mucosal barrier has resulted in bloody diarrhea (hemorrhagic gastroenteritis, canine parvovirus, and feline panleukopenia), and in cases of enterocolitis in which systemic involvement is evidenced by fever, congested mucous membranes, leukocytosis, or leukopenia. The aggressive treatment of such high-risk patients, when septicemia is a potential outcome, should include parenteral antibiotics effective against both gram-negative bacteria and gram-positive anaerobes. A combination of an aminoglycoside such as gentamicin or kanamycin with ampicillin is therapeutically and economically effective. The unpredictable absorption of oral antibiotics by the diseased intestinal mucosa precludes their use by this route. When using aminoglycosides in diarrheic animals especially susceptible to rapid fluid loss, supportive intravenous fluid therapy is necessary to maintain good hydration, thereby reducing the potential of nephrotoxicity. Puppies and kittens are more susceptible to the nephrotoxic effects of aminoglycosides. Spectinomycin is a viable alternative in such cases. This drug has a spectrum similar to the aminoglycosides against gram-negative organisms and is also effective against gram-positive streptococci and staphylococci, as well as mycoplasma. The primary advantage of this drug is its lack of nephrotoxicity.

Infectious Gastroenteritis

The role of enteropathogenic bacteria as a primary cause of canine and feline gastrointestinal disorders is unclear. Potential pathogens capable of causing enteric disease by either invading the mucosal cells or via the release of toxins include enteropathogenic *Escherichia coli, Salmonella* spp., *Yersinia enterocolitica, Campylobacter jejuni, Clostridium* spp., *Bacillus piliformis* (Tyzzer's disease), and *Staphylococcus* spp. Of particular importance to the veterinary practitioner are *Salmonella, Campylobacter,* and *Yersinia,* which are significant human pathogens. Household pets infected with these organisms have been implicated as sources of human infection. Nonsymptomatic and especially diarrheic animals

Table 1. *Selected Antibiotics Used in the Treatment of Gastrointestinal Diseases of Dogs and Cats*

Drug	Suggested Dosage for Dogs (D) and Cats (C)	Comments
Acute Gastroenteritis		
Ampicillin	11 mg/kg every 6 hours IV, IM, SC (D,C)	Combine with aminoglycoside for systemic infections.
Gentamicin	2.2 mg/kg every 8 hours IV, IM, SC (D,C)	Maintain adequate hydration. Evaluate renal function (urinalysis and BUN) every 48 hours. *Campylobacter* and *Yersinia* usually sensitive. Combine with cephalosporin for systemic salmonellosis.
Spectinomycin	5–12 mg/kg every 12 hours IM (D,C)	Possible alternative to aminoglycoside, especially in young animals.
Trimethoprim-sulfadiazine	15 mg/kg every 12 hours IV, IM, PO (D,C)	Long-term (60-day) therapy may eliminate carrier state of salmonellosis. *Yersinia* usually sensitive.
Erythromycin	10 mg/kg every 8 hours PO (D,C)	May cause nausea and vomiting. Five to 7 days of therapy eliminate *Campylobacter* infections.
Chloramphenicol	50 mg/kg every 8 hours IV, IM, SC, PO (D) 50 mg/kg every 8 hours PO (C) 50 mg/kg every 12 hours IV, IM, SC, (C)	*Salmonella, Campylobacter, Yersinia* usually sensitive.
Chronic Enterocolitis		
Sulfasalazine	10–15 mg/kg every 6 hours PO (D)	Safe dosage for cats not established. Adverse effects are uncommon (vomiting, jaundice, keratoconjunctivitis sicca, hemolytic anemia, leukopenia).
Tylosin (powdered)	20–40 mg/kg every 12 hours PO (D) 5–10 mg/kg every 12 hours PO (C)	One teaspoon supplies approximately 400 mg tylosin. Mix thoroughly with food to camouflage bitter taste.
Metronidazole	60 mg/kg every 24 hours PO for 5 days (D,C) 10–15 mg/kg every 12 hours PO (D)	For treatment of giardiasis. For long-term treatment of chronic inflammatory bowel diseases. May cause anorexia and vomiting. Neurologic signs (ataxia, muscular rigidity, seizures) occur if 75 mg/kg/day is given.

harboring these organisms are potential public health risks. Antibiotic therapy should be considered if any one of these organisms is isolated from the feces of a diarrheic dog or cat.

Chronic Enterocolitis

Sulfasalazine (Azulfidine, Pharmacia) is a combination of sulfapyridine and the anti-inflammatory drug 5-aminosalicylate. This drug is the mainstay of therapy in the treatment of active ulcerative and granulomatous colitis in humans and has been used indefinitely to prevent relapse (Korelitz, 1980). Colonic bacteria cleave this compound, liberating the sulfapyridine and the active salicylate. The sulfapyridine is well absorbed in the colon and excreted in the urine and appears to have little therapeutic or antibacterial effect in the treatment of chronic colitis. The 5-aminosalicylate binds to colonic connective tissue, where it exerts an anti-inflammatory effect, presumably by interfering with prostaglandin synthesis. The combination of the sulfa with the salicylate primarily serves as a means of delivering the salicylate to the colon while preventing its absorption in the small intestine. No controlled studies exist on the efficacy of this drug in the treatment of chronic ulcerative colitis in dogs. However, good clinical results with sulfasalazine in the dog have been obtained, and it is considered by most to be the drug of choice in treatment of chronic ulcerative colitis. Response to sulfasalazine is variable and depends on the severity and duration of disease prior to diagnosis. Most dogs have a favorable response within the first 3 to 4 weeks of treatment. Others may require several months of treatment. Extremely severe cases might benefit from the judicious use of corticosteroids, given either systemically or as retention enemas in addition to the sulfasalazine (see later discussion of corticosteroids). Immunosuppressive therapy is potentially harmful to patients with severe ulcerative colitis and should not be used until sulfasalazine and antibiotics have been given an adequate therapeutic trial.

The macrolide antibiotic tylosin has been used empirically to treat a variety of inflammatory diseases of both the large and small bowel (plasmacytic-lymphocytic enteritis, eosinophilic gastroenterocolitis, chronic ulcerative colitis, feline colitis, bacterial overgrowth). Tylosin is effective against a spectrum of gram-positive and gram-negative bacteria in addition to mycoplasma and chlamydia. It is conceivable that any of these microbes could contribute to or perpetuate chronic inflammatory diseases of the intestine, which might explain the reported efficacy of tylosin in such instances. The author's results with the use of tylosin have been extremely unpredictable.

Metronidazole (Flagyl, Searle & Co.) is a unique antibiotic that has also been used in the treatment of nonspecific inflammatory bowel diseases. In addition to its antibacterial action against anaerobes, it is an effective antiprotozoal drug against *Giardia*. Metronidazole also suppresses cell-mediated immune responses and prevents granuloma formation in the bowel. The beneficial effects of this drug in the treatment of inflammatory bowel diseases are most likely related to its action against anaerobes that predominate in the large bowel. Anaerobes have been implicated both as causative organisms and likely secondary invaders perpetuating the inflammatory response of the bowel. Undoubtedly, some chronic small bowel diarrheas successfully treated with metronidazole were caused by undiagnosed *Giardia* infections. *Giardia* in dogs and cats with chronic small bowel diarrhea is difficult to identify. Therefore, clinical response to a 5-day therapeutic trial of metronidazole is a rational diagnostic and therapeutic approach.

Documented efficacy of metronidazole in the treatment of chronic small and large bowel diseases in dogs and cats is lacking. The author has observed therapeutic benefit from metronidazole in the treatment of chronic ulcerative colitis in several dogs that have been refractory to treatment with immunosuppressants, sulfasalazine, antibiotics, and dietary manipulation. In such instances, long-term low-dosage (10 to 15 mg/kg every 12 hours) metronidazole has been used for as long as 8 weeks without significant adverse effects. Metronidazole is also effective in the treatment of bacterial overgrowth syndromes and in the management of perianal abcesses and fistulas when anaerobic bacteria predominate.

ANTIEMETICS

The therapeutic goal in the management of the vomiting animal should always be directed at diagnosis of the primary disorder. Since vomiting is only a clinical sign, pharmacologic control of vomiting may mask the primary disease and delay the diagnosis of potentially fatal disorders such as intestinal obstruction. In general, antiemetics should be used in situations in which the underlying disorder has been diagnosed or when the vomiting is so profuse that fluid, electrolyte, and acid-base balance is difficult to control.

All vomiting is mediated through the vomiting center located in the lateral reticular formation of the brain stem. The vomiting center can be stimulated directly by blood-borne drugs and toxins or indirectly by afferent impulses from the cerebral cortex, the chemoreceptor trigger zone (CRTZ), and through a variety of peripheral receptors located primarily in the pharynx and abdominal viscera.

The importance of input to the vomiting center from the cerebral cortex is poorly understood in domestic animals and probably is of little therapeutic consequence. The CRTZ is located in the floor of the fourth ventricle of the brain and is stimulated by blood-borne chemical substances such as metabolic toxins (ketones, uremic toxins), bacterial toxins, and drugs (cardiac glycosides, antineoplastics, and apomorphine). The CRTZ is also stimulated by impulses from the vestibular apparatus, which is carried to the CRTZ via the eighth cranial nerve as a result of motion sickness or inflammatory vestibular disease. The most abundant peripheral receptors are located in the abdominal viscera, especially the stomach and proximal small intestine, but also in the visceral peritoneum and genitourinary tract. Stimulation of these peripheral receptors occurs primarily in response to inflammation, distension, and rapid changes in osmolality. Afferent impulses from the abdominal viscera to the vomiting center are mediated primarily through the vagus nerve with some sympathetic input (Cornelius, 1982).

Phenothiazines

The centrally acting phenothiazine derivatives are the most effective antiemetics, suppressing both the vomiting center and the CRTZ. At the suggested dosages, these drugs should have minimal tranquilizing effects. The major disadvantages of phenothiazines are (1) their hypotensive effect, caused by alpha-adrenergic blocking and subsequent arteriolar vasodilation and (2) their inability to block visceral afferent (vagal) impulses associated with severe visceral pain and contractions. Phenothiazines should not be included in the therapeutic regimen until adequate fluid therapy has corrected dehydration. Commonly used phenothiazine antiemetics and suggested dosages are listed in Table 2. Phenothiazines can cause some depression in systemically ill animals and potentiate the effects of other central nervous system (CNS) depressants. These drugs also carry a warning suggesting that they might contribute to acute liver failure in children. Accordingly, these drugs should not be used if a hepatopathy is suspected.

Antihistamines

Antihistamines inhibit the CRTZ and depress input from the vestibular apparatus. In general, these compounds seem to be less effective than the phenothiazine antiemetics and are used primarily for motion sickness. Trimethabenzamide (Tigan, Beecham Laboratories) has actions similar to the antihistamines, blocking the CRTZ. This drug is effective against vomiting caused by metabolic toxins and drugs. However, the author's experience with this drug is one of inconsistent responses.

Parasympatholytics

The parasympatholytics are a class of drugs often misused as antiemetics. These drugs do decrease visceral motility, smooth muscle spasms, and gastrointestinal secretions that may contribute to vomiting. However, they can enhance further vomiting and diarrhea by producing gastric atony and ileus. Parasympatholytic drugs are most effective as antiemetics when used in combination with centrally acting phenothiazines in the control of vomiting associated with severe gastrointestinal disease. Darbazine (Norden) combines the parasympatholytic drug isopropamide, which inhibits visceral afferent impulses mediated by the vagus nerve, with the phenothiazine prochlorperazine. Such combinations are especially useful in cases of severe vomiting associated with acute pancreatitis, when the parasympatholytic drug has the additional effect of decreasing pancreatic secretions. Adverse effects other than gastric distension and ileus include urine retention, increased ocular pressures, and constipation. Caution should be used if gastric outlet obstruction, intestinal obstruction, glaucoma, or urinary retention disorders are suspected. Examples and dosages of parasympatholytic drugs and combinations can be found in Table 2.

Metoclopramide

Metoclopramide (Reglan, Robins) is a new antiemetic drug that is rapidly gaining popularity in veterinary gastrointestinal therapeutics. This drug is a derivative of procainamide and has both central and peripheral effects on the gastrointestinal system. Metoclopramide is a potent antiemetic whose effect is believed to be mediated by antidopaminergic actions at the CRTZ. Peripherally, this drug appears to sensitize the smooth muscle of the distal esophagus, stomach, and proximal small intestine to the effects of acetylcholine. These actions result in an increased lower esophageal pressure and increased strength of esophageal contractions, contributing to the competence of the lower esophageal sphincter. Metoclopramide increases gastric antral contractions, promotes relaxation of the pylorus, and increases smooth muscle contraction in the proximal small intestine. This enhances coordination of antral and duodenal contractions, with subsequent acceleration of gastric emptying and small intestinal transit. Metoclopramide has little effect on colonic motility and no effect on emptying of the gallbladder. This drug does not alter gastric or intestinal secretion or intestinal absorption of fluid.

Table 2. Antiemetic Drugs Used in Dogs and Cats

Generic Name	Product (Mfg.)	Suggested Dosage for Dogs (D) and Cats (C)	Comments
Phenothiazines			Block both vomiting center and CRTZ. May cause hypotension. Do not use with hepatopathy. Parenteral, oral, and suppository forms available.
Triethylperazine	Torecan (Sandoz)	0.25 mg/kg every 8 hours IM (D) 0.5 mg/kg every 8 hours rectal (D) 0.125 mg/kg every 8 hours IM (C)	Most effective antiemetic of those listed.
Chlorpromazine	Thorazine (SmithKline Beckman)	0.5 mg/kg every 8 hours IM (D,C) 1.0 mg/kg every 8 hours rectal (D)	
Prochlorperazine	Compazine (SmithKline Beckman)	0.1 mg/kg every 6 hours IM (D,C)	
Antihistamines			Block CRTZ and vestibular input. Effective for motion sickness if given prior to travel.
Diphenhydramine	Benadryl (Parke-Davis)	2.0–4.0 mg/kg every 8 hours PO (D,C) 2.0 mg/kg every 8 hours IM (D,C)	
Dimenhydrinate	Dramamine (Searle)	8 mg/kg every 8 hours PO (D,C)	
Trimethobenzamine	Tigan (Beecham Laboratories)	3 mg/kg every 8 hours IM (D)	No experience with use in cats.
Parasympatholytics			Of questionable efficacy in the control of vomiting; will decrease gastrointestinal spasms and secretions; avoid use for more than 48 hours.
Propantheline	Pro-Banthine (Searle)	0.25 mg/kg every 8 hours PO (D,C)	
Isopropamide	Darbid (SmithKline Beckman)	0.2–1.0 mg/kg every 12 hours PO (D,C)	
Methscopolamine	Pamine (Upjohn)	0.3–1.5 mg/kg every 8 hours PO (D)	Not recommended for cats.
Combination Phenothiazine and Parasympatholytic			
Prochlorperazine and isopropamide	Darbazine (Norden)	0.5–0.8 mg/kg every 12 hours IM, SC, (D,C)	Especially effective if vomiting is associated with severe gastrointestinal pain or spasms.
Procainamide Derivative			
Metoclopramide	Reglan (Robins)	0.2–0.5 mg/kg every 8 hours PO, SC (D,C)	For gastric motility disorders and reflux esophagitis, give 30 minutes prior to meals and at bedtime.
		1–2 mg/kg every 24 hours as a slow IV infusion can be used for severe emesis	Quickly eliminated by IV route. Adverse effects seen at dosage greater than 1 mg/kg (see text).

Metoclopramide is excreted primarily unchanged in the urine (Albibi and McCallum, 1983).

There are numerous clinical applications of metoclopramide in dogs and cats. Generally, it is useful in the management of severe vomiting associated with cancer chemotherapy, acute viral enteritis, or nonspecific gastritis. This drug is particularly useful in the treatment of gastroesophageal reflux and gastric motility disorders. Animals with decreased gastric emptying, which occurs in association with inflammatory gastrointestinal disorders, gastric ulcers and neoplasia, hypokalemia, and chronic gastric dilatation (without volvulus), will benefit from the use of this drug. Metoclopramide enhances recovery in the postoperative gastric volvulus patient with gastric paresis. A good clinical response to metoclopramide supports a diagnosis of pyloric stenosis and is helpful in the medical management of this condition. A canine syndrome has been described, characterized by chronic, intermittent vomiting of bile-tinged fluid, often in the early morning. These dogs are otherwise healthy, and the vomiting is attributed to abnormal gastric motility (Twedt, 1983). A bedtime dose of metoclopramide to stimulate upper gastrointestinal motility and decrease duodenal-gastric reflux of bile has been reported to effectively eliminate the vomiting in such instances (Tams, 1984). Metoclopramide can be used in endoscopic examinations to facilitate passage through the pylorus.

Metoclopramide is contraindicated whenever increased gastrointestinal motility might be harmful, as in gastric outlet obstructions or potential gut perforation. The drug should not be used in epileptics since it may increase the frequency of seizures. Therapeutic dosages of metoclopramide may infrequently result in mental changes ranging from hyperactivity to depression. Cats will infrequently show disoriented or frenzied behavior. Because of the potential for enhanced CNS effects, this drug should not be given with phenothiazines or narcotic analgesics. Most adverse effects resolve when the metoclopramide is discontinued. Anticholinergic drugs such as atropine block the effects of metoclopramide on gastrointestinal motility. Dosages are listed in Table 2.

ANTACIDS AND ANTIULCER MEDICATIONS

The ability of the stomach to withstand the cell-damaging effects of concentrated hydrochloric acid and of the proteolytic enzyme pepsin is attributed to the gastric mucosal barrier. This barrier is composed of the gastric mucosa and its covering mucus layer. It can be damaged by (1) a variety of drugs (aspirin, corticosteroids, phenylbutazone, flunixin), (2) alterations of the gastric mucosal microcirculation (hypotension, shock, sepsis), (3) the reflux of bile and pancreatic enzymes, (4) metabolic toxins (uremia), and (5) hypersecretion of acid (uremia, liver failure, mastocytosis, gastrinoma). Such damage allows luminal acid to diffuse back through the gastric mucosal cells and into the submucosa. Subsequently, tissue mast cells in the submucosa degranulate, releasing histamine. The histamine stimulates more acid production by the gastric parietal cells, enhancing inflammation and edema in the submucosa. The goal of antacid therapy is to reduce the total amount of gastric acid, thereby interrupting this cycle of events. Antacids can also diminish the proteolytic effects of pepsin by inactivating pepsin when gastric pH is 6 or greater. Mild astringent properties of some antacids enhance mucus secretion by the gastric mucosal cells. Generally, antacids are not used in cases of simple acute gastritis. However, they are definitely indicated in the treatment of serious gastric and duodenal bleeding or ulceration (see above). Additionally, antacid therapy is central to the management of reflux esophagitis to neutralize gastric acid, reduce esophageal inflammation, and indirectly increase lower esophageal pressure.

Nonsystemic Antacids

Nonsystemic antacids include a variety of oral preparations containing aluminum hydroxide, calcium carbonate, and magnesium compounds. The efficacy of nonsystemic antacids is determined primarily by the duration of retention in the stomach and by the characteristics of acid secretion (Morrissey and Barreras, 1974). Since acid secretion is more intermittent in dogs than in humans, administration of antacids is probably not indicated at hourly intervals as is suggested for active ulceration in humans. Yet, to be effective and to avoid rebound hypersecretion of acid, administration every 3 to 4 hours is optimal for dogs. The most common side effects of antacids are the constipation caused by the calcium- and aluminum-containing antacids and the laxative effect of the magnesium products. The high absorbability of calcium makes the calcium carbonate products undesirable. Hypercalcemia can occur, resulting in impaired renal function. Dietary calcium also stimulates gastrin secretion. Aluminum-containing products bind phosphate in the gastrointestinal tract, preventing its absorption and increasing fecal excretion of phosphorus. Such aluminum products are especially useful in patients with uremic gastropathy because they reduce the hyperphosphatemia of renal failure in addition to having antacid effects. Most of the nonsystemic antacids have absorbent properties and decrease the bioavailability of concurrently administered drugs.

Systemic Antacids

Gastric parietal cells contain unique receptors for histamine that, when occupied by histamine and in the presence of acetylcholine and gastrin, will stimulate maximal acid secretion. These histamine (H_2) receptors are not affected by common antihistamines but are competitively blocked by the drug cimetidine (Tagamet, SmithKline Beckman), resulting in a 70 to 90 per cent decrease of acid secretion. Cimetidine is most beneficial in the treatment of gastric and duodenal ulceration secondary to renal failure, liver disease, mast cell tumors, and gastrinomas. A combination of cimetidine and metoclopramide is particularly effective in the management of esophagitis associated with persistent vomiting, gastroesophageal reflux, foreign body–induced trauma, and surgical manipulations. Cimetidine is considered an effective adjunct to enzyme replacement therapy in pancreatic exocrine insufficiency, presumably by decreasing gastric acid inactivation of orally administered enzymes (Pidgeon, 1983). There are no specific contraindications to the use of cimetidine in dogs. Cimetidine alters hepatic microsomal enzyme systems, decreasing the hepatic metabolism of warfarin-type anticoagulants, phenytoin, propranolol, and diazepam, resulting in delayed elimination of these drugs. The clinical significance of such interactions in dogs is unknown. The dosage of cimetidine in dogs and cats is 5 to 10 mg/kg every 6 to 8 hours orally. A slow intravenous infusion (30 minutes) of 10 mg/kg every 6 hours can be used if oral dosing is not tolerated. A cimetidine analogue, ranitidine (Zantac, Glaxo), has the treatment advantage of only being required twice daily in dogs.

Sucralfate

Sucralfate (Carafate, Marion) is a relatively new antiulcer drug that has received minimal evaluation in veterinary medicine. This drug accelerates the healing of gastric and duodenal ulcers by local rather than systemic effects. Sucralfate forms a complex with proteinaceous exudates that adheres to the ulcer crater. This complex provides an effective barrier to the penetration of gastric acid. Additionally, sucralfate inhibits pepsin and adsorbs significant amounts of bile acids that can cause gastric mucosal damage. Sucralfate has no acid-neutralizing capacity and reduces the bioavailability of cimetidine, phenytoin, and tetracycline. This binding effect can be avoided by not administering other drugs within 2 hours of treatment with sucralfate. Adverse reactions to this drug in human clinical trials have been infrequent and minor. Constipation is the most frequent complaint. Limited use of this drug in dogs and cats precludes any statement as to efficacy, but this drug may be a valuable adjunct in the management of gastric and duodenal ulcers. The recommended adult human dose is 1 gm, 4 times per day. No significant drug-related toxicity was observed in dogs at a dosage as large as 2 gm/kg/day. One could extrapolate that a dose of 250 mg 4 times per day would be safe for use in a 15-kg (32-lb) dog.

ANTIDIARRHEAL DRUGS

The rational approach to the management of diarrhea requires an understanding of the mechanisms that contribute to increased fecal water content, fecal volume, and frequency of defecations. Most diarrheal syndromes involve combinations of the following mechanisms: (1) altered osmotic gradients resulting from maldigested and malabsorbed nutrients remaining within the lumen of the bowel and exerting marked osmotic and laxative effects, (2) hypersecretion caused by bacterial enterotoxins that stimulate cyclic adenosine monophosphate–mediated secretion of fluid and electrolytes from the enterocyte, (3) increased permeability as a result of structural damage to the gut wall from inflammatory, infectious, and neoplastic diseases, and (4) changes in gut motility that result in decreased transit time of ingesta through the gastrointestinal tract. Motility refers to two types of movements. Peristalsis is the longitudinal wave of constriction that provides the propulsive force to move ingesta in the aboral direction. Segmentation is the concentric contraction of intestinal smooth muscle that functions to mix nutrients and increase resistance to the passage of ingesta. The role of altered motility in the pathogenesis of most diarrheal diseases is not fully defined. However, hypomotility is the usual event associated with diarrhea. This mechanistic classification helps to clarify the rationale of therapeutic manipulations used in the management of diarrhea. Suggested dosages of antidiarrheal drugs are listed in Table 3.

Motility-Modifying Drugs

NARCOTIC ANALGESICS

Narcotic analgesics are the most effective drugs for the symptomatic treatment of diarrhea and include the opiates paregoric and codeine and certain synthetic narcotics such as diphenoxylate (Lomotil, Searle & Co.) and loperamide (Imodium, Ortho Pharmaceutical). The antidiarrheal effects of these drugs are attributed to their direct action on the smooth muscle of the small intestine and colon, causing increased tone and segmentation. This produces increased resistance to luminal transit of ingesta. These drugs effectively relieve abdominal pain and tenesmus and reduce the frequency of stools. No direct effect on electrolyte transport has been reported. However, decreased fecal loss of sodium, potassium, and water has been determined in some human patients, suggesting that these drugs possibly inhibit intestinal secretions and enhance fluid absorption. A variety of antidiarrheal preparations containing narcotics are available. Paregoric is commonly used and contains 2 mg of morphine per 5 ml, making this an especially useful drug when treating dogs weighing less than 10 kg (22 lb). Other antidiarrheal preparations such as Donnagel–PG (Robins; powdered opium, atropine, hyoscyamine, kaolin, and pectin) and Parepectolin (Rorer; paregoric, pectin, and kaolin) are available but offer little benefit over paregoric. The synthetic narcotics diphenoxylate and loperamide have gastrointestinal effects similar to those of the opiates. To decrease the potential for drug abuse, diphenoxylate is marketed in combination with a subtherapeutic amount of atropine, which can cause dry mouth and tachycardia if overdosed. Loperamide reportedly acts more promptly and lasts longer that diphenoxylate and also carries less risk of causing central narcotic effects.

The opiates have limitations as antidiarrheal agents. They are Schedule V drugs subject to controlled substances regulations of the FDA. Adverse effects include constipation, bloating, and sedation. Diphenoxylate in particular has been shown to prolong the diarrhea and systemic symptoms of infectious diarrhea in humans and may also induce toxic dilatation of the colon in patients with inflammatory bowel disease. These drugs may potentiate the effects of barbiturates and tranquilizers. These drugs probably should not be used in cats.

Table 3. Drugs Used to Control Diarrhea in Dogs and Cats

Generic Name	Product (Mfg.)	Suggested Dosage for Dogs (D) and Cats (C)	Comments
Narcotic Analgesics			Contraindicated with infectious diarrheas and with liver disease. NOT recommended for use in cats. Avoid use for more than 48 hours.
Paregoric		0.05–0.06 mg/kg every 8 hours PO (D)	Useful when treating dogs weighing less than 10 kg.
Codeine		0.25–0.5 mg/kg every 8 hours PO (D)	
Diphenoxylate	Lomotil (Searle & Co.)	0.1 mg/kg every 6–8 hours PO (D)	
Loperamide	Imodium (Ortho Pharmaceutical)	0.08 mg/kg every 8 hours PO (D)	Supplied as 2-mg capsules, which are too large for dogs weighing less than 25 kg.
Anticholinergics			Contraindicated in gastrointestinal obstructions, infectious enteritis, glaucoma, obstructive uropathy. Avoid use for more than 48 hours.
Propantheline	Probanthine (Searle & Co.)	0.25 mg/kg every 8 hours PO (D,C)	
Isopropamide	Darbid (SmithKline Beckman)	0.2–1.0 mg/kg every 12 hours PO (D,C)	
Dicyclomide	Bentyl (Merrell-National)	0.15 mg/kg every 8 hours PO (pediatric dosage)	No well-established dosage for dogs.
Combination CNS Depressant and Anticholinergic			
Prochlorperazine and isopropamide	Darbazine (Norden)	0.5–0.8 mg/kg every 12 hours IM, SC (D) 0.2–1.0 mg/kg every 8 hours PO (D)	Similar precautions as for anticholinergics.
Chlordiazepoxide and clidinium	Librax (Roche)	1–2 tabs every 8–12 hours PO (D)	Not recommended for dogs weighing less than 10 kg.
Antisecretory Preparation			
Bismuth subsalicylate	Pepto-Bismol (Norwich-Eaton)	0.25 ml/kg every 4–6 hours PO (D)	May impart dark color to feces; could be misinterpreted as melena.
Combination Antisecretory/Narcotic Analgesic			
Bismuth subsalicylate/paregoric	Corrective Mixture with Paregoric (Beecham Laboratories)	0.25 ml/kg PO initially; then ½ original dose every 4 hours	As above.

ANTICHOLINERGICS AND ANTISPASMODICS

Anticholinergic and related antispasmodic drugs have an uncertain role in the management of diarrhea. Anticholinergics block the effect of acetylcholine, the major neurotransmitter of the gastrointestinal smooth muscle, resulting in both decreased peristalsis and decreased segmentation. Current evidence suggests that most diarrheal diseases are characterized by hypomotility, an effect enhanced by anticholinergics. Although controlled studies on the efficacy of this class of drugs are lacking, these agents may benefit some diarrheic patients by decreasing fluid secretion and improving intestinal absorption.

Naturally occurring belladonna alkaloids such as atropine are generally not used as antidiarrheal drugs because of their short half-life. The synthetic anticholinergics propantheline and isopropamide have a longer duration of effect than the naturally occurring alkaloids. These drugs cause more side effects because they also interfere with the actions of acetylcholine at the autonomic ganglia (nicotinic receptors). Dicyclomine (Bentyl, Merrell-National), an anticholinergic with direct smooth muscle relaxant effects, causes fewer side effects. In general, anticholinergic drugs are probably justified only for short-term symptomatic relief of tenesmus and pain associated with inflammatory diseases of the colon and rectum. Anticholinergics can produce paralytic ileus and subsequently promote bacterial overgrowth of the small intestine.

CNS DEPRESSANTS AND ANTICHOLINERGIC COMBINATIONS

A combination of CNS depressants with anticholinergics (antispasmodics) has been successfully used to treat stress-related gastrointestinal disturbances (irritable bowel syndrome) in humans. This syndrome is characterized by abdominal pain, diarrhea alternating with constipation, and flatulence. It is usually aggravated by stress or anxiety. The primary defect is a functional alteration in gastrointestinal motility in the absence of an underlying disease. This disorder is obviously difficult to document in veterinary medicine, and diagnosis is justified only after the clinician has successfully eliminated organic causes of colonic disease. A history of environmental change or stress from obedience training, showing, and travel is helpful in establishing a diagnosis. Two drugs that may be effective in the symptomatic management of this disorder are Darbazine (Norden) and Librax (Roche). Darbazine combines the sedative effects of the phenothiazine prochlorperazine with the anticholinergic effects of isopropamide to decrease bowel secretions and spasms. Librax combines the centrally active sedative effects of chlordiazepoxide (Librium, Roche) with the anticholinergic effects of clidinium. The same precautions must be observed when using these combinations as when using other anticholinergic drugs.

Absorbents and Protectants

The value of the time-honored role of compounds such as *kaolin* and *pectin* in the management of diarrhea is uncertain. These drugs have been used because of their supposed ability to coat the intestinal wall and absorb various bacteria, viruses, and enterotoxins. Although these preparations are widely used, their efficacy for the symptomatic treatment of diarrhea has never been proved in controlled clinical trials. Although the feces may be more formed when products such as Kaopectate (Upjohn) are used, the fecal loss of water and electrolytes may indeed be increased. This effect can further compromise an already dehydrated patient. Kaolin-containing compounds also impair the absorption of concurrently administered drugs. It should be emphasized that the antidiarrheal effects of drugs such as Parepectolin (Rorer) and Donnagel–PG (Robins) are derived from their narcotic component. Since kaolin is a potent activator of coagulation, it has been suggested that kaolin-containing compounds may be of some benefit in the treatment of gastrointestinal diseases with significant mucosal damage and hemorrhage (Greene, 1984). However, the unproven efficacy and difficult administration of these compounds preclude their routine use in the management of diarrheal syndromes.

Antihypersecretory Drugs

Experimental studies in dogs and cats and clinical studies in humans indicate that salicylates interfere with enterotoxin-induced intestinal hypersecretion. This effect is attributed to a combination of the antiprostaglandin effects of the salicylate and a direct inhibition of cyclic adenosine monophosphate (cAMP) formation (Finck and Katz, 1972). Pepto-Bismol (Norwich-Eaton) and Corrective Mixture (Beecham Laboratories) both contain *bismuth subsalicylate*, which has proven efficacy in the management of hypersecretory diarrhea. These preparations decrease fecal water loss and may help reduce the pain of inflammatory diseases. Corrective Mixture also contains paregoric, making it easy to dose small dogs with gastroenteritis. Oral bismuth preparations are reported to be free of acute or chronic toxic effects in animals and humans. Caution should be used in cats because of their increased sensitivity to aspirin. When given orally, these compounds are essentially unabsorbed and are excreted in the feces.

ANTI-INFLAMMATORY DRUGS

Corticosteroids

Corticosteroids exert a wide range of physiologic effects on most body tissues and can have profound effects on the normal and diseased digestive system. The principal value of corticosteroids in the treatment of gastrointestinal disease is their anti-inflammatory and immunosuppressive effects. These actions are related to corticosteroid inhibition of the synthesis and metabolism of chemical mediators of inflammation and impairment of cellular immune functions. Experimentally, corticosteroids increase electrolyte and water absorption in the small and large intestine (Bastl et al., 1980). They also increase small intestinal brush-border enzyme activity and enhance nutrient absorption (Scott, 1981). These effects on electrolyte, water, and nutrient absorption may be beneficial to the maintenance of water and nutrient balance in certain malabsorptive diseases.

Corticosteroids have few clinically proven indications in the treatment of gastrointestinal diseases. They are beneficial in the initial management of acute gastroenteritis if shock and endotoxemia are a potential. The only specific indication for the use of corticosteroids is in the treatment of documented eosinophilic gastroenteritis-colitis. The cause of this disease is speculated to be an allergic response to dietary, parasitic, or bacterial antigens. In most instances, however, dietary manipulations and anthelmintic and antibiotic therapy are unsuccessful in controlling the disease. Eosinophilic gastroenteritis-colitis in dogs responds well to corticosteroids. An initial dosage of 0.5 to 1.0 mg/kg twice daily of prednisolone for 5 to 7 days usually results in resolution of the clinical signs. The dosage can then be decreased to 0.5 mg/kg/day for an additional 5 to 7 days. The length and intensity of maintenance therapy will depend on the severity of disease and on individual response. Tapering the dosage of prednisolone to alternate-day therapy for 3 to 4 additional weeks is often necessary. Relapses may occur.

There is evidence that immune factors are important in the pathogenesis of both ulcerative colitis and granulomatous enterocolitis in humans. Antibodies to colonic epithelial antigens can be detected in certain patients, and these antigens cross-react with some intestinal *E. coli*. Additionally, the colonic mucosa in colitis usually has increased numbers of plasma cells, eosinophils, and degranulating mast cells. It is thought that antigens entering the mucosa from the gut lumen may induce an immediate-type hypersensitivity reaction, producing or perpetuating the ulcerative colitis. For these reasons, corticosteroids are used to treat chronic inflammatory bowel diseases in humans. Clinical experience with dogs indicates that chronic ulcerative colitis responds best to sulfasalazine. However, a combination of sulfasalazine and prednisolone is recommended in severe cases of histologically documented ulcerative colitis that has not responded to a 7- to 14-day therapeutic trial of sulfasalazine alone. Colonic histoplasmosis and protothecosis must be ruled out before starting corticosteroid therapy. An initial prednisolone dosage of 0.5 mg/kg twice daily for 7 to 10 days is useful in achieving therapeutic control of active disease. If the clinical response is favorable, prednisolone should be tapered over a 2- to 3-week period. Some dogs can then be controlled with sulfasalazine alone, whereas others require longer-term alternate-day prednisolone to maintain remission. Steroid retention enemas may be useful if the distal colon and rectum are the primary locations of disease. These preparations provide high local concentrations of corticosteroids while decreasing systemic effects. As much as 50 per cent of the rectally administered steroid can be absorbed and can potentially cause adrenal suppression (Scott, 1981). Hydrocortisone retention enemas (Cortenema, Rowell) are available as a 60-ml enema providing 100 mg of hydrocortisone. The use of this preparation in a limited number of dogs with distal proctocolitis has given a favorable therapeutic response, especially when used as an adjunct to sulfasalazine. No dosage schedule is established for dogs; however, a suggested guideline is to administer a volume that provides approximately 2 mg/kg body weight per day on an alternate-day basis until the symptoms are controlled. The enema is most effective if given at bedtime.

The cause of most malabsorptive syndromes such as plasmacytic-lymphocytic enteritis and villous atrophy in dogs and cats remains obscure. Immune-mediated reactions to dietary and bacterial antigens have a likely role in these diseases, but this is yet to be proved. Corticosteroids may have a therapeutic immunosuppressive effect in some malabsorptive diseases, in addition to producing enhanced absorption of nutrients, electrolytes, and water. These malabsorptive diseases are generally best managed by a combination of dietary, antimicrobial, and corticosteroid therapy. However, even the most aggressive therapy is often unrewarding, and the prognosis for recovery must be guarded.

Corticosteroids suppress the hypothalamus-pituitary-adrenal axis, increase susceptibility to infection, and may have adverse effects on the gastrointestinal system. They are ulcerogenic to both the normal and diseased gastrointestinal tract. Prostaglandins have a normal cytoprotective effect on gastric, intestinal, and colonic mucosa. This effect is impaired by corticosteroids, predisposing the patient to mucosal injury by drugs, chemicals, and infectious agents (Robert, 1979). Corticosteroids further predispose to ulceration by inhibiting the normal replication of mucosal cells. Corticosteroids can induce acute pancreatitis and steroid hepatopathy in dogs, complicating diagnostic and therapeutic management of gastrointestinal disease. The immunosuppressive effects of glucocorticoids predispose patients to bacterial, fungal, protozoal, and parasitic infections. Subclinical parasitic infections especially can be activated by the use of corticosteroids.

Other immunosuppressive drugs used in the treatment of chronic inflammatory diseases of the gastrointestinal tract in humans have not been well evaluated in dogs and cats. The purine antagonist azathioprine (Imuran, Burroughs Wellcome) has been used with variable results in the treatment of chronic ulcerative and granulomatous enterocolitis in humans. A case of plasmacytic-lymphocytic enteritis unresponsive to dietary, antimicrobial, and corticosteroid therapy promptly resolved when treated with the alkylating agent cyclophosphamide (Cytoxan, Mead Johnson) (Legendre, 1985). These drugs should be used with extreme caution and only as a last resort in the treatment of chronic inflammatory diseases of the gastrointestinal tract until more information is available from controlled studies in dogs and cats.

References and Supplemental Readings

Albibi, R., and McCallum, R. W.: Metoclopramide: Pharmacology and clinical application. Ann. Intern. Med. 98:86, 1983.

Bastl, C. P., Binder, H. J., and Hayslett, J. P.: Role of glucocorticoids and aldosterone in maintenance of colonic cation transport. Am. J. Physiol. 238:F181, 1980.

Chiapella, A. M.: Treatment of intestinal disease. Vet. Clin. North Am. 13:567, 1983.

Cornelius, L. M.: Vomiting. *In* Ettinger, S. J. (ed.): *A Textbook of Veterinary Internal Medicine*. Philadelphia: W. B. Saunders, 1982, p. 51.

Finck, A. D., and Katz, R. L.: Prevention of cholera-induced intestinal secretion in the cat by aspirin. Nature 238:273, 1972.

Greenburger, N. J., Awantakis, C. A., and Hurvitz, A.: *Drug Treatment of Gastrointestinal Disorders*. Vol. 3. New York: Churchill-Livingstone, 1978.

Greene, C. E.: Gastrointestinal, intra-abdominal, and hepatobiliary infections. *In* Greene, C. E. (ed.): *Clinical Microbiology and Infectious Diseases of the Dog and Cat*. Philadelphia: W. B. Saunders, 1984, p. 247.

Kirsner, J. B., and Shorter, R. G.: Recent developments in "non-specific inflammatory bowel disease." Parts I and II. N. Engl. J. Med. 306:775 and 837, 1982.

Korelitz, B.: Therapy of inflammatory bowel disease, including use of immunosuppressive agents. Clin. Gastroenterol. 9:331, 1980.

Legendre, A. L.: Personal communication, 1985.

Morrisey, J. F., and Barreras, R. F.: Antacid therapy. N. Engl. J. Med. 290:550, 1974.

Pidgeon, G. L.: Chronic disorders of the exocrine pancreas, small bowel, and large bowel. Vet. Clin. North Am. 13:541, 1983.

Robert, A.: Cytoprotection by prostaglandins. Gastroenterology 77:761, 1979.

Roe, F. J.: Metronidazole: Review of its uses and toxicity. J. Antimicrob. Chemother. 3:205, 1977.

Scott, J.: Physiological, pharmacological and pathological actions of glucocorticoids on the digestive system. Clin. Gastroenterol. 10:627, 1981.

Simon, G. L., and Gorback, S. L.: Intestinal microflora. Med. Clin. North Am. 66:557, 1982.

Tams, T. R.: Reglan—Clinical applications in GI disorders. Proceedings of the 51st Annual Meeting of the American Animal Hospital Association. 1984, p. 207.

Twedt, D. C.: Differential diagnosis and therapy of vomiting. Vet. Clin. North Am. 13:503, 1983.

Wilson, R. C.: Antimotility drugs used in treatment of diarrhea. J.A.V.M.A. 180:776, 1982.

BACTERIAL ENTERITIS

RAY DILLON, D.V.M.

Auburn, Alabama

THE INTESTINAL FLORA

The microorganisms populating the lumen of the alimentary canal not only are the center of a host-versus-environment reaction but also influence the structure and function of the small bowel mucosa; the metabolism of drugs and nutrients, and the intraluminal metabolism of cholesterol, bile salt, and steroidal hormones. The endogenous flora of the intestines is involved in diseases other than primary gastrointestinal infections, such as hepatoencephalopathy and uremia. An accurate assessment of the types and number of organisms within the alimentary canal and associated with infections is limited by the methods available for collection, isolation, culture, and enumeration of these microbes. The microflora of the gastrointestinal tract is a complex ecosystem of both aerobic and anaerobic microbes, and 500 different bacterial species can exist within a single individual (Table 1).

Although the microbial population of the alimentary tract varies in individuals, generalizations can be made about bacterial numbers and location (Table 2). In healthy dogs and cats, the stomach and small bowel contain relatively low concentrations of bacteria. One third of healthy humans have no bacterial growth from duodenal cultures. When organisms are present in the proximal small bowel, gram-positive aerobes or facultative anaerobes are present in concentrations of 10^4 organisms per gram of content, and anaerobic bacteroides are not found. The lack of organisms in this area is related to gastric acidity, bowel motility, and the pH and redox potentials (mV) of the lumen. However, the distal small bowel generally has a higher pH and the redox potential is reduced, resulting in a zone of transition from a sparse population of aerobic flora to the dense bacterial population of anaerobic organisms found in the colon. In the ileum, the concentration of microorganisms is increased to 10^5 to 10^9 microorganisms per gram of content.

The bacteria, which are only transiently found in the proximal bowel, are regular inhabitants of the ileum. Strict anaerobes generally cannot survive in the jejunum but may colonize the ileum. The ileocolic area is a significant transition point, where the number (10^8 to 10^{12} bacteria per gram of colon content) becomes markedly increased and the flora is dominated by fastidious organisms (bacteroides, anaerobic lactobacilli, and clostridia). The clinician should remember that these microorganisms are difficult to culture and outnumber aerobic and facultative anaerobes by 1000 or 10,000 to 1 within the lumen of the colon. Thus routine stool cultures represent a sampling of only a few of the intestinal flora.

Because the alimentary canal of a host is sterile at birth, animals raised in a gnotobiotic environment have no bacteria in the gut lumen. The enteric flora is derived from the environment, and the enteric bacteria colonize the tract in an oral-to-anal direction. Although there are age-related changes, the host flora is usually established by approximately 3 to 4 weeks after birth and, except in unusual circumstances, does not change thereafter.

In addition to the longitudinal distribution of

Table 1. *Major Microflora of the Gastrointestinal Tract of Dogs and Cats*

	Oral Cavity	Stomach	Small Bowel Proximal	Small Bowel Distal	Cecum/Colon	Feces
Total Counts†						
Fasting	10^7	10^1–10^2	10^1–10^2	10^3–10^7	10^9–10^{10}	10^{10}–10^{11}
Postprandial	10^7	10^4–10^5	10^2–10^3	10^3–10^7	10^9–10^{10}	10^{10}–10^{11}
Aerobic Organisms						
Gram-positive organisms						
Streptococcus	+	10^1	10^1–10^2	10^3–10^4	10^8–10^9	10^9
Staphylococcus	+	$10^{0.4}$	$10^{0.4}$	$10^{1.4}$	10^4–10^5	10^4–10^5
Bacillus	+				$10^{5.4}$	+
Corynebacterium	?				$10^{8.7}$	+
Gram-negative organisms						
Enterobacteriaceae (primarily *Escherichia coli, Enterobacter, Klebsiella*)	+	10^1–10^2	10^2	10^2–10^6	10^7–10^8	10^7–10^8
Pseudomonas	+				+	+
Proteus	+					
Neisseria	+				+	+
Moraxella	+					
Anaerobic Organisms						
Gram-positive organisms						
Clostridium	+	$10^{0.3}$–10^2	$10^{0.1}$	10^4	10^7–10^9	10^7–10^9
Lactobacillus	+	10^1–10^2	10^1–10^3	10^2–10^6	10^8–10^9	10^9–10^{10}
Propionibacterium	+	+			+	+
Bifidobacerium			+	+	$10^{6.6}$	10^6–10^7
Gram-negative organisms						
Bacteroides	+		+	10^1	10^6–10^{10}	10^8–10^{10}
Fusobacterium	+					
Veillonella	+				$10^{5.9}$	$10^{5.9}$
Other Organisms						
Spirochetes	+	+	+	+	+ + +	0
Mycoplasma	+					
Yeasts	+				10^5	+

*Key: + = present but absolute quantity uncertain; + + + = present in large number; 0 = normally absent; blank space = absent or data not available.

†Values expressed as organisms/ml or gram of intestinal contents.

Derived from Greene: *Clinical Microbiology and Infectious Diseases of Dogs and Cats.* Philadelphia: W. B. Saunders, 1984.

bacteria in the bowel, there is also a cross-sectional arrangement. Part of the microflora within the lumen adhere to the mucus layer and form a bacterial "coating," which resists colonization by other bacterial species. In dogs, bacteria do not localize on the epithelial surface of the stomach or proximal small bowl but do localize in the distal ileum, cecum, and colon. The distribution and species of organism do not usually change significantly. Dogs kept in a continuously isolated environment will develop a more complex and anaerobic flora. Antibiotics, diet, and environmental stress can change the composition, attachment, and layering of the flora.

Table 2. *Factors Limiting Intestinal Bacterial Proliferation*

1. pH of lumen—gastric acidity
2. Redox potential in lumen—oxygen needs of flora
3. Bowel motility
4. Bacterial interaction—cross-sectional and longitudinal ecosystem, each with a niche
5. Mucosal resistance—intact epithelium plus IgA (which does not fix complement) and surface indigenous bacteria

Since coliforms replicate every 20 minutes in optimal conditions in the laboratory, it would be anticipated that *in vivo* rapid bacterial overgrowth would overwhelm the host. However, replication time in the intestinal tract in animals is on the order of 1 to 4 divisions per day; the number of microorganisms is controlled by normal peristalsis, gastric acid production, enteric secretions, and microbial interactions. The microbial interaction, especially in the densely populated colon, is important in influencing the endogenous microflora. Facultative bacteria (those that can grow either aerobically or anaerobically) maintain the reduced environment of the colon by using oxygen that diffuses into the colon, allowing the more oxygen-sensitive organisms to survive. Further, other bacteria produce substances that control their own growth in an autoregulatory manner. For example, *Escherichia coli* and anaerobic microbes produce short-chain fatty acids, which suppress bacterial populations. This "trench war" among bacteria limits the number and types of microflora present and can be altered by antibiotic therapy. Although antibiotic suppression of enteric flora may be marked, depending on the luminal concentration of bacteria and drugs used, the effects are usually transient.

The Flora in Diarrhea

During an episode of acute diarrhea, the colonic flora changes to become less anaerobic, regardless of the cause of diarrhea. Because of the rapid transit, the anaerobic bacteria are decreased in number and an increase in coliforms may occur. In the new order, the pathogen itself may rise to ascendancy in the flora and may be the major isolate from the feces.

A survey of fecal cultures from dogs with spontaneous clinical diarrhea revealed no significant difference in the total number of viable bacteria during diarrhea compared with that after recovery. Further, the flora of the diarrheal feces was similar to that in diarrhea experimentally induced with magnesium sulfate in control dogs. Changes during experimental and spontaneous diarrhea included a decrease in *Lactobacillus* and *Bifidobacterium* and an increase in *Bacteroides* and *Enterobacteriaceae*. In both spontaneous and experimental diarrhea, the altered flora persists after clinical recovery from diarrhea.

CLASSIFICATION OF BACTERIAL DIARRHEA

Acute bacterial diarrhea is classified into toxigenic types (in which an enterotoxin is the major pathogenic mechanism) and invasive types (in which the organism penetrates the mucosal surface as the primary event) (Table 3). The enterotoxigenic organisms elaborate toxins, causing fluid and electrolyte secretion in the gut. The ability of an organism to produce an enterotoxin is established *in vivo* with the use of the rabbit ileal loop model and the suckling mouse model, or *in vitro* with the use of tissue cultures. The enterotoxins are classified as cytotonic (activating the intracellular enzymes, such as adenylate cyclase, without any damage to the epithelial cells) and cytotoxic (causing injury to the mucosal cells and producing a lesion).

Table 3. *Examples of Primary Diarrheogenic Bacteria of Dogs and Cats*

Enterotoxigenic
- Cytotonic—hypersecretory
  - Ex.: Toxigenic *Escherichia coli*
- Cytotoxic—mucosal injury
  - Ex.: *Clostridium* spp.

Invasive
- Mucosal invasion—inflammatory
- ??Cytotonic component—hypersecretory
  - Ex.: *Salmonella* spp.
    - *Yersinia enterocolitica*
    - *Campylobacter jejuni*
    - *Bacillus piliformis*

Toxigenic Organisms

Although the prototype organisms in this group are *Vibrio cholerae* and enterotoxigenic *E. coli*, their role in small animal enteritis and the incidence of secretory disease is of unknown clinical importance. The enterotoxin results in rapid irreversible binding of the toxin to the surface of the epithelial cell wall. A portion of the subunit migrates through the cell and stimulates activity of adenosine monophosphate (cAMP). The receptor for the enterotoxin is present in all mammalian cells, but the gut mucosal cell has about 1 million potential binding sites, and occupation of 50,000 by cholera enterotoxin will stimulate maximal gut fluid secretion. Thus, increased cAMP causes increased sodium-dependent chloride secretion of the crypt cells and prevents the sodium chloride cotransport absorption across the brush border of the rest of the villi. Thus the isotonic fluid loss is massive; there is a bicarbonate concentration twice that of plasma and a potassium concentration five times that of plasma.

After experimental oral ingestion of *V. cholerae* toxin or virulent organisms by dogs, severe diarrhea develops, but the subsequent mucosal immunity protects against later challenge.

Invasive Organisms

Although the toxigenic organisms classically involve the secretory portion of the upper intestine, the invasive pathogens target the lower bowel, particularly the distal ileum and colon, and have the ability to invade the intestinal epithelium. The histologic findings include mucosal ulceration, with an acute inflammatory reaction in the lamina propria. Although different pathogens (*Salmonella*, *Campylobacter*, *E. coli*, *Yersinia*) have differing sites and clinical courses, the initial event is mucosal invasion. The diarrhea and initial fluid production may be caused by the concomitant release of enterotoxin. The invasive organisms may increase the local synthesis of prostaglandins at the site of inflammation, and the damaged epithelium may not resorb fluids from the lumen. In fluid loss, normal secretion and decreased ability for resorption is more likely than a mass transudation or exudation of fluid from mucosa. However, in chronic severe infiltrative disease, prolonged disease and loss of mucosal epithelium and function may result in a protein-losing enteropathy.

PATHOGENESIS OF BACTERIAL ENTERITIS

Ingestion and Colonization

The primary diarrheogenic agents are orally ingested. Normally, the low pH of the stomach, the rapid transit time of the small bowel, and the antibody-producing cells in the lamina propria of the small bowel are adequate to keep the jejunum and proximal ileum relatively free (not sterile) of microorganisms. The ileocecal valve partially prevents the proximal migration of the large bowel bacteria, which are primarily slow-growing faculative anaerobes.

In order to pass through the hostile environment of the stomach, diarrheogenic organisms must be acid-resistant (e.g., *Shigella*), occur in large numbers that allow for a few survivors (e.g., *V. cholerae* or *E. coli*), or be ingested with food that provides a neutralized environment.

Once in the small bowel, the organisms must either colonize or invade the mucosa of the jejunum or pass into the terminal ileum (*Salmonella*) or colon (*Shigella*) to colonize and invade the mucosa. The active motility of the small bowel is an effective deterrent to the successful colonization of most organisms entering from the stomach. The organisms (*V. cholerae, E. coli*) that are able to colonize this area have developed special colonization factors such as fimbriae (hairlike projections from the bacterial cell wall surface) or lectins (special proteins that attach to specific carbohydrate-binding sites), which allow these bacteria to associate intimately with the mucosal cell surface and not be "washed" downstream.

Most organisms without special colonization factors pass into the terminal ileum and colon and must then compete with the established flora for an ecologic niche before invading the mucosa. The flora with cross-sectional and longitudinal distribution produce substances (fatty acids, colicins) that inhibit new "foreign" bacteria and prevent proliferation. The ability of diarrheogenic organisms to invade mucosa and thus elude the other inhibiting organisms may account for their more rapid preferential multiplication.

Enterotoxigenic Diarrhea

Most bacteria that colonize the small bowel do not invade mucosal cells but proliferate, and some may produce enterotoxins. The enterotoxins bind to the mucosal cells and cause hypersecretion of isotonic fluid at a rate that overwhelms the reabsortive capacity of the adjacent villi and the reserve capacity of the colon. The enterotoxin may be ingested directly in food, as with staphylococcal food poisoning, rather than be produced in the small intestine. The classic model for secretory diarrhea is *V. cholerae* infection with a watery voluminous stool. Since there is an absence of significant histologic bowel lesions and an absence of clinical signs of systemic illness with this infection, it is evident that the host does not initiate an inflammatory response. Loss of this diarrheal fluid results in a predictable saline depletion, base-deficit acidosis, and potassium deficiency, and the clinical signs are determined by the amount and rate of loss. The electrolyte pattern in the stool is remarkably constant in humans whenever voluminous diarrhea is caused by any of the enterotoxigenic pathogens. Thus, severe voluminous diarrhea can occur without alteration of the mucosa of the bowel.

Some enterotoxigenic bacteria may, in addition to stimulating the secretory mechanism of the small bowel, also produce an enterotoxin that is cytotoxic, thus damaging the gut mucosa and producing a diarrhea in which the volume is small and the protein content is high (*Clostridium perfringens*).

Enterotoxigenic *E. coli* strains are a common cause of diarrhea in young calves, pigs, sheep, and humans; yet the serotypes and colonization factors seem to be species specific. Hypersecretory diarrhea in dogs and cats is of uncertain significance.

Invasive Diarrhea

An inflammatory diarrhea may be caused by invasion of the mucosa in addition to cellular damage from a cytotoxin. Most organisms in this group invade primarily the lower ileum (*Salmonella*) or the large bowel (*Shigella, Yersinia enterocolitica,* and *Campylobacter jejuni*). There is an inflammatory response to invasion, and the stool contains inflammatory cells, large quantities of protein, and often gross blood. Organisms may on rare occasions invade the blood stream and produce mesenteric lymphadenitis (*Salmonella*). The systemic signs depend on the site of invasion and host response but are typical of any acute gastroenteritis, including fever, abdominal pain, and tenesmus. The intestinal invasion may cause hypersegmentation, and the resultant diarrhea is often watery but not perfuse. Although certain strains of invasive bacteria in humans also have the capacity to produce enterotoxins *in vitro* (*Shigella* spp., nontyphoidal *Salmonella, Y. enterocolitica,* and *C. jejuni*), the invasive capacity is of paramount importance in their ability to produce disease.

BACTERIAL ENTERITIS OF DOGS AND CATS

Although several bacterial species are capable of invading the mucosal barrier (*Salmonella* spp., *Shigella* spp., *Campylobacter* spp., and invasive *E. coli*) and other pathogens are known to produce enterotoxins (toxigenic *E. coli, Klebsiella* spp., *V. cholerae*, and staphylococci), the clinical documentation of bacterial pathogens causing diarrhea in dogs and cats is minimal. The enterotoxigenic bacterial toxins can induce secretory diarrhea (adenyl cyclase-cAMP mechanism) experimentally in dogs, but the clinical significance is not established in dogs and cats. Bacteria that are associated with primary bacterial enteritis of dogs and cats include *Salmonella* spp., *Y. enterocolitica, C. jejuni*, and *Bacillus piliformis*. The evidence for *E. coli, Clostridium* spp., staphylococci, *Shigella* spp., and *Chromobacterium* spp. as primary pathogens in dogs and cats is inconclusive.

THERAPY FOR BACTERIAL ENTERITIS

Antimicrobial Drugs

The strategies for use of antibiotics in gastroenteritis can be related to idiopathic causes, specific infective causes, and bacterial overgrowth. Several antimicrobial agents are used for properties other than their antibiotic activities. Sulfasalazine is an effective drug for chronic colitis because the 5-aminosalicylate decreases the inflammatory response through inhibition of prostaglandins. Metronidazole has antiprotozoal activity, suppresses cell-mediated immune reactions, and has activity against anaerobes. The efficacy of metronidazole in chronic diarrhea may be linked to one or all of these actions.

Antibiotic therapy is not indicated for the routine nonspecific acute or chronic gastrointestinal disease of dogs or cats. Irrational use of antibiotics in noninfectious diarrhea may alter the flora to allow a pathogen to proliferate and induce a secondary bacterial complication. Dogs with spontaneous and experimental diarrhea have demonstrated no significant difference in viable organisms in fecal samples during diarrhea and after recovery. Thus, the only specific indication for the use of antibiotics in acute diarrhea is the primary invasive bacterial infection. This general guideline, however, has been compromised by the findings of mixed microbial infections of *C. jejuni* and *Salmonella* in parvovirus infections. Even the use of antibiotics for specific infections is not always indicated. *Salmonella*, frequently isolated from feces of normal dogs and cats, can invade the mucosa and produce a self-limiting gastroenteritis. Antimicrobial agents, especially oral nonabsorbable antibiotics, will in most species of animals increase the incidence and duration of intestinal carriage of salmonellosis. In some dogs with chronic nonspecific diarrhea, tylosin, tetracycline, chloramphenicol, and ampicillin are reportedly effective.

Table 4. *Antimicrobial Agents Recommended for Bacterial Infections in Dogs and Cats*

Gram-Negative Bacteria	Gram-Positive Bacteria
Aminoglycosides	Cephalosporins
Chloramphenicol*	Clindamycin*
Cephalosporins	Lincomycin*
Clindamycin*	Erythromycin*
Lincomycin*	Penicillins*
Penicillins*	Vancomycin*
Polymyxin B, E	
Sulfonamides	
Tetracycline	

*Antibiotics that also have activity against anaerobes and have the potential for altering the normal intestinal flora.

When damage to the intestinal mucosa is suspected because of hemorrhagic diarrhea and in those animals in which leukocytosis, specifically with a left shift (greater than 1000 nonsegmented neutrophils/μl) or leukopenia or fever is documented, systemic antibiotic therapy may be indicated. Mucosal damage and loss of the protective barrier may allow penetration of the normal flora into the portal circulation, which would be an indication for parenteral antibiotic therapy. However, experimental induction in dogs of a systemic septicemia (aerobic or anaerobic) of intestinal origin by intestinal hypoxia or ischemia is difficult. With mucosal erosion, endotoxin migration rather than bacterial invasion and proliferation is a more probable cause of endotoxemia.

When infection caused by the indigenous flora is suspected because of increased bowel permeability, the infections are generally mixed, with a predominance of gram-positive organisms or anaerobes if the stomach or proximal bowel is involved and facultative gram-negative organisms or anaerobes if the small bowel or colon is involved (Table 4). Thus a combination of penicillin derivatives or chloramphenicol and aminoglycosides is recommended. The use of antibiotic combinations that affect both gram-negative bacteria and anaerobic bacteria (gentamicin and clindamycin, respectively) would be the best choice when septicemia of bowel origin is suspected.

Fluid Therapy

Intravenous fluid therapy is probably the most important symptomatic treatment of the dog or cat with severe diarrhea. Hypotension, endotoxemia, shock, and severe dehydration are best corrected by lactated Ringer's solution with volumes calculated to compensate for loss in the stool. Many dogs and cats can be supported with oral fluids if the diarrhea is not voluminous.

Oral solutions containing glucose and sodium, as promoted by the World Health Organization for treating human cholera, are designed to promote the absorptive capacity of the tips of the villi but are designed for hypersecretory diarrhea from enterotoxin when the structure of the bowel is normal. The use of hypertonic oral antidiarrheal solutions in cases with disrupted intestinal mucosal integrity (blood, protein, and polymorphonuclear leukocytes in the stool) may cause an osmotic diarrhea and hyperosmolarity. Oral hyperosmolar solutions should not be used in place of isotonic fluids, either orally or parenterally, in dehydrated dogs and cats.

Motility Modifiers

Controversy continues to surround the treatment of infectious diarrhea with drugs (opiates) that increase segmentation and thus decrease transit time by increasing resistance. Although the clinical signs may improve, the infection may persist longer. In *Shigella* enteritis in humans, the morbidity increases when these drugs are used. The use of drugs (diphenyloxylate, paregoric) that decrease the animal's ability to remove the toxin or decrease the bacterial concentration should be avoided.

Intestinal Protectants

Depending on the type of bacterial diarrhea in dogs and cats, agents that bind endotoxin are of limited value. Kaolin, however, may be useful as a coagulation activator when severe mucosal ulceration has occurred. Similarly, nonsteroidal anti-inflammatory drugs (aspirin) are beneficial because they (1) interfere with enterotoxin-induced hypersecretion by blocking cAMP and (2) decrease fluid loss from the bowel through antiprostaglandin activity. Bismuth subsalicylate may have similar activity and thus is commonly recommended in acute diarrhea.

SPECIFIC CAUSES IN DOGS AND CATS

Escherichia coli

E. coli is a part of the normal enteric flora and has its highest concentrations in the lower ileum and large bowel. Resident and transient strains undergo dynamic changes continuously. More than 100 serotypes of *E. coli* have been found to produce enterotoxin or have invasive properties. The invasive strains of *E. coli* have been suggested as a cause of diarrhea in dogs. Neonatal colibacillosis in dogs would appear to be more related to host resistance than bacterial pathogenicity. Although the enterotoxin of *E. coli* isolated from a human with secretory diarrhea does stimulate adenyl cyclase activity in the dog jejunum, the role of enterotoxic *E. coli* as a classic cause of spontaneous disease of dogs and cats has not been definitively documented. Since inoculation studies are required to document invasive *E. coli* and enterotoxigenic *E. coli* are identified by specific *in vivo* or *in vitro* studies, the separation of nonpathogenic *E. coli* from pathogens is difficult. The isolation of *E. coli* from a diarrheic stool is expected and not significant.

The *E. coli* septicemia of the neonatal puppy develops in the first 2 weeks after birth as a result of the increased intestinal permeability immediately after birth or as a result of insufficient colostrum. The septicemia causes hemorrhagic lesions on serosa of all body cavities and the gastrointestinal tract and results in a high mortality.

The role of *E. coli* as a cause of diarrhea in dogs remains to be defined. The presence of a relatively slow-acting heat-labile enterotoxin of *E. coli* origin was demonstrated in two dogs with diarrhea. The toxin was not typical of that of human or porcine strains and raises the possibility of a new class of weaker enterotoxin of dogs. The role of this endotoxigenic *E. coli* as a concurrent intestinal infection or even as a primary pathogen may be clinically important. Previous surveys for the classic heat-labile toxin in dogs were negative. Since most pathologic *E. coli* are host specific, the zoonotic importance is probably low.

Salmonella

Salmonella is the genus of a large group of gram-negative bacilli with approximately 1700 serotypes and variants with potential pathogenicity for animals and humans. Many serotypes are restricted to narrow host preferences. Species of *Salmonella* are frequently isolated from the feces of normal dogs and cats. The implication that pet animals are asymptomatic carriers is supported by culture surveys revealing approximately a 10 per cent prevalence in the United States canine population. Higher incidence is found in many areas where overcrowding or unsanitary conditions occur. *Salmonella* is acquired via the mouth and gastrointestinal tract and is unique in attacking the ileum and, to a lesser extent, the colon. The infectivity of a specific strain is related to serotype and the inoculum size. A dose-response curve has been determined for certain strains. Since human studies have shown that 10^7 bacteria caused a 50 per cent infection rate compared with a 90 per cent infection rate with 10^9 bacteria, it is likely that the ability of *Salmonella* to induce disease is based on a balance among host resistance, competing enteric bacteria, and number of infective organisms. Thus, *Salmonella* causes clinical disease in young and debilitated animals, animals undergoing stressful procedures, animals exposed to unsanitary environments, and animals administered drugs that alter the normal enteric flora. Further, in view of the size of the inoculum, direct contamination of ingesta by feces is generally not a sufficient inoculum to induce clinical signs, and a period of incubation for bacterial replication is required before the numbers are sufficient to cause disease.

Clinical salmonellosis can be limited to mucosal invasion with typical signs of acute enterocolitis or can develop into a potentially fatal septicemia with signs of systemic illness and even disseminated intravascular coagulation. The mild forms are usually self-limiting, and the infection is localized to the mucosa and mesenteric lymph nodes. In dogs or cats that die from salmonellosis, the organism is often cultured from the mesenteric lymph nodes at necropsy. Certain strains are capable of invading the mucosa, but studies have shown that cAMP can be stimulated by some strains that produce a more profuse fluid accumulation. The clinical incidence of the organism as an opportunist is reflected in the frequent finding of *Salmonella* sp. in dogs with parvovirus infections. With the variable clinical features and the predisposition to be a secondary complication of stress or systemic disease, the zoonotic aspect is frequently overlooked. Humans can become chronic carriers as a consequence of either symptomatic or asymptomatic infections. When an outbreak occurs in a kennel, the dogs, the human caretakers, the sanitary procedures, and the diet should be examined.

The use of antibiotics in salmonellosis is controversial. The local self-limiting disease of the mucosa is probably unaltered by treatment, and the shedding of organisms and production of a chronic carrier state are made more likely by therapy, especially with oral nonabsorbable antibiotics. The chronic carrier state is probably not affected by oral or systemic antibiotics. If systemic signs of septicemia develop in severe cases, then systemic antibacterial therapy is advocated. Although chloramphenicol, gentamicin, and trimethoprim-sulfadiazine are often effective, because of the increasing incidence of antibiotic resistance, treatment is best when based on culture and sensitivity testing.

Yersinia

In animals and humans *Y. enterocolitica* causes a spectrum of clinical illness ranging from simple gastroenteritis to invasive ileitis and colitis. The organism can be found in water sources and has been isolated from dogs, cats, cattle, chickens, and horses. Although it has been isolated in 6 per cent of normal dogs, a different serotype from that involving humans may be involved. Animals kept as pets or used as a food source are believed to be involved in the transmission of this gram-negative rod. The enterocolitis in humans has been reported more frequently in Scandinavia and Europe than in the United States. The pathogenesis involves the production of enterotoxin, cytotoxin, and the ability of the organism to invade the mucosa. Although the most frequent sign in infected humans is enterocolitis, the disease can become systemic, and bacteremia can develop in debilitated patients. The role and incidence of disease in pet animals remains to be defined, but the zoonotic potential is important.

The incidence of dogs carrying *Y. enterocolitica* is lower in North America than in dogs in Japan and Scandinavia. However, the isolation of almost pure cultures of *Y. enterocolitica* from two dogs with mucoid enterocolitis indicates the possible role as a primary pathogen. The organism is common enough in dogs to warrant public health consideration. In humans, transmission can occur by person-to-person contact, environmental sources, or infected foods, and even the rat flea is speculated as a vector. In view of the increasing incidence of this disease in humans, awareness is important. The strains of porcine origin frequently belong to the serogroup closer to human strains than the dog strains. The disease in dogs is probably self-limiting, although response to antibiotics has been reported in two dogs.

The organism prefers colder temperatures than most enteric bacteria. Culture at both 25°C and 37°C requires special conditions, and cold enrichment with subculture is recommended. The organism is relatively sensitive to many antibiotics, including aminoglycosides, trimethoprim-sulfadiazine, chloramphenicol, tetracycline, and colistin. The penicillins, cephalosporins, and lincomycin are not usually effective. Culture and sensitivity testing are recommended. However, there is no substantial evidence in humans that antibiotics alter the course of the gastrointestinal infections, the chronic relapsing forms, or the septicemias. Clinical improvement after cephradine was reported in two dogs.

Bacillus piliformis

B. piliformis (Tyzzer's disease) is an intracellular, filamentous, spore-forming, gram-negative bacillus that is difficult to culture on artificial media. The organism causes a chronic hemorrhagic enterocolitis and is demonstrated by special stains (Giemsa and periodic acid–Schiff [PAS]) in the macrophages along necrotic foci and abscesses of the intestine and liver. The disease is usually well advanced before diagnosis is made because of difficulty in diagnosis. The disease can involve an animal of any age, although young puppies and cats, especially those with systemic illness (distemper, parvovirus, parasitism), are at greater risk. Since the major reservoirs of *B. piliformis* are rodents, dogs and cats exposed to these animals, and especially dogs fed raw rabbits as a routine dietary supplement, are the more likely candidates. When the appropriate history is present, special stains are warranted of surgical biopsies of chronic diffuse bowel disease. Unfortunately, the disease is usually fatal in most dogs because of the delayed diagnosis.

Campylobacter

Although in humans relatively few *C. jejuni* organisms (500 bacteria orally) can cause enteric disease, the primary pathogenicity is not as defined in dogs and cats. This motile, fastidious, microaerophilic bacteria can be isolated from the stools of both normal and diarrheic adult dogs at about the same frequency. Differences in the animal's age, degree of sanitation, and environment may explain the wide discrepancies in the reported rate of infection. Obviously the animal at greatest potential for exposure is the young puppy in a concentrated population with poor sanitation, such as an ill-kept kennel. The isolation rates range from less than 5 per cent to as high as 75 per cent in puppies, and diarrheic young dogs or cats have the greatest chances of infection. The organism is invasive, and bacteremia can result. The organism is frequently found in dogs with parvovirus infections, suggesting a synergistic effect. In 108 dogs with severe enteritis, *C. jejuni* was isolated 22 times, parvovirus 46 times, and 13 cases had both organisms. The ability of species of *Salmonella* and *C. jejuni* to be concurrent infections with parvovirus and the potential zoonosis emphasizes the importance of good sanitation in dogs and cats with diarrhea.

The organism is almost ubiquitous. In mammals, *C. jejuni* has been isolated from healthy cattle, sheep, horses, pigs, goats, dogs, cats, rodents, and monkeys and from diarrheic calves, lambs, dogs, cats, and monkeys. In the avian species, *C. jejuni* has been isolated from 30 to 100 per cent of fecal samples. Since small numbers (500) of *C. jejuni* potentially can cause infection in humans, the possibility of acquiring an infection from contact with feces from an infected or carrier pet animal is real and would appear to be more probable than with species of *Salmonella,* which usually require large numbers (10^5 to 10^7) of organisms for human infection. But if both pet and owner are infected, the most likely scenario would be the exposure of both pet and owner to a common source.

Although experimenters were initially unsuccessful in producing diarrhea in puppies with *Campylobacter* of human origin, a mild diarrhea was produced in gnotobiotic beagle puppies by either human or dog isolates. Compared with humans, dogs seem to have less severe disease and to require more infective organisms as primary pathogens. Feces from infected puppies becomes increasingly fluid at the peak of clinical signs, including tenesmus, lassitude, and mild anorexia. Enteritis in puppies appears to have a 7- to 10-day course of semiformed to watery stools with mucus and occasional blood, tenesmus, and occasional vomiting. As in humans, involvement of the jejunum and ileum was noted in spontaneous infections in dogs rather than just the colitis, as in the gnotobiotic dogs. The isolation of the organisms in clinically normal dogs and the absence of serologic studies in dogs and cats complicate a simple cause-and-effect relationship. In dogs, the occurrence of acute enteritis that is erythromycin-responsive after supportive therapy fails seems to support a role of this or a similar organisms in clinical diarrhea.

Because of the slow growth and microaerophilic nature of the organism, isolation of *C. jejuni* from the stool is difficult and requires special selective media and techniques. Examination of the stool by darkfield or phase-contrast microscopy by an untrained observer can be misleading. Administration of erythromycin, the drug of choice in humans, results in remission of clinical signs and disappearance of the organism from the stool.

The high incidence and possible synergism of *C. jejuni* in dogs with parvovirus indicates that treatment for a suspected *Campylobacter* infection may be included in unresponsive parvovirus disease. Erythromycin, clindamycin, gentamicin, and chloramphenicol but not penicillins are usually effective *in vitro*. Owing to potential public health concern, culture with special selective media should precede therapy.

Bacterial Food Poisoning

Consumption of food contaminated with bacteria or bacterial toxins can cause diarrhea in dogs and cats. Some bacteria may produce enterotoxins in the food, but these may not have the capacity to colonize or invade the bowel. Studies in humans show that the major recognized causes of bacterial food poisoning include *C. perfringens, Staphylococcus aureus, Bacillus cereus, Salmonella, V. cholerae, Shigella, Clostridium botulinum, Vibrio parahaemolyticus,* and toxigenic *E. coli.* Although secretory diarrhea can be experimentally induced in dogs with enterotoxins, clinical confirmation of bacterial food poisoning is rarely documented. Enterotoxigenic staphylococci were isolated from 5.8 per cent of normal dogs, and a canine source for direct or indirect food contamination may be possible.

Minor Bacterial Enteritis

Identification of other pathogenic bacteria, either as primary or concurrent infections, may await the development of new diagnostic methods. Enteropathogenicity in dogs and cats has not been established for invasive species of *Shigella, Proteus, Klebsiella*, or spirochetes, all of which can be cultured from canine stools. Diarrhea of any cause may dislodge spirochetes from the crypts and increase the number observed in the stool. *Chromobacterium violaceum* and *Clostridium perfringens* are potential causes of gastroenteritis.

Bacterial Overgrowth

When the normal bacteria proliferate within the small bowel lumen, the metabolic consequences are malabsorption and, consequently, malnutrition. The small bowel abnormalities conducive to local stasis or recirculation of bowel contents (blind loop syndrome) are accompanied by intraluminal proliferation of microorganisms. Human evidence shows that gastric atrophy and gastric surgery that prevent gastric acid secretion also increase the number of microorganisms residing in the small bowel lumen. In bacterial overgrowth, the small bowel flora resembles that of the colon, and the concentration may approach 10^{10} viable organisms per gram of small bowel content. Bacteroides and anaerobic *Lactobacillus* spp. often predominate, but *Enterobacter enterococcus* and species of *Clostridium* may also be present. Altered biosalt metabolism (primarily deconjugation of bile by anaerobes) is the primary cause of fat malabsorption and steatorrhea. The clinical incidence of bacterial overgrowth is not well defined in dogs, but the identification of chronic small bowel diarrhea associated with malabsorption and a decreased D-xylose absorption test would be compatible with this syndrome. Elevated serum folate concentrations and decreased serum Vitamin B_{12} levels are consistent findings with bacterial overgrowth and are excellent screening tests. The use of nitroso-indole-nitrate test, serum folate, and B_{12}, and the culture of duodenal contents by flexible fiberoptic endoscopy are methods for diagnosis of bacterial overgrowth that may justify the subsequent use of oral tylosin or tetracycline. The efficacy of antibiotics in chronic nonspecific diarrhea may be linked to bacterial overgrowth. Alterations in mucosal enzymes rather than achlorhydria and the presence of simple bacteria are implicated in the diarrhea of exocrine pancreatic insufficiency.

Antibiotic-Induced Enteritis

Pseudomembranous colitis is attributed to toxin production from an overgrowth of *Clostridium difficile* in the colon due to antimicrobial suppression of the normal flora. In humans, the antibiotics most commonly involved include clindamycin, lincomycin, ampicillin, and cephalosporins. This anaerobic infection is successfully treated with vancomycin, although metronidazole and bacitracin also seem to be effective. A similar pseudomembranous colitis was reported in a dog that had been treated with clindamycin. The role of toxin-producing *Clostridium* and perhaps other concomitant infections in antibiotic-associated diarrhea of dogs and cats remains to be carefully demonstrated.

C. difficile, both cytotoxigenic and noncytotoxigenic strains, was isolated from 23 per cent of dogs and 30 per cent of cats. Although the carriage seems to be transient and not associated with enteritis, the carriage was higher in animals with previous antibiotic treatment. The common use of several of the above antibiotics and the seeming absence of resulting gastroenteritis implies a low incidence of antibiotic-induced enteritis. However, in humans the condition may occur 2 to 10 weeks after completion of antibiotic therapy.

References and Supplemental Reading

Batt, R. M., Needham, J. R., and Carter, M. W.: Bacterial overgrowth associated with a naturally occurring enteropathy in the German shepherd dog. Res. Vet. Sci. 35:42, 1983.

Burrows, C. F., and Jezyk, P. F.: Nitrosonapathol test for screening of small intestinal diarrhea disease in the dog. J.A.V.M.A. 183:318, 1983.

Dillon, A. R.: Strategic use of antibiotics in gastrointestinal disease in dogs and cats. J.A.V.M.A. 185:1169, 1984.

Dillon, A. R., and Wilt, G.: The role of *Campylobacter* species in dogs and cats: A cause for concern? Vet. Clin. North Am. 13:647, 1983.

Greene, C. E.: *Clinical Microbiology and Infectious Diseases of Dogs and Cats.* Philadelphia: W. B. Saunders, 1984.

Hirsch, D. C., and Enos, L. R.: The use of antimicrobial drugs in the treatment of diseases of the gastrointestinal tract. *In* Kirk, R. W. (ed.): *Current Veterinary Therapy VII.* Philadelphia: W. B. Saunders, 1983, p. 794.

Ishiwaka, H., Baba, E., and Matsumoto, H.: Studies on bacterial flora of the alimentary tract of dogs. III. Fecal flora in clinical and experimental cases of diarrhea. Jpn. J. Vet. Sci. 44:343, 1982.

Kato, E., Yoshifumi, K., and Kaneko, K.: Enterotoxigenic staphylococci of canine origin. J.A.V.M.A. 39:1771, 1978.

Olson, P., Hedhammar, A., and Wadstrom, T.: Enterotoxigenic *Escherichia coli* infection in two dogs with acute diarrhea. J.A.V.M.A. 184:982, 1984.

Papageorges, M., Higgins, R., and Gosselin, Y.: *Yersinia enterocolitica* enteritis in two dogs. J.A.V.M.A. 182:618, 1983.

Pierce, N. F., Cary, W. C., and Engel, P. E.: Antitoxic immunity to cholera in dogs immunized orally with cholera toxin. Infect. Immun. 27:632, 1980.

Prescott, J. F., Hohnson, J. A., Patterson, J. M., et al.: Haemorrhagic gastroenteritis in the dog associated with *Clostridium welchii.* Vet. Record 103:116, 1978.

Prescott, J. F., and Munroe, D. L.: *Campylobacter jejuni* enteritis in man and domestic animals. J.A.V.M.A. 181:1524, 1982.

Powers, T., and Mercer, H. D.: Antimicrobial drugs. *In* Anderson, N. V. M. (ed.): *Veterinary Gastroenterology.* Philadelphia: Lea & Febiger, 1980.

Sherding, R. G.: Diseases of the small bowel. *In* Ettinger, S. J. (ed.): *Textbook of Veterinary Internal Medicine,* 2nd ed. Philadelphia: W. B. Saunders 1983, 1278–1346.

Simon, G. L., and Gorbach, S. L.: Intestinal microflora. Med. Clin. North Am. 66:557, 1982.

Skirrow, M. B.: *Campylobacter* enteritis: The first five years. J. Hyg. (Camb.) 89:175, 1984.
Strombeck, D. R.: *Small Animal Gastroenterology*. Davis, CA: Stonegate, 1979.
Tedesco, F. J.: Pseudomembranous colitis: Pathogenesis and therapy. Med. Clin. North Am. 66:655, 1982.
Vantrappen, G., Agg, H. O., Beboes, K., et al.: *Yersinia* enteritis. Med. Clin. North Am. 66:639, 1982.

FELINE INFLAMMATORY BOWEL DISEASE

TODD R. TAMS, D.V.M.
West Los Angeles, California

The term *inflammatory bowel disease* (IBD) describes a group of chronic intestinal disorders characterized by a diffuse infiltration of the mucosa by various populations of inflammatory cells including lymphocytes, plasma cells, eosinophils, and neutrophils. This morphologic feature is not exclusive to idiopathic IBD, however. Disorders such as *Giardia* and *Campylobacter* infections may cause a mixed inflammatory cell infiltration in the lamina propria. The term IBD is used here to describe a chronic disorder in which no definitive causative agent can be determined. Subclassifications of chronic inflammatory bowel diseases include lymphocytic-plasmacytic enteritis, feline eosinophilic enteritis, and colitis. These inflammatory disorders may involve only the small intestine or alternatively may involve the stomach and colon as well. This article will cover primarily lymphocytic-plasmacytic enteritis, a disorder now recognized as a common cause of chronic vomiting and diarrhea in cats.

The cause of IBD is currently unknown. Many of the current theories invoke a chronic antigenic challenge and the subsequent development of a cytopathic immunologic response. Although the gut is exposed to an infinite number of antigens, microbial agents and food antigens are highly suspected to be primarily involved.

HISTORY AND CLINICAL SIGNS

One of the most common clinical signs observed in cats with idiopathic small intestinal inflammatory disease is vomiting. Vomiting is most often recognized as an intermittent occurrence for weeks, months, or years. Often as the disorder progresses there is an increased frequency of vomiting and other clinical signs that lead the owner to seek veterinary attention. Alternatively, some cats with even moderate to severe inflammatory changes on biopsy may be presented with clinical signs limited to an acute onset of vomiting and lethargy, with no past history of gastrointestinal signs. Vomiting episodes are usually associated with retching, are nonprojectile, and may produce clear fluid, bile, or food, either fresh or partially digested. A key point is that most often the vomiting and associated nonspecific signs are cyclic in nature. Clinical signs may be evident on one or several days and then spontaneously disappear, indicating that untreated IBD runs a course usually characterized by exacerbations and remissions.

In the author's experience, the second most common sign observed in feline IBD is diarrhea. Diarrhea may be the sole clinical sign or may occur in conjunction with intermittent vomiting. Diarrhea may be acute or chronic. Small bowel diarrhea is most often characterized by large quantities of soft formed, bulky, or watery stool. Steatorrhea may be evident, and more chronic cases are often accompanied by weight loss and listlessness. In contrast, large bowel diarrhea in cats most often has a loose, stringy consistency due to increased mucus content, and intermittent streaks of fresh blood may be present. Other signs include increased frequency of attempts to defecate (which owners commonly misinterpret as attempts to urinate), defecating in abnormal places, and hiding. If the disease is limited to the large intestine, most cats remain active and alert, have a normal appetite, and do not lose weight. Some cats have both small and large intestinal disease (enterocolitis), with similar histologic changes, yet only small intestine or large intestine signs predominate. In some cats with chronic IBD, diarrhea does not occur until some stressful episode (e.g., change in environment, queening) causes an exacerbation of clinical signs.

In addition to vomiting and diarrhea, other clinical signs that may be observed in feline IBD include changes in attitude or activity, altered appetite, and weight loss. Activity level changes are often cyclic. Appetite changes vary from intermittent anorexia to ravenous behavior. Inappetence most commonly seems to cycle with vomiting and listlessness. A ravenous appetite may occur in the face of weight loss and is usually observed in cats in which chronic diarrhea is the predominant sign. Differential diagnosis for this combination of signs includes pancreatic exocrine insufficiency and hyperthyroidism. Weight loss usually occurs only in chronic IBD cases in which episodes of vomiting or diarrhea have been protracted.

INCIDENCE

IBD usually develops in middle-aged and older cats (more than 8 years); however, the author has observed severe inflammatory bowel disease in several cats as young as 5 months. These young cats often are presented with the complaint of never having passed a normal stool. No breed predilection for feline IBD has been identified.

PHYSICAL EXAMINATION

Physical examination may reveal diffusely thickened and firm intestinal loops, but the absence of this finding does not rule out IBD. In some cases of severe IBD, the bowel loops may be quite rigid. Some cats exhibit increased abdominal sensitivity. Occasionally, only localized areas are painful, suggesting the possibility of a foreign body. The intestines may seem doughy or contain increased fluid. If there is concurrent large intestine involvement, the colon may be easily palpable and there may be blood evident on rectal examination or adhered to the end of the thermometer. Mesenteric lymphadenopathy is rarely present and is more commonly found with lymphosarcoma or eosinophilic syndrome.

Routine physical examination of any cat with chronic vomiting or diarrhea should include thorough examination for thyroid lobe enlargement. Many hyperthyroid cats have variable degrees of vomiting or diarrhea or both as part of their history. Gastric and duodenal biopsies in some hyperthyroid cats have significant inflammatory infiltrates, probably as a result of thyrotoxicosis.

Nonspecific signs of a sick cat such as dehydration and unkempt appearance may be evident. However, some cats with IBD remain active, alert, and well fleshed. By no means do these findings rule out a significant feline intestinal disorder. Thorough history and physical examination technique in conjunction with indicated diagnostic procedures remain the cornerstone of an early and accurate diagnosis of IBD.

LABORATORY FINDINGS

Baseline laboratory tests include a complete blood count, serum biochemical profile, feline leukemia virus (FeLV) test, urinalysis, and fecal exam for parasites. Occasionally, changes in the hemogram or profile occur in chronic, moderate to severe cases. There may be a mild nonregenerative anemia (anemia of chronic inflammatory disease), which can also be complicated by blood loss from an inflamed intestinal lining. Leukocytosis of 22,000 to 50,000 cells/mm^3 is sometimes observed in chronic, severe IBD cases and suggests that the inflammatory process is active. There is usually no left shift.

Most cases of severe inflammatory bowel disorders in cats do not result in hypoproteinemia (protein-losing gastroenteropathy syndrome). If hypoproteinemia does occur in conjunction with gastrointestinal signs, the albumin and globulin fractions are usually proportionately decreased. Hypoproteinemia with predominant hypoalbuminemia is usually due to protein-losing nephropathy disorders (increased loss of albumin through glomeruli) or liver disease (decreased albumin production). If hypoproteinemia (less than 6.0 gm/dl is considered significant in the cat) is detected in a mature cat with gastrointestinal signs, a detailed workup to determine cause should be performed as soon as possible. Hypoproteinemia indicates that the disorder is chronic and severe.

Elevated levels of liver enzymes (alanine aminotransferase, alkaline phosphatase) may be seen in cases of IBD with inflammatory hepatopathy. Hypocholesterolemia may result from decreased intestinal absorption, and hypokalemia from a combination of anorexia, vomiting, and chronic diarrhea. Most cats with IBD are FeLV-negative.

Xylose absorption is usually decreased in infiltrative bowel diseases (IBD, lymphoma, histoplasmosis) and stagnant loop syndrome (bacterial overgrowth). Unfortunately, this test is difficult to evaluate accurately in cats because it involves timed blood samples and depends on uniform gastric emptying of test reagents for absorption from the proximal duodenum. Accurate interpretation is difficult in cats because of erratic gastric emptying times, which may often be related to stress.

In most cases of feline IBD, the entire baseline examination is unremarkable. These tests are still quite useful, however, because they help to rule out other disorders. The next step should involve contrast radiographic studies and biopsies, prefera-

Table 1. Differential Diagnosis of Disorders Resembling Feline IBD

Hyperthyroidism
Eosinophilic enteritis (eosinophilic syndrome)
Lymphosarcoma
Exocrine pancreatic insufficiency
Stagnant loop (secondary intestinal obstruction; e.g., adenocarcinoma)
Idiopathic colitis
Functional bowel disorders

bly to include the stomach, duodenum, and colon. Definitive diagnosis of IBD is made only by biopsy.

Plain abdominal radiographs in cats with IBD are usually unremarkable. Abnormal findings on barium contrast examinations in feline IBD may include diffuse mucosal irregularities or spiculated small intestinal mucosal changes and thickened bowel segments, which may be evidenced by narrow dye columns. Although barium studies may show no abnormalities in these cases, this does not rule out an infiltrative bowel disorder.

DEFINITIVE DIAGNOSIS

A definitive diagnosis of IBD can only be made by intestinal biopsy, the single most important diagnostic procedure in the evaluation of intestinal disease. Biopsies can be obtained either under fiberoptic endoscopic control or at exploratory laparotomy. Endoscopy offers a minimally invasive means of examining the stomach and proximal small intestine in cats. The duodenal lumen may appear completely normal grossly in IBD, or alternatively there may be variable degrees of erythema or mucosal irregularity. Severe IBD is often associated with a "cobblestone" appearance of the duodenal mucosa. Multiple biopsies (4 to 8) should always be obtained at endoscopy because of the small sample size that is routinely taken. Biopsies of small intestine as well as stomach should always be obtained in cats with chronic vomiting that are undergoing endoscopy. It is not uncommon for cats with inflammatory changes involving only the small intestine to be presented with signs limited to chronic intermittent vomiting. If only gastric biopsies are obtained, the diagnosis may be missed.

Disadvantages of endoscopy include limitation to visualization, biopsy no further in the small intestine than the duodenum, and collection of samples usually no deeper than the muscularis mucosa. Most cases of idiopathic feline IBD, however, involve the entire small intestine, and inflammatory changes always involve the mucosa. Duodenal endoscopic biopsies, then, are reliably representative of the disorder that is present.

If a laparotomy is performed, any area that appears abnormal should be biopsied. In many cases of IBD, the entire small intestine appears grossly normal. Regardless of gross appearance, if the clinical course has led to the necessity of exploratory laparotomy, biopsies must be obtained because normal appearance does not rule out IBD. Biopsies from the duodenum or jejunum and the ileum should be obtained. Full-thickness intestinal biopsy complications include dehiscence secondary to poor technique or hypoproteinemia (rare in cats); alternatively, extremely thickened intestine may form a stricture at the biopsy site.

PATHOLOGY

In inflammatory bowel disorders, increased numbers of inflammatory cells (plasma cells, lymphocytes, eosinophils, and neutrophils) are present in the lamina propria. Either single cell type or mixed cell infiltrations may be involved. Normally no inflammatory cells are present in gastric mucosa, and only a few inflammatory cells are normally found in the villous lamina propria of the duodenum. Most commonly, these are mature small lymphocytes or plasma cells. Eosinophils are not observed in normal duodenal tissue.

In IBD cases, histologic inflammatory changes are usually reported as mild, moderate, moderate to severe, or severe, and the percentages of various inflammatory cells are noted. Often in severe cases, one or two cell types predominate and the other cell types are scattered (e.g., lymphocytic-plasmacytic enteritis with mild accumulation of eosinophils). Neutrophils are not commonly identified in IBD but when present probably indicate inflammatory response to a microbial component of the disorder. Deeper involvement or small erosions or ulcers may potentiate microbial invasion. Mucosal atrophy with villous blunting or fibrosis indicates chronic disease. Reactive inflammatory changes may occur in the stomach secondary to vomiting (usually a mild change if it does occur) or in the stomach or intestine from the presence of a foreign body or other cause of trauma. Secondary reactive changes are best differentiated in light of an accurate history.

Severe lymphocytic enteritis occasionally is difficult to differentiate from lymphosarcoma. Obviously, serious implications arise as to what type of therapy to prescribe in these cases. Differentiating factors of lymphosarcoma include absolute uniformity of lymphocyte population, mitotic cells, pleomorphism, and attendant ablation of villous arches. In severe lymphocytic enteritis, there is usually at least a scattering of other types of inflammatory cells and the villous arch is not ablated. It is therefore important that several full-thickness biopsies or multiple endoscopic biopsies be submitted to pathologists to facilitate more accurate diagnosis.

TREATMENT

Clinical management of cats with IBD is tailored for each individual case, based on a correlation between clinical signs, laboratory findings, and degree of histopathologic changes. Corticosteroids are the drugs of choice for small intestinal inflammatory diseases. In most cases, prednisone is started at 1 to 2 mg/kg/day divided into two doses. Cats with inflammatory changes characterized as mild to moderate usually respond well to the lower dose. If biopsies reveal disease that is moderate to severe, a dose of 2 mg/kg/day is used for 2 to 4 weeks or until clinical signs resolve. Occasionally, in severe cases characterized by chronic diarrhea, weight loss, and anorexia, an initial dose of 4 mg/kg/day for 2 weeks is required. This dose of corticosteroid is usually well tolerated in cats.

Most cats respond quickly, and it is not unusual for vomiting and diarrhea to subside within the first 3 to 5 days of therapy. Activity level and appetite in previously listless and inappetant cats improve quickly. Occasional vomiting episodes related to IBD are not an unexpected occurrence during early therapy.

If there has been a good response, the initial prednisone dose is decreased by half after 2 weeks and again by half at 4 weeks. Usually, a once-daily medication schedule can be achieved by 4 weeks. Alternate-day therapy should be maintained for 3 months. In cats with intestinal biopsy changes described as mild and in which disease was considered to be primary, corticosteroids can often be discontinued after 3 months. However, if signs recur within 2 to 4 weeks, long-term, low-dose therapy will likely be necessary. Cats with moderate to severe IBD usually require long-term therapy (months to years). After 2 to 3 months, treatment every second to third day with 2.5 mg prednisone usually is sufficient for control.

Cats that have had chronic diarrhea, weight loss, hypoproteinemia, leukocytosis greater than 30,000 cells/mm^3 with neutrophilia, or biopsy changes described as severe IBD usually require lifelong therapy. If attempts to decrease the level of prednisone are unsuccessful or if clinical signs cannot be controlled adequately on 2 mg/kg/day of prednisone, concurrent metronidazole (Flagyl, Searle & Co.) therapy should be started.

Metronidazole's mechanism of action includes an antiprotozoal effect, an inhibition of cell-mediated immune responses, and anaerobic antibacterial activity. A dosage of 10 to 20 mg/kg twice or three times daily is used for IBD. Ideally, at least several months of metronidazole therapy is given once it is started, but if compliance is a problem, shorter terms of 2 to 4 weeks at a time to rescue remissions may be sufficient. Metronidazole is supplied in 250-mg and 500-mg tablets; most cats are given one fourth of a 250-mg tablet twice or three times daily. Side effects at this dose other than occasional nausea or vomiting are uncommon.

Methylprednisone acetate (Depo-Medrol, Upjohn) can be used to treat feline IBD, but consistent control of clinical signs in moderate to severe IBD is more difficult to maintain with this drug. Initially, 20 mg is given subcutaneously or intramuscularly and is repeated at 1- to 2-week intervals for 2 to 3 doses. Injections are then given every 2 to 4 weeks as needed for control. In some cases of chronic diarrhea, there is an excellent but transient response for several days to a week or two. This route of therapy is usually reserved for cases in which it is very difficult for the client to administer oral medication.

The question of how long and at what dosage corticosteroids should be continued is most accurately answered by obtaining follow-up intestinal biopsies 3 months after initial diagnosis. This is most easily accomplished if endoscopic equipment is available. Many cases initially diagnosed as severe IBD show only slight to moderate histologic improvement despite an acceptable resolution of clinical signs on therapy. Maintenance therapy must be continued in these cases. The client must realize that resolution of clinical signs is not synonymous with cure in feline IBD. The majority of feline IBD cases are manageable but not curable. Alternatively, if follow-up biopsies show considerable improvement or complete resolution of inflammatory changes, one should attempt to discontinue therapy.

Antibiotics are uniformly ineffective when used as sole treatment for IBD. In most cases, antibiotics are only indicated if histologic changes include a neutrophilic component. This usually suggests a deeper inflammatory process with subsequent invasion by intestinal flora. Amoxicillin (Beecham Laboratories), a bactericidal antibiotic that is absorbed after oral administration, or metronidazole is most frequently used in these instances for 2 to 4 weeks.

Poor responses to therapy usually result from (1) inadequate initial corticosteroid dosage, (2) poor client compliance, or more commonly (3) treatment for only small intestinal inflammatory disease when colitis is present as well. Some cats with concurrent IBD and colitis may show minimal or no clinical signs of colitis. Initiation of treatment specific for colitis (sulfasalazine [Azulfidine, Pharmacia], for 7 to 10 days and increased dietary fiber) usually results in dramatic improvement in cases of enterocolitis.

Because dietary allergens may play a role in the cause of IBD, specific dietary therapy may be beneficial. Usually, primary IBD is either temporarily responsive or only minimally responsive to careful dietary manipulations. However, long-term control of IBD with as minimal a drug administration schedule as possible may be aided by specific dietary management. This should be started as soon as a diagnosis is made and continued as drug therapy is decreased later. Low-gluten diets such as Iams Feline (Iams Food Co.), Science Feline (Hill's Pet Products), or boiled lamb or chicken may be of benefit. Prescription Diet c/d (Hill's Pet Products), may also be used. The semimoist food Tender Vittles (Ralston Purina) has proved to be an excellent adjunct to the control of chronic diarrhea in cats. Use of Tender Vittles or bran supplementation (e.g., Miller's Bran) often minimizes the need for use of specific medication for feline colitis.

References and Supplemental Reading

Cotter, S. M.: Treatment of lymphoma and leukemia with cycophosphamide, vincristine, and prednisone: II. Treatment of cats. J. Am. Anim. Hosp. Assoc. 19:166, 1983.

Grove, D. I., Mahmoud, A. F., and Warren, K. S.: Suppression of cell-mediated immunity by metronidazole. Int. Arch. Allergy Appl. Immunol. 54:422, 1977.

Hendrick, M.: A spectrum of hypereosinophilic syndromes exemplified by 6 cats with eosinophilic enteritis. Vet. Pathol. 18:188, 1981.

Moore, R. P.: Feline eosinophilic enteritis. *In* Kirk, R. W. (ed.): *Current Veterinary Therapy VIII*. Philadelphia: W. B. Saunders, 1983, p. 791.

Sherding, R. G.: Diseases of the small bowel. *In* Ettinger, S. J. (ed.): *A Textbook of Veterinary Internal Medicine*. Philadelphia: W. B. Saunders, 1982, pp. 1278–1346.

Sherding, R. G., Stradley, R. P., Rogers, W. A., et al: Bentiromide: Xylose test in healthy cats. Am. J. Vet. Res. 43:12, 1982.

INTESTINAL LYMPHANGIECTASIA

ROBERT G. SHERDING, D.V.M.
Columbus, Ohio

Lymphangiectasia is a chronic protein-losing enteropathy of dogs that is characterized by marked dilatation of intestinal lymphatics (Campbell et al., 1968; Finco et al., 1973; Mattheeuws et al., 1974; Flesja and Torstein, 1977; Olson and Zimmer, 1978; Barton et al., 1978). Obstruction to the flow of lymph and distension of intestinal lymphatics lead to rupture of dilated lacteals and leakage of lymph fluid into the gut lumen. The constituents of intestinal lymph—plasma proteins, lymphocytes, and lipid (chylomicrons)—are subsequently depleted through loss into the feces. In addition, the delivery phase of fat absorption is impaired. Thus, the functional consequences of lymphangiectasia (Fig. 1) are panhypoproteinemia, lymphocytopenia, hypocholesterolemia, and fat malabsorption (steatorrhea, fat-soluble vitamin deficiency). Intestinal lymphangiectasia is the most common protein-losing enteropathy in dogs (Tams and Twedt, 1981).

The typical lesion of canine lymphangiectasia is a ballooning distortion of villi caused by markedly distended lacteals. Dilated lymphatics are also seen in the submucosa, serosa, and mesentery. Because of the abnormal villous architecture, the surface texture of the mucosa may appear grossly coarsened like a shag carpet; endoscopically, the whitish tips of swollen villi may be observed. A weblike network of milky white dilated lymphatic channels can usually be seen in the mesentery and on the serosal surface of the small intestines.

Lymphangiectasia can result from a number of causes: (1) congenital malformation of the lymphatic system; (2) infiltration or obstruction of intestinal lymphatics due to an inflammatory, fibrosing, or neoplastic process; (3) obstruction of lymph flow through the thoracic duct; and (4) elevated lymphatic hydrostatic pressure from functional impedence to flow caused by portal vein thrombosis, constrictive pericarditis, or chronic congestive heart failure (Waldman, 1966; Jeffries, 1983).

In canine lymphangiectasia, it appears that generalized inflammatory disease of the intestinal lymphatic network plays an important role in pathogenesis of the condition. Obstructing granulomatous lesions, sometimes referred to as lipogranulomas, are often found in and adjacent to lymphatics. These may be grossly visible as yellow-white nodular infiltrations and granular foamy deposits associated with mesenteric lymphatics or on the intestinal serosa along the mesenteric border. In addition, canine lymphangiectasia is usually accompanied by a lymphocytic-plasmacytic infiltrate in the lamina propria. The cause of these lesions remains to be determined; however, the frequent responsiveness of this disorder to corticosteroids further suggests that canine lymphangiectasia is in some way secondary to an inflammatory process.

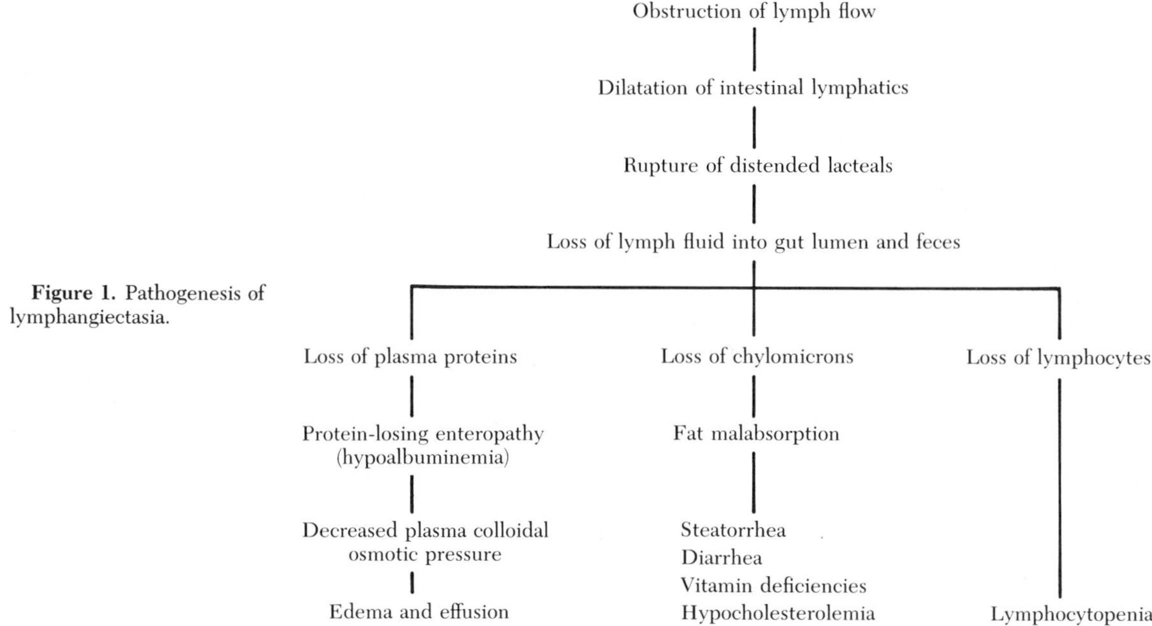

Figure 1. Pathogenesis of lymphangiectasia.

CLINICAL MANIFESTATIONS

The clinical manifestations of lymphangiectasia are attributable mainly to the secondary effects of enteric loss of lymph constituents, particularly albumin, more so than to any effect the disease has on the function of the intestine itself. In fact, hypoproteinemia may be the only apparent manifestation of intestinal disease; affected animals may pass normal-appearing feces and be free of any other signs usually expected with disease of the small intestine.

The excessive enteric loss of plasma proteins in lymphangiectasia leads to hypoalbuminemia and reduced colloidal osmotic pressure of plasma. This promotes fluid transudation from capillaries, resulting in the typical clinical features of severe protein-losing enteropathy: generalized peripheral edema and abdominal or pleural cavity effusion or both. Consequently, presenting signs may include dependent pitting edema of the subcutis and limbs, fluid distension of the abdomen (ascites), and respiratory distress (hydrothorax).

In addition to albumin loss, there is excessive loss of other plasma proteins in lymphangiectasia, including globulins, fibrinogen, clotting factors, lipoproteins, alpha$_1$-antitrypsin, transferrin, ceruloplasmin, and hormone-binding proteins (Jeffries, 1983). Although the plasma levels of these substances decline, they generally are not depleted sufficiently to cause significant functional impairment or clinical signs.

Primary intestinal manifestations may be observed in lymphangiectasia, but they are usually relatively mild. Chronic intermittent diarrhea of a watery to semisolid consistency is a variable finding. Steatorrhea can often be demonstrated, but not in all cases. Weight loss and progressive emaciation are commonly associated with long-standing protein-losing enteropathy.

Two breeds of dogs are reported to be predisposed to lymphangiectasia and protein-losing enteropathy—the lundehund and the basenji (Flesja and Torstein, 1977; Breitschwerdt et al., 1984). The author has observed a high prevalence of the disease in the Yorkshire terrier. In the basenji, lymphangiectasia occurs secondary to a unique intestinal disease that has been referred to as immunoproliferative enteropathy of basenjis (Breitschwerdt et al., 1984). This disorder appears to have a genetic basis and is characterized by chronic intermittent diarrhea, weight loss, hypoalbuminemia, hyperglobulinemia (an unusual finding in protein-losing enteropathy), and the hallmark of the disease—widespread lymphocytic-plasmacytic infiltration of the gastrointestinal tract. Studies have suggested the possibility of defective immunoregulation in the pathogenesis of basenji enteropathy.

DIAGNOSIS

A diagnosis of lymphangiectasia should be considered in animals manifesting hypoproteinemia, with or without edema or effusion, and particularly when accompanied by lymphocytopenia, hypocholesterolemia, or hypoglobulinemia. Lymphangiectasia must be distinguished from other protein-losing enteropathies (Table 1) (Waldman, 1966; Tams and Twedt, 1981; Jeffries, 1983). Also, the nonenteric

Table 1. Differential Diagnosis of Chronic Hypoproteinemia in the Dog

Protein-Losing Gastroenteropathy
Intestinal lymphangiectasia
Congenital malformation of lymphatics
Intestinal lymphatic obstruction (acquired)
Secondary to inflammation
Secondary to fibrosis
Secondary to intra-abdominal neoplasia
Thoracic duct obstruction
Portal vein thrombosis
Congestive heart failure (constrictive pericarditis)
Chronic inflammatory bowel disease
Lymphocytic-plasmacytic enteritis
Granulomatous enteritis
Eosinophilic gastroenteritis
Immunoproliferative enteropathy of basenjis
Gastrointestinal histoplasmosis
Gastrointestinal neoplasia (lymphosarcoma, carcinoma)
Chronic gastritis
Protein-Losing Glomerulopathy
Glomerulonephritis
Renal amyloidosis
Impaired Protein Synthesis
Liver failure
(impaired hepatic synthesis of albumin; body fluid retention)
Severe protein malnutrition
Prolonged starvation or anorexia
Intestinal malabsorption
(usually accompanied by protein-losing enteropathy)

causes of hypoalbuminemia—liver failure (impaired hepatic synthesis of albumin) and renal disease (protein-losing glomerulonephropathies)—should be ruled out through liver function testing and urine protein determinations, respectively. In hypoproteinemia due to liver or kidney disease, it is usually only albumin that is decreased, whereas serum levels of both albumin and globulins are depleted in most protein-losing enteropathies, including lymphangiectasia. The unique exception to this is immunoproliferative enteropathy of basenjis. In this disorder, hyperglobulinemia is usually found along with hypoalbuminemia (Breitschwerdt et al., 1984).

Compared with other protein-losing enteropathies, diarrhea is generally milder and found less consistently in lymphangiectasia. Laboratory studies of intestinal absorptive function, such as fecal fat determinations and the xylose absorption test, may be abnormal in dogs with lymphangiectasia, but not consistently. Since dilated lacteals leak chylomicron-laden lymph into the lumen and they prevent the normal assimilation of dietary fat, steatorrhea is a more likely finding than carbohydrate malabsorption.

Hypocalcemia is a frequent finding in lymphangiectasia. A number of factors are probably responsible: decreased protein-bound fraction of calcium associated with hypoalbuminemia, vitamin D malabsorption, and malabsorption of calcium that is complexed in the intestinal lumen with fatty acids and proteins.

Ancillary diagnostic procedures that may be indicated include (1) cardiac evaluations (auscultation, thoracic radiography, electrocardiography, echocardiography, central venous pressure) to rule out a cardiac cause of lymphangiectasia, (2) radiography to detect or confirm ascites and pleural effusion, and (3) fluid analysis of body cavity effusions. The effusion associated with lymphangiectasia is usually a transudate. Chylous ascites is sometimes found, apparently resulting from leakage of chylous lymph fluid from distended or diseased mesenteric and serosal lymphatics.

The gastrointestinal loss of plasma proteins can be measured by the fecal excretion of intravenously administered radiolabeled proteins and macromolecules (such as ^{51}chromium-labeled albumin); however, these procedures are too impractical for use in the clinical setting. The clearance of alpha$_1$-antitrypsin, a natural plasma protein, has been a simple and reliable method for measuring enteric protein loss in human patients without the use of radioisotopes (Bernier et al., 1978). This test needs to be evaluated in canine protein-losing enteropathy.

Diagnostic mesenteric lymphangiography can be used to evaluate the intestinal lymphatic system and to delineate sites of obstructed lymph flow within the thoracic duct. Since canine lymphangiectasia has been associated with portal vein thrombosis, there may be a role for angiographic evaluation of the portal system.

The diagnosis of lymphangiectasia is established by histologic confirmation of the characteristic mucosal lesion in intestinal biopsies. This also is often the best means of differentiating the various other chronic protein-losing and malabsorptive enteropathies. Biopsies may be obtained via laparotomy, or less invasively by endoscopy or peroral suction biopsy capsule. Surgery in those dogs with severe hypoproteinemia or emaciation should not be taken lightly—chronic protein depletion and the catabolic state may severely impair wound healing. The greatest risk in full-thickness surgical biopsy of the intestine is dehiscence of the enterotomy incision, which leads to subsequent bowel leakage and postoperative peritonitis. Thus, when less invasive biopsy methods such as endoscopy or suction biopsy capsule are unavailable, the diagnosis should be made whenever possible from gross appearance and biopsy of serosal and mesenteric lymphatic lesions without risking invasion of the gut for a full-thickness specimen. In severely hypoproteinemic animals, preoperative plasma infusions are also advisable.

TREATMENT

The major aim of therapy for intestinal lymphangiectasia is to decrease the enteric loss of plasma proteins so that normal plasma protein levels can be restored and edema and effusions controlled. Dietary manipulation and anti-inflammatory therapy are the chief components of treatment (Tams and Twedt, 1981).

The absorption of dietary long-chain triglyceride (LCT) is a major stimulus for intestinal lymph flow. Restriction of dietary intake of LCT reduces the protein loss in lymphangiectasia (Holt 1964; Jeffries et al., 1964). This is presumably because reduction of lymph flow and lymphatic hydrostatic pressure decreases the distension and rupture of lacteals. Fat restriction may also ameliorate diarrhea by reducing steatorrhea.

The ideal diet for the dog with lymphangiectasia should contain minimal fat (LCT) and provide an ample quantity of high-quality protein. Special commercial diets that fulfill these requirements are generally adequate and convenient in most cases (Prescription Diet r/d and Prescription Diet i/d, Hill's Pet Products). Because of the fat malabsorption that occurs in lymphangiectasia, these diets should be supplemented with fat-soluble vitamins. Daily food intake should be divided into two or three feedings.

Homemade diets are another alternative; for example, one part low-fat cottage cheese or yogurt as the protein source expanded with three to four parts rice or potatoes as the carbohydrate source. Homemade diets are not balanced, so vitamin-mineral supplements should be added, again, with extra fat-soluble vitamins.

Low-fat diets are inherently low in calories; yet, another goal of therapy is to reverse the weight loss and malnutrition that usually accompany chronic intestinal disease. Therefore, medium-chain triglycerides (MCTs) can be added to the diet to replace the calories lost by removal of conventional fat (LCT) from the diet. MCTs are useful as a source of calories in states of fat malabsorption because they are hydrolyzed more rapidly and efficiently than LCTs and then are absorbed directly into the portal venous system, bypassing chylomicron formation and the diseased, nonfunctional lymphatic transport system. Commercially available MCTs are derived from coconut oil and can be added to the daily ration as an oil (MCT Oil, Mead Johnson; 8.3 kcal/gm; 1 tbs weighs 14 gm and contains 115 kcal) at 1 to 2 ml/kg body weight, or as a powdered elemental diet mixture (Portagen, Mead Johnson); 1½ cups added to water to make 1 quart of mixture with 30 kcal/fluid oz). This latter mixture is hypertonic and may cause vomiting or aggravate diarrhea.

The plasma protein loss and diarrhea of lymphangiectasia can often be improved by anti-inflammatory doses of corticosteroids, such as oral prednisolone at an initial dosage of 2 to 3 mg/kg/day. Once a remission has been achieved, this dosage should be adjusted to a lower maintenance level. Anti-inflammatory therapy may help resolve obstructing inflammatory lesions of intestinal lymphatics, as well as reduce the lymphocytic-plasmacytic lamina propria infiltrate. However, not all cases of lymphangiectasia are steroid responsive.

Other measures should be considered in the unique enteropathy of the basenji. In addition to dietary management and corticosteroids, reduction of stress and antibiotics for control of bacterial overgrowth have been recommended.

When lymphangiectasia occurs secondary to an identifiable anatomic lymphatic obstruction or portal vein thrombosis, surgical intervention for relief of the obstruction should be considered. In cardiac-associated lymphangiectasia, the emphasis of therapy should be directed toward control of congestive heart failure. Pericardiectomy is usually indicated for the rare case of constrictive pericarditis.

In conclusion, the combination of dietary and anti-inflammatory therapy can be effective for many months or even years at maintaining remission of clinical signs, sustaining normal plasma protein levels, and eliminating effusions in many cases of canine lymphangiectasia. Some animals, however, fail to respond. Many of those dogs that do respond eventually worsen and finally succumb to severe protein-calorie depletion, incapacitating effusions, or intractable diarrhea.

References and Supplemental Reading

Barton, C. L., Smith, C., Troy, G., et al.: The diagnosis and clinicopathological features of canine protein-losing enteropathy. J. Am. Anim. Hosp. Assoc. 14:85, 1978.

Bernier, J. J., Florent, C., Desmazures, C., et al.: Diagnosis of protein-losing enteropathy by gastrointestinal clearance of alpha$_1$-antitrypsin. Lancet 2:763, 1978.

Breitschwerdt, E. B., Ochoa, R., Barta, M., et al.: Clinical and laboratory characterization of the Basenji dog with immunoproliferative small intestinal disease. Am. J. Vet. Res. 45:267, 1984.

Campbell, R. S. F., Brobst, D., and Bisgard, G.: Intestinal lymphangiectasia in a dog. J.A.V.M.A. 153:1050, 1968.

Finco, D. R., Duncan, J. R., Schall, W. D., et al.: Chronic enteric disease and hypoproteinemia in 9 dogs. J.A.V.M.A. 163:262, 1973.

Flesja, K., and Torstein, Y. R. I.: Protein-losing enteropathy in the lundehund. J. Small Anim. Pract. 18:11, 1977.

Holt, P.: Dietary treatment of protein loss in intestinal lymphangiectasia. Pediatrics 34:629, 1964.

Jeffries, G. H.: Protein-losing gastroenteropathy. *In* Sleisenger, M. H., and Fordtran, J. S., (eds.): *Gastrointestinal Disease*, 3rd ed. Philadelphia: W. B. Saunders, 1983, pp. 280–288.

Jeffries, G. H., Chapman, A., and Sleisenger, M. H.: Low-fat diet in intestinal lymphangiectasia: Its effect on albumin metabolism. N. Engl. J. Med. 270:761, 1964.

Mattheeuws, D., DeRick, A., Thoonan, H., et al.: Intestinal lymphangiectasia in a dog. J. Small Anim. Pract. 15:757, 1974.

Olson, N. C., and Zimmer, J. F.: Protein-losing enteropathy secondary to intestinal lymphangiectasia in a dog. J.A.V.M.A. 173:271, 1978.

Tams, T. R., and Twedt, D. C.: Canine protein-losing gastroenteropathy syndrome. Comp. Cont. Ed. Pract. Vet. 3:105, 1981.

Waldman, T. A.: Protein-losing enteropathy. Gastroenterology 50:422, 1966.

EVALUATION AND MANAGEMENT OF CARBOHYDRATE MALASSIMILATION

ROBERT J. WASHABAU, V.M.D.,
C. A. BUFFINGTON, D.V.M.,
and DONALD R. STROMBECK, D.V.M.
Davis, California

Malassimilation of dietary nutrients is usually expressed in terms of fat malassimilation, so that steatorrhea is sought as evidence of the problem. Accurate evaluation for steatorrhea requires quantitation of fecal fat excretion during a 72-hour period when the patient is fed a "standard" diet containing a measured amount of fat. This procedure is seldom done because of the complexity of fat analysis and the cost and length of the study. Steatorrhea is most commonly identified by staining fecal smears with fat stains and examining them for fat droplets. This procedure is not reliable, since fat droplets may not be found in some cases of steatorrhea. Since fat constitutes a small and variable part of the available calories in most commercial dog foods, finding steatorrhea provides only indirect and not always reliable evidence for concurrent malassimilation of carbohydrates and proteins.

Malassimilation of dietary protein is probably not very important in clinical cases, because proteins represent a small part of most diets and ample amounts of gastric and pancreatic enzymes are available for their digestion. Even with the loss of pancreatic enzyme activity, gastric pepsin activity remains to digest proteins. In addition, it is unnecessary for protein digestion to be complete, since dietary nitrogen is absorbed more efficiently in the form of peptides rather than as amino acids.

To the patient with chronic pancreatic or small intestinal disease, malassimilation of carbohydrates is more important than that of fat and protein for the following reasons: (1) carbohydrate is the most abundant nutrient in most commercial diets for dogs, (2) part of dietary carbohydrates are in a form that is not digested in the normal small intestine, and (3) maldigestion of carbohydrates may develop before that of fats and proteins, as the activity of pancreatic enzymes is reduced in the small intestine. That is supported by research (Pidgeon and Strombeck, 1982) showing marked improvement in protein and fat assimilation afforded by pancreatic enzyme replacement therapy in dogs with ligated pancreatic ducts but only partial improvement in fecal dry weight. The increased fecal dry weight represented mostly unabsorbed carbohydrates with only a small amount of fat and protein. Thus, it becomes important to evaluate the patient with chronic weight loss and diarrhea for malassimilation of carbohydrates and to consider the carbohydrate component of the diet when planning dietary management.

Malassimilation of carbohydrates can result in primary problems such as weight loss and diarrhea, or it may produce only secondary signs such as borborygmus or flatulence. Most cases do not show steatorrhea. Weight loss does not appear unless carbohydrate assimilation is marked, such as with pancreatic exocrine insufficiency (where weight loss is the most consistent sign) or moderate to severe small intestinal mucosal disease. Colonic fermentation of unassimilated carbohydrate produces short-chain carbon metabolites that can produce an osmotic diarrhea. Alternately, the diarrhea may be merely an increased volume of formed feces caused by increased amount of unassimilated carbohydrate solutes that were not fermented. Secondary signs of borborygmus and flatulence are also produced by colonic fermentation of carbohydrate that escapes assimilation in the small intestine. Production of hydrogen, carbon dioxide, and, in some cases, methane by colonic bacteria has long been implicated in the genesis of flatulence. Not all gas in the colon is produced by bacterial fermentation, however. Some represents swallowed air.

The digestion of carbohydrates is determined by (1) intestinal activity of pancreatic amylase, (2) the integrity of the intestinal mucosa, and (3) the digestibility of the carbohydrates in the diet. The intestinal activity of pancreatic amylase is determined not only by the amount secreted by the pancreas but also by its rate of disappearance, which is directly related to the number of bacteria in the small intestine. Increases in the number of small intestinal bacteria result in an increased rate of degradation of all digestive enzymes, including amylase. The brush-border enzymes of the small intestinal mucosa (disaccharidases) complete carbohydrate digestion. Only monosaccharides can be absorbed, and they require a special transport mechanism for absorption on the villous surface, which is lost with mucosal disease. The digestibility of carbohydrates is determined by (1) the degree that dietary starch is gelatinized, (2) the amount rendered soluble by cooking, and (3) the source or type of starch. Commercial processing of dry dog food is designed to gelatinize 80 per cent of the starch in the diet. Ungelatinized starch may escape assimilation and produce diarrhea, flatulence, or borborygmus following colonic fermentation.

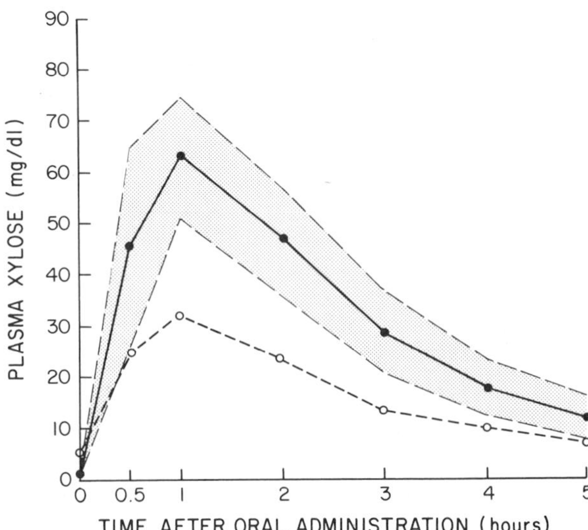

Figure 1. Xylose absorption in 32 normal dogs (filled circles represent means and shaded area denotes standard deviation) and in one dog with bacterial overgrowth of the small intestine (open circles).

EVALUATION OF CARBOHYDRATE MALASSIMILATION

Until recently there has been no reliable means of evaluating patients for carbohydrate malassimilation. Xylose absorption testing, which relies on the measurement of plasma concentrations of xylose at timed intervals after its oral administration, has been used most frequently. The rate of appearance of xylose in the blood is determined by its rate of absorption from the small intestine (Fig. 1). Small intestinal mucosal disease must be moderate to severe in order for the xylose absorption test to be abnormal, and even then the abnormalities are modest. Thus, the xylose absorption test is at best a poor indicator of mucosal disease causing malabsorption. Since xylose is a smaller sugar that does not require a special transport mechanism for absorption and moves across the brush border by passive diffusion, it cannot predict a malabsorption of glucose, the digestive product of starch. The greatest abnormalities in xylose absorption occur in patients with bacterial overgrowth of the small bowel. The bacteria metabolize xylose to such a degree that much less is available for absorption, and lower blood levels of xylose are found (Fig. 1). Bacterial overgrowth is confirmed by treating the patient with an unabsorbed antibiotic, after which the xylose absorption test is repeated and normal results are found. Other tests of carbohydrate malabsorption include those for glucose absorption, galactose absorption, lactose tolerance, and starch tolerance (Strombeck, 1979; Bond and Levitt, 1976). These tests are much less reliable.

A recently developed method to evaluate carbohydrate absorption is based on measurement of breath hydrogen excretion (Levitt, 1969; Levitt and Donaldson, 1970; Bond and Levitt, 1972; Bond and Levitt, 1975; Perman et al., 1984). Hydrogen, produced from the metabolism of carbohydrates by bacteria in the colon, is absorbed from the colon and excreted in expired air. The rate of production of hydrogen is determined by the type and number of colonic bacteria and the amount of available carbohydrate. Few bacteria are present in the normal small intestine, so breath hydrogen does not increase until unassimilated carbohydrate begins to enter the colon, a matter of approximately 6 hours after feeding. Breath hydrogen analysis is relatively simple, involving use of thermal conductivity gas chromatographic analysis of exhaled breath by means of an interval sampling technique (Metz et al., 1976).

Measurement of breath hydrogen provides a tool that is helpful in answering two questions. Is bacterial overgrowth of the small intestine a problem? And is a patient properly assimilating the carbohydrates in its diet? Breath hydrogen increases due to catabolism of carbohydrates by normal colonic microflora are shown in Figure 2. The increases do not begin until 6 hours after feeding, the time required for nutrients to pass through the stomach and small intestine. Breath hydrogen increases due to degradation of food by bacterial overgrowth in the small intestine are also illustrated in Figure 2. Increases appearing at 60 to 90 minutes identify

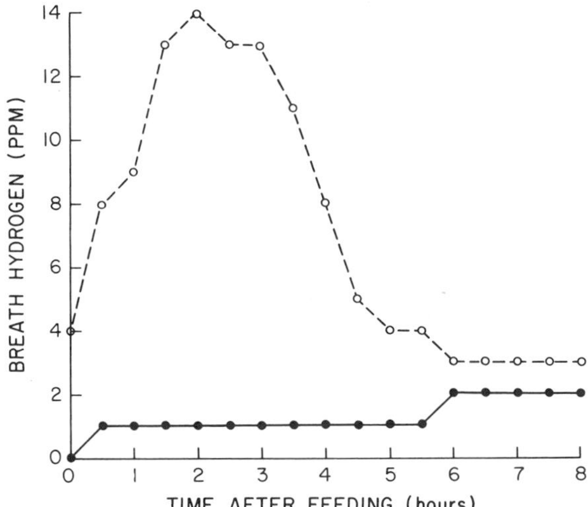

Figure 2. Increase in breath hydrogen caused by catabolism of carbohydrates by normal colonic microflora (filled circles). Increases due to degradation of food by bacterial overgrowth in the small intestine are noted by open circles.

the small intestine as the site of hydrogen production. Diseases that change the rate of gastric emptying or transit of a meal through the small intestine result in the appearance of breath hydrogen from the colon at some time other than after 6 hours. The measurement of breath hydrogen can thus be used to evaluate small intestinal transit time. No other clinical tool (including radiographic studies using positive contrast medium) can be used as reliably to provide this information.

A premature increase in breath hydrogen following a meal occurs in a variety of small bowel diseases: pancreatic exocrine insufficiency, chronic enteritis (which may be characterized by both bacterial overgrowth and villous changes including atrophy and infiltration by lymphocytes, plasma cells, and eosinophils), lymphosarcoma of the intestinal mucosa, stasis in the small intestine caused by a stricture or motility disorder, and many other diseases resulting in bacterial overgrowth. Following the use of breath hydrogen measurement to identify a small intestinal cause of carbohydrate malassimilation, the test can be used to evaluate the patient's response to management.

Patients with carbohydrate malassimilation may have increases in breath hydrogen at 6 hours after feeding in the absence of pancreatic or small intestinal disease. The causes of this finding include excess fiber in the diet, excess digestible carbohydrate in the diet, presence of undigestible carbohydrate in the diet, rapid transit of a meal through the small intestine (unlikely unless the small intestine has severe disease), and dietary allergies that reduce brush-border amylase activities without showing morphologic evidence of disease. The 6-hour increase in breath hydrogen is used to attribute the patient's diarrhea, flatulence, or borborygmus to carbohydrate malassimilation.

MANAGEMENT OF CARBOHYDRATE MALASSIMILATION

The medical management (other than diet) of specific disease entities such as pancreatic exocrine insufficiency and chronic lymphocytic-plasmacytic enteritis will not be discussed here. The medical management of these and other small intestinal diseases is presumed to have been instituted.

The initial consideration in the management of carbohydrate malassimilation is the selection of the carbohydrate that is most likely to be completely digested and absorbed in the small intestine. The addition of wheat or corn sources of starch to a commercial canned food (Prescription Diet d/d, Hill's Pet Products) results in an increase in breath hydrogen 6 hours after feeding (Fig. 3). The addition of an equal amount of rice results in a minimal increase in breath hydrogen 6 hours after feeding. The added starches were cooked so that 80 per cent were gelatinized, which is the percentage of gelatinization achieved in the usual processing of commercial dry dog food. These findings indicate that diets containing wheat or corn can produce signs of carbohydrate malassimilation. These cereals are the most important source of calories in most commercial pet foods. If such foods are processed more rapidly because of time constraints, much of the starch will fail to solubilize, resulting in carbohydrate malassimilation. It is possible that this problem can also occur by feeding other wheat products, such as baked bread and cooked macaroni, which are known to be incompletely assimilated in humans. It is estimated that 10 to 20 per cent of the carbohydrate in gluten-containing flour is not assimilated. The failure to achieve complete assimilation is attributed to incomplete removal of the gluten-protein coating that surrounds the inner core of

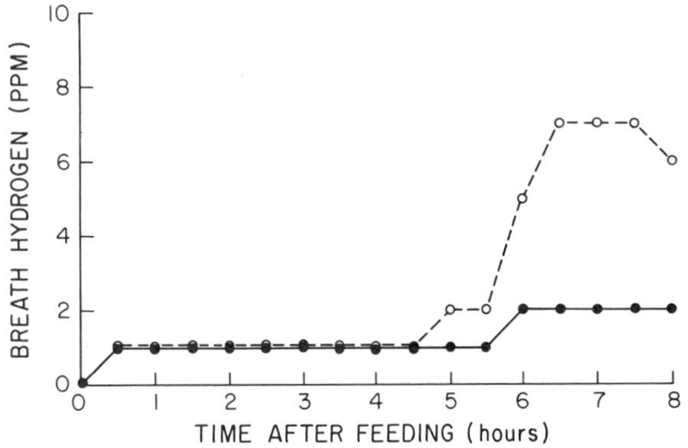

Figure 3. Increases in breath hydrogen after dogs were fed Prescription Diet d/d (Hill's Pet Products) with or without rice added (filled circles) and with wheat or corn added (open circles).

starch granules. This may explain the malassimilation of other gluten-containing cereal flours such as barley and oats. In summary, the starch in rice flour is more completely assimilated than starches in the flours from other common cereal sources. Rice should be selected for the patient with signs of carbohydrate malassimilation. The form of rice to feed may also be important. Instant rice as the only starch source is sometimes not completely digested, since grains of unaltered rice are seen in the feces. If its digestibility is in doubt, the rice may be ground into a flour before it is cooked and offered as food.

The amount of rice fed is seldom recognized to be important for the remission of signs in dogs with evidence of pancreatic or small intestinal problems, but the amount of starch in the diet is often important in cats with diarrhea. It is not unusual to find chronic diarrhea persisting in cats that are fed chicken or turkey and rice, and remission does not occur until the starch (rice) is removed from the diet. These observations suggest that cats have a lower carbohydrate tolerance than dogs. Currently, the authors recommend feeding a balanced diet with poultry meat protein without starch as the initial approach to management of persistent unexplained diarrhea in cats.

Malassimilation of carbohydrates is also determined by the fiber content of the diet. Digestion and absorption of carbohydrate is reduced in diets abundant in fiber. Natural fiber reduces carbohydrate digestion by inhibiting pancreatic amylase activity in the intestine. Fiber also decreases transit time in the intestine so that contents pass through more rapidly. Faster transit may not allow enough time for carbohydrate assimilation to be completed. A high-fiber diet could, therefore, contribute to carbohydrate malassimilation and cause signs of diarrhea and flatulence. Therefore, a low-fiber diet is recommended for animals with carbohydrate malassimilation. The primary indication for fiber in the management of gastrointestinal diseases is based on the observation that some dogs with colitis seem to benefit from the use of bran or commercially prepared fiber products such as Siblin (Parke-Davis). Undigested polysaccharides (mostly fiber) are the most important substrate for colonic bacterial growth and metabolic activity. Their action on fiber may be responsible for flatulence, and it may be possible to document this with persistent increases in breath hydrogen that begin to appear after 6 hours.

Although carbohydrate fermentation in the colon is directly determined by the number of bacteria in the colon, reduction in their numbers can never be realized with the use of orally administered antibiotics. Therefore, the routine use of antibiotics is not recommended.

References and Supplemental Reading

Bond, J. H., and Levitt, M. D.: Use of pulmonary hydrogen (H_2) measurements to quantitate carbohydrate absorption: Study of partially gastrectomized patients. J. Clin. Invest. 51:1219, 1972.

Bond, J. H., and Levitt, M. D.: Investigation of small bowel transit time in man utilizing pulmonary hydrogen (H_2) measurements. J. Lab. Clin. Med. 85:546, 1975.

Bond, J. H., and Levitt, M. D.: Quantitative measurement of lactose absorption. Gastroenterology 70:1058, 1976.

Levitt, M. D.: Production and excretion of hydrogen gas in man. N. Engl. J. Med. 281:122, 1969.

Levitt, M. D., and Donaldson, R. M.: Use of respiratory hydrogen excretion to detect carbohydrate malabsorption. J. Lab. Clin. Med. 75:937, 1970.

Metz, G., Gassull, M. A., and Leeds, A. R.: A simple method of measuring breath hydrogen in carbohydrate malabsorption by end-expiratory sampling. Clin. Sci Molec. Med. 50:237, 1976.

Perman, J. A., Modler, S., Barr, R. G., et al.: Fasting breath hydrogen concentration: Normal values and clinical applications. Gastroenterology 87:1358, 1984.

Pidgeon, G., and Strombeck, D. R.: Evaluation of treatment for pancreatic exocrine insufficiency in dogs with ligated pancreatic ducts. Am. J. Vet. Res. 43:461, 1982.

Strombeck, D. R.: Maldigestion and Malabsorption. *Small Animal Gastroenterology*. Davis, CA: Stonegate Publishing, 1979, pp. 201–222.

WHEAT-SENSITIVE ENTEROPATHY IN IRISH SETTERS

ROGER M. BATT, B.V.Sc.
Liverpool, United Kingdom

New procedures have been introduced for the investigation of dogs with suspected malabsorption, and it now seems likely that chronic small intestinal disorders may be much more common than previously realized (Batt, 1984). Erroneous diagnosis of exocrine pancreatic insufficiency has undoubtedly been a major contributory factor, compounded by the considerable difficulties to be overcome in order to achieve an accurate diagnosis of small intestinal disease. These difficulties include the limitations of routine screening procedures such as the xylose absorption test, the relative inaccessibility of the small intestine to biopsy and, not infrequently, the absence of obvious histologic changes in the mucosa. Predominantly biochemical criteria have now been applied to the analysis of peroral jejunal biopsies, and this new approach has facilitated the detection and characterization of a wheat-sensitive enteropathy in Irish setters.

CLINICAL DESCRIPTION

A specific enteropathy was initially identified in a series of ten Irish setters, one 7 years old and the others between the ages of 7 months and 2 years (Batt et al., 1984a). The main clinical sign was poor weight gain or weight loss, accompanied in eight dogs by intermittent chronic diarrhea, with an onset typically between 4 and 7 months of age. Figure 1 shows that serum folate was reduced in only four dogs, three of which also had reduced xylose absorption, findings consistent with disease of the proximal small intestine. However, this indirect evidence of functional disturbance was not a feature of the majority of the affected animals, reflecting the severity and patchy nature of the morphologic changes discussed below. Normal serum folate was unlikely to have been maintained in spite of defective folate transport by folate of bacterial origin, since no marked bacterial overgrowth (more than 10^5 organisms/ml) was demonstrated in the duodenal juice obtained from seven of these dogs. Bacteria may have contributed to the elevated serum folate concentrations found in two dogs; however, duodenal juice from one of these dogs was cultured and failed to confirm this possibility. Further evidence against long-standing overgrowth was provided by the demonstration of normal serum vitamin B_{12} concentrations in all cases, in marked contrast to the reduced levels in German shepherd dogs with bacterial overgrowth (Batt, 1984). The normal serum vitamin B_{12} concentrations also suggested that the enteropathy was likely to be confined to the proximal small intestine, although a patchy disease of the ileum that did not interfere significantly with vitamin B_{12} absorption could not be ruled out.

MUCOSAL ABNORMALITIES

Morphologic changes in the mucosa were variable and appeared to be patchy within individual animals. The most consistent abnormality was partial villous atrophy (Fig. 2) with no remarkable alterations in the cellular complements of the lamina propria. One biopsy from one dog did exhibit a much more severe subtotal villous atrophy, which is a typical feature of celiac disease (gluten-sensitive enteropathy) in humans. However, this appearance is not pathognomonic for celiac disease since similar changes have been observed occasionally in other disorders, including cows' milk protein intolerance and soybean intolerance in children. Indeed, this extremely flat mucosa is a rare manifestation of the disease in these dogs, and the spectrum of morphologic changes bears a more striking resemblance to that in children with celiac disease who do not maintain a strict gluten-free diet.

Quantitative biochemical assessment of organelles demonstrated that there were specific brush-border

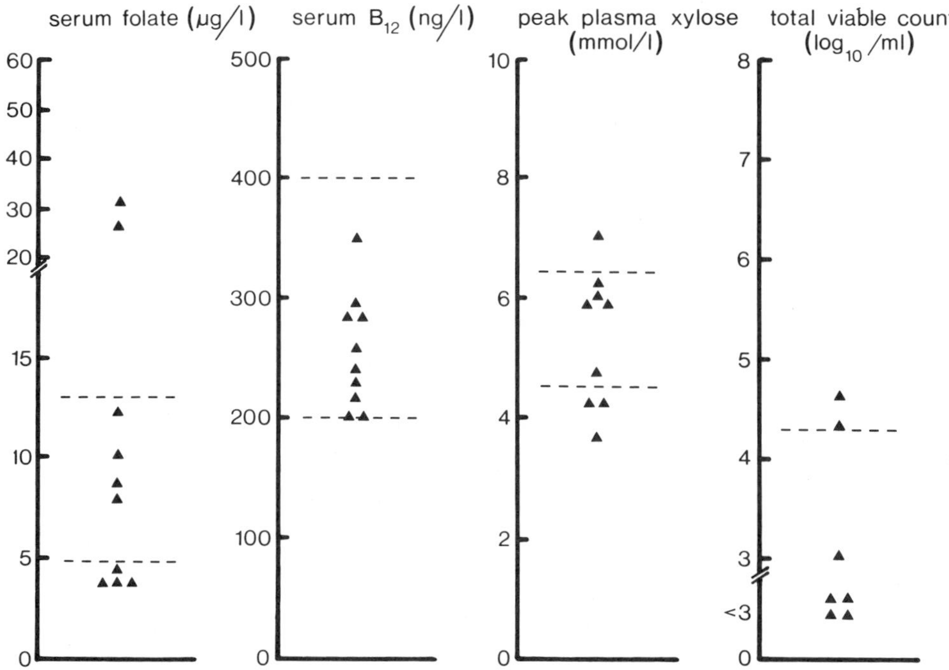

Figure 1. Serum folate and vitamin B_{12} concentrations, results of xylose absorption test, and total bacterial counts in duodenal juice from Irish setters with small intestinal disease. Dotted lines define control ranges or the upper control value for total bacterial counts. (Data from Batt et al.: Res. Vet. Sci. 37:339, 1984.)

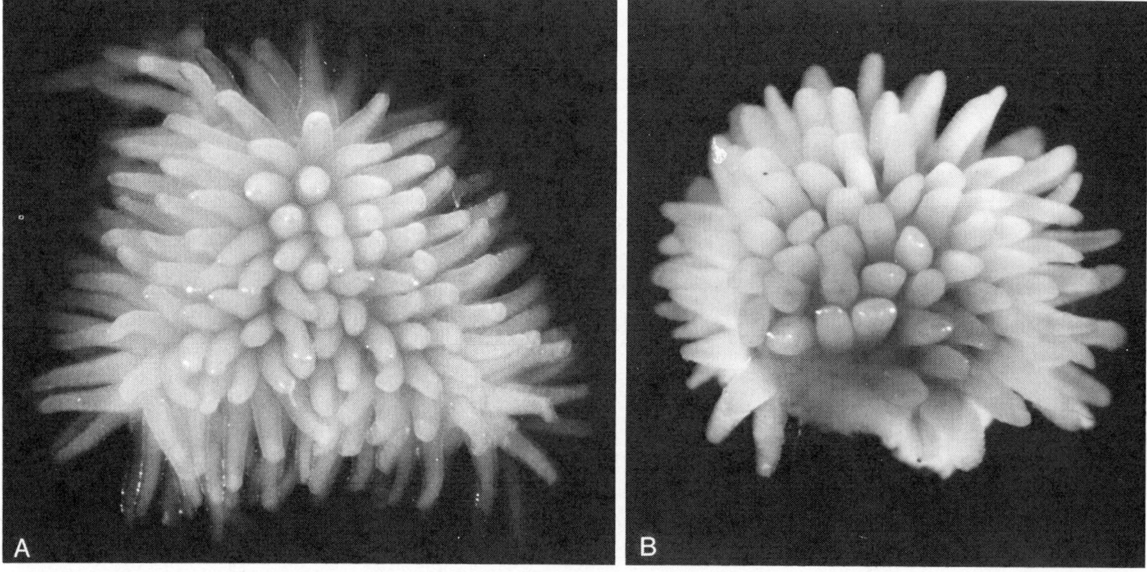

Figure 2. Appearance of jejunal biopsy material through a dissecting microscope. *A*, Jejunum from a normal dog shows long, fingerlike villi; *B*, jejunum from an Irish setter with small intestinal disease shows partial villous atrophy (× 20). (Reprinted with permission from Batt et al.: Res. Vet. Sci. 37:339, 1984.)

abnormalities in jejunal biopsies from affected animals. Table 1 shows that the specific activities of alkaline phosphatase and of aminopeptidase N were selectively decreased, whereas activities of the disaccharidases and of γ-glutamyl transferase were unaltered. These changes contrast markedly with the generalized brush-border abnormalities associated with more severe morphologic damage to the mucosa, for example in the canine enteropathy resembling chronic tropical sprue in humans (Batt, 1984).

DEMONSTRATION OF WHEAT SENSITIVITY

The possibility that this condition might be a wheat-sensitive enteropathy was supported by the considerable clinical improvement in the six dogs treated with a cereal-free diet, a finding pursued by breeding a litter from two affected dogs (Batt et al., 1984b). In all eight progeny, who were fed a normal diet containing meat and cereals including wheat, jejunal biopsies revealed partial villous atrophy and age-related biochemical abnormalities. In biopsies from the first four dogs at 8 months of age, activities of alkaline phosphatase and of aminopeptidase N were almost undetectable, whereas disaccharidases were unaltered. In contrast, biopsies obtained from the second four dogs at 9 months of age showed that there was a selective loss of brush-border alkaline phosphatase, but the activity of brush-border aminopeptidase N was normal.

Further investigation of the first four dogs demonstrated restoration of normal morphologic and biochemical characteristics after 5 months on a cereal-free diet. Relapse on subsequent challenge with wheat flour for 3 months was characterized by patchy partial villous atrophy, intraepithelial blebs, edema of the lamina propria, and a severe but selective loss of brush-border alkaline phosphatase activity.

PATHOPHYSIOLOGIC MECHANISMS

These findings document a wheat-sensitive enteropathy in Irish setters and suggest that this may be an inherited disorder associated with delayed development of specific brush-border enzymes. An abnormality of aminopeptidase N, the most abundant brush-border peptidase, could be particularly important during a critical growth phase and might result not only in protein malabsorption but also in defective degradation of potentially toxic gliadin (wheat protein) peptides. The latter might pemit development of hypersensitivity, perhaps mediated by the mast cell as suggested for celiac disease (Marsh, 1984), so that despite the subsequent appearance of peptidase activity, relatively small concentrations of peptide might be adequate to trigger enterocyte damage and cause villous atrophy. However, at present this possibility is speculative and the pathogenesis of this wheat-sensitive enteropathy has yet to be defined.

PRACTICAL APPROACH TO DIAGNOSIS AND TREATMENT

The diagnosis of this condition is not straightforward, either by the use of indirect functional tests or by the routine morphologic examination of intestinal biopsies. In addition, although the biochemical studies have permitted a detailed characterization of mucosal abnormalities in order to help achieve a better understanding of the pathogenesis of the enteropathy, it seems unlikely that biochemical examination of intestinal biopsies will become a routine diagnostic procedure.

As a practical approach to the investigation of all dogs presented with clinical signs suggestive of chronic malabsorption, the first steps should include the accurate assessment of exocrine pancreatic function, preferably by use of the *N*-benzoyl-L-tyrosyl-*p*-aminobenzoic acid test (Rogers et al., 1980; Batt and Mann, 1981) or, when generally available, by the assay of serum trypsin-like immunoreactivity

Table 1. *Activities of Brush-Border Marker Enzymes in Jejunal Biopsies from Irish Setters with Intestinal Disease and from Controls*

	Alkaline Phosphatase EC 3.1.3.1	Aminopeptidase N EC 3.4.11.1	Maltase EC 3.2.1.20	Sucrase EC 3.2.1.48	Lactase EC 3.2.1.23	γ-Glutamyl Transferase EC 2.3.2.2
Intestinal disease	83.7 ± 18 (9)	66.5 ± 9.1 (10)	306 ± 19 (10)	69 ± 7.0 (10)	23.5 ± 3.4 (10)	11.0 ± 1.3 (10)
Control	134 ± 9.8 (15)	102 ± 8.5 (16)	329 ± 25 (12)	67 ± 5.1 (12)	33.5 ± 3.8 (12)	10.9 ± 0.5 (15)
Statistical significance	$p<0.02$	$p<0.02$	NS	NS	NS	NS

Data (m units/mg protein) are expressed as mean ± SEM with number of animals in parenthesis. Statistical analysis by Student's *t*-test. NS: not significant ($p > 0.05$).

Data from Batt et al.: Res. Vet. Sci. 37:339, 1984.

(Williams and Batt, 1983). Subsequently, estimations of serum folate and vitamin B_{12} concentrations can provide useful information not only to assist the identification of small intestinal disease but also to provide an initial assessment of the likely nature of the mucosal changes (Batt and Morgan, 1982; Batt, 1984). The possibility of a wheat-sensitive enteropathy should then be explored by treatment with an exclusion diet, for example boiled chicken or cottage cheese with either boiled rice or potato, or a prescription diet such as d/d (Hill's Pet Products). Improvement of diarrhea should be relatively rapid, but recovery of normal body weight may take many weeks to achieve. In refractory cases, oral prednisolone (0.5 mg/kg repeated every 12 hours for a month, then a reducing dose) may be helpful, since this treatment is effective in human patients with so-called nonresponsive celiac disease. Beneficial effects may be a consequence of immunosuppression or may be due to the direct action of glucocorticoids to increase the digestive and absorptive capacities of the enterocytes by the induction of specific brush-border proteins (Batt and Scott, 1982). Finally, supplementation with vitamins, particularly oral folate (e.g., 5 mg/day for 1 to 6 months) may be of value, since in some cases a folate deficiency may contribute to villous atrophy by interfering with crypt cell turnover. In the long term, it may prove possible to prevent the development of the disease by the exclusion of cereal from the diet for the first few months of life.

References and Supplemental Reading

Batt, R. M.: Techniques for single and multiple peroral jejunal biopsy in the dog. J. Small Anim. Pract. 20:259, 1979.

Batt, R. M.: Chronic small intestinal disease in the dog. J. Small Anim. Pract. 25:707, 1984.

Batt, R. M., Carter, M. W., and McLean, L.: Morphological and biochemical studies of a naturally occurring enteropathy in the Irish setter dog: A comparison with coeliac disease in man. Res. Vet. Sci. 37:339, 1984a.

Batt, R. M., McLean, L., and Loughran, M.: Specific brush border abnormalities associated with a wheat-sensitive enteropathy (WSE) in the Irish setter dog. Gastroenterology 86:1021, 1984b.

Batt, R. M., and Mann, L. C.: Specifity of the BT-PABA test for the diagnosis of exocrine pancreatic insufficiency in the dog. Vet. Rec. 108:303, 1981.

Batt, R. M., and Morgan, J. O.: Role of serum folate and vitamin B_{12} concentrations in the differentiation of small intestinal abnormalities in the dog. Res. Vet. Sci. 32:17, 1982.

Batt, R. M., and Scott, J.: Response of the small intestinal mucosa to oral glucocorticoids. Scand. J. Gastroenterol. 17:(Suppl 74):75, 1982.

Marsh, M. N.: Morphologic expression of immunologically-mediated change and injury within the human small intestinal mucosa. *In* Batt, R. M., and Lawrence, T. L. J. (eds.): *Function and Dysfunction of the Small Intestine*. Liverpool: Liverpool University Press, 1984, pp. 167–198.

Rogers, W. A., Stradley, R. P., Sherding, R. G., et al.: Simultaneous evaluation of pancreatic exocrine function and intestinal absorptive function in dogs with chronic diarrhea. J.A.V.M.A 1177:1128, 1980.

Williams, D. A., and Batt, R. M.: Diagnosis of canine exocrine pancreatic insufficiency by the assay of serum trypsin-like immunoreactivity. J. Small Anim. Pract. 24:583, 1983.

DIAGNOSIS AND MANAGEMENT OF CHRONIC COLITIS IN THE DOG AND CAT

ANNE CHIAPELLA, D.V.M.
Gaithersburg, Maryland

DIAGNOSIS OF CHRONIC COLITIS

Chronic colitis is an inflammation of the colon that leads to chronic diarrhea, which may be intermittent or continuous in nature. In colitis, the inflammation of the colonic wall disrupts the normal absorptive and secretory patterns of the colon so that net secretion occurs. In addition, the colon, usually a site of rhythmic segmentation that provides resistance to aboral movement of feces, is hypomotile in colitis. The diarrhea that occurs in colitis is due to three major mechanisms: (1) decreased segmentation, which allows the normal peristalsis to move feces more rapidly aborally, (2) increased secretion of water and electroytes, and (3) an increased urge to defecate due to inflammation in the colonic rectal wall. There may also be abnormal microbial digestion in colonic disease. Unfortunately, the cause of most cases of chronic colitis is probably multifactorial and certainly is poorly defined. Only in rare cases is the cause of colitis pinpointed.

The first step in the diagnosis of chronic diarrhea is determining whether it originates in the small intestine or large intestine. Basically, this can be done through historic and physical examination. Radiographs and laboratory data are helpful in ruling out other more serious diseases that may cause signs similar to those of disease of the small or large intestines. Characteristically, the diarrhea in colitis is described as a high-frequency, low-volume stool with tenesmus, dyschezia, and urgency. Mucus, blood, or both are commonly seen in the stool. Frequent vomiting, weight loss, and other clinical signs are usually absent in all but the most severe cases of colitis. Small intestinal diarrhea, on the other hand, is usually characterized by voluminous, watery stools with a slight increase in the frequency of defecation. Weight loss, a variable appetite, and vomiting may accompany small intestinal disease. Tenesmus is uncommon, expect in dysentery.

Unfortunately, a "secondary" colitis is often associated with disease of the small intestines. There is inflammation of the colon by nonabsorbed intraluminal contents such as fatty acids. An animal that has diarrhea characterized as both small intestinal and colonic in origin may actually have small intestinal disease with secondary colitis or diffuse bowel disease involving both areas, such as is seen with lymphosarcoma or histoplasmosis. The clinician must be aware that biopsy of the colon *may not* identify the entire problem and laboratory studies may at times be needed to rule out small intestinal disease.

Results of physical examination of animals with chronic colitis are usually normal except for the presence of mucus and possibly blood in the stools. A rectal examination is critical for elimination of diseases such as rectal carcinoma, perianal fistulas, and others. A corrugated mucosa on rectal examination might indicate the possibility of colonic carcinoma or an infiltrative colitis. Combined rectal and abdominal palpation can rule out abdominal masses and other signs of systemic diseases. Only animals with severe mucosal or transmural colitis will show signs of weight loss and debilitation.

Laboratory studies in cases of chronic colitis are used to eliminate more serious systemic or small intestinal diseases. Most animals with chronic colitis will have a normal hemogram and blood chemistry profile; however, depending on the cause of the colitis, eosinophilia may be noted. Anemia, hypoproteinemia, and other abnormal laboratory results more commonly indicate that the small intestine is involved in the disease process. However, severe forms of colitis such as granulomatous or histiocytic ulcerative colitis may be accompanied by iron deficiency anemia, neutrophilia, and hypoproteinemia. Fungal colitis may also be associated with numerous laboratory abnormalities, depending on the degree of systemic involvement.

Multiple fecal examinations for parasites and microscopic examination of colonic mucus are integral parts of the diagnostic workup for chronic diarrhea. Fecal mucus stained with new methylene blue may identify leukocytes. Fecal leukocytes indicate a break in the mucous membrane of the bowel. A wet preparation of feces is indicated to check for *Giardia*. Hookworms, whipworms, and *Giardia* may all cause chronic colitis in dogs. Bacterial cultures should be performed when the diarrhea is bloody or when signs of infection (fever, leukoytosis, and fecal leukocytes) are an integral part of the history. Unfortunately, routine aerobic cultures provide little information about the significance of the organisms cultured. Many organisms, including *Escherichia coli* and *Staphylococcus aureus* may be cultured even though they do not *necessarily* play a pathogenic role in the diarrhea. *Salmonella* and *Campylobacter* are more likely to be true pathogens in the cause of bloody diarrhea. However, the value of aerobic and anaerobic culture or cultures specifically for *Campylobacter* must await extensive study in cases of chronic colitis in dogs.

Radiographs of the abdomen should be performed in most cases of chronic colitis primarily to rule out other abdominal conditions. This is especially important if the clinician is not certain whether the diarrhea is of small or large bowel origin. An upper gastrointestinal series should not be used to evaluate the cecum and colon because of ineffective filling and subsequent "artifacts" due to residual fecal material. Barium enemas tend to be difficult to interpret unless the animal's colon is very clean, and they are also time-consuming compared with proctoscopy. They *are* recommended when cecal diseases, proximal segmental colitis, or colonic masses are suspected.

Once a tentative diagnosis of chronic colitis is made, protoscopy and colonic biopsy should be undertaken for definitive diagnosis. Colitis is usually a diffuse process, so the results of proctoscopy and biopsies of the distal colon are usually representative of the entire colon. Exceptions to this include cecal diseases, proximal segmental colitis, or colonic masses. Proctoscopic equipment, preferably fiberoptic, is available in various sizes for animals from 4.5 to 7 kg (10 to 15 lb) to larger animals. The colon is cleansed with a combination of oral laxatives and warm-water enemas if necessary over a 24- to 72-hour period; animals with severe bloody diarrhea should be examined without enemas. Most dogs are examined proctoscopically while standing; cats are sedated lightly. The colonic wall is evaluated for color, distensibility, and the presence of erosions, ulceration, and lymph follicles. The normal colon is pale pink in color, is easily distensible, and has a scattering of lymph follicles in the wall. Clinicians should be aware that warm-water enemas induce hyperemia of the colonic wall.

Three to five biopsies should be taken to determine the type of process occurring in the distal colon. Although a variety of instruments are available, the Quinton Multipurpose Suction Biopsy Instrument (Quinton Instrument Co.) has been used safely to obtain excellent biopsies. Biopsies are placed on pieces of cardboard and inserted into formalin fixative. Due to their small size, they must be processed by a pathologist experienced in interpreting such tissue. Occasionally a biopsy must be taken with a biopsy forceps. This provides larger, more easily processed tissue; however, there is a risk of hemorrage and perforation associated with this technique.

Biopsies may yield information that causes the clinican to search elsewhere for the diagnosis. For example, the finding of a normal colon or colonic hyperplasia often indicates that the lesions are higher in the colon or cecum or within the small intestine. The clinician should then review the clinical signs and laboratory and radiographic findings. Further diagnostic tests on the animal might include colonoscopic examination and biopsy or a barium enema, if the signs are still colonic in nature. Occasionally, exploratory laparotomy and biopsy of the colon, cecum, and ileum may be necessary for diagnosis. The author has, at times, recommended cecal removal in cases of chronic bloody diarrhea in which numerous therapies for colitis have failed. This has cured the diarrhea in a limited number of cases.

Dogs with chronic diarrhea of colonic origin but normal colonic biopsy findings may have a stress-related component to their condition. These animals can be identified through a careful history and by ruling out other diseases with laboratory work and colonic biopsy. These commonly are nervous, hyperactive animals that in the owner's opinion are sensitive to changes in their environment. Thunderstorms, family disputes, and the introduction of new animals or persons into the environment can commonly trigger the diarrhea. Parallels exist between this condition and a stress-related colonic motility disorder in humans, irritable bowel syndrome. Veterinarians must be cautious to rule out more serious disease before assuming a stress-related component to the diarrhea in animals.

Biopsies of animals with chronic colitis usually reveal mild fibrosis with goblet cell hyperplasia and infiltration by a variety of different inflammatory cells. These cells may aid in the identification of some factors thought to initiate the colitis. An eosinophilic infiltrate is commonly associated with a parasitic or allergic cause. Such a diagnosis should stimulate a search for hookworms and whipworms and possibly a therapeutic worming for both. Dietary allergy must also be considered. Plasmocytic and lymphocytic infiltrates in the colon may indicate stimulation of the immune system by a variety of antigens, including dietary components, parasites, and colonic bacteria and their by-products. Lymphoid hyperplasia may be seen in a variety of diseases, including whipworm infestations, early lymphoma, and certain small intestinal diseases.

Histiocytic ulcerative colitis and granulomatous colitis are fortunately rare, as they represent a group of idiopathic diseases with a guarded prognosis. In the case of "boxer" histiocytic ulcerative colitis, the disease may be hereditary in origin. These forms of colitis tend to be severe and respond poorly to therapy. Infectious colitis, such as histoplasmosis and protothecosis, may also be diagnosed by colonic biopsy. The prognosis of these diseases depends very much on the primary disease state. Lymphosarcoma and rectal carcinoma may also be documented by biopsy. *Biopsy of the colonic wall is critical, since differentiation of these various processes is not always possible by proctoscopy alone.*

MANAGEMENT OF COLITIS

The practitioner should explain that treatment is commonly aimed at *control* of this disease process and not necessarily at a cure. This will save a great deal of time and energy on the part of the practitioner and places the client's expectations for the animal at a reasonable level. The veterinarian must impress on the client that chronic colitis is made up of many factors. The diarrhea that results from colitis is probably a threshold phenomenon. Numerous factors including dietary sensitivities, parasitic invasion, bacterial flora alterations, and psychogenic factors are interrelated components in the induction of chronic colitis. Other factors as yet undefined may also be involved.

Initial therapeutic decisions regarding animals with chronic colitis are based on clinical impressions, proctoscopic examination of the colon, and prior dietary and pharmacologic successes or failures. Further treatment is determined by the biopsy diagnosis, the severity of the clinical signs, and the client's tolerance for the animal's disease process. Basically, therapy is a combination of dietary alterations, antimicrobial administration, and the occasional use of motility modifiers and corticosteroids. Anthelmintic therapy is used as needed for treatment of parasites.

Dietary Therapy in Chronic Colitis

Dietary therapy for chronic colitis produces quite variable results; however, the concept of "resting the gastrointestinal tract" is basically sound. Small, multiple meals may decrease the gastrocolic reflex, thereby decreasing the diarrhea. A bland, hypoallergenic diet that may decrease antigenic stimulation of the bowel and reduce the number of bacteria in the bowel is ideal. Anaerobes such as *Clostridium perfrigens* are implicated in the origin of experimental colitis, and high-starch diets have been shown to decrease clostridia in the feces of dogs.

A combination of rice and potatoes with low-fat cottage cheese, plain yogurt, skinned chicken, or mutton will be tolerated by most patients. The ratio of carbohydrate to protein should be 4:1 or 3:1. A commercial diet may be used as an alternative. The diet chosen may depend on the disease process diagnosed by the veterinarian. Prescription Diets i/d and r/d (Hill's Pet Products) are both low in fat, gluten free, and probably not indicated unless the colitis is thought to be secondary to a small intestinal problem. Prescription Diet d/d (Hill's Pet Products), which contains mutton and rice, is a hypoallergenic diet indicated when a dietary allergy or food intolerance is suspected. In such cases, a mild eosinophilic or a plasmacytic-lymphocytic infiltrate may be seen in colonic biopsies.

The ideal fiber content in diets today is a point of contention in gastroenterology. Low-residue diets such as the cottage cheese, yogurt, and rice diets are advisable when the intestine is narrowed or ulcerated. However, fiber is now known to alter intestinal motility in a beneficial way. It slows the intestinal transit time, increases stool bulk and water content, and decreases intracolonic pressure. Since rhythmic segmentation is stimulated by distension of the colon, the addition of fiber may help animals with a variety of colonic diseases.

Crude fiber content corresponds to the cellulose, hemicellulose, and pectin content of food. Most bulking agents consist of either a purified fiber or a natural preparation such as bran. Unprocessed bran contains 2.4 gm of fiber per teaspoon. The recommended dietary fiber content is 2.4 gm of fiber per 10 to 15 kg of body weight per day. Cereals such as Kellog's Bran, Bran Buds, and Nabisco bran contain 1 to 2 gm of crude fiber per ounce (½ cup). Unfortunately, such products contain high levels of sugar as well as gluten and may lead to increased flatulence. Over-the-counter dietary supplements such as Siblin (Parke-Davis) or Metamucil (Searle & Co.) can be used instead of the natural fiber products, if such side effects occur. One to 8 tsp per day can be mixed with the food, depending on the size of the dog. Ironically, such products are used for both constipation and diarrhea because of their water-retaining properties and the effect of fecal bulk on colonic motility. In diarrhea, the addition of fiber causes increased fecal bulk, which slows intestinal transit. Fiber can be used in most cases of mild colitis in dogs, as well as in those cases of diarrhea in which the first stool of the day is formed but successive ones are pudding-like stools, perhaps indicating less contact with the colonic mucosa.

In the hospital, decreased physical activity due to cage confinement will automatically decrease the diarrhea in animals with colitis, making evaluation of therapy difficult, so only animals with severe and uncontrolled diarrhea should be hospitalized for any length of time. Instead, routine re-examinations of these animals at 14-day intervals are suggested to evaluate the effectiveness of dietary and drug therapy and to determine the necessity of continuing such therapy. Such examinations also reinforce owners' compliance with the diet. Owners or members of the household who add foods or treats to a controlled diet make it difficult to determine the success or failure of any prescribed diet. Owner education will also aid in identification of individual food or environmental changes that may trigger the colitis.

Once clinical signs improve with the restricted diet, foods can be slowly added, one at a time, every 7 to 10 days. This period allows adequate evaluation of each new additional ingredient. Owners may also begin to add treats that meet the guidelines of the diet, such as rice cookies. The goal of dietary therapy is eventually to switch the animal back to a commercially available diet. The most common commercial diets used in colitis are Eukanuba (Iams Food Co.), Cycle IV (chicken, General Foods), and Chicken Recipe (Champion Valley Farms). If the diarrhea is going to recur, it will most often do so when one third to one half of the diet has been replaced by the new diet. If these dietary changes cannot be attained, the diet should be made better balanced with the addition of a wider variety of foods. Vitamin supplements should be added as needed.

In cats, the most common colitis is a plasmacytic-lympocytic colitis that is thought to be immune mediated. These cats have a bloody mucoid stool and fecal accidents and urgency in the house. Such cats have been reported to respond to cooked horsemeat supplemented with vitamins, although c/d (Hill's Pet Products, liver, meat by-products, horsemeat, ground corn, animal fat, dried skimmed milk, and brewer's yeast) and mutton and rice have also been given with some success. Due to the difficulty of obtaining horsemeat and general client aversion to it, other therapy such as corticosteroids is usually needed to control this form of colitis.

At times, diet alone will stabilize an animal's clinical signs, but additional therapy is commonly required. Usually this therapy just controls the clinical signs, without necessarily effecting a cure. Much of what is written about therapy of chronic colitis is based on clinical impression, not on well-controlled studies of animals with a diagnosis of chronic colitis. However, a constant feature of veterinary medicine is the need to make treatment decisions in the absence of a definitive diagnosis. Treatment, however, must be individualized for each animal and must keep certain goals in mind. The goals of drug therapy in colitis are to return motility and secretion to normal and to decrease the reflexive urge to defecate. Drugs used in the therapy of chronic colitis include antimicrobial agents, motility modifiers, and immunosuppressive drugs.

Antimicrobial Agents Used in Chronic Colitis

Studies in humans indicate that the colonic bacterial population is disrupted by the primary inflammatory response in acute colitis. It returns to normal only after this inflammatory response is resolved. Similar studies in dogs are lacking, but it is well known that the *routine use of antimicrobial agents is discouraged in the therapy of most diarrhea* (Strombeck, 1980). Major disadvantages are inherent in the use of antimicrobial agents in diarrhea. They impair the adhesion of normal organisms to the intestinal epithelium, and this disruption of bacterial flora exposes the host to more pathogenic bacteria, delaying the return of normal intestinal homeostasis. The best-known example of this is the colitis that occurs in humans on antibiotics as a result of the overgrowth of a toxin-producing clostridium.

Chronic colitis in animals is one of the few exceptions to this general principle regarding antimicrobials in diarrhea. Bacteria, especially anaerobes, are important in the development of experimentally induced colitis in various species. Bacterial antigens also may trigger some immunologic reactions encountered in inflammatory bowel disease in humans. These mechanisms have not been studied in the development of naturally occurring colitis in dogs and cats; however, clinical experience suggests some therapeutic efficiency of antimicrobial agents in these conditions. Antimicrobial therapy used in chronic colitis generally consists of the use of three drugs, sulfasalazine, tylosin, and metronidazole. Sulfasalazine and metronidazole are used successfully in treating colitis in humans, whereas the use of tylosin is based on empirical treatment and clinical impression in small animal medicine.

SULFASALAZINE

The major drug used clinically in the treatment of chronic colitis is sulfasalazine (Azulfidine, Pharmacia). Although comparable studies do not exist for dogs, this drug is efficacious in the therapy of ulcerative colitis and granulomatous enterocolitis (Crohn's disease) in humans. Sulfasalazine is a combination of sulfapyridine and 5-aminosalicylic acid (ASA) joined by an azo bond. This drug is cleaved in the colon by colonic bacteria and the sulfa is subsequently absorbed, leaving the ASA, which is excreted in the feces. The ASA is most likely the active ingredient, having possible antiprostaglandin activity within the colonic wall. Its exact mechanism of action is not known, however. The use of this drug should be limited to dogs that both clinically and by biopsy have a fairly severe colitis.

Side effects of this drug include keratoconjunctivitis sicca (KCS), vomiting, allergic dermatitis, and cholestatic jaundice in dogs. KCS is the most serious side effect of the drug; its occurrence is not common but is related to intermittent administration of the drug. The diminished tear flow is probably secondary to hypersensitivity of the lacrimal gland to the sulfonamide. Since this side effect can be irreversible, owners should be warned to look for dryness of the cornea, bilateral mucopurulent ocular discharges, and blepharospasm. If these signs are seen, the drug should be discontinued and oral pilocarpine drops instituted. Incidence of this side effect can be decreased by careful client education and the judicious use of the drug in documented colitis.

Sulfasalazine is available as 500-mg tablets and is administered at a dosage of 35 to 50 mg/kg/day divided into three to four equal doses (limit 4 gm/day). Most dogs with colitis respond to a 2- to 4-week course of this drug. Re-evaluation at this time will allow the clinician to determine the next course of therapy for the animal. Many dogs will only require proper dietary or anthelmintic therapy. Others may need continued drug therapy, in which case tylosin or metronidazole is a preferable maintenance drug. Only those animals with severe forms of colitis such as ulcerative colitis require prolonged therapy with sulfasalazine. Even then, control of severe colitis is less than satisfactory.

Sulfasalazine has been used in cats at one-half the lowest dosage in dogs, but there is some concern about salicylate toxicity. Therefore, it should be used only as a last measure in cats with colitis that is not responding to other adjunctive therapy.

TYLOSIN

Tylosin is a macrolide antibiotic similar to erythromycin and lincomycin. It is reported to inhibit certain bacterial species, some mycoplasma, spirochetes, and chlamydia. Some of these organisms have been implicated in the cause of chronic colitis in humans as well as in experimentally induced colitis in animals; however, their exact role in canine and feline colitis is not known.

Clinical impression would seem to indicate that tylosin is effective in colitis in animals, although its exact mechanism of action is unknown. It is most effective in the powder form, Tylan-Plus Vitamins (Elanco; approximately 470 mg/tsp). In fact, it may be ineffective in the oral tablet form, for reasons not completely understood. The dosage used by the author in dogs is 40 to 80 mg/kg/day in two to three divided doses. Since its taste is quite bitter, it can be either mixed with food or given as a bolus mixed with water. Cats and some dogs may refuse the food with the drug in it, even when used at the lower dosage of 10 to 20 mg/kg/day (1/8 to 1/4 tsp twice daily) for cats. Ideally, the recommended dose is used for 2 weeks and is gradually tapered as the clinician adjusts the animal's diet. Unfortunately, there are a number of animals in which the diarrhea will recur if the tylosin is discontinued; usually these animals have normal colonic biopsies or colonic hyperplasia. They may actually have small intestinal disease with bacterial overgrowth.

This drug can be used in chronic canine colitis when it is undesirable to continue sulfasalazine therapy and when dietary therapy is insufficient to control the symptoms. Side effects have not been seen even when the drug is used over a long period of time. Unfortunately, the overall effects of tylosin on bacterial resistance and gastrointestinal flora are largely unknown in small animals and may represent a cause for concern.

METRONIDAZOLE

Metronidazole (Flagyl, Searle & Co.) has been used in the treatment of chronic colitis in dogs and cats. This drug's mechanism of action is not known but probably includes the following: an antiprotozoal effect against *Giardia*, an alteration of immune-mediated reactions in the bowel, and an antibacterial action against anaerobes. Its effect on anaerobes is not completely understood but is probably related to altered oxidation-reduction ratios that occur in these organisms as a result of the drug. This may be important, since anaerobes are implicated as a source of antigens that may induce immune-mediated bowel disease. Metronidazole's immunomodulating effects are also poorly understood but may be important because of its effectiveness in immune-mediated colitis in humans and animals. The dosage in dogs is 30 to 60 mg/kg/day and 15 mg/kg/day in cats in a once-a-day dose. Animals should be treated for giardiasis for 5 days; however, longer treatment may be necessary in some forms of colitis. Side effects include nausea, vomiting, and dose-related neurologic signs. Ataxia, muscular rigidity, and seizures are seen in the dog at 75 mg/kg/day; these signs are reversed when the drug is discontinued.

Needless to say, certain disadvantages are inherent in the use of all antimicrobial drugs. Since the cause of most chronic bowel diseases is unknown, the use of antimicrobials is based on clinical judgment, often a notoriously poor measure of therapeutic effectiveness. Besides the disruption of the bowel flora, the major disadvantages of antimicrobials are the expense and inconvenience for the owner. They do not represent a cure, only a means of controlling clinical signs, and therefore they are not an ideal solution. For this reason, every effort should be made to accurately diagnose and specifically treat the diarrhea before committing the owner and animal to chronic antimicrobial therapy.

Motility Modifiers

In the normal colon, segmentation and retrograde peristalsis provide resistance to the flow of feces in the cranial colon. This action results in water and salt absorption, with the subsequent formation of feces. Mass movements of the colon effectively empty the entire distal colon of dogs and cats. This movement is partially stimulated by the entry of food into the stomach (the gastrocolic reflex) and by the distension of the colon.

Colonic inflammation not only disrupts the normal absorptive and secretory pattern but also changes the normal colonic motility pattern. Segmentation is decreased in most cases of colitis, making the colon hypomotile. Peristalsis remains normal or may be slightly reduced. These factors, combined with an accentuated defecation reflex owing to irritation of the colonic-rectal wall, result in the diarrhea encountered in colitis.

The goals of motility modifiers should be to restore the normal defecation pattern and provide relief from colonic spasm due to colonic inflammation or ulcerations. In general, the use of motility modifiers in chronic colitis should be limited to cases with acute exacerbation of the diarrhea, cases of severe colitis, and when stress-related colonic disease is suspected. Client intolerance for the pet's diarrhea is another reasonable justification for motility modifiers.

In most cases of chronic colitis, dietary therapy and the addition of bulking agents to the diet will restore the normal motility pattern of the colon. Bran, Metamucil, or Siblin will help distend the colon and stimulate segmentation. However, bulking agents are contraindicated in cases of severe colitis when the colonic wall is severely inflamed or constricted.

Basically there are three different classes of motility modifiers that may be used, with innumerable drugs in each class. These include (1) anticholingeric drugs, (2) narcotic analgesics, and (3) antispasmodic–central nervous system (CNS) depressant drug combinations. All these drugs are contraindicated in cases of invasive and toxigenic bacterial infections of the bowel and gastric outlet obstruction associated with atony. The category of drug that is used in chronic colitis depends on the severity of the clinical signs, the client's intolerance for the pet's

Table 1. *Dosage of Motility Modifiers Commonly Used in Chronic Colonic Diseases in Small Animals*

Drug	Dosage	Frequency
Propantheline bromide (Pro-Banthine, Searle & Co.)	0.5 mg/kg	b.i.d. to t.i.d.
Dicyclomine (Bentyl, Merrell-National)	0.15 mg/kg	t.i.d. to q.i.d.
Codeine†	0.25–0.50 mg/kg	t.i.d. to q.i.d.
Powder opium† (in Donnagel-PG, Robins)	½ tsp/5 kg	q.i.d.
Paregoric† (in Parepectolin, Rorer)	¼ tsp/5 kg	q.i.d.
Diphenoxylate† (Lomotil, Searle & Co.)	0.05–0.1 mg/kg	b.i.d. to t.i.d.
Loperamide† (Immodium, Ortho Pharmaceutical)*	0.1 mg/kg	b.i.d. to t.i.d.
Clidinium bromide and chlordiazepoxide*	0.3–0.5 mg/kg	b.i.d.
Isopropamide-prochlorperazine (Darbazine, Norden)	#1 capsule for <10 kg body weight	b.i.d. to t.i.d.
	#3 capsule for >10 kg body weight	

*Not for use in dogs weighing less than 20 kg.
†Narcotic analgesics should not be used in cats.

diarrhea, and historic evidence of a stress-related component to the diarrhea. The dosages of the commonly used motility modifiers are given in Table 1.

ANTICHOLINERGICS

Anticholinergics are probably the most commonly used class of drugs in gastroenterology. They decrease large intestinal tone and propulsion by blocking the effects of acetylcholine, the major neurotransmitter for both the circular and longitudinal muscle of the intestine. However, since the diarrhea in colitis is probably due to hypomotility, the effect of anticholinergics is contrary to the effect desired—that is, to stimulate segmentation.

Anticholinergic drugs, although not altering the course of diarrhea, may decrease bowel spasm and the tenesmus accompanying inflammatory diseases of the colon and rectum. They may also decrease the diarrhea that occurs in animals under acute stress; such diarrhea may be due to cholinergic mechanisms. Anticholinergics are also frequently used in combination with CNS sedatives for gastrointestinal problems with a stress-related component. Long-acting anticholinergics are the drugs of choice in such cases. Propantheline bromide (Pro-Banthine, Searle & Co.) and isopropamideprochlorperazine (Darbazine, Norden) are included in this category. Anticholinergics such as dicyclomine (Bentyl, Merrell-National) act directly to relax the intestinal smooth muscle. Side effects of such drugs include ileus (which can mask electrolyte and fluid losses), xerostomia, tachycardia, urinary retention, and glaucoma.

NARCOTIC ANALGESICS

Narcotic analgesics are useful in symptomatic therapy of colitis since they increase segmentation by a direct action on the circular smooth muscle of the intestine. They slow intestinal transit time by increasing segmentation, therefore allowing time for water absorption from the stool. These drugs may also provide some analgesia.

The principal narcotic alkaloids that affect gastrointestinal function are morphine and codeine. Tincture of opium and paregoric are typical of this category of drug. Paregoric contains the equivalent of 2 mg of morphine in each 5-ml dose, and tincture of opium is a solution adjusted to contain 1 per cent morphine. These drugs are especially useful when dealing with dogs less than 10 kg (20 lb). The action of various antidiarrheal preparations is primarily due to their narcotic content. These preparations include Donnagel-PG (Robins; powdered opium, atropine, hyoscyamine, kaolin, and pectin), and Parepectolin (Rorer; paregoric, pectin, and kaolin). Codeine is also an effective antidiarrheal agent.

Loperamide and diphenoxylate are narcotic analgesics used in dogs heavier than 10 kg (20 lb), although there is a liquid form of diphenoxylate available for small dogs. Diphenoxylate (2.5 mg) is a narcotic drug combined with atropine (0.025 mg) in a preparation called Lomotil (Searle & Co.). In humans, this combination has the effect of stimulating segmentation of the smooth muscle with the diphenoxylate while possibly inhibiting peristalsis with the atropine. Loperamide (Imodium, Ortho Pharmaceutical) is a synthetic antidiarrheal drug whose action is claimed to be more rapid and prolonged than that of Lomotil. Loperamide may also increase absorption of water by the bowel wall while alternatively decreasing secretion. Although studies in animals are lacking, the duration of action in humans averages 10 hours. Unlike Lomotil, loperamide is no longer a federally controlled drug. Unfortunately, loperamide is not safe for use in small dogs (less than 10 kg). Side effects of narcotic analgesics include constipation, ileus, and sedation; they are contraindicated in liver disease, intestinal obstruction, and invasive or toxigenic bowel disease. They are not recommended for use in cats. The author's preference is loperamide for larger dogs and paregoric for smaller dogs; however, this entire class of drugs should only be used in chronic colitis that cannot be controlled by other means.

CNS DEPRESSANTS AND ANTISPASMODICS

This category of motility modifiers is indicated for animals with diarrhea of colonic origin that is thought to have a stress-related component. These animals may be helped *significantly* by a CNS depressant with or without an antispasmodic drug. In fact, this may be the most successful mode of therapy in some animals. Although definitive evidence of a psychomotor diarrhea is lacking in veterinary medicine, clinical experience has indicated that this type of combination drug has therapeutic value. When environmental changes trigger the diarrhea, a stress-related cause must be considered; colonic biopsies on such animals tend to be normal.

Librax (Roche) and Darbazine (Norden) are common drugs in this category. Librax is a combination of 5 mg of chlordiazepoxide (a centrally acting sedative) and 2.5 mg of clidinium (an anticholinergic); it is used in the irritable bowel syndrome in humans, a colonic motility disorder with a psychomotor basis. Xerostomia, sedation, constipation, bloating, and centrally mediated polydipsia and polyuria are commonly noted side effects of this drug. Darbazine is a combination of phenothiazine tranquilizer (prochlorperazine) and an anticholinergic (isopropamide iodide). Besides centrally mediated sedative and antiemetic effects, the phenothiazine may act peripherally on smooth muscle of the bowel wall by interfering with acetylcholine or serotonin. It may also decrease secretion into the bowel, although the significance of this effect remains to be determined. Side effects of this drug include ileus, hypotension, and CNS abnormalities.

Immunosuppressive Agents

Corticosteroids have long been used in the treatment of certain forms of colitis in humans. Unfortunately, their efficacy in the treatment of colitis in animals remains unproved because of the lack of cases that have been closely followed after biopsy diagnosis. Nevertheless, due to their anti-inflammatory effects they remain a commonly used drug in chronic colitis in animals. They are definitely indicated in eosinophilic colitis when dietary and parasitic infestations have been eliminated or when appropriate therapy is unsuccessful. They have been helpful in controlling diarrhea in cats with plasmacytic-lympocytic colitis and in some dogs with severe colitis when other therapy such as sulfasalazine has been unsuccessful. In the above diseases, prednisolone is usually given in immunosuppressive doses (0.5 to 1 mg/kg twice daily) and tapered gradually over a 3- to 4-week period to the lowest dose of the drug that will control the disease process. Unfortunately, not all cases of granulomatous and histiocytic ulcerative colitis will improve with the use of corticosteroids, and some cases may actually get worse. These forms of colitis are notoriously difficult to control, and a guarded prognosis must be given.

Many of the adverse reactions due to corticosteroids cannot be dissociated from their pharmacologic effects. Besides causing suppression of the pituitary-adrenal axis and increased susceptibility to infection, steroids have ulcerogenic properties, a serious problem in an already damaged intestinal tract. They also increase the negative nitrogen balance in animals already compromised by malnutrition. For these reasons, alternate-day steroid therapy is ideal. Corticosteroids will commonly provide some alleviation of clinical signs but may not help the animal maintain normal intestinal motility. In chronic colitis, normal defecation habits may not be possible or may be attained only with significant side effects from the drugs used to control the colitis, as occurs with corticosteroid use.

References and Supplemental Reading

Burrows, C. F.: Diseases of the colon, rectum and anus in the dog and cat. *In* Andersen, N. (ed.): *Veterinary Gastroenteology*. Philadelphia: Lea & Febiger, 1980, pp. 553–592.

Floch, M. H.: Nutrition and Dietary Therapy in Gastrointestinal Disease. New York: Plenum Publishing, 1981, Chapters 4, 13–15, 17, and 20.

Greenberger, N. J., Arvantakis, C. A., and Hurvitz, A.: Drug Treatment of Gastrointestinal Disorders. Vol. 3. New York: Churchill Livingstone, 1978, Chapters 1, 3, 4, and 11.

Pietrusko, R. G.: Pharmacotherapy of diarrhea. J. Maine Med. Assoc., 70:192, 1979.

Ridgway, M. D.: Management of chronic colitis in the dog. J.A.V.M.A. 185:804, Oct., 1984.

Strombeck, D. R.: Diet and nutrition in management of gastrointestinal problems. *In* Kirk, R. W. (ed.): *Current Veterinary Therapy VII*. Philadelphia: W. B. Saunders, 1980, pp. 919–929.

Strombeck, D. R.: Management of diarrhea: Motility modifiers and adjunct therapy. *In* Kirk, R. W. (ed.): *Current Veterinary Therapy VII*. Philadelphia: W. B. Saunders, 1980, pp. 914–919.

Van Kruiningen, H. J., Clinical efficacy of tylosin in canine inflammatory bowel disease, J. Am. Anim. Hosp. Assoc. 12:198, 1976.

CONSTIPATION

COLIN F. BURROWS, B. VET. MED.
Gainesville, Florida

Constipation, defined as infrequent or absent defecation, excessively hard or dry feces, increased straining to defecate, or a reduced fecal volume, is relatively common in small animal patients. Constipation must also be differentiated from obstipation, a condition of intractable constipation that occurs when feces are retained in the colon and rectum for a prolonged period of time and become excessively hard and dry. Under these circumstances, defecation becomes progressively more difficult until it is virtually impossible. Unlike constipation, obstipation is inevitably associated with a guarded or grave prognosis since degenerative changes in the colon wall are usually irreversible.

Constipation is sometimes used synonymously with the term *megacolon,* a condition of extreme dilatation of the colon. The two terms are not synonymous, however, since animals with megacolon are always constipated but constipated animals do not necessarily have megacolon. Constipation, moreover, is a sign, whereas megacolon is a disorder of both structure and function. Megacolon may be either primary or secondary. The cause of primary megacolon is unknown in dogs and cats but in most instances is probably due to a defect in colonic innervation. Secondary megacolon may occur as a sequel to any lesion or disease that prevents normal defecation for a prolonged period of time.

PATHOPHYSIOLOGY OF CONSTIPATION

Constipation can occur in association with any disorder that impairs the passage of fecal material through the colon. Defects in muscle or nerve function, luminal obstruction, or suppression of the urge to defecate all delay fecal transit. This increased contact time allows the mucosa to remove additional salt and water and produce harder and drier feces. Thus, the final common denominator of constipation is *time.*

In dogs and cats, the colon is small and relatively simple compared with that in other domestic species, and it has but two major functions: (1) the absorption of electrolytes and water from luminal contents and (2) storage, with periodic expulsion of resulting fecal material. Absorption takes place primarily in the proximal colon and storage in the distal part of the organ, but there is some overlap so that in constipated patients all segments can function interchangeably.

Sodium and chloride are actively absorbed from luminal contents by colonic mucosal cells, whereas water follows passively by solvent drag. Coupled absorption of sodium with volatile fatty acids accounts for additional water absorption. Colonic epithelial cell junctions are tight, preventing backdiffusion of sodium against a concentration gradient. The barrier is disrupted in inflammatory disease to reduce absorptive capacity. Disruption and exudation also occur in the constipated patient owing to fecal concretions that irritate the mucosa and cause secretion. Exuded fluid is insufficient to break down the mass and is often passed as liquid feces, explaining the paradoxical complaint of diarrhea in some obstipated patients.

Colonic contents must undergo continual mixing for optimal electrolyte and water absorption. The orderly distal movement of luminal contents together with their regular elimination is achieved by organized and complex patterns of colonic smooth muscle activity. Mixing is achieved by phasic contractions of colonic circular muscle, and propulsion occurs by linked phasic contractions of both the circular and longitudinal layers to form a peristaltic wave. All movements are controlled by the enteric nervous system and modulated by extrinsic nerves.

Both phasic and peristaltic contractions are increased in constipated patients, but motility diminishes as megacolon develops. Colonic smooth muscle degenerates and becomes hypomotile in most animals with megacolon. The hypomotile colon may contain large volumes of either soft or hard feces that are evacuated infrequently or with difficulty. The major cause of a hypomotile megacolon is the primary neuromuscular degeneration that occurs in older cats.

Systemic signs of constipation vary. Feces appear to have to be retained in the colon for a considerable period of time before any deleterious effects are observed. Severely constipated patients frequently exhibit depression, inappetence, and weakness, signs that have been attributed to the absorption of toxins produced by bacterial metabolism of retained fecal material. However, if liver function is normal, it is more probable that these signs are attributable to an underlying disease. Vomiting may also occur in severely constipated animals and may be due to either the effect of these putative "toxins" on the chemoreceptor trigger zone or, more likely, to afferent vagal stimulation of the emetic center subsequent to colonic distension.

CAUSES OF CONSTIPATION

The major causes of constipation in dogs and cats are listed in Table 1. A variety of circumstances and diseases predispose animals to constipation, but these can be categorized into six groups: (1) dietary and environmental, (2) painful, (3) obstructive, (4) neurogenic, (5) metabolic and endocrine, and (6) drug induced.

DIETARY AND ENVIRONMENTAL CONSTIPATION. When mixed with feces, ingested bones, foreign material, or hair can form hard masses that the patient eliminates only with difficulty. Much of this material can be retained to form gradually enlarging masses, which may cause obstipation if unnoticed or untreated.

Psychologic factors may also play a role in the pathogenesis of constipation. Defecation is a routine act for some animals, requiring the appropriate environment and conducive circumstances. For a dog, this may mean a regular daily walk or clean papers if it is paper-trained; cats may require a clean litter box or other suitable location. A change in environment, such as occurs when an animal is hospitalized, can inhibit the stimulus to defecate and can cause constipation. Lack of exercise, dietary change, and some medications exacerbate the situation.

PAINFUL DEFECATION. Constipation frequently occurs in association with diseases that cause painful lesions in the anorectum. Examples include anal sacculitis or abscess, perianal fistula, rectal stricture, rectal tumors, and pseudocoprostasis. After a few initial painful attempts to defecate, the dog or cat with anorectal disease may inhibit or ignore the normal stimulus and severe constipation or obstipation may result.

Constipation may also result if the animal is unwilling or unable to defecate because of the pain and decreased mobility associated with such conditions as fractured pelvis, dislocated hip, or broken leg. Defecation may not be attempted in such patients until the pain has subsided and stabilization has occurred, by which time the feces may be very hard.

OBSTRUCTIVE CONSTIPATION. Intraluminal or extraluminal lesions that obstruct fecal transit frequently cause constipation. This occurs, for example, in association with such disorders as perineal hernia, pelvic fractures that have healed to leave a narrow pelvic canal, severe prostatic hypertrophy or paraprostatic cysts, or rectal, colonic, pelvic, prostatic, or anal tumors. Pseudocoprostasis is another cause of constipation in long-haired breeds when feces matted in the perianal hair impede fecal passage and cause dyschezia.

NEUROGENIC CONSTIPATION. A few neurologic disorders can also cause constipation, either because of an animal's inability to adopt the normal defecatory position or as a result of a disturbance of colonic innervation. Constipation may also occur in spinal cord disease; disc disease is the most frequent cause. Signs may be particularly severe if the animal has undergone corrective surgery. High doses of corticosteroids in combination with laminectomy or fenestration may predispose the animal to constipation, colonic perforation, and peritonitis.

Disruption of colonic innervation with subsequent derangements in colonic motility have been poorly documented in dogs and cats. Young animals presenting with constipation and megacolon probably have some type of congenital neuromuscular dysfunction. Aganglionosis, such as occurs in Hirschsprung's disease in humans, would result in narrowing of a colonic segment and has not yet been documented in dogs and cats. The idiopathic megacolon that occurs in the middle-aged or older cat is also believed to be neurogenic in origin.

METABOLIC AND ENDOCRINE CONSTIPATION. Constipation is an infrequent consequence of hypothyroidism and hyperparathyroidism in the dog. In both instances, however, constipation is induced

Table 1. *Classification of the Causes of Constipation*

Dietary and environmental
Dietary: bones, hair, or foreign material mixed with feces and impacted in the colon
Lack of exercise, change of habit or environment: no litter box, dirty litter box, or hospitalization
Painful defecation
Anorectal disease: anal sacculitis, anal abscesss, perianal fistula, anal stricture, anal spasm, rectal foreign body, pseudocoprostasis
Trauma: fractured pelvis, fractured limb or dislocated hip, bite wounds, or abscess in the perineum
Mechanical obstruction
Extraluminal obstruction: healed fractured of the pelvis with narrowed pelvic canal, prostatic hypertrophy, prostatitis, prostatic tumor, intrapelvic tumor, pseudocoprostasis
Intraluminal obstruction: colonic or rectal tumor, rectal diverticulum, perineal hernia
Neurologic disease
Central nervous system dysfunction: paraplegia, spinal cord disease, disc disease
Intrinsic colonic nerve dysfunction: idiopathic megacolon of the cat
Metabolic and endocrine
Interference with colonic smooth muscle function: hyperparathyroidism, hypothyroidism, hypokalemia
Debility: general muscle weakness and dehydration
Drug-induced
Anticholinergics, antihistamines, opiates, barium sulfate, diuretics

through abnormal smooth muscle function. Hypokalemia also inhibits normal smooth muscle function and may have a similar result. Dehydration and debility from any cause can also be associated with constipation, either through excessive water absorption from the feces in response to dehydration or from generalized muscle weakness.

DRUG-INDUCED CONSTIPATION. Anticholinergics, antihistamines, barium sulfate, diuretics, and opiates can all cause constipation. A history of recent drug therapy is therefore important in the evaluation of the constipated patient.

TREATMENT

Treatment has four basic components: (1) removal or amelioration of the underlying cause, (2) restoration of electrolyte and fluid balance, (3) administration of laxatives or cathartics, and (4) enemas. After successful treatment, the possibility of recurrence is minimized by client education, dietary manipulation, and, if necessary, long-term medication. A guide to treatment is given in Table 2.

There are two types of constipated patients: (1) those that have severe colonic impaction or obstipation when presented for initial evaluation and treatment and (2) those with a known tendency to constipation or with a predisposing underlying disease that may require long-term medical therapy. The first type often needs heroic efforts in an attempt to remove impacted feces and restore normal bowel function, whereas the second type requires long-term dietary management and appropriate medical therapy.

THE SEVERELY CONSTIPATED PATIENT. After fluid and electrolyte balance are restored, the severely impacted patient can be treated with oral laxatives and enemas or by manual removal of fecal concretions while the patient is under general anesthesia. The specific treatment selected depends on the severity of impaction. Fecal concretions can be removed from the anesthetized animal with whelping or sponge forceps. Rapid instillation of enema fluid can induce emesis even in the anesthetized patient, and the possibility of aspiration should be prevented by use of a cuffed endotracheal tube. In the obstipated cat, 30 to 40 ml of water are instilled into the rectum and the bowel is kneaded through the abdominal wall. This breaks down and loosens feces, which can then be milked distally for removal with forceps. Breakdown and removal of these fecal masses should be accomplished as slowly and gently as possible. In severely impacted patients, the outcome is usually better if feces are broken down and removed over a 2- to 3-day period.

MODERATE IMPACTION. Most of these patients can be treated as outpatients with soapy water or phosphate enemas. Dietary supplementation with either bran or one of the other bulk formers is the mainstay of subsequent therapy; laxatives can be given as needed. Regular grooming, strict diet control, and providing the opportunity for regular defecation are mandatory.

Table 2. *Specific Treatment of Constipation*

Contributing Factors	Specific Therapy
Dietary and environmental	
Ingestion of hair, bones, and foreign material	Soften feces with enemas, remove bone fragments manually if necessary; use fecal softeners; prevent recurrence by grooming, dietary modification, and appropriate exercise
Environmental	Correct underlying cause; provide opportunity for defecation; use enemas, suppositories, or laxatives, depending on severity.
Painful defecation	
Anal sac disease	Empty, drain, use antibiotics
Perianal fistula	Surgical correction
Anal stricture	Dilation or excision
Anal spasm	Dilation or pudendal nerve section
Rectal foreign body	Remove
Ulcerating tumor	Remove
Pseudocoprostasis	Clip hair, apply topical corticosteroid, treat myiasis
Obstructive	
Healed pelvic fracture with narrow lumen	Surgical correction if possible, fecal softeners
Prostatitis	Medical therapy
Prostatic hypertrophy	Castration
Prostatic tumor	Symptomatic therapy or surgical therapy
Intrapelvic tumor	Surgical correction
Perianal adenoma	Castration
Rectal adenocarcinoma	Resection, symptomatic therapy
Perineal hernia	Herniorrhaphy, castration, fecal softeners
Neurogenic	
Spinal cord disease	Supportive care
Disc disease	Steroids, surgical correction
Idiopathic megacolon	Enemas, fecal softeners, stimulant laxatives, colectomy
Metabolic and endocrine	
Hypothyroidism	Thyroid replacement, stool softeners
Hyperparathyroidism	Treat hypercalcemia and underlying condition
Hypokalemia	Treat underlying condition, potassium supplementation
Drug-induced	Change drugs or decrease dosage if possible

Medications

Drugs that relieve constipation have traditionally been divided into laxatives and cathartics. Laxatives are milder in effect and usually cause elimination of formed feces, whereas cathartics (or stimulant laxatives) cause a more liquid evacuation. The effect depends on dosage; major drugs and dosages are summarized in Table 3.

EMOLLIENTS (WETTING AGENTS OR SURFACTANTS)

Emollients such as dioctyl sodium sulfosuccinate (DSS) (Colace, Mead Johnson; Doxinate or Surfak, Hoechst-Roussel) act in the same manner as detergents to alter surface tension of liquids and promote emulsification and softening of the feces by facilitating the mixture of water and fat. Laxatives containing DSS are recommended for the treatment of constipation associated with hard, dry feces and are also useful in conditions that require the avoidance of straining. A solution of DSS can be added to the enema fluid in cases of fecal impaction. DSS and its congeners are claimed to be nonsoluble, nontoxic, and pharmacologically inert. Patients should be well hydrated before these drugs are administered, since they decrease jejunal absorption and promote colonic secretion. They should not be administered in conjunction with mineral oil.

LUBRICANTS

Mineral oil (liquid petrolatum) and white petrolatum, the ingredients of some commercial veterinary laxatives, are nondigestible and poorly absorbed products of petroleum. These materials soften feces by coating them to prevent colonic absorption of fecal water and promote easy expulsion. These compounds are widely used to treat hairballs, to relieve minor constipation, and to facilitate defecation in patients with painful anal lesions. A small amount of oil absorption does take place, but with mineral oil the major danger is lipoid aspiration pneumonia due to its lack of taste. These drugs may interfere with fat-soluble vitamin absorption and should be administered only between meals.

BULK-FORMING AGENTS

Bulk-forming laxatives are nonabsorbable synthetic or natural polysaccharide and cellulose derivatives. Because they are hydrophilic and are not absorbed, they swell in the intestinal tract, soften the feces, normalize transit time, and provide bulk. Many, such as Metamucil (Searle & Co.), contain natural *psyllium*, and others contain semisynthetic derivatives. Bran is a cheaper, equally effective, and natural substitute. Such compounds, when mixed with the food, form the basis for the long-term treatment of constipation.

STIMULANT LAXATIVES

Stimulant laxatives differ widely in their mode and site of action and therefore afford a degree of specificity that may be useful in treating specific types of constipation. These compounds increase the propulsive peristaltic activity of the intestine

***Table 3.** Classification and Properties of Laxatives*

Class and Drug	Dosage Form	Dosage/Range	Site of Action	Time Required for Action (Hours)
Emollients (wetting agents)				
Dioctyl sodium sulfosuccinate (e.g., Colace, Mead Johnson)	50- and 100-mg capsules, 1% liquid, 4 mg/ml syrup	1 50-mg capsule once daily for cats, 1–4 for dogs	Small and large intestine	12–72
Dioctyl calcium sulfosuccinate (e.g., Surfak, Hoechst-Roussel)	50- and 240-mg tablets	Cats, 1–2 50-mg tabs; dogs, 2–3 50-mg tabs or 1 240-mg tab once daily	Small and large intestine	12–72
Lubricants				
Mineral oil	Liquid (oral)	5–25 ml b.i.d.	Colon	6–12
White petrolatum (e.g., Laxatone, Evsco)	Paste	1–5 ml once daily	Colon	12–24
Bulk-forming laxatives				
Psyllium (e.g., Metamucil, Searle & Co.)	Powder	1–3 tsp mixed with food once or twice daily	Small and large intestine	12–24
Bran	Powder	1–2 tbsp 400 gm canned food	Small and large intestine	12–24
Stimulant laxatives				
Bisacodyl (e.g., Dulcolax, Boehringer Ingelheim)	Tablet, 5 mg suppository	1 5-mg tablet once daily for cats; 1 10-mg tablet for dogs	Colon	6–12

either by a local effect on the mucosa or by a more selective action on the intramural nerve plexuses.

Castor oil, the best known stimulant, produces a rapid catharsis that is useful in the preparation of the bowel for procedures such as colonoscopy and radiography. The laxative action of castor oil is due to ricinoleic acid, which is produced when the oil is hydrolyzed in the small intestine by pancreatic lipase. The drug irritates mucosal cells to cause secretion, and it is contraindicated in chronic constipation.

Anthraquinones (cascara and senna) are widely used in human medicine but are seldom prescribed in veterinary practice. Phenolphthalein and bisacodyl are the most widely used of the diphenylmethane laxatives; bisacodyl is the most useful in dogs and cats. Bisacodyl (e.g., Dulcolax, Boehringer Ingelheim) produces its effect by stimulating colonic smooth muscle and the myenteric plexus to bring about fairly well-organized peristaltic contractions. The drug is well tolerated, but long-term use in high doses can damage the myenteric plexus. After rehydration and enemas to soften the feces, bisacodyl is the drug of choice for the treatment of severe impaction in dogs and cats.

SALINE LAXATIVES

The active constituents of the saline laxatives are nonabsorbable anions and cations such as the magnesium and sulfate ions. The intestinal wall acts as a semipermeable membrane to the magnesium, sulfate, tartrate, phosphate, or citrate ions, which promotes osmotic retention of water in the intestinal lumen. Increased intraluminal pressure is believed to exert a mechanical stimulus that increases intestinal motility, but other mechanisms such as local gut hormone release and stimulation of the myenteric plexus are also involved. Saline laxatives are rarely used routinely in dogs and cats because of their unavailability in convenient dosage forms. Magnesium citrate is used to prepare the colon before fiberoptic endoscopy. Magnesium-containing laxatives are contraindicated in renal failure because some magnesium can be absorbed and can predispose a patient to hypermagnesemia.

ENEMAS

Enemas act by softening feces in the distal colon and rectum and stimulating colonic motility and the urge to defecate. Their rapid action accounts for their major use in preparing patients for diagnostic procedures.

The enema fluid (warmed or at room temperature) determines the mechanism by which defecation is produced. Tap water, normal saline, and sodium biphosphate add bulk; oils soften, lubricate, and promote the passage of hardened fecal matter; and soapsuds promote defecation by their irritant action.

Saline or plain water enemas are preferred initially in animals with any type of colonic mucosal disease. If ineffective, a soapy water solution should be used after ensuring that the patient is well hydrated. Mineral oil (5 to 30 ml) can be instilled directly into the rectum if feces are very hard.

About 5 ml/kg body weight of a *mild* soap (e.g., Ivory Flakes) solution (3 oz of soap to 1 qt water) should be slowly instilled through a lubricated rectal tube. Better results are usually obtained if the process is repeated several times using smaller volumes of fluid than if large volumes are rapidly instilled in the expectation of rapid results. Large volumes stimulate defecation and are rapidly expelled. Small volumes are retained for longer periods, allowing time to soften and break down fecal impactions. Hexachlorophene soap should not be used since it can cause central nervous system damage.

Sodium phosphate retention enemas (Fleet) are a convenient over-the-counter preparation for the relief of mild constipation. One pediatric enema is sufficient for most medium- to large-sized dogs. In that they have been associated with hyperphosphatemia, hypernatremia, and hypocalcemia, phosphate enemas are contraindicated in small animals with moderate to severe constipation (see page 212). They are also contraindicated in patients with renal insufficiency.

SUPPOSITORIES

Glycerin suppositories are used as laxatives to relieve constipation, but bisacodyl or DSS suppositories are more effective and can be used as a replacement for enemas when the distal colon needs to be emptied. One or two pediatric suppositories are a useful alternative to enemas in the constipated cat.

References and Supplemental Reading

Burrows, C. F.: Diseases of the colon, rectum and anus. *In* Anderson, N. V. (ed.): *Veterinary Gastroenterology*. Philadelphia: Lea & Febiger, 1980, pp. 553–592.

Darlington, R. C., and Curry, C. E.: Laxative products. *In Handbook of Non-Prescription Drugs*, 6th ed. Washington, D.C.: American Pharmaceutical Association, 1979, pp. 37–54.

NUTRITIONAL MANAGEMENT OF GASTROINTESTINAL DISEASES

JAMES F. ZIMMER, D.V.M.
Ithaca, New York

Diseases affecting the gastrointestinal tract produce a commonly recognized spectrum of clinical signs, which include regurgitation, dysphagia, vomiting, diarrhea, constipation, and flatulence. These primary clinical signs are often accompanied by secondary or associated signs, such as weight loss, muscle weakness, anemia, pneumonia, melena, and others. Although the clinical significance and severity of these secondary signs may overshadow the presence of the primary problem, they often aid in defining which portion of the gastrointestinal tract is affected and may suggest potential diagnoses. These clusters of both primary and secondary clinical signs are helpful in identifying, diagnosing, and treating diseases affecting the gastrointestinal tract.

As a result of these diseases, aberrations from normal function of the gastrointestinal tract may also result in compromised nutritional status. Thus, there are two major objectives of the nutritional management of patients with gastrointestinal diseases. The first and broader goal is to provide adequate nutritional intake to sustain the animal during the course of the disease. The plane of nutrition provided should supply the raw materials needed for the reparative process. The second and more direct objective of dietary therapy is to lessen the severity of the disease and the resultant clinical signs and thus foster healing by reducing trauma or further injury to the digestive system.

The major goal of this article is to describe practical aspects of the nutritional management of patients manifesting signs of gastrointestinal diseases. The further characterization of clinical signs, the techniques for establishing appropriate diagnoses, and the other facets of treatment are described elsewhere. The forms of nutritional management described here should be combined with other aspects of therapy for maximal benefit to the patient.

ACUTE GASTROENTERITIS

Dietary management is perhaps the single most effective tool in the symptomatic treatment of animals showing signs of acute gastroenteritis. The intensity of the symptomatic and supportive therapy of these patients is dictated by the severity of the presenting signs. Without historic or physical evidence of more serious problems, the great majority of animals presented with signs suggestive of acute gastroenteritis can be treated symptomatically. The goals of dietary management are to rest the inflamed intestinal tract and prevent ingestion of materials that would exacerbate the clinical signs.

All food is withheld for 12 to 24 hours or longer, depending on the age and size of the animal. If vomiting has been severe, water is also withheld. Warm electrolyte solutions (Resorb, Beecham Laboratories; Life-Guard, Norden; or Gatorade, Stokley-Van Camp) may be given by mouth if vomiting is not a problem. During this fast, the animal's activity and access to food, garbage, and foreign bodies must be restricted. Dogs and cats with gastrointestinal upsets often develop pica and ingest substances that worsen their signs. Restriction of activity also facilitates observation for further clinical signs.

At the end of the fast, small amounts of a warm, bland diet should be offered frequently. This diet should be low in fat, low in fiber, and easily digested and absorbed. The diet must also be palatable to the patient and acceptable to the owner. Commercially available bland diets (Prescription Diet, i/d, Hill's Pet Products) meet most of these criteria and are convenient to prescribe. A homemade bland diet of cottage cheese and boiled rice can also be used (see *Current Veterinary Therapy VII*, pages 919–929). The recipe for another bland diet is provided in Table 1. The nutrient contents of this

*Table 1. Homemade Diets**

Soft bland diet
½ cup Cream of Wheat cooked to make 2 cups
1½ cups uncreamed cottage cheese
1 large egg, hard cooked
2 tbsp brewer's yeast
3 tbsp table sugar
1 tbsp vegetable oil
1 tbsp potassium chloride (salt substitute)
2 tsp dicalcium phosphate
Vitamin-mineral supplement
Hypoallergenic diet
4 oz cooked lamb
1 cup cooked rice
1 tsp corn oil
1½ tsp dicalcium phosphate
Vitamin-mineral supplement

*With slight modification from Lewis, L. D., and Morris, M. L., Jr.: *Small Animal Clinical Nutrition.* Topeka: Mark Morris Associates, 1984.

diet and of other diets and foods are compared in Table 2. When the patient is to be fed, a small amount of either a warm, salted meat broth or a warm puree of a bland diet should be offered. If the animal ingests this meal and does not show a recrudescence of signs, frequent small meals of a bland diet should be offered with the amount fed gradually increased so that after 2 or 3 days the caloric needs are met. If the animal continues to do well, the regular diet can be reintroduced gradually over an additional 3 to 4 days. At the end of that time, the patient should be back on a normal diet on a normal schedule.

If clinical signs do develop again during this process, re-examination and re-evaluation of the patient are warranted. Starting the fast again and repeating the previously described steps may resolve the problems successfully. Alternatively, further diagnostic evaluation and more intensive supportive therapy may be necessary.

ESOPHAGEAL DISEASE

Esophageal motor dysfunction, manifested clinically as regurgitation, is a common clinical problem. The great majority of animals presented because of regurgitation suffer from congenital or acquired megaesophagus. The age of the patient and other aspects of the clinical history help distinguish between these two entities. If the diagnosis is established early and appropriate dietary therapy initiated, the prognosis for young dogs with congenital megaesophagus is favorable. The standard recommendation is to feed these animals from an elevated platform and train them to stay in that position for 10 to 20 minutes after eating. This places the esophagus in a vertical position, adding the effect of gravity to any peristaltic activity present in the esophagus and thus facilitating passage of food through the dilated esophagus. The animal's calculated daily caloric need should be divided and offered in three or more equal feedings. Clinical experience indicates that each affected animal differs in its ability to tolerate various consistencies of food. For some patients with megaesophagus, dry bulky foods stimulate esophageal peristalsis more effectively than do slurries and thereby tend to reduce esophageal overloading. Those animals with little or no peristaltic activity along the length of the esophagus generally fare better on gruels or slurries of food. However, there may be a greater incidence of aspiration pneumonia among animals fed these more liquid diets. After experimenting with diets of various consistencies, the owners of animals with megaesophagus often deduce which consistency produces the least severe signs. This information should be gleaned from the history. Fluoroscopic examination of these patients swallowing diets of varying consistency to which barium sulfate has been added provides the same information.

Treatment of an underlying metabolic disorder that can produce signs of acquired megaesophagus generally lessens to some degree the severity and frequency of the regurgitation. Animals for which such a cause of esophageal dysfunction cannot be identified should be treated as described above. However, in either case, the prognosis for return of normal esophageal function is not favorable.

For a small proportion of animals presenting with

Table 2. Nutrient Content of Diets and Foods (gm per 100 gm as fed)*

Diet or Food	Calories	Moisture	Protein	Fat	Carbohydrate
Prescription Diet i/d	137	71	8	4	15
Prescription Diet d/d	131	73	7	6	12
Prescription Diet r/d	73	74	7	2	9
Soft bland diet	95	78	7	2	10
Hypoallergenic diet	175	65	10	8	15
Boiled rice	109	73	2	trace	24
Cooked spaghetti or macaroni	148	64	5	0.5	30
Lean ground beef, boiled	200	65	25	5	0
Uncreamed cottage cheese	86	79	17	0.3	3

*From Lewis, L. D., and Morris, M. L., Jr.: *Small Animal Clinical Nutrition.* Topeka: Mark Morris Associates, 1984; and United States Department of Agriculture: *Handbook of the Nutritional Contents of Foods.* New York: Dover Publications, Inc., 1975.

regurgitation, the esophageal motor dysfunction reflects the presence of active esophagitis. The esophagitis may have resulted from an esophageal foreign body, reflux of gastric contents into the esophagus, or ingestion of caustic material. In turn, the esophagitis causes reduced tone in the gastroesophageal junction and reduced efficiency of peristalsis along the esophagus. These sequelae predispose the animal to a steady progression of the esophagitis to stricture formation. Temporarily withholding food and water and providing parenteral fluids diminishes the frequency of local mechanical trauma and hastens healing. Minimizing trauma to the inflamed or necrotic esophageal mucosa may also reduce the fibroblastic reaction that normally occurs and thus reduce the tendency for stricture formation. This enforced fast is generally continued for 3 to 5 days, at which time small volumes of slurried food are offered frequently. The diet offered to animals with esophageal motor dysfunction due to esophagitis should be rich in protein and carbohydrate and low in fat. Such a diet will increase tone in the lower esophageal sphincter and reduce the propensity for gastroesophageal reflux. One diet filling these criteria is Prescription Diet i/d to which 2 cups of boiled lean ground beef are added per pound of canned food. This mixture is made into a gruel or slurry with bouillon, broth, or warm water. If the animal continues to do well clinically, this mixture is offered frequently for several days. Thereafter, the diet is gradually changed back to normal. The use of a pharyngostomy tube to feed an animal with esophagitis has been advocated to minimize trauma to the ulcerated esophageal mucosa. However, this procedure has been associated with delayed epithelial healing and is not currently recommended.

The end stage of untreated esophagitis is esophageal stricture, which results in regurgitation, dysphagia, and weight loss. In the treatment of animals with esophageal stricture, medical therapy for the ongoing esophagitis should accompany the dietary regimen for esophagitis described above. The mixture of Prescription Diet i/d and boiled lean ground beef can be made into a liquid by adding adequate volumes of bouillon or broth and running the mixture through a kitchen blender. An aggressive attempt to manage patients with esophageal stricture with medical and dietary therapy should be made before either surgical intervention or bougienage is considered.

GASTRIC DISEASE

Chronic vomiting, the major clinical manifestation of gastric dysfunction, results from either a primary gastrointestinal disease or an underlying metabolic disease that indirectly induces vomiting. A stepwise but thorough diagnostic evaluation is often required to distinguish between these two possibilities and to define the specific cause of the vomiting. Therapy directed at an underlying disease may significantly reduce the frequency and severity of vomiting. When such therapy is not effective in allaying the vomiting, depending on the nature of the underlying disease, medical and nutritional therapy for chronic vomiting due to primary gastrointestinal diseases may be applied.

At the risk of oversimplifying the principles of gastric pathophysiology, the broad spectrum of primary gastrointestinal diseases manifested clinically as chronic vomiting can be divided into two groups: those that primarily affect the mucosa and those that involve the muscular layers of the stomach. Diseases affecting the mucosa generally produce an inflammatory infiltrate, alter the permeability of the mucosa, and may progress to ulceration or atrophy of the mucosa. These changes may result in altered gastric motility and delayed gastric emptying, as well as chronic vomiting. Direct involvement of the muscular layers of the stomach with inflammatory or infiltrative diseases directly alters gastric motility and is manifested as chronic vomiting and either rapid or delayed gastric emptying. Abnormal gastric motor function without an organic lesion produces signs similar to those seen with involvement of the muscle layer.

The goals of the nutritional management of diseases primarily affecting the gastric mucosa are to minimize physical trauma to the damaged mucosa, reduce gastric secretion, and facilitate gastric emptying. These goals are accomplished by providing the diet in the form of a slurry. Mixing and mincing the diet described below with an adequate volume of broth or bouillon in a kitchen blender easily allows one to adjust the consistency and texture.

Ingesta in the form of a fine suspension minimizes abrasive trauma to the inflamed gastric mucosa. Providing the diet in this form also hastens gastric emptying, since the rate of movement of ingesta from the dog's stomach is inversely related to the size of the particulate matter in the food. The liquid portion of a meal empties readily and rapidly from the stomach. Normally, most particles of solid food leaving the dog's stomach are less than 1 mm in diameter. The fineness of this suspension of ingesta entering the small bowel reflects the normal efficiency of the pyloric antrum and canal in grinding the ingesta and regulating the rate of egress of solids from the stomach. (After the liquid and triturated solid ingesta have left the stomach, gastric peristalsis changes in character so that solid objects, such as foreign bodies, are forcefully expelled from the stomach into the small bowel.) The ingestion and retention of a liquid diet also assist in maintaining normal hydration of patients with chronic vomiting.

Reducing physical abrasion of the gastric mucosa and enhancing the rate of gastric emptying also indirectly reduce the stimuli for gastric secretion. Distension of the stomach by ingesta is a potent stimulus of gastrin, gastric acid, and pepsinogen secretion. The persistence of ingesta in the stomach prolongs gastric acid and pepsinogen secretion and increases the total amounts secreted.

The biochemical characteristics of the ingesta also affect the rate and composition of gastric secretion and the rate of gastric emptying. The secretory response to food in the stomach is determined chiefly by the protein content of the ingesta for two reasons: protein digestion products are the most powerful stimulants for the release of gastrin, and protein is the major buffer in foods. Thus, there is a strong direct linear correlation between the protein content of the diet and the total amount of gastric acid secreted by the dog's stomach. Protein digestion products also liberate cholecystokinin from the intestinal mucosa and thereby delay gastric emptying. However, dietary fat is the most potent of the nutrients that slow gastric motility. This effect of fat is also mediated by cholecystokinin release, which in turn delays gastric emptying and leads to increased gastric acid and pepsinogen secretion.

Therefore, on the basis of these principles of physiology, the diet deemed optimal for treating gastric disease is one that is relatively low in fat and protein and rich in carbohydrates. Carbohydrates and their products of digestion do not stimulate gastric acid secretion, nor do they delay gastric emptying. These concepts of physiology and nutrition translate into the pragmatic recommendation that animals with primary gastric disease be fed a bland diet, rich in carbohydrates, offered in the form of a slurry. Specifically, this diet can consist of either canned Prescription Diet i/d, canned Prescription Diet d/d (Hill's Pet Products), or the soft bland diet defined in Table 1, to each of which is added an equal volume of plain cooked spaghetti noodles, cooked macaroni, or boiled rice. This mixture is homogenized in a kitchen blender while broth, bouillon, or warm water is added to produce a liquid slurry. This diet should be fed at room temperature or slightly warmed. Small amounts are offered frequently. The combination of this dietary therapy with medical therapy consisting of a histamine H_2-receptor blocker (cimetidine or ranitidine) and an antiemetic that stimulates gastric peristalsis (metoclopramide) enhances the effectiveness of both modes of therapy.

Implicit in the above description of the physiology, pathophysiology, and nutritional management of gastric mucosal diseases is the concept that gastric secretion and gastric motility are closely interrelated and interdependent. The stimuli for one often affect the other, either directly or indirectly. Thus, for those animals in which the primary gastrointestinal disease involves the muscle layers of the stomach, either functionally or physically, the protocol for nutritional therapy described above may be beneficial. For these patients, minimizing the ingestion of fiber is essential for prevention of the formation of gastric concretions that could further alter gastric secretion and motility. For maximum effectiveness, the concurrent medical therapy for these patients may be different from that for animals with mucosal disease.

Unfortunately, with our incomplete understanding of the origin and pathogenesis of gastric dilation and volvulus ("bloat"), it is difficult to recommend definitive preventive dietary measures for the dogs of large breeds prone to develop this problem. Frequent feedings of small quantities of a well-balanced, highly digestible diet may be helpful. Providing the calculated daily caloric intake in the form of a liquid slurry will hasten gastric emptying and minimize the risk of dilation and volvulus. Unlimited volumes of tepid water should be available with meals. These dogs should be fed alone in a quiet location. Restricting postprandial exercise and excitement may also be beneficial. Since protein in the diet enhances gastric secretion and delays gastric emptying, avoiding the high-protein diets currently touted may help reduce the risk of dilation and volvulus.

Another dietary factor that may contribute to the development of "bloat" is prolonged excessive dietary calcium intake. Calcium ingestion is known to stimulate gastrin secretion, and excessive calcium intake over a prolonged period results in chronically increased gastrin secretion. Gastrin reduces gastric motility and causes hyperplasia of the gastric mucosa. These changes may interfere with gastric emptying and predispose an animal to dilation and volvulus. Additional support for this hypothesis is the observation that large breeds of dogs prone to developing this problem commonly receive calcium supplementation during much of their lives. Objective clinical evaluation of these two postulates is needed.

INTESTINAL DISEASE

The most common clinical manifestation of significant intestinal disease is diarrhea, the presence of which reflects disruption of normal intestinal digestive or absorptive functions. Various schemes and algorithms have been described for the classification and evaluation of patients with diarrhea. A complete history and a thorough physical examination generally provide a basis for deciding whether signs of small bowel disease or large bowel disease predominate. For animals with primarily small bowel signs, the history and examination combined with simple laboratory evaluation often suggest the presence of either maldigestion or malabsorption. Since the diseases and their effects on intestinal function and the nutritional status of the animal vary greatly, each of these major categories will be discussed separately.

Small Bowel Disease: Malabsorption

Malabsorption results from a metabolic or an organic abnormality producing failure of the normal absorptive processes of the small intestine. This failure of absorption may reflect damage or destruction of the intestinal mucosa produced by acute or chronic infectious diseases or idiopathic villous atrophy. Infiltration of the submucosa and lamina propria with eosinophils, lymphocytes and plasma cells, or malignant lymphoblasts can also cause malabsorption and may result in excessive loss of plasma proteins into the lumen of the intestines (a protein-losing enteropathy). Congenital or acquired abnormalities of lymph drainage from the small bowel can also produce malabsorption of fat and a concurrent protein-losing enteropathy.

The dietary management of acute gastroenteritis as described above can be used for treatment of dogs and cats with acute infectious enteritides (such as induced by parvovirus, coronavirus, and bacteria). The bland diet can be started when the animal is able to tolerate oral intake. Patients with chronic infectious enteritis, most commonly parasite-induced (giardiasis, infestation with other protozoal agents and common intestinal parasites), warrant appropriate medical management and may also require temporary therapy with a diet designed for treating malabsorption. Animals with idiopathic villous atrophy should be treated for malabsorption as described below.

Treatment of animals with malabsorption due to infiltrative diseases of the small bowel consists of medical therapy and concurrent dietary management. The form and intensity of medical therapy will be dictated by the histologic findings made on examination of full-thickness biopsies of the small intestine. The dietary therapy of these patients is based on three clinical observations. First, elevated fecal nitrogen levels do not produce detrimental effects in patients that have normal liver function. Second, large dietary carbohydrate loads are generally well tolerated by most patients with malabsorption. However, the lactose content of the diet must be minimized since small bowel brush-border lactase activity may be deficient. Lactose fed to an animal with deficient lactase activity will persist in the gut, be broken down in the large bowel, and produce flatulence and an osmotic diarrhea. Third, reduction of dietary fat (mostly long-chain triglycerides) generally reduces the severity of the diarrhea by decreasing steatorrhea. Therefore, the diet of an animal with malabsorption should be high in protein and carbohydrate, low in fat, and low in lactose.

Providing large quantities of protein of high biologic value may prevent protein malnutrition, may facilitate intestinal adaptation to enteric dysfunction or disease, and may hasten recovery. Diets rich in high-quality protein are also generally quite palatable. The biologic value of the protein in milk is high. During the processing of cottage cheese, nearly all of the lactose in milk is removed. Thus, uncreamed cottage cheese is a good source of protein of high biologic value with little lactose and little fat present. Lean ground beef from which much of the fat is removed by boiling is another potential source of protein of high biologic value. Carbohydrate can be provided easily and inexpensively in the form of boiled rice, cooked macaroni, and cooked spaghetti noodles. Adequate caloric intake in the form of carbohydrates is necessary to spare dietary protein from being used as an energy source. A diet composed of one can of Prescription Diet i/d mixed with one pound (3 cups) of uncreamed cottage cheese and 2½ cups of cooked rice fulfills these objectives.

The overall process of the digestion and absorption of the long-chain triglycerides that represent most of the dietary fat is more complicated and more dependent on the full integration of intestinal, pancreatic, and hepatic function than is either protein or carbohydrate digestion and absorption. Also, fat malabsorption produces clinical signs that are more pronounced and persistent than those of malabsorption of other dietary components. The reduction in caloric intake resulting from restricted fat intake can be offset by the addition of medium-chain triglycerides (MCTs) to the diet. MCTs are a mixture of triglycerides distilled from coconut oil and contain fatty acids with carbon chains that are six to twelve atoms long. MCTs are hydrolyzed more rapidly and efficiently in the lumen of the small intestine than are long-chain triglycerides. The products of digestion of the MCTs are absorbed directly into the portal venous system, bypassing the lymphatic drainage of the gut. The indications for the use of MCTs are (1) fat malabsorption of any cause, (2) abnormalities of intestinal lymphatic drainage (i.e., intestinal lymphangiectasia, either congenital or acquired), and (3) malabsorption for which there is no specific therapy. The aim of their use is to provide calories lost by restriction of fat in the diet. MCTs are available commercially in two forms: (1) a powdered formula containing 30 kcal per fluid ounce (Portagen, Mead Johnson Nutritional), and (2) an oil that is liquid at room temperature and contains 230 kcal/30 ml (MCT Oil, Mead Johnson Nutritional). Since the palatability of MCTs is limited, treatment is started with only 1 tsp of oil per meal and slowly increased to a maximal tolerated dose or 30 ml/lb of food. Side effects include nausea and vomiting, bloating, flatulence, and diarrhea. These side effects may be transient, and long-term administration may be feasible.

Vitamin supplementation of the diet, especially with the fat-soluble vitamins (A, D, E, and K), is also recommended. Commercially available vitamin-mineral supplements for dogs and cats will generally suffice.

In summary, the basal diet for treating veterinary patients with malabsorption can consist of either Prescription Diet i/d, Prescription Diet d/d, or the bland diet described in Table 1. To to one pound of this diet is added a source of protein (3 cups of uncreamed cottage cheese or 2 cups of boiled lean ground beef) and a source of carbohydrate (2½ cups of cooked rice, macaroni, or spaghetti). MCT Oil is added at the rate described. A vitamin-mineral supplement is provided. The calculated daily intake is divided into three or four warm meals of equal size to avoid overload of the intestinal digestive-absorptive capacity. The body weight and condition of the patient are monitored regularly, and the amount of diet fed is adjusted to maintain normal body weight and condition. Depending on the cause of the malabsorption and the animal's response to medical and dietary therapy, it may be possible to gradually change the diet to a well-balanced, commercially available diet.

Patients that show signs of small bowel dysfunction and that are suspected of having a food allergy or sensitivity may respond to a hypoallergenic diet such as Prescription Diet d/d or the diet described in Table 1. These diets contain ingredients not commonly present in most commercial dog foods. If the animal responds to dietary modification, it is fed only this diet and water and is exposed to other foods, one at a time, to identify offending foods. The goal of this provocative exposure is to determine which foods the patient can tolerate, from which a balanced diet can be compounded.

Dogs and cats are occasionally presented because of intermittent or persistent diarrhea characteristic of small bowel malabsorption. Although the cause often is inapparent, there may be a historic indication that the animal is unable to tolerate common commercial diets. For dogs so affected, Eukanuba (Iams Food Co.) or Science Diet Performance (Hill's Pet Products) may successfully control the diarrhea. For cats, Tender Vittles (Ralston Purina) or Prescription Diet c/d (Hill's Pet Products) may be beneficial.

Small Bowel Disease: Maldigestion

Maldigestion is most commonly caused by exocrine pancreatic insufficiency (EPI), which results from either pancreatic atrophy or recurrent bouts of pancreatitis. Both dietary management and pancreatic enzyme supplementation (Viokase V powder, Robins) are needed for optimal response. A study of different modes and combinations of therapy for dogs with experimentally induced exocrine pancreatic insufficiency demonstrated that feeding a highly digestible diet was of greater benefit than any other single treatment. Feeding a highly digestible, low-fiber, moderate-fat diet was essential for the best therapeutic response to supplementation with pancreatic enzymes. The bland diet defined in Table 1, Prescription Diet i/d, or diets of similar composition meet these criteria. Even with concurrent appropriate medical therapy, the net digestion of such diets by some dogs with EPI does not return to a normal range. Thus, a 15 per cent caloric excess has been recommended. The calculated daily caloric need should be fed in three or four meals of equal size to which is added pancreatin supplementation. The animal's body weight and condition are monitored regularly, and caloric intake is adjusted accordingly. Supplementation with fat-soluble vitamins is also recommended.

Large Bowel Disease: Diarrhea

The frequent, small-volume, mucoid stools characteristic of large bowel disease or dysfunction represent the clinical manifestation of altered colonic motility and absorption. In normal dogs and cats, ingesta is retained in the upper half of the colon by segmental and orally directed peristalsis. Absorption of fluid and electrolytes from the retained ingesta produces stool of normal consistency. With alteration of these functions, the liquid ileal effluent traverses the colon more rapidly than normal and is passed as the stool characteristic of large bowel disease. With infiltrative or inflammatory diseases or functional abnormalities of the large bowel, there is a concurrent stimulation of the large population of goblet cells in the colonic mucosa, resulting in the excess mucus production evident in these stools. These pathologic changes in the colon also cause a sensation of a need to defecate, which contributes to the frequent defecation and tenesmus.

The goal of dietary management of patients with acute colitis is to reduce the volume of ingesta reaching the large bowel and thus reduce the stimulation of abnormal motility and reduce the need for efficient colonic absorption. This goal is most easily attained by applying the protocol for treating acute gastroenteritis, which was described above. Resting the intestinal tract by fasting the animal, then feeding a highly digestible, bland diet minimizes demands on the colon and reduces the signs of acute colitis.

The optimal dietary management of patients with chronic colitis is uncertain and must be defined and adjusted for each patient. Initial therapy with the highly digestible, bland diets described above will often allay the clinical signs of most patients with chronic colonic disease. Appropriate concurrent medical therapy is also provided. If the patient does not show satisfactory response, a high-fiber diet may be beneficial. Some dogs with large bowel diarrhea respond more favorably to this type of diet than to a highly digestible diet. Increasing dietary fiber reduces the rate of transit of ingesta through the intestinal tract.

A high-fiber diet is produced simply by adding bran or other bulk-forming agents (Metamucil, Searle Consumer Products; Siblin, Parke-Davis) to the diets described above. Bran can generally be purchased at a health-food store, is less expensive than the other products, and is equally effective. The amount of bran added to the diet is empirical; the ideal amount for each patient must be determined by assessing response to an initial dose of 1 tbsp of bran added to each meal. The amount is then altered as needed. An alternate method of providing a high-bulk diet is feeding a reducing diet such as Prescription Diet r/d for dogs or cats (Hill's Pet Products). Since these diets have a low caloric density (300 to 350 kcal/lb of food), caution must be exercised to provide adequate caloric intake for the animal to maintain normal body weight.

CONSTIPATION

Constipation and obstipation (recurrent or intractable constipation) result from prolonged retention of material in the colon with excessive absorption of electrolytes and water. Physical or functional obstruction of the flow of ingesta through the colon may produce prolonged retention. Efforts must be made to diagnose and treat directly those abnormalities resulting in physical obstruction of the colonic lumen; e.g., foreign material, obstructive neoplasia, or reduced diameter of the pelvic canal. When such therapy is not possible or beneficial, and in those patients with functional abnormalities producing retention of colonic contents, dietary management may help reduce the frequency and the severity of constipation.

The goals of dietary management of animals with (recurrent) constipation are to hasten transit of material through the colon and reduce colonic absorption of electrolytes and water. Increased volume of ingesta in the upper portion of the colon is a major stimulus for waves of peristalsis that move the ingesta into the lower colon. Such movement of material into the descending colon and rectum produces a sensation of a need to defecate. Feeding a high-fiber diet increases the volume of undigestible material reaching the colon and increases the frequency of evacuation of the upper large bowel. Undigestible fiber also inherently retains water and thus tends to produce a softer stool. A high-fiber diet can be produced by adding bran or bulk-forming agents to the highly digestible diets described above. Alternatively, Prescription Diet r/d for dogs or cats can be fed. In general, the dry dog and cat foods tend to have higher fiber content than do the canned or semimoist foods.

Another means of enhancing the retention of water and electrolytes within the lumen of the colon and producing softer stools is to include in the diet other substances that are not digestible. As mentioned above, animals that are deficient in small bowel brush-border lactase activity will have an osmotic diarrhea when fed diets containing lactose. Many middle-aged and older animals have decreased small bowel lactase activity either as a result of prior small intestinal diseases or as a result of the aging process itself. Offering lactose in the form of whole cow's milk may alleviate a problem of obstipation if it develops in such an animal. The amount of milk to be offered daily must be adjusted to produce stools that are passed easily. For those dogs and cats that have a problem with obstipation and do have adequate small bowel lactase activity (as indicated by no response to ingestion of milk), lactulose, a synthetic disaccharide, can be added to the food. Since there is no enzyme capable of hydrolyzing this disaccharide present in the small intestine, it persists in the gut and enters the large intestine, where it is broken down by the action of the bacteria. This results in an increase in osmotic pressure and causes an increase in stool water content, which softens the stool. The amount to be added to the food varies with each patient. Older cats with recurrent obstipation are started at a dose of 1 ml added to each of three meals of high-fiber diet per day. Thereafter, the dose is adjusted as needed to produce soft stools.

Patients with obstipation are also encouraged to consume more water. This can be accomplished by feeding canned foods that contain approximately 75 per cent water. The palatability of the canned foods can be used to mask the addition of bran or lactulose. Reducing the caloric intake by these animals may facilitate passage of stools by minimizing the fat accumulated within the pelvic canal. This fat may narrow the rectal lumen and produce a functional stricture. Physical exercise of patients with obstipation may also be beneficial by inducing more frequent evacuation of soft material from the upper colon. This will produce more frequent passage of soft stool.

FLATULENCE

Although the cause of chronic flatulence in pets is not established in most cases, there are several factors that can contribute to this offensive problem that should be considered. Most gas present in the intestinal tract results from swallowing air during eating or panting. Some intestinal gas is formed by bacterial fermentation of undigestible carbohydrates and fiber in the large bowel. Beans and soybeans contain large amounts of undigestible short-chain carbohydrates, which are partially broken down by the colonic bacteria. Malabsorption and maldigestion also predispose to colonic fermentation of residual nutrients. Therefore, the dietary management of animals exhibiting excessive flatulence should consist of (1) feeding a highly digestible, low-bulk diet either free choice or in two or three meals per day, (2) feeding the animal alone in a quiet location to minimize aerophagia, and (3) avoiding diets that contain beans and soybean meal. If dietary management is not successful in controlling the flatulence, the patient should be evaluated for the presence of diseases that produce malabsorption or maldigestion.

References and Supplemental Reading

Chiapella, A. M.: Treatment of intestinal disease. Vet. Clin. North Am. 13:567, 1983.

Floch, M. H.: *Nutritional and Diet Therapy in Gastrointestinal Disease.* New York: Plenum Medical Book Co., 1981.

Lewis, L. D., and Morris, M. L., Jr.: *Small Animal Clinical Nutrition.* Topeka: Mark Morris Associates, 1984, pp. 7–1 to 7–56.

Lorenz, M. D.: Diseases of the large bowel. *In* Ettinger, S. J. (ed.): *Textbook of Veterinary Internal Medicine. Diseases of the Dog and Cat.* Philadelphia: W. B. Saunders, 1983, pp. 1346–1372.

Pidgeon, G.: Effects of diet on exocrine pancreatic insufficiency in dogs. J.A.V.M.A. 181:232, 1982.

Sherding, R. G.: Diseases of the small bowel. *In* Ettinger, S. J. (ed.): *Textbook of Veterinary Internal Medicine. Diseases of the Dog and Cat.* Philadelphia: W. B. Saunders, 1983, pp. 1278–1346.

Twedt, D. C., and Wingfield, W. E.: Diseases of the stomach. *In* Ettinger, S. J. (ed.): *Textbook of Veterinary Internal Medicine. Diseases of the Dog and Cat.* Philadelphia: W. B. Saunders, 1983, pp. 1233–1277.

Zimmer, J. F.: Examination of the gastrointestinal system. Vet Clin. North Am. 11:561, 1981.

Zimmer, J. F.: Clinical Management of acute gastroenteritis including virus-induced enteritis. *In* Kirk, R. W. (ed.): *Current Veterinary Therapy VIII.* Philadelphia, W. B. Saunders, 1983, pp. 1171–1177.

Zimmer, J. F.: Canine esophageal foreign bodies: Endoscopic, surgical, and medical management. J. Am. Anim. Hosp. Assoc. 20:669, 1984.

DISEASES OF THE ANUS AND RECTUM

HOWARD B. SEIM III, D.V.M.
Fort Collins, Colorado

Disorders involving the anus and rectum occur frequently in small animal practice. In order to appropriately diagnose and treat these disorders, knowledge of the regional anatomy, physiology, and common clinical signs they produce are mandatory, along with proper physical examination techniques.

PHYSIOLOGY

The rectum has little importance in digestion and acts as a reservoir for undigested waste. The most important physiologic function of the rectum and anus is in the controlled act of defecation (continence).

CLINICAL SIGNS

Common clinical signs associated with diseases of the anus and rectum include dyschezia, hematochezia, anal licking, ribbon-like stools, matting of anal hair, anal discharge, scooting, excessive flatulence, and diarrhea.

PHYSICAL EXAMINATION

A complete physical examination should be performed on all patients with clinical signs specific for anorectal disease in order to rule out systemic disorders that manifest themselves with anorectal abnormalities (e.g., pemphigus). Specific examination of the anorectal region should include close visual examination of the perineum, circumanal area, and base of the tail, as well as careful digital rectal palpation. When a more detailed examination is needed, the use of an anal dilator or proctoscope may be indicated. Heavy sedation or general anesthesia may be needed to perform these techniques adequately. Epidural anesthesia has proved to be the most effective anesthetic for examination of the anus and rectum. Excellent muscle relaxation allows easy anal sphincter dilation and visualization of the anal canal and rectal mucosa.

CONGENITAL DISEASES OF THE ANUS AND RECTUM

Imperforate Anus

Three classifications of imperforate anus (types I, II, III) have been described. Treatment is surgical, and the technique varies with each type of imperforate anus.

In imperforate anus type I, a membrane is left covering the anal opening. Treatment consists of simply rupturing the membrane and trimming off the excess tissue. A rectal thermometer is used to ensure that the opening is sufficient. The prognosis is excellent.

Imperforate anus type II (also referred to as atresia ani) results from a failure of the cloacal membrane to rupture, leaving a relatively thick membrane covering the anal orifice. Treatment is directed at locating the anal dimple, dissecting the membrane to the level of the rectal mucosa, and suturing the mucosa to the subcutaneous tissue and skin. The prognosis is favorable, as the anal sphincter is usually intact and functional.

Imperforate anus type III (also referred to as rectal agenesis) differs anatomically from imperforate anus type II in that the rectum ends blindly a variable distance from the anal membrane. It is critical that the two conditions (types II and III) be differentiated, because the surgical technique differs, as does the prognosis. A lateral abdominal x-ray with the hind end slightly elevated will allow visualization of gas in the termination of the rectum. The distance from the rectum to the anal membrane will allow differentiation between types II and III. Treatment for imperforate anus type III requires an abdominal-perineal surgical approach. The distal rectum is exposed abdominally and then delivered through the pelvic canal to an opening made in the anal dimple. Rectal mucosa is then sutured to the subcutaneous tissues and skin in the perianal region. The prognosis is guarded, and patients may remain incontinent postoperatively.

Rectovaginal Fistula

This disorder occurs much less frequently than imperforate anus. Clinical signs include fecal material passed from the anus and vulva, or just the vulva, if imperforate anus occurs concurrently. Barium enemas demonstrate contrast material in the rectum and vaginal vault. Treatment is surgical, requiring obliteration of the fistulous tract and primary closure of the rectum and vagina. The prognosis is guarded.

ACQUIRED DISEASES OF THE ANUS AND RECTUM

Anal Stricture (Stenosis)

Anal stenosis most commonly occurs secondary to surgery of the anus for the treatment of perianal disorders. Trauma and infection in the anal region have also been reported to cause a secondary stenosis. Treatment with periodic digital dilation and anti-inflammatory medication (steroids) has been unsuccessful in most cases. Surgical correction is directed at the removal of excessive scar tissue in the anal area and uniting rectal mucosa with the subcutaneous tissue and skin with simple interrupted sutures. The prognosis for return to normal function is favorable.

Anal Sacculitis

Anal sac impaction and abscessation is the most common anorectal disorder diagnosed. Diagnosis is confirmed by clinical signs and by visual and digital rectal examination. Relief of impaction by digitally expressing the anal sacs is easily performed during rectal examination. If abscessation is present, cauterization with silver nitrate and infusion of an antibiotic preparation are sufficient to eliminate the infection. If abscessation becomes a chronic recurrent problem, surgical excision of both anal sacs is the treatment of choice. Surgery should be delayed, however, until the immediate infection or abscess has been controlled medically as described above. If the entire anal sac is removed and the external anal sphincter muscle preserved, the prognosis is excellent.

Anal Ulceration (Anusitis)

Anal ulceration is a superficial, nonfistulating ulceration involving 360 degrees of the perianal skin. This disorder occurs most commonly in German shepherds but has been diagnosed in other breeds. Clinical signs include anal licking and pain on manipulation of the tail. Visual examination reveals a 360-degree portion of the perianal skin that is inflamed, moist, and painful. Treatment by lightly cauterizing the ulcerated area with silver nitrate applicators (Medisco-Federal, 75 per cent silver nitrate and 25 per cent potassium nitrate) is generally effective. Three to 5 minutes after application of the silver nitrate, the area is rinsed with 0.9 per cent sodium chloride solution. This precipitates the silver ion and stops the cauterizing effect. Re-epithelialization occurs in 10 to 14 days. If the lesion is still ulcerated in 10 days, the area should be recauterized. Dogs that have an associated abnormal anal sac secretion should also have a bilateral anal sacculectomy performed.

Perianal Fistula

Perianal fistulas are chronic suppurating sinus tracts involving the perianal and perirectal tissues of dogs. The tracts may involve the mucosa of the anal canal, perineal skin, external anal sphincter, internal anal sphincter, and anal sacs. German shepherds are the most commonly affected, but Irish setters, black Labrador retrievers, and other large breeds are also affected.

The cause of perianal fistula is unknown. The most commonly accepted theory is that the fistulas originate from infected circumanal glands. The breeds most commonly affected either have a broad tail base or a low tail carriage or both, allowing a fecal film to develop over the perianal area. The low tail carriage results in poor ventilation. These "conformational defects" can lead to infection and abscessation of the circumanal glands and hair follicles in the perianal skin, resulting in sinus tract formation.

The most common clinical signs are dyschezia, hematochezia, diarrhea, and anal licking. Examination reveals multiple fistulous tract openings in the perianal skin. Involvement ranges from one single tract to extensive 360-degree ulceration.

Medical management including systemic antibiotics, topical antibiotics, chemical cauterization of fistulous tracts, povidone-iodine flush, and elevation of the tail may temporarily control the problem but will not result in a cure. It is generally accepted that some form of surgical management is necessary to treat perianal fistulas successfully.

Several surgical techniques are available for treatment of perianal fistula. These include anoplasty, electrosurgical débridement and fulguration, cryosurgery, and tail amputation as a last resort. No single technique has been uniformly successful in all cases. Predictably successful treatment may require any one or a combination of the above techniques, depending on the severity of the perianal fistulas.

Mild perianal involvement (up to 90 degrees) can be successfully managed by any of the above techniques. If the fistula is in the area of the anal sac, an anal sacculectomy is also performed.

Moderate involvement (90 to 180 degrees) can be initially managed by surgical excision of the involved tissue, including anal sacculectomy and reuniting the rectal mucosa to the remaining perianal skin. If recurrence of one or two fistulous tracts occurs, cryosurgical treatment can be attempted as a second procedure. Care is taken to preserve the external anal sphincter muscle by careful direction.

Moderately involved cases also respond favorably to electrosurgical débridement and fulguration. In this technique, if the anal sacs are involved in the fistulous tissue an anal sacculectomy is performed. Each fistulous tract is carefully explored and opened by using an electroscalpel. All chronic granulation tissue and scar tissue is resected. Diseased tissue involving the external anal sphincter muscle or deep in the pararectal region is either fulgurated with electrocautery or cauterized with Lugol's iodine or 80 per cent liquefied phenol solution. Care is taken to cauterize only diseased tissue. The wounds are left open to heal by contraction and epithelialization. Recurrent fistulas should be treated immediately by débridement and fulguration.

Severely involved cases (360-degree involvement) are either treated by a two-stage electrosurgical débridement and fulguration procedure or cryosurgical therapy. The two-stage débridement is accomplished by operating on 180 degrees of the involved area at 1-month intervals as described above. Cryosurgical therapy requires deep and superficial freezing of all diseased tissue. These procedures often result in enough scar tissue formation that anal stenosis may occur. Correction is as described above for anal stenosis.

The most common postoperative complications are stenosis, incontinence, and recurrence. Careful dissection of fistulous tracts will prevent destruction of the external anal sphincter muscle and the caudal rectal nerve, thus decreasing the chance of incontinence. Anal stenosis is treated by resection of excessive scar tissue. Recurrent episodes must be treated aggressively and as early as possible.

Rectocutaneous Fistula

Rectocutaneous fistulas can occur secondary to external trauma (e.g., bite wound, missile wound), internal trauma (fractured pelvis, rectal foreign body), pararectal abscess, or pararectal surgery (perineal hernia repair, resection of pararectal mass). Diagnosis is based on the observation of fecal material passing through the anus and pararectal wound. A simplified surgical approach has been developed that produces excellent results. The rectum and wound are evacuated of all fecal material. The cranial edge of the defect is grasped and gently undermined sufficiently to retract it to the mucocutaneous junction. The interposed mucous membrane is then removed, and the cranial edge of the fistula is sutured to the mucocutaneous junction.

Rectal Stricture

Rectal strictures are most commonly due to trauma (internal or external) or neoplasia, occur secondary to surgical manipulation, or are idiopathic. Diagnosis is based on clinical signs, digital rectal palpation, and barium enema. Most strictures can be managed surgically by distal rectal resection. The anocutaneous junction is incised for 360 degrees. The dissection progresses pararectally until the rectum is freed to the level of the stricture. Dissection does not include the anal sphincter muscles or caudal rectal nerve, thus preserving continence. The involved rectum is then amputated proximal to the stricture. The rectal mucosa is sutured to the subcutaneous tissues and perianal skin, completing the procedure. The prognosis for return to function is favorable.

Rectal Diverticulum, Rectal Sacculation, Rectal Deviation

These defects in rectal anatomy are most commonly associated with perineal hernia in dogs. In rectal deviation, the intact rectum curves within the herinal sac. This type of defect responds to perineal hernia repair. Rectal sacculation is a defect in the full thickness of the rectal wall, whereas rectal diverticulum is an outpouching of the rectal mucosa through a defect in the muscularis. Repair of rectal sacculation and rectal diverticulum involve cross-clamping of the defect with intestinal forceps, excising the defect, and suturing the incision with a double layer, continuous inverting suture pattern. The prognosis for return to function is favorable.

Rectal Prolapse

Rectal prolapse is a sign, not a disease. Some of the underlying causes include intestinal parasitism, chronic diarrhea, dystocia, or any disease that causes dyschezia, stranguria, or abdominal pressing. Diagnosis is made by visual observation of a tubelike protrusion of rectal mucosa.

Rectal prolapse must be differentiated from a prolapsed intussusception. This can be done by placing a finger or blunt instrument between the prolapsed mucosa and mucocutaneous junction. If the finger or instrument is easily passed, an intussusception is present; if resistance is met, a rectal prolapse has occurred.

Rectal prolapse can be managed by several methods, including reduction and purse-string suture, amputation, or colopexy. The technique selected depends on the viability of the prolapsed tissue, the size and reducibility of the prolapse, and recurrence after a previous technique has failed. Patients with rectal prolapse are often presented early, before significant mucosal necrosis occurs. Therefore, initial management generally involves reduction and placement of a purse-string suture. This is accomplished by general anesthesia, application of 50 per cent dextrose or granulated sugar to reduce mucosal edema, gentle reduction of the prolapsed tissue, and placement of the purse-string suture. Topical anesthetic ointment with 1 per cent dibucaine (Nupercainal Ointment, Ciba) is instilled in the rectum postoperatively and continued for 2 to 3 days after purse-string removal. The purse-string suture remains for 2 to 3 days. Diagnosis and treatment of the underlying cause aid in the ultimate success.

A nonreducibile viable prolapse or a recurrent rectal prolapse may be treated by celiotomy and colopexy. Scarified surfaces of the colon and the sublumbar body wall are sutured together with simple interrupted sutures, completing the colopexy. Topical anesthetic ointment is instilled rectally after surgical correction and continued for 5 to 6 days postoperatively. A nonreducibile rectal prolapse with nonviable mucosa should be treated by amputation.

NEOPLASMS OF THE ANUS AND RECTUM

Perianal Adenoma

Perianal gland adenomas generally occur in middle-aged to older intact male dogs. The tumor can occur wherever perianal (circumanal) glands are located, in the anal ring, tail head, prepuce, and ventral midline. The adenoma is hormone dependent (testosterone). Diagnosis is based on visual examination of the perianal region. Perianal adenomas may be single or multiple and range in size from a small BB-sized mass to a large, ulcerated, hemorrhagic mass of 3 to 5 cm in diameter.

The most effective forms of therapy for perianal adenomas include surgical excision, electrocautery, cryosurgery, and castration. Because of the hormone-dependent nature of the tumor, castration should be recommended in all cases. It has been reported that castration alone is adequate in most cases; however, patients that present with painful, ulcerated, or hemorrhagic tumors should have an excision performed at the time of castration for palliation. Also, definitive diagnosis can be established only by incisional or excisional biopsy of the tumor. Cytologic testing has not proved to be accurate in differentiating perianal gland adenomas from perianal gland adenocarcinomas.

Perianal Adenocarcinoma

Perianal gland adenocarcinomas are malignant neoplasms of perianal (circumanal) glands. They can occur wherever circumanal glands are located but are most commonly found in the perianal area of middle-aged and older dogs. Males are more commonly affected than females. The tumors are firm, often ulcerated, hemorrhagic, and invasive. They must be differentiated from perianal gland adenomas by histopathologic examination. Complete excision is often difficult because of the invasive nature of the tumor. The recommended therapy is cytoreduction (debulking) by surgical excision and local radiation therapy. Castration does not affect the prognosis, as the neoplasm does not seem to be hormonally dependent. Metastasis is generally to the sublumbar lymph nodes and may be present at the time of diagnosis. Routine abdominal x-rays are taken prior to therapy to assess tumor metastasis and determine the prognosis. Local recurrence after therapy is common but may take as long as 5 to 8 months. Multiple surgical procedures for local excision are warranted for palliation, as distant metastasis generally takes a protracted course. The long-term prognosis is unfavorable because of local recurrence and metastasis.

Anal Sac Apocrine Adenocarcinoma

Adenocarcinomas of anal sac origin are malignant neoplasms of apocrine glands in the wall of the anal sac, occurring most commonly in older spayed females. The tumor often secretes a parathyroid hormone-like substance resulting in a hypercalcemia. The most common presenting signs are those of hypercalcemia (anorexia, depression, polyuria, polydipsia, weight loss, and weakness). Careful visual and digital rectal examination of the anal sac region will often reveal the tumor. Careful examination is necessary, as the tumor can be quite small (2 to 5 mm in diameter). Metastasis to regional lymph nodes often is present at the time of diagnosis. Abdominal radiographs are recommended to help determine proper therapy. Treatment is aimed at controlling the hypercalcemia (see Primary Hyperparathyroidism in *Current Veterinary Therapy VIII*), removing the tumor load, and controlling recurrence. Surgical excision of the primary and metastatic lesions is performed in a two-stage procedure. A guarded prognosis must be given for dogs with this neoplasm.

Rectal Polyps

Rectal polyps are infrequently seen in small animal practice. They appear as lobulated, grape-like clusters with a pedunculated or sessile base. They are very friable and bleed easily when manipulated. They arise from the rectal mucosa and are generally found as solitary masses but can be multiple. They are most often located in the terminal portion of the rectum, generally within 3 and 8 cm of the anal orifice. The most common clinical signs are hematochezia and appearance of the polyp as it prolapses through the anus during defecation. Diagnosis is based on digital rectal examination and excisional biopsy.

Rectal polyps located 1 to 3 cm from the anal orifice can be treated by digitally exteriorizing the polyp and excising it. If the polyp is pedunculated, scalpel, cautery, or cryosurgical excision can be easily performed. If the polyp has a sessile base, cautery or cryosurgical therapy is preferred.

Rectal polyps located 3 to 8 cm from the anal orifice require iatrogenic rectal prolapse for adequate exposure. Epidural anesthesia, because it causes excellent muscle relaxation, is the anesthetic of choice. The anus is digitally dilated, exposing the folds of rectal mucosa. Three to four stay sutures are placed in the mucosal folds equidistant around the rectum. Gentle traction on the stay sutures allows prolapse of the rectal mucosa. The procedure is repeated until the polyp has been completely prolapsed. Excision of the polyp is performed as described above. When excision is complete, the prolapse is reduced, a tampon is inserted for hemostasis, and a purse-string suture is placed in the anus to keep the tampon in place and to prevent recurrence of the prolapse. The purse-string suture is removed in 12 to 24 hours, and the patient is allowed to pass the tampon. The prognosis is excellent if the tumor is completely removed. Recurrence is most common with sessile polyps. Malignant transformation has recently been documented.

Rectal Adenocarcinoma

Rectal adenocarcinoma is a malignant neoplasm arising from the rectal mucosa and generally affecting older dogs (8 to 9 years). The most common clinical signs include dyschezia and hematochezia. A presumptive diagnosis is based on digital rectal palpation and proctoscopy. Contrast radiography (barium enema) may be helpful in establishing the extent of the tumor. Definitive diagnosis is based on incisional biopsy. Rectal adenocarcinomas are one of two types: proliferative or invasive. Proliferative adenocarcinomas involve the rectal mucosa but rarely invade beyond the submucosa until late in the disease. These can be surgically excised with a guarded prognosis. Distal rectal resection (as described under rectal stricture) is the procedure of choice.

Invasive rectal adenocarcinomas hold a grave prognosis, as they are often inoperable at the time of presentation because of deep invasion and metastasis. Diversion procedures (ileovesical fistula) have been attempted for palliative treatment only.

References and Supplemental Reading

Christie, T. R.: Perianal fistula in the dog. Vet. Clin. North Am. 5:353, 1975.

Dee, J. F.: Surgery of the cecum, colon, and rectum. Vet. Clin. North Am. 5:421, 1975.

Elkins, A. D., and Hobson, H. P.: Management of perianal fistula. A retrospective study of 23 cases. Vet. Surg. 11:110, 1982.

Engen, M. H.: *Management of Rectal Prolapse in Current Techniques in Small Animal Surgery,* 2nd ed. Philadelphia: Lea & Febiger, 1983.

Hause, W. R., et al.: Pseudohyperparathyroidism associated with adenocarcinomas of anal sac origin in four dogs. J. Am. Anim. Hosp. Assoc. 17:373, 1981.

Krahwinkel, D. J.: Rectal diseases and their role in perineal hernia. Vet. Surg. 12:160, 1983.

Liska, W. D.: Anorectal and perianal cryosurgery. Vet. Clin. North Am. 10:803, 1980.

Liska, W. D., and Withrow, S. J.: Cryosurgical treatment of perianal gland adenomas in the dog. J. Am. Anim. Hosp. Assoc. 14:457, 1978.

Vasseur, P. B.: Perianal fistulas in dogs: a retrospective analysis of surgical techniques. J. Am. Anim. Hosp. Assoc. 17:177, 1981.

Vasseur, P. B.: Results of surgical excision of perianal fistulas in dogs. J.A.V.M.A. 185:60, 1984.

Wilson, G. P., and Hayes, H. M., Jr.: Castration for treatment of perianal gland neoplasms in the dog. J.A.V.M.A. 174:130, 1979.

TREATMENT OF GASTROINTESTINAL PARASITISM

LARRY M. CORNELIUS, D.V.M.,
and EDWARD L. ROBERSON, D.V.M.
Athens, Georgia

Gastrointestinal parasites continue to be major problems in dogs and cats in most areas of the world. Several safe and highly effective anthelmintics have become available during the past few years, and these should be used instead of older, more toxic drugs. The purpose of this article is to present, in a concise table format, clinically useful drugs for treating common canine and feline gastrointestinal parasites. The reader is referred to *Current Veterinary Therapy VII* and *VIII* for details of diagnosis, pathogenesis, supportive treatment, prevention, and control.

Table 1. *Intestinal Protozoal Drugs for Dogs and Cats*

Organism	Drug	Dosage	Comments
Coccidia, *Cystoisospora*	Bactrovet (sulfadimethoxine*) (Pitman-Moore)	Dogs and cats: 50 mg/kg once daily the first day; 25 mg/kg once daily for 14–20 days thereafter	Sulfas are coccidiostatic; supportive care, including fluids and good nutrition, is important
	Corid (amprolium) (Merck Sharp & Dohme)	*Capsule or feed:* 6-week-old pups of small breeds, one 100-mg capsule containing 20% amprolium soluble powder daily for 7–10 days; 200 mg for pups of larger breeds; capsule contents can be added to feed *Drinking water:* 7.8 ml of 9.6% amprolium solution is mixed in 1.0 L drinking water for 7–10 days; no other source of water is provided	Either regimen can be used for treatment or prevention (especially before stress when shipping kennel pups); amprolium is a thiamine inhibitor; side effects (neural disturbances, anorexia, diarrhea) are rare
	Rovamycin (spiramycin) (Rhone-Poulenc, Denmark)	Not established in dogs and cats	No experience with this drug
Giardia	Atabrine (quinacrine) (Winthrop)	Dogs: 9 mg/kg once daily for 6 days	*Giardia* of dogs and cats may be of public health significance; control of *Giardia* requires improvement in kennel sanitation
	Flagyl (metronidazole) (Searle & Co.)	Dogs and cats: 65 mg/kg once daily for 5 days	

*Other intestinal sulfas are reported to be effective against coccidia.

Table 2. Anthelmintics for Dogs and Cats

Trade Name	Generic Name	Efficacy*: Hookworms	Efficacy*: Ascarids	Efficacy*: Whipworms	Efficacy*: Tapeworms	Efficacy*: *Strongyloides*	Dosage†	Comments
Canopar	Thenium closylate (Burroughs Wellcome)	89%	±	—	—	—	1 tablet (500 mg) for dogs over 5 kg (10 lb) regardless of weight; ¼ tablet (125 mg) 2.5- to 5-kg (5- to 10-lb) dogs	Some emesis; cannot use in nursing pups or those less than 2.5 kg (5 lb); occasional deaths (collies and Airedales)
Caricide	Diethylcarbamazine (American Cyanamid)	—	80%	—	—	—	6.6 mg/kg/day PO as a heartworm preventative	Substantial adult ascarid burden is eliminated when DEC is given as a heartworm preventive; contraindicated if microfilariae present
DNP	Disophenol (American Cyanamid)	95%	—	—	—	—	10 mg/kg SC	36 mg/kg is fatal; weigh pups and kittens accurately and use 1-ml syringe; do not administer to overheated animals or those with respiratory problems; can be used on nursing young; takes 24 hours for hookworm expulsion
Droncit	Praziquantel (Haver Lockhart)	—	—	—	100% T,D,E*	—	Dogs: 5 mg/kg, single PO or IM dose Cats: 11 mg total (1–3 lb) 22 mg total (3–11 lb) 33 mg total (> 11 lb)	10 mg/kg required for *Echinococcus* juveniles; effective against tapeworm larvae in many intermediate hosts; no effect on nematodes
Nemex-2	Pyrantel pamoate (Pfizer)	95%	95%	±	—	—	15 mg/kg in tablet or suspension (Nemex-2, Strongid-T, Imathal) 30 min after light meal	Used in dogs and cats all ages, including nursing young; no contraindications; current FDA approval is for dogs, not cats
Panacur	Fenbendazole (American Hoechst)	98%	99%	100%	88–100% T* 0% D*	Estimated 100% with 5-day treatment	50 mg/kg/day for 3 consecutive days (dogs and cats) In valuable pregnant bitches, 50 mg/kg/day from day 40 of gestation until 2 weeks after parturition—90 to 99% reduction in transmission of hookworm and ascarid larvae to pups	Suspension (horses) or granules (added to moist food); single dose, even at 150 mg/kg, is not effective in dogs or cats; current FDA approval is for dogs, not cats
	Piperazine	—	52–100%	—	—	—	45–65 mg base/kg PO; maximum of 150 mg for pups under 2.5 kg and for cats and kittens	No contraindications except long-standing renal or liver disease
Scolaban	Bunamidine HCl (Burroughs Wellcome)	—	—	—	100% T* 56– 90% D* 85–100% E*	—	25–50 mg/kg on empty stomach; feed lightly in 3 hours	Occasional idiosyncratic reaction (sudden death in larger dogs); do not use simultaneously with Styquin; do not crush tablets before administration

Styquin	Butamisole HCl (American Cyanamid)	92%	—	99%	—	—	2.4 mg/kg SC	A fourfold overdose is lethal; approved for dogs; do not use simultaneously with Scolaban, in heartworm-positive or debilitated dogs, or in pups less than 8 weeks old; dogs often show evidence of pain for about 1 hour after injection
Styrid-Caricide	DEC + styrylpyridinium chloride (American Cyanamid)	80%	80%	—	—	—	6.6 mg DEC and 5.5 mg styryl. cl./kg/day PO	Used as a heartworm preventive and as an aid in control of ascarids and hookworms; contraindicated if microfilariae present
Task	Dichlorvos (Squibb)	95%	95%	90%	—	—	Dogs: 27–33 mg/kg Puppies and cats: 11 mg/kg	Contraindications include heartworm disease, liver or kidney damage, and severe diarrhea accompanied by anemia and listlessness in pups with hookworms; do not use in conjunction with other cholinesterase inhibitors; split dosage b.i.d. for debilitated animals; takes 8 hours for hookworm expulsion
Telmintic	Mebendazole (Pitman-Moore)	95%	95%	95%	95% T* 0% D*	—	22 mg/kg in food daily for 3 days (nematodes) or 5 days (*Taenia*)	Approved for dogs; experimental in cats; evidence suggests occasional drug-induced acute hepatic necrosis in dogs
Thenatol	Thenium closylate and piperazine (Burroughs Wellcome)	96%	89%	—	—	—	2 doses, 8 hours apart; each dose: 0.9–2.3 kg (2–5 lb), ½ tab; 2.3–4.5 kg (5–10 lb), 1 tab; 4.5 kg (10 lb), 2 tabs 1st dose AM before feeding; feed between 1st and 2nd doses; no milk or fatty foods	
Vercom Paste	Febantel and praziquantel (Haver-Lockhart)	>91%	98%	100%	100% T* 100% D*	—	Adult dogs, cats: 10 mg feb. and 1.0 mg praz./kg for 3 consecutive days Puppies, kittens: 15 mg feb. and 1.5 mg praz./kg for 3 consecutive days	Can administer to adults by mouth or in food without regard to feeding schedule Administer only by mouth on full stomach to pups and kittens (<6 mos)
Vermiplex	Toluene and dichlorophene (Pitman-Moore)	82%	90%	—	72% T* 85% D*	—	Size capsule as directed by manufacturer	Incoordination, emesis, muscular tremors when overdosed
Yomesan	Niclosamide (Chemagro)	—	—	—	80% T* 18–56% D*	—	100–157 mg/kg PO	Heavy mucus interferes with elimination of scolex

*Percentages in "Tapeworms" column refer to percentage of dogs cleared of infection; all others refer to percentage of nematodes expelled. T = *Taenia* sp.; D = *Dipylidium caninum; E* = *Echinococcus* sp.

†Retreatment is usually advisable to kill mature worms that were immature larvae during earlier treatments; re-treatment schedule: (1) hookworms—for litter from a bitch that previously lost pups from hookworm anemia, treat weekly for 5–6 weeks, beginning at 1 week of age; others—retreat in 2 weeks; (2) ascarids (especially *Toxocara*)—for pups or kittens with heavy ascarid infection, treat every other week for three or four treatments, beginning at 2 weeks of age; for mature animals; re-treatment is not usually necessary; (3) whipworms—for severe infections, re-treat in 1–2 weeks; recheck at 3-month intervals; (4) tapeworms—re-treatment is not necessary unless reinfection occurs; and (5) *Strongyloides*—repeated treatment monthly if needed.

In addition to drugs used to treat the adult stage of canine intestinal parasites (Table 2), the FDA-approved heartworm preventive drug, diethylcarbamazine (DEC), when given at a continuous daily dosage of 6.6 mg/kg, is effective not only in preventing the establishment of ascarid infections but also in eliminating approximately 80 per cent of patent ascarid adults. Combination drugs containing DEC and styrylpyridinium chloride (Styrid-Caricide, American Cyanamid) or oxibendazole (Filaribits Plus, Norden) provide protection also against the establishment of hookworm infections in dogs. At continuous low daily dosages, the latter drugs are not known, however, to eliminate existing burdens of adult hookworms. Specific treatment to expel the adult worms is recommended before starting the daily preventive regimen.

BIOCHEMICAL EVALUATION OF HEPATIC FUNCTION IN THE DOG AND CAT

SHARON A. CENTER, D.V.M.
Ithaca, New York

Biochemical screening profiles and liver function tests useful in small animal practice have received increasing attention in the past decade. Tests customarily used include activities of serum enzymes of liver origin and the measurement of serum and urine concentrations of other substances synthesized, regulated, or excreted by the liver. The results of the serum and urine tests collectively provide evidence of hepatic synthetic and excretory functions, the integrity of hepatocellular and biliary plasma membranes, and exposure to microsomal enzyme-inducing substances. This article concentrates on the biochemical indicators of hepatobiliary disorders that are useful to the small animal clinician. Differences in test sensitivities, pitfalls in test interpretation, and expected test abnormalities in different hepatobiliary disorders are discussed.

LIVER ENZYMES

Abnormalities in serum activities of liver enzymes are commonly encountered in small animal practice. Although they are considered sensitive indicators of hepatobiliary disturbances, they lack specificity as to the nature or severity of the disorder. Increases in serum enzyme activities may be due to reversible or irreversible alterations in cell membrane permeability, microsomal enzyme induction, or to structural injury associated with hepatocellular ischemia, necrosis, or cholestasis. Various pathologic processes involving the liver can cause proportionately different increases in liver enzymes owing to variation in the distribution of each particular enzyme within the hepatic lobule. Severe liver disease can exist in the absence of significant increases in serum enzyme activity. Use of serum enzyme activities as prognostic indicators of the severity of liver disease cannot be recommended.

ALANINE AMINOTRANSFERASE AND ASPARTATE AMINOTRANSFERASE

The hepatic transaminase alanine aminotransferase (ALT, formerly SGPT) is regarded as a liver-specific enzyme in the dog and cat. The highest cellular concentrations of ALT are located in the cytosol. Following severe, acute, diffuse hepatocellular necrosis, serum ALT values sharply increase up to 20- to 40-fold normal and sometimes higher. If the injurious agent or disorder quickly resolves, serum ALT values decline to normal values within 1 to 3 weeks. A persistent increase in ALT activity suggests continued hepatocellular enzyme liberation, since the serum half-life is less than 24 hours.

Extrahepatic bile duct obstruction is associated with increased ALT of lesser initial magnitude than that associated with acute necrosis. Within 1 week of complete duct obstruction, levels of ALT may increase 40 to 80 times normal in dogs, and to values 15 to 40 times normal in cats.

In dogs, microsomal enzyme inducers such as anticonvulsant drugs and glucocorticoids cause smaller increases in ALT activity than those typical of necrosis or bile duct obstruction. The administration of glucocorticoids to dogs often results in ALT values 3 to 5 times normal within 1 week, and up to 10 times normal within 30 days.

Increases in ALT from 3 to 30 times normal have been observed in dogs with hepatocellular carcinoma. Metastatic hepatic neoplasia may be associated with slight to moderate increases in serum ALT in dogs and in cats.

In cats, ALT values are increased from 2 to 40 times normal in cholangitis, cholangiohepatitis, or hepatitis. Two to 10-fold increases occur in idiopathic feline lipidosis, and values 2 to 5 times normal occur in severe acute anemia, septicemia, and in feline leukemia virus–associated diseases (lymphosarcoma, myeloproliferative disease).

Aspartate aminotransferase (AST, formerly SGOT) is present in substantial quantities in many tissues and therefore is not liver specific in dogs or cats. Increased serum AST values in the absence of abnormal ALT activity indicate an extrahepatic enzyme origin. Hepatic AST is located in the cytosol and also is associated with mitochondria. Highest serum values of AST are associated with hepatic necrosis and inflammation. In cats, AST may be a more sensitive indicator of hepatobiliary disorders than it is in dogs, but this is controversial. Serum values of AST have been more markedly increased than ALT values in some cats with cholangiohepatitis, myeloproliferative disease, hepatic lymphosarcoma, and chronic bile duct obstruction.

ALKALINE PHOSPHATASE

Alkaline phosphatase (ALP) is a membrane-bound enzyme present in many tissues. Only four serum isoenzymes are identifiable in dogs, including bone, liver, corticosteroid-induced, and one of unknown origin and significance. Hepatic origin of the corticosteroid isoenzyme has been proved. In cats, liver and bone ALP isoenzymes are detectable in serum. The serum ALP half-life in cats is very short as compared with that of the dog, and this, in conjunction with the much smaller hepatic ALP content in cats than in dogs, explains the subtle ALP increases that develop in cholestatic disorders in the cat. There is no corticosteroid ALP isoenzyme detectable in cats and there is only limited information regarding ALP induction in this species.

The ALP bone isoenzyme increases during osteoblast activity, and therefore serum activity may be increased in young growing animals, animals with primary bone tumors, and in secondary renal hyperparathyroidism. The increase in the bone isoenzyme is minor (2- to 3-fold) compared with increases possible with liver or corticosteroid ALP isoenzymes in dogs. In cats, however, the serum activity of the bone isoenzyme may simulate those ALP increases associated with hepatobiliary disease.

The hepatic isoenzyme of ALP may increase as a result of primary or secondary hepatocellular disorders, or, in dogs, as the direct result of hepatic ALP synthesis induced by drug treatment. In acute hepatocellular necrosis, serum ALT values typically are markedly increased; in contrast, ALP is not, since it is not readily released. Largest ALP increases are associated with diffuse or focal cholestatic disorders, primary hepatic neoplasms, and, in dogs, with drug induction. In general, serum ALP values increase as a result of increased hepatic enzyme synthesis rather than immediate cellular release.

Following acute hepatic necrosis, ALP values increase 2 to 5 times normal in dogs and as much as 3 times those in cats and then gradually decline over 2 to 3 weeks. Extrahepatic bile duct obstruction in dogs results in ALP values that reach 30 times normal in 2 days and as much as a 100-fold increase within 1 to 2 weeks. In cats, ALP values following extrahepatic bile duct obstruction show a 2-fold increase within 2 days and as much as a 6-fold increase within 2 weeks. Serum ALP values stabilize and then gradually decline in prolonged obstruction.

Any hepatic parenchymal inflammation may cause secondary hepatocellular changes leading to intrahepatic cholestasis. Any involvement of biliary structures results in increased ALP values, largely as a result of increased synthesis, although regurgitation of enzyme into the serum is also contributory. It is probable that bile salts that locally increase in cholestasis alter the permeability of cellular membranes and thereby facilitate the release of newly synthesized ALP. Increases in ALP activity owing to secondary hepatic changes appear to be especially common in dogs and result in ALP values up to 5 times normal.

A unique ALP isoenzyme develops in dogs affected with hyperadrenocorticism and in dogs treated with glucocorticoids. Serum enzyme values show 10- to 30-fold and as great as 100-fold increases in dogs treated with glucocorticoids. The electrophoretic separation of ALP isoenzymes only infrequently provides information of diagnostic importance in the small animal patient. On occasion, however, an increased corticosteroid ALP has been the only strong indication of hyperadrenocorticism on screening tests in some canine patients. The production of the glucocorticoid isoenzyme does not mean that a dog treated with glucocorticoids has hyperadrenocorticism, a suppressed pituitary adrenal axis, or a glucocorticoid hepatopathy. This isoenzyme may also increase in some chronically ill dogs. Liver biopsy in some chronically ill dogs has shown a glucocorticoid-like (vacuolar) hepatopathy in spite of the absence of glucocorticoid treatment or spontaneous hyperadrenocorticism.

The liver ALP isoenzyme induced by anticonvulsant medications often increases 2 to 6 times normal. With combination treatments of primidone and phenytoin, ALP may be increased to 12 times normal, and with high-dose phenobarbital, 40-fold increases have been observed. Increases of ALP up to 100 times normal have been identified in dogs with hepatocellular carcinoma.

GAMMA GLUTAMYL TRANSFERASE

Gamma glutamyl transferase (gamma glutamyl transpeptidase, GGT) is a membrane-bound enzyme with highest tissue activity in the dog and cat in the kidney and pancreas, with lesser amounts in the liver, spleen, heart, and lungs. The renal and pancreatic isoenzymes contribute negligible serum GGT activity. Hepatic GGT is located in the plasma membrane of hepatocytes, in bile canaliculi, and in luminal borders of bile duct epithelium. The GGT of hepatic origin is primarily responsible for the serum GGT increases observed in dogs and cats.

Serum GGT activity increases as a result of intrahepatic or extrahepatic cholestasis and pancreatitis in dogs and cats. In dogs, increases in serum GGT typically are associated with increases in ALP. Corticosteroid and microsomal enzyme–inducing drugs stimulate GGT production similar to what occurs with ALP. Values of GGT may be more markedly increased in some cats with certain hepatic disorders than are ALP values. Some cats with cirrhosis, major bile duct obstruction, or intrahepatic cholestasis have been observed to have larger increases in GGT than in ALP.

Serum GGT activity has increased 10 times greater than normal or higher in some dogs with hepatocellular carcinoma. In humans with hepatocellular carcinoma, increased serum GGT values are associated with increased GGT activity originating within the hepatic tumor. This is suspected but has not been proved in dogs. The major clinical value of GGT in humans is in the evidence it provides regarding tissue specificity of increased ALP, since increased GGT activity is absent when bone origin ALP increases exist. A similar application seems appropriate for dogs and cats.

MISCELLANEOUS CAUSES OF INCREASED SERUM LIVER ENZYME ACTIVITY

Miscellaneous conditions associated with increased serum liver enzyme activity are numerous in dogs and cats. Disorders associated with endotoxemia, septicemia, anoxia, hyperthermia, thromboembolism, alterations in hepatic perfusion, and microsomal enzyme induction may be associated with increased values of ALT, AST, ALP, and GGT. In most instances, magnitudes of enzyme increase do not exceed 2 to 3 times normal and are usually much smaller. Hyperthyroidism in cats is typically characterized by increases in serum liver enzyme values, particularly serum alkaline phosphatase (SAP) but also ALT and AST. Liver function testing in these animals has not indicated significant hepatobiliary dysfunction. The origin of the ALP activity in hyperthyroidism has not been substantiated. It is speculated that it may be the bone isoenzyme, as reported in humans with hyperthyroidism, owing to bone mobilization and osteoblast activity. Serum GGT activity is usually normal in hyperthyroid cats.

The anticonvulsant drugs primidone and phenytoin are associated with variable increases in liver enzyme activity. Although only a small number of dogs on anticonvulsants develop drug-associated liver disease, caution is warranted in disregarding abnormal values as nonsignificant. Liver function tests are essential in differentiating dogs with hepatic dysfunction from those with anticonvulsant-induced liver enzyme activity. Primidone is more consistently associated with increased serum liver enzyme activity than is phenytoin, perhaps owing to the ultrashort half-life of phenytoin in dogs. Combination therapy with primidone and phenytoin or primidone and phenobarbital more consistently induces enzyme activity and to larger magnitudes than does primidone alone. Transaminase values increase moderately, up to 2-fold, with each drug used alone. There exists a significant linear association between primidone dose and the magnitude of the serum ALT increase. Combination anticonvulsant therapy may induce transaminase values that are 3 to 5 times normal. Serum ALP appears to be more remarkably and consistently increased by anticonvulsants than are the transaminases. Values up to 4 times normal are common with primidone and combination therapy, and up to 2 times normal values occur with phenytoin alone. Values up to 40 times normal occasionally develop with primidone or combination therapy in the absence of substantial liver disease. There is a significant linear relationship between the dose and magnitude of ALP with either primidone or phenytoin. The GGT activity is infrequently altered in dogs receiving phenytoin, but values up to 2 times normal are common with primidone and combination treatment.

ARGINASE

Arginase is a major enzyme in the urea cycle, and large quantities are present in the cytosol of the hepatocyte. This enzyme is considered to be liver specific in dogs and cats. It has been used to differentiate acute necrosis from continuing necrosis because of its very short serum half-life. Accordingly, continued increases in serum arginase values suggest progressive hepatocellular necrosis.

PLASMA PROTEINS

Albumin is the major plasma protein synthesized in the liver, and it is principally responsible for the plasma colloid osmotic pressure. The normal half-life of serum albumin in dogs is approximately 23 days, but this may be extended by decreased catabolism during periods of hypoalbuminemia. The normal liver has a tremendous reserve capacity for albumin synthesis. Insufficient albumin synthesis occurs in hepatic failure (70 to 80 per cent reduction in functional hepatic mass) or severe protein malnutrition. Marked hypoalbuminemia is a characteristic of chronic, severe hepatocellular insufficiency owing to the prolonged half-life of serum albumin. Other causes of hypoalbuminemia, including losses incurred through cutaneous, gastrointestinal, or urinary routes, severe malabsorption, or iatrogenic hypoalbuminemia following overzealous fluid therapy, must be considered before failure of hepatic synthesis is assumed. Hypoalbuminemia ranging from 1.5 to 2.5 gm/dl may develop secondary to albumin accumulation within the peritoneal space unassociated with liver disease. In this circumstance, total body albumin is unchanged, but its volume of distribution is increased, resulting in a diminution of the serum albumin value.

Albumin is essential as an intravascular transport vehicle for various endogenous and exogenous substances. Clinical signs associated with altered sensitivities to therapeutic agents and endogenous substances may therefore occur in conjunction with hypoalbuminemia, owing to changes in serum protein binding.

The extent of hypoalbuminemia may be obscured by concomitant dehydration or hyperglobulinemia. Plasma protein fractionation should therefore be obtained to reveal the actual albumin concentration. Albumin values of less than 2.0 gm/dl are variably associated with anasarca, ascites, pleural effusion, or localized peripheral edema. Postural impingement of venous and lymphatic drainage increases the intravascular hydrostatic pressure and potentiates extravascular fluid accumulation. The formation of peripheral edema is a problem that develops in hypoalbuminemic patients allowed only limited exercise and confined to a cage.

Most of the serum globulins are synthesized in the liver, with the exception of the immunoglobulins. Globulin values may be normal to increased in generalized hepatic parenchymal disease, hepatic failure, or portosystemic vascular anastomosis. Systemic antigenic challenge develops whenever the hepatic reticuloendothelial system is bypassed or is otherwise dysfunctional. In this circumstance, increased serum globulins represent immunoglobulin production in response to systemic antigenic stimulation from antigenemia of enteric origin. Immunocompetent cells in the spleen, lymph nodes, and elsewhere are believed to be the origin of the increased serum globulins. Compensatory increases in serum globulins also occur in the presence of severe hypoalbuminemia as a homeostatic regulatory mechanism adjusting the intravascular colloid osmotic pressure. Although interesting, evaluation of serum proteins by electrophoresis provides limited practical information for the differential diagnosis of liver disease in the small animal patient.

BLOOD UREA NITROGEN

Urea is synthesized in the liver as the major metabolic end product of ammonia detoxification. Decreased urea production occurs in acquired hepatic failure, portosystemic vascular anastomosis, and rarely, in urea cycle enzyme deficiencies. Although compatible with hepatic insufficiency, decreased blood urea nitrogen (BUN) values may be the result of fluid diuresis or reduction in protein intake. Caution should be exercised in the use of a decreased BUN as an indicator of impaired hepatobiliary function.

Since urea excretion depends on glomerular filtration, reduced renal function in conjunction with decreased hepatic urea production can complicate the interpretation of BUN values. In this circumstance, serum creatinine provides a more reliable measure of renal function.

AMMONIA

Ammonia is a major waste product of protein catabolism. It is produced primarily by microbial degradation of endogenous urea and dietary amines within the intestinal tract. Ammonia is detoxified primarily in the liver by conversion to urea, and normally the liver has a large reserve capacity for this process. The ability of the liver to regulate blood ammonia concentrations reflects the integrity of the hepatic portal circulation as well as the functional hepatic mass.

Blood ammonia has been used as a direct indicator of hepatic failure in dogs and in cats with hepatic encephalopathy. Animals with portosystemic venous anastomosis or acquired hepatocellular insufficiency demonstrate hyperammonemia inconsistently following a prolonged fast or after meals. Hyperammonemia is more consistent in these patients following the oral administration of ammonium chloride. The ammonia tolerance test (ATT) is a provocative test of hepatic ammonia detoxification. Following a 12-hour fast, a dose of 0.1 gm/kg of ammonium chloride (not to exceed 3 gm total dose) is given by mouth or stomach tube. Dilute solutions (no more than 20 mg/ml ammonium chloride) are recommended because hypertonic solutions may induce vomiting. Blood is collected into a heparinized Vacutainer before and 30 minutes after the administration of ammonium chloride and is stored on ice until the plasma is separated. If laboratory determinations cannot be immediately completed, the separated plasma may be frozen at −20°C for 24 hours without causing alterations in the ammonia values. The metabolic generation of ammonia in improperly managed whole blood can invalidate the blood ammonia test. It is therefore wise to collect a control sample from a fasted, healthy animal to provide evidence of appropriate sample management. Many clinical laboratories provide blood ammonia analysis. Unfortunately, because ammonia is so labile, coordination of clinical testing and laboratory analysis is essential. Although this test is a sensitive and specific indicator of hepatic insufficiency and abnormal hepatoportal circulation, it is inconvenient in many clinical settings. Furthermore, normal values vary considerably between laboratories, necessitating careful documentation of normal ranges for each clinical situation. The administration of ammonium chloride to clinical patients with hepatic insufficiency produces relatively few adverse effects, perhaps because many other toxins are involved in the generation of the encephalopathic signs.

Blood ammonia concentrations remain unchanged or increase up to twice those of fasting values in healthy animals 30 minutes after the oral administration of ammonium chloride. Comparatively, blood ammonia concentrations following ATT in animals with portosystemic shunts or acquired hepatic insufficiency increase from normal to elevated fasting values (2- to 10-fold increase), to concentrations ranging from 3 to 10 times greater than ATT values in normal animals. The magnitude of ammonia increase following the ATT in animals with hepatic insufficiency or portosystemic shunts ranges between 1.5 and 10 times greater than their baseline values. The magnitude of ammonia increase in a particular patient is less diagnostically useful than comparison with the normal range.

Animals with hyperammonemia frequently develop ammonium biurate or urate crystalluria. Recurrent ammonium biurate crystalluria may result in the formation of urate calculi. It is important to remember that normal Dalmatians may also have urate crystalluria and consequentially urate calculi in the absence of hepatocellular functional insufficiency.

COAGULATION FACTORS

The liver is essential for maintenance of normal coagulation homeostasis. It is the major site of synthesis for many of the plasma procoagulants including Factors I (fibrinogen), II (prothrombin), V, VII, IX, and X. It is probable that the liver is the origin of the remaining plasma coagulation factors, with the exceptions of Factor VIII and calcium. The prothrombin coagulant Factors II, VII, IX, and X are dependent on vitamin K for activation and are thus influenced by bile duct obstruction or other disorders causing fat malabsorption. The liver is also a major source of synthesis of other regulators of coagulation, including plasminogen, the precursor of the fibrinolytic protease plasmin, and antithrombin III. The liver provides additional coagulation regulatory functions in the removal of activated coagulation factors and fibrin degradation products (FDPs) from the circulation.

Tests evaluating coagulation factors (prothrombin time [PT], activated coagulation time [ACT], and activated partial thromboplastin time [APTT]), provide a measure of hepatic function. The prothrombin time evaluates the extrinsic coagulation system, whereas the ACT and APTT evaluate the intrinsic coagulation system. Each test will reflect abnormalities in the common pathway. During synthetic failure, the extent of factor deficiency is determined by factor utilization and factor half-life. The factor half-lives vary from hours to days; the shortest-lived factor is VII, having a half-life of 7 hours. Factor consumption can exceed the rate of factor synthesis, even in the presence of a normal liver, and coagulation tests quickly reflect this balance.

Although the PT and APTT are sensitive indicators of hepatic dysfunction, they are not practically useful in the differential diagnosis of liver disease. The exception is in cholestatic disease owing to extrahepatic bile duct obstruction in which vitamin K responsiveness can be shown. Typically, the PT is prolonged but the APTT and ACT may also be abnormal. Following the administration of 5 to 15 mg of active vitamin K (K_1, AquaMEPHYTON, Merck Sharp & Dohme), correction of the PT prolongation by greater than 30 per cent is expected within 24 hours. Vitamin K deficiency develops following bile duct obstruction from the fat malabsorption, owing to the absence of intestinal bile acids. Although the liver normally stores large amounts of vitamin K, these stores are quickly depleted without continued replenishment. Large doses of vitamin K may improve coagulation abnormalities in patients with severe diffuse liver disease, but correction of abnormal coagulation is less dramatic than that observed in major cholestasis.

Laboratory demonstration of PT or APTT prolongation occurs when one or more of the involved coagulants are reduced below 30 per cent. The sensitivity of these tests can be improved by using dilutions of the patient's citrated platelet-poor plasma. Quantitative or semiquantitative assays can be performed for each clotting factor. Estimation of specific factor activity has been shown to have discriminant value in the differential diagnosis of hepatobiliary disease, but such measurements are neither practical nor expediently accomplished in most clinical settings.

Coagulation abnormalities in liver disease may be complicated by thrombocytopenia owing to splenic sequestration, increased platelet destruction, or decreased platelet production and survival. Qualitative platelet defects may also develop. Often the pathogenesis of hemorrhage in liver disease remains obscure, since decreased factor synthesis, increased factor consumption, excessive fibrinolysis, thrombocytopenia, and thrombasthenias may coexist in various combinations.

It is important that coagulation function be assessed prior to hepatic biopsy. The PT, APTT or ACT, fibrinogen, and platelet count should be evaluated. Deficiencies should be corrected using fresh whole blood or plasma transfusions, as appropriate. It is wise to remember that marked factor deficiency (but not less than 30 per cent) may occur in the presence of normal coagulation tests. Fresh whole blood or plasma should therefore be an anticipated need of any animal with liver disease undergoing biopsy, despite the results of coagulation profiles. Blood should not be indiscriminately administered to patients with hepatic insufficiency. Blood stored for prolonged intervals should be avoided, as it may contain large amounts of ammonia, which along with other proteinaceous substances may invoke an encephalopathic crisis.

GLUCOSE

Blood glucose values are insensitive indicators of hepatobiliary disease, since less than 30 per cent of the liver is sufficient to maintain euglycemia. Acute toxic and ischemic insults or infections can cause diffuse hepatic injury capable of disrupting normal hepatic glucose regulation. After complete hepatectomy, dogs develop hypoglycemia within hours, prior to other evidences of hepatic insufficiency.

There appear to be diminished hepatic glucose production, decreased hepatic glycogen stores, and decreased responsiveness to glucagon in animals with portosystemic vascular anastomosis. The reduced hepatic glycogen stores have been attributed to the absence of normal high insulin concentration in the hepatic portal circulation. In some dogs and cats with portal vein anomalies, hypoglycemia has been recognized as a clinical problem. Deficient delivery of insulin to the liver resulting in decreased insulin degradation may also be an important factor in the development of hypoglycemia in these patients. Hypoglycemia should be anticipated as a problem in any patient with hepatic insufficiency that is undergoing a prolonged fast or anesthetic or surgical procedures. Intravenous dextrose supplementation is advised in such patients.

CHOLESTEROL

Serum cholesterol is regulated in normal dogs by dietary intake, by the rate of hepatic synthesis, and by biliary excretion. The bile acids are synthesized from cholesterol, and this represents the primary pathway for cholesterol degradation. Several metabolic disorders and major organ system dysfunctions may be associated with substantially increased or decreased serum cholesterol values (see Table 1).

Acute cholestatic disorders may be associated with increased serum cholesterol concentrations up to 2 or 3 times normal. An increase in hepatic synthesis of cholesterol and a decrease in the incorporation into bile acids are principally responsible for this hypercholesterolemia. In extrahepatic cholestasis, cholesterol values may decrease to the normal range or become mildly reduced after 1 to 2 weeks. Serum cholesterol values may become markedly reduced in hepatic failure, and this indicates a grave prognosis. The ratio of esterified to nonesterified cholesterol has not yet been shown to be diagnostically beneficial in dogs or cats.

Spur cell anemia has been observed in humans and in dogs with hypercholesterolemia associated with cholestatic liver disease. It is speculated that abnormal erythrocyte membrane lipids or abnormal serum lipids are responsible for the formation of these acanthocytes.

BILIRUBIN

Bilirubin is synthesized during hemoprotein degradation. Most of the heme pigments metabolized to bilirubin in reticuloendothelial cells are derived from senescent erythrocytes (80 to 90 per cent), and smaller amounts are derived from other heme moieties (e.g., myoglobin and cytochromes). Free bilirubin is taken up by the liver and conjugated with glucuronide in a complex series of steps and is then excreted in the bile. Within the intestinal tract, bilirubin undergoes degradation to urobilins (urobilinogen), which may undergo enterohepatic circulation and provide evidence of bile duct patency.

The total serum bilirubin is composed of unconjugated and conjugated moieties. Unconjugated bilirubin is avidly bound to albumin in the circulation, is insoluble in water, and is not excreted by glomerular filtration. It does not react directly with the Ehrlich diazo reagent used for bilirubin esti-

Table 1. Biochemical Indicators of Liver Disease

	Basis for Test	Sensitivity*	Specificity*	Liver Diseases Associated With Abnormal Test Values†	Causes for Abnormal Test Values in the Absence of Clinically Significant Liver Disease‡
Liver Enzyme					
Alanine aminotransferase (ALT)	Large amounts in hepatocyte; increased release following reversible or irreversible membrane injury or microsomal enzyme induction	+ + + + (↑ ALT)	+ +	Necrosis: mild to moderate (2–10×); severe diffuse (20–40×); cholestasis (up to 80× dog, 40× cat); hepatic neoplasia (2–30×); cirrhosis (N–100×); inflammation (2–40×); idiopathic feline lipidosis (2–10×)	In the dog, microsomal enzyme induction; primidone (up to 4× or higher); phenobarbital (4–6× or higher); phenytoin (up to 4×); glucocorticoids (3–10×); thiacetarsamide (2–10×); feline hyperthyroidism (N–2×)
Aspartate aminotransferase (AST)	Large amounts in hepatocyte; increased release following reversible or irreversible membrane injury or microsomal enzyme induction	+ + (↑ AST)	+ +	Severe diffuse necrosis (up to 40× dog, 16× cat); cirrhosis (N–10×); cholestasis (2–40×); larger magnitude of increase in AST than in ALT in some cats with cholangiohepatitis, lymphosarcoma, and myeloproliferative disease (2–20×); hepatic lipidosis (2–10×); and extrahepatic bile duct obstruction (10–20×)	Substantial AST in other tissues: skeletal and cardiac muscles; in the dog, microsomal enzyme induction: phenobarbital (2×); primidone (2×); feline hyperthyroidism (N–2×)
Serum alkaline phosphatase (SAP)	Bound to membranes of bile canaliculi and bile ducts; values increase owing to increased synthesis, regurgitation from biliary system into serum and microsomal enzyme induction	+ + + (↑ SAP)	+	Severe necrosis (2–5×); cholestasis (dog 30–100×, cat 2–6×); secondary cholestatic disorders (dog 2–5×, cat N–2×); steroid hepatopathy (dog 2–100×); primary hepatic or biliary cancer (dog up to 100×)	Increase in SAP owing to various isoenzymes; bone (2–3×); microsomal enzyme induction in dogs: primidone (3–6×); phenobarbital (3–5× up to 40×); phenytoin (3–6×); glucocorticoid isoenzyme (10–30× up to 100×); feline hyperthyroidism (2× up to 12×)
Gamma glutamyl transferase (GGT)	Bound to membranes of bile canaliculi and bile ducts; values increase owing to increased synthesis, regurgitation from biliary system into serum; and microsomal enzyme induction	+ + (↑ GGT)	+ +	Severe necrosis (2–3×); cholestasis (dog 5–30×, cat 2–15×); steroid hepatopathy (dog 7–10×); primary hepatic or biliary cancer (dog 2–10×); larger magnitude of increased GGT than in SAP in some cats with cirrhosis or cholestasis	Microsomal enzyme induction in dogs: primidone (N–2×); glucocorticoids (2–10×); feline hyperthyroidism (usually N but up to 5×)
Arginase	Major urea cycle enzyme present in large amounts within hepatocytes; increased after severe hepatocellular membrane injury	+ (↑ arginase)	+ + + +	Severe diffuse active necrosis (increased 1000×); major bile duct obstruction (increased 2×)	Unknown
Synthetic Function					
Albumin	Synthesized only in the liver; large reserve synthetic capacity	+ (↓ albumin)	+	Decreased synthesis with severe, diffuse hepatic insufficiency; (≥ 70% compromised function); cirrhosis, portosystemic vascular anomaly, severe diffuse necrosis	Other conditions associated with hypoalbuminemia: protein-losing nephropathy, protein-losing enteropathy, severe chronic blood loss, cutaneous losses (burns); decreased synthesis in severe protein malnutrition
Globulins	Synthesized in liver and other organs containing immunocomponent cells (i.e., lymph nodes, bone marrow)	+ (↑ globulins)	+ +	Increased values in inflammatory liver disease or when hepatic RE system is compromised	Any systemic or focal inflammatory condition may increase globulins
Fibrinogen	Synthesized only in liver; large reserve synthetic capacity; is an acute phase reactant	+ (↑ or ↓ fibrinogen)	+ +	Decreased synthesis with severe, diffuse hepatic insufficiency; may increase in inflammatory or cholestatic liver disorders	Any systemic inflammatory condition may increase fibrinogen; accelerated fibrinogen consumption (DIC) or fibrinolysis may decrease fibrinogen

Coagulation factors	Most coagulation factors are synthesized in liver; Factors II, VII, IX, X are vitamin K dependent	+ +	+ + (↑ PT, ↑ APTT)	Decreased factor synthesis causing increase in PT and APTT with severe hepatic insufficiency; increase in PT and/or APTT with vitamin K malabsorption in bile duct obstruction	Increase in PT and/or APTT (ACT): accelerated factor consumption (DIC), congenital factor deficiency, warfarin toxicity, anticoagulant therapy
Urea	Synthesis from ammonia in the liver	+	+ (↓ BUN)	Decreased synthesis with severe hepatic insufficiency (≥70% compromised function): cirrhosis, diffuse necrosis, portosystemic vascular anomaly	Decreased BUN: fluid diuresis, anabolic steroids, low-protein diets, normal animals
Cholesterol	Hepatic synthesis inversely proportional to dietary intake; hepatobiliary excretion	+ + + +	+ + + (↓ cholesterol) + + + (↑ cholesterol)	Decreased synthesis with severe hepatic insufficiency Increased synthesis and decreased excretion with acute bile duct obstruction	Cholesterol increased (2–4×): pancreatitis, diabetes mellitus, hyperadrenocorticism, nephrotic syndrome, hypothyroidism, postprandial periods, idiopathic hyperlipidemia (beagles, schnauzers); decreased cholesterol: intestinal lymphangiectasia
Metabolic and Excretory Functions					
Glucose	Blood glucose regulation; glycogenolysis and other hormones regulating blood glucose	+	+ (↓ glucose)	Decreased gluconeogenesis and abnormal glucagon responsiveness in severe hepatic insufficiency, cirrhosis, diffuse necrosis, portosystemic vascular anomaly	Hypoglycemia: pancreatic beta cell tumor, nonpancreatic neoplasia, hunting dog collapse, glycogen storage disease, iatrogenic (insulin therapy), septic stock, pregnancy, starvation, and neonatal distress
Ammonia	Urea cycle ammonia detoxification in the liver; a large reserve capacity	+ +	+ + + + (↑ ammonia)	Decreased NH_3 regulation in severe hepatic insufficiency (≥70% compromised function): cirrhosis, diffuse necrosis, portosystem vascular anomaly, and rarely in urea cycle enzyme deficiencies	Increased NH_3: increase in NH_3 or amine ingestion; gastrointestinal hemorrhage, transfusion of stored blood
Total bilirubin	Synthesis from heme pigments; glucuronide conjugation, storage and biliary excretion determine serum values	+ +	+ + + (↑ bilirubin)	Decreased uptake, decreases in conjugation or biliary excretion in severe diffuse liver disease or cholestasis	Increased heme pigment release: accelerated erythrocyte destruction, hemolytic anemia, post-transfusion
Sulfobromophthalein (BSP)	Hepatic perfusion, uptake, storage, glutathione conjugation, and biliary secretion influence plasma dye disappearance	+ +	+ + + (↓ clearance)	Decreased clearance with decreases in perfusion, conjugation, and biliary excretion: diffuse parenchymal disease, portosystemic vascular anomaly, or cholestasis	Decreased BSP clearance: systemic circulatory impairment, hypotension, competitive clearance delay caused by hyperbilirubinemia; increased clearance with hypoalbuminemia; invalid per cent retention with inappropriate dose: failure to adjust dose to lean body weight
Indocyanine green (ICG)	Hepatic perfusion, uptake, storage, and biliary secretion influence plasma dye disappearance	+ +	+ + + (↓ clearance)	Decreased clearance with decrease in hepatic perfusion, decreased biliary excretion: diffuse parenchymal disease; portosystemic vascular anomaly; or cholestasis	Decreased ICG clearance: systemic circulatory impairment, hypotension, competitive clearance delay caused by hyperbilirubinemia; increased clearance with hypoalbuminemia; invalid per cent retention with inappropriate dose: failure to adjust dose to lean body weight
Bile acids	Hepatic perfusion, uptake, storage, biliary excretion and efficiency of enterohepatic circulation determine serum values	+ +	+ + + + (↑ serum bile acids)	Decreased clearance with decrease in hepatic perfusion, diffuse parenchymal disease or cholestasis	Increased bile acids: improper sampling interval (too soon after test meal: 2 hours is the optimal postprandial interval); decreased bile acids following a prolonged fast longer than 12 hours, too late after test meal, ileal disease

*Increasing number of plus signs (+) denotes increasing sensitivity or specificity.
†Numbers in parentheses denote increases over normal values; N indicates no change.

mation but requires the addition of alcohol for the coupling reaction. Increased values indicate increased heme pigment release or delayed hepatic bilirubin uptake, storage, or conjugation. Acute hemolytic disorders are principally responsible for unconjugated hyperbilirubinemia in dogs and cats.

Conjugated bilirubin is less avidly bound to protein than is unconjugated bilirubin, is water soluble, and can be excreted by glomerular filtration. It reacts with the diazo reagent directly. Conjugated hyperbilirubinemia indicates hepatic parenchymal or cholestatic disorders or increased hemoprotein degradation. Conjugated hyperbilirubinemia is the principal form of hyperbilirubinemia associated with jaundice in dogs and cats, and it rapidly develops after an acute hemolytic crisis. The differentiation of relative quantities of unconjugated and conjugated bilirubin provides little information of practical clinical importance that is not already apparent from hematologic, physical, and other biochemical examinations.

Although less sensitive than the serum activities of liver enzymes in identifying hepatobiliary disorders, bilirubin values interpreted in conjunction with the serum liver enzyme activities improve the specificity of enzymes in the diagnosis of liver disease.

Jaundice develops when bilirubin values exceed 1.5 to 2.0 mg/dl. When liver disease is responsible for jaundice, a severe diffuse disorder or major bile duct obstruction is suspected. When primary cholestatic disorders are responsible for hyperbilirubinemia, jaundice develops earlier in the disease process than with parenchymal disease. Bilirubinuria is present before jaundice becomes apparent and has therefore been acknowledged as a useful screening test, although not specific, for liver disease. Bilirubin is normally present in the urine of dogs, albeit in small amounts. There is evidence that dogs can produce bilirubin from hemoglobin in the renal tubular epithelium. Detection of urine bilirubin in cats is a strong indication of hyperbilirubinemia, since normal cats do not have bilirubinuria. Even trace amounts of bilirubin in concentrated urine are considered to be abnormal in cats. Although the specificity is high, the sensitivity of urine bilirubin for the detection of liver disease in cats is unknown.

The use of the tablet method (Ictotest, Ames) for the detection of bilirubin in urine is more sensitive and reliable than the reagent strip method and is therefore the preferred procedure.

BILE ACIDS

The primary serum bile acids, cholic acid and chenodeoxycholic acid, are synthesized in the liver from cholesterol. The secondary bile acids, deoxycholic acid and lithocholic acid, are produced in the intestines by bacterial dehydroxylation of the primary bile acids. After hepatic conjugation to the amino acid taurine or glycine, bile acids are transported through the biliary system to the gallbladder, where they are concentrated and stored. At mealtime, numerous neurohumoral and hormonal factors induce bile secretion and gallbladder contraction, resulting in the passage of bile acids into the intestines.

In the intestines, the detergent action of bile acids facilitates lipid digestion and absorption. Most of the bile acids are reabsorbed in the ileum by an active transport process and then rapidly extracted by the liver from the portal circulation. In the normal animal, the enterohepatic bile acid circulation is extremely efficient, resulting in the fecal loss of only 2 to 5 per cent of the total circulating pool of bile acids each day. During and after meals, the total pool of bile acids recycles between three and five times, depending on the efficiency of the enterohepatic circulation. After a 12-hour fast and in the presence of normal hepatic perfusion, hepatobiliary and gallbladder function, only small amounts of bile acids are present within the systemic circulation. The normal enterohepatic circulation of bile acids is illustrated in Figure 1. Fasting values of serum bile acids in healthy dogs and cats should not exceed 5.0 μmol/L and 2.0 μmol/L, respectively.

The serum bile acid concentration can be altered by interruption in the enterohepatic circulation at any of several steps. Impaired ileal absorption of bile acids may cause decreased fasting and postprandial serum bile acid values. Otherwise, abnormalities in hepatic uptake, storage, excretion, or hepatic perfusion delay bile acid extraction from serum and result in increased serum values. Endogenous challenge of the regulators naturally occurs during the postprandial interval. A 2-hour postprandial sampling time has been shown to be suitable in humans, dogs, and cats for assessment of the enterohepatic bile acid circulation. Values for healthy dogs and cats 2 hours after feeding should not exceed 15.5 μmol/L and 10.0 μmol/L, respectively.

Animals with substantial hepatic insufficiency such as that resulting from portosystemic venous anomalies and cirrhosis usually have increased fasting serum bile acid values, but they may have normal or only moderately increased values after a prolonged fast. Two-hour postprandial concentrations are markedly increased and clearly differentiate these animals from normal animals (Fig. 2). Patterns typical for some other forms of hepatobiliary disorders are also illustrated in Figure 2.

Although bile acid formation depends on hepatic synthesis, hepatic failure does not limit the serum bile acid concentrations. The liver maintains a tre-

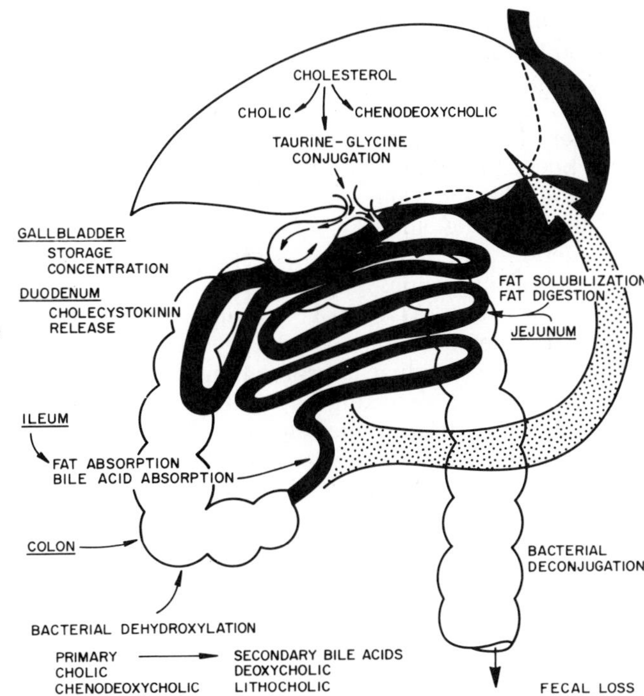

Figure 1. Illustration of the synthesis, enterohepatic circulation, and excretion of bile acids.

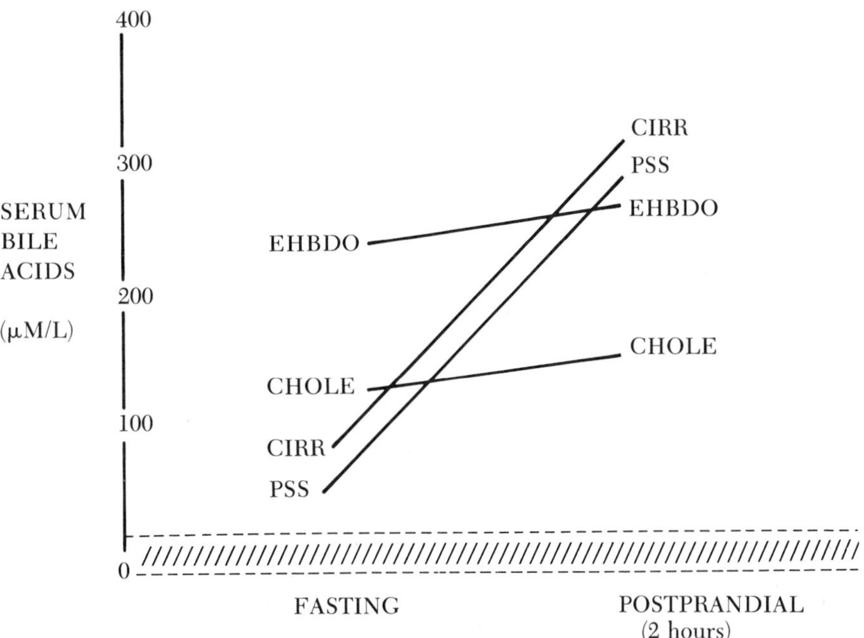

Figure 2. Typical patterns of serum bile acid values in dogs and cats with various hepatobiliary disorders. Values are given for both fasting and 2-hour postprandial conditions; hatched area denotes normal range. Key: EHBDO, extrahepatic bile duct obstruction; CHOLE, intrahepatic cholestasis; CIRR, cirrhosis; PSS, portosystemic venous anastomosis. Values shown are from clinical patients at the New York State College of Veterinary Medicine, 1984.

mendous reserve capacity for bile acid synthesis, and this reserve is never maximally utilized since only very small quantities of bile acids are required for physiologic purposes. Shortcomings of the postprandial test include delays in gastric emptying and gallbladder contraction and variation in the rate of intestinal transit delaying ileal presentation of bile acids for absorption. In addition, ileal disease can cause bile acid malabsorption.

Serum bile acid values have been shown to be very useful in the clinical assessment of hepatobiliary function and, hence, in the diagnosis of liver disease. Fasting values improve the specificity of routine liver tests (ALT, ALP, bilirubin, and albumin) in the detection of hepatobiliary dysfunction. Although the individual interpretation of bile acid values is useful in detecting impairment of hepatobiliary function, these values alone are not reliable in determining a definitive diagnosis. It is suggested that liver biopsy be sought when fasting or postprandial bile acid values consistently exceed 30 μmol/L in the dog and 20μmol/L in the cat.

Serum bile acid values are more sensitive than sulfobromophthalein (BSP) and equivalent in sensitivity to the ATT in the diagnosis of portosystemic venous anastomosis and cirrhosis. The convenience of the bile acid test to the clinician and patient surpasses that of the ATT or organic anion dye retention tests. Bile acids are stable in serum at room temperature for many hours, for months when frozen at 0°C, and for years at −20°C. They can be conveniently mailed to the laboratory for analysis in a nonfrozen condition. Contrasted to the difficulties encountered in obtaining blood ammonia measurements, the serum bile acid test provides a welcome alternative.

Use of postprandial serum bile acid values necessitates standardization of the test meal to eliminate variations in gastric emptying and cholecystokinin-invoked gallbladder contraction. Diets used in the author's clinic consist of commercial canned dog food (Prescription Diet p/d, Hill's Pet Products) and cat foods (Prescription Diet c/d, Hill's Pet Products). In patients in which encephalopathic effects of protein are anticipated, low-protein meals mixed with a small amount of corn oil (1 to 2 tbsp) are recommended to ensure adequate gallbladder contraction and bile release.

The availability of bile acid analysis is currently limited, as this is a new diagnostic test (Gastroenterology Laboratory, New York State College of Veterinary Medicine). Care must be taken that methodologies used have been validated for use with dog and cat sera, especially when radioimmunoassay is employed. Methods directed at the measurement of total serum bile acids are preferable to those measuring specific individual bile acids.

SULFOBROMOPHTHALEIN AND INDOCYANINE GREEN

The cholephilic organic anions sulfobromophthalein (BSP) and indocyanine green (ICG) (Cardio-Green, Hynson, Westcott & Dunning) are water-soluble substances that are bound to proteins in circulation and excreted by the liver into bile. Hepatobiliary excretion of these substances requires a complex series of steps including circulatory transport and delivery to the hepatocyte, uptake into the cell, binding to cytosolic carrier proteins, cytosolic storage, biotransformation (in the case of BSP), passage into the canalicular network, and finally biliary excretion. Abnormalities in any excretory step will alter the plasma dye disappearance. Plasma dye clearance is a sensitive yet nonspecific indicator of hepatobiliary dysfunction and is mainly considered a function of hepatic circulation and metabolism. Protein binding normally restricts dye distribution to within the vascular compartment, more so for ICG than for BSP, which is less avidly protein bound. In the presence of hypoalbuminemia, plasma dye disappearance is accelerated owing to extravascular dye dispersal. Uptake by soft tissue structures, glomerular excretion, and diffusion into edema or ascites may each contribute to accelerated clearance. Test results in the presence of hypoalbuminemia, therefore, warrant careful scrutiny since they underestimate the extent of hepatobiliary dysfunction.

Impairment of 60 to 70 per cent of the functional hepatic mass or cholestasis results in delayed dye clearance. Any disorder causing decreased liver perfusion causes delayed extraction of dye from the circulation (e.g., congestive heart failure, pericardial tamponade, heartworms, hypotension, or severe dehydration).

The use of BSP or ICG as function tests is inappropriate in the presence of hyperbilirubinemia when a diagnosis of liver dysfunction is already apparent. Increased serum bilirubin concentrations (greater than or equal to 3.0 mg/dl) competitively delay BSP or ICG plasma clearance. The principal value of these tests is for the detection of occult liver disease and for the subsequent reassessment of hepatobiliary function once functional impairment has been recognized.

Dye dose adjustments are necessary when marked obesity, edema, or ascites exist, since normal dye retention and clearance values rely on the proportionality of liver mass to body mass. Phenobarbital may accelerate plasma dye clearance by increasing the hepatic uptake and excretion of organic anions. Normal values for BSP and ICG retention tests and the specifics of test performance are given in Table 2.

Table 2. Liver Function Tests

Test	Dose	Route	Procedure	Precautions	Normal Value
Ammonia tolerance test	0.1 gm/kg NH_4Cl (not to exceed 3 gm)	PO	Collect blood (heparinized) following a 12-hour fast Administer NH_4Cl (20 mg/ml solution) Collect blood 30 minutes after NH_4Cl administration	Blood must be stored on ice Improper blood storage results in metabolic generation of ammonia and invalid results Evaluate a control animal concurrent with patient for quality control of sample management Animals may vomit hypertonic NH_4Cl solutions, invalidating test Possible (rare) encephalopathic signs if severe hepatic insufficiency	Must be determined in each laboratory for particular assay used and for each species
Sulfobromophthalein (BSP)	5 mg/kg	IV	Inject BSP Collect blood (heparinized plasma or serum) 30 minutes after BSP injection from a different vein for per cent retention	BSP solution is irritating if injected extravascularly Hypoalbuminemia accelerates dye clearance Dose should be calculated on the basis of lean body weight Improper dose causes invalid results Hyperbilirubinemia competitively delays clearance Extravascular BSP injection precludes further dye studies for 24 hours Systemic allergic reactions possible, but rare	30-minute per cent retention: dog ≤ 5.0% cat ≤ 3.0%
Indocyanine green (ICG)	1.0 mg/kg (dog) 1.5 mg/kg (cat)	IV	Mix freeze-dried ICG with special diluent to make 5 mg/ml solution—*ONLY IMMEDIATELY PRIOR TO USE* Collect a preinjection blood sample (heparinized) Inject ICG Collect blood 30 minutes after ICG injection for per cent retention For clearance study collect blood at 0, 5, 10, and 15 minutes	Hypoalbuminemia accelerates dye clearance Dose should be calculated on the basis of lean body weight Improper dose causes invalid 30 minute % retention Hyperbilirubinemia competitively delays clearance Extravascular ICG injection precludes further dye studies for 24 hours Storage of ICG solution or use of improper diluent results in aggregates that cause embolization	30-minute per cent retention: dog 14.7 ± 5.0 cat 7.3 ± 2.9 Clearance (ml/min/kg): dog 3.7 ± 0.7 cat 8.6 ± 4.1
Bile acids	Endogenous test (test meal)	NA‡	Collect blood following a 12-hour fast (serum) Feed dogs p/d,* cats c/d* to stimulate bile flow and gallbladder contraction Collect blood 2 hours after food ingestion	Delayed gastric emptying or intestinal transit may alter the mechanics of the enterohepatic bile acid circulation (uncommon) Severe ileal disease (malabsorption, resection) decreases mesenteric bile acid resorption resulting in a decreased hepatic bile acid challenge Radioimmunoassays† must be validated for dog and cat sera and normal values determined for each laboratory In animals with hepatic encephalopathy, use diets having a smaller protein content supplemented with corn oil	Fasting values (μM/L): dog ≤ 5.0 cat ≤ 2.0 2-hour postprandial values (μM/L): dog ≤ 15.5 cat ≤ 10.0

*Prescription diet p/d, prescription diet c/d—Hill's Pet Products.
†Procedure validated for dogs and cats = conjugated bile acids solid-phase radioimmunoassay kit ^{125}I, Becton-Dickinson Immunodiagnostics.
‡NA = not applicable.

Recently the availability of BSP has been limited owing to its discontinuation as a test of liver function in humans. Popularity declined following reports of lethal anaphylactoid reactions and of severe perivascular inflammation and cellulitis resulting from inadvertent extravascular dye injection. Similar inflammatory reactions to extravasated BSP occur in dogs and cats. The author has observed an anaphylactoid reaction in one dog following BSP injection that resolved after immediate corticosteroid and epinephrine therapy.

Studies in normal cats suggest that BSP is too rapidly excreted to be a sensitive indicator of hepatobiliary function at the recommended 5.0 mg/kg dose. Although BSP and ICG are similar in many respects, ICG is considered the preferred substance for testing hepatobiliary function in the cat. Compared to BSP, ICG is less convenient to use for clinical testing. The chemical analysis of ICG is more difficult than that of BSP. Additionally, ICG is supplied in freeze-dried form and must be dissolved only in a specific diluent, immediately prior to injection. Storage of ICG in solution form results in the formation of macromolecular aggregates that can embolize a patient on intravenous injection.

URINALYSIS

Urine concentration is prohibited in hepatic insufficiency because of limited urea production, increased renal medullary blood flow, and abnormal water retention. These factors interact to diminish the renal medullary concentration gradient.

As already mentioned, urine bilirubin provides useful information regarding serum conjugated bilirubin values, and this appears to be especially important in cats. Bilirubin is unstable in urine and is oxidized to other pigments following storage (especially when exposed to light), and these are not reactive with the standard tests for bilirubin.

Positive urine urobilinogen indicates bile duct patency and intact enterohepatic bilirubin circulation. Urobilinogen is a colorless product of enteric bacterial degradation of conjugated bilirubin. Most of the urobilinogen is excreted in the feces, but small amounts (10 to 15 per cent) are normally absorbed into the portal circulation. Most of this absorbed urobilinogen undergoes enterohepatic circulation, and most is reexcreted into the intestines and lost in the feces. Only small amounts of urobilinogen are excreted in the urine, of which the oxidation products (urobilins) are yellow. The greatest clinical importance of urobilinogen is its absence from the urine during jaundice. The absence of urobilinogen suggests, but does not confirm, the absence of intestinal bile delivery. Numerous endogenous factors, including prolonged fasting, oral antibiotic therapy, altered intestinal transit time, and malabsorption syndromes, may complicate the interpretation of urine urobilinogen. Reduced amounts of urine urobilinogen may also occur from urine dilution (polyuria), in the presence of acid urine, and following prolonged urine storage. During complete bile duct obstruction, when undetectable values of urine urobilinogen are expected, alternate routes of bilirubin entry into the intestines may develop, thereby allowing some urobilinogen production.

Certain crystals when present in urine indicate major changes in hepatic regulatory or synthetic functions. Tyrosine or leucine crystals reflect aminoaciduria, which may occur in severe hepatic necrosis or hepatic insufficiency of any origin. Bilirubin crystals are yellow and indicate conjugated hyperbilirubinemia. Ammonium biurate crystals are classically described as thorn apple in configuration, are golden in color, and reflect hyperammonemia or a metabolic problem causing abnormal urate excretion.

References and Supplemental Reading

Badylak, S. F., and Van Vleet, J. F.: Alterations of prothrombin time and activated partial thromboplastin time in dogs with hepatic disease. Am. J. Vet. Res. 42:2053, 1981.

Badylak, S. F., Dodds, J. W., and Van Vleet, J. F.: Plasma coagulation factor abnormalities in dogs with naturally occurring hepatic disease. Am. J. Vet. Res. 44:2336, 1983.

Braun, J. P., Benard, P., Burgat, V., et al.: Gamma glutamyl transferase in domestic animals. Vet. Res. Commun. 6:77, 1983.

Bunch, S. E., Baldwin, B. H., Hornbuckle, W. E., et al.: Compromized hepatic function in dogs treated with anticonvulsant drugs. J.A.V.M.A. 184:444, 1984.

Bunch, S. E., Center, S. A., Baldwin, B. H., et al.: Validation of a solid phase radioimmunoassay for the measurement of total conjugated bile acids in dogs and cats. Am. J. Vet. Res. 45:2051, 1984.

Center, S. A., Baldwin, B. H., de Lahunta, A., et al.: Evaluation of serum bile acid concentrations for the diagnosis of portosystemic venous anomalies in the dog and cat. J.A.V.M.A. 186:1090, 1985.

Center, S. A., Baldwin, B. H., Erlo, H. N., et al.: Bile acid concentrations in the diagnosis of hepatobiliary disease in the dog. J.A.V.M.A. 187:935, 1985.

Center, S. A., Bunch, S. E., Baldwin, B. H., et al.: Comparison of sulfobromophthalein and indocyanine green clearances in the cat. Am. J. Vet. Res. 44:727, 1983.

Cornelius, L. M., and DeNovo, R. C.: Icterus in cats. *In* Kirk, R. W. (ed.): *Current Veterinary Therapy VIII*. Philadelphia: W. B. Saunders, 1983, pp. 822–829.

Feldman, B. F.: Clinical pathology of the liver. *In* Kirk, R. W. (ed.): *Current Veterinary Therapy VII*. Philadelphia: W. B. Saunders, 1980, pp. 875–885.

Hardy, R. M.: Diseases of the liver. *In* Ettinger, S. J. (ed.): *Textbook of Veterinary Internal Medicine—Diseases of the Dog and Cat*. Philadelphia: W. B. Saunders, 1983, pp. 1372–1434.

Lees, G. E., Hardy, R. M., Stevens, J. M., et al.: Clinical implications of feline bilirubinuria. J. Am. Anim. Hosp. Assoc. 20:765, 1984.

Magne, M. L., and Macy, D. W.: Intravenous glucagon challenge test in the diagnosis and assessment of therapeutic efficacy in dogs with congenital portosystemic shunts. Abstract, ACVIM Scientific Proceedings, 1984, p. 36.

Meyers, D. J., Stombeck, D. R., Stone, E. A., et al.: Ammonia tolerance in clinically normal dogs and in dogs with portosystemic shunts. J.A.V.M.A. 173:378, 1978.

Prasse, K. W., Bjorling, D. E., Holmes, R. A., et al.: Indocyanine green clearance and ammonia tolerance in partially hepatectomized and hepatic devascularized anesthetized dogs. Am. J. Vet. Res. 44:2320, 1983.

Roberts, H. R., and Cederbalm, A. I.: The liver and blood coagulation: Physiology and pathology. Gastroenterology 63:297, 1972.

Soeters, P. B., Weir, G., Ebeid, A. M., et al.: Insulin, glucagon, portal systemic shunting and hepatic failure in the dog. J. Surg. Res. 23:183, 1977.

Strombeck, D. R.: *Small Animal Gastroenterology*. Davis, CA: Stonegate Publishing, 1979.

CHRONIC HEPATITIS IN DOBERMAN PINSCHERS

DENNIS A. ZAWIE, D.V.M.
New York, New York

Over the past few years, there have been several reports in the veterinary literature of inflammatory hepatopathy in Doberman pinschers (Crawford et al., 1984; Johnson et al., 1982). Additionally, in two studies evaluating canine chronic active hepatitis in 15 dogs, 6 of the 15 were Doberman pinschers (Doige and Lester, 1981; Meyer et al., 1980).

Although the cause of this disease is unknown, several important features have become evident. First, the disease primarily affects females; in fact, female Doberman pinschers account for 39 of 41 reported cases. Second, hepatic biopsy specimens from clinically ill animals show histologic changes characteristic of chronic active hepatitis and intrahepatic cholestasis. Progression of the inflammatory process eventually leads to cirrhosis (Johnson et al., 1982). Third, hepatic copper concentrations in affected Doberman pinschers are two to seven times higher than those of normal dogs (Johnson et al., 1982).

Whether the term *chronic active hepatitis* should be used to describe this disease is controversial. In humans, certain clinical, biochemical, immunologic, and histologic criteria must be met before a diagnosis of chronic active hepatitis can be made. Similar criteria for evaluating canine inflammatory liver disease have not been established.

The role that potentially causative agents such as drugs and viruses play and how genetic, immunologic, and hormonal factors influence the pathogenesis of this disease are unknown.

CLINICAL SIGNS AND PHYSICAL FINDINGS

Middle-aged (average age, 6.7 years) female Doberman pinschers are affected most often (Johnson et al., 1982). Common clinical signs include polyuria and polydipsia, anorexia, weight loss, and vomiting. With progression of the disease, jaundice and ascites often are noted. Petechial and ecchymotic hemorrhages, melena, epistaxis, and other signs of coagulation abnormalities also might develop. Signs of hepatic encephalopathy usually are associated with terminal stages of the disease. Splenomegaly, a common physical finding, probably results from portal hypertension.

The veterinary clinician should be aware that acute hepatic failure in a previously asymptomatic dog can occur following anesthesia and surgery. Presumably, the stress of surgery and use of intravenous, short-acting barbiturates for anesthetic induction contribute to the decompensation.

CLINICAL PATHOLOGY AND RADIOGRAPHY

Increased serum alkaline phosphatase activity is the most consistent biochemical abnormality in clinically ill dogs; it probably results from intrahepatic cholestasis encountered in hepatic biopsy specimens (Crawford et al., 1984; Hardy, 1985; Johnson et al., 1982). Serum alanine aminotransferase activity is generally increased, but the magnitude of elevation varies. Increased sulfobromophthalein (BSP) retention time after 30 minutes, hyperbilirubinemia, hypoalbuminemia, and hyperammonemia frequently are noted in patients with end-stage liver disease.

Thrombocytopenia secondary to hypersplenism caused by portal hypertension, mild normocytic, normochromic, nonregenerative anemia, and leukocytosis (20,000 to 45,000 WBC/mm^3) are common hematologic abnormalities. If present, coagulation abnormalities can range from increased prothrombin time alone to changes consistent with disseminated intravascular coagulation. Analysis of ascitic fluid usually reveals a modified transudate compatible with chronic obstructive effusion.

Liver size generally is reduced on routine abdominal radiographs. Moderate splenomegaly might be visualized, unless the presence of ascitic fluid obscures radiographic detail.

HEPATIC BIOPSY

Hepatic biopsy is necessary to differentiate this disease from other causes of jaundice and hepatic dysfunction. It must be remembered that anesthesia can pose considerable risk to dogs with liver disorders. In our experience, the intravenous administration of oxymorphone (Numorphan, Endo) followed by intubation and general anesthesia with halothane is a safe anesthetic regimen. *Intravenous, short-acting barbiturates should be avoided.* At our hospital, laparoscopy is performed routinely to obtain liver biopsy specimens, but other liver biopsy techniques are acceptable.

Grossly, the livers of severely affected Doberman pinschers are smaller than normal with mottled, dark brown, or tan capsular surfaces. The surfaces are smooth and have accentuated, lobular patterns or are coarsely nodular (Johnson et al., 1982).

Histopathologic changes depend on the stage and severity of the disease process. Variable degrees of periportal hepatocyte degeneration, necrosis, and fibrosis are seen. Typically, normal hepatic architecture is lost, and destruction of limiting plates is evident. Fibrosis can be extensive and outline nodules of hepatocytes. Intracellular accumulation of bile pigment and intracanalicular bile stasis are characteristic of the disease in its advanced stages (Johnson et al., 1982).

Abnormally high copper concentration is a prominent feature of this disease. Hepatic copper concentration in normal dogs is approximately 200 μg/gm dry tissue (Twedt et al., 1979). In these Doberman pinschers, copper accumulation is greatest in the periportal zones of hepatocyte degeneration and necrosis. Concentrations of 1400 to 1700 μg/gm dry tissue are not uncommon (Johnson et al., 1982).

Iron accumulation in macrophages and Kupffer's cells also is noted in biopsy specimens and is attributed to the increased erythrocyte destruction that can occur in the presence of severe liver disease and coagulation abnormalities. This is unlike iron accumulation in idiopathic hemochromatosis in humans and experimentally induced iron toxicosis in dogs, in which iron is seen primarily in hepatocytes (Pedro, 1971).

Several histochemical methods for staining copper are available. The technique using rhodanine, which stains copper granules red-orange, is a simple, reliable method for demonstrating tissue copper in dogs with cholestatic syndromes (Sternlieb, 1980).

COPPER METABOLISM

Copper is an element essential to several enzymes in mammals; however, accumulation of excess copper can cause severe tissue injury. Excessive hepatic copper can alter hepatic membrane permeability, interfere with normal hepatocyte transport of proteins and triglycerides, deplete hepatic glutathione reserves resulting in necrosis, and stimulate fibrogenesis (Sternlieb, 1980). Known genetic diseases that affect copper metabolism in humans (e.g., Wilson's disease) and dogs (copper toxicosis in Bedlington terriers) illustrate the detrimental effect excess copper can have on the liver.

Proper maintenance of copper balance in the body depends on the amount of copper that leaves the liver in the bile. Intra- and extrahepatic diseases that disrupt normal bile flow (cholestatic syndromes) can lead to copper accumulation in periportal hepatocytes.

As previously stated, intrahepatic cholestasis is a common histologic finding in these Doberman pinschers. Although this might explain copper accumulation in periportal hepatocytes in these dogs, a recent report documented elevated hepatic copper concentrations in two Doberman pinschers with subacute hepatitis (Thornburg et al., 1984). According to the authors, cholestasis was not present in these biopsy specimens, leading to speculation that a genetic defect in copper metabolism might be the primary cause of the liver disease.

PROGNOSIS

No laboratory test is available that detects this disease in asymptomatic Doberman pinschers. Occasionally, routine biochemical testing might reveal abnormal liver enzyme activity before clinical signs are apparent. If histologic changes in the liver are mild to moderate, appropriate dietary and medical therapy might be effective. In such cases, the prognosis is fair (mean survival, 12 months) (Crawford et al., 1984). A majority of dogs with the disease are clinically ill, however, and biopsy shows histologic evidence of advanced disease. Despite vigorous supportive care, most dogs die within several weeks to months after diagnosis.

Bile acid determination is a much more sensitive indicator of hepatic disease in humans than routine biochemical tests used to evaluate hepatic function. Recently, an assay for canine bile acids has been developed and normal values have been established (Center et al., 1984). Although no data are available, this assay might allow earlier detection of the disease.

TREATMENT

Appropriate treatment of these Doberman pinschers depends on the stage and severity of disease. If cirrhosis has developed, therapy is largely supportive. Maintenance of proper fluid, electrolyte, and acid-base balance is important. Administration of broad-spectrum antibiotics and parenteral administration of vitamin K might be necessary. Patients with hepatic encephalopathy might require the addition of enemas and oral lactulose (Cephulac, Merrell-National). Additionally, the administration of oral aminoglycosides, with or without metronidazole (Flagyl, Searle), aids in the reduction of colonic bacteria that contribute to hyperammonemia. Low-protein dietary therapy is essential; this has been reviewed extensively (Hardy, 1985; Strombeck, 1979).

No controlled studies evaluating the use of corticosteroids in canine chronic active hepatitis have been performed; however, there might be some rationale for their use in the early stages of this disease. The recommended dosage of oral prednisone in dogs is 1 to 2 mg/kg daily until remission of disease. The drug is then tapered gradually to 0.4 mg/kg daily (Hardy, 1985). Optimal duration of corticosteroid therapy is unknown.

D-Penicillamine (Cuprimine, Merck Sharp & Dohme) has been effective in reducing hepatic copper concentration in human patients with Wilson's disease (Sternlieb, 1980) and primary biliary cirrhosis (Vierling, 1982), and in Bedlington terriers with copper toxicosis (Twedt et al., 1979). One report of its use in Doberman pinschers shows similar results (Hardy, 1985). The recommended oral dosage for dogs is 10 to 15 mg/kg twice daily. Common side effects include anorexia and vomiting. Therapy must be continued for a minimum of several months or longer before hepatic copper concentrations return to normal.

In addition to chelating copper, D-penicillamine can modulate immune responses and alter collagen maturation. These properties of the drug might be more beneficial in managing this disease as well as other chronic inflammatory liver diseases (Vierling, 1982).

References and Supplemental Reading

Center, S. E., Leveille, C. R., Baldwin, B. H., et al.: Direct spectrometric determination of serum bile acids in the dog and cat. Am. J. Vet. Res. 45:2043, 1984.

Crawford, M. A., Jensen, R. K., and Schall, W. D.: Hepatopathy in 24 Doberman pinscher dogs. ACVIM Scientific Proceedings, 1984, p. 34 (abs.).

Doige, C. E., and Lester, S.: Chronic active hepatitis in dogs—a review of 14 cases. J. Am. Anim. Hosp. Assoc. 17:725, 1981.

Hardy, R. M.: Chronic hepatitis: An emerging syndrome. Vet. Clin. North Am. 15:135, 1985.

Johnson, G. F., Zawie, D. A., Gilbertson, S. R., et al.: Chronic active hepatitis in Doberman pinschers. J.A.V.M.A. 180:1438, 1982.

Meyer, D. J., Iverson, W. O., and Terrell, T. G.: Obstructive jaundice associated with chronic active hepatitis in a dog. J.A.V.M.A. 176:41, 1980.

Pedro, E. L.: Experimental hepatic cirrhosis in dogs caused by chronic massive iron overload. Gut 12:363, 1971.

Sternlieb, I.: Copper and the liver. Gastroenterology 78:1615, 1980.

Strombeck, D. R.: *Small Animal Gastroenterology.* Davis, CA: Stonegate Publishing, 1979, pp. 450–463.

Thornburg, L. P., Rottinghaus, G., Koch, J., et al.: High liver copper levels in two Doberman pinschers with subacute hepatitis. J. Am. Anim. Hosp. Assoc. 20:1003, 1984.

Twedt, D. C., Sternlieb, I., and Gilbertson, S. R.: Clinical, morphologic, and chemical studies on copper toxicosis of Bedlington terriers. J.A.V.M.A. 175:269, 1979.

Vierling, J. M.: Primary biliary cirrhosis. *In* Zakim, D., and Boyer, T. (eds.): *Hepatology.* Philadelphia: W. B. Saunders, 1982, pp. 646–657.

CHRONIC HEPATIC DISEASE IN DOGS

ROBERT M. HARDY, D.V.M.

St. Paul, Minnesota

The origin, pathogenesis, prognosis, and therapy of chronic hepatitis in dogs are just beginning to be defined. There has been a tendency to consolidate an etiologically diverse group of chronic inflammatory liver diseases under the common term *chronic active hepatitis* (CAH). Although this may be semantically correct, it can lead to inappropriate therapeutic decisions. CAH in dogs has become synonymous with steroid-responsive hepatitis. In all likelihood, many inflammatory canine liver diseases are not steroid responsive, and, in some cases, steroids may worsen the disease.

CHRONIC HEPATITIS IN DOGS

The full spectrum of chronic hepatitis in dogs is only beginning to be appreciated (Table 1). During the past several years, a number of different causative agents have been identified as leading to

Table 1. *The Spectrum of Chronic Hepatitis in Dogs*

Cause Known or Suspected	Cause Unknown
1. Copper-associated hepatitis in Bedlington terriers	1. Idiopathic CAH
2. Copper-associated hepatitis in Doberman pinschers	2. Lobular dissecting hepatitis
3. Copper-associated hepatitis in West Highland white terriers	
4. Leptospirosis-associated CAH	
5. Infectious canine hepatitis virus-associated CAH	
6. Drug-induced chronic hepatitis	
a. Anticonvulsants (primidone, phenytoin)	
b. Glucocorticoids	
Lesions That Resemble Those in Human CAH	
1. Copper-associated hepatitis in Bedlington terriers	
2. Copper-associated hepatitis in Doberman pinschers	
3. Leptospirosis-associated CAH	
4. Infectious canine hepatitis virus–associated CAH	
5. Idiopathic canine CAH	

chronic hepatitis in dogs (Bishop et al., 1979; Bunch et al., 1984; Gocke et al., 1967; Hardy et al., 1975). In addition, several breeds of dogs appear to have genetic predispositions to develop chronic inflammatory liver disease (Hardy et al., 1975; Johnson et al., 1982). Lastly, numerous articles have appeared describing an entity in dogs considered similar to human idiopathic or autoimmune CAH (Barton, 1977; Bishop et al., 1979; Doige and Lester, 1981; Meyer and Burrows, 1982; Meyer et al., 1980; Strombeck and Gribble, 1978; Strombeck et al., 1976; Thornburg et al., 1981). As will be seen, there is considerable overlap of these three areas.

Canine Chronic Active Hepatitis

CAH appears to be the popular diagnosis of the 1980s in veterinary hepatology. Unfortunately, this "diagnostic" designation is applied indiscriminately to virtually any inflammatory liver disease that persists for a few weeks and has lesions even remotely resembling those seen in human CAH.

Caution concerning overzealous use of this disease designation has been recommended by one author who questions whether CAH (as it is defined in humans) exists at all in dogs (Thornburg, 1982). Reasons for this lack of diagnostic specificity are partly due to semantics, poor definition of diagnostic criteria, unknown specificity of diagnostic criteria, lack of availability of supportive laboratory methods, and lack of any controlled therapeutic trials.

Diagnostic criteria that are used in humans and that are considered reasonable to apply to the canine disease include (1) clinical data supporting active (necroinflammatory) hepatic disease for 6 months or longer, (2) the presence of multiple abnormal immunologic findings, and most importantly, (3) biopsy confirmation. Biopsy not only helps to differentiate CAH from other types of chronic active liver disease but allows morphologic staging of the disease process. Biopsy material is best interpreted by individuals knowledgeable about the histopathologic spectrum of this disorder. Since immunosuppressive therapy is indicated in some forms of CAH, diagnostic accuracy is especially important. If needle biopsies are used, they should be at least 2 cm in length to reduce sampling errors (Whitcomb, 1979). When cirrhosis is present, diagnostic inaccuracies increase (Whitcomb, 1979).

What is the situation regarding CAH in dogs as it stands today? The designation of a canine liver disease as chronic can be based on history (often unreliable), repetitive biochemical evaluations (usually not obtained), or histopathologic findings supporting chronicity (fibrosis). How long does a disease need to be present for a "chronic" designation? Twelve weeks of active illness has been suggested by one report (Strombeck and Gribble, 1978) as a reasonable length of time for this designation to be applied. Present information in veterinary medicine is inadequate to determine how long *nonprogressive* idiopathic inflammatory liver diseases persist in dogs if only supportive care (without steroids) is given. There are no controlled clinical trials involving idiopathic inflammatory hepatic diseases in dogs, substantiating the value or lack thereof of any therapeutic modality as specific therapy.

What is "active" liver disease? Activity means evidence of continuing inflammation or necrosis or both. This is most easily determined by laboratory evaluations of aminotransferases. It has been suggested that serum alanine aminotransferase (ALT) concentrations average 15 times normal in canine CAH (Strombeck and Gribble, 1978). However, several cases of presumed canine CAH reportedly had normal ALT concentrations (Barton, 1977; Doige and Lester, 1981; Strombeck et al., 1976). In humans, transaminases 5 to 10 times normal are considered compatible with CAH. No definite range of transaminases in canine CAH cases has been established.

There are no data supporting the assertion that immunologic mechanisms induce hepatic injury in canine CAH, although reference is made to elevated IgG concentrations in some case reports. Hypergammaglobulinemia is a nonspecific change noted in many inflammatory liver diseases in dogs. Although occasional patients have titers against nucleoprotein (ANA) or have abnormal LE cells, the significance of such findings is unknown. No measurements of antibodies against smooth muscle or mitochondria have been performed, and techniques to identify liver-specific antigens or antibodies directed against such antigens have not been developed for dogs. All this, of course, does not mean that such abnormalities are not present and important in terms of disease pathogenesis; the work has just not been done.

The most specific information for diagnosing CAH has been through histopathologic study. In fact, the diagnosis cannot be made without it. Biopsy changes compatible with human criteria for CAH have been used by most investigators to substantiate this diagnosis in dogs (Barton, 1977; Doige and Lester, 1981; Meyer et al., 1980; Strombeck and Gribble, 1978; Strombeck et al., 1976; Thornburg et al., 1981). This is in spite of the fact that biopsy alterations are not pathognomonic for CAH in humans and great care must be taken not to "overinterpret" histologic findings in animals, as well.

Morphologic features typical of human and canine CAH include piecemeal necrosis, bridging necrosis, and active cirrhosis (Whitcomb, 1979). Piecemeal necrosis describes a specific pattern of periportal necrosis and inflammation typical of CAH. Although this lesion was at one time considered "pathognomonic" for CAH, it is also now known to occur in other nonprogressive hepatic diseases (Whitcomb, 1979). Inflammation begins in the portal triad and extends outward into hepatic lobular parenchyma. In this process of expansion, the limiting plate (a row of hepatocytes that is one cell thick and surrounds the portal triad) is obscured or destroyed. Typically, most of the inflammatory cells inducing necrosis are lymphocytes and plasma cells, although variable numbers of neutrophils may also be present. Small groups or islands of hepatocytes tend to be isolated and surrounded by inflammatory cells. Other pathologic changes that may accompany piecemeal necrosis, but are more variable, include bile duct proliferation, bile stasis, fatty change, lobular collapse, and ultimately cirrhosis (Thornburg, 1982).

As this destructive process progresses deeper into hepatic parenchyma, bands of inflammatory cells and necrotic hepatocytes will connect one portal tract to another or extend from portal tract to central vein, forming a "bridge" between adjacent hepatic lobules. This progressive change is termed *bridging necrosis* (Thornburg, 1982; Whitcomb, 1979). The resultant collapse of normal hepatic tissue results in adjacent portal areas and central veins that are in much closer proximity than normal. Bridging necrosis is considered a much more serious prognostic finding, as such patients often progress to cirrhosis and death. Although bridging necrosis is typical of CAH, as with piecemeal necrosis, it is not pathognomonic and is seen in some cases of acute (viral) hepatitis as well (Whitcomb, 1979).

The final pathologic stage of CAH is active cirrhosis (Whitcomb, 1979). Inflammatory cells are replaced by fibrosis in areas of bridging necrosis, regenerative nodules are widespread, and marked architectural distortion is evident. In some cases, patients are first diagnosed in this advanced stage and confirmation that these changes resulted from CAH is difficult. For accurate assessment of the severity of fibrosis accompanying inflammation, stains such as Mallory's trichrome should be used in conjunction with routine hematoxylin-eosin preparations. A combination of clinical signs, biochemical profiles, immunodiagnostics, and biopsy can lead to a diagnosis of CAH in most cases.

CAH-LIKE SYNDROMES IN DOGS

The following disease entities or syndromes exist in dogs, produce chronic hepatitis, and have lesions compatible with CAH but are likely not autoimmune in nature: Bedlington hepatitis (Hardy et al., 1975; Twedt et al., 1979), copper-associated hepatitis in West Highland white terriers (Thornburg, personal communication), chronic hepatitis in Doberman pinschers (Crawford et al., 1984; Johnson et al., 1982), leptospirosis-associated hepatitis (Bishop et al., 1979), anticonvulsant-induced hepatitis (Bunch et al., 1982), lobular dissecting hepatitis (Bennett et al., 1983), and infectious canine hepatitis (Gocke et al., 1967). In addition, a population of dogs exists with chronic hepatitis, histologic lesions compatible with CAH, and no identified cause for their illness. This group may have autoimmune CAH.

Copper-Associated Hepatitis in Bedlington Terriers

Chronic hepatitis in Bedlington terriers was first described in 1975. The disease may present as acute fulminant hepatitis, chronic hepatitis, or cirrhosis. It is an inherited disorder (autosomal recessive), and liver damage is caused by progressive copper accumulation. Histopathologic changes in certain stages (subacute to chronic) have features compatible with a diagnosis of CAH (Twedt et al., 1979). Specific therapy is directed at mobilizing stored hepatic copper with D-penicillamine (250 mg/day). D-Penicillamine chelates copper in the circulation and promotes its elimination in urine. "Decoppering" requires months to years of continuous (daily) treatment. There is no evidence that steroids serve any useful purpose in this disorder.

Chronic Hepatitis in West Highland White Terriers

West Highland white terriers also appear to have a copper-associated hepatitis (Thornburg, personal communication). A number of dogs have been evaluated histologically, and all have similar lesions of centrolobular hepatitis associated with significant copper accumulation. There is so little data on this disease, other than histologic, that the purpose in mentioning it here is to sensitize veterinarians to its presence. Any West Highland white terrier with hepatic disease of undefined cause should undergo a biopsy, and the material should be assessed for excessive copper accumulation. No therapeutic trials have been conducted, but D-penicillamine would be a rational choice.

Chronic Hepatitis in Doberman Pinschers

Chronic hepatitis in Doberman pinschers is a fascinating disease about which very little is known. Only two published accounts of this disease have appeared (Crawford et al., 1984; Johnson et al., 1982). Interestingly, Dobermans accounted for 6 of 15 cases of CAH in two reports of idiopathic CAH (Doige and Lester, 1981; Meyer et al., 1980). This disease has several unique features. Affected females strongly outnumber males. Of 41 reported cases, 39 were female. Clinical signs are typical of liver failure, and polyuria, polydipsia, weight loss, ascites, and icterus predominate. Most dogs are in advanced hepatic failure by the time they are examined. Prominent biochemical abnormalities are increases in alkaline phosphatase, ALT, and bilirubin, and evidence of hypoalbuminemia, coagulopathies, and thrombocytopenia (Crawford et al., 1984; Johnson et al., 1982). Liver size is most often very reduced on survey abdominal radiographs. Histopathologic features are those of CAH, but in addition, significant accumulations of copper and iron are present. The copper accumulation may be primary (cause of the disease) or secondary (due to prolonged cholestasis). Therapeutic success using varying combinations of D-penicillamine, nutritional therapy, prednisone, and low-copper diets have not been reported to enhance survival significantly (Crawford et al., 1984; Johnson et al., 1982). The author has treated one dog with early lesions by using 250 mg D-penicillamine twice daily. Hepatic copper concentrations returned to normal range after 3.5 months of therapy. Most dogs die in a few weeks to a few months after diagnosis, regardless of therapeutic attempts. Early detection in presymptomatic stages is likely to be the only way to improve therapeutic success. Clinical evaluations of asymptomatic Dobermans is currently under way to determine the prevalence of occult (biochemical) liver disease in the breed. No data on the nature of inheritance of this presumed genetic disorder are available at this time.

Lobular Dissecting Hepatitis

Recently, an unusual form of chronic hepatitis termed *lobular dissecting hepatitis* was described in six dogs (Bennett et al., 1983). Primary clinical features were ascites and portal hypertension in each dog. Biochemical abnormalities included in all dogs hypoalbuminemia, increased BSP retention (greater than 23 per cent), and increased fasting blood ammonia (1.5 to 6 times normal). ALT and alkaline phosphatase concentrations were normal to moderately increased.

Lesions were characterized microscopically by a mild, mixed inflammatory reaction. Cells were mostly neutrophils, lymphocytes, and macrophages. Reticulin and fine collagen fibers dissected lobular parenchyma. Limiting plates were disrupted by this process, but portal inflammation was inconstant and seldom marked. Lesions were described as different from those of CAH in dogs and other chronic hepatitides in humans. No cause was identified.

Leptospirosis-Associated Chronic Hepatitis

An outbreak of chronic active hepatitis associated with leptospirosis in five American foxhounds has been reported (Bishop et al., 1979). Biochemical data were taken on only one of these dogs, and mild increases in concentrations of serum alkaline phosphatase, ALT, BSP, and gamma globulin were reported. Spirochetes were identified histologically in four of five dogs by using special staining techniques (Warthin-Starry stains). Other lesions identified in the liver were compatible with CAH.

Virus-Induced Chronic Hepatitis

The adenovirus responsible for infectious canine hepatitis (ICH) has been associated with the production of chronic hepatitis and periportal mononuclear infiltrates in dogs with low concentrations of antibody to ICH virus (Gocke et al., 1967). Lesions were compatible with those of CAH. Virus was not identifiable except in the very early stages of infection. What role canine hepatitis virus may play in inducing CAH in clinical patients is unknown.

Drug-Induced Chronic Hepatitis

Chronic anticonvulsant therapy has recently been implicated as a cause of chronic hepatitis and cirrhosis in dogs (Bunch et al., 1984; Bunch et al., 1982). It has long been known that anticonvulsants, particularly primidone and phenytoin, induce alterations in hepatic biochemical profiles. Only recently has it been appreciated that some dogs with biochemical abnormalities will progress from chronic hepatitis to cirrhosis. It was estimated in one survey that as many as 15 per cent of dogs given long-term anticonvulsant therapy (primidone or combinations of primidone and phenytoin) are at risk to develop serious hepatotoxicity (Bunch et al., 1984). Although histopathologic changes in these dogs are not typical of CAH, the presence of long-term biochemical abnormalities and severe liver lesions may result from these dogs having been given anticonvulsants. What is needed is a change in anticonvulsant medications (decrease dosages, eliminate, or switch to alternatives).

Idiopathic CAH in Dogs

Lastly, there is left a group of dogs that have biochemical evidence of chronic hepatitis but no known cause is identified and biopsies resemble those from dogs with CAH (Barton, 1977; Doige and Lester, 1981; Meyer and Burrows, 1982; Meyer et al., 1980; Strombeck and Gribble, 1978; Thornburg et al., 1981). What should the disease be called and how should the dogs be treated?

The veterinarian's first goal should be to confirm the diagnosis. Establishing a diagnosis of idiopathic CAH in dogs should involve the following steps. First, it must be established that active liver disease exists. This will be done by using the clinical history and appropriate biochemical tests, ALT in particular. If no identifiable cause can be found and the patient's signs are mild or intermittent, it is likely only supportive care will be necessary (no steroids). If the patient's signs worsen, or if there is evidence biochemically of a continuing necroinflammatory process or that the disease is chronic, a liver biopsy should be taken. Biopsies should be sent to pathologists familiar with the features of CAH. If the biopsy findings are compatible with those for CAH, a diagnosis of CAH of undefined cause, possibly autoimmune, may be made.

Recommendations regarding specific therapy for idiopathic CAH in dogs are purely speculative at this time. No controlled clinical trials using steroids have been performed. Clinical data supporting their efficacy remain to be confirmed. Initial dosages recommended for dogs are 1 to 2 mg/kg daily until clinical remission is evident (Strombeck and Gribble, 1978). Steroids are gradually decreased until maintenance levels of 0.4 mg/kg/day are attained. The steroid chosen should be prednisone or prednisolone. Optimal duration of therapy is unknown. Patients should be monitored biochemically at least monthly. If hepatic enzyme and functional data suggest that complete remission exists, steroids may be stopped. Patients should be re-evaluated for evidence of relapse.

Because of the sensitivity of dogs to steroid-induced hepatopathy, it will be difficult to assess improvement other than by clinical status and hepatic histopathologic signs. Patients that appear to be improving should undergo another biopsy during therapy to assess whether morphologic recovery is also occurring. When both biochemical and histopathologic results support recovery, medications should be slowly tapered off; the ultimate goal is complete drug elimination. There are no long-term studies of idiopathic CAH in dogs to support the effectiveness of these recommendations.

D-Penicillamine (Cuprimine, Merck Sharp & Dohme) has been used as an antifibrotic agent in human CAH. Preliminary evidence indicates it may be more effective than steroids in reversing or delaying hepatic fibrosis in CAH. The recommended canine dosage is 10 to 15 mg/kg twice daily. Vomiting and anorexia are common complaints when the drug is first administered.

Polyunsaturated phosphatidylcholine (PPC, lecithin) has been used experimentally in human CAH and is thought to modify the immune injury in this disease. PPC therapy at 3 gm/day significantly reduced histologic severity, and no relapses were encountered in one human study. This drug was recommended for adjunctive therapy when steroids and azathioprine were inadequate to control the disease.

Colchicine is another drug that may be useful in advanced (cirrhotic) stages of CAH. Colchicine has been advocated as a drug with potential for inhibiting or reversing hepatic fibrosis. Significant reductions in hepatic fibrosis have been observed in human cirrhotic patients given this drug. Canine dosages are not firmly established, but 0.03 mg/kg/day has recently been recommended for control of hepatic fibrosis (Boer et al., 1984). Use of this drug in clinical patients should only be undertaken with full understanding by the owner of its experimental nature.

Even though a number of drugs have been discussed as possible "specific" therapies for idiopathic canine CAH, they have yet to be proved beneficial. Supportive and symptomatic care remain the backbone of any therapeutic regimen for patients in hepatic failure. Such therapy will often reduce the severity of clinical signs, improve the quality of life for the patient, and provide optimal conditions for hepatic repair and regeneration. These benefits may be obtained even in progressive, fatal disorders.

Dietary therapy is the single most important means of modifying the course of the majority of spontaneous liver diseases. Dietary therapy tends to be most useful in slowly progressive diseases, since these animals will often feel well enough to voluntarily eat reasonable quantities of calories. Intake of nutrients is adjusted to match the patient's ability to metabolize them in a failing liver.

The type and quantity of protein ingested are the most important considerations when a diet for dogs in hepatic failure is formulated. If appropriate adjustments are made, reduction in blood ammonia concentrations and normalization of altered circulating amino acid ratios will occur. Cottage cheese can serve as a beneficial sole protein source for dogs with hepatic failure. Cottage cheese has a high biologic value, is easily digested, contains no chemical additives, and has a good ratio of branched chain to aromatic amino acids. Initially, protein should be supplied at a level of 2 gm/kg body weight per day. Normal adult maintenance requirements are 4.8 gm/kg/day. If hypoalbuminemia is present, restricted protein intake may not allow for adequate protein synthesis by the liver. If clinical signs improve but hypoalbuminemia persists or worsens, protein intake should be slowly increased. Increase dietary protein by increments of 0.5 gm/kg/day for a week at a time, until clinical signs worsen or protein anabolism is evident. It is not necessary to increase total daily protein intake beyond 4.8 gm/kg/day. Commercial, balanced, reduced-protein diets such as Prescription Diet k/d (Hill's Pet Products) will work well for many dogs. If dogs will eat enough of this diet to meet their caloric needs, it will supply approximately 2 gm/kg body weight per day of high-biologic-value protein. If protein malnutrition is evident on this diet, it may be supplemented with cottage cheese.

Carbohydrates should provide the bulk of the calories in diets made for patients with hepatic failure. Carbohydrate sources should be easily digestible so that minimal residues reach the colon. This will reduce colonic bacterial production of volatile fatty acids, substances implicated in the pathogenesis of hepatic encephalopathy. Boiled white rice is an inexpensive, useful carbohydrate source.

Fats should be provided in sufficient quantities to supply essential fatty acids and fat-soluble vitamins, as well as improve palatability. Fats should be added so that they constitute 6 per cent of the dry weight of the diet (1.32 gm/kg/day). Excessive fat intake may worsen clinical signs. Certain fatty acids have been shown to aggravate signs of encephalopathy, and cholestatic liver diseases can be associated with impaired fat assimilation and resulting steatorrhea.

Vitamin and mineral supplementation should only be necessary if home-formulated diets are used. Hypovitaminosis is common in hepatic failure. Vitamins most often deficient in human hepatic failure are B_6, B_{12}, thiamine, A, E, riboflavin, nicotinic acid, pantothenic acid, and folic acid. The most common mineral deficiencies are zinc and cobalt. When home-made diets are used, a good quality, high-potency vitamin and mineral supplement should be added to the daily ration (Centrum, Lederle Labs).

Lipotropic drugs have long been a mainstay in veterinary therapeutics for patients with hepatic disease. Since these drugs invariably contain methionine, they should *not* be given to animals in hepatic failure. Oral methionine will consistently induce hepatic coma in dogs in hepatic failure. Methionine metabolites also act synergistically with short-chain fatty acids and ammonia to induce hepatic encephalopathy.

Formulations for two well-balanced homemade diets for dogs with hepatic insufficiency have recently been published (Strombeck et al., 1983). Some owners prefer to make their own diets for their pets, and these formulations are quite similar to commercially available dry k/d diet.

An improved awareness and understanding of chronic inflammatory hepatic diseases in dogs is occurring in veterinary practice. It is hoped that more specific recommendations concerning the diagnosis, origin, pathogenesis, and therapy of chronic hepatitis in dogs will be forthcoming in the near future.

References and Supplemental Reading

Barton, C.: Chronic active hepatic disease with cirrhosis in a dog. Missouri Vet., 28:17, 1977.

Bennett, A. M., Davies, J. D., Gaskell, C. J., et al.: Lobular dissecting hepatitis in the dog. Vet. Pathol. 20:179, 1983.

Boer, H. H., Nelson, R. W., and Long, G. G.: Colchicine therapy for hepatic fibrosis in a dog. J.A.V.M.A. 185:303, 1984.

Bishop, L., Strandberg, J. D., Adams, R. J., et al.: Chronic active hepatitis in dogs associated with leptospires. Am. J. Vet. Res. 40:839, 1979.

Bunch, S. E., Baldwin, B. H., Hornbuckle, W. E., et al.: Compromised hepatic function in dogs treated with anticonvulsant drugs. J.A.V.M.A. 184:444, 1984.

Bunch, S. E., Castleman, W. L., Hornbuckle, W. E., et al.: Hepatic cirrhosis associated with long-term anticonvulsant drug therapy in dogs. J.A.V.M.A. 181:357, 1982.

Crawford, M. A., Jensen, R. K., and Schall, W. D.: Hepatopathy in 24 Doberman pinscher dogs. ACVIM Scientific Proceedings, 1984, p. 34.

Doige, C. E., and Lester, S.: Chronic active hepatitis in dogs—a review of 14 cases. J. Am. Anim. Hosp. Assoc. 17:725, 1981.

Gocke, D. J., Presig, R., Morris, T. D., et al.: Experimental viral hepatitis in the dog: Production of persistent disease in partially immune animals. J. Clin. Invest. 46:1506–1517, 1967.

Hardy, R. M., Stevens, J. B., and Stowe, L.: Chronic progressive hepatitis in Bedlington terriers associated with elevated liver copper concentrations. Minn. Vet. 15:13, 1975.

Johnson, G. F., Zawie, D. A., Gilbertson, S. R., et al.: Chronic active hepatitis in Doberman pinschers. J.A.V.M.A. 180:1438, 1982.

Meyer, D. J., and Burrows, C. F.: The Liver. II. Biochemical diagnosis of hepatobiliary disorders in the dog. Comp. Cont. Ed. Pract. Vet. 4:706, 1982.

Meyer, D. J., Iverson, W. O., and Terrell, T. G.: Obstructive jaundice associated with chronic active hepatitis. J.A.V.M.A. 176:41, 1980.

Strombeck, D. R., and Gribble, D. G.: Chronic active hepatitis in the dog. J.A.V.M.A. 173:380, 1978.

Strombeck, D. R., Rogers, W., and Gribble, D.: Chronic active hepatic disease in a dog. J.A.V.M.A. 169:802, 1976.

Strombeck, D. R., Schaffer, M. L., and Rogers, Q. R.: Dietary therapy for dogs with chronic hepatic insufficiency. *In* Kirk, R. W. (ed.): *Current Veterinary Therapy VIII*. Philadelphia: W. B. Saunders, 1983, pp. 817–821.

Thornburg, L. P.: Chronic active hepatitis. What is it, and does it occur in dogs? J. Am. Anim. Hosp. Assoc. 18:21, 1982.

Thornburg, L. P.: Personal communication. College of Veterinary Medicine, Department of Veterinary Pathology, University of Missouri, Columbia, MO, 1985.

Thornburg, L. P., Moxley, R. A., and Jones, B. D.: An unusual case of chronic active hepatitis in a Kerry blue terrier. Vet. Clin. North Am. [Small Anim. Pract.] 76:363, 1981.

Twedt, D. C., Sternlieb, I., and Gilbertson, S. R.: Clinical, morphologic and chemical studies on copper toxicosis of Bedlington terriers. J.A.V.M.A. 175:269, 1979.

Whitcomb, F. F.: Chronic active liver disease. Definition, diagnosis and management. Med. Clin. North Am. 63:413, 1979.

ACUTE HEPATIC FAILURE

SUSAN E. JOHNSON, D.V.M.
Columbus, Ohio

Acute hepatic failure occurs whenever a sudden, severe insult to the liver compromises at least 70 to 80 per cent of the functional hepatic mass. The resulting clinical and laboratory features of acute hepatic failure are not specific for the inciting cause but reflect disruption of one or more major hepatic functions: metabolism of carbohydrates, fat, and protein; synthesis of plasma proteins and coagulation factors; detoxification and excretion of drugs, toxins, and metabolites; and formation and elimination of bile.

Management of the patient with acute hepatic failure is first directed toward symptomatic and supportive treatment for control of the impending metabolic derangements, thus allowing time for specific diagnostic and therapeutic measures. When the cause remains undetermined or specific therapy is unavailable, supportive care may allow time for hepatic regeneration and eventual recovery.

ETIOLOGY

Causes of acute hepatic failure include hepatotoxins, infectious or parasitic agents, and metabolic disturbances (Table 1). In many clinical cases, however, the inciting cause is not identified. A liver biopsy is usually required for complete evaluation of the causes of liver failure. An etiologic diagnosis may be obtained for diseases with characteristic histopathologic features such as systemic fungal infections, toxoplasmosis, and feline infectious peritonitis (coronavirus). When the microscopic evaluation is not diagnostic for a specific cause, descriptive morphologic characteristics such as acute necrosis, acute hepatitis, or steatosis aid in classification of the hepatic disorder. Acute, diffuse hepatic necrosis is the lesion that most consistently produces acute hepatic failure.

A liver biopsy is also useful to differentiate acute and chronic hepatic disease. In occult chronic liver disease, the clinical signs may be vague and go unrecognized by the owner until the final phase of hepatic decompensation, thus mimicking acute hepatic failure. This is an important distinction to make, since the intensive supportive care indicated in acute hepatic failure may not be warranted in chronic end-stage liver disease.

Diseases of the extrahepatic biliary tract should also be considered in the differential diagnosis of acute hepatic failure accompanied by jaundice. This distinction is particularly important, since surgical intervention is indicated in some of these disorders (e.g., rupture of the biliary tract and cholelithiasis).

CLINICAL RECOGNITION AND DIAGNOSIS

The clinical findings in acute hepatic failure tend to be nonspecific and overlap those of other systemic disorders. These historic and physical abnormalities reflect general hepatic dysfunction rather than the specific underlying cause. However, signs of extrahepatic or systemic disease often provide important diagnostic clues in liver failure associated with septicemia or endotoxemia, pancreatitis, hemolytic disease, and many of the infectious diseases. When the clinical findings are vague, hepatic failure may not be suspected until the results of laboratory tests, such as increased liver enzyme activity or hyperbilirubinemia, indicate that liver disease is present. After the presence of hepatic dysfunction is identified, an attempt is made to determine the inciting cause by further historic questions, ancillary laboratory tests, and, ultimately, liver biopsy.

History and Clinical Signs

The signs most frequently observed include anorexia, depression, vomiting, and diarrhea that may be accompanied by polydipsia and polyuria. The owner will often describe an acute onset of these signs in a previously healthy animal. Occasionally, an observant owner will note overt jaundice and bilirubinuria (dark or orange-colored urine). When

Table 1. Causes of Acute Hepatic Failure

Hepatotoxins
Therapeutic Agents
Acetaminophen (feline)
Anticonvulsants (phenytoin, primadone, diphenylsilanediol)
Aprindine
Azathioprine
Halothane
Ketoconazole
Mebendazole
Methotrexate
Methoxyflurane
Phenazopyridine (feline)
Sulfonamides (sulfadiazine and trimethoprim)
Tetracycline
Thiacetarsamide
Tolbutamide
Chemicals
Arsenic
Carbon tetrachloride
Chlordane
Chlorinated biphenyls, hydrocarbons, naphthalenes
Dieldrin
Dimethylnitrosamine
Heavy metals (copper, iron, mercury)
Phosphorus
Selenium
Tannic acid
Biologic Substances
Aflatoxin (hepatitis X)
Blue-green algae endotoxin
Amanita mushroom toxin
Zamia floridana seeds (cycads)
Pyrrolizidine alkaloids
Bacterial endotoxin

Infectious and Parasitic Agents
Bacterial
Gram-negative septicemia/endotoxemia
Leptospira spp.
Salmonella spp.
Clostridium spp.
Bacillus piliformis (Tyzzer's disease)
Viral
Infectious canine hepatitis (adenovirus I)
Canine herpesvirus
Feline infectious peritonitis (coronavirus)
Fungal
Histoplasmosis
Coccidioidomycosis
Blastomycosis
Others
Protozoal
Toxoplasmosis
Canine heartworm disease
Postcaval syndrome

Miscellaneous
Acute pancreatitis
Acute hemolytic anemia (AIHA)
Heat stroke
Surgical hypotension or hypoxia
Trauma
Inflammatory bowel disease—colitis

severe hepatocellular dysfunction is present, the signs of hepatic encephalopathy may dominate the clinical picture. These include depression, behavioral changes, dementia, ataxia, pacing, circling, blindness, hypersalivation, seizures, and coma. Clinical evidence of a bleeding tendency, such as melena, hematemesis, cutaneous and mucosal hemorrhage, or hematuria, is uncommon except in fulminant acute hepatic necrosis.

When hepatic dysfunction is suspected, the owner should be asked further history pertaining to (1) recent drug therapy (especially those agents listed in Table 1), (2) recent anesthetic procedures, (3) current vaccination status (especially leptospirosis and infectious canine hepatitis), and (4) potential exposure to toxins or infectious agents.

Physical Examination

As with the historic signs of acute hepatic failure, the physical findings tend to be nonspecific. Key findings that may suggest the presence of hepatobiliary disease include hepatomegaly, hepatodynia (liver pain), acholic feces, and icterus. Causes of a smooth, generalized hepatomegaly include infiltration of the liver (e.g., neoplasia, lipid, corticosteroid-induced vacuolization, inflammation, reticuloendothelial hyperplasia, and extramedullary hematopoiesis), hepatic congestion (e.g., right-sided heart failure, pericardial disease, postcaval syndrome of heartworms), and cholestasis (e.g., intra- or extrahepatic biliary obstruction).

Asymmetric hepatomegaly and localized hepatic masses are caused by hepatic neoplasms, fungal granulomas, or benign regenerative nodules. The finding of hepatodynia also aids in localizing a problem to the liver and suggests acute hepatic swelling with stretching of the liver capsule. The presence of acholic feces implies complete obstruction of the common bile duct, with failure of bile pigments to enter the intestine. The clay-colored appearance of acholic feces must be differentiated from the light tan color caused by severe steatorrhea.

Jaundice of the skin and mucous membranes, in the absence of pallor, is suggestive of primary hepatic or posthepatic disruption of normal bilirubin metabolism. However, further laboratory evaluation is necessary to eliminate prehepatic (hemolytic) causes of jaundice. Bilirubinuria (bright yellow or orange urine) accompanies overt icterus caused by hepatobiliary disease but may also be noted before jaundice is detectable.

In severe acute hepatic failure, signs of encephalopathy may predominate. On neurologic examination, findings such as altered consciousness, personality changes, motor disturbances, and seizures suggest diffuse cerebral dysfunction. When the underlying hepatic disease is chronic rather than acute, the severity of the signs may wax and wane and be interspersed with periods of apparently normal neurologic function.

Clinical evidence of a bleeding diathesis is occasionally noted on physical examination. Petechial and ecchymotic hemorrhages of the skin, subcutaneous tissues, and mucous membranes may be detected. Gastrointestinal hemorrhage is suggested by the findings of hematemesis or melena. When hemorrhage is severe, the resulting anemia causes pallor and weakness.

Extrahepatic manifestations of systemic diseases that concurrently affect the liver may provide important diagnostic clues to the underlying disorder; for example, the finding of coexisting renal involvement (leptospirosis), ocular disease (mycoses, feline infectious peritonitis, toxoplasmosis), pulmonary involvement (mycoses, heartworms, toxoplasmosis), cranial abdominal pain (pancreatitis, cholecystitis, peritonitis), pale mucous membranes (hemolytic anemia), and fever (infectious, inflammatory, or neoplastic diseases). Concurrent findings of liver disease and a severe bacterial infection (e.g., pyometra) or other disease likely to be associated with endotoxemia (e.g., parvoviral enteritis) suggest hepatic damage secondary to septicemia or endotoxemia. The findings of cachexia, emaciation, ascites, or edema suggest a more protracted illness and are characteristic of chronic rather than acute liver failure.

Table 2. *Ancillary Evaluations Used to Diagnose Acute Hepatic Failure Due to Extrahepatic or Multisystemic Disease*

Diagnostic Evaluation	Intended Diagnosis (Rule Out)
Bacterial cultures:	
Liver and bile	Bacterial invasion of the liver
Blood, feces, infected tissues	Sepsis, endotoxemia
Serologic tests (antibody titers)	Mycoses (histoplasmosis, coccidioidomycosis, blastomycosis) Toxoplasmosis Leptospirosis Feline infectious peritonitis (FIP)
Urine darkfield exam (for spirocheturia)	Leptospirosis
Lymph node aspiration cytologic exam	Mycoses Lymphoid neoplasia
Microfilaria exam	Heartworm disease
Serum amylase and lipase	Acute pancreatitis
Coombs' test	Autoimmune hemolytic anemia
Thoracic radiography	Mycoses Toxoplasmosis Heartworm disease
Abdominal radiography	Hepatic abscesses Emphysematous cholecystitis Cholelithiasis Pancreatitis
Abdominal ultrasonography	Pancreatic disease Hepatic abscesses or neoplasia Biliary or gallbladder disease

Modified from Sherding, R. G.: Acute hepatic failure. Vet. Clin. North Am. 15:119, 1985.

Laboratory Evaluation

Acute hepatic failure is potentially associated with a number of abnormal findings on standard laboratory tests such as the complete blood count, serum chemistry profile, urinalysis, hemostasis screen, blood gas analysis, and liver function tests. These abnormalities and their clinical significance are discussed in the article entitled Biochemical Evaluation of Liver Function in the Dog and Cat. Additional ancillary test results (Table 2) may also be abnormal when specific extrahepatic or multisystemic diseases are present.

SERUM ENZYME ACTIVITY

Increased serum activity of enzymes originating from hepatic tissue occurs frequently in patients with acute hepatic failure and may be the first indication of hepatobiliary disease. The traditional serum enzymes monitored for hepatobiliary disease are alanine aminotransferase (ALT, formerly SGPT) and alkaline phosphatase (AP).

Increased serum activity of ALT results when excessive release of the enzyme from the hepatocyte cytoplasm occurs during hepatocellular necrosis or altered cell metabolism. This is the most consistent laboratory finding in acute hepatic necrosis (Strombeck, 1979). The magnitude of ALT increase does not correlate with morphologic changes except in the period immediately following the hepatic insult. For example, despite a half-life of 2.5 hours, serum ALT activity in dogs given a single dose of carbon tetrachloride is persistently increased for 2 to 3 weeks, suggesting continued enzyme leakage even during the reparative process (Meyer, 1982). Furthermore, serum ALT activity may decline following an initial insult despite persistence of extensive necrosis (Strombeck, 1979). Nonetheless, increased serum ALT activity is a useful test for clinical detection of acute hepatic damage. Another liver enzyme, aspartate aminotransferase (AST, formerly SGOT) tends to parallel changes in ALT activity but is less liver-specific in dogs and cats.

Increased serum AP activity occurs when intrahepatic or extrahepatic cholestasis stimulates an increased production of this enzyme (Meyer, 1982).

Since acute hepatic necrosis and hepatocyte swelling cause intrahepatic obstruction to bile flow, AP is usually also increased in acute hepatic injury. Extrahepatic sources of AP (e.g., bone, intestine, and certain neoplasms) may also contribute to increased total serum AP activity in other conditions. Of particular importance in dogs is the steroid-induced increase in serum AP that accompanies endogenous or exogenous hypercortisolism (Hardy, 1983). Analysis of the specific isoenzyme is useful in differentiating the origin of the AP activity. Species differences also influence interpretation of increased serum AP activity. In cats, AP has a shorter half-life and the liver has less AP activity, resulting in a lower magnitude of increase than would be expected in dogs with diseases of similar severity (Hardy, 1983).

HEPATIC FUNCTION TESTS

Total serum bilirubin concentration is frequently increased in acute hepatic failure as a result of impaired hepatic uptake, conjugation, and excretion of bilirubin (Meyer, 1982). Overt jaundice is not detected until the total bilirubin concentration exceeds 2 to 3 mg/dl. The detection of bilirubin pigment and crystals in the urine indicates an increased concentration of conjugated bilirubin in the plasma. Although fractionation of the total serum bilirubin into unconjugated and conjugated components has been advocated to distinguish prehepatic, hepatic, and posthepatic causes of hyperbilirubinemia, fractionation patterns overlap considerably. In primary hepatocellular disease, a mixed pattern of hyperbilirubinemia is present. Unconjugated bilirubinemia may predominate early in the course of a hemolytic anemia; however, with time, a mixed pattern prevails. In this case, evaluation of red blood cell morphology for spherocytes and parasites, along with other clinical measurements of hemolysis, is usually adequate to distinguish prehepatic from hepatobiliary jaundice. Acute liver failure is occasionally a complication of primary immune-mediated hemolytic anemia. Posthepatic obstruction should be considered when greater than 90 per cent of the total bilirubin is conjugated, and further evaluation should include urinalysis for the presence of urobilinogen. However, it must be emphasized that intrahepatic and extrahepatic biliary obstruction cannot be reliably distinguished by any single test or combination of biochemical tests.

The liver is the major site for production of most coagulation factors, including Factors I, II, V, VII, VIII, IX, X, XI, and XII (Strombeck, 1979). The liver also synthesizes activators and inhibitors of the fibrinolytic system and catabolizes activated procoagulant factors and fibrin degradation products. Consequently, it is not surprising that hepatic disease often disrupts the normal hemostatic mechanisms (Badylak and Van Fleet, 1981). Hemostatic defects associated with hepatobiliary disease may be attributed to disseminated intravascular coagulation (DIC), primary failure of the liver to synthesize clotting factors, or vitamin K deficiency caused by biliary obstruction. In acute hepatic failure, the first two mechanisms are probably the most important. The complication of DIC has been reported in infectious canine hepatitis, acute hepatic necrosis, aflatoxicosis, and leptospirosis. A prolonged one-stage prothrombin time (OSPT), activated partial thromboplastin time (APTT), or activated clotting time (ACT) suggests impaired hemostatic capabilities as a result of one or more of the previously mentioned mechanisms. When DIC is present, additional findings of thrombocytopenia, circulating fibrin degradation products, and hypofibrinogenemia may be detected. Hematologic evidence of blood loss anemia and hypoproteinemia may be consequences of excessive hemorrhage due to coagulopathy. Bleeding gastric ulcers are another mechanism for blood loss anemia associated with liver failure in dogs.

The most specific laboratory test available to confirm that neurologic signs are attributable to hepatic encephalopathy is the determination of blood ammonia concentration. Increased resting plasma ammonia levels or intolerance of an oral ammonia load in the clinical setting of acute hepatic failure implies severe diffuse hepatocellular damage. The formation of ammonium biurate crystals in the urine indirectly suggests hyperammonemia.

Additional tests of hepatic function that frequently yield abnormal results in acute hepatic failure include sulfobromophthalein (BSP) dye excretion and serum bile acid concentration. In addition, hypoglycemia may occur when hepatic damage is severe, presumably the result of impaired hepatic gluconeogenesis. Hypoglycemia induced by endotoxemia should also be considered in the clinical setting of acute hepatic failure, since this mechanism has a different prognostic and therapeutic significance. The metabolic consequences of acute hepatic failure may also include hypokalemia and acid-base imbalances. The findings of decreased serum albumin, urea nitrogen, and cholesterol concentrations suggest chronic hepatic dysfunction; however, these tests are also influenced by extrahepatic disorders.

Radiographic Procedures

Abdominal radiographs are useful to confirm alterations in liver size that are suspected on physical examination. A normal or large liver is compatible with an acute hepatic disorder, whereas a small liver may suggest chronic liver disease (e.g., portocaval shunt or cirrhosis). Occasionally, massive hepatic necrosis causes collapse of normal hepatic architecture and results in microhepatia. Radiolucent densities in the area of the liver or gallbladder suggest hepatic abscesses or emphysematous cholecystitis. Mineralized densities may represent choleliths or benign mineralization of hepatic or biliary tissue. Both abdominal and thoracic radiographs may suggest the presence of systemic or extrahepatic diseases (Table 2). Abdominal ultrasonography appears to be the preferred method for distinguishing intrahepatic from posthepatic cholestasis and provides information concerning abnormalities of the biliary tract and pancreas and mass lesions of the liver (Nyland and Gillett, 1982; Nyland and Park, 1983).

Liver Biopsy

A liver biopsy should be performed when the cause of acute hepatic failure is not suggested by preliminary ancillary tests. Histologic examination of hepatic tissue is useful to eliminate known causes of acute hepatic failure and to distinguish between acute and chronic liver disease. If extrahepatic biliary obstruction is suspected, an exploratory laparotomy should be performed so that the biliary tract may be examined at the same time that liver tissue is obtained for histopathologic evaluation. This procedure allows for both diagnostic and therapeutic intervention. Other methods of liver biopsy include percutaneous Menghini needle aspiration biopsy, keyhole needle biopsy (Tru-Cut, Travenol Labs), and laparoscopy. Although the presence of a coagulopathy is not an absolute contraindication for liver biopsy, extreme caution is recommended and a blood transfusion may be required if postbiopsy bleeding is excessive. The author prefers to use laparoscopy to obtain a liver biopsy when a coagulopathy is present.

TREATMENT

Management of the patient with acute hepatic failure is first directed toward symptomatic and supportive therapy of the metabolic derangements and complications of general hepatic failure (Table 3). Ideally, specific treatment of the underlying cause should be instituted when appropriate—for example, antibiotics for leptospirosis and amphotericin B or ketoconazole for systemic mycoses. Although specific antidotal therapy is not available for drug-induced liver damage, discontinuing the suspect drug will prevent further hepatocellular damage. In many cases, the cause remains unidentified or specific therapy is unavailable; however, supportive care alone may provide adequate time for hepatic regeneration and eventual recovery. Strict attention to fluid, electrolyte, and acid-base balance is the cornerstone of supportive therapy. Preventing

Table 3. *General Therapy for Acute Hepatic Failure*

Goals of Therapy	Therapeutic Regimen
1. Facilitate hepatic regeneration and reduce hepatic pain	Cage rest, exercise restriction
2. Maintain fluid and acid-base balance	0.9% or 0.45% saline or Ringer's solution IV Use $NaHCO_3$ IV if severe metabolic acidosis is present (caution: avoid alkalosis in the presence of HE)
3. Prevent hypokalemia	Add 10–15 mEq KCl to each 500 ml of IV maintenance fluids Monitor serum potassium every 24–48 hours and adjust potassium supplementation according to sliding scale (see text)
4. Prevent hypoglycemia	Add dextrose to IV fluids to make a 2.5–5% concentration
5. Control hepatic encephalopathy	
a. Avoid use of CNS depressants (e.g., anticonvulsants, tranquilizers, sedatives, anesthetics)	If anticonvulsant therapy is required, use IV diazepam or phenobarbital or oral phenobarbital (at reduced dosage)
b. Prevent production and absorption of enteric toxins	Cleansing enemas every 6 hours Retention enemas every 6 hours with: (1) Neomycin 15 mg/kg (2) Lactulose diluted 1:2 in water (50–200 ml total) OR Oral therapy: (1) Neomycin 10–20 mg/kg every 6 hours (2) Lactulose 5–30 ml every 6 hours
c. Restrict diet	Low-protein, low-fat, high-carbohydrate (e.g., Prescription Diet k/d or u/d; cottage cheese, boiled rice)
d. Control gastrointestinal hemorrhage	Correct coagulopathy (see below) Eliminate concurrent GI parasites Treat for gastric ulcers (see below)
6. Control coagulopathy	Vitamin K_1 5–20 mg IM every 12 hours Fresh plasma or blood transfusion DIC: Heparin 5–10 units/kg SC every 8 hours May incubate initial dose with plasma for 30 minutes before transfusion
7. Control gastric ulcers	Cimetidine 10 mg/kg every 8 hours PO or IV Sucralfate 1 gm tablets, 1 tablet/25 kg every 8 hours PO
8. Prevent or control endotoxemia	Systemic antibiotics: penicillin, ampicillin, cephalosporins, gentamicin, kanamycin Enteric antibiotics: neomycin Enteric toxin binders: cholestyramine

or controlling complications such as hypoglycemia, hepatic encephalopathy, coagulopathy, and endotoxemia is also important.

When drugs are administered to patients with hepatic failure, it is important to consider the potential for impaired hepatic metabolism and subsequent accumulation of the drugs. Although specific drug and dose modifications are unavailable, the veterinarian should attempt to determine whether the liver is important for metabolism of that particular drug and decrease the dose accordingly.

Fluid, Electrolyte, and Acid-Base Balance

The first step in treating the patient with acute hepatic failure is to correct dehydration and ensure that normal hydration is maintained. A reasonable fluid choice is saline (0.9 or 0.45 per cent) or Ringer's solution supplemented with dextrose (2.5 to 5 per cent) and potassium chloride (10 to 15 mEq/500 ml bottle of fluid). Maintenance volumes of fluid (40 to 60 ml/kg/24 hours) and additional amounts to replace ongoing fluid losses from vomiting and diarrhea should be provided. Fluid therapy is important in acute hepatic failure because it preserves the hepatic microcirculation, aids in renal excretion of potential hepatotoxins, and helps prevent complications such as DIC, hepatic encephalopathy, renal failure, and shock.

Hypokalemia is the most consistent electrolyte disturbance that occurs in acute hepatic failure. Hypokalemia usually results from anorexia (lack of potassium intake) or vomiting (excessive potassium loss). Urinary loss of potassium may be augmented by secondary hyperaldosteronism caused by liver failure. Metabolic alkalosis, a common acid-base disturbance in acute hepatic failure (see below), also contributes to hypokalemia by shifting potassium intracellularly. Proposed guidelines (Greene and Scott, 1975) for administration of intravenous potassium chloride are as follows:

Serum Potassium (mEq/L)	mEq KCl Added to 250 ml Fluid*
<2.0	20
2.1–2.5	15
2.6–3.0	10
3.1–3.5	7

*Not to exceed 0.5 mEq/kg/hour.

The serum potassium concentration should be monitored every 24 to 48 hours and potassium supplementation adjusted accordingly.

Acute hepatic failure may be accompanied by disorders of acid-base balance (Twedt and Grauer, 1982). Respiratory alkalosis most commonly accompanies hepatic encephalopathy and has been attributed to direct stimulation of the respiratory center by toxins. Ammonia has been suspected, since the intravenous administration of ammonium acetate induces hyperammonemia and respiratory alkalosis in dogs (Roberts et al., 1956). In addition, metabolic alkalosis may be precipitated by excessive loss of hydrogen ion from the gastrointestinal tract (vomiting) or urinary tract (hyperaldosteronism) and by intracellular shifting of hydrogen ion as a result of hypokalemia. Alkalosis is particularly deleterious since it can potentiate signs of hepatic encephalopathy by converting ammonium ion to ammonia, which freely diffuses into cells. On the other hand, metabolic acidosis may develop when circulatory collapse and lactic acidosis complicate hepatic failure. When alkalosis or a normal acid-base status is present, fluids without alkali, such as 0.9 or 0.45 per cent saline or Ringer's solution, are indicated. Bicarbonate rather than lactate (e.g., lactated Ringer's solution) should be used for treatment of severe metabolic acidosis since the alkalinizing properties of lactate are dependent on its *in vivo* metabolism by the liver, and in liver failure, unmetabolized lactate may accumulate.

Hypoglycemia

Hypoglycemia may complicate liver failure and hepatic encephalopathy. It may be caused by impaired hepatic gluconeogenesis or endotoxemia. Dextrose should be added to the intravenous fluids to make a 2.5 to 5 per cent concentration, thus preventing hypoglycemia, providing caloric supplementation, and possibly increasing uptake of ammonia by glutamate. When hypoglycemia is detected, a solution of 50 per cent dextrose is infused slowly intravenously, to effect (about 1.0 mg/kg). Dextrose is then added to the intravenous fluids (5 per cent) to maintain normoglycemia.

Hepatic Encephalopathy

Hepatic encephalopathy (HE) is a syndrome of altered central nervous system (CNS) function resulting from hepatic insufficiency (Hardy, 1983; Schenker et al., 1974; Sherding, 1981). The precise cellular mechanisms responsible for HE remain unknown despite considerable research. Postulated mechanisms include interference with brain energy metabolism, disturbance of neuronal membrane function, and impaired synaptic transmission caused by a derangement in the balance of neurotransmitters. Of clinical importance is the concept that the principal lesion of HE is a biochemical and not a structural alteration in the CNS. Consequently, the clinical signs of HE are potentially reversible if hepatic function can be improved or if the metabolic imbalances or accumulation of toxins can be reversed.

Interactions between a variety of toxins and the metabolic imbalances of liver failure are probably responsible for the clinical manifestations of HE. Inadequate hepatic clearance of enteric toxins has long been suspected to cause HE. The clinical improvement observed in patients treated with intestinal antibiotics suggests that enteric bacteria do play a role in this syndrome. Potential toxins thought to originate from the gut include ammonia, mercaptans, short-chain fatty acids (SCFA), indoles, skatoles, biogenic amines, and γ-aminobutyric acid.

The toxin most frequently incriminated in HE is ammonia, which is generated by urease-producing colonic bacteria. The primary substrate is intestinal urea, although dietary amino acids also contribute to ammonia production. Normally, ammonia is absorbed into the portal blood and converted to urea in the liver by the Krebs-Henseleit urea cycle and is then excreted in the urine. In acute hepatic failure, impaired hepatic extraction or metabolism of ammonia results in excessive accumulation of ammonia in the blood, brain, and cerebrospinal fluid. However, plasma ammonia levels do not correlate well with the degree of encephalopathy, indicating that other factors may influence intracerebral ammonia concentrations, such as alkalosis and hypokalemia.

The basis of many of the recommendations for preventing and treating hepatic encephalopathy is directed toward eliminating protein, and thus indirectly, ammonia, from the system. Many factors can increase ammonia production in the gut; for example, high-protein diets, gastrointestinal hemorrhage, and constipation. Prevention and control of HE necessitates detection and treatment of these precipitating events. When HE accompanies acute hepatic failure, dietary protein is initially deleted from the diet. When signs of HE are absent, a diet restricted in protein (e.g., Prescription Diet k/d, Hill's Pet Products) is used. Since protein is required for hepatocellular regeneration, additional protein is introduced cautiously in the recovery phase of acute hepatic failure to a level that is well tolerated and does not precipitate signs of HE.

Hypovolemia should be detected and treated, since it causes azotemia and retention of nitrogenous wastes, precipitating hepatic decompensation. Moreover, the direct depressive effects of uremia on the cerebrum may potentiate signs of HE. Consequently, correction of volume deficits and maintenance of normal hydration will improve signs of HE. Bacterial infections are treated with appropriate antibiotic therapy, since infection has a catabolic effect and increases endogenous nitrogen load.

Dogs with liver disease should not be administered stored blood, which contains 170 μg of NH_3 per 100 ml after just 1 day, and the amount increases progressively with further storage.

The use of antibiotics (e.g., neomycin or metronidazole) is recommended to reduce the numbers of urea-splitting bacteria in the colon and thus inhibit ammonia production. The nonabsorbable, nonmetabolizable synthetic disaccharide lactulose is used to lower blood ammonia concentrations in HE. The means by which this is accomplished include (1) acidification of the colon with ionic trapping of ammonium, (2) catharsis, (3) alteration of colonic bacterial flora, and (4) increasing stool nitrogen content. Lactulose may also exert a beneficial antiendotoxin effect. Although objective data are lacking, orally administered lactulose, alone or in combination with neomycin, seems to be effective in dogs with HE. When severe dementia or coma precludes oral administration of neomycin and lactulose, these drugs can be administered as a retention enema.

Mercaptans are produced by bacterial degradation of dietary methionine and have also been implicated as toxins of encephalopathy. As with ammonia, inadequate hepatic clearance of mercaptans leads to excess plasma accumulation. Mercaptans can induce a reversible coma in dogs. Furthermore, the administration of methionine-containing lipotropic drugs has been associated with worsening of encephalopathy in dogs. Thus, methionine should not be empirically administered to dogs with severe liver disease, since this amino acid may potentiate the development of HE.

In addition to toxins of gut origin, imbalances of CNS neurotransmitters and their precursor amino acids have also been suspected to contribute to encephalopathy. Dogs with acute hepatic failure have increases of most plasma amino acids. This has been attributed to excessive hepatocellular release and impaired hepatic clearance. The ratio of branched-chain amino acids (BCAA) to aromatic amino acids (AAA) in normal dogs is 3:1 to 4:1, whereas ratios of 1:1 to 1.5:1 or less are detected in dogs with hepatic insufficiency. Alterations in amino acid ratios generally correlate with the degree of encephalopathy in dogs. Moreover, normalization of the amino acid ratio by administration of BCAA is associated with improvement of clinical signs in dogs with experimentally induced hepatic insufficiency. These derangements probably alter intracerebral amino acid metabolism and synthesis of neurotransmitters. Although these findings suggest that intravenous administration of tailored solutions of amino acids would be useful in the treatment of HE, the cost of these solutions precludes their clinical use at this time.

The inability of dogs with liver disease to tolerate

recommended doses of CNS-depressant drugs (i.e., tranquilizers, anticonvulsants, and anesthetics) may be attributed partly to impaired hepatic metabolism but also to increased "cerebral sensitivity" to such drugs. Increased cerebral sensitivity is more likely to occur with chronic hepatic failure; however, these drugs should be used cautiously in patients with acute hepatic failure, as they may potentiate signs of encephalopathy. When seizures cannot be controlled by the previously outlined methods for treatment of hepatic encephalopathy, intravenous diazepam or phenobarbital may be administered at reduced dosages.

Disorders of Hemostasis

Primary failure of hepatocytes to synthesize clotting factors must be differentiated from biliary obstruction causing impaired production of the vitamin K–dependent Factors II, VII, IX, and X. Administration of vitamin K_1 intramuscularly should correct the coagulopathy caused by biliary obstruction in 24 to 48 hours. A fresh blood or plasma transfusion may temporarily improve coagulopathies due to hepatocyte damage; however, the long-term prognosis is poor. If DIC is present, mini- or low-dose heparin therapy in conjunction with a blood or plasma transfusion may be attempted, but response to therapy is usually poor.

Gastrointestinal Bleeding

Gastric ulceration and bleeding may complicate hepatic disorders (Strombeck, 1979). The pathogenesis of gastric ulceration in liver disease is unknown but may involve elevated plasma gastrin concentrations with enhanced gastric acid secretion. Blood lost into the gastrointestinal tract is a substrate for ammonia production; thus there is potential for precipitation of encephalopathy. If gastric bleeding is suspected (hematemesis and melena or blood loss anemia with positive fecal occult blood), cimetidine therapy should be instituted to decrease gastric acidity and promote mucosal healing. Other causes of gastrointestinal bleeding, such as intestinal parasites (hookworms, whipworms) or coagulopathies, should be identified and treated if possible.

Endotoxemia

Impaired hepatic reticuloendothelial cell function may predispose the patient with liver disease to developing endotoxemia (Hardy, 1983). Removal of bacteria and endotoxins from the portal blood is a necessary hepatic function. Endotoxemia may in turn cause such extrahepatic signs of liver disease as hypergammaglobulinemia, hypoglycemia, renal vasoconstriction, acute tubular necrosis, DIC, fever, and myocardial depression. Furthermore, these toxins have been implicated in the pathogenesis of hepatocellular injury. Oral antibiotics or toxin-absorbing drugs such as cholestyramine have been recommended to decrease endotoxin production.

PROGNOSIS

The prognosis for recovery from acute hepatic failure is dependent on the severity of the insult and whether the inciting cause can be eliminated. The prognosis is poor when acute, widespread hepatic necrosis results in severe hepatic dysfunction (e.g., coagulopathy and HE). When milder degrees of hepatic damage occur, hepatocellular regeneration may result in complete recovery. Widespread hepatic necrosis that is not immediately fatal may eventually lead to postnecrotic cirrhosis characterized by collapse of necrotic lobules and severe hepatic fibrosis. Persistent hepatic inflammation may also lead to chronic hepatitis and subsequent cirrhosis. In order to detect persistent hepatic damage and progressive deterioration of hepatic function, serum enzymes and liver function tests should be evaluated at 2- to 3-week intervals for the next 2 months. If abnormalities persist after this period of time, a follow-up liver biopsy should be considered. Histologic evidence of chronic hepatitis may be an indication for corticosteroid therapy; however, it is not known whether this will prevent progression to cirrhosis.

References and Supplemental Reading

Badylak, S. F., and Van Vleet, J. F.: Alterations of prothrombin time and activated partial thromboplastin time in dogs with hepatic disease. Am. J. Vet. Res. 42:2053, 1981.

Greene, R. W., and Scott, R. C.: Lower urinary tract disease. *In* Ettinger, S. F. (ed.): *Textbook of Veterinary Internal Medicine.* Philadelphia: W. B. Saunders, 1975, p. 1572.

Hardy, R. M.: Diseases of the liver. *In* Ettinger, S. F. (ed.): *Textbook of Veterinary Internal Medicine: Diseases of the Dog and Cat,* 2nd ed. Philadelphia: W. B. Saunders, 1983, p. 1372.

Meyer, D. J.: The liver. I. Biochemical tests for the evaluation of the hepatobiliary system. Comp. Cont. Ed. Pract. Vet. 4:663, 1982.

Nyland, T. G., and Gillett, N. A.: Sonographic evaluation of experimental bile duct ligation in the dog. Vet. Radiol. 23:252, 1982.

Nyland, T. G.,and Park, R. D.: Hepatic ultrasonography in the dog. Vet. Radiol. 24:74, 1983.

Roberts, K. E., Thompson, F. G., Poppell, J. W., et al.: Respiratory alkalosis accompanying ammonium toxicity. J. Appl. Physiol. 9:367, 1956.

Schenker, S., Breen, K. J., and Anastacio, M. H., Jr.: Hepatic encephalopathy: Current status. Gastroenterology 66:121, 1974.

Sherding, R. G.: Hepatic encephalopathy in the dog. Comp. Cont. Ed. Pract. Vet. 3:55, 1981.

Strombeck, D. R.: *Small Animal Gastroenterology.* Davis, CA: Stonegate Publishing, 1979.

Twedt, D. C., and Grauer, G. F.: Fluid therapy for gastrointestinal, pancreatic, and hepatic disorders. Vet. Clin. North Am. 12:463, 1982.

Section 11

ENDOCRINE AND METABOLIC DISORDERS

MARK E. PETERSON, D.V.M.
Consulting Editor

***Additional Pertinent Information Found in* Current Veterinary Therapy VIII:**

Chew, D. J., and Meuten, D. J.: Primary Hyperparathyroidism, p. 880.
Mulnix, J. A.: Diabetes Insipidus, p. 850.

***Additional Pertinent Information Found in* Current Veterinary Therapy VII:**

Andersen, G. L., and Lewis, L. D.: Obesity, p. 1034.
Martin, S. L., and Capen, C. C.: Puerperal Tetany, p. 1027.
Schwartz-Porsche, D.: Diabetes Insipidus, p. 1005.

PRINCIPLES OF GLUCOCORTICOID THERAPY IN NONENDOCRINE DISEASE

ROBERT J. KEMPPAINEN, D.V.M.
Auburn, Alabama

Glucocorticoids are undoubtedly one of the most commonly used group of drugs in veterinary medicine. Their popularity can be attributed to the fact that they are capable of influencing virtually all body tissues and that they are potent inhibitors of the inflammatory, allergic, and immune responses frequently encountered in the clinical setting. The temporary use of glucocorticoids, usually in conjunction with other therapeutic measures, plays an important role in effective control of many disease conditions. However, unwarranted and injudicious use of these drugs may be associated with myriad side effects that can prove more deleterious to the patient than the primary disease process. The following discussion of the physiology and pharmacology of glucocorticoids presents an attempt to provide guidelines for their use in clinical veterinary medicine.

PHYSIOLOGY OF GLUCOCORTICOIDS

Control of Secretion

The inner two zones of the adrenal cortex are the principal sources of the endogenous glucocorticoids, hydrocortisone (cortisol) and corticosterone. In dogs and cats, cortisol is the predominant glucocorticoid. Control of both the synthesis and release of glucocorticoids depends on the release of an anterior pituitary protein hormone, adrenocorticotropin (ACTH) (Fig. 1). ACTH also has a vital role in maintaining the responsiveness of the adrenal cortex. If ACTH is removed from the system, the adrenal gland will rapidly lose the ability to respond to ACTH. If the deprivation continues, the glucocorticoid-secreting zones of the cortex will atrophy. The production and release of ACTH appear to depend in large part on the positive influences of a protein from the hypothalamus, corticotropin-releasing factor (CRF). This substance, isolated and characterized in 1981, has been synthetically produced and is currently being examined as a diagnostic tool in human medicine. The neurons producing and releasing CRF receive input from humoral and neural sources, which provide a balance of stimulatory and inhibitory influences. This system can respond extremely rapidly to stressful events (hemorrhage or surgery, for example) by increasing CRF output and thus ACTH and cortisol levels (as much as 5- to 10-fold increase) in minutes.

Cortisol levels in blood follow quite closely the pattern of pituitary ACTH secretion (Fig. 2). Release of these two hormones occurs in a dynamic or episodic fashion—dogs in one study averaged about 10 episodes of ACTH and cortisol secretion during the day (Kemppainen and Sartin, 1984). The rapidly changing nature of the normal hormonal profile demonstrates one reason why measurement of baseline levels of these hormones often provides little useful information in evaluation of pituitary-adrenocortical function. It is estimated that a dog normally secretes approximately 1.0 mg/kg/day of cortisol from the adrenal glands. Although it has often been stated that dogs have a circadian or diurnal rhythm in the pattern of pituitary-adrenocortical activity,

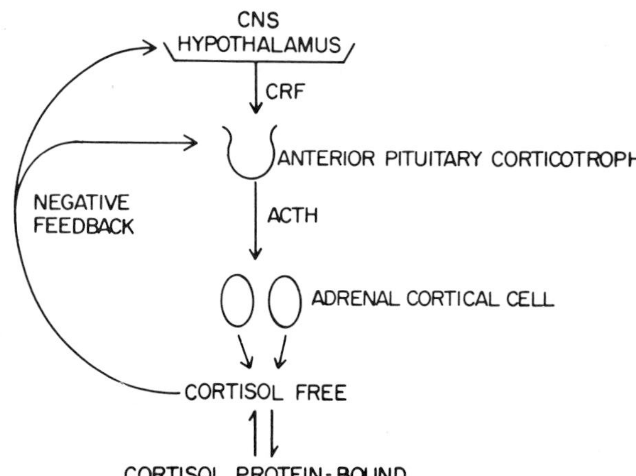

Figure 1. The hypothalamic-pituitary-adrenocortical (HPA) axis. CNS, central nervous system; CRF, corticotropin-releasing factor; ACTH, adrenocorticotropin. (From Kemppainen: Vet. Clin. North Am. 14:721, 1984, with permission.)

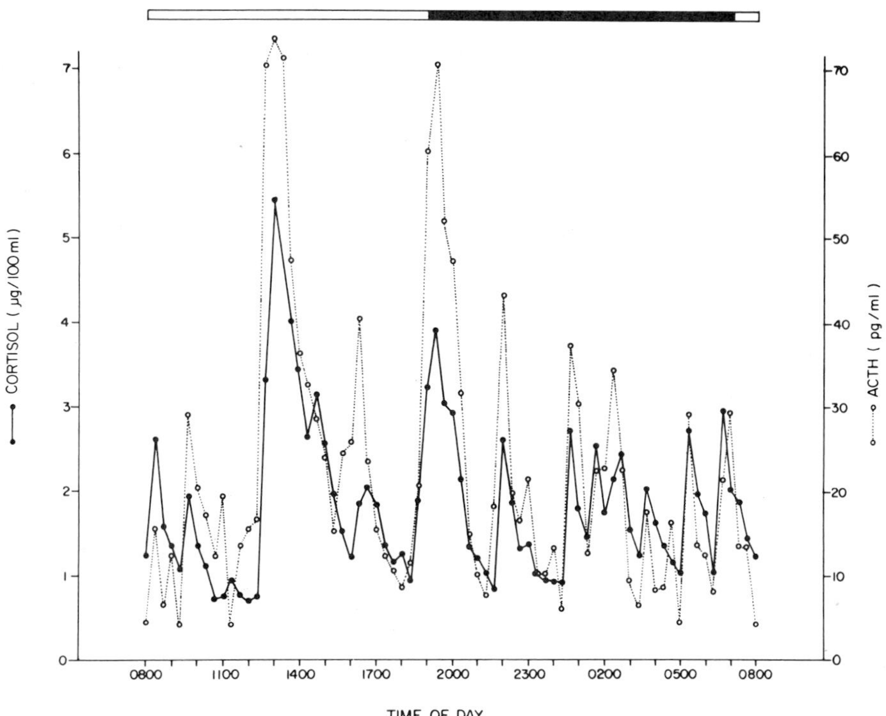

Figure 2. Plasma levels of cortisol and ACTH determined in samples obtained through a venous cannula from a dog at 20-minute intervals throughout the day. Note the episodic pattern of secretion and the close correlation in the levels of the two hormones. The dark bar shows the period of darkness. (From Kemppainen and Sartin: J. Endocrinol. 103:219, 1984, with permission.)

several studies have been unable to document this, and it appears that dogs either lack or have only a very subtle rhythm.

Much of the endogenous glucocorticoid released by the adrenal gland circulates bound to transport proteins, whereas a small fraction circulates unbound or free (Fig. 1). It is this free portion that is considered available for cellular entry and thus able to mediate biologic effects. As levels of glucocorticoids in circulation increase, a negative feedback effect is exerted at the hypothalamic-pituitary level. This results in a decline in ACTH secretion and consequently a fall in cortisol levels (Fig. 1). Recent research has shown that this negative feedback action is a complex process, involving two temporally distinct signals. A rapid-onset, rate-sensitive type of feedback occurs when blood levels of glucocorticoids are increasing, whereas a slower-onset, dose-sensitive feedback occurs later and inhibits ACTH release for variable periods depending on the type and amount of glucocorticoid reaching the hypothalamic-pituitary unit. Exogenously administered glucocorticoids are effective at activating these negative feedback signals, and the magnitude and duration of this feedback inhibition varies with the agent used, the dose, and the frequency and route of administration. Continued use of exogenous glucocorticoids will therefore result in a variable activation of the dose-sensitive feedback system, resulting in a reduction in ACTH and cortisol secretion and a decline in adrenocortical responsiveness to ACTH (hypothalamic-pituitary-adrenocortical [HPA] axis suppression).

The HPA axis described above serves to secrete metabolically important glucocorticoids under basal or resting conditions and is also capable of rapidly increasing cortisol secretion in response to a variety of physical or psychologic stresses. It should be noted that this system plays only a minor role in the control of the release of the mineralocorticoid hormones (principally aldosterone) from the outermost zone of the adrenal cortex. Instead, mineralocorticoid secretion is primarily controlled by the renin-angiotensin system and plasma potassium concentrations. Consequently, long-term glucocorticoid therapy resulting in even severe HPA suppression (and possibly clinical signs of secondary adrenocortical insufficiency) is not accompanied by alterations in plasma electrolyte concentrations.

Mechanism of Action

Glucocorticoids are thought to participate in the physiologic regulation of most body tissues. The principal mode for their mechanism of action is via specific receptor proteins in the cytoplasm of responsive cells. The unbound glucocorticoid is readily able to penetrate the cell membrane and bind to the receptor, and this binding directs the hormone-receptor complex to move to the nucleus. In the nucleus, the receptor complex attaches to the chromatin and activates the transcription process of DNA into messenger RNA formation. The messenger RNA is then translated into a new protein (e.g., enzyme) on ribosomes in the cytoplasm. Although it is likely that some of the effects of glucocorticoids occur without the need for cellular entry, it is generally held that most metabolic effects occur by nuclear activation of protein synthesis.

The scheme described above allows for the possible explanation of clinically relevant events observed when animals are treated with glucocorticoid hormones. First, it is known that an administered dose of a glucocorticoid may influence a biologic process for a time greater than the plasma life of the hormone. Activation of protein synthesis in responsive cells may continue for a time after the glucocorticoid leaves the cell; also, newly formed proteins may have relatively prolonged metabolic half-lives. Alterations in receptor numbers would be postulated to have a marked effect on the response to glucocorticoid therapy. In humans, certain patients showing an abnormal resistance to glucocorticoid treatment have been found to have low numbers of or biochemical defects in their glucocorticoid receptors. The phenomenon of steroid tachyphylaxis, in which an initial favorable response to a glucocorticoid wanes, may in part be explained on the basis of changing receptor number or activity.

PHYSIOLOGIC AND PHARMACOLOGIC EFFECTS OF GLUCOCORTICOIDS

Glucocorticoids were first employed to a large extent in medicine in the 1950s because of their ability to ameliorate the clinical signs of rheumatoid arthritis. Today, they continue to enjoy widespread use in the treatment of disorders or conditions in which inflammation or immune phenomena play a central role. Although the exact nature of the beneficial effects of glucocorticoids in reducing the inflammatory response is unknown, it appears that these drugs influence this process in a number of ways: reducing the accumulation and action of phagocytes at the inflamed site, maintaining capillary integrity, stabilizing lysosomal membranes, inhibiting the formation of vasoactive substances (e.g., kinins, prostaglandins), and, later, causing a decrease in collagen production and fibrous scar formation. Glucocorticoids are nonspecific in their anti-inflammatory effects; therefore, use of these agents may mask the clinical signs of bacterial, viral, fungal, or parasitic diseases or potentiate the spread of these diseases. The antagonistic actions of glucocorticoids in immune-mediated responses also appear to be multifold in nature, by the inhibition of factors such as the processing of antigens and the proliferation and differentiation of immune-competent cells. The administration of glucocorticoids is associated with a decline in lymphocyte numbers, and thymus-derived (T) cells are apparently more sensitive than bone marrow–derived (B) cells. In large doses, glucocorticoids are effective inhibitors of cell-mediated immune processes, as evidenced by their usefulness in the treatment of organ transplant rejection. Antibody production, particularly during anamnestic responses, is relatively resistant to glucocorticoid inhibition. Instead, the actions of glucocorticoids in suppressing antibody-mediated disease are likely through indirect effects on the inflammatory response subsequent to antigen-antibody formation.

As is obvious from their name, glucocorticoids modify the metabolism of glucose, generally favoring the sparing of glucose at the expense of protein and fat. The acute administration of a glucocorticoid is followed by the inhibition of glucose uptake in tissues such as skin and fat and the enhanced breakdown of protein in these tissues and muscle, resulting in increased levels of amino acid precursors for hepatic gluconeogenesis. Fat breakdown is also enhanced, leading to increases in plasma free fatty acids and glycerol, the latter also used as a gluconeogenic substrate. In the liver, glucocorticoids stimulate gluconeogenic capacity and glycogen formation both by increasing the levels of necessary precursors and by enhancing the levels and activity of key enzymes involved in the biochemical processes. After longer periods of glucocorticoid exposure, pancreatic insulin secretion increases to counter many of the catabolic and antianabolic actions of glucocorticoids. Therefore, under conditions of exogenous or endogenous glucocorticoid excess, insulin levels are generally elevated and glucose tolerance is often reduced. The redistribution of fat observed in animals exposed to long-term glucocorticoid excess may be a result of regional differences in the adipose tissue response to elevations in insulin and glucocorticoid levels.

Many other alterations in body tissues have been associated with glucocorticoid administration, and the number and magnitude of these effects increase directly with the dose, potency, and duration of glucocorticoid treatment. Table 1 lists some of the reported side effects of glucocorticoids, with particular emphasis on changes noted in dogs. Cats are apparently more resistant to development of many of these side effects than are dogs. It should be noted that a considerable amount of individual variation in the appearance of these side effects is not uncommon.

GLUCOCORTICOID PHARMACOLOGY

Most commonly used glucocorticoids are synthetic derivatives of the cortisol molecule with

Table 1. *Reported Side Effects of Glucocorticoid Treatment in Dogs*

Blood and blood chemistry	
Increases in:	Decreases in:
Neutrophils	*Eosinophils
Erythrocytes	Lymphocytes
Monocytes	Blood urea nitrogen
Platelets	
*Alkaline phosphatase	
Cholesterol	
Glucose	
Alanine aminotransferase	
Central nervous system	
Behavioral and mood changes (depression, increased irritability)	
Lethargy	
Panting	
Endocrine	
Iatrogenic Cushing's disease, *HPA suppression, secondary adrenocortical insufficiency	
Reduced thyroid hormone (T_4 and T_3) levels	
Reduced gonadotropin and sex steroid levels	
Anestrus, testicular atrophy, reduced libido	
Elevated insulin levels, carbohydrate intolerance	
Reduced vitamin D levels	
Elevated parathyroid hormone levels	
Gastrointestinal	
*Polyphagia	Hepatomegaly
Anorexia (rare)	Hepatopathy
Diarrhea (may be bloody)	Pancreatitis
	Colonic perforation
Increased gastric acid secretion	
Kidney	
*Polyuria with secondary polydipsia	
Increased urinary calcium excretion	
Musculoskeletal	
Muscle atrophy	
Weakness, exercise intolerance	
Myotonia (rare)	
Osteoporosis	
Skin	
Calcinosis cutis	
Thin skin	
Bilateral hair loss	
Increased bruising	
Other	
Increased risk of infection	
Enhanced spread of infection	
Poor wound healing	
Redistribution of body fat	
Reduced growth	

*Relatively common findings

chemical modifications that enhance the anti-inflammatory potency while reducing the less desirable mineralocorticoid (sodium retention) effects. Fortunately, excessive sodium retention and potassium excretion are relatively uncommon side effects of glucocorticoids in dogs and cats. Increasing in parallel with increased anti-inflammatory potency, however, are undesirable effects such as the ability to suppress the activity of the HPA axis or to elicit other catabolic side effects listed in Table 1. Part of the increased potency of the synthetic glucocorticoids is due to a reduced degree of plasma protein binding (greater percentage of free hormone), slower metabolic clearance rate, and probably enhanced interaction with the cytoplasmic receptor in responsive cells. Table 2 lists some of the glucocorticoids in common use in veterinary medicine.

Of major chemical importance in maintaining glucocorticoid activity is a hydroxyl group on carbon 11 of the steroid ring. Two agents, cortisone and prednisone, do not possess this structure and must be converted to their active metabolites, cortisol and prednisolone, respectively, before they become active. This conversion largely occurs in the liver. Therefore, these precursor glucocorticoids are unwise choices for therapy in patients with compromised hepatic function and also are of questionable value in local therapy such as topical, intra-articular, or intralesional administration.

A variety of chemical compounds have been linked to the parent glucocorticoid molecule to alter characteristics such as solubility and rate of absorption. These constituents are always separated from the base glucocorticoid before cellular entry and initiation of the physiologic event. The combination of a glucocorticoid with a water-soluble acid such as phosphoric or succinic results in a compound with greater aqueous solubility, an increased rate of absorption from injection sites, and an enhanced rate of distribution to tissues and often allows for intravenous administration. In contrast, the addition of an acetate or acetonide ester to a glucocorticoid base reduces aqueous solubility, slowing absorption from injection sites and allowing for a prolonged release effect. The more lipid-soluble compounds (such as acetate esters) also penetrate certain tissues

Table 2. *Comparison of the Biologic Potency and Duration of Action of Commonly Used Glucocorticoids*

Duration of Action of Base	Relative Potency (mg)	Equivalent Anti-inflammatory Potency* (mg)
Short		
Not suited for alternate-day use:		
Hydrocortisone (cortisol)	1.0	20
Cortisone	0.8	25
Suited for alternate-day use:		
Prednisone	4.0	5
Prednisolone	4.0	5
Methylprednisolone	5.0	4
Intermediate		
Triamcinolone	5.0	4
Long		
Flumethasone	15.0	1.5
Betamethasone	25.0	0.6
Dexamethasone	30.0	0.75

*Approximates the duration of HPA suppression, although longer-acting glucocorticoids tend to cause disproportionately longer periods of HPA suppression.

such as the cornea better than aqueous soluble forms. Other ester forms, particularly acetonide and valerate, apparently enhance the topical activity of certain glucocorticoid compounds (triamcinolone acetonide, betamethasone-17-valerate, fluocinolone acetonide) possibly by sequestering the glucocorticoid in the affected skin tissue.

THERAPEUTIC USES OF GLUCOCORTICOIDS

Glucocorticoids as therapeutic agents are unparalleled in their range of use in veterinary medicine. Major uses are to suppress inflammation in various tissues and in the treatment of the different forms of shock and trauma. Table 3 lists a number of nonendocrine diseases and conditions for which glucocorticoids are used in small animal medicine.

It is important to realize that considerable individual variation exists in the clinical responses to glucocorticoids. For this reason, the type, dose, and duration of glucocorticoid therapy must be tailored to the needs of each patient. Of course, fundamental goals in the proper use of glucocorticoids are to use the lowest dose for the shortest possible time that allows for adequate control of the clinical signs. Alternative forms of therapy (e.g., nonsteroidal anti-inflammatory drugs, hyposensitization of the allergic patient) should always be considered before or during the use of glucocorticoids, for they may permit a reduction in dose or even discontinuance of the drug. Glucocorticoid treatment should not be used as a substitute for establishing a diagnosis.

Table 3. *Examples of Nonendocrine Conditions in Small Animals Treated, at Least in Part, with Glucocorticoids*

System	Condition
Hemolymphatic	Immune-mediated hemolytic anemia
	Lymphosarcoma
	Thrombocytopenia
Musculoskeletal	Polyarthritis (nonseptic)
	Polymyositis
Nervous	Edema
	Trauma
	Tumors
	Vestibular disorders
Ophthalmic	Blepharitis
	Conjunctivitis
	Keratitis
	Pannus
	Uveitis
Pulmonary	Inhalation injury
Skin	Allergic dermatitis (atopy, contact, parasitic)
	Feline eosinophilic granuloma complex
	Immune-mediated dermatitis (pemphigus complex)
	Pyotraumatic dermatitis
	Seborrheic dermatitis
Multisystemic	Heat stroke
	Shock
	Systemic lupus erythematosus

FORMS OF GLUCOCORTICOID THERAPY

Local

In certain situations, the delivery and maintenance of relatively high concentrations of glucocorticoids at a restricted area proves effective in therapy and reduces the systemic side effects. Examples include topical administration of betamethasone-17-valerate to treat acute contact dermatitis, intralesional (or sublesional) injection of triamcinolone acetonide to treat a mast cell tumor, or application of a dexamethasone phosphate solution to treat nonulcerative keratitis. To maximize the effects of topically (skin) applied glucocorticoids, it is often necessary to clip the hair in and around the affected area and apply the glucocorticoid frequently (two to four times per day). Occlusive dressings (such as a plastic wrap) offer a very effective method to increase skin penetration but are difficult to maintain in many instances. Although the more potent glucocorticoids (betamethasone, triamcinolone, dexamethasone) are recommended for topical use in the acute phases of a condition, less potent agents such as cortisol (hydrocortisone) are recommended when chronic topical use is desired. Systemic effects from the local application of glucocorticoids cannot be discounted, particularly when the agents are used frequently, when the area of application is large, when the integrity of the treated area is compromised, or when potent agents are used. Other situations in which systemic effects are likely occur when the patient ingests the glucocorticoid or when repeated intralesional injections are administered.

Short-Term Systemic Therapy

Glucocorticoids are often used in moderate to high doses for short periods (generally less than 72 hours) for the treatment of a variety of acute conditions such as shock, brain and spinal cord trauma, and inhalation injury. The more aqueous soluble preparations (succinates, phosphates) are compatible with intravenous administration and, at least theoretically, are more rapidly distributed to cellular sites than less aqueous soluble forms (such as dexamethasone in polyethylene glycol). The efficacy of high-dose glucocorticoid therapy in conditions such as hypovolemic shock or brain edema following trauma has not been clearly documented. However, the clinical impression from use of these drugs in most circumstances is positive. All studies demonstrating beneficial effects of glucocorticoids in these acute crisis situations show that the drugs must be given as early as possible after the insult and in high doses, which often need to be repeated (every 4 to 12 hours). Glucocorticoids are of benefit in these instances when used as supportive treatment with the documented, specific forms of therapy (e.g., fluid therapy in hypovolemic shock).

Examples of glucocorticoid doses recommended as adjunctive therapy for various forms of shock are as follows: dexamethasone sodium phosphate, 4 to 6 mg/kg; prednisolone or methylprednisolone sodium succinate, 30 to 35 mg/kg; and hydrocortisone sodium succinate, 150 mg/kg (Haskins, 1983). Fortunately, side effects from such high-dose short-term therapy appear minimal, although colonic perforation and death were reportedly associated with large-dose dexamethasone therapy in four dachshunds with neurologic disease (Toombs et al., 1980). There is little risk of prolonged suppression of the HPA axis when even large doses of glucocorticoids are given for short periods, and it appears that there is little need to taper the dose when treatment is terminated.

Long-Term Systemic Therapy

Glucocorticoids are clearly capable of improving the clinical signs in a variety of conditions that require relatively long-term (weeks to months) treatment. Before instituting glucocorticoids in these cases, certain questions should be addressed: What is the likelihood that this treatment may produce side effects that are more deleterious than the disease itself? Are there alternative types of treatment that provide a reasonable chance for control of the disease? If the decision is made to use glucocorticoids, several recommendations can be given concerning longer periods of use. First, although higher doses and more frequent administration of glucocorticoids are often necessary to control the initial stages of many inflammatory processes, maintenance of remission often is attained by considerably lower levels of the drugs. Second, oral administration of glucocorticoids provides a considerable advantage to parenterally administered treatment, since the dose can more easily be adjusted or altered quickly if adverse reactions occur. Alternate-day treatment is the best method to reduce the development of adverse side effects (including HPA suppression) and should be attempted whenever courses of therapy with a duration of over 2 weeks are anticipated (Chastain and Graham, 1979). Finally, long courses of glucocorticoid therapy will inevitably cause some biochemical and morphologic changes, which will vary among individuals. HPA suppression is one of the most common side effects that should be suspected and monitored in any dog receiving long-term glucocorticoid treatment.

Because of the variability in diseases and in the response of individual animals to glucocorticoids, it is impossible to give exact guidelines for dosages of these drugs in clinical situations. Immunologic-based disorders often require two to four times as much glucocorticoid as compared with purely inflammatory-based conditions to initially suppress the acute phase and to maintain remission. Table 4 describes *approximate* guidelines for initial and maintenance glucocorticoid therapy in a dog treated for an inflammatory condition. If the initial glucocorticoid treatment is rapidly effective in suppressing the clinical signs, conversion to alternate-day therapy may begin more quickly without the need to consolidate the dose to once every morning. Cats require approximately double the initial and maintenance doses of glucorticoids needed for dogs (Scott, 1980). The short-acting glucocorticoids, prednisone, prednisolone, and methylprednisolone (Table 2) are best suited to alternate-day therapy because of the duration of their biologic and HPA suppressive effects. Even if "equivalent" doses (Table 2) of intermediate (triamcinolone) or long-acting (dexamethasone) glucocorticoids are substituted for these agents in alternate-day treatment, the chances of development of side effects, including profound HPA suppression, are markedly increased. However, certain patients requiring long courses of steroids become refractory to the "standard" glucocorticoids, and it may be necessary to use one of the more potent, long-acting drugs to control their disease. Data from humans indicate that the HPA suppressive effect of glucocorticoids can be minimized by administering the drugs in the morning hours, at a time coincident with the greatest level of HPA activity. In dogs, evidence of such a circadian rhythm in the HPA axis is scant; however, until studies are conducted in dogs comparing the HPA suppressive effects of glucocorticoids administered at different times of the day, morning administration is still recommended. In cats, a circadian rhythm in HPA activity opposite to that in humans or dogs has been reported (Scott, 1980). Based on these findings, it has been recommended to administer oral glucocorticoids to cats in the evening or on alternate evenings. However, until more studies

Table 4. *Guidelines for Initial and Maintenance Glucocorticoid Therapy in a Dog with an Inflammatory Condition*

1. Suppress the active inflammatory process using 1 to 2 mg/kg/day of prednisone, prednisolone, or methylprednisolone divided b.i.d. or t.i.d. for 5 to 10 days.
2. After suppressing the clinical signs, consolidate the dose to 1 to 2 mg/kg given once a day between 7 and 10 A.M. Continue for 1 week, then reduce dose to 0.5 to 1.0 mg/kg/day once per day for 5 to 7 days.
3. Convert to alternate-day therapy by giving 1 to 2 mg/kg on alternate mornings.
4. Reduce dose by half each week until a minimally effective dose is reached.

document the existence of such a rhythm or demonstrate the benefits of nighttime glucocorticoid treatment in cats, the exact value of such a practice is unknown.

Parenterally administered depot forms of glucocorticoids are attractive from a clinical standpoint because they negate the need for client administration of medication and reputedly provide for a prolonged duration of action. When compared with orally administered forms, however, these depot agents provide less daily glucocorticoid activity with a more profound HPA suppression. Dogs given a single intramuscular dose of methylprednisolone acetate (2.5 mg/kg) showed evidence of HPA suppression for at least 5 weeks, whereas a single dose of triamcinolone acetonide (0.22 mg/kg) suppressed the axis for approximately 4 weeks (Kemppainen et al., 1981, 1982). Adverse reactions developing after administration of these long-acting agents are obviously more difficult to control than those occurring during treatment with orally administered glucocorticoids. Although single doses of these agents are unlikely to alter the health of an individual dog, they should not be employed repeatedly for long-term treatment. Repeated use, particularly if administered more frequently than once every 6 weeks, will likely result in profound HPA suppression and possibly iatrogenic Cushing's disease. Methylprednisolone acetate is an effective glucocorticoid for a variety of conditions in cats (dose of 5.5 mg/kg; Scott, 1980), and this species is relatively resistant to development of severe systemic side effects.

The goal for every patient on long-term glucocorticoid treatment should be to find the lowest dose that need be administered at the least frequent interval to effectively control clinical signs. In most patients, the drugs can be discontinued after the causative factor is brought under control from other types of therapy or if the factor is temporary in nature (e.g., atopy). Termination of glucocorticoid therapy is generally associated with few problems in dogs. Possible complications, however, are remission of the underlying disease process, the "steroid withdrawal syndrome," or iatrogenic secondary adrenocortical insufficiency. If clinical signs of the original condition reappear after terminating glucocorticoid therapy, it is often necessary to increase the dose and frequency of drug treatment to again induce remission of the disorder and then begin the tapering process at a slower rate. A steroid withdrawal syndrome has been documented in humans taken off long-term glucocorticoid therapy, and these patients exhibit signs such as lethargy, weakness, anorexia, nausea, and fever but show normal function of the HPA axis. It is possible that their tissues became adapted to the higher levels of glucocorticoids and the decline associated with termination of treatment triggered the onset of their symptoms. Although a similar syndrome has not been documented in dogs, it is likely that it occurs. Treatment would require institution of daily low (physiologic) doses of a short-acting glucocorticoid, such as hydrocortisone, with a gradual tapering. Iatrogenic secondary adrenocortical insufficiency occurs in association with HPA suppression, and animals exhibit signs such as lethargy, depression, anorexia, or acute circulatory collapse after sudden withdrawal from glucocorticoid treatment or after exposure to an acutely stressful event.

IATROGENIC SECONDARY ADRENOCORTICAL INSUFFICIENCY AND HPA SUPPRESSION

Although HPA suppression is one of the most common sequelae to glucocorticoid therapy, most affected dogs show no clinical abnormalities. However, clinical cases of dogs with documented HPA suppression have been reported, showing the clinical signs of adrenocortical insufficiency described above. Figure 3 shows a photomicrograph of the adrenal cortices from both a healthy dog and a dog given four injections of methylprednisolone acetate at weekly intervals. The atrophied adrenocortical tissue in the glucocorticoid-treated dog correlated with the total absence of a response of plasma cortisol to ACTH stimulation and a failure to elicit a cortisol increase after a moderate hemorrhage, in contrast to that of the healthy dog. Coincident with the lack of a cortisol response to the hemorrhage stimulus was a reduced ability to restore circulating blood volume. This demonstrates one potential role of the "stress" response of the HPA axis and the possible consequences of HPA inactivity subsequent to long-term glucocorticoid treatment.

Probably the best method to detect and monitor HPA suppression in the canine or feline patient is to use the ACTH stimulation test. Examples of the progression of responses to ACTH stimulation that may be observed in an animal before, during, and after glucocorticoid therapy are shown in Figure 4. The baseline cortisol level must be compared with the post-ACTH level, since some glucocorticoids (i.e., hydrocortisone, cortisone, prednisone, prednisolone) cross-react in many assays measuring cortisol. Such interference would falsely elevate the baseline level of cortisol, but the post-ACTH level would show little increase if HPA suppression were present. It is best to stop glucocorticoid therapy at least 48 hours before performing ACTH stimulation testing to minimize these influences. It has also been reported that animals recovering from glucocorticoid therapy may exhibit an abnormal (reduced) response to low-dose dexamethasone suppression testing (Stolp and Meijer, 1983).

No currently available forms of treatment will

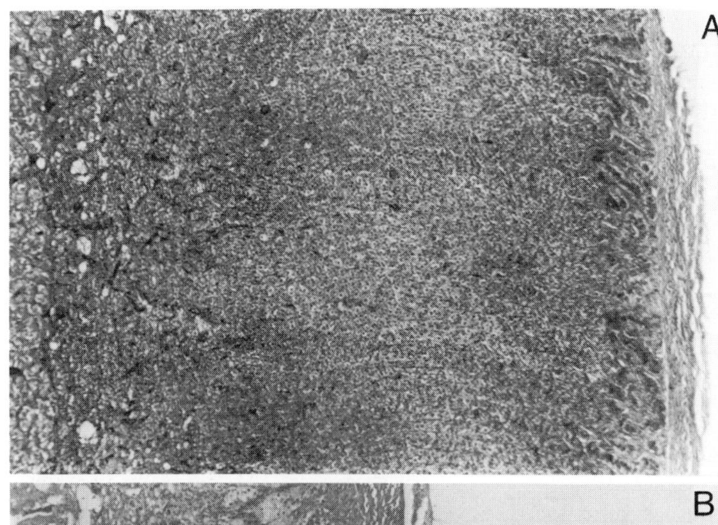

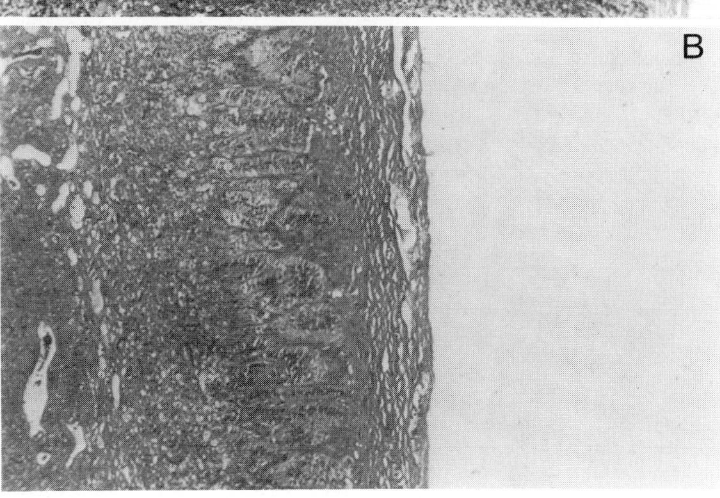

Figure 3. Cross-section of normal (*A*) and atrophied (*B*) canine adrenocortical tissue. The atrophy resulted from four injections of methylprednisolone acetate (2.5 mg/kg, IM) given at weekly intervals.

hasten the return of function in cases of HPA suppression. ACTH therapy will restore adrenal responsiveness, but since the origin of inhibition is in the anterior pituitary and higher brain centers, ACTH therapy may actually hinder recovery by providing continued activation of negative feedback. Fortunately, dogs appear to regain HPA function faster than humans, who may require as long as a year to regain activity after prolonged glucocorticoid treatment. Animals exhibiting mild to moderate signs of glucocorticoid deficiency should be given low, physiologic doses of a short-acting glucocorticoid (prednisolone or prednisone, 0.2 mg/kg every other day; hydrocortisone or cortisone, 0.2 to 0.5 mg/kg every day), and the adrenal responsiveness to ACTH should be monitored at 4- to 6-week intervals until both baseline and post-ACTH cortisol levels are within normal limits. These patients, as well as those exhibiting no clinical signs of glucocorticoid deficiency but having HPA suppression, should be given higher doses of glucocorticoids (hydrocortisone sodium succinate, 4 to 5 mg/kg; dexamethasone, 0.1 to 0.2 mg/kg; prednisolone sodium succinate, 1.0 to 2.0 mg/kg) just before and after stressful events such as major surgery, and lower doses should be continued at least until the third postoperative day (Peterson et al., 1984). Clients should also have access to an aqueous-soluble form of a glucocorticoid (such as hydrocortisone sodium phosphate or methylprednisolone sodium succinate), which can be administered to the patient if a sudden episode of collapse occurs.

CONCLUSIONS

The supportive use of glucocorticoids in the treatment of a variety of common conditions in veterinary medicine is well justified. Use of these drugs, however, cannot serve as a substitute for an accurate diagnosis. General guidelines to follow while using glucocorticoids are to administer the lowest effective doses for the shortest allowable times and to use alternate-day therapy if longer periods of treatment are anticipated. Especially in patients on long-term therapy, careful biochemical and physical monitoring at periodic intervals is necessary to avoid potentially serious side effects. It is advisable for clinicians to become more familiar with the actions of a few glucocorticoid agents and to initiate their use in

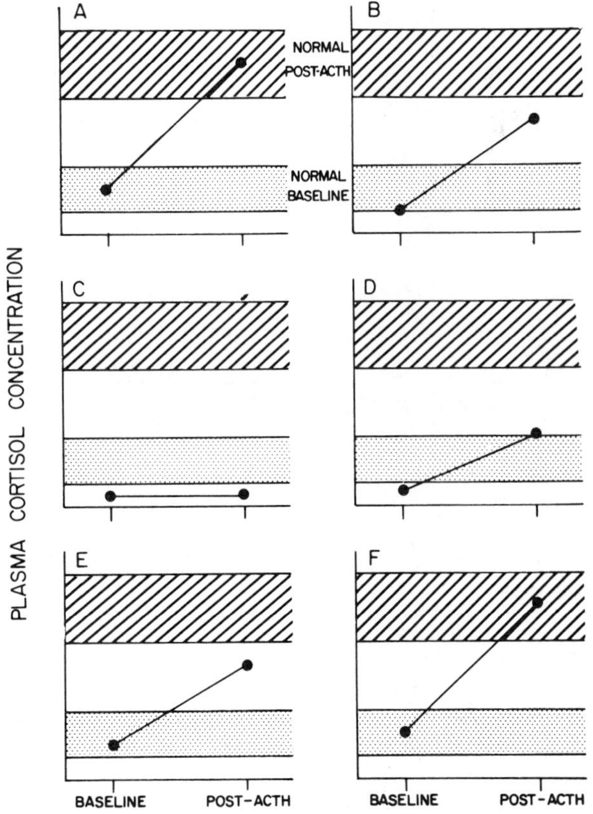

Figure 4. Patterns of baseline and post-ACTH stimulated plasma cortisol levels in a dog before, during, and after relative long-term glucocorticoid therapy. *A*, Normal response to ACTH stimulation. *B* and *C*, Glucocorticoid therapy is ongoing; early loss of adrenocortical response to ACTH (*B*) is observed as low to normal baseline levels fail to reach the normal post-ACTH range. As treatment continues, both baseline and post-ACTH levels may decline to below the normal baseline range (*C*). *D* and *E*, Glucocorticoid therapy is discontinued, and adrenocortical responsiveness returns. Generally, baseline levels of cortisol return to normal range before post-ACTH concentrations. *F*, Eventual recovery to normal response.

most patients requiring glucocorticoid treatment. Side effects accompanying glucocorticoid therapy are directly related to potency, dose, and duration of use; however, individual variation in the development of adverse effects is not uncommon.

References and Supplemental Reading

Azarnoff, D. L. (ed.): *Steroid Therapy*. Philadelphia: W. B. Saunders, 1975.

Baxter, J. D., and Forsham, P. H.: Tissue effects of glucocorticoids. Am. J. Med. 53:573, 1972.

Chastain, C. B., and Graham, C. L.: Adrenocortical suppression in dogs on daily and alternate-day prednisone administration. Am. J. Vet. Res. 40:936, 1979.

Fauci, A. S.: Glucocorticosteroid therapy. *In* Wyngaarden, J. B., and Smith, L. H. (eds.): *Textbook of Medicine*. Philadelphia: W.B. Saunders, 1982, pp. 86–91.

Haskins, S. C.: Shock (The pathophysiology and management of the circulatory collapse states). *In* Kirk, R. W. (ed.): *Current Veterinary Therapy VIII*. Philadelphia: W. B. Saunders, 1983, pp. 2–27.

Keller-Wood, M. E., and Dallman, M. F.: Corticosteroid inhibition of ACTH secretion. Endocr. Rev. 5:1, 1984.

Kemppainen, R. J., Lorenz, M. D., and Thompson, F. N.: Adrenocortical suppression in the dog after a single dose of methylprednisolone acetate. Am. J. Vet. Res. 42:822, 1981.

Kemppainen, R. J., Lorenz, M. D., and Thompson, F. N.: Adrenocortical suppression in the dog given a single intramuscular dose of prednisone or triamcinolone acetonide. Am. J. Vet. Res. 43:204, 1982.

Kemppainen, R. J., and Sartin, J. L.: Evidence for episodic but not circadian activity in plasma concentrations of adrenocorticotrophin, cortisol and thyroxine in dogs. J. Endocrinol. 103:219, 1984.

Melby, J. C.: Clinical pharmacology of systemic corticosteroids. Ann. Rev. Pharmacol. Toxicol. 17:511, 1977.

Peterson, M. E., Birchard, S. J., and Mehlhaff, C. J.: Anesthetic and surgical management of endocrine disorders. Vet. Clin. North Am. 14:911, 1984.

Rosenthal, R. C., and Wilcke, J. R.: Glucocorticoid therapy. *In* Kirk, R. W. (ed.): *Current Veterinary Therapy VIII*. Philadelphia: W. B. Saunders, 1983, pp. 854–863.

Scott, D. W.: Feline dermatology 1900–1978: A monograph. J. Am. Anim. Hosp. Assoc. 16:331, 1980.

Scott, D. W.: Dermatologic uses of glucocorticoids: Systemic and topical. Vet. Clin. North Am. 12:19, 1982.

Stolp, R., and Meijer, J. C.: Differential diagnosis and laboratory evaluation of hyperadrenocorticism in dogs. Proc. Kal Kan Symposium for the Treatment of Small Animal Diseases, 1983, pp. 9–14.

Toombs, J. P., Caywood, D. D., Lipowitz, A. J., et al.: Colonic perforation following neurosurgical procedures and corticosteroid therapy in four dogs. J.A.V.M.A. 177:68, 1980.

CANINE HYPERADRENOCORTICISM

MARK E. PETERSON, D.V.M.
New York, New York

Spontaneous canine hyperadrenocorticism (Cushing's syndrome) is a disorder caused by the excessive production of cortisol by the adrenal cortex. In 85 to 90 per cent of dogs, the underlying cause of the sustained hypercortisolism is the excessive secretion of adrenocorticotropic hormone (ACTH) by the pituitary gland, which results in bilateral adrenocortical hyperplasia (pituitary-dependent hyperadrenocorticism, or PDH). In the remaining dogs, unilateral tumors of the adrenal cortex that secrete cortisol independent of endogenous ACTH control are responsible for cortisol overproduction.

CLINICAL FEATURES

AGE, BREED, AND SEX. Spontaneous canine hyperadrenocorticism usually develops in middle-aged to old dogs; however, PDH may occur in dogs as young as 1 year. PDH develops most frequently in poodles, dachshunds, and boxers but can affect any breed. Although no breed predilection occurs in dogs with functional adrenal tumors, larger breeds are affected more frequently than the toy breeds. Both sexes are affected equally in dogs with PDH, whereas 70 to 75 per cent of dogs with adrenal tumors are female.

CLINICAL SIGNS. Table 1 lists the common clinical and historic signs observed in dogs with naturally occurring hyperadrenocorticism. Because of the multisystemic effects of long-term glucocorticoid excess, dogs with hyperadrenocorticism usually develop clinical signs that reflect dysfunction of many organ systems. In many dogs, however, one clinical sign (e.g., polyuria, lethargy, or hair loss) may predominate, making the clinical diagnosis of hyperadrenocorticism more difficult. In addition to cortisol excess, the compressive effects of a pituitary or adrenal neoplasm (and its metastases) may also contribute to the clinical signs seen in some dogs with hyperadrenocorticism.

The clinical manifestations of canine hyperadrenocorticism may be mild to severe and can be modified by the duration and cause of the disorder. The course of hyperadrenocorticism is usually insidious and slowly progressive; in a few of these dogs with mild disease, clinical signs may be intermittent with periods of remission and relapse. Other dogs, however, especially those with adrenocortical carcinoma, may have a rapid onset and progression of disease; many of these dogs fail to develop the prominent dermatologic signs commonly observed in hyperadrenocorticism.

ROUTINE LABORATORY FINDINGS

COMPLETE BLOOD COUNT. The hemogram may show mature leukocytosis, eosinopenia, and lymphopenia; however, these findings are inconsistent. The most common hematologic abnormality in canine hyperadrenocorticism is absolute eosinopenia, which occurs in about 80 per cent of cases. Dogs with hyperadrenocorticism frequently have high normal values of hemoglobin, packed cell volume

Table 1. *Incidence of Historic and Clinical Signs of Naturally Occurring Canine Hyperadrenocorticism*

Sign	Approximate Percentage of Cases
Polyuria and polydipsia	85
Pendulous abdomen	70
Hepatomegaly	70
Hair loss	65
Lethargy	60
Polyphagia	60
Muscle weakness	60
Anestrus	55
Obesity	50
Muscle atrophy	35
Comedones	35
Increased panting	30
Testicular atrophy	30
Hyperpigmentation	20
Calcinosis cutis	10
Facial nerve palsy	5

(PCV), and erythrocyte count; mild to moderate erythrocytosis (PCV = 52 to 65 per cent) develops in about 15 per cent of dogs.

SERUM BIOCHEMICAL TESTS. The most common serum biochemical abnormality in dogs with hyperadrenocorticism is an elevation in the concentration of alkaline phosphatase. Such increases are caused by glucocorticoid induction of a specific hepatic isoenzyme of alkaline phosphatase. Other findings may include mild to marked elevations in serum cholesterol, alanine aminotransferase, glucose, and total carbon dioxide.

URINALYSIS. In dogs with marked polyuria and polydipsia, the urine specific gravity may be very low (less than 1.010). These dogs, however, usually have the ability for urinary concentration when deprived of water. Bacteriuria, hematuria, and urine sediment changes compatible with a urinary tract infection are also common findings in dogs with hyperadrenocorticism.

EVALUATION OF PITUITARY-ADRENOCORTICAL FUNCTION

Once hyperadrenocorticism is suspected (based on clinical signs and routine laboratory findings), additional laboratory investigations should proceed through two stages. The objective of the first or "screening" stage is to confirm (or rule out) the diagnosis of hyperadrenocorticism. Once the diagnosis is confirmed, the second stage is to differentiate PDH from that caused by an adrenal tumor. Figure 1 shows a flow sheet of diagnostic tests useful in evaluating dogs with suspected hyperadrenocorticism.

Tests to Diagnose Hyperadrenocorticism

RESTING CORTISOL CONCENTRATIONS

Single basal plasma or serum cortisol determinations are of little diagnostic value in distinguishing normal dogs from those with hyperadrenocorticism. When several basal cortisol samples are collected throughout the day, average cortisol concentrations in dogs with hyperadrenocorticism are higher than normal; however, about half of dogs with hyperadrenocorticism have random cortisol values that lie within the normal range.

In both normal dogs and dogs with hyperadrenocorticism, bursts of cortisol secretion (episodic secretion) occur throughout the day, with frequent fluctuations in circulating cortisol concentrations. Such episodic secretion results in a pattern of peaks and troughs of cortisol concentration; peak cortisol levels may be five to six times higher than the lowest concentrations. Although the amplitude of these cortisol peaks in dogs with hyperadrenocorticism is higher than normal, peak concentrations in normal dogs frequently will overlap with the trough levels in dogs with hyperadrenocorticism. Hyperadrenocorticism is difficult to diagnose accurately based on single basal cortisol concentrations because of these fluctuating and overlapping values.

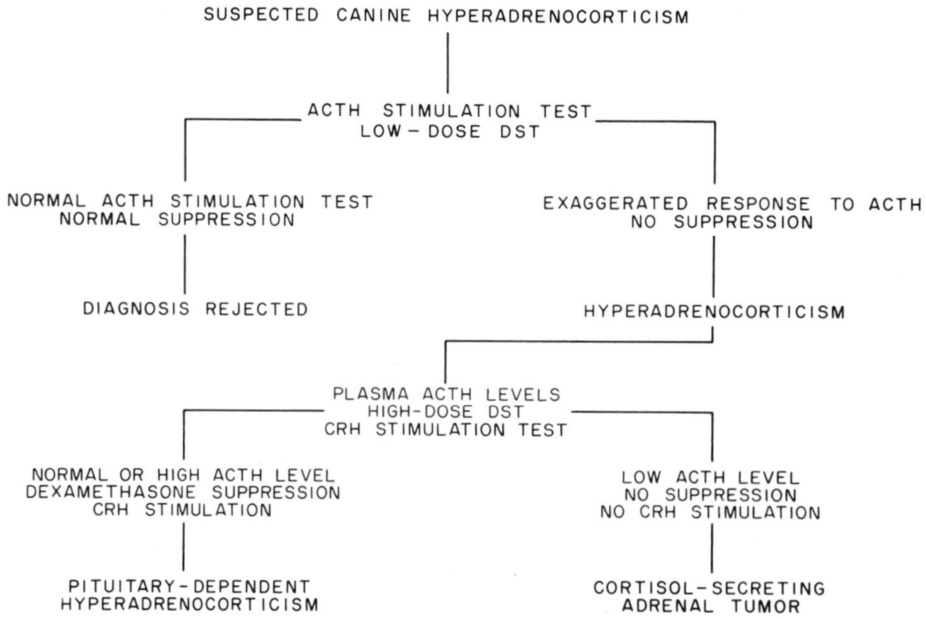

Figure 1. Flowchart for evaluation of dogs with suspected hyperadrenocorticism. DST = dexamethasone suppression test; CRH = corticotrophin-releasing hormone.

ACTH STIMULATION TEST

A useful test for diagnosing hyperadrenocorticism is the ACTH stimulation test. Several ACTH preparations are available, and many regimens for ACTH stimulation testing have been described. One method is to collect plasma or serum samples for cortisol determination before and 2 hours after intramuscular administration of ACTH gel (20 U). With this regimen, maximum rise in cortisol concentrations occurs 2 hours after administration of ACTH; cortisol concentrations usually return to basal levels within 10 hours of injection.

Post-ACTH cortisol concentrations in normal dogs are at least two to three times higher than basal levels. Results of an ACTH stimulation test are diagnostic for hyperadrenocorticism when the post-ACTH cortisol concentration exceeds the upper limit of normal, indicating a greater than normal adrenal response. Approximately 85 per cent of dogs with PDH have an excessive response to ACTH stimulation. Over half of dogs with adrenocortical tumors hyperrespond; of these, dogs with adrenal carcinoma tend to hyperrespond more frequently and have higher responses than do dogs with adenomas.

The ACTH stimulation test is a valuable screening test for canine hyperadrenocorticism because it tests the functional capacity of the adrenal glands to secrete cortisol. The ACTH stimulation test is, however, limited in its usefulness. If hyperadrenocorticism is suspected clinically, the diagnosis should not be excluded based on normal ACTH stimulation test results, since many dogs with adrenal tumors respond normally to ACTH stimulation. The test is also limited because it cannot be used to reliably distinguish PDH from hyperadrenocorticism caused by adrenal tumors, since the majority of dogs with PDH and approximately half of dogs with functional adrenocortical tumors have an exaggerated response.

LOW-DOSE DEXAMETHASONE SUPPRESSION TEST

An excellent test for diagnosing canine hyperadrenocorticism is the low-dose dexamethasone suppression test. In normal dogs, pituitary ACTH secretion is regulated by the central nervous system (CNS). Neurotransmitters such as serotonin, dopamine, and norepinephrine direct the hypothalamus to produce corticotropin-releasing hormone (CRH), which travels to the pars distalis via the hypophyseal portal system and stimulates ACTH secretion. The canine pituitary pars intermedia also secretes ACTH, but unlike the pars distalis is avascular and is controlled by serotonergic and dopaminergic fibers from the brain. Pituitary ACTH is the major regulator of cortisol secretion. Normally, rising circulating cortisol concentrations decrease secretion of ACTH through CNS and pituitary negative feedback inhibition; as ACTH secretion decreases, cortisol secretion also decreases and physiologic levels of circulating cortisol are maintained. Potent synthetic analogues of cortisol such as dexamethasone also inhibit pituitary ACTH release through negative feedback inhibition. In hyperadrenocorticism, the pituitary-adrenal axis controlling ACTH and cortisol secretion is abnormally resistant to suppression by dexamethasone.

The recommended protocol for the low-dose dexamethasone suppression test is to collect a baseline morning plasma or serum sample for cortisol determination, administer dexamethasone (0.015 mg/kg IM or IV), and collect additional samples 2, 4, 6, and 8 hours after injection. Others have suggested a similar sampling protocol but using a slightly smaller dose of dexamethasone (0.010 mg/kg IV). With either regimen, the samples drawn 4 and 8 hours after dexamethasone injection are most important for interpretation of the test.

In normal dogs, the low dose of dexamethasone consistently suppresses cortisol concentration to less than 1.0 μg/dl for the 8-hour test period, whereas dogs with PDH and adrenal tumors are resistant to suppression with this dose. Figure 2 shows the five patterns of cortisol responses that are seen in dogs with hyperadrenocorticism. No cortisol suppression occurs in most dogs with adrenal tumors and in 25 per cent of those with PDH (Fig. 2*A*). In other dogs with either adrenal tumors or PDH, 50 per cent suppression of baseline cortisol concentrations occurs during the testing period, but all cortisol values remain greater than 1.0 μg/dl (Fig. 2*B* and *C*); in dogs that have partial suppression 2 to 6 hours after injection, cortisol again increases to presuppression levels by the eighth hour (Fig. 2*C*). In about a third of dogs with PDH, cortisol is suppressed to normal concentrations 2 to 4 hours after injection, but escape from suppression occurs at the sixth to eighth hour, with cortisol rising to the presuppression level (Fig. 2*D*). With this pattern, further testing to define the cause of hyperadrenocorticism (see below) is unnecessary since it is diagnostic of PDH. Finally, in a few dogs with early, mild PDH, normal cortisol suppression is observed (Fig. 2*E*); these dogs usually develop abnormal test results when retested 2 to 4 months later.

It can be difficult to diagnose hyperadrenocorticism in dogs with concurrent diabetes mellitus on clinical grounds alone, since many clinical signs (polyuria, polydipsia, polyphagia, and hepatomegaly) are common to both disorders. Underlying hyperadrenocorticism should be suspected in any diabetic dog that has or develops hair loss, abdominal distension, calcinosis cutis, or other clinical signs suggestive of glucocorticoid excess. In many diabetic dogs with untreated hyperadrenocorticism,

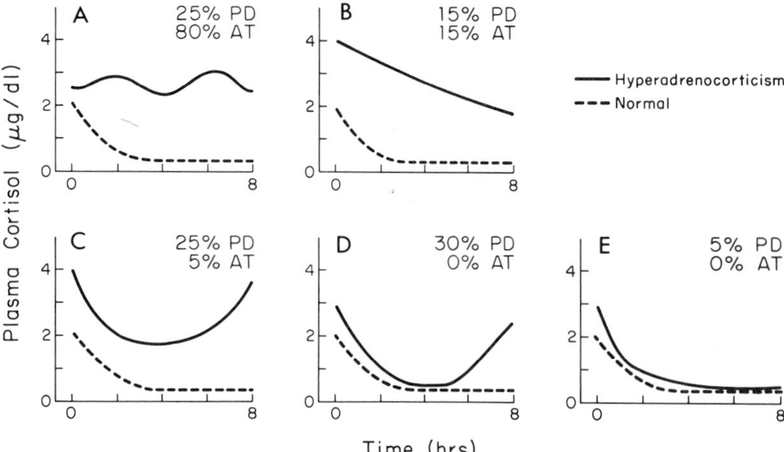

Figure 2. Patterns of plasma cortisol responses during low-dose dexamethasone testing in normal dogs and dogs with hyperadrenocorticism. PD = pituitary-dependent hyperadrenocorticism; AT = adrenal tumor.

resistance to the glucose-lowering effects of exogenous insulin therapy also develops; concurrent hyperadrenocorticism should be excluded in any diabetic dog that has sustained hyperglycemia and glycosuria despite high daily insulin doses (greater than 2.2 U/kg). In the diabetic dog with suspected hyperadrenocorticism, however, caution must be used when interpreting the results of ACTH stimulation and low-dose dexamethasone suppression tests, since the "stress" associated with poorly controlled diabetes mellitus alone could produce false-positive test results. Dogs with diabetes should not be evaluated for hyperadrenocorticism with these testing procedures until azotemia and ketoacidosis have resolved and diabetic control with insulin has stabilized. In general, the low-dose dexamethasone suppression test is the preferred screening test in these dogs, since many diabetic dogs *without* concomitant hyperadrenocorticism will show slightly exaggerated cortisol responses with ACTH stimulation testing. It is imperative, however, to monitor serial blood glucose concentrations during low-dose dexamethasone suppression testing, especially in dogs receiving high daily insulin doses, which may produce hypoglycemia with rebound hyperglycemia (the Somogyi overswing effect) (see the article on Canine Diabetes Mellitus). Hypoglycemia is a potent stimulus of ACTH and cortisol secretion. If low blood glucose concentrations (less than 65 mg/dl) develop during the low-dose dexamethasone suppression test, the stimulatory effects of hypoglycemia may override the suppressive effects of dexamethasone to produce a false-positive test result for hyperadrenocorticism. In general, if only slightly abnormal test results suggestive of hyperadrenocorticism are obtained, it is usually wise to withhold treatment for hyperadrenocorticism and reconfirm the abnormal test results 1 to 3 months later to prevent unnecessary and potentially dangerous treatments.

Tests to Differentiate the Cause of Hyperadrenocorticism

HIGH-DOSE DEXAMETHASONE SUPPRESSION TEST

A useful test to determine the cause of canine hyperadrenocorticism is the high-dose dexamethasone suppression test. The low-dose dexamethasone suppression test, discussed earlier, is a screening test for hyperadrenocorticism; the low dose of dexamethasone suppresses ACTH and subsequently cortisol in normal dogs but does not adequately suppress cortisol secretion in dogs with either PDH or functional adrenal tumors. In dogs with functional adrenal tumors, dexamethasone, no matter how high the dosage, will not adequately suppress cortisol levels, because ACTH secretion has been suppressed by high circulating concentrations of cortisol from the tumor. In PDH, the threshold for glucocorticoid negative feedback of ACTH is higher than normal. ACTH secretion is relatively resistant to glucocorticoid suppression, but high doses of dexamethasone can suppress ACTH secretion in dogs with PDH.

The recommended protocol for the high-dose dexamethasone suppression test is to collect samples for plasma or serum cortisol assay before and 2, 4, 6, and 8 hours after administration of dexamethasone (1.0 mg/kg IV or IM). Although others have suggested using a similar protocol with a dexamethasone dose of 0.1 mg/kg, we have found this smaller dose to be less reliable in suppressing cortisol secretion in dogs with PDH.

Regarding interpretation of the results of a high-dose dexamethasone suppression test, it has been suggested that 50 per cent suppression of baseline cortisol concentration is diagnostic for PDH. We have found this criterion to be unreliable, however, since 50 per cent suppression occasionally occurs in dogs with adrenal tumors (see below). In our laboratory, we have established that suppression of cortisol concentration below 1.5 μg/dl is diagnostic for PDH, whereas cortisol values remain above 1.5 μg/dl at all sampling times in dogs with adrenal tumors (Fig. 3). This cortisol value, however, may not necessarily be the same for other cortisol radioimmunoassays, and similar criteria for suppression must be established in each individual laboratory.

Four patterns of cortisol responses are seen with the high-dose dexamethasone suppression test in dogs with hyperadrenocorticism (Fig. 3). In most dogs with PDH, cortisol concentrations are suppressed diagnostically (Fig. 3*A*); in these dogs, the 6- and 8-hour samples are most important for the interpretation of the test because suppression is greatest at these times. In a few dogs with PDH, cortisol is suppressed at 2 to 4 hours after injection but rises to presuppression levels by the eighth hour (Fig. 3*B*). Although the test reveals PDH reliably in most cases, adequate cortisol suppression does not occur in approximately 15 per cent of dogs with PDH (Figs. 3*C* and *D*). In some of these dogs, adequate cortisol suppression occurs with a higher dose of dexamethasone, but in other dogs suppression may not occur even with dexamethasone doses as high as 2.0 mg/kg. In the majority of dogs with adrenal tumors, no cortisol suppression occurs (Fig. 3*D*). About 20 per cent of dogs with adrenal tumors, however, show a 50 per cent decrease in basal cortisol concentrations (Fig. 3*C*), but all values remain above those considered adequate for suppression (1.5 μg/dl).

The major limitation of the high-dose dexamethasone suppression test is its inability to differentiate dogs with adrenal tumors from the 15 per cent of dogs with PDH that do not demonstrate adequate cortisol suppression. Therefore, before surgical exploration of the adrenal glands is performed in these dogs, additional testing procedures such as determination of endogenous ACTH (see below) should be undertaken. Alternatively, if additional testing cannot be performed, the results of short-term treatment with *o,p'*-DDD can also be used to aid in diagnosis. In most dogs with nonsuppressible PDH, loading therapy with *o,p'*-DDD (see Treatment, below) effectively reduces both basal and post-ACTH cortisol concentrations to low or normal resting levels; in contrast, administration of usual loading doses of *o,p'*-DDD has little to no effect on adrenal reserve in most dogs with functional adrenal tumors.

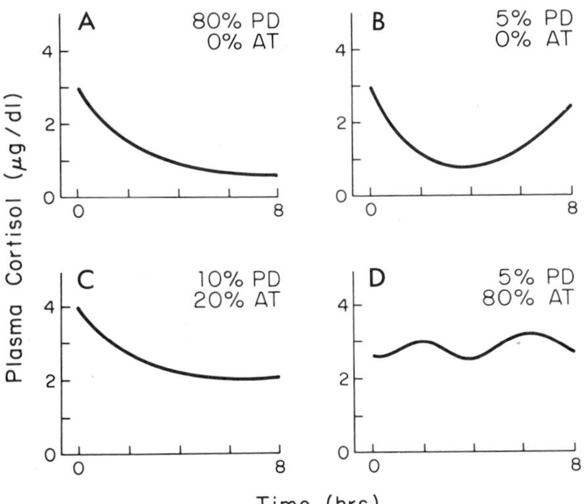

Figure 3. Patterns of plasma cortisol responses during high-dose dexamethasone suppression testing in dogs with hyperadrenocorticism. PD = pituitary-dependent hyperadrenocorticism; AT = adrenal tumor.

PLASMA ACTH DETERMINATIONS

Endogenous plasma ACTH concentrations are extremely useful in determining the cause of canine hyperadrenocorticism, especially when interpreted together with the results of a high-dose dexamethasone suppression test. Plasma ACTH concentrations are normal to elevated in dogs with PDH and are low to low-normal in dogs with adrenocortical tumors. Determination of single basal plasma ACTH concentrations is not useful as a screening test for hyperadrenocorticism because, like cortisol, ACTH is secreted episodically with overlapping values in normal dogs and those with hyperadrenocorticism.

The normal to high plasma ACTH concentrations in dogs with PDH indicate secretion of inappropriate and excessive amounts of ACTH by a pituitary tumor or a defect in the CNS negative feedback mechanism. Low to undetectable concentrations of ACTH in dogs with adrenal tumors reflect normal negative feedback control of pituitary ACTH secretion; high circulating cortisol concentrations suppress ACTH secretion through the negative feedback system to low or undetectable levels.

Accurate determination of plasma ACTH requires proper collection and handling of the specimen and a carefully performed, difficult radioimmunoassay technique. ACTH is unstable in unfrozen plasma and can be inactivated at room temperature. Therefore, for reliable results, blood for ACTH assay should be collected in either heparin- or EDTA-containing tubes that are filled to the full draw of the Vacutainer (Becton, Dickinson) volume. If the Vacutainer tubes are inadequately filled, the resulting relative excess of anticoagulant per volume of plasma might interfere with the ACTH assay and produce spurious results. After collection, the blood should be spun *immediately* for 10 to 15 minutes (ideally at 4°C). The plasma (at least 1.0 ml is required for assay) should then be promptly separated into plastic or polypropylene tubes and kept frozen until assayed. Because plasma ACTH assays are technically difficult to perform, many commercial laboratories may be unable to provide dependable results. Therefore, we strongly recommend use of a veterinary laboratory that offers a reliable, validated assay for canine ACTH (Kemppainen and Sartin, 1984).* Again, because ACTH is unstable in unfrozen plasma, it is imperative that the samples be packed with adequate quantities of dry ice in a Styrofoam container and be sent by air express to ensure reliable results.

CRH STIMULATION TEST

CRH is a 41–amino acid polypeptide produced in the hypothalamus that modulates the secretion of ACTH by the pituitary gland. The recent isolation and synthesis of CRH offers an additional diagnostic test to differentiate the two causes of canine hyperadrenocorticism. In normal dogs, administration of ovine CRH (1.0 μg/kg IV) produces significant elevations of the plasma concentrations of both ACTH and cortisol, with peak levels occurring by 15 to 30 minutes after injection. Similarly, dogs with PDH respond to CRH injection with prompt increases in both plasma ACTH and cortisol concentrations. In contrast, no rise in the circulating concentrations of either ACTH or cortisol occurs in dogs with adrenal tumors following a single-bolus injection of CRH because pituitary ACTH secretion has been chronically suppressed. Therefore, using plasma cortisol determinations alone, the CRH stimulation test appears to clearly differentiate PDH from hyperadrenocorticism caused by adrenal tumors in most dogs.

The advantage of the CRH stimulation test in determining the cause of hyperadrenocorticism is that the test can be completed over a period of 1 to 2 hours and that only four to six cortisol determinations are needed for diagnostic interpretation. Although CRH is available commercially as a powder preparation (Bachem), it is expensive and must be dissolved, sterilized, lyophilized, and finally aliquoted into sterile vials before injection. Therefore, until a relatively inexpensive, single-dose, sterilized CRH preparation becomes available, the CRH stimulation test appears to be of limited usefulness for most veterinarians.

TREATMENT

The cause of hyperadrenocorticism determines treatment. PDH can be treated surgically with bilateral adrenalectomy or hypophysectomy, or it can be managed medically with the adrenocorticolytic agent *o,p'*-DDD. Unilateral adrenocortical tumors should be surgically removed, especially since about half are carcinomas that will metastasize unless resected. Regardless of the treatment method chosen, canine hyperadrenocorticism cannot be treated easily, inexpensively, or without close monitoring and follow-up. Without treatment, hyperadrenocorticism is usually a progressive disorder with an unfavorable prognosis. In some dogs with PDH, however, the disease may be relatively mild in severity and be very slowly progressive; observation alone may be best for these dogs.

Pituitary-Dependent Hyperadrenocorticism

PDH can be treated with either bilateral adrenalectomy or hypophysectomy; both require a skilled surgeon, intensive monitoring during and after surgery, and lifelong hormone replacement therapy. Surgical techniques and management are described in *Current Veterinary Therapy VII* (Lubberink, 1980).

PDH can also be managed with drugs that act on the pituitary gland and CNS (cyproheptadine [Periactin, Merck, Sharp & Dohme] and bromocriptine [Parlodel, Sandoz]), or directly on the adrenal cortex (*o,p'*-DDD [Lysodren, Bristol]). Cyproheptadine and bromocriptine lower plasma ACTH concentrations and produce remission in some dogs with PDH; however, because of their frequent side effects and infrequent success, these drugs appear to have limited usefulness in the management of canine PDH.

The drug most frequently used in the treatment of canine PDH is *o,p'*-DDD. It decreases cortisol production by selective necrosis and atrophy of the adrenocortical zona fasciculata and zona reticularis. Because the zona glomerulosa (arcuosa) is relatively resistant to the cytotoxic effects of *o,p'*-DDD, normal secretion of aldosterone is usually maintained. Initial dosage of *o,p'*-DDD is 30 to 50 mg/kg daily for 10 days; glucocorticoid supplementation with oral prednisone (0.2 mg/kg/day), prednisolone (0.2 mg/kg/day), or cortisone (1.0 mg/kg/day) reduces many side effects associated with acute glucocorticoid withdrawal in the initial phase. In dogs with concomitant diabetes mellitus that develop exogenous insulin resistance (daily insulin requirements greater than 2.2 U/kg), treatment with *o,p'*-DDD removes the cause of insulin resistance (i.e., cortisol excess) and reduces the daily insulin requirement. A serious complication associated with the standard *o,p'*-DDD loading protocol in these diabetic dogs, however, may be a rapid decrease in daily insulin requirements, predisposing to insulin overdosage and hypoglycemia. Use of a lower initial dose of *o,p'*-DDD (25 mg/kg/day) and a higher daily main-

---

*Endocrine Diagnostic Laboratory, Department of Physiology and Pharmacology, School of Veterinary Medicine, Auburn University, AL 36849.

tenance dose of prednisone (0.4 mg/kg), prednisolone (0.4 mg/kg), or cortisone (2 mg/kg) prevents the rapid reductions in circulating glucocorticoid levels and daily insulin requirements and allows for easier regulation of the diabetic state. With adequate instruction, most owners can manage this treatment successfully at home.

The most common side effects observed during initial *o,p'*-DDD therapy include lethargy, vomiting, weakness, anorexia, and diarrhea. About 25 per cent of dogs develop one or more side effects during initial *o,p'*-DDD treatment, but they are relatively mild in most dogs. Adverse signs develop when plasma cortisol concentrations either decrease below normal resting range (less than 1.0 μg/dl) or drop too rapidly into normal range (glucocorticoid withdrawal syndrome) and resolve promptly with increased glucocorticoid supplementation. If adverse signs occur during initial *o,p'*-DDD treatment, the drug should be stopped and the glucocorticoid dosage doubled until the dog can be evaluated. If clinical signs persist longer than 3 hours after increasing the glucocorticoid dosage, other medical problems should be considered (Fig. 4).

All dogs should be evaluated after the *o,p'*-DDD induction period. In general, most dogs are stronger and more active; signs of polyuria and polydipsia will have usually decreased in severity but may not completely resolve during initial *o,p'*-DDD treatment because of renal medullary washout. There are many means of assessing the effectiveness of *o,p'*-DDD therapy, including measurement of daily water consumption and eosinophil and lymphocyte cell counts. All of these measurements can be misleading since they only indirectly reflect circulating cortisol concentrations. A more direct approach to determine the effectiveness of *o,p'*-DDD is to perform an ACTH stimulation test (Fig. 4). Since prednisone, prednisolone, and cortisone all cross-react in most cortisol assays and falsely elevate the measurement of endogenous cortisol concentration, glucocorticoid supplementation should not be given on the morning of ACTH stimulation testing. During *o,p'*-DDD therapy, decrease in circulating cortisol concentration results in loss of negative feedback inhibition of pituitary ACTH secretion; therefore, the normal to elevated endogenous plasma ACTH concentrations found in untreated dogs with PDH rise to even higher levels (Fig. 5). Unless adrenocortical reserve is decreased below normal, such elevated plasma ACTH concentrations still cause resting plasma cortisol concentrations to rise above normal range at frequent intervals throughout the day. To ensure adequate control of hyperadrenocorticism with *o,p'*-DDD both basal and post-ACTH cortisol concentrations should remain within normal resting range (Fig. 5). Following *o,p'*-DDD induction therapy and ACTH stimulation testing, it is wise to withhold *o,p'*-DDD and to continue daily glucocorticoid supplementation until cortisol results are available (Fig. 4).

Initial daily *o,p'*-DDD treatment decreases both resting and post-ACTH plasma cortisol concentra-

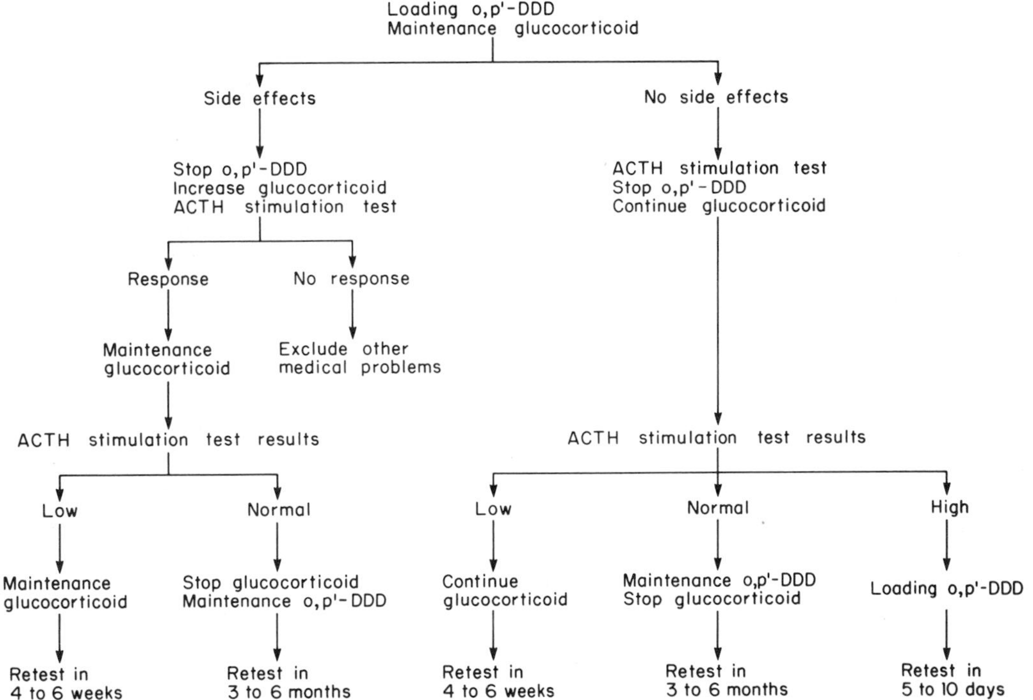

Figure 4. Flowchart for management of dogs with pituitary-dependent hyperadrenocorticism after initial *o, p'*-DDD treatment.

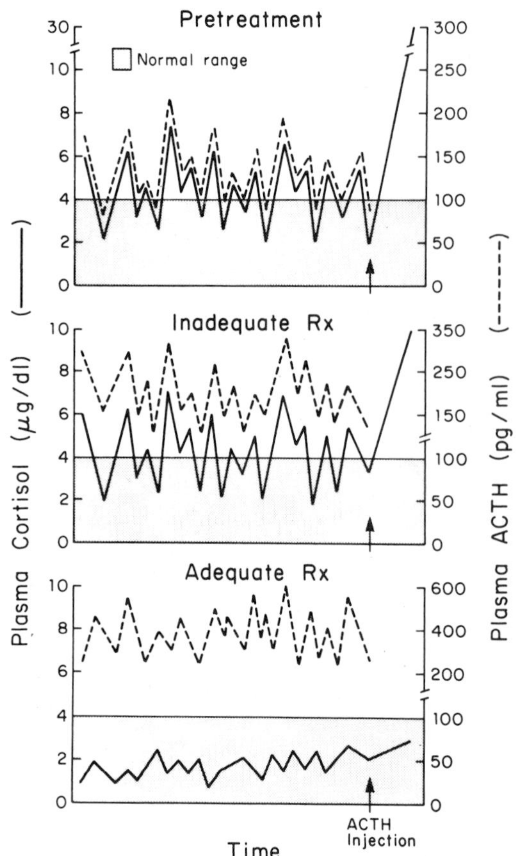

Figure 5. Concentrations of plasma ACTH and cortisol in canine pituitary-dependent hyperadrenocorticism, before and after treatment with *o, p'*-DDD. Before treatment (top panel), both ACTH and cortisol are secreted in a pattern of peaks and troughs, with frequent fluctuations above normal range throughout the day. During therapy with *o, p'*-DDD, decreased cortisol secretion results in loss of negative feedback inhibition of pituitary ACTH secretion; therefore, ACTH concentrations rise to extremely high levels. Unless adrenocortical reserve is decreased below normal (adequate treatment, bottom panel) with both basal and post-ACTH cortisol concentrations within normal *resting* range, such elevated endogenous ACTH concentrations still cause cortisol to rise above normal ranges at frequent intervals (inadequate treatment, middle panel).

tions into normal resting range in most dogs with PDH. About 15 per cent of dogs, however, still respond to exogenous ACTH with plasma cortisol concentrations above normal resting range (greater than 4 to 5 μg/dl). In these dogs, daily *o,p'*-DDD treatment should be continued and ACTH stimulation tests repeated at 5- to 10-day intervals until cortisol concentrations remain within normal resting range (Fig. 4); this may require as long as 30 to 60 days in a few dogs. In contrast, basal and post-ACTH cortisol concentrations fall below normal resting range (less than 1.0 μg/dl) in about one-third of dogs following the initial 10-day *o,p'*-DDD treatment. In these dogs, the drug should be stopped and glucocorticoid therapy continued as needed until circulating cortisol levels normalize. Although low cortisol concentrations usually increase spontaneously to normal resting range within 2 to 6 weeks, levels may remain subnormal for months in some dogs.

Once normal plasma cortisol concentrations are documented by ACTH stimulation testing, *o,p'*-DDD should be continued at a maintenance dosage of 50 mg/kg weekly in two to three divided doses. During maintenance therapy with *o,p'*-DDD, glucocorticoid supplementation rarely is required; however, daily glucocorticoid therapy should be continued together with *o,p'*-DDD in those dogs that frequently develop mild side effects despite normal plasma cortisol concentrations. In addition, during periods of stress, appropriate dosages of glucocorticoid should always be administered. Complete remission of all clinical signs may take from 3 to 5 months in some dogs. Although serious side effects rarely occur during maintenance treatment with *o,p'*-DDD, mild side effects will develop in about 30 per cent of dogs at some time during treatment. If adverse signs occur during maintenance *o,p'*-DDD therapy, the drug should be stopped and glucocorticoid supplementation given. In most cases, maintenance *o,p'*-DDD can be resumed 2 to 6 weeks later when low plasma cortisol concentrations have again increased into the normal resting range (Fig. 4). If adverse signs persist for longer than 3 hours after glucocorticoid therapy, the dog should be immediately re-evaluated to exclude other medical problems, including mineralocorticoid deficiency. About 5 per cent of dogs treated with maintenance *o,p'*-DDD dosage develop iatrogenic hypoadrenocorticism, characterized by low basal and post-ACTH cortisol concentrations and electrolyte changes of hyperkalemia and hyponatremia. Such mineralocorticoid deficiency may develop weeks to months after good control with maintenance *o,p'*-DDD therapy has been achieved. Adverse clinical signs in dogs with iatrogenic hypoadrenocorticism resolve after stopping *o,p'*-DDD and supplementing with appropriate dosages of glucocorticoid and fludrocortisone acetate (Florinef, Squibb). These dogs usually require permanent daily corticosteroid replacement therapy; further *o,p'*-DDD administration is not required unless hypoadrenocorticism resolves and basal and post-ACTH cortisol concentrations increase above normal resting range (1 to 5 μg/dl).

Despite initial control of hyperadrenocorticism with *o,p'*-DDD, excessive pituitary ACTH secretion continues in dogs with PDH. As the disorder progresses, pituitary ACTH secretion usually increases to progressively higher levels; such sustained elevations in circulating ACTH concentrations tend to overcome the adrenocortical suppressive effects of maintenance *o,p'*-DDD therapy, and relapse of hyperadrenocorticism commonly occurs. In addition, *o,p'*-DDD may induce the hepatic microsomal enzymes involved in its biotransformation, which would increase the degradation and therefore decrease the adrenocorticolytic effects of the drug. About 50 per cent of dogs treated with initial loading and maintenance dosages of *o,p'*-DDD relapse within 12 months of treatment, as evidenced by recurrence of clinical signs and elevated basal and post-ACTH cortisol concentrations. To ensure continued control and prevent serious relapse during *o,p'*-DDD therapy, ACTH stimulation testing should be repeated after 3 and 6 months of maintenance therapy and every 6 months thereafter (Fig. 4). If basal and post-ACTH cortisol concentrations rise above normal range (4 to 5 μg/dl), the *o,p'*-DDD dosage should be increased to 30 to 50 mg/kg daily for 5 days, and the weekly maintenance dosage should be increased by approximately 50 per cent to help prevent further relapse. Because of multiple relapses, some dogs eventually require maintenance *o,p'*-DDD dosages as high as 100 to 300 mg/kg/week to control hyperadrenocorticism.

Adrenocortical Tumors

If possible, adrenocortical tumors should be surgically removed. Adrenalectomy can be performed via a retroperitoneal approach (flank incision) or a ventral midline celiotomy. We prefer the ventral midline approach since it enables the surgeon to inspect both adrenal glands and search for possible metastasis. With unilateral adrenocortical tumors, the contralateral adrenal gland atrophies and may be difficult to identify. If both adrenals are enlarged, nonsuppressible PDH should be suspected; biopsy of one adrenal gland confirms this diagnosis. After the unilateral adrenal tumor is located, the ventral midline incision can be extended paracostally for better exposure. Because the unaffected adrenal gland is chronically suppressed and atrophied, removal of a unilateral adrenal tumor will result in a precipitous drop in circulating cortisol concentrations. Therefore, large doses of glucocorticoid must be administered before and immediately after surgery. An appropriate regimen is to administer soluble hydrocortisone (4 to 5 mg/kg), dexamethasone (0.1 to 0.2 mg/kg), or prednisolone sodium succinate (1.0 to 2.0 mg/kg) IV either 1 hour prior to surgery or at time of induction of anesthesia. Alternatively, the glucocorticoid can be added to the intravenous fluids and infused during the surgical procedure. On completion of the operation, one should again administer the preoperative dose of a soluble glucocorticoid preparation either intravenously or intramuscularly. During the first postoperative day, glucocorticoid supplementation should be continued at five times maintenance dosage as prednisone (0.5 mg/kg twice a day), prednisolone (0.5 mg/kg twice a day), cortisone acetate (2.5 mg/kg twice a day), or dexamethasone (0.1 mg/kg once a day). Unless postoperative complications arise, the glucocorticoid dosage should be gradually tapered to maintenance levels over the first 7 to 10 postoperative days. Should fever or other complications develop, however, the glucocorticoid supplementation should be maintained at or be increased to a dosage of five times the maintenance dose until such problems subside. Once the glucocorticoid has been tapered to a maintenance dosage of prednisone (0.2 mg/kg once a day), prednisolone (0.2 mg/kg once a day), or cortisone (0.5 mg/kg twice a day), supplementation should be continued until the remaining adrenal gland is functioning normally, based on ACTH stimulation testing. In most dogs, glucocorticoids can be discontinued within 2 months of surgery.

If the adrenal tumor is malignant, if the owner refuses surgery for the animal, or if the dog is considered to be an unsuitable surgical candidate, medical adrenalectomy with *o,p'*-DDD should be attempted. Although treatment with *o,p'*-DDD reduces cortisol production by some adrenal adenomas, only limited success has been obtained in the treatment of adrenal carcinomas. In general, when *o,p'*-DDD is used as chemotherapy for adrenocortical neoplasia, the drug should be administered at the daily dosage of 50 to 150 mg/kg and ACTH stimulation testing repeated at 2-week intervals. If *o,p'*-DDD is effective in reducing cortisol secretion by the tumor, it should be continued at such high daily dosages until both basal and post-ACTH plasma cortisol concentrations fall to normal or low levels (less than 4 to 5 μg/dl). Subsequent dosage adjustments should be based on results of periodic ACTH stimulation tests. If remission does occur, maintenance glucocorticoid supplementation is recommended, since *o,p'*-DDD may also destroy the normal contralateral adrenal cortex.

PROGNOSIS

Without treatment, canine hyperadrenocorticism is generally a progressive disorder with an unfavorable prognosis. Many factors, however, influence the prognosis in hyperadrenocorticism, including the rate of progression, severity, and cause of the disorder. In untreated hyperadrenocorticism, death may result from metastasis of an adrenocortical carcinoma, growth of a pituitary tumor, or most commonly from complications associated with sustained hypercortisolism itself such as hypertension, cardiovascular disease, thromboembolism, glucose intolerance, and increased susceptibility to infection.

Although the morbidity and mortality of adrenalectomy must be considered, the prognosis for dogs with adrenocortical adenoma is usually excellent. In contrast, the outcome with adrenal carcinoma is generally poor, and death usually occurs shortly after diagnosis. Medical treatment with *o,p'*-DDD appears to improve the prognosis of PDH, especially in dogs with moderate to severe clinical signs of disease. In a few dogs with mild, slowly progressive PDH, however, the prognosis is usually good to excellent even without *o,p'*-DDD therapy. Until unacceptable or moderate signs develop, observation may be the treatment of choice in these dogs. Since hyperadrenocorticism is a disorder of older dogs, most will die or be euthanized within 2 years of diagnosis because of diseases (e.g., renal disease, heart failure, malignancies) unrelated to either PDH or *o,p'*-DDD therapy. About 10 per cent of dogs with PDH, however, can be successfully managed with *o,p'*-DDD for periods greater than 4 years. In those dogs with PDH that fail to demonstrate diagnostic cortisol suppression during high-dose dexamethasone suppression testing, the long-term prognosis is extremely guarded since many will eventually develop neurologic signs as a result of an expanding, invasive pituitary tumor.

References and Supplemental Reading

Feldman, E. C.: Comparison of ACTH response and dexamethasone suppression as screening tests in canine hyperadrenocorticism. J.A.V.M.A. 182:506, 1983.

Feldman, E. C.: Distinguishing dogs with functioning adrenocortical tumors from dogs with pituitary-dependent hyperadrenocorticism. J.A.V.M.A. 183:195, 1983.

Johnston, D. E.: Adrenalectomy via retroperitoneal approach in dogs. J.A.V.M.A. 170:1092, 1977.

Kemppainen, R. J., and Sartin, J. L.: Evidence for episodic but not rcadian activity in plasma concentrations of adrenocorticotrophin, cortisol, and thyroxine in dogs. J. Endocrinol. 103:219, 1984.

Lubberink, A. A. M. E.: Therapy for spontaneous hyperadrenocorticism. *In* Kirk, R. W. (ed.): *Current Veterinary Therapy VII*. Philadelphia: W. B. Saunders, 1980, pp. 979–983.

Peterson, M. E., Nesbitt, G. H., and Schaer, M.: Diagnosis and management of concurrent diabetes mellitus and hyperadrenocorticism in 30 dogs. J.A.V.M.A. 178:66, 1981.

Peterson, M. E., and Drucker, W. D.: Advances in the diagnosis and treatment of canine Cushing's syndrome. Proc. 31st Gaines Veterinary Symposium, 1981, pp. 17–24.

Peterson, M. E.: Hyperadrenocorticism. Vet. Clin. North Am. [Small Anim. Pract.] 14:731, 1984.

Peterson, M. E., Altszuler, N., and Nichols, C. E.: Decreased insulin sensitivity and glucose tolerance in spontaneous canine hyperadrenocorticism. Res. Vet. Sci. 36:177, 1984.

Peterson, M. E., Birchard, S. J., and Mehlhaff, C. J.: Anesthetic and surgical management of endocrine disorders. Vet. Clin. North Am. (Small Anim. Pract.) 14:911, 1984.

Peterson, M. E., and Orth, D. N.: Corticotropin-releasing hormone stimulation test: An aid to the differential diagnosis of canine Cushing's syndrome. ACVIM Scientific Proceedings, 1985, p. 151.

Stolp, R., and Meijer, J. C.: Differential diagnosis and laboratory evaluation of hyperadrenocorticism in dogs. Proc. Kal Kan Symposium for the Treatment of Small Animal Diseases, 1982, pp. 9–14.

HYPOADRENOCORTICISM

LEE ANN SCHRADER, D.V.M.

New York, New York

Adrenocortical insufficiency, or hypoadrenocorticism, results from deficient production of glucocorticoid, mineralocorticoid, or both. Primary adrenocortical insufficiency (Addison's disease) is a result of bilateral atrophy or destruction of all layers of the adrenal cortex, leading to both glucocorticoid and mineralocorticoid deficiency. Most cases of Addison's disease are believed to be idiopathic (probably immune-mediated), although adrenocortical destruction can be secondary to infectious or granulomatous diseases, tumors, infarctions, and the drug *o,p'*-DDD (mitotane). Secondary adrenocortical insufficiency is characterized by inadequate pituitary ACTH production resulting in decreased circulating concentrations of adrenal glucocorticoids. Mineralocorticoid production is not significantly affected by inadequate circulating ACTH. Most commonly, secondary adrenocortical insufficiency develops after abrupt withdrawal of long-term or high-dose exogenous corticosteroid therapy; however, any lesion of the hypothalamus or pituitary gland can decrease ACTH production.

So-called atypical hypoadrenocorticism (signs of adrenocortical insufficiency with normal electrolyte concentrations) is being recognized with increasing frequency, but it cannot be categorized into either primary or secondary adrenal failure without tests designed to differentiate the two types of hypoadrenocorticism, such as plasma ACTH concentrations or prolonged ACTH stimulation testing (see below).

Spontaneous hypoadrenocorticism is a relatively uncommon abnormality in dogs, with young to middle-aged females most commonly affected. There is no breed predilection. The disease is extremely rare in cats.

PATHOGENESIS

A large number of metabolic and physiologic derangements can be attributed to inadequate adrenal corticosteroid production. Cortisol deficiency can lead to many abnormalities, including decreased gluconeogenesis and glycogenolysis, gastrointestinal signs such as anorexia and vomiting, impaired renal ability to excrete a water load, decreased vascular sensitivity to catecholamines, and depressed mentation. Effects of mineralocorticoid deficiency are related primarily to renal sodium, chloride, and water wasting, with potassium and hydrogen ion retention. Renal sodium wasting, vomiting, and diarrhea lead to depletion of circulating blood volume, which combines with poor vascular tone to result in hypotension and reduced cardiac output. Decreased tissue perfusion follows and is seen clinically as weakness, depression, prerenal azotemia, and eventually shock. Decreased excretion of potassium and hydrogen ions secondary to mineralocorticoid deficiency and decreased glomerular filtration results in hyperkalemia and metabolic acidosis. The most well-known effect of hyperkalemia is decreased myocardial excitability and a slowed cardiac conduction rate. Hyperkalemia also contributes to muscular weakness. The hyponatremia associated with Addison's disease can be attributed to dilution of extracellular sodium. Antidiuretic hormone is released in response to reduced extracellular volume and mediates free-water resorption in the distal tubules and collecting ducts. Hyponatremia can result in central nervous system disturbances and exacerbates the effects of hyperkalemia on the myocardium.

HISTORY AND CLINICAL SIGNS

A high index of suspicion is necessary for the early diagnosis of hypoadrenocorticism, because most of the clinical signs are not specific and are present in numerous other disorders. In most cases of primary adrenocortical insufficiency, gradual, progressive, adrenocortical destruction initially produces relative adrenocortical deficiency with normal basal corticosteroid secretion. Clinical signs may be apparent only under stressful conditions, when the ability of the adrenal cortex to respond to ACTH and angiotensin II is blunted. As adrenocortical destruction progresses, clinical signs become more persistent. Similarly, clinical signs are often intermittent in patients with secondary adrenocortical insufficiency, as relative and then complete ACTH deficiency results in inadequate concentrations of adrenal glucocorticoid.

In dogs with chronic adrenocortical insufficiency, historic findings include intermittent anorexia, weight loss, occasional bouts of vomiting and diarrhea, muscle weakness, lethargy, depression, and occasionally hematochezia or melena. These signs may have been present for weeks to months and may have transiently responded to administration of fluid or corticosteroids or both.

On physical examination, a patient might be in acute adrenal failure and have minimal or very recent historic signs, which may be associated with a stressful incident. Clinical findings vary from mild lethargy and weakness to severe bradycardia and shock. The most common findings are depression and weakness. Dehydration, bradycardia, weak femoral pulses, prolonged capillary refill time, and melena are encountered less commonly.

LABORATORY EVALUATION

The lack of specificity of historic and clinical findings in animals with adrenocortical insufficiency makes laboratory evaluation necessary to confirm the diagnosis.

In more than one third of dogs with hypoadrenocorticism, the hemogram shows a mild normocytic, normochromic, nonregenerative anemia, although this may be masked by concurrent hemoconcentration. With fluid expansion of the vascular compartment, mild anemia may become apparent. Normal to elevated eosinophil and lymphocyte counts in an ill dog are significant, because the expected adrenocortical response to stress would result in eosinopenia and lymphopenia. Adrenocortical insufficiency therefore should be suspected in any dog with signs suggestive of hypoadrenocorticism and normal to elevated absolute eosinophil and lymphocyte numbers.

In dogs with primary adrenocortical insufficiency, blood chemistry abnormalities most commonly seen are hyponatremia and hyperkalemia, with a sodium:potassium ratio of less than 27:1. However, early in the course of Addison's disease, in patients recently given parenteral fluids, or in animals with secondary adrenocortical insufficiency, serum electrolyte values might be normal. Hypercalcemia has been reported in approximately 25 per cent of dogs with hypoadrenocorticism, and the severity of hypercalcemia seems to correlate with the severity of the disease. Hypercalcemia might be caused by increased renal tubular calcium resorption.

Decreased renal perfusion often results in prerenal azotemia, which in most cases normalizes with adequate parenteral fluid therapy. Occasionally the blood urea nitrogen (BUN) and creatinine do not rapidly return to normal, which might indicate inadequate fluid administration or primary renal involvement secondary to prolonged ischemia. Often the pretreatment urine specific gravity is more dilute (1.016 to 1.028) than would be expected in an animal with prerenal azotemia (i.e., greater than 1.030). The cause of this apparent loss of renal concentrating ability is poorly understood, but it might be secondary to renal sodium loss with resultant medullary washout or decreased efficiency of the countercurrent mechanism resulting from decreased renal blood flow. The findings of urine specific gravity less than that considered concentrated, together with azotemia that may not immediately respond to fluid administration, might lead the veterinary clinician to the erroneous diagnosis of primary renal disease.

Blood chemistry findings in dogs with atypical hypoadrenocorticism are less specific in that changes in electrolyte concentrations are not seen initially, although a large number of these patients will develop hyperkalemia and hyponatremia, usually within several weeks of the initial diagnosis. In several of such dogs the authors have treated, the most consistent finding has been mild to moderate azotemia with dilute urine (1.016 to 1.028). Dogs with primary renal failure would be expected to have a urine specific gravity in the isosthenuric range (1.008 to 1.014), which underscores the importance of obtaining a urine sample prior to fluid therapy.

Hypoglycemia is an unusual finding in dogs with hypoadrenocorticism. Mild to moderate metabolic acidosis is a frequent finding that results from loss of the aldosterone effect on the secretion of renal tubular hydrogen ions.

When electrolyte abnormalities are present, the electrocardiogram can be of significant value in diagnosing Addison's disease. Earliest findings (potassium greater than 5.5 mEq/L) include increased amplitude of the T waves, which can progress to decreased R wave amplitude, prolongation of QRS complexes and P-R intervals, and ST segment depression. At serum potassium concentrations greater than 8.5 mEq/L, the P waves might disappear and a slow sinoventricular rhythm with atrial standstill can develop. Eventually this is replaced by a sine wave pattern, ventricular flutter, fibrillation, or asystole. Although the electrocardiogram is useful in both diagnosing and in estimating the degree of hyperkalemia, there is a poor correlation between the degree of hyperkalemia and electrocardiographic changes in dogs with primary adrenocortical insufficiency. The toxic effects of hyperkalemia on the myocardium are exacerbated by both hyponatremia and acidosis, common findings in patients presented in an addisonian crisis.

RADIOGRAPHIC FINDINGS

Radiographs might show a decrease in the size of the cardiac silhouette (microcardia) secondary to hypotension and volume depletion in dogs in an acute adrenal crisis. The caudal vena cava and descending aorta might appear narrow, along with a decreased density of the lung fields secondary to hypoperfusion. Esophageal dilation, or megaesophagus, also has been reported as a rare complication of hypoadrenocorticism.

DIAGNOSIS

Definitive diagnosis of hypoadrenocorticism requires the demonstration of inadequate cortisol response to exogenous ACTH. The procedure for an ACTH stimulation study using either natural or synthetic ACTH is quite simple and has been previously described (Feldman and Peterson, 1984). The test should be performed immediately in a patient with suspected acute adrenal crisis. Many synthetic glucocorticoids including prednisolone, prednisone, and cortisone will cross-react in the cortisol assay, falsely elevating values. Dexamethasone has little effect on cortisol measurement and can be used in the initial treatment of acute adrenal failure without interfering with the testing procedure. If prednisolone, prednisone, or cortisone has been used, it should be discontinued 36 to 48 hours prior to ACTH stimulation testing.

Dogs with either primary or secondary adrenocortical insufficiency show a subnormal response with the ACTH stimulation test. The resting cortisol concentration is usually but not always well below normal, and the post-ACTH value is similar to or only slightly above the basal concentration.

In dogs with normal serum sodium and potassium concentrations (atypical hypoadrenocorticism), ACTH concentrations can be used to differentiate primary and secondary adrenocortical insufficiency. Absence of the negative feedback effect of cortisol on the hypothalamus and pituitary in cases of primary adrenal failure results in extremely elevated ACTH concentrations. In contrast, secondary hypoadrenocorticism is the result of pituitary failure to secrete adequate concentrations of ACTH. Blood for determination of endogenous ACTH levels should be drawn prior to exogenous corticosteroid administration and must be handled quickly, because the half-life of ACTH in fresh whole blood is approximately 25 minutes. Samples should be kept at low temperatures and separated immediately using only plastic containers, as ACTH is known to adhere to glass.

An alternate method of differentiating primary and secondary adrenocortical insufficiency involves twice-daily administration of ACTH gel (20 U) for 4 to 5 days, followed by a repeat ACTH stimulation test. Response to ACTH will remain subnormal in cases of primary adrenal failure, whereas the trophic effect of exogenous ACTH results in a nearly normal response in animals with secondary hypoadrenocorticism.

TREATMENT OF ACUTE ADRENOCORTICAL INSUFFICIENCY

Acute adrenal failure constitutes a medical emergency requiring immediate therapy. If the history, clinical signs, and electrocardiogram are suggestive of glucocorticoid or mineralocorticoid deficiency, appropriate therapy should be instituted pending the results of laboratory values and specific diagnostic tests. Initial therapeutic aims include restoration of circulating blood volume, correction of hyperkalemia and hyponatremia, correction of acidosis, provision of an immediate source of glucocorticoid, and correction of hyperkalemic myocardial toxicity, if present.

An indwelling intravenous catheter should be placed, preferably in the jugular vein, to allow for the administration of large volumes of isotonic fluids. Blood should be collected prior to treatment for blood chemistry and resting cortisol determinations, to be followed by ACTH administration. Urine also should be collected at this time. The intravenous fluid of choice is normal (0.9 per cent) saline, which should be administered at a rate of 40 to 80 ml/kg/hour during the first 1 to 2 hours. If hypoglycemia is present and the animal is not dehydrated, 50 per cent dextrose can be added to the initial isotonic fluids to result in a final concentration of 2.5 per cent dextrose. If clinical signs of hypoglycemia are present, 50 per cent dextrose can be given as a slow (over 10 to 20 minutes) bolus at the rate of 0.5 to 1.0 ml/kg. Rate of fluid administration is dependent on the degree of hypotension and dehydration and clinical signs such as skin turgor, membrane moistness, capillary refill time, and urine output. As these monitored values return to normal, the rate of fluid administration should be decreased, because the animal deficient in glucocorticoid or mineralocorticoid or both has a reduced ability to excrete a water load. The rate of fluid administration can then be lowered to 60 to 70 ml/kg/day, divided evenly over two or three treatments. Azotemic animals require increased amounts of intravenous fluids (up to 5 per cent of body weight), because obligatory diuresis results from excretion of retained solute. Fluid administration is tapered when hydration, sodium, potassium, BUN, and creatinine levels become normal. Tapering of intravenous fluid administration usually can be initiated after 48 to 72 hours and can be accomplished over an additional 24 to 48 hours, depending on the animal's clinical status and results of laboratory tests.

Rapid intravenous administration of a glucocorticoid is extremely important in the initial management of acute adrenocortical collapse. In most cases, intravenous dexamethasone (0.5 to 1.0 mg/kg) is adequate and will not interfere with concurrent ACTH stimulation testing. In critical cases, the more rapidly acting dexamethasone sodium phosphate (Tech America Group, 2.0 to 4.0 mg/kg) should be used.

In addition to glucocorticoid, initial therapy should include desoxycorticosterone acetate (DOCA; Percoten acetate, Ciba) given intramuscularly; this will not interfere with the results of ACTH stimulation testing. The mineralocorticoid effects of this drug enhance renal potassium excretion and sodium resorption. The initial dosage ranges from 1 mg in small dogs to 5 mg in giant breeds, once daily. The dosage is adjusted on the basis of daily serum electrolyte determinations and is continued until oral fludrocortisone acetate (Florinef, Squibb) can be initiated.

Severe acidosis, if present, should be treated by the addition of sodium bicarbonate to intravenous fluids. If determination of blood gases is not possible, total venous carbon dioxide (CO_2) can be used to approximate the base deficit by subtracting the patient's venous CO_2 from normal venous CO_2 (approximately 22 mEq/L). Total milliequivalents of bicarbonate necessary can be calculated by using the following formula:

$$\text{Deficit in mEq} = (\text{body weight in kg})\ (0.3)\ (\text{base deficit})$$

One half of this calculated amount should be added to the intravenous fluids during the first 12 hours, at which time the dog's acid-base status should be re-evaluated. Rarely do animals treated appropriately with parenteral fluids and corticosteroids require further bicarbonate therapy. Sodium bicarbonate administration should be based on results of serial laboratory testing and should not be performed empirically.

TREATMENT OF HYPERKALEMIC MYOCARDIAL TOXICITY

The early electrocardiographic changes associated with mild to moderate hyperkalemia, such as peaking of the T wave and widening and flattening of the P wave, usually resolve spontaneously with corticosteroid and intravenous saline administration. If no P waves are seen, QRS complexes are wide or bizarre, or the heart rate is slow, one can assume that severe hyperkalemia (greater than 7.5 mEq/L) is present. Specific therapy aimed at lowering the serum potassium often is necessary because intravenous saline, intravenous glucocorticoid, and intramuscular DOCA may not bring about rapid resolution of the hyperkalemia. Rapid and effective therapy for severe hyperkalemia involves the intravenous administration of regular crystalline insulin and dextrose. This effects rapid (usually within 15 minutes) lowering of serum potassium via insulin-mediated intracellular movement of potassium. The intravenous dosage of regular insulin is a bolus of 0.5 U/kg body weight, followed by administration of 2.0 to 3.0 grams dextrose (as 50 per cent dextrose) per unit of insulin. Half of the dextrose is given as an intravenous bolus; the other half is added to the intravenous fluids over the following 4 to 6 hours. Care should be taken to avoid hypoglycemia, because patients with adrenocortical insufficiency are highly sensitive to the glucose-lowering effects of insulin. Other treatments that may be used include 10 per cent calcium gluconate at the rate of 0.5 to 1.0 ml/kg body weight, given intravenously over 10 to 20 minutes. Calcium ion antagonizes the effects of potassium ion on the myocardium but does not lower the serum potassium concentration. Sodium bicarbonate enhances the intracellular movement of potassium and can be given at the rate of 1.0 to 2.0 mEq/kg body weight intravenously over 10 to 20 minutes.

These emergency therapies can be given alone or in combination in cases of life-threatening hyperkalemia, and they usually need to be administered only once. Bicarbonate should not be mixed in calcium-containing fluids because a precipitate will form. The electrocardiogram should be monitored frequently during treatment until the rhythm and complexes return to normal.

TREATMENT OF CHRONIC ADRENOCORTICAL INSUFFICIENCY

Many dogs with chronic primary adrenocortical insufficiency have only mild to moderate changes in electrolytes, BUN, and creatinine, whereas the expected findings in patients with atypical hypoadrenocorticism and secondary hypoadrenocorticism range from normal blood chemistry values to moderate azotemia. These dogs do not require the aggressive therapy previously described. Intravenous saline (or lactated Ringer's in cases of normal potassium concentration) should be administered if azotemia is present, the sodium:potassium ratio is greater than 27:1, or if there is anorexia, vomiting, or diarrhea. The importance of intravenous fluid therapy in the maintenance of vascular volume and tissue perfusion in patients with adrenocortical insufficiency should not be underestimated, and most patients will benefit from fluid therapy during the early phase of treatment. If the patient is vomiting, intramuscular DOCA should be initiated at a dosage of 1.0 to 5.0 mg once daily, along with parenteral prednisone (or prednisolone) at a dosage of 0.2 mg/kg once daily or given in divided doses. When oral intake is possible, prednisone (or prednisolone) can be given orally, and fludrocortisone acetate, which is available in 0.1-mg tablets, can be substituted for DOCA at an initial dosage of 0.1 to 0.3 mg once daily or in divided doses, based on the size of the dog. Small incremental increases can be made in the dosage of DOCA or fludrocortisone acetate based on daily monitoring of electrolyte concentrations during the hospitalization period.

MAINTENANCE THERAPY

Maintenance therapy for the patient with primary adrenocortical insufficiency consists of mineralocorticoid and, in most cases, glucocorticoid supplementation, along with the addition of sodium chloride to the diet.

The dosage of mineralocorticoid supplementation is adjusted based on serial electrolyte determinations. One of the advantages of daily administration of fludrocortisone acetate is the ease of dosage adjustment. Initially, sodium and potassium concentrations should be determined every 1 to 2 weeks and the dosage adjusted by 0.05 to 0.1 mg/day. Once the serum electrolyte concentrations have stabilized in the normal range, BUN, creatinine, and serum electrolytes should be re-evaluated every 3 to 4 months. Many patients will require increasing amounts of fludrocortisone acetate during the initial 6 to 18 months of treatment; thereafter the dosage usually stabilizes. Most patients in which Addison's disease is controlled require approximately 0.1 mg fludrocortisone acetate per 5 kg body weight. Some dogs develop resistance to fludrocortisone acetate, and in these animals, as well as in those in which daily oral medication is difficult or inconvenient, injectable repositol mineralocorticoid can be employed. Desoxycorticosterone pivalate (DOCP) (Percorten pivalate, Ciba), is injected intramuscularly every 3 to 4 weeks at a dosage of 25 to 100 mg, depending on the patient's size; 25 mg of DOCP is approximately proportional to 1 mg DOCA or 0.1 mg fludrocortisone. Many dogs that have a decreased sensitivity to fludrocortisone do well on a proportionately lower dosage of DOCP.

Sodium chloride supplementation is also useful in dogs with Addison's disease. The tablets are administered at the rate of 1 to 5 gm daily.

Many patients do well on mineralocorticoid and salt supplementation alone. This may be due to the glucocorticoid activity of fludrocortisone acetate. About one half of all dogs with primary adrenocortical failure, however, require additional glucocorticoid supplementation to prevent the development of signs consistent with glucocorticoid deficiency such as weakness, lethargy, and anorexia. Some animals also may become mildly azotemic secondary to inadequate glucocorticoid concentrations. In these cases, prednisone or prednisolone (0.1 to 0.3 mg/kg body weight per day) or cortisone (1.0 mg/kg body weight per day) should be added to the treatment regimen. In all cases, the owner should have glucocorticoid on hand to give during times of illness or stress. Clinicians also must remember that dogs with adrenocortical insufficiency must be supplemented with large doses (two to ten times basal levels) of parenteral glucocorticoids during surgical procedures and medical or traumatic illnesses.

Patients with documented secondary adrenocortical insufficiency usually do not require mineralocorticoid or sodium chloride supplementation. The daily dose of glucocorticoid, as described previously, is usually sufficient to control clinical signs. The veterinarian, however, must carefully monitor serum electrolytes during the early weeks of therapy; some animals believed to have secondary adrenocortical insufficiency later develop electrolyte changes consistent with primary hypoadrenocorticism and require mineralocorticoid supplementation.

References and Supplemental Readings

Feldman, E. C., and Peterson, M. E.: Hypoadrenocorticism. Vet. Clin. North Am. (Small Anim. Pract.) 14(4):751, 1984.
Peterson, M. E., and Feinman, J. M.: Hypercalcemia associated with hypoadrenocorticism in sixteen dogs. J.A.V.M.A. 181:802, 1982.
Rogers, W., Straus, J., and Chew, D.: Atypical hypoadrenocorticism in three dogs. J.A.V.M.A. 179:155, 1981.
Willard, M. D., Shall, W. D., McCaw, D. E., et al.: Canine hypoadrenocorticism: Report of 37 cases and review of 39 previously reported cases. J.A.V.M.A. 180:59, 1982.

CANINE PHEOCHROMOCYTOMA

STEVEN L. WHEELER, D.V.M.
Fort Collins, Colorado

Pheochromocytomas in dogs are rare and often functional endocrine tumors arising from the adrenal medulla. The clinical signs result both from the excessive production of catecholamines and by local invasive spread of the tumor. The pharmacologic effects of catecholamine stimulation are many; thus, the signs associated with this condition can be vague and may be confused with many more common clinical disorders. Frequently, the diagnosis is missed clinically and is only made at necropsy. Awareness of the pathophysiologic alterations and common presenting signs should improve the chances of the clinical diagnosis of canine pheochromocytoma.

CLINICAL PRESENTATION

The common manifestations of pheochromocytomas may result directly from the physical presence of the tumor but more often are related to its production of increased amounts of catecholamines, resulting in hypertension. These hypertension-associated signs may be sustained or paroxysmal, depending on the secretion characteristics of the tumor. As in human patients with pheochromocytoma, episodic hypertension separated by symptom-free intervals resulting from paroxysmal secretion of catecholamines from the tumor appears to be more common in dogs with pheochromocytoma. The length of the episodes is quite variable, and the duration of these signs prior to diagnosis ranges from days to years. The paroxysmal nature of the historic events is a diagnostic key worth remembering when forming a differential diagnosis. Other dogs show acute fulminating signs associated with a hypertensive crisis and may die from shock, pulmonary edema, ventricular fibrillation, or cerebral hemorrhage.

The clinical signs associated with pheochromocytomas are quite variable and often subtle (Table 1). Respiratory signs characterized by episodic panting or dyspnea are common and may result either from pulmonary congestion or from a direct action

Table 1. *Common Clinical Signs of Pheochromocytomas*

Respiratory signs (panting, dyspnea, coughing)
Weakness or exercise intolerance
Tremors or shaking
Restlessness or irritability
Polydipsia or polyuria
Anorexia
Neurologic signs (e.g., seizures, ataxia)
Epistaxis
Cyanosis
Flushing
Abdominal distention
Diarrhea
Collapse

of catecholamines on the central nervous system to stimulate hyperventilation. Another common sign reported in dogs with pheochromocytoma is episodic or acute weakness, which may range in severity from mild exercise intolerance to overt collapse. Other signs that may occur include muscle tremors, polydipsia, polyuria, and anorexia. Episodic restlessness, reluctance to sleep, tachycardia, and flushing of the pinnae have also been reported by observant owners (Table 1). If the paroxysmal release of catecholamines produces severe hypertension, epistaxis, seizures, or a cerebrovascular accident may occur. Dogs may also be presented for acute collapse and hypovolemic shock secondary to intra-abdominal hemorrhage from a ruptured vascular tumor.

PHYSICAL EXAMINATION

Pheochromocytomas most often occur in older dogs. There appears to be no breed or sex predilection for this tumor. The physical examination findings are relatively nonspecific and are frequently unrewarding in the diagnosis. Because of the episodic pattern of tumor catecholamine secretion, neither hypertension nor the resulting clinical signs may be present during the physical examination.

In about one fourth of cases, the tumor is large enough to be detected on abdominal palpation. Because this tumor is locally invasive, invasion of the posterior vena cava by a tumor thrombus occurs in about one third of all cases. Complete or partial obstruction of the vena cava by the tumor thrombus may produce ascites, edema of the rear legs, or distention of the caudal epigastric veins.

Auscultation of the thorax often reveals abnormalities including abnormal breath sounds and cardiac disturbances. Frequently, dogs with pheochromocytoma have tachypnea with harsh or increased bronchial sounds. Alveolar sounds can also be ausculted in those dogs with pulmonary congestion and edema. Cardiac abnormalities are also commonly detected in dogs with pheochromocytomas. Catecholamines can directly cause myocarditis or conduction abnormalities, probably as a result of catecholamine-induced vasoconstriction and secondary myocardial ischemia. Tachycardia, various arrhythmias, or cardiac murmurs are found in about 15 per cent of dogs with pheochromocytoma.

Catecholamine release can produce either flushing or blanching of the mucous membranes, which may be continuous or intermittent. Most dogs, however, are reported to have normal membrane color and perfusion. An elevated body temperature may also be detected. Ophthalmoscopic examination may reveal hypertensive retinopathies such as retinal hemorrhage.

Neurologic findings that occur in dogs with pheochromocytoma are generally nonspecific. Dilated pupils secondary to excess sympathetic input may be seen. Other neurologic abnormalities include seizures, head tilts, nystagmus, and strabismus. In most cases, focal neurologic deficits appear to result from cerebral vascular hemorrhage.

DIAGNOSTIC PROCEDURES

The presence of a pheochromocytoma may be suspected on the basis of the history and physical examination. The diagnosis of pheochromocytoma, however, is usually dependent on the clinician's awareness of the subtleties of the disease, since confirmation of this disorder rests on laboratory tests that document excess catecholamine secretion.

Routine Laboratory Tests

There are no consistent abnormalities encountered in the routine laboratory tests of dogs with pheochromocytoma. The hematocrit and total solids may be increased because of a decrease in the plasma volume and relative increase in red cell mass. Although the exact mechanism of hemoconcentration with this tumor is unknown, production of an erythropoietin-like substance by the tumor has been postulated. Affected dogs may also be anemic either from blood loss or "chronic disease." Catecholamine release can cause demargination of neutrophils from blood vessels and result in a transient neutrophilia in normal dogs. Neutrophilia is observed in about one half of all dogs with pheochromocytoma. However, since catecholamine release is usually quite paroxysmal and often does not occur at the time of the examination, it is possible that the neutrophilia occurs because of other causes.

Increased fasting glucose and free fatty acid levels may develop in human patients with pheochromocytoma, some of whom are initially suspected as having primary diabetes mellitus. Although high-normal serum glucose concentrations have been noted, overt hyperglycemia has not been documented in dogs with pheochromocytoma. Proteinuria and hematuria are found in many cases and may be the result of glomerulopathies secondary to hypertension. The remainder of the laboratory tests are quite variable and do not help in the diagnosis of a pheochromocytoma.

Blood Pressure Determinations

Sustained or intermittent hypertension in humans is the characteristic manifestation of pheochromocytoma. The presence of hypertension, together with its related clinical signs, is the principal signal to perform further diagnostic screening tests to rule out pheochromocytoma. However, due to paroxysmal release of catecholamines by the tumor, normal arterial blood pressure values do not eliminate pheochromocytoma as a diagnosis. If pheochromocytoma is suspected, multiple blood pressure determinations may be necessary to document the presence of hypertension.

Radiology

Radiographic studies are some of the most important diagnostic procedures used to localize a pheochromocytoma. Routine radiographs of the chest may reveal cardiac enlargement and pulmonary congestion or edema. Scout films of the abdomen will identify an adrenal mass in about 35 per cent of cases. The tumor may result in caudal displacement of the adjacent kidney, and calcified tumors may be radiographically apparent. Left adrenal tumors are easier to detect on radiographs because the right adrenal is closely associated with the liver and is not as easily visualized. Peritoneal infusion of gas (pneumoperitoneography) may aid in the visualization of the tumor.

Contrast intravenous urograms may also aid in the diagnosis of a pheochromocytoma. The nature of the tumor will often cause either displacement or invasion of the cranial pole of the kidney. Although it will identify an adrenal mass in fewer than 10 per cent of the cases, the intravenous urogram should still be included in the diagnostic workup. Selective arteriography has also been used in humans to demonstrate adrenal tumors and is often successful because of the highly vascular nature of the tumor. However, the most diagnostic radiographic procedure in this disease is vena caval venography, which should be performed in all suspected cases. Since tumor thrombus invading the posterior vena cava is common in pheochromocytomas, outlining such a thrombus will support a presumptive diagnosis. A vena caval study is simply performed by a rapid hand injection of contrast media into the lateral saphenous vein, followed by a series of abdominal films. Compression, deviation, or occlusion of the vena cava is seen in about 80 per cent of cases. There also is often reflux of contrast media into the caudal superficial epigastric veins, segmental spinal veins, and renal veins.

Chemical Tests

Although routine procedures are usually useful in locating an adrenal tumor, they are still not specific for identifying a pheochromocytoma. Certain chemical tests, however, provide unequivocal data for a definitive diagnosis. These include the measurement of catecholamines in the blood or the determination of the urinary excretion of catecholamines or their metabolites. The availability, technical difficulty, and considerable expense of these tests, however, have limited their use in veterinary medicine. Information is still needed to determine normal values and to specify those assays that are the most reliable for detecting pheochromocytomas in dogs.

Theoretically, dogs with functional secretory pheochromocytomas should have increased levels of catecholamines in the blood. Determination of plasma concentrations of total catecholamines is extremely difficult. In addition, since the release of catecholamines in pheochromocytomas can be quite episodic, plasma catecholamine concentrations may not be elevated at the time of evaluation. Finally, although levels are usually very high in pheochromocytomas, there can be some overlap with values that may occur with the stress or excitement of venipuncture in normal dogs. Because of these factors, the measurement of urinary concentrations of catecholamines and metabolites is usually more reliable in the diagnosis of canine pheochromocytomas. For determinations on urine, 24-hour samples are collected in 15 ml of 6 N hydrochloric acid. Concentrations of catecholamines (epinephrine and norepinephrine) and the catecholamine metabolites (metanephrine, normetanephrine, and vanillylmandelic acid) should be measured. Because a variety of tests exist and because the methods used in each laboratory differ in specificity, normal values should be determined for dogs in the particular laboratory used.

Provocative Tests

In most cases, the demonstration of increased levels of plasma or urinary catecholamines and their metabolites should suffice to confirm the diagnosis of pheochromocytoma. However, when the biochemical tests are equivocal and the diagnosis is still open to question, a pharmacologic approach can be used. Several pharmacologic tests have been devised to block the effects of catecholamines or to stimulate their release. These tests are useful in the diagnosis of pheochromocytoma because they usually cause profound changes in blood pressure as compared with normal dogs, which respond with only moderate blood pressure alterations. It is important, however, to recognize the limitations and potential hazards of these tests.

The phentolamine (Regitine, Ciba) suppression test is based on the principle that alpha-adrenergic blocking agents will lower elevated blood pressure by blocking the alpha (vasoconstrictor) effects of catecholamines. When this alpha-blocking drug is injected into a hypertensive dog with pheochromocytoma, a significant and sustained fall in blood pressure usually occurs. The animal must, however, be hypertensive before the test can be performed. To perform this test, a dose of 0.5 to 1.5 mg of phentolamine is given intravenously and blood pressure is measured at 1- to 2-minute intervals for 10 minutes. The phentolamine suppression test is considered diagnostic for pheochromocytomas if the fall in the systolic pressure (greater than 35 mm Hg) lasts for at least 4 minutes. A profound fall in blood pressure and shock may be produced as a result of inhibition of the alpha-mediated vasoconstrictor effects, leaving the beta-mediated vasodilatative effects of the catecholamines unopposed. Phenylephrine (Neo-Synephrine, Winthrop), an alpha-agonist, and intravenous isotonic fluids should be given in such a crisis.

The administration of clonidine (Catapres, Boehringer Ingelheim), which suppresses the release of catecholamines in normal subjects but fails to decrease catecholamine secretion in human patients with pheochromocytomas, has also been recently advocated as a reliable suppression test for diagnosis of this tumor. Use of clonidine, however, has yet to be evaluated in dogs with pheochromocytoma.

If the animal is normotensive, stimulatory agents can be administered to provoke release of catecholamines. As compared with a normal animal, the histamine test will cause a marked rise in blood pressure in dogs with pheochromocytoma. The intravenous injection of 5 to 25 μg of histamine base is considered positive for a pheochromocytoma if the blood pressure rises more than 40 mm Hg. False-positive and negative responses, however, are reported in approximately 30 per cent of human patients with this tumor. Because of the possible precipitation of a severe hypertensive crisis following histamine administration, phentolamine (an alpha-adrenergic blocker) should be available for prompt intravenous administration. The exact mechanism of action by histamine is unknown, but it appears that histamine causes a direct release of catecholamines from the tumor. In addition to measuring changes in blood pressure after histamine administration, catecholamine levels in the blood and urine can also be determined, and significant increases in catecholamine levels following the provocative administration of histamine are diagnostic for pheochromocytoma.

Two other provocative agents used in humans with suspected pheochromocytomas include tyramine and glucagon. Tyramine is an indirectly acting sympathomimetic agent that produces hypertension in patients with pheochromocytomas without causing many of the side effects noted with histamine. Glucagon also induces a marked rise in both blood pressure and plasma catecholamine concentrations in patients with pheochromocytomas, compared with normal subjects. Neither tyramine nor glucagon has been evaluated in dogs with pheochromocytoma.

TREATMENT

The therapy of choice for pheochromocytoma in dogs is surgery. The major role of medical therapy in this disease is to normalize the cardiovascular and metabolic status of the patient prior to surgery in order to reduce the risk involved with anesthesia and surgery. Medical therapy is also indicated for the chronic management of dogs with inoperable malignant pheochromocytoma. The two classes of drugs used include the alpha- and beta-adrenergic blocking agents. Both inhibit the effects of catecholamines but do not alter their synthesis or degradation. Phenoxybenzamine hydrochloride (Dibenzyline, Smith Kline & French), an alpha-adrenergic blocking agent, should be administered at a dosage of 0.2 to 1.5 mg/kg orally twice daily for 10 to 14 consecutive days prior to surgery. It is suggested to initiate phenoxybenzamine at the low end of the dosage range and gradually increase the dosage until the desired reduction in blood pressure is observed. Postoperatively, residual effects of this agent do not usually cause sustained hypotension that is unresponsive to pressor agents and fluid administration. Phenoxybenzamine will dampen but not totally inhibit diagnostic increases in blood pressure that may occur as the surgeon palpates the tumor mass.

The beta-adrenergic blocking agents are used to control cardiac arrhythmias and hypertension that persists despite alpha-blocker therapy. Relatively low doses of propranolol (Inderal, Ayerst; 0.15 to 0.5 mg/kg orally three times daily) should be used. Propranolol should not be initiated without concomitant phenoxybenzamine therapy, however, or severe hypertension could be precipitated.

New agents that act to decrease catecholamine production by the pheochromocytoma are currently being investigated. One such drug, alpha-methyltyrosine, acts to inhibit tyrosine hydroxylase, the rate-limiting step in catecholamine biosynthesis.

When planning an anesthetic regimen, care must be given to the choice of preanesthetic, induction, and maintenance agents. Phenothiazines such as acepromazine should be avoided because they possess alpha-blocking effects and can result in unopposed beta-adrenergic effects, leading to vasodilation and hypotensive crisis. Because dogs with pheochromocytomas may show a pronounced tachycardia after treatment with atropine, this agent should also be avoided as a preanesthetic. Narcotic agents combined with glycopyrrolate (Robinol, Robins) are generally used in the preanesthetic regime. Ultrashort-acting barbiturates may be used for induction because they do not cause the release of catecholamines; however, they do have the drawback of being arrhythmogenic. For this reason, narcotic agents may be a better choice for induction. There is considerable controversy involving the choice of maintenance agents. Halothane potentiates catecholamine-induced arrhythmias, and for this reason, methoxyflurane or enflurane is probably a better choice. Concurrent use of nitrous oxide will allow decreased amounts of maintenance anesthetic agents to be used.

As important as the type of anesthesia is the close monitoring of the patient during surgery. Prior to induction, an intra-arterial catheter for measuring blood pressure and a jugular catheter to monitor central venous pressure (CVP) should be inserted. The cardiac rhythm should also be monitored with an electrocardiogram. Close monitoring will ensure adequate blood volume, blood pressure, and tissue oxygenation. Hypertension can develop with anesthetic induction, intubation, peritoneal incision, or manipulation of the tumor. These hypertensive episodes are best treated with repeated intravenous boluses of phentolamine (0.02 to 0.1 mg/kg), a short-acting alpha-adrenergic blocking agent. CVP is used to assess blood volume and to direct fluid replacement during surgery. Extrasystoles, bigeminy, and ventricular tachycardia are the most common arrhythmias that develop during anesthesia and surgery and should be managed with intravenous administration of propranolol (0.03 to 0.1 mg/kg). Tumor removal may result in a pronounced decline in blood pressure, which appears to result primarily from a reduction in blood volume secondary to chronic vasoconstriction rather than a decrease in circulating catecholamine levels. Therefore, hypotension is more successfully managed with vigorous fluid administration than with pressor administration. Monitoring the CVP is essential when administering intravenous fluids to these patients.

The potential for surgical success in complete resection of pheochromocytomas in dogs is dependent on the invasive nature of the adrenal tumor. Tumors without local invasive spread can often be completely resected. Great care must be taken in the dissection of the tumor mass, since it is quite vascular and can bleed profusely when incised. Invasive tumors, especially involving thrombus growth into the vena cava, carry a guarded prognosis.

The majority of pheochromocytomas in dogs are associated with only one adrenal gland. It is, however, still very important for the surgeon to completely explore the abdomen to look for multicentric disease. The vast majority of tumors lie within the retroperitoneal space either in or around the adrenals, or they arise in chromaffin rests along the aorta and its main branches. Location of the tumor can be aided by observing an elevation in arterial blood pressure when the tumor is palpated by the surgeon. This will usually occur even if the dog has been pretreated with alpha-blockers. Because it is difficult to judge the malignancy of a pheochromocytoma on histologic evidence alone, the surgeon should look for signs of local invasiveness or evidence of spread of the tumor to local lymph nodes and other tissues. For optimal histologic characterization of the tumor, biopsy specimens should be placed in Zenker's fixative without acetic acid rather than in formalin. If no drop in blood pressure is observed following removal of the tumor, there is a strong possibility that additional tumor tissue is present. Several days after surgery, urinary excretion of catecholamines and metabolites should be re-evaluated to ascertain if resection was complete. If catecholamine concentrations are still elevated, further evaluation is indicated and re-exploration should be considered.

References and Supplemental Reading

Bravo, E. L., and Gifford, R. W.: Pheochromocytoma: Diagnosis, localization, and management. N. Engl. J. Med. 311:1298, 1984.

Melmon, K. L.: The endocrinologic functions of selected autocoids: Catecholamines, acetylcholine, serotonin, and histamine. *Textbook of Endocrinology*. Philadelphia: W. B. Saunders, 1981.

Schaer, M.: Pheochromocytoma in a dog: A case report. J. Am. Anim. Hosp. Assoc. 16:583, 1980.

Twedt, D. C., Tilley, L. P., et al.: Grand rounds conference: Pheochromocytoma in a canine. J. Am. Anim. Hosp. Assoc. 11:491, 1975.

Twedt, D. C., and Wheeler, S. L.: Pheochromocytoma in the dog. Vet. Clin. North Am. 14:767, 1984.

HYPOGLYCEMIA

CONNIE E. LEIFER, D.V.M.*
New York, New York

Hypoglycemia is an abnormal depression of extracellular glucose concentration that manifests as central nervous system (CNS) signs. It is a biochemical abnormality rather than a disease. Tumors of both pancreatic and extrapancreatic origin, failure of endocrine or nonendocrine organs, derangements of gastrointestinal anatomy, drugs, and severe infection all can produce hypoglycemia.

The brain is the most important obligate consumer of glucose. Cerebral cells have limited stores of glycogen and a limited ability to utilize protein and amino acid pools for energy. Other relatively obligate users of glucose are red and white blood cells, platelets, peripheral nerves, and the renal and adrenal medulla. Other tissues, however, exhibit considerable flexibility, deriving energy from free fatty acids and lesser amounts from ketone bodies in addition to glucose.

Maintenance of a euglycemic state in a fasting animal depends on three major factors: (1) a hormone milieu characterized by normal or reduced circulating insulin concentrations and normal or increased circulating concentrations of glucagon, growth hormone, epinephrine, and cortisol; (2) a healthy liver with intact glycogen synthesis, gluconeogenesis, and glycogenolytic processes; and (3) an availability of the precursors of hepatic gluconeogenesis. The mechanisms for the maintenance of euglycemia are the subject of several recent reviews (Davidson, 1981; Leifer and Peterson 1984).

CLINICAL SIGNS

Blood glucose concentration is normally maintained in the range of 70 to 110 mg/dl. Manifestations of hypoglycemia usually are not apparent until the blood glucose concentration has fallen below 45 mg/dl. Because the brain is the organ most sensitive to glucose deprivation, the signs of hypoglycemia on examination are neurologic and are related to the rate of fall of blood glucose, the concentration of glucose attained, and the duration of hypoglycemia.

Clinical signs of hypoglycemia can be roughly divided into two categories: (1) adrenergic manifestations, caused by increased tone of the sympathetic nervous system, and (2) neuroglucopenic manifestations, which result from glucose deprivation of the CNS. Since hypothalamic glucoreceptors sense a rapidly falling glucose concentration, the animal might show adrenergic signs of pupillary dilatation, heart rate acceleration, nervousness, vocalization, and irritability. If the decline of the blood glucose is gradual enough so that activation of the autonomic nervous system does not occur, only neuroglucopenic effects will appear. Signs of hypothermia, visual disturbances, mental dullness, confusion, seizures, and bradycardia might progress to decerebrate rigidity, miotic pupils, absence of deep tendon reflexes, and coma. The degree to which a given area of the brain is affected by hypoglycemia depends on the order of phylogenetic evolution, rostral to caudal. From the neocortex, which has the greatest dependence on glucose, the subcortex, diencephalon, mesencephalon, and myelencephalon are affected in decreasing order of dependency. A prolonged period of hypoglycemia can produce irreversible neurologic damage, with histologic changes in the cortex, basal ganglia, and rostral medulla. Although most of the damage due to hypoglycemia occurs above the foramen magnum, peripheral nerve degeneration and demyelination also have been documented.

LABORATORY DOCUMENTATION

The laboratory documentation of hypoglycemia is subject to several errors. Since glycolysis by red and white blood cells decreases blood glucose by 7 mg/dl/hour, the results of blood glucose testing might be falsely low if samples are left at room temperature prior to clot separation. Also, a variety of reducing methods are not specific for glucose and occasionally might give falsely elevated results. Assays for glucose oxidase or a combination of hexokinase and glucose-6-phosphate dehydrogenase are methods of analysis that are sufficiently free from error. It is recommended that the blood be stored

*Deceased 1985.

in sodium fluoride if a delay in separating serum or plasma is anticipated.

CAUSES OF HYPOGLYCEMIA

Classification of the causes of hypoglycemia is given in Table 1.

Functional Hypoglycemia

NEONATAL HYPOGLYCEMIA. The fetus is provided with a continuous infusion of glucose from the placenta and is therefore not dependent on its own gluconeogenic capacity. The canine neonate might develop hypoglycemia after only 12 hours of fasting, as opposed to adult dogs, which can undergo weeks of starvation without hypoglycemia. Between meals, the neonate relies on glycogenolysis and gluconeogenesis. Glycogen stores are rapidly depleted, at which time gluconeogenesis becomes the sole support for glucose homeostasis. In the neonate, however, a small muscle mass, lack of adipose tissue, and possible lack of gluconeogenic enzymes all limit gluconeogenesis. In addition, decreased use of free fatty acids as an alternative energy source and a brain:body mass ratio two to four times that of the adult place severe stress on neonatal glucose homeostasis.

The majority of human infants who develop hypoglycemia within the first 24 hours of life have a pertinent prenatal history (mothers with diabetes mellitus or toxemia) or physical findings (premature birth or small size for age). In dogs, stresses such as dystocia, trauma by the bitch, hypothermia, hypoxia, dehydration, diarrhea, early maternal rejection, and poor maternal nutrition can lead to neonatal hypoglycemia.

Table 1. *Differential Diagnosis of Hypoglycemia*

Functional hypoglycemia (no recognizable lesion)
- Neonatal hypoglycemia
- "Toy breed" hypoglycemia (juvenile hypoglycemia)
- "Hunting dog" hypoglycemia
- Starvation

Hepatic enzyme deficiencies
- Von Gierke's disease (type I glycogen storage disease)
- Cori's disease (type III glycogen storage disease)
- Other enzyme defects

Exogenous agents
- Insulin excess
- Sulfonylurea administration
- Ethanol
- Salicylate ingestion
- Propranolol

Bacterial shock

Organic hypoglycemia (recognizable lesion)
- Severe hepatic disease
- Adrenocortical insufficiency
- Renal failure
- Cardiac disease–induced hypoglycemia
- Extrapancreatic tumor–induced hypoglycemia
- Hyperinsulinism secondary to islet cell tumor of the pancreas

Because dehydration, hypothermia, and hypoglycemia commonly occur together in the canine neonate, the therapeutic approach has three aspects. Ideally, the blood glucose concentration should be determined, although blood sampling from a small, stressed patient might be difficult. A semiquantitative determination of glucose can be made by using Chemstrips bG (Boehringer Mannheim Diagnostics) and blood from a clipped nail. Subcutaneous administration of warmed half-strength lactated Ringer's solution in 2.5 per cent dextrose (0.04 ml/gm body weight) followed by oral administration of 5 to 10 per cent (0.01 ml/gm) glucose will correct dehydration and hypoglycemia. Often, intravenous therapy is difficult. Nursing should recommence as soon as possible, and hand rearing is necessary if the bitch dies or rejects the pup. An ambient temperature of 29.4 to 32.2°C should be maintained by means of body heat, incubators, heating pads, or hot water.

TOY BREED HYPOGLYCEMIA (JUVENILE HYPOGLYCEMIA). The most common form of childhood hypoglycemia, ketotic hypoglycemia, seems similar in some respects to the hypoglycemia observed in small breeds of pups less than 6 months old. This disorder classically affects children between the ages of 18 months and 5 years, with spontaneous remissions occurring between 8 and 9 years of age. Low blood glucose concentrations with ketonuria, ketonemia, and neurologic signs of hypoglycemia are characteristic of these children. A diet high in fats and low in carbohydrates and calories precipitates hypoglycemic episodes. The children, like the pups, are small for their age. Gluconeogenic substrate deficiency appears to be responsible for this syndrome. Any modest compromise in the supply of endogenous gluconeogenic substrate from muscle mass can lead to hypoglycemia. The defect is probably present at birth, although it is not manifested until the child is stressed with caloric restriction. As the supplies of endogenous substrates increase relative to the demand for glucose, spontaneous remission occurs.

Canine juvenile hypoglycemia, usually seen in puppies less than 6 months of age and most often in toy breeds, can be precipitated by stress (shipping, exposure to cold), infectious disease, parasitism, fasting, or gastrointestinal disturbances. Signs on examination are related to effects of hypoglycemia on the CNS. Diagnosis is made by documenting low blood glucose concentration and by the immediate clinical response to glucose administration (either oral or 1 ml/kg 50 per cent dextrose IV). Until oral intake can be re-established, an intravenous infusion of glucose sufficient to maintain the blood glucose concentration greater than 40 mg/dl should be administered through a central venous catheter. The owner should be advised to give frequent high-protein, high-carbohydrate feedings and told that the problem will probably resolve as the pup matures.

"HUNTING DOG HYPOGLYCEMIA." This syndrome has been reported but poorly described. The typical dog is a lean, high-strung, eager hunter that, several hours after beginning to work, appears confused and weak and might have grand mal seizures. Although the pathogenesis remains unknown, hunting dog hypoglycemia might be similar to the hypoglycemia of marathon runners or healthy human patients exercised to exhaustion. With prolonged exercise, liver glycogen stores are depleted and glucose production cannot keep pace with the rate of glucose use. Pathogenesis of this condition might include a limited epinephrine response.

Owners of affected hunting dogs should be advised to feed a moderate meal of protein, fat, and complex carbohydrates several hours prior to exercise to provide a pool of gluconeogenic precursors and alternate energy sources. Snacks in the form of candy bars can be given every 4 hours during the hunt. If hypoglycemia signs occur, a source of glucose (syrup, honey, candy, dextrose solution) should be given. Other preventives include prednisone, sedatives, and tranquilizers.

STARVATION. Hypoglycemia in severely malnourished patients has been reported. As discussed, both children and juvenile animals are affected more severely than adults. Such dogs are not hyperinsulinemic, and gluconeogenic mechanisms remain intact. Reasons for hypoglycemia include decreased hepatic glycogen and decreased fat stores.

Hepatic Enzyme Deficiencies

The glycogen storage diseases are inherited defects. Enzymes involved in the degradation of glycogen are either deficient or defective.

Type I glycogen storage disease, or von Gierke's disease, is typically seen in young animals and is characterized by severe hypoglycemia that responds to glucose administration. No glycemic response is noted in animals tested with glucagon. Hepatic enzymatic analysis shows low or absent glucose-6-phosphatase. No confirmed cases have been reported in dogs, although a series of toy breed dogs have been suspected. Type III glycogen storage disease (amylo-1,6-glucosidase deficiency) has been documented in puppies with clinical signs of massive hepatomegaly, failure to thrive, and muscle weakness. Because the gluconeogenic enzymatic system is still intact, spontaneous hypoglycemia is less common. Massive glycogen stores are present on histologic examination of the liver, cardiac and skeletal musculature, and brain. Very low (0 to 7 per cent of normal) concentrations of amylo-1,6-glucosidase in the liver and muscle confirm the diagnosis. Other enzymatic defects (e.g., in the phosphorylase system, gluconeogenesis, and glycogen synthesis) might lead to hypoglycemic conditions, but these have not been documented in dogs.

Exogenous Agents

Hypoglycemia reactions can occur following administration or accidental ingestion of a variety of drugs. Any insulin-treated animal can have hypoglycemic episodes. Predisposing causes include failure to eat, unaccustomed exercise, and inadvertent overdose of insulin.

Sulfonylurea compounds (tolbutamide, acetohexamide, tolazamide, chlorpropamide) are oral hypoglycemic agents that stimulate islet cells to secrete insulin by degranulation of beta cells. Tolbutamide causes a rapid decrease in blood sugar that remains low for several hours and is used as a diagnostic test for islet cell tumor.

Other exogenous agents that can precipitate hypoglycemia include ethanol, salicylates, and propranolol.

Bacterial Shock

Classically, clinical bacterial sepsis is accompanied by hyperglycemia, possibly caused by catecholamine inhibition of insulin secretion. However, overwhelming sepsis has been recognized as a cause of hypoglycemia in both humans and dogs; depletion of glycogen stores, increased peripheral utilization of glucose, decreased gluconeogenesis, and circulatory factors might contribute. Hypotension with decreased tissue perfusion can cause a shift to anaerobic metabolism, requiring 18 times more glucose to produce the same number of adenosine triphosphate (ATP) as aerobic metabolism. Concurrent metabolic acidosis impairs gluconeogenesis.

Fluid therapy is imperative because the generalized endothelial damage and shock of endotoxemia create acidosis, regional abnormalities in blood flow, and organ dysfunction. Administration of glucose, insulin, and potassium has been shown to reverse the hemodynamic, renal, and metabolic derangements, allowing recovery of dogs in lethal endotoxic shock. Administration of a combination of corticosteroids and bactericidal antibiotics, if used early enough, has been shown to prevent death from endotoxic shock. Bacterial sepsis carries a guarded to poor prognosis—death is caused by disseminated intravascular coagulation and shock lung.

Organic Hypoglycemia

Organic hypoglycemia, which is caused by a histologically recognizable lesion, might be caused by imbalance of the hormone milieu of insulin and its counter-regulatory hormones, malfunction of the liver (with faulty glycogenolytic or gluconeogenic processes), and unavailability of substrates for gluconeogenesis. Severe hepatic disease, adrenocortical insufficiency, renal failure, and cardiac disease–induced hypoglycemia are generally identified by physical examination, laboratory testing, and radiography. Treatment of the hypoglycemic aspect of the disease necessitates treatment of the primary disorder. The two major causes of organic hypoglycemia include extrapancreatic tumor and insulin-secreting islet cell tumor.

EXTRAPANCREATIC TUMOR HYPOGLYCEMIA. Tumors arising outside the pancreatic islet cells can cause severe hypoglycemia by several mechanisms: (1) secretion of insulin, an insulin-like substance, or an insulin potentiator; (2) utilization of glucose at an accelerated rate; and (3) inhibition of the liver's ability to release glucose, possibly by suppression of counter-regulatory hormones. In humans, hypoglycemia has been reported in a variety of mesenchymal, epithelial, and hematopoietic tumors. Hypoglycemia is more common in the later stages of disseminated malignancy but might occasionally develop early in the course of the disease and therefore dominate initial clinical signs. Hypoglycemia associated with non-islet cell tumor also has been recognized in dogs; a variety of tumor types have been reported, and hepatic tumors are the most frequent. Dogs, regardless of tumor type, are examined because of signs of hypoglycemia, and in most cases a mass lesion is identifiable on physical examination and can be confirmed radiographically. In hepatic tumors, high serum alanine aminotransaminase and serum alkaline phosphatase activities are often encountered. Serum insulin concentrations tend to be low to low-normal. This contrasts to cases of islet cell tumor in which physical examination, radiography, and routine laboratory testing are generally noncontributory except for hypoglycemia and elevations of serum insulin concentration. Supportive care for the hypoglycemia state might be necessary, but removal of the mass lesion (i.e., surgical resection, radiation, or chemotherapy) represents the only long-term control.

INSULIN-SECRETING ISLET CELL TUMOR. Insulin-secreting tumors frequently have been described in dogs. These neoplasms have been named beta cell tumors, islet cell tumors, islet cell adenocarcinomas, insulinomas, and insulin-producing pancreatic tumors. They are rarely encapsulated, are often associated with proliferative adenomatous changes that make identification of normal tissue margins difficult, possess a histologic appearance common to other endocrine tumors that belies malignancy, and have a high rate of metastasis to regional lymph nodes and liver.

Islet cell tumors develop in dogs of middle to old age. No sex predilection is apparent. Clinical signs are related to the rate of fall of blood glucose, the concentration of blood glucose attained, and the duration of hypoglycemia. The most common signs include grand mal seizures, posterior paresis, collapse, shaking, trembling, generalized weakness, ataxia, focal facial seizures, polyphagia, polyuria, polydipsia, behavior change (hysteria, apathy), and status epilepticus. Occasionally, discovery of the tumor may be accidental. Signs may occur episodically or be provoked by fasting, feeding, or exercise. Most dogs exhibit multiple signs, which tend to become more frequent and severe as the disease progresses.

To diagnose an insulin-secreting tumor of the pancreas, the rational steps are as follows: (1) Demonstrate that the animal's signs are caused by hypoglycemia, (2) demonstrate that the hypoglycemia is caused by inappropriately elevated serum insulin concentrations, and (3) rule out other causes of hyperinsulinemia. Results of radiography, hematologic testing, and biochemical testing, with the exception of glucose concentrations, are noncontributory.

Nonfasting glucose concentrations often are below normal (less than 70 mg/dl). Simultaneous determinations of serum glucose and insulin after an overnight fast are diagnostic in most dogs with islet cell tumors. Alternately, the dog can be fed in the morning and blood collected every 2 to 4 hours during the day until the glucose concentration has fallen below 60 mg/dl. When adequate clinical or biochemical hypoglycemia develops, a blood sample for glucose and insulin determinations is drawn and the fast terminated. Although hypoglycemia will develop in many dogs within 8 hours of fasting, others must be fasted 24 to 72 hours to suppress blood glucose concentrations. When absolute elevations in serum insulin concentrations do not develop, other criteria can be used to evaluate the presence of inappropriate insulin secretion, including the glucose:insulin and insulin:glucose ratios and the amended insulin:glucose ratio (AIGR). The AIGR is based on the assumption that in a "normal" human or dog, the circulating insulin is undetectable when the circulating glucose falls to 30 mg/dl. Although this ratio provides fewer false-negative results than that of elevation in serum insulin concentrations, it appears less specific and has yielded false-positive results in other conditions in which the blood glucose concentrations are very low (e.g., sepsis, extrapancreatic tumor hypoglycemia). Therefore, the AIGR should not be used as the sole criterion for diagnosis of insulin-secreting tumor unless other causes of hypoglycemia have been ruled out, especially when blood glucose concentrations are less than 40 mg/dl.

If even prolonged fasting does not produce clinical or biochemical hypoglycemia but suspicion of islet cell tumor persists, provocative testing with glucagon, glucose, leucine, tolbutamide, or calcium to elicit excess insulin secretion can be performed. Caution is needed because islet cell tumors vary in their responsiveness to these secretagogues, false-negative results are common, and some of these agents can precipitate severe, prolonged hypoglycemia.

Once diagnostic testing has demonstrated absolute or relative (inappropriate) hyperinsulinemia, the treatment of choice is resection of the primary pancreatic mass and, if possible, any metastatic disease (enlarged duodenal, hepatic, splenic, and greater mesenteric nodes and focal hepatic involvement). Although most islet cell tumors in dogs are malignant, surgery offers the best chance of control. Careful visual inspection and palpation are required. Neoplastic tissue is often buried between lobules, and, in 14 per cent of the dogs reported by Mehlhaff and colleagues, masses were found in more than one pancreas lobe. Because islet cell tumors most often are not encapsulated, wide resection of the mass (partial pancreatectomy) might result in longer hypoglycemia-free survival periods than with local resection of the mass.

Hypoglycemia must be controlled preoperatively. In some dogs, frequent feeding is sufficient. In others, continuous glucose infusions through a central jugular catheter are necessary, adjusting the infusion as needed to maintain euglycemia.

Postoperatively, food and water are withheld for 3 to 5 days to avoid exacerbating presumed iatrogenic pancreatitis. Intravenous administration of balanced electrolyte solutions are provided to maintain fluid, glucose, and electrolyte balance. Serum concentrations of glucose, electrolytes, amylase, and lipase are monitored daily until the dog is stable.

If the insulin-secreting tumor has unresectable metastasis, if the owner declines surgical intervention, if no pancreatic tumor can be located at surgery, or if hypoglycemia recurs at any time postoperatively, medical methods of controlling hypoglycemia are recommended.

In many dogs with islet cell tumor, frequent feedings may control clinical hypoglycemia. If this fails, diazoxide, a nondiuretic benzothiadizene antihypertensive agent, might be successful. The mechanism of action of diaxozide is not known, but the drug directly inhibits pancreatic insulin secretion, enhances epinephrine-induced glycogenolysis, and inhibits glucose uptake by the tissues. Diazoxide successfully controls hypoglycemic episodes in about 70 per cent of dogs with islet cell tumor. The recommended dosage is 10 mg/kg/day initially, gradually increasing to 40 mg/kg/day as needed to control hypoglycemia. The most common adverse side effects are vomiting and anorexia.

Other forms of medical management include glucocorticoids to enhance hepatic gluconeogenesis and decrease peripheral tissue utilization. The use of diphenylhydantoin, which has hyperglycemic properties in humans, has not been studied well in dogs. Streptozocin, a nitrosurea antibiotic and antineoplastic agent that destroys islet cells, has been evaluated in a few dogs with islet cell tumor, but it caused severe side effects of hepatic damage and renal tubular destruction.

Prolonged hypoglycemia might be the most serious complication of islet cell tumor, causing focal or laminar and pseudolaminar necrosis of the cerebral cortex and acquired epilepsy. If seizures persist despite correction of hypoglycemia, cerebral edema might occur; antiedema doses of corticosteroids as well as mannitol, diazepam, and phenobarbitol might be necessary, in addition to continuing the glucose infusions. The clinician must identify the cause of the seizures, since acquired epilepsy can be managed with long-term oral anticonvulsants whereas hypoglycemic seizures indicate recurrence of the insulin-secreting tumor.

Polyneuropathy has been documented in some dogs with islet cell tumor and accompanying hypoglycemia. Clinical signs include extreme weakness and absence of patellar, gastrocnemius, and cranial tibial reflexes. The neuropathy is usually symmetric, involving distal motor nerves, and is usually reversible once hypoglycemia and hyperinsulinemia are corrected.

Transient or permanent diabetes mellitus might develop after surgical removal of the islet cell tumor. Excessive insulin secretion by the tumor may suppress the activity of normal beta cell tissue, resulting in insulin deficiency. In most dogs with postoperative hyperglycemia, the diabetic state is transitory and resolves in 2 to 4 days. In a smaller number of dogs, however, the hyperglycemia is severe and is accompanied by ketoacidosis. These patients require exogenous insulin therapy. In such a case, if the diabetic state resolves or if hypoglycemia develops while the dog is on insulin therapy, it should be re-evaluated for recurrence of the insulin-secreting tumor.

Iatrogenic pancreatitis, as previously discussed, might develop as a sequela to surgical manipulation of the pancreas, usually within a few days after surgery, although clinical and biochemical evidence of pancreatitis has been observed as late as 2 to 3 weeks postoperatively.

In dogs, most insulin-secreting tumors are malignant. Even if metastasis is not detected at surgery, it is difficult to completely excise the tumor, and recurrence is likely. Partial pancreatectomy may be a superior procedure to local excision. Surgical removal, offering the best means to control hypoglycemia, might control signs of hypoglycemia for months to years. In dogs with recurrence, surgical treatment has been shown to produce a second prolonged remission, unless there is widespread metastasis. In such cases, medical management should be considered. With close monitoring and surgical and medical management, excellent survival times are possible.

References and Supplemental Reading

Davidson, M. B.: *Diabetes Mellitus: Diagnosis and Treatment*. New York: John Wiley & Sons, 1981, p. 420.

Fajans, S. S., and Floyd, J. C.: Fasting hypoglycemia in adults. N. Engl. J. Med. 294:766, 1976.

Kahn, C. R.: The riddle of tumour hypoglycaemia revisited. Clin. Endocrinol. Metab. 9:335, 1980.

Kruth, S. A., Feldman, E. C., and Kennedy, P. C.: Insulin-secreting islet cell tumors: Establishing a diagnosis and the clinical course for 25 dogs. J.A.V.M.A. 181:54, 1982.

Leifer, C. E., and Peterson, M. E.: Hypoglycemia. Vet. Clin. North Am. [Small Anim. Pract.] 14:873, 1984.

Leifer, C. E., Peterson, M. E., and Matus, R. E.: Insulin-secreting tumor: Diagnosis and medical and surgical management in 55 dogs. J.A.V.M.A. 188:60, 1986.

Leifer, C. E., Peterson, M. E., Matus, R. E., et al.: Hypoglycemia associated with nonislet cell tumor in 13 dogs. J.A.V.M.A. 186:53, 1985.

Mehlhaff, C. J., Peterson, M. E., Patnaik, A. K., et al.: Insulin producing islet cell neoplasms: Surgical considerations and general management in 35 dogs. J. Am. Anim. Hosp. Assoc. 21:607, 1985.

Pagliara, A. S., Karl, I. E., Haymond, M., et al.: Hypoglycemia in infancy and childhood: Part II. J. Pediatr. 82:558, 1973.

DIABETIC KETOACIDOSIS

MARGARETHE HOENIG, DR. MED. VET.

Ithaca, New York

Diabetic ketoacidosis is a severe alteration of metabolism caused by an absolute deficiency of insulin or a defect in insulin action. Diabetic ketoacidosis is characterized by acidemia, ketonemia, hyperglycemia, and depletion of intracellular and extracellular water and electrolytes. Most diabetic ketoacidotic animals are previously undiagnosed diabetics, whereas the remainder have already been receiving insulin treatment for diabetes. It has been well established in humans that diabetic ketoacidosis is closely associated with an increased secretion of the stress-related hormones (catecholamines, glucagon, cortisol, and growth hormone) and is often precipitated by concurrent infections or endocrinologic disorders. This also seems to be the case in animals, in which other illnesses often complicate the diabetic ketoacidotic state.

PATHOGENESIS

Hyperglycemia

In diabetes, glucose production in the liver is increased because the low ratio of insulin to glucagon activates hepatic enzymes necessary for gluconeogenesis. Cortisol and catecholamines have permissive and possibly synergistic effects to increase hepatic glucose production. Insulin is not required for glucose uptake in the liver. This is contrary to the situation in many peripheral tissues, where glucose cannot be normally utilized without the presence of insulin. The resulting high plasma glucose concentrations soon exceed the renal threshold for maximal reabsorption of glucose. An osmotic diuresis ensues with concomitant loss of large amounts of water and salt. Unless there is adequate replacement of water and electrolytes, a vicious circle occurs: intravenous volume depletion leads to poor perfusion of the kidneys, resulting in decreased clearance of glucose and an increase in stress hormones, causing a further rise in plasma glucose concentrations.

Ketoacidosis

Hepatic ketogenesis has been extensively studied, and excellent reviews are available (McGarry and Foster, 1980). Briefly, insulin deficiency and glucagon excess accelerate lipolysis from fat depots and increase delivery of free fatty acids (FFA) to the liver. In the liver, FFA are converted to their coenzyme A derivatives and either re-esterified in the cytosol of the hepatocyte or oxidized to acetyl coenzyme A (acetyl-CoA) in the mitochondria. The rate at which the FFA enter mitochondria in the hepatocyte determines whether FFA will be re-esterified to triglycerides or oxidized to ketone bodies. The entry into mitochondria is dependent on the activity of carnitine acetyl transferase (CAT

I), an enzyme located on the inner mitochondria membrane. In diabetes, CAT I is activated and FFA readily enter the mitochondria and are oxidized to acetyl-CoA. Normally, high concentrations of malonyl-CoA, an intermediate in the conversion of glucose into fat, inhibit CAT I and therefore favor re-esterification of FFA. In diabetes, however, the conversion of glucose into fat is inhibited because hepatic concentrations of both malonyl-CoA and glycogen are depleted. Therefore, fatty acid oxidation is enhanced, resulting in the production of large amounts of acetyl-CoA that are converted to acetoacetate, β-hydroxybutyrate, and acetone. Since the liver cannot utilize these ketone bodies, they are released into the bloodstream and rapidly dissociate, thereby causing an increase in arterial hydrogen concentration. In addition, utilization of ketones by peripheral tissues is impaired in diabetes mellitus. The resulting ketoacidosis leads to a decrease in the serum bicarbonate concentration and a widening of the anion gap. As organic anions, ketoacids bind both sodium and potassium. They are excreted by the kidneys together with sodium and potassium, thereby contributing to the electrolyte and water loss in diabetic ketoacidosis and aggravating hypovolemia and dehydration. As systemic acidosis develops, a compensatory hyperventilation may develop (Kussmaul's breathing), and persisting acidosis may ultimately lead to a depression of the respiratory center.

CLINICAL FEATURES

The most common historic findings associated with diabetic ketoacidosis include polyuria, polydipsia, weight loss, anorexia, vomiting, and weakness. Few animals will actually present in coma.

Physical findings include moderate to severe dehydration, hepatomegaly, and hyper- or hypoventilation, depending on the severity of the acidosis. Some clinicians may be able to detect a fruity breath odor, which is caused by acetone. Other signs pertaining to concomitant illnesses may be present and should be thoroughly investigated.

LABORATORY FINDINGS

Glucose

Plasma glucose concentrations usually range between 400 and 800 mg/dl in diabetic ketoacidosis. However, glucose values approaching the renal threshold for maximal glucose reabsorption (approximately 200 mg/dl) and levels of greater than 1000 mg/dl may be encountered.

Ketones

The diagnosis of diabetic ketoacidosis is confirmed by the findings of increased blood or urine ketone concentrations. Ketones can be measured in a qualitative manner in blood using nitroprusside tablets (Acetest, Ames) and in urine with Multistix (Ames) or Keto-Diastix (Ames). Since β-hydroxybutyrate, although grouped together with the other ketones, does not contain a ketogroup, it is not measured by routine methods and, until now, could only be detected by specific enzymatic assays. Recently, however, a semiquantitative method has been developed for the routine detection of β-hydroxybutyrate (Hasrano et al., 1984). Determination of the concentration of β-hydroxybutyrate is important because it is the ketone body present in highest amounts in diabetic ketoacidosis. It predominates because of a shift in the cellular redox potential, which increases the reduction of acetoacetate to β-hydroxybutyrate. Therefore, even accurate measurements of acetoacetate and acetone can be misleading in the estimate of the degree of ketonemia.

Electrolytes

The serum sodium concentration is usually either low or normal in diabetic ketoacidosis. Several factors affect serum sodium levels in diabetes mellitus. Hyperglycemia and hyperosmolarity lead to a dilutional hyponatremia by transfer of water from the intracellular to the extracellular space. Insulin increases tubular reabsorption of sodium, whereas glucagon is a natriuretic hormone; therefore, the lack of insulin and excess of glucagon associated with diabetic ketoacidosis results in an increased loss of sodium into the urine. The osmotic diuresis of diabetic ketoacidosis, together with the excretion of ketoacids in forms of sodium salts, may also lower the serum sodium concentration; however, since water is usually lost in excess of sodium, this tends to increase rather than decrease serum sodium concentrations. A spurious lowering of the serum sodium concentration (pseudohyponatremia) may occur if the animal is hyperlipemic. Although the sodium concentration in plasma water remains normal, the sodium concentration, expressed as milliequivalents per total volume of serum (which in ketoacidosis contains a large nonaqueous phase), is low.

Serum potassium concentrations are usually normal in diabetic ketoacidosis, but very low or high levels may be seen. The serum potassium concentrations do not reflect the status of the body stores. Body potassium stores are commonly depleted in diabetic ketoacidosis as a consequence of the acidosis, diuresis, and vomiting. Serum potassium concentrations, however, may be increased as a result of volume contraction and acidosis. A low or normal serum potassium concentration is therefore almost always indicative of total body potassium depletion.

Serum phosphorus concentrations may range from very low to very high but are usually normal or elevated. Again, as is true for potassium, serum phosphorus levels are not representative of body stores, and phosphorus depletion may occur in diabetic ketoacidosis as a consequence of the acidosis and osmotic diuresis.

Hematology

Although the effects of diabetic ketoacidosis on hemostatic values have not been investigated in dogs or cats, hemostasis is abnormal in human diabetic patients. Increased platelet aggregation and increased concentrations of coagulation factors, together with diminished fibrinolytic activity, have been described. These may lead to disseminated intravascular coagulation (DIC).

It has also been shown in dogs and other species that neutrophil function is abnormal in diabetes. This may predispose diabetics to bacterial infections.

TREATMENT

Diabetic ketoacidosis constitutes an acute, life-threatening condition that requires aggressive and immediate therapy. Treatment involves the administration of regular (crystalline) insulin, fluids, and electrolytes.

Insulin Therapy

Treatment with regular insulin should be initiated as soon as the diagnosis of diabetic ketoacidosis has been established. Regular insulin can be administered in one of three different regimens, which include the continuous low-dose intravenous method, the low-dose intramuscular method, and the high-dose intravenous or subcutaneous bolus method.

Overall, best results are usually obtained using the continuous insulin infusion method. The initial insulin dosage employed is 2.2 U/kg/day for dogs and 1.1 U/kg/day for cats. Insulin can be administered quite accurately intravenously when added to fluids and delivered with a pediatric intravenous set. It should be remembered that insulin binds to glass and plastic surfaces. Saturation of these nonspecific binding sites can be achieved by flushing the intravenous set with the insulin-containing fluid prior to its use.

With the continuous insulin infusion method, plasma glucose concentrations should be monitored at least every 2 hours, and preferably hourly. Blood glucose levels can either be determined by routine laboratory methods or estimated by visual inspection using glucose-impregnated strips (Dextrostix, Ames; Chemstrip bG, Bio-Dynamics). Very accurate glucose measurements can be achieved by reading the test strips with a reflectance colorimeter (Dextrometer, Ames).

Once the glucose concentration reaches 250 mg/dl, intravenous fluids are changed to a dextrose-containing solution (2.5 per cent dextrose in 0.45 per cent saline or 5 per cent dextrose in water) in order to avoid hypoglycemia; such dextrose supplementation also provides a continuous substrate for insulin in the absence of oral caloric intake. Regular insulin is then continued either by IV infusion or administered as bolus subcutaneous injections every 6 hours until the animal is able to eat without vomiting. At that time, the animal is treated as an uncomplicated diabetic with an intermediate or long-acting insulin preparation.

If insulin resistance is detected during treatment of diabetic ketoacidosis, the rate of the continuous insulin infusion should be increased accordingly until blood glucose concentrations decrease to less than 250 mg/dl. For example, if a significant decrease in glucose levels is not seen after 4 to 6 hours of intravenous regular insulin and fluid therapy, the infused insulin dose should be increased by 25 per cent; if the response is still minimal after another 4- to 6-hour period, the dose is increased by 50 per cent above the original insulin dose. The goal of treatment is to increase the dose as needed to obtain effective insulin concentrations within a reasonable period of time.

Conversely, in animals that develop hypoglycemia during the continuous intravenous infusion, the insulin infusion should be temporarily stopped, and the animal should be maintained on a dextrose-containing solution until the blood glucose concentration again increases to greater than 250 mg/dl. The insulin dose can then be adjusted in an arithmetic fashion, based on the results of blood glucose determinations.

With the low-dose intramuscular method, the protocol for animals weighing less than 10 kg (22 lb) consists of the administration of 2.0 U of regular insulin initially, followed by hourly injections of 1.0 U/hour. Dogs weighing more than 10 kg receive an initial intramuscular dose of 0.25 U/kg followed by hourly injections of 0.1 U/kg. This regimen is continued until blood glucose concentrations fall below 250 mg/dl, at which time regular insulin is administered subcutaneously every 6 hours (Chastain and Nichols, 1981). Once the animal is eating and does not vomit, regular insulin can be discontinued and therapy with an intermediate- or long-acting insulin initiated.

The third regular insulin administration method consists of subcutaneous bolus injections at 6-hour intervals (Schaer, 1983). Administration of regular insulin by intravenous bolus injection at 2- to 3-hour intervals has also been described but is not recommended.

No matter what initial method of insulin administration is used, avoiding hypoglycemia is as important as treating hyperglycemia. A common reason for hypoglycemia in diabetic ketoacidosis is the use of excessive insulin doses because of persisting ketonemia during treatment. Adjustment in insulin dosage should be based on the plasma glucose level and not on the concentration of ketone bodies. As mentioned earlier, β-hydroxybutyrate is present in highest amounts in ketoacidosis, but it is not measured with routine methods. With proper regular insulin and fluid therapy, ketoacidotic animals will soon show an improvement of tissue perfusion and oxygenation. This will lead to a shift from β-hydroxybutyrate to acetoacetate, which is measured by presently available test strips. Therefore, with the initiation of treatment, Ketostix or nitroprusside tablets may actually become more positive for ketone bodies. In addition, acetone, which also gives a positive ketone reaction, is cleared very slowly.

Fluid and Electrolyte Therapy

Appropriate use of fluid therapy is an extremely important aspect of treatment of diabetic ketoacidosis. Animals with ketoacidosis are invariably dehydrated and hypotensive. The initial fluid replacement needed to correct hydration deficits can be calculated according to the following formula:

$$\text{Fluid deficit (ml)} = \text{per cent dehydration} \times \text{kg body weight} \times 1000$$

Initially, fluid depletion should be replaced aggressively by intravenous administration of 20 to 40 ml/kg/hour until rehydration is complete. If possible, central venous pressure should be closely monitored. It is also recommended that urinary output be quantitated either by inserting a urinary catheter or by using a metabolic cage that pools voided urine. Maintenance fluid therapy after correction of dehydration is calculated on the volume of urine output plus the daily insensible fluid loss. Usually 50 to 60 ml/kg are administered daily; however, this dose may have to be raised if urine output is increased.

Initially, isotonic saline should be used as the replacement fluid to maintain intravascular volume and restore the sodium deficit. The use of fluids containing lactate (i.e., lactated Ringer's solution) is not recommended during the initial treatment of diabetic ketoacidosis. Although the coexistence of lactic acidosis in diabetic ketoacidosis has not been examined in dogs and cats, lactate may not be utilized by the liver in the animal with ketoacidosis because of the reduction of the redox potential associated with poor tissue perfusion and acidosis. The initial use of hypotonic fluids, which may result in a rapid decrease in serum osmolarity, should be avoided. Use of hypotonic fluid solutions may produce large fluid shifts from the extracellular to the intracellular space, irreversible shock, and cerebral edema in diabetic ketoacidosis if the plasma osmolarity is decreased too rapidly.

In diabetic ketoacidosis, assessment of the serum electrolyte levels and correction of any abnormalities are extremely important. The most common electrolyte disturbances associated with ketoacidosis include hypokalemia and hypophosphatemia. If hypokalemia is detected, potassium should be supplemented in the intravenous fluids and infused at a rate not exceeding 0.5 mEq/kg/hour; 20 to 40 mEq of potassium chloride or phosphate are added to each liter of fluids administered. The serum potassium concentrations should be monitored on a daily basis during intravenous potassium supplementation in order to further adjust electrolyte therapy. As soon as the animal has recovered from the ketoacidotic state, oral potassium supplementation (4 to 6 mEq orally three times daily) can be substituted for the intravenous replacement. As is routinely done in human patients, it may be advisable to administer potassium orally for 1 week following the recovery from diabetic ketoacidosis to allow the gradual restoration of the total body potassium deficit.

If hypophosphatemia is detected during treatment of diabetic ketoacidosis, phosphate can be administered together with potassium as potassium phosphate solution at a dose of 2.5 mg phosphate/kg/day. Phosphate should be infused slowly over a period of several hours and should only be given in animals with adequate renal function. As soon as the animal is eating, phosphate depletion will resolve. Phosphate replacement is important in diabetic ketoacidosis in view of erythrocyte 2,3-diphosphoglycerate (2,3-DPG) levels; when serum phosphate concentrations are low, 2,3-DPG levels decrease, causing an increase in the hemoglobin affinity for oxygen, thereby impairing oxygen delivery to tissues. This effect is counterbalanced by the opposite effect of acidosis on the oxygen dissociation of hemoglobin. As soon as the acidosis is corrected, however, low 2,3-DPG levels will shift the oxygen dissociation curve to the left, resulting in impaired oxygen delivery to tissues. Phosphate depletion may also change cellular energy potentials and can lead to insulin resistance by altering membrane proteins.

The administration of bicarbonate in the treatment of diabetic ketoacidosis is controversial. In general, the use of bicarbonate is discouraged, however, because a rapid correction of the acidosis by bicarbonate may lead to severe tissue hypoxia by changing the oxyhemoglobin dissociation curve. It can also cause a paradoxical central nervous system acidosis and may lead to the complications associated with postcorrection alkalosis. Proper insulin therapy leads to regeneration of bicarbonate when ketone bodies become oxidized, and the administration of isotonic saline solution supplies the body with fixed base, which is necessary to correct the ketoacidotic state.

In summary, ketoacidosis is a life-threatening complication of diabetes mellitus. Early recognition of diabetic ketoacidosis, together with aggressive and proper treatment, will drastically reduce the mortality rate.

References and Supplemental Reading

Chastain, C. B., and Nichols, C. E.: Low-dose intramuscular insulin therapy for diabetic ketoacidosis in dogs. J.A.V.M.A. 178:561, 1981.

Church, D. B.: Diabetes mellitus. *In* Kirk, R. W. (ed.): *Current Veterinary Therapy VIII.* Philadelphia: W. B. Saunders, 1983, p. 838.

Clements, R. J., Jr., and Vourganti, B.: Fatal diabetic ketoacidosis: Major causes and approaches to their prevention. Diabetes Care 1:314, 1978.

Hasrano, Y., Suzuki, M., Kojima, H., et al.: Development of paper-strip test for 3-hydroxybutyrate and its clinical application. Diabetes Care 7:481, 1984.

McGarry, J. D., and Foster, D. W.: Regulation of hepatic fatty acid oxidation and ketone body production. Ann. Rev. Biochem. 49:395, 1980.

Schaer, M.: Insulin treatment for the diabetic dog and cat. Comp. Cont. Ed. Pract. Vet. 5:5789, 1983.

CANINE DIABETES MELLITUS

RICHARD W. NELSON, D.V.M.,
West Lafayette, Indiana

and EDWARD C. FELDMAN, D.V.M.
Davis, California

CLASSIFICATION

Diabetes mellitus is an extremely complex disorder. In humans, diabetes mellitus usually appears as one of two recognized clinical pictures—the juvenile (growth-onset, usually young, ketosis-prone, hypoinsulinemic, insulin-dependent) type (Type I) or the more common adult-onset (ketosis-resistant, noninsulin dependent, noninsulinopenic, obese, middle-aged) type (Type II). The essential abnormalities in juvenile diabetes are related to absolute insulin deficiency, whereas those of adult-onset diabetes are more often the result of a delayed release of endogenous insulin in response to a carbohydrate challenge and a reduction in functional insulin receptors. In addition, some patients with adult-onset, ketosis-resistant diabetes have a subnormal capacity for insulin synthesis. In humans, there exists a third broad category of diabetes mellitus composed of patients with carbohydrate intolerance induced by medication. Usually, the inciting medications are thiazide diuretics, oral contraceptives, or glucocorticoids. In most instances, this form of diabetes is transient, reversing itself with withdrawal of the drug.

With the development and use of insulin assays in dogs, comparisons have been made between canine and human types of diabetes mellitus. On the basis of fasting plasma glucose and insulin concentrations, in addition to results of glucose tolerance tests, Kaneko and colleagues (1978) proposed three categories for classification of canine diabetes: Type I, comparable to the insulin-dependent form of human diabetes; Type II, comparable to the noninsulin-dependent form of human diabetes; and Type III, which was compared with subclinical or impaired glucose tolerance diabetes in humans.

The most common form of canine diabetes mellitus closely resembles human Type I, insulin-dependent diabetes. Some dogs may have a severe form of Type II diabetes, but that remains speculative. Most diabetic dogs have an absolute or relative hypoinsulinemia, impaired insulin secretion following a glucose challenge, a necessity for insulin injections, and a tendency to develop ketoacidosis.

Canine diabetes can occur at any age but is most common in middle-aged to older dogs. A juvenile form of canine diabetes mellitus described by Atkins and colleagues (1979, 1983) closely resembles human maturity-onset diabetes of the young, a subclassification of Type II, maturity-onset diabetes mellitus. These dogs also tend to require exogenous insulin therapy.

Hormonally induced diabetes mellitus is well documented in dogs and, depending on the degree of insulin antagonism, may fall into the Type II or Type III categories proposed by Kaneko and colleagues (1978). Increased plasma concentrations of any of the diabetogenic hormones (i.e., glucocorticoids, epinephrine, glucagon, or growth hormone) due to excessive secretion, impaired degradation, or exogenous administration could result in a diabetic condition. Progesterone may result in insulin antagonism due to stimulation of growth hormone secretion (Eigenmann, 1981).

HISTORY AND CLINICAL SIGNS

Hypoinsulinemia and peripheral cell insensitivity to insulin actions result in decreased peripheral tissue utilization of amino acids, triglycerides, and glucose, as well as a modest increase in hepatic gluconeogenesis and glycogenolysis. Glucose obtained from the diet or from hepatic gluconeogenesis accumulates in the circulation, causing hyperglycemia. As the plasma glucose concentration increases, the ability of the renal tubular cells to resorb glucose from the glomerular ultrafiltrate is exceeded, resulting in glycosuria. This occurs when the plasma glucose concentration exceeds 180 to 220 mg/dl. Glycosuria creates an osmotic diuresis, causing polyuria. Compensatory polydipsia prevents hypovolemia. The diminished capacity for peripheral utilization of glucose results in a catabolic state. Both fat and muscle are broken down during the formation of substrates for gluconeogenesis. This catabolism goes unchecked in diabetes mellitus, resulting in significant or severe weight loss. Loss of calories in the form of glycosuria further complicates the body's inability to utilize calories in the blood. Polyphagia results from an inability of blood glucose to enter the cells of the satiety center in the hypothalamus when there is a relative or absolute lack of circulating insulin. As a result, hunger is not inhibited but the increased caloric intake does nothing to reverse the catabolic state.

Thus, the history in virtually all diabetics includes the classic alterations of polydipsia, polyuria, polyphagia, and weight loss. Owners will often bring a previously housebroken pet to the veterinarian because they notice that it is urinating in the home. The other signs are established by further questioning of the owner. A complete anamnesis is extremely important even in the so-called obvious diabetes, because the clinician must be aware of any complicating or concurrent problem in the patient. In many instances, these dogs may have been borderline or latent diabetics and developed overt diabetes secondary to drug therapy, pancreatitis, congestive heart failure, estrus, urinary tract infections, or myriad other potential causes.

Occasionally an owner will bring a dog (ultimately found to be diabetic) to the veterinarian because of blindness caused by cataract formation. The classic signs of diabetes mellitus may have gone unnoticed or been considered insignificant by the owner. Cataract formation is the most common secondary complication in the diabetic dog and is directly related to the severity and duration of hyperglycemia.

PHYSICAL EXAMINATION

There are no classic physical examination findings for nonketotic diabetes mellitus. Most diabetic dogs are obese but are otherwise in good physical condition. Dogs with prolonged untreated diabetes may lose a significant amount of weight but are rarely thin. Secondary to mobilization of fats with resultant hepatic lipidosis, hepatomegaly may be found on palpation of the abdomen. Cataracts are another common clinical finding in canine diabetes.

The physical examination remains an extremely important tool in evaluating dogs with diabetes, despite the lack of pathognomonic abnormalities. A simple diagnosis of diabetes mellitus falls short of revealing the entire picture in any animal. The incidence of concurrent medical problems is so common that we again point out the value and necessity of performing a thorough physical examination on these dogs prior to treatment or hospital admission.

CLINICAL PATHOLOGY

A thorough laboratory evaluation is recommended for all dogs with diabetes. The clinician must be aware of any disease that might be causing or contributing to the carbohydrate intolerance, such as hyperadrenocorticism, infection, pancreatitis, congestive heart failure, liver or renal disease, and others. In addition, the practitioner should be searching for abnormalities that are a result of the diabetic state, such as prerenal uremia, urinary tract infection, or ketoacidosis.

The minimum laboratory evaluation to assess a candidate for long-term insulin therapy should include a urinalysis, fasting blood glucose, complete blood count, renal function test (blood urea nitrogen [BUN] or creatinine), total serum protein, serum albumin, serum alanine transaminase (SGPT), and serum alkaline phosphatase. Dogs with vomiting, diarrhea, anorexia, and dehydration should be evaluated for pancreatitis as well as electrolyte and acid-base imbalance. After the anamnesis is obtained and the physical examination is completed, other tests may be warranted.

DIAGNOSIS

Diabetes mellitus should be suspected whenever there is a history of polydipsia, polyuria, polyphagia, and weight loss or the sudden development of blindness due to cataract formation. The diagnosis is confirmed by the finding of persistent fasting hyperglycemia. The normal fasting plasma glucose concentration in dogs is 70 to 110 mg/dl, and the finding of fasting values greater than 200 mg/dl is usually considered diagnostic of overt diabetes in the absence of complicating factors. Complicating factors include exogenous administration of diabetogenic medications or excessive endogenous secretion of diabetogenic hormones.

Hyperglycemia in the range of 120 to 200 mg/dl may be the result of recent consumption of a meal high in sugar (semimoist dog foods) and can be caused by excessive secretion or exogenous administration of any of the diabetogenic hormones. Mild hyperglycemia may also be associated with azotemia and can be indicative of a subclinical diabetic animal with impaired ability to secrete insulin, especially if tested in the postprandial state. Postprandial hyperglycemia does not occur in normal dogs fed canned or kibbled dog food. Remember, clinical signs of polyuria, polydipsia, and weight loss do not develop until glycosuria and the resultant osmotic diuresis occur. A dog with polyuria and polydipsia probably does *not* have diabetes mellitus if the blood glucose is less than 180 mg/dl and glycosuria is not present.

When the blood glucose concentration exceeds the renal threshold, glycosuria results; this is easily detected with Diastix (Ames Division, Miles Labs) paper strips. In dogs, glycosuria begins to occur when the blood glucose concentration is 180 to 220 mg/dl. The urinalysis cannot be used as the sole test in diagnosing diabetes mellitus because of the rare cases of primary renal glycosuria, a tubular defect involving the reabsorption of glucose, resulting in persistent glycosuria with euglycemia. The syndrome has been reported in many breeds but appears to be most common in the basenji and Norwegian elkhound. It may be mistaken for diabetes mellitus if only a urinalysis is evaluated.

TREATMENT

Oral Hypoglycemic Agents

These drugs have commonly been used in humans with noninsulin-dependent diabetes mellitus, but they are not often employed in veterinary practice. The sulfonylureas have several antidiabetic actions, including the acute stimulation of insulin secretion by beta cells, the chronic enhancement of muscle and adipose tissue carbohydrate transport, a direct effect on the liver to decrease hepatic glucose output, and the potentiation of insulin action on the liver.

Two sulfonylureas (glipizide [Glucotrol, Roerig], 0.25 to 0.5 mg/kg twice daily, and glibenclamide [Diabeta, Hoechst-Roussel; Micronase, Upjohn], 0.2 mg/kg daily) have been recommended for diabetic dogs that have a measurable insulin response to a glucose challenge (Type III and some Type II diabetics) (Church, 1983). However, chronic treatment with some of the sulfonylureas, including glibenclamide, may result in decreased insulin content in beta cells and decreased nutrient-stimulated insulin secretion in normal animals (Lebovitz and Feinglos, 1983). Therefore, caution must be used in the long-term treatment of canine diabetes with these oral hypoglycemic agents. In addition, many Type II and III diabetic dogs have insulin antagonism as a result of hyperadrenocorticism or excessive growth hormone secretion. Insulin-antagonistic drug therapy must also be ruled out as a cause of hyperglycemia and carbohydrate intolerance. Identification and correction of insulin antagonism may resolve the diabetic state.

Insulin

Commercial insulin is categorized by promptness, duration, and intensity of action after subcutaneous administration (Table 1). The solubility of insulin is determined by the size of the insulin crystals, the zinc content, and the nature of the buffer in which it is suspended. Commonly used insulins for the long-term management of diabetics include isophane (NPH), lente, and protamine zinc (PZI) insulins.

INITIAL HOSPITAL MANAGEMENT. Insulin therapy is usually begun with NPH isophane insulin as a single morning injection. Small dogs (less than 15 kg [33 lb]) receive approximately 1 U/kg of body weight, and large dogs (greater than 25 kg [55 lb]) receive 0.5 U/kg. The dose of insulin, like that of many medications, is better based on the animal's size in square meters (m^2) than simply on its body weight. Usually, the larger the animal, the smaller

Table 1. *Properties of Beef-Pork Insulin Preparations Used in Dogs and Cats**

Type of Insulin	Route of Administration	Onset of Effect	Time of Maximum Effect *Dog*	Time of Maximum Effect *Cat*	Duration of Effect *Dog*	Duration of Effect *Cat*
Regular crystalline	IV	Immediate:	¼–2 hours		½–4 hours	
	IM	10–30 minutes	1–2 hours		1–4 hours	
	SC	10–30 minutes	1–5 hours		4–10 hours	
NPH (isophane) insulin	SC	Immediate: 3 hours	2–10 hours	2–8 hours	8–24 hours	6–12 hours
PZI insulin	SC	1–4 hours	5–20 hours	3–12 hours	8–30 hours	12–24 hours
Lente insulin	SC	Immediate	2–10 hours	?	8–24 hours	?
IZS-P insulin	SC	Immediate	2–10 hours	?	8–20 hours	?

*Purified-pork regular, NPH, and PZI insulins appear to be more potent, act faster, and have a shorter duration of action than beef-pork insulins.

This chart is derived primarily from personal experience, Church (1981), and Moise and Reimers (1983). Time sequences relate to plasma glucose concentrations, not plasma insulin concentrations.

the dose needed per kilogram. It is preferable to begin therapy at these relatively low doses, since it is easier to adjust for hyperglycemia than to deal with a hypoglycemic crisis. After insulin therapy is initiated, these dogs are fed canned and kibbled dog food based on ideal body weight. Small dogs receive approximately 75 kcal/kg of body weight per day, and large dogs are given 40 kcal/kg/day. They are fed approximately half of their caloric allotment after the insulin injection and the remainder 6 to 12 hours later.

A dog requires 2 to 4 days for glucose homeostasis to equilibrate after initiation of insulin or after any change in insulin dosage or preparation. Therefore, dogs initially receiving insulin are not critically monitored for the first 2 or 3 days. Blood glucose concentrations are determined once or twice in the afternoon during this time to identify significant sensitivity to these conservative doses. Alternatively, one could teach the owner to administer the insulin and send the newly diagnosed animal home for this equilibration period. However, we prefer and recommend hospitalization in order to complete the dog's medical assessment and the initial therapy simultaneously.

After completing the first few equilibration days, critical monitoring of the blood glucose response to exogenous insulin is imperative. The blood glucose concentration should be checked immediately prior to insulin administration and every 1 or 2 hours thereafter for a minimum of 10 to 12 hours, but preferably for a complete 24-hour period. Dogs can be transferred to an emergency clinic for the evening glucose determinations in hospitals that are staffed for typical working hours only.

Checking only one or two blood glucose concentrations in a 24-hour period is not recommended because of the remarkable variation in onset, peak, and duration of effect of NPH and PZI insulins. Evaluating multiple blood glucose values will allow the clinician to determine both these factors, as well as the degree of fluctuation in blood glucose concentrations. Alterations in the dosage and type of insulin, frequency of administration, and time of feeding may be necessary to achieve satisfactory control.

Knowing precise glucose concentrations is not necessary, and the expense of laboratory glucose measurements requiring 2 to 3 ml of blood per assay is considered excessive. Instead, we have used the new reagent strips (Chemstrip bG, Bio-Dynamics), which require only one drop of whole blood and are excellent aids for the in-hospital management of diabetics. Checking urine glucose concentrations is also helpful but is not recommended as the sole method of monitoring therapy.

An ideal graph of the serial glucose concentrations shows the lowest blood glucose concentration of 80 to 110 mg/dl occurring 10 to 12 hours after insulin administration. The duration of insulin effect should be 20 to 24 hours, and the highest blood glucose concentration of 200 to 240 mg/dl is 24 hours after the insulin injection. As would be expected, the well-controlled diabetic pet will produce urine free of glucose for most of each 24-hour period, which is imperative in eliminating polydipsia and polyuria.

Adjusting the insulin dosage will usually affect the lowest blood glucose concentration obtained without significantly altering the duration of effect of the insulin. If the duration of effect of NPH insulin is less than 20 hours, either PZI administered once daily or NPH insulin administered twice daily may be necessary. If insulin is administered twice a day, similar doses should be given at 12-hour intervals. Twice-daily administration of PZI may be needed but should be based on serial blood glucose determinations in order to avoid excessive overlapping of insulin action.

Determining the time of peak insulin effect will help establish an ideal feeding schedule. Feeding one half of the total daily caloric intake at the time of the insulin injection and the remainder approximately 2 hours before the peak effect of the insulin appears to be an excellent protocol. For most diabetic dogs, the second meal is given 6 to 10 hours postinjection. With twice-daily insulin administration, the owner's schedule must be considered and the treatment protocol altered to comply with what is feasible. Most clients who are administering insulin twice a day feed their pets two equal meals, one meal immediately after each insulin injection.

When the initial blood glucose curve is generated in the hospital, the dog should be fed the same amount and type of dog food that it receives at home. A curve generated without feeding the dog may identify the time of peak insulin action but will not allow adequate evaluation of the dosage or duration of action. If the lowest blood glucose value occurs before the dog receives its evening meal, the time interval between insulin injection and the evening feeding should be shortened accordingly. If the effects of the insulin are dissipating at the time of the evening feeding, a dramatic increase in the blood glucose concentration will occur after feeding the dog. This is an indication of rapid metabolism of the insulin, and either a switch to PZI or administration of NPH insulin twice a day should be considered.

Fine control of the blood glucose concentrations and determination of the exact insulin dose should not be the objective of hospital regulation. Diet and exercise are two important variables that affect insulin requirements once the dog is at home. The main objective of hospital regulation is to determine a "ballpark" insulin-treatment regimen.

HOME MANAGEMENT. Once the type of insulin, frequency of administration, approximate dosage, and feeding schedule have been determined in the hospital, the diabetic dog can be sent home. Insulin requirements will often change at home because of differences in caloric intake and exercise. The goals of home therapy are to maintain plasma glucose concentrations as close to euglycemia as possible, thereby preventing both the recurrence of clinical signs and the long-term complications associated with poorly controlled diabetes mellitus.

The vast majority of dogs in our experience develop complications associated with insulin under- or overdosage as a result of owners' being misled by urine glucose concentrations. Therefore, we recommend that owners monitor urine glucose levels but not use this information in changing the insulin dose at home. As will be detailed below (see Complications), persistent morning glycosuria may suggest an underdosage but will also occur with a poor insulin administration technique, a problem with the insulin potency, rapid metabolism of insulin, insulin-induced hyperglycemia, diestrus, hyperadrenocorticism, steroid administration, an improper feeding schedule or diet, insulin antibodies, or other factors. Thus, marked glycosuria is correct in suggesting underdosage in only a minority of cases. The appropriate therapy to re-establish blood glucose control is different for each of these situations. In addition, persistent negative urine glucose readings will be suggestive of a well-controlled diabetic more often than an insulin overdosage. Therefore, daily adjustments in insulin dose based on the urine glucose measurements should be done with caution and an understanding of potential pitfalls. This method should be discontinued at the slightest indication of a problem.

An alternative method for monitoring the diabetic patient at home is to use a combination of owner observance for recurrence of clinical signs, urine glucose determinations, and periodic in-hospital re-evaluation of blood glucose responses. Most important is the owner's subjective opinion of water intake and urine output. If these factors are normal, the pet is usually well controlled. They should have a good, but not ravenous, appetite. We do have our owners check the urine daily for glucose and ketones. Ideally, the urine should be negative for glucose prior to feeding if the animal is responding properly to the injections. At least once a week, owners are also encouraged to check the urine glucose concentration as many times during the day as possible. All urine test results should be recorded in a daily diary. Numerous negative urine glucose values in a dog that is doing well suggest adequate control. Persistent glycosuria suggests a problem that requires evaluation by in-hospital blood glucose determinations at the owner's earliest convenience, regardless of the dog's condition. Occasional ketonuria in a clinically healthy dog is not worrisome. However, if ketonuria persists for longer than 2 consecutive days, the dog should be re-evaluated.

Initially, re-evaluation of the diabetic dog is recommended once every 7 to 14 days until satisfactory glycemic control is achieved. The owner should administer insulin and feed the pet as usual that morning. The animal should then be brought to the veterinary hospital soon after the insulin injection to monitor hourly blood glucose concentrations throughout the day. Adjustments in therapy are based on the results of these studies. These blood glucose determinations not only check the dog's response to insulin but they also assess the owner's ability to administer insulin. If the pet is reasonably controlled, subsequent rechecks every 2 to 4 months are recommended. These rechecks should consist of a thorough history, physical examination, body weight check, review of insulin and syringes used, and determination of hourly blood glucose concentrations for at least 10 to 14 hours. The owner should have administered the insulin at home and should bring insulin and syringes to the hospital to be certain that correct materials are in use.

Veterinary assessment should take place prior to the scheduled rechecks if any of several situations develop. Dogs with signs of hypoglycemia, persistent glycosuria, anorexia, ravenous appetite, polydipsia, polyuria, persistent ketonuria, or any illness are easier to understand and properly manage with one veterinary evaluation than with repeated changes in treatment instructions given over the telephone. If there is doubt as to an animal's control, serial blood glucose determinations are recommended.

Glycosylated hemoglobin determination has been touted as an excellent tool to assess blood glucose control during a period of several weeks preceding the test. Glycosylation of hemoglobin represents a nonenzymatic reaction between glucose and hemoglobin, the extent of glycosylation being directly related to the plasma glucose concentration. Measurement of this hemoglobin should aid in determining the success of any particular insulin regimen, since good diabetic control should result in normal or near normal glycosylated hemoglobin concentrations. Unfortunately, the concentration of glycosylated hemoglobin can be affected by the age of circulating red blood cells and the occurrence of recent acute hyperglycemia for whatever reason, depending on the glycosylated hemoglobin assay technique. In addition to insulin underdosage, hyperglycemia can also result from improper owner injection techniques, rapid metabolism of insulin, insulin-induced hyperglycemia, and several other factors. Therefore, it appears that periodic determinations of serial blood glucose levels are of greater value in the continuing management of diabetic pets than is measurement of glycosylated hemoglobin concentration.

The signs of uncomplicated diabetes mellitus (i.e., polyuria, polydipsia, polyphagia, and weight loss) should resolve with proper insulin therapy. In addition, results of urine glucose testing should be negative for glycosuria during most of the day. Occasionally, a diabetic dog will have persistent morning glycosuria (1 to 2 per cent) or continued polyuria, polydipsia, or polyphagia despite insulin therapy. Owners may also observe afternoon weakness, lethargy, or convulsions. These signs indicate a potential problem with the insulin therapy, and an investigation should be undertaken to determine its cause (Table 2).

An effort to eliminate the simple or obvious causes of poor diabetic control should be undertaken before expensive, sophisticated, or time-consuming studies are performed. A thorough review of the owner's injection method is extremely important. Lack of a satisfactory response to therapy may involve improper insulin administration by the owner, inadequate mixing of the insulin prior to withdrawal into the syringe, use of outdated insulin, inactivated insulin from improper storage, or outdated urine glucose test strips. The veterinarian must compare the syringes used with the type of insulin administered (i.e., U-100 insulin requires the use of U-100 syringes). Owners should be routinely asked to carry their syringes and insulin when they bring their dog to the hospital. We may then ask them to administer insulin (or saline) so that their technique can be observed and evaluated. The method of mixing is checked, and storage habits are reviewed. Only when these obvious potential problems are demonstrated not to be responsible for poor diabetes control should the dog be hospitalized for further evaluation.

***Table 2.** Common Differential Diagnosis for Persistent Hyperglycemia Despite Insulin Therapy in the Diabetic Dog and Cat*

- Improper insulin administration
- Inactive, outdated insulin
- Rapid insulin metabolism
- Insulin-induced hyperglycemia (Somogyi overswing)
- Hyperadrenocorticism
  - Spontaneous
  - Iatrogenic
- Elevation in progesterone
  - Spontaneous (diestrus)
  - Iatrogenic
- Improper feeding schedule
- Improper food
- Stress
  - Infection
  - Recurrent pancreatitis
  - Renal failure
  - Cancer
- Insulin antibodies

Our approach to the *problem diabetic* dog is to determine the effects of the current insulin dose regimen and feeding schedule prior to recommending alterations in therapy. Beginning at the normal time for insulin injection, the home insulin and current dose should be administered, and the pet's daily feeding schedule (using its own food) followed. Blood glucose concentrations (usually using Chemstrip bG reagent strips) are determined every 1 or 2 hours for 10 to 24 hours after the injection of insulin. A graph of the serial blood glucose determinations will then help define the problem. The following are common disturbances that have been identified by using serial blood glucose determinations.

Insulin-Induced Hyperglycemia ("Somogyi Overswing"). Insulin-induced hyperglycemia, or the Somogyi overswing, results from excessive insulin administration. The overdose causes the blood glucose concentration to decrease below 65 mg/dl, which stimulates the release of diabetogenic hormones, especially epinephrine and glucagon. These hormones promote hepatic gluconeogenesis and glycogenolysis and decrease peripheral tissue utilization of glucose. As a result, the blood glucose concentration begins to increase, usually preventing a hypoglycemic convulsion. However, because these dogs are diabetic, sufficient endogenous insulin cannot be secreted to dampen the rising blood glucose concentration. Within 12 hours, the blood glucose concentration can be extremely elevated (400 to 800 mg/dl), and the morning urine glucose is consistently 1 to 2 gm/dl as measured with urine glucose test strips. If the owners are adjusting the daily insulin dose based on the morning glucose concentration, they can interpret these readings as indicating that the dog received insufficient amounts of insulin, especially if hypoglycemic signs (e.g., weakness, ataxia, bizarre behavior, or convulsions) are not observed. Therefore, owners may increase the insulin dose the following morning, and a continuous cycle of worsening insulin-induced hyperglycemia occurs.

Insulin-induced hyperglycemia is a common problem when daily insulin adjustments are based on morning urine glucose concentrations but can also occur in diabetic dogs receiving a fixed insulin dosage. The dosage of insulin that will induce posthypoglycemic hyperglycemia is variable and can be relatively low (less than 1 U/kg). Insulin-induced hyperglycemia should be suspected when there is persistent morning glucosuria (greater than 1 gm/dl on urine glucose test strips), continued polyuria and polydipsia, late afternoon signs of hypoglycemia, and high daily insulin dosages (greater than 2 U/kg of body weight).

The confusion surrounding this complex disorder may be compounded if the veterinarian elects to obtain only one late afternoon blood glucose determination. In most dogs with insulin-induced hyperglycemia, this physiologic rebound has commenced prior to 2 to 3 P.M. Thus, hyperglycemia may be noted after this time, further supporting the incorrect diagnosis of insulin underdosage.

Diagnosis of insulin-induced hyperglycemia requires demonstration of hypoglycemia (less than 65 mg/dl) followed by hyperglycemia (greater than 300 mg/dl) within one 24-hour period after insulin administration. Therapy involves reducing the insulin dosage 50 to 75 per cent, allowing 3 or more days for the dog to equilibrate on this new dose and then reassessing the dog's blood glucose concentrations. Further adjustments in the insulin dose should be made after reviewing these results.

Unrecognized rapid insulin metabolism (see below) is a common cause of the induction of the Somogyi phenomenon. Therefore, re-evaluation of serial glucose determinations 1 or 2 weeks after the insulin dosage is reduced is extremely important. Insulin dosage adjustments based on the morning concentration of glucose in the urine should be discontinued, and a fixed insulin dosage with afternoon urine checks initiated.

Rapid Metabolism of Insulin. In some diabetic dogs, the duration of effect of PZI or NPH insulin is considerably less than 24 hours. As a result, significant hyperglycemia (greater than 200 mg/dl) occurs for prolonged periods each day. This hyperglycemia begins as early as 6 to 8 hours following insulin administration in some dogs. Diabetic dogs that rapidly metabolize insulin will have persistent morning glycosuria (greater than 1 gm/dl on urine glucose test strips). Owners of these pets usually mention continuing problems with evening polyuria and polydipsia.

A diagnosis of rapid insulin metabolism is made by demonstrating significant hyperglycemia (greater than 200 mg/dl) within 18 hours or less of the insulin injection while the lowest blood glucose concentration is maintained above 80 mg/dl. If owners are adjusting the daily insulin dosage based on the morning urine glucose concentration, they may unnecessarily increase the insulin dosage and cause insulin-induced hyperglycemia. Veterinarians obtaining single afternoon blood glucose determinations may find normal glucose concentrations as well as mild or severe hyperglycemia. Therefore, diabetic dogs that may not have an ideal duration of insulin action can only be diagnosed by serial blood glucose concentrations.

There are two possible treatments for the diabetic dog metabolizing insulin too rapidly. If the duration of NPH insulin is longer than 12 to 14 hours but less than 18 hours, NPH can be administered twice daily or PZI can be used. PZI theoretically has a longer duration of action when compared with NPH insulin; however, many diabetic dogs will metabolize PZI in a similar manner to NPH insulin. As a general rule, the dose of PZI is approximately 25 per cent greater than NPH to achieve the same degree of effect. Therefore, the correct dosage should be based on serial blood glucose determinations. The duration of effect and time of peak effect can thus be determined and the insulin dosage and feeding schedule adjusted accordingly.

If the effect of NPH insulin is less than 12 hours, NPH given twice a day or PZI used once or even twice a day should be considered. If insulin is administered twice each day, it is recommended that similar doses be given at 12-hour intervals initially. Most of our owners who administer insulin twice daily give two equal-sized meals, one immediately following each injection.

Twice-daily insulin injections can be crudely monitored by checking urine glucose concentrations before each insulin injection. Well-controlled diabetic dogs treated with this regimen may have test results that are persistently negative for urine glucose. If a dog is clinically well and not symptomatic for hypoglycemia, we recommend serial blood glucose determinations every 2 to 4 months. Dogs with persistent 1 or 2 per cent glycosuria may be over- or underdosed and should be brought to the veterinarian. Those with 1/10, 1/4, or 1/2 per cent glucosuria are considered "adequately" controlled if they are not polyphagic, polyuric, and polydipsic.

These dogs can have serial blood glucose levels monitored at the scheduled recheck examination. However, if such dogs are not believed to be well controlled by the owner, an earlier recheck is always advisable.

Insulin Antagonism/Resistance. Insulin resistance implies peripheral antagonism to the effects of insulin. As a result, there is persistent hyperglycemia (greater than 300 mg/dl) and glycosuria, as well as continued polyuria, polydipsia, polyphagia, and weight loss despite insulin therapy. Increasing the insulin dosage is relatively ineffective in controlling these signs. Diabetic dogs with this problem will often be receiving more than 2 U of insulin/kg body weight. Recognized common causes of insulin resistance in dogs are listed in Table 2.

A diagnosis of insulin resistance is made by demonstrating either persistent hyperglycemia (greater than 300 mg/dl) on serial blood glucose studies despite increasing the insulin dosage above 2.5 U/kg body weight, or unusually high dose requirements to obtain desired blood glucose concentrations. Endogenous hyperinsulinemia rather than hypoinsulinemia may be found, depending on the underlying cause. If both insulin resistance and hyperinsulinemia are present and the cause of the insulin resistance can be corrected, permanent insulin-requiring diabetes mellitus may not develop.

It must be remembered that problems with the handling of insulin and owner administration can result in serial blood glucose concentrations that resemble insulin resistance. The same is true if the animal is markedly underdosed. These causes should be adequately investigated before embarking on a diagnostic evaluation for insulin resistance. If an adequate dose of new insulin administered by the veterinarian (rather than the old insulin given by the owner) is still ineffective in decreasing the blood glucose concentration, a diagnostic evaluation for a cause for insulin resistance is justified.

If insulin resistance is diagnosed in an intact diabetic bitch, estrus or diestrus (with or without pregnancy) should be suspected. The serum progesterone concentration will be increased above anestrus levels for 2 to 3 months after standing heat. This may stimulate the secretion of growth hormone, an insulin antagonist (Eigenmann, 1981). Exogenous administration of a progestin, such as medroxyprogesterone acetate, may also stimulate secretion of growth hormone. Increased circulating growth hormone concentrations appear to decrease the number of insulin receptors in cell membranes, alter the affinity of cell receptors for insulin, and possibly alter or inhibit postreceptor cellular reactions normally stimulated by insulin. The resultant insulin antagonism may result in poor control of a previously well-controlled diabetic or may result in the appearance of signs of diabetes mellitus in a previously undiagnosed bitch.

If the owners are not certain of recent estrus activity, a serum progesterone determination will identify the presence of a functioning corpus luteum or lutea. Ovariohysterectomy will result in a rapid decline in both the serum progesterone and growth hormone concentrations and subsequent loss of insulin resistance. An occasional diabetic bitch may no longer require insulin therapy either after being spayed or at the end of diestrus.

Glucocorticoids promote hepatic gluconeogenesis, decrease peripheral tissue utilization of glucose, and inhibit cellular receptor affinity for insulin. The resultant insulin resistance can occur with spontaneous hyperadrenocorticism or exogenous steroid administration. Careful questioning of the owner for recent glucocorticoid administration or recent "unknown" shots given by another veterinarian may explain the difficulties in diabetes control.

Unfortunately, polyuria, polydipsia, and polyphagia are common owner complaints in both diabetes mellitus and hyperadrenocorticism. Some dogs with both diseases will not initially have other clinical signs consistent with hyperadrenocorticism (i.e., truncal alopecia, abdominal distension, thin skin, or obesity). Therefore, a high index of suspicion for hyperadrenocorticism should be maintained in a diabetic dog requiring large doses of insulin (greater than 2 U/kg/day). An adrenocorticotropic hormone (ACTH) stimulation test or low-dose dexamethasone screening test or both should be performed to diagnose or rule out hyperadrenocorticism.

With appropriate medical or surgical therapy, as well as discontinuation of exogenous glucocorticoid administration, plasma glucocorticoid concentrations will decline, insulin antagonism will resolve, and the daily insulin dosage will decrease.

Hyperglucagonemia may be associated with bacterial infections, trauma, congestive heart failure, azotemia, and functional tumors of the alpha cells of the pancreatic islets or gastrointestinal tract. Glucagon stimulates gluconeogenesis, glycogenolysis, and ketogenesis and decreases the affinity of cell receptors for insulin. With correction of the underlying problem, plasma glucagon concentrations should decline and the insulin antagonism resolve.

Because insulin is a protein, prolonged administration may result in anti-insulin antibody production and insulin resistance. The most common commercially available insulin preparations are a combination of beef and pork insulins. The amino acid sequence of pork and dog insulin is identical; however, the amino acids at position 8 and 10 of the A chain are different in the cow and the dog. The immunogenic sites on the insulin molecule are amino acids 8 through 11 on the A chain and 3 and 30 on the B chain. Therefore, beef insulin injected into the dog is potentially antigenic and could result in antibody production and the development of insulin resistance, whereas pure pork insulin may not be antigenic.

Insulin antibody production was evaluated by radioimmunoassay in spontaneous, insulin-dependent diabetic dogs receiving only either purified pork insulin or beef-pork insulin (Feldman et al., 1983). Insulin antibodies were not detected in dogs receiving pork insulin, whereas antibody production was consistently documented in dogs receiving beef-pork insulin. However, the degree of antigenicity associated with beef-pork insulin is rarely significant. Insulin resistance was not present in dogs receiving beef-pork insulin in which insulin antibody production was documented. In fact, we have found pork insulin to be more potent and quicker in onset but briefer in duration of action than its beef-pork counterpart. It has been suggested that low titers of insulin antibodies induced in animals on beef-pork insulin mixtures act as a buffer to prolong the effects of insulin by lessening insulin's immediate availability and prolonging its biologic half-life.

Hypoglycemia. One of the most common complications associated with insulin therapy is hypoglycemia. If the diabetic dog receives too much insulin or exercises too strenuously, severe hypoglycemia may occur before the diabetogenic hormones (e.g., glucagon, cortisol, epinephrine, and growth hormone) are able to compensate for and reverse the low blood glucose level. Signs of hypoglycemia include weakness, lethargy, shaking, head tilt, ataxia, convulsions, and coma. Occurrence of clinical signs is thought to be dependent on the rate of decline of plasma glucose levels as well as the degree of hypoglycemia. As plasma glucose decreases, areas of the brain with the highest metabolic rate (e.g., cerebral cortex) are affected first, whereas areas with the slowest metabolic rate (e.g., brain stem nuclei) are affected last. Therefore, the initial clinical signs are cortical in origin and include disorientation, weakness, and hunger. With progressive hypoglycemia, convulsions and coma occur. If hypoglycemia is prolonged, death may result from depression of the respiratory centers.

If mild signs of hypoglycemia develop, the animal should be fed its normal food. If severe signs are present or if convulsions occur, intravenous dextrose or sugar water (Karo syrup) rubbed on the buccal mucosa should be continued until the convulsions stop. Fluid should not be forced down the mouth of a convulsing animal, nor should fingers be placed inside the mouth. Once the animal is conscious and placed in sternal recumbency, food should be offered. Whenever signs of hypoglycemia occur, the insulin dose needs to be decreased. Serial blood glucose concentrations should be used to make appropriate insulin dosage adjustments.

References and Supplemental Reading

Atkins, C. E., and Chin, H.: Insulin kinetics in juvenile canine diabetics after glucose loading. Am. J. Vet. Res. 44:596, 1983.

Atkins, C. E., Hill, J. R., and Johnson, R. K.: Diabetes mellitus in the juvenile dog: A report of four cases. J.A.V.M.A. 175:362, 1979.

Church, D. B.: The blood glucose response to three prolonged-duration insulins in canine diabetes mellitus. J. Small Anim. Pract. 22:301, 1981.

Church, D. B.: Diabetes mellitus. *In* Kirk, R. W. (ed.): *Current Veterinary Therapy VIII*. Philadelphia: W. B. Saunders, 1983, pp. 838–845.

Eigenmann, J. E.: Diabetes mellitus in elderly female dogs: Recent findings on pathogenesis and clinical implications. J. Am. Anim. Hosp. Assoc. 17:805, 1981.

Feldman, E. C., Nelson, R. W., and Karam, J. H.: Reduced immunogenicity of pork insulin in dogs with spontaneous insulin-dependent diabetes mellitus (abstr). Diabetes 32(Suppl. 1):153A, 1983.

Kaneko, J. J., Mattheeuws, D., Rottiers, R. P., et al.: Glucose tolerance and insulin response in diabetes mellitus of dogs. J. Small Anim. Pract. 118:85, 1978.

Lebovitz, H. E., and Feinglos, M. N.: The oral hypoglycemia agents. *In* Ellenberg, M., and Rifkin, H. (eds.): *Diabetes Mellitus: Theory and Practice*, 3rd ed. New York: Medical Examination Publishing Co., 1983, pp. 591–608.

Moise, N. S., and Reimers, T. J.: Insulin therapy in cats with diabetes mellitus. J.A.V.M.A. 182:158, 1983.

FELINE DIABETES MELLITUS

EDWARD C. FELDMAN, D.V.M.,
Davis, California

and RICHARD W. NELSON, D.V.M.
West Lafayette, Indiana

Diabetes mellitus is a common endocrine disorder of small animals; however, it occurs less frequently in cats than in dogs. Diabetes mellitus presents a difficult challenge both diagnostically and therapeutically, because the pathogenesis of the disease in cats is not well understood. However, comparisons with humans and dogs are not only inevitable but potentially provide insight into some of the unique features regarding this endocrinopathy in the cat.

Within the past few years, it has become clear that diabetes mellitus is a heterogeneous disease. In humans it has been classified into two main categories: insulin-dependent diabetes mellitus (IDDM) and noninsulin-dependent diabetes mellitus (NIDDM) (Waife, 1980). Insulin-dependent diabetes mellitus is the easily recognized classic form of the illness, associated with severe relative or absolute insulin deficiency. This condition is difficult to manage despite exogenous insulin injections. Noninsulin-dependent diabetes mellitus is the more recently identified form of the disease. In humans it has an insidious onset, may be difficult to distinguish from a normal state, and usually is easier to treat (diet, oral hypoglycemics). It is now suggested that an overlap in pathophysiology exists in persons with mild IDDM and those with severe NIDDM (Porte et al., 1982). Individuals with severe NIDDM develop ketoacidosis during severe stress and require exogenous insulin, but with proper care of the diabetes mellitus and treatment of underlying illnesses, they may not require insulin injections permanently.

Different diabetic states may exist in cats, corresponding with those in diabetic humans. Cats with IDDM require lifelong therapy and have clinical signs similar to those seen in humans and dogs. The majority of cats, however, may have NIDDM. These cats may exist for prolonged periods of time in a compensated state without signs and may not require therapy. They probably develop clinical signs of diabetes mellitus, requiring insulin therapy, during episodes of severe stress. However, these cats often are not difficult to manage on a day-to-day basis. With resolution of the stress or illness, they may spontaneously recover from their insulin dependence (Moise and Reimers, 1983) as they revert back toward a milder form of NIDDM.

Insulin resistance due to concurrent illness may also result in the diabetic state in cats. Hyperadrenocorticism and acromegaly represent spontaneous conditions that may result in insulin resistance. Administration of various drugs may also create insulin resistance and hyperglycemia.

HISTORY AND PHYSICAL EXAMINATION

Diabetes mellitus may be diagnosed in cats of any age or breed, although most diabetic cats are 6 years of age or older and the disease appears to be more common in males.

Classic signs of diabetes mellitus begin when the blood glucose concentration exceeds the renal tubular capacity for glucose reabsorption. Associated with the osmotic diuretic effects of glycosuria is an increase in urine volume and secondary hypovolemia, stimulating in turn an increased fluid intake. The owner sees an animal with polydipsia and polyuria. Polyphagia is caused by an inability of the satiety center in the hypothalamus to recognize calories in the blood. The inability of peripheral tissues to utilize calories ultimately causes loss of weight. Stress, usually in the form of a concurrent illness such as cystitis, cardiomyopathy, pancreatitis, or any other serious illness or disease, is seen in many of these cats. Underlying illnesses such as these may alter the classic signs of polydipsia, polyuria, polyphagia, and weight loss, causing a cat to exhibit some of the other signs seen in diabetics: anorexia, dyspnea, coughing, lethargy, vomiting, diarrhea, stranguria, or weakness (Schaer, 1977;

Moise and Reimers, 1983). The presence and severity of all these signs are highly variable and are dependent, in part, on how quickly an owner seeks veterinary care after a pet's illness begins and what, if any, underlying disorder exists. Diabetic cats with a history of being abnormal for days to months may be brought to a veterinarian.

On physical examination, there are no pathognomonic alterations with diabetes mellitus. Obesity and hepatomegaly are common. Icterus, coat abnormalities, and dehydration are often noted. Diabetic cats may develop a plantigrade posture (i.e., the hocks touch the ground when the cat walks). However, this posture, possibly caused by diabetic neuropathy, is not common, and such a gait or stance has also been observed in cats with chronic polyarthritis. A majority of diabetic cats have some concurrent illness. Recognition of problems in other organ systems is quite important and will be discussed in the next paragraphs.

DIFFERENTIAL DIAGNOSIS

Cats with polydipsia, polyuria, polyphagia, and weight loss, with or without any of the other signs mentioned above, are likely to have diabetes mellitus. However, the signs of several diseases mimic all or some of the signs of diabetes mellitus. Besides diabetes mellitus, there are two major disease states in cats that are associated with weight loss despite normal or increased food consumption. These are hyperthyroidism and gastrointestinal lymphosarcoma. Hyperthyroidism is an extremely important differential because the disease is quite common, the signs of the two disorders (diabetes and hyperthyroidism) can be virtually identical, and cats can be afflicted with both disorders simultaneously. Gastrointestinal neoplasia, especially lymphosarcoma, is a common cause of polyphagia, diarrhea, and weight loss. Although a tentative diagnosis can be formulated after a thorough physical examination (including careful abdominal palpation), and perhaps a response to glucocorticoid therapy, the definitive diagnosis requires histologic evaluation of an intestinal biopsy sample.

Hyperadrenocorticism and acromegaly appear to be rare conditions in cats but may be associated with severe hyperglycemia and insulin resistance. Iatrogenic glucocorticoids also impair insulin action and may cause deterioration in the control of diabetic cats. Megestrol acetate therapy, used in a variety of conditions in feline practice, does not commonly lead to a diabetic state, but diabetes is well recognized as a potential transient or, rarely, permanent side effect of megestrol acetate treatment. It can be hypothesized that megestrol acetate may cause the occasional mild NIDDM cat to have an episode of secondary (iatrogenic) severe NIDDM.

Other differential diagnoses of feline diabetes mellitus are diseases that result in weight loss and inappetence. Renal disease can result in polydipsia, polyuria, and weight loss. Liver disease can have a multitude of signs, including weight loss. Pancreatitis is not diagnosed with the same frequency as in diabetic dogs, but this inflammatory process is a potential cause of weight loss, as well as of gastrointestinal problems.

CLINICAL PATHOLOGY

Blood and Urine Glucose

Cardinal features of diabetes mellitus include persistent fasting hyperglycemia and glycosuria. Both of these basic abnormalities have rather unique features in the cat.

Fasting hyperglycemia (greater than 200 mg/dl) is a constant finding in diabetic cats. Hyperglycemia, with glucose reaching levels in the range of 300 to 400 mg/dl, may also be seen in stressed cats. Unfortunately, stress is a subjective factor that cannot be measured, is not always easily recognized, and may evoke inconsistent responses among cats. Hyperglycemia in ill or frightened cats is usually stress induced. Stress-induced acute hyperglycemia is likely to have strong roots in the evolution of cats; acute stress can be compared with the sudden exertion associated with hunting, an activity with potent and sustained bursts of action. Stress-induced hyperglycemia is thought to be the result of sudden secretion of epinephrine, causing both a release of glucose and a simultaneous inhibition of insulin action at the level of the cell membrane (Hamburg et al., 1980). Epinephrine is a potent cause of hyperglycemia, making the diagnosis of feline diabetes mellitus anything but routine.

The diagnosis of diabetes mellitus is reserved for hyperglycemic, glycosuric cats observed by the owner to have at least three of the four major signs encountered in this disturbance: polydipsia, polyuria, polyphagia, and weight loss. Hyperglycemic cats receiving megestrol acetate and those that are ketoacidotic can also be assumed to have diabetes mellitus. A diagnosis of diabetes is questionable in all other hyperglycemic cats that do not have typical signs. However, the owner and veterinarian should be aware of the hyperglycemia, and extra care should be taken in observing these animals for onset of the classic signs. By admitting a hyperglycemic cat to the hospital overnight in order to adjust it to the environment and then by performing another blood glucose determination the next day, one can often separate stress-induced from diabetic-associated hyperglycemia. A more aggressive option would be to place an intravenous catheter into a jugular vein 12 to 24 hours prior to rechecking the blood glucose concentration in order to avoid the stress associated with venipuncture. One could also recheck the urine for persistence of the glycosuria either in the hospital or at home.

When the blood glucose concentration exceeds the renal tubular capacity for total reabsorption, glycosuria results. Diabetic cats subjectively appear to have a renal threshold for glucose of approximately 200 mg/dl (similar to dogs); however, the reported mean threshold for normal cats is 290 mg/dl (Kruth and Cowgill, 1982). Diabetic cats, at the time of diagnosis, always have glycosuria and occasionally have ketonuria. Glycosuria without hyperglycemia can result from isolated renal tubular disorders in cats. A transient elevation in blood glucose concentration may not consistently result in measurable glycosuria. Although the presence or absence of glycosuria is easily identified, the interpretation of any finding may not be straightforward. In cats, there is no common cause of ketonuria other than decompensation of diabetes mellitus, since cats appear to be relatively resistant to development of significant ketonemia or ketonuria associated with starvation.

Blood Chemistry Abnormalities

As cellular glucose utilization diminishes in the diabetic animal, fat mobilization becomes excessive and frank lipemia develops. Insulin deficiency may also lead to impaired lipoprotein lipase activity, the enzyme system responsible for the intracellular transport of plasma fatty acids. The fatty changes in the liver lead to hepatomegaly, the most common radiographic abnormality. Alanine transaminase (SGPT) and alkaline phosphatase concentrations are usually mildly or moderately elevated in association with the hepatic lipidosis in feline diabetes. The catabolic state associated with diabetes mellitus leads to fat breakdown and may cause mild increases in serum cholesterol. Ten to 20 per cent of diabetic cats have elevated total bilirubin concentrations, perhaps caused by hepatic lipidosis, thickened bile, a bile duct disorder, or pancreatitis with obstruction of the bile ducts. Mild to severe dehydration frequently results in prerenal azotemia, relative erythrocytosis, hyperproteinemia, and hyperalbuminemia. Serum electrolytes should be monitored in cats with protracted histories and those with inappetence or anorexia, since decreases in serum potassium or sodium concentration may require specific therapy in the anorexic, polyuric, diabetic cat.

Urinalysis

Urine must be examined not only for glucose but for specific gravity and signs of infection. Renal azotemia can occasionally be distinguished from prerenal azotemia with a check of the specific gravity, although cats with renal disease may maintain some capacity for urine concentration. Pyuria, proteinuria, and hematuria are suggestive of urinary tract infections. Routine culture of urine obtained by cystocentesis from diabetic animals is warranted, because infection is so common.

Stool Examination

Cats with diabetes mellitus are not commonly afflicted with bulky, foul-smelling stools. If such stools are seen, either hyperthyroidism, pancreatic exocrine insufficiency, or primary intestinal disorders should be considered.

Glucose Tolerance Tests

Glucose tolerance tests (oral or intravenous) are unnecessary diagnostic tests in cats with overt diabetes mellitus. They may ultimately prove useful in cats that are difficult to diagnose (borderline or "latent" diabetics) or in differentiating IDDM from NIDDM. These tests are rarely performed because these two situations are not often encountered in clinical practice. Simple rechecks of the fasting blood glucose concentration usually distinguish the diabetic from the stressed cat, and the need to recognize NIDDM has not been well defined.

Intravenous glucose tolerance tests can be performed after an overnight fast by using a glucose dose of 500 mg/kg. The 50 per cent solution is injected over a period of 45 to 75 seconds. Through another vein, usually using an indwelling venous catheter, blood samples are collected before and 5, 15, 25, 35, 45, and 60 minutes after the glucose infusion. In normal cats, the blood glucose concentration returns to preinjection levels by 45 to 60 minutes (Hsu and Hembrough, 1982). In general, the longer it takes for a glucose concentration to return to normal (beyond 60 minutes), the more severe the carbohydrate intolerance. Various anesthetic agents may adversely affect the glucose metabolism (Hsu and Hembrough, 1982). If chemical restraint is needed, it is useful to place an indwelling catheter while the cat is under anesthesia and then wait until the animal has completely recovered from anesthesia before the glucose tolerance test is performed.

TREATMENT

Oral Hypoglycemia Agents

Oral medications are used in the treatment of a large percentage of humans with NIDDM. There has been little mention of their use in spontaneous feline diabetes. The authors have had little or no response in three treated cats. Detailed work regarding differentiation of IDDM from NIDDM in cats, in addition to the application of oral hypoglycemic drugs, is yet to be reported.

Insulin Therapy

INITIAL TREATMENT. The use of insulin in the treatment of feline diabetes mellitus is well accepted in veterinary practice. However, the type of insulin, monitoring techniques, and number of injections per day are controversial.

Diabetic cats can usually be controlled with insulin doses of 0.2 to 1.0 U/kg/body weight. The average cat is started on 1 to 3 U of protamine zinc insulin (PZI) per cat, once daily at 8 A.M. (Table 1). The cat is treated for 3 days in the hospital, but blood glucose levels are not monitored critically until the fourth day of hospitalization. The initial 3 days allow the animal a chance to equilibrate on its new treatment. If the cat is stable and an evaluation for concurrent illness is complete, the pet need not remain hospitalized. The owners can be taught to administer insulin, and the cat can be monitored after several days of treatment at home. They are usually fed at 8 A.M. and again at 6 P.M.; equal-sized meals consisting of canned cat food or food provided by the owner are adequate. On the fourth day of hospitalization, or after several days at home, the easily handled cat has its blood glucose levels monitored before and at hourly intervals after receiving insulin. Monitoring is usually decreased to checks every 2 or 3 hours between 6 P.M. and 8 A.M. the following morning. This generally is a well-tolerated, easy, and inexpensive approach to treatment. For practitioners, cats can be sent to emergency clinics for the overnight testing. A 25-gauge needle is used for venipunctures, and only one or two drops of blood are withdrawn for each test. Blood glucose levels are determined by using Chemstrip bG sticks (Bio-Dynamics), which can be split into halves or thirds. These sticks are reliable, inexpensive, easy to use, and provide a most convenient tool for monitoring diabetic cats. The fractious cat must either have an indwelling catheter placed during anesthesia or simply be monitored at home by the owners, who must assess clinical signs and test for urine glucose concentrations.

Table 1. *Initial Hospital Treatment Protocol for Uncomplicated Feline Diabetes Mellitus*

1. Administer 1 to 3 U of PZI insulin once daily.
2. Feed the cat two equal meals of canned or kibble food (once in the morning, once in the afternoon).
3. Do not critically monitor diabetes mellitus for the initial 2 or 3 days of therapy, except for periodic blood and urine glucose checks.
4. On day 4 of hospitalization:
   - Obtain blood glucose concentration with Chemstrip bG at 8:00 A.M.
   - Administer insulin and feed.
   - Check blood glucose values hourly until 5 or 6 P.M.
   - Decide whether to continue monitoring throughout night.
5. Review serial blood glucose results. Adjust the dose and frequency of insulin administration, if necessary.
6. Send the cat home. Recheck with serial blood glucose values and owner appraisal in 7 days.

INSULINS. In the past several years, NPH insulin has been commonly recommended for use in diabetic pets. NPH, an intermediate-acting insulin, is known to have an immediate or rapid onset of action, reach a peak effect in 2 to 6 hours, and last 4 to 10 hours in most cats (Moise and Reimers, 1983). Even when administered twice daily, this insulin often causes wide fluctuations in blood glucose concentrations from hour to hour (Fig. 1*A*). Thus, this insulin is not usually satisfactory in gaining good control of blood glucose in diabetic cats, and its use is not recommended.

Long-acting insulins appear to be best suited for cats. PZI begins to lower blood glucose concentrations in 1 to 3 hours, has its peak effect at 4 to 10 hours, and has a duration of action of 12 to 30 hours. There is significant individual variation (Fig. 1*B*, *C*). Approximately two thirds of our diabetic cats receive PZI (beef-pork mixture) once daily, and the remaining cats receive this insulin twice daily. More cats would be best treated with twice-daily injections, but owner or cat willingness may not allow frequent administration. Serial blood glucose values usually determine if a cat is metabolizing insulin rapidly and therefore indicate whether the animal would be better controlled with two injections. In this situation, the blood glucose levels reach 80 to 150 mg/dl and then begin to rise to concentrations greater than 250 mg/dl within 10 to 20 hours of the injection. With both once- or twice-daily insulin injections, cats are fed equal-sized meals twice daily. In some households, cats have food available at all times, but this does not appear to be advantageous.

In a large series of diabetic cats, each has responded somewhat differently to insulin. There is no consistent typical time for peak insulin effect or for the duration of insulin action. Thus, the need for serial blood glucose determinations is apparent. As seen in Figures 1 and 2, obtaining a single blood glucose concentration at some time during the day has a greater chance of misleading the practitioner than of providing usable information. A blood glucose value of 80 to 120 mg/dl may mistakenly suggest good control, when only 2 hours earlier the blood glucose may have been at 40 mg/dl, or it may be in excess of 250 mg/dl 2 hours later. Defining the pattern throughout the day provides useful information and makes the added work worthwhile.

TREATMENT GOALS. There are two primary goals

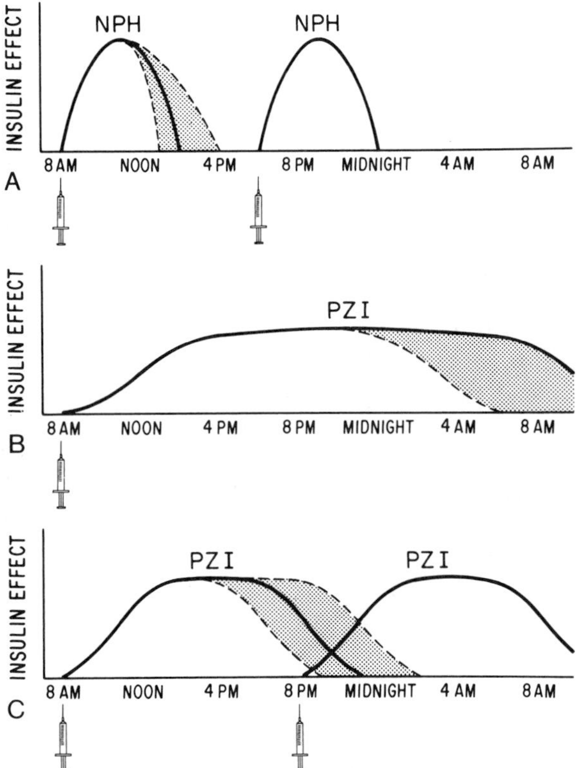

Figure 1. The effects of NPH (*A*) and PZI insulins (*B* and *C*) in the diabetic cat. Note the variability in effect seen with each type of insulin; serial glucose monitoring is required to assess response to therapy in each cat.

in treating diabetic cats, both of equal importance. First is to maintain blood glucose concentrations between 100 mg/dl (at the lowest) and 200 to 250 mg/dl (at the highest) during each 24-hour period. The second is to have the owner report resolution or improvement of the signs caused by diabetes mellitus. It is assumed that to attain the goals set forth, one must achieve constant, albeit varying, blood levels of insulin at all times (Fig. 1).

HOME MANAGEMENT. Cats can usually be sent home after the initial set of serial blood glucose values is obtained. Any dosage adjustments or alterations in frequency of administration can be made at home after those glucose values are assessed. Subsequent rechecks should be performed after the *owner* has administered the insulin and fed the cat. The first recheck should be performed 5 to 7 days after the initial series of glucose determinations. At that time, any of the owner's questions can be answered, and both the owner's ability to administer insulin and the cat's response to this hormone can be assessed. This and all subsequent recheck evaluations should include hourly blood glucose determinations beginning within an hour of insulin injection (regardless of the time used by the owner) and continuing for 10 to 24 hours postinjection. The shorter testing periods are reserved for cats that are doing well, and the longer evaluation times are used for cats that have not responded satisfactorily. Dose adjustments are made only by the veterinarian. The stable cat should be reassessed every 1 to 3 months according to the initial protocol outlined above. Any dosage adjustment should be followed by a 4- to 7-day equilibration period before serial blood glucose concentrations are rechecked. These recommendations may seem excessively strict to some clinicians, but this is the method that has evolved as most successful in both canine and feline diabetics and is one accepted by most owners of diabetic pets.

MANAGEMENT MADE EASIER. The size and personality of most cats make treating them a significant challenge for their owners. These people need all the help and support possible from their veterinarians if success is to be achieved. Several suggestions may simplify matters. Specific diluting solutions for each type of insulin are available. Diluting U-100 solution 1:10 creates an insulin concentration that is manageable. Owners are instructed to purchase 0.5 ml, U-100 syringes with 27-gauge needles (Monoject, Sherwood). These syringes measure to 50 U with bold, easy-to-read numbers. An owner administering 3.5 U draws out 35 U on the syringe when using 10-fold diluted insulin. Satisfactory dilutions can be made with saline, but the most consistent results are obtained by using the specific diluting solutions. After 6 to 8 weeks, any unused diluted insulin should be discarded and a fresh insulin dilution should be made up.

Owners must be carefully taught proper injection technique. Instruction should include use of the syringe, sites of injection (usually neck or lumbar area), pinching up the skin, and delivery of insulin

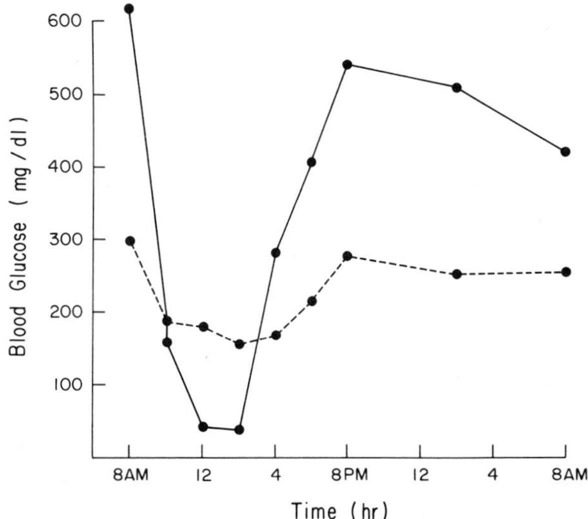

Figure 2. Serial blood glucose values from a cat receiving excessive amounts of NPH insulin (solid line) versus the proper dose of protamine zinc insulin.

(Stogdale, 1984). Owners may wish to make a bag out of one or two towels into which the cat can be placed. Slits for the neck area allow insulin injection without harm to owner or cat.

Diabetic cats should not be fed semimoist foods because of their high sugar content. Observation of appetite, water intake, urine output, and body weight are extremely helpful. A thorough explanation of what is done during rechecks and how these studies improve a cat's control is helpful. When owners understand what their money is going toward, they are much more likely to allow frequent rechecks, which in turn result in better patient care.

Hypoglycemia and its clinical manifestations should be described. Owners should have a sugar-containing syrup available for emergencies. Replacing cat litter with shredded newspaper or covering the litter with plastic wrap to obtain a small amount of urine gives the owner a chance to check urine for glucose and ketones. This information should be tabulated by the owner and provided to the veterinarian in a daily log. Urine glucose concentrations, however, should not be used by the client for adjusting insulin dose. The properly controlled pet does not have glycosuria. Those that are always glycosuric should be re-evaluated in the hospital. Male cats should be castrated and females spayed in order to improve control as well as life expectancy.

POOR CONTROL. Cats may not respond to insulin injections for various reasons. Due to the independent nature of many cats, a common cause for poor control is the inability of an owner to administer insulin. If blood glucose concentrations fail to decline despite increases in insulin dosage, the veterinarian should administer fresh insulin from a new bottle. If response is then achieved, the owner's insulin may need to be discarded. Additionally, owners should be evaluated on how they mix and store the insulin, how well they can withdraw and measure insulin within a syringe, and how they inject insulin into the animal. It is important to actually observe an owner's technique in administering insulin (or saline) to the pet. If technique problems are not discovered, other causes of poor control must be investigated. These may include improper diet, rapid metabolism of insulin, insulin overdosage (insulin-induced hyperglycemia [see *Current Veterinary Therapy VII*]), insulin underdosage, or insulin resistance (due to hyperadrenocorticism, acromegaly, hyperthyroidism, pregnancy, megestrol acetate, exogenous glucocorticoids, or pseudopregnancy). Evaluation of serial blood glucose concentrations should enable the clinician to determine the next diagnostic or therapeutic step (see Canine Diabetes Mellitus).

References and Supplemental Reading

Hamburg, S., Hendler, R., and Sherwin, R. S.: Influence on small increments of epinephrine on glucose tolerance in normal humans. Ann. Intern. Med. 93:566, 1980.

Hsu, W. H., and Hembrough, F. B.: Intravenous glucose tolerance test in cats: Influenced by acetylpromazine, ketamine, morphine, thiopental, and exylazine. Am. J. Vet. Res. 43:2060, 1982.

Kruth, S. A., and Cowgill, L. D.: Renal glucose transport in the cat. ACVIM Scientific Proceedings, 1982 (abs.), p. 78.

Moise, N. S., and Reimers, T. J.: Insulin therapy in cats with diabetes mellitus. J.A.V.M.A. 182:158, 1983.

Porte, D., Jr., Pfeifer, M. A., Halter, J. B., et al.: Impaired B-cell function in noninsulin-dependent diabetes mellitus: The essential lesion? *In* Skyler, J. S. (ed.): *Insulin Update: 1982*. Princeton: Excerpta Medica, 1982, pp. 1–24.

Schaer, M.: A clinical survey of thirty cats with diabetes mellitus. J. Am. Anim. Hosp. Assoc. 13:23, 1977.

Stogdale, L.: Diabetes mellitus: An owner information guide. Kal Kan Forum 3:16, 1984.

Waife, S. O.: *Diabetes Mellitus*. Indianapolis: Eli Lilly, 1980, pp. 1–11.

DISORDERS ASSOCIATED WITH GROWTH HORMONE OVERSECRETION: DIABETES MELLITUS AND ACROMEGALY

J. E. EIGENMANN, D.V.M.
Philadelphia, Pennsylvania

PHYSIOLOGY OF GROWTH HORMONE ACTION AND REGULATION

Growth hormone (GH) is a single-chain polypeptide of pituitary origin. In most species, including the dog, it has a molecular weight of approximately 22,000 daltons. In contrast to other pituitary hormones, GH is not confined in its action to one single target, and the hormone displays diametrically opposed intrinsic anabolic and catabolic activities (Fig. 1). Its catabolic activity (enhanced lipolysis and restricted glucose transport caused by insulin resistance) is directly caused by the peptide. It is now widely accepted that the anabolic effects of GH are mediated by insulin-like growth factors or somatomedins.

In normal animals, an increase in plasma insulin concentration acutely leads to an increase in glucose transport by adipose tissue. In hypophysectomized GH-deficient animals, however, basal glucose transport occurs at a maximal rate, and adipose tissue glucose transport in such animals is insensitive to the action of insulin. Administration of GH in this animal model reduces glucose transport back to normal. Thus, GH normally restricts glucose transport, and this transport can be acutely modulated by insulin. Hence, insulin appears to inhibit a GH-controlled "glucose transport limiting factor". The glucose transport limiting factor may be the high-affinity Ca^{2+}-ATPase found in fat cell membranes. Insulin decreases and GH increases Ca^{2+}-ATPase activity. Additionally, it has been suggested that the high affinity Ca^{2+}-ATPase of isolated fat cells may be involved in early metabolic steps influenced by insulin, which regulates intracellular Ca^{2+} levels. This concept is in keeping with the finding that excessive GH produces insulin resistance at a site distal to the insulin binding site by modifying one or several intracellular processes involved in insulin action.

The regulation of GH secretion is complex. GH secretion is governed by a dual system of hypothalamic hypophyseotropic hormones, one inhibitory and the second stimulatory. In humans, substances or situations leading to GH secretion include hypoglycemia, amino acids, peptides, monoamines (levodopa, dopamine agonists), α-adrenergic substances such as epinephrine or clonidine, serotonin precursors, and melatonin. The situation is slightly different in dogs. Hypoglycemia and amino acids are very weak and undependable stimuli of GH secretion in dogs, whereas dopamine or α-adrenergic substances

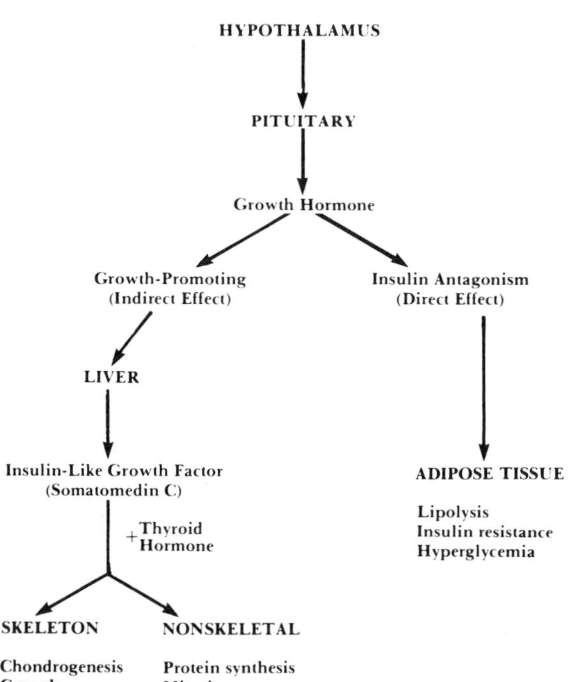

Figure 1. The main actions of growth hormone (GH) are depicted. Direct catabolic diabetogenic actions are shown on the right side of the figure; indirect anabolic actions are shown on the left side. (From Eigenmann *in* van Marthens (ed.): Proceedings of the Kal Kan Symposium 6:107, 1983, with permission.)

such as clonidine are potent stimulators of GH secretion. An appreciable amount of attention has been given to a long-suspected hypothalamic GH-releasing factor (GRF). Recently, a peptide with a potent intrinsic GH-releasing activity was isolated from pancreatic tumors of two human patients suffering from acromegaly. These patients did not suffer from primary GH overproduction but from primary GRF overproduction. This peptide thus is called hp (human pancreatic) GRF. In both reports, the GH-releasing effects of hp-GRF were highly specific both *in vivo* and *in vitro*. It is highly likely that α-adrenergic substances or α-adrenergic impulses stemming from the central nervous system (CNS) act to increase GH secretion by increasing hypothalamic GRF secretion. These drugs do not act directly on the pituitary. Additionally, in some patients suffering from "isolated GH deficiency" as diagnosed by a failure of GH to increase in response to classic stimuli (hypoglycemia, clonidine), hp-GRF can cause release of GH. The hypothalamic system inhibiting pituitary GH release is represented by somatostatin, variably called GH-inhibiting factor (GIF) or somatotropin release inhibiting factor (SRIF). In the dog, SRIF inhibits the GH surge normally provoked by levodopa administration.

Separate lines of research, initially perceived as nonrelated, have converged to form the present field of the insulin-like growth factors or somatomedins. In one series of studies, it was demonstrated that GH exerts *in vivo* growth-promoting activity but fails to do so when incubated *in vitro* with cartilage. In the presence of serum, however, cartilage was found to be highly responsive to a GH-dependent serum factor (sulfation factor), which eventually was named somatomedin. A second major line of research on this subject was derived from the investigation of a serum fraction whose insulin-like activity, as assessed by glucose uptake in adipose tissue, could not be abolished by anti-insulin antibodies. Five factors or groups of factors meeting the criteria of insulin-like growth factors have been found thus far: insulin-like growth factors I and II (IGF I and II), somatomedin A, somatomedin C, and multiplication-stimulating activity (MSA). The principal properties of insulin-like growth factors and somatomedins include the following: (1) single-chain polypeptides having molecular weights of 5000 to 10,000, (2) weak *in vitro* insulin-like activity in adipose tissue, (3) stimulation of sulfate uptake by cartilage *in vitro*, (4) stimulation of nucleic acid, protein, and glycogen synthesis in calvaria cells, (5) preferential enhancement of myoblast differentiation in chicken embryonic cells, and (6) interaction with cell surface receptors specific for somatomedins and some interaction with insulin receptors.

The regulation of insulin-like growth factors appears to be governed by multifactoral processes. Recent studies have shown that the peptides are synthesized and promptly released from the liver into the circulation under the influence of GH. The findings that insulin-like growth factor levels are low in some catabolic and high in some anabolic *in vivo* situations suggest an important growth-promoting role for these factors. The question as to whether GH, insulin-like growth factors, or both are primarily responsible for body growth remains unclear. Although small size in GH-deficient patients is associated with low levels of insulin-like growth factors, no conclusion can be drawn since concentrations of both GH and insulin-like growth factor are low. Similarly, in acromegaly levels of both GH and insulin-like growth factor are elevated. Some light has been shed on this problem recently. Insulin-like growth factors given to hypophysectomized rats provoke body growth similar to that obtained by GH administration. This supports the hypothesis that the action of growth hormone is mediated by insulin-like growth factors.

GROWTH HORMONE–INDUCED DIABETES MELLITUS

Diabetes mellitus is the metabolic disorder characterized by disturbances of carbohydrate, lipid, and protein metabolism. Diabetes mellitus may be either overt (frank, persistent hyperglycemia) or chemical in nature (normal or slightly elevated blood glucose concentrations accompanied by abnormal glucose tolerance). The hyperglycemia of diabetes mellitus results from either an absolute or relative lack of insulin or a defect in insulin action at the target tissues. In the latter situation, where a diminished responsiveness of tissues to the action of insulin action exists, circulating insulin concentrations may be subnormal, normal, or even elevated. Therefore, the hyperglycemia associated with diabetes mellitus is not always the result of a lack of insulin. Hyperglycemia associated with high levels of insulin (characteristic of an insulin-resistant state at target tissues) may develop in association with other endocrine disorders (such as GH excess) and may be reversible if the underlying cause of the insulin resistance is detected and treated.

In humans, primary or idiopathic diabetes can be divided into two main types. Type I (insulin-dependent, ketosis-prone) diabetes mellitus usually occurs in young people, whereas Type II (insulin-dependent, non-ketosis-prone) diabetes mellitus occurs primarily in mature individuals and is usually associated with obesity. Diabetes mellitus may also develop secondary to pancreatic disease or hypersecretion of hormones with actions antagonistic to those of insulin. Compared with the idiopathic (Types I and II) forms of diabetes mellitus, however, secondary diabetes is a less common cause of human diabetes mellitus.

In dogs, diabetes mellitus is a relatively frequent disease, but because of a lack of comprehensive endocrinologic, pathologic, immunologic, and genetic studies, data on canine diabetes mellitus are less complete than in humans. In a epizootiologic study of diabetes in dogs, its prevalence was estimated to range from 1:100 to 1:500 dogs presented to veterinary hospitals. The risk was found to be lowest in young dogs, with about 2 to 3 per cent of affected animals being 1 year of age or younger. In young animals, the risk is approximately equal for males and females, but in older dogs, females are at greater risk.

Although diabetes mellitus similar to juvenile-onset Type I does occur, the majority of cases of diabetes mellitus develop in mature dogs. As opposed to mature-onset (Type II, noninsulin dependent) diabetes of humans, however, most adult diabetic dogs require insulin therapy to survive. In addition, insulin levels, a prerequisite for categorizing cases into Type I or Type II diabetes, have been measured infrequently in diabetic dogs, and conflicting results have been obtained. In one study, investigators demonstrated that diabetic dogs brought to a veterinary clinic had very low circulating insulin levels, suggesting that canine diabetes mellitus generally is associated with hypoinsulinemia, similar to Type I diabetes mellitus of humans. In another study, dogs with diabetes were classified into several groups by measuring the insulin response to a glucose load. These investigators showed that insulin levels in diabetic dogs may be low, normal, or elevated. They also attempted to compare dogs having undetectable insulin levels with human beings affected by Type I diabetes, and dogs having normal or elevated insulin levels with human beings affected by Type II diabetes. However, a classification based on plasma insulin levels alone seems questionable, because it provides no clues as to the pathogenesis or origin of the disorder. Moreover, regardless of the diabetes-inducing principle, insulin levels may be high, normal, or undetectable depending on the stage of the disease. For instance, if normal dogs are rendered diabetic by GH treatment, diabetes mellitus can be transient or permanent, depending on the duration of treatment. Insulin levels in such dogs are initially high and later become normal and eventually subnormal. If the administration of GH is stopped after a few days, the disease reverses. However, if GH therapy is continued for several days and then stopped, the disease persists and insulin levels decline steadily, despite cessation of the treatment. This process occurs over a period of several months, and affected dogs survive for months even if no insulin is given.

There are few known causes of diabetes mellitus in mature dogs. It is known, however, that several underlying disturbances can be associated with canine diabetes mellitus, and it is possible that secondary diabetes mellitus may be the most common form of the disease in mature dogs. Although it is well recognized that severe pancreatic disease can produce secondary diabetes in dogs, pancreatitis appears to be an uncommon cause of diabetes mellitus in this species. A more important cause of secondary diabetes in dogs, however, appears to be endogenous GH excess.

When factors precipitating diabetes mellitus in dogs are evaluated carefully, it becomes clear that the disease occurs frequently in aged females and is manifested during the corpus luteum phase (diestrus) of the estrous cycle, when the synthesis of progesterone is maximal. This is in keeping with the findings from epizootiologic studies that indicate that intact female dogs are at higher risk than males. Thus, it appears that progesterone may induce diabetes mellitus in some dogs. However, progesterone alone cannot be responsible for the precipitation of the disease, because only a minor fraction of intact females develop diabetes mellitus. Thus, progesterone in conjunction with a genetically determined predisposition or another progesterone-controlled diabetogenic factor must be responsible for the induction of the disease.

Despite the known relationship between the development of diabetes and the period following estrus (progesterone phase), the pathogenesis involved in the disorder has remained obscure. Recent studies of mammary tumor induction by progestagens revealed that progestagens, in addition to their tumor induction potency in some dogs, induced diabetes mellitus and soft tissue changes reminiscent of human acromegaly. From the latter observations, the hypothesis was derived that both conditions (i.e., diabetes and acromegalic changes) could have been caused by progestagen-induced GH overproduction. This could explain why some intact female dogs develop diabetes during their progesterone phase.

GH, especially in carnivores (dogs, cats), exerts a powerful diabetogenic action. There is ample evidence that the diabetogenic action of GH is mainly brought about by induction of insulin resistance on insulin targets such as adipose tissue. GH appears to induce insulin resistance at a site on the insulin receptor distal to the insulin-binding site (i.e., transduction) or at one or more of the intracellular reactions important in insulin action. It has been shown that GH-induced diabetes in dogs may be reversible or permanent, depending on the dose of GH administered, the duration of GH treatment, and an animal's individual response to GH. At any rate, during the early stage of treatment, circulating insulin levels increase approximately 20-fold whereas a 90 per cent decrease in pancreatic insulin content occurs. This striking shift of pancreatic insulin toward peripheral insulin is likely to be the result of the appreciable insulin resistance GH can

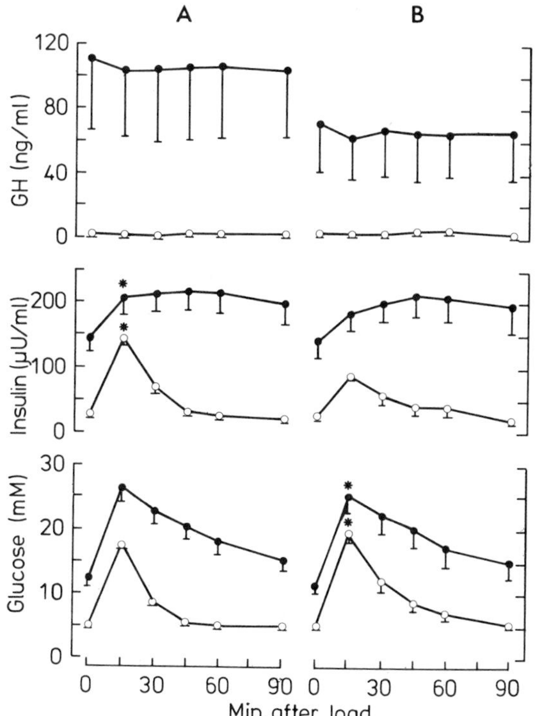

Figure 2. *A*, Plasma levels of glucose, insulin, and GH during an intravenous glucose tolerance test (IVGTT) in 21 dogs with signs of diabetes mellitus or acromegaly. (Filled circles denote 10 dogs during a natural progesterone phase and 11 during treatment with low doses of MPA.) Open circles represent IVGTT in 20 normal dogs. *B*, Plasma levels of glucose, insulin, and GH during IVGTT in 14 dogs during a stage of GH elevation (filled circles) and again when GH levels were lowered after ovariohysterectomy (open circles); note improvement in glucose tolerance and normalization of GH levels in face of a weaker insulin secretion after ovariohysterectomy. (From Eigenmann et al.: Acta Endocrinol. (Copenh.) 104:167, 1983; with permission.)

induce. Yet the rate of secretion of insulin is elevated over the rate of formation of insulin, thus explaining the final exhaustion of pancreatic B cells taking place in GH diabetes.

Historic Signs and Laboratory Findings in Dogs with GH Excess

Female dogs with either glucose intolerance or frank diabetes mellitus were investigated to determine the relationship to progesterone or progestagen excess. Some dogs developed glucose intolerance or diabetes mellitus during diestrus, whereas others were affected after treatment with medroxyprogesterone acetate (MPA), an estrus-repressing agent. More than half of the dogs also showed, at least to some degree, signs of acromegaly (see below).

Laboratory findings revealed that about half of the dogs studied had frank hyperglycemia (plasma glucose concentration greater than 10 mM, or greater than 180 mg/dl), whereas the remainder had fasting basal glucose levels that ranged from 5.4 to 7.7 mM (95 to 140 mg/dl). In addition, despite extreme elevation of basal insulin levels, these dogs exhibited glucose intolerance during intravenous glucose tolerance testing, as well as drastic elevation of GH levels when compared with results obtained in normal dogs (Fig. 2*A*). Thus, as expected from the initial hypothesis, GH levels are high and diabetes in such animals is characterized by hyperinsulinemia rather than hypoinsulinemia; this is consistent with insulin resistance. If such animals are subjected to progestagen withdrawal or ovariohysterectomy, GH levels drop and, despite appreciably lowered insulin levels, glucose tolerance improves (Fig. 2*B*). Diabetes mellitus, however, may not disappear in some animals (see Treatment, below). The trend for development of associated acromegalic changes appears to be higher in animals with only moderate glucose intolerance, whereas dogs with frank diabetes mellitus appear to develop acromegaly less commonly.

Dogs exhibiting signs of glucose intolerance (with or without acromegaly) during a natural progesterone phase (diestrus) have progesterone levels within the normal range but elevated GH levels. In animals developing signs during diestrus, ovariohysterectomy or a spontaneous reduction in progesterone levels is followed by a slight but inevitable drop in GH levels (Fig. 2). In animals who develop signs after MPA administration, plasma levels of the compound at the time of presentation are usually low. GH levels in pregnant dogs who are invariably under the influence of progesterone are only occasionally elevated.

Pathogenesis of GH-Induced Glucose Intolerance

The finding of hyperinsulinemia in these dogs with GH excess points to insulin resistance as the factor responsible for their hyperglycemia or glucose intolerance or both. This is further supported by the fact that despite elevated endogenous insulin levels, the insulin requirement of diabetic dogs with GH elevation is appreciably higher than the insulin requirement of diabetic dogs not having GH elevations (see Treatment, below). These findings are compatible with GH-induced diabetes. GH causes glucose intolerance mainly by inducing insulin resistance. In contrast to other species such as the rat, carnivores are particularly sensitive to the diabetogenic action of GH. Administration of GH to dogs can within a matter of days produce a diabetic state that initially is characterized by hyperinsulinemia. If exposure to high GH levels persists, exhaustion of pancreatic B cells and hypoinsulinemia may ensue. It is important to note that in affected dogs there is generally no correlation between the degree of GH elevation and the degree of hyperglycemia. The fact that GH is elevated in animals exhibiting diabetes during progestagen exposure but not in dogs developing diabetes independently of such exposure precludes the possibility that GH elevation may be caused by hyperglycemia or the diabetic state as such.

The fact that GH levels drop after ovariohysterectomy and progestagen withdrawal is evidence for a progestagen-GH interrelationship. Compared with these dogs with high GH concentrations, most pregnant dogs have normal GH levels. This suggests that GH production in some dogs is paradoxically controlled by natural levels of progesterone.

The mechanism by which the GH axis becomes responsive to progesterone remains unknown. The disorder may be present at birth or develop later in life. The fact that GH levels in some diabetic dogs were already elevated to an extent certainly sufficient to induce diabetes earlier in life suggests that the condition, for some unknown reason, only develops in older age. In this context, it is important to realize that dogs, in contrast to other species, exhibit almost identically high postestrus progesterone concentrations whether pregnant or not. Additionally, a dog's reproductive cycles do not cease in old age. Whether such lifelong exposure to "pregnancy progesterone levels" contributes to or provides the necessary environment for the development of the disorder is unknown but remains an interesting possibility.

Treatment

In dogs with glucose intolerance resulting from GH excess, the following diagnostic and therapeutic points are emphasized: (1) prompt recognition of hyperglycemia or impaired glucose intolerance, (2) prompt correction of hyperglycemia, and (3) performance of ovariohysterectomy or cessation of progestagen treatment or both in order to lower plasma GH levels and insulin output and preserve most of the remaining β-cell activity.

Recognition of Hyperglycemia or Glucose Intolerance. In any intact female dog presenting with signs of acromegaly or diabetes (respiratory stridor, increased number of skin folds, increased abdominal size, fatigue, polyuria, polydipsia) either during progestagen treatment or during a natural progesterone phase, the plasma glucose level should be evaluated immediately. Testing only the urine for glucose is insufficient for the diagnosis, since a number of animals affected by the disorder may have mild elevations of fasting plasma glucose. These animals, however, because of their glucose intolerance, may readily spill some glucose in the urine after food ingestion. If the fasting plasma glucose is only moderately elevated (less than 150 mg/dl), the most appropriate means of diagnosing glucose intolerance is with an intravenous glucose tolerance test. Although normal animals generally have glucose assimilation coefficient (k) values greater than 3, affected animals have glucose intolerance manifested by k values of less than 2. In normal dogs, plasma glucose levels should return to a preload concentration within 60 minutes of the glucose load.

Ovariohysterectomy. It has proved practical to ovariohysterectomize affected intact females as soon as possible regardless of whether the animal has developed the disease when treated with progestagens or during a luteal phase. Even in dogs in which the chance for recovery from diabetes is minimal, ovariohysterectomy is recommended. Intact female dogs that have developed diabetes because of progesterone-induced GH excess will invariably have an increased insulin demand during the following progesterone phase. Progesterone at that time will again lead to high GH levels; the resulting resistance to insulin may develop abruptly and be extreme. It is impossible to predict the degree of insulin resistance, and the owners of such dogs are often unable to cope with the changes in insulin requirement. It is also possible that such dogs, because of insufficient insulin administration, may develop ketoacidosis. Treatment at that time may be frustrating, especially if the animal is also affected by pyometra or renal failure. The recommendation to ovariohysterectomize dogs as soon as possible, provided the animal is not ketotic, appears to have only advantages. The advantages are that early ovariohysterectomy in dogs that still suffer from appreciable GH elevation leads to a rapid decrease in plasma GH levels and, thus, to an amelioration of the insulin resistance. Moreover, if ovariohysterectomy is performed early, the time course for the decrease in insulin requirement becomes more predictable.

Finally, it must be emphasized that suppression of estrus (chemical ovariohysterectomy) in such animals is contraindicated. Some veterinarians have the notion that estrus and diestrus are somehow involved in the pathogenesis of diabetes in intact females and attempt to eliminate cycles by administering estrus-suppressing agents such as MPA. By doing this, they obviously directly provoke the hormonal situation (e.g., progestagen-induced GH excess) that is responsible for the development and dysregulation of diabetes in such animals. The safety of testosterone derivatives such as mibolerone (Cheque-Drops, Upjohn) remains unknown. Although testosterone derivatives are C_{19} steroids, it is conceivable that by cross-reacting with progesterone receptors they may have progestagen-like activities.

Insulin Treatment. A crucial question is at which blood glucose level to start insulin replace-

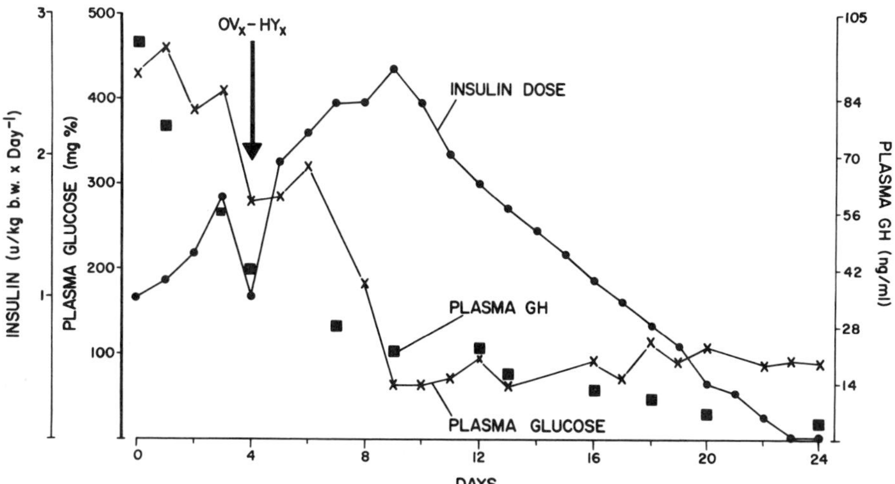

Figure 3. Plasma glucose levels, insulin dose, and plasma GH concentrations in a dog with spontaneous GH-induced diabetes. Note the decrease in plasma GH concentrations and eventual fall in insulin requirements after ovariohysterectomy. (From Eigenmann and Peterson: Vet. Clin. North Am. [Small Anim. Pract.] 14:837, 1984.)

ment. This question is complex and, in a clinical setting, has no straightforward answer. The reason is that, in general, the clinician does not have data concerning the dog's actual plasma insulin, GH, and progesterone concentrations. Even if these determinations are available, they do not always indicate the actual pancreatic insulin reserve or the degree of insulin resistance. Plasma insulin concentrations, however, should be measured whenever possible. The finding of a high plasma insulin concentration indicates that the dog has a fair chance of recovery from the diabetic state if adequately treated; in contrast, a subnormal plasma insulin level indicates that the chance of recovery is minimal. In a dog that has a fair chance for recovery, strict control of the blood glucose concentration is warranted because of its positive influence on recovery from the diabetic state.

In general, a longer duration of clinical signs lessens the chance for recovery. By questioning owners carefully, one can often learn that the dog has had similar signs during earlier progesterone phases. The frequency of episodes is likely to provide an additional negative influence on the chance of recovery from the diabetic state.

It is important to know whether the dog has developed diabetes following estrus or during progestagen medication. In dogs treated with progestagens, plasma GH concentrations can remain elevated for prolonged periods of time, thus decreasing the chance of recovery. Progestagens, probably because of their depot effect, appear to influence GH secretion more profoundly. As a rule, one should initiate insulin therapy if the fasting plasma glucose concentration is greater than 150 mg/dl in the progestagen-treated dog and when the plasma glucose level is greater than 200 mg/dl in dogs that develop diabetes during the progesterone phase.

Both GH-induced insulin resistance and the functional recovery of the residual pancreatic beta cells play significant roles in determining the dog's initial and subsequent insulin requirements. Plasma GH concentrations usually normalize within a matter of days after ovariohysterectomy. Recovery of residual beta-cell function, however, may take days to weeks. After ovariohysterectomy, it is recommended to keep such dogs in the hospital for a few days and to adjust their daily insulin requirement by monitoring serial blood glucose concentrations. As soon as the blood glucose concentrations begin to decrease, the daily insulin dose should be decreased accordingly. In some dogs, the insulin requirement may drop to zero during the initial postoperative period. In other dogs, the daily insulin requirement may initially decrease, then plateau, and finally continue to gradually decrease over a longer period of time. Figure 3 illustrates the insulin adjustments before and after ovariohysterectomy in a dog that developed diabetes mellitus during the progesterone phase.

If a dog does not recover from the diabetic state during its hospital stay, it is discharged and the insulin requirement is adjusted at home. Diabetic monitoring is slightly more complicated at home because blood glucose measurements cannot be easily performed. During this time, blood glucose concentrations should be evaluated at least once a week and the daily insulin dose lowered if necessary. In a number of dogs, however, weekly blood glucose monitoring becomes insufficient and the

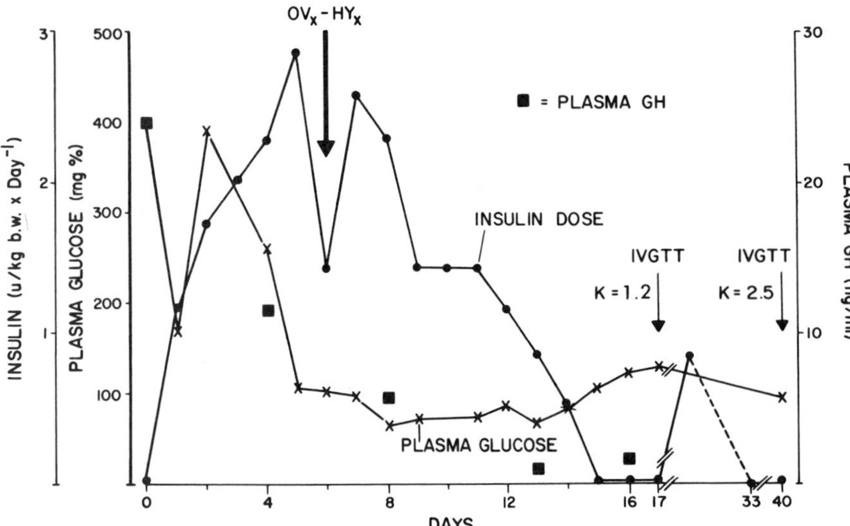

Figure 4. Plasma glucose levels, insulin dose, and plasma GH concentrations in a dog with spontaneous GH-induced diabetes. Note the initial increase in insulin requirement and eventual drop after ovariohysterectomy, the fall of elevated plasma GH levels, the increase in resting plasma glucose levels after insulin withdrawal and glucose intolerance (K = 1.2) and improved glucose tolerance (K = 2.5) after again giving insulin for two more weeks. (From Eigenmann and Peterson: Vet. Clin. North Am. [Small Anim. Pract.] 14:837, 1984.)

insulin dose has to be lowered according to clinical signs of mild hypoglycemia. Although hypoglycemia is undesirable, it is still the best biologic indicator of improving beta-cell function. The owners should be advised to observe the dog closely and to take action as soon as mild signs of hypoglycemia develop. At that time, the dog must be given carbohydrates orally, and several smaller meals should be offered subsequently throughout the day. The daily insulin dosage should also be lowered the following morning. Tapering of the insulin dose should be continued until it reaches another plateau or drops to zero.

It is recommended that insulin therapy not be withdrawn simply on the basis of negative morning urine glucose concentrations. Although complete insulin withdrawal may be appropriate in some cases, there is no way to predict this possibility since urine glucose measurements are an insensitive way of assessing glucose tolerance. Even basal plasma glucose measurements may be insensitive (Fig. 4). After appropriate insulin treatment and ovariohysterectomy in a dog with GH-induced diabetes, the insulin dose was lowered according to afternoon blood glucose readings until it was totally discontinued (Fig. 4). Over a period of 2 days off insulin treatment, the afternoon glucose started to rise again. An intravenous glucose tolerance test performed at that time revealed that the dog was still diabetic. Over the next 2 weeks, the dog was again treated with decreasing amounts of insulin. Another glucose tolerance test performed 7 days later showed greatly improved glucose tolerance, and insulin therapy was permanently discontinued (Fig. 4). This is compatible with the known fact that recovery of the beta cells may take time and that strict control of blood glucose levels is important if total recovery is to occur.

ACROMEGALY

In humans, acromegaly is a chronic endocrine disorder characterized by overgrowth of the soft tissues and bony structures in adulthood. The disorder is caused by excessive GH secretion, usually resulting from a pituitary tumor or hyperplasia of pituitary acidophils. Patients suffering from the disorder exhibit profound soft tissue increases of their face, hands, and feet. Fatigue, headache, amenorrhea, loss of libido, and diabetes mellitus may also occur. There is no sex predilection in human patients.

In dogs, spontaneous acromegaly was first con-

***Table 1.** History and Clinical Findings in 22 Acromegalic Dogs**

Age (years)	4–11 (range); 8.4 (mean)
Progestagen treatment (No. dogs)	15
Spontaneous occurrence during luteal phase (No. dogs)	7
Breeds (No. dogs)	Dachshund (4); American cocker spaniel (3); Crossbreed (4); Dalmatian (3); German shepherd (2); English cocker spaniel (2); springer spaniel, French bulldog, beagle, poodle (1 each)
Inspiratory stridor (No. dogs)	19
Polyuria and polydipsia (No. dogs)	10
Visible increase in soft tissue mass (No. dogs)	19
Enlargement of interdental spaces (No. dogs)	13

*With permission from Eigenmann, J. E.: Naturally occurring and iatrogenic acromegaly in the dog. *In* van Marthens, E. (ed.): Proc. Kal Kan Symposium for the Treatment of Small Animal Diseases, 6:81, 1983.

firmed in 1980 (Rijnberg et al.), although an intact female dog with clinical signs suggestive of acromegaly had previously been reported. Recently, the results of high-dose long-term toxicity studies with progestagens such as MPA have also been reported in dogs. Although these studies were primarily aimed at the elucidation of mammary gland tumor induction by these compounds, they showed that some dogs treated with progestagens developed signs of acromegaly or diabetes. Therefore it appeared that acromegaly might occur spontaneously in female dogs during the progesterone phase (diestrus) or in dogs treated with progestagens.

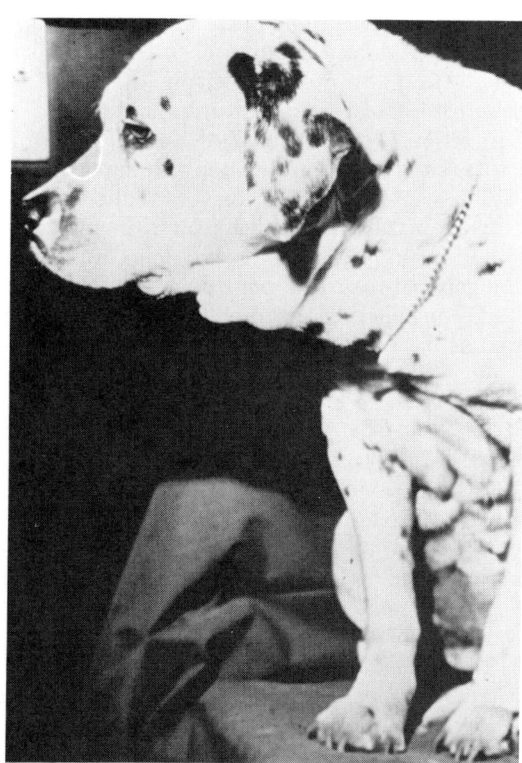

Figure 6. Dalmatian dog with severe spontaneous acromegaly. Note increase in skin folds on head and neck. (From Eigenmann and Vender-van Haagen: J. Am. Anim. Hosp. Assoc. 17:813, 1983.)

Historic Findings and Clinical Signs Encountered in Canine Acromegaly

All dogs thus far diagnosed as having acromegaly have been intact females. Some of the dogs develop acromegaly during MPA treatment for estrus suppression. In other dogs, acromegaly develops during diestrus (progesterone phase). In one study of 22 acromegalic dogs, clinical signs included inspiratory stridor, polydipsia and polyuria, fatigue, increased abdominal size, prominent skin folds, and mammary gland tumors (Table 1). Respiratory stridor, a prominent sign in these dogs, occurs because of excessive soft tissue proliferation in the orolingual, pharyngeal, and laryngeal regions. On physical examination, increased interdental spaces can also be observed (Fig. 5). Frequent abnormalities in laboratory data include elevated serum alkaline phosphatase, hyperglycemia, and a slightly lowered packed cell volume. In some dogs, the increase in soft tissue of the head, neck, and trunk is dramatic (Fig. 6), but only subtle changes may be observed in other dogs.

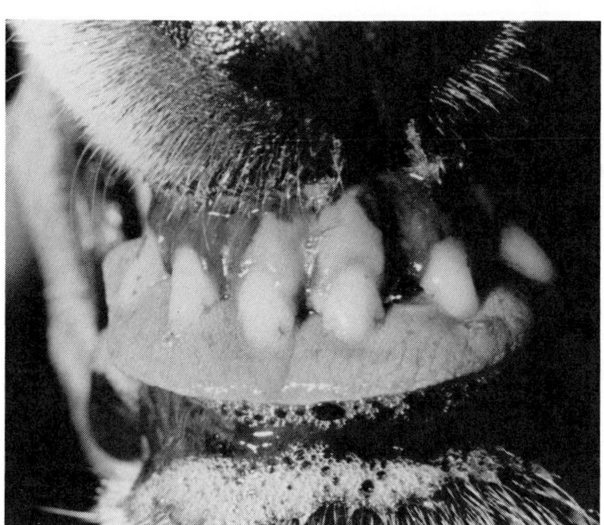

Figure 5. Dog exhibiting acromegaly and diabetes mellitus during a natural progesterone phase. Note the soft tissue changes in the tongue. (From Eigenmann et al.: Acta Endocrinol. (Copenh.) 104:167, 1983, with permission.)

Diagnosis of Acromegaly

A tentative diagnosis of acromegaly can be made based on the dog's history, clinical signs, and laboratory findings. Radiographs of the head and neck can be helpful in establishing the diagnosis. In most dogs with acromegaly, there is diffuse proliferation of the soft tissues of the orolingual, oropharyngeal, and laryngeal regions. In a dog with inspiratory stridor, it must be determined whether the respiratory distress (particularly in brachycephalic, intact female dogs) is caused by acromegaly or simply by an elongated soft palate. The comparison of pictures taken of the dog early in life and again during the disease state has also proved particularly helpful in recognizing changes typical of acromegaly.

A conclusive diagnosis of acromegaly requires the demonstration of persistent elevations of plasma GH concentrations. Basal GH levels in acromegalic dogs vary greatly, and there is no correlation between the degree of GH elevation and the extent of acromegaly. In addition, basal GH concentrations may be elevated in conditions other than acromegaly. Therefore, to definitively diagnose acromegaly, one must demonstrate that plasma GH concentrations remain elevated during a suppression test, such as the intravenous glucose tolerance test (1 gm of glucose/kg body weight). Finally, measurement of insulin-like growth factors or somatomedin can also be helpful in diagnosing canine acromegaly. Since these peptides are GH dependent, acromegalic dogs have elevated plasma levels, compared with normal animals.

Treatment

Canine acromegaly may be diagnosed in dogs under MPA treatment and in dogs under the influence of progesterone during diestrus. Since the GH elevations in acromegalic dogs are induced by progestagen exposure, treatment should include withdrawal of progestagens or ovariohysterectomy or both. After treatment (progestagen withdrawal), circulating GH concentrations again normalize and soft tissue abnormalities resolve.

GROWTH HORMONE EXCESS IN THE FELINE

We recently studied an old, castrated, male domestic short-haired cat with insulin-resistant diabetes mellitus. Despite extremely elevated levels of endogenous insulin, the cat exhibited hyperglycemia. In order to control the animal's hyperglycemia adequately, insulin (lente) doses as high as 70 U/day had to be administered. GH levels were approximately 100 times normal. In multiple samples obtained over a period of 1 year, GH concentration was persistently elevated. Lesions in the endocrine pancreas were compatible with GH-induced diabetes. In addition to diabetes, the cat exhibited signs of acromegaly (enlarged abdomen, prognathia inferior). A mass in the pituitary region was diagnosed by computerized axial tomography and gamma camera imaging. A pituitary tumor was confirmed at necropsy.

Besides this cat, we have seen similar extreme plasma GH elevations in a few other diabetic cats with high insulin requirements. Furthermore, pathology reports support the view that GH may be involved in the development of the disease in cats. Gembardt and Loppnow (1976) described an adenoma of pituitary acidophil cells that was presumed to produce GH in two diabetic cats.

References and Supplemental Reading

Eigenmann, J. E.: Diabetes mellitus in elderly female dogs: Recent findings on pathogenesis and clinical implications. J. Am. Anim. Hosp. Assoc. 17:805, 1981.

Eigenmann, J. E.: Diabetes mellitus in dogs and cats. Proc. Kal Kan Symposium for the Treatment of Small Animal Diseases, 1982, pp. 51–58.

Eigenmann, J. E., and Eigenmann, R. Y.: Radioimmunoassay of canine growth hormone. Acta Endocrinol. (Copenh.) 98:514, 1981.

Eigenmann, J. E., and Rijnberk, A.: Influence of medroxyprogesterone acetate (Provera) on plasma growth hormone levels and on carbohydrate metabolism. I. Studies in the ovariohysterectomized bitch. Acta Endocrinol. (Copenh.) 98:599, 1981.

Eigenmann, J. E., and Eigenmann, R. Y.: Influence of medroxyprogesterone acetate (Provera) on plasma growth hormone levels and on carbohydrate metabolism. II. Studies in the ovariohysterectomized, oestradiolprimed bitch. Acta Endocrinol. (Copenh.) 98:603, 1981.

Eigenmann, J. E., Eigenmann, R. Y., Rijnberk, A., et al.: Progesterone-controlled growth hormone overproduction and naturally occurring canine diabetes and acromegaly. Acta Endocrinol. (Copenh.) 104:167, 1983.

Eigenmann, J. E., Patterson, D. F., Zapf, J., et al.: Insulin-like growth factor I in the dog: A study in different dog breeds and in dogs with growth hormone elevation. Acta Endocrinol. (Copenh.) 105:294, 1984.

Eigenmann, J. E., and Venker-van Haagen, A. J.: Progestagen-induced and spontaneous canine acromegaly due to reversible growth hormone overproduction. Clinical picture and pathogenesis. J. Am. Anim. Hosp. Assoc. 17:813, 1981.

Eigenmann, J. E., Wortman, J. A., and Haskins, M. E.: Elevated growth hormone levels and diabetes mellitus in a cat with acromegalic features. J. Am. Anim. Hosp. Assoc. 20:747, 1984.

Gembardt, C., and Lopponow, H.: Zur Pathogenese des spontanen Diabetes mellitus der Katz. II. Mitteilung: Azidophile Adenome des Hypophysenvorderlappens und Diabetes mellitus in zwei Fallen. Berl. Munch. Tierarztl. Wochenschr. 89:336, 1976.

Rijnberk, A., Eigenmann, J. E., Belshaw, B. E., et al.: Acromegaly associated with transient overproduction of growth hormone in a dog. J.A.V.M.A. 177:534, 1981.

GROWTH HORMONE–DEFICIENT DISORDERS ASSOCIATED WITH ALOPECIA IN THE DOG

J. E. EIGENMANN, D.V.M.
Philadelphia, Pennsylvania

Endocrine alopecia is an important clinical condition that must be distinguished from nonendocrine hair loss. Well-known causes of endocrine alopecia include hypothyroidism and hyperadrenocorticism (Cushing's syndrome). Other poorly understood causes of endocrine alopecia include the "gonadal imbalances," such as those associated with testicular tumors and with cases of hair loss in female dogs. One approach to diagnosing endocrine alopecia is to rule out disorders that can be diagnosed definitively, such as hypothyroidism and Cushing's syndrome. Another frequently employed approach in alopecias of suspected "gonadal origin" is evaluation of the response following gonadectomy or replacement of sex steroids.

Recently, the availability of canine growth hormone (GH) assays has enabled veterinarians to definitively diagnose alopecia resulting from GH deficiency. This chapter will discuss the etiologic, diagnostic, and therapeutic aspects of alopecias caused by GH deficiency.

PHYSIOLOGY OF GH ACTION ON THE SKIN

The general aspects of GH physiology are discussed in the article Disorders Associated with Growth Hormone Oversecretion: Diabetes Mellitus and Acromegaly. Although most effects of GH on various tissues (including the skin) are mediated through the production of insulin-like growth factors, GH also appears to have a direct action on the skin. This is supported by findings in both humans and dogs. In humans, two separate disorders can produce dwarfism associated with GH or insulin-like growth factor deficiency. These include primary GH deficiency and primary insulin-like growth factor deficiency (also called Laron dwarfism). Primary GH deficiency is characterized by low plasma concentrations of both GH and the insulin-like growth factors, whereas primary insulin-like growth factor deficiency is characterized by subnormal insulin-like growth factor but normal GH concentrations. In patients with primary GH deficiency, the number of skin elastin fibers is reduced; in contrast, the number of skin elastin fibers remains normal in Laron dwarfism. Therefore, GH itself appears to have a direct effect on the maintenance of normal numbers of skin elastin fibers.

Other evidence for a direct effect of GH on the skin has been obtained by measuring the plasma concentrations of an insulin-like growth factor (IGF I) in dogs of various sizes. In general, there is a parallel relationship between body size and plasma IGF I levels; the larger dogs have the highest IGF I concentrations. Within the poodle breed, there are three genetic subgroups—the standard, miniature, and toy. All three groups of poodles secrete similar amounts of GH, but circulating IGF I levels parallel body size; the miniature or toy subgroups are relatively deficient in insulin-like growth factors. However, the fact that miniature and toy poodles do not develop alopecia due to relative IGF I deficiency provides evidence for a direct effect of GH on the skin.

ALOPECIAS RELATED TO GH DEFICIENCY

Two subgroups of GH deficiency must be distinguished: (1) primary GH deficiency and (2) GH deficiency secondary to another cause such as hypothyroidism, hyperadrenocorticism, or zinc deficiency. In the latter circumstance, however, specific treatment is not needed because GH secretory capacity becomes normal as the primary cause is treated.

Primary GH Deficiency

Skin changes observed in primary GH deficiency include hyperpigmentation and loss of primary (guard) hairs, which can result in total body alope-

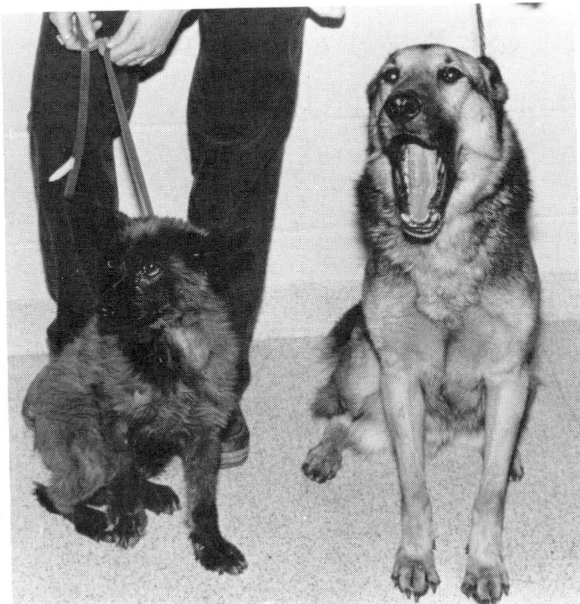

Figure 1. Normal adult German shepherd and German shepherd dwarf.

cia. Generally, the skin is fragile, and on histologic examination there is a diminished number of elastin fibers.

GH DEFICIENCY IN DWARF GERMAN SHEPHERDS. This disorder is encountered in young dogs that become stunted at a few weeks of age (Fig. 1). Owners usually do not complain that the dog is undersized but rather that the dog is losing hair. Hair loss in some dogs can be observed early in the course of their disease; others retain their puppy coat for several years. There is no apparent sex predilection for the disease. The most common endocrine abnormality encountered in this disorder is lack of GH. Basal plasma thyroxine (T_4) concentrations may be subnormal, but there is usually a clear-cut increase in T_4 levels in response to administration of thyroid-stimulating hormone (TSH). Injection of adrenocorticotropic hormone (ACTH) generally produces a normal increment in plasma cortisol concentration.

It is believed that this disorder is genetically transmitted by a simple recessive mode of inheritance. In most dwarf dogs studied at necropsy, a colloid-filled pituitary cyst can be identified, suggesting that the cyst may induce pituitary hypofunction by exerting pressure on the surrounding tissues. This hypothesis is questionable, however, because a number of normal adult dogs have pituitary cysts (as many as 7 per cent of mongrels). It is possible that the primary defect involves cells of the hypophysis, which fail to differentiate normally and therefore secrete nonsense proteins into Rathke's cleft. These nonsense proteins may attract water and thereby produce progressive enlargement of the cystic Rathke's pouch.

GH DEFICIENCY IN MATURE DOGS. Isolated GH deficiency occurs in mature dogs and leads to skin changes including hyperpigmentation and partial or total alopecia. Affected animals are usually young adults (Lhasa apso, Pomeranian, poodle, terriers, and chow chow). When the GH secretory capacity is assessed, subnormal responses are noted (Fig. 2). Although most dogs have complete GH deficiency, others exhibit only partial GH deficiency. Adrenal and thyroid function studies in these dogs are normal. The skin changes are reversible with GH treatment.

The underlying defect leading to the GH deficiency in these dogs remains unknown, and necropsy results are not available. Further, it has not been determined whether the GH deficiency is caused by primary pituitary or primary hypothalamic dysfunction. Future studies employing GH releasing factor may be helpful both diagnostically and therapeutically. In addition, the question as to whether the condition has a familial background remains unknown. The fact that a large number of affected dogs belong to a particular breed (e.g., Pomeranian) suggests the possibility that the condition may indeed have a familial background in some breeds.

Secondary GH Deficiency

HYPOTHYROIDISM. Thyroid hormone appears to have a profound positive influence on pituitary GH

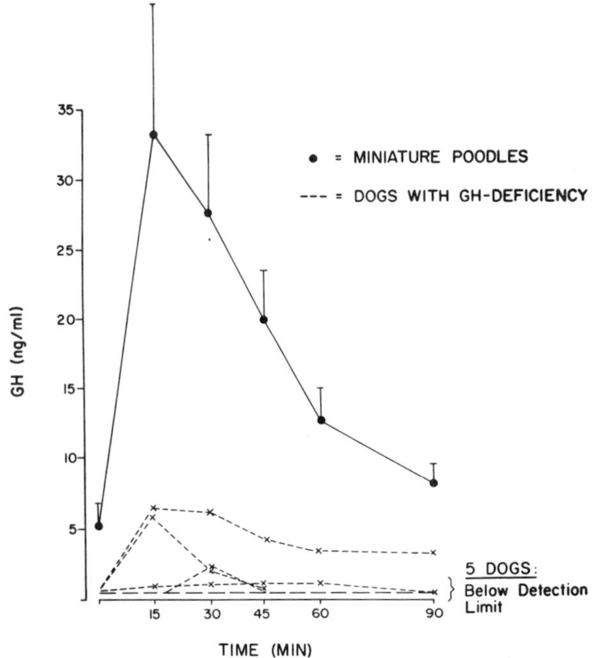

Figure 2. Growth hormone secretory response after intravenous administration of clonidine in normal poodles and dogs with growth hormone (GH) deficiency.

secretion. Thyroid hormone is required for normal messenger RNA synthesis and GH production in pituitary GH cells. Therefore, a decreased GH secretory capacity may develop secondarily to the hypothyroid state. The skin changes associated with hypothyroidism may be related to various degrees of GH deficiency, as well as to lack of thyroid hormones.

We recently investigated a young bullmastiff affected by secondary hypothyroidism with typical signs of juvenile hypothyroidism such as dwarfism, mental dullness, and bilateral symmetrical alopecia. The GH secretory capacity in this dog was severely impaired during the diseased state. Following thyroxine replacement, the GH secretory response became normal.

HYPERADRENOCORTICISM (CUSHING'S SYNDROME). Both spontaneous and iatrogenic glucocorticoid excess may impair GH secretion. Similarly, impaired GH responses to provocative stimuli may develop after treatment with medroxyprogesterone acetate, a progestagen agent with intrinsic glucocorticoid activity. After correction of glucocorticoid excess, the impaired GH secretory capacity returns to normal in most of these patients.

Although the pathogenesis of alopecia produced by glucocorticoid excess is unclear, it is possible that GH deficiency, as well as hyperadrenocorticism, contributes to the skin changes associated with spontaneous and iatrogenic Cushing's syndrome. Both GH and the insulin-like growth factors appear to have an anabolic effect on cutaneous tissues, whereas glucocorticoids have catabolic effects on both skin and connective tissue. Therefore, alterations in skin and hair growth during a state of glucocorticoid excess may result from the loss of the anabolic effects of GH and the insulin-like growth factors, as well as the catabolic effects of hyperadrenocorticism. In support of this concept, glucocorticoid excess generally produces less severe signs of skin disease in larger dogs as compared with dogs of the smaller breeds; this may be related to the higher concentrations of circulating insulin-like growth factor normally found in the larger breeds.

GH-RESISTANT STATES. A classic example of resistance to the effects of circulating GH is one of the human types of familial dwarfism (Laron dwarfism), as discussed above. Clinically, this disorder is indistinguishable from the dwarfism caused by isolated GH deficiency, and both types can be associated with sparse hair. It is possible that a similar form of GH resistance accounts for the congenital alopecia that occurs in the Chinese crested dog and the Mexican hairless breeds.

Resistance to the cutaneous effects of GH may also be involved in the pathogenesis of hair loss encountered with zinc deficiency. In rats, production of zinc deficiency induces a state of GH resistance that is reversible with zinc supplementation.

DIAGNOSIS OF GH DEFICIENCY

In dogs with suspected GH deficiency, routine laboratory determinations (e.g., complete blood count, serum biochemical analysis) should be performed before proceeding with any endocrine testing. This is of particular importance in dwarf dogs in order to rule out hepatic, renal, or gastrointestinal disease, all of which could cause dwarfism. If primary GH deficiency is suspected in an adult dog with endocrine alopecia, hypothyroidism and Cushing's syndrome must be ruled out before GH testing is performed, since these disorders may produce various degrees of reversible GH deficiency. At this point, a diagnostic dilemma may arise when the clinician is left with the differential diagnosis of alopecia related to either gonadal imbalance or GH deficiency. Unless the history and clinical signs unequivocally point to gonadal imbalance, testing for GH deficiency is recommended.

To diagnose GH deficiency, plasma GH concentrations should be determined in samples obtained before and during a stimulation test. Measurement of basal GH levels alone cannot distinguish between normal dogs and dogs with GH deficiency, since many normal dogs have resting GH concentrations that are low. Both clonidine (Catapres, Boehringer Ingelheim) and xylazine (Rompun, Haver-Lockhart) are potent provocative stimuli of GH secretion in dogs, and either agent can be used for the stimulation test. To perform the test, blood (2 to 4 ml) should be collected in edetate (EDTA) tubes before and 15, 30, 45, 60, and 90 minutes after the intravenous injection of either clonidine (10 μg/kg) or xylazine (100 μg/kg). After collection, the blood should be promptly centrifuged and the plasma frozen until assayed for GH.

Canine GH should be measured using a species-specific, homologous radioimmunoassay, since it will not cross-react in assays devised for determination of human GH. Although measurements of insulin-like growth factors are possible, these assays are difficult and time-consuming; in addition, levels are normally low in small-sized dogs and therefore might not distinguish between normal and GH-deficient dogs.

TREATMENT

Limited information is available concerning the treatment of GH deficiency in dogs. GH is difficult to obtain and is expensive. Although GH of nonprimate origin is biologically inactive in humans, human GH appears to be active in phylogenetically lower animals such as dogs. The growth hormones of nonprimate origin (e.g., feline, canine, porcine, ovine, bovine) are immunologically interrelated, and all appear to be effective for treatment.

The recommended dose of GH is 0.1 U/kg, administered subcutaneously three times a week.

Treatment should be continued for up to 5 weeks, at which time hair regrowth should be evident. If alopecia again develops, the GH treatment can be repeated. Some dogs may become nonresponsive or refractory to treatment, possibly because of the development of antibodies against GH, which decrease its biologic activity. In German shepherd dwarf dogs, thyroxine (20 μg/kg/day) should also be given if concurrent hypothyroidism is present.

Synthetic human GH, manufactured by recombinant DNA techniques, is currently available to a limited extent. Although synthetic human GH appears to be effective for treatment of human GH-deficient disorders, long-term results are not yet available. A possible future treatment includes the use of GH-releasing factor in dogs with primary hypothalamic disease resulting in GH deficiency.

References and Supplemental Reading

Andrensen, E., and Willeberg, P.: Pituitary dwarfism in German shepherd dogs: Genetic investigations. Nord. Vet. Med. 16:692, 1974.

Eigenmann, J. E.: Diagnosis and treatment of dwarfism in a German shepherd dog. J. Am. Anim. Hosp. Assoc. 17:798, 1981.

Eigenmann, J. E.: Diagnosis and treatment of pituitary dwarfism in dogs. Proc. 6th Kal Kan Symposium, 1982, pp. 107–110.

Eigenmann, J. E.: Growth hormone and insulin-like growth factor I in the dog: Clinical and experimental investigations. Domestic Anim. Endocrinol. 2:1, 1985.

Eigenmann, J. E., and Eigenmann, R. Y.: Radioimmunoassay of canine growth hormone. Acta Endocrinol. (Copenh.) 98:514, 1981.

Eigenmann, J. E., Zanesco, S., Arnold, U., et al.: Growth hormone and insulin-like growth factor I in German shephard dwarf dogs. Acta Endocrinol. (Copenh.) 105:289, 1984.

Eigenmann, J. E., and Patterson, D. F.: Growth hormone deficiency in the mature dog. J. Am. Anim. Hosp. Assoc. 20:741, 1984.

Eigenmann, J. E., Patterson, D. F., and Frosch, E. R.: Body size parallels insulin-like growth factor I levels but not growth hormone secretory capacity. Acta Endocrinol. (Copenh.) 106:448, 1984.

Eigenmann, J. E., Patterson, D. F., Zapf, J., et al.: Insulin-like growth factor I in the dog: A study in different dog breeds and in dogs with growth hormone elevation. Acta Endocrinol. (Copenh.) 105:294, 1984.

Hampshire, J., and Altszuler, N.: Clonidine or xylazine as provocative tests for growth hormone secretion in the dog. Am. J. Vet. Res. 42:1073, 1981.

Parker, W. H., and Scott, D. W.: Growth hormone responsive alopecia in the mature dog: A discussion of 13 cases. J. Am. Anim. Hosp. Assoc. 16:824, 1980.

Peterson, M. E., and Altszuler, N.: Suppression of growth hormone secretion in spontaneous canine hyperadrenocorticism and its reversal after treatment. Am. J. Vet. Res. 42:1882, 1980.

THYROID HORMONE REPLACEMENT THERAPY

DUNCAN C. FERGUSON, V.M.D.
Ithaca, New York

As suggested by the term *replacement therapy*, the goal of hormone administration in an endocrine deficiency state is the reversal of the pathophysiologic effects of deficiency in a manner that mimics the natural pattern of secretion and metabolism of that hormone. This goal is an ideal that is rarely achieved; however, rational replacement therapy is based on a compromise between practicality and the metabolic requirements of the patient.

The major indication for thyroid hormone replacement therapy is the treatment of hypothyroidism, either spontaneous, as commonly encountered in dogs, or surgically induced, a potential sequela to bilateral thyroidectomy as therapy for hyperthyroidism in cats. (A review of the causes, breed incidence, physical findings, and diagnosis of hypothyroidism appears in *Current Veterinary Therapy VIII*, pp. 869–875, together with a detailed listing of the commercially available thyroid hormone products.) For more details on thyroid physiology and function testing, the reader is referred to recent reviews of these subjects (Rosychuk, 1982a; Ferguson, 1984). This discussion will emphasize the physiologic bases for choice of appropriate thyroid hormone products and replacement regimens.

REVIEW OF RELEVANT PHYSIOLOGY

The metabolically active thyroid hormones are the iodothyronines L-thyroxine (L-T_4) and 3,5,3′-L-triiodothyronine (L-T_3). Thyroxine is the main secretory product of the normal thyroid gland. However, T_3, which is about three to five times more potent than T_4, as well as smaller amounts of 3,3,′,5′-L-triiodothyronine (rT_3), a thyromimetically inactive product, and further deiodinated metabolites have been found to be secreted by the canine thyroid. Thyrotropin (thyroid-stimulating hormone, TSH), a glycoprotein secreted by the anterior pituitary gland, increases the secretion of T_4 and T_3 from the thyroid gland. The ratio of T_4:T_3 is lower in the venous effluent of the thyroid (about 6:1) than it is in the canine thyroid gland itself (about 12:1), demonstrating that thyroidal deiodination of T_4 to T_3 is also stimulated by TSH (Laurberg, 1980). The synthesis and secretion of TSH are regulated primarily through negative feedback by plasma T_4 and T_3 in the free or unbound form. The pituitary rapidly and completely deiodinates T_4 from the plasma to T_3, which acts via pituitary nuclear receptors to inhibit TSH synthesis and secretion. Thus, although T_3 is the active hormone intracellularly in suppressing TSH release, plasma T_4 is the preferred and less variable source of intrapituitary T_3 (Larsen et al., 1981). In rats, there is now also some direct evidence that thyroid hormones may have negative feedback action on the hypothalamus to inhibit the release of thyrotropin-releasing hormone (TRH), the modulator of pituitary TSH release.

It is clinically important to recognize that thyroid hormones are highly bound to plasma proteins. In dogs, about 0.1 per cent of total serum T_4 is unbound or free, whereas about 1 per cent of T_3 is free. Most evidence suggests that it is the free hormone fraction that is available to tissues. The bound fraction acts as a reservoir of hormone that buffers against rapid increases or decreases of hormone delivery to tissue. The proportion of free hormone is also a primary determinant of the rate of fractional metabolic and excretory turnover. Humans, in contrast to dogs, have thyroxine binding globulin (TBG) in plasma, with a high affinity for T_4, and the fractional free T_4 is one-third to one-fifth that in dogs. In dogs, the plasma half-life of T_4 has been estimated to be between 10 and 16 hours, compared with about 7 days in humans, and the plasma half-life of T_3 is estimated to be 5 to 6 hours in dogs (Fox and Nachreiner, 1981). It should be emphasized that these figures reflect plasma disappearance and do not indicate the extent or duration of biologic action.

Certain organs, particularly the liver and kidneys, can concentrate thyroid hormones and may exchange hormone rapidly with the plasma. Therefore, these organs serve also as reservoirs of hormone that may "buffer" against rapid changes in serum concentrations, which might have detrimental cellular effects. Although clinical measurements of serum concentrations of thyroid hormone are limited to the plasma compartment, approximately 50 to 60 per cent of the body's T_4 and 90 to 95 per cent of the T_3 are intracellular. Therefore, because T_3 is primarily an intracellular hormone, measurement of its serum concentration is a less meaningful estimate of the total body T_3 pool than is measurement of total serum T_4 concentration in estimating the body T_4 pool.

Although all T_4 is secreted by the thyroid, a considerable amount (40 to 60 per cent in dogs) of T_3 is derived from extrathyroidal deiodination of T_4 by the enzyme T_4-5′-deiodinase. Therefore, T_4 can be considered to be a "prohormone," and its "activation" to the more potent T_3 is a step regulated individually by peripheral tissues. Such a control mechanism may serve as a safeguard against tissue T_3 deficiency in critical tissues; for example, in hypothyroidism in rats, the conversion of T_4 to T_3 increases in the brain but decreases in the liver, as well as in most other tissues. Through this type of regulation, the brain may continue to obtain adequate cellular T_3 levels necessary to prevent or delay dysfunction due to T_4 deficiency, whereas the liver reduces its production of T_3, thereby leading to a diminished metabolic rate. Although most tissues are able to deiodinate T_4 to T_3, the liver and kidneys appear to be the most active. Muscle and skin, although they have low enzyme activity, may produce a significant amount of the body's T_3 solely because of their large mass (Wartofsky and Burman, 1982; Larsen et al., 1981).

In addition to deiodinative pathways, conjugation and fecal excretion are significant routes of thyroid hormone metabolism and loss. It is important to note that dogs lose in the feces more than half of the T_4 secreted daily by the thyroid gland. Fecal wastage of T_3 is also significant (about 30 per cent of daily disposal); this route accounts for 20 times more loss than in humans. As a result, in dogs, the extrathyroidal body stores of T_4 are metabolized or excreted and replaced in slightly less than 1 day, whereas stores of T_3 are lost and replaced twice daily. In dogs, it is likely that the fractional loss of orally administered thyroid hormones is even greater because of the first-pass effect of bolus amounts of hormone taken up from the hepatoportal system, metabolized by the liver, and excreted into the bile—although no data are available to support this hypothesis. It is possible that, in some animals, dividing the daily dose may serve to reduce the loss of hormone due to the first-pass effect, resulting in a more consistent clinical response.

DETERMINANTS OF BIOAVAILABILITY AND CLINICAL EFFICACY OF THYROID HORMONE PREPARATIONS

The ultimate determinants of bioavailability and efficacy of administered thyroid hormone preparations include the following: (1) route of administration, (2) absorption, (3) peripheral metabolism, (4) persistence of cellular stores, and (5) persistence of biologic effects. All of these factors bear on the clinician's design of a rational thyroid replacement regimen.

Route of Administration and Absorption

Although the daily thyroidal secretion of T_4 has been estimated to be 2.5 μg/kg in dogs, approximately twice the rate in humans, the administration of this dose once or divided twice daily subcutaneously or intravenously to surgically thyroidectomized dogs did not normalize serum T_4 concentrations; serum T_4 concentrations did not become normal until the divided intravenous daily dose of 10 μg/kg was reached (Hulter et al., 1984). This study suggests that if normalization of serum T_4 is a desirable therapeutic goal (it is a therapeutic ideal but is probably not necessary, as discussed below), then parenterally administered doses of hormone must greatly exceed the amounts secreted physiologically. With the clinical use of oral thyroid hormone products, the additional variability of gastrointestinal absorption is introduced. Although systematic studies have not been performed in dogs, comparison of oral T_4 doses necessary to create normal serum T_4 concentrations (20 to 40 μg/kg/day) with parenteral doses (2.5 to 10 μg/kg/day) suggests that net gastrointestinal absorption is probably in the range of 10 to 50 per cent. In humans, absorption of T_4 preparations varies from 50 to 80 per cent, whereas T_3 absorption is close to 100 per cent. Intraluminal contents, including plasma protein, dietary factors, and intestinal flora, may bind T_4 and make it less available for diffusion.

Metabolism

As mentioned, T_4 is deiodinated to T_3 in peripheral tissues by a regulated pathway. This conversion is impaired in acute and chronic starvation, surgery, diabetes, most chronic illnesses, and hepatic and renal disease in humans. Changes in thyroid hormone metabolism in these conditions are less well characterized in dogs than in humans; however, it appears that the "euthyroid sick syndrome" also occurs in dogs as characterized by decreases in serum T_3 and T_4. Decreases in serum T_3 can also likely be attributed to depressed conversion of T_4 to T_3, whereas decreased total serum T_4 may be associated with an increase in the free fraction of T_4 in serum due to serum binding inhibitors. It is unclear whether the "euthyroid sick syndrome" is associated with tissue hypothyroidism. The bulk of evidence suggests that this change is not detrimental but that a decrease in the production of the more potent T_3 may be an adaptive mechanism to limit the catabolic state of illness or malnutrition.

Many drugs are known to influence thyroid hormone metabolism. Drugs that might inhibit the conversion of T_4 to T_3 and limit the response to T_4 replacement therapy include glucocorticoids, quinidine, nonsteroidal anti-inflammatory drugs, and iodinated radiocontrast agents such as iopanoic acid (Telepaque, Winthrop), diatrizoate (Cardiografin, Cystografin, Gastrografin, Renografin, Squibb; Hypaque, Winthrop), ipodate (Oragrafin, Squibb), tyropanoate (Bilopaque, Winthrop), and metrizamide. Agents that induce drug-metabolizing enzyme systems also increase the rate of thyroid hormone metabolism. Barbiturates, carbamazepine, and diphenylhydantoin enhance the deiodinative metabolism of thyroid hormones. Therefore, greater doses of T_4 might be necessary when these drugs are administered concurrently.

Cellular Effects

The ultimate determinant of efficacy is the persistence of the cellular effects of thyroid hormone. Many of its effects are mediated by nuclear thyroid hormone receptors, subsequent DNA synthesis, ribosomal translation, and new protein synthesis. The overt responses include growth, differentiation, proliferation, and maturation. The chronicity of these effects contributes to the possibility of observing adequate responses to therapy even when serum concentrations are not in the normal range at all times during the day. An analogy might be the clinical responses to glucocorticoids, which have biologic half-lives that are significantly longer than serum half-lives.

INDICATIONS

The major indications for thyroid hormone replacement therapy, in order of prevalence, are primary hypothyroidism (spontaneous and post-thyroidectomy) and irreversible secondary or pituitary hypothyroidism.

NON-INDICATIONS

Low serum T_4 or T_3 concentrations do not, by themselves, confirm the diagnosis of hypothyroidism. As mentioned, concentrations can be low in nonthyroidal illness (NTI; "euthyroid sick syndrome") and with certain drugs. Replacement therapy to "normalize" serum hormone concentrations is not indicated and may be contraindicated in these situations. These possibilities can usually be distinguished by the history (including careful drug history), physical examination, and standard diagnostic tests. At the present time, the TSH stimulation test remains the best test to distinguish primary hypothyroidism from secondary hypothyroidism, NTI, or the effect of drugs. In primary hypothyroidism, the post-TSH increase in serum T_4 is usually minimal or absent; in NTI, drug-induced lowering of serum thyroid hormone concentrations, or secondary and tertiary hypothyroidism, the basal T_4 concentrations are low but a normal thyroid reserve is demonstrated by a post-TSH rise in serum T_4 concentration that parallels the normal response.

PREPARATIONS

Thyroid hormone preparations can be classified into the following groups: (1) crude hormones prepared from animal thyroid, (2) synthetic L-thyroxine, (3) synthetic L-triiodothyronine, and (4) synthetic combinations of L-T_4 and L-T_3. (An extensive list of the available commercial preparations is included in *Current Veterinary Therapy VIII.*) Each group will be discussed individually with recommended or reported treatment protocols.

Crude Thyroid Products

Thyroid hormone products derived from thyroidal tissue from hogs, sheep, or cattle are available in the forms of desiccated thyroid (e.g., Thyroid USP, Lilly; Armour Thyroid, USV Pharmaceutical) and thyroglobulin (e.g., Proloid, Parke-Davis; S-P-T, Fleming). Although desiccated thyroid accounted for 40 per cent of the sales of thyroid replacement products in 1982, there appear to be no good reasons to continue to use these products for replacement therapy. Their variable T_4 and T_3 content, unphysiologically low ratios of T_4:T_3 (2:1 to 4:1), and poor shelf life are problems that outweigh the lower cost of these products. The newer standards listed in the United States Pharmacopoeia for control of hormone content (see below) may improve the reproducibility of these products but are unlikely to eliminate the other disadvantages.

Synthetic L-Thyroxine

Thyroxine is the compound of choice for most indications. It is generally formulated and used as levothyroxine sodium for oral administration. Examples include generic levothyroxine sodium, USP (Thyro-Tab, Vet-A-Mix; Soloxine, Daniels Pharmaceutical; other manufacturers include Boots Pharmaceuticals, Pharmaceutical Basics, Heather Drug Co., Chelsea Laboratories, Spencer-Mead), Synthroid (Flint Laboratories), Levothroid (Armour), and Levoid (Nutrition Control). Injectable forms are available from Flint Laboratories (Synthroid injection) and Nutrition Control Products (Levoid).

Thyroxine is the treatment of choice for hypothyroidism for the following reasons:

1. L-Thyroxine is the main secretory product of the thyroid gland.
2. L-Thyroxine is the physiologic "prohormone"; administration of L-T_4 does not bypass the cellular regulatory processes controlling the production of the more potent T_3 from T_4 (5′-deiodination). The therapeutic goal should be to achieve normal concentrations of both tissue and serum T_4 and T_3, and this is accomplished in the most physiologic manner with exogenous T_4 administration.
3. The pituitary appears to regulate TSH release primarily according to serum T_4 concentrations. In humans, therapy is often tailored to normalize serum TSH as well as average T_4 and T_3 concentrations, and this can only be accomplished with the administration of T_4. With administration of T_3, the serum T_3 concentrations must be higher than normal to normalize serum TSH.
4. In general, variability among the bioavailability of preparations is less than for crude products. Bioavailability is, however, significantly variable from animal to animal.
5. It is less expensive than other synthetic preparations.

In 1982, the United States Pharmacopoeial Convention adopted a new method for the assay of hormone content in thyroid hormone preparations. The old, less accurate determinations based on iodine content were replaced by high-pressure liquid chromatographic (HPLC) determination. With the change of the assay, Flint Laboratories changed the formulation of the most widely used T_4 product, Synthroid. Some controversy ensued over the bioavailability of this commercial T_4 preparation. With the change to the reformulated preparation, human patients maintained on Synthroid had increases in serum T_4, and in some cases, signs of thyrotoxicosis developed. It seems well documented that the old formulation had less than 80 per cent of the listed amount of active ingredient (Sawin et al., 1984). Flint Laboratories, in an open letter to clinical endocrinologists, stated that the change in formulation of Synthroid was designed to improve stability characteristics and claimed that the bioavailability of the new preparation was no greater but that a change from tablets near the expiration date to the new formulation may have led to the increase in serum T_4 concentrations. To the author's knowledge, similar observations have not been made in domestic animals; however, this experience points out the potential for an alteration of clinical response when the thyroid hormone preparation is altered or an old preparation is changed to a newer one. Dogs are very resistant to the development of thyrotoxic signs and require 10 to 20 times the replacement dose chronically in order to consistently demonstrate signs. This is likely the result of the dog's capacity to efficiently clear thyroid hormone through biliary and fecal excretion. However, the change to a product with significantly decreased bioavailability might lead to an eventual return of the clinical signs of hypothyroidism.

DOSAGE SCHEDULES FOR L-THYROXINE. With very few exceptions, thyroid hormone replacement therapy will be continued for the remainder of the animal's life. Therefore, careful initial diagnosis and tailoring of treatment are essential. A variety of dosage regimens for T_4 therapy have been recommended in the literature. This variability probably reflects the variations in hormone absorption and metabolism among animals, the variable degree of remaining endogenous hormone secretion by the failing thyroid, the possible effect of circulating anti-T_4 antibodies in a subgroup of animals, the resistance to the development of thyrotoxicity with overdoses in the dog, and the vague and variable criteria by which clinical improvement is judged.

In general, reported replacement doses for T_4 range from *0.02 mg/kg to 0.04 mg/kg daily*. Probably, a more logical approach is to dose according to body surface area (BSA) (*0.5 mg/m² daily*), which is proportional to the metabolic rate (Chastain, 1982). This method accounts and corrects for the tendency of some large dogs to develop thyrotoxicosis, or at least elevated serum T_4 concentrations, when the dose is determined according to body weight. For example, according to body surface area, a 5-kg (0.29 m^2 BSA) dog would start on a dose of 0.15 mg L-T_4 daily, or 0.03 mg/kg. A 50-kg dog (1.36 m^2 BSA) would start on 0.70 mg/day, or less than half the dose according to body weight, 0.014 mg/kg. There are no reported studies to confirm the validity of this dosing method, however.

It is common practice to administer T_4 in single or divided doses. Although the protocol should be tailored to each animal, it is becoming more widely recognized that once-daily administration of T_4 leads to clinical improvement in a significant number of animals. Because of the significant intracellular capacity for storage of T_4 and T_3, bolus oral doses of thyroid hormone may be substantially distributed into tissue. During the initial days to weeks of replacement therapy in a hypothyroid animal, the hormone stores of the liver and kidney are repleted to euthyroid levels and then can serve to "buffer" serum concentrations when the circulating hormone "store" bound to binding proteins begins to be depleted. Probably for this reason, many hypothyroid animals can be maintained on once-daily T_4 therapy despite the fact that the serum half-life of T_4 in normal dogs is 10 to 16 hours. In addition, in chronic hypothyroidism, the serum half-life of T_4 may also be longer than in normal dogs because T_4 metabolism is reduced. In humans, it seems that clinical improvement and suppression of serum TSH can be maintained by any replacement regimen that, over the course of a day, leads to a normal average serum concentration without leading to the acute toxic effects of thyroid hormone. For example, the serum T_4 concentration might be high at one time of the day and low at another; however, the tissue response "integrates" the serum concentration throughout the day, thereby reflecting the average concentration. For these reasons, it may not be necessary to maintain serum hormone concentrations in the normal range throughout the day. It is also important to note that once-daily administration probably leads to greater compliance by owners.

Nonetheless, it is the common clinical impression that some animals require twice-daily therapy to achieve an optimal clinical response. Dividing the dose has the advantage that it more closely mimics the constant serum T_4 levels; in addition, it might be advantageous during the initial weeks of therapy in order to replete intracellular hormone stores and minimize fecal hormone loss, as well as to avoid the adverse effects of periodically high serum concentrations on previously hypothyroid tissues. Gradual introduction of hormone is ideal, particularly in individuals with decreased ability to metabolize T_4 and increased risk of the development of thyrotoxicosis, such as in hypoadrenal, aged, cardiac, or diabetic patients. In these animal groups, it is recommended to use divided-dose protocols and to increase the daily dose in 20 to 25 per cent increments (e.g., 0.1 mg/m², 0.2 mg/m², 0.3 mg/m², 0.4 mg/m², 0.5 mg/m² twice daily) over a period of 4 to 8 weeks. Glucocorticoid replacement should begin prior to thyroid replacement therapy in patients with concomitant hypoadrenocorticism (e.g., hypopituitarism). This assures steroid replacement prior to the increase in metabolic demand for endogenous steroids that follows correction of hypothyroidism. In all cases, because the metabolism of thyroid hormone changes with correction of hypothyroidism, dosage regimens should be reassessed by clinical or laboratory criteria after 6 to 12 weeks of initial therapy.

Although no conclusive studies have been performed, dosing regimens for cats have followed those in dogs (for most cats, 0.05 to 0.20 mg once or twice daily). The major indication for thyroid hormone replacement in cats is following bilateral thyroidectomy for therapy of spontaneous hyperthyroidism, since about 70 per cent have bilateral toxic nodular goiter (Peterson et al., 1983). Cats with unilateral disease likely will recover function of the suppressed normal thyroid lobe. Replacement therapy is only recommended in these cases if recovery of serum T_4 is prolonged or if clinical signs of hypothyroidism intervene. If therapy is chosen, it should eventually be tapered to allow full recrudescence of endogenous thyroid function. In a series of 19 cats receiving bilateral thyroidectomy, only three had recovered normal thyroid function 6 weeks after surgery, probably because of the function of ectopic thyroid tissue or incomplete thyroidectomy. Therefore, it is recommended to replace thyroid hormone in cats following bilateral thyroidectomy (Hoenig et al., 1982). In some cases, it may be possible to successfully withdraw replacement therapy at a later date. The experience at veterinary referral institutions with ^{131}I-radioiodine therapy for hyperthyroidism has shown that the incidence of posttreatment hypothyroidism is significant, particularly with regimens using higher ablative doses.

Synthetic L-Triiodothyronine

Although T_3 is the active intracellular hormone, there are few valid reasons to use this product for replacement therapy and some good reasons not to use it. Triiodothyronine "replacement" is not physiologic and bypasses the final cellular regulatory step of 5′-deiodination of T_4. Thyroxine does have intrinsic thyromimetic activity. Its role is particularly important for central nervous system and pituitary function. Treatment with T_3 alone may provide amounts sufficient for organs like the liver, kidneys, and heart, which derive a high proportion of T_3 from plasma. However, the brain and pituitary, which derive a majority of their T_3 from T_4, may be deficient in thyroid hormone. Conversely, T_3 therapy adequate for the brain and pituitary may be excessive for the liver, kidneys, and heart.

There is no evidence at this time that T_3 therapy is indicated in the "low-T_3 syndrome" associated with NTI. Because of its higher oral bioavailability, it may be used to improve the clinical response in an animal with demonstrated or suspected poor T_4 absorption. In such cases, "post-pill" serum T_4 and T_3 concentrations would be low following reasonable oral dose regimens. In animals that have serum antibodies to T_4 (and not T_3), the total serum T_4 concentration would be normal or high, the fractional free T_4 concentration would be low, and consequently the serum T_3 concentration would be low. In both situations, increasing the T_4 dose above the commonly used range is also a reasonable step and may be safer than T_3 therapy. The latter situation might be mimicked by concomitant NTI, for which T_3 therapy might be detrimental. Triiodothyronine therapy may be indicated when thyroid replacement is necessary with the simultaneous administration of drugs that inhibit the conversion of T_4 to T_3; an important example is pharmacologic doses of glucocorticoids.

Anecdotal reports suggest that a small fraction of hypothyroid dogs convert T_4 to T_3 poorly and therefore do not respond to L-thyroxine therapy. Two possible cellular mechanisms could be the basis for this observation: (1) The entrance of T_4 into tissue and, therefore, its subsequent deiodination to T_3 may be reduced, or (2) there is a true decrease in all or isolated tissues of the 5′-deiodinase enzyme, which converts T_4 to T_3. Triiodothyronine therapy has been recommended in these cases as an adjunct to T_4 or as sole therapy. The response to T_3 in these purported "poor converters" following the failure of T_4 therapy does not constitute sufficient evidence of a selective 5′-deiodinase defect. Other more likely possibilities include concomitant NTI, greater oral bioavailability of T_3 than of T_4, or increased serum T_4 binding, possibly due to T_4 antibodies, resulting in decreased T_4 uptake into tissue. If indeed a selective tissue or generalized 5′-deiodinase defect exists in some dogs not suffering from NTI, these animals would provide an important and unique model that should be studied further, because similar defects have not been described in humans.

DOSAGE SCHEDULE FOR L-TRIIODOTHYRONINE. The commercial T_3 (Liothyronine, L-triiodothyronine sodium) preparations include Cytomel (Smith Kline & French) and Cytobin (Norden). A regimen of *4 to 6 μg/kg three times* or possibly twice daily appears necessary to maintain serum T_3 concentrations without high peaks, which appear to be associated with signs of thyrotoxicosis.

Synthetic Combinations

The use of synthetic thyroid hormone combinations should be limited in veterinary medicine. Commercial combinations of synthetic L-T_4 and L-T_3 in the ratio of 4:1 are available (generic liotrix; Thyrolar, Armour; Euthroid, Parke-Davis). These preparations were intended to mimic the ratio of T_4:T_3 in thyroidal secretion (about 6:1 in dogs), and tablets are designed to provide the equivalent of 1 grain (65 mg) of desiccated thyroid (Thyrolar, 50 μg T_4/12.5 μg T_3; Euthroid, 60 μg/15 μg). A variety of dosage schemes have been proposed, but the most common suggests dosing according to the T_4 content and division of the dose to account for the shorter serum half-life of T_3. Administration of these preparations will commonly lead to a low-normal to normal serum T_4. Increasing the dose to normalize serum T_4 can result in high serum T_3 concentrations and can potentially produce thyrotoxicosis due to the T_3 content. These preparations share the disadvantages of the commercial T_3 preparations Cytobin (Norden) and Cytomel (Smith Kline & French): increased cost, increased complexity of dosing regimes, and a higher incidence of thyrotoxic signs. Perhaps most importantly, they do not reliably succeed in their goal—physiologic delivery of thyroid hormone to tissue.

POTENTIAL FACTORS AFFECTING DOSE

Clinically adequate doses of thyroid hormone can be quite variable from animal to animal. In addition to the mentioned effects of concomitant drug therapy on thyroid hormone metabolism, increased doses of T_4 appear to be necessary in hypothyroid humans during the colder months of winter. Although similar studies have not been performed in animals, it is possible that an animal housed outdoors might require a higher dose of T_4 than an animal predominately in the house, particularly during the colder months. In dogs, basal serum concentrations of T_4 decrease with age as they do in elderly humans. In addition, it has been observed that older hypothyroid human patients require lower doses of T_4 for adequate replacement, and they are more apt to develop the adverse effects of slight thyroid hormone overdoses.

SIGNS OF OVERDOSE (THYROTOXICOSIS)

Animals on replacement therapy, particularly with a product containing T_4 or T_3, can develop signs of thyrotoxicosis; however, the incidence at recommended doses is rare. Animals should be monitored for signs suggesting an overdose, including polyuria, polydipsia, nervousness, weight loss, increase in appetite, panting, and fever. Diagnosis is confirmed by elevated serum levels of T_4 or T_3.

THERAPEUTIC TRIAL FOR DIAGNOSIS OF HYPOTHYROIDISM

The institution of thyroid replacement therapy in the absence of confirmatory laboratory evidence (serum T_4 or TSH stimulation test) has been suggested as a valid diagnostic step in an animal suspected to be hypothyroid. Although the major factor cited in defense of this practice is the cost of the diagnostic testing for the owner, it should be emphasized to an owner that replacement therapy is generally necessary for the remainder of the animal's life. Therefore, incorrect diagnosis can also be quite expensive, and a delayed diagnosis of another disease could be detrimental. Diagnostic procedures following a therapeutic trial with equivocal results can be quite difficult to interpret because secretion of the normal thyroid gland is inhibited by this procedure.

MONITORING THERAPY

The success of thyroid replacement therapy should be judged primarily on clinical grounds. With successful replacement therapy, changes in the animal's activity and alertness may be noticed within the first week or two. Such effects are probably the clinical expression of the rapid cellular actions of thyroid hormone such as enhancement of mitochondrial oxygen utilization and membrane transport functions. The clinical changes that take a longer time to be manifested during the development of hypothyroidism, such as alopecia, alterations in cutaneous lipid and keratin metabolism, and weight gain, are typical of the cellular effects mediated via binding to nuclear thyroid hormone receptors leading to changes in protein synthesis. The reversal of these changes should be noted clinically over a period of 1 to 5 months. Therefore, careful observation by the owner and clinician can successfully monitor therapy in the majority of cases.

In cases in which clinical improvement is marginal or signs of thyrotoxicosis are seen, the clinical observations can be supported by measurement of serum thyroid hormone concentrations, so-called post-pill testing. Clearly, the documentation of elevated serum T_4 concentrations following T_4 administration and elevated serum T_3 concentrations following T_3 administration, concomitant with signs of thyrotoxicosis, confirm an overdose.

Much confusion has resulted about the interpretation of post-pill serum thyroid hormone concentrations in cases of suspected underdosing. Several reasonable approaches can be outlined. Such therapeutic monitoring should not be attempted until steady-state conditions are reached, probably minimally 1 month after the initiation of therapy. With once-daily T_4 administration, the peak serum concentrations of T_4 generally should be in the normal to high-normal range 4 to 8 hours after dosing and should be low-normal to normal 24 hours after dosing. Given the dog's resistance to signs of thyrotoxicosis, it may be reasonable and adequate to check serum T_4 only at 24 hours after the previous day's dose and expect it to still be in the normal range. Animals on twice-daily administration probably can be checked at any time, but peak concentrations can be expected at the middle of the dosing interval (4 to 8 hours), with the nadir just prior to the next dose. Once the animal's dose is stabilized, once- or twice-yearly checks of serum T_4 (with or without T_3) concentrations will guard against impending therapeutic failure or toxicosis.

If serum T_3 concentrations are to be measured following T_4 administration, something not routinely recommended, they should be interpreted carefully together with the serum T_4 results and, most importantly, the clinical response. Serum T_3 radioimmunoassays are subject to greater artifactual problems than T_4 assays; it is therefore particularly important that the assay be validated for the species of animal and that the normal ranges be well established. It should be remembered that the vast majority of the body's T_3 is intracellular, where it cannot be easily measured. A low serum T_3 and T_4, together with a poor clinical response, suggests an underdose or inadequate bioavailability (absorption). A low serum T_3 with a normal or high serum T_4 concentration may suggest several possibilities. In order of highest to lowest likelihood, they are (1) concomitant NTI or drug effects, (2) serum antibodies to T_4 and not T_3 (antithyroglobulin antibodies described in the dog [Gosselin et al., 1982] may be of sufficient titer and specificity to bind T_4), and (3) decreased 5′-deiodination of T_4 to T_3 unassociated with NTI (as yet, poorly documented). The development of routinely available measurements of serum free T_4 concentrations and thyroglobulin antibody should help to distinguish these possibilities. In addition, the measurement of serum reverse T_3, which likely would be decreased in underdosing or with T_4 antibodies and increased in NTI and in poor converters, is already available in a limited number of veterinary diagnostic and research laboratories.

With T_3 administration, serum concentrations are reported to peak 2 to 3 hours after administration. Serum T_4 concentrations are routinely low or undetectable; any remaining endogenous thyroidal T_4 secretion is inhibited because of the suppression of pituitary TSH secretion by T_3.

REASONS FOR THERAPEUTIC FAILURE

If clinical signs of hypothyroidism remain despite thyroid hormone therapy, the following possibilities must be considered, in approximate order of likelihood: (1) The dose or frequency of administration is improper, (2) the owner is not complying with instructions or is not successfully administering the product, (3) the animal may not be absorbing the product well or is metabolizing or excreting it too rapidly, (4) the product is outdated, (5) the diagnosis is incorrect, (6) the animal has serum antibodies to T_4 or T_3, (7) the animal has a tissue 5′-deiodinase defect (not yet documented), or (8) there is peripheral tissue resistance to the effects of thyroid hormone (not yet documented).

References and Supplemental Reading

Chastain, C. B.: Canine hypothyroidism. J.A.V.M.A. 181:349, 1982.

Ferguson, D. C.: Thyroid hormone function test in the dog: Recent concepts. Vet. Clin. North Am. [Small Anim. Pract.] 14:783, 1984.

Fox, L. E., and Nachreiner, R. F.: The pharmacokinetics of T_3 and T_4 in the dog. Proc. 62nd Conference of Research Workers in Animal Disease, 1981, p. 13.

Gosselin, S. J., Capen, C. C., Martin, S. L., et al.: Autoimmune lymphocytic thyroiditis in dogs. Vet. Immunol. Immunopathol. 3:185, 1982.

Hoenig, M., Goldschmidt, M. H., Ferguson, D. C., et al.: Toxic nodular goiter in the cat. J. Small Anim. Pract. 23:1, 1982.

Hulter, H. N., Gustafson, L. E., Bonner, E. L., et al.: Thyroid replacement in thyroparathyroidectomized dogs. Miner. Electrolyte Metab. 10:228, 1984.

Larsen, P. R., Silva, J. E., and Kaplan, M. M.: Relationships between circulating and intracellular thyroid hormones: Physiological and clinical implications. Endocr. Rev. 2:87, 1981.

Laurberg, P.: Iodothyronine release from the perfused canine thyroid. Acta Endocrinol. [Suppl.] (Copenh.) 236:1, 1980.

Peterson, M. E., Kintzer, P. P., Cavanagh, P. C., et al.: Feline hyperthyroidism: Pretreatment clinical and laboratory evaluation of 131 cases. J.A.V.M.A. 183:103, 1983.

Rosychuk, R. A. W.: Thyroid hormones and antithyroid drugs. Vet. Clin. North Am. [Small Anim. Pract.] 12:111, 1982a.

Rosychuk, R. A. W.: Treatment of hypothyroidism. *In* Kirk, R. W. (ed.): *Current Veterinary Therapy VIII*, 1983, pp. 869–875.

Sawin, C. T., Surks, M. I., London, M., et al.: Oral thyroxine: Variation in biologic action and tablet content. Ann. Intern. Med. 100:641, 1984.

Wartofsky, L., and Burman, K. D.: Alterations in thyroid function in patients with systemic illness: The "euthyroid sick syndrome." Endocr. Rev. 3:164, 1982.

FELINE HYPERTHYROIDISM

MARK E. PETERSON, D.V.M.,
New York, New York

and JANE M. TURREL, D.V.M.
Davis, California

Hyperthyroidism (thyrotoxicosis) is a multisystemic disorder resulting from excessive circulating concentrations of the thyroid hormones, thyroxine (T_4) and triiodothyronine (T_3). Feline hyperthyroidism occurs in middle-aged to old cats; there is no breed or sex predilection. Functional thyroid adenoma (adenomatous hyperplasia) involving one or both thyroid lobes is the most common cause of feline hyperthyroidism. Thyroid carcinoma, the primary cause of canine hyperthyroidism, rarely causes hyperthyroidism in cats. Although first described only 7 years ago, hyperthyroidism has become a common and extremely important disorder of cats.

CLINICAL FINDINGS

The clinical manifestations of feline hyperthyroidism may be mild to severe and are modified by the duration of hyperthyroidism, the presence of concomitant abnormalities in various organ systems, and the inability of a body system to meet the demands imposed by thyroid hormone excess. Because of the multisystemic effects of hyperthyroidism, most cats have clinical signs that reflect dysfunction of many organ systems; in some, however, clinical signs of one body system predominate and may obscure other features of hyperthyroidism. Since clinical signs of feline hyperthyroidism are so variable, the presence or absence of one sign can neither confirm nor exclude hyperthyroidism. In addition, hyperthyroidism in cats might be misdiagnosed because of its resemblance to many other feline diseases.

The most common signs of feline hyperthyroidism include weight loss, hyperexcitability or irritability, and increased appetite (Table 1). Although the cause is unclear, about 20 per cent of hyperthyroid cats also have short periods of decreased appetite that alternate with longer periods of normal to increased appetite.

Polydipsia and polyuria are also frequent clinical signs in feline hyperthyroidism (Table 1). Although concurrent primary renal disease contributes to polyuria and polydipsia in some cats with hyperthyroidism, these signs also occur in many cats without evidence of renal dysfunction and resolve after treatment of hyperthyroidism. The exact cause of these signs in hyperthyroidism is unknown. The hyperthyroid state may, however, impair urine concentrating ability by increasing total renal blood flow and thereby decreasing renal medullary solute concentration; such medullary washout may cause polyuria with secondary polydipsia. Alternatively, in cats with normal renal concentrating ability, a hypothalamic disturbance caused by thyrotoxicosis may produce compulsive polydipsia with secondary polyuria.

Gastrointestinal signs that occur in feline hyperthyroidism include vomiting, diarrhea, increased frequency of defecation, and increased volume of feces (Table 1). Rapid overeating, common in hyperthyroid cats, appears to contribute to vomiting since it usually occurs shortly after eating. Intestinal hypermotility appears to be responsible for the increased frequency of defecation and diarrhea. Malabsorption with increased fecal fat excretion also develops in some cats with hyperthyroidism; al-

Table 1. *Historic and Clinical Findings in Feline Hyperthyroidism*

Clinical Finding	Percentage of Cats
Weight loss	95
Thyroid gland enlargement	85
Polyphagia	75
Hyperactivity	65
Tachycardia	60
Polyuria and polydipsia	50
Vomiting	50
Cardiac murmur	50
Diarrhea	30
Increased fecal volume	25
Anorexia	25
Polypnea (panting)	25
Muscle weakness	20
Muscle tremor	15
Congestive heart failure	15
Dyspnea	15

though the exact cause is unknown, it is likely that excessive fat intake resulting from polyphagia is a contributing factor.

Cardiovascular signs, including tachycardia, systolic murmurs, gallop rhythm, dyspnea, cardiomegaly, and congestive heart failure are common in cats with hyperthyroidism (Table 1). Electrocardiographic changes include tachycardia, increased R-wave amplitude in lead II, atrial and ventricular arrhythmias, and intraventricular conduction disturbances. Echocardiographic changes frequently found in cats with hyperthyroidism include left ventricular hypertrophy and evidence of increased contractility (manifested by increased shortening fraction and velocity of circumferential fiber shortening). Most cats with hyperthyroidism will develop a form of reversible hypertrophic cardiomyopathy, which may or may not be associated with congestive heart failure (see the article entitled Hyperthyroid Heart Disease in Cats). Although the exact pathogenesis of cardiac abnormalities associated with hyperthyroidism is unclear, direct action of thyroid hormones on the heart, interactions with the sympathetic nervous system, and cardiac changes that compensate for altered peripheral tissue function caused by thyrotoxicosis all appear to be factors that influence cardiac function in hyperthyroidism.

Apathetic or masked hyperthyroidism is a clinical form of thyrotoxicosis that develops in about 10 per cent of cats with hyperthyroidism. In these cats, hyperexcitability or restlessness is replaced by extreme depression and weakness as the dominant clinical feature. Weight loss remains a common clinical sign but is usually accompanied by anorexia rather than increased appetite. Affected cats also frequently have cardiac abnormalities, including arrhythmia and congestive heart failure.

On physical examination, enlargement of one or both thyroid lobes can be detected in about 85 to 90 per cent of cats with hyperthyroidism. The normal thyroid gland is not palpable in cats. To palpate an enlarged thyroid gland, the cat's neck should be slightly extended with the head tilted backward. Using the thumb and index finger, one should gently pass the fingers over both sides of the trachea, starting at the laryngeal area and moving ventrally toward the thoracic inlet. Since the thyroid lobes of the cat are loosely attached to the trachea, the enlarged lobes frequently descend ventrally from their normal location adjacent to the larynx. Many cats in which thyroid gland enlargement is not palpable have affected lobes that have descended into the thoracic cavity.

LABORATORY FINDINGS

Complete Blood Count

Mature leukocytosis and eosinopenia are common hematologic findings in feline hyperthyroidism and probably reflect a stress response to thyroid hormone excess. Mild to moderate erythrocytosis, characterized by concurrent increases in packed cell volume (PCV), red blood cell (RBC) count, and hemoglobin concentration, develops in 15 to 20 per cent of cats with hyperthyroidism. The erythrocytosis of hyperthyroidism appears to result from both a direct effect of thyroid hormones on erythroid marrow and an increased production of erythropoietin. Despite these stimulatory effects of thyroid hormone excess on RBC formation, a small number of cats with severe hyperthyroidism develop mild anemia, which probably reflects a deficiency of one or more hematopoietic nutrients.

Serum Biochemical Tests

The most common serum biochemical abnormalities, which occur in 50 to 75 per cent of cats with hyperthyroidism, include elevations in concentrations of alanine aminotransferase (ALT), aspartase aminotransferase (AST), alkaline phosphatase (SAP), and lactic dehydrogenase (LDH). Histologic examination of the liver usually reveals only modest and nonspecific changes, including centrilobular fatty infiltration and mild hepatic necrosis. The causes of hepatic damage and elevation in liver enzyme concentrations in thyrotoxicosis are unclear; malnutrition, congestive heart failure, infections, hepatic anoxia, and direct toxic effects of thyroid hormone on the liver may all contribute. Since only ALT is specific for hepatic necrosis in the cat, it is likely that other organs may also contribute to the elevations of SAP, AST, and LDH concentrations. Whatever the cause, elevated concentrations of ALT, AST, SAP, and LDH normalize with treatment of hyperthyroidism.

Serum Thyroid Hormone Concentrations

Increased serum thyroid hormone concentrations are the biochemical hallmarks of hyperthyroidism. Resting serum concentrations of T_4 and T_3 are increased above normal range in most cats with hyperthyroidism. A few hyperthyroid cats with elevated T_4 concentrations, however, have normal T_3 levels. Although the cause is unclear, most hyperthyroid cats with normal serum T_3 concentrations have only mild clinical signs of hyperthyroidism; therefore, it is likely that the normal T_3 levels found in these cats would eventually increase into the thyrotoxic range if the disorder were allowed to progress untreated.

In hyperthyroid cats with severe concurrent nonthyroidal illness (e.g., renal disease, diabetes mellitus, primary hepatic disease, and other chronic illnesses), high-normal or only slightly elevated total serum thyroid hormone concentrations may be found at time of initial evaluation. It is likely that the normal serum T_3 concentrations in these hyperthyroid cats with nonthyroidal illness result from impaired peripheral conversion of T_4 to T_3, whereas the normal total serum T_4 values result from inhibition of T_4 binding to plasma proteins. Despite such normal total serum T_4 concentrations, free levels of T_4 remain elevated in these cats. Since severe nonthyroidal illness would be expected to decrease total serum thyroid hormone concentrations into the subnormal range, concomitant hyperthyroidism should be suspected in any middle-aged to old cat with severe nonthyroidal illness and high-normal total serum T_4 and T_3 concentrations, especially if signs of hyperthyroidism are also present. On stabilization of or recovery from the concurrent nonthyroidal disorder, serum thyroid hormone concentrations will increase into the "diagnostic" thyrotoxic range in these cats with hyperthyroidism.

THYROID IMAGING

In cats with hyperthyroidism, thyroid imaging is an extremely useful procedure to determine the extent of thyroid gland involvement (Peterson and Becker, 1984). In about 70 per cent of hyperthyroid cats, thyroid imaging reveals enlargement and increased radionuclide accumulation in both lobes, whereas involvement of only one lobe is seen in the remaining cats. With unilateral thyroid lobe involvement, the normal contralateral lobe is completely suppressed and cannot be visualized. Thyroid imaging is also helpful in the hyperthyroid cat in which no enlargement of the thyroid gland can be palpated; in many of these cats, thyroid imaging demonstrates that an affected lobe has descended into the thoracic cavity. Finally, scanning is of value in detecting regional or distant metastasis of functional thyroid carcinoma causing feline hyperthyroidism.

TREATMENT

The underlying etiology of the thyroid adenomatous hyperplasia that causes feline hyperthyroidism is not known. Since spontaneous remission of the disorder does not occur, the aim of treatment is to control the excessive secretion of thyroid hormone from the adenomatous thyroid gland. Feline hyperthyroidism can be treated in three ways—with surgical thyroidectomy, use of radioactive iodine (^{131}I), or chronic administration of an antithyroid drug. Antithyroid drugs are also extremely useful as short-term treatment (3 to 6 weeks) in the preoperative preparation of the hyperthyroid cat prior to thyroidectomy. The advantages and disadvantages of each form of treatment are summarized in Table 2 and should always be weighed when selecting the most appropriate treatment. The treatment of choice for an individual cat depends on several factors, including the presence of associated cardiovascular disease or other major medical problems, availability of an experienced thyroid surgeon or nuclear medicine department, and the owner's willingness to accept the form of treatment advised. Of the three forms of treatment available, it must be emphasized that only surgery and radioactive iodine "cure" the hyperthyroid state. Antithyroid drugs block thyroid hormone synthesis; however, since these drugs do not destroy adenomatous thyroid tissue, relapse of hyperthyroidism invariably occurs within 24 to 72 hours after the medication is discontinued.

Table 2. *Advantages and Disadvantages of Treatment Modalities for Feline Hyperthyroidism*

	Antithyroid Drugs	Surgery	Radioiodine
Persistent hyperthyroidism	Low (dose-related)	Rare	Low (dose-related)
Complications			
Hypoparathyroidism	Never	Common	Never
Permanent hypothyroidism	Never	Intermediate	Rare
Other	Common* (anorexia, vomiting, hematologic complications)	Low (but significant morbidity and mortality)	Rare
Time until euthyroid	1–3 weeks	1–2 days	1–12 weeks
Relapse or recurrence	High	Intermediate	Low
Hospitalization time	None	2–5 days	1–4 weeks
Ease of treatment	Simple (but daily administration essential)	Most difficult	Simple (but not readily available)

*Much less common for methimazole than for PTU.

Antithyroid Drugs

Methimazole (Tapazole, Lilly) and propylthiouracil (PTU) are the two thioureylene antithyroid drugs available for use in the United States. After administration, these drugs are actively concentrated by the thyroid gland, where they act to inhibit the synthesis of thyroid hormones through the following mechanisms: (1) by blocking the incorporation of iodine into the tyrosyl groups in thyroglobulin; (2) by preventing the coupling of iodotyrosyl groups (mono- and diiodotyrosines) into T_4 and T_3; and (3) through direct interactions with the thyroglobulin molecule. Antithyroid drugs do not interfere with the thyroid gland's ability to concentrate, or "trap," inorganic iodine, nor do they block the release of stored thyroid hormone into the circulation. Several factors can influence the antithyroid drug dosage and duration of treatment needed to restore euthyroidism in cats with hyperthyroidism. These variables include bioavailability (gastrointestinal absorption) of the drug, amount of absorbed drug that is concentrated within the thyroid gland, initial degree of hyperthyroidism, amount of preformed (stored) thyroid hormone, thyroid hormone secretory rate, and extent to which thyroid hormone production is inhibited.

In cats, methimazole appears to be at least 10 times more potent than PTU in blocking thyroid hormone synthesis. Therefore, antithyroid drug therapy is usually initiated at a daily dosage of 150 mg of PTU or 15 mg of methimazole, as previously described (Peterson, 1981; Peterson, 1984). Although both antithyroid drugs are effective in restoring euthyroidism, we recently reported that administration of PTU is associated with a high incidence of both mild and serious adverse effects, including anorexia, vomiting, lethargy, immune-mediated hemolytic anemia, and thrombocytopenia in both normal and hyperthyroid cats (Aucoin et al., 1985; Peterson, 1984). Because of the prevalence of these severe hematologic complications, use of PTU for control of feline hyperthyroidism can no longer be recommended. Over the past 3 years, we have evaluated the efficacy and safety of methimazole in more than 200 cats with hyperthyroidism; methimazole appears to be better tolerated and safer than PTU and is therefore favored over PTU in the preoperative and long-term medical management of feline hyperthyroidism.

Initially, methimazole should be administered at a dose of 15 mg/day. Although single daily doses may be adequate in some cats, divided doses (administered every 8 to 12 hours) usually provide a more reliable response. Methimazole is available as 5-mg and 10-mg tablets; however, the 5-mg tablets are smaller and easier for most owners to administer. During the first 3 months of therapy, serum T_4 concentrations and complete blood and platelet counts should be monitored at 2-week intervals. In most hyperthyroid cats treated with a daily methimazole dose of 15 mg, serum T_4 concentrations fall to normal or low values within 2 weeks of treatment. If little to no decrease in serum T_4 concentrations occurs during this initial period, the methimazole dose should be increased to 20 to 25 mg/day, after it is determined that the owner administered the medication as directed. Euthyroidism can be restored in virtually all cats with adequate methimazole therapy. Although a few cats appear to be "resistant" to the effects of the drug, such resistance is usually the result of difficulty in administering the medication or poor owner compliance. If the drug is given as preoperative preparation, surgical thyroidectomy can be performed and drug administration discontinued once euthyroidism is restored.

Mild side effects associated with methimazole treatment are uncommon and include anorexia, vomiting, and lethargy. In most cats, these adverse signs are transient and resolve despite continued administration of the drug. Adverse gastrointestinal signs persist in some cats, however, necessitating discontinuation of the antithyroid drug. Drug allergy, manifested by skin rash and pruritus, also develops in a few cats treated with methimazole. Mild hematologic findings that appear to be induced rarely by methimazole administration include transient leukopenia with a normal differential count, eosinophilia, and lymphocytosis. Drug-induced leukopenia is not a harbinger of agranulocytosis (see below), is not associated with infection, and is not ordinarily a reason to discontinue therapy. More serious reactions that develop in fewer than 5 per cent of cats treated with methimazole include agranulocytosis (severe leukopenia with a total granulocyte count less than 250/mm^3) and severe thrombocytopenia (platelet count less than 75,000/mm^3). Immune-mediated hemolytic anemia, a major side effect associated with PTU treatment, has not been observed with methimazole therapy. Because of the potential for granulocytopenia or thrombocytopenia, however, complete blood and platelet counts should be monitored at 2-week intervals, especially between the second and twelfth week of therapy, when these side effects usually appear to occur. If serious hematologic reactions develop, drug administration should be discontinued and supportive therapy instituted. These adverse reactions should resolve within 5 days after the methimazole is withdrawn.

During methimazole therapy, serum antinuclear antibodies (ANA) also develop in a substantial number of cats receiving the drug. The incidence of methimazole-induced ANA increases with the duration of treatment; ANA develops in more than a third of cats treated for longer than 6 months. Drug-induced ANA also commonly develops during chronic PTU treatment of normal or hyperthyroid cats (Aucoin et al., 1985; Peterson et al., 1984b). In humans, a variety of drugs can induce ANA and produce a lupus-like disease; however, the prevalence of ANA is considerably higher than clinical signs of lupus. After long-term treatment with hydralazine or procainamide, the two major drugs associated with lupus-like syndromes in humans, more than half of the patients develop ANA but fewer than 10 per cent of these develop overt signs of lupus. Similarly, despite the high prevalence of

ANA in cats receiving chronic methimazole or PTU treatment, associated clinical signs suggestive of lupus (polyarthritis, glomerulonephritis) appear to be extremely rare.

In cats in which long-term methimazole treatment is planned, the drug dosage should be decreased from 15 mg to 10 mg/day once euthyroidism is restored (usually 2 to 4 weeks). Although this reduced methimazole dosage is adequate to maintain euthyroidism in most hyperthyroid cats, a rise of circulating thyroid hormone concentrations into the thyrotoxic range will occur in some cats, necessitating a return to the initial daily methimazole dosage of 15 mg. In other cats that developed subnormal serum thyroid hormone concentrations during initial therapy, serum T_4 values remain low despite the reduction in methimazole dosage to 10 mg/day; however, these cats usually maintain normal serum concentrations of T_3, which may explain why clinical evidence of hypothyroidism only rarely develops during treatment with this reduced methimazole dosage. Further reduction in the daily methimazole dosage is not recommended unless clinical signs suggestive of hypothyroidism develop, since relapse of hyperthyroidism will almost always occur if the maintenance dosage is decreased to 5 mg/day.

Poor owner compliance in reliably administering the medication is the most common reason for failure of long-term methimazole therapy to control hyperthyroidism. In cases in which owner compliance is difficult to achieve because of an inconvenient dosage schedule, the total daily methimazole dose can be administered as a single daily dose rather than as two or three divided doses. Methimazole must be given at least once daily, however, or serum thyroid hormone levels will again rise into the thyrotoxic range.

Although serious adverse effects of methimazole treatment usually develop during the first few weeks of drug administration, side effects can potentially occur at any time during treatment. Therefore, to maintain circulating thyroid hormone concentrations below thyrotoxic levels and to monitor for serious adverse reactions during long-term treatment, complete blood and platelet counts, serum ANA determinations, and serum thyroid hormone measurements should be repeated at 2- to 3-month intervals and methimazole dosage adjustments made as necessary. If serum ANA develop during long-term treatment, periodic monitoring of serum biochemical values and urinalyses are also recommended. Although methimazole-induced lupus appears to be extremely rare, drug administration should be stopped and alternate therapy used for hyperthyroidism (see below) if signs consistent with a lupus-like syndrome (polyarthritis, glomerulonephritis, and dermatitis) do develop.

Surgery

Surgical thyroidectomy is a highly effective treatment for feline hyperthyroidism, but it can be associated with significant morbidity and mortality. Although thyroidectomy in itself is a relatively simple procedure, hyperthyroidism is a systemic illness that affects all body systems; resultant cardiovascular, hepatic, and gastrointestinal dysfunctions greatly increase the anesthetic and surgical risk in cats with hyperthyroidism. All hyperthyroid cats should therefore be prepared for surgery by administration of an antithyroid drug, propranolol, or iodide to decrease the metabolic and cardiac complications associated with hyperthyroidism.

PREOPERATIVE PREPARATION. Use of an antithyroid drug (methimazole or PTU), as described above, is the method of choice for the preoperative preparation of a hyperthyroid cat. After antithyroid drug treatment has maintained euthyroidism for 1 to 3 weeks, most systemic dysfunctions associated with hyperthyroidism will have improved or resolved, and the anesthetic and surgical complications will be minimized. The last dose of methimazole or PTU should be administered on the morning of surgery.

In hyperthyroid cats that cannot tolerate antithyroid drug treatment, alternate preoperative preparation with propranolol or stable iodine, alone or in combination, should be used. Although propranolol, a β-adrenergic blocker, does not lower elevated serum thyroid hormone concentrations, this drug blocks many of the cardiovascular and neuromuscular effects of excess thyroid hormone and controls the tachycardia and hyperexcitability associated with feline hyperthyroidism. Propranolol should be administered for 7 to 14 days before surgery at a dosage of 2.5 to 5.0 mg three times daily as required to decrease resting heart rate to within normal range and control hyperexcitability. In cats that have developed congestive heart failure secondary to chronic thyroid hormone excess, propranolol should be used with extreme caution, since the drug depresses myocardial function.

Large doses of stable iodine block the release of T_4 and T_3 from the thyroid gland and lower serum thyroid hormone concentrations. Iodine has major limitations as antithyroid therapy, however, since serum T_4 and T_3 concentrations may not ever completely normalize during iodine treatment, and the drug often loses its antithyroid effect within a few weeks. Therefore, iodine should not be used as sole therapy in preparation for thyroidectomy but can be given in conjunction with propranolol or an antithyroid drug. Iodine should be administered as either oral potassium iodide or intravenous sodium iodide at a dosage of 50 to 100 mg/day for 7 to 14 days prior to surgery. Common side effects of oral potassium iodide treatment include excessive salivation and decreased appetite; such adverse signs appear to result from the unpleasant taste of iodine.

ANESTHESIA. Because of altered metabolism, cats with hyperthyroidism tend to be highly sensitive to all preanesthetic and anesthetic agents. Therefore, anesthesia should be carefully induced and the cat must be closely monitored during surgery. Since arrhythmias commonly occur during surgery in cats with hyperthyroidism, electrocardiographic monitoring is advisable.

SURGICAL CONSIDERATIONS. Techniques for unilateral and bilateral thyroidectomy have been reported for cats with hyperthyroidism (Birchard et al., 1984; Peterson et al., 1984a). About 30 per cent of hyperthyroid cats have disease in only one thyroid lobe, whereas the remaining 70 per cent have bilateral thyroid lobe involvement. In cats with unilateral thyroid tumors, the contralateral lobe is normal in position and either normal or small in size when inspected at surgery. Hemithyroidectomy corrects the hyperthyroid state in these cats, and relapse, resulting from the development of adenomatous changes in the remaining "normal" thyroid lobe, is extremely rare and takes years to develop. In cats with bilateral thyroid adenomas (adenomatous hyperplasia), removal of both lobes with preservation of parathyroid function is necessary to control hyperthyroidism and avoid postoperative hypocalcemia. With bilateral thyroid tumors, enlargement of both lobes can easily be identified at surgery in most cats; about 15 per cent of cats with bilateral lobe involvement, however, have one lobe that is only slightly enlarged and may be mistaken as normal. Preoperative thyroid imaging is helpful in defining the extent of thyroid lobe involvement in these cases (Peterson and Becker, 1984). If thyroid imaging is not feasible, we recommend removal of the obviously enlarged lobe with preservation of the associated external parathyroid gland in all cats with suspected unilateral lobe involvement. If bilateral lobe involvement was initially present, relapse of hyperthyroidism will usually occur within 9 months of surgery. Preservation of the external parathyroid gland during hemithyroidectomy minimizes the risk of hypoparathyroidism should removal of the contralateral lobe be required.

POSTOPERATIVE COMPLICATIONS. There are many potential complications associated with thyroidectomy, including hypoparathyroidism, Horner's syndrome, and vocal cord paralysis. The most serious complication is hypocalcemia, which develops after the parathyroid glands are injured, devascularized, or inadvertently removed in the course of bilateral thyroidectomy. Since only one parathyroid gland is required for maintenance of normocalcemia, hypoparathyroidism develops only in cats treated with bilateral thyroidectomy. After bilateral thyroidectomy, the serum calcium concentration should be monitored on a daily basis until it has stabilized within the normal range. In most cats with iatrogenic hypoparathyroidism, clinical signs associated with hypocalcemia will develop within 1 to 3 days of surgery. Although mild hypocalcemia (6.5 to 7.5 mg/dl) is common, laboratory evidence of hypocalcemia alone does not require treatment; however, if accompanying signs of muscle tremors, tetany, or convulsions develop, therapy with vitamin D and calcium is indicated (see the article entitled Hypoparathyroidism). Although hypoparathyroidism may be permanent in some cats, spontaneous recovery of parathyroid function may occur weeks to months after surgery. In most cases, such transient hypocalcemia probably results from reversible parathyroid damage and ischemia incurred during surgery. Alternatively, accessory parathyroid tissue may compensate for the damaged parathyroid glands and maintain normocalcemia.

LONG-TERM MANAGEMENT. Following hemithyroidectomy for unilateral thyroid lobe involvement, serum thyroid hormone concentrations fall to subnormal levels for 2 to 3 months postoperatively; however, thyroxine supplementation is rarely required during this period. If total thyroidectomy has been performed, thyroxine (0.1 mg/day) should be started 24 to 48 hours after surgery. Although thyroxine supplementation at this low dosage can be safely continued indefinitely, the low serum concentrations of T_4 and T_3 that develop 24 to 48 hours after bilateral thyroidectomy may spontaneously increase to within normal range weeks to months postoperatively; thyroxine administration can then be discontinued. It can be difficult to remove all abnormal thyroid tissue while concurrently preserving parathyroid function. Small remnants of thyroid tissue that remain attached to the capsule may regenerate and produce normal amounts of circulating T_4 and T_3. In some cats, such regeneration of residual adenomatous thyroid tissue continues until recurrent hyperthyroidism develops. Therefore, all cats treated with surgical thyroidectomy should have serum thyroid hormone concentrations monitored at 6- to 12-month intervals to ensure that relapse does not occur.

Radioactive Iodine

Radioactive iodine provides a simple, effective, and safe treatment for cats with hyperthyroidism. The basic principle for treatment of hyperthyroidism with radioiodine is that thyroid cells do not differentiate between stable and radioactive iodine; therefore, radioiodine, like stable iodine, is concentrated by the thyroid gland after administration. In cats with hyperthyroidism, radioiodine is concentrated primarily in the hyperplastic or neoplastic thyroid cells, where it irradiates and destroys the hyperfunctioning tissue. Normal thyroid tissue, however, tends to be protected from the effects of radioiodine, since the uninvolved thyroid tissue is suppressed and receives only a small dose of radiation.

The radioisotope most frequently used to treat hyperthyroidism is ^{131}I, which has a half-life of 8 days and emits both beta particles and gamma radiation. The beta particles, which produce 80 per cent of the tissue damage, travel a maximum of 2 mm in tissue and have an average path length of 400 μm. Therefore, beta particles are locally destructive but spare adjacent hypoplastic thyroid tissue, parathyroid glands, and other cervical structures.

Various methods, derived primarily from human medicine, have been used to estimate the activity of ^{131}I required to destroy the hyperfunctioning thyroid tissue in cats with hyperthyroidism. The goal of these methods is to restore euthyroidism with a single dose of radiation without producing hypothyroidism.

With the first method of ^{131}I dose determination, various measurements of thyroid kinetics are determined with a small "tracer" dose of radioiodine. Using an estimated desired radiation dose of 15,000 to 20,000 rads/gm of thyroid tissue (Turrel et al., 1984), the therapeutic dose of ^{131}I is calculated from the following values: (1) the effective half-life of ^{131}I (which accounts for both the physical half-life and duration of radioiodine retention by the thyroid), (2) the fraction of ^{131}I deposited in the thyroid gland (the percentage of thyroid uptake), and (3) the estimated thyroid gland weight. With this method, the calculated ^{131}I dose may range from 1 to 10 mCi, which can be administered either orally or by a single intravenous injection. In our experience in treating more than 300 hyperthyroid cats with this ^{131}I-dose method, over 90 per cent of the cats become euthyroid within 3 months after a single dose of radioiodine, and the remaining cats are successfully cured with a second ^{131}I treatment. With this regimen, very few cats develop hypothyroidism from ^{131}I overdosage and require thyroid hormone supplementation.

The second method of dose determination is to select a fixed, relatively low dose of ^{131}I without determining thyroid gland kinetics. Administration of 2 to 4 mCi of ^{131}I will produce euthyroidism in most cats with hyperthyroidism. However, use of this approach will also result in under- or overtreatment of a significant number of cats, resulting in persistent hyperthyroidism or hypothyroidism, respectively. The advantage of this method is that nuclear medicine equipment is not needed and the time required to determine thyroid kinetics is eliminated.

The third method of radioiodine therapy is to administer extremely large doses of radioiodine (10 to 30 mCi). These doses of ^{131}I will almost always totally destroy the normal as well as hyperplastic thyroid tissue. Thus, this method is effective in curing the hyperthyroidism in almost all cats but also has the disadvantage of inducing hypothyroidism in the majority of cases. In general, we recommend use of such large doses of ^{131}I only in cats with hyperfunctioning thyroid adenocarcinoma to ensure complete destruction of the malignant tissue.

Regardless of the method of dose determination selected, there are certain radiation safety restrictions and procedures that must be followed. These cats should be confined to restricted areas of the hospital that have minimal traffic and should be housed in metabolic cages so that urine and feces can be collected safely. All personnel handling the cats, cages, food dishes, and excreta should wear long laboratory coats, disposable plastic gloves, and film badges. All material removed from the cage must be handled as radioactive waste and should be disposed of accordingly. These cats are dismissed from the hospital when the radiation dose rate has decreased to a safe level that has been determined by the state radiation control office (usually after a 2- to 3-week period). The owners are advised prior to radioiodine therapy that their cat will be radioactive when discharged and are given instructions to minimize their risk.

Overall, use of radioiodine may be the optimal treatment for feline hyperthyroidism when nuclear medicine facilities are available. Radioactive iodine treatment involves a single, nonstressful procedure that is without associated morbidity or motality. Untoward systemic effects have not been observed. Anesthesia is not required. A single ^{131}I treatment will induce euthyroidism in most cats with hyperthyroidism, whereas cats that remain persistently hyperthyroid can be successfully retreated with radioiodine and those that become hypothyroid can be supplemented readily with thyroxine. At present, the major disadvantage of radioiodine therapy is the unavailability of facilities that can safely handle ^{131}I and accurately determine the ideal dose to administer.

References and Supplemental Reading

Aucoin, D. P., Peterson, M. E., Hurvitz, A. I., et al.: Propylthiouracil-induced immune-mediated disease in cats. J. Pharmacol. Exp. Ther. 234:13, 1985.

Birchard, S. J., Peterson, M. E., and Jacobson, A.: Surgical treatment of feline hyperthyroidism: Results of 85 cases. J. Am. Anim. Hosp. Assoc. 20:705, 1984.

Peterson, M. E.: Propylthiouracil in the treatment of feline hyperthyroidism. J.A.V.M.A. 179:485, 1981.

Peterson, M. E.: Feline hyperthyroidism. Vet. Clin. North Am. 14:809, 1984.

Peterson, M. E., and Becker, D. V.: Radionuclide thyroid imaging in 135 cats with hyperthyroidism. Vet. Radiol. 25:23, 1984.

Peterson, M. E., Birchard, S. J., and Mehlhaff, C. J.: Anesthetic and surgical management of endocrine disorders. Vet. Clin. North Am. 14:911, 1984a.

Peterson, M. E., Hurvitz, A. I., Leib, M. S., et al.: Propylthiouracil-associated hemolytic anemia, thrombocytopenia, and antinuclear antibodies in cats with hyperthyroidism. J.A.V.M.A. 184:806, 1984b.

Peterson, M. E., Kintzer, P. P., Cavanaugh, P. G., et al.: Feline hyperthyroidism: Pretreatment clinical and laboratory evaluation of 131 cases. J.A.V.M.A. 183:103, 1983.

Turrel, J. M., Feldman, E. C., Hays, M., et al.: Radioactive iodine therapy in cats with hyperthyroidism. J.A.V.M.A. 184:554, 1984.

CANINE THYROID TUMORS

ANDREW S. LOAR, D.V.M.
Hermosa Beach, California

Benign and malignant tumors of thyroid tissue constitute a small fraction of neoplastic diseases in dogs. Relative to all forms of canine thyroid disease, however, neoplasia of the gland is not an uncommon clinical problem. Benign thyroid tumors are often found incidentally and rarely disrupt normal endocrine function. Malignant neoplasia of the thyroid gland generally shows an aggressive clinical behavior, frequently resulting in death of the dog. The clinical outcome (prognosis) of an animal with thyroid cancer is dependent on the stage, and particularly the size, of the tumor at the time of diagnosis. Clearly, the prediction of tumor recurrence or metastasis is useful to the clinician in selecting the most appropriate treatment. In recent years, studies have examined the value of several antitumor treatment modalities for thyroid carcinoma, including the use of surgical resection, radiation therapy, and cytotoxic chemotherapy. Moreover, a review of significant tumor characteristics in these studies shows a distinction between the responses in dogs with favorable and unfavorable prognoses.

INCIDENCE AND EPIDEMIOLOGY

In the dog, neoplasia of thyroid origin causes 10 to 15 per cent of all primary tumors in the head and neck region and accounts for as many as 2 per cent of all canine tumors. Malignant thyroid neoplasms appear to be more common than benign tumors, probably because the latter are generally small, often nonpalpable, and rarely cause clinical abnormalities. The average age of dogs with thyroid adenomas is 10 years, whereas that for thyroid carcinomas is 9 years. Although thyroid tumors have been reported in dogs as young as 3 years, such tumors are extremely rare in animals less than 5 years old.

In contrast to the higher incidence of thyroid tumors in women than in men, no sex predilection is noted in dogs. However, in one study (Hayes and Fraumeni, 1975), the risk of thyroid carcinoma rose in older, neutered bitches as compared with older males, suggesting that ovarian hormones may protect against the development of thyroid malignancy. Compared with other breeds, the boxer is at a significantly increased risk of developing adenomas of the thyroid. The golden retreiver, beagle, and boxer appear to have an increased incidence of carcinomas.

The majority of palpable thyroid tumors will be unilateral, although bilateral malignant and benign involvement are not uncommon. Neoplasms originating in ectopic thyroid tissue accounts for a small portion of all thyroid tumors. These aberrant sites include the mediastinum and, rarely, the ventral cervical regions anterior or posterior to the thyroid gland.

The term *goiter* implies enlargement of the thyroid gland; in dogs, goiter is generally secondary to hyperplasia, neoplasia, or inflammation. In North America during the previous 50 years, hyperplasia has been an uncommon cause of goiter; however, in regions of the world with iodine deficiency, it is reported more frequently. It is believed that mammals (including humans) in these iodine-deficient regions produce decreased levels of thyroid hormone, resulting in chronic secretion of thyroid-stimulating hormone (TSH) and eventually a compensatory increase in thyroid size. Interestingly, animals and persons in these locations have a higher risk of thyroid malignancies than is found in the United States. In addition, laboratory studies have shown that animals given antithyroid drugs, as well as those fed iodine-deficient diets, have a marked increase in thyroid tumors. Thus, these studies suggest that chronic thyroid stimulation from elevated levels of TSH may be tumorigenic. However, the decline of hyperplastic goiter in the United States because of the inclusion of iodized salt in both human and canine diets has not been associated with a decrease in the incidence of reported thyroid carcinoma in either species.

A significant number of dogs with thyroid neoplasms develop additional primary tumors during their lifetime. The tumor types reported most frequently include chemodectoma, perianal gland adenoma, mast cell tumor, lipoma, and adrenal adenoma (Hayes and Fraumeni, 1975). The epidemiologic significance of this data is not clear. A dog with multiple endocrine neoplasia (MEN), consisting of medullary carcinoma, pheochromocytoma, and parathyroid hyperplasia, has been reported (Peterson et al., 1982). In humans, syndromes of MEN are familial and rare, but it is not known if this is an inherited condition in dogs. Ionizing radiation to the head and neck region in humans is a well-documented cause of thyroid tumors, but it has not been implicated in canine thyroid neoplasms.

PATHOLOGY

The histologic criteria and nomenclature used to classify canine thyroid tumors may not be clear to the clinician evaluating the biopsy report. The histopathologist examines the thyroid mass for the following: (1) the size, shape, and colloid content of the cells; (2) the general pattern in which the cells are arranged (i.e., the formation of follicles, papillae, or densely packed or compact sheets); (3) the presence of a capsule surrounding the tumor and evidence of tumor invasion through this capsule; (4) the presence of cystic areas within the tumor; and (5) evidence of tumor invasion into blood and lymphatic vessels.

Adenomas typically contain well-differentiated cells arranged in compact and follicular groupings. Cavities are commonly present and contain necrotic debris and blood. A fibrous connective tissue capsule demarcates the tumor from adjacent normal thyroid tissue. Capsular or vessel invasion is usually absent in thyroid adenomas.

Carcinomas contain cells with variable nuclear morphology; anaplasia and mitotic figures are infrequent features in the majority of thyroid cancers in the dog. In most carcinomas, the cells form prominent follicular patterns in addition to having compact arrangements. Less commonly, a predominantly compact or predominantly follicular pattern is noted in the tumor. The presence of capsular or vessel invasion is strongly suggestive of carcinoma. Malignant neoplasms arising from the parafollicular cells (C cells) are known as medullary carcinomas, and in humans and some dogs they have been associated with excessive production of calcitonin. These neoplasms are rare, accounting for fewer than 5 per cent of all canine thyroid tumors. Histologically, medullary carcinomas are difficult to distinguish from thyroid tumors not of C-cell origin, particularly those showing a compact cellular pattern.

The most important aspect of a histologic grading system is its value in predicting the biologic behavior of a tumor. Obviously, the distinction between benign and malignant tumor types is important prognostically. With the exception of extremely anaplastic tumors, however, the several different histologic forms of thyroid malignancies, described above, do not appear to correlate with a specific prognosis. At least one group of researchers (Leav et al., 1976) suggested that malignant thyroid tumors showing a follicular pattern followed a more rapid, less favorable course than those in which a compact pattern predominated. Unfortunately, more recent studies have not supported this.

NATURAL BEHAVIOR AND CLINICAL FEATURES

Functional Aspects

In contrast to their behavior in cats, most thyroid masses in dogs are not capable of iodine uptake and thyroid hormone secretion and thus are not likely to cause signs of hyperthyroidism. Evaluation of thyroid radioiodine turnover and uptake, as well as measurement of serum thyroid hormone concentrations, is the most accurate method of determining the functional status of a thyroid tumor. More than a decade ago, Rijnberk and his colleagues in the Netherlands demonstrated that nearly one third of a large series (N = 55) of dogs with thyroid masses showed uptake of radioiodine by their tumors; about 20 per cent of all the dogs exhibited signs of hyperthyroidism. Histologically, only one of these hyperfunctional tumors was an adenoma; the remainder were malignant neoplasms (Rijnberk, 1971).

It has been shown that most of these functional tumors are responsive to TSH administration, although they are not influenced by normal negative feedback mechanisms. Moreover, hormone secretion from these tumors often suppresses the function of the normal thyroid tissues by inhibiting the production of TSH from the pituitary gland. Further studies suggest that a functional thyroid tumor is less efficient at producing and secreting hormone than an equal volume of normal thyroid tissue. Therefore, a thyroid neoplasm capable of secreting sufficient thyroid hormone to suppress T_4 and T_3 production by the remaining tissue, and ultimately cause clinical signs of hyperthyroidism, is likely to be at least as large as the animal's normal thyroid gland.

Canine hyperthyroidism (thyrotoxicosis) clinically appears similar to the condition in the cat, and clinical signs of polyuria, polydipsia, polyphagia, and weight loss are the most common. Dogs presented with signs suggestive of thyrotoxicosis should initially be evaluated for swelling in the ventral cervical region and for laboratory findings of increased serum levels of thyroid hormones. Generally these animals have elevated circulating levels of both T_4 and T_3.

Dogs seldom show evidence of hypothyroidism secondary to thyroid tumors. When hypothyroidism does occur, it may be due to one of several possible causes: First, in the case of a nonfunctional, bilateral carcinoma, tumor invasion may result in destruction of both thyroid glands. Second, large thyroid tumors can potentially produce high levels of inactive thyroid hormones; although these iodoproteins do not cause signs of hyperthyroidism, they may suppress TSH secretion, eventually resulting in atrophy of normal thyroid tissues. Last, in animals with bilateral carcinoma treated with bilateral thyroidectomy, clinical hypothyroidism is likely. In the case of a dog presenting with a unilateral thyroid tumor and showing signs of hypothyroidism, the clinician should consider that the loss of thyroid function may have preceded the occurrence of the neoplasm. Indeed, some authors have suggested that chronic TSH elevation secondary to primary hypothyroidism may predispose to subsequent tumor development (Branham et al., 1982).

Adenomas

Dogs presenting with thyroid adenomas generally have histories of progressive enlargement of the thyroid gland and a duration of signs ranging from a few weeks to as long as 5 years. Occasionally, fluid accumulation into cavitated lesions of the tumor will result in rapid swelling. These tumors are rarely attached to the overlying skin and typically are freely movable. The solid tissue portion of thyroid adenomas varies in size from microscopic to more than 100 cm^3; however, most will be smaller than their associated thyroid lobe. Nodules composed of hyperplastic rather than adenomatous tissue are occasionally found; however, the diagnosis of thyroid hyperplasia must be a histologic rather than a clinical one.

Unless thyroid dysfunction occurs, the clinical course of dogs with thyroid adenomas is related to the presence of the mass. Small nodules within or on the surface of the gland should cause no problems. If the tumors are large, particularly when significant cystic fluid accumulates, laryngotracheal compression may result. With complete mass resection, recurrence is extremely unlikely.

Adenocarcinomas

As in dogs with thyroid adenomas, most animals with carcinomas are initially presented for a swelling or palpable mass in the neck. Other signs may include coughing or dyspnea, dysphagia, voice changes, regurgitation, and weight loss. In animals with a functional thyroid tumor, signs of thyrotoxicosis (polyuria, polydipsia, polyphagia, and weight loss) may predominate. In a series of 38 dogs with thyroid carcinoma seen at the Animal Medical Center (AMC, New York, NY), 20 per cent were initially examined for the evaluation of problems other than goiter, as described above.

The duration of signs varies considerably between different studies, ranging from 1 week to 24 months. Generally, these malignant tumors grow rapidly and become fixed to adjacent tissues, including the overlying skin. Moreover, these masses may compress and invade the larynx, trachea or esophagus, surrounding lymphatic tissues, and large blood vessels such as the jugular vein. Relatively few dogs are presented for veterinary examination while their tumors are still small. In the AMC series, about 10 per cent of the dogs had a primary tumor volume of 2 cm in diameter (8 cm^3) or less when the initial diagnosis was made. The majority presented with tumor volumes in excess of 100 cm^3.

When palpated, a thyroid carcinoma feels like a firm, irregular mass. Formation of cysts within the tumor may result in a nonuniform consistency and shape. Examination of the remainder of the ventral cervical area may reveal lymphadenopathy of the mandibular, retropharyngeal, or superficial cervical (prescapular) nodes. Cording of local lymphatic and blood vessels due to tumor extension or obstruction may also be noted. As many as a third of all tumors may involve both thyroid glands by the time of diagnosis. Most of these represent massive primary disease, so it is not clear if the carcinoma originated in both thyroid lobes or spread from one to the other (Leav et al., 1976).

In addition to the local aggressiveness of these cancers, regional and distant metastases frequently occur. In dogs dying as a result of their tumors, 60 to 80 per cent show dissemination of the disease at necropsy. The tumor spreads most commonly to the lungs, probably by hematogenous routes, and to the regional lymph nodes. Other metastatic sites include the adrenal glands, kidneys, myocardium, liver, brain, and, rarely, bone. Clinical evidence of metastases to these areas is often present antemortem and, again, may be the reason for the animal's initial presentation. The total volume of the primary tumor mass at the time of necropsy appears to correlate with the presence of metastases (Leav et al., 1976). Dogs whose thyroid carcinomas are less than 20 cm^3 show less than a 20 per cent incidence of metastatic disease. Three fourths of those whose tumors are 21 to 100 cm^3 will have metastases, whereas virtually all dogs whose tumors are larger than 100 cm^3 have metastases. These data should have tremendous prognostic significance, especially regarding the initial surgical management of the primary thyroid mass.

Tumors occurring in ectopic thyroid tissues are uncommon and generally are associated with a primary unilateral carcinoma of a thyroid lobe. Rarely, an ectopic neoplasm may develop without evidence of tumor elsewhere. The most frequent sites involved are cranial to the heart and within the pericardial sac (Leav et al., 1976). In these cases, mediastinal enlargement and compression of adjacent structures may occur. A much less frequently reported site of aberrant thyroid neoplasia is the remnant of the thyroglossal duct, located either just cranial or caudal to the thyroid gland. Cysts or tumors of this embryonic structure may cause swelling in the ventral midcervical region (Harkema et al., 1984).

Malignant neoplasms of the parafollicular cells (medullary carcinoma) appear to have a similar biologic behavior as those originating from follicular cells. Medullary carcinomas have been reported to grow rapidly and may be very large when the animals are first presented. Metastatic lesions have been reported in regional lymph nodes and in more distant sites. Tumors of C-cell origin are capable of producing calcitonin as well as other biologically active amines such as serotonin and 5-hydroxytryptophan. Assays for these substances in tumor tissues suspected to be of parafollicular cell origin may be useful in confirming a diagnosis of medullary carcinoma. A few studies have reported mild to moderate hypocalcemia in dogs with these tumors (Leav et al., 1976). However, hypocalcemia is not characteristic of medullary carcinoma and appears to occur rarely in both dogs and humans.

DIAGNOSTIC MANAGEMENT

The differential diagnosis for an enlarging mass in the ventral midcervical region of a dog should include inflammatory conditions such as abscessation, granuloma formation, and cellulitis, as well as neoplasia. Nonthyroid tumors that may result in cervical lymphadenopathy include tonsillar carcinoma and other oral malignancies, regional soft tissue sarcomas, and lymphosarcoma. Disorders that may cause soft tissue masses in the pericardium or anterior mediastinum include various infectious and granulomatous diseases, neoplasms of the chemo- and baroreceptor organs, hemangiosarcoma, mesothelioma, lymphosarcoma, and tumors of aberrant thyroid tissue.

The physical examination must include palpation of both thyroid lobes as well as the regional lymph nodes. On visual examination, the lack of movement of the thyroid nodule with swallowing and its fixation to surrounding tissues strongly suggest malignancy and indicate an unfavorable prognosis for complete surgical resection. Occasionally, large thyroid masses not attached to deeper tissues may migrate in a dependent direction toward the thoracic inlet. Data from hematologic evaluation and biochemical and urine analyses are generally unremarkable in dogs with thyroid neoplasms but are useful as part of the preanesthetic data base. Thoracic radiography will aid in demonstrating advanced disease; however, metastatic nodules smaller than 3 mm in diameter are not visible radiographically. Determination of serum thyroid hormone concentrations and other thyroid function studies are indicated to confirm hypo- or hyperthyroidism.

The imaging of canine thyroid tumors (scintigraphy) is valuable for diagnosis and staging and is similar to its use in the management of feline hyperthyroidism. To perform scintigraphy on an animal with a suspected thyroid neoplasm, either sodium pertechnetate ($Na^{99m}TcO_4$) or one of the various forms of radioactive iodine (^{131}I, ^{123}I) is administered; a scintillation (gamma) camera or a rectilinear scanner is subsequently used to obtain an image of the thyroid region and thorax. A functional tumor shows a high uptake of the radioisotope and appears as a radiodense ("hot") area. In addition, the metastatic sites from a functional thyroid carcinoma may be visible as radiodense nodules in nearby tissues and nodes and in the lungs. A nonfunctional thyroid tumor, such as that with a solid (compact) tissue structure and a medullary carcinoma, will appear as a less radiodense ("cold") area adjacent to or surrounded by normal, active thyroid tissue. A scintigraph may also be used to evaluate normal thyroid function and to determine the response to antitumor therapy (Mitchell et al., 1979).

Accurate diagnosis and staging of thyroid tumors can only be achieved through histologic examination of tissue samples. Cytologic evaluation of material obtained from fine-needle aspiration techniques is useful in supporting a diagnosis of thyroid malignancy but does not provide information concerning cellular architecture, and it occasionally will result in a false-negative diagnosis (Thompson et al., 1980). Incisional biopsy of a thyroid mass will generally provide a histologic diagnosis and grade and may be the only management option in dogs with large, inoperable tumors. Whenever possible, excision of all gross evidence of disease and submission of representative specimens for histopathologic analysis are the most reliable methods for the diagnosis, staging, and treatment of thyroid neoplasia.

The stage of a tumor represents the extent of disease involvement. It is calculated by accumulating specific clinical and histologic data from a patient and choosing the characteristics that are of the most prognostic significance. The clinical characteristics that show the highest influence on disease outcome include the total volume of the primary tumor, the degree of local invasion, the number and extent of regional lymph node involvement, and the presence of distant metastatic disease. This tumor-node-metastasis (TNM) system has been developed for staging most of the common neoplasms of companion animals and was offered to veterinary clinicians several years ago by the World Health Organization (WHO) (Owen, 1980). The WHO staging protocol for canine thyroid tumors (Table 1) lists four stages of thyroid malignancy. None of the reports in the literature have used this staging protocol in an attempt to correlate the stage of disease with a specific prognosis; however, the unpublished AMC study (see Prognosis, below) revealed that tumor staging is a valuable prognostic guide.

Table 1. *Clinical Staging of Canine Thyroid Tumors*

T: *Primary tumor*
- T0 No evidence of tumor
- T1 Tumor < 2 cm maximum diameter: T1a—not fixed, T1b—fixed
- T2 Tumor 2–5 cm maximum diameter: T2a—not fixed, T2b—fixed
- T3 Tumor > 5 cm maximum diameter: T3a—not fixed, T3b—fixed

N: *Regional lymph nodes (RLN)**
- N0 No evidence of RLN involvement†
- N1 Ipsilateral RLN involved: N1a—not fixed, N1b—fixed
- N2 Bilateral RLN involved: N2a—not fixed, N2b—fixed

M: *Distant metastasis*
- M0 No evidence of distant metastasis
- M1 Distant metastasis detected

Stage Grouping	T	N	M
I	T1a,b	N0	M0
II	T0	N1	M0
	T1a,b	N1	
	T2a,b	N0 or N1a	
III	Any T3	Any N	M0
	Any T	Any Nb	
IV	Any T	Any N	M1

*The RLN are the mandibular and the superficial cervical lymph nodes.

†Involvement implies histologic evidence of tumor invasion.

Modified from Owen, L. N. (ed.): *The TNM Classification of Tumours in Domestic Animals.* Geneva: World Health Organization, 1980.

THERAPEUTIC MANAGEMENT

Surgery

The initial treatment of thyroid neoplasia is surgical resection. The primary goal of therapy is complete removal of all visible tumor tissue, although this may not be possible in all dogs. Diffuse local invasion or the presence of nodal or distant metastases may result in incomplete resection. When available, scintigraphy may reveal foci of tumor not evident on clinical or radiographic examination. Small malignant tumors as large as 2 to 3 cm in diameter, and sometimes larger, can generally be excised without difficulty. Patients whose carcinomas have invaded regional nodes probably will not be benefited by more aggressive surgery such as radical neck dissection and *en bloc* node removal. Additionally, at least one study showed that large, firm, nonmobile tumors were correlated with a high degree of invasiveness and were seldom completely resectable (Mitchell et al., 1979). In the AMC study, 40 per cent of dogs had unresectable tumors at initial surgery.

The major complications of aggressive tumor removal are related to the surgical wound. Highly invasive carcinomas often infiltrate local blood vessels, resulting in significant blood loss during attempts at surgical resection. Not infrequently, massive intraoperative hemorrhage cannot be controlled and the dogs must be euthanized. If large tumors are removed without incident, acceptable wound closure may be difficult because of the large dead space. In addition, when the tumor is attached to the overlying skin, this area should be excised also.

The surgeon should always attempt to obtain adequate normal tissue margins (1 to 2 cm) during surgical resection of thyroid carcinoma. Whenever a massive dissection is anticipated, the surgeon must be familiar with the many vital structures of the cervical region. In cases of bilateral involvement, bilateral thyroidectomy is indicated; however, postoperatively these animals are likely to develop signs of hypoparathyroidism as well as hypothyroidism and must be monitored carefully.

Chemotherapy

Dogs with bulky, inoperable, or disseminated disease (i.e., stage III or stage IV tumors, Table 1) and those with carcinomas that can be removed by surgery but have a high likelihood of lymph node involvement or metastasis (i.e., stage II or stage III tumors) may be candidates for cytotoxic drug treatment. In the former group, animals that respond to chemotherapy will have some decrease in tumor volume. In some of these dogs with massive local disease, preoperative reduction of tumor volume may decrease the potential morbidity of the surgical procedure and improve the chances of a complete resection. In the latter group, postoperative (adjuvant) chemotherapy may reduce the number of microscopic tumor foci and thus prolong the duration of remission. In humans and dogs, doxorubicin (Adriamycin, Adria) appears to be the most effective agent against thyroid carcinoma. The addition of other drugs to a doxorubicin-based protocol, including vincristine and cyclophosphamide, has rarely shown added antitumor benefit.

Doxorubicin is administered intravenously at a dose of 30 mg/m^2 of body surface area (see Appendix for table for converting kilograms to square meters) every 3 weeks. At least two treatments are necessary to evaluate for response; if the tumor volume decreases, as many as four additional doses may be administered. The drug should be discontinued if progression of disease occurs. Doxorubicin should be diluted with normal saline and given either in short intravenous boluses or as a continuous infusion during a 15- to 30-minute period. Potentially severe toxicities include neutropenia, anorexia, vomiting, diarrhea, and, with high cumulative doses, congestive cardiomyopathy. These problems are uncommon and, with the exception of the cardiac toxicity, are generally self-limiting. Less serious reactions are facial swelling and urticaria associated with drug administration and, occasionally, focal or generalized alopecia. Doxorubicin-induced cardiomyopathy is an irreversible condition, and it may occur weeks to months after the last treatment. The condition has occurred in dogs that have received cumulative doses of as little as 135 mg/m^2 (five total treatments) (Loar and Susanek, in press). The problem appears to be more common in dogs than in humans given equivalent amounts of the drug. Currently, there is no reliable method to predict which patients are at high risk of developing this unique toxicity.

In a limited number of dogs treated by the author and others (Jeglum and Whereat, 1983) with two or more doses of doxorubicin, between 40 and 50 per cent responded with at least a 50 per cent decrease in tumor size. Probably, animals responding in this fashion will show an improved attitude and increased appetite and activity. Unfortunately, the objective effects of doxorubicin therapy on the quality of life and the duration of survival have not been determined. In animals whose tumors have been surgically excised, the benefits of chemotherapy are also not clear. Theoretically, cytotoxic drugs may greatly reduce or eliminate microscopic disease; however, this effect is difficult to demonstrate, and it is unknown if this form of therapy will subsequently delay or prevent recurrence. Nevertheless, in the face of a high incidence of subclinical metastatic disease, particularly in animals with large primary tumors, the use of adjuvant chemotherapy is justifiable.

In addition to the use of antineoplastic agents, thyroid hormone therapy may be of value after tumor excision or debulking procedures are performed. As described earlier, thyroid tumor growth may be enhanced by high circulating levels of TSH. The administration of maintenance doses of T_4 (L-thyroxine, 20 to 40 μg/kg/day, orally) is recommended to suppress pituitary production and release of TSH. Thyroid hormone replacement is also indicated in dogs rendered hypothyroid from tumor invasion or surgery.

Radiotherapy

External beam radiation (teletherapy) consisting of cobalt radiation or administration of large doses of radioiodine (^{131}I) may be useful against thyroid tumors. As is true with many canine carcinomas, thyroid cancer appears to be relatively radiosensitive. However, these treatments are generally offered only at large referral centers and may be restricted because of their cost or toxicities.

External beam radiation is most commonly used to decrease the size of nonresectable primary tumors. It may also be valuable as postoperative therapy when directed against the surgical site; in this way, small populations of residual tumor cells may be reduced in an effort to delay or prevent tumor recurrence. Successful teletherapy in the treatment of canine thyroid tumors, however, has not been well documented.

Radioactive iodine produces antitumor effects by emission of beta particles when the radioisotope undergoes decay. Because this form of radiation is most potent over extremely short distances, the best responses would be expected in those tumors that show avid uptake of iodine. In addition, normal thyroid tissues compete for uptake of the isotopes and are susceptible to the cytotoxic effects of the radiation. Therefore, information derived from scintigraphy may be predictive of the positive and negative results of ^{131}I therapy. Other disadvantages of this form of treatment are strict federal regulation concerning the procurement and use of the radioisotopes (e.g., animals receiving the material must be maintained in a radiation isolation facility for several weeks after therapy) and the fact that normal tissues adjacent to sites of high radioisotope uptake may sustain intense damage (e.g., radiation pneumonitis in an animal with diffuse pulmonary metastases). Although relatively few dogs with thyroid cancer have been treated with ^{131}I, most have shown impressive objective responses (Mitchell et al., 1979).

PROGNOSIS

The long-term prognosis for dogs with thyroid adenomas, irrespective of their functional status, is generally good with surgical removal. As suggested earlier, however, the outcome for dogs with malignant tumors is more variable. Patients with small carcinomas showing no evidence of regional or distant spread may achieve prolonged disease-free intervals after surgical resection. In the AMC study, of the 10 dogs treated with surgery alone for primary carcinomas less than 5 cm in diameter (stage I and II tumors), eight (80 per cent) remained free of tumor for more than 7 months postoperatively. Thus, it appears that early detection and resection will significantly benefit some animals with thyroid carcinoma. Given the high incidence of metastatic disease in dogs with primary tumors greater than 21 cm^3, the use of adjuvant chemotherapy or radiotherapy or both, when available, may further improve the prognosis.

In dogs with large, invasive carcinomas, the likelihood for a surgical cure is slim. In the AMC group, of 26 dogs with tumors larger than 5 cm in diameter, with or without nodal invasion (i.e., stage III), 19 (73 per cent) had a recurrence or died as a result of their tumors within 7 months of surgery. Few of these dogs were offered adjuvant chemo- or radiotherapy postoperatively. From this and other studies, animals with advanced local disease as well as those with distant metastases (stage IV) would be expected to have a grim, short-term prognosis in spite of attempts to debulk their tumors surgically. The use of cytotoxic agents or radiotherapy or both may be helpful in the short-term control of these tumors. Modifications in the recommended therapeutic management of canine thyroid carcinoma should occur only after comparing responses to different treatments in large groups of dogs with similar stages of disease.

References and Supplemental Reading

Branham, J. E., Leighton, R. L., and Hornof, W. J.: Radioisotope imaging for the evaluation of thyroid neoplasia and hypothyroidism in a dog. J.A.V.M.A. 180:1077, 1982.

Harkema, J. R., King, R. R., and Hahn, F. F.: Carcinoma of the thyroglossal duct cysts: A case report and review of the literature. J. Am. Anim. Hosp. Assoc. 20:319, 1984.

Hayes, H. M., and Fraumeni, J. F.: Canine thyroid neoplasms: Epidemiologic features. J. Natl. Cancer Inst. 55:931, 1975.

Jeglum, K. A., and Whereat, A.: Chemotherapy of canine thyroid carcinoma. Compend. Cont. Ed. Pract. Vet. 5:96, 1983.

Leav, I., Schiller, A. L., Rijnberk, A., et al.: Adenomas and carcinomas of the canine and feline thyroid. Am. J. Pathol. 83:61, 1976.

Loar, A. S., and Susanek, S. J.: Doxorubicin-induced cardiomyopathy in five dogs. J.A.V.M.A., in press.

Mitchell, M., Hurov, L. I., and Troy, G. C.: Canine thyroid carcinomas: Clinical occurrence, staging by means of scintiscans, and therapy of 15 cases. Vet. Surg. 8:112, 1979.

Owen, L. N.: Clinical stages (TNM) of canine tumours of the thyroid gland. *In* Owen, L. N. (ed.): *TNM Classification of Tumours in Domestic Animals.* Geneva: World Health Organization, 1980.

Peterson, M. E., Randolph, J. F., Zaki, F. A., et al.: Multiple endocrine neoplasia in a dog. J.A.V.M.A. 180:1476, 1982.

Rijnberk, A.: Iodine metabolism and thyroid disease in the dog. (Doctoral dissertation) Utrecht, The Netherlands: Drukkerij Elinkwijk, 1971.

Rijnberk, A., and Leav, I.: Thyroid tumors. *In* Kirk, R. W. (ed.): *Current Veterinary Therapy VI.* Philadelphia: W. B. Saunders, 1976.

Theilen, G. H., and Madewell, B. R.: Tumors of the endocrine glands. *In* Theilen, G. H., and Madewell, B. R. (eds.): *Veterinary Cancer Medicine.* Philadelphia: Lea and Febiger, 1979.

Thompson, E. J., Stirtzinger, T., Lumsden, J. H., et al.: Fine needle aspiration cytology in the diagnosis of canine thyroid carcinoma. Can. Vet. J. 21:186, 1980.

HYPOPARATHYROIDISM

MARK E. PETERSON, D.V.M.
New York, New York

Hypoparathyroidism is a metabolic disorder characterized by hypocalcemia and hyperphosphatemia and either transient or permanent parathyroid hormone (PTH) insufficiency. The most common cause of hypoparathyroidism is iatrogenic injury or removal of the parathyroid glands during thyroid surgery. This form of postoperative hypoparathyroidism has become relatively common in cats because of the recent increased use of thyroidectomy for treatment of hyperthyroidism; the incidence of feline hypoparathyroidism following total thyroidectomy is approximately 10 per cent at our institution. Postoperative hypoparathyroidism also frequently develops in dogs after excision of a parathyroid tumor for treatment of primary hyperparathyroidism; this type of PTH insufficiency is usually temporary and occurs because the remaining "normal" parathyroid glands atrophy as a result of the hypersecretion of PTH by the tumor. Finally, spontaneous (idiopathic) hypoparathyroidism is a rare disorder that most commonly affects mature, female dogs of small breeds. Immune-mediated destruction of parathyroid tissue appears to play a role in the pathogenesis of spontaneous canine hypoparathyroidism, since the parathyroid parenchyma is typically replaced by an extensive lymphocytic-plasmocytic cellular infiltrate and fibrous connective tissue. Most dogs with idiopathic hypoparathyroidism have complete parathyroid destruction and atrophy and therefore require lifelong therapy to maintain normocalcemia.

PATHOGENESIS OF CALCIUM AND PHOSPHATE ALTERATIONS IN HYPOPARATHYROIDISM

Normally, the integrated actions of PTH and vitamin D maintain circulating concentrations of calcium and phosphate within relatively narrow physiologic ranges. Parathyroid hormone acts to promote renal calcium resorption and phosphate excretion and to increase the rate of bone resorption. Vitamin D raises serum calcium concentrations primarily by stimulating the absorption of calcium from the intestinal tract. Although the metabolic derangements of hypoparathyroidism might be ascribed to reduced PTH action alone, it is becoming increasingly clear that full expression of the hypoparathyroid state requires the concurrent deficiency of 1,25-dihydroxyvitamin D, the active renal metabolite of vitamin D (Favus, 1978).

Vitamin D is obtained from dietary sources and is produced endogenously in the skin (Fig. 1). Ultraviolet irradiation of ergosterol, a sterol found in certain plants and yeast, produces ergocalciferol (vitamin D_2). In addition, certain animal tissues, fish-liver oils, and irradiated milk contain cholecalciferol (vitamin D_3). Vitamin D_3 is also produced endogenously in the skin, where natural ultraviolet light converts 7-dehydrocholesterol, a by-product in the synthesis of cholesterol, to cholecalciferol. The term *vitamin D* without subscript is nonspecific and refers to both vitamin D_2 and D_3; although vitamin D_2 is relatively inactive in birds and New World monkeys, vitamins D_2 and D_3 are equipotent in other mammals. Vitamin D itself is biologically inactive, however, and must undergo further *in vivo* metabolic transformation to exert its effects.

Once formed in the skin or absorbed by the intestine, vitamin D, the biologically inactive prohormone, is transported to the liver, where it is hydroxylated at the 25 position to form 25-hydroxyvitamin D, a partially active metabolite (Fig. 1). This substance is transported to the kidneys, where it is hydroxylated either at the 1 position to produce 1,25-dihydroxyvitamin D, the most potent vitamin D metabolite, or at the 24 position to produce 24,25-dihydroxyvitamin D, an inactive compound of unclear biologic significance (Fig. 1). The activities of renal 1-hydroxylase and 24-hydroxylase are separately and reciprocally regulated, such that conditions that favor the synthesis of one dihydroxylated metabolite inhibit the formation of the other dihydroxylated product. Both PTH and phosphate play key roles in regulating the activities of these renal hydroxylase enzymes. Elevated PTH concentrations and hypophosphatemia enhance formation of active 1,25-dihydroxyvitamin D, whereas decreased secretion of PTH, with resultant hyperphosphatemia, increases the rate of 24,25-dihydroxyvitamin D synthesis and impairs the production of the active metabolite (Fig. 1). Therefore, in hypoparathyroidism resulting from diminished or absent PTH secretion, a deficiency of active vitamin D also develops, contributing to the hypocalcemia characteristic of hypoparathyroid states.

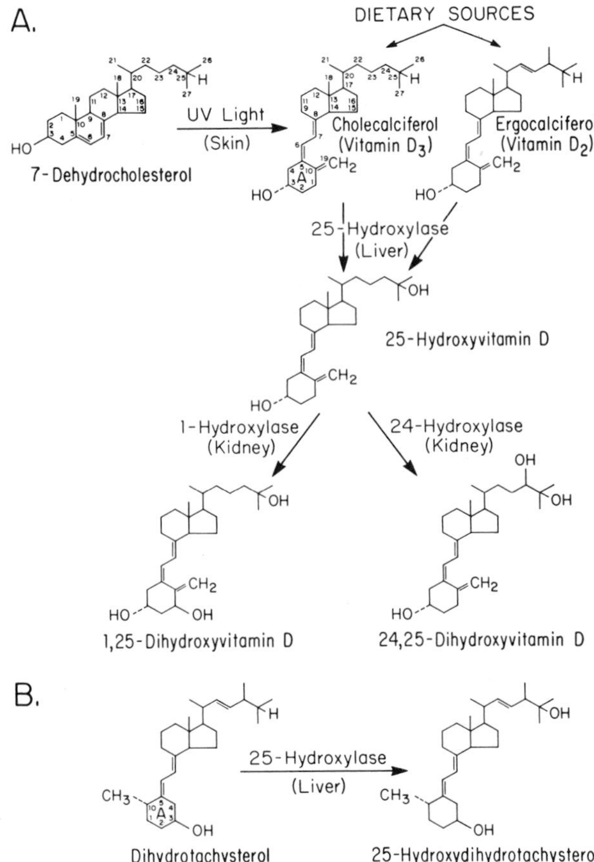

Figure 1. Chemical structures of the major vitamin D metabolites and analogues. The numbering system is based on that of cholesterol, and the A ring of cholecalciferol is so designated. *A*, Metabolism of vitamin D_2 and D_3. Note that vitamin D_2 differs from D_3 only in that it has a 24-methyl group and a 22-23 double bond in the side chain. *B*, Metabolism of the vitamin D analogue, dihydrotachysterol. Note that the A-ring is rotated 180 degrees so that the hydroxy group in the 3 position serves as a pseudo-1-hydroxyl group.

The biochemical hallmarks of hypoparathyroidism include hypocalcemia and hyperphosphatemia. Hypocalcemia results from inadequate PTH-mediated calcium mobilization from bone and decreased calcium reabsorption from the renal tubule, as well as reduced intestinal calcium absorption due to the impaired formation of 1,25-dihydroxyvitamin D. The serum phosphate concentrations rise in hypoparathyroidism because of increased renal tubular reabsorption of phosphate; however, hyperphosphatemia may be limited because of decreases in both the bone resorption and intestinal absorption of phosphate.

CLINICAL SIGNS

Hypocalcemia (decreased serum ionized calcium concentration) causes the major clinical manifestations of hypoparathyroidism by increasing the excitability of both the peripheral and central nervous systems. Peripheral neuromuscular signs classically include muscle tremors, twitches, and tetany. Generalized convulsions, resembling those of an idiopathic seizure disorder, is the predominant central nervous system manifestation of hypoparathyroidism. Unlike classic grand mal convulsions, however, hypocalcemic seizures are usually not associated with loss of consciousness or incontinence. Other central nervous system signs of hypocalcemia may include weakness, a stiff gait, ataxia, and behavioral changes (lethargy, restlessness, disorientation, or aggression).

Gastrointestinal, renal, and cardiac signs may also occur in animals with hypoparathyroidism. Anorexia, vomiting, abdominal pain, polydipsia, and polyuria have all been observed. The classic electrocardiographic correlate of hypocalcemia that might be detected is prolongation of the Q-T interval; this results from a lengthened S-T segment rather than an altered QRS complex and returns to normal rapidly after hypocalcemia is corrected.

In iatrogenic feline hypoparathyroidism resulting from parathyroid damage or excision during thyroid surgery, initial clinical signs may include lethargy, generalized weakness, anorexia, vomiting, and prolapse of the third eyelids. Without treatment, muscle tremors, tetany, or seizures will also develop, usually within the first three postoperative days.

Dogs with idiopathic hypoparathyroidism can have either an acute or chronic type of clinical presentation. The acute form is characterized by an abrupt onset of tetany or seizures. In contrast, dogs with the chronic type of presentation have protracted clinical courses characterized by intermittent episodes of less severe neuromuscular or behavioral signs, sometimes progressing to tetany or convulsions. Dogs with chronic untreated hypoparathyroidism may initially be misdiagnosed as having epilepsy or other neurologic disorders.

DIAGNOSIS

Diagnosis of hypoparathyroidism is based on history, clinical signs, laboratory evidence of hypocalcemia and hyperphosphatemia, and the exclusion of other causes of hypocalcemia including hypoproteinemia, malabsorption, vitamin D deficiency, pancreatitis, and renal failure (Juan, 1979). In general, nonhypoparathyroid hypocalcemic conditions are associated with secondary hyperparathyroidism; consequently, as long as the glomerular filtration rate is not severely depressed, the serum phosphate concentration will be normal or low in these disorders. Both hypocalcemia *and* hyperphosphatemia occur only in hypoparathyroidism and renal insufficiency, and these two conditions can usually be easily differentiated on clinical grounds and by routine evaluation of renal function (blood urea nitrogen [BUN] or serum creatinine determinations).

Idiopathic hypoparathyroidism is a reasonable tentative diagnosis in any dog that has clinical signs of hypocalcemia together with laboratory evidence of hypocalcemia, hyperphosphatemia, and normal renal function. This diagnosis can be confirmed by demonstrating absolute or relative lack of circulating PTH; however, valid assays for canine PTH are expensive and not widely available. Suspected hypoparathyroidism can also be confirmed by biopsy and examination of parathyroid glands. Since the parathyroid glands are usually not grossly evident in dogs with hypoparathyroidism, a unilateral thyroparathyroidectomy should be performed to ensure that adequate parathyroid tissue is removed for examination. Careful histologic examination may reveal a remnant of parathyroid tissue containing an infiltrate of lymphocytes and plasma cells, consistent with parathyroiditis.

After thyroid or parathyroid surgery, the potential development of hypoparathyroidism should be anticipated. Postoperatively, the serum calcium concentration should be monitored on a daily basis until it has stabilized within the normal range. A mild degree of suppression of the serum calcium level appears to be a nonspecific response to surgery and requires no treatment. However, if severe hypocalcemia and accompanying signs of heightened neuromuscular irritability develop, therapy with vitamin D and calcium is indicated. In most animals that require treatment for iatrogenic hypoparathyroidism, clinical signs associated with severe hypocalcemia (less than 6.0 mg/dl) will develop 24 to 72 hours after surgery.

TREATMENT

Treatment of hypoparathyroidism includes the use of calcium supplements and vitamin D. Parathyroid hormone has a short half-life, is expensive, and must be given parenterally; therefore, it is not a practical treatment for hypoparathyroidism. In addition, PTH replacement therapy is ineffective on a long-term basis because of the development of neutralizing antibodies, which diminish the efficacy of the hormone.

Calcium Preparations

Although many parenteral calcium preparations are available (Table 1), calcium gluconate is generally preferred for intravenous use. Calcium chloride solution, also commonly employed for use during cardiopulmonary resuscitation, is more irritating to veins and subcutaneous tissues than other preparations; therefore, if calcium chloride is administered intravenously, care must be taken to avoid extravasation, or extensive inflammation and sloughing may result. If intravenous therapy is unfeasible, some calcium formulations can be administered intramuscularly or subcutaneously with minimal irritation at the injection site (Table 1). Calcium gluconate, however, should not be given intramuscularly for treatment of hypoparathyroidism because of the large volume of solution required and the risk of abscess formation. Similarly, calcium chloride should only be given intravenously because severe tissue necrosis results from intramuscular injection. Although Calphosan (Carlton) is widely available and can be given either intramuscularly or subcutaneously, the high phosphate content of this product makes it a less than ideal preparation for treatment of hypoparathyroidism.

Oral calcium supplements are available as the gluconate, lactate, chloride, carbonate, and glubionate salts (Table 2). Calcium lactate or gluconate tablets are usually the preparations of choice, but they may be poorly dissolved and absorbed in some animals. To circumvent this problem of inadequate tablet dissolution, calcium lactate and chloride are also available in powder preparations that can be put into solution and given orally. Alternatively, Neo-Calglucon (Dorsey), a commercially available oral liquid preparation that contains 23 mg of elemental calcium per milliliter, is convenient but expensive. All calcium preparations can produce gastrointestinal disturbances, especially when administered in high doses. In addition, the chloride and carbonate salts can potentially induce acid-base alterations that are undesirable. Whatever oral calcium preparations are used, frequent small doses are more effective than fewer large doses.

The most common mistake in the use of calcium preparations is thinking in terms of weight of salt rather than the quantity of elemental calcium. There are large differences in calcium content between one salt and another (Tables 1 and 2) but little difference in effect when prescribed in equimolar amounts.

Vitamin D Preparations

The three major vitamin D preparations available include vitamin D_2, dihydrotachysterol, and 1,25-dihydroxyvitamin D (Table 3). Although all vitamin D preparations raise serum calcium concentrations primarily by increasing the gastrointestinal absorption of calcium, there are important differences in the doses of the three preparations needed to achieve normocalcemia in hypoparathyroidism, as well as differences in the times of maximal onset of effect and duration of action for each form of vitamin D.

The main practical advantage of therapy with vitamin D_2 is the drug's low cost. A theoretic advantage is that this parent compound serves as a precursor to all possible metabolites, since metabolites other than 1,25-dihydroxyvitamin D may be required for all of the actions of vitamin D to be expressed. A major disadvantage of vitamin D_2 is its instability. With storage, significant loss of strength can occur as a result of oxidation and photochemical decomposition. Another disadvantage of vitamin D_2 in initial treatment of hypoparathyroidism is the long onset of action—approximately 4 weeks. The lag period results from extensive tissue storage and time needed for conversion into active metabolites. Use of a loading dose of vitamin D_2, however, shortens the time needed to attain stable normocalcemia to 1 to 2 weeks. Because of the extreme individual variations in vitamin D_2 dosage required, the exact maintenance dosage cannot always be predicted and overdosage may occur during either initial or long-term maintenance therapy. Vitamin D_2 has a long

Table 1. *Parenteral Calcium Preparations*

Salt	Formulation of Compound	Elemental Calcium Content (mg/ml)	Route of Administration
Calcium gluconate	10% solution in 10-ml vials	9.2	IV
Calcium gluceptate	22% solution in 5-ml vials	18.0	IV, IM
Calcium chloride	10% solution in 10-ml vials	27.2	IV
Calcium glycerophosphate and lactate (Calphosan, Carlton)	1% solution in 60-, 125-, and 250-ml vials	1.9	IM, SC
	10% suspension in 30- and 240-ml vials	18.7	IM

Table 2. Oral Calcium Preparations

Salt	Dosage Forms	Elemental Calcium Content (%)
Calcium gluconate	325-, 500-, 650-, and 1000-mg tablets	9.2
Calcium lactate	325- and 650-mg tablets; powder preparation	13.0
Calcium chloride	Powder preparation	27.2
Calcium carbonate	500-, 650-, and 1250-mg tablets	40.0
Calcium glubionate	Neo-Calglucon syrup, 360 mg/ml	6.4

half-life; if overdosage occurs, hypercalcemia may persist for days to weeks after discontinuing therapy.

Dihydrotachysterol has major advantages over vitamin D_2 in that it raises serum calcium more rapidly and its effects are dissipated more quickly when the drug is discontinued. This drug is also much more potent than vitamin D_2 because 1.0 mg of dihydrotachysterol is equivalent to 3.0 mg (120,000 U) of vitamin D_2. Dihydrotachysterol is an A-ring analogue of vitamin D_2 in which the A ring is rotated 180 degrees so that the hydroxyl group in the 3 position serves as a pseudo-1-hydroxyl group (Fig. 1). After administration, this drug requires hepatic 25-hydroxylation for maximal biologic activity, but it does not undergo renal 1-hydroxylation, presumably because of the similarity of the pseudo-1-hydroxyl group to the 1α-hydroxyl group of 1,25-dihydroxyvitamin D. This ability to bypass renal 1-hydroxylation explains the rapidity of action

Table 3. Vitamin D Preparations

Product	Dosage Forms	Commercial Names
Vitamin D_2	Capsules, tablets (25,000 U, 50,000 U)*	Calciferol (Kremers-Urban), Drisdol (Winthrop), Deltalin (Lilly)
	Oral solution (8000 U/ml)	Drisdol (Winthrop), Calciferol (Kremers-Urban)
	IM injectable (500,000 U/ml)	Calciferol (Kremers-Urban), Vitadee (Gotham)
Dihydrotachysterol	Tablets (0.125 mg, 0.2 mg, 0.4 mg)	Dihydrotachysterol (Philips Roxane)
	Capsules (0.125 mg)	Hytakeral (Winthrop)
	Oral solution (0.25 mg/ml)	Hytakeral (Winthrop)
1,25-Dihydroxyvitamin D_3	Capsules (0.25 μg, 0.50 μg)	Rocaltrol (Roche)

*40,000 U of vitamin D_2 has an activity of 1.0 mg.

and potency of dihydrotachysterol therapy in hypoparathyroidism, a syndrome associated with deficient renal 1-hydroxylase activity. Thus, in animals with hypoparathyroidism, this compound has biologic activity intermediate between that of 1,25-dihydroxyvitamin D and 25-hydroxyvitamin D. In addition, the polarity and lower dosage requirements of dihydrotachysterol limit its storage in fat, making significant or prolonged vitamin D intoxication unlikely.

Finally, 1,25-dihydroxyvitamin D (Calcitriol, Table 3) offers the advantage of rapid onset of action (1 to 4 days) and short half-life (less than 1 day). If hypercalcemia results from overdosage, it can be rapidly corrected by discontinuing the drug for 24 to 48 hours. Because 1,25-dihydroxyvitamin D does not require activation by the kidney, physiologic dosages will maintain normocalcemia in hypoparathyroidism, a state in which renal 1-hydroxylase activity is low; in contrast, pharmacologic dosages of vitamin D_2 must be used to overcome this block in renal 1-hydroxylation. In humans, the dose of 1,25-dihydroxyvitamin D ranges from 0.03 to 0.06 μg/kg/day, about a thousandth of the dose of vitamin D_2 needed to achieve the same effect. A similar dosage would likely be effective in dogs and cats; in one study of normal dogs, calcium concentration remained normal when the drug was administered at a dosage of 0.06 μg/kg/day for 4 weeks, but hypercalcemia developed within 4 weeks of treatment in dogs given a dosage of 0.12 μg/kg/day (Caywood et al., 1979). The major disadvantage of this agent is its cost—about 20 times that of vitamin D_2 for equivalent therapeutic effects.

Treatment of Acute Hypocalcemia

Hypocalcemic tetany or convulsions are indications for the immediate intravenous administration of calcium; a dose of elemental calcium, 10 to 15 mg/kg of body weight, should be slowly infused over a 10- to 20-minute period. Calcium preparations appropriate for initial intravenous administration (Table 1) include calcium gluconate (1.0 to 1.5 ml/kg), calcium gluceptate (0.5 to 0.8 ml/kg), or calcium chloride (0.4 to 0.6 ml/kg). Electrocardiographic monitoring is advisable during this calcium infusion; if bradycardia or shortening of the Q-T interval occurs, the intravenous injection should be slowed or temporarily discontinued.

Once the life-threatening signs of hypocalcemia have been controlled, calcium can be added to the intravenous fluids and administered as a slow infusion of 60 to 90 mg/kg/day of elemental calcium (e.g., 2.5 ml/kg 10 per cent calcium gluconate every 6 to 8 hours). Serum calcium concentration should be determined once to twice daily during this treatment. The rate of calcium administration should be adjusted as necessary to maintain a normal serum calcium concentration, and the infusion should be continued for as long as necessary to prevent recurrence of hypocalcemia. Although this continuous calcium infusion will maintain normocalcemia, its effects are short-lived; hypocalcemia will recur within hours of stopping the infusion unless other treatment is given. Therefore, oral calcium and vitamin D should be initiated as soon as oral medication can be tolerated.

During initial treatment, large doses of vitamin D should be administered concomitantly with oral and intravenous calcium supplementation. Of the three major vitamin D preparations (Table 3), dihydrotachysterol is usually preferred over vitamin D_2 in the treatment of hypoparathyroidism because of its rapid onset of action and more reliable response. Although 1,25-dihydroxyvitamin D may be the ideal preparation for therapy of hypoparathyroidism, its use in veterinary medicine is limited because of the drug's considerable expense. With either dihydrotachysterol or vitamin D_2, use of a loading dose shortens the time needed to attain stable normocalcemia. By administering dihydrotachysterol at the approximate dosage of 0.03 to 0.06 mg/kg/day for 2 to 3 days, then 0.02 to 0.03 mg/kg/day for 2 to 3 days, and finally 0.01 mg/kg/day until further dosage adjustments are indicated, stable serum calcium concentrations (8.5 to 9.5 mg/dl) can usually be achieved within a week. Similarly, if vitamin D_2 is used, administration of high initial dosages (4000 to 6000 U/kg/day) will usually restore stable normocalcemia within 1 to 2 weeks; vitamin D_2 should then be reduced to the approximate maintenance dosage of 1000 to 2000 U/kg/day. During this initial treatment period, oral calcium supplements that provide 50 to 100 mg/kg/day of elemental calcium should be administered in three to four divided daily doses to ensure that sufficient calcium is available for increased intestinal calcium absorption resulting from the action of the vitamin D preparation. After near-normal serum calcium concentrations are maintained with the combined treatment of parenteral calcium infusion, oral calcium, and vitamin D for 1 to 2 days, the dose of intravenous calcium should be reduced and finally discontinued if tolerated. It may be necessary, however, to reinitiate parenteral calcium therapy for an additional 24 to 48 hours if the serum calcium concentration again falls to less than 7.0 mg/dl. Whatever vitamin D and calcium regimen is chosen, serum calcium should be determined once to twice daily during this initial treatment period until levels have stabilized in the low-normal range.

Maintenance Therapy for Hypoparathyroidism

The chronic treatment of hypoparathyroidism requires the administration of a maintenance dosage of a vitamin D preparation together with an adequate dietary or supplemental calcium intake. In contrast to acute hypoparathyroidism, in which control of signs of hypocalcemia is paramount, the aim of chronic treatment is to maintain serum calcium concentrations within the low-normal range (8.0 to 9.5 mg/dl). This calcium level is high enough to control signs of hypocalcemia while minimizing both the degree of hypercalciuria as well as the risk of overt hypercalcemia from vitamin D overdosage. In the absence of PTH, renal tubular resorption of calcium is decreased, and much of the calcium absorbed from the gastrointestinal tract is lost in the urine. If serum calcium is normalized to concentrations of 10 to 11 mg/dl with vitamin D and calcium therapy, urine calcium excretion may be dangerously high, leading to nephrocalcinosis and deterioration of renal function.

The ingestion of adequate amounts of calcium is an important component of the therapeutic regimen for hypoparathyroidism, since vitamin D (whatever preparation is used) raises serum calcium concentrations predominantly by increasing intestinal calcium absorption. Although animals receiving a well-balanced commercial diet may not require an additional source of calcium, it may be wise to supplement the diet with approximately 25 mg/kg/day of elemental calcium to ensure an adequate calcium intake for vitamin D action. Additional calcium can be provided by supplementation with appropriate amounts of calcium-rich foods (Table 4). Alternatively, calcium supplements (Table 2) can be given in three to four divided daily doses if the animal cannot obtain the desired amount of calcium by dietary means because of lactose intolerance or distaste for foods rich in calcium. Whatever calcium regimen is used, a constant daily calcium intake should be maintained; large changes in dietary calcium ingestion could potentially produce hyper- or hypocalcemia.

Specific therapy for hyperphosphatemia is generally not required in hypoparathyroidism, since restoration of normocalcemia tends to decrease the renal threshold for phosphate excretion and lower serum phosphate concentrations. If moderate to severe hyperphosphatemia persists despite control of hypocalcemia, however, ingestion of all phosphorus-rich dairy products should be discontinued and

Table 4. *Calcium-Rich Foods*

Food	Amount	Elemental Calcium (mg)
Cheddar cheese	¾-inch cube	110
Cottage cheese (creamed)	1 tbsp	25
Macaroni and cheese	1 cup	400
Milk (whole or skim)	8 oz	300
Swiss cheese	1 oz	260
Yogurt	1 cup	280

calcium salt supplements added to the therapeutic regimen to bind phosphate in the intestinal tract. An alternate but less desirable approach is to reduce intestinal phosphate absorption by administering aluminum-containing antacids (e.g., aluminum hydroxide).

Vitamin D maintenance therapy must be strictly individualized, and dose adjustments are based on frequent determinations of the serum calcium concentrations. With either dihydrotachysterol or vitamin D_2, the serum calcium should be monitored at weekly intervals after initial stabilization, and the dosage should be adjusted by 15 to 20 per cent increments until a dosage level is found that maintains serum calcium concentration in the low-normal range. Thereafter, calcium should be measured every 3 to 4 months and further dosage adjustments made as needed. With both dihydrotachysterol and vitamin D_2, small dosage changes can be achieved most readily by using a high-potency preparation of vitamin D in liquid form, which is administered into the animal's mouth with a tuberculin syringe.

The major complication associated with treatment of hypoparathyroidism is hypercalcemia, which develops as a consequence of overtreatment with calcium and vitamin D. Owners should frequently be reminded of the clinical signs of hypercalcemia (e.g., polyuria, polydipsia, anorexia) so that prompt treatment can be initiated to prevent hypercalcemic nephropathy and soft tissue calcification (Chew and Capen, 1980). If elevated serum calcium concentrations develop during the course of treatment, calcium and vitamin D therapy should be temporarily discontinued. In addition, diuresis induced by saline and furosemide administration may be indicated if severe hypercalcemia is present. Once normocalcemia has been restored, vitamin D therapy should be reinstituted at a lower maintenance dosage (approximately 20 per cent less than that previously administered). In animals with hypoparathyroidism that might be transient (e.g., after thyroidectomy), however, vitamin D and calcium treatment should be reinstated only if significant hypocalcemia (less than 8.0 mg/dl) again develops.

With iatrogenic hypoparathyroidism, spontaneous recovery of parathyroid function may occur weeks to months after surgery (Birchard et al., 1984). After 2 to 3 months of therapy, one should attempt to taper the dosage of vitamin D and wean the animal from medication. This can be safely accomplished by first reducing the vitamin D dosage by 25 to 50 per cent and monitoring calcium concentration at weekly intervals. After cessation, the effects of dihydrotachysterol and vitamin D_2 persist for approximately 2 and 4 weeks, respectively; therefore, if serum calcium concentration remains within normal range when rechecked at these times, gradual dosage reduction is continued until the vitamin D can finally be stopped completely.

References and Supplemental Reading

Birchard, S. J., Peterson, M. E., and Jacobson, A.: Surgical treatment of feline hyperthyroidism: Results of 85 cases. J. Am. Anim. Hosp. Assoc. 20:705, 1984.

Caywood, D. D., Wallace, L. J., Olson, W. G., et al.: Effects of 1α, 25-dihydroxycholecalciferol on disuse osteoporosis in the dog: A histomorphometric study. Am. J. Vet. Res. 40:89, 1979.

Chew, D. J., and Capen, C. C.: Hypercalcemic nephropathy and associated disorders. *In* Kirk, R. W. (ed.): *Current Veterinary Therapy VII.* Philadelphia: W. B. Saunders, 1980, pp. 1067–1072.

Favus, M. J.: Vitamin D physiology and some clinical aspects of the vitamin D endocrine system. Med. Clin. North Am. 62:1291, 1978.

Juan, D.: Hypocalcemia: Differential diagnosis and mechanisms. Arch. Intern. Med. 139:1166, 1979.

Kornegay, J. N.: Hypocalcemia in dogs. Comp. Cont. Ed. Pract. Vet. 4:103, 1982.

Okano, K., Furukawa, Y., Morii, H., et al.: Comparative efficacy of various vitamin D metabolites in the treatment of various types of hypoparathyroidism. J. Clin. Endocrinol. Metab. 55:238, 1982.

Pierides, A. M.: Pharmacology and therapeutic uses of vitamin D and its analogues. Drugs 21:241, 1981.

Sherding, R. G., Meuten, D. J., Chew, D. J., et al.: Primary hypoparathyroidism in the dog. J.A.V.M.A. 176:439, 1980.

Spangler, W. L., Gribble, D. H., and Lee, T. C.: Vitamin D intoxication and the pathogenesis of vitamin D nephropathy in the dog. Am. J. Vet. Res. 40:73, 1979.

CANINE HYPERLIPEMIAS

CAROLE A. ZERBE, D.V.M.

East Lansing, Michigan

Although lipemic serum is frequently encountered by the veterinarian, there is relatively little information concerning the diagnostic approach and management of hyperlipidemia in dogs. Lipemias are important because they alert the clinician to the possibility of underlying metabolic derangements, whereas hyperlipemia itself can lead to significant, sometimes fatal disease. The terms lipemia, hyperlipemia, hyperlipidemia all refer to increased concentrations of lipids or lipoproteins in the serum. Dyslipoproteinemia refers to an abnormal distribution of lipoproteins with normal total concentration of lipids.

LIPID CLASSES

An understanding of lipids and lipid metabolism is essential to the evaluation and treatment of hyperlipidemia. The major classes of lipids found in serum are fatty acids, phospholipids, cholesterol (free and esterified), and triglycerides. These can be thought of as divided into polar and nonpolar lipids. The nonpolar lipids are cholesteryl esters and triglycerides, and the polar lipids are cholesterol, fatty acids, and phospholipids.

Free fatty acids are present only in minute concentrations in plasma and cells, but they are constituents of most lipid classes. Although they can be free (nonesterified), free fatty acids (FFA) most commonly exist as esters of naturally occurring alcohols such as glycerol. Fatty acids constitute 95 per cent of triglycerides by weight and are released from adipose tissue by hydrolysis of stored triglycerides.

Phospholipids are found in most body tissues and fluids. They have an important role in oxidative phosphorylation and the energy-linked transport of ions across membranes. In addition, they are important structural components of membranes.

Triglycerides are the most abundant form of lipid in animal tissues and serve as an important reservoir of energy. They can be formed in the intestinal mucosa from dietary lipids (exogenous triglycerides) or they can be synthesized in the liver from nonlipid precursors (endogenous triglycerides). Triglycerides are transported in the blood as chylomicrons or very low-density lipoproteins. They are stored in adipose tissue and are readily hydrolyzed to glycerol and fatty acids.

Cholesterol exists in two forms—cholesteryl ester, which is the storage form of cholesterol, and free or unesterified cholesterol, which is the more metabolically active form. Cholesterol serves three major functions. It is a required structural component of the plasma membrane of cells and acts as a precursor for both the steroid hormones and bile acids. Cholesterol can be dietary in origin (exogenous) or it can be synthesized in the liver (endogenous).

LIPOPROTEINS

Since lipids are insoluble in water, they must be transported in association with plasma proteins. The polar lipids generally are bound to albumin, whereas the nonpolar lipids are transported in much larger macromolecular complexes, called lipoproteins. These spherical lipoproteins are composed of two basic parts, an inner core and an outer surface coat. Varying proportions of nonpolar lipids (primarily triglycerides and cholesteryl esters) make up the larger hydrophobic core. Surrounding the core is a polar surface coat that stabilizes the lipoprotein particle so it can remain in solution in the plasma. It is composed of a mixed monolayer of lipids (phospholipids, cholesterol) and a group of proteins called apolipoproteins (also called apoproteins). The apolipoproteins are very important, as they bind to specific enzymes or transport proteins on cell membranes, thus directing the lipoprotein to its site of metabolism.

On the basis of size, density, and electrophoretic mobility, four classes of lipoproteins have been recognized in dogs (Table 1). These include the chylomicrons, very low-density lipoproteins (VLDL), low-density lipoproteins (LDL), and high-density lipoproteins (HDL).

Chylomicrons

The largest lipoproteins, chylomicrons, are formed in the intestinal mucosa from dietary fats (Fig. 1). They are composed almost entirely of triglycerides and are located at the origin region on the electrophoretic pattern of lipoprotein assay. The major apoproteins in chylomicrons are Apo B and Apo C (Table 1). Since chylomicrons are derived exclusively from dietary fat, they are often called *exogenous triglycerides*. Normally, they are cleared from the bloodstream within 12 hours after a meal and are not present in the fasting state.

Very Low-Density Lipoproteins

Very low-density lipoproteins are synthesized in the liver and are also composed predominantly of triglycerides (Fig. 1). They contain apoproteins B and C (Table 1). Since VLDLs are derived from within the body, they are known as endogenous triglycerides.

Low-Density Lipoproteins

Low-density lipoproteins are a degradation product of VLDL. They are composed mainly of cholesterol (Table 1). LDLs supply cholesterol to hepatic and extrahepatic tissues (Fig. 1). Apo B is the major apolipoprotein in LDL.

High-Density Lipoproteins

Protein-rich lipoproteins, HDLs, are formed by the hepatocytes. There are two subclasses, HDL_1 and HDL_2, both of which contain Apo A. Because they recycle lipids from peripheral tissues, they are considered "scavengers" for cholesterol. HDL is the primary lipoprotein in dogs.

***Table 1.** Composition and Characteristics of Canine Lipoproteins*

Lipoprotein* Class	Composition (%)				Major Apoprotein	Electrophoretic Mobility	Chylomicron Test	
	Triglyceride	*Cholesterol*	*Phospholipids*	*Protein*			*Cream*	*Turbidity*
Chylomicron	80–95	2–7	3–6	1–2	Apo A Apo B Apo C	Origin	+	–
VLDL	59	15	16	10	Apo B Apo C Apo E	Pre-beta	–	+
LDL	30	22	24	23	Apo B	Beta	–	–
HDL_1	2	35	40	22	Apo A	Alpha2	–	–
HDL_2	1	20	36	42	Apo A	Alpha1	–	–

*HDL = high-density lipoprotein; LDL = low-density lipoprotein; VLDL = very low-density lipoprotein.

Other Lipoproteins

Two other lipoprotein classes, which include beta-VLDL and HDL cholesterol (HDLc), have also been noted in dogs. The HDLc migrates in the alpha range on the electrophoretic pattern, as do HDL_1 and HDL_2; however, its major apolipoprotein is Apo E rather than Apo A. It can be produced in dogs fed diets high in cholesterol. Some investigators believe that HDLc may represent HDL_2 that has become overloaded with cholesterol. Beta-VLDLs have Apo E and the density characteristic of normal VLDL, but during electrophoresis they migrate in the beta range instead of the pre-beta range. Since their properties are intermediate between VLDL and LDL, they probably represent remnant particles generated from VLDL catabolism. Beta-VLDLs have only been recognized in dogs given very high-cholesterol diets.

LIPOPROTEIN METABOLISM

It is useful to think of the lipoproteins in two broad categories—triglyceride-rich lipoproteins (chylomicrons and VLDL), and cholesterol-rich lipoproteins (LDL and HDL); these two classes of lipoproteins are, in turn, acted on by two different enzyme systems—lipoprotein lipase (LPL) and lecithin cholesterol acyltransferase (LCAT), respectively (Fig. 1). LPL hydrolyzes triglyceride and is responsible for clearing chylomicrons and VLDLs from the plasma. LCAT is responsible for esterification of cholesterol and acts on HDL and LDL.

The triglyceride-rich lipoproteins, chylomicrons and VLDLs, both contain Apo C, which activates the enzyme LPL. LPL is attached to capillary endothelial cells and is particulary dense in the capillaries of skeletal muscle and adipose tissue. When LPL is activated, the core triglycerides are hydrolyzed into FFA and glycerol, which are removed from the lipoprotein. The outer surface coat also undergoes changes and decreases in size. The transformed lipoprotein, a remnant particle, is rich in cholesterol esters and apoproteins B and E (Fig. 1). Many of these remnant particles formed from VLDL catabolism, however, undergo further transformation to form LDL.

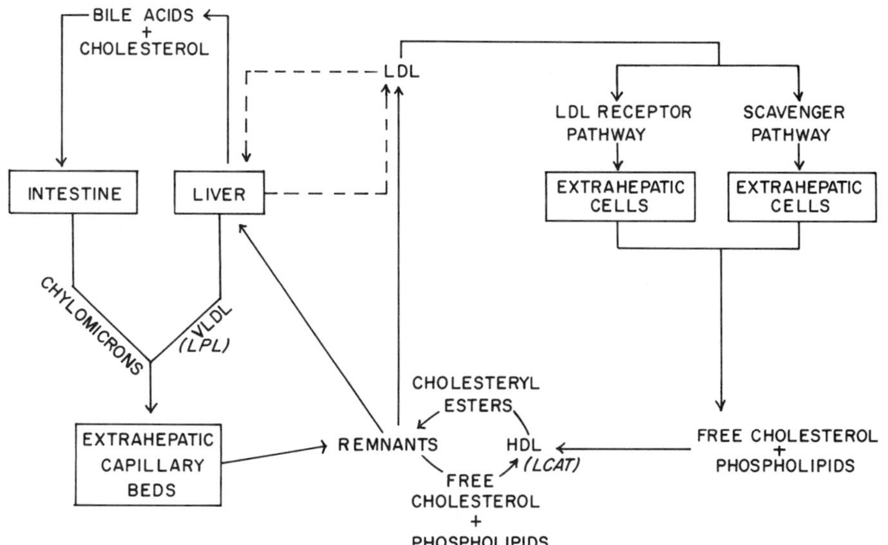

Figure 1. Model for plasma triglyceride and cholesterol transport in humans. The details of this model are discussed in the text. VLDL = very low-density proteins; LDL = low-density lipoproteins; HDL = high-density lipoproteins; LPL = lipoprotein lipase; LCAT = lecithin-cholesterol acyltransferase. (From Havel et al. *in* Bondy and Rosenberg (eds.): *Metabolic Control and Disease.* 8th ed. Philadelphia: W.B. Saunders, 1980, pp. 393–494, with permission.)

Plasma LDL and HDL are the cholesterol-rich lipoproteins. Plasma LDL functions as a storage depot for cholesterol, whereas HDL functions as a cholesterol scavenger. When extrahepatic cells, such as adrenocortical cells, need cholesterol, they form an LDL receptor (receptor pathway), which allows uptake of the lipoprotein by the cell (Fig. 1). Once inside the cell, the cholesteryl esters of LDL are hydrolyzed by the enzyme LCAT. Cholesterol is then available for membrane synthesis and as a precursor for steroid hormone synthesis. When plasma LDL exceeds the cholesterol needs of extrahepatic cells, it is phagocytized by reticuloendothelial cells by a receptor-independent (scavenger) pathway (Fig. 1).

As cells undergo turnover, unesterified cholesterol is released into the plasma. This cholesterol binds to HDL (the cholesterol scavenger) and is esterified through the action of the LCAT (Fig. 1). The resultant cholesteryl esters on HDL are either returned to the liver with the remnant particles or become part of the LDL. Thus, a cycle is established by which LDL delivers cholesterol to extrahepatic cells and by which cholesterol is returned to LDL from extrahepatic cells via HDL.

DIAGNOSTIC TOOLS

Several useful and inexpensive tests are available to veterinarians for evaluation of hyperlipidemias. These include (1) total serum triglyceride and cholesterol concentration determinations, (2) the chylomicron test, and (3) lipoprotein electrophoresis. Other tests are available for use in humans but have not yet been adopted for use in dogs.

Total Serum Triglyceride and Cholesterol

If a serum sample obtained after a 12-hour fast is grossly lipemic, it is important to determine if the lipemia is caused by increased concentrations of triglyceride, cholesterol, or both. For example, an increase in the VLDL (endogenous triglyceride) fraction is always accompanied by hypercholesterolemia, since VLDLs contain approximately 15 per cent cholesterol. On the other hand, hyperchylomicronemia (exogenous triglyceride) is not necessarily accompanied by increased cholesterol concentration, since chylomicrons contain relatively little cholesterol. Total serum triglyceride and cholesterol concentrations are included as part of the serum biochemical profile by many laboratories. If an abnormality is noted, it can serve as an important clue to underlying disease.

Not all hyperlipemias have grossly lipemic serum. For example, hypercholesterolemia in the absence of hypertriglyceridemia will not have grossly lipemic serum, since cholesterol is not opalescent.

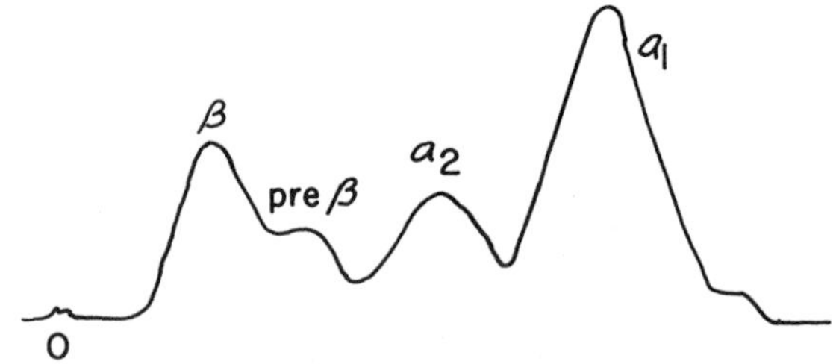

Figure 2. Normal canine lipid profile. Values depicted represent the accepted normal ranges for triglycerides and cholesterol. O = origin. (From Ford: Gaines Veterinary Symposium, Gaines Dog Research Center, 1977, pp. 12–16, with permission.)

Chylomicron Test

This test, also referred to as the refrigeration test, is easily performed by allowing the serum sample obtained after a 12-hour fast to stand in the refrigerator for 12 to 14 hours. The serum is then evaluated for the presence or absence of a cream layer and serum lactescence. Care should be taken not to freeze the sample, however, since freezing damages the lipoprotein structure and makes the serum useless for subsequent lipoprotein electrophoretic analysis (see below).

At cool temperatures, chylomicrons rise to the surface to form a creamy layer. VLDLs, when present, remain in stable dispersion and diffract light, which causes the serum to appear turbid. The smaller lipoprotein particles such as LDLs cannot be detected by this test since they are not large enough to diffract light (Table 1).

Lipoprotein Electrophoresis

This test is similar to protein electrophoresis and separates lipoprotein classes on the basis of electric charge and molecular diameter. Since this test provides only qualitative data, it should be used in conjunction with quantitative tests such as triglyceride and cholesterol determinations.

Five major bands may be identified with lipoprotein electrophoresis (Fig. 2). Chylomicrons remain at the origin region of the electrophoretic pattern. Serum LDLs move the slowest and have beta-band mobility, whereas VLDLs migrate at the pre-beta band. The HDL_1 migrates as the $alpha_2$ band, and HDL_2 moves the fastest, migrating as the $alpha_1$ band. As indicated earlier, however, if beta-VLDL is present it will migrate in the beta range with the LDL fraction. Because it provides only qualitative data, the application of lipoprotein electrophoresis is limited.

Other Tests

LPL activity can be assessed by administration of heparin. When given intravenously, heparin releases LPLs from the capillary endothelium, which in turn causes hydrolysis of the triglycerides of chylomicrons and VLDLs. Serum for triglyceride and cholesterol concentrations and lipoprotein electrophoresis determination should be collected prior to and 15 minutes after the intravenous administration of heparin (90 IU/kg body weight). If there is no change in the serum lipid concentrations or the lipoprotein electrophoretic pattern, an absent or defective LPL enzyme system should be suspected. Assays of canine lipoprotein lipase are being investigated but are not presently available.

Another test, lipoprotein ultracentrifugation, separates lipoproteins into the various classes and provides both qualitative and quantitative data. However, its application to the evaluation of hyperlipidemia in dogs has only recently begun to be investigated.

Test Combinations

By evaluating the total serum triglyceride and cholesterol concentrations and by performing the chylomicron test, a great deal of information can be gained inexpensively and simply. For example, a hyperlipidemic dog with severe hypertriglyceridemia, mild hypercholesterolemia, and lactescent serum would be evaluated as having increased VLDL concentrations. This pattern would be consistent with the lipid profile associated with diabetes mellitus.

In addition, it is useful to get a qualitative or quantitative assessment of the lipoprotein fractions. Lipoprotein ultracentrifugation would be preferred to lipoprotein electrophoresis since it provides quantitative data. However, until ultracentrifugation becomes available to the veterinary clinician, lipoprotein electrophoresis will remain a useful procedure for assessing lipoprotein fractions.

DIAGNOSTIC APPROACH

When lipemic serum is encountered, three major situations should be considered. The first and by far the most common is that the animal has not fasted for 12 hours. Second, the lipemia may be secondary to an underlying disorder. Finally, and least commonly, the lipemia may be primary or idiopathic in origin (Table 2).

Table 2. *Major Causes of Hyperlipemia*

Postprandial hyperlipemia

Secondary hyperlipemia
- Most common:
  - Hypothyroidism
  - Diabetes mellitus
  - Pancreatitis
- Less common:
  - Hyperadrenocorticism
  - Liver disease
  - Pregnancy
  - Drug-induced
  - Obesity
  - Nephrotic syndrome
  - Gram-negative sepsis

Primary hyperlipemia
- Idiopathic hyperlipemia of the miniature schnauzer
- Idiopathic hyperchylomicronemia

Hyperlipemia after a 12-hour fast should always be considered abnormal. Any animal suspected of having postprandial hyperlipemia should be fasted for 12 hours and re-evaluated (Fig. 3). If lipemia persists, primary or secondary hyperlipidemia is present.

Secondary Hyperlipidemia

Secondary hyperlipidemia refers to increased concentrations of lipoproteins that occur secondary to an underlying metabolic alteration. Metabolic disorders that can cause hyperlipidemia include pancreatitis, hypothyroidism, diabetes mellitus, liver disease, hyperadrenocorticism, and others (Table 2).

Diabetes Mellitus. The hyperlipidemia that frequently occurs in diabetic dogs results primarily from hypertriglyceridemia, but hypercholesterolemia may also contribute. In humans, the degree, type, and pathogenesis of the hyperlipidemia depend on the type of diabetes mellitus (i.e., noninsulin-dependent or insulin-dependent diabetes) and with the degree to which the diabetes is regulated.

Type I, or insulin-dependent diabetes mellitus, is the most common type of diabetes in dogs. Insulin is required for lipoprotein lipase synthesis; therefore, in insulin-deficient states there is impaired lipoprotein lipase activity. This results in decreased catabolism and thus increased concentrations of chylomicrons and VLDLs. In Type I diabetes, there is also decreased hepatic production of VLDLs. However, there is an overall increase in serum VLDL concentrations, since the decrease in hepatic production occurs to a lesser extent than does the decrease in catabolism.

Patients with type II, or noninsulin-dependent

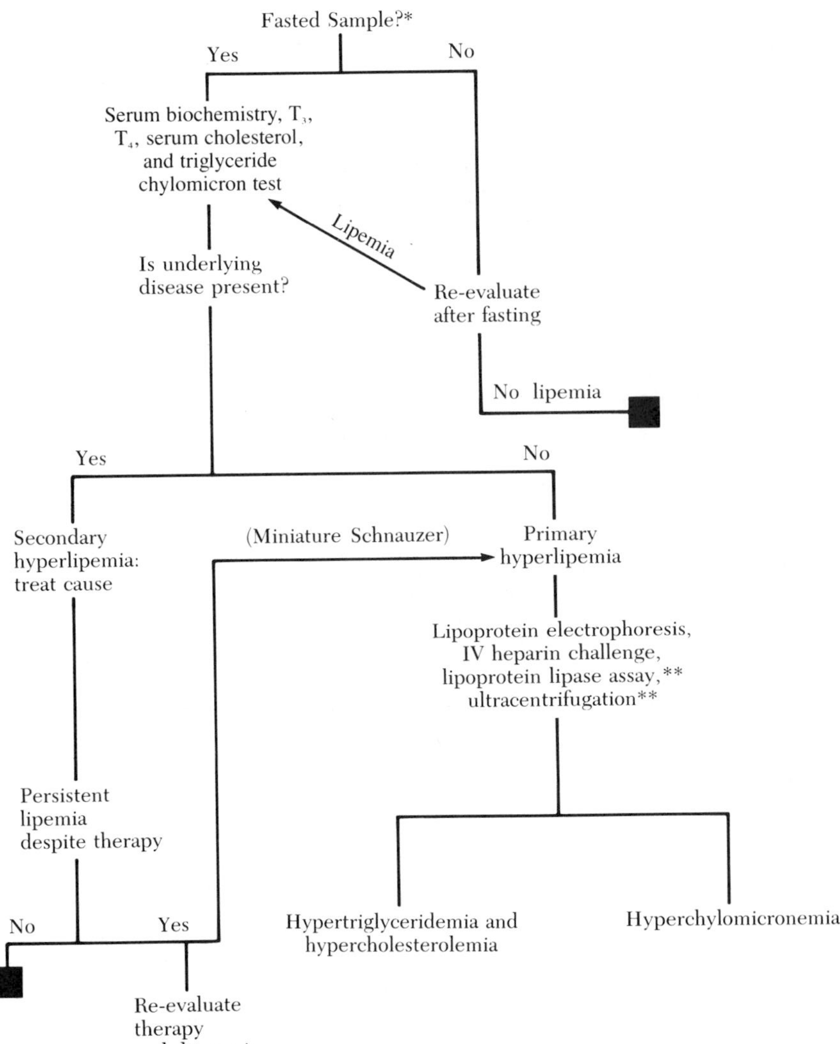

Figure 3. Approach to hyperlipemia. Note that not all hyperlipemias will be grossly apparent in the serum. * = fasting should be a minimum of 12 hours; ** = not currently available for routine clinical use in the dog; solid box = no further work-up is required for hyperlipemia.

diabetes, also have hypertriglyceridemia as a result of increased VLDL concentrations, but it occurs secondary to increased synthesis of VLDLs by the liver.

Hypercholesterolemia can also develop in diabetes mellitus and may be the result of increases in the serum concentrations of VLDL, LDL, or both. Increases in either lipoprotein would result in a secondary increase in serum cholesterol concentrations, since VLDLs and LDLs contain about 15 and 22 per cent cholesterol, respectively.

Therefore, the hyperlipidemia secondary to diabetes mellitus is characterized primarily by hypertriglyceridemia with less severe hypercholesterolemia. Serum lactescence with or without a cream layer is found by using the chylomicron test. The lipoprotein electrophoretic pattern shows increased origin, pre-beta, and beta ranges (Fig. 4). The hyperlipidemia usually resolves with improved control of the diabetic patient.

HYPOTHYROIDISM. Thyroid hormones regulate cholesterol synthesis and enhance the hepatic degradation of cholesterol to bile acids. They may also increase the sensitivity of adipose tissue to the lipolytic effects of several hormones. In addition, thyroid hormones may be necessary for activation of lipoprotein lipase. In hypothyroidism, lipid breakdown is diminished to a greater degree than is synthesis.

Severe degrees of hypothyroidism are commonly accompanied by severe hypercholesterolemia. Serum triglyceride levels are less consistently increased. Lipoprotein electrophoresis may reveal increases in the pre-beta, beta, and $alpha_2$ regions (Fig. 5). There may be a slight cream layer, serum lactescence, or clear serum on the chylomicron test. These abnormalities will usually disappear with therapy.

PANCREATITIS. The association of pancreatitis and hyperlipidemia has long been recognized. Recent

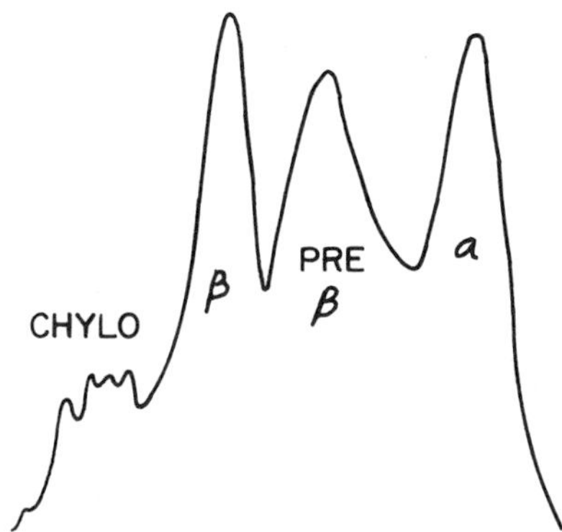

Figure 4. Lipid profile from a dog with diabetes mellitus. Note the increased intensity at the origin (β) and pre-β ranges on electrophoresis as well as the presence of a cream layer and serum lactescence on the chylomicron test. These results indicate that the hypertriglyceridemia is due to increases in both chylomicrons and VLDLs. The hypercholesterolemia is due to increased LDL and VLDL.

studies in humans suggest that hypertriglyceridemia precedes the development of pancreatitis, and may be responsible for precipitating acute pancreatitis. Although the mechanism of hyperlipidemia-induced pancreatitis remains unknown, high concentrations of triglyceride in and around the pancreas may be hydrolyzed by pancreatic lipase, resulting in the local release of large quantities of FFA. Generally, FFA are not toxic because they are bound to albumin; however, if the binding capacity of albumin is exceeded, the unbound FFA would be very

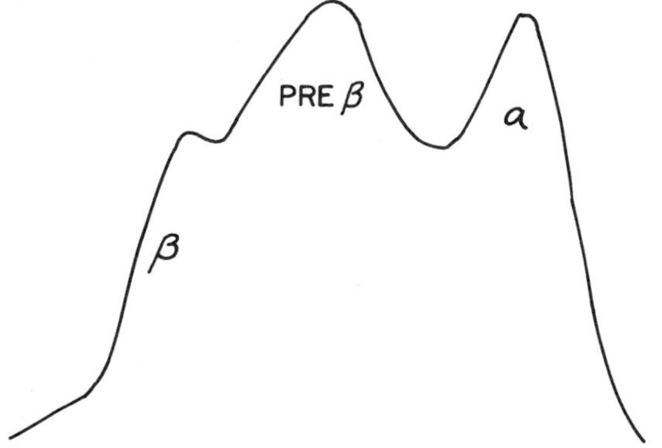

Figure 5. Lipid profile from a dog with hypothyroidism. Note that the serum is clear and there is increased intensity at the β, pre-β, and α ranges. The hypercholesterolemia is associated with increased LDL and HDL fractions.

toxic to tissues and could result in vascular injury and acute pancreatitis.

In cases of pancreatitis, the serum may be either lipemic or clear. Hypercholesterolemia with an increased alpha$_2$ or beta-lipoprotein band may be observed on lipoprotein electrophoresis. Thus, it appears that the hypercholesterolemia of pancreatitis may result from increases of both LDL and HDL classes. Hypertriglyceridemia may be noted in some dogs with pancreatitis, but this is a less common finding than hypercholesterolemia.

OTHERS. Other causes of secondary hyperlipidemia include hyperadrenocorticism, liver disease, nephrotic syndrome, pregnancy, and obesity. Glucocorticoids are thought to induce lipemia by increasing the secretion of VLDL by the liver and by decreasing LPL activity; both hypertriglyceridemia and hypercholesterolemia may develop in hyperadrenocorticism. The liver plays a major role in both cholesterol synthesis and excretion. Therefore, if hyperlipemia occurs in liver disease, it is usually caused by hypercholesterolemia, whereas serum triglyceride concentrations remain normal. Hypercholesterolemia is also a common finding in the nephrotic syndrome. In late pregnancy, serum concentrations of VLDL, LDL, and HDL all increase in women. In humans, obesity also appears to increase the hepatic synthesis of VLDL and produce hyperlipidemia.

IDIOPATHIC OR PRIMARY HYPERLIPOPROTEINEMIAS

Every effort should be made to rule out secondary forms of hyperlipoproteinemia before the primary or idiopathic hyperlipidemias are considered. In humans, the term *primary hyperlipidemia* refers to lipemias that result from heritable defects in lipoprotein metabolism. Since the hereditary aspects of hyperlipidemia have not been determined in dogs, the term *idiopathic* rather than *primary* is preferred. Two forms of idiopathic hyperlipidemia have been recognized in dogs: (1) idiopathic hyperlipoproteinemia and (2) idiopathic hyperchylomicronemia.

Idiopathic hyperlipoproteinemia, first reported in the miniature schnauzer in 1975, has become a well-recognized clinical entity in that breed. Affected dogs may be clinically asymptomatic or have seizures, an acute onset of blindness, cloudy eyes, or signs referable to pancreatitis, such as abdominal pain and vomiting. Hepatomegaly may be detected on physical examination.

Although the pathogenesis of idiopathic hyperlipoproteinemia in the miniature schnauzer remains poorly understood, hypertriglyceridemia appears to be the major abnormality, and serum triglyceride concentrations sometimes exceed 100 times the normal value. Serum cholestrol concentrations are also moderately increased, but rarely to the extent of the triglycerides. Affected dogs have increased serum levels of chylomicrons, VLDLs, and LDLs, as suggested by the presence of a cream layer (chylomicronemia), serum lactescence (from VLDL), hypertriglyceridemia, and intense staining of the beta electrophoretic band. Increased serum HDL_1 concentrations are also occasionally increased, as reflected by intense staining of the $alpha_2$ electrophoretic band.

Administration of heparin to miniature schnauzers with idiopathic hyperlipidemia tends to clear serum lactescence, markedly decrease serum triglyceride concentrations, and shift the lipoprotein electrophoretic pattern toward the alpha region. Since these findings are compatible with activation of lipoprotein lipase activity, an absolute deficiency of lipoprotein lipase is an unlikely cause of this syndrome. However, after administration of heparin, the prominent beta band is still usually visible with lipoprotein electrophoresis. Therefore, it is possible that these dogs have a beta-VLDL that migrates with the LDL in the beta region on electrophoresis and contributes to the hyperlipoproteinemia. This may be similar to a disease in humans, familial dyslipoproteinemia, in which there is increased beta-VLDL secondary to a defect in Apo E. Further studies must be performed, however, to elucidate the underlying defect that is responsible for idiopathic hyperlipidemia in the miniature schnauzer.

Idiopathic hyperchylomicronemia has been reported in two dogs. It is characterized by marked lipemia with serum lactescence and a cream layer on the chylomicron test. This gives the plasma a characteristic appearance of cream of tomato soup. In one case, there was negligible change in the hyperlipidemia after heparin administration, whereas there was some response in the other. The cause of this disorder remains unknown.

THE IMPORTANCE OF HYPERLIPEMIAS

The presence of fasting hyperlipemia can provide a clue to the presence of an underlying disease process. Of equal importance, however, is that the presence of persistent or severe hyperlipemia may predispose the dog to other diseases that can ultimately be fatal. Severe lipemia can also spuriously alter many serum biochemistry results.

Diseases That Result from Hyperlipemia

Diseases that develop as a consequence of hyperlipemia can be thought of as divided into those occurring secondary to hypertriglyceridemia and those that are secondary to hypercholesterolemia.

Diseases that result from hypertriglyceridemia include ocular abnormalities, central nervous system (CNS) disturbances, and pancreatitis. The ocular abnormalities include lipid-laden aqueous humor and lipemia retinalis. Dogs with lipid-laden aqueous humor may present with photophobia, cloudy eyes, or an acute onset of blindness. Management should include treatment for anterior uveitis and diet change to a low-fat diet. The lipid-laden aqueous humor usually clears with correction of serum hyperlipoproteinemia. Lipemia retinalis, characterized by cream-colored retinal vessels, is usually noted as an incidental finding during physical examination, since vision appears to be unaffected. CNS abnormalities, usually manifested by seizure activity, can also be produced by hyperlipemia. Such CNS dysfunction appears to develop most commonly in schnauzers with idiopathic hyperlipoproteinemia. Pancreatitis is the most serious problem associated with hypertriglyceridemia (pathogenesis is discussed earlier in this chapter) and is frequently a recurrent, severe, and sometimes fatal complication. The diabetic miniature schnauzer appears to have an unusually high incidence of recurrent pancreatitis, which, at least in some cases, may be related to an underlying primary or idiopathic hyperlipidemia.

Hypercholesterolemia may result in atherosclerosis and corneal arcus. Dogs, unlike humans, appear to be highly resistant to the development of atherosclerosis; however, atherosclerosis has been observed in beagles with naturally occurring hypothyroidism. Corneal arcus refers to arclike patterns of lipid deposition in the cornea and has also only been reported in hypothyroid dogs. Although the lipid deposition became less dense with thyroid hormone supplementation, it did not resolve.

Effect on Serum Biochemistries

Hyperlipemia interferes with many serum biochemical tests. Most notably, it produces a falsely low estimate of the serum sodium concentration (pseudohyponatremia). Lipids and water exist in separate phases in the circulation. When the lipid phase is appreciably increased, as in hyperlipidemia, the aqueous sodium concentration remains normal, but the sodium concentration expressed as milliequivalents per total volume of serum (which now contains a large nonaqueous phase) will be low. Potassium concentrations will also be low. Values for serum bilirubin, total protein, albumin, calcium, phosphorus, and glucose will be falsely increased. Depending on the method employed, amylase levels may be falsely low, an especially important consideration in a patient in which pancreatitis is suspected. There is also a tendency for *in vitro* hemolysis to occur in lipemic serum. The degree of biochemical abnormalities present will depend on the severity of the lipemia.

TREATMENT

In most secondary hyperlipoproteinemias, the first step is to treat the underlying disorder. In some instances, lowering of lipid levels may be facilitated by modifying the diet. If obesity is present, weight reduction may also be of benefit.

There is very little information available on the treatment of canine idiopathic hyperlipoproteinemias. This, in part, reflects the lack of characterization of the underlying defects for these lipid abnormalities. Dietary alterations and the use of lipid-lowering drugs are two modes of therapy that may be of value in the management of idiopathic hyperlipoproteinemia in dogs.

Since hypertriglyceridemia appears to be the major abnormality associated with idiopathic lipid disorders of dogs, therapy should be directed at lowering serum triglyceride levels by changing the fat content of the diet. This can be accomplished by feeding low-fat diets such as Prescription Diet r/d (Hill's Pet Products). Such low-fat diets will reduce serum triglyceride levels and cause clearing of the serum in many miniature schnauzers with idiopathic hyperlipoproteinemia. If concurrent hyperchylomicronemia is noted, medium-chain triglycerides (MCTs), which contain fatty acids with no more than 10 carbons, may also be beneficial, since they provide calories without promoting triglyceride and chylomicron synthesis by the intestine. MCTs are commercially available as MCT Oil (Mead Johnson) and should be administered at the dosage of 0.5 ml/kg/day. Since MCT Oil does not provide essential fatty acids, a small amount of vegetable oil should also be given. Alternatively, Portagen (Mead Johnson), a powdered preparation with both MCT and corn oil, can be used in cases of hyperchylomicronemia.

The drugs most commonly used to decrease serum triglyceride levels in human patients include clofibrate (Atromid-S, Ayerst), gemfibrozil (Lopid, Parke-Davis), and niacin. Clofibrate and gemfibrozil reduce plasma VLDLs presumably by decreasing hepatic synthesis. Niacin, one of the B vitamins, lowers both triglycerides (VLDLs) and cholesterol (LDLs). At present, these drugs cannot be recommended for use in dogs until their safety and efficacy have been further established.

References and Supplemental Reading

Consensus Conference: Treatment of Hypertriglyceridemia. J.A.M.A. 251:1196, 1984.

Crispin, S. M., and Barnett, K. C.: Arcus lipoides (corneae secondary to hypothyroidism in the Alsatian). J. Small Anim. Pract. 19:127, 1978.

Ford, R.: *Clinical Application of Serum Lipid Profiles in the Dog.* College Station, Texas: Gaines Veterinary Symposium, 1977, pp. 12–16.

Havel, R. J., Goldstein, J. L., and Brown, M. S.: Lipoproteins and lipid transport. *In* Bondy, P. K., and Rosenburg, L. E. (eds.): *Metabolic Control and Disease,* 8th ed. Philadelphia: W.B. Saunders, 1980, pp. 393–494.

Mahley, R. W., and Weisgraber, K. H.: Canine lipoprotein and atherosclerosis. I. Isolation and characterization of plasma lipoproteins from control dogs. Circ. Res. 35:713, 1974.

Manning, P. J.: Thyroid gland and arterial lesions of beagles with familial hypothyroidism and hyperlipoproteinemia. Am. J. Vet. Res. 40:820, 1979.

Olin, D. D., Rogers, W. A., and MacMillan, A. D.: Lipid-laden aqueous humor associated with anterior uveitis and concurrent hyperlipemia in two dogs. J.A.V.M.A. 168:861, 1976.

Rogers, W. A.: Lipemia in the dog. Vet. Clin. North Am. 7:637, 1977.

Rogers, W. A., Donovan, E. F., and Kociba, G. J.: Idiopathic hyperlipoproteinemia in dogs. J.A.V.M.A. 166:1087, 1975.

Rogers, W. A., Donovan, E. F., and Kociba, G. J.: Lipids and lipoproteins in normal dogs and dogs with secondary hyperlipoproteinemia. J.A.V.M.A. 166:1092, 1975.

Sloan, R. W.: Hyperlipemia. Am. Fam. Physician 28:171, 1983.

Section 12

INFECTIOUS DISEASES

FREDRIC W. SCOTT, D.V.M.
Consulting Editor

***Additional Pertinent Information Found in* Current Veterinary Therapy VIII:**

Attleberger, M. H.: Actinomycosis, Nocardiosis, and Dermatophilosis, p. 1184.
Attleberger, M. H.: Practical Diagnostic Procedures for Mycotic Diseases, p. 1157.
Attleberger, M. H.: Subcutaneous and Opportunistic Mycoses, p. 1177.
Attleberger, M. H.: Systemic Mycoses, p. 1180.
Baldwin, S.: Feline Enteric Viruses, p. 1168.
Fowler, M. H.: Immunoprophylaxis in Nondomestic Carnivores, p. 1129.
Pollock, R. V. H.: Canine Viral Enteritis, p. 1164.
Shin, S. J., and McDonough, P. L.: Practical Diagnostic Procedures for Bacterial Diseases, p. 1148.
Weiss, R. C.: Practical Diagnostic Procedures for Viral Diseases, p. 1143.

UNIFYING CONCEPTS OF FELINE LEUKEMIA VIRUS INFECTION

GARY L. COCKERELL, D.V.M.*
Ithaca, New York

Feline leukemia virus (FeLV) represents a common, serious infection in cats and a common problem for interpretation and handling by clinical veterinarians and for decision-making by cat owners. Over the past several years we have learned a great deal more about the pathogenesis of this infection, have recognized the diverse nature of diseases associated with the virus, and have begun to formulate methods for its treatment and prevention. It is pertinent, therefore, to review some of the basic premises of FeLV infection in the context of more recent findings. More in-depth articles on specific aspects of FeLV infection are also present in this edition and are referred to in the following text.

PATHOGENESIS AND FREQUENCY OF INFECTION

A thorough understanding of the pathogenesis of FeLV infection is essential in order that the veterinarian make sound recommendations on all aspects of the cat that is exposed to or infected by FeLV. After FeLV is inhaled or ingested (the usual natural routes of exposure), the virus first replicates locally in oropharyngeal lymphoid tissue. This is quickly followed by a transient mononuclear leukocyte–associated viremia that serves to distribute the virus to systemic lymphoid tissue, where it undergoes additional replication. The infection then spreads to bone marrow precursor cells and intestinal crypt epithelium. Finally, infected neutrophils and platelets emanate from the bone marrow, persistent viremia is established, mucosal and glandular epithelium become infected, and virus is excreted.

FeLV is readily shed from infected cats; it occurs principally in the saliva, but lesser amounts of virus are present in the urine, feces, and other body excretions or secretions. Relatively prolonged and close contact between infected and uninfected cats, however, is required for effective viral transmission and is most likely to occur under conditions of close intermingling, when animals share water, feed, and litter pans and groom each other. Distant aerosol transmission is not an important vector, since infected and uninfected cats can be maintained in the same household as long as they are physically separated and there is no direct transfer of infectious material by the handlers (via clothing or footwear) to the uninfected cats. Less frequent means of infection of kittens include *in utero* transfer of virus across the placenta or ingestion of FeLV excreted in colostrum and milk from infected queens. FeLV is very labile in the environment, dies within several hours after desiccation, and is easily destroyed by most routine household detergents and disinfectants.

Under conditions of limited or unknown exposure to FeLV, as many as 70 per cent of healthy cats show evidence of previous infection by the presence of serum antibodies either against virion antigens or FOCMA (feline oncornavirus-associated cell membrane antigen). These cats undergo the transient viremia stage and may even develop infection of bone marrow precursor cells and intestinal crypt epithelium but thereafter mount an effective humoral immune response, and the infection becomes self-limiting after several days to weeks. The infection progresses to the essentially irreversible bone marrow stage of infection with circulating mature FeLV-infected leukocytes and platelets in less than 2 per cent of cats under similar conditions; these cats are persistently viremic and susceptible to the development of FeLV-related disease. This situation changes dramatically in FeLV-exposed multicat households, where continued exposure to the virus results in 30 to 50 per cent of the cats becoming persistently viremic. Important modifying factors under both conditions include dose and duration of virus exposure, age of the cat (young kittens are more susceptible), immunocompetence, and poorly

*Present address: Department of Pathology, College of Veterinary Medicine and Biomedical Sciences, Colorado State University, Fort Collins, Colorado.

defined factors in the genetic susceptibility of the cat.

METHODS OF DETECTION AND INTERPRETATION OF RESULTS

The two most common methods in use for the direct detection of FeLV are an indirect fluorescent antibody test (IFAT), which demonstrates viral protein antigen (p27) in leukocytes or platelets in fixed blood smears, and an enzyme-linked immunosorbent assay (ELISA), which demonstrates free viral protein antigen (p27) in serum. In addition, serum can be analyzed for the presence of anti-FeLV or anti-FOCMA antibodies to demonstrate previous exposure to the virus. These latter tests, as well as techniques for direct isolation of FeLV, are more laborious or require specialized reagents and techniques, and they are usually applied only in an experimental setting (see article entitled Immunodiagnosis of Feline Leukemia Virus Infection).

A positive IFAT indicates that the FeLV infection has reached the bone marrow; these cats are usually also ELISA-positive. However, IFAT-positive, ELISA-negative cases may rarely occur, possibly as a result of viral reactivation (see Latency, below). The opposite situation—an ELISA-positive, IFAT-negative result—may occur during the incubation period of the disease, when virus is released into the circulation prior to reaching the bone marrow; if an efficient immune response is made, the ELISA result will revert to negative, whereas if the infection progresses, the ELISA will remain positive and the IFAT will also become positive. It is interesting that a certain group of cats may remain repeatedly ELISA-positive, IFAT-negative, indicating a persistent source of infection without circulating virus-expressing neutrophils or platelets. The biologic significance of this type of FeLV infection, including the eventual development of the disease and its role as a source of infectious virus for other cats, remains unknown.

A positive IFAT or ELISA indicates that a current FeLV infection exists and should generally be equated with viremia and active shedding of virus, but it does not indicate the current health or disease status of the infected cat. A positive result may be obtained from healthy cats or those with a variety of neoplastic or non-neoplastic diseases. It is difficult to render a prognosis on the basis of a single positive test, especially with the ELISA, and positive cats should be retested at 1- to 3-month intervals. Although a small number of persistently viremic cats can remain healthy (while continuing to shed virus) for years, less than 5 per cent of cats that remain ELISA- or IFAT-positive with repeated testing are able to reject the virus, and up to 80 per cent will succumb to a FeLV-related disease within 3.5 years.

FeLV-RELATED DISEASES

The original impetus for the study of FeLV, and indeed its appellation, came from its association with lymphoid (and also myeloproliferative) malignancies. Approximately 70 per cent of cats with lymphoid tumors, usually solid tissue lymphosarcomas, are actively infected with FeLV. There is additional epidemiologic and other evidence that the remaining 30 per cent of cases are associated with past exposure to FeLV, suggesting that even these FeLV-negative cases are etiologically related to FeLV.

Besides these classic oncogenic effects of FeLV, the virus has more recently been associated with a wide variety of non-neoplastic diseases. These non-oncogenic manifestations of FeLV are related to its ability to infect many different types of rapidly dividing cells or to interfere with normal immunological reactivity, thereby inducing a severe immunosuppression. (See the articles Feline Acquired Immunodeficiency Syndrome (FAIDS) Induced by the Feline Leukemia Virus, and Hematologic Consequences of Feline Leukemia Virus Infection.) These diseases include nonregenerative anemia, a panleukopenia-like enteric syndrome, premature thymic involution, reproductive problems (such as fetal resorptions, abortions and infertility), and increased susceptibility to secondary diseases such as toxoplasmosis, hemobartonellosis, feline infectious peritonitis, chronic stomatitis, recurrent abscesses and nonhealing skin lesions, and chronic upper respiratory disease. Characteristically, these diseases, many of which may be of minimal medical significance in normal cats, are difficult to resolve with treatment and terminate fatally in FeLV-infected cats. More FeLV-infected cats are presented clinically and die as a result of these nononcogenic manifestations of FeLV than die of lymphosarcoma. The immunologic deficits and resultant secondary diseases in FeLV-infected cats share many biologic similarities to acquired immune deficiency syndrome (AIDS) in humans. There is, however, no known association of FeLV-infection in cats with the human AIDS condition or any other disease in humans.

LATENCY

The potent anti-viral or anti-FOCMA antibody titers frequently observed in healthy FeLV-negative cats have been interpreted as the result of an early immune-mediated abrogation of the viral infection prior to the establishment of bone marrow infection and persistent viremia. Recent findings, however, suggest that FeLV may not be totally eliminated from these cats, but generally remain in an unexpressed form in certain cells within bone marrow and lymph nodes. Specifically, it has been possible to reactivate virus expression from as many as 80 per cent of these FeLV-negative cats either by culturing their bone marrow or lymph node cells *in vitro* or by treating the cats with corticosteroids *in vivo*. Since these cats usually have high antibody titers, reactivated viral antigen released into the circulation may form antigen-antibody complexes and be removed by phagocytosis to extravascular tissue, thereby explaining the rare IFA-positive, ELISA-negative cases that are sometimes observed. It has also been possible to reactivate FeLV from bone marrow cells but not tumor cells of at least some cats with FeLV-negative lymphosarcoma, thereby providing additional evidence that the virus is etiologically involved in the development of these tumors.

To date, studies on the latency and reactivation of FeLV have been conducted primarily under experimental conditions, and it is difficult to judge the true clinical significance of this phenomenon. However, the experimental reactivation of FeLV with corticosteroids, which are commonly used clinically, suggests that a similar event could occur in a clinical setting (although the doses of corticosteroids used experimentally have been higher than common therapeutic doses). Further, the natural release of endogenous glucocorticoids associated with common stressful situations in a cat's life, such as changes in ownership or nutrition, parturition, fighting, surgery, or intercurrent disease, must be considered as a potential cause of FeLV reactivation in previously FeLV-exposed cats. Some cats with reactivated FeLV infections will revert to FeLV-negative status when steroid treatment is stopped, but the eventual development of disease in cats experiencing reactivated infections has been incompletely studied. Other results suggest that latent FeLV infections disappear and that virus can no longer be reactivated 6 to 8 months after the occurrence of a transient viremia. Cats with FeLV infections that can be reactivated do not appear to be highly infectious sources of virus for other cats, but few cases have been studied. It seems certain that not all FeLV-exposed but FeLV-negative cats are truly virus-free, but our knowledge of viral latency is too limited at this point to make further conclusions about these cats.

***Table 1.** VMTH Policy for Chemically Inactivated FeLV Vaccine (Leukocell)*

1. *Prior to or at time of first vaccination:* Cat should be tested for FeLV (ELISA). Ideally, the test should be done prior to the first vaccination; alternatively, a blood sample for the test may be taken at the time of the first vaccination.
2. *Vaccinate:* Show cats, shelter cats, negative cats going into multiple-cat households, outdoor cats, cats in multiple-cat households with mobile population.
3. *Give:* Three IM injections (local or systemic reactions may occur)
   (1) at 9 weeks or older
   (2) 3 weeks later
   (3) 3 months later
   Give annual booster thereafter.
4. *Other concerns:* If initial blood test is positive, either do not vaccinate or discontinue vaccination program and retest in one (1) month. (Also, do not vaccinate cats that are pregnant, blood donors, isolated cats in single-cat households).
   (a) If second test is negative, the cat has experienced a transient viremia and may now be naturally immune; however, vaccination should be initiated or resumed to further boost immunity.
   (b) If second test is positive, cat is persistently viremic and should be handled accordingly. Vaccination of positive cats has neither detrimental nor beneficial effects.

Vaccination against FeLV can proceed simultaneously with accepted vaccination regimens against other feline diseases such as panleukopenia, viral rhinotracheitis, caliciviral disease, pneumonitis, and rabies.

TREATMENT AND PROPHYLAXIS

Treatment of FeLV-infected cats is symptomatic and directed toward general medical support and alleviation of clinical signs. It is imperative that owners be informed that such treatment is palliative, that there is no readily available and reliable treatment to resolve the underlying FeLV infection, and that infected cats continue to shed virus during treatment. Effective chemotherapeutic regimens and surgical procedures have been developed for the neoplastic effects of FeLV, and general clinical improvement can often be achieved for many of the nononcogenic manifestations, but in the face of a persistent viremia, relapses almost invariably occur with the same or another FeLV-related disease. Recurrence of neoplastic disease may be due to incomplete elimination of the original tumor cells and their subsequent regrowth, the development of tumor clones resistant to chemotherapy, or additional foci of newly transformed cells. Treatment of FeLV-immunosuppressed cats can be particularly frustrating since immune defense mechanisms are crippled and normally effective antibiotic therapy for secondary infectious diseases results in incomplete clearing of microorganisms or prompt return of clinical signs after cessation of therapy.

Several novel forms of experimental therapy for FeLV-induced lymphoid tumors in cats have recently been described, including plasmapheresis (which may remove circulating immunosuppressive factors such as blocking antibodies or antigen-antibody complexes), administration of normal feline plasma constituents (such as fibronectin), or specific immunotherapy with anti-FeLV or anti-FOCMA antibodies. In some cases, persistent viremias have been reversed and cats have remained free of clinically detectable tumors for months. It will be important to follow these and additional cases for longer periods in order to determine the possible presence of latent virus and to solve a variety of practical considerations before these newer therapeutic modalities can be considered for general clinical use. Overall, the prognosis for FeLV-infected cats remains guarded, depending primarily upon initial presenting signs. The decision of whether or not to treat or even maintain such cats should be based upon a thorough knowledge of the pathobiology of FeLV and the circumstances involved in individual cases.

The first federally licensed FeLV vaccine (Leukocell, Norden Laboratories) became commercially available in January 1985, and it provides for the first time the possibility of preventing FeLV infection by any practical means other than environmental isolation of susceptible cats. Since little information on this product, as finally prepared for clinical use, has appeared in the scientific literature, the following information is based principally upon data made available by the manufacturer.

Leukocell is a subunit vaccine consisting of soluble antigens, including a virion glycoprotein envelope antigen (gp70) and FOCMA, to induce both a virus neutralizing (anti-gp70) and anti-FOCMA immune response. These antigens are harvested from the supernatant of a FeLV-infected and transformed lymphoblastoid cell line maintained in tissue culture and are then chemically inactivated. The vaccine is free of infectious FeLV, as evidenced by failure to induce viremia in vaccinated cats when administered at 50 times the recommended dose and failure to induce transformed foci in susceptible cells *in vitro*. The final product is compounded with a combined adjuvant and is indicated for intramuscular administration.

Norden Laboratories have reported efficacy studies in vaccinated cats experimentally challenged with a large inoculum of FeLV in conjunction with corticosteroid treatment to enhance susceptibility to virus. Approximately 80 per cent of vaccinated cats experienced an asymptomatic transient viremia lasting for up to 2 months after challenge, and 20 per cent (five out of 25) of these cats remained persistently viremic and died of a FeLV-related disease or lymphosarcoma during the 2-year period of observation. By comparison, 70 per cent (seven out of ten) of nonvaccinated controls that received a similar challenge became persistently viremic and died during the same period. This is undoubtedly a more serious FeLV exposure than cats experience under natural environmental conditions, but little data are currently available from controlled clinical trials when vaccinated cats are returned to FeLV-infected, multicat households. These trials, published earlier by the research group that discovered the vaccine, used an adjuvant and vaccination regimen that differed from those of the final commercial product; these data therefore are not directly applicable. Vaccinated but nonchallenged cats did not suffer the immunosuppressive consequences of virulent FeLV infection, but approximately 13 per cent developed adverse reactions (including local pain and discomfort at the vaccination site) or transient systemic reactions such as lethargy and fever.

The efficacy of Leukocell and circumstances under which vaccination should or should not be recommended in natural settings will become more clear in the next several years as results of vaccination of cats in household and cattery populations become known. To aid in the collection and interpretation of these results, the working policy shown in Table 1 has been developed for the use of Leukocell at the Veterinary Medical Teaching Hospital (VMTH) at the New York State College of Veterinary Medicine.

Several points within this vaccination policy deserve additional consideration. First, in view of the limited information on vaccine efficacy in the field, it is considered imperative to test for the presence of FeLV prior to vaccination. In the case of a cat of unknown FeLV status that was vaccinated and subsequently found to be FeLV-positive, it would be impossible to know whether the cat was viremic prior to vaccination, or the vaccine induced the viremia, or the vaccine failed to prevent infection by FeLV exposure after vaccination. Second, the ELISA is recommended as the prevaccination screening test for FeLV because it can detect cats in the incubation period of the infection prior to a positive IFAT. Third, vaccination should be reserved for those cases in which there is a high risk of exposure to FeLV rather than as a standard immunization similar to those that provide protection against other common but more easily transmitted feline diseases. Finally, vaccination should add to, but not replace, existing test and removal or isolation programs for FeLV-infected cats.

References and Supplemental Reading

Hardy, W. D., Jr.: Immunopathology induced by the feline leukemia virus. Springer Semin. Immunopathol. 5:75, 1982.

Hayes, A. A., MacEwen, E. G., Matus, R. E., et al.: Antileukemic activity of plasma cryoprecipitate therapy in the cat. *In* Hardy, W. D., Jr., Essex, M., and McClelland, A. J. (eds.): *Feline Leukemia Virus.* New York: Elsevier North Holland, 1980, pp. 245–252.

Jones, F. R., Yoshida, L. H., Ladiges, W. C., et al.: Treatment of feline lymphosarcoma by extracorporeal immunosorption. *In* Hardy, W. D., Jr., Essex, M., and McClelland, A. J. (eds.): *Feline Leukemia Virus.* New York: Elsevier/North Holland, 1980, pp. 235–244.

FELINE INFECTIOUS PERITONITIS AND OTHER FELINE CORONAVIRUSES

FREDRIC W. SCOTT, D.V.M.
Ithaca, New York

The feline coronaviruses cause some of the most frustrating feline infectious diseases that the small animal practitioner encounters. These viruses produce disease by unique methods, many are difficult to isolate or diagnose in the laboratory, the disease often is difficult to accurately diagnose clinically, there is no effective treatment or vaccine, and generalized clinical disease usually results in death of the cat. There is little wonder that clinicians feel totally frustrated in attempting to deal with some of these viruses effectively.

ETIOLOGY

A number of coronaviruses can infect cats. The most important of these viruses are those that cause feline infectious peritonitis (FIP). Although much more research is needed for clarification, it appears that there are at least two general types of feline infectious peritonitis viruses (FIPV). Type 1 is very difficult to isolate in cell culture and produces a severe, usually fatal disease. Type 2 is a common enteric virus similar to canine coronavirus. It is easily isolated from infected cats and generally produces a mild or subclinical disease. However, on occasion type 2 can produce fatal FIP. Evidence is contradictory concerning the antigenic relationship of type 1 and type 2 FIPV. Certainly these two types behave differently in cell cultures, but both can produce clinical and fatal FIP. Some cats with FIP do not develop detectable antibody titers to the standard commercial feline coronavirus antibody tests, and this therefore lends credence to the concept of multiple types of FIPV.

The feline enteric coronavirus (FECV) was isolated by Pedersen and coworkers (1981) from kittens with mild enteritis. Morphologically and antigenically it is indistinguishable from FIPV. The question then must be asked, Is this a distinct coronavirus of cats or merely an intestinally adapted strain of FIPV? There are arguments for both positions, and only further research will determine the true relationship.

At least three other coronaviruses of the FIPV antigenic cluster group have been shown, at least experimentally, to infect cats. These infections result in shedding of virus from the respiratory tract, oropharynx, or the gastrointestinal tract and seroconversion as evidenced by the coronavirus antibody tests. Transmissible gastroenteritis virus (TGEV) of swine results in asymptomatic infections of cats that shed virus for several weeks. Canine coronavirus (CCV) produces asymptomatic infections and virus shed from the oropharynx; a similar asymptomatic infection occurs with human bronchitis coronavirus serotype 229E. Both CCV and 229E produce seroconversion in the coronavirus antibody tests; however, neither creates sensitization in the cat or produces protection against virulent FIPV exposure.

HOST RANGE

In addition to infecting the domestic cat, FIPV naturally infects many if not all species of the family Felidae. It produces devastating effects in breeding colonies of cheetahs.

From time to time there occurs an FIP-like disease in other species of animals. To date none of these cases has been shown to be associated with FIPV.

PATHOGENESIS OF FIPV INFECTION

The generalized infection of cats with FIPV is antibody-mediated and complement-dependent. Thus, previous exposure and antibody formation to a nonvirulent or cross-sensitizing strain of FIPV or other coronavirus may not produce protection but instead a state of enhanced susceptibility.

In the initial infection, FIPV apparently replicates in the epithelial cells of the oropharynx or upper respiratory tract. Infection is generally subclinical or may produce mild respiratory signs. Once antibodies appear, there is aggregation of viral-antibody complexes and subsequent uptake by and infection of monocytes. The exact mechanism of this immune enhancement of viral uptake into the mononuclear cells is not understood, but it is assumed that the Fc portions of the gamma globulins bind to the mononuclear cells; this enables attachment and, therefore, uptake of the virus. The virus is then transmitted throughout the body in the monocytes and enters the perivascular areas after the monocytes attach to and migrate through the walls of the veins. The resulting perivasculitis is the initial lesion observed in histopathologic sections of clinical FIP. This lesion is an intense, destructive, inflammatory process that may damage the vessel walls in such a way that the protein-rich serum can escape from the vessels into the body cavities (e.g., peritoneum or pleural cavity). This produces the characteristic protein-rich fluid of high specific gravity that is present in the effusive form of FIP.

In most infections there is little or no fluid accumulation; instead, multiple perivascular pyogranulomatous inflammations, characteristic of the noneffusive form of FIP, occur.

In both the effusive and noneffusive forms of FIP, the tissue reactions continue unabated and almost invariably result in death within a few days or a few weeks.

CLINICAL SIGNS

Infection of cats with the enteric coronavirus may result in a mild enteritis of a few days' duration that generally has no severe adverse consequences. There are strains of FIPV that produce as their main early signs a somewhat severe gastrointestinal involvement with enlarged and palpable mesenteric lymph nodes. Cases of these strains usually progress into disseminated fatal FIP.

In "primary" infection with FIPV, some cats may develop mild upper respiratory clinical signs, characterized by sneezing and watery discharges of the eyes and nose. It appears that most of these "primary" infections are transient; the cats recover but may be persistently infected and shedders of virus. There is some indication that some of the so-called chronic upper respiratory problems frequently encountered in multiple-cat households and catteries may be associated with one or more of these coronaviruses.

In those cats in which a disseminated FIP results, the onset of clinical disease is usually quite insidious, with a gradual onset of fever, anorexia, weight loss, rough hair coat, and possibly fluid accumulation in the peritoneal or thoracic cavities or both areas. The fever is persistent and nonresponsive to antibiotic therapy.

Clinical signs resulting from specific lesions in various parts of the body may occur. These include central nervous signs, ocular involvement, and enteritis. Neurologic signs can vary widely, depending on the specific site of the lesions. Chronic ocular involvement is not uncommon and should be specifically looked for in any cat with a persistent fever of unknown origin. Other organs of involvement, and the corresponding clinical signs associated with disease of those organs, include the liver, pancreas, and kidney. FIP is probably the most common cause of liver disease in cats.

FIPV may be associated with reproductive failure and kitten mortality, although this has not been proved.

DIAGNOSIS OF FIP

Some cases of FIP can be diagnosed relatively easily, based upon the presenting clinical signs, fluid analysis, and clinical pathologic findings. However, other cases provide a real diagnostic challenge, and some noneffusive FIP cases will defy accurate antemortem diagnosis.

If fluid is present, its color (light amber or straw-colored), consistency (sticky, egg-white), and specific gravity (generally greater than 1.018) should be noted.

Serum chemistries usually reveal elevated levels of total serum proteins and liver enzymes. Results of total and differential blood counts are quite variable and cannot be used as diagnostic signs for FIP.

Several types of serum antibody tests for coronavirus are available, but unfortunately none of these alone is diagnostic of FIP. There is considerable need for an accurate assay for detection of specific FIP virus in the blood of cats. Until such a test is available, clinicians should continue to use the coronavirus antibody assay as an aid—but only an aid—in diagnosis of FIP.

Coronavirus antibody assays include viral neutralization (VN), indirect immunofluorescence (IFA), and various enzyme-linked immunosorbent assay (ELISA) tests, including kit tests and the KELA, or kinetics ELISA, test. Various antigens used in these tests include frozen sections of liver from FIP-infected cats and virus from TGE-, CCV-, or FIPV-infected cell cultures. All of these tests when positive merely indicate that the animal had a previous infection with a cornavirus of the FIP antigenic group of viruses; the agent of infection could possibly be but is not necessarily FIPV.

The height of the titer has some relevance in clinically ill cats, since clinical cases of FIP tend to have titers of serum anticoronavirus antibody of 1:400 or higher. However, it should be clearly understood that not all clinical cases of FIP have high titers; in fact, there have been numerous well-documented clinical cases of FIP in which the coronavirus antibody titer was either negative or very low. If this conflict does occur, one should ignore the antibody titer and rely upon the clinical diagnosis if the signs and clinical pathologic findings indicate FIP.

Some laboratories have stated that the only reliable means of diagnosing FIP in the laboratory is by detecting a rising antibody titer over a few days or weeks. In our experience, some cases may indeed have a rising titer, but more often there is a declining antibody titer, especially in the terminal stages of the disease. We believe that this is due to an aggregation of virus and antibody and a removal of the aggregates from the circulation.

It appears that there may be more than one serotype of FIP virus, which may account for negative or low antibody titers in some cats with clinical FIP.

One should also be aware that recent vaccination with any vaccine of cell-culture origin may produce a transient (up to 3 months) false-positive coronavirus antibody test. Cats develop antibodies against bovine serum that may be present in the vaccine. Bovine serum is commonly used in cell cultures as a nutrient for growing both the vaccine viruses and the antigen used in the antibody tests. A low-positive antibody test against coronaviruses should be viewed with some caution when it occurs within 3 months after vaccination with any of the commercially available vaccines.

At present, the only definitive method for the laboratory diagnosis of FIP is by histopathologic examination of biopsy or necropsy tissues.

TREATMENT

Undoubtedly many mild or subclinical cases of FIP occur. These cats require either no treatment or only general symptomatic treatment.

Cases of FIP that are restricted to the eyes generally respond relatively well to local (subconjunctival) treatment with corticosteroids. These cats often have extremely high antibody titers, and these titers will gradually decline as the treatment progresses.

Once general or disseminated infection and clinical signs develop, it is generally accepted that treatment is not going to produce a cure or significant remission. Most of these animals will progress through the course of the disease and ultimately die. The prognosis must be very guarded once an accurate diagnosis of disseminated effusive or noneffusive FIP has been made.

Various treatment regimens have been advocated for FIP from time to time, but none of these as yet has been shown to produce consistent beneficial results. Antibiotics have no effect on the virus, and the only rationale for their use is an attempt to prevent secondary bacterial infection. However, bacterial infection rarely plays any role in the outcome of FIP.

The use of various anti-inflammatory or chemotoxic drugs has been advocated because FIP is an immune-mediated disease that causes an increase in the production of gamma globulin; therefore, it is hypothesized that if overproduction of antibody could be reduced, the cat might be able to overcome the infection. There are little if any data to support this hypothesis. In fact, it is commonly accepted that the immunosuppressive viral infection of feline leukemia predisposes cats to develop clinical FIP. Therefore, one must question the value of immunosuppressive drugs in treating FIP.

There is some indication that the use of certain immunomodulators early in the disease may have some beneficial results. Unfortunately, there are no controlled studies in which these immunomodulators have been evaluated and shown to be beneficial against clinical FIP.

There are no antiviral compounds that have been shown to have antiviral activity against FIPV. Interferon treatment for FIP has not been reported as of this writing.

IMMUNIZATION AGAINST FIP

As of this writing there is no vaccine available to protect cats against FIP. Studies have been underway for several years to develop such a vaccine, but because of the sensitization without protection that is produced by the antibody response, all attempts to date to develop an effective vaccine have been fruitless.

Attempts to use other cross-reacting coronaviruses in the FIP antigenic group (such as TGEV, CCV, and human bronchitis virus 229E) as heterotypic vaccines have failed to produce protection against FIP virus challenge, even though the resulting vaccine antibody titers were not sensitizing.

There have been implications that successful vaccination against feline leukemia virus (FeLV) will greatly reduce or eliminate clinical FIP. It is the view of the author that while there probably will be some reduction of clinical FIP if the cat population is adequately immunized against FeLV, FeLV immunization will not eliminate or even substantially reduce the problem of FIP. It is true that the early clinical reports of FIP showed that up to 50 per cent of clinical cases of FIP were also positive for FeLV. These were generally effusive cases. In the author's experience in recent years, the incidence of FeLV-positive cases of FIP is far below 50 per cent. Many severe outbreaks of FIP have occurred in catteries where FeLV has not occurred.

References and Supplemental Reading

Barlough, J. E.: Serodiagnostic aids and management practice for feline retrovirus and coronavirus infections. Vet. Clin. North Am. [Small Anim Pract.] 14:955, 1984.

Barlough, J. E., and Weiss, R. C.: Feline infectious peritonitis. *In* Kirk, R. W., ed.: *Current Veterinary Therapy VIII*. Philadelphia: W. B. Saunders, 1983, pp. 1186–1193.

Horsinek, M. C., and Osterhaus, A. D. M. E.: The virology and pathogenesis of feline infectious peritonitis. Arch. Virol. 59:1, 1979.

Ott, R. L.: Feline infectious peritonitis. *In* Pratt, P. W. (ed.): *Feline Medicine*. Santa Barbara: American Veterinary Publications, 1983, pp. 116–123.

Pedersen, N. C.: Feline infectious peritonitis and feline enteric coronavirus infections. Feline Pract. 13(4):13, and 13(5):5, 1983.

Pedersen, N. C., Boyle, J. F., Floyd, K., et al.: An enteric coronavirus infection of cats and its relationship to feline infectious peritonitis. Am. J. Vet Res. 42:368, 1981.

Weiss, R. C., and Scott, F. W.: Laboratory diagnosis of feline infectious peritonitis. Feline Pract. 10(2):16, 1980.

Weiss, R. C., and Scott, F. W.: Pathogenesis of feline infectious peritonitis: Nature and development of viremia. Am. J. Vet Res. 42:382, 1981.

CALICIVIRUS INFECTIONS OF SMALL ANIMALS

JEFFREY E. BARLOUGH, D.V.M.

Corvallis, Oregon

The caliciviruses are a group of small (35 to 40 nm), nonenveloped, single-strand RNA viruses with an unusual surface structure characterized by geometrically arranged cup-shaped depressions (Latin *calix*, cup or goblet). Although classified originally as a provisional genus of the family Picornaviridae, the caliciviruses possess a number of unique features of polypeptide composition, genome structure, and replication strategy that have prompted their reclassification as a separate virus family, the Caliciviridae (Schaffer et al., 1980). A growing body of evidence now supports the concept that the spectrum of infectivity and pathogenicity of the caliciviruses is unusually broad, encompassing a constellation of host species and disease manifestations (Smith, 1983). To date, caliciviruses have been isolated from a wide variety of mammalian species, including pigs, pinnipeds (California sea lions, northern fur seals, northern elephant seals, walruses), dolphins, mink, dogs, cats, cattle, subhuman primates, and humans (Barlough et al., in press). In addition, caliciviruses or "calicilike" viruses have been recovered from ocean fish, reptiles, amphibians, and insects. Vesiculation, ulceration, respiratory disease, gastroenteritis, encephalitis, and reproductive disorders are among the many clinical disease entities to which caliciviruses have been linked in a number of animal species.

Caliciviruses are relatively heat-stable agents and are quite insensitive to the action of most lipid solvents and quaternary ammonium compounds (Schaffer et al., 1980). Under favorable environmental conditions, virion infectivity can be retained outside the host for 8 to 10 days. However, viral particles are destroyed by formaldehyde, most phenolic disinfectants, and sodium hypochlorite (bleach). For feline caliciviruses (FCVs), household bleach (Clorox) diluted 1:32 in water has been shown to be effective for the rapid inactivation of calicivirus particles (Scott, 1980).

FELINE CALICIVIRUS INFECTIONS

A number of clinical entities associated with FCV infections have been described over the years, and most of these have involved manifestations of respiratory disease. The spectrum of pathogenicity of these caliciviruses is quite wide, ranging from asymptomatic infection with seroconversion to life-threatening pneumonia. Thus, although most FCV isolates appear to belong to a single serotype (Povey, 1974; Kalunda et al., 1975), the variability of individual strains in the production of disease can be striking (Hoover and Kahn, 1973).

Clinical signs of infection with FCVs of low or moderate virulence generally are restricted to the oral cavity, nasal passages, and conjunctiva. The incubation period usually is short (2 to 5 days), and early signs consist of variable degrees of anorexia, pyrexia, and malaise. Profound depression tends to be rare. Mild serous oculonasal discharges frequently develop but, in contrast to feline herpesvirus 1 infection (feline viral rhinotracheitis), coughing and sneezing are minimal and ulcerative keratitis is not seen. Vesicles that rapidly rupture to produce well-defined, ulcerated lesions can be found variably on the surface of the tongue and hard palate, on the nasal philtrum, and, rarely, on the paws. Ulceration without oculonasal involvement may also occur. The course of disease in uncomplicated cases is generally short, and recovery can be expected within 7 to 10 days. Morbidity may be high but mortality is usually low.

Clinical signs of infection with more virulent (pneumotropic) strains of FCV include pyrexia, anorexia, severe depression, and pneumonia (polypnea, dyspnea, moist rales). This form of caliciviral disease can be especially virulent in young kittens, which may show signs suggestive of acute parvovirus infection (feline panleukopenia), including vomiting, diarrhea, profound depression, and sometimes sudden death (Love and Baker, 1972). Morbidity in severe pneumonic caliciviral disease is usually high and mortality may be substantial (up to 100 per cent), especially among very young kittens. Mortality may be especially high when complications due to secondary bacterial pneumonia occur.

Transmission of FCVs and their maintenance in the feline population are accomplished primarily by direct contact with oropharyngeal secretions of diseased animals, by virus persistence (8 to 10 days) in favorable environments and on fomites (litter pans, feeding bowls, toys, blankets, grooming instruments, hands, and clothing), and by persistent excretion of virus by asymptomatic carrier cats. Asymptomatic carriers appear to be widespread in the general feline population. A period of asymptomatic virus excretion apparently is a normal sequela to FCV infection (Wardley and Povey, 1977). Virus is harbored primarily in tonsillar tissue, and, in contrast to the intermittent excretion associated with feline herpesvirus 1 infection, is excreted more or less continuously from the oropharynx and to some extent in feces. Excretion of FCV by some asymptomatic carriers may persist for years (Wardley, 1976). There is some indication that persistent FCV infections may in some cats be associated with either chronic gingivitis or pharyngitis or both conditions (Thompson et al., 1984), which may be especially severe if complicated by secondary bacterial infection or by persistent feline leukemia virus infection.

The clinical diagnosis of FCV disease is made by evaluation of history and presenting signs (e.g., respiratory illness without severe coughing or sneezing, presence of oronasal vesiculation or ulceration). A definitive diagnosis in the living animal is dependent upon isolation in monolayer cell culture of FCV taken from the oropharynx during clinical illness. Actually, isolation of virus is infrequently attempted, except in catteries, where severe, chronic respiratory disease (often complicated by secondary bacterial infections) may be of significant concern. Under such circumstances, isolation of FCV from pulmonary lesions of kittens that have succumbed to pneumonic disease is important in confirming the presence of a virulent, pneumotropic strain of FCV. Postmortem diagnosis in the absence of virus isolation requires histopathologic examination of formalin-fixed lung tissue and immuofluorescent antibody testing of frozen lung sections for caliciviral antigen.

Current treatment regimens for FCV disease, in the absence of effective antiviral therapy, are purely supportive in nature. Animals with mild respiratory signs should be treated as outpatients whenever possible, primarily to prohibit the spread of calicivirus on hospital premises but also to avoid the stress of forced hospitalization on the patient. Administration of a broad-spectrum antibiotic such as ampicillin (20 mg/kg t.i.d. PO for 7 to 10 days) is recommended for control of secondary bacterial infections. Multivitamin supplementation (vitamins A and B-complex, including B_{12}) may be helpful for anorectic patients. Whenever possible, liquid or pediatric preparations and parenteral injections should be given in preference to tablets or capsules, because pharyngitis and lymphoid hyperplasia may make swallowing difficult and painful. Treatment of oral ulcerations usually is not indicated because most of these lesions will resolve spontaneously within a few days. Patients should be maintained in a clean, warm, draft-free environment. Ocular and nasal discharges should be gently cleansed away at frequent intervals. Warm humidification by steam vaporizers is recommended to help loosen accumulated mucus and open clogged airways. In order to encourage them to eat, cats should be provided strongly flavored, aromatic foods (smoked turkey, chicken, bacon, fish), preferably in liquid or paste form for easy swallowing. Human infant food products containing meat can be especially helpful in this regard.

Cases of severe pneumonic caliciviral disease in young kittens may require hospitalization and intensive supportive care. Administration of balanced electrolyte solutions, bronchodilators, and mucolytics and nebulization with oxygen therapy may be required in individual cases. Again, broad-spectrum antibiotics are recommended for control of secondary bacterial infections. Severely debilitated, anorectic patients may require the use of a stomach or pharyngostomy tube. The veterinarian should always remember that severe pneumonic caliciviral disease in young kittens is a potentially life-threatening situation, and owners of affected animals should be counselled accordingly.

Immunization against FCV disease can be accomplished by the use of combination vaccines containing feline herpesvirus 1 and, frequently, feline parvovirus fractions in addition to FCV. Chlamydial immunogens also may be included in some preparations. Currently both modified-live and inactivated FCV vaccines are available. Vaccine-strain FCVs generally are good immunogens, and most vaccinated animals produce significant titers of circulating antibody after exposure. Intranasal FCV vaccines have also been developed that are capable of producing local (secretory) immunity at mucous membrane surfaces as well as systemic immunity. In general, available FCV vaccines, in combination with proper management practices, provide reasonably good protection against FCV disease. Side effects sometimes seen with the intranasal preparations are mild, and they include sneezing and a watery ocular discharge. General recommendations for FCV immunization call for initial inoculation at 8 to 10 weeks of age (all vaccines) and a booster at 12 to 14 weeks (parenteral vaccines only) (Scott, 1983). *Annual re-vaccination is recommended for all animals regardless of the type of vaccine administered and the route of inoculation.* In addition, extra boosters have been recommended for animals at particular risk of stress and FCV exposure (e.g., boarders in catteries or veterinary hospitals, show and stud cats, etc.) (Gaskell and Gaskell, 1980).

Colostral antibody to FCV is detectable often for up to 3 months after birth, and in many cases exposure to FCV during the later stages of maternal antibody decline may actively immunize kittens without producing serious disease (Johnson and Povey, 1984). Under other conditions, however, kittens may develop severe clinical signs. Unfortunately, even kittens with high levels of maternal antibody may develop life-threatening pneumonic caliciviral disease when exposed to a highly virulent, pneumotropic strain. This situation may be frequently encountered in cattery environments, where both stress and levels of exposure to virus can be severe. In addition, conditions of forced crowding may also predispose kittens to development of clinical signs of disease with milder strains of FCV. It is obvious that routine immunization schedules may need modification in situations in which FCV problems such as these are found. One strategy for strengthening protection of young kittens in these cases is to vaccinate with an intranasal preparation at a very early age (even younger than 1 week), and then at regular intervals (every 3 to 4 weeks) afterward until cats are about 4 months of age (Gaskell and Gaskell, 1980; Ott, 1983). Such early mucosal vaccination is designed especially to help provide local immunity at mucous membrane surfaces where penetration by FCV would be expected to occur. Such inoculations should be performed *only* with vaccine preparations licensed for intranasal use. Although it may not be successful in every case, early use of intranasal vaccines in this way has undoubtedly been of benefit in the prevention of many cases of severe caliciviral disease in kittens and thus may be helpful when the threat of disease is great. An alternative approach for protecting kittens is to first rear them with the queen in isolation and then to wean them at an early age (4 to 5 weeks) away from their mother in the event that she is actively excreting virus (Gaskell and Gaskell, 1980). The kittens should be maintained in isolation and then vaccinated at the usual times before they are introduced into the general cattery population. Unfortunately, this may be an impractical procedure for many owners, and the risk of mechanical transmission of such a resistant agent as FCV to the isolated kittens may be substantial.

Caliciviruses also have been associated with several clinical entities in cats other than respiratory disease. In the feline urologic syndrome (FUS), the Manx calicivirus has been postulated as a possible potentiating agent for feline herpesvirus 2 in the induction of obstructive struvite urolithiasis (Fabricant, 1979). However, several additional noninfectious factors also appear to be important in the development of FUS in individual cats, and further studies are required in order to elucidate the exact role of caliciviruses in this disease. Calicivirus isolations have been made also from cats with diarrheal disease (Hoshino et al., 1981). Although several caliciviruses have been implicated as the cause of gastroenteritis in a number of species (including humans), their role, if any, in feline gastrointestinal disease is still unclear. It is uncertain whether the reported isolates represent enteric-adapted viruses or simply FCVs excreted through the gut. Diarrhea associated with FCV-induced respiratory disease has been reported previously (Wardley and Povey, 1977). Infrequently, caliciviruses have been associated with neurologic disease (Love and Baker, 1972; Love, 1975) and with jaundice and abortion (Ellis, 1981). More recently, a transient febrile "limping" syndrome associated with two new strains of FCV has been described (Pedersen et al., 1983). This interesting disorder is characterized clinically by pyrexia, depression, generalized stiffness, and lameness in kittens in the absence of distinctly recognizable histopathologic changes. The course of the illness varies from 2 to 4 days. Of special significance is the observation that one of the two causative FCV strains is not neutralized by FCV vaccine–induced antibody. Such a finding should not be totally surprising, however, considering that in both swine (vesicular exanthema virus) and pinnipeds (San Miguel sea lion virus), multiple calicivirus serotypes are the rule rather than the exception (Smith, 1983; Barlough et al., in press). Hence, the concept of "one FCV serotype, many FCV strains" may soon require revision.

CANINE CALICIVIRUS INFECTIONS

More than 30 years ago, Bankowski and Wood (1953) demonstrated that lingual inoculation of dogs with vesicular exanthema virus of swine produced epithelial erosion and extension at the sites of injection and frequently a slight febrile response. Since that time, relatively little additional information concerning calicivirus infectivity for dogs has been added to the veterinary literature. Recently, however, interesting reports have begun to appear describing natural canine infections with caliciviruses of various types.

Vesiculation and ulceration of the tongue and gingiva of two dogs originating from a single household have been reported (Evermann et al., 1981, 1983). A calicivirus antigenically related to FCV was subsequently isolated from the lesions of one of these dogs. Neither animal had been housed at any time with cats nor had any other known exposure to cats occurred, although both were apparently allowed to run outside for varying periods of time. Thus, the possibility of natural transmission of FCV from cats could not be ruled out entirely, and it seems probable that these cases do indeed represent aberrant infection of dogs with FCV. Additional caliciviruses antigenically similar to FCV have been isolated from two young dogs and a coyote kit with gastrointestinal disease (Evermann et al., 1982). *Salmonella* was also isolated from one of these dogs, and rotavirus antigen was detected in the feces of the other. The etiologic significance of these FCV-like viruses is currently unclear, but without doubt their presence in canids warrants further investigation.

Of great interest is a very recent report by Schaffer and coworkers (1985) that describes the isolation from diarrheic canine feces of a calicivirus antigenically unrelated to any other recognized mammalian calicivirus. This canine calicivirus (CaCV) originated from an adult dog in Tennessee that had bloody diarrhea and neurologic signs. Concurrent infection with canine parvovirus could not be demonstrated. Subsequent serologic studies indicate that CaCV has been relatively widespread in the canine population in Tennessee since at least 1976. However, to date it has not been possible to conclusively link CaCV etiologically with either gastrointestinal or neurologic disease or with any other distinct disease condition in dogs. Another virus with the morphologic appearance of a calicivirus has recently been isolated from vaginal lesions of an adult dog with vesicular vaginitis (Crandell, 1984). Preliminary studies have thus far failed to demonstrate an antigenic relationship between this virus and either FCV or CaCV.

Taken together, these data indicate that at least three immunologic types of calicivirus (one of which is probably FCV) appear to be actively circulating within the current American canine population. Further research obviously will be required before the full spectrum of calicivirus infectivity and pathogenicity in this species can be revealed.

References and Supplemental Reading

Bankowski, R. A., and Wood, M.: Experimental vesicular exanthema in the dog. J.A.V.M.A. 123:115, 1953.

Barlough, J. E., Berry, E. S., Skilling, D. E., et al.: Sea lions, caliciviruses, and the sea. Avian/Exotic Pract., in press.

Crandell, R. A.: Personal communication, 1984.

Ellis, T. M.: Jaundice in a siamese cat with *in utero* feline calicivirus infection. Austral. Vet. J. 57:383, 1981.

Evermann, J. F., Bryan, G. M., and McKeirnan, A. J.: Isolation of a calicivirus from a case of canine glossitis. Canine Pract. 8(2):36, 1981.

Evermann, J. F., Stann, S., DiGiacomo, R. F., et al.: Epizootiologic and diagnostic features of canine diarrheal disease in high and low risk dog populations. Proc. 25th Ann. Meet. Am. Assoc. Vet. Lab. Diagnos. 1982, p. 229.

Evermann, J. F., Smith, A. W., Skilling, D. E., et al.: Ultrastructure of newly recognized caliciviruses of the dog and mink. Arch. Virol. 76:257, 1983.

Fabricant, C. G.: Herpesvirus-induced feline urolithiasis—A review. J. Comp. Immunol. Microbiol. Infect. Dis. 1:121, 1979.

Gaskell, C., and Gaskell, R.: Respiratory diseases of cats. In Pract. 2(6):5, 1980.

Hoover, E. A., and Kahn, D. E.: Lesions produced by feline picornaviruses of different virulence in pathogen-free cats. Vet. Pathol. 10:307, 1973.

Hoshino, Y., Baldwin, C. A., and Scott, F. W.: New insights in gastrointestinal viruses. Cornell Feline Health Center News 2:2, 1981.

Johnson, R. P., and Povey, R. C.: Feline calicivirus infection in kittens borne by cats persistently infected with the virus. Res. Vet. Sci. 37:114, 1984.

Kalunda, M., Lee, K. M., Holmes, D. F., et al.: Serologic classification of feline caliciviruses by plaque-reduction neutralization and immunodiffusion. Am. J. Vet. Res. 36:353, 1975.

Love, D. N.: Feline calicivirus associated with convulsions in a cat. Austral. Pract. 5:29, 1975.

Love, D. N., and Baker, K. D.: Sudden death in kittens associated with a feline picornavirus. Austral. Vet. J. 48:643, 1972.

Ott, R. L.: Feline calicivirus infection. *In* Pratt, P. W. (ed.): *Feline Medicine*. Santa Barbara: American Veterinary Publications, 1983, pp. 97–99.

Pedersen, N. C., Laliberte, L., and Ekman, S.: A transient febrile "limping" syndrome of kittens caused by two different strains of feline calicivirus. Feline Pract. 13(1):26, 1983.

Povey, R. C.: Serological relationships among feline caliciviruses. Infect. Immun. 10:1307, 1974.

Schaffer, F. L., Bachrach, H. L., Brown, F., et al.: Caliciviridae. Intervirology 14:1, 1980.

Schaffer, F. L., Soergel, M. E., Black, J. W., et al.: Characterization of a new calicivirus isolated from feces of a dog. Arch. Virol., 84:181, 1985.

Scott, F. W.: Virucidal disinfectants and feline viruses. Am. J. Vet. Res. 41:410, 1980.

Scott, F. W.: Feline immunization. *In* Kirk, R. W. (ed.): *Current Veterinary Therapy VIII*. Philadelphia: W. B. Saunders, 1983, pp. 1127–1129.

Smith, A. W.: Focus on. . .caliciviral disease. *U.S.D.A. Foreign Animal Disease Report*, no. 11–3, 1983, pp. 8–16.

Thompson, R. R., Wilcox, G. E., Clark, W. T., et al.: Association of calicivirus infection with chronic gingivitis and pharyngitis in cats. J. Small Anim. Pract. 25:207, 1984.

Wardley, R. C.: Feline calicivirus carrier state: A study of the host/virus relationship. Arch. Virol. 52:243, 1976.

Wardley, R. C., and Povey, R. C.: The clinical disease and patterns of excretion associated with three different strains of feline caliciviruses. Res. Vet. Sci. 23:7, 1977.

RABIES

DENNIS R. HOWARD, PH.D.
Manhattan, Kansas

Rabies is an infectious viral disease characterized by encephalitis. The disease affects primarily carnivores and bats, but all warm-blooded animals, including humans, are susceptible. Skunks, foxes, and raccoons are the major carnivore hosts in the United States and remain sources of rabies for dogs and cats.

Dogs and cats are incidental hosts for rabies, and the disease is a result of spillover from other reservoir animals. Epizootics of canine rabies that involve dog-to-dog transmission have occurred along the border of the United States and Mexico.

Canine rabies is the major reservoir in most parts of the world, and dog and cat bites constitute the main source of infection for humans. Since 1966, the only cases of human rabies in the United States that could be attributed directly to canine bites occurred in persons who were exposed to the disease in other countries. One case of human rabies has been attributed to cat exposure since that date. The decreased incidence of rabies in dogs and cats is directly related to the widespread immunization and control measures against the disease.

ETIOLOGY

Rabies virus belongs to the rhabdovirus group. It is approximately 75 by 180 μm in size and has a spiked outer envelope containing a helical RNA nucleocapsid. It is a neutrotropic virus found primarily in nerve tissue and salivary glands, but many studies have shown that rabies virus may be found in any tissue.

The virus is quite labile and easily destroyed by sunlight and heat. It is inactivated with common disinfectants such as 70 per cent ethanol, 0.1 per cent quaternary ammonium compounds, organic iodine compounds, and 5 per cent chlorine bleach.

Rabies viruses were considered to be very closely related antigenically. Recently, techniques have made it possible to differentiate strains of rabies virus by nucleocapsid and glycoprotein antigens. Virus preparations have been shown to be antigenically different when studied by immunoassays with rabies-specific monoclonal antibodies.

Rabies has been reported in several species after they were vaccinated with modified-live virus (MLV) rabies vaccine. Virus isolates from vaccine-induced rabies have been shown to have monoclonal antibody reactivity patterns identical to those of the vaccines administered to dogs, cats, and one fox. Monoclonal antibodies can differentiate MLV rabies vaccines marketed in the United States and can determine the origin of virus isolates from vaccines or from circulating rabies virus in the wild.

Monoclonal antibodies are now used to group isolates of strains of rabies virus from humans and animals. Strains of rabies virus can be classified into distinct groups related to animal species and geographic location. In a recent case of human rabies in the United States, the virus isolated from the patient was similar to that obtained from insectivorous bats common to the United States. This monoclonal study suggested that a bat was the source of exposure.

INCUBATION

The incubation period of rabies is extremely variable: it usually averages between 3 and 8 weeks and is influenced by many factors such as host susceptibility, virus strain, dose, and inoculation site. In dogs, rabies incubation can be as short as 10 days, and some reports suggest it can be as long as 6 months. The excretion of virus in saliva usually occurs after onset of clinical signs of the disease.

CLINICAL SIGNS

The clinical signs of rabies in carnivores are variable, but the disease is usually classified as furious rabies or dumb rabies, depending on the most prominent signs.

The clinical course of the disease can be divided into three phase: the prodromal, the excitative, and the paralytic. The prodromal stage usually lasts 2 to 3 days, and the clinical signs include a slight rise in temperature and a subtle change in temperament. In the excitative phase, signs of furious rabies are frequent, and exposure to man and other animals is more likely to occur. Dogs are easily irritated, are restless, and have a tendency to be aggressive and bite anything that is in their path or that moves. Dogs may exhibit pica. Dumb rabies progresses quickly to the paralytic phase, in which death occurs 1 to 3 days later.

The clinical signs of rabies in cats are similar to that of dogs, but aggressiveness is more commonly seen.

DIAGNOSIS

Many factors should be considered in the diagnosis of rabies, but a definitive diagnosis requires demonstration of the virus. Laboratory diagnosis may involve more than one type of examination. The fluorescent rabies antibody (FRA) test is the best single examination available for a rapid diagnosis and is now the test of choice in the United States. The FRA test is based on direct microscopic observation of a specific antigen-antibody reaction. In the hands of competent, well-trained technicians, the FRA can establish a diagnosis of rabies within a few hours.

Several laboratory animals can be used to isolate and identify rabies virus. Albino mice are most commonly used in laboratories still utilizing animal inoculation in the United States. Brain tissue and salivary glands are usually used for diagnosis by animal inoculation. Mice are injected intracerebrally with 0.3 ml of tissue suspended in diluent and are observed throughout 28 days for signs of rabies.

The FRA test has also been used to detect rabies in living animals. Numerous investigators have reported the presence of virus in a variety of tissues other than the traditional areas, the brain and salivary glands. Virus has been identified in frozen section of skin biopsies. The usefulness of this technique has been demonstrated in naturally infected animals and humans.

FRA examination of skin specimens obtained by surgical biopsy has had a great effect on the traditional diagnostic technique of examining brain tissue.

Centrifugal dissemination of virus occurs through the cranial nerves to the facial areas. The lateral sensory papillae on the cheek of a dog are surrounded by a nerve plexus, and these are examined for the presence of virus. The biopsy technique allows the physician an additional tool to evaluate the possibility of rabies exposure. This technique for rabies diagnosis could conceivably save the bite victim from taking rabies treatment.

The Centers for Disease Control (CDC) currently use skin biopsies for antemortem diagnosis of human rabies. The Veterinary Diagnostic Laboratory at Kansas State University has been conducting rabies examination of skin tissue for several years.

PREVENTION

The most effective prevention of rabies depends on quarantine, immunization of dogs and cats, and control of strays.

Immunization of Dogs and Cats

Effective vaccines are available; see the compendium of animal rabies vaccines in the Appendices.

Immunization of Humans

Exposure to rabies is an occupational hazard for veterinarians. It is strongly recommended that veterinarians, staff, and all others who have frequent contact with animals be immunized against rabies. A human vaccine against rabies is available, and its product insert is shown in Figure 1.

Many studies involving reduced dosage have shown that intradermal immunization with 0.1 ml Human Diploid Cell Rabies Vaccine has been effective in producing an amount of rabies-neutralizing antibodies much greater than the minimum accepted level of 1:5 (as determined by the rapid fluorescent focus inhibition test, [RFFIT]), even two years after immunization.

Many references concerning the RFFIT have been made by CDC publications and the manufacturers of rabies vaccines. The RFFIT is currently available from the Veterinary Diagnostic Laboratory, College of Veterinary Medicine, Kansas State University, Manhattan, KS 66506.

POSTEXPOSURE TREATMENT

Dogs and Cats

Unvaccinated dogs and cats bitten by or exposed to a rabid animal should be destroyed immediately. If the owner is unwilling to have this done, the unvaccinated animal should be placed in isolation for 6 months and vaccinated 1 month prior to release. Dogs and cats with a current vaccination status should be revaccinated immediately, leashed, and confined for 90 days.

Humans

The decision to treat a person for possible rabies exposure is a difficult task for a physician. Many factors should be considered in this decision*:

1. The nature of exposure.

Text continued on page 1071

*See also Rabies Vaccine Imovax insert, Figure 1.

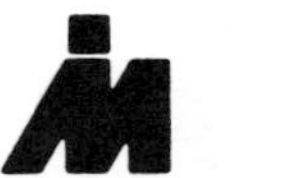

RABIES VACCINE IMOVAX® RABIES
Wistar Rabies Virus Strain PM-1503-3M
Grown in Human Diploid Cell Cultures

DESCRIPTION

The IMOVAX® RABIES Vaccine produced by Institut Merieux is a sterile, stable, freeze-dried suspension of rabies virus prepared from strain PM-1503-3M obtained from the Wistar Institute, Philadelphia, PA.

The virus is harvested from infected human diploid cells, MRC-5 strain, concentrated by ultrafiltration and is inactivated by beta propiolactone. One dose of reconstituted vaccine contains less than 100 mg albumin, less than 150 μg neomycin sulfate and 20 μg of phenol red indicator. The vaccine is for intramuscular use.

The vaccine contains no preservative or stabilizer. It should be used immediately after reconstitution.

The potency of Merieux IMOVAX RABIES Vaccine is equal to or greater than 2.5 international units of rabies antigen.

CLINICAL PHARMACOLOGY

Pre-Exposure Immunization

High titer antibody responses of the Merieux IMOVAX RABIES Vaccine made in human diploid cells have been demonstrated in trials conducted in England (1), Germany (2,3), France (4) and Belgium (5). Seroconversion was often obtained with only one dose. With two doses one month apart, 100% of the recipients developed specific antibody and the geometric mean titer of the group was approximately 10 international units. In the U.S., Merieux IMOVAX RABIES Vaccine resulted in geometric mean titers (GMT) of 12.9 I.U./ml at Day 49 and 5.1 I.U./ml at Day 90 when three doses were given intramuscularly during the course of one month. The range of antibody responses was 2.8 to 55.0 I.U./ml at Day 49 and 1.8 to 12.4 I.U. at Day 90. The definition of a minimally acceptable antibody titer varies among laboratories and is influenced by the type of test conducted. CDC currently specifies a 1:5 titer by the rapid fluorescent-focus inhibition test (RFFIT) as acceptable. The World Health Organization (WHO) specifies a titer of 0.5 I.U.

Post-Exposure Immunization

Post-exposure efficacy of Merieux IMOVAX RABIES Vaccine was successfully proven during clinical experience in Iran (7) in conjunction with antirabies serum. Forty-five persons severely bitten by rabid dogs and wolves received Merieux vaccine within hours of and up to 14 days after the bites. All individuals were fully protected against rabies.

INDICATIONS AND USAGE

I. Rationale of Treatment

Physicians must evaluate each possible rabies exposure. Local or state public health officials should be consulted if questions arise about the need for prophylaxis. (8)

In the United States and Canada, the following factors should be considered before antirabies treatment is initiated.

Species of Biting Animal

Carnivorous wild animals (especially skunks, raccoons, foxes, coyotes, and bobcats) and bats are the animals most commonly infected with rabies and have caused most of the indigenous cases of human rabies in the United States since 1960. Unless an animal is tested and shown not to be rabid, post-exposure prophylaxis should be initiated upon bite or nonbite exposure to the animals. (See definition in "Type of Exposure" below.) If treatment has been initiated and subsequent testing in a competent laboratory shows the exposing animal is not rabid, treatment can be discontinued. (8)

The likelihood that a domestic dog or cat is infected with rabies varies from region to region; hence the need for post-exposure prophylaxis also varies. (8)

Rodents (such as squirrels, hamsters, guinea pigs, gerbils, chipmunks, rats and mice) and lagomorphs (including rabbits and hares) are rarely found to be infected with rabies and have not been known to cause human rabies in the United States. In these cases, the state or local health department should be consulted before a decision is made to initiate post-exposure antirabies prophylaxis. (8)

Circumstances of Biting Incident

An UNPROVOKED attack is more likely than a provoked attack to indicate the animal is rabid. Bites inflicted on a person attempting to feed or handle an apparently healthy animal should generally be regarded as PROVOKED.

Type of Exposure

Rabies is transmitted by introducing the virus into open cuts or wounds in skin or via mucous membranes. The likelihood of rabies infection varies with the nature and extent of exposure. Two categories of exposure should be considered:

Bite: Any penetration of the skin by teeth.

Nonbite: Scratches, abrasions, open wounds, or mucous membranes contaminated with saliva or other potentially infectious material, such as brain tissue, from a rabid animal. Casual contact, such as petting a rabid animal (without a bite or nonbite exposure as described above), does not constitute an exposure and is not an indication for prophylaxis. There have been two instances of airborne rabies acquired in laboratories and two probable airborne rabies cases acquired in a bat-infested cave in Texas. (8,9)

The only documented cases for rabies from human-to-human transmission occurred in four patients in the United States and overseas who received corneas transplanted from persons who died of rabies undiagnosed at the time of death. (9,10) Stringent guidelines for acceptance of donor corneas should reduce this risk.

Bite and nonbite exposure from humans with rabies theoretically could transmit rabies, although no cases of rabies acquired this way have been documented. Each potential exposure to human rabies should be carefully evaluated to minimize unnecessary rabies prophylaxis. (8,11)

II. Pre- and Post-Exposure Treatment of Rabies

A. Pre-Exposure—See Table 1

Pre-exposure immunization may be offered to persons in high risk groups, such as veterinarians, animal handlers, certain laboratory workers, and persons spending time (e.g. 1 month or more) in foreign countries where rabies is a constant threat. Persons whose vocational or avocational pursuits bring them into contact with potentially rabid dogs, cats, foxes, skunks, bats, or other species at risk of having rabies should also be considered for pre-exposure prophylaxis. (8)

Vaccination is recommended for children living in or visiting countries where exposure to rabid animals is a constant threat. Worldwide statistics indicate children are more at risk than adults.

Pre-exposure prophylaxis is given for several reasons. First, it may provide protection to persons with inapparent exposure to rabies. Secondly, it may protect persons whose post-exposure therapy might be expected to be delayed. Finally, although it does not eliminate the need for additional therapy after a rabies exposure, it simplifies therapy by eliminating the need for globulin and decreasing the number of doses of vaccine needed. This is of particular importance for persons at high risk of being exposed in countries where the available rabies immunizing products may carry a higher risk of adverse reactions.

Pre-exposure immunization does not eliminate the need for prompt prophylaxis following an exposure. It only reduces the post-exposure treatment regimen. (8)

PRE-EXPOSURE RABIES TREATMENT GUIDE

1. **Pre-Exposure Immunization:** Consists of three doses of HDCV, 1.0 ml, intramuscularly (i.e. deltoid area), one each on Days 0, 7, 21 or 28. Administration of routine booster doses of vaccine depends on exposure risk category as noted in Table 1. Pre-exposure immunization of immunosuppressed persons is not recommended. (8)

Table 1 (8) Criteria for Pre-Exposure Immunization

Risk category	Nature of risk	Typical populations	Pre-exposure regimen
Continuous	Virus present continuously, often in high concentrations. Aerosol, mucous membrane, bite, or nonbite exposure possible. Specific exposures may go unrecognized.	Rabies research lab workers.* Rabies biologics production workers.	Primary pre-exposure immunization course. Serology every 6 months. Booster immunization when antibody titer falls below acceptable level.*
Frequent	Exposure usually episodic, with source recognized, but exposure may also be unrecognized. Aerosol, mucous membrane, bite, or nonbite exposure.	Rabies diagnostic lab workers,* spelunkers, veterinarians, and animal control and wildlife workers in rabies epizootic areas.	Primary pre-exposure immunization course. Booster immunization or serology every 2 years.†
Infrequent (greater than population-at-large)	Exposure nearly always episodic with source recognized. Mucous membrane, bite, or nonbite exposure.	Veterinarians and animal control and wildlife workers in areas of low rabies endemicity. Certain travelers to foreign rabies epizootic areas. Veterinary students.	Primary pre-exposure immunization course. No routine booster immunization or serology.
Rare (population-at-large)	Exposure always episodic, mucous membrane, or bite with source recognized.	U.S. population-at-large, including individuals in rabies-epizootic areas.	No pre-exposure immunization

*Judgment of relative risk and extra monitoring of immunization status of laboratory workers is the responsibility of the laboratory supervisor (see U.S. Department of Health and Human Service's *Biosafety in Microbiological and Biomedical Laboratories,* 1984).

† Pre-exposure booster immunization consists of one dose of HDCV, 1.0 ml/dose, IM (deltoid area). Acceptable antibody level is 1:5 titer (complete inhibition in RFFIT at 1:5 dilution) See Clinical Pharmacology. Boost if titer falls below 1:5.

B. Post Exposure—See Table 2

The essential components of rabies post-exposure prophylaxis are local treatment of wounds and immunization, including administration, in most instances, of both globulin and vaccine (Table 2). (8,13)

Figure 1. Product insert for human rabies vaccine. Reproduced with the permission of Dr. Pinya Cohen, Merieux Institute, Miami, Florida.

Illustration continued on opposite page

1. **Local Treatment of Wounds:** Immediate and thorough washing of all bite wounds and scratches with soap and water is perhaps the most effective measure for preventing rabies. In experimental animals, simple local wound cleansing has been shown to reduce markedly the likelihood of rabies. (8,11)

Tetanus prophylaxis and measures to control bacterial infection should be given as indicated.

2. **Specific Treatment:** Post-exposure antirabies immunization should always include administration of both antibody (preferably RIG) and vaccine, with one exception: persons who have been previously immunized with the recommended pre-exposure or post-exposure regimens with HDCV or who have been immunized with other types of vaccines and have a history of documented adequate rabies antibody titer should receive only vaccine. The combination of globulin and vaccine is recommended for both bite exposures and nonbite exposures regardless of the interval between exposure and treatment.(14,15) The sooner treatment is begun after exposure, the better. However, there have been instances in which the decision to begin treatment was made as late as 6 months or longer after the exposure due to delay in recognition that an exposure had occurred. (8,13)

3. **Treatment outside the United States:** If post-exposure is begun outside the United States with locally produced biologics, it may be desirable to provide additional treatment when the patient reaches the U.S. State health departments should be contacted for specific advice in such cases. (8)

POST-EXPOSURE TREATMENT GUIDE

The following recommendations are only a guide. In applying them, take into account the animal species involved, the circumstances of the bite or other exposure, the vaccination status of the animal, and presence of rabies in the region. Local or state public health officials should be consulted if questions arise about the need for rabies prophylaxis. (8)

Table 2 (8)

	Animal species	Condition of animal at time of attack	Treatment of exposed person*
DOMESTIC	Dog and cat	Healthy and available for 10 days of observation	None, unless animal develops rabies†
		Rabid or suspected rabid	RIG§ and HDCV
		Unknown (escaped)	Consult public health officials. If treatment is indicated, give RIG§ and HDCV
WILD	Skunk, bat, fox, coyote, raccoon, bobcat, and other carnivores	Regard as rabid unless proven negative by laboratory tests ¶	RIG§ and HDCV
OTHER	Livestock, rodents and lagomorphs (rabbits and hares)	Consider individually. Local and state public health officials should be consulted on questions about the need for rabies prophylaxis. Bites of squirrels, hamsters, guinea pigs, gerbils, chipmunks, rats, mice, other rodents, rabbits, and hares almost never call for antirabies prophylaxis.	

**All bites and wounds should immediately be thoroughly cleansed with soap and water.* If antirabies treatment is indicated, both rabies immune globulin (RIG) and human diploid cell rabies vaccine (HDCV) should be given as soon as possible, *regardless* of the interval from exposure. Local reactions to vaccines are common and do not contraindicate continuing treatment. Discontinue vaccine if flourescent-antibody tests of the animal are negative.

†During the usual holding period of 10 days, begin treatment with RIG and HDCV at first sign of rabies in a dog or cat that has bitten someone. The symptomatic animal should be killed immediately and tested.

§If RIG is not available, use antirabies serum, equine (ARS). Do not use more than the recommended dosage.

¶ The animal should be killed and tested as soon as possible. Holding for observation is not recommended.

CONTRAINDICATIONS

For post-exposure treatment there are no known specific contraindications to the use of Merieux IMOVAX RABIES Vaccine. In cases of pre-exposure immunization, there are no known specific contraindications other than situations such as developing febrile illness, etc.

WARNINGS

In both pre-exposure and post-exposure immunization, the full 1.0 ml dose should be given intramuscularly.

In the case of pre-exposure immunization, recently a significant increase has been noted in "immune complex-like" reactions in persons receiving booster doses of HDCV. (16) The illness characterized by onset 2-21 days post-booster, presents with a generalized urticaria and may also include arthralgia, arthritis, angioedema, nausea, vomiting, fever, and malaise. In no cases were the illnesses life-threatening. Preliminary data suggest this "immune complex-like" illness may occur in up to 6% of persons receiving booster vaccines and much less frequently in persons receiving primary immunization. Additional experience with this vaccine is needed to define more clearly the risk of these adverse reactions. (8,17)

Two cases of neurologic illness resembling Guillain-Barre syndrome (18,19), a transient neuroparalytic illness, that resolved without sequelae in 12 weeks and a focal subacute central nervous system disorder temporally associated with HDCV, have been reported. (20)

All serious systemic neuroparalytic or anaphylactic reactions to a rabies vaccine should be immediately reported to the state health department or the Division of Viral Diseases, Center for Infectious Diseases, CDC, 404-329-3095 during working hours, or 404-329-2888 at other times. (8)

PRECAUTIONS

General

When a person with a history of hypersensitivity must be given rabies vaccine, antihistamines may be given; epinephrine (1:1000) should be readily available to counteract anaphylactic reactions, and the person should be carefully observed after immunization.

While the concentration of antibiotics in each dose of vaccine is extremely small, persons with known hypersensitivity to any of these agents could manifest an allergic reaction. While the risk is small, it should be weighed in light of the potential risk of contracting rabies.

Drug Interactions

Corticosteroids, other immunosuppressive agents, and immunosuppressive illnesses can interfere with the development of active immunity and predispose the patient to developing rabies. Immunosuppressive agents should not be administered during post-exposure therapy, unless essential for the treatment of other conditions. When rabies post-exposure prophylaxis is administered to persons receiving steroids or other immunosuppressive therapy, it is especially important that serum be tested for rabies antibody to ensure that an adequate response has developed. (8)

Usage in Pregnancy

Pregnancy Category C. Animal reproduction studies have not been conducted with IMOVAX RABIES Vaccine. It is also not known whether the product can cause fetal harm when administered to a pregnant woman or can affect reproductive capacity. Rabies vaccine should be given to a pregnant woman only if clearly needed.

Because of the potential consequences of inadequately treated rabies exposure and limited data that indicate that fetal abnormalities have not been associated with rabies vaccination, pregnancy is not considered a contraindication to post-exposure prophylaxis. (8,21) If there is substantial risk of exposure to rabies, pre-exposure prophylaxis may also be indicated during pregnancy. (8)

Pediatric Use

Both safety and efficacy in children have been established.

ADVERSE REACTIONS

ALSO SEE WARNINGS AND CONTRAINDICATIONS SECTIONS FOR ADDITIONAL STATEMENTS

Once initiated, rabies prophylaxis should not be interrupted or discontinued because of local or mild systemic adverse reactions to rabies vaccine. Usually such reactions can be successfully managed with anti-inflammatory and antipyretic agents (e.g. aspirin).

Reactions after vaccination with HDCV are less common than with previously available vaccines. (12,16,17) In a study using five doses of HDCV, local reactions, such as pain, erythema, and swelling or itching at the injection site were reported in about 25% of recipients of HDCV, and mild systemic reactions such as headache, nausea, abdominal pain, muscle aches and dizziness were reported in about 20% of recipients. (8)

Serious systemic anaphylactic or neuroparalytic reactions occurring during the administration of rabies vaccines pose a dilemma for the attending physician. A patient's risk of developing rabies must be carefully considered before deciding to discontinue vaccination. Moreover, the use of corticosteroids to treat life-threatening neuroparalytic reactions carries the risk of inhibiting the development of active immunity to rabies. It is especially important in these cases that the serum of the patient be tested for rabies antibodies. Advice and assistance on the management of serious adverse reactions in persons receiving rabies vaccines may be sought from the state health department or CDC. (8)

DOSAGE AND ADMINISTRATION

Parenteral drug products should be inspected visually for particulate matter and discoloration prior to administration, whenever solution and container permit.

Reconstitute the freeze-dried vaccine in its vial with the 1.0 ml of diluent supplied in the disposable syringe using the longer of the two needles. Gently swirl the contents until completely dissolved and withdraw the total amount of dissolved vaccine into the syringe by setting the vial in an upright position on the table. Remove the reconstitution needle and replace it with the smaller needle.

The reconstituted vaccine should be used immediately.

After preparation of the injection site, immediately inject the vaccine intramuscularly, preferably into the deltoid muscle or into the upper and outer quadrant of the buttocks. In infants and small children, the mid lateral aspect of the thigh may be preferable. Care should be taken to avoid injection into or near blood vessels and nerves. After aspiration, if blood or any suspicious discoloration appears in the syringe, do not inject but discard contents and repeat procedure using a new dose of vaccine, at a different site.

NOTE: The freeze-dried vaccine is creamy white to orange.
After reconstitution it is pink to red.

A. Pre-Exposure Dosage

1. **Primary Vaccination:** In the United States, the Immunization Practices Advisory Committee (ACIP) recommends three injections of 1.0 ml each, one injection on Day 0 and one on Day 7 and one either on Day 21 or 28. (8)
2. **Booster Dose:** Persons working with live rabies virus in research laboratories and in vaccine production facilities should

Illustration continued on following page

have rabies antibody titers checked every six months and boosters given as needed to maintain an adequate titer. (For Definition of Adequate Titer, See Clinical Pharmacology.) Only laboratory workers, such as those doing rabies diagnostic tests, spelunkers and veterinarians, animal control and wildlife officers in areas where rabies is epizootic should have boosters every 2 years or have their serum tested for rabies antibody every 2 years and, if the titer is inadequate, have a booster dose. Veterinarians and animal control and wildlife officers, if working in areas of low rabies endemicity, do not require routine booster doses of HDCV after completion of primary pre-exposure immunization (Table 1). (8)

Persons who have experienced "immune complex-like" hypersensitivity reactions should receive no further doses of HDCV unless they are exposed to rabies or they are truly likely to be inapparently and/or unavoidably exposed to rabies virus and have unsatisfactory antibody titers.

B. Post-Exposure Dosage

The World Health Organization established a recommendation for six intramuscular doses of human diploid cell vaccine (HDCV) based on studies in Germany and Iran. (3,7) Used in this way, a total of 6 injections of a 1.0 ml dose of vaccine are given according to the following schedule: on Day 0, 3, 7, 14, 30 and 90. The first dose should be accompanied by Rabies Immune Globulin (RIG) or Antirabies Serum (ARS). Studies conducted at the CDC in the United States have shown that a regimen of 1 dose of Rabies Immune Globulin (RIG) and 5 doses of HDCV induced an excellent antibody response in all recipients. Of 511 persons bitten by proven rabid animals and so treated, none developed rabies. (8)

Based on these data, the ACIP recommends a 5-dose regimen for post-exposure situations. Five 1.0 ml doses are given intramuscularly on Days 0, 3, 7, 14 and 28 in conjunction with RIG on Day 0. (8)

Because the antibody response following the recommended vaccination regimen with HDCV has been so satisfactory, routine post-vaccination serologic testing is not recommended. Serologic testing is indicated in unusual circumstances, as when the patient is known to be immunosuppressed. Contact state health department or CDC for recommendations. (8)

C. Post-Exposure Therapy of Previously Immunized Persons

When an immunized person who was vaccinated by the recommended regimen with HDCV or who had previously demonstrated rabies antibody is exposed to rabies, that person should receive two I.M. doses (1.0 ml each) of HDCV, one immediately and one 3 days later. RIG should not be given in these cases. If the immune status of a previously vaccinated person who did not receive the recommended HDCV regimen is not known, full primary post-exposure antirabies treatment (RIG plus 5 doses of HDCV) may be necessary. In such cases, if antibody can be demonstrated in a serum sample collected before vaccine is given, treatment can be discontinued after at least two doses of HDCV. (8)

HOW SUPPLIED

IMOVAX RABIES Vaccine is supplied in a tamper-proof unit dose plastic box with:
—One vial of freeze-dried vaccine containing a single dose.
—One disposable needle and syringe containing diluent for reconstitution.
—One smaller disposable needle for administration.

STORAGE

The freeze-dried vaccine is stable if stored in the refrigerator between 2°C and 8°C (36°F to 46°F). Do not freeze.

REFERENCES

1. Aoki FY, Tyrrell DAJ, Hill LE. Immunogenicity and acceptability of a human diploid cell culture rabies vaccine in volunteers. The Lancet, March 22, pp 660-2 (1975)
2. Cox JH, Schneider LG. Prophylactic immunization of humans against rabies by intradermal inoculation of human diploid cell culture vaccine. J Clin Microbiol 3: 96-101 (1976)
3. Kuwert EK, Marcus I, Werner J, Iwand A, Thraenhart O. Some experiences with human diploid cell strain—(HDCS) rabies vaccine in pre- and post-exposure vaccinated humans. Develop Biol Standard 40: 79-88 (1978)
4. Ajjan N, Soulebot J-P, Stellmann C, Biron G, Charbonnier C, Triau R, Merieux C. Resultats de la vaccination antirabique preventive par le vaccin inactive concentre souche rabies PM/WI38-1503-3M cultives sur cellules diploides humaines. Develop Biol Standard 40: 89-199 (1978)
5. Costy-Berger F. Vaccination antirabique preventive par du vaccin prepare sur cellules diploides humaines. Develop Biol Standard 40: 101-4 (1978)
6. Bernard KW, Roberts, MA, Sumner J, Winkler WG, Mallonee J, Baer GM, Chaney R. Human diploid cell rabies vaccine. JAMA 247: 1138-42 (1982)
7. Bahmanyar M, Fayaz A, Nour-Salehi S, Mohammadi M, Koprowski H. Successful protection of humans exposed to rabies infection. JAMA 236: 2751-4 (1976)
8. CDC. Recommendations of the Immunization Practices Advisory Committee (ACIP). Rabies Prevention—United States, 1984. MMWR 33: 393-402, 407-8 (1984)
9. Anderson LJ, Nicholson KG, Tauxe RV, Winkler WG. Human rabies in the United States, 1960 to 1979: epidemiology, diagnosis and prevention. Ann Intern Med 100: 728-35 (1984)
10. WHO. Sixth report of the Expert Committee on Rabies. Geneva Switzerland: World Health Organization. (WHO technical report no. 523) (1973)
11. Baer GM, ed. The natural history of rabies. New York: Academic Press. (1975)
12. Greenberg M, Childress J. Vaccination against rabies with duck-embryo and Semple vaccines. JAMA 173: 333-7 (1960)
13. Helmick CG. The epidemiology of human rabies postexposure prophylaxis. JAMA 250: 1990-6 (1983)
14. Devriendt J, Staroukine M, Costy F, Vanderhaegen J-J. Fatal encephalitis apparently due to rabies. JAMA 248: 2304-6 (1982)
15. CDC. Human Rabies—Rwanda. MMWR 31: 135 (1982)
16. CDC. Systemic allergic reactions following immunization with human diploid cell rabies vaccine. MMWR 33: 185-7 (1984)
17. Rubin, Hattwick MAW, Jones S, Gregg MB, Schwartz VD. Adverse reactions to duck embryo rabies vaccine. Ann Intern Med 78: 643-9 (1973)
18. Boe E, Nyland H. Guillain-Barre syndrome after vaccination with human diploid cell rabies vaccine. Scand J. Infect Dis 12: 231-2 (1980)
19. CDC. Adverse reactions to human diploid cell rabies vaccine. MMWR 29: 609-10 (1980)
20. Bernard KW, Smith PW, Kader FJ, Moran MJ. Neuroparalytic illness and human diploid cell rabies vaccine. JAMA 248: 3136-8 (1982)
21. Varner MW, McGuinness GA, Galask RP. Rabies vaccination in pregnancy. Am J of Obst and Gyn 143: 717-8 (1982)
22. CDC. Recommendation of the Immunization Practices Advisory Committee (ACIP). Supplementary statement on rabies vaccine and serologic testing. MMWR 30: 535-6 (1981)

Distributed by
Merieux Institute, Inc.
Miami, Florida 33126
800-327-2842
305-593-9577

Manufactured by
INSTITUT MERIEUX
Lyon—France
U.S. License No. 384

Revised September 1984

2. The presence of rabies in the area from which the biting animal came.
3. The species of animal.
4. The clinical status of the animal.
5. The availability of the animal for observation or laboratory testing.

PUBLIC HEALTH ASPECTS

Dogs and cats (unvaccinated) still pose a threat to people who may be exposed to rabies when "spillover" from wild animals occurs. Veterinarians play an important role in public health by encouraging maintenance of an immunized pet population.

References and Supplemental Reading

Baer, G. M.: *The Natural History of Rabies.* New York: Academic Press, 1975.

Fischman, H. R.: Rabies. *In* Last, J. M. (ed.): *Public Health and Preventive Medicine,* 11th ed. New York: Appleton-Century-Crofts, 1984.

Tierkel, E. S.: Rabies. *In* Hull, T. G. (ed.): *Diseases Transmitted from Animals to Man.* Springfield, IL: Charles C Thomas., 1963.

Whetstone, C. A., Bunn, T. O., Emmons, R. W., et al.: Use of monoclonal antibodies to confirm vaccine-induced rabies in ten dogs, two cats, and one fox. J.A.V.M.A. 185:285, 1984.

World Health Organization: *WHO Expert Committee on Rabies.* Seventh Report. Geneva, 1984.

PSEUDORABIES IN DOGS AND CATS

DENNIS R. HOWARD, PH.D.
Manhattan, Kansas

Pseudorabies (PR), also known as Aujeszky's disease, infectious bulbar paralysis, or "mad itch," is an acute, infectious, fatal, naturally occurring virus disease primarily affecting swine. It occurs in a wide variety of domestic and wild animals including dogs, cats, cattle, sheep, and rats.

The disease was first reported in 1902 by Aladár Aujeszky as a fatal disease in cattle and dogs. PR occurs most often in dogs and cats in areas where swine are raised. Swine are the natural hosts and principal reservoir of the virus. The incidence of PR in dogs and cats is directly related to the prevalence of the disease in swine, and in many cases its occurrence may be the only indication that the virus is present.

ETIOLOGY

Pseudorabies is casued by a herpesvirus measuring approximately 150 to 180 μm in diameter. PR has the ability to persist in the host species as a latent infection. The virus may survive for 2 to 7 weeks in an infected environment and for up to 5 weeks in meat. It can be readily inactivated with chloroform, ether, 1 per cent sodium hydroxide, and 5 per cent phenol. PR virus is susceptible to heat, ultraviolet light, and gamma radiation.

TRANSMISSION

Dogs and cats serve as monitors of inapparent pseudorabies infections in swine. The primary mode of transmission to dogs and cats is the consumption of virus-contaminated tissues of swine. In the laboratory, these animals have also been infected with pseudorabies by subcutaneous, intramuscular, intracranial, and intraocular routes.

Studies have shown that dogs appear to be less susceptible to oral infection than cats. Cats invariably die after eating food contaminated with pseudorabies virus.

It appears that direct viral spread from infected to noninfected dogs and cats does not occur as it does in swine, but it is possible that other modes of exposure to pseudorabies virus exists.

CLINICAL SIGNS AND FINDINGS

Pseudorabies in dogs and cats occurs as an acute clinical infection and has a rapid, fatal course. The incubation period ranges from 2 to 10 days, and in most naturally occurring cases the range is between 3 and 6 days. Death usually occurs within 24 to 48 hours after initial clinical signs of the disease appear.

Pseudorabies in dogs begins with an excitement phase, characterized by fever, restlessness, vomiting, and salivation. Intense pain, convulsions, facial tremors, and paresis also occur. Intense pruritus with scratching or chewing to the point of severe self-mutilation is the most common clinical sign. Vocalization due to discomfort often occurs during the infection. Most dogs become progressively more incoordinated and the encephalitis progresses to depression, coma, and death within 24 hours.

Pseudorabies in cats manifests itself differently than in dogs. Cats usually die within 24 hours after onset of symptoms. The cat first appears to be sluggish and becomes progressively more agitated. The fur is usually matted with viscid saliva. Intense pruritus may occur and can be localized on one side of the head. Anisocoria often accompanies the pruritus. Self-mutilization from scratching is apparent, and mewing is persistent. Respiration becomes labored and heart rate increases. These signs of PR soon diminish and the encephalitis progresses to convulsions, coma, and death. Atypical cases of PR occur in the cat and are more difficult to interpret.

The PR virus travels along peripheral nerves and upon reaching the dorsal root causes a very intense pruritus. Pseudorabies virus in both peripheral and central nervous tissue causes one of the most severe forms of pruritus. The finite mediator of the pruritus is unknown; however, it is believed to be proteolytic enzymes released at the skin site.

Clinical laboratory findings are of little value since the course of the disease is so short. Pseudorabies in dogs may lead to an acid-base imbalance. Vomiting causes loss of hydrochloric acid, resulting in metabolic alkalosis. This may result in elevated levels of carbon dioxide in the blood. Hypokalemia may also occur. Total serum protein may be elevated. Fibrinogen levels may increase because of dehydration or the presence of inflammation.

DIAGNOSIS

A presumptive diagnosis of PR can be made by the occurrence of the classical clinical signs of pruritus and self-mutilation accompanied by salivation and sudden death.

A clinical diagnosis of PR can be confirmed in the laboratory by the fluorescent antibody test (FAT). Tonsil, brain, and brain stem are the tissues of choice for the FAT. Pruritic areas of skin may also be examined for the presence of virus. Histopathologic examination of fixed tissue shows a nonspecific viral encephalitis. Diagnostic inclusion bodies occur but are hard to find. Pseudorabies virus can also be isolated in cell culture and identified by virus neutralization.

A diagnosis of PR can be confirmed by subcutaneous inoculation of laboratory animals with tissue suspensions. Rabbits are highly sensitive to the virus, and inoculation with infected tissue causes intense local pruritus in 4 to 6 days, followed by death.

TREATMENT

There is no known treatment that will reverse the course of the disease after its clinical signs appear. Animals with severe pruritus, pain, and convulsions should be given a central nervous system depressant, or euthanasia may be elected since the prognosis is grave. Topical therapy to alleviate intense pruritus associated with PR is of little value.

PROPHYLAXIS

Studies indicate that dogs vaccinated with an inactivated virus vaccine and challenged were not protected against PR even though they had high titers of antibody in the blood. Protection of dogs against PR with inactivated vaccine may be difficult to achieve. Vaccines are available for swine but are not recommended for use in other animals. Live-virus vaccine may cause the disease in dogs and cats. Antiserum has been used in swine, but studies of use in dogs and cats have not been encouraging.

References and Supplemental Reading

Chrisman, C. L., and Averill, D. R., Jr.: Diseases of peripheral nerves and muscles. *In* Ettinger, S. J. (ed.): *Veterinary Internal Medicine*, 2nd ed. Philadelphia: W. B. Saunders, 1983, p. 643.

Crandell, R. A.: Pseudorabies (Aujeszky's disease). *In* Howard, J. L. (ed.): *Current Veterinary Therapy. Food Animal Practice*. Philadelphia: W. B. Saunders, 1981, pp. 604–607.

Gustafson, D. P.: Pseudorabies. *In* Dunne, H. W., and Leman, A. D. (eds.): *Diseases in Swine*, 4th ed. Ames, IA: Iowa State University Press, 1975, pp. 391–410.

Gustafson, D. P.: Pseudorabies in dogs and cats. *In* Kirk, R. W. (ed.): *Current Veterinary Therapy VII*. Philadelphia: W. B. Saunders, 1980, pp. 1296–1298.

Ihrke, P. H.: Pruritus. *In* Ettinger, S. J. (ed.): *Veterinary Internal Medicine*, 2nd ed. Philadelphia: W. B. Saunders, 1983, pp. 115–121.

Muller, G. H., Kirk, R. W., and Scott, D. W.: *Small Animal Dermatology*, 3rd ed. Philadelphia: W. B. Saunders, 1983, pp. 40–42.

Pensaert, M. B., Commeyne, S., and Andries, K.: Vaccination of dogs against Pseudorabies (Aujeszky's disease), using an inactivated-virus vaccine. Am. J. Vet. Res. 41:2016, 1980.

Shell, L. G., Ely, R. W., and Crandell, R. A.: Pseudorabies in a dog. J.A.V.M.A. 178:1159, 1981.

CANINE AND FELINE CAMPYLOBACTERIOSIS

JAMES G. FOX, D.V.M.
Cambridge, Massachusetts

Species of *Campylobacter (Vibrio)* have been known as pathogenic and commensal bacteria in domestic farm animals for decades; however, only recently has *Campylobacter jejuni* been listed in the differential diagnosis of bacterial diarrheas in humans and companion pet animals. Dogs and the cats are increasingly cited as reservoir hosts of *Campylobacter* organisms, although host animals may or may not have diarrhea. It is now recognized that diarrheal disease caused by *Campylobacter* can occur in dogs and cats and that the organism can spread to the pet's owner, resulting in illness. There has been a dramatic increase in the number of both pet stores and animal shelters and pounds that care for feral animals and stray pets, and these facilities may serve as a nidus where animals become infected with *Campylobacter* through contact with other animals shedding the organism in feces.

ETIOLOGIC AGENT

Organisms of the genus *Campylobacter* are now classified as gram-negative, slender, curved, motile bacteria that have microaerophilic growth requirements. The probable reason why *Campylobacter* has not been associated with diarrheal disease until recently is that a special cultural milieu is required for its cultivation. Some species of *Campylobacter* are thermophilic, can be grown at 42°C, are isolated on commercially available selective growth media containing various antibiotics, and can be defined biochemically (Skirrow and Benjamin, 1980). Most isolates from dogs and cats (like those from humans) are hippurate positive and therefore classified as *Campylobacter jejuni.* In considering *Campylobacter* enteritis, the microscopic examination of feces from animals with diarrhea can yield important information. The presence of leukocytes or erythrocytes in feces, found commonly in *Campylobacter* infection in humans, is supporting evidence of an acute inflammatory process. Dark-field or phase-contrast microscopy can be used to obtain a presumptive diagnosis of *Campylobacter* enteritis or colitis, provided that fresh feces are examined and substantial numbers of organisms are present in diarrheic stool. *Campylobacter* organisms can be recognized by their rapid, darting motility and oscillating appearance.

EPIZOOTIOLOGY

Investigations of the prevalence of *Campylobacter jejuni* indicate that appreciable numbers of dogs and cats maintained in pounds and shelters, both in the United States and elsewhere, shed the organism in their feces. Infection rates in dogs and cats with and without diarrhea from these sources have been reported to range from 0 to 45 per cent (Fox et al., 1983b). Puppies and kittens appear more likely to acquire infection and therefore may more commonly shed the organism. As with most enteric pathogens, fecal-oral spread and food-borne and water-borne transmission appear to be the principal avenues for infection; these include ingestion of contaminated meat products, particularly poultry, and unpasteurized milk. Nosocomial infections are also a possible mode of transmission, as is exposure to other pets (ferrets, hamsters, birds, rabbits) and rural farm animals that may shed the organism (Fox, 1982).

The most widely adopted serotyping scheme in use today is the passive hemagglutination assay; to date, approximately 55 serotypes have been recognized in both animals and humans (Penner et al., 1980). Unfortunately, the serotypes most commonly isolated from dogs and cats are unknown.

ZOONOSES

C. jejuni is now included with shigellae and salmonellae as a leading cause of diarrhea in humans. Previously, the organism was relegated to the role of a pathogen or commensal in domestic animals. Investigators in 1961 were the first to suspect a positive association between *Campylobacter* infection in humans and in dogs. With the heightened interest in *Campylobacter* as a human pathogen, several articles linking the disease in humans to pet animals recently have appeared (Blaser et al., 1980). Many of these were dogs, puppies, and kittens recently purchased from animal shelters or pounds. Clinical signs in pets preceded the onset of diarrhea in humans who lived in the same household and who also had *C. jejuni* isolated from their feces.

Although *C. jejuni* appears to be prevalent among dogs and cats, it is not known whether all serotypes found in dogs and cats cause diarrhea in humans. Increased awareness of the potential of infection from dogs and cats to humans and the utilization of a reliable serotyping system (now in use for isolates from humans) will allow a more complete understanding of the role that animal hosts play in the epidemiology of *Campylobacter* infection in humans.

CLINICAL SYNDROME

As in cases of *Salmonella* infection, many dogs and cats can be asymptomatic carriers of *Campylobacter*. The clinical disease occurs most frequently in animals less than 6 months of age. In addition, animals may be more susceptible to clinical infection if stressed by hospitalization, concurrent disease, pregnancy, shipment, or surgery. The pathogenic mechanisms responsible for the clinical alterations and laboratory changes found in infected animals is poorly understood. However, the typical presenting clinical signs, in the author's experience, include mucus-laden watery or bile-streaked diarrhea (with or without blood and leukocytes) of 3 to 7 days duration, partial anorexia, and occasional vomiting (Fox et al., 1983a). Elevated temperature and leukocytosis may also be present. In certain cases, diarrhea can persist for more than 2 weeks, be intermittent, and in some dogs be present for several months (Fox et al., 1984b; Fleming, 1983; Davies et al., 1984). Occasionally, pet dogs with canine parvovirus also harbor *C. jejuni* (Sandstedt and Wierup, 1980). Apparently, however, in some animals gastroenteritis associated with *Campylobacter* but not parvovirus infection can mimic a parvovirus infection, and the bacterium should be considered in the differential diagnosis along with parvovirus and *Salmonella* in dogs with acute-onset gastroenteritis, vomiting, and bloody diarrhea.

In cats, the clinical symptomatology is less well defined. In a recent survey of 159 cats from pound sources, 17 (10.7 per cent) shed *C. jejuni*, whereas three (2.0 per cent) had *Salmonella typhimurium* isolated from their feces. Only two of 17 shedding *C. jejuni* had bloody, mucus-laden diarrhea; *Giardia* was present in both, combined with *Isospora* in one cat and *Toxacara* in the other. One cat dually infected with *S. typhimurium* and *C. jejuni* was depressed and anorectic but not diarrheic. Recultures of the two cats' diarrheic feces after antibiotic therapy were negative for *C. jejuni* (Fox et al., 1985).

PATHOLOGIC FINDINGS

The exact pathogenesis of *Campylobacter*-induced bowel disease is unknown. Blood and leukocytes in the feces, congestion, edema, ulcers of the mucosa, and occasional sepsis in humans suggest that the organism can be invasive. Enterotoxin recently has been isolated from *C. jejuni* that was isolated from diarrheal patients and may be responsible for certain clinical features of the disease (Ruiz-Palacios et al., 1983).

Attempts to induce enteritis in seven puppies and three kittens with *C. jejuni* isolated from humans have been equivocal; only one orally inoculated pup developed transient diarrhea, and *C. jejuni* was not recovered from its feces (Prescott and Karmali, 1978). Gnotobiotic pups also were inoculated with *C. jejuni* by the same scientists (Prescott et al., 1981). Two days after inoculation, the pups were depressed and had loose feces and tenesmus. Grossly the colon was congested and edematous, and the colonic contents were abnormally fluid. Microscopically, the colon and cecum showed reduction in epithelial cell height, loss of brush border, and reduced numbers of goblet cells. The hyperplastic epithelial glands resulted in a thickened mucosa. Subepithelial congestion, hemorrhage, and inflammatory infiltrate also were observed.

Similar microscopic changes to those documented in gnotobiotic beagles experimentally infected with *C. jejuni* also have been noted in naturally occurring cases of campylobacteriosis in puppies (Collins et al., 1983). Other investigators have isolated *C. jejuni* from dogs with naturally occurring enteric disease and have orally inoculated these organisms into adult dogs. Watery, mucoid diarrhea was produced in the experimentally inoculated dogs. Necropsy findings were similar to those noted in some dogs with natural campylobacteriosis: stunting of intestinal villi, infiltration by inflammatory cells of the lamina propria, and enlarged Peyer's patches. Stunting and fusing of intestinal villi and mononuclear cell infiltrate in lamina propria have been noted in subacute stages of parvovirus infection and also were noted on intestinal biopsy samples from a dog with protracted *Campylobacter*-associated diarrhea (Davies et al., 1984).

It must be stressed, however, that infection with coronavirus, parvovirus, or other enteric pathogens must also be ruled out in dogs with *Campylobacter*-associated diarrhea. The pathogenesis of *C. jejuni* infection in dogs requires further study. The underlying mechanism by which diarrhea is induced in some animals but not in others that shed the organism in their feces is unknown.

THERAPY

Isolation of *C. jejuni* from the feces of dogs or cats is not necessarily an indication for antibiotic therapy; however, there is increasing evidence that diarrhea produced by *C. jejuni* (in dogs and cats) may warrant antimicrobial therapy. Because it is now established that both dogs and cats pose a potential zoonotic threat for the spread of *C. jejuni* to humans, antibiotic treatment of infected animals also may be indicated to eliminate potential sources of infection to household members exposed to an animal shedding the organism. Isolates of *C. jejuni* from both dogs and cats have recently been screened for susceptibility to several antimicrobial agents by an agar dilution technique; the findings were in general agreement with those found in isolates obtained from human populations (Fox et al., 1984a). Gentamicin and furazolidone were the most active of the drugs examined. The strains tested were frequently sensitive to two other aminoglycoside antibiotics, neomycin and kanamycin. Erythromycin, the drug of choice for *Campylobacter*-induced diarrhea in humans, also was effective at levels achievable in serum. Doxycycline and chloramphenicol also were active against most strains. The minimal inhibitory concentrations were high for penicillin, ampicillin, tetracycline, metronidazole, and sulfadimethoxine.

It is generally accepted that the β-lactam antibiotic, ampicillin, is relatively inactive against most strains of *Campylobacter*. Penicillin shows little activity as well, and most strains are resistant at therapeutically achievable drug levels. Resistance of human *C. jejuni* strains to penicillin also commonly occurs. *Campylobacter* strains may produce a β-lactamase, which accounts for their resistance to penicillin and, in some cases, ampicillin. Tetracycline resistance of strains of *C. jejuni* in humans and nonhuman primates was demonstrated to be plasmid-mediated and transmissible within the species of *C. jejuni*. Isolates with tetracycline resistance encountered in pets may also be plasmid-mediated. Efficacy of sulfadimethoxine and sulfa combinations in dogs and cats and in human isolates is variable, as reflected by therapeutic response and various *in vitro* studies. Isolates of *C. jejuni* from dogs and cats are sensitive to many antimicrobial agents of potential therapeutic value. However, the susceptibility of *C. jejuni* to other antibiotics can be variable, and many strains are resistant to drugs commonly used to treat diarrhea in dogs and cats. Before therapy for diarrhea in dogs and cats is instituted, attempts at *Campylobacter* isolation should be performed, and if *C. jejuni* organisms are identified, appropriate *in vitro* antibiotic testing should be undertaken.

Because *C. jejuni* is only beginning to emerge as a pathogen in dogs and cats, efficacy of antibiotic therapy in infected animals has been reported infrequently. Initial clinical results indicate that most dogs and cats with *Campylobacter*-associated diarrhea will respond favorably to appropriate antibiotic therapy. However, in limited cases, dogs or cats may be refractory to antibiotic therapy and may continue to shed the organism in feces. Another type of antibiotic therapy may be instituted, and the presence of intercurrent disease states in the animal should be determined. Careful attention to the management of fluid and electrolyte balance will aid in successful recovery of clinically affected animals, particularly puppies and kittens.

CONCLUSIONS

Nonspecific enteritis in dogs and cats is a common finding, and all too often its origin is not ascertained. It is now recognized that *C. jejuni* is a leading cause of diarrhea in humans. Commercial availability of selective culture media and simplification of culture techniques make isolation of *C. jejuni* feasible in dogs and cats encountered in veterinary practice, particularly those recently procured from pet stores or pound sources. Inclusion of *C. jejuni* in the list of potentially pathogenic microorganisms in these animals will help further our understanding of its role in diarrheal diseases of pets and humans, its epidemiology, and its potential zoonotic importance.

References and Supplemental Reading

Blaser, M. J., LaForce, F. M., Wilson, N. A., et al.: Reservoirs for human campylobacteriosis. J. Infect. Dis. 141:665, 1980.

Collins, J. E., Libal, M. C., and Brost, D.: Proliferative enteritis in two pups. J.A.V.M.A. 183:886, 1983.

Davies, A. P., Gebhart, C. J., and Meric, S. A.: *Campylobacter*-associated chronic diarrhea in a dog. J.A.V.M.A. 184:469, 1984.

Fleming, M. P.: Association of *Campylobacter jejuni* with enteritis in dogs and cats. Vet. Rec. 113:372, 1983.

Fox, J. G.: Campylobacteriosis—A "new" disease in laboratory animals. Lab. Anim. Sci. 32:625, 1982.

Fox, J. G., Ackerman, J. I., and Newcomer, C. E.: The prevalence of *Campylobacter jejuni/coli* in random source cats used in biomedical research. J. Infect. Dis., 151:743, 1985.

Fox, J. G., Dzink, J. L., and Ackerman, J. I.: Antibiotic sensitivity patterns of *Campylobacter jejuni/coli* isolated from laboratory animals and pets. Lab. Anim. Sci. 34:264, 1984a.

Fox, J. G., Moore, R., and Ackerman, J. I.: *Campylobacter jejuni*-associated diarrhea in dogs. J.A.V.M.A. 183:1430, 1983a.

Fox, J. G., Moore, R., and Ackerman, J. I.: Canine and feline campylobacteriosis: Epizootiology, clinical and public health features. J.A.V.M.A. 183:1420, 1983b.

Fox, J. G., O'Neill-Maxwell, K., and Ackerman, J. I.: *Campylobacter jejuni* associated diarrhea in commercially reared beagles. Lab. Anim. Sci. 34:151, 1984b.

Macartney, L., McCandlish, I. A. P., Al-Masat, R. R., et al.: Natural and

experimental infections with *Campylobacter jejuni* in dogs. *In* Newell, D. G. (ed.): Campylobacter: *Epidemiology, Pathogenesis and Biochemistry*. Lancaster, England: M.T.P. Press, 1982, p. 172 (abs.).
Penner, J. L., and Hennessy, J. N.: Passive hemagglutination technique for serotyping *Campylobacter fetus* subsp. *jejuni* on the basis of soluble heat-stable antigens. J. Clin. Microbiol. 12:732, 1980.
Prescott, J. F., Barker, I. K., Manninen, K. I., et al.: Campylobacter colitis in gnotobiotic dogs. Can. J. Comp. Med. 45:377, 1981.
Prescott, J. F., and Karmali, M. A.: Attempts to transmit campylobacter enteritis to dogs and cats. Can. Med. Assoc. J. 119:1001, 1978.
Ruiz-Palacios, G. M., Torres, J., Torres, N. I., et al.: Cholera-like enterotoxin produced by *Campylobacter jejuni*. Lancet 2:250, 1983.
Sandstedt, K., and Wierup, M.: Concomitant occurrence of *Campylobacter* and parvovirus in dogs with gastroenteritis. Vet. Res. Commun. 4:271, 1980.
Skirrow, M. B., and Benjamin, J.: 1001 Campylobacters: Cultural characteristics of intestinal campylobacters from man and animals. J. Hyg. (Cambridge) 85:427, 1980.

COCCIDIOIDOMYCOSIS

DENNIS W. MACY, D.V.M.
Fort Collins, Colorado

Coccidioidomycosis (valley fever, San Joaquin Valley fever) is caused by a saprophytic fungi, *Coccidioides immitis*. The organism was named *Coccidioides* because its spherules with endospores looked like protozoan parasites (coccidia-like). Because the first cases described were fatal, the species name *immitis* was given. The term *valley fever* is sometimes used to describe cases of coccidioidomycosis and refers to the San Joaquin Valley in California, from which many of the first described human cases were acquired.

ETIOLOGY

Coccidioides immitis is a highly specialized saprophytic fungus that lives in the soils of semiarid geographic areas in the Western Hemisphere. The fungus is dimorphic and grows as a mold in the soil and in artificial media. In this form, it grows as a filamentous septate mycelium and produces spores (arthrospores). These arthrospores (about 2 by 5 μm) are readily airborne and represent the infective form of the organism. When inhaled into the host's tissues and held at a temperature of 37°C, the arthrospores develop into spherules that gradually enlarge to 20 to 100 μm in diameter. The nuclei within the spherules divide to form numerous endospores 2 to 3 μm in diameter. These are eventually released and may enter lymphatics or adjacent tissues. The endospores then develop into new mature spherules and repeat the above process. When cultured at less than 37°C, the organisms revert to the mycelial phase.

EPIZOOTIOLOGY

Coccidioides immitis has specialized growth requirements and is limited to geographic regions with sandy alkaline soils, low altitude, hot summers, mild and moderately wet winters, and infrequent freezes. These conditions are met in the area called the lower Sonoran life zone. In the United States, this area includes parts of the southwestern United States (California, Arizona, New Mexico, Texas, and southern portions of Nevada and Utah). Outside the United States, in portions of Mexico, Central America (Guatemala and Honduras), and South America (Colombia, Venezuela, Paraguay, and Argentina), the distribution and relative concentration of *Coccidioides immitis* in soils of endemic areas varies; some focal areas are the continual source of infections. In these endemic areas, during the prolonged periods of low soil moisture and high temperatures, *Coccidioides immitis* is present deep below the soil surface. During the rainy season, the fungi return to the soil surface, the mycelial phase proliferates, and the arthrospores are produced and eventually released and spread by the wind. Since the organism is contained in the soil surface, exposure is increased as a result of movement of the soil through digging and windstorms. Because of the frequently chronic nature of the disease, coccidioidomycosis is diagnosed year-round. Most cases of the disease are identified in the endemic regions; however, because of the mobility of the population and their pets, more and more cases are now diagnosed outside the endemic areas. Taking a travel history is therefore especially important in the diagnosis of a possible case of coccidioidomycosis outside of endemic areas.

Animal-to-animal transmission is rare, apparently because spherules are too large and endospores are too fragile to survive this type of transmission; likewise, spread of the disease from humans to animals has not been documented. *In utero* transmission has been reported in the horse. In humans, direct transmission occurred after aerosolization of cast material contaminated by drained exudate from cutaneous coccal lesions. Laboratory accidents during culturing of *Coccidioides immitis* have resulted in infection (over 200 cases reported). Culture of this agent should not be attempted in clinical laboratories unless personnel have received special training and a biohazard safety hood is available.

Burial of animals infected with coccidioidomycosis in soils capable of supporting the growth of the mycelial form of this organism should be avoided, since experimental studies have shown that this practice has rendered the surrounding soils positive for *Coccidioides immitis* for many years.

Animals living in endemic areas usually are exposed to the organism and either become immune or develop the disease at a very early age. Infection rates for those animals living in endemic areas is high and probably is greater than 80 per cent. Most dogs found to have the disseminated form of *Coccidioides immitis* are between the ages of 1 and 4 years. Young, male, large dogs, particularly those used for hunting, appear to be at highest risk of exposure to endemic rural environments. Several reports have indicated that boxers and Doberman pinschers run a higher risk of developing disseminated disease. However, other studies have failed to support this breed predilection (Millman et al., 1979, Selby et al., 1981). Cats appear to be relatively more resistant to the development of disseminated disease than are dogs.

PATHOGENESIS

The pathogenesis of infection with *Coccidioides immitis* is similar to that of histoplasmosis and blastomycosis. After arthrospores are inhaled, there is phagocytosis by alveolar macrophages. *Coccidioides immitis* is a facultative intracellular parasite, and as the arthrospore grows and metabolizes, it transforms into spherules within 48 to 72 hours. They enlarge to 20 to 100 μm in diameter. This process terminates in the endosporulation, rupture, and release of endospores, which disseminate into adjacent interstitial lung tissues in airways and spread by way of the lymphatics and blood to many regions of the body.

In some individuals, in addition to the granulomas formed by cell-mediated immunity, a microabscess characterized by polymorphonuclear infiltration is observed. Theories about these two findings suggest that spherules and endospores differ in their abilities to attract inflammatory cells and that spherules are associated with granuloma formation and endospores with a polymorphonuclear response.

In the vast majority of patients, early appearance of cell-mediated immunity to the infection is associated with granuloma formation and a minimal antibody response, presumably owing to the prompt destruction of relatively few organisms. In a small percentage of patients, cell-mediated immunity apparently is minimal and antibody production is exuberant. In these patients the host responds with large numbers of polymorphonuclear leukocytes. In the latter situation, the host usually succumbs to disseminated disease. In clinical practice, the response of patients may range between the two extremes of the spectrum.

CLINICAL MANIFESTATIONS

Coccidioidomycosis is usually classified as either a primary or disseminated disease. Primary coccidioidomycosis may be cutaneous (rare) or pulmonary. Primary cutaneous coccidioidomycosis has been described in both dogs and cats. The criteria for primary cutaneous coccidioidomycosis have been described by Wilson (1953) and Wolf (1979) and include the following: (1) no history of pulmonary disease immediately preceding the lesion; (2) history suggestive of inoculation through a break in the skin at the site of the lesion; (3) short period of time between suspected inoculation and the time the lesion is first noticed (1 to 3 weeks); (4) lesion resembling a relatively painless, firm, indurated nodule with central ulceration; (5) lymphadenitis and lymphadenopathy present but only in the region of the draining lesion; (6) precipitin developed to coccidioidin. Complement fixation antibodies, if developed, should be detected in only low titers (less than 1:16).

Pulmonary coccidioidomycosis may be asymptomatic and result in mild infection or may be symptomatic, characterized by tracheal bronchitis and, on radiographs, by infiltration of nodular densities, lung consolidation, and transitory cavitation. Primary lung disease may be confirmed serologically. Few cases of primary lung disease are recognized in the dog. If it does not resolve, primary pulmonary coccidioidomycosis may develop in two ways. In the first, it may remain localized (persist as a primary disease or progress as a primary lung disease characterized by local extension into adjacent lobes) or regress with healing characterized by local fibrosis, bronchiectasis, and, occasionally, calcification. It may also develop by dissemination to lungs, extrapulmonary sites, bones, joints, viscera, and the central nervous system (CNS).

The vast majority of patients undergoing complete resolution develop a degree of cell-mediated immunity that prevents the development of lesions. Unfortunately, probably because of spontaneous resolution of primary disease and owner procrastination, many dogs presented to veterinarians have the disseminated form of the disease. Dissemination rate in humans is reported to be one case in about

1,000. Although definitive studies have not been done, the dissemination rate in dogs appears to be higher than that observed in humans. The time from initial infection to dissemination may vary from 2 weeks to several years. The disseminated form has been defined as having hilar lymphadenopathy, bone lesions, pericardial effusion, or peripheral lymphadenopathy, but essentially any organ may be involved in the dissemination process.

Clinical signs associated with disseminated coccidioidomycosis reflect the organs and tissues infiltrated. Coughing, dyspnea, and dysphagia are common presenting complaints and are associated with enlargement of tracheobronchial lymph nodes. Vague signs such as inappetence and progressive weight loss are frequently reported. Bone involvement is usually associated with painful swellings of long bones or joint enlargement and may involve one or more sites. The bone lesions are usually located in long bones and may be present in the distal diaphyseal, metaphyseal, or epiphyseal regions. Radiographic evaluation is usually consistent with osteomyelitis; however, negative radiographic findings may be seen early in the disease. Axial skeletal lesions occur less frequently. Skin lesions in the form of draining tracts are frequently associated with underlying bony lesions. A fever that is partially responsive to antibiotic therapy is common but may not be present in the more chronic cases. Orchitis, prostatitis, peripheral lymphadenopathy, and ocular and CNS signs are less commonly observed.

Radiographic signs of lung lesions may be found in 80 per cent of the disseminated cases of coccidioidomycosis (Millman et al., 1979). These lesions are most frequently characterized by a mixture of either interstitial, bronchial, or alveolar patterns. Fifty per cent of the cases will have isolated pulmonary infiltrates, cavitating lesions, or circumscribed radiodense nodules. None of the radiographic features of coccidioidomycosis are pathognomonic for the disease. The intrathoracic radiographic sign seen most frequently with coccidioidomycosis is hilar lymphadenopathy, which is most frequently observed in lymphosarcoma and mycotic diseases in the dog. It was observed in 75 per cent of cases of coccidioidomycosis and is a result of lymphatic spread of the organism from the lung to the tracheobronchial lymph nodes and subsequent lymph node inflammation. Mild pleural effusion as a result of direct extension of the infection from the hilar lymph nodes is present in approximately half of the cases of disseminated coccidioidomycosis. Pericardial effusion or restrictive pericarditis is a frequent finding on necropsy (40 per cent) and occasionally may be detected radiographically or by electro- or echocardiography.

DIAGNOSIS

Disseminated coccidioidomycosis is associated with a variety of clinical, environmental, radiographic, hemotologic and biochemical changes that may highly suggest the presence of the disease but are not in themselves pathognomonic. Diagnosis should be confirmed by demonstrating typical endosporulating spherules in body fluids or tissue sections, by serologic testing, or by fungal culture. The clinical and radiographic features have been discussed. The hematologic features in dogs with disseminated coccidioidomycosis include increased erythrocyte sedimentation rate, mild anemia, and, in about one third of the cases, a leukocytosis. Eosinophilia commonly seen in human patients with disseminated disease only occasionally is reported in dogs. Hypergammaglobulinemia may occur with chronic antigenic stimulation. Hypercalcemia associated with coccidioidomycosis osteomyelitis has been reported in humans but has not been reported in dogs.

Cytology

The most productive body fluid for demonstrating the presence of *Coccidioides immitis* is the material drained from cutaneous tracts. Lymph node aspirates have also been reported to exhibit the organisms. Tracheal washes are not as productive as they are in humans with the disease. The organism may be seen in unstained preparations under reduced lighting; it appears as a round, double-walled structure 10 to 80 μm in diameter with endospores. Young spherules without endospores may be confused with other fungi or artifacts. Ten per cent potassium hydroxide can be applied to clear unstained preparations. Specimens may be stained after air drying with Grocott-Gomori's methenamine silver (GMS) or periodic acid-Shiff (PAS) stain. With GMS stain, the refractile capsule wall is black in color, the endospores are red to brown, and the cytoplasm usually stains yellow. With PAS stain, the spherule wall is not stained and the endospores are bright red in color.

Biopsy

Occasionally, excisional biopsy may be necessary to demonstrate the organisms. Lymph nodes, lungs, and skin are the most frequently sampled tissues. Organisms may be easily demonstrated in microabscesses, but they are scarce in granulomas. Routine hematoxylin and eosin stains are considered inferior to special stains such as PAS or GMS stains.

Culture

Because of the hazards associated with culturing *Coccidioides immitis*, in-house isolation of this organism is not recommended, and samples should be submitted to outside laboratories equipped to handle such hazardous materials. Swabs are usually not adequate means of collection; suspect material should be inoculated on Sabouraud's agar and sent to the laboratory. *Coccidioides immitis* grows well on this and other fungal culture media at room temperature in about 3 to 4 days; sporulation occurs by day 10 to 14.

Serology

Probably the most widely used method for confirming a diagnosis of coccidioidomycosis is the serologic test. Antibody response to *Coccidioides immitis* is of diagnostic significance but appears to have no protective effect for the host. After the animal is exposed to the organism, the first antibodies to appear are IgM. They may be detected by tube precipitation test, latex particle agglutination test, and immunodiffusion to precipitation tests. In dogs, IgM usually appears between 2 and 6 weeks after infection, and most of the dogs that develop clinical signs will develop precipitins. The precipitin tests are qualitative tests and fade quickly after resolution of the primary disease but may persist in severe disseminated coccidioidomycosis. A positive precipitin test with clinical signs associated with coccidioidomycosis indicates presence of the disease. IgG antibody follows IgM response and usually appears 8 to 10 weeks after infection. Unlike the case in the IgM response, a qualitative rise in titer usually correlates with the extent of the disease.

Complement fixation (CF) titers of 1:4 are considered negative. Titers greater than 1:8 are considered suspicious, and titers equal to or greater than 1:16 are positive. The CF titer has prognostic significance in that the more severe the disease, the higher the titer; likewise, a rise in titer suggests progression of the disease. Clinical improvement usually results in a significant fall in CF titer. Tests for titers may be run every 6 to 8 weeks in order to monitor therapy, but caution should be exercised in interpreting titers, since one dilutional change is probably not significant. CF titers may remain elevated long past clinical resolution of the disease process. The anticomplementary nature of some canine serum and cross-reactivity with histoplasmosis and blastomycosis organisms may limit the usefulness of the CF titer. The anticomplementary nature of some canine serum is due to the ability to fix complement in the absence of antigen. This may be caused by immune complexes or bacterial contamination in the tested serum. Serum that is found to be anticomplementary may be tested by double electroimmunodiffusion, but this test should be considered qualitative only. CF titers have not been reliable indicators of infections in the few reported cases of disseminated disease in cats. Skin testing has little diagnostic significance for clinical disease and is seldom employed in veterinary medicine except for epidemiologic studies.

TREATMENT

Although amphotericin B is still the treatment of choice in humans with disseminated coccidioidomycosis, it has been replaced by ketoconazole in the treatment of the disease in dogs and cats. Ketoconazole is an imidazole derivative that inhibits biosynthesis of ergosterol, the main sterol in the membranes of fungi. Usual doses in experimental and clinical studies suggest that ketoconazole is fungistatic rather than fungicidal. The drug appears to stabilize the infection while the host's cell-mediated immunity walls it off. Because of this property, prolonged treatment periods are usually necessary to control disseminated coccidioidomycosis. The duration of therapy is at least 6 months to 1 year, and some animals with bony lesions may never be weaned off the drug without relapsing. Despite the drug's limitation, it has many advantages over other treatments. It is readily absorbed from the gastrointestinal tract after oral administration, and this absorption may be enhanced by feeding. Ketoconazole does not cross the blood-brain barrier in sufficient quantities to be therapeutically effective at usual dosages. However, because of its low toxicities, large doses (1200 mg/day) have been used to obtain therapeutic levels in the CSF in humans.

In addition to its advantage or oral administration, ketoconazole is associated with minimal toxicity. In the author's experience, 90 per cent of dogs show no toxic side effects. The side effects reported to occur in dogs include inappetence, vomiting, hepatotoxicity, and a temporary lightening of the coat. The most severe of its effects is hepatotoxicity, which is reported most frequently in cats. The mechanism of this toxicity is unknown, but in humans it is believed to be due to a metabolic idiosyncratic reaction. Because the duration of therapy for disseminated coccidioidomycosis is prolonged, bimonthly monitoring of liver enzymes has been suggested.

Ketoconazole is supplied in 200-mg tablets that should be administered orally with meals in a dosage of 5 to 10 mg/kg twice daily. The duration of therapy will depend on the response of the patient. The decision to reduce the dose or terminate therapy should be based upon radiographic and clinical evidence of resolution of the disease process. Serologic testing may be helpful in determining treatment progress; however, CF titers may remain high for a long period of time after resolution of clinical disease. Despite apparent clinical cures after many months of treatment, some dogs relapse when the drug is discontinued. Continual low-dose administration of ketoconazole may be required in some patients to prevent relapse. Apparently, control rather than complete eradication of *Coccidioides immitis* organisms occurs in some cases, especially those with bone lesions.

PROGNOSIS

The prognosis of dogs with disseminated coccidioidomycosis should be considered guarded. Dogs with the respiratory form of the disease should be treated to decrease the chance of dissemination. Although up to 90 per cent of dogs have been reported to improve on ketoconazole, they may require lifelong therapy. Despite the prolonged therapy associated with ketoconazole, the prognosis with this drug is better than that reported with amphotericin B, in which a recovery rate of only 20 per cent can be expected.

References and Supplemental Reading

Armstrong, P. J., and DiBartola, S. P.: Canine coccidioidomycosis: A literature review and report of eight cases. J. Am. Anim. Hosp. Assoc. 19:937, 1983.

Barsanti, J. A., and Jeffery, K. L.: Coccidioidomycosis. *In* Greene, C. E. (ed.): *Clinical Microbiology and Infectious Diseases of the Dog and Cat.* Philadelphia: W. B. Saunders, 1984, pp. 710–719.

Catanzaro, A., Einstein, H., Levine, B., et al.: Ketoconazole for treatment of disseminated coccidioidomycosis. Ann. Intern. Med. 96:436, 1982.

Macy, D. W., and Small, E.: Coccidioidomycosis. *In* Ettinger, S. J. (ed.): *Textbook of Veterinary Internal Medicine*, 2nd ed. Philadelphia: W. B. Saunders, 1983, pp. 242–248.

Millman, T. M., O'Brien, T. R., Suter, P. F., et al.: Coccidioidomycosis in the dog: Its radiographic diagnosis. J. Am. Vet. Radiol. Soc. 20:50, 1979.

Selby, L. A., Becker, S. V., and Hayes, H. W.: Epidemiologic risk factors associated with canine systemic mycoses. Am. J. Epidemiol. 113:133, 1981.

Wilson, J. W., Smith, C. E., and Plunkett, O. H.: Primary cutaneous coccidioidomycosis: Criteria for diagnosis and report of a case. Calif. Med. 79:233, 1953.

Wolf, A. M.: Primary cutaneous coccidioidomycosis in a dog and a cat. J.A.V.M.A. 174:504, 1979.

ROCKY MOUNTAIN SPOTTED FEVER AND EHRLICHIOSIS

CRAIG E. GREENE, D.V.M.
Athens, Georgia

Rocky Mountain spotted fever (RMSF) and ehrlichiosis are two tickborne rickettsial diseases that affect dogs. Both diseases have many clinical features in common that make them difficult to differentiate during the acute stages, although they can be distinguished with appropriate serologic testing.

ETIOLOGY

Rickettsia rickettsii, the cause of RMSF, and *Ehrlichia canis*, the primary agent of canine ehrlichiosis, are both obligate intracellular parasites in the family Rickettsiaceae. *R. rickettsii* belongs to a larger antigenically related group known as the spotted fever rickettsiae, which infect people in various parts of the world and cause similar febrile illnesses. The group of spotted fever organisms are antigenically distinct from the typhus group of rickettsiae, which primarily infect humans, and the less closely related rickettsiae such as *Neorickettsia helminthoeca* and *E. canis*, which infect dogs. *R. rickettsii* or antigenically related organisms infect a wide variety of mammals and birds because many vertebrates have detectable antibodies to the spotted fever group of rickettsiae. *E. canis* only infects carnivores of the family Canidae and thus poses no public health hazard. *E. equi*, one of the causes of equine ehrlichiosis, has been associated with ehrlichiosis in dogs. The wide host range of this organism includes dogs, sheep, goats, cats, and nonhuman primates. It is not known whether *E. risticii*, the newly discovered agent of Potomac fever in horses, can infect dogs. Another closely related but antigenically distinguishable rickettsia, *E. platys*, has been isolated from dogs with cyclic thrombocytopenia. This disease appears to be much milder than canine ehrlichiosis caused by either *E. canis* or *E. equi*.

Dogs in the United States have been reported to

be naturally infected with *R. rickettsii*, based upon their seropositivity in surveys from many states. Similar surveys of the disease in humans indicate that eastern states have the highest prevalence, although the disease has been reported from all states except Maine, Vermont, Alaska, and Hawaii. It is also known to occur in western Canada, Mexico, Panama, Colombia, and Brazil.

In contrast, epizootiologic and serologic studies in the United States of dogs infected with *E. canis* have indicated that ehrlichiosis occurs in most southern states. Throughout the world, the disease is seen in tropical and semitropical regions, and in the Northern Hemisphere it has been recognized primarily in countries below the 45th parallel.

Clinical cases of RMSF in dogs in the United States have been recognized mostly during the months of April through September, whereas ehrlichiosis has been reported throughout the year. The strict seasonal prevalence of RMSF (compared with ehrlichiosis) probably relates to two factors. The incubation period and duration of illness prior to examination of dogs with RMSF are relatively shorter and more self-limiting than those of dogs with ehrlichiosis, and thus most cases of RMSF occur during the tick season. Furthermore, the ticks *Dermacentor variabilis* and *D. andersoni*, which have been most commonly implicated in the transmission of RMSF in the United States, are outdoor ticks, whereas *Rhipicephalus sanguineus*, the vector of ehrlichiosis, remains active in the colder months and survives indoors or in kennels wherever dogs are kept.

Table 1. *Comparison of Clinical Findings in Rocky Mountain Spotted Fever and Canine Ehrlichiosis**

RMSF		Ehrlichiosis
	Common Findings	
89	Fever >102° F	66
86	Fever >104° F	33
93	Listlessness, depression	53
75	Anorexia	60
43	Lymphadenopathy	13
57	Ticks on history or physical examination	22
18	Petechiae or hemorrhagic diathesis	22
36	Dyspnea	11
32	Neurologic deficits other than depression	10
28	Lumbar or abdominal hyperesthesia	11
21	Edema of extremities	33
21	Diarrhea, vomiting	11
11	Splenomegaly, hepatomegaly	33
	Unique Findings	
25	Stiffness, abnormal gait	—
18	Scleral congestion	—
14	Polydipsia, polyuria	—
—	Anterior uveitis	33
—	Pale mucosa	67
—	Weight loss	30

*For both diseases, values are percentages of affected animals that have the specified clinical findings.

Data taken from Greene et al.: J.A.V.M.A., 186:465, 1985; and Troy et al.: J. Am. Anim. Hosp. Assoc. 16:181, 1980.

CLINICAL FINDINGS

Although dogs of any age can contract either disease, most of those with RMSF tend to be younger (less than 2 years) than those with ehrlichiosis. Purebred dogs, especially German shepherds, appear to be more susceptible to either disease than are crossbred dogs.

Listlessness, depression, fever, and anorexia are among the most common clinical signs observed in dogs with RMSF; however, they are less common in dogs with ehrlichiosis (Table 1). Fever occurs in up to 90 per cent of dogs with RMSF but only in 66 per cent of those with ehrlichiosis. The fever is usually greater than 40°C (104°F) in three fourths of the dogs with RMSF, whereas this occurs in only one third of those with ehrlichiosis. Ticks are found on physical examination or are mentioned in the history of approximately 50 per cent of dogs with RMSF and approximately 20 per cent of those with ehrlichiosis. Generalized lymphadenopathy, dyspnea, neurologic abnormalities, and abdominal or paralumbar hyperesthesia, diarrhea, and vomiting can be present in both diseases, but they are more common with RMSF. Hepatosplenomegaly can be found in both diseases but more frequently accompanies ehrlichiosis. Petechial or ecchymotic hemorrhages or other evidence of a hemorrhagic diathesis are observed in only 20 per cent or less of affected animals with either disease. Edema of the extremities is found in dogs with either disease, and acronecrosis can occur if diagnosis and appropriate therapy are delayed. Certain features such as stiffness of gait, scleral congestion, and a history of polydipsia are primarily seen in RMSF, whereas anterior uveitis, pale mucosae, and weight loss are more typically signs of ehrlichiosis.

Depression is a consistent neurologic finding in dogs with either RMSF or ehrlichiosis. Neurologic signs other than depression can be observed in up to one third of dogs having either disease. Paraparesis or tetraparesis and ataxia, caused by dysfunction of upper motor neurons, are commonly observed findings. Acute central or peripheral vestibular dysfunction and generalized or localized hyperesthesia are often found. Seizures, cranial nerve deficits (in addition to vestibular), and coma are seen in dogs with RMSF and may occur just prior to death. Anisocoria from unilateral mydriasis can be seen in RMSF but is more common in ehrlichiosis; its presence is probably related to the severe retinal lesions found in the latter disease. Dogs with RMSF may have focal retinal hemorrhage or chorioretinal exudate, whereas those with ehrlichiosis often have extensive hemorrhage and exudation with retinal detachment.

LABORATORY FINDINGS

Hematologic findings are generally different in the two diseases, although many cases require additional diagnostic testing for positive identification of the disease that is present. Dogs with RMSF generally have higher hematocrits than those with ehrlichiosis, which often have anemia. Depression of erythrocytic and leukocytic elements in the blood of dogs with chronic ehrlichiosis parallels the suppressive effects of this infection on the function of bone marrow. In contrast, leukocytosis, a more common finding in chronic cases of RMSF, increases in magnitude proportionally to the duration of illness. Thrombocyte counts cannot always be used to distinguish dogs with RMSF from those with ehrlichiosis, since animals with either disease have overlapping ranges of low platelet counts. Platelet counts in dogs with RMSF range from 23,000 to 209,000/μl (mean of 95,000/μl). Platelet counts tend to be lower in dogs with ehrlichiosis and range from 1,000 to 200,000/μl (mean of 50,000/μl). In general, animals with RMSF have higher platelet counts but show external signs of hemorrhage at a frequency similar to that of dogs with ehrlichiosis. This probably relates to the fact that petechiae in RMSF are produced primarily as a result of the vasculitis, and the thrombocytopenia is secondary to vascular disruption. In any case, the presence of thrombocytopenia appears to be important as a reliable indicator for either disease, although a small proportion of affected dogs can have normal numbers of platelets.

Hypoalbuminemia is a frequent finding in dogs with either disease. Despite the fact that serum globulin concentrations in dogs with RMSF remain normal, their levels of serum protein are often reduced. In contrast, dogs with ehrlichiosis commonly have increased concentrations of serum globulin, which offset hypoalbuminemia and produce relatively normal concentrations of mean total protein. The serum alkaline phosphatase activity of dogs with RMSF is usually greater than that in dogs with ehrlichiosis. In contrast, the activity of alanine transaminase (SGPT) is often increased in dogs with ehrlichiosis but not in those with RMSF. Serum calcium concentration may be low as a result of hypoalbuminemia, but the reduction of this concentration is usually mild. Serum cholesterol concentration is high in most dogs with RMSF but not in those with ehrlichiosis. Concentrations of muscle enzymes such as creatine kinase may be increased in sera from dogs with RMSF.

Lymphadenopathy is associated with both diseases, and reactive hyperplasia is the cytologic pattern noted on fine-needle aspiration. The results of coagulation testing, other than platelet counting, are usually normal, although dogs with severe RMSF and hemorrhage may have prolonged coagulation times if they develop disseminated intravascular coagulation (DIC). Tests for serum antinuclear antibody, lupus erythematosus cells, erythrocyte autoantibodies, platelet autoantibodies, and rheumatoid factor usually produce negative findings in both diseases. Abnormal synovial fluid can be found in dogs with RMSF, and there is usually an increase in leukocytes, predominantly nondegenerate neutrophils, similar to that seen in immune-mediated polyarthritis. Reported findings of cerebrospinal fluid (CSF) analyses have been limited in both diseases; however, if the analysis reveals pleocytosis, in dogs with RMSF it consists primarily of neutrophils and in dogs with ehrlichiosis it primarily shows lymphocytes. Diffuse interstitial density in the lung field may be found in dogs showing signs of cough or dyspnea with either disease.

SEROLOGIC TESTING

This appears to be a relatively specific means of differentiating RMSF and ehrlichiosis, since minimal cross-reaction has been found in sera from dogs with either disease. The disadvantages of serologic testing are that the results are often not available until after a course of therapy has been instituted and that in the case of RMSF, follow-up samples must be taken because a rising titer must be demonstrated. The most reliable and specific test for RMSF is the microimmunofluorescent method, which is species-specific and can be performed by several veterinary diagnostic laboratories in the United States.* The high antibody titers to *R. rickettsii* that develop in actively infected dogs generally decrease after 3 to 5 months, although some remain elevated (greater than 1:128) for at least 10 to 12 months, making single titers unreliable in the confirmation of active infection. Although a fourfold rise is needed for confirmation, actively infected dogs may already have an elevated titer when the first serum sample is taken, and thus the magnitude of the increase in titer will be reduced.

Direct fluorescent antibody staining of skin biopsy

---

*C. E. Greene, RMSF Laboratory, Department of Small Animal Medicine, College of Veterinary Medicine, University of Georgia, Athens, GA 30602.

Pathologists' Service Professional Associates, Inc., P. O. Box 50122, Federal Annex, Atlanta, GA 30302.

RMSF Project, c/o E. Breitschwerdt, Department of CASS, School of Veterinary Medicine, North Carolina State University, 4700 Hillsborough Street, Raleigh, NC 27606.

GJL Medical Labs, Inc., Veterinary Division, 15 Ireland Place, Amityville, NY 11701.

Texas Veterinary Medical Diagnostic Laboratory, Drawer 3040, College Station, TX 77840.

samples from infected dogs appears to be a valuable test for rapid diagnosis of RMSF, since it is positive in up to 80 per cent of dogs tested.* Skin biopsy samples should be taken from the inguinal region prior to institution of antimicrobial chemotherapy, whether or not petechial hemorrhages are present and regardless of the duration of clinical signs prior to examination. These samples can be fixed in formalin, since the antigen that is detected is not denatured by this procedure. The presence of relatively high titers of serum antibody in dogs does not appear to confirm the finding of rickettsiae in skin.

An indirect fluorescent serum antibody test is used to diagnose ehrlichiosis.† The test is highly sensitive and specific for *E. canis*. A positive result at the lowest measured titer of 1:10 on a single serum sample is considered diagnostic because, unlike RMSF, *Ehrlichia* infections are persistent unless they are treated. However, animals having questionable or low (up to 1:20) antibody titers should have their sera resubmitted in 30 days because the antibody titer to *Ehrlichia* after infection is not usually increased until at least 20 days and the titers in untreated dogs do not peak until 80 days. Serum antibody titers to *E. canis* decrease gradually within 3 to 9 months after the elimination of infection with tetracycline. The persistence or increase in titer to *E. canis* may be useful in distinguishing chronic carriers from those successfully treated and cleared of infection.

Although the detection of intracellular inclusions in peripheral blood samples has been used to diagnose ehrlichiosis, serologic testing is the best means of detecting the disease in practice because of its ambiguous clinical signs and the brief persistence of the organism in peripheral blood. Unfortunately, serologic tests detecting *E. canis* infection do not cross-react with those for detecting infection with *E. equi*, *E. platys*, or *E. risticii*. Dogs that have clinical signs and laboratory findings consistent with RMSF or canine ehrlichiosis and that are seronegative for either disease might be infected with these or perhaps other as yet undiscovered rickettsiae.

THERAPY

The response to therapy when most dogs with RMSF are treated with tetracycline (22 mg/kg, given three times daily for 2 weeks) is rapid and dramatic. Most dogs without neurologic deficits improve within 24 to 48 hours, although in some cases the response takes up to 5 days. Chloramphenicol (15 mg/kg, given three times daily for 2 weeks) is recommended in pups less than 5 months of age because of the risk of staining their dental enamel with tetracycline. Chloramphenicol may also be used in the rare case that may relapse.

Dogs with neurologic deficits have variably prolonged recovery periods. Much of the delayed response is related to residual neurologic deficits that persist despite resolution of the other systemic signs. These deficits, which may never resolve in some cases, indicate the presence of permanent brain damage. The rapidly progressive neurologic form of RMSF, characterized by seizures, coma, and cardiovascular collapse, is usually fatal despite immediate institution of antimicrobial therapy.

The time interval for response to therapy with tetracycline (22 mg/kg, given three times daily for 2 weeks) in dogs with ehrlichiosis is more variable than in those with RMSF. Prolonged recovery periods are common in animals with long-standing infection because of severe bone marrow damage that results in pancytopenia. Dogs with mild clinical signs, normal leukocyte counts, or acute stages of illness show dramatic improvement in clinical and hematologic measurements within 24 to 48 hours after therapy is instituted; this response is similar to that seen in dogs with RMSF. Dogs with chronic pancytopenia may not respond to therapy for a period of up to 120 days. The prognosis in such cases is poor because of the risk of fatal hemorrhage or infection developing prior to recovery. These cases require therapy with androgenic steroids, antimicrobial therapy when secondary infection develops, and repeated fresh whole-blood transfusions when necessary.

Several drugs have become available for more effective treatment of cases of ehrlichiosis that are refractory to tetracycline. Relapses and reinfections are more common in dogs with this disease than in those with RMSF. Imidocarb dipropionate (5 to 7 mg/kg IM, divided twice daily for 1 to 2 days) has been used to treat ehrlichiosis, and dogs receiving this drug have had fewer relapses than those treated with tetracycline. Unfortunately, this agent may produce transient toxic effects such as salivation, serous nasal discharge, dyspnea, and diarrhea. Despite clinical recovery, up to 10 per cent of treated dogs may have relapses after therapy. This drug is not currently available in the United States. Doxycycline or minocycline, lipid-soluble tetracyclines, readily penetrate the intact cell and are therefore more effective than tetracycline or oxytetracycline. Oral dosages of 5 mg/kg are given once daily for 7 to 10 days in acute ehrlichiosis, and 10 mg/kg is

*Pathologists' Service Professional Associates, Inc., P. O. Box 50122, Federal Annex, Atlanta, GA 30302.

†Veterinary Diagnostic Laboratories, P. O. Box U, University of Illinois, Urbana, IL 61801.

given once daily for 7 to 10 days in chronic cases. Intravenous administration of doxycycline may be used in dogs that vomit the medication.

PREVENTION

Dogs are immune to reinfection after they recover from RMSF. The best means of preventing infection in dogs is to eliminate their exposure to wooded areas and to remove attached ticks rapidly and safely. *R. rickettsii*, which becomes avirulent in overwintering ticks, becomes reactivated (infectious) after the ticks attach to a mammalian host and take their first meal of blood in the spring. In addition, ticks must remain attached for 5 to 20 hours before the rickettsiae within them become virulent. Presumed zoonotic spread occurs when humans remove engorged infected ticks from dogs and come into contact with tick hemolymph. When newly attached ticks are removed promptly from dogs or humans they are less likely to be a source of infection. Tick eradication in the environment is an impossible method of controlling RMSF because the rickettsial life cycle is maintained by ticks feeding on rodents and other wild reservoir hosts.

Unlike RMSF, canine ehrlichiosis can be prevented with treatment of the vertebrate host and by adequate tick control. This difference in vector control is possible because the tick *R. sanguineus* only feeds on dogs and it primarily survives in areas where dogs are kept. Attempts to control the tick population in households or kennels where infected dogs are identified should be made by spraying the living quarters and dipping the animals at 1- to 2-week intervals. New dogs entering a tick-free kennel should be dipped, and they should be quarantined until they have been found to be seronegative for *E. canis* infection. Epizootics in a kennel can be successfully controlled or contained by long-term tetracycline prophylaxis (6.6 mg/kg given once daily). Dogs should be given tetracycline for at least 4 to 6 months so that ticks will pass through a generation cycle and so that already infected ticks will die off without infecting new hosts. Therapy for as long as 1 to 2 years may be required in highly endemic areas. *E. canis*, unlike *R. rickettsii*, does not appear to produce lasting immunity to infection after treatment, and dogs are always susceptible to reinfection. Although inactivated vaccines have been developed for use in humans, their efficacy has been poor. It is uncertain whether or not suitable vaccines will be developed for either disease in dogs.

References and Supplemental Reading

Greene, C. E., and Philip, R. N.: Rocky Mountain spotted fever. *In* Greene, C. E. (ed.): *Clinical Microbiology and Infectious Diseases of the Dog and Cat.* Philadelphia: W. B. Saunders, 1984, p. 562.

Greene, C. E., and Harvey, J. W.: Canine ehrlichiosis. *In* Greene, C. E. (ed.): *Clinical Microbiology and Infectious Diseases of the Dog and Cat.* Philadelphia: W. B. Saunders, 1984, p. 545.

Greene, C. E., Burgdorfer, W., Cavagnolo, R., et al.: Rocky Mountain spotted fever in dogs and its differentiation from canine ehrlichiosis. J.A.V.M.A., 186:465, 1985.

Troy, G. C., Vulgamott, J. C., and Turnwald, G. H.: Canine ehrlichiosis: A retrospective study of 30 naturally occurring cases. J. Am. Anim. Hosp. Assoc. 16:181, 1980.

BACTERIAL ANTIBIOTIC RESISTANCE

GARY M. DUNNY, Ph.D.
Ithaca, New York

Antibiotics are the primary weapons available to veterinary practitioners in the treatment of infectious diseases. In the proper circumstances, these agents are extremely effective in controlling bacterial infections. Unfortunately, there are a number of factors that can preclude a successful course of antibiotic therapy. One of these factors is the expression of antibiotic resistance by the pathogenic microorganisms responsible for the infection. In this article, the mechanisms and genetics of microbial antibiotic resistance will be discussed along with some of the ways in which inappropriate antibiotic use can contribute to the spread of resistance. Finally, some principles to guide practitioners in the prudent use of antibiotics will be suggested.

ANTIBIOTICS AND ANTIBIOTIC SUSCEPTIBILITY

Antibiotics are compounds produced by microorganisms. They generally act by inhibiting macromolecular biosynthesis (of either nucleic acids, proteins, or cell walls) in bacteria. There are both naturally occurring antibiotics and "semisynthetic" antimicrobial agents produced by pharmaceutical companies. These manufactured compounds have the same mechanisms of action as the antibiotics from which they were derived, but they have modified chemical structures that improve their stability, their effectiveness of interaction with the target organism, or their pharmacologic properties.

Antibiotic susceptibility is measured in the laboratory by inoculating identical aliquots of the culture to be tested into a series of vessels containing a standardized volume of culture medium and increasing concentrations of the antibiotic of interest. The lowest concentration of antibiotic that prevents growth of the organism is called the minimum inhibitory concentration, or MIC. MIC values can be influenced by the inoculum size, the type of medium used, whether the assay is carried out in liquid or agar, and other factors.

In order for an antibiotic to be clinically effective, the concentration of the antimicrobial agent at the site of the infection must equal or exceed the MIC for the organism growing in the specific environment of the infection. Because it is impossible to measure MICs *in vivo* on a routine basis, predictions of the clinical efficacy of antimicrobial agents have been made by comparing the laboratory MIC value of an antimicrobial agent with the serum concentration of the drug obtained during therapy. In the case of sensitivity tests carried out with antibiotic discs, the size of zones of inhibition around the discs have been correlated with MIC values.

From this brief discussion, it should be obvious that even under the best of circumstances, laboratory determinations of sensitivity represent estimates of the absolute clinical susceptibility of a pathogen to antibiotic therapy. These estimates can be greatly influenced by conditions in both the patient and the laboratory. Nevertheless, properly performed culture and sensitivity testing of clinical material obtained prior to the administration of a drug can provide extremely useful information to confirm the initial choice of antimicrobial agents and to suggest alternate courses of therapy in the event of a lack of clinical response to the initial treatment. This is particularly important in the case of infections caused by staphylococci or gram-negative enteric bacteria, in which the incidence of antibiotic resistance tends to be very high.

MICROBIAL ANTIBIOTIC RESISTANCE

As noted previously, several factors can interfere with the clinical effectiveness of an antibiotic to which an organism is sensitive. The inherent, or basal, level of resistance of microorganisms to antibiotics varies with the organism and the antimicrobial agent. This variability is due mainly to differences from species to species in bacterial structures such as cell walls and membranes. In the laboratory, it is often possible to obtain antibiotic-resistant mutants from sensitive parent strains. These mutant derivatives may display a considerable increase over the basal level of the MIC for the antibiotic in question, but they often show reduced pathogenicity and defects in growth properties in the absence of the antibiotic. In many cases, several successive, independent mutations are required to generate mutants with very high levels of resistance. Furthermore, these mutants do not typically exhibit cross-resistance to other antibiotics, except for those closely related to the antibiotic used to select the mutant.

When the first therapeutic failures of antibiotic treatment due to resistant microbes were reported, the initial speculation was that the resistant strains were mutants that had been selected for by the antibiotic treatment. Although this type of selection can occur in clinical situations, it quickly became apparent that most of the resistant clinical isolates contained unique extrachromosomal DNA elements called resistance plasmids, or R-factors. The antibiotic-resistant genes carried by these plasmids were completely different from the genes of laboratory mutants.

Whereas laboratory mutants generally show alterations in structural genes for the targets of antibiotics (such as ribosomal proteins), resistance plasmids often carry genes that code for enzymes that break down or modify antibiotics to inactive forms. Examples of such enzymes include β-lactamases, which attack penicillins and cephalosporins; phosphotransferases, which inactivate aminoglycosides such as kanamycin and streptomycin; and acetyltransferases, which inactivate chloramphenicol. Alternatively, certain enzymes mediate resistance by modifying the bacterial cell. An example of this type of resistance is the "MLS" phenotype. In this case, a plasmid-encoded enzyme modifies bacterial ribosomal RNA and renders the microbe completely resistant to a variety of macrolide, lincosamide, and streptogramin antibiotics, including erythromycin, clindamycin, lincomycin, and tylosin. Thus, plasmid-mediated antibiotic resistance can be thought of as a metabolically active form of resistance, in contrast to the type of "passive" resistance resulting from mutations in structural genes. An important clinical consequence of the type of enzymatic resistance associated with plasmids is that the host bacterium is often rendered resistant to an extremely high level of the compound; this precludes the possibility of overcoming the microbe by using an increased dose of the antibiotic.

Bacterial plasmids are chemically identical to bacterial chromosomes and consist of double-stranded DNA in a circular form. Generally, the genes carried by plasmids are not necessary for the basic growth and metabolism of the host cell. Instead, genes found on plasmids often confer certain special properties, such as resistance to antibiotics, or heavy metals, on the host cell. Under the proper conditions, such properties can have tremendous survival value. In addition to resistance, plasmid-linked genes sometimes confer properties such as toxin production or the ability to colonize a mucosal surface. One of the most important genetic properties of plasmids is their ability to transfer horizontally between cells in bacterial populations. This type of transfer often occurs across species barriers and between nonpathogenic and pathogenic organisms. Several different mechanisms of plasmid transfer have been demonstrated, including conjugal transfer by direct cell-to-cell contact. Conjugal transfer is actually mediated by genes carried on the plasmid, although not all plasmids carry such genes. It has also been shown that many resistance genes can transpose from one plasmid to another within a bacterial cell by a novel mechanism of genetic recombination. This type of transposition can also facilitate the dissemination of the gene through microbial populations.

Since the resistance genes carried by plasmids seem to be different from genes produced in the laboratory by mutation, the question arises as to their origin. Although the origin of many of these determinants is unknown, in some cases identical resistance determinants have been found in both bacteria from clinical infections and from the microorganisms that produce antibiotics. It is quite conceivable that resistance genes originated in the producing organisms and, through a series of genetic transfers, made their way into clinical isolates. These data suggest that for every new antibiotic that may be discovered, there is already a resistance gene present in the microbial world. A resistant strain encountered in a patient represents a selection for a gene that existed prior to treatment of the patient. Thus, the probability that a resistant strain will be encountered is dependent on the amount of previous exposure of the microbial flora of the patient and the environment to the antibiotic. The best way to preserve the effectiveness of antibiotics is to avoid their indiscriminate use when they are unnecessary or contraindicated.

The genetic and biochemical properties of plasmid-mediated drug resistance have several important clinical implications of which practitioners should be aware. Table 1 shows several undesirable outcomes of antibiotic therapy that may result from the exposure of a microbial population containing plasmids to antibiotic selection pressure. Since some plasmids can carry 50 or more genes, the ominous possibility of selecting for a single plasmid carrying multiple resistance and virulence genes by using a single antimicrobial agent should never be forgotten.

Table 1. *Undesirable Effects of Antibiotic Use on Microbial Populations*

1. Use of a single antibiotic may select for multiply resistant strains.
2. Conversion of normal to resistant flora through heavy treatment provides a reservoir of resistance that can be transmitted subsequently to pathogens.
3. If a plasmid carrying both resistance determinants and virulence determinants is present in a microbial population, use of antibiotics may select directly for more virulent strains.

GUIDELINES FOR THE USE OF ANTIBIOTICS

Detailed discussions of the microbiologic techniques and therapeutic practices essential for the correct use of antibiotics in a veterinary practice can be found in *Current Veterinary Therapy VIII*. The following list, based upon the current state of knowledge of microbial drug resistance, summarizes the most important principles to guide decisions regarding antibiotic use.

1. Avoid routine prescription of antibiotics in cases in which the clinical signs are inconsistent with a bacterial infection.
2. Avoid prescribing antibiotics in situations in which therapeutic compliance is unlikely.
3. Make every attempt to back up diagnoses with culture and sensitivity testing, particularly when gram-negative enteric organisms or staphylococci are the suspected pathogens.
4. Be aware that the extent of antibiotic resistance is constantly changing. In general, organisms are becoming more resistant. Therefore, it is not always safe to assume that the treatment that worked last year, or even last week, will be effective tomorrow.

Adherence to these principles will almost surely help to preserve the effectiveness of antimicrobial agents, which are the most important weapons available to control infectious diseases.

References and Supplemental Reading

Broda, P.: *Plasmids*. Oxford, UK: W. H. Freeman, 1979.
Linton, A. H.: Antibiotic resistance in veterinary practice. In Pract. 4:11, 1982.
Monaghan, C., Tierney, U., and Colleran, E.: Antibiotic resistance and R-factors in the fecal coliform of urban and rural dogs. Antimicrob. Agents Chemother. 19:266, 1981.

POTENTIAL AND NEWLY RECOGNIZED PET-ASSOCIATED ZOONOSES

JANET M. SCARLETT KRANZ, D.V.M.
Ithaca, New York

Several diseases have emerged in recent years as zoonotic or potentially zoonotic as a result of the development of new culture and diagnostic techniques, the application of analytic epidemiologic study designs to human diseases of unknown cause, and the accumulation of further data regarding the prevalence of certain infections in domestic animals and wildlife. Many of these diseases have been associated with exposure to companion animals. This article is designed to provide the practitioner with a brief synopsis of the data implicating dogs and cats as reservoirs for agents or potential agents of several human diseases including cryptosporidiosis, *Campylobacter* enteritis, giardiasis, alveolar hydatid disease, multiple sclerosis, amyotrophic lateral sclerosis, and leukemia. In view of the reports these studies often generate in the popular press, it is important for the practitioner to keep apprised of the current status of research regarding pet-associated zoonoses so that interested clients may also be kept informed.

CRYPTOSPORIDIOSIS

Cryptosporidiosis, a protozoan disease caused by *Cryptosporidium*, has been recognized in turkeys, chickens, calves, lambs, pigs, goats, and numerous other species for many years. Before 1976, however, the disease had not been described in humans. Since that time over 50 human patients with *Cryptospordium* infections have been reported (Navin and Juranek, 1984), and there now seems little doubt that the organism is zoonotic.

The majority of human infections to date have been documented in immunodeficient humans (e.g., patients with AIDS, or hypogammaglobulinemia) in which the organism has produced a profuse, irreversible, watery diarrhea, and contributed to several deaths. There is no known treatment. Immunocompetent people, on the other hand, have developed either inapparent infections or, more often, a self-limiting, watery diarrhea associated with low-grade fever, nausea, abdominal cramps, general malaise, and headache.

Humans have acquired infection after direct contact with infective *Cryptosporidium* oocysts in the fecal material of infected calves (and probably from other species, including humans) and indirectly, after consumption of contaminated food or water. Although it was once believed that there were 11 species of *Cryptosporidium*, each host-specific for a different mammalian species, it now appears that there is considerably less host specificity in this organism.

The role of dogs and cats in the epidemiology of the disease is, as yet, unclear. Experimental studies have demonstrated that both puppies and kittens are susceptible to infection with *Cryptosporidium* from human feces and will shed oocysts in their stools (Navin and Juranek, 1984). "Natural" infections in cats have been reported, and a recent report of *Cryptosporidium* infection in a human with clinical and laboratory evidence of AIDS strongly suggests that the cryptosporidial infection was acquired from the patient's cat. This raises questions about the importance of pets as reservoirs for human infection.

Much remains to be learned about *Cryptosporidium* infections in dogs and cats. The few experimental studies conducted suggest that infections remain asymptomatic and that oocysts are shed only transiently, but further work is essential. In human medicine, a modification of the traditional Sheather's sugar flotation test, viewed under phase-contrast microscopy, is currently the favored method of diagnosis. This method has also been used to diagnose infection in experimentally infected dogs and cats. Many other questions must be addressed regarding the prevalence of this infection, the magnitude of the risk to humans, whether the organism can produce clinical disease in pets, whether there are age, sex, or breed differences in susceptibility, and so forth, before specific recommendations can be made to veterinary practitioners regarding the diagnosis, prevalence, and importance of this parasite in small animals.

GIARDIASIS

Infection with *Giardia lamblia* is now recognized as a major cause of human diarrhea. At one time, it was believed that only people traveling outside the United States were at high risk of infection with this protozoan parasite. In recent years, after several outbreaks of human giardiasis traced to contaminated municipal water supplies, the beaver and other wildlife species have been implicated in the transmission of *Giardia* to humans.

These outbreaks have renewed interest in the zoonotic potential of *Giardia* and, as in the case with *Cryptosporidium*, data now exist documenting the cross-species transmission of some *Giardia* species. The organism is transmitted in the cyst stage by the fecal-oral route, and in humans it produces diarrhea, abdominal cramping, bloating, and sometimes fever and nausea. Inapparent infections are common.

Clinical giardiasis can occur in dogs and cats, or the infection may be asymptomatic. Young animals seem to be at highest risk of infection. Clinically affected animals exhibit a soft, light-colored, diarrheic stool and often have a history of signs lasting for weeks or months. Aside from demonstration of the organism in the stool, there is no way to distinguish giardiasis from other conditions or agents causing diarrhea in companion animals. Methods of diagnosis have been described by Kirkpatrick and Farrell (1982). Several studies of the prevalence of *Giardia* infection in dogs and cats have been published and provide a range of estimates from 1 to 36 per cent. These data must be interpreted cautiously since fecal examinations (even zinc sulfate flotation) can fail to detect infected animals, and the characteristics of the dogs surveyed (e.g., the percentage of immature animals) probably differ.

Although dogs have been infected experimentally with *Giardia lamblia* of human origin, their role as reservoirs of human infection is as yet poorly understood. The diagnosis of giardiasis in five family members in Fort Collins and the isolation of a large number of *Giardia* cysts from the feces of the family cat, as well as the identification of *Giardia* cysts in the stool of another cat and that of its owner and the owner's boyfriend, provide strong circumstantial evidence of the zoonotic potential of this parasite.

Until further, more definitive studies are conducted both to ascertain the prevalence of infection with *Giardia* among companion animals and to assess the potential for spread to human owners, it seems prudent to actively consider the diagnosis of giardiasis in dogs and cats with chronic, unresponsive diarrhea and to treat all infected animals. It is certainly not unreasonable to examine the stools of animals owned by families suffering from giardiasis.

It is also probably wise to note that parakeets can be infected with *Giardia* both symptomatically and asymptomatically, and they can shed cysts into their environment. The zoonotic potential of this infection is unknown (Panigrahy et al., 1979).

CAMPYLOBACTER ENTERITIS

Before selective techniques for stool culture made it possible to isolate *Campylobacter* species easily, these gram-negative organisms were largely believed to be confined to cattle and sheep, in which they were known to cause abortion (and were formerly called *Vibrio fetus*). After the widespread adoption of new culture techniques, *Campylobacter jejuni* has been recognized as a major cause of human enteritis, and prevalence estimates in industrialized countries range from 7 to 15 per cent of patients with diarrhea. *C. jejuni* (formerly *C. fetus* subsp. *jejuni*) and *C. coli* cause disease in humans. Because these organisms differ only slightly, and because *C. jejuni* is the species most commonly associated with human disease, they are often collectively referred to as *C. jejuni* (Blaser and Reller, 1981).

The disease in humans fortunately is usually self-limiting, characterized by cramps and diarrhea of 24 to 72 hours' duration and accompanied by fever, general malaise, headache, and muscle soreness. The disease is usually not severe, although deaths have been reported among elderly or debilitated persons, and before recognition of this agent, several patients underwent unnecessary abdominal surgery (Prescott and Munroe, 1981). Erythromycin is the treatment of choice for humans. Untreated, infected patients can shed the organism in their feces for as long as 1 year.

A knowledge of this organism, its zoonotic potential, its mode of transmission, and its prevalence is important to the veterinary practitioner because the principal reservoirs are animals (dogs, cats, pigs, goats, cattle, sheep, horses, chickens, and other species). The disease can apparently result from consumption of a very small number of organisms. Most infections occur after direct contact with the feces of infected animals or the consumption of contaminated food and water.

Naturally occurring infections in dogs and cats have been well-documented (Dillon and Wilt, 1983). Likewise, in view of the numerous reports of human infection acquired from both dogs and cats, there is little doubt regarding the zoonotic potential of *Campylobacter jejuni* in these species. The magnitude of the role these animals play as reservoirs of human infection, however, is unclear. A recent report from Great Britain estimated that no more than 5 per cent of all human *Campylobacter* infections were associated with dogs and cats, and most of those resulted from exposure to dogs. The authors, however, readily admit that accurate data regarding the true relative importance of these species as reservoirs are lacking. Most human infections (acquired from dogs and cats) have been associated with puppies and kittens, newly introduced into the household and displaying diarrhea shortly before the human illness occurred. This is probably the result of a higher prevalence of infection among young animals, as well as close contact with them. Often the affected humans have been infants or other young children, whose sanitary habits put them at high risk of infection. In addition to the higher prevalence of infection observed in young animals, stray and kennelled dogs also appear to have a high prevalence of infection.

The pathogenicity of *Campylobacter jejuni* in dogs and cats is not well understood (Skirrow, 1981). Although clinical enteritis has been observed, particularly among infected puppies and kittens in households with human illness, experimental infections have failed to produce clinical disease or have produced only mild enterocolitis. Studies of the prevalence of *C. jejuni* in dogs with and without diarrhea have produced conflicting results; some demonstrate a significant difference in infection rates and others fail to do so. Prevalence of infection is not a good measure of risk of clinical disease, however, and there is a need to assess whether disease is produced when animals are infected initially. Preliminary evidence suggests that *Campylobacter* infections are less common in cats, but the pattern of occurrence is probably similar to that observed in dogs (Skirrow, 1981).

From the data available, it can be concluded that the risk of human infection from contact with dogs and cats is low, but clients owning animals with diarrhea should be cautioned to separate the affected animal from very young children and to observe good hygienic practices, particularly washing hands after handling or cleaning up after dogs and cats with diarrhea.

ALVEOLAR HYDATID DISEASE

Alveolar hydatid disease in humans is caused by infection with the larval stage of the parasite *Echinococcus multilocularis*. The infection is insidious and potentially fatal if not recognized in its early stages. The cestode parasite, whose intermediate hosts are small rodents and whose natural definitive host is the fox (but whose hosts can also be dogs and cats), has a wide geographic distribution. It was not until the 1950s, however, that it was described in North America, and not until 1964 was it recognized in North Dakota. The parasite deserves brief mention since it has now been documented to occur in wild rodents and foxes in several of the North Central States, and several recent surveys of farm cats in North Dakota have demonstrated infection rates ranging from 1 to 5 per cent (Gamble et al., 1979).

The sylvatic cycle (involving wild rodents and foxes) is probably of little concern from the standpoint of human health, but the potential for the evolution of a cycle involving wild mice and cats or dogs has far-reaching public health implications. Several investigators have expressed concern that a cycle in house mice and cats may become established and put both urban and rural children playing with cats at high risk of contracting the infection (Gamble et al., 1979).

Fortunately, within the 48 contiguous United States only one human case of alveolar hydatid disease has been reported in which the infection was apparently acquired from pet exposure. Practitioners from the North Central States should monitor further research regarding this parasite.

HUMAN DISEASES IMPLICATED WITH EXPOSURE TO DOGS OR CATS

In recent years, several studies of human diseases (including multiple sclerosis, leukemia, and amyotrophic lateral sclerosis) have implicated exposure to animals as part of the etiology of these disorders.

Since experimental studies in humans are impossible to conduct for ethical reasons, much of the data collected to evaluate these hypotheses have been gathered by using observational, epidemiologic study designs. Although it is beyond the scope of this article to discuss the strengths and weaknesses inherent to these research designs (see Schwabe et al., 1977), it is important to understand that without the closely controlled conditions of the laboratory, it is far more difficult to establish a definitive causal link between disease and a hypothesized exposure. A brief summary of the current findings regarding each of these diseases is included to facilitate the veterinarian's discussions with interested clients.

Multiple Sclerosis

In 1977 two neurologists identified a statistical association between ownership of small dogs (less than 25 lbs) and the development of multiple sclerosis (MS). A subsequent study by the same researchers appeared to confirm the existence of this relationship and sparked numerous additional investigations. The subsequent studies (employing the same case-control design) have almost unanimously failed to identify a relationship.

To understand the intense interest at first generated by the early results, it is important to consider the biologic feasibility of the suggested hypothesis. An infectious cause for MS has long been entertained. The suggestion of an infectious agent of canine origin prompted speculation regarding the canine distemper virus (CDV) because of its documented proclivity for nervous tissue and the demyelinating lesions it produces (with some similarities to those observed in MS); likewise, its apparent ability to remain latent in nervous tissue for years and sometimes produce a fatal encephalitis (old dog encephalitis), and its morphologic and antigenic similarities to the human measles virus, an agent consistently associated with the origin of MS, made the CDV hypothesis attractive.

Subsequent studies of the frequency of CDV antibodies in the sera of MS patients, compared with controls, have failed to demonstrate a difference between the two groups. Likewise, veterinarians, who are at high risk of exposure to the canine distemper virus, have not been found to have an unusually high risk of MS, although this may reflect the fact that the putative exposure must be experienced before the mid-teenage years.

Further impetus for the distemper-MS link was provided by studies of the temporal occurrence of distemper and MS epidemics in several island populations. Unusually high frequencies of MS have been described in populations of the islands of Sitka (Alaska), Iceland, and the Faroes after epidemics of canine distemper. Although these observations are provocative, their significance has been questioned on various grounds (depending on the study), including the possibility of introduction of other agents concurrently with the distemper virus, the failure to identify accurately all MS patients prior to the distemper outbreaks, and the sometimes incomplete geographic overlap between two "outbreaks."

To summarize, there is currently no conclusive scientific data to support a causal relationship between dog ownership or the canine distemper virus and multiple sclerosis. On this basis, there is currently no reason for clients to fear contracting multiple sclerosis from their dogs and no evidence to support any intervention on the part of veterinary practitioners.

Amyotrophic Lateral Sclerosis

After the publication of the studies associating multiple sclerosis with dog exposure, a case-control study of amyotrophic lateral sclerosis (ALS) also demonstrated an increased exposure to small dogs among ALS patients, compared with controls. Until further data are forthcoming, the meaning of this association cannot be assessed.

Leukemia

Studies evaluating the risk of human infection with the feline leukemia virus (FeLV) and the risk of development of human leukemia after exposure to FeLV-infected cats have been reviewed elsewhere (Burridge, 1979). One recent study at the Sloan-Kettering Institute for Cancer Research is of interest, since the researchers tested patients with various cancers (including rare soft-tissue sarcomas and hematologic cancers) for the presence of FOCMA (feline oncovirus-associated cell membrane antigen) on the membranes of the tumor cells; they also tested for FeLV antigen and FeLV and FOCMA antibodies. They could find no evidence of active FeLV infection or a history of previous infection in any of the patients tested (Sordillo et al., 1982).

Although these results do not definitively rule out transmission of FeLV to humans, they, together with evidence from most earlier studies, fail to support the hypothesis suggesting the zoonotic spread of this virus to humans.

SUMMARY

Other diseases, such as systemic lupus erythematosus and rheumatoid arthritis, have also been linked with pet exposure, but the data supporting the proposed associations are unconvincing. Hypotheses of similar associations will undoubtedly continue to be advanced because of the close relationship of humans to pet animals and our ignorance regarding the causes of many human diseases.

Likewise, it is conceivable that as more is learned about agents such as *Campylobacter*, *Cryptosporidium*, and others, veterinary practitioners may have to be more explicit in identifying the causes of diarrhea in their patients and more careful in their recommendations to clients.

For ethical and legal reasons, small animal practitioners must be familiar with the current status of research regarding zoonoses and potential zoonoses in companion animals.

References and Supplemental Reading

Blaser, M. J., and Reller, L. B.: Campylobacter enteritis. N. Engl. J. Med. 305:1444, 1981.

Burridge, M. J.: Canine and feline diseases of controversial zoonotic potential. Comp. Cont. Ed. Pract. Vet. 1:529, 1979.

Dillon, A. R., and Wilt, G. R.: Campylobacter species in the dog and cat. A cause for concern? Vet. Clin. North Am. [Small Anim. Pract.] 13:647, 1983.

Gamble, W. G., Segal, M., Schantz, P. M., et al.: Alveolar hydatid disease in Minnesota: First human case acquired in the contiguous United States. J.A.V.M.A. 241:904, 1979.

Kirkpatrick, C. E., and Farrell, J. P.: Giardiasis. Comp. Cont. Ed. Pract. Vet. 4:367, 1982.

Navin, T. R., and Juranek, D. D.: Cryptosporidiosis: Clinical, epidemiologic and parasitologic review. Rev. Infect. Dis. 6:313, 1984.

Panigrahy, B., Grimes, J. E., Rideout, M. I., et al.: Zoonotic diseases in psittacine birds: Apparent increased occurrence of chlamydiosis (psittacosis), salmonellosis, and giardiasis. J.A.V.M.A. 175:359, 1979.

Prescott, J. F., and Munroe, D. L.: *Campylobacter jejuni* enteritis in man and domestic animals. J.A.V.M.A. 181:1524, 1982.

Schantz, P. M.: Emergent or newly recognized parasitic zoonoses. Comp. Cont. Ed. Pract. Vet. 5:163, 1983.

Schwabe, C. W., Riemann, H. P., and Franti, C. E.: *Epidemiology in Veterinary Practice.* Philadelphia: Lea & Febiger, 1977, pp. 172–191.

Skirrow, M. B.: Campylobacter enteritis in dogs and cats: A "new" zoonosis. Vet. Res. Commun. 5:13, 1981.

Sordillo, P. P., Markovich, R. P., and Hardy, W. D.: Search for evidence of feline leukemia virus infection in humans with leukemia, lymphomas or soft tissue sarcomas. J. Natl. Cancer Inst. 69:333, 1982.

IMMUNOMODULATORS

JAMES V. DESIDERIO, PH.D.,
Syracuse, New York

and BRUCE M. RANKIN, B.A.
Ithaca, New York

The immune system of higher animals has evolved for the primary purpose of providing host defense against the myriad of potential threats from parasitic, infectious, and neoplastic diseases. However, for a long time the underlying mechanisms that direct and regulate immune mechanisms have, for the most part, been poorly defined. Today, our understanding of the immune system, albeit incomplete, has progressed to the point where we now know sufficiently enough to influence many of the mechanisms that govern immune function and thus may manipulate them to the advantage of the host. This concept forms the basis of "immunomodulation"; that is, the enhancement or augmentation of immune response mechanisms (specific or nonspecific) in favor of the host.

The pharmacologic manipulation of immune mechanisms offers intriguing possibilities in diverse areas of clinical immunology, including the control of hypersensitivities, the treatment of autoimmune diseases, and the prevention of transplant rejection. However, the clinical use of immunomodulators has, thus far, focused primarily on their role as a therapeutic modality in human medicine for the treatment of cancer. In comparison, the use of immunomodulators in the treatment or prevention of infectious diseases has received less attention. It is becoming increasingly evident that immunomodulators will find significant applications in the augmentation of host defenses in infectious diseases. Numerous lines of evidence have shown that immunomodulators have the ability to (1) potentiate the immune response to vaccines, (2) restore immune competence in immunocompromised animals, (3) nonspecifically enhance resistance to infection, and (4) increase the effectiveness of conventional chemotherapy.

There is a growing concern among clinicians regarding the pitfalls of antimicrobial chemotherapy. First, conventional chemotherapy is optimally effective only in animals with fully intact and functional immune systems. Its effectiveness can be severely hampered in immunosuppressed or immune-deficient animals. Second, despite the existence of powerful antimicrobial drugs, there still remain a substantial number of life-threatening bacterial and fungal infections, and there still is no drug that is broadly effective against viral infections. Finally, the overuse of antimicrobial drugs can be associated with toxic side effects, hypersensitivity reactions, selection of resistant organisms, and even predisposition to secondary infections. As a result, the therapeutic potential of agents capable of stimulating existing host immune mechanisms is being realized.

This chapter will deal with recent information regarding the potential role of immunomodulators in veterinary medicine. Emphasis will be placed on the augmentation of host defenses for the prevention and treatment of infectious diseases.

CELLULAR INTERACTIONS IN THE IMMUNE RESPONSE

Figure 1 illustrates some of the cellular interactions involved in the network of immunologic communication and cooperation. It is not within the scope of this chapter to review in detail the numerous mechanisms governing the immune response. However, it is clear, even from this oversimplified diagram, that the immune system is far more complex than was thought only a decade ago. Within this system exist numerous subpopulations of immunocompetent cells, each with distinct characteristics and functions. The maturation, differentiation, and effector functions of the individual cells composing each subpopulation are under the influence of multiple control mechanisms. For example, more than 100 soluble factors have been identified that serve as communication signals in the regulation and coordination of events involved in the immune response. In theory, the goal of immunomodulation is to selectively influence individual cell populations or regulatory signals in the immune network so that host defense is reinforced or enhanced. Since the various immunomodulators influence different mechanisms of defense, the choice of a particular immunomodulator will depend upon the desired effect. This requires a certain amount of knowledge about individual host-pathogen interactions. For example, the principal effector mechanism responsible for the elimination of virally infected cells is believed to be the cytotoxic T-lymphocyte, whereas negation of exotoxins from toxigenic bacteria is effectively accomplished by specific antibody. Similarly, the activated macrophage is the key defense against facultative intracellular bacteria. This means

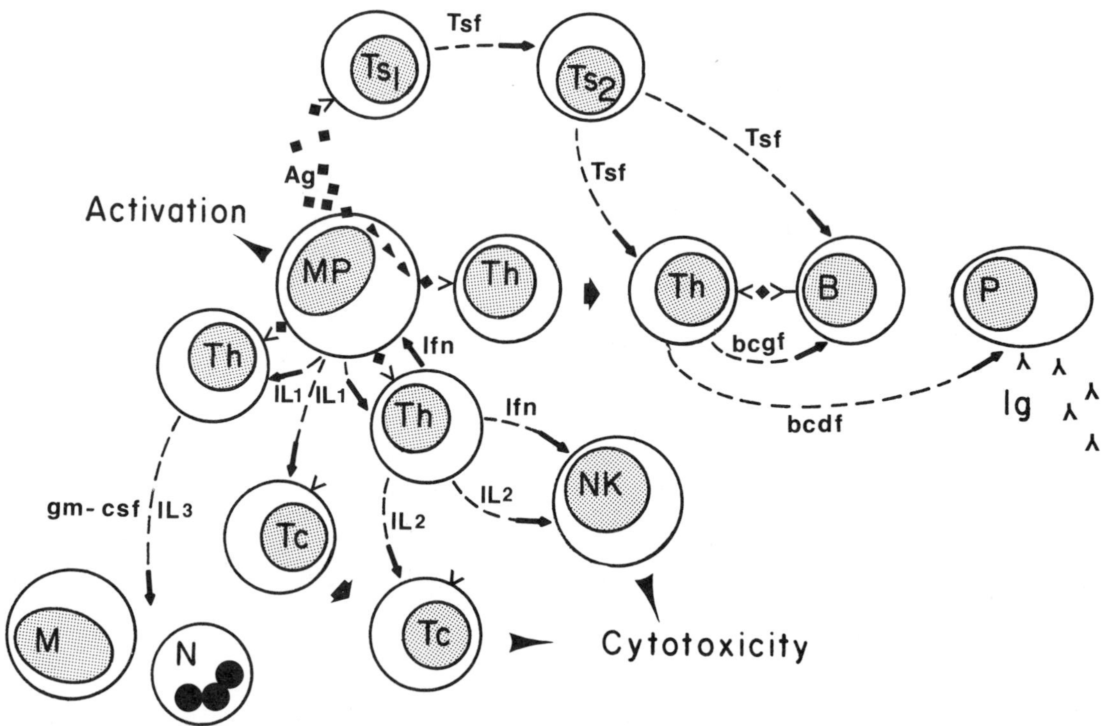

Figure 1. *Cellular Interactions in the Immune Response.* The macrophage (MP) is an important cell in the immunologic network because of its dual role in both the inductive and effector ends of the immune response. Macrophages and other antigen-presenting cells trap foreign antigens (e.g., virus particles) and "process" them for presentation to antigen-specific helper T-lymphocytes (Th). The release of interleukin 1 (IL1) (formerly, lymphocyte-activating factor) by macrophages stimulates Th to produce, among other mediators, interleukin 2 (IL2) (formerly, T cell growth factor). IL1 also induces the expression of the IL2 receptor on other effector lymphocytes. Th cells, in turn, regulate the function of other cells. The presentation of antigen to B-lymphocytes is accompanied by the release of B cell growth factor (bcgf), which induces the clonal expansion of the antigen-stimulated B cell. Under the influence of B cell differentiation factor (bcdf), subsequent development of B cells into plasma cells (P) producing immunoglobulin (IG) occurs. IL2 also initiates clonal expansion of antigen-stimulated cytotoxic T-lymphocytes (Tc) which, along with natural killer cells (NK), can kill virally infected host cells. The release of gamma interferon (Ifn) from Th cells is a potent macrophage activator. Interleukin 3 (IL3) and granulocyte/monocyte colony stimulating factor (gm-csf) induce the maturation and production of monocytes (M), neutrophils (N), and other cells in the bone marrow. Suppressor T-lymphocytes (Ts) inhibit the activity of other lymphocytes, thereby slowing down immune responses.

that the effectiveness of an immunomodulator against a particular disease depends upon the ability of the immunomodulator to stimulate the appropriate mechanism of defense.

Table 1 represents a partial list of substances with documented immunomodulatory activity either in experimental models or in human clinical trials. One immediately recognizes the wide diversity of compounds that can exert immunomodulatory influences on immune function. There is apparently no single characteristic that can be associated with the ability to enhance immune mechanisms. This is explained in part by the fact that there are a vast number of sites in the immune system at which a given immunomodulator may exert its influence. For the most part, the target and mechanisms of action of most immunomodulators are still unclear. It is widely agreed, however, that agents that stimulate macrophage function, either directly or through lymphocyte activation, hold the broadest potential for the enhancement of host defense to infectious disease. Thus, in the majority of experimental investigations, the level of macrophage activation was well correlated with resistance to infection by a variety of infecting agents.

The dose, timing, and route of administration are important factors that influence the action of immunomodulators on host defense mechanisms. Most immunomodulators exert their effects when administered *prior to* antigenic challenge. Such agents would find application as prophylactic measures, for example, in animals at risk of opportunistic infections (e.g., surgical patients or animals on cancer chemotherapy or prolonged steroid therapy). Those immunomodulators that are most effective when administered *simultaneously* with antigens may prove to be good immunologic adjuvants for the potentiation of the specific immune response to vaccines. Immunomodulators that influence immune function *after* antigenic challenge could potentially be used in the treatment of infections by stimulating and mobilizing the appropriate effector mechanisms. This last group of immunomodulators may be useful against infectious agents for which no vaccine or satisfactory therapy exists (e.g., canine coronaviral enteritis or feline infectious peritonitis), diseases that are associated with immune suppression (feline leukemia or canine distemper), and those diseases resistant or refractory to conventional chemotherapy.

The following is a summary of what is known about several immunomodulators that have attracted a considerable amount of attention and that have potential use in veterinary medicine.

SYNTHETIC COMPOUNDS

Levamisole

Levamisole, the levo-isomer of tetramisole, is widely used in veterinary medicine as an anthelmintic drug. Recently, levamisole has been shown to possess immunostimulatory properties in certain situations. Given orally or parenterally in doses of 2 to 15 mg/kg, levamisole restored normal immune function in animals with impaired cell-mediated mechanisms. However, in animals with normally functioning defense mechanisms, the effect of levamisole was marginal. Animals suffering from recurrent or chronic infections were shown to benefit from levamisole therapy. The drug reduced the frequency, duration, and severity of disease episodes. Levamisole has been shown to stimulate the production of precursor T-lymphocytes, increase DNA synthesis in mitogen-stimulated lymphocytes, and increase the ratio of helper to suppressor cells. Restoration of cellular immunity by levamisole was shown to reverse the anergy associated with some chronic infectious diseases. Although levamisole exerts no direct effect on antibody production, it does increase the B cell proliferative response to mitogens. The drug has also been shown to enhance many functions of macrophages and granulocytes, including chemotaxis, phagocytosis, and intracellular killing, possibly as an indirect consequence of lymphokine action. The mechanism of action of levamisole in the restoration of immune competence is not entirely known, but it is probably related to

Table 1. *Substances with Reported Immunomodulatory Activity*

Biologically Derived		Synthetic	
Muramyl dipeptide	Vaccinia virus	Isoprinosine	Azimexon
Lipopolysaccharide	Interleukins	Pyrimidinoles	Thiazolylbenzimidazoles
Trehalose dimycolate	Tuftsin	Levamisole	Diethyldithiocarbamate
Propionibacterium acnes	Thymic hormones	Cimetidine	Oligonucleotides
Bacillus Calmette-Guérin (BCG)	Glucan	Indomethacin	Cyclophosphamide
Nocardia cell wall skeleton	Levan	Lipoidal amines	Adenosine arabinoside
OK-432 (picibanil)	Lentinan	Aclacinomycin	Lysophospholipids
Interferon	Mannozym	Pyran copolymer (MVE-2)	
Ubiquinones	Schizophyllan		
Forphenicine	Bestatin		
Vitamin A	Zymosan		

the influence the drug exerts on levels of cyclic nucleotides in leukocytes.

Methisoprinol

Methisoprinol (Isoprinosine, Newport) is a molecular complex consisting of inosine and the *p*-acetamidobenzoate salt of *N,N*-dimethylamino-2-propanol (1:3 molar ratio). Methisoprinol exerts its influence primarily on T-lymphocyte populations and has been shown to potentiate lymphoproliferative responses both *in vitro* and *in vivo* and to enhance cell-mediated responses to a variety of viral and fungal agents *in vivo*. The mechanism of action of this agent is unclear, although enhanced production of interleukin 2 and gamma interferon by antigen-stimulated helper cells and of interleukin 1 by macrophages has been demonstrated. As a result of its effect on the production of lymphokines by lymphocytes, methisoprinol exerts indirect influence on macrophage function. In controlled clinical trials, oral doses of Isoprinosine (50 mg/kg/day for 4 days) resulted in increased resistance to infection by influenza virus and restoration of immune competence in elderly patients.

Cimetidine

The mechanism of action of cimetidine, a drug used clinically as an antigastritis agent, is to block cell receptors for histamine (H_2 receptors). Recent evidence has demonstrated that suppressor T cells (Ts) possess H_2 receptors and that binding of histamine to these receptors results in Ts activation and immune suppression. In well-defined model systems, oral administration of cimetidine (10 to 25 mg/kg, twice daily for 6 days) was shown to abrogate antigen-specific Ts function and to result in the enhancement of the immune response to the antigen. Cimetidine treatment was found to reverse the generalized immunosuppression in patients with chronic mucocutaneous candidiasis and to restore specific cell-mediated immune responses against fungal antigens. Thus, cimetidine acts as an immunomodulator by reversing Ts-mediated immune suppression that is often associated with some chronic infectious diseases.

LYMPHOKINES AND CYTOKINES

Interferon

The interferons are a family of glycoproteins originally identified for their ability to inhibit viral replication in infected cells. One class of this substance, type II (immune) interferon (or gram interferon), is produced by antigen-stimulated T-lymphocytes. Gamma interferon (gIFN) exhibits a multiplicity of effects on the immune system and, in this respect, is classified as an immunomodulator. An important biological effect of this lymphokine is its ability to significantly enhance macrophage antimicrobial activity. In fact, most recent evidence suggests that the lymphokine called macrophage-activating factor (MAF) and gamma interferon are one and the same molecule. Gamma interferon has also been shown to directly influence the activity of B cells, cytotoxic T cells, and natural killer (NK) cells. The stimulation of macrophages by gIFN may have important applications in the elimination of intracellular parasites, the destruction of virus-infected cells, and the elimination of multicellular organisms. Although gIFN could have profound influences on the course of infectious diseases, several factors have thus far prevented its use in small animal medicine. Most importantly, host cell receptors for gIFN are highly species-specific. Recombinant gIFN of mouse, bovine, and human origin is available, but these show no activity in heterologous systems. Second, the effect of gIFN on host immune mechanisms is observed only after a continuous level is attained by administration of repeated high doses. An attractive alternative is the use of interferon inducers. These are agents which, upon administration, result in the production of endogenous interferon by host cells. Oligonucleotides, pyrimidinoles, and many nonpathogenic viruses are good inducers of interferon *in vivo*. Studies indicate that induced endogenous interferon in the animal persists for a longer time than does administered recombinant gIFN. Additionally, the whole spectrum of host interferons would presumably be produced by interferon inducers.

Interleukins

Recombinant interleukin 1 (lymphocyte-activating factor) and interleukin 2 (T cell growth factor) are presently available. An absolute requirement for interleukin 2 has been demonstrated for the long-term maintenance of lymphocytes *in vitro* and for normal T cell responses to antigen *in vivo*. In fact, the mechanism of action of the potent immunosuppressive drug, cyclosporine A, is the inhibition of the production of interleukin 2 by helper cells.

Interleukins are currently under clinical investigation in patients with various immune-deficiency disorders. Unlike interferon, the interleukins do not appear to express strict species specificity and therefore may be of potential value in small animal medicine for the enhancement of T cell functions in immunosuppressed patients.

BIOLOGICALLY DERIVED MOLECULES

Lentinan

Lentinan is a beta (1,3) glucan extracted from the edible mushroom *Lentinus edodes*. It is a fully purified, neutral polysaccharide with a molecular weight of 10^5 to 10^6 daltons. Lentinan is a potent stimulator of the retuculoendothelial system and induces macrophage activation *in vivo* but not *in vitro*, a property shared by other microbial polysaccharides (e.g., glucan and levan). As a result, numerous experimental models demonstrate that pretreatment with lentinan (1 mg/kg IV) confers nonspecific protection against a variety of infectious agents, most notably the facultative intracellular parasites. The mechanisms responsible for this are unclear but are believed to result from the phagocytic load caused by the polysaccharide, since mammalian systems are deficient in enzymes effective on beta (1,3) glucans. In addition to the macrophage-stimulating ability of lentinan, this immunomodulator also induces the production of interleukin 1 by macrophages and exerts stimulatory effects on some T-lymphocyte populations.

Muramyl Dipeptide

N-acetylmuramyl L-alanyl D-isoglutamine (MDP) is the minimum structure that can substitute for the adjuvanticity of *Mycobacterium bovis* in Freund's complete adjuvant. The molecule, which has been synthesized, and many of its derivatives exert several stimulatory effects on the immune system. MDP is most well known as a powerful macrophage activator and stimulator of the reticuloendothelial system. In single doses of 10 to 25 mg/kg daily for 4 days, by either the oral or parenteral route, MDP significantly enhanced host resistance to a wide variety of pathogens including species of *Klebsiella, Streptococcus, Pseudomonas, Salmonella, Listeria, Candida, Trypanosoma*, and *Toxoplasma*. Lipophilic derivatives of MDP were found to be superior to the water-soluble molecule in enhancing host resistance. This is presumably because the derived MDP is retained longer *in vivo* and displays a much higher affinity for macrophages.

IMMUNOMODULATORS LICENSED FOR VETERINARY USE

Recently, several products specifically designated as immunostimulants have received approval for use in veterinary medicine. Ribigen (Fort Dodge) and Immunoregulin (ImmunoVet) are available in the United States. Ribigen is supplied as a lyophilized emulsion consisting of cell wall components of *Mycobacterium* organisms. It is intended for local immunotherapy of equine sarcoid and bovine ocular carcinoma and is under investigation for use in certain canine tumors. It has recently been demonstrated that systemic administration of Ribigen to laboratory animals results in the enhancement of host resistance to a variety of infectious diseases. The mechanism of action appears to be a direct stimulation of reticuloendothelial system (RES) function. Immunoregulin is a suspension of killed *Propionibacterium acnes* (formerly designated *Corynebacterium parvum*). *P. acnes* has been extensively studied in laboratory animals and is well documented as a potent enhancer of many immune mechanisms and, in particular, RES function. Immunoregulin has been shown to be clinically effective as an adjunct in the treatment of chronic secondary infections in the immunocompromised animal. In doses as low as 15 μg/kg, twice a week for 2 to 3 weeks, this immunostimulant has demonstrated clinical efficacy in cases of feline viral rhinotracheitis, pyodermic dermatitis, and feline leukemia–related infections.

Domon-L (Nichibo Labs, Tokyo), an immunostimulant prepared from the bacillus *Achromobacter stenohalis*, is widely distributed for veterinary use in Japan, Korea, and China. As with Ribigen and Immunoregulin, Domon-L has been shown to stimulate nonspecific host immune mechanisms. Additionally, this immunostimulant has been shown to increase neutralizing antibody titer to a variety of viruses and, as a result, has demonstrated clinical effectiveness in cases of canine distemper, parvoviral enteritis, feline viral rhinotracheitis, and feline panleukopenia.

MODULATION OF THE IMMUNE RESPONSE TO VACCINES

Recent views about how the immune system recognizes and responds to foreign antigens has led to several new and intriguing concepts in vaccine development. Whereas traditional approaches to the development or improvement of vaccines focused heavily on defining new or better antigens, newer approaches involve the manipulation of host immune response mechanisms so that vaccine antigens are processed in the vaccinated animal in a predetermined and desired fashion. An example of such a manipulation is the covalent attachment of synthetic, antigenic molecules of low molecular weight with an immunomodulator such as MDP. The resulting water-soluble vaccine complex consists of chemically defined antigenic determinants with built-in adjuvanticity.

Another avenue of research is in the use of recombinant live vaccines. It is now possible to incorporate a defined portion of the nucleic acids from highly pathogenic viruses (e.g., hepatitis B) into the genome of the relatively benign vaccinia virus. Viral replication *in vivo* results in the expression of viral antigens, including the hepatitis B antigens. Experimental animals immunized with this recombinant vaccine were protected from disease after a challenge with the intact hepatitis B virus.

The preferential stimulation of specific immune mechanisms by vaccination is another area of intensive research. For example, protection against facultative intracellular bacteria (e.g., *Salmonella*) is correlated with a specific cell-mediated response and concomitant macrophage activation and is unrelated to the level of specific antibody. Targeting *Salmonella* antigens, in a lipophilic form, to the systemic macrophage population (e.g., by incorporating the antigens in microscopic phospholipid vesicles) favors the generation of cellular immunity over humoral immunity and, in experimental systems, affords better protection against a challenge infection.

Finally, the latest area of vaccine research is in the use of anti-idiotype vaccines. These vaccines are based on the concept that lymphocyte receptors bear unique structural configurations in their antigen binding sites, referred to as idiotypes. Lymphocytes are activated by the binding of antigens to their receptors. In the same manner, antibodies produced against these idiotypes can, upon binding, also activate the lymphocyte of a given antigen specificity. The techniques now exist for production of these reagents.

In summary, the pharmacologic manipulation of host immunologic mechanisms for the purpose of achieving a desired effect is now possible, albeit in early stages of development. With further advances in our understanding of immune function, it may soon be possible to selectively stimulate a predetermined target in the immune network and direct its function, at will, for the treatment or prevention of disease.

References and Supplemental Reading

Chedid, L., Miescher, P. A., and Mueller-Eberhard, H. J. (eds.): *Immunostimulation.* New York: Springer-Verlag, 1980.

Fenichel, R. L., and Chirigos, M. A. (eds.): *Immune Modulation Agents and Their Mechanisms.* New York: Marcel Dekker, 1984.

Fudenberg, H. H., and Whitten, H. D.: Immunostimulation: Synthetic and biological modulators of immunity. Ann. Rev. Pharmacol. Toxicol. 24:147, 1984.

Kende, M., Gainer, J., and Chirigos, M. (eds.): *Chemical Regulation of Immunity in Veterinary Medicine.* New York: Alan R. Liss, 1984.

Roitt, I. M. (ed.): *Immune Intervention: New Trends in Vaccines.* New York: Academic Press, 1984.

CANINE BABESIOSIS

SHEHU U. ABDULLAHI, D.V.M.,
and ABDULRAHIM SANNUSI, D.V.M.
Zaria, Nigeria

Canine babesiosis is clearly one of the most important tick-borne, blood protozoal infections of dogs in the tropical and subtropical regions of the world. The climatic conditions of these areas support the development of the tick vectors, *Rhipicephalus sanguineus* and, to a minor extent, *Haemaphysalis leachi* (Shortt, 1973). In the authors' experience, *R. sanguineus* is by far the more widespread and more important vector of this disease.

The disease has been reported from southern and southwestern United States, southern Europe, Central America, South America, Asia, Africa, and northern Australia (Flyn, 1973). The disease is caused by intraerythrocytic protozoan parasites, *Babesia canis* and *Babesia gibsoni*. *Babesia canis* is far more important and has a wider geographic distribution than *B. gibsoni*. These parasites are highly host-specific and are transmitted by hard ticks of the three-host type. Unlike other forms of babesiosis, canine babesiosis affects young dogs as well as old ones, although in endemic areas the frequency of disease occurrence diminishes with age.

CLINICAL SIGNS

The clinical signs of canine babesiosis are quite variable. The signs are even more complex if the disease is complicated by infections of *Ehrlichia canis* or *Hepatozoon canis*. The authors' experience has been with cases involving *B. canis* infection; however, the clinical signs of infection with either

B. canis or *B. gibsoni* are similar, although they tend to be vague in the case of the latter (Groves and Dennis, 1972). The disease may be hyperacute, acute, or chronic, depending on the degree of parasitemia and the immune status of the patient. In endemic areas, many dogs may have subclinical infections and only exhibit clinical signs when they are stressed.

Hyperacute Cases

Dogs brought to the authors' clinic with this form of the disease are few in number, and they are often presented comatose and in shock or even dead. The common history reported by owners is that the dog was fine the previous day but suddenly became anorectic and lethargic on the day of presentation. "Bloody" urine due to hemoglobinuria may also be reported. Heavy tick infestation is almost invariably associated with this form of babesiosis.

Acute Cases

In the authors' practice, this is the most common form of canine babesiosis. The common history associated with this form of the disease is anorexia and lethargy for 1 to 2 days. In a few of these cases, the owners may report "bloody" urine. The common clinical signs observed include high fever (40 to 41.5°C), severe anemia, hemoglobinuria, icterus, splenomegaly, generalized lymphadenopathy, and emesis resulting in dehydration. Dogs presented early may have congested mucous membranes and bilateral mucopurulent ocular discharge; they resemble cases of acute canine ehrlichiosis. Heavy tick infestation is often observed on affected dogs.

Chronic Cases

Dogs with this form of babesiosis resemble cases of helminthiasis. The common signs observed include inappetence, mild anemia, mild icterus, intermittent fever, emaciation, and reduced activity. The spleen and the superficial lymph nodes may be enlarged.

DIAGNOSIS

Tentative diagnosis of canine babesiosis can be made in dogs presented with the typical signs outlined above. Confirmatory diagnosis can be made by finding *Babesia* organisms in erythrocytes of affected dogs. A blood sample to which about 10 to 20 mg ethylene diamine tetraacetic acid (EDTA) anticoagulant per 10 ml of sample has been added

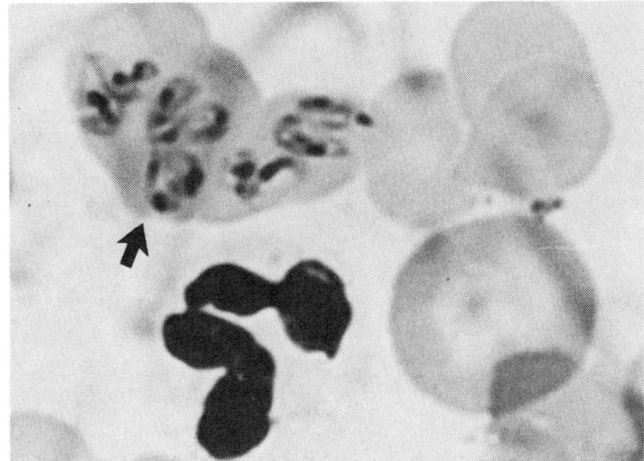

Figure 1. Characteristic multiple infection of *B canis* in three red blood cells (arrow).

is needed for laboratory diagnosis. Thin blood smears should be prepared and stained with Giemsa stain. Detection of *B. canis* is confirmed by the presence of large, paired pyriform bodies and by multiple invasion of single red blood cells (Fig. 1). If fresh postmortem materials are available for investigation, particularly in hyperacute cases in which blood samples have been missed, organ impression smears prepared from the lungs, liver, kidney, and brain will assist in arriving at a confirmatory diagnosis.

Differential Diagnosis

Acute babesiosis may resemble ehrlichiosis; however, icterus is a common feature of babesiosis, whereas epistaxis is commonly observed in ehrlichiosis. Nevertheless, in many instances blood examination is required to differentiate the two diseases or to determine if they occur concurrently. Infection with *Hepatozoon canis* may be confused with babesiosis, but icterus and hemoglobinuria are not features of hepatozoonosis. Hookworm disease in puppies and malnourished, aged dogs may cause anemic signs, but absence of fever and parasitemia coupled with fecal examination will help differentiate such cases from babesiosis. Leptospirosis should be considered, but the vaccination history of the dogs, the disease incidence in the area, and the presence of uremic signs will help in the diagnosis.

MANAGEMENT AND PROGNOSIS

In endemic areas, the aim of specific treatment of canine babesiosis is to achieve a premunitive state in the dogs without sterilizing the infection.

Over the years, three effective drugs have been used in the authors' clinic for such treatment. A single-dose therapy of any of the following drugs has been used: a 7 per cent solution of diminazene aceturate (Berenil, Farbwerke-Hoechst) given at a dose of 3.5 mg/kg intramuscularly or subcutaneously; imidocarb dipropionate (Imizol, Burroughs Wellcome) at 5 mg/kg intramuscularly or subcutaneously; and phenamidine isethionate (Lomadine, May & Baker) at 10 to 15 mg/kg subcutaneously (Aliu, 1983). Although very effective, Berenil has been reported to produce neurotoxic signs in dogs when it is administered at higher or repeated doses (Moore, 1979). It is therefore recommended that the dose of Berenil should never exceed 7 mg/kg, and even when given at 3.5 mg/kg, the dosage should not be repeated in 2 weeks. Imizol is the drug of choice, as it is less toxic and has high curative and prophylactic activity against *Babesia* organisms. Moreover, Imizol is also effective against *E. canis* and *H. canis*, the two other tick-borne blood parasites often associated with canine babesiosis in some endemic areas. The only disadvantage of Imizol is its cost.

In addition to specific treatment, supportive therapy may be essential for the proper management of cases of canine babesiosis. In the authors' experience, failure to administer supportive therapy in hyperacute and some acute cases often led to death of the patients even when specific therapy was given. Cases with severe anemia require blood transfusion, whereas cases with mild to moderate anemia may only require iron supplementation. In endemic areas, the need to keep parasite-free donors should not be overlooked. Administration of iron compounds is particularly important in patients with hemoglobinuria. Dehydrated patients require fluid therapy, and lactated Ringer's solution is very useful for this purpose. To combat metabolic acidosis commonly observed in canine babesiosis, alkalizing agents such as sodium bicarbonate should be administered. Dogs presented in shock should be given glucocorticosteroids and broad-spectrum antibiotics intravenously. The authors also recommend the use of vitamin B complex and improved nutrition in all recovering patients.

Most chronic and acute cases recover after specific and supportive therapy. However, relapses or reinfections are common, especially in cases treated with Berenil. Dogs presented in shock have a poor prognosis, which is compounded if blood is not immediately available for transfusion. Cases with concurrent ehrlichiosis are difficult to treat, particularly if only babecidal drugs are used.

PREVENTION

No commercial vaccine has yet been developed for the control of canine babesiosis. Until this is done, strict tick control by using effective acaricides at regular intervals will remain the only practical means of controlling the disease in endemic areas. The use of 1:400 dilution of chlorfenvinphos (Pfizona, Pfizer Nigeria) in water has been found to be very useful in controlling *R. sanguineus* on dogs. Dogs are given a bath or dip at 2-week intervals when the population of the ticks is high and at monthly intervals when the population is low. The solution can also be used to kill ticks in the immediate environment of the dogs. In addition, the authors recommend regular blood examination and appropriate treatment of dogs in endemic areas.

References and Supplemental Reading

Aliu, Y. O.: Tick-borne diseases of domestic animals in Nigeria: Current treatment procedures. Vet. Bull. 53:233, 1983.

Flyn, R. J.: *Parasites of Laboratory Animals*. Ames, IA: The Iowa State University Press, 1973.

Groves, M. G., and Dennis, G. L.: *Babesia gibsoni*. Field and laboratory studies of canine infections. Exp. Parasitol. 31:153, 1972.

Moore, D. J.: Therapeutic implications of *Babesia canis* infection in dogs. J. S. Afr. Vet. Assoc. 50:346, 1979.

Purnell, R. E.: Babesiosis in various hosts. *In* Ristic M. and Kreier, J. P. (eds.): *Babesiosis*. New York: Academic Press, 1981, pp. 25–63.

Shortt, H. E.: *Babesia canis*: The life cycle and laboratory maintenance in its arthropod and mammalian hosts. Int. J. Parasitol. 3:119, 1973.

Soulsby, E. J. L.: *Helminths, Arthropods and Protozoa of Domesticated Animals*. 7th ed. London: Bailliere Tindall, 1982.

CANINE HEPATOZOONOSIS

SHEHU U. ABDULLAHI, D.V.M.
Zaria, Nigeria

Canine hepatozoonosis is a disease caused by a protozoan blood parasite, *Hepatozoon canis*. The disease has been reported from Italy, France, United States, Middle East, Philippines, India, Malaysia, Sri Lanka, Southeast Asia, and various parts of Africa. The causative agent is transmitted to dogs by the brown dog tick, *Rhipicephalus sanguineus*. The life cycle of *H. canis* is similar to that of coccidia; the sexual stages and sporulation occur in ticks and schizogony and gametogony occur in dogs. The tick becomes infected by ingestion of blood containing gametocytes located in leukocytes of infected dogs. The dog becomes infected by ingestion of a tick containing sporulated oocysts in its hemocoel.

The clinical manifestations of canine hepatozoonosis have not yet been clearly defined. *Hepatozoon canis* used to be considered harmless to dogs. However, there is now increasing evidence that it causes canine disease of varying severity. In the author's practice, the parasite is seen more often in younger dogs than in older ones; however, *H. canis* seems to be more commonly associated with disease in older dogs. The most common clinical signs of canine hepatozoonosis are fever, inappetence, anemia, and emaciation. Other less commonly reported signs include cough, vertebral column stiffness, mucopurulent ocular discharge, and generalized lymphadenopathy.

Diagnosis of canine hepatozoonosis based on clinical signs may be difficult, as the signs are not only variable but also resemble those of other blood parasitic diseases, particularly babesiosis and ehrlichiosis. Moreover, these diseases may occur concurrently with hepatozoonosis in the same dogs in some endemic areas. Cases with severe lymphadenopathy may resemble cases of lymphosarcoma. Diagnosis of the disease is confirmed by detecting gametocytes of *H. canis* in leukocytes, particularly neutrophils, in Giemsa-stained thin blood smears (Fig. 1). Other findings in the blood include evidence of nonregenerative anemia, neutrophilic leukocytosis, and eosinophilia. The author has detected gametocytes of *H. canis* in Giemsa-stained biopsy material from lymph nodes during the course of cytologic examination of suspected cases of lymphosarcoma.

There is no drug known that completely eliminates *H. canis* from blood of infected dogs. However, the author has observed remission of clinical

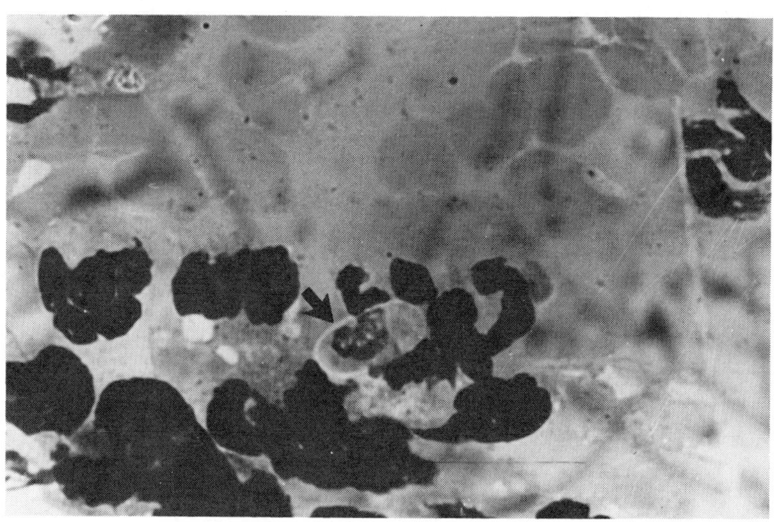

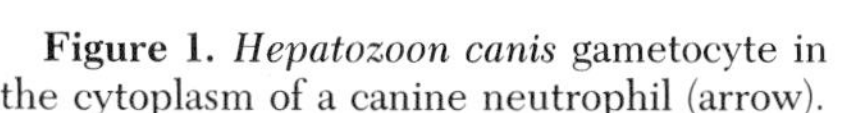

Figure 1. *Hepatozoon canis* gametocyte in the cytoplasm of a canine neutrophil (arrow).

signs and a decrease in the level of parasitemia in dogs treated with a single dose of imidocarb dipropionate (Imizol, Burroughs Wellcome) given at 5 mg/kg intramuscularly. Tetracyclines, sulfonamides, chloramphenicol, or common antiprotozoal drugs such as diminazene aceturate are ineffective (Aliu et al., 1976; Craig et al., 1978). Cautious use of corticosteroids and aspirin has been recommended for dogs with infections in bone (Craig et al., 1978). Severe, chronic cases may require such supportive therapy as fluids, blood transfusion, and vitamin B complex.

Until an effective treatment is evolved, a strict program of tick control will remain the only means of controlling the disease. An effective program will also help in controlling two other important tick-borne diseases of dogs, babesiosis and ehrlichiosis, which are often associated with hepatozoonosis.

References and Supplemental Reading

Aliu, Y. O., Sannusi, A., Ezeokoli, C. D., et al.: Canine hepatozoonosis and its therapeutic management: Selected case reports. Nig. Vet. J. 5:9, 1976.

Craig, T. M., Smallwood, J. E., Knauer, K. W., et al.: *Hepatozoon canis* infection in dogs: Clinical, radiographic, and hematologic findings. J.A.V.M.A. 173:967, 1978.

Ezeokoli, C. D., Ogunkoya, A. B., Abdullahi, R., et al.: Clinical and epidemiological studies on canine hepatozoonosis in Zaria, Nigeria. J. Small Anim. Pract. 24:455, 1983.

Lavine, N. D.: *Protozoan Parasites of Domestic Animals and Man.* Minneapolis, MN: Burgess Publishing Co., 1973.

LYME DISEASE

BARRY A. LISSMAN, D.V.M.
Holbrook, New York

Lyme disease is a tick-borne inflammatory disorder of dogs and humans. The disease has clinical manifestations affecting multiple organ systems, and it is caused by a spirochete (*Borrelia burgdorferi*) that is transmitted by the tick *Ixodes dammini.* It is endemic in the northeastern United States, and human cases have been reported in the Southeast, West, and Midwest.

Arthritis and fever are the predominant clinical findings observed in the dog. The arthritis usually involves the large joints, is often recurrent, and may progress to chronic arthritis. Results of routine hematologic and biochemical profiles are normal. Early disease in humans is usually characterized by an expanding annular skin lesion, erythema chronicum migrans, which may be followed days to months later by chronic or recurrent arthritis and neurologic or cardiac sequelae. It is not known whether dogs develop a skin lesion prior to arthritis.

The diagnosis may be made serologically by indirect immunofluorescence and by blood culture of the spirochete. The differential diagnosis should include all other causes of canine arthritis.

Dogs have been successfully treated with ampicillin at 10 mg/lb orally three times daily or tetracycline at 10 mg/lb orally three times daily.

References and Supplemental Reading

Benach, J. L., Bosler, E. M., Hanrahan, J. P., et al.: Spirochetes isolated from the blood of two patients with Lyme disease. N. Engl. J. Med. 308:740, 1983.

Burgdorfer, W., and Keirans, J. E.: Ticks and Lyme disease in the United States. Ann. Intern. Med. 99:121, 1983.

Lissman, B. A., Bosler, E. M., Camay, H., et al.: Spirochete-associated arthritis (Lyme disease) in a dog. J.A.V.M.A. 185:219, 1984.

Steere, A. C., Bartenhagen, N. H., Craft, J. E., et al.: The early clinical manifestations of Lyme disease. Ann. Intern. Med. 99:76, 1983.

Steere, A. C., Hutchinson, G. J., Rahn, D. W., et al.: Treatment of the early manifestations of Lyme disease. Ann. Intern. Med. 99:22, 1983.

Steere, A. C., Gibofsky, A., Patarroyo, M. E., et al.: Chronic Lyme arthritis: Clinical and immunogenetic differentiation from rheumatoid arthritis. Ann. Intern. Med. 90:896, 1979.

Steere, A. C., Malawista, S. E., Snydman, D. R., et al.: Lyme arthritis: An epidemic of oligoarticular arthritis in children and adults in three Connecticut communities. Arthritis Rheum. 20:7, 1977.

Steere, A. C., Malawista, S. E., Newman, J. M., et al.: Antibiotic therapy in Lyme disease. Ann. Intern. Med. 93:1, 1980.

Section 13

URINARY DISORDERS

JEANNE A. BARSANTI, D.V.M.
Consulting Editor

Continued

Additional Pertinent Information Found in Current Veterinary Therapy VIII: Diagnosis of Urinary Tract Disorders

Lees, G. E., and Osborne, C. A.: Use and Misuse of Intermittent and Indwelling Urinary Catheters, p. 1097.

Disorders of the Urinary Tract

Chew, D. J., and DiBartola, S. P.: Familial Renal Disease in Doberman Pinscher Dogs, p. 975.
Cornelius, L. M.: Fluid Therapy in the Uremic Patient, p. 989.
Finco, D. R., and Barsanti, J. A.: Parenteral Nutrition During a Uremic Crisis, p. 994.
Low, D. G., and Cowgill, L. D.: Emergency Management of the Acute Uremic Crisis, p. 981.

Management of Urinary Tract Disorders

Ling, G. V.: Treatments of Urinary Tract Infections with Antimicrobial Agents, p. 1051.
Ling, G. V., and Hirsh, D. C.: Antimicrobial Susceptibility Tests for Urinary Tract Pathogens, p. 1048.
Osborne, C. A., and Polzin, D. J.: Conservative Medical Management of Feline Chronic Polyuric Renal Failure, p. 1008.

Additional Pertinent Information Found in Current Veterinary Therapy VII: Management of Urinary Tract Disorders

Klausner, J. A., and Osborne, C. A.: Struvite Urolithiasis, p. 1168.
Lage, A. L.: Cystinuria and Cystine Urolithiasis, p. 1175.
Osborne, C. A., et al.: Canine Silica Urolithiasis, p. 1184.
Osborne, C. A., and Klausner, J. S.: Calcium Oxalate Urolithiasis, p. 1177.
Thornhill, J. A.: Urate Urolithiasis, p. 1172.

Diagnosis of Urinary Tract Disorders

ASSESSMENT OF RENAL FUNCTION IN THE DOG AND CAT

LINDA A. ROSS, D.V.M.
North Grafton, Massachusetts

The primary indication for assessment of renal function is the diagnosis of renal disease and renal failure, although it is important to monitor renal function in other clinical settings as well. The administration of fluid therapy requires knowledge of renal function, since the kidneys are primarily responsible for regulating water and electrolyte balance within the body. A number of drugs are excreted primarily by the kidneys, and dosage modifications must be made when renal insufficiency is present. The administration of nephrotoxic drugs also requires monitoring of renal function.

One of the major difficulties in the assessment of renal function is that common clinical tests fail to detect mild to moderate decreases in function. These tests also do not localize abnormalities in function—that is, determine whether renal insufficiency is prerenal, primary renal, or postrenal in origin. The clinician must interpret and correlate the history, physical findings, and laboratory tests in order to obtain the best estimate of renal function. Specialized tests must be performed if the level of renal function must be determined more precisely. Different tests of varying sensitivity and specificity assess the integrity of different parts of the nephron.

GLOMERULAR FUNCTION

The glomerular filtration rate (GFR) is assessed clinically by the determination of blood urea nitrogen (BUN) and serum creatinine concentrations. Both substances are freely filtered through the glomerular basement membrane. Much of the urea that is filtered is reabsorbed as it passes through the renal tubules; the amount reabsorbed is dependent on the rate of flow through the tubules. Blood urea nitrogen (BUN) levels are dependent on several nonrenal factors as well. Since urea is generated by the liver as a breakdown product of protein, the BUN concentration will vary with dietary protein intake. The BUN concentration rises postprandially and may remain elevated for as long as 18 hours after food ingestion; however, the concentration almost always remains within the normal range (Finco, 1984). It may also rise with any condition resulting in increased protein catabolism such as fever, massive muscle trauma, or corticosteroid administration. Low BUN levels may be associated with hepatic insufficiency.

Creatinine is an end product of muscle metabolism. Dogs, but not cats, have a weak proximal tubular secretory mechanism for creatinine. This mechanism is more pronounced in male dogs; however, it does not have a significant effect on the serum creatinine concentration. Some creatinine is also metabolized by bacteria in the intestinal tract. Enteric degradation of creatinine may become proportionately more important as renal function decreases.

The serum creatinine concentration is less dependent on nonrenal factors than is the BUN. Cachexia may occasionally result in decreased creatinine production and a low serum creatinine concentration. Conversely, a muscular working animal may have a slightly higher serum creatinine concentration than a sedentary house pet. In both cases, the values should remain within the normal range.

Both BUN and serum creatinine concentrations are, at best, only crude reflections of GFR. Neither value will rise above the normal range until approximately three fourths of renal function is lost. Conversely, both values will rise under conditions that produce a decrease in GFR despite normal renal function (pre- or postrenal azotemia). Prerenal azotemia is most commonly the result of either hypovolemia secondary to dehydration or blood loss, or decreased renal blood flow due to shock or heart failure. Postrenal azotemia is caused by obstruction to urine outflow or a tear in the ureters, bladder, or urethra.

The serum creatinine concentration is considered to be a more accurate index of GFR than is BUN because it is less dependent on nonrenal factors. The BUN concentration is still useful, however, because of its simplicity, reproducibility, and low cost. Simultaneous measurement of BUN and serum creatinine concentrations yields the most information about renal function. The widespread availability of serum chemistry profiles now makes such measurements convenient and inexpensive. The ratio of BUN to serum creatinine has been used to help determine the pathogenesis of azotemia in humans. However, in dogs it does not differentiate between prerenal, renal, and postrenal causes (Finco, 1980).

BUN and serum creatinine concentrations rise as GFR decreases, although the relationship is not linear. It has been stated that a serum creatinine concentration greater than 5 mg/dl indicates a grave prognosis. This is not true. Serum creatinine concentrations may reach very high levels in animals with obstructive uropathy or postrenal uremia, yet these lesions are readily reversible. Many animals with chronic renal failure and serum creatinine concentrations between 5 and 8 mg/dl can be managed successfully.

In some clinical settings, it may be desirable to obtain a more precise measurement of GFR. Animals that are suspected of having renal disease but have only marginally elevated BUN or serum creatinine concentrations may fall into this category. Such a measurement of GFR may be obtained by measuring the clearance of a substance. The term *clearance* refers to the amount of plasma that is completely cleared of a given substance per unit of time. To provide an accurate estimate of GFR, the substance measured must be freely filtered through the glomerulus and neither reabsorbed nor secreted by the renal tubules. Historically, the two most commonly used substances are inulin and creatinine. Inulin is rarely used in a clinical setting because of technical difficulties in providing a constant intravenous infusion of the chemical and in performing its chemical assay. Since creatinine is a substance normally produced by the body, endogenous creatinine clearances are more practical to perform in clinical situations (Table 1).

All clearance procedures have the inherent disadvantage of requiring the collection of a timed urine sample. This can be difficult or impossible in some patients, particularly small female dogs, and cats of both sexes. Long collection periods (24 hours) minimize the effect of short-term fluctuations in GFR. The relatively large volume of urine collected also minimizes errors in the laboratory determination of urine creatinine levels. Unfortunately, accurate collection of a 24-hour urine sample is difficult. It requires either a metabolic cage, which is not available in most practices, or the use of an indwelling urinary catheter, which carries the risk of inducing a urinary tract infection in the patient. Loss of a portion of the urine sample is still common despite careful technique and will result in inaccurate determination of GFR. Short collection periods (20 minutes) minimize labor time but again require catheterization of the bladder and the risk of infection. The small volume of urine produced during the collection period will potentiate errors caused by failure to collect all the urine that is produced. It is the author's experience that the 24-hour endogenous creatinine clearance test yields more re-

Table 1. *Protocol for Determining Endogenous Creatinine Clearance*

24-hour collection

1. Make sure the urinary bladder is empty, either by voiding or catheterization.
2. Collect all urine produced during a 24-hour period, either by collection in a metabolic cage or periodic voiding or catheterization. Loss of more than a few milliliters of urine will abort the test. The bladder must be emptied at the end of the 24-hour period, preferably by catheterization.
3. Obtain a blood sample for serum creatinine determination approximately 12 hours into the test.

20-minute collection

1. Catheterize the urinary bladder and remove all urine (discard); rinse the bladder with saline. The catheter should be secured in the bladder for the duration of the test.
2. Begin the urine collection period immediately after rinsing the bladder. It is best to clamp the catheter for most of the collection period.
3. Obtain a blood sample for serum creatinine determination halfway through the collection period.
4. Begin collecting the urine in the bladder after approximately 18 minutes. Flush the bladder several times with saline; add the saline flushes to the urine collected. *Make sure that all urine and saline have been removed from the bladder.* If in doubt, extend the collection period; the time is not critical as long as the exact duration of the collection period is recorded.

Calculation of clearance

1. Determine the creatinine concentration of each blood sample and an aliquot of each urine sample.
2. Use the following formula:

$$C_{creat} = \frac{U_{creat} \times V}{SC \times T \times BW}$$

where C_{creat} = creatinine clearance; ml/minute/kg
U_{creat} = urine creatinine concentration, mg/dl
V = urine volume, ml
SC = serum creatinine concentration, mg/dl
T = time of collection period, minutes
BW = body weight, kg

Table 2. *Normal Values for Selected Renal Function Tests in Dogs and Cats*

Test	Dog	Cat
Endogenous creatinine clearance, ml/minute/kg	2.0–4.0	1.6–3.8
Exogenous creatinine clearance, ml/minute/kg	3.2–5.4	2.6–3.3
Sodium sulfanilate excretion, T½, minutes	50–80	48–50
PSP excretion, %	>30*	>50†
PSP plasma disappearance, T½, minutes	18–24	21–28‡
Urine specific gravity§	>1.030	>1.035
Urine osmolality, mOsm/kg§	>1500	>1800

*20 minutes postinjection.
†30 minutes postinjection.
‡Not a specific renal function test in cats.
§Minimum value indicating normal tubular function.
(Data from Finco, 1980; Hardy and Osborne, 1979; Osbaldiston and Fuhrman, 1970; Ross and Finco, 1981)

liable results. Regardless of the length of the collection period, it is best to obtain several collections on a given patient and determine the average clearance (Tables 1 and 2).

The creatinine clearance in female dogs is considered an accurate reflection of GFR. It slightly overestimates GFR in male dogs because of the proximal tubular secretory mechanism. Creatinine clearance determinations slightly underestimate GFR in cats. The exact reason for this is not clear but may be due to the methods used in the determination of serum creatinine concentrations (Finco and Barsanti, 1982).

An alternative method for estimation of GFR is to determine the rate of excretion of a substance known to be excreted primarily by glomerular filtration. Sodium sulfanilate is one such substance whose excretion has been shown to be a valid estimation of GFR in dogs and cats. A 5 per cent solution of sodium sulfanilate (Alfa Products) is injected intravenously at a dose of 0.2 ml/kg. Blood samples are collected after 30, 60, and 90 minutes and analyzed for sodium sulfanilate concentration. The plasma half-life (T½) is then calculated and compared with normal values (Finco, 1980; Ross and Finco, 1981). Neither sodium sulfanilate nor laboratory analyses of the plasma concentration are readily available to practitioners, however. The excretion of other substances such as ^{125}I-iodothalamate have been shown to correlate well with GFR, but their use is usually confined to research.

TUBULAR FUNCTION

Renal tubular function is generally assessed by the ability of the animal to produce a concentrated or dilute urine. Osmolality measures the number of osmotically active molecules in solution. Sodium, chloride, and bicarbonate molecules constitute most of the osmotic activity in urine. Although osmolality provides a more accurate reflection of urine concentrating ability than does specific gravity, the cost of an osmometer (Wescor) precludes its use in most practices. Although there is only a rough correlation between osmolality and specific gravity, the latter provides sufficient information to assess tubular function in most clinical cases. Specific gravity is a reflection of the relative amount of solids in solution, and it may be easily determined by the use of a refractometer (Reichert Scientific Instruments) or urinometer (Clay Adams Division of Becton, Dickinson, and Co.).

The urine specific gravity or osmolality is the only portion of the urinalysis that provides information about renal function. It should always be evaluated with respect to the hydration status of the animal as well as other renal function tests. A normal animal may produce urine that is dilute, isosthenuric, or concentrated, depending on its water balance at that point in time. The production of dilute urine (specific gravity 1.001 to 1.007) requires metabolic work by the tubules and suggests that some tubular function persists. A number of diseases may be associated with hyposthenuria, including hyperadrenocorticism, diabetes insipidus, and pyelonephritis.

Animals with renal insufficiency have been thought to have isosthenuria (urine specific gravity 1.008 to 1.012). This is not strictly true, however. Animals in which glomerular lesions predominate may have renal insufficiency as indicated by an elevated BUN and serum creatinine, yet they may retain some degree of urine concentrating ability. In some cases, they may be able to concentrate urine normally. Cats with renal insufficiency may become azotemic while retaining the ability to concentrate urine, especially in the early stages of the disease (Ross and Finco, 1981). Dogs with renal insufficiency may occasionally produce urine of specific gravity greater than 1.012, although almost never above 1.025 (Osborne and Polzin, 1983). The exact reasons for this are not clear. In cats, it is probably related to their ability to normally produce very concentrated urine.

Normal urine concentrating ability has traditionally been defined as the production of urine of specific gravity greater than 1.025. However, this figure was extrapolated from human beings whose maximal urine specific gravity is approximately 1.040. Since dogs are able to produce urine with a specific gravity of 1.065 and cats 1.080, the figure 1.025 is probably too low for these species. Current recommendations suggest that normal urine concentrating ability is indicated by a urine specific gravity greater than 1.030 in dogs and 1.035 in cats. These values may be seen on either a random urine sample or after a challenge (water deprivation or antidiuretic hormone [ADH] response test). Puppies and kittens are able to concentrate urine to some extent, but not to the same degree as an adult animal (Lage, 1980). The exact age at which the kidneys of immature animals attain normal concentrating ability is not well documented but appears to be approximately 12 to 16 weeks. Tests of urine concentrating ability are therefore difficult to evaluate in young animals.

Calculation of the ratio of urine to plasma osmolality provides information about the ability of the kidneys to concentrate or dilute glomerular filtrate. A ratio of urine to plasma osmolality that is greater than 1 indicates that the kidney is able to concentrate urine to some extent; less than 1 indicates ability to dilute the urine. In normal dogs, the ratio may be 7 or greater. To determine the osmolality ratio, urine and plasma samples should be obtained simultaneously; they can be tested then or frozen for testing at a later date. Many human clinical pathology laboratories can perform osmolality determinations.

Animals may produce dilute urine with subsequent polydipsia and polyuria with renal failure as well as numerous other diseases. An algorithm for the diagnosis of polydipsia and polyuria has been described and is helpful in determining the cause (Hardy and Osborne, 1980).

OTHER TESTS

Phenolsulphonphthalein (PSP; Hynson, Westcott, and Dunning) is a dye that is excreted primarily by proximal tubular secretion in dogs. A PSP excretion test has been described in dogs (Osborne et al., 1972); however, at the dose used, the test reflects renal plasma flow rather than proximal tubular function (Table 2). Low levels of PSP excretion may therefore be encountered in any condition causing a reduction in renal plasma flow. The technique for performing the PSP excretion test in dogs is as follows: (1) Place an indwelling urinary catheter, empty the bladder, and discard this urine. (2) Administer 6 mg of PSP intravenously. (3) Collect all urine produced during the 20 minutes immediately following injection—saline rinses are used to rinse the bladder during the last few minutes of the period and are added to the urine. (4) The urine and saline mixure is analyzed for PSP and the percentage of excretion calculated (Finco, 1980). PSP excretion has also been measured in cats using a 3-mg dose and 30-minute collection period (Osbaldiston and Fuhrman, 1970) (Table 2).

The plasma clearance of PSP has been studied in cats. Plasma half-life of PSP showed a poor correlation with renal plasma flow in cats, indicating that it is not a valid test of renal function in this species (Ross and Finco, 1981). The reason for this is not known but could be due to excretion of PSP by other routes (possibly hepatic) in cats.

SERUM PHOSPHATE CONCENTRATION

Hyperphosphatemia is associated with renal failure, but it is a relatively nonspecific and insensitive indicator of renal function. Phosphate ions are filtered through the glomerular basement membrane and reabsorbed in the renal tubules. In chronic renal failure, hyperphosphatemia will occur when the decrease in GFR exceeds the ability of the tubule to limit its reabsorptive process. In humans, significant hyperphosphatemia is encountered when the GFR falls below 30 ml per minute. No corresponding figure has been determined for dogs and cats. Azotemia may exist without hyperphosphatemia; however, hyperphosphatemia may also be associated with prerenal azotemia. The serum phosphate concentration is affected by several nonrenal factors as well. It will vary with dietary protein intake, since most ingested phosphate is of protein origin. Serum phosphate levels rise postprandially and may exceed the normal range if measured within several hours after a meal.

RADIOGRAPHY

Contrast radiography plays a minor role in the assessment of renal function, since the information it provides is strictly qualitative. Although a poor-quality intravenous urogram may be the result of decreased renal function, it may also be due to decreased renal blood flow from any cause. Intravenous urography may be helpful in determining differences in function between the two kidneys as shown by differences in radiographic density; it may show abnormal size, shape, or contour of the kidneys, and it may illustrate the presence of obstructive uropathy. The most important information that can be gained from contrast radiography is the diagnosis of a tear or rupture in the urinary system. Administration of iodinated contrast media has been associated with acute renal failure in humans, especially those with pre-existing renal insufficiency, volume depletion, or multiple myeloma. Although this does not appear to be a significant problem in dogs and cats, the possibility must be considered. A more practical consideration is the failure to achieve a diagnostic study in animals with renal insufficiency, especially those with serum creatinine values greater than 3.0 mg/dl.

Nuclear medicine has provided yet another means for determining renal function. Studies using radioisotopes are being developed, and these allow quantitative assessment of GFR and renal blood flow (see the article entitled Assessment of Individ-

Table 3. Interpretation of Some Clinical Renal Function Tests

BUN	Serum Creatinine Concentration	Urine Specific Gravity	Possible Causes
Increased*	Increased†	>1.030 dogs >1.035 cats	Prerenal azotemia Primary renal insufficiency (cats only) Postrenal azotemia Rarely primary glomerular disease; if so will have marked proteinuria.
Increased*	N‡	As above	As above Extrarenal azotemia
Increased*	Increased†	1.008–1.030 dogs 1.008–1.035 cats	Primary renal insufficiency Postrenal azotemia Rarely hypoadrenocorticism
N	Increased†	1.008–1.030 dogs 1.008–1.035 cats	Primary renal insufficiency with concurrent low-protein diet or hepatic insufficiency
N	N	1.008–1.030 dogs 1.008–1.035 cats	Primary renal insufficiency Other causes of polydipsia/polyuria§
N	N	1.001–1.006	Rarely renal insufficiency Other causes of dilute urine§

*Normal range 10–30 mg/dl
†Normal range 0.5–1.5 mg/dl
‡Normal.
§Consult Hardy and Osborne, 1980.

ual Kidney Function by Quantitative Renal Scintigraphy). Such studies will be limited to use in large institutions because of the extremely high cost of the equipment.

HISTOPATHOLOGY

Renal biopsy, although essential in determining the pathologic basis for renal disease, is of little benefit in the assessment of function. There is poor correlation between the severity of histopathologic lesions and the degree of renal dysfunction. This disparity may be attributed to several factors, including the compensatory reserve of the kidney; physiologic, rather than pathologic, abnormalities resulting in renal insufficiency; and sampling errors due to the small amount of tissue biopsied.

SUMMARY

The assessment of renal function must be done with care because of the myriad of factors that are involved. Table 3 provides information in a simplified form to guide clinicians in the assessment of renal function. Other sources should be consulted for help in localizing azotemia (Osborne and Polzin, 1983; Osborne et al., 1983) or in determining the cause of dilute urine (Hardy and Osborne, 1980). If the BUN, serum creatinine, and urine specific gravity suggest primary renal disease or insufficiency, the clinician may choose to perform one or more of the tests described above in order to better evaluate the level of renal function. The author's choice in such cases is to determine the endogenous creatinine clearance. In cases of severe renal failure with greatly elevated BUN and serum creatinine levels, these tests will probably not add additional information to the clinical picture.

References and Supplemental Reading

Coles, H.: *Veterinary Clinical Pathology.* Philadelphia: W. B. Saunders, 1980, pp. 217–256.

Finco, D. R.: Clinical evaluation of renal function. *In* Marthens, E. V. (ed.): *Seventh Annual Kal Kan Symposium for the Treatment of Small Animal Diseases Proceedings.* Vernon, California: Kal Kan Foods, Inc; 1984, pp. 95–99.

Finco, D. R.: Kidney function. *In* Kaneko, J. J. (ed.): *Clinical Biochemistry of Domestic Animals.* New York: Academic Press, 1980, pp. 338–400.

Finco, D. R., and Barsanti, J. A.: Mechanism of urinary excretion of creatinine by the cat. Am. J. Vet. Res. 43:2207, 1982.

Hardy, R. M., and Osborne, C. A.: Water deprivation test in the dog: Maximal normal values. J.A.V.M.A. 174:479, 1979.

Hardy, R. M., and Osborne, C. A.: Water deprivation and vasopressin concentration test in the differentiation of polyuric syndromes. *In* Kirk, R. W. (ed.): *Current Veterinary Therapy VII.* Philadelphia: W. B. Saunders, 1980, pp. 1080–1085.

Lage, A. L.: Neonatal clinical nephrology. *In* Kirk, R. W. (ed.): *Current Veterinary Therapy VII.* Philadelphia: W. B. Saunders, 1980, pp. 1085–1087.

Osborne, C. A., Finco, D. R., and Low, D. G.: Pathophysiology of renal disease, renal failure, and uremia. *In* Ettinger, S. J. (ed.): *Textbook of Veterinary Internal Medicine,* vol. II, 2nd ed. Philadelphia: W. B. Saunders, 1983, pp. 1733–1792.

Osborne, C. A., Low, D. G., and Finco, D. R.: *Canine and Feline Urology.* Philadelphia: W. B. Saunders, 1972.

Osborne, C. A., and Polzin, D. J.: Azotemia: A review of what's old and what's new. Part I. Definition of terms and concepts. Comp. Cont. Ed. Pract. Vet. 5:497, 1983.

Osborne, C. A., and Polzin, D. J.: Azotemia: A review of what's old and what's new. Part II. Localization. Comp. Cont. Ed. Pract. Vet. 5:561, 1983.

Osbaldiston, G. W. and Fuhrman, W.: The clearance of creatinine, inulin, para-aminohippurate and phenolsulphonphthalein in the cat. Can. J. Comp. Med. 34:138, 1970.

Ross, L. A., and Finco, D. R.: Relationship of selected clinical renal function tests to glomerular filtration rate and renal blood flow in cats. Am. J. Vet. Res. 42:1704, 1981.

ASSESSMENT OF INDIVIDUAL KIDNEY FUNCTION BY QUANTITATIVE RENAL SCINTIGRAPHY

LARRY D. COWGILL, D.V.M.,
and WILLIAM J. HORNOF, D.V.M.
Davis, California

The detection of unilateral renal disease and quantitation of individual kidney function is a formidable clinical problem. Anatomic constraints may prohibit adequate palpation of each kidney, routine radiography may not allow their complete visualization, and contrast radiography does not quantitate function. Plasma urea nitrogen and creatinine are the major clinical indices of renal function but are too imprecise and insensitive to distinguish subtle or unilateral alterations of renal function. Quantitation of individual kidney function by exogenous inulin or endogenous creatinine clearance is a burdensome procedure requiring catheterization of each ureter and represents an unacceptable risk for any clinical assessment. Thus, unilateral renal dysfunction may be masked entirely or remain uncharacterized by conventional diagnostic approaches until late in its clinical course.

Notwithstanding these technical difficulties and hazards, precise documentation of glomerular filtration rate (GFR) and in particular the size and functional capacity of individual kidneys has clinical merit and could substantially augment the diagnosis and management of renal disease in companion animals.

QUANTITATIVE RENAL SCINTIGRAPHY

Quantitative renal scintigraphy (QRS) is a nuclear diagnostic technique with the capacity to noninvasively image the kidneys and to measure bilateral renal function without the need of urethral or ureteral catheterization. It employs the radiopharmaceutical ^{99m}Tc diethylenetriaminepentaacetic acid (DTPA), which is excreted by the kidney analogous to inulin or creatinine and thus serves as a marker of glomerular filtration. Because it is also a radionuclide, its relative distribution within the body can be detected by a gamma camera to produce an image called a scintigram (Fig. 1A). Because DTPA is preferentially distributed to and concentrated in the kidneys, the scintigram provides a semiquantitative assessment of excretory function similar to kidney density on an excretory urogram. The advantage of QRS, however, lies in the noninvasive capacity to quantitate precisely the accumulation and disappearance of the isotope from each kidney in real time. Mathematic manipulation of the "time-activity" data generated by the gamma camera allows computer determination of the relative size and actual GFR of each kidney.

Estimation of Renal Size

We have developed a computer algorithm that accurately defines the edge of each renal margin regardless of the relative radioactivity within the kidney. This algorithm generates a computer-resolved scintigram that depicts the size and shape of each kidney (Fig. 1*B*). From the edge-detected scintigram, quantitative measurements of each kidney's geometry can be made; this information may

The authors wish to acknowledge the technical expertise and assistance provided by Paul E. Fisher and Larry A. Neal and the Morris Animal Foundation for its generous support in the development of this technology.

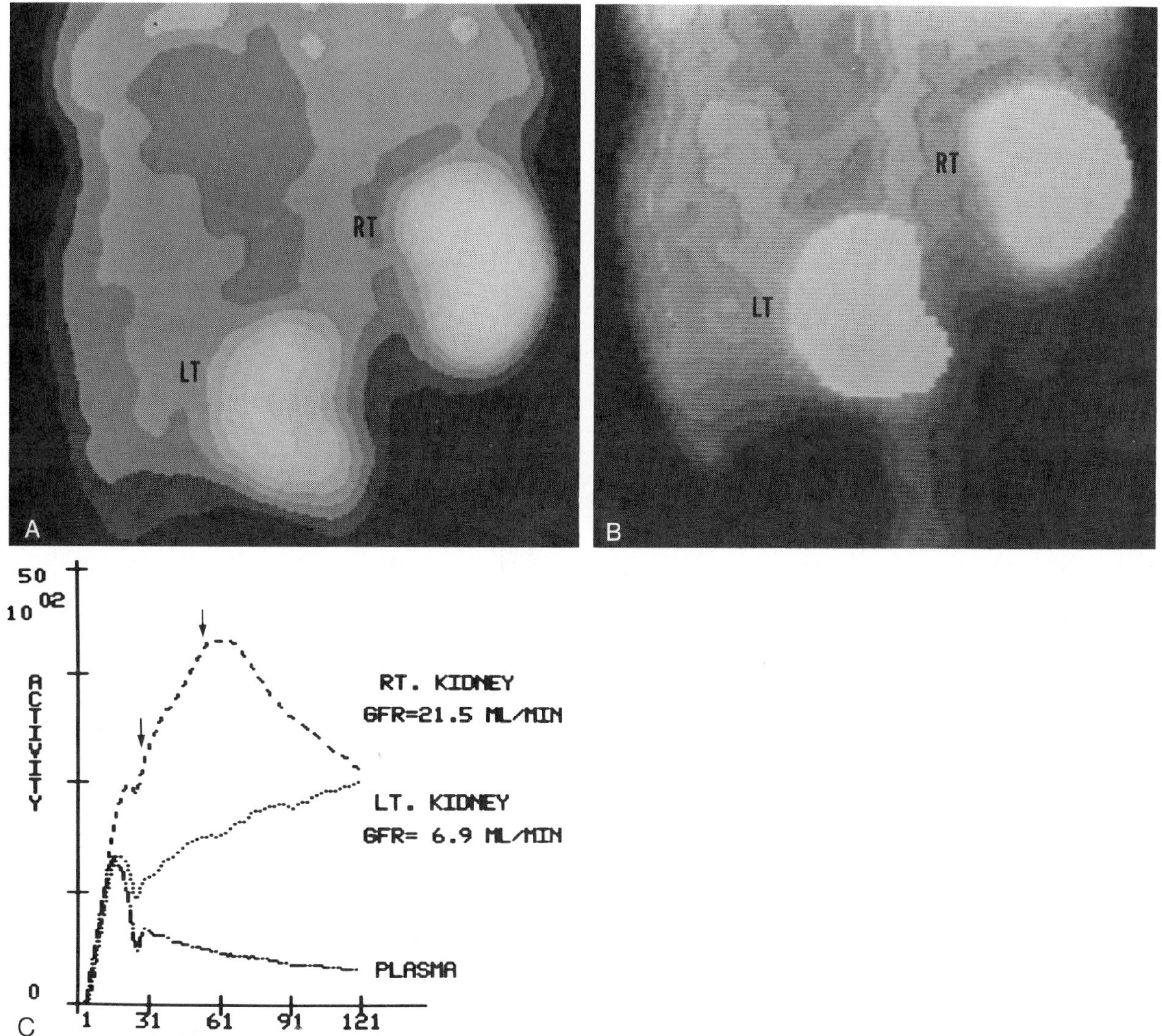

Figure 1. Quantitative renal scintigraphy in the dog. *A*, ^{99m}Tc DTPA scintigram of an anesthetized dog 1 hour after occlusion of the left renal artery for 35 minutes. The figure demonstrates reduced uptake of the DTPA in the compromised left kidney (LT), as compared with the normal right (RT) kidney, and provides a semiquantitative assessment of relative renal function. *B*, Computer-generated renal scintigram from the same dog; edge-detection algorithms have been used to define each kidney's anatomic margins. This process depicts relative renal geometry of each kidney independently of the degree of its excretory function as depicted in *A*. *C*, Time vs. radioactivity curves for right and left kidneys and plasma from the scintigram depicted in *A*. Each kidney's radioactivity was derived from the "region of interest" determined by the edge-detection procedure illustrated in *B*. In this case, the plasma curve was generated from an exteriorized blood source. GFR for each kidney is calculated from the uptake of DTPA during the brief interval (between arrows) after passage of the initial DTPA bolus until the radioactivity leaves the kidney in the urine. Actual GFR values for each kidney are calculated from mathematical treatment of the kidney and plasma curves. The calculated values are in close agreement to simultaneously determined inulin clearances of 24.0 ml/min and 7.2 ml/min for the right and left kidneys, respectively.

not be obtainable with excretory urography when a kidney is functioning poorly.

Measurements of renal geometry are helpful in the differential diagnosis of acute and chronic uremia and renal neoplasia when excretory capacity is severely compromised. This concept is clearly illustrated in Figure 1. The scintigram in Figure 1*A* was obtained from an anesthetized dog 1 hour after occlusion of the left renal artery for 35 minutes. Despite the obvious deterioration of excretory capacity in the left kidney (Fig. 1*A* and *C*), it has normal dimensions in the edge-detected scintigram (Fig. 1*B*) as would be predicted with an acute insult when there has been no loss of renal mass. The nonedge-detected scintigram in Figure 1*A* underrepresents the true size of the occluded kidney because of its reduced ability to excrete the DTPA.

Estimation of GFR

Traditionally, GFR is estimated by inulin or creatinine clearance, which is time-consuming and subject to the inaccuracies of quantitative urine collections. With QRS, it is possible to make rapid GFR determinations of each kidney without the necessity of urine collections. The gamma camera is capable of simultaneously detecting both the plasma concentration and the individual kidney uptake of the DTPA after its intravenous injection. The results are displayed as time versus radioactivity curves for each kidney region on the scintigram, as illustrated in Figure 1*C*. The edge-detection algorithm is used to define precisely each renal "region of interest" and prevents under- or overestimation of renal activity in the calculation of GFR. For the brief interval following passage of the initial DTPA bolus until the radioactivity leaves the kidney in the urine (Fig. 1*C*), the rate of uptake of DTPA by the kidney (slope of time-activity curve) is a direct function of its GFR and the plasma concentration of DTPA. Thus the GFR for each kidney can be calculated from the ratio of the rate of renal uptake to plasma concentration of DTPA at simultaneous times.

This calculation is illustrated in Figure 1*C*, where GFR values for each kidney are displayed with their time-activity curve. The values correlate with the divergent renal uptake curves, the renal intensities in the scintigram (Fig. 1*A*), and the simultaneously determined inulin clearance values for each kidney (Fig. 1*C*). Total renal function is the sum of the individual kidney values and can be used to stage the degree of renal insufficiency or formulate therapy.

The function of each kidney can be expressed in an alternative and less complex manner as the percentage of the injected DTPA taken up by the kidney within a specified time interval. As it happens, this expression is a mathematic function of the ratio of GFR to metabolic body size and is therefore normalized for all animals. The percentage excreted by normal kidneys is a constant; thus, the amount (or percentage) of residual function in a diseased kidney can be readily determined. Even though this measure has no physiologic counterpart, it has definite clinical significance in estimating excretory reserve and can be more simply derived from the scintigraphic measurements.

CONCLUSIONS

Quantitative renal scintigraphy is a new and highly sophisticated diagnostic procedure that allows accurate quantitation of individual kidney function and geometry in a rapid and noninvasive manner in conscious animals. The procedure is completed within 5 minutes of isotope injection and requires neither urethral nor ureteral catheterization or urine collection. Scintigraphic equipment is becoming more widely available at universities, human nuclear diagnostic facilities, and specialty veterinary practices. The primary indications for its use are detection of early renal insufficiency, quantitating differential kidney function, diagnosis of acute and chronic renal failure, and serial monitoring of the progression and response to therapy of renal injury. In addition to its diagnostic utility, QRS provides a powerful tool for the investigation of renal disease and therapy in companion animals. Because it is painless, nontraumatic, and poses no patient risk, its use for clinical research can be highly justified.

ASSESSMENT OF PROTEINURIA IN THE DOG AND CAT

ELIZABETH A. RUSSO, D.V.M.
College Station, Texas

Routine laboratory screening of sick, preoperative, or geriatric small animal patients commonly reveals proteinuria. Accurate assessment of this finding depends on knowledge of the methods used to measure protein in the urine and an understanding of the physiology and pathophysiology of proteinuria.

LABORATORY MEASUREMENT OF URINE PROTEIN

Colorimetric reagent strips used to detect urine protein have an area impregnated with buffered tetrabromphenol blue. The amino groups of protein molecules bind to and change the color of this acid-base indicator without changing its pH. A trace positive reading may indicate a protein concentration as low as 5 to 20 mg/dl. These strips are most sensitive to albumin, thus false-negatives may occur if the urine protein is not predominantly albumin or if the urine is dilute and the concentration of protein is below the level of detection. False-positives may occur if there has been contamination with certain antiseptics such as quaternary ammonium compounds (e.g., Zephiran Chloride, Winthrop) or chlorhexidine, if the reagent strips have not been kept dry, or if the buffer in the strip has been washed away by prolonged contact with an excessive volume of urine. Highly alkaline urine supposedly can also cause false-positives, although one researcher demonstrated that alkaline pH in the physiologic range (up to 9) did not affect test results (Rennie, 1967).

Turbidometric tests rely on the precipitation of protein from urine by various acids such as nitric acid, heat plus acetic acid, and sulfosalicylic acid (SSA). The last is commercially available as Bumintest Tabs (Ames). The quantity of precipitate is subjectively graded 0 to 4+. These tests should be performed on clear urine or supernatant so that urine turbidity will not interfere with their interpretation. The SSA test, although still most sensitive to albumin, will also detect globulins, glycoproteins, and Bence Jones proteins. False-positives can occur because of the presence of radiographic contrast agents, penicillins, cephalosporins, or sulfonamide metabolites in the urine. Gross hematuria may add enough serum protein to urine to cause positive reactions with both reagent strips and turbidometric tests. Highly concentrated urine may also produce positive results with both methods. The SSA test may be more reliable than the reagent strip as it is often negative when the dipstick gives a trace to 1+ reading.

There are numerous quantitative tests used for measurement of protein in urine. They vary considerably in their technical difficulty and their sensitivity to various urine proteins as well as to interfering substances. The protein or mixture of proteins used as a standard in these tests will also affect the results (Barsanti, 1979; Kassirer and Gennari, 1979; Pesce, 1974). Some examples of quantitative tests are the Kjeldahl's, biuret, Lowry, trichloroacetic acid–ponceau S, and Coomassie brillant blue methods. Quantitative tests are usually performed on an aliquot of all urine produced in a 24-hour period.

MECHANISMS OF PROTEINURIA

Proteinuria has been classified as prerenal, postrenal, or renal in origin (Kassirer and Gennari, 1979; DiBartola et al., 1980b). Prerenal or "overproduction" proteinuria is due to elevated serum levels of certain proteins that are able to pass through the glomerular barrier into the urine. Hemoglobin released in intravascular hemolysis will readily pass through the glomerulus if the amount present in the serum exceeds the capacity of the larger haptoglobin molecules to bind it. Myoglobin released in the rare condition of rhabdomyolysis will also pass through the glomerulus and appear in urine. In multiple myeloma, massive production of immunoglobulin by neoplastic plasma cells occurs. The excessive immunoglobulin light-chain monomers and dimers in the serum are readily filtered through the glomerulus and appear in the urine as so-called Bence Jones proteins. A similar phenomenon may occur in macroglobulinemia and in some leukemias. Because Bence Jones proteins are precipitated by SSA but do not produce a reaction with reagent strips, a negative or trace dipstick reaction with a positive SSA test is suggestive of the presence of excessive immunoglobulin light chains in the urine (Abuelo, 1983).

Postrenal proteinuria is due to proteins that have been added to the urine after it has left the kidney—that is, by the lower urinary tract or genital organs. If proteinuria is found on a voided urine sample, a second sample obtained by cystocentesis should be analyzed to confirm that the protein is of urinary and not genital tract origin.

RENAL PROTEINURIA—NORMAL URINE PROTEINS. Urine normally contains small amounts of protein that are usually not detected by qualitative or semiquantitative tests used in routine urinalysis (Barsanti and Finco, 1979). The majority of these are proteins of plasma origin that have filtered through the glomerular barrier. Their passage is inversely related to their size and negative charge but is also dependent on their shape. Small globulin fragments; numerous hormones such as insulin, growth hormone, glucagon, vasopressin, adrenocorticotropic hormone (ACTH), and parathyroid hormone (PTH); other small proteins such as ribonuclease and lysozyme; and some albumin enter the filtrate (Kassirer and Gennari, 1979). These are, with the exception of albumin, largely reabsorbed by endocytosis and degraded by the renal tubular cells. Twenty-five to 70 per cent of normal urine protein in dogs is albumin (Barsanti and Finco, 1979; DiBartola et al., 1980b).

The epithelial cells of Henle's loop, the distal tubule, and collecting ducts also add protein to the urine. This Tamm-Horsfall glycoprotein, also called uromucoid, is present in undetectably low concentrations, 0.5 to 1 mg/dl (DiBartola et al., 1980b). Casts are composed of Tamm-Horsfall protein that has been precipitated by albumin. Another normal urine protein of high molecular weight is IgA that has been secreted from urinary epithelial surfaces. Low-molecular-weight urokinase is another normal urine protein of tubular origin.

FUNCTIONAL PROTEINURIA. In humans, functional proteinuria is detectable proteinuria of renal origin that is considered to be nonpathologic. It often follows a precipitating event such as strenuous exercise, extremes of heat or cold, fever, or stress. It also may accompany essential hypertension or congestive heart failure. The proteinuria is transient and usually mild except in severe venous congestion, when it may be of greater magnitude. It is composed primarily of albumin as it is due to increased glomerular permeability. Idiopathic, transient, benign proteinuria may also occur in humans, especially young males. Functional proteinuria following strenuous exercise has also been reported to occur in dogs (Biewenga et al., 1982).

PATHOLOGIC RENAL PROTEINURIA. This type of proteinuria may be due to (1) a glomerulopathy allowing increased filtration of serum proteins, (2) tubular disease causing decreased reabsorption of normally filtered proteins, or (3) renal parenchymal inflammatory disease causing exudation of protein into urine. Glomerular proteinuria is composed primarily of albumin, although leakage of globulins of higher molecular weight may also occur.

Tubular proteinuria may be due to a reabsorptive defect of the tubular cells as is seen in Fanconi's syndrome or tubular necrosis. It may also be due to leakage of tubular cell proteins into the urine as occurs in tubular necrosis. The urine proteins in these syndromes are composed largely of proteins of smaller molecular weight rather than of albumin and are more readily detected by the SSA test than by dipstick reagent strips.

ASSESSMENT OF PROTEINURIA

On finding proteinuria in a patient, one should first attempt to ascertain (1) whether the protein is of urinary tract origin and (2) whether it is persistent. This is determined by testing a second urine sample obtained by cystocentesis several days later. A turbidometric test as well as a dipstick determination should be performed, and common causes for false-positive results eliminated.

If, in addition to proteinuria, hematuria or pyuria is found on urine sediment examination, it is indicative of hemorrhage or exudation into the urine. These are more commonly but not exclusively associated with lower urinary tract disease. Pyelone-

Table 1. *24-Hour Urinary Protein Excretion in Normal Animals*

Species	Protein Excretion: mg/day — *Range*	mg/day — *Mean ± SD*	mg/kg/day — *Range*	mg/kg/day — *Mean ± SD*	Method of Analysis	Reference
Dog	24–197	70 ± 49			CBB	Barsanti and Finco, 1979
	8–151	38 ± 41			TCA-PS	
Dog		440 ± 64			Lowry	Stuart et al., 1975
Dog	41–317	110	2.7–23.2	6.6	TCA-PS	Biewenga et al., 1982
Dog	48–1040	333 ± 309	4.55–28.3	13.9 ± 7.71	TCA-PS	DiBartola et al., 1980b
Cat	11.65–113.90	52.30 ± 25.70	4.13–42.92	17.43 ± 9.05	CBB	Russo et al., 1985

CBB = Coomassie brilliant blue
TCA-PS = Trichloroacetic acid–ponceau S

Table 2. *24-Hour Urinary Protein Excretion in Dogs with Glomerular Disease*

	Protein Excretion			
	gm/day		*mg/kg/day*	
Light Microscopic Glomerular Lesion	***Range***	***Mean ± SD***	***Range***	***Mean ± SD***
Amyloidosis (n = 6)	4.78–16.1	10.3 ± 4.25	150.3–959.6	506.9 ± 266.9
Glomerulonephritis (n = 11)	0.57–13.2	3.48 ± 3.68	81.23–387.1	164.7 ± 91.08
Glomerular atrophy—secondary to interstitial disease (n = 4)	0.77–3.87	2.40 ± 1.42	31.95–131.2	87.82 ± 44.25

Modified from DiBartola et al.: J.A.V.M.A. 177:73, 1980a.

phritis, other renal inflammatory disease, or neoplasia could also be responsible for such findings. Hematuria does not accompany acute glomerulonephritis in dogs as it does in humans. Urine culture and contrast radiography may be necessary to investigate proteinuria accompanied by hematuria or pyuria. The absence of hematuria, pyuria, or bacteriuria will help to rule out lower urinary tract disease as a cause of the proteinuria.

Significant, persistent proteinuria with a benign sediment most likely indicates a glomerulopathy such as glomerulonephritis or amyloidosis. The triad of clinical pathologic findings including proteinuria, hypoalbuminemia, and hypercholesterolemia is highly suggestive of proteinuria due to glomerular disease.

Although a trace to 1+ proteinuria as detected by semiquantitative methods is more likely to be significant if detected in dilute urine than in a more concentrated sample, the actual magnitude of protein loss is difficult to judge based on analysis of a single sample (Barsanti and Finco, 1979; DiBartola et al., 1980b). A quantitation of 24-hour urinary protein excretion should be performed to investigate or confirm significant proteinuria.

The animal may be catheterized to empty its bladder, or the 24-hour collection of urine may be started after a spontaneous voiding. Complete emptying should be verified by palpation. All urine produced within the 24-hour period may be collected by placing the animal in a metabolic cage, or a similar device may be used (i.e., a container that will catch urine voided into the cage). Dogs may be walked outside several times during the collection period, but all urine must be caught in a pan or bucket. At the end of the collection period, which may be somewhat more or less than exactly 24 hours, the bladder must again be emptied. Urine samples, which have been refrigerated as they are collected, are combined, the total volume is measured, and an aliquot is quantitatively analyzed for protein.

Table 3. *24-Hour Urinary Protein Excretion Typical of Various Urinary Tract Diseases of Humans*

Protein Excretion	**Disease**
<0.5 gm	Lower urinary tract disease
<1 gm	Interstitial disease, pyelonephritis, nephrosclerosis, obstructive disease, neoplasia, hypercalcemic nephropathy, postural proteinuria
1–2 gm	Fanconi's syndrome
1–3.5 gm	Wide variety of conditions including mild glomerulopathies
>3.5 gm	Glomerulopathies (nephrotic syndrome)

Daily urine protein excretion in mg/day may then be calculated by use of the following equation:

$$\text{Urine protein concentration (in mg/dl)} \times \text{Urine volume (in ml)} \div 100\ \frac{\text{ml}}{\text{dl}}$$

If the actual collection period was not exactly 24 hours, a correction must be made by multiplying by the following factor:

$$\frac{\text{Actual number of minutes in the collection}}{\text{1440 (i.e., number of minutes/day)}}$$

A 24-hour urine collection also affords one the opportunity to calculate endogenous creatinine clearance. This may indicate a decrease in the patient's glomerular filtration rate prior to detectable increases in its serum urea nitrogen or serum creatinine.

Normal 24-hour urinary protein excretion has been reported. There is some variation (Table 1), since different quantitative tests and protein standards were used.

The ratio of the urine protein concentration to the urine creatinine concentration of a single urine sample may be used in lieu of a 24-hour urine collection to confirm or rule out significant proteinuria. A ratio of less than 1.0 indicates a proteinuria of less than 1 gm/day. Most normal dogs in one study had a ratio of less than 0.2, which is considered normal for humans; all normal dogs had a ratio of less than 0.6. This test was of value even when dipstick protein determinations were negative in dilute urine samples (White et al., 1984).

Daily protein excretion in several glomerulopathies in dogs has been reported (Table 2). Although there were significant differences among groups, there was considerable overlap in values. There are at present no reports for dogs or cats of quantitation of proteinuria in other renal diseases such as tubular necrosis, Fanconi's syndrome, pyelonephritis, or interstitial inflammatory disease. In humans, less than 150 mg/day is considered normal urine protein excretion. Expected degrees of proteinuria in various pathologic conditions are given in Table 3. Unfortunately there is overlap; mild glomerulopathies may produce the same degree of proteinuria encountered in other conditions.

Urine protein electrophoresis may be used to help determine the origin of abnormal proteinuria. The electrophoretogram of protein of glomerular origin will show an albumin peak. Tubular proteinuria will produce a diffuse increase in globulin fractions. Prerenal proteinuria due to multiple myeloma will cause the appearance of a globulin spike similar to that seen on a serum protein electrophoretogram of the same patient (Kassirer and Gennari, 1979). Urine protein electrophoresis is the best way to confirm the presence of Bence Jones proteins (Pesce, 1974).

A renal biopsy will confirm the diagnosis if laboratory findings do not clearly indicate the type of renal disease. Prognosis may also be made more accurately with the availability of a specific histopathologic diagnosis.

The progression of renal disease (glomerulopathies) may be followed by monitoring urinary protein levels. However, the 24-hour excretion of protein may actually decrease as the disease progresses and the glomerular filtration rate or serum albumin concentration falls.

Changes in the albumin clearance

$$\left(\frac{[\text{albumin}]_{\text{urine}} \times \text{volume of urine}}{[\text{albumin}]_{\text{serum}}}\right)$$

or in the fractional clearance of albumin

$$\left(\frac{[\text{albumin}]_{\text{urine}} \times [\text{creatinine}]_{\text{serum}}}{[\text{albumin}]_{\text{serum}} \times [\text{creatinine}]_{\text{urine}}}\right)$$

may be of more value in assessing the changing magnitude of albuminuria (DiBartola et al., 1980b).

Finally, the absence of proteinuria does not rule out significant renal disease. Amyloidosis in cats, for example, can be primarily medullary in distribution and cause renal failure without proteinuria. Glomerulopathies in their final stages may result in a greatly reduced glomerular filtration rate and loss of urine concentrating ability, so that proteinuria is minimal and below the concentration detectable by common laboratory methods.

References and Supplemental Reading

Abuelo, J. G.: Proteinuria: Diagnostic principles and procedures. Ann. Intern. Med. 98:186, 1983.

Barsanti, J. A., and Finco, D. R.: Protein concentration in urine of normal dogs. Am. J. Vet. Res. 40:1583, 1979.

Biewenga, W. J., Gruys, E., and Henriks, H. J.: Urinary protein loss in the dog: Nephrological study of 29 dogs without signs of renal disease. Res. Vet. Sci. 33:366, 1982.

DiBartola, S. P., Spaulding, G. L., Chew, D. J., et al.: Urinary protein excretion and immunopathologic findings in dogs with glomerular disease. J.A.V.M.A. 177:73, 1980a.

DiBartola, S. P., Chew, D. J., and Jacobs, G.: Quantitative urinalysis including 24-hour protein excretion in the dog. J. Am. Anim. Hosp. Assoc. 16:537, 1980b.

Kassirer, J. P., and Gennari, F. J.: Laboratory evaluation of renal function. *In* Earley, L. E., and Gottschalk, C. W. (eds.): *Strauss and Welt's Diseases of the Kidney*, 3rd ed. Vol. 1. Boston: Little, Brown & Co., 1979, pp. 62–71.

Pesce, A. J.: Methods used for the analysis of proteins in the urine. Nephron 13:93, 1974.

Rennie, I. D. B., and Keen, H.: Evaluation of clinical methods for detecting proteinuria. Lancet 2:489, 1967.

Russo, E. A., Lees, G. E., and Hightower, D.: Am. J. Vet. Res., in press.

Stuart, B. P., Phemister, R. D., and Thomassen, R. W.: Glomerular lesions associated with proteinuria in clinically healthy dogs. Vet. Pathol. 12:125, 1975.

White, J. V., Olivier, N. B., Reimann, R., et al.: Use of protein-to-creatinine ratio in a single urine specimen for quantitative estimation of canine proteinuria. J.A.V.M.A. 185:882, 1984.

THE EFFECT OF RADIOGRAPHIC CONTRAST MEDIA ON THE URINALYSIS

DANIEL A. FEENEY, D.V.M.,
PATRICIA A. WALTER, D.V.M.,
and GARY R. JOHNSTON, D.V.M.
St. Paul, Minnesota

Radiographic contrast media (CM) are often used during the evaluation of small animal patients for urinary tract and cardiovascular diseases. These diagnostic agents are administered both by intravenous and retrograde routes (via the external urethral or the vaginal orifice) depending on the purpose of the study. The routine urinalysis is commonly used both for presurgical evaluation of urinary tract status as well as for the specific evaluation of patients with known or suspected urinary tract disease. During efforts to provide cost- and time-effective patient evaluation, there is a tendency to perform diagnostic procedures on small animal patients in rapid sequence or, when possible, simultaneously. The potential effects of CM on the various components of urinalysis prompted the authors to assemble the following information.

URINE SPECIFIC GRAVITY

The measurement of urine specific gravity is a screening test for the evaluation of renal tubular concentrating capacity. Since urographic and angiographic CM have specific gravity values in the range of 1.200 to 1.350, their presence in urine may introduce significant errors in specific gravity determinations. An obvious ramification of these agents in urine would be overestimation of renal concentrating capacity due to the erroneous increase in urine specific gravity induced by these compounds. This effect occurs when either the refractometer or urinomoter method is utilized (Feeney et al., 1980; Smith et al., 1983). However, a recent report suggests that specific gravity strips (N-Multistix Reagent Strips, Ames) are accurate despite the presence of CM (Smith et al., 1983).

Since the anionic portion (tri-iodinated benzoic acid derivative) of common angiographic/urographic CM is excreted via glomerular filtration essentially unchanged when given systemically, these agents will influence urine specific gravity. It has been reported that, in dogs, if the urinary specific gravity is greater than or equal to 1.040 prior to intravenous CM administration, there will be an identifiable decrease at 15 minutes postinjection. However, if preinjection urine specific gravity is less than 1.040, there will be a detectable increase 15 minutes postinjection (Feeney et al., 1980). Obviously, the latter is the most clinically relevant finding, since the increase in urine specific gravity could be overinterpreted as evidence of adequate renal tubular concentrating capacity, if the presence of CM is not considered. Although no data are available specifically on cats, a somewhat similar effect is expected. However, since cats tend to retain the ability to concentrate urine despite significant renal disease, the influence of the CM adds another variable that must be considered. In humans, the situation is considerably less complex, since it is unlikely that urine specific gravity values greater than or equal to 1.040 will be encountered. Therefore, values of this magnitude are almost invariably due to the presence of CM in the urine (Caraway and Kammeyer, 1972; Henry et al., 1974; McNeeley, 1980). This accounts for the statement in the human literature that the presence of CM will always cause an increase in urine specific gravity (Hurt, 1960). Our observations suggest that urine specific gravity values greater than 1.040 are quite common in dogs and cats without the influence of CM.

CM directly administered for retrograde urethrocystography and possibly vaginography will always increase urine specific gravity (Feeney et al., 1980). The change in urine specific gravity is linear and is directly proportional to the concentration of CM in the final solution (Feeney et al., 1980; Smith et al., 1983). This linear relationship was identified when CM was mixed with either distilled water or urine.

URINE OSMOLALITY

There exists some question in the literature about the effect of CM on measured urine osmolality.

Change in urine osmolality following systemic administration of CM has been reported in humans (Benness, 1968). However, a recent report suggests that osmolality determinations are not affected by CM (Smith et al., 1983). In our opinion, since the osmolality of CM ranges from about 1600 to 2700 mOsm/kg, we recommend that the same precautions be observed for urine osmolality determinations as for urine specific gravity determinations until there is convincing evidence to the contrary (Feeney et al., 1980).

SEMIQUANTITATED TEST FOR URINE CONSTITUENTS

According to available reports, commonly used tests for urine pH, urine ketones, urine bilirubin, and urine hemoglobin (occult blood) are not affected by the presence of CM in the urine (Caraway and Kammeyer, 1972; Hurt, 1960; Koneman and Schlesser, 1965; McNeeley, 1980). However, results of some screening tests for urine glucose, urine protein (particularly albumin), and urine urobilinogen are affected. Table 1 describes the methods used to analyze for these constituents and the observed effects induced by CM. Of potential interpretive significance is that true (apparent transient) proteinuria has been documented in patients following excretory urography and nephroangiography (Feeney et al., 1979; Holtas et al., 1981). This is in addition to that described as false-positive proteinuria due to CM, described in Table 1.

QUANTITATION OF URINE PROTEIN

Several methods can provide accurate quantitation of urine protein. It is difficult to find information about the effects of CM on the results obtained using these methods. Based on available data, both the ponceau-S method (Dilena et al., 1983; McElderry et al., 1982) and the biuret DTC method (Doetsch and Gadsden, 1973) would be affected. The ponceau-S method requires the use of trichloroacetic acid as part of the working reagent. Since CM has induced false-positive reactions when using acid determinations for protein (Bradley and Benson, 1974), caution should be employed until specific laboratory evidence stating otherwise is available. In a specific report describing the biuret DTC method, gross interference by CM was described (Doetsch and Gadsden, 1973).

URINE SEDIMENT

The cytologic evaluation of urine sediment is one method of screening for urinary tract neoplasia. It has been reported that CM will induce urothelial changes such as decreased cell size, nuclear shrinkage, cytoplasmic vacuolation, and fragmentation that are directly proportional to the concentration of these agents in the urine (McClennan et al., 1978). These authors suggested that this may result in incorrect diagnoses of neoplasia when such changes are interpreted without consideration for the potential influence of CM. This effect appeared to be more prominent in retrograde procedures than in excretory urography or angiography. This is most likely due to the local effect of the concentrated CM (administered by retrograde route) directly in contact with the urothelial cells.

Unusual crystals have been observed on microscopic examination of urine sediment in the presence of CM. These have been described as resembling wheat sheaves and have been reported to occur as a result of the precipitation reaction induced when Ehrlich's reagent is added to urine containing CM (Caraway and Kammeyer, 1972; Hurt, 1960; Koneman and Schlesser, 1965). These crystals resemble sulfonamide crystals but are negative when tested with lignin (Koneman and Schlesser, 1965).

There are numerous reports describing the effects of CM on several species of bacteria in both humans and domestic animals (Johansen and Klausen, 1977; Kim and Lachman, 1982; Kuhns et al., 1972; Melson et al., 1974; Narins and Chase, 1971; Ruby et al., 1983). However, there appears to be some disagreement among reports as to the specific effects of CM on determinations for these bacteia. Much of the variation can be related to the methods used for the assessment and interpretation of these effects. Considering the potential variability in methods used by laboratories as well as the apparent variation in sensitivity of the different urinary tract pathogens exposed to urinary contrast agents (despite the fact that they may be cultured in agar that is not contamined with CM), we agree with Ruby and colleagues (1983) that both quantitative and qualitative urine cultures should be obtained before any CM is administered.

RECOMMENDATIONS

Since no species-specific data are available for prediction of the time following either retrograde or systemic administration of CM when the concentration of these agents will no longer affect specific tests, we advocate a conservative approach. Based on available reports in humans, urine specific gravity returns to normal preinjection levels at about 6 to 8 hours after systemic CM administration (Free and Free, 1975), and nearly 100 per cent of the CM is excreted after 24 hours (Cattell et al., 1967). Unless significant urine retention is a factor, as in

Table 1. *Radiographic Contrast Media Effects on Semiquantitated Tests in Routine Urinalysis*

Test	Method	Reported Effect on Determination	References
Protein (primarily albumin)	Tetrabromphenol blue*	No effect	Abuelo, 1983; Caraway and Kammeyer, 1982; Free and Free, 1975; Hurt, 1960; Kark, 1971; McNeeley, 1980;
		False-positive	Sunderman, 1970
	Tetrabromphenophthalein†	No effect	Abuelo, 1983; McNeeley, 1980
	Heat acidification test	False-positive	Abuelo, 1983; Bradley and Benson, 1984; Caraway and Kammeyer, 1972; Kark, 1971; Koneman and Schessler, 1965; McNeeley, 1980
		No effect	Hurt, 1960
	Sulfosalicyclic acid test	False-positive	Abuelo, 1983; Bradley and Benson, 1984; Caraway and Kammeyer, 1982; Hurt, 1960; Kark, 1971; Koneman and Schessler, 1965; Lee and Schoen, 1966; McNeeley, 1980; Sunderman, 1970
	Nitric acid ring test	False-positive	Hurt, 1960; Kark, 1971; Lee and Schoen, 1966
	Bromphenol blue‡	No effect	Bradley and Benson, 1984; Caraway and Kammeyer, 1972; Lee and Schoen, 1966
Glucose	Glucose oxidase rxn†§	No effect	Caraway and Kammeyer, 1972; Free and Free, 1975; Sunderman, 1970
	Copper-reduction‖ (incl. Benedict's reagent)	False-positive (often black or greenish black)	Caraway and Kammeyer, 1972; Free and Free, 1975; Lee and Schoen, 1966; Sunderman, 1970
		No effect	Hurt, 1960
Urobilinogen	Ehrlich's adehyde reagent	White to yellow cloudy ppt. that gives a negative lignin test for sulfonamides	Caraway and Kammeyer, 1972; Hurt, 1960; Koneman and Schessler, 1965

*Albustix, Uristix, Labstix, Bili-Labstix, Multistix, Ames
†Chemstrip G-P, BioDynamics
‡Albutest, Ames
§Tes-Tape, Lilly
‖Clinitest, Ames

outflow obstruction, a 24-hour interval is proposed as a reasonable delay between CM administration and further laboratory evaluation of the urine of companion animals. If possible, we recommend that all tests on the urine be completed prior to administration of CM. This includes quantitative assessments of renal function, since these may be transiently impaired by systemically administered CM.

References and Supplemental Reading

Abuelo, J. G.: Proteinuria: Diagnostic principles and procedures. Ann. Intern. Med. 98:186, 1983.

Benness, G. T.: Urographic excretion study. Australas. Radiol. 12:245, 1968.

Bradley, J. M., and Benson, E. J.: The examination of urine. *In* Davidsohn, I., and Henry, J. B. (eds.): *Clinical Diagnosis by Laboratory and Methods*, 15th ed. Philadelphia: W. B. Saunders, 1974, pp. 15–83.

Caraway, W. T., and Kammeyer, C. W.: Clinical interference by drugs and other substances with clinical laboratory test procedures. Clin. Chim. Acta 41:395, 1972.

Cattell, W. R., Fry, I. K., Spencer, A. G., et al.: Excretion urography, factors determining the excretion of Hypaque. Br. J. Radiol. 40:561, 1967.

Dilena, B. A., Penberthy, L. A., and Fraser, C. G.: Six methods for determining urinary protein compared. Clin. Chim. 29:553, 1983.

Doetsch, K., and Gadsden, R. H.: Determination of total urinary protein, combining Lowry sensitivity and biuret specificity. Clin. Chim. 19:1170, 1973.

Feeney, D. A., Osborne, C. A., and Jessen, C. R.: Effects of radiographic contrast media on the results of urinalysis, with emphasis on alteration and specific gravity. J.A.V.M.A. 176:1378, 1980.

Feeney, D. A., Thrall, D. E., Barber, D. L., et al.: Normal canine excretory urogram: Effects of dose, time, and individual dog variation. Am. J. Vet. Res. 40:1596, 1979.

Free, A. H., and Free, H. M.: *Urinalysis in Clinical Laboratory Practice*. Cleveland: CRC Press, 1975.

Henry, R. J., Cannon, D. C., and Winkelman, J. W. (eds.): *Clinical Chemistry, Principles and Techniques*, 2nd ed. New York: Harper & Row, 1974.

Holtas, S., Billstrom, A., and Tejler, L.: Proteinuria following nephroangiography. IX. Chemical and morphologic analyses in dogs. Acta Radiol. Diag. 22:427, 1981.

Hurt, R.: The effect of radiographic contrast media on urinalysis. Am. J. Med. Technol. 26:122, 1960.

Johansen, J. G., and Klausen, O. G.: Antibacterial effects of metrizoate and metrizimide on bacterial growth in vivo. Acta Radiol. Diag. 18:269, 1977.

Kark, R. M.: Proteinuria II: Diagnosis and management. Hosp. Manage. 6:59, 1971.

Kim, S. K., and Lachman, R.: In vitro effects of iodinated contrast media on the growth of staphylococci. Invest. Radiol. 17:305, 1982.

Koneman, E. W., and Schessler, J.: Unusual urinary crystals. Am. J. Clin. Pathol. 44:358, 1965.

Kuhns, L. R., Baublis, J. W., Gregory, J., and Poznanski, A. K.: In vitro effect of cystographic contrast media on urinary tract pathogens. Invest. Radiol. 7:112, 1972.

Lee, S., and Schoen, I.: Black-copper reduction reaction simulating alkaptonuria—occurrence after intravenous urography. N. Engl. J. Med. 275:266, 1966.

McClennan, B. L., Oertel, Y. C., Malmgren, R. A., et al.: The effect of water soluble contrast material on urine cytology. Acta Cytol. 22:230, 1978.

McElderry, L. A., Tarbit, I. F., and Cassells-Smith, A. J.: Six methods for urinary protein compared. Clin. Chim. 28:356, 1982.

McNeely, M. D. D.: Urinalysis. *In* Sonnewirth, A. C., and Jarett, L.

(eds.): *Gradwohl's Clinical Laboratory Methods and Diagnosis*: Vol. 1. St. Louis: C. V. Mosby, 1980, pp. 478–491.

Melson, G. L., McDaniel, R. C., Southern, P. M., et al.: In vitro effects of iodinated arthrographic contrast media on bacterial growth. Radiology 112:593, 1974.

Narins, D. G., and Chase, R. M.: The effect of Hypaque upon urine culture. J. Urol. 105:433, 1971.

Ruby, A. L., Wing, G. V., and Ackerman, N.: The effect of sodium diatrizoate on in vitro growth of three common canine urinary bacterial species. Vet. Radiol. 24:222, 1983.

Smith, C., Arbogast, C., and Phillips, R.: The effect of x-ray contrast media on results of relative density of the urine. Clin. Chem. 29:730, 1983.

Sunderman, F. W.: Drug interference in clinical biochemistry. *In Critical Reviews in Clinical Laboratory Science*, Cleveland: CRC Press, 1970, pp. 427–449.

DIAGNOSIS AND LOCALIZATION OF URINARY TRACT INFECTION

GEORGE E. LEES, D.V.M.,
and KENITA S. ROGERS, D.V.M.
College Station, Texas

Although a resident population of aerobic bacteria usually colonizes the terminal portion of the urethra, a normal animal's proximal urethra, urinary bladder, ureters, renal pelves, and kidneys do not contain microorganisms. Urinary tract infection (UTI) exists whenever any portion of the urinary tract that is normally sterile is colonized by microbes. By this definition, unequivocal diagnosis of UTI must be based on finding the existence of microbial colonization where it normally is not present. Demonstration of bacteriuria is ordinarily used for this purpose; however, urinary tract tissues rather than urine specimens can also be examined microscopically or microbiologically to diagnose UTI.

Except for bacteriuria, clinical signs and laboratory features of UTI are nonspecific. A variety of noninfectious urinary diseases can produce similar clinical manifestations and laboratory abnormalities. Additionally, infections may exist without producing notable clinical or laboratory changes. Therefore, presence or absence of UTI may be suspected for a number of reasons, but confirmation of the diagnosis usually depends on results of urine culture.

Once existence of a urinary infection has been identified, determination of the anatomic extent of the infection is the next diagnostic step. It is particularly important to identify whether infection extends to the kidneys or is confined to the lower urinary tract (i.e., bladder, urethra, or both). Despite the importance of its prognostic and therapeutic implications, accurate localization of urinary infections is not easily accomplished. Particular tests or procedures that are sufficiently sensitive, specific, safe, and economical to be relied on for localization of urinary infection are not currently available. Judgments about the probable localizations of infections are more reasonably based on clinical correlations and responses to treatments.

With these perspectives, it is apparent that the diagnostic process for UTI has three sequential phases: (1) recognition that infection may be present, (2) confirmation that infection does exist, and (3) localization of infection.

CLINICAL FORMS OF URINARY TRACT INFECTION

When it is initially recognized, an animal's episode of UTI may be categorized as one of four possible clinical forms: (1) asymptomatic bacteriuria, (2) simple urethrocystitis, (3) simple pyelonephritis, and (4) complicated UTI. Before the identifying features of these forms of UTI are described, it is important to point out that the initial categorization of a specific patient may or may not ultimately prove to be correct. It is necessary and sufficient to base this diagnostic judgment on information that is available initially. Subsequent events and findings, including the patient's response to treatment, may indicate that the infection is a different type than was originally suspected. This is not only unavoidable, it is the most cost-effective and reliable way to arrive at an accurate diagnosis of certain types of urinary infections.

Asymptomatic Bacteriuria. Patients with this form of UTI do not exhibit any clinical sign attributable to the infection. Compatible laboratory abnormalities such as pyuria may or may not be present, but results of urine culture clearly indicate that microbes have colonized the urinary tract. In dogs and cats, this form of UTI has been observed sporadically; however, it has not been studied thoroughly, and its importance is uncertain. In contrast, this form of UTI is well characterized in humans, in whom it is found increasingly with advancing age and has specific clinical implications for particular groups of patients.

SIMPLE URETHROCYSTITIS. This form of UTI is characterized by production of clinical signs attributable to inflammation of the bladder or urethra in a patient lacking apparent abnormalities impairing host urinary tract defenses against infection. Affected patients typically exhibit dysuria, increased frequency of urination (pollakiuria), and urgency without fever or constitutional signs. Concomitant abnormalities (e.g., anatomic anomalies, neurologic deficits, calculi, indwelling catheters) that impair host defenses exclude affected patients from this group; such forms of UTI are termed "complicated." Simple urethrocystitis is primarily an episodic disease of females that produces morbidity but little mortality. Patients with urethrocystitis may also have asymptomatic renal infection.

SIMPLE PYELONEPHRITIS. This form of UTI is characterized by production of clinical signs attributable to inflammation of the kidneys in a patient lacking apparent abnormalities that impair host defenses. Clinical signs that are often noted in affected patients include fever, lumbar pain, lethargy, anorexia, nausea, vomiting, and polyuria. Concomitant abnormalities that impair host defenses also exclude affected patients from this group. Pyelonephritis is a serious form of UTI that has greater morbidity and mortality than urethrocystitis and is more difficult to treat successfully. Many patients with pyelonephritis will manifest signs of urethrocystitis simultaneously.

COMPLICATED UTI. This designation is used for episodes of urinary infection that are known or suspected to be associated with abnormalities that impair host defenses against infection. Although there are many specific abnormalities that might "complicate" urinary infection, the two most common categories of complications are (1) causes of urinary retention (i.e., incomplete voiding) and (2) foreign objects (e.g., stones, catheters) in the urinary tract. Lasting improvement in the condition of affected patients generally requires effective treatment of infection and the complicating circumstance.

Outcomes of Urinary Tract Infection

Most episodes of UTI that come to medical attention are treated. Whether or not treatment is instituted, episodes of UTI may have one of only four possible outcomes: (1) cure, (2) persistence, (3) relapse, or (4) reinfection. Of course, therapy is generally intended to produce cure as the outcome, but patterns of recurrent UTI will emerge if any of the other three outcomes are obtained instead. Although clinical manifestations may be similar, each of these three causes of recurrent UTI has distinctive patterns of bacteriuria. These distinctions are important because each pattern has a different diagnostic implication.

CURE. Eradication of all microorganisms from the urinary tract cures an episode of UTI. Although it is also expected that clinical signs subside, verification of cure is provided by urine culture results indicating that the urinary tract remains free of microbial colonization after completion of treatment.

PERSISTENCE. Failure to eradicate infecting organisms from the urine is indicated by sequential urine cultures demonstrating continued presence of the same microbes. To be an effective treatment for UTI, an antimicrobial drug must at least be able to eradicate the organisms from the urine while it is being given. Urine culture results showing persistent infection during antimicrobial therapy usually indicate that the drug regimen chosen for use is inappropriate, but poor owner compliance and inadequate drug excretion are other possible causes. It is important to recognize that signs may subside during drug therapy even though infection persists; mere suppression of bacterial proliferation within the urinary tract can be sufficient to produce a favorable clinical response.

RELAPSE. Urine culture results showing resolution of bacteriuria during antimicrobial therapy verify the selected drug's effectiveness against the infecting organisms. Recrudescence of the same infection after cessation of therapy using an effective drug generally indicates inadequate duration of therapy. Because microbes were eradicated from the urinary space during treatment, relapse indicates that the infection extended to more deep-seated locations such as the kidneys or, in males, the prostate gland. Eradication of infecting organisms from these sites generally requires prolonged treatment.

REINFECTION. Cure of a particular episode of UTI may be followed by development of yet another infection. Although outcome of the initial infection is actually cure, timing of the occurrence of reinfection can produce a clinical pattern of recurrent urinary infection that mimics relapse. Indeed, reinfection may occur during therapy for the initial infection and can mimic persistence. The identifying feature of reinfection, however, is that different microbes are demonstrated by follow-up urine cultures. A pattern of recurrent UTI caused by frequent reinfection implies inadequacy of host urinary tract defenses against infection rather than ineffective treatment of the initial infection.

RECOGNITION THAT URINARY TRACT INFECTION MAY BE PRESENT

The possible existence of UTI is generally recognized because of clinical signs, laboratory abnormalities, or a high index of suspicion prompted by certain clinical findings. Clinical signs and laboratory abnormalities that will be observed vary depending on the location and intensity of tissue reaction induced by the infection and on development of complications.

Alteration in the pattern of behavior associated with micturition is the hallmark of diseases of the urinary bladder and urethra, including those caused by infection. Pollakiuria, urgency and discomfort associated with urination, and continued voiding efforts after the bladder has been emptied are common clinical manifestations of these disorders. Although these findings have localizing value, they are etiologically nonspecific. Indeed, UTI may not be the sole cause of such signs even if it is present. Additionally, UTI that involves renal or prostatic parenchyma may cause fever, lethargy, inappetence, and other systemic signs. However, such signs may also be caused by many other conditions.

Few abnormalities detected by physical examination are particularly suggestive of the existence of UTI. Palpation of inflamed organs such as the kidneys or urinary bladder may produce signs of discomfort. Additionally, palpation of the bladder may stimulate micturition more easily than normal or may reveal thickening of the bladder wall.

Animals that have UTI usually have abnormal urine. Gross abnormalities (e.g., discoloration by blood, lack of normal clarity, malodor) may be apparent, and patients may be brought to medical attention for such reasons. Results of complete urinalysis, however, are more reliably used to detect abnormalities of urine that might be caused by UTI. Hemorrhage or inflammation in the urinary tract causes the urine to be mixed with blood or exudate, producing various amounts of proteinuria, hematuria, and pyuria as revealed by macroscopic and microscopic tests. These abnormalities are etiologically nonspecific and lack intrinsic localizing value.

Clinical signs, physical changes, and laboratory abnormalities that occur in patients with UTI are sometimes produced by conditions that are essentially complications of the infection. Struvite urolithiasis in dogs and acute or chronic renal failure are examples of conditions that may be induced by infection. In affected patients, features of the resulting illness may be more indicative of the complicating condition than of the underlying infection.

Occurrence of UTI in certain types of patients or clinical circumstances is sufficiently frequent to justify having a high index of suspicion of infection regardless of other indicators. Many dogs with chronically excessive corticosteroid hormone activity, whether its origin is endogenous (i.e., hyperadrenocorticism) or exogenous (i.e., corticosteroid drug administration), have UTI. In these patients, asymptomatic infections and lack of notable pyuria occur frequently, possibly because of the anti-inflammatory effects of the concurrent glucocorticoid excess. UTI is also prevalent in animals with diabetes mellitus and in patients with neurogenic disorders of micturition associated with spinal cord disease or injury. Use of urinary catheters, particularly in patients with impaired host urinary tract defenses, is frequently associated with UTI. Indeed, the possible existence of UTI is of concern in virtually all animals with diseases of the urinary system. Even if infection is not the initial cause of disease, impairment of host defenses against infection is produced frequently, and spontaneous or iatrogenic infection may occur secondarily.

Diagnosis of UTI thus begins with consideration of associated history, clinical signs, and laboratory abnormalities; however, conclusive identification of the presence or absence of infection requires use of urine culture results.

CONFIRMATION OF THE EXISTENCE OF URINARY TRACT INFECTION

Accurate diagnosis of UTI based on urine culture results depends on using a suitable specimen, performing the culture with proper techniques, and using appropriate criteria to interpret the results. Confirming or ruling out the diagnosis of a suspected UTI is but one of several purposes that culture of a urine specimen may serve. Results of urine culture may be used to guide selection of an appropriate therapeutic agent. This is sometimes accomplished merely because discovery of the identity of infecting organisms allows selection of predictably effective therapy (see the article entitled Management of Urinary Tract Infections). Alternatively, therapeutic choices may be guided by results of *in vitro* susceptibility testing made possible by cultivation and isolation of the infecting organisms. Efficacy of a therapeutic regimen may also be evaluated by comparing results of urine cultures performed before, during, or after treatment. Finally, urine cultures may be used to characterize the pattern of bacteriuria associated with recurrent UTI and thus differentiate persistence, relapse, and reinfection.

There are three methods for obtaining urine

specimens that are suitable for culture: (1) cystocentesis, (2) catheterization, and (3) voiding. Culture results are only useful if they can be interpreted to reflect presence or absence of bacteriuria *in vivo*; therefore, it is essential to prevent or minimize contamination of the specimen during or after its collection. Urine specimens obtained from normal animals by catheterization or during voiding frequently have been found to contain bacteria, occasionally in large numbers, despite precautions to minimize contamination. Because urine in the bladder of these animals does not contain bacteria, organisms found in specimens obtained by catheterization or voiding presumably come from the terminal portion of the urethra or from surrounding external genitalia or skin. For most patients, properly performed cystocentesis is safe and well tolerated. Specimens obtained for urine culture by cystocentesis entirely avoid the potential sources of contamination that are encountered using other collection methods. Consequently, cystocentesis is the superior way to obtain urine for culture. Results of culture of such specimens can be interpreted without equivocation; the presence of organisms in specimens obtained by cystocentesis indicates bacteriuria *in vivo*. Urine specimens that are properly collected by catheterization are useful for culture, but contamination must be considered a possible explanation for bacteriuria that is found.

A urine specimen that is intended for culture should be placed in a sealed, sterilized container. The culture should be performed while the specimen is as fresh as possible. If more than 30 minutes will elapse before laboratory processing begins, the specimen should be refrigerated. If necessary, the specimen can be stored under refrigeration for 6 to 8 hours without altering the results.

To adequately support diagnostic and therapeutic decision-making in small animal pratice, the urine culture technique that is used should provide (1) a reliable estimate of the abundance of organisms (i.e., bacteria per milliliter of urine) that are present in the specimen, (2) the number and identity of different bacterial isolates that are found in the specimen, and (3) isolated colonies of organisms that can be used for antibacterial susceptibility testing, if needed. Use of quantitative urine culture techniques is especially important when using specimens collected by catheterization because knowledge of the magnitude of bacteriuria is essential to proper interpretation of results that are obtained. Although less critical, quantitation of bacteriuria in specimens obtained by cystocentesis is also highly desirable. Identification of the genus of such isolates is important for at least two reasons. First, great progress toward selection of appropriate therapy can frequently be based on this information alone; the antimicrobial susceptibility of some common urinary pathogens is highly predictable. Second, mixed infections (i.e., simultaneous colonization of the urinary tract by two or more types of microbes) will not be recognized otherwise. These account for a substantial number of UTI (about 20 per cent in dogs). As mentioned, results of susceptibility testing are not always required for selection of effective antimicrobial drug therapy, but such testing is frequently important. The need for antimicrobial susceptibility testing generally arises because the susceptibility of infecting organisms to various drugs is unpredictable or because the infection has failed to respond favorably to the first drug used and another choice must be made.

Several substantial difficulties are encountered if distant laboratories are used for the culture of urine specimens. Attempting delivery of an uncontaminated, refrigerated, and reasonably fresh urine specimen by mail or messenger service can be a formidable (not to mention expensive) task. Possible adulteration of the specimen in transit cannot be completely ruled out when results are interpreted. Additionally, results may not be reported in a timely manner. For these reasons, it is highly desirable to rely on a local laboratory or to perform routine urine culture as an office procedure. Disposable volume-calibrated inoculating loops as well as culture media and a small incubator that are sufficient for routine urine cultures can be acquired without great expense. The seven genera of bacteria that cause most episodes of UTI are not particularly difficult to grow and identify. Results that are available after overnight incubation include all important variables except antimicrobial susceptibility, which may or may not be needed. When necessary, the bacteria that are isolated can be sent to another laboratory to confirm their identity and test their antimicrobial susceptibility. One or two colonies of the isolated organisms can be transferred on a culture swab with comparative ease, even to a quite distant laboratory.

Appropriate criteria must be used to interpret the results of urine cultures. For urine specimens obtained by cystocentesis, interpretation of culture results is not difficult. Bacteriuria in such specimens is unequivocally abnormal. Large numbers of bacteria (greater than 10,000 organisms/ml) are generally found in urine specimens obtained from infected animals before treatment, whereas specimens obtained from uninfected animals yield no bacterial growth. It is unusual to find bacteriuria of an intermediate magnitude, and the most likely explanation for such a result is contamination of the specimen because of technical error. With concomitant or recent antimicrobial therapy, however, a low level of bacteriuria may be an accurate and important indication of the *in vivo* condition (i.e., suppression but not eradication of the infection).

Because false-positive and false-negative results are rarely produced, culture of a urine specimen obtained by cystocentesis is a highly sensitive (virtually all affected patients have a positive test) and specific (virtually all unaffected patients have a negative test) diagnostic procedure for UTI. Using specimens obtained either by catheterization or during voiding, however, unavoidably reduces the sensitivity and specificity of urine culture for diagnosis of infection. This is because similar magnitudes and types of bacteriuria are sometimes found in specimens obtained by these methods from normal and infected animals. Bacteriuria that is associated with infection tends to be of higher magnitude than bacteriuria that is due to contamination in these specimens, but levels of bacteriuria that may be found in normal and infected animals do overlap. Consequently, there is no cutoff value that can be used to define the boundary between positive and negative test results that does not produce false-positives, false-negatives, or both.

Contaminating bacteriuria tends to be of greater frequency and magnitude in voided specimens obtained from normal animals than it is in specimens obtained by catheterization. Therefore, the cutoff value that should be used to define a positive test (i.e., the level of bacteriuria that is indicative of infection) is highest for cultures of voided urine specimens. The cutoff value that has been most widely used for this purpose is 100,000 organisms/ml; bacteriuria equal to or greater than this magnitude in cleanly caught, midstream-voided urine specimens has generally been regarded to be persuasive evidence of infection. In studies of normal animals, this level of bacteriuria has been found in 35 per cent of voided specimens from dogs and 9 per cent of voided specimens from cats. Thus, specificity of the test using this cutoff is 65 per cent for dogs and 91 per cent for cats. For dogs, this poor specificity could be improved by raising the cutoff, but this not only would decrease sensitivity of the test but would be technically difficult. Techniques for quantitative urine culture that are used in most laboratories are not calibrated to accurately measure bacterial concentrations greater than 100,000 organisms/ml. Consequently, it is probably best to continue to use this cutoff (100,000 organisms/ml in voided specimens) for dogs despite its limitations. For cats, however, this excellent specificity is associated with such low sensitivity (57 per cent) that a lower cutoff is needed. Use of 10,000 organisms/ml as the cutoff value for voided specimens obtained from cats is recommended (sensitivity 78 per cent, specificity 86 per cent).

Studies of normal animals have revealed bacteriuria in 26 per cent of specimens obtained by catheterization from dogs and 17 per cent of such specimens from cats. However, the frequency of bacteriuria exceeding 100,000 organisms/ml in specimens obtained from dogs was only 10 per cent, and none of the specimens obtained from cats contained as many as 1000 organisms/ml. Consequently, use of 100,000 organisms/ml as the cutoff value for catheterized specimens obtained from dogs yields excellent specificity (90 per cent). In fact, it may be possible to lower this cutoff to 10,000 organisms/ml for improved sensitivity without an unacceptable loss of specificity, but this alternative has not been studied. For cats, use of 1000 organisms/ml as the cutoff for specimens obtained by catheterization is recommended (sensitivity 82 per cent, specificity 100 per cent).

LOCALIZATION OF URINARY TRACT INFECTION

Information that will contribute to accurate identification of the anatomic extent of a UTI may be obtained in several ways. Results of diagnostic investigations such as history taking, physical examination, complete blood count, urinalysis, and serum biochemistry determinations sometimes include important localizing clues. Fever, leukocytosis, and constitutional signs (e.g., lethargy, depression, poor appetite, weight loss) may suggest renal or prostatic involvement or dissemination of the infection beyond the urinary tract (e.g., septicemia). Suspicion may also arise because the prostate gland or a kidney is palpably abnormal or is an evident source of pain. Polydipsia, polyuria, impaired urinary concentrating ability, or azotemia might also suggest renal infection. In all these instances, however, interpretation of the various findings must be considered carefully; each has numerous possible causes, even in patients with UTI. Observation of leukocyte casts in urine sediment clearly indicates renal involvement, but such casts are so inconsistently observed in animals with kidney infections that their absence means little. Overall, data obtained by routine diagnostic investigations are rarely sufficient to accurately localize UTI.

Special diagnostic procedures intended to identify renal or prostatic involvement in animals with UTI can also be helpful. With regard to the kidneys, contrast radiographic examination such as excretory urography is probably the most widely available and least invasive; however, this method of localizing UTI is not highly sensitive or specific. Dilation of the renal pelvis or ureter and changes in renal size (primarily decreases, but occasionally slight increases with acute infections) are noted in some animals with upper UTI. Studies of other animals with pyelonephritis produce entirely normal findings. Furthermore, active infections are not necessarily present at the sites of anatomic changes even in bacteriuric patients; abnormalities can be consequences of previous or unrelated problems.

Despite its limitations, excretory urography is probably the method of choice for investigation of suspected pyelonephritis in general practice; none of the alternatives is particularly attractive. A renal biopsy specimen may be obtained for microscopic examination and culture, but this method is invasive and is not highly sensitive unless an open biopsy is used so that visibly abnormal portions of the kidney can be selected. Culture of urine obtained directly from a ureter or renal pelvis is informative, but collection of suitable specimens is invasive and technically difficult. Ureteral catheterization requires visualization of the distal ureteral openings either by cystoscopy or cystotomy, and percutaneous nephropyelocentesis requires fluoroscopy. Localizing procedures such as detection of antibody-coated bacteria or the bladder washout technique are used to advantage in humans, but attempts to adapt them for use in animals have been unsuccessful. The fact remains—a satisfactorily sensitive, specific, noninvasive, simple, rapid, and inexpensive method for identifying UTI that involve the kidneys is not available.

Reliable identification of prostatic involvement in males with UTI is nearly as difficult as localizing renal infections. Prostatic secretions can be obtained for culture by ejaculation or prostatic massage techniques, but not without exposure to contamination by bacteria in the urethra or bladder. Therefore, diagnosis of bacterial prostatitis using such specimens requires demonstration that they contain either a number or a type of bacteria that is not attributable to such contamination. Even in males that lack bladder bacteriuria, this has proved to be difficult to do reliably because of resident microflora in the terminal portions of normal urethras. When UTI exists, the interpretive difficulties are compounded. Abundance of bacteria in the urinary tract makes it especially difficult to demonstrate a substantial increment in bacterial numbers when prostatic fluids are added, and the same type of organisms would be expected in both sites if the UTI had extended to involve the prostate. Methods of obtaining specimens from the prostate without contamination from the urethra include aspiration and biopsy. Depending on the position of the prostate, fine-needle aspirates may be obtained by a transabdominal or perineal (pararectal) approach. Biopsy procedures may be open or closed. Candidates for closed aspiration or biopsy procedures must be selected with care because perforation of a prostatic cyst or abscess is contraindicated. Specimens that are obtained by aspiration or biopsy should be cultured and examined microscopically.

The diagnostic utility of observing the course of the patient's disorder and its response to treatment, as displayed over time, should not be overlooked. When evidence to the contrary is lacking, an episode of UTI will be diagnosed and treated as simple urethrocystitis. If the outcome is not cure, appropriate investigation of the pattern of recurrent UTI that emerges will cause the true nature of the problem to be discovered. The first step is to determine that the problem is not merely persistence of the infection because of an inappropriate drug selection or poor compliance with treatment instructions. The next step is reconsideration of whether the patient may have "complicated" UTI. Persistence of clinical signs or abnormal urinalysis results despite eradication of bacteriuria during treatment suggests an underlying abnormality. Finally, recurrence due to relapse must be differentiated from that due to reinfection. If treatment appears to be effective while it is given but relapse occurs promptly when therapy is discontinued, a deep-seated infection that is difficult to eradicate should be suspected. In females with relapse, renal infection is most likely, but in males, prostatic infection should be ruled out before renal infection is pursued. If a pattern of frequent reinfection emerges, inadequacy of normal host defense mechanisms against infection should be suspected.

References and Supplemental Reading

Finco D. R., and Barsanti, J. A.: Localization of urinary tract infection in the dog. Vet. Clin. North Am. [Small Anim. Pract.] 9:775, 1979.

Ling, G. V., Biberstein, E. L., and Hirsh, D. C.: Bacterial pathogens associated with urinary tract infections. Vet. Clin. North Am. [Small Anim. Pract.] 9:617, 1979.

Osborne, C. A., Klausner, J. S., and Lees, G. E.: Urinary tract infections: Normal and abnormal host defense mechanisms. Vet. Clin. North Am. [Small Anim. Pract.] 9:587, 1979.

CYSTOGRAPHY

MARY B. MAHAFFEY, D.V.M.
Athens, Georgia

Cystography is a widely used technique for the study of urinary bladder diseases. Since the lumen and mucosal surface of the bladder have the same radiographic density as urine, contrast media of greater (positive) or lesser (negative) radiographic density than the bladder wall must be inserted into the lumen to provide contrast.

TYPES OF CYSTOGRAMS

There are three basic types of cystograms: positive contrast, double contrast, and negative contrast. The positive contrast cystogram is performed using a water-soluble organically bound iodinated contrast medium diluted with saline. Most of the commercially available contrast media (e.g., Conray, Mallinckrodt; Renografin-76, Squibb) manufactured for intravenous use are acceptable. The double contrast cystogram is performed by using a combination of undiluted positive and negative media. The positive medium forms a puddle in the dependent portion of the bladder while the bladder is further distended with a negative medium such as carbon dioxide, nitrous oxide, or room air. A negative contrast cystogram is performed with negative contrast medium only. A rare potential complication of double and negative contrast cystography is air embolization and death. Carbon dioxide and nitrous oxide are much more soluble in blood than air and are therefore considered safer to use.

The positive contrast cystogram is the procedure of choice for detecting a ruptured bladder and for evaluating bladder location. Positive contrast medium is easily seen within the peritoneal space if a rupture is present, whereas free gas within the peritoneal space is much more difficult to detect. Horizontal beam radiography may have to be performed to definitely rule out the presence of free gas in the peritoneal cavity if a negative contrast cystogram is performed.

Double contrast cystography is the best technique to evaluate the bladder wall and lumen. Calculi and blood clots are seen as filling defects within the positive contrast puddle. Although very small calculi may be overlooked with any cystogram technique, they are less likely to be missed with the double contrast cystogram than with positive or negative contrast cystograms. The medium used in the positive contrast cystogram may obscure small calculi, whereas gas used in a negative contrast cystogram may not provide enough contrast to detect radiolucent calculi. Bladder wall thickness and mucosal margination are better defined with the double contrast cystogram. Positive medium will adhere to mucosal erosions, making them stand out.

The only advantage of the negative contrast cystogram is the ready availability and "low cost" of the contrast medium if room air is the contrast agent used. The use of negative contrast cystograms is not advised, because the other two techniques are diagnostically superior.

TECHNIQUE

PREPARATION. The gastrointestinal tract should be evacuated by overnight fasting and an enema so that the bladder will not be obscured by overlying bowel contents. Radiopaque calculi that could be seen on survey radiographs might be overlooked if superimposed over ingesta in the intestine. Ventrodorsal (VD) and lateral survey radiographs should be made to confirm intestinal evacuation and that radiographic technique is adequate. Also, a diagnosis such as bladder calculi may be made on the survey radiographs, eliminating the need for a cystogram.

The urinary bladder should be aseptically catheterized and emptied. If blood clots are present, the bladder should be flushed with sterile saline. A rubber urethral catheter (Sherwood Medical Industries) may be used in males and females, but a Foley catheter (American Hospital Supply) is preferred in females to prevent reflux of contrast medium around the catheter. Most animals will need to be sedated.

POSITIVE CONTRAST CYSTOGRAMS. If the purpose of cystography is to evaluate the bladder for rupture or for change in location as with a perineal hernia, the contrast medium should be diluted to a 15 to 20 per cent solution with sterile saline. If the bladder is ruptured, contrast medium will be easily seen within the peritoneal space. A small amount of medium (approximately 1.5 ml/kg) should be infused into the bladder initially so that an excessive amount will not leak into the peritoneal space if a large rupture is present. Small tears may be temporarily sealed and may not be detected unless the bladder is fully distended. If a rupture is not seen on the initial radiograph, a second radiograph should be made after the bladder is completely distended (i.e., when the bladder is palpably taut, contrast medium refluxes around the catheter, or increased back-pressure is felt on the syringe plunger).

If a positive contrast cystogram is to be used to evaluate bladder conditions other than rupture or abnormal location, the contrast medium should be diluted to a 5 to 10 per cent concentration so that the chance of mucosal lesions or calculi being obscured will be lessened. Again, the double contrast cystogram is usually better for evaluating such lesions (Fig. 1). Depending on the blackness of the survey radiograph, the film blackness should usually be increased by 50 per cent. This can be done by either increasing the peak kilovoltage by 10 per cent or by increasing the number of milliampere-seconds by 50 per cent.

Double Contrast Cystography. Infuse 0.44 to 0.88 ml/kg of undiluted positive contrast medium into the bladder, then further distend the bladder with carbon dioxide. False-positive findings of bladder disease such as mucosal irregularity and pseudomasses caused by indentation of the bladder by adjacent bowel may occur if the bladder is inadequately distended. It is not necessary to distend the bladder completely to eliminate such false-positive

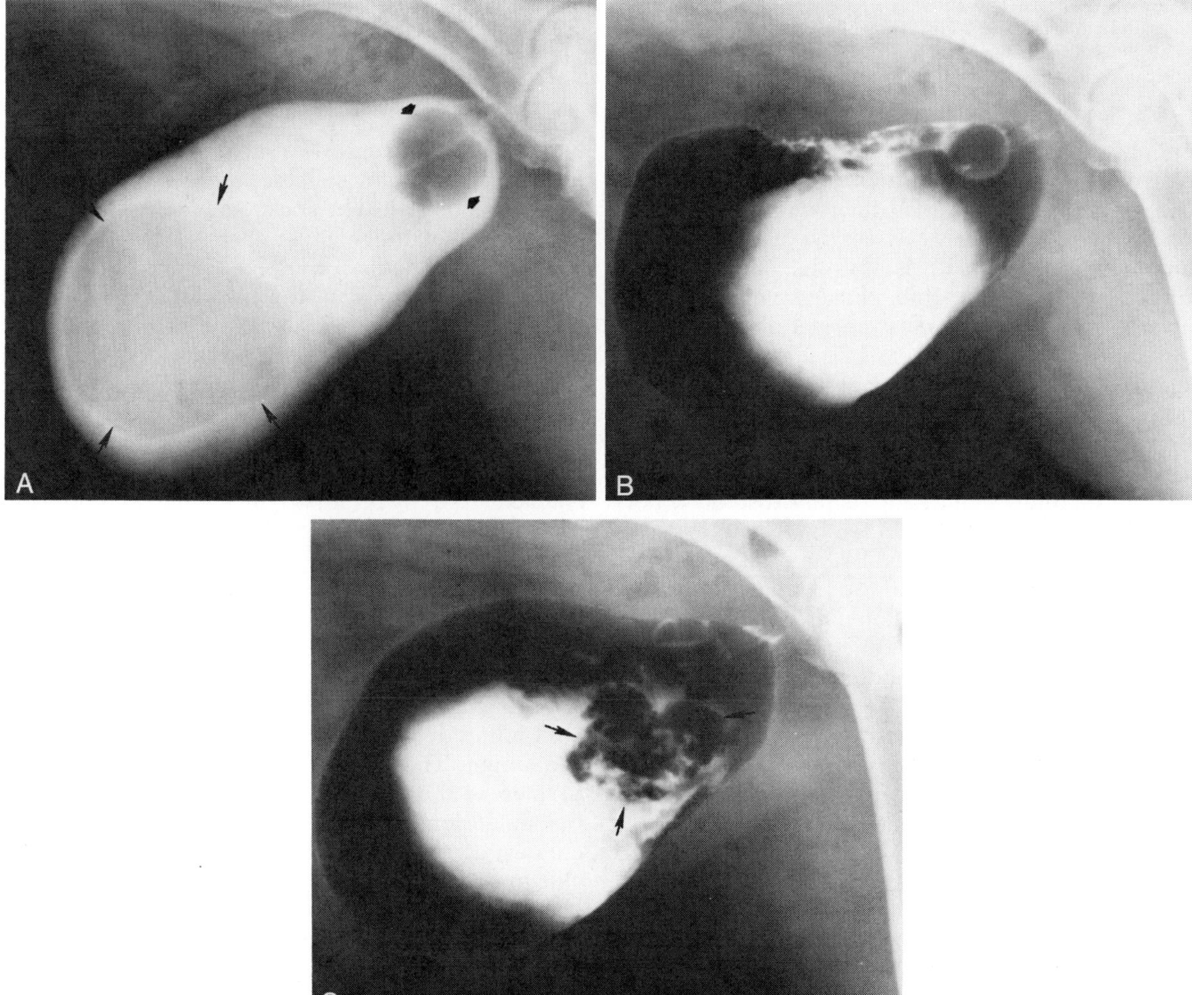

Figure 1. Lateral views of a positive contrast cystogram (*A*) and a double contrast cystogram (*B* and *C*) of a dog with a bladder mass. *A*, Bladder wall appears smooth; the filling defects and mucosal irregularity in *B* and *C* are obscured by the positive contrast medium. A large gas bubble (thin arrows) and the inflated cuff of the Foley catheter (wide arrows) can be seen. *B* and *C*, The radiograph in *B* was made with the dog in right lateral recumbency; in *C* the dog is in left lateral recumbency. The dorsal bladder wall is irregularly marginated, and positive contrast medium adheres to eroded mucosa. A large mass (arrows) is seen in *C* but not in *B*. The radiographs appear different because most of the mass is on the left side, causing a filling defect in the positive contrast puddle when the left side is down. The lesion was not well delineated on the ventrodorsal view. The mass was not examined histologically.

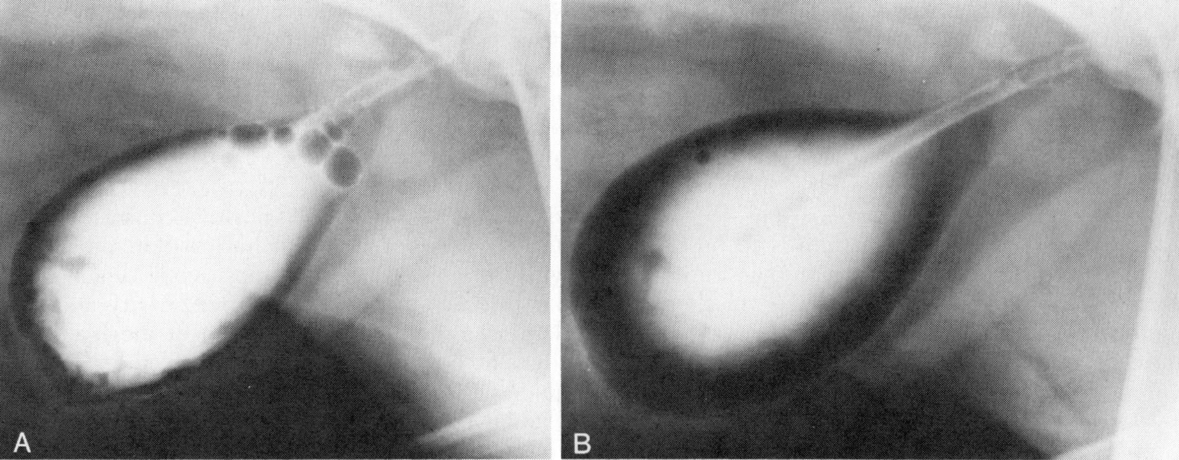

Figure 2. Lateral views of a double contrast cystogram of a dog with cystitis. The bladder wall is thickened, and the mucosa is irregularly marginated cranioventrally. These changes are more obvious when the bladder is mildly distended (*A*) than when it is completely distended (*B*). Positive contrast medium adheres to eroded mucosa in both radiographs. The sharply marginated, round filling defects in the periphery of the positive contrast puddle are air bubbles. There is mild prostatomegaly and urethroprostatic reflux of contrast medium.

findings. Also, mucosal irregularities seen in dogs with mild cystitis may be more obvious when the bladder is mildly distended than when the bladder is fully distended (Fig. 2). Excessive bladder distention may cause hematuria, cystitis, and rupture. Fifty to 100 ml of carbon dioxide will eliminate mucosal irregularity in most normal dogs weighing less than 20 kg. A dose of 5 ml/kg should be adequate for larger dogs. If at that dose bladder indentation mimicking a wall mass is present, the bladder should be further distended. A total dose of 11 ml/kg of carbon dioxide in addition to the positive medium should adequately distend a normal bladder. Since the bladder is usually less distensible in dogs with cystitis, the amount of contrast medium required to distend the bladder adequately may be less. The bladder should always be palpated during infusion of contrast medium, and infusion stopped whenever the bladder is palpably taut or increased back-pressure is felt on the syringe plunger. The above dosages are approximate. The amount of carbon dioxide needed to adequately distend the bladder is variable; there is no dosage that will be adequate for all dogs.

Lateral and VD views should be made. Occasionally, the opposite lateral and VD oblique views are helpful in detecting lesions not seen on the initial radiographs (Fig. 1). Depending on survey film blackness, the peak kilovoltage should be decreased by 8 to 10 per cent.

INTERPRETATION

Normal bladder shape is variable depending on the degree of distension. When nearly empty, it is indented by adjacent intestine and does not assume the characteristic oval shape until intravesical pressure is increased. The location is also variable. In dogs, most of the bladder may be located within the pelvic canal when the bladder is empty, and as much as 35 per cent of the bladder length may be within the pelvic canal when the bladder is full. In cats, the bladder is almost always located within the abdominal cavity even when empty. Bladder wall thickness should be about 1 mm, and mucosal margins should be smooth.

MURAL-MUCOSAL LESIONS. Cystitis is usually characterized by gradual thickening and mucosal irregularity of the cranioventral aspect of the bladder wall. Mucosal irregularity can also be seen at the periphery of the positive contrast puddle. The degree of thickening and mucosal irregularity increases with increasing severity and chronicity of cystitis. Most neoplastic lesions are located in the trigone and are characterized by irregularly marginated filling defects that protrude from the wall into the lumen. The change from normal wall thickness to increased thickness is more abrupt than with benign lesions. Rarely, tumors are located in the cranioventral aspect of the bladder, making it difficult to differentiate them from cystitis. Usually the change in wall thickness is still more abrupt than with non-neoplastic lesions. Biopsy of such lesions will have to be performed for a definitive diagnosis. The mucosa is often eroded in both cystitis and neoplasia. Positive contrast medium will adhere to the eroded areas (Figs. 1 and 2).

INTRALUMINAL FILLING DEFECTS. There are basically three types of intraluminal filling defects: calculi, blood clots, and air bubbles. In the double contrast cystogram, calculi are usually seen as sharply marginated radiolucent filling defects in the center of the positive contrast puddle, which is in the dependent portion of the bladder. Calculi may be rounded or irregularly shaped. Air bubbles will be located in the periphery of the positive contrast puddle and will be seen as sharply marginated, rounded, radiolucent filling defects (Fig. 2). Blood clots may be located anywhere within the bladder and are irregularly shaped with indistinct margins.

References and Supplemental Reading

Mahaffey, M. B., Barber, D. L., Barsanti, J. A., et al.: Simultaneous double-contrast cystography and cystometry in dogs. Vet. Rad. 25:254, 1984.

Mahaffey, M. B., Barsanti, J. A., Barber, D. L., et al.: Pelvic bladder in dogs without urinary incontinence. J.A.V.M.A. 184:1477, 1984.

Park, R.: Radiology of the urinary bladder and urethra. *In* O'Brien, T. R. (ed.): *Radiographic Diagnosis of Abdominal Disorders in the Dog and Cat: Radiographic Interpretation, Clinical Signs, Pathophysiology.* Philadelphia: W. B. Saunders, 1978, pp. 543–614.

RISKS OF URINARY CATHETERIZATION

GEORGE E. LEES, D.V.M.

College Station, Texas

Urethral catheterization is a valuable, sometimes essential, procedure that is used for a variety of diagnostic and therapeutic purposes. However, urinary catheterization can be harmful, and the possible risks of catheterization must be recognized and carefully considered in each case.

Risks associated with use of urinary catheters include direct physical injury and induction of urinary tract infection. The magnitude of these risks and the importance of their consequences are modified by numerous factors. The veterinarian has considerable control over some of these factors, and it is important that every possible precaution be taken to minimize associated risks when catheters are used. However, other factors are intrinsic features of various clinical circumstances and cannot be altered. One must recognize that even the most judicious and careful use of a urinary catheter may produce an adverse effect.

CATHETER-INDUCED PHYSICAL INJURY

Factors that affect the occurrence of urinary tract injury during catheterization are (1) the catheter that is selected for use, (2) the catheterization technique that is employed, and (3) the condition of the urinary tract at the time of catheterization.

Urinary catheters differ with respect to their size, composition, design, and condition. Diameter of a catheter is usually expressed in French units (F), which can be converted to millimeters by dividing by 3. Use of catheters that are too large, either in diameter or length, is a common cause of catheter-induced injury. Urinary catheters are available in a variety of diameters and lengths, and a large assortment of such catheters is required to meet the needs of patients of the diverse sizes that are ordinarily seen in small animal practice.

Urinary catheters have been manufactured from a large number of different materials. Catheters composed of metal or glass are rigid and potentially traumatic. Most urinary catheters are presently made of more flexible materials such as rubber, latex, polypropylene, polyvinyl, or nylon, but catheters composed of some of these materials are considerably less pliable than others. In general, the probability of causing physical injury with a catheter diminishes as its pliability increases.

When a catheter is left indwelling, another aspect of its composition may become important. Many synthetic materials are complex formulations of a variety of materials including dyes, vulcanizers, and stabilizers, as well as the principal material. Some of these compounds might diffuse out of catheters while they are in place and chemically injure surrounding tissues. Unfortunately, little is known about differences between catheter materials with respect to this potential mechanism of injury. In one study, polyvinyl indwelling urinary catheters produced less evidence of urethral injury in cats than did polypropylene indwelling catheters, but the reason for the difference was not determined. The lesser tissue reaction was presumed to be associated with the greater pliability of the polyvinyl catheters, but chemically mediated tissue injury could have contributed to the differences that were observed.

Differences in the design of catheters, particularly their internal or proximal tips, may also affect their potential to cause harm. Many catheters have blunt, rounded, or tapered tips with one or more side holes located near their internal ends. However, others have open ends that could more easily gouge or scrape the inner surface of the urethra if they were not used with sufficient care. Some urinary catheters have inflatable balloons near their internal tips; after the catheter is inserted, inflation of the balloon helps hold the catheter in proper position if it is to be left indwelling. Sometimes, however, the balloon is intentionally positioned in the urethra and inflated to temporarily obstruct the urethral lumen. Because prolonged distention of balloon-tipped catheters in the urethra of dogs and cats produces urethral lesions, improper use of balloon-tipped catheters may cause injury. Excessive traction on an indwelling catheter with an inflated balloon may cause the balloon to become wedged in the urethra, or a balloon that is intentionally inflated within the urethra may be left in place too long.

Regardless of its other attributes, a urinary catheter that is not in good physical condition may be harmful. Discard damaged or defective catheters that have burrs, sharp edges, or rough surfaces that might cause abrasion or laceration of the urinary tract.

Occurrence of urinary tract trauma is greatly affected by catheterization technique. Use of adequate physical or chemical restraint during catheter insertion is essential, or damage may be caused by sudden or forceful movement of the animal against the catheter. Furthermore, having to struggle with an uncooperative or uncomfortable patient prohibits use of the proper gentle touch during catheter insertion, and gentleness is probably the most important single technical consideration. Liberal use of catheter lubricants is necessary to minimize patient discomfort and abrasion of urothelial surfaces. In males, proper positioning of the penis to straighten the course of the urethra is important. Insertion of an excessive length of catheter must always be avoided. Once the catheter is inserted, traumatic injury to the urinary tract may continue, and minimizing the duration of catheterization is the only way to reduce this risk.

The condition of the urinary tract during catheterization also affects whether or not injury occurs. Submucosal inflammation and edema produce swelling that encroaches on the amount of space for the catheter to occupy within the lumen of the bladder or urethra. Inflamed and edematous tissues are also more susceptible to physical injury than are normal tissues. Punctures or lacerations may be more easily produced if the strength and resilience of urinary tract tissues have been impaired by necrosis or excessive distension. Obstructions in the urinary space (e.g., calculi) may deflect the catheter tip so that it strikes adjacent tissues at an unintended angle when the catheter is advanced.

CATHETER-INDUCED INFECTION

Factors that affect the occurrence of urinary tract infection during catheterization are (1) microbial contamination of the urinary tract, (2) the effectiveness of normal urinary tract defenses, and (3) concomitant antimicrobial therapy.

At the time of catheter insertion, microbes may be propelled into previously sterile portions of the urinary tract. Such contamination is minimized by using appropriate materials and techniques. Catheters, lubricants, and irrigating solutions should be sterilized and protected from contamination prior to their use. Preparation for catheter insertion should include removal of hair from the field and cleansing of the penis and prepuce or vulva. Sterilized forceps or gloves should be used to grasp and manipulate the catheters. Regardless of the precautions that are taken, however, contamination at the time of catheter insertion is not often eliminated entirely. The catheter is passed through the distal urethra, where bacteria ordinarily reside even in healthy animals. Consequently, truly aseptic catheterization of the urinary tract is probably not possible. There is a risk of inducing infection with even a single brief catheterization of a healthy patient. Studies of repeated catheterization have generally found that the cumulative risk of infection is proportional to the number of catheterizations.

During indwelling catheterization, microbial contamination of the urinary tract may occur through the catheter lumen or through the space between the urethral mucosa and the outside of the catheter. Connection of the catheter to a sterilized, closed urine collection system minimizes ascent of microbes through the catheter. External surfaces of indwelling catheters and adjacent tissues should be kept clean, but little can be done to prevent migration of bacteria through the urethra outside the catheter. Development of infection during indwelling catheterization is just a matter of time; if the catheter remains in place long enough, infection will occur.

By itself, microbial contamination of the urinary tract does not cause infection. Impairment of normal host defense mechanisms against microbial colonization of the urinary tract must be combined with contamination to produce infection. However, such impairment frequently exists because of antecedent disease or because of effects of the catheter in patients that are catheterized. Patients that have urinary tract disease already are the most susceptible to development of catheter-induced infection, but these are also the patients that most often require frequent or indwelling catheterization. Additionally, the catheter itself bypasses urethral defenses and may impair mucosal defenses by causing physical or chemical injury.

Antimicrobial drugs have frequently been used in conjunction with urinary catheterization with the intention of preventing catheter-induced infection. With brief catheterization, either on a single occasion or when repeated intermittently, instilling an antibiotic or antiseptic solution into the urinary bladder before removing the catheter may be effective. Alternatively, an antimicrobial drug may be given systemically so that it will be present in the urine that fills the bladder after catheterization. With indwelling catheterization, however, the benefits of prophylactic antimicrobial therapy are limited whether it is administered locally or systemically. At best, such therapy delays the onset of infection, and then only for a few days. This prevents infection only if the catheter is removed during the delay. If the catheter is not removed, infection will ultimately develop despite antimicrobial therapy. Furthermore, the infecting organisms will predictably be resistant to the drug in use, and their susceptibility to other antimicrobial drugs may be limited as well.

GUIDELINES FOR USE OF URINARY CATHETERS

An appropriate catheter should be selected for use. With respect to catheter diameter, it is generally better to choose the smallest catheter that will work rather than the largest catheter that will fit. Similarly, the softest and most pliable catheter that can be used successfully is preferred. Such catheters sometimes are more difficult to insert than are stiffer ones, but increased safety for the patient justifies the additional effort that is required.

Optimal catheterization technique should always be used. The catheter, lubricant, and any other materials that may be required should be sterilized. Principles of aseptic technique should be followed, at least so far as avoidable sources of contamination are concerned. Insertion of an excessive length of catheter should be avoided, and a gentle touch must always be used.

When intermittent or indwelling catheterization is needed and either can be used, intermittent catheterization is preferred. If indwelling catheterization is employed, the catheter should be connected to a sterilized, closed urine drainage system whenever such a system can be maintained. Duration of catheterization must be minimized; the catheter should be removed as soon as possible.

Antimicrobial agents should be used judiciously in conjunction with catheterization. Risks of drug side effects and development of infection by organisms resistant to the drug being used must be weighed against the probability of actually preventing infection. In healthy male dogs, for example, risk of infection after a single brief catheterization is minimal and prophylactic antimicrobial therapy is probably not necessary. In other patients, the risk of inducing infection may justify antimicrobial prophylaxis. If an antimicrobial agent is infused before the catheter is removed, several precautions should be taken. The retrograde flow through the catheter should not be allowed to propel organisms into the bladder from contaminated distal sites. Solutions selected for this purpose should not be irritating, and their sterility should be assured. Bacterial colonization of stock supplies of antimicrobial solutions stored in multiple-dose containers has been known to occur and cause infections rather than prevent them. An additional limitation of infusing an antimicrobial solution is that it will be diluted by urine that is formed subsequently. Most of the shortcomings of infusing solutions into the bladder are avoided by using a single dose or short course of a systemic antimicrobial drug such as ampicillin that will reach high levels in the urine following its administration.

With indwelling catheterization, it may sometimes be better to withhold antimicrobial therapy, accept development of infection if it occurs, and treat with an appropriate regimen when the need for catheterization has passed. If systemic antimicrobial therapy is administered during catheterization, the fact that infection may not be prevented must be recognized. Continuing administration of the same drug after the catheter is removed without performing appropriate tests to detect whether infection exists is irrational. An infection, if present, will be caused by organisms that are resistant to that drug.

Finally, adverse effects of catheter use must be recognized and treated appropriately when they occur. Culture of urine specimens should be performed routinely to detect catheter-induced infections, guide their treatment, and verify their eradication.

References and Supplemental Reading

Lees, G. E., and Osborne, C. A.: Urinary tract infections associated with the use and misuse of urinary catheters. Vet. Clin. North Am. [Small Anim. Pract.] 9:713, 1979.

Lees, G. E., and Osborne, C. A.: Use and misuse of indwelling urinary catheters in cats. Vet. Clin. North Am. [Small Anim. Pract.] 14:599, 1984.

Disorders of the Urinary Tract

RENAL HEMATURIA IN DOGS

ELIZABETH A. STONE, D.V.M.
Raleigh, North Carolina

Hematuria can have renal and extrarenal origins. Extrarenal sources include urinary bladder or urethral tumors, urolithiasis, urinary tract infections, and coagulopathies. Causes of renal hematuria include renal trauma, renal neoplasia, nephroliths, glomerulonephritis, polycystic kidneys, renal vascular abnormalities, and idiopathic conditions.

DIAGNOSIS

The initial data base for the problem of hematuria should include a complete history and physical examination, urinalysis, complete blood count, and serum creatinine or urea nitrogen determinations. Further diagnostic tests may include contrast radiography, coagulation tests, and exploratory laparotomy. Extrarenal causes of hematuria should be ruled out first. An absence of dysuria suggests a renal or ureteral lesion. Urinary bladder and urethral neoplasms and calculi may be seen with contrast radiography. However, large blood clots in the urinary bladder may not be distinguishable from other space-occupying masses with contrast radiography. Bleeding times, platelet counts, and activated coagulation times in conjunction with history and physical examination findings give an index of the coagulation status. Clotting profiles identify more subtle coagulopathies.

Traumatic renal hematuria can be caused by a laceration of the renal parenchyma, renal pedicle injury, or rupture of the kidney. The amount of hematuria (gross or microscopic) does not correlate with the degree of renal damage. Trauma-induced renal hematuria is suggested by the case history, physical examination findings of sublumbar pain or swelling, and occasionally from an excretory urogram or arteriogram. Uremia is unlikely unless both kidneys are damaged. Renal bleeding is more frequently discovered during an exploratory laparotomy to determine the source of abdominal bleeding after trauma.

Renal tumors that can cause hematuria include renal cell carcinoma, transitional cell carcinoma, hemangioma, and hemangiosarcoma. Occasionally, tumor cells may be seen during microscopic examination of the urine sediment. Survey radiographs may show a cranial abdominal mass. An excretory urogram may reveal a filling defect within the renal pelvis. Definitive diagnosis is based on cytologic or histologic examination of tumor tissue. Tissue can be obtained percutaneously by a fine-needle aspirate or needle biopsy or during an exploratory laparotomy by wedge biopsy.

Renal calculi may be asymptomatic, but they occasionally induce bleeding. Diagnosis is based on survey radiographs and an excretory urogram. Quantitative analysis of the mineral content of the calculus after surgical removal is essential for postoperative preventive management.

Polycystic kidney disease, a rare disease in dogs, may cause hematuria by erosion of vessels. On excretory urography, the cyst area is radiopaque and is surrounded by areas of radiodense functioning parenchyma. If polycystic kidney disease is suspected, a percutaneous biopsy should not be performed since intra-abdominal hemorrhage and leakage of cyst fluid may occur.

Hematuria associated with glomerulonephropathy is usually accompanied by moderate to severe proteinuria. Hematuria may occur during the early stages of glomerulonephritis, but it is not a frequent finding in dogs and cats. The presence of large numbers of casts, or even a single red cell cast, indicates that the hematuria originated from the kidney rather than from the lower urinary tract and that there is probably glomerular disease. A percutaneous or operative renal biopsy for light, electron, and immunofluorescent microscopy is necessary to determine the specific type of glomerular disease.

Renal vascular abnormalities, such as arteriovenous fistulas, ruptured aneurysms, or communications between the calyces and the venous sinuses, have been found to cause massive hematuria in humans but have not been documented in dogs or cats. The definitive diagnosis would require renal angiography or radionuclide studies of the vascular architecture of the kidneys.

Chronic hematuria associated with renal pelvic blood clots was reported in two dogs (DiBartola et al., 1983). One dog had had a previous nephrotomy, and there was granulation tissue and focal necrosis in the affected kidney. The specific cause of the hematuria was not determined for either dog.

Renal parasities, *Dioctophyma renale* and *Capillaria plica*, may cause renal hematuria. The diagnosis is made by detecting parasitic ova in the urine or by identifying the adult stages during abdominal exploratory surgery.

Massive hematuria of nontraumatic renal origin without an obvious source or mechanism of hemorrhage has been encountered in dogs. In humans, the syndrome has been labeled benign essential hematuria, benign recurrent hematuria, and idiopathic renal hematuria. The criteria for classification into this syndrome include a negative history of bleeding diathesis, renal surgery, radiation therapy, or trauma; a normal urinalysis except for red blood cells; normal renal function; and a normal excretory urogram. The cases reported in dogs fulfilled the criteria except for hydronephrosis and hydroureter seen on the excretory urogram (Stone et al., 1983).

The decision for an exploratory laparotomy to determine the specific cause of renal hematuria is based on several factors. Severe hemorrhagic anemia that cannot be corrected with blood transfusions, inability to locate the source of hemorrhage, or the need to rule out neoplasms may prompt surgical exploration. The finding of hydroureter and hydronephrosis secondary to a blood clot is an indication for surgery. Hydronephrosis secondary to complete obstruction of the ureter is reversible if the obstruction is removed within 6 to 7 days. A large blood clot within the urinary bladder that obstructs the urethra may need surgical removal.

TREATMENT

Intraoperative management of renal hematuria includes gross inspection of the kidneys and the urinary bladder. If only one kidney is grossly abnormal, a biopsy, nephrotomy, or nephrectomy can be performed. Any nephroliths can be removed through a nephrotomy incision. If persistent bleeding can be identified and controlled, the renal incision can be closed. Otherwise, a nephroureterectomy should be performed. If both kidneys are abnormal, biopsies are taken.

Nephroureterectomy is the treatment of choice for unilateral renal tumors with no evidence of metastasis or vascular invasion. The entire ureter should be removed. The efficacy of chemotherapy, radiation therapy, or immunotherapy for the treatment of renal tumors in dogs and cats has not been established.

If the kidneys appear normal, a ventral cystotomy incision is made so the ureteral openings can be inspected and the ureters atraumatically catheterized. Urine is collected separately from each ureter and examined microscopically, if necessary, to determine which kidney is the source of the hemorrhage. Catheters are passed from the urinary bladder into each renal pelvis to check for obstruction.

A nephrotomy is performed to locate correctable causes of hemorrhage. Any hemorrhaging vessels are ligated. Usually, however, the source of the hemorrhage is not apparent. Excision of the affected kidney will prevent recurrence of the hematuria.

References and Supplemental Reading

Crow, S. E.: Hematuria: An algorithm for differential diagnosis. Comp. Cont. Ed. Pract. Vet. 2:941, 1980.

DiBartola, S. P., Myer, C. W., Boudrieau, R. J., et al.: Chronic hematuria associated with renal pelvic blood clots in two dogs. J.A.V.M.A. 183:1102, 1983.

Lage, A. L.: Hematuria, a clinical approach: Its meaning and differential diagnosis in the dog and cat. Bi-Weekly Small Anim. Vet. Med. Update 15:1, 1978.

Stone, E. A., DeNovo, R. C., and Rawlings, C. A.: Massive hematuria of nontraumatic renal origin in dogs. J.A.V.M.A. 183:868, 1983.

GLOMERULAR DISEASE IN THE DOG AND CAT

STEPHEN P. DiBARTOLA, D.V.M.,
and DENNIS J. CHEW, D.V.M.
Columbus, Ohio

The term glomerulopathy refers to a pathologic process that has its primary effect on glomeruli, although other parts of the nephron may be affected secondarily as the disease progresses. In dogs and cats, chronic renal failure secondary to glomerular disease, nephrotic syndrome, and asymptomatic proteinuria have been recognized. The nephrotic syndrome is defined as the presence of moderate to marked proteinuria, hypoalbuminemia, hypercholesterolemia, and ascites or edema. The two major glomerular diseases of dogs and cats are glomerulonephritis and amyloidosis. Amyloidosis is a progressive disease that leads to chronic renal failure in both species. On the other hand, the natural history of glomerulonephritis in dogs and cats is less clear.

PATHOPHYSIOLOGY

The glomeruli function as filters across which an ultrafiltrate of plasma is created by the force of cardiac contraction. The glomerular filter is composed of three major components: the fenestrated endothelial cells of the glomerular capillary, the glomerular basement membrane, and the visceral epithelial cells, or podocytes. The interdigitating foot processes of the podocytes and the slit diaphragms between them are negatively charged owing to the presence of acidic glycoproteins known collectively as glomerular polyanion. The basement membrane and endothelium also contain negatively charged glycoproteins. The basement membrane does not completely surround the capillary loops of the glomerulus, thus creating the mesangial space, which represents the core or stalk of the glomerular tuft. Mesangial cells are of reticuloendothelial origin and contact the endothelium in areas where it is not invested by basement membrane. They provide support for the glomerular tuft and, by virtue of their phagocytic properties, may remove filtration residues that become trapped between endothelial cells and the basement membrane.

The normal glomerulus is both a size-selective and charge-selective filter. Its size-selective properties are thought to reside primarily in the basement membrane and are such that circulating macromolecules greater than 34 nm in diameter are excluded from filtration. Serum albumin with a molecular weight of 69,000 has an effective molecular diameter of 36 nm and is thus normally excluded from filtration. The presence of glomerular polyanion restricts filtration of circulating negatively charged macromolecules.

Glomerulonephritis

Immune-mediated damage is thought to be largely responsible for glomerular injury in glomerulonephritis. Two basic types of immunologic damage to glomeruli have been identified. In one form of injury, soluble circulating immune complexes formed in moderate antigen excess become trapped in the glomerular filter. Glomerular damage results from the activation of the complement system, with the production of anaphylatoxic and chemotactic complement fragments (e.g., C3a, C5a, $\overline{C567}$) and subsequent influx of neutrophils that release lysosomal enzymes and oxygen-derived free radicals, thus damaging the glomerulus. Platelets may adhere to the damaged endothelium and the coagulation system may be activated, resulting in the deposition of fibrin in glomeruli.

The offending antigens are not of glomerular origin, but their source is rarely determined. They may be endogenous (e.g., tumor antigens, nuclear antigens) or exogenous (e.g., infectious agents, drugs) in origin. Disease processes that may be associated with a continuous high level of antigenic exposure include chronic infections, neoplasia, and immune-mediated diseases.

Immunofluorescence studies demonstrate discontinuous granular deposition of immunoglobulins and complement in glomeruli, resulting in the so-called lumpy-bumpy pattern of fluorescence. Electron microscopic studies show electron-dense deposits in subepithelial, subendothelial, and mesangial sites.

In the second type of immune-mediated injury, antibodies react *in situ* with antigens in the glomerulus. These antigens may be intrinsic glomerular antigens (as in antiglomerular basement membrane disease) or may be nonglomerular antigens that have become "planted" in the glomerulus.

In antiglomerular basement membrane disease, antibody attaches to intrinsic antigens along the glomerular basement membrane, and immunofluorescence studies demonstrate a continuous linear pattern of fluorescence. Despite the fact that linear fluorescence suggestive of antiglomerular basement membrane disease has been observed occasionally in dogs, attempts to elute the antibody from the tissue and demonstrate its reactivity with normal renal tissue have not been successful. Glomerular injury due to "planted" antigens results in the same discontinuous granular pattern of fluorescence described above for circulating immune complexes.

Nonimmunologic mechanisms may affect the progression of glomerular disease. For example, glomerular hyperfiltration in remnant nephrons leads to glomerular sclerosis and is believed to be one mechanism explaining the inexorably progressive nature of renal disease after a critical number of nephrons have been destroyed. Hypertension may lead to fibrinoid degeneration and hyalinization of glomerular vessels and thus may also aggravate glomerular damage.

Amyloidosis

Amyloidosis is not a single disease but a group of diseases that have in common the extracellular deposition of fibrillar proteins with a specific biochemical conformation known as the beta-pleated sheet. Amyloid deposits are characteristically green when stained with alkaline Congo red and viewed under polarized light. This property is used in the clinical diagnosis of amyloidosis. Thioflavine-T stains amyloid deposits so that they are yellow-green when studied by fluorescence microscopy, but this stain is not specific for amyloid. Recently, the various amyloid syndromes in humans have been classified as reactive systemic, immunoglobulin-associated, heredofamilial, and localized. Several different precursor proteins have been identified that may ultimately be deposited as amyloid.

Reactive systemic amyloidosis may be associated with chronic infectious, inflammatory, or neoplastic diseases. The amyloidogenic precursor is a serum protein that is elevated in many inflammatory and neoplastic diseases by virtue of its behavior as an acute-phase reactant. The source of this precursor, known as serum amyloid A protein (SAA), is the hepatocyte. In this type of amyloidosis, tissue deposits are composed of amino-terminal fragments of SAA and are called amyloid AA. Many experimental models of amyloidosis (including cyclic neutropenia in gray collies) and spontaneous amyloidosis in dogs and cats are examples of reactive systemic amyloidosis. Although amyloid deposits may occur in several organs, deposits in the kidneys lead to progressive renal disease and death due to uremia in dogs and cats with amyloidosis. In some cases, the underlying inflammatory or neoplastic disease is detected, but in approximately 70 per cent of dogs with amyloidosis, no predisposing disease can be found. Amyloidosis is uncommon in cats, and an underlying predisposing disease is rarely found. In the Abyssinian cat, however, systemic amyloidosis characterized by the presence of amyloid protein AA is a familial disease.

In immunoglobulin-associated amyloidosis (e.g., that associated with multiple myeloma), the amyloid deposits contain amino-terminal fragments from the variable region of immunoglobulin light chains. These light chains originate from plasma cells, and such deposits are designated amyloid AL. Approximately 10 per cent of humans with multiple myeloma develop amyloidosis, but amyloidosis in dogs and cats with multiple myeloma appears to be rare. There is no documentation that such deposits, if they occur, are of light-chain origin.

Amyloidosis develops only in a few human patients with multiple myeloma or chronic inflammatory disease, and hence chronic elevation of the serum precursor proteins is not solely responsible for the disease. Other host-related factors such as genetically determined or acquired defects in proteolysis of the amyloidogenic precursor proteins are likely to be important in the pathogenesis of amyloidosis.

Heredofamilial neuropathic syndromes of amyloidosis in humans have not been recognized in domestic animals. Localized amyloidosis does occur in the pancreatic islets of older domestic cats.

DIAGNOSIS

History

Dogs and cats with either glomerulonephritis or amyloidosis may be presented to the veterinarian for evaluation of signs related to some underlying inflammatory or neoplastic disorder, but this is relatively uncommon. More often, there is no clear history of a predisposing disease process and the major historic findings are those of chronic renal failure (vomiting, lethargy, anorexia, weight loss, polydipsia, and polyuria). When the nephrotic syndrome is present, the animal is usually presented for evaluation of a distended abdomen (ascites) or swollen extremities (subcutaneous edema). Occasionally, asymptomatic proteinuria is detected in the clinical evaluation of another medical problem. Rarely, dogs are presented for signs related to acute thromboembolism, which may complicate glomerular disease.

Physical Findings

Physical findings in dogs and cats with glomerular disease are also variable and are usually related to the presence of renal failure (emaciation, poor coat, oral ulceration, dehydration, irregular kidneys). Ascites or subcutaneous edema may be found if the nephrotic syndrome is present. Occasionally, there may be signs of an underlying inflammatory disease process (e.g., osteomyelitis, bronchopneumonia) or neoplasia. In one study of dogs with glomerular disease, neoplasia was the most common extrarenal finding. Signs of thromboembolism, if present, will depend on the site of involvement. Pulmonary thromboembolism with associated dyspnea is found most frequently, but thrombosis may occur in other vessels as well. Sudden loss of rear limb function may occur with femoral artery thrombosis.

Laboratory Findings

Urinalysis findings in dogs and cats with glomerular disease include proteinuria, isosthenuria, and hyaline cylindruria. Proteinuria in the absence of remarkable sediment findings is the hallmark of glomerular disease (see the article entitled Assessment of Proteinuria in the Dog and Cat). Marked proteinuria is common in dogs with amyloidosis because of the predominant glomerular location of the deposits, but, in cats, glomerular deposition of amyloid is very variable and proteinuria may not be a prominent feature of the disease. Marked medullary deposition of amyloid in cats, however, commonly leads to early interference with urinary concentrating ability. Isosthenuria will also be observed if the glomerular disease has progressed to the extent that there is severe interstitial fibrosis and mononuclear nephritis with loss of more than two thirds of the functional nephrons.

Care must be taken by the clinician to localize the proteinuria (see the article entitled Assessment of Proteinuria in the Dog and Cat). This can be facilitated by considering the history, physical findings, method of urine collection, and urinary sediment findings.

Hematuria and red blood cell casts are common in humans with glomerulonephritis but are rarely observed in dogs and cats with glomerular disease. Hyaline casts are common because of the presence of proteinaceous fluid in the tubules.

Hypoalbuminemia occurs in most dogs with glomerular disease at the time of presentation to the veterinarian. Total serum protein values are variable depending on changes in the globulin fractions. Frequently, animals with glomerulonephritis and amyloidosis have elevations in alpha, beta, or gamma globulins. Serum cholesterol elevations are found in most animals with glomerular disease. There is evidence that increased hepatic synthesis of cholesterol-rich lipoproteins occurs in the presence of hypoalbuminemia and that there is an inverse relationship between serum albumin and cholesterol levels. Animals that have hypoalbuminemia, hypercholesterolemia, proteinuria, and ascites or edema are said to have the nephrotic syndrome. Ascites and edema are the least consistent features of the nephrotic syndrome in dogs. Either glomerulonephritis or amyloidosis can lead to end-stage renal disease and laboratory findings typical of uremia (nonregenerative anemia, azotemia, hyperphosphatemia, and metabolic acidosis).

Renal biopsy is required for the differentiation of glomerulonephritis and amyloidosis. This distinction is important because glomerulonephritis in dogs and cats may have a variable course characterized by clinical remission and stable renal function for several years, whereas amyloidosis is generally progressive. Also, some aspects of therapy may differ between the two diseases.

Routine light microscopic techniques using hematoxylin and eosin, Congo red, and thioflavine-T stains are sufficient for the diagnosis of amyloidosis. Permanganate oxidation techniques will allow presumptive diagnosis of reactive amyloidosis (amyloid AA), because these deposits lose their Congo red affinity after permanganate oxidation. The technique of renal biopsy also should be considered. In dogs, amyloidosis is primarily a glomerular disease, and a cortical biopsy taken by the keyhole technique is sufficient for diagnosis. In cats, however, the predominant medullary distribution of amyloid can make diagnosis difficult. In cats suspected of having amyloidosis, an open wedge biopsy may be of more value, and an attempt should be made to obtain medullary tissue.

The diagnosis of glomerulonephritis often requires immunofluorescence and electron microscopic studies because light microscopic changes may be subtle. For immunofluorescence, samples must be snap-frozen in dry ice and acetone or preserved in Michel's solution. The former is cumbersome, but use of the latter preservative solution is convenient and allows samples to be shipped for processing by regular mail. Samples for electron microscopy should be minced immediately into 1-mm cubes and placed in cold 2 per cent glutaraldehyde for processing.

In animals, glomerulonephritis has not been as clearly subdivided as in humans. In cats, glomerulonephritis is usually described as membranous. Ultrastructurally, there is a loss of foot processes, and electron-dense deposits are usually subepithelial and mesangial in location but occasionally subendothelial. In dogs, membranous, membranoproliferative, and proliferative types of glomerulonephritis have been described most frequently on light microscopic examination, but mesangioproli-

Table 1. *Diseases Associated with Glomerulonephritis in Dogs and Cats*

Dogs	Cats
Infectious	
Canine adenovirus-1	Feline leukemia virus
Ehrlichiosis	Feline infectious peritonitis
Brucellosis	Polyarthritis (*Mycoplasma gateae*)
Leishmaniasis	Other
Bacterial endocarditis	
Pyometra	
Dirofilariasis	
Other	
Inflammatory	
Pancreatitis	Pancreatitis
Systemic lupus erythematosus	Systemic lupus erythematosus
Neoplastic	
Lymphosarcoma	Hemolymphatic neoplasia
Mastocytoma	Other
Other	
Idiopathic	
Many cases	Many cases
Familial	
Doberman pinschers (?)	Glomerulonephritis in sibling cats

ferative and mesangiosclerosing glomerular lesions have occasionally been reported. In addition to loss of foot processes, subendothelial, mesangial, and intramembranous deposits are usually found on electron microscopic examination. Subepithelial deposits have only rarely been described. In both species, immunoglobulins and complement have been found in a discontinuous granular pattern when studied by immunofluorescence techniques.

TREATMENT

General Principles of Treatment

An attempt should be made to identify and eliminate any predisposing infectious, inflammatory, or neoplastic disease. For example, the glomerular lesions in dogs with pyometra resolve after removal of the infected uterus. Dogs with dirofilariasis and glomerulonephritis should have their heartworm infection treated. In amyloidosis, identification and successful treatment of the predisposing disease process may arrest further amyloid deposition and enhance resolution of existing deposits.

If necessary, appropriate fluid therapy should be administered to resolve prerenal azotemia and reestablish normal hydration. Conservative management for chronic renal failure should then be instituted (see the article entitled Update—Conservative Medical Management of Chronic Renal Failure). When formulating low-protein diets for animals with glomerular disease, it is important to include additional protein to replace that lost in the urine. Also, recommendations regarding sodium intake must be given special consideration (see Complications, below).

Specific Treatment

There is debate about the effectiveness of various types of specific therapy for glomerulonephritis in humans. Corticosteroids and other immunosuppressive agents such as cyclophosphamide, azathioprine, and chlorambucil have been tried in the various categories of glomerulonephritis. It is generally agreed that treatment of lipoid nephrosis (minimal change disease) with corticosteroids is beneficial. There is also some evidence that immunosuppressive therapy is helpful in idiopathic membranous nephropathy and lupus nephritis. Immunosuppressive therapy in other types of glomerulonephritis in humans is controversial. There are no controlled studies of the use of corticosteroids in dogs and cats with glomerulonephritis. Individual case reports have suggested transient improvement with steroid therapy, especially in cats. On the other hand, long-term remission of clinical signs without therapy has been reported occasionally in dogs. Until controlled studies of large numbers of animals are available, immunosuppressive therapy cannot be recommended for dogs and cats with glomerulonephritis.

Anticoagulant (heparin and coumadin) and antiplatelet (aspirin, indomethacin, and dipyridamole) therapy has been used in humans for treatment of glomerulonephritis based on the roles of the coagulation system and platelets (see Complications, below). There is no reported experience with this therapy in veterinary medicine, but such drugs may be useful based on the fact that glomerular disease is a hypercoagulable state in dogs as well as in humans.

No specific therapy for amyloidosis is of known benefit. Dimethyl sulfoxide (DMSO) is a highly soluble compound with anti-inflammatory effects. There has been speculation that it may aid in the solubilization of amyloid fibrils and removal of amyloid subunit proteins, decrease levels of the acute-phase reactant SAA, and reduce inflammation and fibrosis in affected kidneys. There is no good evidence that such therapy actually mobilizes amyloid fibrils from the kidneys, but renal function has been shown to improve in human patients with reactive amyloidosis treated with DMSO, suggesting that its anti-inflammatory effects may be of some benefit. It was used in humans at a dosage of 7 to 15 gm divided three times daily.

Colchicine is a compound that blocks secretion of SAA by hepatocytes, and it has been used in human patients with familial Mediterranean fever. These patients have recurrent fever and inflammatory disease involving their serosal surfaces and are predisposed to development of amyloidosis. There is evidence that colchicine therapy reduces the occurrence of amyloidosis in these patients. This therapy is unlikely to be of benefit in veterinary medicine, because animals are usually not presented until their amyloidosis is advanced.

COMPLICATIONS

Hypercoagulability

The nephrotic syndrome is a hypercoagulable state, and affected animals are predisposed to thromboembolism. The pulmonary vessels are most commonly affected, and sudden onset of dyspnea is the major clinical sign. Other vessels that may be involved include the femoral arteries, portal vein, coronary arteries, renal artery or vein, splenic arteries, or mesenteric artery. Occasionally, clinical signs related to thromboembolism may overshadow other signs of the nephrotic syndrome and constitute the major clinical presentation.

The pathogenesis of the hypercoagulable state in the nephrotic syndrome appears to be multifactorial. Clotting Factors I (fibrinogen), V, VII, VIII, and X are increased, whereas Factors IX, XI, and XII are decreased. Mild thrombocytosis and decreased platelet life span may occur, and platelet function is altered. Platelet adhesiveness and spontaneous aggregability are increased owing to increased prostaglandin endoperoxide synthesis. These platelet abnormalities have led to the use of antiplatelet drugs such as aspirin, indomethacin, and dipyridamole in glomerular disease.

Increased serum lipids (including cholesterol and triglycerides), altered fibrinolysis, and uremic vascular lesions have also been considered to play roles in the pathogenesis. Dehydration, shock, infection, and corticosteroid-induced inhibition of fibrinolysis are considered secondary factors contributing to hypercoagulability.

Recently, it has been determined that antithrombin III, a low-molecular-weight (65,000) hemostatic modulator, may be markedly decreased in humans and dogs with the nephrotic syndrome. Normally antithrombin III acts as a serine protease that inactivates activated clotting factors, especially Factor II but also Factors X, IX, XI, and XII. Heparin acts as a cofactor for antithrombin III and increases its affinity for these clotting factors. Antithrombin III is lost in the urine in the nephrotic syndrome to the extent that inactivation of activated clotting factors may be insufficient to prevent thrombosis.

Severe proteinuria leads to hypoalbuminemia and depletion of other serum proteins of low molecular weight, and there is an attempt by the liver to increase protein synthesis and replace the lost proteins. An overall compensatory increase in hepatic protein synthesis (including large-molecular-weight clotting factors) with continued selective loss of albumin and low-molecular-weight globulins (including low-molecular-weight clotting factors and hemostatic modulators such as antithrombin III) in the urine leads to an abnormal distribution of clotting factors and regulatory proteins. Prevailing inflammatory disease may also contribute to an increase in acute-phase reactant proteins such as fibrinogen (Factor I), alpha$_2$ macroglobulin, and Factor VIII.

Recently, plasma antithrombin III levels have been measured and found to be low in dogs with the nephrotic syndrome. It was recommended that dogs with antithrombin III levels less than 70 per cent of normal and with fibrinogen levels greater than 300 mg/dl be considered candidates for anticoagulant therapy. Heparin may be less effective than coumadin in this situation, because the relative deficiency of antithrombin III would lessen the efficacy of heparin.

Sodium Retention and Hypertension

Patients with the nephrotic syndrome may retain sodium, contributing to ascites, edema, hypertension, and weight gain. The classic explanation for the pathogenesis of ascites and edema in the nephrotic syndrome is based on activation of the renin-angiotensin system. Progressive loss of albumin in the urine leads to hypoalbuminemia, decreased oncotic pressure, and loss of water from the extracellular fluid space. Decreased effective circulating volume causes decreased renal blood flow and activation of the renin-angiotensin system. This in turn leads to increased aldosterone production and consequent renal conservation of salt and water. This attempt to restore the extracellular fluid volume to normal is not effective, because hypoalbuminemia prevents retention of water in the vascular space.

Recently, it has been observed that human patients with the nephrotic syndrome who are retaining sodium fall into two categories. Those in one group have low blood volume, high renin levels, and normal to high aldosterone levels. Those in the other group have high blood volume and low to normal renin and aldosterone levels. Administration of captopril (an angiotensin-converting enzyme inhibitor that blocks the formation of angiotensin II) to human patients with the nephrotic syndrome who were retaining sodium led to reduced aldosterone levels but did not prevent sodium retention and weight gain. These findings are thought to be explained by the occurrence of an intrarenal mechanism for sodium retention in the nephrotic syndrome. In those patients with high blood volume, sodium retention through the intrarenal mechanism has led to expansion of the extracellular fluid volume and suppression of the renin-angiotensin system. In patients with low blood volume, it is thought that severe hypoalbuminemia leads to reduced blood volume and subsequent activation of the renin-angiotensin system despite the intrarenal mechanism for sodium retention.

A recent study has shown that hypertension may be more common in dogs with chronic renal failure than has been appreciated in the past. Convenient and accurate methods for estimation of canine blood pressure have not been readily available to practitioners. Measurement of blood pressure by ultrasonic Doppler techniques appears to be most practical. In a study of normal dogs, average systolic blood pressure was 148 ± 16 mm Hg, average diastolic blood pressure was 87 ± 8 mm Hg, and average mean blood pressure was 102 ± 9 mm Hg. These values were determined by direct needle puncture of the femoral artery. These same investigators showed that 60 per cent of dogs with chronic renal failure had hypertension that was independent of the degree of azotemia and that 80 per cent of dogs with glomerular disease had hypertension. This study emphasizes that hypertension may be an important complication of glomerular disease in dogs, as it is in humans. Hypertension may contribute to the retinal detachments and retinal hemorrhages occasionally observed in dogs with the nephrotic syndrome. Also, hypertension represents a potential nonimmunologic mechanism for progression of renal disease by hyalinization and fibrinoid degeneration of small renal vessels.

Sodium retention and hypertension in the nephrotic syndrome may be treated by gradual restriction of salt intake and by administration of diuretics. Animals with renal disease cannot make rapid adjustments in their renal excretion of solutes when dietary intake is abruptly changed. Therefore, sodium intake should be reduced slowly over several weeks. It has been recommended that sodium be restricted to 0.1 to 0.3 per cent of the diet. Animals with the nephrotic syndrome that are retaining sodium and have ascites and edema should not have their dietary sodium intake increased, as is sometimes recommended in the management of dogs with chronic renal failure. Diuretics such as furosemide (2 to 4 mg/kg) may be used to increase excretion of sodium and lower blood pressure. Care should be taken to prevent dehydration, which may superimpose prerenal azotemia and may aggravate the tendency toward thromboembolism.

PROGNOSIS

The prognosis for dogs with glomerular disease depends on the severity of the disease at presentation and the histologic diagnosis. If the animal is already in renal failure at presentation and has severe end-stage renal lesions on biopsy, the prognosis is poor. The rate of progression of renal disease, however, varies considerably from individual to individual, and the clinician should reserve judgment about prognosis until the animal has been carefully rehydrated and placed on appropriate conservative medical therapy.

Renal amyloidosis is an inexorably progressive disease with a poor prognosis. Glomerulonephritis, however, appears to be more variable in its course. It is difficult to speculate on the natural history of glomerulonephritis in dogs and cats. The frequency of asymptomatic proteinuria in the canine and feline population is unknown, as many of these animals will not be presented for veterinary attention. Several pathologic studies have indicated that the frequency of glomerular lesions in apparently normal populations of dogs is quite high. Therefore, animals with proteinuria and glomerulonephritis in the absence of renal failure cannot be regarded as necessarily having a poor prognosis. Most clinical descriptions of glomerulonephritis in dogs and cats suggest that the disease is variably progressive. Some animals remain stable over a period of several years, whereas others develop end-stage renal disease and progress to renal failure.

References and Supplemental Reading

Barsanti, J. A., and Finco, D. R.: Protein concentration in urine of normal dogs. Am. J. Vet. Res. 40:1583, 1979.

Biewenga, W. J., Gruys, E., and Hendriks, H. J.: Urinary protein loss in the dog: Nephrological study of 29 dogs without signs of renal disease. Res. Vet. Sci. 33:366, 1982.

Brenner, B. M., Hostetter, T. H., and Humes, H. D.: Molecular basis of proteinuria of glomerular origin. N. Engl. J. Med. 298:826, 1978.

Brown, E. A., Markandu, N. D., Roulston, J. E., et al.: Is the renin-angiotensin-aldosterone system involved in the sodium retention in the nephrotic syndrome? Nephron 32:102, 1982.

Chew, D. J., DiBartola, S. P., Boyce, J. T., et al.: Renal amyloidosis in related Abyssinian cats. J.A.V.M.A. 181:139, 1982.

Cowgill, L. D., and Kallet, A. J.: Recognition and management of hypertension in the dog. *In* Kirk, R. W. (ed.): *Current Veterinary Therapy VIII*. Philadelphia: W. B. Saunders, 1983, pp. 1025–1028.

Couser, W. G., and Salant, D. J.: In situ immune complex formation and glomerular injury. Kidney Int. 17:1, 1980.

DiBartola, S. P., Chew, D. J., and Jacobs, G.: Quantitative urinalysis including 24-hour protein excretion in the dog. J. Am. Anim. Hosp. Assoc. 16:537, 1980.

DiBartola, S. P., Spaulding, G. L., Chew, D. J., et al.: Urinary protein excretion and immunopathologic findings in dogs with glomerular disease. J.A.V.M.A. 177:73, 1980.

Glenner, G. G.: Amyloid deposits and amyloidosis: The beta fibrilloses. N. Engl. J. Med. 302:1283, 1980.

Green, R. A., and Kabel, A. L.: Hypercoagulable state in three dogs with nephrotic syndrome: Role of acquired antithrombin III deficiency. J.A.V.M.A. 181:914, 1982.

Kauffmann, R. H., Veltkamp, J. J., Van Tilburg, N. H., et al.: Acquired antithrombin III deficiency and thrombosis in the nephrotic syndrome. Am. J. Med. 65:607, 1978.

Kendall, A. G., Lohmann, R. C., and Dossetor, J. B.: Nephrotic syndrome: A hypercoagulable state. Arch. Intern. Med. 127:1021, 1971.

Lewis, R. J.: Canine glomerulonephritis: Results from a microscopic evaluation of fifty cases. Can. Vet. J. 17:171, 1976.

Muller-Peddinghaus, R., and Trautwein, G.: Spontaneous glomerulonephritis in dogs. I. Classification and immunopathology. Vet. Pathol. 14:1, 1977.

Murray, M., and Wright, N. G.: A morphologic study of canine glomerulonephritis. Lab. Invest. 30:213, 1974.

Nash, A. S., Wright, N. G., Spencer, A. J., et al.: Membranous nephropathy in the cat: A clinical and pathological study. Vet. Rec. 105:71, 1979.

Osborne, C. A., and Vernier, R. L.: Glomerulonephritis in the dog and cat: A comparative review. J. Am. Anim. Hosp. Assoc. 9:101, 1973.

Robbins, S. L., Cotran, R. S., and Kumar, V.: *Pathologic Basis of Disease*, 3rd ed. Philadelphia: W. B. Saunders, 1984, pp. 1002–1025.

Rouse, B. T., and Lewis, R. J.: Canine glomerulonephritis: Prevalence in dogs submitted at random for euthanasia. Can. J. Comp. Med. 39:365, 1975.

Simon, N. M., and Rosenberg, M. J.: Medical treatment of glomerular diseases. Med. Clin. North Am. 62:1157, 1978.

Slauson, D. O., and Gribble, D. H.: Thrombosis complicating renal amyloidosis in dogs. Vet. Pathol. 8:352, 1971.

Slauson, D. O., Gribble, D. H., and Russell, S. W.: A clinicopathologic study of renal amyloidosis in dogs. J. Comp. Pathol. 80:335, 1970.

Slauson, D. O., and Lewis, R. M.: Comparative pathology of glomerulonephritis in animals. Vet. Pathol. 16:135, 1979.

Stuart, B. P., Phemister, R. D., and Thomassen, R. W.: Glomerular lesions associated with proteinuria in clinically healthy dogs. Vet. Pathol. 12:125, 1975.

Thomson, C., Forbes, C. D., Prentice, C. R., et al.: Changes in blood coagulation and fibrinolysis in the nephrotic syndrome. Q. J. Med. 43:399, 1974.

White, J. V., Olivier, N. B., Reimann, K., et al.: Use of protein-to-creatinine ratio in a single urine specimen for quantitative estimation of canine proteinuria. J.A.V.M.A. 135:882, 1984.

Wright, N. G., Nash, A. S., Thompson, H., et al.: Membranous nephropathy in the cat and dog: A renal biopsy and follow-up study of sixteen cases. Lab. Invest. 45:269, 1981.

POLYCYSTIC RENAL DISEASE

WAYNE A. CROWELL, D.V.M.
Athens, Georgia

Renal cysts are not all the same—they can vary in size, shape, origin, cause, signs, and prognosis. The term *polycystic renal disease* must be defined at the outset to prevent confusion with other renal cystic diseases. Polycystic renal diseases have been defined as familial disorders in which functionally significant portions of normally differentiated kidneys are replaced by cysts (Gardner, 1976). Two types are recognized in humans—adult polycystic renal disease (APCD) and infantile polycystic renal disease (IPCD). Although there are several case reports of "polycystic" renal disease in dogs and cats, only two have been shown to be familial (McKenna et al., 1980; Crowell et al., 1979), and these two examples appear to be cases of IPCD. The possibility of familial factors in the other cases of polycystic renal disease was not stated, and their cause is unknown. Thus polycystic renal disease is either rare in dogs and cats or is not being recognized and diagnosed. Since there are numerous case reports of renal cysts, it is doubtful the syndrome is being unrecognized but rather that it is indeed rare in dogs and cats. The following information thus was gathered from human as well as canine and feline cases.

INFANTILE POLYCYSTIC RENAL DISEASE

This disease usually causes death during the first 2 months of life, and cysts (or cystlike abnormalities) are found in the liver as well as in the kidneys. It is familial (thought to be autosomal recessive), and siblings are frequently affected. The first clinical sign that is noted is distended abdomen due to markedly enlarged kidneys. Death occurs during the first months of life, because the condition is bilateral and renal function is inadequate. Clinical-pathologic data are sparse for IPCD in puppies and kittens, but available hematologic and serum chemistry data are compatible with those from renal failure and uremia.

Signalment and Signs

The disease has been reported in Cairn terrier puppies and domestic short-hair kittens. Affected puppies and kittens appear normal at birth but develop enlarged abdomens by 2 to 6 weeks of age. The owner may note the enlarged abdomen and seek veterinary advice at that point. Cases may be presented after siblings in a litter have died. Affected Cairn terrier puppies were alert and active at the time of presentation (6 weeks of age). The puppies were euthanized at that time, so other abnormal signs did not develop. Affected kittens that died from the disorder appeared clumsy and incoordinated (because of abdominal distention), became lethargic and anorexic (because of uremia), and later became comatose before death.

Pathology

The abdominal distention encountered in IPCD is due to the enlarged kidneys and to hepatomegaly.

Excess abdominal fluid was not encountered in the affected kittens or puppies. The kidneys are two to three times larger than normal, but since the renal enlargement is symmetric, the kidneys are reniform. On cut surfaces, the renal pelvis appears normal, but the cortex and medulla appear spongiform because of the numerous cysts. The cysts radiate through the cortex and medulla and contain clear fluid. Histologic study reveals that the cysts are perpendicular to the capsular surface and are lined by a single layer of cuboidal epithelium that may be flattened in some areas. The origin of the cysts has not been determined in puppies and kittens but in human cases has been determined to be the collecting ducts.

The liver is enlarged, but proportionally less than the kidney. Histologic examination shows bile duct expansion or cyst formation with an excess of connective tissue around ductules and ducts. The bile duct changes are present throughout the liver but are grossly more apparent on the liver margins, where they appear in an arboriform pattern.

Diagnosis and Treatment

Recognition of abdominal distention and the subsequent identification of its cause are the keys to diagnosis of polycystic renal disease in puppies and kittens. Owing to the rareness of polycystic renal disease in dogs and cats, the diagnosis may be incidental to examination by laparotomy or necropsy. Abdominal palpation and subsequent recognition of grossly enlarged kidneys in a kitten or puppy should alert the practitioner to the possibility of polycystic renal disease. A history of abdominal distention in siblings or in previous litters should increase the practitioner's suspicion that polycystic renal disease may be present. Radiographic examinations may be helpful, and renal biopsy examination should confirm renal cystic disease. A diagnosis of polycystic renal disease should not be made without evidence of familial occurrence and histologic study confirmating liver and kidney lesions.

There is no treatment at present, and the disease is progressive. The owners should be informed of the familial nature and probable genetic cause. Because affected animals are needed for research, appropriate institutions should be informed.

ADULT POLYCYSTIC DISEASE

Although adult polycystic disease has not been reported in dogs or cats, a brief summation of the disease in humans follows to provide information that may facilitate its recognition.

Adult polycystic disease can occur in young individuals but usually does not cause renal insufficiency in humans until the fifth or subsequent decades of life. It is inherited as an autosomal dominant trait with high penetrance and is considered to have a frequency of occurrence of one in every 500 persons. The kidneys are enlarged and cystic but are reniform, even though the cysts vary somewhat in size. Both kidneys are cystic, and other organs (liver, pancreas, spleen, epididymis) may have cysts. Cysts in organs other than the kidney are asymptomatic. Clinical complications of the renal cysts include pain, hematuria, proteinuria, renal calculi, abdominal mass, and perhaps renal neoplasia in addition to eventual uremia. Extrarenal lesions include aneurysms of the cerebral, renal, and splenic arteries and other cardiovascular malformations.

It is likely that this condition is present in dogs and cats but has not been recognized as such. Dogs or cats that have bilateral renal cysts should be examined further for evidence of cysts in other organs, and appropriate tissues should be submitted for histopathologic examination. Owners of such animals should be questioned concerning the offspring, siblings, or parents of the possibly affected animal in order to obtain evidence of similar renal cysts.

References and Supplemental Reading

Crowell, W. A., Hubbell, J. J., and Riley, J. C.: Polycystic renal disease in related cats. J.A.V.M.A. 175:286, 1979.

Gardner, K. D.: *Cystic Diseases of the Kidney.* New York: John Wiley & Sons, 1976.

McKenna, S. C., and Carpenter, J. L.: Polycystic disease of the kidney and liver in the Cairn terrier. Vet. Pathol. 17:436, 1980.

NEPHROGENIC DIABETES INSIPIDUS

EDWARD B. BREITSCHWERDT, D.V.M.
Raleigh, North Carolina

The definition of a disease is to an extent arbitrary and in general reflects the current state of knowledge regarding the pathophysiology of the disease process. Nephrogenic diabetes insipidus is characterized by defective responsiveness of distal tubules and collecting ducts to vasopressin (antidiuretic hormone). Lack of responsiveness to exogenous vasopressin distinguishes nephrogenic diabetes insipidus from pituitary-dependent (central) diabetes insipidus, which is caused by a deficiency of vasopressin. Based on current concepts regarding renal concentrating mechanisms, it seems appropriate to restrict the diagnosis of nephrogenic diabetes insipidus to diseases in which structural or functional hormone receptor or end-organ abnormalities alter vasopressin-induced cell-membrane permeability to water in the distal tubule and collecting duct.

PATHOPHYSIOLOGY

Vasopressin is synthesized in the supraoptic and paraventricular nuclei of the hypothalamus and is subsequently transported down the neurohypophyseal tract for storage in the posterior pituitary. Hypertonicity and volume depletion represent the major stimuli for vasopressin release. After release into the blood, vasopressin binds to the basolateral membrane of the cortical and medullary collecting ducts, thereby activating adenylate cyclase, which through a series of intracellular events increases tubular permeability to water. Water deprivation in a normal animal induces volume depletion and blood hypertonicity. Vasopressin is released into the systemic circulation, to enhance distal tubule and collecting duct permeability, with subsequent water reabsorption and production of a highly concentrated urine. It is important to recognize that medullary hypertonicity, produced by the countercurrent mechanism, is necessary for renal tubular water reabsorption following the enhancement of vasopressin-induced tubular permeability. Thus, medullary washout (loss of the medullary concentration gradient) can complicate the diagnostic evaluation of a patient with defective urine-concentrating ability.

Glomerular filtrate is isotonic with plasma, and osmolality changes as fluid passes through different parts of the nephron. Tubular fluid becomes hypotonic on entry into the distal tubule. The final concentration of the urine is determined by the permeability of the collecting ducts to water. When the blood concentration of vasopressin is high, water permeability of the collecting duct is increased, resulting in net water reabsorption and increased urine concentration. When concentration of blood vasopressin is low, water reabsorption is minimal, and dilute urine is produced. Nephrogenic diabetes insipidus is characterized by dilute urine, despite the production and release into the circulation of normal or elevated amounts of vasopressin.

DISEASE SYNDROMES

Nephrogenic diabetes insipidus is classified as either congenital or acquired. The defect in urine-concentrating ability may be characterized as partial or complete, reflecting the degree of severity of the renal tubular concentrating defect. Animals with a complete lack of responsiveness to antidiuretic hormone (ADH) will not concentrate urine after water deprivation or administration of exogenous vasopressin. Animals with partial defects in ADH responsiveness produce less than maximally concentrated urine, despite the administration of exogenous vasopressin.

Congenital nephrogenic diabetes is a rare canine disease, characterized by polyuria, dehydration, vomiting, and stunted growth. Vomiting occurs as a result of chronic overdistention of the stomach with water. Polyuria and nocturia are noted shortly after weaning. The mechanism responsible for ADH nonresponsiveness in congenital nephrogenic diabetes insipidus is not well defined.

The acquired forms of nephrogenic diabetes insipidus can be divided into three major categories: (1) metabolic disorders, (2) intrinsic renal disease, and (3) drug-induced. Hyperadrenocorticism and hypercalcemia represent the most frequently encountered and well-documented metabolic causes of acquired nephrogenic diabetes insipidus. Hypokalemia, elevated blood prostaglandin E, and *Escherichia coli* endotoxins may also inhibit ADH-dependent membrane permeability to water. Binding of *E. coli* antigens to renal tubular epithelium may contribute to the alteration in urine concentration in some bitches with pyometra. Amyloidosis, polycystic renal disease, myeloma, ureteral obstruction, and pyelonephritis represent documented intrinsic renal causes of nephrogenic diabetes insipidus in humans and are likely to cause tubular unresponsiveness to vasopressin in dogs and cats. Although poorly understood, hyposthenuria may be documented during the early course of chronic renal failure in dogs. A multifactorial mechanism is likely; however, a uremic toxin that antagonizes the action of ADH has been proposed. Renal tubular insensitivity to ADH is reported to contribute to the polyuric phase of acute renal failure. The severe obligatory water loss associated with the polyuric phase of acute renal failure should be anticipated to prevent life-threatening volume depletion. Drug-induced nephrogenic diabetes insipidus in humans has been associated with the use of glucocorticoids, demeclocycline, methoxyflurane, colchicine, lithium, vinblastine, and various arteriographic contrast agents. The role of these drugs in canine and feline nephrogenic diabetes insipidus is poorly defined. Hyperadrenocorticism appears to interfere with vasopressin-mediated water reabsorption in dogs.

Despite clinical consideration of the above causative factors, the cause of nephrogenic diabetes insipidus is not identified in some animals. This suggests that other factors interfere with vasopressin-mediated water reabsorption. Since there are altered hormone-receptor mechanisms in other endocrine diseases, other causes of nephrogenic diabetes insipidus to investigate would include abnormal vasopressin amino acid content, antivasopressin antibodies, antivasopressin-receptor antibodies, agents that block vasopressin-receptor binding, and interference with intracellular cyclic AMP-mediated tubular permeability to water.

DIAGNOSIS

Diagnostic criteria for nephrogenic diabetes insipidus include lack of response to (1) water deprivation, (2) exogenous administration of vasopressin, or (3) hypertonic saline infusion. Because of complications associated with the hypertonic saline infusion test (Hickey-Hare test), the modified water deprivation test is now the preferred diagnostic test. Although not readily available at this time, concurrent measurement of vasopressin by radioimmunoassay markedly enhances interpretation of the water deprivation test for differentiation of the various causes of polyuria.

Animals with complete nephrogenic diabetes insipidus have severe polyuria with secondary polydipsia. Urine is generally hyposthenuric (urine specific gravity 1.001 to 1.007), reflecting an adequate number of functional nephrons to alter glomerular filtrate so as to generate solute-free water. When an animal fails to respond to endogenous or exogenous vasopressin after water deprivation, hyposthenuria reflects a disease process that interferes with water permeability in the distal tubule and collecting duct.

The initial diagnostic goal is to characterize the animal's renal function, since a water deprivation test should not be performed if renal function is compromised. At least three urinalyses should be evaluated to establish a trend for urine-concentrating ability and to rule out intrinsic renal disease, such as pyelonephritis. Renal function tests such as serum urea nitrogen, serum creatinine, and creatinine clearance should be performed to rule out serious renal dysfunction.

The second diagnostic goal, using the modified water deprivation test, is to establish whether vasopressin-induced water reabsorption is altered. In order to interpret the modified water deprivation test properly, it is important to collect sequential data. This enables accurate evaluation of urine concentration during maximal endogenous vasopressin release and following exogenous vasopressin administration. Determination of body weight, serum osmolality, and urine osmolality, monitored at least every 2 hours, is important to prevent dehydration and profound serum hyperosmolality in patients with nephrogenic diabetes insipidus. (A detailed discussion of the modified water deprivation test for differentiation of various polyuric stages appears in *Current Veterinary Therapy VII*, p. 1080.) It is important to recognize that a variety of diseases can result in a partial concentrating response to water deprivation; however, lack of urine concentration after subsequent administration of exogenous vasopressin implicates medullary washout or partial nephrogenic diabetes insipidus. Failure to concentrate urine during partial or gradual water restriction with concurrent administration of exogenous vasopressin has been used to rule out the possibility of medullary washout. As discussed previously, concurrent measurement of vasopressin levels in blood in conjunction with water deprivation would represent a superior diagnostic approach. The initial concentrating response to water deprivation may be related to the fact that hypophysectomized dogs can concentrate urine to 550 mOsm/L (approximately 1.016 specific gravity) in the absence of vasopressin.

Having established the diagnosis of nephrogenic diabetes insipidus by using the modified water deprivation test, the third diagnostic goal is to determine the cause of impaired water reabsorption in the distal tubules and collecting ducts. Congenital nephrogenic diabetes insipidus is implicated historically in young, potentially stunted animals that have been polyuric since birth. In animals with acquired nephrogenic diabetes insipidus, historic, physical, and laboratory abnormalities suggestive of hyperadrenocorticism, hypercalcemic states, hypokalemia, pyometra, or intrinsic renal disease should be explored. Hypercalcemia should be eliminated from the differential list early in the course of patient evaluation, since sustained elevations in serum calcium can cause rapidly progressive renal damage and deterioration of renal function. Unlike nephrogenic diabetes insipidus, chronic renal failure is generally characterized by isosthenuria (specific gravity 1.008 to 1.012) secondary to solute diuresis. Creatinine clearance, excretory urography, renal biopsy, or other diagnostic procedures may be necessary to rule out intrinsic renal disease such as chronic pyelonephritis, amyloidosis, and others. The animal's history of drug administration should be reviewed to identify drugs that might interfere with the action of vasopressin.

TREATMENT

Management of patients with nephrogenic diabetes insipidus involves two major therapeutic modalities. When the predisposing cause can be established, treatment should be directed toward eliminating the causative factor. Chemotherapy for lymphosarcoma-associated hypercalcemia, ovariohysterectomy for pyometra, and antimicrobial therapy for pyelonephritis are examples of therapeutic correction of the predisposing cause that may result in total remission of diabetes insipidus. In some instances, more than one factor may contribute to polydipsia and polyuria. For example, cortisol induces a primary polydipsia, inhibits release of vasopressin from the posterior pituitary, and interferes with vasopressin-mediated water permeability in the distal tubule and collecting duct. The degree to which each of these mechanisms contributes to polydipsia and polyuria appears to vary in canine hyperadrenocorticism, perhaps explaining the variation in response to the modified water deprivation test in these dogs. Asymptomatic urinary tract infection is also frequently encountered in dogs with hyperadrenocorticism. Cortisol excess, pyelonephritis, and *E. coli* endotoxin could contribute to nephrogenic diabetes insipidus in these dogs.

By definition, animals with nephrogenic diabetes insipidus will not respond to vasopressin challenge therefore exogenous vasopressin is not a beneficial form of therapy. Control of congenital nephrogenic diabetes insipidus with a salt-restricted diet and chlorothiazide has reportedly reduced the severity of polyuria by 50 to 85 per cent. Chlorothiazide diuretics decrease polyuria by blocking the generation of solute-free water, thereby allowing excretion of urine that is more concentrated. Prostaglandin inhibitors such as aspirin, indomethacin, tolmetin, or ibuprofen, used in conjunction with chlorothiazide diuretics and a low-sodium diet, further decrease urine volume in humans. Although the mechanism is poorly understood, prostaglandin inhibition causes increased proximal tubular reabsorption of sodium and water and enhanced vasopressin-induced collecting duct permeability. Side effects associated with chronic administration of prostaglandin inhibitory drugs should be carefully monitored.

References and Supplemental Reading

Bovee, K. C.: Pathophysiology of water metabolism. *In* Bovee, K. C. (ed.): *Canine Nephrology*. Philadelphia: Harwal Publishing, 1984, pp. 327–338.

Breitschwerdt, E. B.: Clinical abnormalities of urine concentration and dilution. Comp. Cont. Ed. Pract. Vet. 3:414, 1981.

Breitschwerdt, E. B., Verlander, J. W., and Hribernik, T. N.: Nephrogenic diabetes insipidus in three dogs. J.A.V.M.A. 179:235, 1981.

Chevalier, R. L., and Rogol, A. D.: Tolmetin sodium in the management of nephrogenic diabetes insipidus. J. Pediatr. 101:787, 1982.

Hardy, R. M.: Disorders of water metabolism. Symposium on fluid and electrolyte balance. Vol. 12. Philadelphia: W. B. Saunders, 1982, pp. 353–373.

Lage, A. L.: Urinary concentration and dilution. *In* Bovee, K. C. (ed.): *Canine Nephrology*. Philadelphia: Harwal Publishing, 1984, pp. 175–190.

Singer, I., and Forrest, J. N.: Drug-induced states of nephrogenic diabetes insipidus. Kidney Int. 10:82, 1976.

NEPHROTOXICITY OF AMPHOTERICIN B

STANLEY I. RUBIN, D.V.M.

Saskatoon, Saskatchewan

For more than 20 years amphotericin B has been the most effective treatment for systemic mycoses. Therapy usually involves the administration of multiple doses of amphotericin until either an arbitrary cumulative dose is achieved or the disease process is in remission. The renal toxicity of this drug represents the most serious limitation of its use for treatment of invasive fungal infections.

CLINICAL PHARMACOLOGY

Amphotericin is lipophilic and forms complexes with membrane sterols. Binding causes membrane deformation and increased permeability, resulting in leakage of cytosolic constituents with subsequent cell lysis and death. The increased susceptibility of fungi to amphotericin is due to its strong binding affinity to ergosterol, the principal sterol of fungal cell membranes. Cholesterol, the main sterol in animal cell membranes, binds less avidly to amphotericin.

Amphotericin B is poorly absorbed across the skin or gastrointestinal mucosa and must be administered intravenously to evoke a systemic effect. After administration, most of the drug is bound initially to cell membranes throughout the body. Some of the amphotericin is gradually released back into the blood as serum concentrations fall. In dogs, about one fifth of the dose is excreted in the bile and a further one fifth in the urine. The remainder may be metabolized locally at various tissue sites. Penetration of amphotericin into the crebrospinal fluid and ocular media is poor. Blood concentrations of amphotericin B persist for a long time because of the gradual release from the tissue stores.

PATHOPHYSIOLOGY

Nephrotoxicity is the most serious complicating factor in amphotericin therapy. Most of the adverse effects of the drug are probably related to disruption of the mammalian cell membrane. Renal tubular toxicity may be a reflection of this general membrane disruption. Butler and colleagues (1964) performed experiments in dogs in which the kidneys were observed both grossly and by arteriography during and after infusion of amphotericin into the renal artery. During infusion, the kidney blanched, softened, and became smaller, and the renal veins collapsed. Arteriograms after infusion revealed an absence of contrast media throughout most of the cortex of the kidney. These findings were consistent with a sudden reduction of renal blood flow (RBF) caused by vasoconstriction of both afferent and efferent arterioles. Reduced RBF would explain the decrease in glomerular filtration rate (GFR) and the development of azotemia.

Amphotericin nephrotoxicity may be explained on the basis of a phenomenon called tubuloglomerular feedback. When the distal tubule is presented with a chloride load, a feedback inhibition of GFR to the nephron occurs. Amphotericin causes an increase in permeability to chloride ions, and excess chloride is presented to the distal tubule. This initiates a tubuloglomerular feedback response with resultant reduction in GFR and RBF. An excessive response would have the potential to cause renal ischemia resulting in renal parenchymal damage. The responsiveness of this reflex is influenced by sodium status; salt depletion enhances and salt loading decreases the vasoconstrictor responses.

Other functional renal abnormalities include renal tubular acidosis, hypokalemia, and hyposthenuria. The majority of these effects appear to be abnormalities of the distal nephron; defects in proximal tubular function have not been demonstrated. Amphotericin binding to sterols in cell membranes may increase permeability of renal tubular epithelial cells to potassium, sodium, chloride, hydrogen ions, water, and solutes of low molecular weight.

Renal tubular acidosis after amphotericin administration has been described in both humans and rats; however, it has yet to be documented in dogs. Renal tubular acidosis is a defect in urinary acidification, so urine pH is not lowered in response to oral acid loading, and many patients become acidotic. In some patients, the acidifying defect may occur without systemic acidosis (i.e., incomplete renal tubular acidosis). This acidification defect is due to increased permeability of the luminal membrane and increased back-diffusion of hydrogen ions.

Defects of urine-concentrating ability have been noted in both humans and dogs. Amphotericin may in some way alter the distal tubular membrane to make it unresponsive to the action of antidiuretic hormone.

Hypokalemia is a frequently reported sequela to amphotericin therapy in humans; however, its frequency and clinical significance in dogs and cats are unknown at this time.

Figure 1 summarizes the renal pathophysiologic effects associated with amphotericin B nephrotoxicity.

PATHOLOGY

The severity of the lesions is generally related to the dose of the drug received. Glomerular lesions include thickening and fragmentation of basement membranes, hypercellularity, fibrosis, and hyalinization. Tubular lesions include infraglomerular tubular reflux, focal and generalized degeneration of epithelium, and intratubular and interstitial calcium deposits. The mechanism by which amphotericin induces tubular damage and calcification is not well understood. Tubular necrosis may result from either direct toxic effects on the epithelium or decreased RBF.

DIAGNOSIS

Nephrotoxicity is a predictable event in both animal and human patients receiving amphotericin

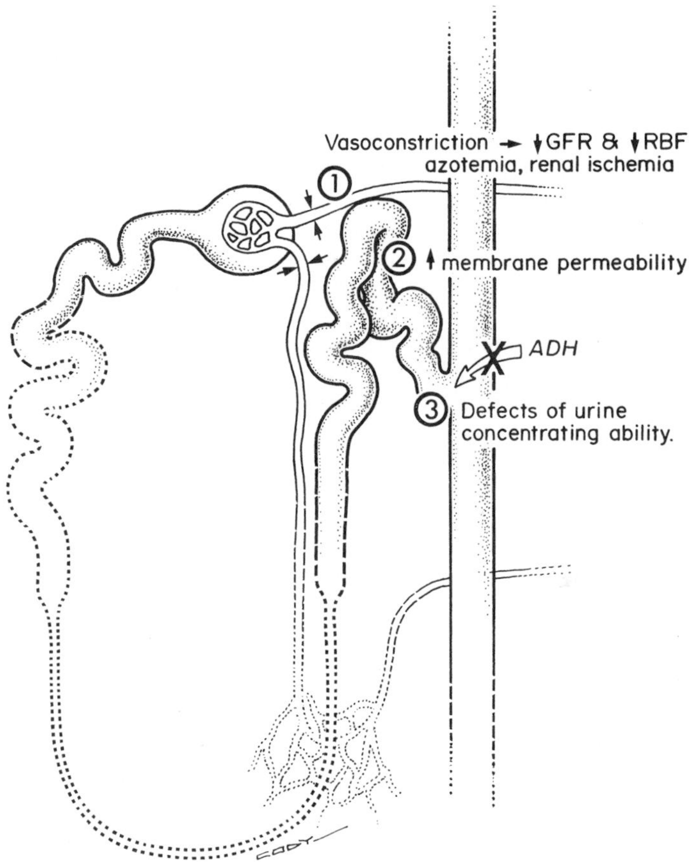

Figure 1. Pathophysiology associated with amphotericin B nephrotoxicity. Amphotericin acts on several sites of the nephron. At site 1 there is vasoconstriction, either as the result of direct action of the drug on the vessels or by reflex mechanisms. This results in decreased renal blood flow and azotemia; it may increase renal damage by causing renal ischemia. At site 2 the membranes of the distal tubule cells show altered permeability. This may initiate reflex mechanisms to decrease GFR (by tubuloglomerular feedback) and may cause excessive loss of electrolytes, producing hypokalemia and distal renal tubular acidosis. At site 3 the action of ADH is antagonized, which produces defects in urine concentration.

B. The degree of toxicity is dependent on the daily and cumulative dose, rate of administration, a wide range of individual sensitivities to the nephrotoxic effects of the drug, and the presence of pre-existing renal lesions.

The earliest renal abnormality observed following the administration of amphotericin is the development of an abrupt decrease in urine specific gravity and osmolality with polydipsia and polyuria.

Decreases in GFR also occur. The onset of azotemia after initiation of treatment is variable and to a great extent is dependent on individual variation, dose of drug, rate of administration, and presence of pre-existing renal dysfunction. Serum creatinine determination appears to be a better means of assessing renal function clinically than serum urea nitrogen. These patients are often anorectic, and their serum urea nitrogen may inadequately reflect GFR because of the lowered protein intake.

Abnormalities in the urine sediment have been described in humans and dogs receiving amphotericin; these include hematuria, pyuria, proteinuria, and cylindruria.

Renal function usually improves after cessation of amphotericin therapy. This improvement may, however, be very gradual, taking weeks or months. Permanent (residual) renal dysfunction is possible, and it is usually a reflection of the total dose received.

Other toxic effects of amphotericin B include fever, chills, nausea, vomiting, diarrhea, anorexia, phlebitis, weight loss, and nonregenerative anemia.

PREVENTION

Many attempts have been made to reduce the toxic effects of amphotericin by the simultaneous administration of other compounds. Early attempts to alleviate amphotericin-induced vasoconstriction with vasoactive drugs were not successful. The acute renal toxicity was not alleviated by the use of quinidine, tolazoline (alpha-adrenergic antagonist), hydralazine, and trimethaphan camsylate (ganglionic blockade). Mannitol also had equivocal benefits in reducing nephrotoxicity.

Although renal tubular acidosis may follow amphotericin administration, experimental studies in dogs have indicated that sodium bicarbonate does not reduce the nephrotoxic effects. Bicarbonate-treated dogs developed more severe azotemia and more severe renal lesions than did animals treated with amphotericin alone.

Gerkens and Branch (1980) investigated the pos-

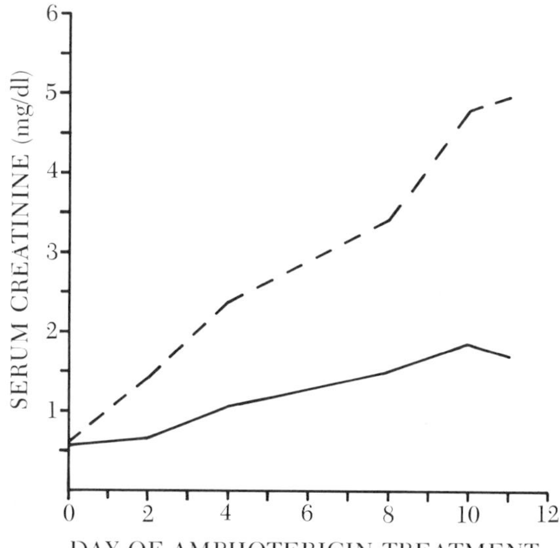

Figure 2. Comparison of slow intravenous administration of amphotericin (solid line) and a rapid IV bolus (dashed line) in 20-kg dogs. Amphotericin B (1 mg/kg) was administered on alternate days (days 1, 3, 5, 7, 9, and 11) to two groups of six dogs. Mean serum creatinine was significantly lower in the group receiving the amphotericin in a slow infusion over 5 hours in 1 L of D5W, compared with the group receiving the amphotericin as a rapid bolus in 20 ml of D5W over 5 minutes.

sibility that amphotericin nephrotoxicity may be mediated by tubuloglomerular feedback, which results in vasoconstriction and a decreased GFR. In acute studies, beneficial effects were obtained when furosemide or normal saline solution was given just prior to the administration of amphotericin. Furosemide was thought to act by blocking tubular reabsorption of chloride and inhibiting the tubuloglomerular feedback reflex. In addition, sodium loading was associated with an improvement of renal function due to the amphotericin nephrotoxicity in sodium-depleted human patients. If tubuloglomerular feedback is a mediator of the nephrotoxic response to amphotericin, then the sodium status of the patient receiving amphotericin might be expected to have a profound effect on the ability of this drug to impair renal function. It is not known whether a high salt intake (orally or parenterally) before amphotericin treatment might confer a prophylactic benefit on patients with normal sodium balance. However, it is likely that many dogs are sodium depleted as a result of the anorexia that often accompanies either amphotericin therapy or the underlying disease.

Well-defined dosage schedules for the clinical use of amphotericin in either human or veterinary medicine have not been well established. Critical factors such as rate of administration, optimal daily dose, optimal total dose, and optimal duration of therapy are not well defined.

The usual method of administration of amphotericin in human patients is to dissolve the drug in 500 ml of 5 per cent dextrose in water (D5W), which is infused intravenously over a period of 2 to 6 hours. In veterinary medicine, the dosage schedules and methods of administration have been developed empirically. They are based on a combination of convenience, limits of toxicity, clinical experience, and data obtained from work in humans. There is no general agreement on the best procedure for dogs. The two most popular methods of administration include a rapid bolus of amphotericin, diluted in 20 to 30 ml of D5W and given intravenously over 1 to 3 minutes, or diluting the amphotericin in 500 or 1000 ml of D5W and administering it by slow infusion over 4 to 6 hours. (Greene et al., 1984). In the author's experience (Rubin, 1984), the slow infusion method causes significantly less toxicity than the bolus method. Slow infusion reduces GFR to a lesser degree (Fig. 2) and causes less histopathologic damage.

SPECIFIC RECOMMENDATIONS FOR THE CLINICAL USE OF AMPHOTERICIN B

Prior to the administration of amphotericin B, laboratory tests (BUN, serum creatinine, electrolytes, packed cell volume [PCV], total plasma protein [TPP], and urinalysis) should be obtained to determine if pre-existing renal dysfunction exists and to serve as a baseline to assess toxicity during therapy.

A flow sheet should be prepared to include the following variables: body weight, BUN, serum creatinine, electrolytes, PCV, TPP, urinalysis, cumulative amphotericin dose to date (mg/kg), and amphotericin dose administered on that particular day (mg).

It may be prudent to start intravenous sodium loading prior to administration of the amphotericin. Approximately 50 ml/kg of 0.9 per cent sodium chloride solution may be administered intravenously over a period of 1 to 3 hours before the delivery of amphotericin. Care must be taken not to allow any of the amphotericin to mix with the saline solution, as the amphotericin will precipitate. Alternatively, the animal may be given supplemental sodium chloride simply by salting its food. In animals with debilitating systemic fungal infections, it is important to ensure that the patient is well hydrated prior to the administration of amphotericin.

Amphotericin B stock solution (Fungizone, Squibb)* is then diluted to 500 to 1000 ml of D5W

*Stock solution is prepared by adding 10 ml of sterile water to a vial to produce a solution with a concentration of 5 mg/ml.

and administered over a period of 4 to 6 hours on alternate days. In smaller dogs and cats, the daily dose may be diluted in smaller amounts of D5W (125 to 250 ml). The recommended daily dose varies from 0.15 to 1.0 mg/kg. The higher dosage is associated with an increased risk of nephrotoxicity and should only be used in life-threatening and particularly resistant infections. A dose of 0.5 mg/kg on alternate days is a reasonable dose for many dogs. Cats are more sensitive to the nephrotoxic effects of amphotericin. Doses recommended for cats have varied from 0.1 to 0.5 mg/kg. The author recommends a dose of 0.15 mg/kg.

The body weight, PCV, TPP, BUN, and serum creatinine level should be checked before each subsequent therapy. Supplemental fluids should be given as necessary to prevent dehydration. In patients with impaired renal function, the daily dose may need to be reduced to prevent worsening of renal insufficiency. Therapy should be discontinued if the BUN becomes abnormal (greater than 30 to 40 mg/dl) or if severe systemic toxic signs appear, such as severe depression or vomiting. Therapy is then reinstituted, often at a reduced dosage, after the azotemia or systemic signs resolve.

Electrolytes should be monitored periodically (once weekly). If hypokalemia is identified, then oral potassium supplementation should be instituted.

Serious attention should be given to the patient's nutritional status, as the amphotericin toxicity may exacerbate the anorexia that is present secondary to the debilitating disease.

References and Supplemental Reading

Appel, G. B., and Neu, H. C.: The nephrotoxicity of antimicrobial agents. III. N. Engl. J. Med. 296:784, 1977.

Butler, W. T., Hill, G. J., Szweed, C. F., et al.: Amphotericin B renal toxicity in the dog. J. Pharmacol. Exp. Ther. 143:47, 1964.

Codish, S. D., Tobias, J. S., and Monaco, A. P.: Recent advances in the treatment of systemic mycotic infections. Surg. Gynecol. Obstet. 148:435, 1979.

Craven, P. C., et al.: Excretion pathways of amphotericin B. J. Infect. Dis. 140:329, 1979.

Gerkens, J. F., and Branch, R. A.: The influence of sodium status and furosemide on canine acute amphotericin B nephrotoxicity. J. Pharmacol. Exp. Ther. 214:306, 1980.

Greene, C. E., O'Neal, K. G., and Barsanti, J. A.: Antimicrobial Chemotherapy. *In* Greene, C. E. (ed.): *Clinical Microbiology and Infectious Diseases of the Dog and Cat.* Philadelphia: W. B. Saunders, 1984, pp. 172–178.

Heidemann, H. T., Gerkens, J. F., Spickard, W. A., et al.: Amphotericin B nephrotoxicity in humans decreased by salt repletion. Am. J. Med.. 75:476, 1983.

Legendre, A. M., Selcer, B. A., Edwards, D. F., et al.: Treatment of canine blastomycosis with amphotericin B and ketoconazole. J.A.V.M.A. 184:1249, 1984.

Macy, D. W.: The effects of bicarbonate and mannitol on amphotericin B nephrotoxicity in the dog. M.S. Thesis, University of Illinois at Urbana-Champaign, 1977.

Medoff, G., and Kobayashi, G. S.: Strategies in the treatment of systemic fungal infections. N. Engl. J. Med. 302:145, 1980.

Richardson, R. C.: Treatment of systemic mycoses in the dog. J.A.V.M.A. 183:335, 1983.

Rubin, S. I.: Nephrotoxicity of amphotericin B in the dog: Comparison of rapid intravenous bolus versus slow intravenous administration. M.S. Thesis, Univesity of Illinois at Urbana-Champaign, 1984.

Pyle, R. L.: Clinical pharmacology of amphotericin B. J.A.V.M.A. 179:83, 1981.

GENTAMICIN NEPHROTOXICOSIS IN THE DOG

SCOTT A. BROWN, V.M.D.,
and JEANNE A. BARSANTI, D.V.M.
Athens, Georgia

Gentamicin is frequently necessary for the treatment of serious gram-negative infections. Its usefulness, however, is limited by nephrotoxicosis, defined clinically as a reduction in glomerular filtration rate (GFR) and evidenced by a rise in serum creatinine or blood urea nitrogen (BUN). This toxicity is difficult to predict and often is recognized only in the late stages of renal failure.

PATHOGENESIS

Gentamicin is eliminated from the body almost exclusively through the process of glomerular filtration. After filtration, most gentamicin remains in the renal tubular fluid and reaches high concentrations in the urine. Some gentamicin binds to the proximal tubule luminal membrane and enters the cell through a process of pinocytosis similar to that responsible for protein reabsorption. Storage in the cells results in accumulation of gentamicin in the renal cortex, where drug levels can reach 20 to 50 times the serum concentration and can persist for weeks.

The mechanism of toxicity of gentamicin remains to be completely elucidated but probably involves alterations in membrane phospholipids, Na-K ATPase (sodium-potassium adenosine triphosphatase), and intracellular calcium concentrations and damage to mitochondria and lysosomes. The high cortical concentrations damage the proximal tubular cells and result in loss of glomerular filtration through the nephron. Since gentamicin excretion depends on glomerular filtration, a vicious circle exists, with toxicosis leading to drug retention leading to further toxicosis.

Gentamicin nephrotoxicity follows four sequential stages, each of which may be more or less evident in a particular case. In some cases, the stages will appear to occur simultaneously because of the insensitive clinical tools available to detect toxicosis.

Stage I involves functional changes, evidenced by decreased ability to concentrate urine, polyuria, proteinuria, and sometimes glucosuria. The second stage is proximal renal tubular cell death, which is usually heralded clinically by the presence of casts in the urine. Stage III is reduction in GFR, identified clinically as elevated serum creatinine and BUN concentrations. Stage IV is regeneration, which begins as soon as cell necrosis is complete. Nearly all patients treated with gentamicin will have some nephrons in each of the various stages during any point in therapy. The kidney will behave as a sum of the function of its nephrons. Kidney damage with gentamicin therapy is often subclinical, but it should be remembered that this is a function of the tremendous reserve capacity present, since even one dose of gentamicin will produce functional and structural alterations in the kidney.

DIAGNOSIS

Diagnosis of gentamicin nephrotoxicosis is aided by urinalysis and determinations of BUN and serum creatinine. Evaluation of the patient's medical and drug history, and consideration of other possible causes of renal failure, may give adequate information to tentatively diagnose gentamicin-associated acute renal failure. If there is doubt about the cause or a lack of response to therapy, a percutaneous renal biopsy is indicated. The early histologic change is cloudy swelling, which progresses to severe cellular vacuolation and flattening with luminal casts. Interstitial changes include edema, white blood cell infiltration, and later fibrosis. Because each nephron will progress through the four stages at a characteristic rate, histopathologic changes typically are patchy in distribution. There are no glomerular changes detectable by light microscopy.

Acute renal failure due to gentamicin administration is often not evident until 3 to 5 days after discontinuation of gentamicin therapy (5 to 10 days from the start of therapy). Nonoliguric acute renal failure occurs most often and has a better prognosis than oliguric renal failure.

THERAPY

Therapy of acute renal failure due to gentamicin should be managed in ways similar to those for other forms of acute renal failure. However, loop diuretics (furosemide) must be avoided, since they enhance the toxicity of gentamicin. Patients with nephrotoxicosis have prolonged drug retention, and, if elevated serum levels of gentamicin are suspected or documented, dialysis should be considered. Eight hours of hemodialysis or 36 hours of peritoneal dialysis will significantly reduce the serum concentration of gentamicin.

Gentamicin nephrotoxicosis is often reversible, although long-term therapy may be required. Since patients treated with gentamicin are generally hospitalized for their primary problem before development of renal failure, economic constraints may make lengthy hospitalization difficult. For canine patients, response to therapy is delayed, and a decline in serum creatinine often is not seen until 5 to 7 days after initiation of therapy for renal failure. The delay is due to the persistence of gentamicin in serum and tissue and the continuation of kidney damage for several days following discontinuation of the antibiotic.

Other pertinent findings typical of the clinical course of gentamicin-associated acute renal failure include electrolyte abnormalities. Hypokalemia due to the combination of renal potassium wasting and lack of dietary potassium intake is common, and serum potassium levels must be monitored and potassium provided to maintain eukalemia (see Fluid Therapy, *Current Veterinary Therapy VIII*, pp. 28–40). Disorders of calcium homeostasis with elevations or reductions in serum calcium levels are possible. Hypercalcemia is of particular concern, since concurrent hyperphosphatemia due to renal failure will predispose the patient to soft tissue mineralization. Phosphate binders should be instituted in this situation. No specific therapy is generally necessary for hypocalcemia, since clinical signs are rare and calcium supplementation during hyperphosphatemia is contraindicated. Because of the chronic nature of the disease and the presence of pre-existing negative protein and calorie balance in many patients, weight loss and hypoalbuminemia are common. Food intake should be encouraged as soon as vomiting has been controlled.

Table 1. Program for Gentamicin Therapy

1. Reserve gentamicin for treatment of serious infections, when gram-negative or highly resistant gram-positive bacteria are involved.
2. Dose appropriately, generally 2.2 mg/kg every 8 hours subcutaneously. Minimize the length of therapy.
3. Avoid dehydration, hypokalemia, furosemide, and other nephrotoxins. Avoid the use of gentamicin in patients with pre-existing renal disease.
4. Obtain a baseline serum creatinine or BUN measurement and a urinalysis with sediment exam prior to initiation of gentamicin treatment. Repeat the urinalysis every other day and the serum creatinine and BUN every fourth day. Continue monitoring for 7 days after discontinuing the antibiotic.
5. Discontinue gentamicin use if any sign of toxicosis is detected or if culture and sensitivity testing indicate that a less toxic antibiotic may be effective.

PROGNOSIS

Prediction of which dogs will respond to therapy for renal failure is difficult. From clinical experience at the University of Georgia Veterinary Medical Teaching Hospital (UGAVMTH), it appears that those dogs not monitored with sequential urinalyses and serum creatinine determinations during gentamicin therapy have a worse prognosis, implying that early detection and treatment of toxicosis are advantageous.

A renal biopsy may provide prognostic information, since increased numbers of granular casts and extensive interstitial fibrosis and mineralization appear to be associated with a poor prognosis for recovery.

Long-term prognosis is fair; some dogs remain azotemic, whereas others regain enough renal function to concentrate urine and resolve the azotemia. Improvement in renal function is gradual, often requiring 2 months or longer to reach a maximum.

PREVENTION

Since gentamicin toxicosis may be fatal, prevention is important. Clinical and experimental studies have identified several factors that increase the likelihood of gentamicin nephrotoxicosis. It also is important to evaluate the patient's renal function throughout therapy and for several days afterward. Thus, each veterinary clinician should develop a program for use of gentamicin. The cornerstones of this program must be to minimize risk factors and monitor the patient carefully (Table 1). Failure to institute such a program places the patient at an unjustifiable risk.

Risk Factors for Gentamicin Toxicosis

Of the species commonly treated in veterinary medicine, dogs appear to be relatively sensitive to gentamicin nephrotoxicosis. Cats are relatively resistant, although less is known about aminoglycoside pharmacokinetics in this species. Advanced age may predispose an animal to toxicosis, whereas neonatal puppies younger than 30 days are less susceptible.

The patient's state of hydration has an influence on the development of complications from gentamicin therapy. Dehydration increases serum and tissue drug concentrations by reducing the volume of distribution of the drug, enhancing toxicity. Dietary sodium restriction, by reducing the volume of distribution, will enhance toxicity. Patients with Addison's disease, with similar fluctuations in extracellular volume status, will be at risk.

The use of furosemide potentiates the nephrotoxicity of gentamicin and makes the development of acute renal failure more likely and more devastating if it occurs. Furosemide may act by reducing the volume of distribution of gentamicin or enhancing renal cortical concentration of the antibiotic. Alternatively, furosemide may have a synergistic toxic effect on the proximal tubular cells. Thus, furosemide should not be used in conjunction with gentamicin.

Potassium depletion potentiates toxicosis. Gentamicin therapy may cause renal potassium wasting, which exacerbates the often pre-existing negative whole-body potassium balance in these patients. Serum potassium levels should be carefully monitored and the patient supplemented orally or parenterally in order to maintain serum levels above 3.5 mEq/L. Eukalemic patients with inadequate dietary intake of potassium during gentamicin therapy should be supplemented with 1 to 2 mEq/kg of potassium daily to prevent development of potassium depletion. Patients who become hypokalemic during gentamicin therapy should receive two to three times this amount on a daily basis.

Septicemia and fever, when present, are factors that place patients at risk, but these are often the reason for gentamicin therapy. If other less toxic antibiotics cannot be chosen, these risk factors are generally beyond the control of the clinician.

The presence of pre-existing renal disease affects the renal clearance and deposition of gentamicin, making prediction of both therapeutic efficacy and toxicity difficult. Since BUN and serum creatinine determinations do not detect renal dysfunction until about 75 per cent reduction in glomerular filtration rate, their concentrations will not be a reliable indicator of renal clearance of gentamicin. Basing dosage on creatinine clearance (CCl) measurements may be reliable, if stable renal function is present. The following formula should be used:

1. Maintain the same dosage (in milligrams).
2. Increase the interdose interval by a factor of normal CCl ÷ patient's CCl.

A related, less reliable formula based on serum creatinine is as follows:

1. Maintain the same dosage (in milligrams).
2. Increase the interdose interval by a factor of patient's serum creatinine ÷ normal serum creatinine.

The above fixed-dose, increased interval regimen is less nephrotoxic in dogs and is preferred over the alternate choice of dose reduction at constant interval.

Several other variables may exist in canine patients with pre-existing renal disease. Acute canine glomerulonephritis and possibly other renal diseases are associated with an increased volume of drug distribution, resulting in subtherapeutic levels of gentamicin at normal doses. Correction for this factor is not possible on a clinical basis. Patients with pyelonephritis are at risk to develop nephrotoxicosis possibly due to a local synergism between bacterial toxins and gentamicin. Therapy of pyelonephritis with gentamicin may be unrewarding, since higher gentamicin concentrations exist in the renal cortical tissue, and infection is predominantly medullary. It is evident that alternative antibiotic choices should be considered in patients with pre-existing renal disease because of the many complicating factors present.

Factors associated with drug administration that modulate toxicity include dose, frequency of administration, duration of therapy, and concurrent use of other nephrotoxins. The manufacturer's recommended dose for dogs is 4.4 mg/kg twice the first day, then 4.4 mg/kg once daily thereafter, a regimen that has proven efficacy in lower urinary tract infections. However, available pharmacokinetic data indicate that a dose of 2 to 4 mg/kg repeated every 6 to 8 hours is required to maintain adequate serum levels of the drug for systemic infections. The dose most frequently employed at the UGAVMTH is 2.2 mg/kg subcutaneously repeated every 8 hours. Overdosage, particularly common in small dogs, will lead to nephrotoxicosis, often within a few days of therapy. Increased frequency of dosage has been associated with increased toxicity, and some have recommended once-daily dosing. Once-daily dosing may result in higher levels of gentamicin in bronchopulmonary secretions, fibrin, and interstitial fluid. However, prolonged interdose intervals have been associated with the development of bacteremia. Information available at this time is inadequate to recommend increasing normal interdose intervals.

Increasing the duration of gentamicin therapy increases the likelihood of developing nephrotoxicosis. Development of toxicosis does not commonly occur in canine clinical patients treated with an appropriate dose for less than 5 days. Most frequently, the toxicosis develops after therapy of 5 to 10 days. Consideration of a magic figure of 10 days for safe therapy is thus inaccurate.

Because of the prolonged tissue half-life, prior administration of any aminoglycoside may increase the likelihood of development of nephrotoxicosis. This risk probably diminishes 30 days after cessation of prior treatment. As mentioned previously, furosemide should be avoided in patients treated with gentamicin. Other nephrotoxins, such as amphotericin B or chemotherapeutic agents, may exert synergistic toxicity. Although not yet substantiated in dogs, gentamicin toxicity may be enhanced when used in conjunction with cephalosporins or nonsteroidal anti-inflammatory agents.

Other less toxic aminoglycosides are now being introduced, but their expense may limit their usefulness in veterinary medicine in the near future. Of the commonly used aminoglycosides in veterinary medicine, only streptomycin has limited nephrotoxicity, and development of resistance to this antibiotic renders it a poor therapeutic choice for most infections.

Monitoring Gentamicin Therapy

It is necessary to develop a monitoring scheme, because nephrotoxicosis is gradual in onset, progressive through several stages, and occurs unpredictably. Early recognition of toxicosis and withdrawal of the drug will improve the prognosis.

Serum aminoglycoside determinations and measurement of renal excretion of enzymes and β_2-microglobulin have been used in human medicine and experimental studies. Though useful, they do not replace measurements commonly available to veterinarians, namely serial urinalyses and determinations of BUN and serum creatinine.

The most reliable monitoring method is serial urinalyses with careful examination of urinary sediment, preferably in a quantitative manner, for the presence of casts. Urinalyses should be performed before initiation of gentamicin therapy in order to establish a baseline, and they should be repeated every other day throughout gentamicin administration. Any increase in the number of casts suggests that a significant number of nephrons have progressed through stage II (proximal tubular cell death), and gentamicin therapy should be discontinued in favor of a less toxic antibiotic. The presence of proteinuria heralds the development of significant nephrotoxicosis but may also be due to contamination during urine collection. The presence of normoglycemic glucosuria is a reliable indicator of toxicosis, and the drug should be withdrawn. Once there is an indication of toxicosis, the antibiotic should be discontinued. The patient should be maintained in a well-hydrated state. Diuresis is probably of little benefit. Continued monitoring will be essential, since toxicosis will continue to progress for several days after discontinuation of gentamicin because of persisting high renal cortical concentrations.

Uncommonly, the urinalysis of a dog progressing rapidly to stage III (reduction in GFR) may not show the abnormalities noted above. This is believed to be because of a rapid shutdown in glomerular filtration; consequently, tubular casts, protein, and other solutes will not reach the urine. In these patients, identification of toxicosis may only be possible by serial measurements of serum creatinine and BUN. In all other patients, use of the urine sediment examination is more reliable and will detect toxicosis several days earlier than determinations of serum creatinine and BUN.

Even if toxicosis was not evident during gentamicin administration, the dog should be monitored after discontinuation of therapy, since nephrotoxicosis is often not evident until this time. Determination of serum creatinine or BUN concentrations every 2 to 3 days for 7 days is an adequate monitoring program once the drug has been discontinued.

PROTECTION

Recently, efforts have turned to measures that will protect patients from nephrotoxicosis. Dietary sodium, potassium, and calcium loading and thyroid hormone administration have shown some promise, but further investigation will be necessary before the clinical use of these agents can be advocated.

References and Supplemental Reading

Brown, S. A., Barsanti, J. A., and Crowell, W. A.: Gentamicin associated acute renal failure in the dog. J.A.V.M.A. 186:686, 1985.

Raisbeck, M. F., Hewitt, W. R., and McIntyre, W. B.: Fatal gentamicin nephrotoxicosis associated with furosemide and gentamicin therapy in a dog. J.A.V.M.A. 183:892, 1983.

Riviere, J. E., and Davis L. E.: Renal handling of drugs in renal failure. In Bovee, K. C. (ed.): *Canine Nephrology*. Philadelphia: Harwal Publishing, 1984, pp. 643–685.

Riviere, J. E., Traver, D. S., and Coppoc, G. L.: Gentamicin toxic nephropathy in horses with disseminated bacterial infection. J.A.V.M.A. 180:648, 1982.

Schentag, J. J.: Aminoglycoside pharmacokinetics as a guide to therapy and toxicology. *In* Whelton, A., and Neu, H. C. (eds.): *The Aminoglycosides*. New York: Marcel Dekker, 1982, pp. 143–168.

BACTEREMIA OF URINARY TRACT ORIGIN (UROSEPSIS)

JEANNE A. BARSANTI, D.V.M.,
and DELMAR R. FINCO, D.V.M.
Athens, Georgia

There are two potentially life-threatening complications of urinary tract infection (UTI): chronic renal failure secondary to chronic pyelonephritis and bacteremia. In human medicine, the urinary tract, when infected, is recognized as the most common site of origin of transient or intermittent bacteremias. In one study in veterinary medicine, the skin and urinary tract were the most frequent sites of origin of bacteremia (Calvert and Greene, 1984). The purpose of this article is to review some of the literature on bacteremia associated with UTI in both veterinary and human medicine and to review the pathophysiology, signs, and management of UTI.

PATHOPHYSIOLOGY

A transient bacteremia can arise from manipulation of infected tissues during procedures such as urinary catheterization or during tissue manipulation such as prostatic massage or urinary tract surgery. These bacteria are usually efficiently cleared from the blood by phagocytes of the reticuloendothelial system. Often no signs result, but in some humans and animals, tremors and fever occur 30 to 90 minutes after the procedure. An intermittent bacteremia may also occur with chronic UTI, especially if it is associated with partial obstruction or urine stasis.

The possible consequences of such bacteremias include septic shock, endocarditis, and abscess formation in other parts of the body. Sepsis in which the organism arises from the urinary tract (urosepsis) occurs in about 20 per cent of persons who become bacteremic from UTI. Signs of sepsis usually develop 12 to 18 hours after bacteremia begins. Sepsis results in death in approximately 10 per cent of persons who become bacteremic from UTI (Bryan and Reynolds, 1984). Most of these individuals also have severe underlying disease such as neoplasia, diabetes mellitus, or liver or renal failure.

Approximately 5 to 10 per cent of humans with bacteremia from UTI develop abscesses or foci of infection in bone, brain, liver, or lungs. The most frequent site of spread in humans is the skeleton (60 per cent), with the heart second (30 per cent) (Siroky et al., 1976). The latency period from an episode of bacteremia to obvious bone lesions is a mean of 54 days. The most common type of skeletal infection in humans and dogs is diskospondylitis, which has been associated with dissemination of bacteria from a distant site, often the urinary tract. In one survey, 10 of 23 dogs with diskospondylitis had positive urine cultures and five of these had the same organism isolated from urine and blood or disk space (Kornegay and Barber, 1980). One of the dogs had recurrent staphylococcal cystitis prior to radiographic diagnosis of diskospondylitis.

Traumatized uroepithelium loses its ability to resist bacterial invasion. Bacteria can enter the systemic circulation through an injured bladder or urethral wall, from a diseased prostate, or from a diseased kidney. Damage to the urinary tract can occur through chemical injury (e.g., cyclophosphamide), trauma (e.g., catheterization), pressure (e.g., retrograde urethrography or cystography with the bladder distended, urethral or ureteral obstruction), or from infection alone. Infection of the renal pelvis, especially when associated with calculi, has been postulated to result in bacteremia through microruptures of urothelium and movement of infected urine into the renal parenchyma. Interestingly, bacteremia was not found after cystocentesis in children with UTI, although numbers sampled and number of blood samples checked were small (Mustonen and Uhari, 1978).

In one survey of dogs, the kidney and prostate were the most frequent sites of UTI to result in septicemia. Dogs receiving glucocorticoids were especially susceptible. In one experimental study in healthy dogs, bacteremia resulted from injection of *Escherichia coli* under pressure into the prostatic urethra (Barsanti et al., 1982). We have had dogs with bacterial prostatitis become septicemic after prostatic massage or aspiration. We have also noted death from sepsis in a cat after urethral catheterization and perineal urethrostomy. In humans, bacteremia most commonly results from lower urinary tract infection associated with indwelling catheterization of the urinary bladder, with partial urethral obstruction related to prostatic disease, or with transurethral prostatic resection.

In urosepsis, the UTI precedes the bacteremia, and the same organism is isolated from urine and blood. The organisms involved are usually gram-negative. Bacteriuria may also develop subsequent to bacteremia through renal embolization of bacteria or through a currently unknown mechanism in which bacteria enter urine from blood in the absence of gross or microscopic renal lesions. The organism usually implicated is *Staphylococcus aureus*. *S. aureus* can also cause UTI that may result in bacteremia. Whether bacteriuria or bacteremia develops first when *S. aureus* is the causative organism can be difficult to determine without sequential cultures and a thorough history.

CAUSATIVE ORGANISMS

The most common causative organisms in human UTI are gram-negative rods; their order of frequency is as follows: *E. coli*, *Klebsiella* or *Enterobacter*, *Proteus*, and *Pseudomonas*. *E. coli* is most frequent in both community- and hospital-acquired bacteremic UTI. It is the most likely organism to enter blood from urine. Combination *Klebsiella* and *Enterobacter* infections most frequently occur in patients on antibiotic therapy and in those with obstructive urinary tract disease. *Proteus* infections occur most frequently as chronic infections associated with obstructive disease, chronic catheterization, or repeated antibiotic therapy. *Pseudomonas* infections occur either in patients who have had repeated surgery or catheterization or in those who have obstructive disease. *Pseudomonas* is a particularly common hospital pathogen, since it can survive in water, antiseptic solutions, and certain antimicrobials, such as penicillin.

Gram-positive organisms and anaerobes in the urinary tract also can cause bacteremia but do so less frequently with gram-negative bacteria. Gram-positive bacteremias are less life-threatening than gram-negative ones. Anaerobes are the least common and are usually associated with severe obstructive disease or abscessation.

The same genera (*E. coli*, *Proteus*, *Staphylococcus*) are the most common causes of UTI in small animals. We have noted a trend toward infection with *Klebsiella* and *Pseudomonas* in dogs with chronic indwelling bladder catheters, even when closed systems are used. Two of the most common organisms associated with sepsis in dogs are also staphylococci and *E. coli* (Calvert and Greene, 1984).

CLINICAL SIGNS

The most common signs associated with acute bacteremia are fever and tremors. Other signs include depression, anorexia, nausea, hyperventilation, and diarrhea. Signs of lower UTI, such as dysuria, are often absent in humans and in dogs. Hypotension develops with septic shock. Signs of metastatic infection are referable to the organ involved (e.g., spinal pain with diskospondylitis).

At laboratory evaluation, leukocytosis may be present. With sepsis, the white blood cell count may initially rise and then fall, resulting in leukopenia. Acidemia, prerenal azotemia, electrolyte abnormalities, hypoglycemia, and coagulation defects associated with disseminated intravascular coagulation (DIC) can also be found in a septic animal.

Upon urinalysis, hematuria, proteinuria, pyuria, and bacteriuria indicate UTI. In an animal with suspected sepsis, a urinalysis should always be performed. If urinalysis results suggest UTI, a urine culture as well as blood cultures are indicated. To confirm a diagnosis of urosepsis, blood and urine should contain the same organism. The diagnosis is often difficult to confirm, since the bacteremia may be intermittent and blood cultures at any one time may be negative.

If the urinary tract is suspected as the site of origin of the bacteremia, the underlying cause of the UTI should be investigated. Survey and contrast radiography are indicated to identify calculi or anatomic abnormalities.

MANAGEMENT

When a dog or cat presents with septicemia or bacteremia, a urinalysis should be performed. If UTI is suspected on the basis of the urinalysis or in any animal in which the cause of sepsis is undetermined, a culture of a properly collected urine sample is indicated. Treatment of sepsis includes fluid therapy, antimicrobials, glucocorticoids, and in some cases management for DIC with anticoagulants such as heparin. Treatment of sepsis has recently been reviewed (Hardie and Rawlings, 1983). Antimicrobial therapy should be based on culture and sensitivity tests once these are returned. Pending culture results, therapy should be started with bactericidal antibiotics. Our usual first choices are intravenous ampicillin or cephalosporins because, unlike the aminoglycosides, they are not nephrotoxic. However, if *Pseudomonas* is suspected, gentamicin or carbenicillin or both are required. In one study in humans, patient outcome was not related to initial antimicrobial choice but was related to appropriate antibiotic therapy once the causative organism was identified. Veterinarians must remember that no antimicrobial agent is effective against all pathogens. Thus, placing an animal on antibiotics does not prevent all infections. In fact, antibiotic use will select resistant bacteria and encourage transfer of resistance. Use of antimicrobials is most important in treatment of sepsis, but a specific diagnosis based on cultures is important to guide antimicrobial choice.

Effort should be made to identify and correct the underlying urinary tract disorder that predisposed the patient to UTI, such as uroliths, abscessation, anatomic defects, inability to urinate, or obstructive lesions. Animals that become septic during indwelling or intermittent bladder catheterization should have the urine cultured at the time bacteremia is identified, even if previous cultures have been performed, since organisms associated with bladder catheterization change frequently, even in the same animal.

Animals with UTI or prostatic infection that are to have surgery should have the causative organism and its antimicrobial sensitivity identified before surgery if time allows. Also, UTI should be controlled (negative urine cultures while on therapy) before surgery if the patient's condition permits. If not, parenteral antibiotic therapy should be begun a few hours prior to surgery and continued for 48 hours thereafter.

References and Supplemental Reading

Barsanti, J. A., Crowell, W. A., Finco, D. R., et al.: Induction of chronic bacterial prostatitis in the dog. J. Urol. 127:1215, 1982.

Bryan, C. S., and Reynolds, K. L.: Community-acquired bacteremic urinary tract infection: Epidemiology and outcome. J. Urol. 132:490, 1984.

Bryan, C. S., and Reynolds, K. L.: Hospital-acquired urinary tract infection: Epidemiology and outcome. J. Urol. 132:494, 1984.

Calvert, C. A., and Greene, C. E.: Cardiovascular infections. *In* Greene, C. E. (ed.): *Clinical Microbiology and Infectious Diseases of the Dog and Cat.* Philadelphia: W. B. Saunders, 1984, pp. 220–237.

Hardie, E. M., and Rawlings, C. A.: Septic Shock. II. Prevention, recognition, and treatment. Comp. Cont. Ed. Pract. Vet. 5:483, 1983.

Kornegay, J. N., and Barber, D. L.: Diskospondylitis in dogs. J.A.V.M.A. 177:337, 1980.

Mustonen, A., and Uhari, M.: Is there bacteremia after suprapubic aspiration in children with urinary tract infection? J. Urol. 119:822, 1978.

Riff, L. J.: Bacteremia arising from the urinary tract. Urol. Clin. North Am. 2:521, 1975.

Siroky, M. B., Moylan, R. A., Austen, G., et al.: Metastatic infection secondary to genitourinary tract sepsis. Am. J. Med. 61:351, 1976.

PARASITES OF THE URINARY TRACT

SCOTT A. BROWN, V.M.D.,
and ANNIE K. PRESTWOOD, D.V.M.
Athens, Georgia

Three species of nematode parasites—*Capillaria plica*, *Capillaria feliscati*, and *Dioctophyma renale*—infect the urinary tracts of domesticated small animals. Infections are often asymptomatic and may be discovered incidentally through the identification of ova in the urine sediment. Appropriate management and therapeutic measures are dependent on an understanding of the life cycle and pathogenicity of these parasites.

Capillaria plica

C. plica infects the urinary bladder of the dog, wolf, fox, raccoon, otter, marten, and badger. The fox and raccoon may be the natural hosts, and there are reported prevalences of 23.5 per cent in wild foxes in the Netherlands and more than 50 per cent in raccoons in the southeastern United States. The adults are threadlike and yellow, reaching a length of 60 mm. This trichurid nematode has a widespread geographic distribution. The prevalence may exceed 75 per cent in certain kennel situations where soil or grass surfaces are employed.

The bipolar ova of *C. plica* (Fig. 1) are passed in the urine and embryonate. Ova containing the first-stage larva are ingested by earthworms and develop to the infective stage. Ingestion of the infected earthworm will result in a patent infection in dogs in 61 to 88 days. Other intermediate hosts have been postulated but not yet identified.

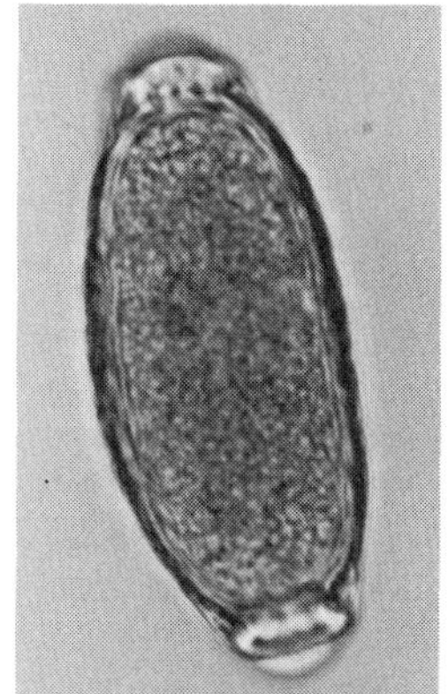

Figure 1. *Capillaria plica* ovum (63 μm × 27 μm). Note the bipoplar plugs.

C. plica adults invade the renal pelvis, urinary bladder, and ureteral submucosa, producing a mild superficial inflammatory response. Clinical signs in dogs are rare. In cases of heavy infestations, clinical signs of cystitis with dysuria and pollakiuria may be present. Secondary bacterial cystitis is uncommon. Infection with this parasite should be considered in cases of chronic cystitis unresponsive to antibiotics.

Diagnosis relies on finding the characteristic ova in the urine sediment of affected dogs. Pyuria and hematuria are common findings. If urine is obtained by cystocentesis, fecal contamination from inadvertent rectal puncture may yield a false-positive result due to *Trichuris vulpis* ova. There is no information available on the prevalence of occult infection.

Control of this parasite in kennels in which a high prevalence exists relies on discontinuation of the use of soil and grass surfaces. Sand, gravel, and concrete are alternatives.

The infection is usually self-limiting, since affected animals will often develop negative ovum counts if held in isolation for 12 weeks. Occasionally an affected dog will maintain a prolonged patent infection despite these control measures. If clinical signs are present, anthelmintic therapy may be considered. Successful treatment has been reported with fenbendazole (50 mg/kg daily for 3 to 10 days). Albendazole (50 mg/kg b.i.d. for 10 to 14 days) is an alternative, although it frequently causes anorexia at this dose.

Capillaria feliscati

C. feliscati is a trichurid nematode that infects the bladder of the domestic cat. It has been reported in North and South America, Europe, Africa, and Australia. The adults are small threadlike worms; females range from 28 to 45 mm in length and males reach 13 to 30 mm. Identification of the adults may be difficult with the unaided eye. Details of the life cycle are unknown.

The adult worms are found in the urinary bladder, partially embedded in the superficial bladder wall. There is a very mild inflammatory response seen on histologic examination.

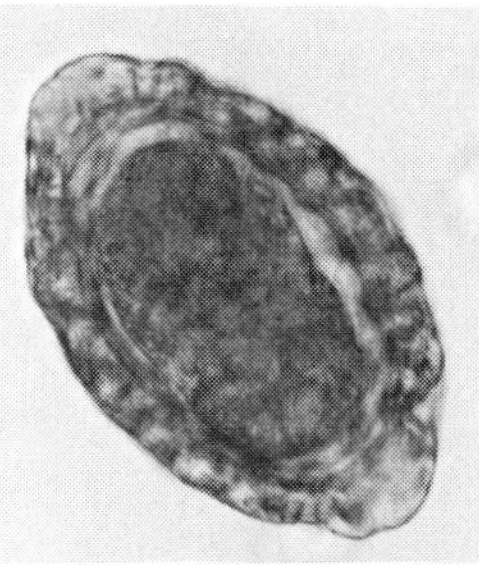

Figure 2. *Dioctophyma renale* ovum (74 μm × 46 μm). Note the absence of mammillations at the poles. The ova are brownish-yellow in color.

Clinical signs are usually absent, although stranguria, hematuria, and dysuria have been attributed to the parasite. Affected cats rarely develop bacterial cystitis.

Affected cats are almost always older than 8 months. Reports in Australia indicate an 18 to 34 per cent prevalence of infection. However, reports of this parasite have been uncommon in the United States.

Diagnosis requires identification of either the adults in the urinary bladder or the ova passed in the urine. The ova are present in the urine sediment of most, if not all, affected cats. Ova are similar morphologically to those of *C. plica*, measuring 50 to 68 μm long by 22 to 32 μm wide. Urine contamination of feces may result in a positive fecal result.

Treatment is not necessary unless clinical signs are present. Successful treatment has been reported with methyridine (200 mg/kg orally, single dose), which is unavailable in this country. One case responded to levamisole, but potential toxicosis limits the use of this agent in cats. Fenbendazole (25 mg/kg b.i.d. for 3 to 10 days) has been suggested as an alternate treatment.

Dioctophyma renale

D. renale parasitizes the kidneys of dogs. It has also been reported to afflict cats, pigs, horses, mink, and humans. It is the largest known nematode. In dogs, females may reach a length of more than 100 cm and males, 45 cm. In mink, the natural definitive host, adult worms are smaller, generally 15 to 45 cm in length. The parasite has a worldwide distribution and has been reported in most states. The prevalence rate is very low, although several dogs in the same environment may be affected.

Unembryonated ova are passed in the urine of hosts with infected kidneys (Fig. 2). The first-stage larva develops within the ovum over 1 to 7 months and is resistant to environmental factors. The ovum may persist in the environment for 2 to 5 years. The larvated ovum is ingested by the intermediate host, an aquatic oligochaete annelid *Lumbriculus variegatus*, in which the first-stage larva develops into an infective third-stage larva in 2 to 3 months. The annelid is then ingested by a definitive or a paratenic host. Fish (catfish, pike, and others) and frogs are the most common paratenic hosts. The third-stage larvae encyst in muscles and viscera of the transport host. After the infective larvae are ingested, either directly or through a paratenic host, the larvae rapidly excyst and penetrate the stomach wall (within 1 hour), at which time vomiting has been noted experimentally. The larvae migrate to the liver, where they remain for approximately 50 days, when they undergo their final migration to the kidney or peritoneal cavity. Ova appear in the urine 3.5 to 6 months after ingestion of the infective larvae. Adult worms may live for 1 to 3 years. The entire life cycle requires as much as 2 years.

Although the parasite has been reported in the urinary bladder, urethra, ovary, uterus, and pericardium, it most commonly is located in the peritoneal cavity or kidneys. More than 75 per cent of canine infections involve the peritoneal cavity, frequently as the only site (60 per cent). Forty per cent of the time kidney infection is present, with a predilection for the right kidney by a 7:1 factor. Simultaneous left and right kidney infections occur less than 3 per cent of the time. The teleologic advantage to the parasite of avoiding bilateral renal infections with resultant renal failure in the host is apparent. The predilection for the right kidney remains an unexplained phenomenon. Explanations offered include the proximity of the right kidney to the liver and duodenum, both potential access points for migrating larvae to reach the right kidney. However, the homing mechanism may involve more than anatomic clues, since larvae placed free in the abdominal cavity preferentially penetrate the right renal parenchyma. Parasites found free in the peritoneal cavity frequently occupy the fossa between the right kidney and caudate lobe of the liver.

Dogs may be an abnormal host, as witnessed by the number of "dead-end" infections involving a single parasite, a single sex, or infection not involving the kidneys. In the mink, the natural definitive host, the parasite has an 85 per cent prevalence for right kidney infection alone.

Clinical signs are usually absent unless there is bilateral renal infection or unilateral infection with concurrent disease in the contralateral kidney, in which case signs compatible with the degree of renal insufficiency will be encountered. Ascites and hemoperitoneum have been reported rarely. Gross hematuria and associated dysuria due to blood clots may be seen. Signs referable to an abnormal site of infection may be present.

Diagnosis depends on demonstration of ova in the urine sediment, although these will be found only if gravid females are present in a kidney (40 per cent or less of affected dogs). Urinalysis may demonstrate hematuria, proteinuria, and pyuria in addition to ova. Because of the high prevalence of infections involving only the peritoneal cavity, abdominocentesis and peritoneal lavage have been used to identify affected animals in some cases. Eosinophilia, basophilia, and hyperglobulinemia are usually noted in affected dogs, regardless of site of infection. Despite marked gross and histopathologic hepatic changes, liver function and enzymes are generally unaffected. An excretory urogram will localize the affected kidneys. Hydronephrosis or a contracted remnant kidney may be seen. Pyelonephritis has been reported in affected kidneys; consequently, antibiotics where indicated by urine culture and sensitivity tests should be instituted. The pelvic mucosa of infected kidneys undergoes metaplastic change to a stratified squamous epithelium. Connective tissue metaplasia resulting in bone formation and calcification is frequent and is occasionally apparent radiographically.

The only definitive therapy is surgical. If renal infection is present, nephrectomy (nephrotomy for bilateral infections) is indicated. Marked peritonitis due to the inflammatory response to ova and excretory products of the worms will be present. Masses of ova embedded in granulation tissue with reactive mesothelium may be found within the abdominal cavity. Adhesions make the performance of a nephrectomy technically difficult. A complete exploratory operation to identify and remove all parasites is imperative.

Control is difficult. Prevention of ingestion of raw fish and frogs may be beneficial, but ingestion of water from an infected area may also be a concern. Although uncommon, infections of humans have been reported, and the parasite remains a public health concern.

References and Supplemental Reading

Gillespie, D.: Successful treatment of canine *Capillaria plica* cystitis V.M./S.A.C. 78:682, 1983.

Harris, L. T.: Feline bladderworm. V.M./S.A.C. 76:844, 1981.

Mace, T. F., and Anderson, R. C.: Development of the giant kidney worm, *Dioctophyma renale*. Can. J. Zool. 53:1552, 1975.

Osborne, C. A., Stevens, J. B., Hanlon, G. F., et al.: *Dioctophyma renale* in the dog. J.A.V.M.A. 155:605, 1969.

Senior, D. F., Solomon, G. B., Goldschmidt, M. H., et al.: *Capillaria plica* infection in dogs. J.A.V.M.A. 176:901, 1980.

Waddell, A. H.: Further observations on *Capillaria feliscati* infections in the cat. Aust. Vet. J. 44, 33, 1968.

URINARY TRACT TRAUMA

ROBERT D. ZENOBLE, D.V.M.,
Auburn, Alabama

and ROBERT D. PECHMAN, JR., D.V.M.
Baton Rouge, Louisiana

Urinary tract injuries occur frequently in dogs and cats after severe blunt trauma, usually caused by motor vehicles. Approximately 25 per cent of dogs with traumatic pelvic injuries are found to have urinary tract injuries. In a prospective study of dogs suffering pelvic trauma, 40 per cent showed evidence of urinary tract injury, including self-limiting mucosal hemorrhage (Selcer, 1982). Urologic injuries in the acutely traumatized patient are usually overshadowed by more obvious orthropedic and soft tissue injuries. The clinician must be an accurate observer and investigate the urinary system when certain subtle signs are noted. If the possibility of damage to the urinary system is considered from the outset and the diagnosis is pursued, an early assessment can be made before severe metabolic complications arise. Urinary tract injury should be considered when fractures of the caudal ribs, vertebrae, or pelvis are seen in survey radiographs. Less commonly, urologic injuries result without orthopedic injuries or from penetrating wounds of the abdomen. Because signs of urologic injury are often vague and overshadowed by more obvious injuries, investigation of the urinary tract should be based on history, magnitude, and location of the traumatic injuries rather than on specific signs.

Diagnosis and treatment of traumatic injuries of the urinary system must not take precedence over treatment of shock, respiratory distress, or ongoing hemorrhage. Many urologic injuries are mild and self-limiting; even potentially fatal urologic injuries do not require emergency correction. Leakage of urine into the peritoneal cavity, retroperitoneal space, or pelvic and perineal tissues is not rapidly fatal. The extravasation of sterile urine is relatively harmless for 24 to 36 hours. Experimentally, death occurs about 3 days after urinary bladder rupture in dogs (Bjorling, 1984), and total nephrectomy in dogs results in death after 3 to 6 days.

The most common severe traumatic urinary tract injury is a ruptured urinary bladder. This is typically associated with pelvic fractures. Traumatic urinary bladder rupture occurs equally in male and female dogs that sustain severe pelvic trauma (Selcer, 1982). Ruptures can occur at any location on the bladder, but the most common site for traumatic rupture is in the fundic region. Rupture of the bladder can also result from forceful digital compression of a distended inflamed bladder during an attempt to dislodge a urethral obstruction in a dog or cat. Other causes of bladder rupture are falls from heights, any forceful blow to the abdomen, penetrating wounds of the abdomen, and forceful bladder catheterization. A displaced or herniated urinary bladder may occur in male or female patients. Although there is no leakage of urine into a body cavity with urinary bladder herniation, there is usually total urinary outflow obstruction resulting in severe postrenal azotemia. The bladder usually herniates through the abdominal musculature and is noted as an undefined subcutaneous mass. Additionally, the bladder cannot be palpated in its normal position in the caudal abdomen (Bjorling, 1984).

Rupture of the urethra occurs most commonly in male dogs with pelvic fractures. Less common causes of urethral rupture include bite wounds, gunshot injuries, and forceful catheterization of obstructed male cats. Dysuria, stranguria, and local swelling after trauma suggest the need to investigate the lower urinary tract.

Traumatic injuries to the kidneys are not common. The kidneys are mobile, surrounded by fat, and covered by a thin, fibrous capsule. They are protected by the rib cage, lumbar musculature, and spine. Bruising and ecchymoses are the most common renal lesions resulting from trauma. Transient hematuria may occur, but bleeding stops spontaneously and the subcapsular blood is absorbed. A hematoma occurs when the fibrous capsule is torn and blood accumulates in the perinephric area. Bleeding usually stops spontaneously, and the noninfected hematoma is eventually absorbed without impairment of renal function. A laceration of the renal parenchyma can occur from severe blunt trauma. If the tear involves the renal hilus and pelvis, extravasation of both blood and urine into the retroperitoneal space ensues. Marked hematuria occurs. Severe injury to other abdominal organs is common in such cases and often warrants exploratory laparotomy.

Blunt trauma causing injury to the ureters is rare in dogs and cats. The site of injury is usually close to the kidney or near the bladder. A severed ureter may allow urine to empty directly into the peritoneal cavity. If the avulsion is unilateral and there are no other urologic injuries, recognition of the problem awaits signs of peritonitis. The degree of azotemia will be modest because of the remaining functional kidney.

DIAGNOSIS OF UROLOGIC INJURIES

The likelihood of urologic injuries is related more to the history and the extent of trauma than to any specific physical finding. Physical abnormalities that suggest urologic injury are limited. A subcutaneous fluid-filled mass could be a herniated bladder. The intact urinary bladder should be filled with urine and readily palpable after emergency stabilization of the patient with fluid therapy. Inability to identify the bladder by palpation could suggest underhydration, oliguria, or a displaced or ruptured bladder. Distention of the bladder without passage of urine can result from disruption of the urethra. Accumulation of urine in the peritoneal cavity will usually cause abdominal tenderness, fever, malaise, and vomiting in 24 to 72 hours. The spontaneous passage of urine does not rule out the possibility of a ruptured bladder or laceration of the urethra. A ruptured bladder may be overlooked because a patient voids urine or urine is returned through a catheter. Urine may be collected from a bladder with a laceration or urine may be collected directly from the abdominal cavity if the urinary catheter passes through the torn bladder. A positive contrast cystogram or urethrogram must be performed if the integrity of the bladder or urethra is in doubt.

No routine clinical pathologic finding can substantiate a disruption of the urinary tract. Although azotemia usually accompanies urinary tract disruption, it is nonlocalizing and is often encountered with severe metabolic disorder (previous renal disease, hypovolemia, dehydration). Hematuria secondary to mucosal hemorrhage is the most common finding in urinary tract injury and often resolves spontaneously. In contrast, severe injuries such as a ruptured bladder can be present without hematuria. The presence of free urine in the abdominal cavity indicates disruption of the urinary tract. Abdominal paracentesis with a syringe and needle may retrieve fluid, but the use of a peritoneal dialysis catheter is more accurate in the detection of intra-abdominal fluid. Abdominal paracentesis and diagnostic peritoneal lavage will not detect retroperitoneal urine accumulation. To determine if peritoneal fluid contains urine, the urea nitrogen and creatinine of the fluid must be compared with those from the patient's plasma. The urea molecule is small and rapidly equilibrates by diffusion across the peritoneal membranes. In contrast, the creatinine molecule is larger and is slowly removed from the peritoneal cavity. When urine freely enters the abdominal cavity, the concentration of both urea and creatinine of the abdominal fluid are greatly elevated. However, urea rapidly diffuses into the circulation, and the peritoneal fluid and plasma concentration of urea will be similar. The creatinine concentration in the urine-contaminated peritoneal fluid will be approximately twice that of the plasma concentration. When urine is detected in peritoneal fluid, the source must be identified (Bjorling, 1984; Burrows and Bovee, 1974).

RADIOGRAPHIC SIGNS OF URINARY TRACT TRAUMA

Plain radiographs are rarely diagnostic of urinary tract injury. Orthopedic injuries in the areas of the urinary tract raise the index of suspicion for urologic injury. Radiographic signs that strongly suggest urinary tract injury include the following: nonvisualization, displacement, or asymmetry of one or both kidneys; increased density in the sublumbar region; loss of normal intra-abdominal contrast; and reduced size or absence of the urinary bladder shadow (Pechman, 1982).

Renal shadows may appear asymmetric as a result of rupture of the kidney and its capsule or intracapsular hemorrhage or urine accumulation due to renal parenchymal injury. The kidneys and colon may be displaced from their normal positions if there is hemorrhage or extravasted urine in the retroperitoneal space. Nonvisualization of the kidney shadows can be caused by retroperitoneal fluid accumulation. Retroperitoneal fluid also produces increased opacity of the retroperitoneal space. Streaky, hazy, irregularly shaped areas of increased opacity in the retroperitoneal space, with or without ventral displacement of the colon or effacement of the kidney margins, are highly suggestive of upper urinary tract injury.

Normal intra-abdominal contrast will be reduced by fluid accumulation within the peritoneal cavity. Serosal surfaces of abdominal organs, normally seen because of the natural contrast with intra-abdominal fat, are not well seen when fluid of any sort accumulates in the abdomen. Abdominal fluid can be associated with injuries to organs other than those of the urinary system, but urinary tract injury should be considered whenever abdominal fluid is recognized in a traumatized patient. Urinary bladder rupture, ureteral rupture near the bladder trigone, and urethral rupture may lead to fluid accumulation in the peritoneal cavity.

Nonvisualization of the urinary bladder or marked reduction in the size of this organ may be noted with urinary system trauma. When either sign is noted, along with signs of intra-abdominal fluid, a ruptured urinary bladder or other traumatic injury of the lower urinary system is strongly suggested. Abdominocentesis and fluid analysis must be attempted to substantiate the presence of urine outside the urinary tract.

Contrast examination of the urinary system will dramatically increase the accuracy of diagnosis of urinary system trauma. Urinary contrast studies are the most reliable noninvasive method of establishing the exact site, nature, and extent of the traumatic injury to the urinary tract.

CONTRAST EXAMINATION OF THE URINARY SYSTEM

The urinary system is quickly and easily accessible to evaluation by radiographic contrast examinations. This is particularly important in traumatized patients, as significant data can be gained without resorting to complex or time-consuming procedures. With excretory urography, cystography, and urethrography, the entire urinary system can be examined to determine the nature and extent of the urinary system injury.

Excretory Urography

A variety of techniques for excretory urography are available: slow drip infusion of a high dose of contrast material; slow injection of contrast material; and rapid injection of contrast material. All these techniques involve intravenous administration of aqueous organic iodide contrast agents. Rapid administration of high doses of contrast media is the method of choice for examination of the upper urinary system. A contrast dosage of iodine (880 mg/kg) will yield the best results. Any of a wide variety of organic iodide contrast agents suitable for intravascular use can be used. The time after injection that radiographs are made is important in evaluation of the upper urinary system. Recommended times are as follows: immediately postinjection to observe a nephrogram; 5 minutes postinjection to best observe the ureters; 20 minutes postinjection to observe the renal pelvis and ureters; and 40 minutes postinjection to best observe the renal pelvic diverticula. These times are appropriate under most circumstances; however, to reach an accurate diagnosis in a traumatized patient it is rarely necessary to make radiographs beyond 20 minutes postinjection. Abdominal compression devices may improve visualization of the upper urinary structures, but these devices are not needed in traumatized patients and may be contraindicated.

Ventrodorsal and recumbent lateral projections should be made throughout the course of the excretory urogram. The ventrodorsal view is usually the most helpful projection, since both kidneys and ureters will be seen without the superimposition of upper urinary tract structures as occurs in lateral views. Oblique projections can be helpful in some cases to improve definition of the site of a urinary tract injury. Although familiarity with the normal appearance of an organ or structure is always important in radiographic interpretation, most traumatic injuries of the urinary system are readily apparent; it is usually not necessary to search for subtle anatomic alterations from normal to arrive at a diagnosis of traumatic injury of the upper urinary system.

Extravasation of contrast material is the most common finding on excretory urograms of patients with upper urinary tract trauma. Contrast material may accumulate diffusely within the renal capsule if there is parenchymal injury with an intact renal capsule. If the renal capsule is also disrupted, contrast will accumulate in the retroperitoneal space. Laceration of the renal pelvis or proximal ureter also results in contrast accumulation in the retroperitoneal space. The location and nature of the injury is, in most cases, easily identified. Rupture of the distal portions of the ureters may lead to contrast accumulation in the retroperitoneal space or within the peritoneal cavity, depending on the exact site of ureter injury. The traumatized ureter proximal to the site of the rupture and the renal pelvis on the affected side will be enlarged.

Nonvisualization of a kidney on an excretory urogram of a traumatized patient may indicate disruption of the renal vascular pedicle. Renal arteriography is the contrast study of choice to evaluate the blood supply to the kidney. This need not be a complex selective procedure but may be performed by rapidly injecting a bolus of contrast medium into a large vein and making two or three radiographs at 5- or 6-second intervals after the start of the injection. In many cases, this technique will permit an evaluation of the renal vascular pedicle.

Cystography

Contrast cystography can be performed by using negative, positive, or double contrast techniques (see also article entitled Cystography). Positive contrast cystography is the most reliable examination used to evaluate bladder integrity. Bladder integrity may also be determined in the late stages of an excretory urogram; this technique may be helpful in animals that are difficult to catheterize.

Cystography is performed by passing a catheter into the bladder and withdrawing all the urine. If blood clots are present, flushing the bladder with sterile water or saline may aid in their removal. Any of the aqueous organic iodide contrast agents for intravenous administration can be used for cystography. Less expensive agents, specifically for cystography and not suitable for intravenous administration, are equally effective. The contrast medium should be diluted to a final concentration of 10 to 15 per cent prior to instillation into the bladder. The urinary bladder should be fully distended with contrast material, and four views should be made: recumbent lateral, ventrodorsal, and two ventrodorsal obliques. If no resistance to filling of the bladder with contrast material is encountered during the procedure, a lateral radiograph of the abdomen should be made to determine if there is contrast material free in the peritoneal cavity.

Positive contrast cystography in a patient with urinary bladder rupture will show the contrast medium free in the abdominal cavity. The contrast material will coat and outline other abdominal organs. In animals with small perforations of the bladder, free contrast will be seen in the abdomen, and the site of contrast leakage from the bladder may be identified. Mucosal lacerations and separations of the muscular layer of the bladder wall will be identified as convex protrusions of the bladder wall on positive contrast cystograms. Most bladder ruptures occur in the fundic region of the bladder; mucosal lacerations and disruptions of the muscular layers are most common in the same region.

Intraluminal material is less easily identified on positive contrast cystograms. If the positive contrast cystogram is normal, the contrast should be aspirated from the bladder and a negative contrast medium (carbon dioxide or nitrous oxide) introduced into the bladder to produce a double contrast cystogram. Blood clots and the intraluminal solid material will be seen as radiolucent filling defects in the puddle of positive contrast remaining in the bladder.

Urethrography

Positive contrast urethrography is the examination of choice to evaluate urethral injury. Aqueous organic iodide contrast agents should be used. The contrast material should be diluted to 10 to 15 per cent concentration with sterile water or saline. Sterile aqueous lubricant may be used as a diluent but is not necessary for evaluation of traumatic injuries. Air should not be used as a negative contrast agent; urethrocavernous reflux can occur, and embolization of instilled air may be fatal.

Retrograde positive contrast urethrography is performed by placing a balloon-tipped catheter in the urethra and inflating the balloon to prevent contrast reflux. Ten to 20 ml of contrast medium is injected and a radiograph made while the last few milliliters are being injected. Complete urethral evaluation requires a lateral and two ventrodorsal oblique radiographs; in nearly all cases, a lateral view is sufficient to reach a diagnosis.

The most common site of urethral rupture is the urethrovesicle junction. Contrast material will be found in the abdominal or pelvic cavity when urethrography is performed. Urethral trauma at other sites will permit extravasated contrast medium to accumulate in the soft tissues around the site of injury. Urethrocavernous reflux with opacification of pelvic veins and the caudal vena cava by contrast material may be seen in some patients. Areas of urethral stricture can be clearly demonstrated by positive contrast urethrography.

CONCLUSIONS

Evaluation of the urinary tract should progress in an orderly manner. The history and physical examination may suggest injury to the abdominal area. Fractures or abnormal findings on abdominal palpation should be pursued with radiographs. The nature and source of abdominal fluid should be determined by paracentesis and careful evaluation of the fluid obtained. Diagnostic peritoneal lavage will increase the chance of obtaining fluid and cells representative of those present in the abdomen. If continued malaise (depression, nausea, vomiting, anorexia) can be observed 2 to 3 days after urinary tract trauma and is associated with continued or rising azotemia, the urinary tract should be investigated carefully. If urine is present in the abdominal cavity, the urethra and bladder should be examined with retrograde urethrography and cystography. Should contrast studies of the urethra and bladder fail to identify the source of urine entering the abdominal cavity or if survey radiographs indicate the presence of retroperitoneal fluid, excretory urography should be performed. All of these diagnostic tests are not required for evaluation of the urinary tract in every traumatized animal. However, surgical exploration without adequate preoperative examination can be frustrating and does not ensure that the function and integrity of the urinary tract have been satisfactorily assessed.

References and Supplemental Reading

Bjorling, D. E.: The urogenital system. Vet. Clin. North Am. 14:61, 1984.

Burrows, C. F., and Bovee, K. C.: Metabolic changes due to experimentally induced rupture of the canine urinary bladder. Am. J. Vet. Res. 35:1083, 1974.

Pechman, R. D.: Urinary trauma in dogs and cats: A review. J. Am. Anim. Hosp. Assoc. 18:33, 1982.

Selcer, B. A.: Urinary tract trauma associated with pelvic trauma. J. Am. Anim. Hosp. Assoc. 18:75, 1982.

FELINE URINARY INCONTINENCE

JEANNE A. BARSANTI, D.V.M.,
and DELMAR R. FINCO, D.V.M.
Athens, Georgia

This article will present an approach to the medical problem of incontinence in cats. We define incontinence as involuntary passage or leakage of urine. As a basis for understanding treatment recommendations, the normal mechanism of micturition will first be reviewed briefly. Differential diagnoses based on whether or not the bladder is distended are listed. A diagnostic plan will be presented for each of these subcategories. Finally, specific and symptomatic treatments will be recommended.

PHYSIOLOGY OF FELINE MICTURITION

The neuromuscular integration of normal micturition is complex, and only a greatly simplified summary will be presented here in order to coordinate physiology with treatment.

Normal micturition requires storage and emptying phases. During the storage phase, the bladder gradually distends, with little increase in intravesicular pressure. The smooth muscle of the urethral sphincter maintains tone, causing intraurethral pressure to exceed bladder pressure and preventing urine leakage from the bladder. The striated muscle of the urethral sphincter assists in maintaining urethral pressure, especially during stress such as coughing or sneezing. The neuronal control of the storage phase involves both α- and β-adrenergic control. Stimulation of α-adrenergic fibers causes increased tone in the smooth muscle of the urethra, whereas β-adrenergic stimulation facilitates bladder filling by causing relaxation of the detrusor muscle. The hypogastric nerve carries both of these fiber types. The striated urethral muscle that extends distally from the prostate gland is supplied by the pudendal nerve.

The emptying phase begins when stretch receptors in the bladder wall detect bladder fullness. This information is relayed by the pelvic nerves to the sacral spinal cord and then to the brain stem, where higher brain centers can control the voluntary act of micturition. The efferent phase involves impulse transmission back down the spinal cord to the sacral segments. The pelvic nerve (parasympathetic) relays the command to the detrusor muscle to contract. At the same time, the sympathetic input is inhibited, decreasing urethral tone. The striated muscle sphincter of the urethra also relaxes. A voluntary abdominal press and pelvic muscle relaxation may also be involved in initiating urination.

DIAGNOSTIC PLAN

The first step in diagnosing the cause of incontinence in a cat is to obtain a thorough history. One must be sure that the problem is incontinence, a lack of voluntary control of urination, and not inappropriate urination, dysuria, polyuria, or nocturia caused by polyuria. The client should be asked certain questions to obtain as precise a description of the problem as possible. When does the problem occur? What exactly happens? Does the cat urinate voluntarily? Does the cat strain or show any discomfort when urinating or when urine leaks? How long has the problem existed? Is it getting better or worse? Is the cat on any medication? Does the cat have any other abnormal signs? With the problem of incontinence, a precise history is one of the most valuable tools in reaching a diagnosis. If a good history can be obtained, it is possible to determine if incontinence actually exists and to establish its duration, severity, association with any other problem, and whether urination ever occurs normally.

After the history is obtained, a physical examination including a brief neurologic assessment should be performed. This should include evaluation of the perineal reflex, since this reflex involves the sacral spinal cord, as do reflexes involved with urinary continence. If neurologic abnormalities are detected, a complete neurologic examination is indicated to localize the lesion. Further testing such as radiographs, cerebrospinal fluid evaluation, and myelogaphy should be based on lesion localization and most likely differential diagnoses. This article will concentrate on urinary incontinence unassociated with other neurologic abnormalities.

The urinary tract should be carefully palpated, and special attention should be paid to the size of the bladder. If possible, the act of micturition should be observed. The bladder should be repalpated after attempted urination to determine the effectiveness of bladder emptying. Based on the physical examination, the problem of incontinence should be further defined as associated with bladder distention or with an empty bladder.

INCONTINENCE ASSOCIATED WITH A FULL BLADDER

Incontinence associated with a full bladder is due to the overflow of urine from a bladder whose capacity for storage has been exceeded. Such incontinence can be due to failure of stretch receptors in the bladder wall to detect bladder fullness; failure of nerve impulse transmission between the bladder, the sacral spinal cord, and reflex center in the brainstem; or failure of the detrusor muscle to contract or the urethral muscle to relax in response to nerve impulses. Incontinence also occurs in association with partial occlusion of the outflow tract.

Diagnostic Plan

The diagnostic plan for incontinence associated with a full bladder should first be directed toward determining whether urethral obstruction is present. This may require any or all of the following: gentle attempts at bladder expression, attempted passage of a urinary catheter, survey radiography of the urethra, retrograde or antegrade urethrography, and urethral pressure profiles. If an obstruction is found, the cause should be identified and removed if possible. The most common cause in male cats is thought to be a conglomeration of mucus and struvite crystals (feline urologic syndrome). Other causes such as uroliths, neoplasia, connective tissue swelling, or strictures are also possible.

Once an anatomic urethral obstruction is ruled out, in the absence of other neurologic signs, the cause of incontinence with a full bladder may be bladder wall dysfunction (detrusor atony) or urethral dysfunction (reflex dyssynergia). Detrusor dysfunction causes incontinence because intravesicular pressure cannot overcome normal urethral pressure. By contrast, failure of the urethral muscle to relax will prevent voiding of urine in spite of normal detrusor contraction. These can be difficult to differentiate. Determining (1) whether the cat consciously detects bladder fullness and tries to urinate and (2) the degree of urethral resistance to urine flow as the bladder is manually expressed is the only diagnostic method short of sophisticated electrodiagnostic testing. A cystometrogram may be performed in referral centers to determine whether detrusor muscle contraction is normal.

In primary bladder dysfunction, both the afferent and efferent limbs may be affected since they are closely related anatomically. One of the more common causes of detrusor dysfunction is loss of detrusor tight junctions from prolonged overdistention due to urethral obstruction. Other causes include neurologic diseases anywhere along the urinary pathway. The lesion site should be localized by a complete neurologic examination. Some specific causes include trauma, congenital defects as in the Manx cat, neoplasia, infection, or inflammation. One cause of bladder dysfunction described in Great Britain is an autonomic polyganglionopathy, first identified by Key and Gaskell (1982) and now referred to as feline dysautonomia (Sharp et al., 1984; Rochlitz, 1984). The bladder dysfunction in this syndrome consists of apparent inability to contract the bladder in spite of efforts to do so, but the bladder can be easily expressed manually. Other signs such as persistent pupillary dilation, decreased tear production, chronic regurgitation due to megaesophagus, and constipation are more common than bladder atony in this syndrome.

Detrusor-urethral sphincter dyssynergia consists of failure to relax either the smooth or striated urethral sphincter when the detrusor muscle contracts. This is characterized clinically by inability of the cat to empty its bladder in spite of efforts to do so and difficulty in manually expressing urine. Yet no anatomic obstruction can be identified, and detrusor contraction is present on cystometrography. A form of dyssyneregia occurs with neurologic lesions cranial to the sacral segments, and the condition is then referred to as an upper motor neuron bladder. Reflex dyssynergia unassociated with upper motor neuron paralysis has been described briefly in dogs (Oliver, 1983) but has not been well described clinically in cats, although its existence has been referred to in a recent review (Lees and Moreau, 1984). Reflex dyssynergia was described in experimental cats during electrophysiologic testing (Abdel-Rahman et al., 1981). It has been described in humans as associated with various neurologic problems, especially multiple sclerosis (DeGroat and Booth, 1980).

Therapeutic Plan

The therapeutic plan for cats unable to empty their bladders will vary with the cause of the problem. If the cause is an intraluminal or extraluminal urethral obstruction, this obstruction must be removed or bypassed. If the cause is primary detrusor dysfunction, specific treatment is aimed at any identifiable cause of the neurologic dysfunction. If the cause is bladder overdistention or is a neurologic disorder that is not specifically treatable (such as spinal cord trauma, congenital defects, or autonomic polygangionopathy), symptomatic treatment is indicated. The most effective symptomatic treatment is to keep the bladder empty so the tight junctions of the detrusor muscle can reform or be maintained. This can be done by manually expressing urine frequently, by using an indwelling urinary catheter, or by use of cholinergic drugs.

Manually expressing urine several times a day can be used to keep the bladder empty. Use of an α-adrenergic blocking agent such as phenoxybenzamine or a striated muscle relaxant such as diazepam to reduce urethral tone and thus outflow resistance may make bladder emptying easier (Scott and Morrow, 1978). Unfortunately, these drugs have not been evaluated thoroughly for use in cats and should be used cautiously; animals should be observed for possible adverse effects. The recommended dosage of phenoxybenzamine is 0.5 mg/kg orally per day (Moreau, 1982). For most cats, this will be about 2.5 mg. The dosage can be increased gradually by 2.5 mg to a maximum daily dosage of 10 mg (Moreau, 1982). Each dose should be given for approximately 5 days before ineffectiveness is concluded, since the drug's activity is relatively slow in onset. Phenoxybenzamine should not be used in cats with cardiovascular disease, since possible side effects include tachycardia and hypotension. The recommended dose of diazepam is 2.5 to 5.0 mg given 15 to 30 minutes before expression of urine. Diazepam's activity is short in duration, and possible side effects include behavioral changes such as depression. Perineal urethrostomy, a surgical method to reduce urethral resistance, has also been used to manage irreversible bladder dysfunction in a cat (Edwards, 1979). One interesting observation in experimental cats used to study spinal cord injury was that reflex urination stimulated by wetting the perineal area (as occurs in neonatal kittens) returned in cats with spinal cord transection (DeGroat, 1975). This reflex is normally lost as kittens reach 7 to 12 weeks of age and is replaced by an inhibitory response to perineal stimulation. Whether this reflex could be used therapeutically in clinical cases with traumatic spinal cord injury remains to be evaluated.

An indwelling urinary catheter can also be used to keep the bladder empty. A closed system should be employed to reduce the incidence of urinary tract infection. Even with a closed system, the likelihood of urinary tract infection increases progressively with time (Smith et al., 1981). Use of antibiotics will reduce the incidence of infection, but infection can still occur with bacteria resistant to the antibiotic used (Lees et al., 1981). For this reason, we use antibiotics only after the catheter is removed and urination is restored unless a systemic infection requiring antibiotics exists.

The cholinergic drug bethanechol has been recommended to stimulate bladder contraction. This drug is contraindicated if urethral obstruction is present. The efficacy of bethanechol in humans has been questioned (Light and Scott, 1982). Studies of efficacy in stimulating detrusor contraction in clinical cases in small animals are not available. Bethanechol given to cats unable to urinate due to dysautonomia stimulated urination 30 to 60 minutes after an oral dose of 0.125 or 0.25 mg (Rochlitz, 1984). Side effects included salivation, vomiting, abdominal straining, and bradycardia. Drugs to decrease urethral outflow resistance such as phenoxybenzamine can be used in conjunction with bethanechol (Moreau, 1982).

Treatment for reflex dyssynergia is directed toward decreasing urethral outflow resistance. To accomplish this, phenoxybenzamine or diazepam or both are recommended at dosages discussed previously.

INCONTINENCE WITH THE BLADDER EMPTY

Diagnostic Plan

Several possible causes exist for incontinence when the bladder is small or normal in size. These include hormone-responsive incontinence, incontinence apparently associated with feline leukemia virus infection, ectopic ureters, incontinence after perineal urethrostomy, and incontinence associated with inability of the bladder to expand (urge incontinence).

Incontinence that developed after neutering was reported in two of 214 female cats that underwent ovariohysterectomy (David and Rajendran, 1980). The type of incontinence was not well described, but both cats apparently responded to oral estrogen supplementation (1 mg/day for 10 days). However, one of the cats had signs of hyperestrogenism at this dosage. This clinical description is similar to "spay" incontinence in dogs, which appears to be due to urethral incompetence. Diagnostic tests to confirm this cause of incontinence include response to therapy and perhaps the testing of urethral pressure, although this technique requires standardization in female cats.

An incontinence that clinically resembles spay incontinence but that occurs in cats of either sex, neutered or not, seems to be related to feline leukemia virus infection (Barsanti and Downey, 1984). Incontinence in these middle-aged (2 to 6 years) cats consisted of intermittent dribbling of urine while resting or sleeping but normal urination otherwise. Physical examination of the bladder was normal, but an associated clinical sign in six of the 11 cats was an intermittent anisocoria. Besides the typical history and physical examination, diagnostic techniques should include testing for feline leukemia virus. This type of incontinence needs to be further characterized in clinical cases by radiography, cystometography, and measurements of urethral pressure.

Ectopic ureters result in incontinence by providing a passage for urine that bypasses the urethral sphincter mechanism. Incontinence is noted early in life in cats with congenitally ectopic ureters. In contrast to its distribution in dogs, in cats, incontinence due to ectopic ureters has been described as often in males as in females. Hydroureter and hydronephrosis commonly have been associated with the ectopic ureter. Acquired ectopic ureters have been described in two female cats as a consequence of ovariohysterectomy or cesarean section with marked adhesions, hydroureter, and hydronephrosis (Allen and Webbon, 1980). Diagnosis of ectopic ureters most often has been accomplished in cats by excretory urography. In the cases reported, excretory urography for ectopic ureters was easier to interpret in cats than in dogs because the affected ureters bypassed the bladder completely and did not tunnel through the submucosa.

Incontinence due to decreased urethral resistance after perineal urethrostomy in male cats has been mentioned (Gregory, 1984). Diagnosis was by urethral pressure profiles.

Another possible complication of repeated urethral obstruction or of any severe cause of lower urinary tract inflammation is loss of bladder distensibility, or urge incontinence. Urge incontinence is the inability to control micturition between the time of the urge to urinate and actual voiding. Urine volume is usually small, because the decreased bladder capacity triggers the urge to urinate. Diagnostic tests should include urinalysis, urine culture, survey radiographs of the bladder, and contrast cystography to identify the cause of bladder inflammation.

Therapeutic Plan

The specific therapeutic plan will depend on the cause of the incontinence. In incontinence that is secondary to ovariohysterectomy, supplemental estrogen therapy has been reported to be successful. Because of the very limited number of cases, duration and dosage are empirical, but the minimum amount and the least frequent administration that control the signs is recommended. Other drugs that have been used in dogs to increase urethral tone are α-adrenergic stimulants such as ephedrine or phenylpropanolamine. These drugs have not been evaluated for ovariohysterectomized cats.

Only a few cats with incontinence associated with feline leukemia virus infection have been treated. One of three neutered males treated seemed to respond to 5 to 10 mg of testosterone propionate administered intramuscularly. One neutered male responded to phenylpropanolamine, either 7 mg three times daily or 12.5 mg twice daily. However, the owner discontinued treatment because of the cat's resistance to repeated oral dosing.

Surgical reimplantation has been successful in congenital ectopic ureter. Resolution of hydroureter and hydronephrosis occurred in one cat (Smith et al., 1983), whereas other cats have had persistence of hydroureter and dilated renal pelves (Biewenga et al., 1978). Unilateral nephrectomy was performed in cats with acquired ectopic ureters (Allen and Webbon, 1980).

Recommended therapy for urge incontinence is to control the underlying cause of bladder irritation. As symptomatic therapy in conjunction with specific therapy or in cases in which the cause of the bladder hyperactivity cannot be identified, the anticholinergic drug propantheline has been recommended. However, the dosage and effectiveness have not been studied in cats. One recommended dosage is 7.5 mg every 72 hours (Osborne et al., 1984). Possible side effects include constipation and urine retention after voiding. Profuse salivation is possible if the cat bites the tablet during administration. Alpha-adrenergic blockers such as phenoxybenzamine are used in conjunction with anticholinergic drugs in humans (Khanna, 1976).

References and Supplemental Reading

Abdel-Rahman, M., Galeano, C., Lamarche, J., et al.: A new approach to the study of voiding cycle in the cat. Invest. Urol. 18:475, 1981.

Allen, W. E., and Webbon, P. M.: Two cases of urinary incontinence in cats associated with acquired vagino-ureteral fistula. J. Small Anim. Pract. 21:367, 1980.

Barsanti, J. A., and Downey, R.: Urinary incontinence in cats. J. Am. Anim. Hosp. Assoc. 20:979, 1984.

Bebko, R. L., Prier, J. E., and Biery, D. M.: Ectopic ureters in a male cat. J.A.V.M.A. 171:738, 1977.

Biewenga, W. J., Rothuizen, J., and Voorhout, G.: Ectopic ureters in the cat—a report of two cases. J. Small Anim. Pract. 19:531, 1978.

David, G., and Rajendran, E. I.: The after-effects of spaying in bitches and cats. Cheiron 9:193, 1980.

DeGroat, W. C.: Nervous control of the urinary bladder of the cat. Brain Res. 87:201, 1975.

DeGroat, W. C., and Booth, A. M.: Physiology of the urinary bladder and urethra. Ann. Intern. Med. 92:312, 1980.

Edwards, L. E.: Manual expression of urine in a male cat. Feline Pract. 9:43, 1979.

Grauer, G. F., Freeman, L. F., and Nelson, A. W.: Urinary incontinence associated with an ectopic ureter in a female cat. J.A.V.M.A. 182:707, 1983.

Gregory, C. R.: Electromyographic and urethral pressure profilometry. Vet. Clin. North Am. 14:567, 1984.

Key, T. J. A., and Gaskell, C. J.: Puzzling syndrome in cats associated with pupillary dilatation. Vet. Rec. 110:160, 1982.

Khanna, O. P.: Disorders of micturition. Urology 8:316, 1976.

Lees, G. E., and Moreau, P. M.: Management of hypotonic and atonic urinary bladders in cats. Vet. Clin. North Am. 14:641, 1984.

Lees, G. E., and Osborne, C. A.: Use and misuse of indwelling urinary catheters in cats. Vet. Clin. North Am. 14:599, 1984.

Lees, G. E., Osborne, C. A., and Stevens, J. B.: Adverse effects of open indwelling urethral catheterization in clinically normal cats. Am. J. Vet. Res. 42:825, 1981.

Leipold, H. W., Huston, K., Blauch, B., et al.: Congenital defects of the caudal vertebral column and spinal cord in Manx cats. J.A.V.M.A. 164:520, 1974.

Light, J. K., and Scott, F. B.: Bethanechol chloride and the traumatic cord bladder. J. Urol. 128:85, 1982.

Moreau, P. M.: Neurogenic disorders of micturition in the dog and cat. Comp. Cont. Ed. Pract. Vet. 4:12, 1982.

Oliver, J. E.: Dysuria caused by reflex dyssynergia. *In* Kirk, R. W. (ed.): *Current Veterinary Therapy VIII*. Philadelphia: W. B. Saunders, 1983, pp. 1088–1089.

Oliver, J. E., and Lorernz, M. D.: *Handbook of Veterinary Neurologic Diagnosis*. Philadelphia: W. B. Saunders, 1983, pp. 90–105.

Osborne, C. A., Polzin, D. J., Klausner, J. S., et al.: Medical management of male and female cats with nonobstructive lower urinary tract disease. Vet. Clin. North Am. 14:617, 1984.

Rochlitz, I.: Feline dysautonomia (the Key-Gaskell or dilated pupil syndrome): A preliminary review. J. Small Anim. Pract. 24:587, 1984.

Scott, M. B., and Morrow, J. W.: Phenoxybenzamine in neurogenic bladder dysfunction after spinal cord injury. J. Urol. 119:480, 1978.

Sharp, N. J. H., Nash, A. S., and Griffiths, I. R.: Feline dysautonomia (the Key-Gaskell syndrome): A clinical and pathological study of 40 cases. J. Small Anim. Pract. 25:599, 1984.

Smith, C. W., Burke, T. J., and Froehlich, P.: Bilateral ureteral ectopic in a male cat with urinary incontinence. J.A.V.M.A. 182:172, 1983.

Smith, C. W., Schiller, A. G., and Smith, A. R.: Effects of indwelling catheters in male cats. J. Am. Anim. Hosp. Assoc. 17:427, 1981.

OBSTRUCTIVE UROPATHIES

DELMAR R. FINCO, D.V.M.,
and JEANNE A. BARSANTI, D.V.M.
Athens, Georgia

Obstructive uropathy refers to impingement on normal urine outflow and the deleterious consequences of such impingement. Many diseases cause outflow obstruction, and the prognoses for the disease vary widely. However, given the same site, degree, and location of obstruction, different diseases result in a common pattern of body responses to the obstruction. One pitfall to avoid in managing problems of obstructive uropathy is considering obstruction a disease instead of a sign of disease.

CAUSES OF OBSTRUCTIVE UROPATHY

In male cats, urethral obstruction is commonly observed. Although exhaustive studies have not been conducted to enumerate the frequency of different causes, it appears that most cats have obstructions because of impaction of the urethra with crystals and amorphous debris. However, other causes (inflammatory diseases of the urethra, uroliths, stenosis secondary to trauma, neoplasia of the urethral or periurethral structures, functional abnormalities of the urethra as in reflex dyssynergia, obstruction associated with bacterial infection) should be considered. Although uncommon, urethral obstruction may occur in female cats as a result of the same causes.

Urinary outflow obstruction that occurs higher in the tract than the level of the urethra apparently occurs rarely in cats. Bladder trigone neoplasms, ureteral neoplasms, and ureteroliths are rare in this species.

In dogs, the male most commonly develops urethral obstruction because of lodging of uroliths. However, all the other causes previously listed for cats have been described in dogs. Prostatic hyperplasia occurs in many older male dogs, but impingement on the urethral lumen is uncommon with this disease. Prostatic cysts or abscesses may cause the gland to assume an abdominal position because of a marked increase in size. Pinching or twisting of the urethra in this circumstance may interfere with urine outflow. In contrast to the situation with hyperplasia, prostatic neoplasia often causes urethral obstruction, even when external gland size is not markedly altered.

Ureteral obstruction in dogs has been encountered most frequently in cases of bladder trigone neoplasia. Obstruction secondary to ureteroliths, trauma, ureteral neoplasms, and surgical procedures such as ovariohysterectomy also have been reported.

CONSEQUENCES OF OBSTRUCTION

Several variables influence both the clinical signs of and the pathophysiologic responses to obstruction. These include the site, degree, and duration of obstruction, the presence or absence of concomitant bacterial infection, and whether upper tract obstruction is unilateral or bilateral. With regard to site, urethral obstruction causes the animal to attempt to urinate either beause of the distention of the urethra itself or because of bladder distention that occurs as urine accumulates. With complete urethral obstruction, anuria, azotemia, and uremia occur because of pathophysiologic mechanisms (see below). The interval between obstruction and azotemia varies with factors such as bladder capacity and rate of urine production. It was found that cats had few clinical signs of abnormalities in blood chemistry during the first 48 hours of urethral obstruction but that both signs and chemical abnormalities developed rapidly between 48 and 72 hours.

The bladder can undergo both morphologic and functional changes secondary to total urethral obstruction. Morphologic changes include hemorrhage into the bladder wall during obstruction. Functionally, the bladder may lose its impermeable character so that urine constituents are resorbed back into the body. On release of obstruction, the detrusor muscle may not be able to contract adequately to expel urine (bladder atony).

Partial urethral obstruction may or may not be complicated by the changes described for complete obstruction, depending on the quantity of urine passing by the obstructed site.

Acute bilateral total ureteral obstruction does not cause lower urinary tract abnormalities (dysuria) but will result in uremia. The onset of abnormalities is more rapid than for urethral obstruction, because the ureters and renal pelvis lack the compliance to accommodate urine. Because uremia develops rapidly and is fatal if obstruction is not resolved, dramatic morphologic changes do not develop in the kidneys. Acute total bilateral ureteral obstruction appears to occur uncommonly in dogs and cats.

Incomplete or partial bilateral ureteral obstruction may occur in association with lesions in the bladder trigone. Transitional cell carcinoma of the urinary bladder of dogs is the most common cause. Such animals may develop lower urinary tract signs (dysuria, hematuria, incontinence) that are directly related to the neoplasm but in addition may also develop polyuria or uremia by the mechanisms discussed below.

Abrupt unilateral ureteral obstruction (e.g., a renolith passing into the ureter) may cause intense pain because of dilatation of the ureter or pelvis and swelling of the kidney associated with accumulation of urine proximal to the obstruction. If renal infection exists, fever also may occur. Gradual unilateral ureteral obstruction is less obvious; renal enlargement occurs secondary to urinary retention and destruction of renal parenchyma. A mere shell of the kidney may remain in cases of partial unilateral ureteral obstruction.

PATHOPHYSIOLOGY OF RENAL DYSFUNCTIONS

Renal Blood Flow and Glomerular Filtration

The effects of obstruction on renal functions are important in treatment and prognosis. Alterations both during and after release of obstruction are known to occur. Experimentally, dogs and rats have been used extensively to determine these effects.

With total abrupt ureteral obstruction, renal blood flow (RBF) increases for a few hours but then undergoes a progressive, severe decrease. Glomerular filtration rate (GFR) decreases in parallel with RBF. Until recently, the increase in RBF was unexplained and the decrease in RBF and GFR was attributed to increased intratubular pressure associated with urine retention. However, studies in dogs revealed that the increase in intratubular pressure that occurs after obstruction does not persist; after 24 hours, it is normal with unilateral complete obstruction and only slightly elevated with bilateral complete obstruction. The persistence of depressed RBF and GFR after this time is a consequence of both afferent and efferent glomerular arteriolar constriction. The arteriolar constriction appears to be due to angiotensin II initially and thromboxane A later in the course of obstruction. The initial vasodilation that occurs is probably due to the effects of prostaglandin E_2.

The duration of complete ureteral obstruction is a very significant factor in resumption of renal function after the obstruction is corrected. Older studies in dogs suggest that unilateral obstruction of 1 week or less results in return of renal function to normal in the involved kidney, whereas obstruction for 4 weeks leaves inadequate functional tissue for survival.

Postobstruction Diuresis

In obstruction in which both kidneys are involved, a diuresis may occur following release of the obstruction. This diuresis may be due to several factors, including volume expansion associated with continued fluid intake after onset of anuria, solute diuresis because of increased blood and tissue levels of urea and other compounds, a defect in the renal concentrating mechanism, or the presence of a humoral agent as a natriuretic factor that enhances salt and water excretion. The contribution of each of these factors may vary from animal to animal, depending on individual factors.

It is of interest that postobstruction diuresis (POD) does not occur after release of unilateral ureteral obstruction. There is evidence to suggest that single nephron tubuloglomerular feedback plays a role in this difference. The tubuloglomerular feedback system normally operates so that when flow rate in the distal tubule increases, GFR is decreased to counter this potential loss of fluid. With bilateral ureteral obstruction, this feedback response is blunted so that GFR is maintained, distal delivery of fluid persists, and diuresis ensues. By contrast, the tubuloglomerular feedback system is more sensitive with unilateral ureteral obstruction and so diuresis is inhibited.

Concentrating Defect

Animals with partial urinary obstruction are known to develop a urine-concentrating defect. This defect may be different in pathogenesis from that of renal failure. In children, inability to resorb free water often results in hyposthenuria and hypernatremia. The pathogenesis of this concentrating defect is not entirely known, but the condition is unresponsive to vasopressin and is associated with a decrease in renal medullary hyperosmolality.

Other Defects

Obstruction causes other defects in renal function. Acidosis may occur as a consequence of development of a distal tubule acidifying defect and, possibly, a proximal tubular bicarbonate leak. Magnesium excretion increases inappropriately after release of both unilateral and bilateral ureteral obstruction. Correction of bilateral obstruction results in increased phosphorus excretion, whereas resolution of unilateral obstruction results in less excretion of phosphorus by the obstructed kidney. The precise mechanisms by which some of these alterations in function are brought about are current topics of investigation.

MANAGEMENT OF OBSTRUCTIVE UROPATHIES

Emergency Treatment of Anuria

Anuria due to any cause is known to produce certain biochemical alterations in both dogs and cats because of interference with normal renal excretory functions. For example, cats with urethral obstruction may have water loss, hyperproteinemia, metabolic acidosis, mild hyponatremia, hyperkalemia, hypermagnesemia, hypocalcemia, hyperphosphatemia, hyperglycemia, and azotemia. The most life-threatening abnormalities in acute, total urinary outflow obstruction are hyperkalemia and acidosis. Since acute total urinary tract obstruction results in development of clinical signs within a few days of its onset, renal damage usually is minimal and removal of obstruction results in correction of potassium and hydrogen ion abnormalities by the kidneys. However, in cases with more severe clinical signs (dehydration, depression, hypothermia), additional steps should be taken to reduce extracellular concentrations of potassium and hydrogen. In cats with urethral obstruction, removal of obstruction coupled with intravenous administration of an alkaline multiple electrolyte solution resulted in markedly improved survival compared with cats with similar biochemical abnormalties that did not receive fluid therapy. Treated cats had a marked reduction in serum potassium concentration in 4 hours and correction of acidosis in 24 hours. The reduction in the concentration of serum potassium was attributable to hemodilution, increased GFR and renal potassium excretion, and an extracellular-to-intracellular shift of potassium associated with correction of acidosis. A specific protocol for emergency treatment of urethral obstruction of cats has been published previously (see *Current Veterinary Therapy VII*, pp. 1188–1190).

Re-establishment of Urine Outflow

Removal of obstruction is an obvious approach to obstructive uropathies. For some conditions, this may be accomplished effectively and may be the sole therapy required for return of the patient to a state of health. Many male cats that have urethral obstruction but no signs of uremia require only removal of the obstructing debris by back-flushing for temporary resolution of the problem.

Removal of obstructing urethroliths in male dogs by hydropropulsion (see *Current Veterinary Therapy VI*, pp. 1194–1197) is an effective way to manage a severely uremic patient that may not tolerate general anesthesia. With re-establishment of urine outflow and improvement in the patient's clinical condition, surgery may be performed if required to remove cystoliths or renoliths.

Unfortunately, some causes of obstruction are less easily managed. In humans, partial bilateral ureteral obstruction due to invasive neoplasia warrants urinary diversion. A popular method for elimination of urine is to implant the ureters in an isolated loop of ileum that has its sole opening to the external abdominal wall. Surgical and chemical treatment of the neoplasm also is performed. In dogs, a variety of methods for urinary diversion have been used, but none has been free of problems. Ileal conduits in dogs may result in at least transient blood chemical imbalances because of resorption of urinary components by the loop. Transplantation of the ureters or bladder trigone to the colon may result in diarrhea; development of bacterial pyelonephritis also is a potential problem. In instances of urethral obstruction (i.e., prostate carcinoma) or focal bladder neoplasia, creating a bladder stoma may be feasible for urinary diversion (Lage, 1985). However, considering all of these alternatives, it is accurate to state that an effective method of urinary diversion that has a high rate of client acceptance remains to be developed for dogs and cats.

On some occasions, it may be helpful to divert temporarily urine from the renal pelvis to the exterior. A technique for pyelonephrostomy in dogs has been described (Ling et al., 1979) that entails percutaneous insertion of a needle through the abdominal wall and renal parenchyma into the renal pelvis. For the procedure, visualization of the kidney by fluoroscopy after intravenous injection of a renal contrast agent is required.

Management of POD and Renal Damage

POD can potentially lead to water and electrolyte depletion. Such depletion is particularly likely in patients that do not resume oral alimentation once obstruction is relieved. In all cases, it is advisable to monitor body weight, urine output, and both food and water intake after removal of obstruction in order to determine if nutritional balance exists. Animals that refuse food and water should receive these materials by gavage unless vomiting is a problem.

Although POD is often a transient event, some animals with prolonged obstruction may suffer from more lasting renal dysfunction. In acute total obstruction that has resulted in azotemia, relief of obstruction results in return of blood urea nitrogen and plasma creatinine concentrations to normal in 48 to 96 hours unless complicating factors exist. Complicating factors include poor renal perfusion because of hypovolemia (prerenal factor) and primary renal dysfunction as a consequence of the obstruction. The former circumstance is correctable with adequate hydration, whereas the same treatment does not resolve the azotemia if it is primarily renal in origin. Since experimental data indicate that renal damage from obstruction for periods as long as 1 week is almost totally reversible, symptomatic and supportive therapy after removal of obstruction usually results in gradual resolution of the renal dysfunction. In view of the potential defects in renal function previously described, attention should be directed toward the patient's water balance and plasma concentrations of urea, creatinine, potassium, bicarbonate, and, perhaps, magnesium.

References and Supplemental Reading

Finco, D. R., and Cornelius, L. M.: Characterization and treatment of water electrolyte, and acid-base imbalances of induced urethral obstruction in the cat. Am. J. Vet. Res. 38:823, 1977.

Klahr, S.: Pathophysiology of obstructive nephropathy. Kidney Int. 23:414, 1983.

Lage, A.: Personal communication. South Weymouth, MA, 1985.

Ling, G., Ackerman, N., Lowenstine, L. J., et al.: Percutaneous nephropyelocentesis and nephropyelostomy in the dog: A description of the technique. Am. J. Vet. Res. 40:1605, 1979.

Wahlberg, J., Stenberg, A., Wilson, D. R., et al.: Tubuloglomerular feedback and interstitial pressure in obstructive nephropathy. Kidney Int. 26:294, 1984.

UPDATE—CONSERVATIVE MEDICAL MANAGEMENT OF CHRONIC RENAL FAILURE

DAVID J. POLZIN, D.V.M.,
and CARL A. OSBORNE, D.V.M.
St. Paul, Minnesota

Conservative medical management of chronic renal failure (CRF) is designed to minimize clinical and pathologic consequences of reduced renal function. Components of conservative medical management and their indications are outlined in Table 1. Many of these recommendations are empirical. They have been extrapolated from studies in human beings and other species. Some of these recommendations have been re-examined recently in dogs, cats, and other species. It is the purpose of this article to revise, edit, and update current recommendations for conservative medical management of CRF in dogs and cats in light of the results of recent studies. Refer to References and Supplemental Reading for detailed information concerning application of these principles and other aspects of therapy for chronic renal failure (Cowgill and Kallet, 1983: Osborne and Polzin, 1979; Osborne and Polzin, 1983; Polzin and Osborne, 1979; Polzin and Osborne, 1980; Polzin and Osborne, 1983).

DIETARY PROTEIN RESTRICTION

The rationale and specific recommendations for nutritional therapy of CRF have been reviewed in detail (Osborne and Polzin, 1979; Polzin and Osborne, 1979; Polzin and Osborne, 1980). Consumption of excessive quantities of dietary protein by dogs with CRF is associated with increased morbidity and mortality (Polzin et al., 1984). Studies documenting the effects of high-protein diets on cats with CRF have not been reported.

It is generally agreed that reduced dietary protein intake may be beneficial in ameliorating clinical signs of uremia; however, controversy continues as to the timing and substance of nutritional therapy.

Table 1. *Conservative Medical Management of Chronic Polyuric Renal Failure*

Treatment	Indications
Avoid stress	Renal failure of any severity
Unlimited access to water	Polyuria and polydipsia
Diet therapy	See text
Water-soluble vitamins	Polyuria, polydipsia, and anorexia
Sodium supplementation	See text
Oral sodium bicarbonate	Documented metabolic acidosis; consider substituting calcium lactate or calcium carbonate if sodium must be restricted*
Phosphate binders	See text
Calcium supplements	Hypocalcemia or renal osteodystrophy after hyperphosphatemia has been corrected (USE CAUTION)*
Vitamin D supplements	Hypocalcemia and/or renal osteodystrophy after hyperphosphatemia has been corrected (USE CAUTION)*
Anabolic steroids	See text
Antihypertensive agents	Use only when blood pressure and response to therapy can be monitored (see text and supplemental reading)†
Adjust drug dosages	Depends on drug and severity of renal dysfunction; consult reference material*

*See Osborne and Polzin, 1983; Polzin and Osborne, 1983.
†See Cowgill and Kallet, 1983.

Issues of major concern are (1) the extent to which dietary protein should be restricted (i.e., How much protein should be fed to renal failure patients?) and (2) when during the course of CRF should protein restriction be initiated.

DIETARY PROTEIN REQUIREMENTS FOR DOGS WITH RENAL FAILURE

Optimal dietary protein requirements for dogs and cats with CRF have not been established. However, when dogs with moderate CRF were fed a daily diet containing 1.25 gm of cooked egg protein/kg body weight for 40 weeks, clinical and laboratory evidence of malnutrition characterized by hypoalbuminemia, anemia, weight loss, and reduced body tissue mass developed (Polzin et al., 1983). In this same study, dogs fed daily 3.6 gm of protein/kg body weight did not develop clinical or biochemical evidence of protein malnutrition. Both reduced-protein diets were beneficial in ameliorating clinical and biochemical effects of uremia as compared with a daily diet providing 9.7 gm of protein/kg body weight. Results of this study indicate that diets deficient in protein and diets containing excessive protein may be deleterious for patients with CRF.

The effects of diets providing 0.7, 1.3, and 2.0 gm of protein/kg body weight on nutrition and retention of proteinaceous waste products has been examined in dogs with moderate CRF (Polzin and Osborne, 1985). Reduction of daily dietary protein intake from 2.0 to 0.7 gm of protein/kg body weight caused varying degrees of protein malnutrition, the severity of which was related to the degree of protein restriction. However, reduced consumption of dietary protein consistently resulted in a proportional reduction of serum urea nitrogen concentrations. In a subsequent study, dogs with moderate renal failure (mean serum creatinine concentration, 3.2 mg/dl) were fed 2.0 gm of protein/kg body weight daily for 16 weeks without developing detectable evidence of protein malnutrition (Polzin and Osborne, 1985).

We currently recommend that dogs with mild to moderate CRF (mean serum creatinine concentration, 1.5 to approximately 4.5 mg/dl) be fed approximately 2.0 to 2.2 gm of high-biologic-value protein/kg body weight each day. One protein-restricted diet designed for dogs with renal failure provides approximately this quantity of protein (Prescription Diet k/d, Hill's Pet Products). However, we emphasize the intrinsic variability of protein requirements of normal dogs and the probable varied influence of uremia on protein requirements of uremic dogs. Therefore, dietary protein intake should be individualized to meet patient needs. If evidence of protein malnutrition (hypoalbuminemia, anemia, weight loss, or loss of body tissue mass) occurs, dietary protein should gradually be increased until these abnormalities are corrected.

If diets designed to provide daily 2.0 gm of protein/kg body weight do not result in amelioration of the clinical and biochemical manifestations of uremia, dietary protein intake may be cautiously reduced further. One protein-restricted diet has been designed to provide 1.3 gm of protein/kg of body weight each day to patients with advanced uremia (Prescription Diet u/d, Hill's Pet Products). The goal of therapy in patients with advanced uremia should be to achieve the best attainable compromise between dietary control of the biochemical and clinical manifestations of uremia and prevention of malnutrition.

DIETARY PROTEIN INTAKE FOR CATS WITH RENAL FAILURE

Cats have significantly higher dietary protein requirements than dogs. Dietary protein requirements for adult cats have been estimated to be approximately three times the protein requirement for adult dogs (12.5 per cent of diet calories as protein for cats versus 4 per cent of diet calories as protein for dogs) (Burger et al., 1984). This higher protein requirement for cats is not solely the result of a higher requirement for one or more essential amino acids. Rather, it appears to reflect reduced efficiency of anabolic utilization of dietary protein in cats compared with other species. A significant portion of the protein in their diets is used as a source of calories.

Dietary protein requirements of cats with renal failure are not known; studies documenting the safety and efficacy of reduced-protein diets in treatment of feline renal failure have not been reported. In the absence of these data, we cautiously recommend that cats with CRF be fed diets containing approximately 20 per cent of calories as protein (equivalent to 3.3 to 3.5 gm of high-biologic-value protein/kg body weight each when feeding 70 to 80 kcal/kg/day) (Osborne and Polzin, 1983).

INITIATION OF DIET THERAPY

There are at least three potential benefits that may result from restriction of dietary protein intake: (1) the quantity of proteinaceous waste products in the body will be reduced, (2) progression of CRF may be slowed or stopped, and (3) abnormalities of divalent ion metabolism leading to renal secondary hyperparathyroidism and renal osteodystrophy may be minimized as a result of reduced dietary phosphate. The major disadvantage of dietary protein restriction is potential protein malnutrition. In addition, reduced-protein diets may be less palatable to the cat and inconvenient for the owner. These benefits and risks should be weighed carefully when one determines the time to initiate nutritional therapy.

Influence of Reduced-Protein Diets on Progression of Renal Failure

THE PROGRESSIVE NATURE OF RENAL FAILURE. In several mammalian species, it appears that once a threshold of renal dysfunction has occurred, progression to end-stage renal failure invariably follows, regardless of whether the initiating cause of renal dysfunction has been resolved or eradicated. Removal of approximately three quarters or more of the functional renal tissue in rats results in a syndrome of progressive azotemia, proteinuria, arterial hypertension, and eventual death due to uremia. In human beings with renal disease, renal insufficiency regularly progresses to end-stage renal failure without apparent regard to the initiating cause of renal damage.

Clinical impression suggests that canine CRF spontaneously progresses in much the same way as that observed in rats and humans. It appears that most dogs with CRF eventually die or are euthanized as a result of uremic complications. However, conclusive data documenting the progressive nature of spontaneous canine renal failure are not yet available. Long-term studies of dogs with experimental renal disease failed to document progressive deterioration of renal function during periods of 40 weeks to 42 months (Bovee et al., 1979; Polzin et al., 1984). Therefore, the question as to whether spontaneous deterioration of renal function in dogs occurs in a fashion analogous to that observed in rats with renal failure remains unresolved.

DIETARY MODIFICATION OF THE PROGRESSIVE NATURE OF RENAL FAILURE. Recent studies in rats suggest that the progressive nature of renal failure may be modified by at least two dietary factors: (1) dietary protein intake and (2) dietary phosphate intake. Consumption of "normal" or high-protein diets by rats with experimental renal failure was associated with altered renal function and renal structure and proteinuria. These physiologic and pathologic changes were associated with progressive deterioration of renal function and, ultimately, death due to complications of the uremic syndrome. In contrast, development of proteinuria, renal structural lesions, and progressive deterioration of renal function was largely prevented in rats fed reduced-protein diets.

Considerable data have been gathered in an attempt to ascertain the influence of dietary protein on progression of renal failure in humans with CRF. Although results of these studies are not yet conclusive, available data strongly support a beneficial role of dietary modification in slowing or preventing progression of CRF. In virtually every study in patients with renal failure, when low-protein diets were prescribed there appeared to be a reduction in the rate of progression of renal failure.

Data on the influence of diet on progression of renal failure in dogs and cats are lacking. However, data are available that demonstrate that some of the physiologic effects of protein restriction recognized in rats and humans, including reduced glomerular hyperfiltration (see below) and reduced proteinuria, also occur in an analogous fashion in dogs.

THE HYPERFILTRATION THEORY. Studies in a variety of species including dogs have demonstrated that dietary protein intake has a direct effect on renal function. Increased dietary protein intake is associated with enhanced renal blood flow and glomerular filtration rate (GFR), whereas reduced protein intake is associated with reductions in these functions. Dietary enhancement of renal function appears to be mediated by hormonal mechanisms.

It has been shown that dietary protein intake also influences filtration rates in remaining functional nephrons of dogs and rats with experimental renal failure. Single-nephron GFR (SNGFR) is enhanced when dietary protein intake is increased and reduced when dietary protein intake is reduced. When SNGFR exceeds levels found in normal kidneys, the increase is termed "hyperfiltration." When high-protein diets are fed to dogs or rats with chronic renal failure, SNGFR of many functional nephrons exceeds levels found in normal kidneys, yet total GFR remains reduced from normal because the total number of nephrons contributing to overall GFR is reduced.

It has been hypothesized that hyperfiltration may be responsible for development of proteinuria and glomerular lesions in rats with reduced renal mass and thereby serves as a link between high dietary protein intake and progression of renal failure. It is thought that sustained hyperfiltration resulting from consumption of high-protein diets may damage the glomerular microvasculature, leading to increased passage of macromolecules into the glomerular mesangium and urinary space. The net result is proteinuria and mesangial proliferation leading to glomerular sclerosis. Hyperfiltration may therefore serve as the final common pathway for progression of renal failure after a threshold reduction in renal mass. Low-protein diets are thought to protect against progression of renal failure by mitigating the hemodynamic alterations resulting from high protein intake.

HIGH-PROTEIN DIETS AND THE CANINE KIDNEY. It has been proposed that "normal" and even high-protein diets are beneficial for dogs with early renal failure because they sustain maximum renal function. However, there is no clinical or experimental evidence to support the contention that sustaining maximum renal function by feeding high-protein diets is necessary or beneficial. In fact, studies indicate that consumption of high-protein diets by patients with early to moderate renal failure may be associated with increased retention of some "uremic toxins" despite enhancement of renal function.

In contrast to studies in rats, long-term studies of dogs with experimentally reduced renal function have generally not demonstrated progressive deterioration of renal function, regardless of whether high- or low-protein diets were fed. These findings have been interpreted to mean that dogs differ from rats in that no obvious association exists between consumption of high-protein diets and progressive deterioration of renal function. However, these studies failed to rule out the possibility that progressive nephron destruction occurred and that renal function remained stable as a result of functional modification (increased hyperfiltration) in remaining nephrons. If this were the case, progressive deterioration in overall GFR might not occur until the capacity of residual nephrons to undergo compensatory hyperfiltration were exceeded.

There is evidence that beneficial effects of reduced protein intake similar to those observed in rats with diminished renal function may also occur in dogs. As previously described, dogs fed reduced-protein diets have reduced glomerular hyperfiltration and reduced proteinuria. In addition, studies in our laboratory have demonstrated that glomerular lesions similar to those observed in uremic rats fed high-protein diets occur in dogs with reduced renal function. Furthermore, these lesions are more severe in dogs with demonstrable hyperfiltration.

In summary, available data do not conclusively demonstrate a protective effect of dietary protein restriction against progression of CRF. However, a beneficial role for dietary protein restriction is suggested by physiologic and pathologic findings in dogs with CRF. Additional studies are required before firm conclusions can be stated regarding the beneficial role of dietary protein restriction in preventing spontaneous progression of canine and feline CRF.

Recommendations

Reduced-protein diets are clearly indicated for dogs with moderate to severe CRF that are azotemic, hyperphosphatemic, and not anorectic. Justification for use of these diets in this category of patients is based primarily on the need to control clinical signs of uremia. Prescribing modified-protein diets for dogs with CRF that do not require reduction in their dietary protein intake for control of uremia remains controversial. The decision as to whether modified protein diets should be considered for use based solely on their potential for slowing progression of renal functional deterioration remains a matter of personal opinion.

Potential benefits of early protein (and phosphate) restriction in dogs with CRF include (1) slowing or prevention of progression of renal structural and functional deterioration and (2) slowing or prevention of renal osteodystrophy. The potential disadvantage of reduced protein intake in early renal failure is unncessary induction of protein malnutrition as a result of excessive protein restriction. It is not yet known to what extent protein intake must be restricted to maximally retard progression of renal disease. The goal of diet therapy in early to moderate renal failure should be to minimize progression of renal dysfunction (if possible) and normalize divalent ion balance while maintaining adequate nutrition.

Before initiating protein restriction, the patient's renal function and nutritional status should be evaluated. Minimum patient evaluation should include the following: physical examination; subjective evaluation of nutritional status and hydration; determination of body weight; assessment of serum creatinine, urea nitrogen, albumin, calcium, and phosphate concentrations; complete blood count; and urinalysis. This evaluation should be repeated at appropriate intervals. Initially, the authors routinely recommend monthly evaluations. Signs of protein malnutrition include (1) reduced muscle mass, (2) progressive loss of body weight, and (3) progressive reductions in packed cell volumes or serum albumin concentrations or both. If malnutrition is detected, consideration should be given to increasing dietary protein intake. Reductions in dietary protein intake, however, should be undertaken only after considering the potential nutritional effects of this action.

DIETARY PHOSPHATE RESTRICTION

Adverse Effects of Dietary Phosphate

Dietary phosphate is absorbed from the gastrointestinal tract and excreted primarily by the kidneys through glomerular filtration. In patients with CRF, reduced GFR results in phosphate retention and subsequent hyperphosphatemia. Hyperphosphatemia is a primary cause of renal secondary hyperparathyroidism, which in turn promotes renal osteodystrophy and soft tissue calcification. In addition, parathyroid hormone (PTH) appears to be a uremic toxin that may contribute to neurotoxicity, anemia, hemorrhagic diathesis, susceptibility to infection, and a variety of other disorders characteristic of the uremic syndrome (Massry, 1983).

Effects of Dietary Phosphate on Progression of Renal Failure

Excessive dietary phosphate intake has also been proposed as a factor predisposing to progression of renal failure. In studies performed in rats with experimentally induced CRF, dietary phosphate restriction prevented proteinuria, renal calcification, renal histologic alterations, renal functional deterioration, and death due to uremia (which occurred when higher phosphate diets were fed). However, results of recent studies in rats have led to a re-evaluation of the validity of these results. The value of phosphate restriction in preventing deterioration of renal function is currently controversial.

Studies performed in cats with experimentally induced renal failure revealed that normal dietary phosphate intake was associated with microscopic evidence of renal mineralization, fibrosis, and mononuclear cell infiltration (Ross et al., 1982). These abnormalities were prevented when dietary phosphate intake was reduced. However, evidence of renal functional deterioration was not detected, regardless of dietary phosphate intake.

The role of phosphate in progression of renal failure in dogs is unclear. Results of long-term studies of dogs with mild to moderate renal failure indicate that "normal" dietary phosphate intake does not appear to be associated with progressive renal dysfunction (Bovee et al., 1979; Polzin et al., 1984).

Recommendations

It is desirable to attempt to normalize phosphate balance in patients with CRF in order to minimize hyperparathyroidism (and possibly to retard progression of renal failure). Therapeutic options include (1) maintaining body fluid balance, blood vascular volume, and renal perfusion; (2) feeding reduced-protein, reduced-phosphate diets; (3) enhancing intestinal loss of phosphate by administration of nonabsorbable phosphate-binding agents; or (4) a combination of these measures.

The authors prefer to use reduced-protein, reduced-phosphate diets in properly hydrated patients. This therapy is supplemented with phosphate-binding agents if diet alone fails to normalize serum phosphate concentrations. We do not recommend use of intestinal phosphate-binding agents unless dietary restriction has failed to reduce serum phosphate concentrations to normal. Our preference for dietary management is related to the fact that most oral phosphate-binding agents (except capsules) are poorly tolerated by dogs and owners. In addition, use of oral phosphate-binding agents requires greater patient monitoring to prevent hypophosphatemia (severe hypophosphatemia can lead to debility, weakness, and anorexia) and other complications. Some phosphate-binding agents may be less effective in normalizing phosphate balance in dogs than was initially thought. A recent study performed in dogs with moderate renal failure revealed that a dose of 1500 to 2500 mg of a phosphate-binding agent (aluminum carbonate) failed to consistently correct hyperphosphatemia when dogs were fed diets containing greater than 1.0 per cent phosphate (dry weight) (Finco et al., 1985). Aluminum oxide has been found to be a more effective phosphate-binding agent in dogs (Rutherford et al., 1973); however, this product is not currently available because of production and marketing difficulties.

Phosphorus restriction should be employed to achieve normal serum phosphate concentrations; however, the degree to which dietary phosphate must be restricted to prevent the adverse effects of phosphate retention is unknown. Some nephrologists have suggested that perhaps phosphate intake should be reduced sufficiently to maintain a normal renal tubular reabsorption of phosphate. This magnitude of reduction would require extremely low intake of phosphate, which could result in phosphate depletion. Pending the results of further studies, we prefer to attempt to normalize serum phosphate concentration. Phosphate consumption or the dosage of oral phosphate binder should be adjusted in response to results of serial determinations of serum phosphate concentrations. Samples obtained for determinations of serum phosphate concentration should be collected after a 12-hour fast to avoid postprandial influence.

Available oral phosphate-binding agents include aluminum hydroxide (Amphojel Tablets and Suspension, Wyeth; Dialume Capsules, Armour) and aluminum carbonate (Basaljel Tablets, Capsules, and Suspension, Wyeth). Dosage of these drugs should be individualized to patient needs. An initial dose of 30 to 90 mg/kg/day may be instituted and the effect monitored by serial evaluation of serum phosphate concentrations at 10- to 14-day intervals until the desired effect is achieved. Constipation, a common side effect, may require laxative therapy.

ANABOLIC STEROIDS

Anabolic steroids (AS) have been recommended for treatment of the nonregenerative anemia of CRF. Studies in a number of animal species have suggested that certain AS (including nandrolone decanoate, testosterone enanthate, and fluoxymesterone) may increase red blood cell mass by enhancing renal and nonrenal production of erythropoietin and by recruiting undifferentiated bone marrow stem cells to erythroid precursors. Other AS (oxymetholone and stanozolol) act solely by enhancing erythropoietin production and therefore may be less effective in treatment of uremic anemia because erythropoietin production in these patients is already maximized.

AS may also increase concentrations of 2,3-diphosphoglycerate in red blood cells, thereby enhancing delivery of oxygen to tissues. In addition to their potential benefit for treatment of uremic anemia, AS have been hypothesized to stimulate appetite, promote anabolism, and enhance skeletal calcium deposition in uremic humans.

The efficacy of AS in dogs and cats with CRF has not been documented. In a recent study evaluating the effects of an AS in dogs with experimentally induced acute renal failure, AS did not appear to stimulate appetite or enhance anabolism (Finco et al., 1984). Because the study was limited to a 6-week period and because the dogs were not anemic, the influence of AS on nonregenerative anemia of CRF could not be assessed.

Anabolic steroids have been reported to be associated with a variety of potentially adverse effects in humans, including hepatotoxicity, elevated serum triglyceride concentrations, prostatomegaly, sodium and fluid retention, and premature epiphyseal closure when administered to immature individuals.

The authors are unable to endorse AS therapy for dogs and cats with CRF because of the dearth of data validating their clinical efficacy. Therapy with AS may be carefully considered in patients with moderate to severe anemia of renal failure. Response to therapy may require from 1 to 3 months or more to occur. It may be characterized by maintenance of stable packed cell volume or by a reduction in the rate of decline of the packed cell volume.

SODIUM INTAKE AND HYPERTENSION

Rationale for Sodium Supplementation. In past years, oral supplementation with sodium chloride and high-sodium diets were recommended for dogs and cats with CRF on the basis of the following hypotheses: (1) sodium-induced diuresis minimizes tubular reabsorption of potential uremic toxins, (2) obligatory urinary sodium loss as a result of generalized nephron dysfunction predisposes uremic patients to negative sodium balance, and (3) reduced sodium intake may promote metabolic acidosis in dogs with CRF by reducing renal tubular capacity to reabsorb bicarbonate. Pilot studies performed in our laboratory have suggested that high intakes of sodium (approximately 1200 mg sodium/100 gm dry weight) may enhance urinary excretion of nitrogenous waste products.

It has recently been shown that increased fractional excretion of sodium in urine in dogs with one form of experimentally induced CRF is a compensatory response to sodium intake rather than an obligatory loss of sodium associated with renal dysfunction. Whether or not these data can be extrapolated to dogs with all forms of spontaneously occurring renal failure has not yet been determined. However, certain forms of renal disease recognized in humans (especially diseases that affect primarily the renal medulla) may be associated with a "sodium-wasting" tendency. Pilot studies performed in our laboratory did not reveal substantial metabolic acidosis when diets containing 250 mg sodium/100 gm of dry food were fed to dogs with moderate experimental CRF (typical sodium content for commercial canned dog foods is 750 mg sodium/100 gm dry weight). Whether or not clinically significant metabolic acidosis would result from more profound dietary sodium restriction is unknown.

Sodium and Hypertension. In humans, hypertension is an established cause of renal dysfunction and may aggravate the polysystemic signs of uremia. In addition, hypertension may be a major factor involved in self-perpetuation of renal failure. It has recently been recognized that high sodium intake may contribute to hypertension in dogs with CRF (Cowgill and Kallet, 1983). Similar studies have not been reported for cats, in part because of difficulty in obtaining accurate, reproducible blood pressure values.

RECOMMENDATIONS—SODIUM INTAKE. Because of the apparent link between sodium intake and hypertension, it is generally recommended that dogs and cats with CRF be fed "normal" (as opposed to high) or restricted-sodium diets. Establishment of sodium requirements for dogs and cats with polyuric CRF must be based on future controlled experimental and clinical studies designed to evaluate sodium balance and its impact on hypertension and hypertension-related complications in dogs and cats with primary renal failure. Until such data become available, dietary sodium intake should be individualized on the basis of knowledge of current disease processes (e.g., hypertension, congestive heart failure, hypoproteinemia, edema) and response to modification of dietary sodium intake.

Dietary sodium intake may be modified in an attempt to achieve the following goals: (1) minimize or prevent sodium-associated hypertension, (2) prevent negative sodium balance and volume depletion, and (3) avoid inducing metabolic acidosis. Changes in sodium intake should be made gradually. Patients with CRF may adapt to a wide range of dietary consumption patterns; however, such adaptation occurs gradually. Abrupt changes in sodium intake may be associated with a transient imbalance between intake and urinary loss. Sudden reduction in dietary sodium may cause reduction in extracellular fluid volume, which in turn may lead to poor renal perfusion and further reduction in renal function. We recommend that changes in dietary sodium be made over at least a 2-week period.

Response may be determined by monitoring body weight, hydration, renal function, and acid-base status during and for several weeks after the reduction in dietary sodium. Progressive loss of body weight, progressive azotemia, or dehydration suggests that the patient may be unable to adapt to reduced sodium intake. In this event, a more gradual and lesser reduction of sodium intake may be considered.

RECOMMENDATIONS—HYPERTENSION THERAPY. Controlled studies designed to evaluate the efficacy of various therapeutic regimens for hypertension in dogs and cats with CRF have not been reported. Empirical recommendations for combined drug therapy of hypertension in dogs with CRF include sodium restriction, diuretics, sympatholytic drugs, and vasodilator drugs (Cowgill and Kallet, 1983). Use of diuretics, sympatholytic agents, and vasodilator drugs is advisable only if blood pressure can be serially monitored to evaluate response to therapy. No specific recommendations are available for therapy of hypertension in cats because of technical difficulties in obtaining reliable blood pressure values in this species.

References and Supplemental Reading

Bovee, K. C., Kronfeld, D. S., Bomberg, C., et al.: Long-term measurement of renal function in partially nephrectomized dogs fed 56, 27, or 19% protein. Invest. Urol. 16:378, 1979.

Burger, I. H., Blaza, S. E., Kendall, P. T., et al.: The protein requirement of adult cats for maintenance. Feline Pract. 14:8, 1984.

Cowgill, L. D., and Kallet, A. J.: Recognition and management of hypertension in the dog. *In* Kirk, R. W. (ed.): *Current Veterinary Therapy VIII*. Philadelphia: W. B. Saunders, 1983, pp. 1025–1028.

Finco, D. R., Barsanti, J. A., and Adams, D.: Effects of an anabolic steroid on acute uremia in the dog. Am. J. Vet. Res. 45:2285, 1984.

Finco, D. R., Crowell, W. A., and Barsanti, J. A.: Effects of three diets on dogs with induced chronic renal failure. Am. J. Vet. Res. 46:646, 1985.

Massry, S. G.: The toxic effects of parathyroid hormone in uremia. Semin. Nephrol. 3:306, 1983.

Osborne, C. A., and Polzin, D. J.: Strategy in the diagnosis, prognosis, and management of renal disease, renal failure, and uremia. Proc. 46th Ann. Meet. Am. Anim. Hosp. Assoc. 1979, pp. 559–630.

Osborne, C. A., and Polzin, D. J.: Conservative medical management of feline chronic polyuric renal failure. *In* Kirk, R. W. (ed.): *Current Veterinary Therapy VIII*. Philadelphia: W. B. Saunders, 1983, pp. 1008–1019.

Polzin, D. J., and Osborne, C. A.: Management of chronic primary polyuric renal failure with modified protein diets: Concepts, questions, and controversies. Proc. 29th Ann. Gaines Veterinary Symposium, White Plains, NY, 1979, pp. 24–35.

Polzin, D. J., and Osborne, C. A.: Conservative management of polyuric primary renal failure. Diet therapy. *In* Kirk, R. W. (ed.): *Current Veterinary Therapy VII*. Philadelphia: W. B. Saunders, 1980, pp. 1097–1101.

Polzin, D. J., and Osborne, C. A.: Conservative medical management of canine chronic polyuric renal failure. *In* Kirk, R. W. (ed.): *Current Veterinary Therapy VIII*. Philadelphia: W. B. Saunders, 1983, pp. 997–1007.

Polzin, D. J., and Osborne, C. A.: Unpublished data. 1985.

Polzin, D. J., Osborne, C. A., Hayden, D. W., et al.: Influence of reduced protein diets on morbidity, mortality, and renal function in dogs with induced chronic renal failure. Am. J. Vet. Res. 45:506, 1984.

Polzin, D. J., Osborne, C. A., Stevens, J. B., et al.: Influence of modified protein diets on the nutritional status of dogs with induced chronic renal failure. Am. J. Vet. Res. 44:1694, 1983.

Ross, L. A., Finco, D. R., and Crowell, W. A.: Effect of dietary phosphorus restriction on the kidneys of cats with reduced renal mass. Am. J. Vet. Res. 43:1023, 1982.

Rutherford, W. E., Mercado, A., Hruska, K., et al.: An evaluation of a new and effective phosphorus binding agent. Trans. Am. Soc. Artif. Intern. Organs 19:446, 1973.

MANAGEMENT OF URINARY TRACT INFECTIONS

GERALD V. LING, D.V.M.
Davis, California

Bacterial infection of the urinary tract is one of the most common infectious diseases of dogs. In terms of incidence, it may be predicted that about 10 per cent of all canine patients seen by veterinarians *for any reason* have this infection (often unrecognized) in addition to the problems for which they were presented. Fever, malaise, backache, dysuria, and pollakiuria accompany most episodes of urinary tract infection (UTI) in women, but dogs usually do not manifest any clinical signs or physical findings that indicate that UTI is present. Diagnosis, therefore, *must* be made in the laboratory by examination of urine sediment and results of bacterial culture (see the article entitled Diagnosis and Localization of Urinary Tract Infection).

The consequences of UTI are similar whether or not clinical signs are present. Pyelonephritis with scarring and eventual kidney failure is a possible sequela to long-standing or recurrent UTI. UTI caused by coagulase-positive staphylococci is a causal factor in the formation of struvite urinary calculi in dogs. UTI in male dogs frequently extends to the prostate gland. From this site, bacteria may reinfect the urinary tract after treatment, they may spread distantly to infect other parts of the body, or they may cause an acute or chronic infection locally within the prostate, with or without eventual abscess formation. Infections of the urinary tract may extend to the spermatic cords and testicles of male dogs and may be a cause of infertility in both sexes. Septicemia may result if large doses of immunosuppressive agents (corticosteroids, anticancer drugs) are given to dogs with unrecognized UTI. Diskospondylitis may be secondary to UTI in certain instances (see the article entitled Bacteremia of Urinary Tract Origin). There is need, therefore, to be aware of the incidence of UTI, to take steps to screen patients for its presence, and to properly treat animals that have the disease. Because UTI is so common in both sexes of dogs and because the serious consequences of canine UTI are nearly always preventable, proper procedures of diagnosis and management of UTI should be understood and routinely used by anyone engaged in small animal practice.

Bacterial infection of the urinary tract is an uncommon occurrence in cats. Cats with dysuria, pollakiuria, and pink urine—signs that have been characterized as "feline urologic syndrome (FUS)"—usually have bacteriologically sterile bladder urine (see the article in this section entitled Medical Management of Feline Urologic Syndrome).

SELECTION OF AN ANTIMICROBIAL AGENT

It is generally accepted that urine concentrations of antimicrobial agents are more important than blood concentrations in the successful treatment of UTI. All of the antimicrobials commonly used in the treatment of UTI will be present in urine in active form at concentrations that may exceed 100 times their peak blood concentrations. To aid in the success of therapy, the amount of antimicrobial agent in the patient's urine should be maintained at high concentrations during each treatment interval. Most antimicrobial agents that are used in the treatment of canine UTI have short therapeutic half-lives (i.e., rapid absorption and rapid excretion of the active compound and its metabolites into the urine). Because most household dogs are able to retain urine without voiding for at least 8 hours, owners of dogs with UTI should routinely be instructed to allow their pets freedom to urinate only just before they are due to receive the next dose of medication. Because of short therapeutic half-lives and the natural (frequent) voiding patterns of most dogs, it is desirable to administer most antimicrobial agents three times each day to dogs with UTI.

The critical antimicrobial concentration in the treatment of any urinary tract infection is called the minimum inhibitory concentration (MIC), defined as the least amount of an antimicrobial agent that will cause complete inhibition of growth of the infecting species or strain of bacteria. Understanding the relationship of bacterial inhibition to the concentration of antimicrobial agent in urine is of prime importance, since it is the basis for effective use of drugs such as penicillin in the treatment of many gram-negative infections (*Escherichia coli*, *Proteus mirabilis*, and others) encountered in the urinary tract that are typically "resistant" to penicillin in other organs or tissues of the body.

When planning treatment of UTI, one should choose an antimicrobial agent that (1) is easy for the client to administer, (2) has few (if any) undesirable or toxic side effects, (3) is relatively inexpensive, and (4) will result in urine concentrations that exceed by at least fourfold the MIC for the infecting species or strain of bacteria. The drug should be administered frequently enough to *maintain* inhibitory urine concentrations and long enough to rid the urinary tract of the infecting agent. The optimal duration of antimicrobial therapy for canine UTI is unknown. However, there is ample precedence for a 2-week course of treatment for uncomplicated infections.

In human medicine, it is customary for physicians to begin antibacterial therapy for single episodes of UTI on the basis of the patient's symptoms alone or on the basis of symptoms and the result of a urine sediment examination. This is an acceptable custom in this setting because *E. coli* is the causative bacterial species in more than 80 per cent of human UTI and because human beings are rarely exposed to antimicrobial agents that may alter the predictable susceptibility of the infecting agent. This approach is *not* the author's recommended procedure in dogs for three reasons: (1) diagnosis is more difficult because most dogs do not manifest clinical signs of UTI; (2) seven bacterial genera commonly cause UTI in dogs, whereas only two genera commonly cause UTI in women; (3) bacterial isolates from the urine of dogs, especially *E. coli, Klebsiella* spp., and *Enterobacter* spp., may be resistant to one or more drugs because of a dog's more frequent exposure to antimicrobials or to antimicrobial residues.

In order to initiate proper management of canine UTI, one must first identify the bacterial species causing the infection by culture of the patient's urine. Selection of an appropriate antimicrobial agent may often be made with great accuracy, *without* the need for susceptibility testing, when the species of the infecting bacteria is known. The reason for this is that most canine urinary pathogens have highly predictable susceptibility to one or more antibiotics. The common bacterial species associated with canine UTI (species that cause more than 3 per cent of infections), the approximate frequency of occurrence of each species, and an oral antimicrobial agent of choice for each are summarized in Table 1. The information in this table may be used routinely for single episodes of UTI or for multiple episodes that are widely separated in time (several months apart).

Daily doses and recommended frequency of administration of penicillin G, ampicillin, trimethoprim-sulfa, cephalexin, and tetracycline are also listed in Table 1. There are many other antimicrobial agents available for treatment of UTI in animals. These five drugs are mentioned specifically because they are given orally, they seem to offer the best chance of therapeutic success at the least cost to the client and the least risk to the patient, and because clinical trials substantiating their efficacy have been conducted in dogs.

Table 1. In Vivo *Susceptibility of Common Canine Urinary Tract Bacterial Pathogens to Certain Oral Antimicrobial Agents*

	Frequency of Occurrence
Approaching 100 per cent susceptibility	
Staphylococcus spp. (penicillin)*	15%
Streptococcus spp. (penicillin)	10%
About 80 per cent susceptibility	
Escherichia coli (trimethoprim-sulfa)†	38%
Proteus mirabilis (penicillin)	14%
Pseudomonas aeruginosa (tetracycline)‡	3%
Klebsiella pneumoniae (cephalexin)§	8%
Enterobacter spp. (trimethoprim-sulfa)†	3%

*Penicillin G given orally at the rate of 110,000 U/kg (50,000 U/lb) in three divided doses daily. Ampicillin given orally at the rate of 77 mg/kg (35 mg/lb) in three divided doses daily.

†Tribrissen (Burroughs Wellcome), Septra (Burroughs Wellcome), or Bactrim (Roche) given orally at the rate of 26.4 mg/kg (12 mg/lb) in two divided doses daily.

‡Tetracycline given orally at the rate of 55 mg/kg (25 mg/lb) in three divided doses daily.

§Keflex (Dista) given orally at the rate of 30 mg/kg (13.6 mg/lb) in three divided doses daily.

The MIC of oral penicillin G, ampicillin, and other penicillins for virtually all urinary streptococci and staphylococci, including penicillinase-producing strains, is less than 10 μg/ml, whereas the mean 8-hour urine concentration of these agents is about 350 μg/ml at recommended urinary dosages. It may be assumed with almost 100 per cent confidence, therefore, that these antimicrobials will be effective in the treatment of UTI caused by species of *Streptococcus* and *Staphylococcus* (Table 1).

Approximately 80 per cent of single-episode UTI caused by *E. coli* may be treated successfully with oral trimethoprim-sulfa based on information obtained by testing this drug combination against urinary isolates of *E. coli* and on results of treatment of dogs with UTI caused by *E. coli.* After similar studies, it has been determined that oral penicillin G or ampicillin may be used to successfully treat about 80 per cent of canine UTI caused by *P. mirabilis*, oral cephalexin may be used to successfully treat about 80 per cent of canine UTI caused by *Klebsiella pneumoniae*, and oral tetracycline may be used in the treatment of UTI caused by *Pseudomonas aeruginosa* with a success rate of about 80 per cent. The success of oral tetracycline is due to the fact that the MIC of tetracycline for most canine urinary isolates of *Pseudomonas* is less than 40 μg/ml, whereas the mean 8-hour urine concentration of tetracycline given orally to dogs at standard dosage is about 150 μg/ml.

Appropriate antimicrobial susceptibility tests *must* be conducted when treatment failures or recurrences of infection occur, especially those involving bacterial pathogens of the *E. coli*, *Klebsiella*, or *Enterobacter* groups. In response to antibiotic exposure, bacteria within a population of any of these three species are able to change their antimicrobial susceptibility very rapidly by means of transfer among themselves of small pieces of extrachromosomal DNA called R plasmids. These pieces of genetic information are incorporated into the bacterial genome and act to code for resistance on the part of the progeny of these bacteria in a variety of ways to any one or more of several classes of antimicrobial agents. An entire bacterial population can acquire resistance by this method of genetic transfer within a few hours after exposure to *one dose* of an antimicrobial agent. Therefore, it is necessary to conduct frequent urine cultures, definitive species identifications, and susceptibility testing when attempting to treat unresponsive or recurrent UTI caused by members of these three groups of bacteria.

In order for treatment decisions to be made, results of susceptibility testing are also needed in situations in which more than one bacterial species are isolated from the urine. Susceptibilities of each species must be determined for each antimicrobial agent tested so that the antimicrobial agent selected is effective against all isolates.

Approximately 18 per cent of canine UTI are associated with more than one bacterial species. In these situations, selection of an antimicrobial agent depends on the species of the bacteria encountered and on their susceptibilities. For example, if *E. coli* or *P. mirabilis* occurs in any combination with a species of *Streptococcus* or *Staphylococcus* (a gram-negative and a gram-positive species), trimethoprim-sulfa is a logical choice. If *Streptococcus* and *Staphylococcus* are the associated organisms (two gram-positive species), penicillin is the logical choice. If two gram-negative species (e.g., *E. coli, P. mirabilis, Enterobacter*, or *Klebsiella*) occur together, trimethoprim-sulfa or cephalexin is a logical first choice. Penicillin is a poor choice, because fewer than 20 per cent of UTI isolates of *Klebsiella* organisms are susceptible to penicillin. If the combination of infecting bacteria includes *Pseudomonas*, an effective oral antimicrobial may not be available. In this situation, two options are available: (1) treat the non-*Pseudomonas* isolate with the most effective agent and then treat the *Pseudomonas* isolate with tetracycline after the other species is eliminated; or (2) use one of the injectable aminoglycoside antimicrobials (gentamicin, tobramycin, or amikacin). The author favors the first option because of the risk of nephrotoxicity of these latter agents, their higher cost, the general inconvenience associated with the use of injectable drugs, and the fact that species of *Pseudomonas* are *not* difficult to eradicate from the urinary tract.

It may be tempting at times to initiate treatment by administering two or more antimicrobial agents simultaneously, especially when two or more causative bacterial species are isolated from the urine of a single animal. When two antimicrobials are indiscriminately administered simultaneously, the effect of the combination on the infecting bacterial population may be additive, synergistic, antagonistic, or one of indifference and may vary unpredictably with the antimicrobials administered, the bacterial species involved, and the site of infection in the body. Therefore, combining two or more antimicrobial agents without in-depth knowledge of their interaction in each specific set of circumstances for which therapy is being given is contraindicated. Mixtures of antimicrobial agents have been shown to be superior to a single agent on the basis of controlled clinical trials in only a few instances.

MANAGEMENT OF SINGLE EPISODES OF UTI

After identification of the infecting bacteria, an appropriate antimicrobial agent may be selected by using the information presented in Table 1 or on the basis of results of antimicrobial susceptibility testing.

A urine specimen for bacterial culture should routinely be taken between the fourth and seventh days of therapy. If bacterial growth is not observed, the medication should be continued for a total of 14 days. A second follow-up urine culture should be conducted on a urine specimen collected 2 to 4 days after completion of the therapeutic course.

If growth of the same or of a different species of bacteria is observed in a urine specimen taken between the fourth and seventh days of therapy, the treatment has failed and another antimicrobial agent must be substituted immediately, using a new susceptibility test as a guideline for selection. Culture of urine should then be conducted 4 to 7 days after beginning the substitute antimicrobial and 2 to 4 days after completion of the therapeutic course.

Culture of all follow-up urine specimens in patients with UTI is strongly recommended over urine sediment examination for two reasons. First, if the numbers of infecting bacteria in a follow-up specimen are less than 10,000/ml, a false impression of cure may be given, since bacteria cannot usually be demonstrated in sediment examination if their numbers are below this figure. Second, the number of white blood cells may unpredictably decrease to normal during treatment of a UTI, even when the antimicrobial agent used is ineffective in eradicating the infecting organism. Examination of urine sediment is, therefore, unreliable for assessment of success or failure of antimicrobial therapy of UTI.

MANAGEMENT OF MULTIPLE EPISODES OF UTI

Preliminary evidence indicates that recurrence of UTI in dogs is caused by bacterial reinfection (a different strain or species) rather than bacterial relapse (the same strain or species) in about 80 per cent of cases. When reinfection occurs only once or twice each year, administration of the appropriate oral antimicrobial agent for 7 to 14 days as described previously is the best approach to management. When reinfection occurs more than three times in a single year, long-term antimicrobial administration may be necessary to prevent reinfection.

Use of trimethoprim-sulfa, cephalexin, or nitrofurantoin in dogs with histories of gram-negative or gram-mixed infections and penicillin G or ampicillin in dogs with histories of gram-positive infections is effective in reducing the incidence of reinfection to about one-tenth its former frequency. The dosage given is about one third of the total daily dose administered once daily for 6 months. Urine specimens collected only by cystocentesis are cultured once each month. If bacteria cannot be cultured from urine collected during follow-up evaluation, the regimen should be continued unchanged. If bacteria are cultured from a follow-up urine specimen, the appropriate oral antimicrobial agent should be given three times daily as previously described for individual infections. If at the end of 2 weeks of this type of therapy urine is once again culture-negative, the once-daily regimen is resumed with monthly follow-ups for 6 months. At the end of 6 consecutive months of bacteria-free urine cultures, the once-daily antimirobial therapy is discontinued. Most animals receiving this regimen do not have additional episodes of bacteriuria.

As noted above, follow-up urine specimens taken from these patients should be collected *only* by cystocentesis. Introduction of a urinary catheter in these patients, regardless of how carefully and aseptically the procedure is conducted, will introduce urethral bacterial contaminants that may colonize the uroepithelium and initiate UTI.

MEDICAL DISSOLUTION AND PREVENTION OF CANINE STRUVITE UROLITHS

CARL A. OSBORNE, D.V.M.,
DAVID J. POLZIN, D.V.M.,
JOHN M. KRUGER, D.V.M.,
St. Paul, Minnesota

and SHEHU U. ABDULLAHI, D.V.M.
Zaria, Nigeria

OVERVIEW OF ETIOPATHOGENESIS

Mineral Composition

The most common type of mineral encountered in uroliths of dogs is magnesium ammonium phosphate hexahydrate (MAP), or struvite (Table 1). MAP uroliths have also been called phosphate calculi, infection stones, urease stones, and triple-phosphate stones. Triple-phosphate is a misnomer that originated because quantitative chemical analyses of uroliths often revealed a combination of calcium, magnesium, ammonium, and phosphate (three cations and one anion). The name is incorrect, since struvite does not contain calcium. However, canine struvite uroliths are frequently impure, containing minor quantities of calcium phosphate (also called calcium apatite) and carbonate apatite. Car-

Table 1. *Mineral Composition of 839 Canine Uroliths Analyzed by Quantitative Methods**

Predominant Mineral Type	Number of Uroliths	%
Magnesium ammonium phosphate (•$6H_2O$)		
100%	312	37
70–99%†	250	30
Magnesium hydrogen phosphate (•$3H_2O$)	1	<1
Calcium oxalate		
Calcium oxalate monohydrate		
100%	13	2
70–99%†	34	4
Calcium oxalate dihydrate		
100%	3	<1
70–99%†	7	<1
Calcium phosphate		
Calcium phosphate		
100%	14	2
70–99%†	6	<1
Calcium hydrogen phosphate (•$2H_2O$)		
100%	4	<1
70–99%†	1	<1
Uric acid and urates		
Ammonium acid urate		
100%	25	3
70–99%†	14	2
Sodium acid urate		
100%	2	<1
70–99%†	2	<1
Uric acid	1	<1
Cystine	20	3
Silica		
100%	19	2
70–99%†	5	<1
Mixed‡	42	5
Compound§	58	<1
Matrix	7	<1
Total	839	100%

*Analysis performed by optical crystallography and x-ray diffraction.

†Uroliths composed of 70–99% of mineral type listed; no nucleus and shell detected.

‡Uroliths did not contain at least 70% of mineral type listed; no nucleus and shell detected.

§Uroliths contained an identifiable nucleus and one or more surrounding layers of different mineral type.

bonate apatite may be a minor constituent in uroliths that form in patients with urinary tract infections (UTI) caused by urease-producing microbes (especially staphylococci, *Proteus* spp., and ureaplasmas). Generation of carbonate ion (CO_3^{2-}) as a consequence of hydrolysis of urea by microbial urease is sometimes associated with displacement of some phosphate anions in calcium apatite molecules. Canine struvite uroliths may also contain minor quantities of ammonium acid urate (Table 2).

Causative Factors

Urine must be supersaturated with MAP for struvite uroliths to form. Supersaturation of urine with MAP may be associated with several factors, including UTI with urease-producing microbes, alkaline urine, genetic predisposition, and diet.

INFECTION-INDUCED STRUVITE

When UTI with urease-producing microbes (especially species of *Staphylococcus*, *Proteus*, and *Ureaplasma*) occurs in animals forming urine with a sufficient quantity of urea, the unique combination of concomitant elevation in the concentrations of ammonium and carbonate (CO_3^{2-}) in an alkaline environment may develop. These conditions favor formation of uroliths containing struvite ($MgNH_4PO_4 \cdot 6H_2O$), calcium apatite [$Ca_{10}(PO_4)_6(OH)_2$], and carbonate apatite [$Ca_{10}(PO_4)_6CO_3$]. The following mechanisms are involved:

Table 2. *Common Characteristics of Canine Struvite Uroliths*

Chemical Name
Magnesium ammonium phosphate hexahydrate
Crystal Name
Struvite
Formula
$MgNH_4PO_4 \cdot 6H_2O$
Variations in Composition
Struvite only
Struvite mixed with lesser quantities of calcium apatite and ammonium acid urate
Nucleus of a different mineral surrounded by variable layers composed primarily of struvite. Small quantities of calcium apatite and ammonium acid urate may also be present.
Physical Characteristics
Color: Struvite uroliths are usually white, cream, or light brown in color. The surface of uroliths is commonly red because of concomitant hematuria, and it may be green (caused by bile pigments).
Shape: Variable, commonly round, elliptic, or pyramidal; rapidly growing uroliths with a large quantity of matrix may form a cast of the lumen (renal pelvis, ureter, bladder, urethra) in which they formed.
Nuclei and laminations: Common in infection-induced uroliths.
Density: Variable; soft if they contain a large quantity of matrix; dense and harder to cut if little matrix is present. A combination of hard and soft internal density may occur within the same urolith. Radiodense compared with nonskeletal tissue on survey radiographs. Degree of radiodensity is related to the quantity of matrix (inversely proportional) and other minerals, especially calcium apatite (more proportional).
Number: Single or multiple.
Location: May be located in the kidney, ureter, urinary bladder, and urethra. Most occur in the urinary bladder.
Size: Microscopic to a size limited by the capacity of the structure (kidney and urinary bladder) in which they form.
Predisposing Factors
Urinary tract infections with urease-producing microbes in patients whose urine contains a large quantity of urea.
Alkaline urine pH
Unidentified factors
Characteristics of Affected Canine Patients
Mean age: 6 years (range < 1 to > 16 years)
Especially common in miniature schnauzers, dachshunds, poodles, Scottish terriers, beagles, Pekingese, and Welsh corgis; any breed may be affected.
More common in females (70 per cent) than males (30 per cent).

1. Urease (a metalloenzyme containing nickel) produced by bacteria or *Ureaplasma* hydrolyzes urea to form two molecules of ammonia and a molecule of carbon dioxide.

2. The ammonia molecules react spontaneously with water to form ammonium and hydroxyl ions (pK of NH_3 = 9.03), which alkalinizes urine by reducing its hydrogen ion concentration. The solubility of struvite and calcium apatite decreases in alkaline urine. The newly generated ammonium ion is available for formation of MAP crystals.

3. The newly generated molecule of carbon dioxide combines with water to form carbonic acid, which in turn dissociates to form bicarbonate (pK = 6.33) and hydrogen ion. In an extremely alkaline environment, bicarbonate may lose its proton to become carbonate (pK = 10.1). Anions of carbonate may displace anions of phosphate in calcium apatite crystals to form carbonate apatite crystals.

4. In the progressively alkaline environment induced by microbial hydrolysis of urea, dissociation of monobasic hydrogen phosphate ($H_2PO_4^-$) results in an increased concentration of dibasic hydrogen phosphate (HPO_4^{2-}) and anionic phosphate (PO_4^{3-}). Given a constant concentration of total phosphate, a change in pH from 6.80 to 7.40 increases the PO_4^{3-} concentration by a factor of approximately 6. Anionic phosphate is then available in increased quantities to combine with magnesium and ammonium to form struvite, or with calcium to form calcium apatite.

5. Ammonium ions may combine with urates to form ammonium acid urate.

The quantity of dietary protein catabolized for energy influences formation and dissolution of infection-induced struvite uroliths. Consumption of dietary protein in quantities that exceed daily protein requirements for anabolism results in the formation of urea from catabolism of amino acids. Hyperammonuria, hypercarbonaturia, and alkaluria mediated by microbial urease is dependent on the quantity of urea (the substrate of urease) in urine.

Abnormal urinary excretion of minerals as a result of enhanced glomerular filtration rate, reduced tubular reabsorption, or enhanced tubular secretion is not required for initiation and growth of infection-induced struvite uroliths. However, metabolic and anatomic abnormalities may indirectly induce struvite uroliths by predisposing to UTI.

STERILE STRUVITE

Clinical studies indicate that microbial urease is not involved in formation of struvite uroliths in some dogs. Several observations suggest that dietary or metabolic factors may be involved in the genesis of sterile struvite uroliths in these species. Pilot studies of clinical cases of struvite uroliths in dogs revealed a population of patients (9 of 20) whose urine was frequently alkaline but did not contain identifiable bacteria and did not contain detectable quantities of urease. Microscopic examination of demineralized Gram-stained sections of some struvite uroliths removed from dogs with bacteriologically sterile urine revealed no gram-positive bacteria. Whereas infection-induced human struvite uroliths frequently contain calcium apatite or carbonate apatite (these minerals occur as a consequence of urease-positive bacterial infections), a large number of canine sterile uroliths were 100 per cent struvite (an observation that supports their noninfectious origin).

Although struvite is less soluble in alkaline than in acidic urine, the mechanism of sterile struvite urolith formation in dogs is not clear. Under physiologic conditions associated with alkaluria, urine contains low concentrations of ammonia (and thus ammonium ion). Thus alkaline urine formed in absence of ureolysis would not be expected to favor formation of crystals that contain ammonia ion (such as MAP).

DIAGNOSIS

Uroliths are usually suspected on the basis of typical findings obtained by history and physical examination. Urinalyses, urine culture, and radiography may be required to differentiate uroliths from UTI, diverticula of the bladder, inflammatory polyps, neoplasia, or other disorders. Since many struvite uroliths in dogs occur as sequelae to UTI, and since UTI occur as sequelae to abnormalities in local or systemic host defense mechanisms, appropriate effort should be directed toward defining the underlying problem. A problem-specific data base for urolithiasis has been developed (Table 3).

Various methods have been used to evaluate the mineral composition of uroliths, including gross appearance, crystalluria, radiographic appearance, qualitative analysis, quantitative analysis, and uroith culture. Of these, quantitative analysis provides the most definitive diagnostic, prognostic, and therapeutic information.

MEDICAL DISSOLUTION OF CANINE STRUVITE UROLITHS

Indications

Surgery has been a time-honored approach for management of all types of urolithiasis in dogs. Although surgery has been an effective method that provides immediate elimination of uroliths, it is associated with several limitations. These include (1) persistence of underlying causes and a high rate

Table 3. Problem-Specific Data Base for Urolithiasis

1. Obtain appropriate history and perform physical examination, including rectal examination of urethra.
2. Perform complete urinalysis; save aliquot for possible determination of mineral concentrations.*
3. Perform complete blood count.
4. Freeze aliquot of serum collected at time of venipuncture to obtain complete blood count for possible determination of urea nitrogen, creatinine, calcium, uric acid, chloride, and potassium concentration.
5. Obtain quantitative urine culture and determine urine urease activity; obtain antimicrobial susceptibility if bacterial pathogens are identified. Consider attempts to isolate ureaplasmas if urease-positive urine is bacteriologically sterile.
6. Obtain radiographs.
   a. Take survey radiographs of entire urinary system.
   b. Consider IV urography for patients with renal or ureteral calculi.
   c. Consider IV urography or contrast cystography for patients with bladder calculi.
   d. Consider contrast urethrography for patients with urethral calculi.
   e. Ultrasonography is recommended if equipment is available.
7. Remove bladder or kidney biopsy specimens for microscopic examination if nephrolithotomy or cystolithotomy is performed.
8. Correct any anatomic defects during surgical procedure performed to remove uroliths.
9. Compare number of uroliths removed during surgery with number of uroliths identified by radiography; if necessary, postsurgical radiographs should be obtained to evaluate completeness of urolith removal.
10. Save all uroliths for quantitative analysis.
11. Initiate therapy to promote dissolution or arrested growth of uroliths, if necessary.
12. Initiate therapy to eradicate UTI, if necessary.
13. Initiate therapy to prevent recurrence of uroliths.
14. Formulate follow-up protocol with clients.

*The patient should be consuming the same food as at time of urolith formation. Alternatively, a standardized diet designed to promote reproducible excretion of minerals in the urine of normal animals may be used.

of recurrence of uroliths despite surgery, (2) patient factors that enhance adverse consequences of general anesthesia or surgery, and (3) inability to remove all uroliths or fragments of uroliths during surgery. In addition, situations occasionally arise in which owners of companion animals will not consent to surgical therapy but will consider medical therapy. For these and other reasons (e.g., if the urolith is asymptomatic), medical dissolution of struvite uroliths may be considered.

Despite the feasibility of dissolution of struvite uroliths, it is emphasized that this form of therapy is associated with potential hazards. Uroliths always represent a predisposing cause of UTI and always predispose to obstructive uropathy. Both risks and benefits of medical versus surgical therapy must be considered for each patient.

Objectives

The objectives of medical management of uroliths are to arrest further urolith growth and to promote urolith dissolution by correcting or controlling underlying abnormalities. For therapy to be effective, it must induce undersaturation of urine with calculogenic crystalloids by (1) increasing the solubility of crystalloids in urine, (2) increasing the volume of urine in which crystalloids are dissolved or suspended, and (3) reducing the quantity of calculogenic crystalloids in urine. For example, attempts to increase the solubility of crystalloids in urine often include administration of medications designed to change urine pH in order to create a less favorable environment for crystallization. Likewise, induction of diuresis is a method commonly used to increase the volume of urine in which crystalloids are dissolved or suspended. Change in diet is an example of a method to reduce the quantity of calculogenic crystalloids in urine.

These objectives may be difficult to achieve, because uroliths are not homogeneous in composition. This has not been a significant problem in dogs with uroliths composed primarily of MAP with lesser degrees of calcium phosphate, because the solubility characteristics of the two minerals are similar. However, it is logical to expect difficulty in attempting to induce dissolution of a urolith with a nucleus of cystine or silica and a shell of struvite, because the solubility characteristics of these two minerals are dissimilar. This phenomenon should be considered if medical therapy seems to become ineffective after the size of a urolith is initially reduced.

Definition of Urolith Composition

Formulation of therapy to reduce the composition of specific calculogenic crystalloids in urine is dependent on knowledge of the composition of uroliths. For example, administration of D-penicillamine would be of no benefit to patients with struvite uroliths. Likewise, administration of ascorbic acid, a commonly used acidifer, might potentiate calcium oxalate urolithiasis, since it is a precursor of oxalic acid. In situations in which consideration is being given to medical therapy but uroliths are not available for analysis, one may be forced to make an educated guess about their composition (Table 4).

Recommendations

Current recommendations include (1) eradication or control of UTI with appropriate antimicrobial agents, (2) use of calculolytic diets, and (3) administration of urease inhibitors (acetohydroxamic acid)

Table 4. *Checklist of Factors that May Aid in "Guesstimation" of Mineral Composition of Uroliths*

1. Radiographic density and physical characteristics of uroliths
2. Urine pH
   a. Struvite and calcium apatite uroliths—usually alkaline in dogs
   b. Ammonium urate uroliths—variable
   c. Cystine uroliths—acidic
   d. Calcium oxalate—variable
   e. Silica—variable
3. Identification of crystals in uncontaminated fresh urine sediment, preferably at body temperature
4. Type of bacteria, if any, isolated from urine
   a. Urease-producing bacteria, especially staphylococci and less frequently *Proteus* spp. are typically associated with canine struvite uroliths. *Ureaplasma* may cause struvite uroliths.
   b. UTI often is absent in patients with calcium oxalate, cystine, ammonium urate, and silica uroliths.
   c. Calcium oxalate, cystine, ammonium urate, and silica uroliths may predispose patients to UTI; if infections are caused by urease-producing bacteria, struvite may precipitate around metabolic uroliths.
5. Serum chemistry evaluation
   a. Hypercalcemia may be associated with calcium-containing uroliths.
   b. Hyperuricemia may be associated with uric acid or urate uroliths.
   c. Hyperchloremia, hypokalemia, and acidemia may be associated with distal renal tubular acidosis and calcium phosphate uroliths.
6. Urine chemistry evaluation
   a. Patient should be consuming a standardized diagnostic diet or the diet consumed when uroliths formed.
   b. Although no controlled studies have been performed in dogs, excessive quantities of one or more minerals contained in the urolith are expected.
7. Breed of animal and history of occurrence of uroliths in patient's ancestors or littermates
8. Analysis of uroliths fortuitously passed and collected during micturition

to patients with *persistent* UTI caused by urease-producing microbes (Table 5).

ERADICATION OR CONTROL OF UTI

The importance of UTI with urease-producing bacteria in the formation of most struvite uroliths in dogs emphasizes the need for therapy to eliminate or control them. Because of the quantity of urease produced by bacterial pathogens, it may be impossible to acidify urine with urine acidifiers administered at dosages that prevent systemic acidosis. Therefore, sterilization of urine appears to be an important objective in creating a state of struvite undersaturation that may prevent further growth of uroliths or that promotes their dissolution.

Appropriate antimicrobial agents selected on the basis of susceptibility or minimum inhibitory concentration tests should be used at therapeutic dosages. The fact that diuresis reduces the urine concentration of the antimicrobial agent should be considered when formulating antimicrobial dosages. Antimicrobial agents should be administered as long as the uroliths can be identified by survey radiography. This recommendation is based on the fact that bacterial pathogens harbored inside uroliths may be protected from antimicrobial agents. Although the urine and surface of calculi may be sterilized after appropriate antimicrobial therapy, the original infecting organisms may remain viable below the surface of the urolith. Discontinuation of antimicrobial therapy may result in relapse of bacteriuria and infection.

Table 5. *Summary of Recommendations for Medical Dissolution of Canine Struvite Uroliths*

Adult Dogs With UTI

1. Perform appropriate diagnostic studies including complete urinalyses, quantitative urine culture, and diagnostic radiography. Determine precise location, size, and number of uroliths. The size and number of uroliths are not a reliable index of probable efficacy of therapy.
2. Determine mineral composition of available uroliths. If unavailable, estimate their composition by evaluation of appropriate clinical data (Table 4).
3. Consider surgical correction if uroliths are obstructing urine outflow, or if correctable abnormalities predisposing to recurrent UTI are identified by radiography or other means.
4. Eradicate or control UTI with appropriate antimicrobial agents. Maintain antimicrobial therapy during, and for 3 to 4 weeks following, urolith dissolution.
5. Initiate therapy with calculolytic diets. No other food or mineral supplements should be fed to the patient. Compliance with dietary recommendations is suggested by reduction in serum urea nitrogen concentration (usually $\leq$ 10 mg/dl.)
6. Feed patients calculolytic diet for 1 month after disappearance of uroliths as detected by survey radiography.
7. If possible, avoid diagnostic follow-up studies requiring urinary tract catheterization.
8. Consider administration of acetohydroxamic acid (25 mg/kg/day divided into two equal doses) to patients with persistent urease-producing microburia despite use of antimicrobial agents and calculolytic diets.
9. Devise a protocol for periodic follow-up including the following:
   a. Serial urinalyses. Urine pH, specific gravity, and microscopic examination of sediment for crystals are especially important. Remember, crystals formed in urine stored at room or refrigeration temperatures may represent artifacts.
   b. Serial radiography at monthly intervals to evaluate stone locations, number, size, density, and shape.
   c. Quantitative urine culture when indicated.

Adult Dogs With Sterile Urine

1. Follow the protocol described above, but do not administer antimicrobial agents or acetohydroxamic acid.
2. Periodically culture urine specimens obstained by cystocentesis to detect secondary UTI. If UTI develops, initiate antimicrobial therapy.

Immature Dogs

1. Use caution in consideration of use of protein-restricted diets in growing pups.
2. Short-term therapy with calculolytic diets may be considered. If initiated, monitor the patient for evidence of nutritional deficiencies (especially protein malnutrition).
3. Acetohydroxamic acid has not been evaluated in growing pups.
4. Pending further studies, surgery remains the safest means of removing uroliths from immature dogs.

Although use of antimicrobial agents alone may result in dissolution of struvite uroliths in some patients, experimental studies in rats and dogs and clinical studies in humans indicate that this phenomenon represents the exception rather than the rule. In addition to the unpredictable response to this form of therapy, the time required to induce urolith dissolution with antimicrobial agents is usually measured in multiples of months rather than weeks.

CALCULOLYTIC DIETS

The goal of dietary modification for patients with struvite uroliths is to reduce urine concentration of urea (the substrate of urease), phosphorus, and magnesium. A calculolytic diet (Prescription Diet Canine s/d, Hill's Pet Products) was formulated that contains a reduced quantity of high-quality protein (1.6 per cent) and reduced quantities of phosphorus (0.648 per cent) and magnesium (0.006 per cent). The diet was supplemented with sodium chloride to stimulate thirst and induce compensatory polyuria. Reduction of hepatic production of urea from dietary protein reduces concentration of urea in the renal medulla and further contributes to diuresis.

The efficacy of this diet in inducing dissolution of infected struvite uroliths has been confirmed by controlled experimental studies in dogs. The calculolytic diet was highly effective in inducing struvite urolith dissolution in five of six experimental dogs despite persistent infection with urease-producing bacteria. The uroliths underwent dissolution in about 3.5 months (range, 8 to 20 weeks). The urolith in the remaining dog decreased to less than half its pretreatment size at the termination of the study, 6 months after initiation of dietary therapy. UTI persisted in these dogs until the uroliths dissolved, at which time they underwent remission in three dogs. In the corresponding control group fed a maintenance diet (10 per cent protein, 0.19 per cent phosphorus, and 0.06 per cent magnesium), calculi increased in size by a mean of 5.5 times their pretreatment size (range, 3 to 8 times). A urolith developed in the renal pelvis of one of these dogs. UTI persisted in control dogs throughout the 6-month study.

In a related experimental study of sterile struvite uroliths, consumption of the calculolytic diet induced urolith dissolution in a mean of 3.3 weeks (range, 2 to 4 weeks). In a corresponding control group fed a maintenance diet, uroliths in four dogs dissolved over a mean period of 14 weeks (range, 2 to 5 months). In the remaining two control dogs, uroliths were one fifth of their initial size at the termination of the study.

Consumption of calculolytic diets by dogs with experimentally induced staphylococcal UTI and struvite uroliths was associated with a marked reduction in the serum concentration of urea nitrogen (baseline = 21.8 mg/dl ± 2.9; post-treatment = 3.5 mg/dl ± 2.4) and mild reductions in the serum concentrations of magnesium (baseline = 2.2 mg/dl ± 0.2; post-treatment = 1.8 mg/dl ± 0.2), phosphorus (baseline = 4.6 mg/dl ± 0.6; post-treatment = 3.8 mg/dl ± 0.8), and albumin (baseline = 3.1 gm/dl; post-treatment = 2.1 gm/dl ± 0.3). A mild increase in the serum activity of hepatic alkaline phosphatase isoenzyme (baseline = 3.1 μl/ml ± 1.50; post-treatment = 147.7 μl/ml ± 48.1) also was observed. These alterations in serum chemistry values were of no detectable clinical consequence during 6-month experimental studies or during clinical studies. However, they underscore the fact that the diet is designed for short-term (weeks to months) dissolution therapy rather than long-term (months to years) prophylactic therapy. Changes in serum urea nitrogen concentrations may be used as one index of client and patient compliance with dietary recommendations.

Since development and evaluation of the initial calculolytic diet, the quantity of high-quality protein (previously 1.5 per cent) has been increased (2.2 per cent) (Prescription Diet Canine s/d, Hill's Pet Products). Clinical evaluation of the calculolytic diet containing somewhat higher protein has revealed that it has comparable calculolytic value to the original prototype with less effect on serum alkaline phosphatase activity and serum albumin concentration.

UREASE INHIBITORS

Clinical studies in humans and experimental and clinical studies in dogs have revealed that administration of microbial urease inhibitors in pharmacologic doses is capable of inhibiting struvite urolith growth and promoting struvite urolith dissolution. Hydroxamic acids are specific inhibitors of urease. They apparently owe at least a portion of their inhibitory activity to their molecular structure, which is similar to that of urea. The terminal –CO–NHOH structure of acetohydroxamic acid may noncompetitively block the active site of urease molecules because its similarity to the amide groups of urea allows access to the active site. Because hydroxamic acids also chelate nickel, they may bind to nickel atoms in urease, thereby interfering with urease activity. Of the variety of hydroxamic acids, acetohydroxamic acid (AHA) combines an acceptable level of toxicity with a relatively rapid inhibitor effect against urease.

AHA is rapidly and completely absorbed from the gastrointestinal tract of dogs and is excreted and concentrated in urine. When given orally at pharmacologic doses, AHA retards alkalinization of urine caused by urease-producing microbes. Its urease-inhibiting activity is effective between urine pH of 5 and 9 but is most effective at pH 7. AHA has been reported to have a dose-related bacteriostatic effect against some gram-positive and gram-negative bacteria. It may also potentiate the antimicrobial effect of antibiotics (especially trimethoprim and sulfamethoxazole) and urine antiseptics (methenamine).

In an experimental study of dogs with normal renal function, a dose-related ability of AHA to inhibit further struvite urolith growth and to induce struvite urolith dissolution was observed. Administration of AHA at a dosage of 50 to 100 mg/kg body weight each day caused detectable reduction of urine urease activity, urine pH, and crystalluria and either inhibited urolith growth (50 mg/kg) or induced urolith dissolution (100 mg/kg). Although administration of AHA at a daily dosage of 25 mg/kg did not cause a detectable reduction in urine pH, it did reduce urease activity and crystalluria and inhibited further urolith growth. These events occurred despite persistent UTI with urease-producing *Staphylococcus aureus*. The fact that infected dogs treated with AHA had less severe dysuria, bacteriuria, pyuria, hematuria, and proteinuria and had less severe lesions of the urinary tract than positive-control dogs indicates that the drug reduced the pathogenicity of staphylococci. Reduction in the quantity of ammonia produced by the action of bacterial urease on urea may have minimized the degree of chemically induced damage to tissues of the urinary tract, with an associated reduction in the magnitude of the inflammatory response.

When AHA was given to dogs in sufficient quantity to dissolve experimentally induced struvite uroliths, a reversible hemolytic anemia and blood dyscrasia occurred. Prolonged administration of AHA at large doses induced abnormalities in bilirubin metabolism in some dogs. The exact mechanism responsible for these abnormalities was not determined. AHA has been reported to inhibit DNA synthesis and cell division and has the capacity to chelate metallic ions. Reduction of the quantity of AHA to a dosage that did not cause adverse reactions eliminated its ability to induce struvite urolith dissolution under the conditions of this study. However, nontoxic doses of AHA were effective in prolonged inhibition of further urolith growth.

In a study performed at the University of Minnesota, oral administration of AHA at a daily dose of 25 mg/kg to pregnant female beagle dogs induced developmental anomalies of the heart, skeletal system, and ventral midline of pups. Cardiac anomalies included atrial septal defects (20 per cent), ventricular septal defects (3 per cent), and atrial and ventricular septal defects (3 per cent). Skeletal anomalies included coccygeal hemivertebrae and fused coccygeal vertebrae (50 per cent), supernumerary vertebrae (67 per cent), supernumerary ribs (50 per cent), duplicated sternebrae (3 per cent), and lumbar hemivertebrae (3 per cent). Defects of the ventral midline of the abdominal wall occurred in 20 per cent of pups exposed to AHA *in utero*. Other abnormalities observed included retarded growth, high neonatal mortality, and a decreased number of circulating erythrocytes compared with that in control dogs. These observations indicate that AHA should not be given to pregnant females.

COMBINATION THERAPY

The struvolytic effect of various combinations of antibiotics (ampicillin given orally at a dosage of 16 mg/kg/day), AHA (given orally at a dosage of 25 mg/kg/day), and calculolytic diet were studied in dogs with staphylococcus-induced struvite uroliths. After 5 months of therapy, four uroliths increased in size and two dissolved in six dogs given ampicillin and a maintenance diet. Four of six uroliths dissolved and two decreased in size in six dogs given ampicillin and calculolytic diet. All uroliths in six dogs dissolved 6 weeks after initiation of therapy with a combination of calculolytic diet, ampicillin, and AHA.

When a combination of calculolytic diet and antimicrobial agents were given to 11 dogs with naturally occurring urease-positive UTI and urocystoliths presumed to be composed of struvite, similar results were obtained. Likewise, use of a calculolytic diet to induce dissolution of urocystoliths presumed to be struvite in nine dogs without UTI has also been effective. The mean time required to induce urocystolith dissolution in these 20 dogs was 2.26 months (range, 2 weeks to 7 months). The mean urine pH of the 20 patients at the time of diagnosis was 7.6; the mean serum urea nitrogen concentration was 19.5 mg/dl. The mean urine pH of these dogs during calculolytic therapy was 6.9; the mean serum urea nitrogen concentration was 7.1 mg/dl.

Pretreatment mean serum alkaline phosphatase activity ($\bar{x}$ = 70.5 mU/ml) tripled during calculolytic diet therapy ($\bar{x}$ = 245 mU/ml) but rapidly returned to normal values ($\bar{x}$ = 55 mU/ml) after discontinuation of therapy. Likewise, mean serum albumin concentration ($\bar{x}$ = 3.3 gm/dl) at the time of diagnosis dropped ($\bar{x}$ = 2.58 gm/dl) during calculolytic therapy but returned to normal values ($\bar{x}$ = 3.35 gm/dl) after cessation of treatment.

Results of clinical and experimental studies have revealed that the size and number of uroliths per se do not dictate the probable response to therapy. Likewise, there is no rigid therapeutic time interval after which response is unlikely. As long as uroliths progressively reduce in size at monthly intervals, therapeutic response is satisfactory. If two monthly intervals lapse without any change in urolith size or if uroliths increase in size and number at any time, the therapeutic protocol should be re-evaluated.

Because calculolytic diets stimulate thirst and promote diuresis, the magnitude of pollakiuria in dogs with urocystoliths may increase for a variable time after initiation of dietary therapy. Pollakiuria and the abnormal odor of urine caused by bacterial degradation of urea usually subside as infection is controlled and uroliths decrease in size. Reduction in ammonia-induced chemical inflammation as a result of ureolysis may also be involved in remission of these clinical signs.

Precautions

We have successfully induced dissolution of large bilateral renoliths presumed to be infection-induced struvite in a 6-year-old female bassett hound. Although the dog had impaired renal concentrating capacity (urine specific gravity was 1.016 during clinical dehydration) as a consequence of pyelonephritis, she was not azotemic (serum urea nitrogen = 11 mg/dl; serum creatinine = 0.7 mg/dl) at the time therapy of calculolytic diet and antimicrobial agents was initiated. This point is emphasized since dogs with moderate to severe primary renal failure require a greater than normal quantity of dietary protein for anabolism. The calculolytic diet used in our studies could induce protein malnutrition if given for prolonged periods to dogs with moderate azotemic primary renal failure.

Diuresis induced by augmenting water consumption appears to be a logical method to decrease the urine concentration of struvite and other calculogenic substances. However, additional salt is not recommended for dogs fed the previously described calculolytic diet, which has been formulated to contain supplemental sodium chloride. The mean urine specific gravity values of dogs fed the calculolytic diet were 1.008 ± 0.003, compared with baseline values of 1.028 ± 0.01. The mean 24-hour urine volume of dogs fed the calculolytic diet was 549 ml ± 223 compared with baseline values of 352 ml ± 107.

Because acidification of urine dramatically increases the solubility of struvite, it is an important therapeutic goal. A pH change of only 0.6 units (from 7.4 to 6.8) will result in a 75 per cent increase in apparent solubility of struvite. Since dogs fed calculolytic diet developed aciduria, however, supplemental use of urine acidifiers is not recommended. The mean urine pH of dogs with experimentally induced staphylococcal UTI and fed calculolytic diet was 6.2 ± 0.7, compared with baseline values of 7.6 ± 0.5. A similar response was observed in clinical trials (mean baseline urine pH = 7.6; mean treatment urine pH = 6.9).

Monitoring Response to Therapy

The size of uroliths should be periodically monitored by survey radiography. We recommend that radiographs be taken at monthly intervals (Figs. 1 and 2). Survey radiography is usually preferable to retrograde contrast radiography, since use of catheters during retrograde radiographic studies may result in iatrogenic UTI. Alternatively, intravenous urography may be considered.

Periodic evaluation of urine sediment for cystalluria also may be considered. Struvite crystals should not form if therapy has been effective in promoting formation of urine that is undersaturated with MAP.

UTI may persist despite antimicrobial therapy in patients with infection-induced struvite uroliths consuming the calculolytic diet. However, in most patients the magnitude of bacteriuria is usually reduced substantially (i.e., from more than 10^5 bacteria/ml of urine to 10^2 or 10^3 bacteria/ml of urine), and the associated inflammatory response progressively subsides. Difficulty in eradication of infection while uroliths persist may be related to persistence of viable microbes harbored within the stones. Diet-induced diuresis should be considered when formulating dosages of antimicrobial agents that will achieve minimum inhibitory concentrations in urine. Despite persistent bacteriuria during antimicrobial and dietary treatment of infected patients with struvite uroliths, we have had excellent success in inducing urolith dissolution. Concomitant use of calculolytic diets, antimicrobial agents, and AHA in this situation provided the most effective method of inducing urolith dissolution.

Urine collected by cystocentesis should be quantitatively cultured during therapy and 5 to 7 days after discontinuation of antimicrobial therapy. It is emphasized that results of urine culture may not be the same as results obtained prior to therapy or from cultures of the interior of uroliths. Rapid recurrence of UTI caused by the same type of organism (relapse) or a different type of bacterial pathogen (reinfection) after withdrawal of antimicrobial therapy may indicate residual calculi within the urinary tract or other abnormalities in local host defense mechanisms that predisposed the patient to UTI and subsequent urolithiasis.

Since small uroliths may escape detection by survey radiography, we recommend that the calculolytic diet and (if necessary) antimicrobial agents be continued for at least 1 month after radiographic documentation of urolith dissolution.

If uroliths increase in size during therapy or do not begin to decrease in size after approximately 8

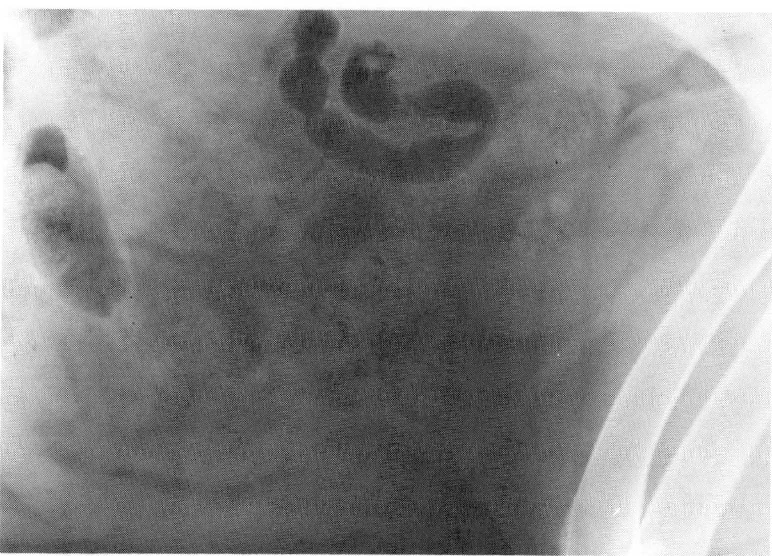

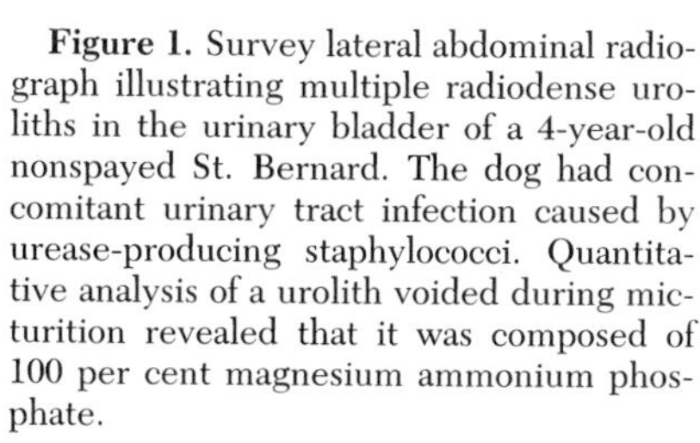

Figure 1. Survey lateral abdominal radiograph illustrating multiple radiodense uroliths in the urinary bladder of a 4-year-old nonspayed St. Bernard. The dog had concomitant urinary tract infection caused by urease-producing staphylococci. Quantitative analysis of a urolith voided during micturition revealed that it was composed of 100 per cent magnesium ammonium phosphate.

weeks of appropriate medical therapy, alternative methods of management should be considered. Small uroliths that become lodged in the urethra of male or female dogs during therapy may be readily returned to the urinary bladder lumen by urohydropropulsion. Complete obstruction of a ureter or renal pelvis, especially with concomitant UTI, is an absolute indication for surgical intervention.

Difficulty in inducing complete dissolution of uroliths by creating urine that is undersaturated with the suspected calculogenic crystalloid should prompt consideration that (1) the wrong mineral component was identified (Figs. 3 and 4), (2) the nucleus of the urolith is of different mineral composition than outer portions of the urolith, and (3) the owner or the patient is not complying with therapeutic recommendations.

SURGICAL AND MEDICAL MANAGEMENT

Detection of uroliths is not, in itself, an indication for surgery. However, along with medical management, surgical intervention has a vital role in therapy of urolithiasis. Surgical candidates include (1) patients with urolith-induced obstruction in urine outflow that cannot be corrected by nonsurgical techniques, especially in patients with concomitant UTI, (2) patients with uroliths that are refractory to current methods of medical dissolution (e.g., silica, calcium oxalate, calcium phosphate, and probably cystine uroliths), (3) patients with uroliths that are increasing in size or number despite medical therapy designed to inhibit their growth or cause their dissolution (especially if they are causing obstruction to urine outflow or progressive deterioration in renal

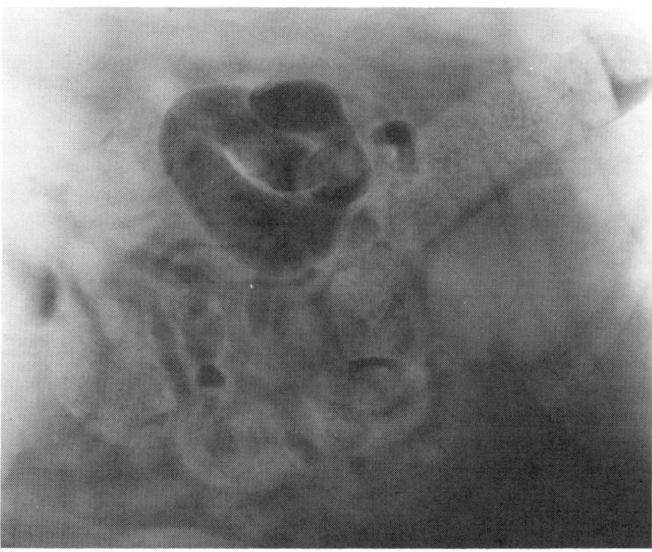

Figure 2. Survey lateral abdominal radiograph of the dog described in Figure 1. Radiographs obtained 32 days after initiation of therapy revealed only three uroliths. There are no detectable uroliths in the urinary tract in this radiograph, obtained 53 days after initiation of calculolytic therapy.

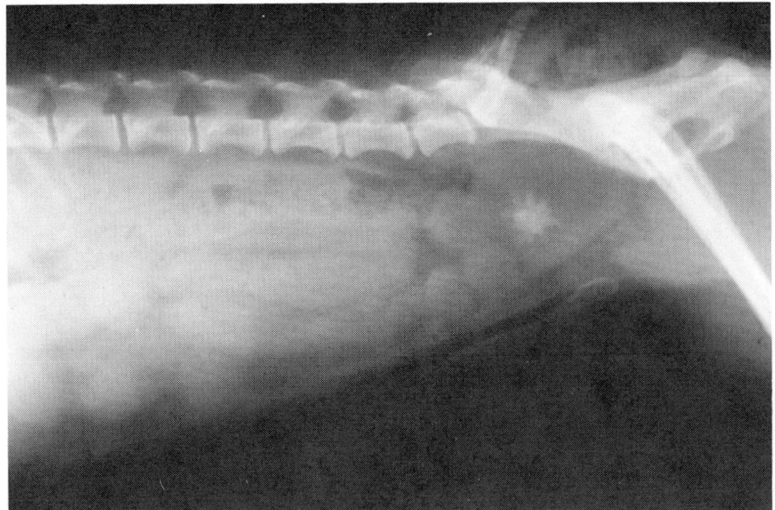

Figure 3. Survey lateral abdominal radiograph of a 7-year-old male Yorkshire terrier. The radiograph was obtained 98 days after initiation of calculolytic therapy. There is no change in the size or number of uroliths from those seen in a pretreatment radiograph.

function), (4) patients with nephroliths and renal dysfunction of such nature that the time required to induce medical dissolution is likely to be associated with more renal dysfunction than that associated with surgical procedures, (5) patients with anatomic defects of the urogenital tract that predispose to recurrent UTI and urolithiasis and are amenable to surgical correction at the time uroliths are removed, and (6) patients unable to respond to medical management because of poor client or patient compliance with therapeutic recommendations.

Complete obstruction to urine outflow caused by uroliths in patients with concomitant UTI should be regarded as a surgical emergency. In this situation, rapid spread of infection and associated damage to the urinary tract, especially the kidneys, are likely to induce septicemia and peracute renal failure caused by a combination of obstruction and pyelonephritis.

Unilateral renoliths or ureteroliths that have caused outflow obstruction and substantial impairment of function of the associated kidney should be managed by surgical intervention or (if possible) percutaneous nephropyelonephrostomy. Medical therapy designed to induce urolith dissolution during a period of several weeks in patients with poorly draining kidneys is unlikely to be effective, since the uroliths will not be continually bathed with newly formed urine modified to induce litholysis. The same concept applies to urethroliths that cannot be removed by nonsurgical methods.

Combined use of surgical removal of struvite uroliths followed by medical calculolytic protocols may be of value in some patients. Examples include patients in which uroliths or fragments of uroliths remain after surgery and patients with struvite cystalluria of a character and magnitude that indicate that rapid recurrence is likely. In this circumstance, meticulous procedure should be used in

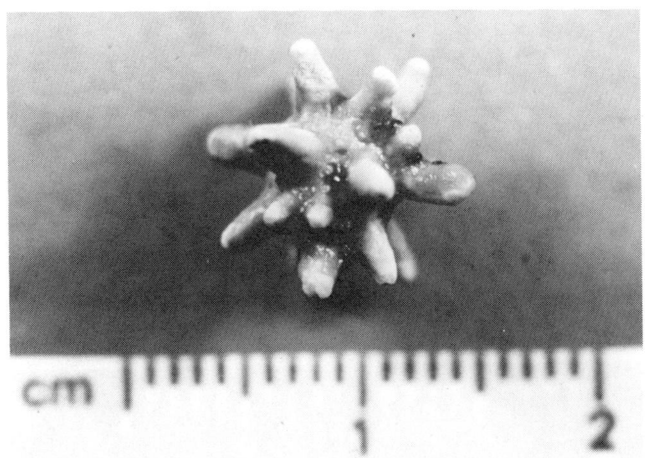

Figure 4. Amorphous silica jackstone removed from the urinary bladder of the dog described in Figure 3.

repairing surgical incision in dogs, since canine calculolytic diets are restricted in proteins.

PREVENTION OF CANINE STRUVITE UROLITHS

Eradication or control of UTI due to urease-producing bacteria is the most important factor in preventing recurrence of most infection-induced struvite uroliths. If recurrent UTI persists, indefinite therapy with prophylactic dosages of antimicrobial agents eliminated in high concentration in urine is indicated. These include nitrofurantoin, ampicillin, and trimethoprim-sulfa.

Because dietary modification is effective in inducing struvite urolith dissolution, its use in preventing recurrence of uroliths is logical and feasible. However, further studies must be performed to evaluate the long-term effects of low-protein calculolytic diets in dogs before reliable recommendations can be established. Because these diets induce polyuria, varying degrees of hypoalbuminemia, and mild alterations in hepatic enzymes and morphology, their long-term use is recommended only if patients develop recurrent urolithiasis despite augmented fluid intake and urine acidification. Preliminary results of a clinical trial in progress at the University of Minnesota indicate that diets for animals with renal failure (Prescription Diet u/d, Hill's Pet Products) containing less salt and more protein are good alternatives for prevention of canine struvite uroliths. Studies to evaluate the effectiveness of AHA in prevention of struvite urolithiasis in dogs with persistent UTI caused by urease-producing bacteria have been encouraging. Administration of 25 mg of AHA/kg/day to dogs with urinary bladder foreign bodies (zinc disks) and experimentally induced urease-positive staphylococcal UTI has been effective in preventing urolith formation and minimizing the rate of urolith growth. AHA has also been reported to be effective in prevention of struvite uroliths induced by urease-producing mycoplasma in rats.

Caution must be used in deciding whether or not to induce prophylactic diuresis in patients with struvite uroliths induced by recurrent UTI. Although formation of dilute urine tends to minimize supersaturation of urine with calculogenic crystalloids, it tends to counteract innate antimicrobial properties of urine. Experimental studies performed in rats and cats indicate that diuresis tends to minimize pyelonephritis but enhance lower urinary tract infections.

If the urine pH of patients with previous struvite urolithiasis remains alkaline despite antimicrobial and dietary therapy, administration of urine acidifiers should be considered.

References and Supplemental Reading

Abdullahi, S. U., Osborne, C. A., Leininger, J. R., et al.: Evaluation of a calculolytic diet in female dogs with induced struvite urolithiasis. Am. J. Vet. Res. 45:1508, 1984.

Boistelle, R., Abbona, F., Berland, Y., et al.: Growth and stability of magnesium ammonium phosphate (struvite) in acidic sterile urine. Urol. Res. 12:79, 1984.

Boyce, W. H., and Garvey, F. K.: The amount and nature of the organic matrix in urinary calculi. J. Urol. 76:213, 1956.

Burns, J. R., and Finlayson, B.: Solubility product of magnesium ammonium phosphate hexahydrate at various temperatures. J. Urol. 128:426, 1982.

Coe, F. L., and Favus, M. J.: Disorders of stone formation. *In* Brenner, B. M., and Rector, F. C. (eds.): *The Kidney*, 2nd ed., Vol. 2. Philadelphia: W. B. Saunders, 1981, pp. 1950–2007.

Fishbein, W. N.: Urease inhibitors in the treatment of infection induced stones: Some chemical, pharmacologic, and clinical considerations. *In* Smith, L. H., et al. (ed.): *Urolithiasis: Clinical and Basic Research*. New York: Plenum, 1981, pp. 209–214.

Grant, A. M. S., Baker, L. R. I., and Neuberger, A.: Urinary Tamm-Horsfall glycoprotein in certain kidney diseases and its content in renal and bladder calculi. Clin. Sci. 44:377, 1973.

Griffith, D. P.: Struvite stones. Kidney Int. 13:372, 1978.

Griffith, D. P., and Klein, A. S.: Infection-induced urinary stones. *In* Roth, R. A., and Finlayson, B. (eds.): *Clinical Management of Urolithiasis*. International Perspectives in Urology 6:210, 1983.

Griffith, D. P., Moskowitz, P. A., and Carlton, C. W.: Adjunctive chemotherapy of infection-induced staghorn calculi. J. Urol. 70:25, 1979.

Klausner, J. S., Osborne, C. A., O'Leary, T. P., et al.: Struvite urolithiasis in a litter of miniature schnauzer dogs. Am. J. Vet. Res. 40:712, 1980.

Klausner, J. S., Osborne, C. A., O'Leary, T. P., et al.: Experimental induction of struvite uroliths in miniature schnauzer and beagle dogs. Invest. Urol. 18:127, 1980.

Krawiec, D. R., Osborne, C. A., Leininger, J. R., et al.: Effect of acetohydroxamic acid on dissolution of canine uroliths. Am. J. Vet. Res. 45:1266, 1984.

Krawiec, D. R., Osborne, C. A., Leininger, J. R., et al.: Effect of acetohydroxamic acid on prevention of canine struvite uroliths. Am. J. Vet. Res. 45:1276, 1984.

Lamm, D. L., Johnson, S. A., Friedlander, A. M., et al.: Medical therapy of experimental infection stones. Urology 10:418, 1977.

Osborne, C. A., Abdullahi, S. U., Polzin, D. J., et al.: Current status of medical dissolution of canine and feline uroliths. Proc. 7th Kal Kan Symposium. Vernon, Calif. Kal Kan Foods Inc. 1984, pp. 52–79.

Osborne, C. A., Klausner, J. S., Krawiec, D. R., et al.: Canine struvite urolithiasis. Problems and their dissolution. J.A.V.M.A. 179:239, 1981.

Rosenstein, I. J. M., and Hamilton-Miller, J. M. T.: Inhibitors of urease as chemotherapeutic agents. Crit. Rev. Microbiol. 11:1, 1984.

Senior, D. G., Thomas, W. C., Gaskin, J. M., et al.: Relative merit of various strategies of nonsurgical treatment of infection stones in dogs. Urol. Res. 12:39, 1984.

Spector, A. R., Gray, A., and Prien, E. L.: Kidney stone matrix. Differences in acidic protein composition. Invest. Urol. 13:387, 1976.

MEDICAL DISSOLUTION AND PREVENTION OF FELINE STRUVITE UROLITHS

CARL A. OSBORNE, D.V.M.,
JOHN M. KRUGER, D.V.M.,
DAVID J. POLZIN, D.V.M.,
and MICHAEL F. McMENOMY, D.V.M.
St. Paul, Minnesota

TERMINOLOGY

In the past, confusion has occurred as a result of the variety of terms used to describe precipitates that form in feline urine. Depending on the size and consistency of the precipitates, they have been referred to as crystals, sand, sabulous plugs, gravel, pebbles, stones, rocks, uroliths, or calculi.

The world *crystal* is derived from the Greek word *krystallos*, which means "ice," and is used to refer to the solid phase of substances having a specific internal structure and enclosed by symmetrically arranged planar surfaces. The term *sabulous* is derived from the Latin word *sabulosus*, meaning "sand." The word *sand* refers to stones that range in diameter from 0.06 to 2 mm. The Latin word *calculus* means "pebble." The Greek word *lithos* means "stone," and *–uria* is a suffix derived from a Greek word (*ouron*) meaning "urine." The preferred terminology for abnormal microscopic precipitates in urine is *crystalluria*, whereas macroscopic concretions are called *uroliths* (e.g., nephroliths, urocystoliths). Plugs are defined as objects of any composition that close or obstruct passageways or ducts. Pending further studies, feline urethral plugs should be described with terminology that reflects their approximate proportion of minerals and matrix.

FELINE URETHRAL PLUGS VERSUS FELINE STRUVITE UROLITHS

Feline Urethral Plugs (Table 1)

GROSS APPEARANCE. Urethral plugs that form in male cats often resemble toothpaste that is forced through the narrowed circular opening of a toothpaste tube (Fig. 1). Typical soft, pastelike, compressible plugs sometimes have a cylindric shape when they are forced out of a male cat's external urethral orifice. At other times, they form a shapeless gelatinous mass. It is probable that their cylindric shape, when present, is influenced by the distended urethral lumen and the shape of the external urethral orifice. Although urethral plugs may be readily distorted and compressed by external pressure, classic uroliths are rocklike in consistency.

RADIOGRAPHIC APPEARANCE. The radiodensity of urethral plugs compared with that of soft tissue has not been evaluated in a large population of male cats with confirmed urethral disorders associated with intraluminal plugs. The radiodensity of urethral plugs formed *in vivo* may be influenced by a variety of factors: (1) their size, (2) their location

Table 1. *Characteristics of Feline Struvite Urethral Plugs*

Chemical name
Magnesium ammonium phosphate hexahydrate
Crystal name
Struvite
Formula
$MgNH_4PO_4{\cdot}6H_2O$
Variations in composition
Struvite only
Struvite mixed with relatively small quantities of calcium apatite
Physical characteristics
Color: Struvite urethral plugs are typically white, cream, or light brown in color
Shape: Often have a cylindrical shape; sometimes they form a shapeless gelatinous mass
Nuclei and laminations: None grossly visible
Density: Soft and easily compressible
Number: Apparently single
Size: Diameter conforms to diameter of urethra. Length varies from a few millimeters to several centimeters
Predisposing factors
Reduced diameter of the penile urethra
Locally produced matrix?
Factors affecting struvite crystalluria?
Characteristics of affected feline patients
Mean age = 3.8 yrs (range, < 1 to > 12 yr)
No obvious breed disposition
Consistently in males

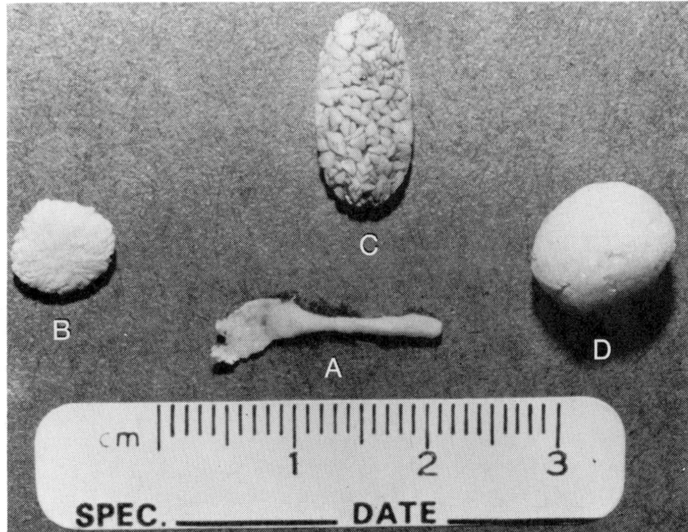

Figure 1. Concretions removed from the urinary tracts of male cats. *A*, Crystalline-matrix urethral plug; *B* and *C*, two waferlike, sterile struvite urocystoliths; *D*, an infected struvite urocystolith.

(within or exterior to the bony pelvis), (3) their ratio of mineral to matrix, (4) the quantity of tissue that must be penetrated by x-rays, and (5) the radiographic technique used to evaluate them. Uroliths that are composed primarily of matrix are radiolucent.

MICROSCOPIC APPEARANCE. Microscopic examination of a limited number of fresh matrix-crystalline plugs removed from the urethra of male cats during the initial episode of dysuria, when fixed in formalin and stained with hematoxylin and eosin or Gram stain, failed to demonstrate gram-positive bacteria within their matrix. This observation suggests that urease-producing staphylococci were not involved in initiation of their formation.

MATRIX COMPOSITION. When typical male feline urethral plugs are allowed to soak in solutions that are not supersaturated with calculogenic materials (water, physiologic saline solution, formalin, lactated Ringer's solution), a portion of their crystalline components frequently migrates into the surrounding medium, leaving behind varying quantities of gelatinous substances that are presumed to be matrix. When classic uroliths are allowed to soak in such solutions, they occasionally become more friable, but there is no perceptible visible change in their composition.

The specific composition and origin (urine and tissue surrounding the lumen of the urinary tract) of the matrix in urethral plugs has not been identified, nor has it been established whether or not matrix components of different plugs are consistently similar. The fact that many urethral plugs are typically constructed with a pastelike consistency and the fact that they have poor radiodensity indicate that they contain a substantially greater quantity of matrix than classical uroliths.

MINERAL COMPOSITION. Although it has been generally accepted that male feline urethral plugs are composed of varying quantities of minerals and matrix, there have been only a few reports of evaluation of the mineral composition of a limited number of plugs. Quantitative mineral analysis of 266 male feline urethral plugs submitted to the University of Minnesota by colleagues in private practice in North America revealed that 78 per cent (205) were composed of 100 per cent struvite, 13 per cent (35) were composed primarily (greater than 70 per cent) of struvite, less than 2 per cent (4) were composed primarily of calcium phosphate, less than 2 per cent (3) were composed of calcium oxalate, and less than 1 per cent (1) were composed of ammonium acid urate. About 4 per cent (10) were composed almost entirely of matrix, and less than 2 per cent were composed of a mixture of minerals. The infrequency with which nonstruvite minerals were recognized in urethral plugs suggests that they are not of great clinical importance. However, they are of great conceptual importance because they suggest that any type of crystal may become trapped in plug matrix. The importance of this observation is that it suggests that matrix may play an important primary role in the formation of some urethral plugs, whereas crystals may play a secondary role in their development.

MALES VERSUS FEMALES. Although females develop naturally occurring classical uroliths almost as often as male cats, available evidence indicates that urethral plugs composed of a large quantity of matrix and variable quantities of minerals are extremely uncommon in females (if they occur). The reason for this difference is unknown. Although it is possible that plugs form in female cats and are voided during micturition, lack of detection of pluglike material in the lower urinary tract of female felines makes this explanation improbable. We are consid-

Table 2. Common Characteristics of Feline Struvite Uroliths

Chemical name
Magnesium ammonium phosphate hexahydrate
Crystal name
Struvite
Formula
$MgNH_4PO_4 \cdot 6H_2O$
Variations in composition
Struvite only (most common).
Struvite mixed with lesser quantities of calcium apatite, ammonium acid urate, or uric acid.
Nucleus of a different mineral surrounded by variable layers composed primarily of struvite. Small quantities of calcium apatite or ammonium acid urate or both may also be present.
Physical characteristics
Color: Struvite uroliths are usually white, cream, or light brown in color. The surface of uroliths is commonly red because of concomitant hematuria, and it may be green (caused by bile pigments).
Shape: Sterile struvite uroliths obtained from the urinary bladder of cats commonly have a wafer or disc shape; they are typically thicker at their center than at the periphery. Sterile feline struvite uroliths may also have a rough, jagged, quartz-like appearance.
Nuclei and laminations: Common in infection-induced uroliths in all species. Uncommon in sterile struvite uroliths of cats.
Density: Variable; soft if they contain a large quantity of matrix; dense and harder to cut if little matrix is present. A combination of hard and soft internal density may occur within the same urolith. Radiodense compared with nonskeletal tissue on survey radiographs. Degree of radiodensity is related to the quantity of matrix (inversely proportional) and other minerals, especially calcium apatite (more proportional).
Number: Single or multiple.
Location: May be located in the kidney, ureter, urinary bladder, and urethra in all species. Most occur in the urinary bladder of cats.
Size: Microscopic to a size limited by the capacity of the structure (kidney and urinary bladder) in which they form.
Predisposing factors
Urinary tract infections with urease-producing microbes in patients whose urine contains a large quantity of urea.
Alkaline urine pH.
Staphylococci may cause struvite uroliths in cats, but most feline struvite uroliths form in sterile urine.
Characteristics of affected patients
No obvious breed disposition in cats.
No apparent sex predisposition in cats.

ering an alternative explanation related to sex differences in periurethral glandular tissue.

Feline Uroliths (Table 2)

GROSS APPEARANCE AND LOCATION. The gross appearance and consistency of classic struvite uroliths encountered in male and female cats are unquestionably different from feline urethral plugs that occur in male cats (Fig. 1). Unlike urethral plugs, uroliths are composed of organized crystal aggregates with a complex internal structure.

The majority of uroliths observed in cats have occurred in the urinary bladder; however, on occasion small uroliths formed in the bladder have passed through or obstructed the urethra. Renoliths are less common than bladder uroliths in cats; ureteroliths have been rarely encountered.

Although uroliths removed from the urinary tract of cats may assume any of a variety of shapes, many sterile struvite uroliths located in the urinary bladder of cats have been shaped like wafers or disks (Fig. 1). Such uroliths are typically thicker at their center than at the periphery. The gross appearance of some of these uroliths resembles those induced with calculogenic diets supplemented with magnesium.

RADIOGRAPHIC APPEARANCE. Spheric uroliths with a diameter greater than 3 mm are usually radiodense when evaluated by survey radiography. However, since smaller uroliths frequently occur in the urinary bladders of cats, double contrast radiography may be required to detect their presence. Flattened circular uroliths are also commonly encountered in the urinary systems of cats and are less radiodense than spheric uroliths of similar maximum circumference.

MINERAL COMPOSITION. Uroliths similar in appearance to those encountered in dogs and other species have frequently been observed in the urinary system of male and female cats. Struvite uroliths are the most common form of feline uroliths; ammonium urate, uric acid, calcium phosphate, and calcium oxalate uroliths occur less frequently (Table 3).

In humans and dogs, uroliths predominantly composed of struvite commonly contain smaller quantities of calcium apatite and carbonate apatite (refer to the article entitled Medical Dissolution and Prevention of Canine Struvite Uroliths for additional information). However, the majority of struvite uroliths in cats are pure (100 per cent) magnesium ammonium phosphate (Table 1). This observation supports the hypothesis that the initiation of one type of struvite urolith in cats is not linked to infection with urease-producing bacteria.

MICROSCOPIC APPEARANCE. The microscopic appearance of the matrix of uroliths removed from cats is influenced by whether or not they were formed in association with urinary tract infection (UTI). Gram-positive bacteria cannot be identified in the inner portions of struvite uroliths formed in bacteriologically sterile urine. In contrast, large numbers of gram-positive bacteria can be readily identified in the inner portions of struvite uroliths formed in infected urine, especially those associated with urease-producing staphylococci. On occasion, a combination of a gram-negative struvite nidus surrounded by infected struvite laminations may occur.

Table 3. *Mineral Composition of 494 Feline Uroliths Analyzed by Quantitative Methods**

Predominant Mineral Type	Number of Uroliths	Percentage
Magnesium ammonium phosphate (•$6H_2O$)	420	85.0
100%	(329)	(66.6)
70–99%†	(91)	(18.4)
Calcium oxalate	15	3.0
Calcium oxalate monohydrate		
100%	(4)	(0.8)
70–99%†	(8)	(1.6)
Calcium oxalate dihydrate		
70–99%†	(3)	(0.6)
Calcium phosphate	10	2.0
Calcium phosphate		
100%	(4)	(0.8)
70–99%†	(5)	(1.0)
Calcium hydrogen phosphate (•$2H_2O$)		
100%	(1)	(0.2)
Uric acid and urates	9	1.8
Ammonium acid urate		
100%	(6)	(1.2)
Uric acid		
100%	(2)	(0.4)
70–99%†	(1)	(0.2)
Cystine	0	0
Silica	0	0
Mixed‡	19	3.8
Compound§	7	1.4
Matrix	14	2.8
Totals	494	100%

*Analysis performed by optical crystallography and x-ray diffraction.

†Uroliths composed of 70 to 99 per cent of mineral type listed; no nucleus and shell detected.

‡Uroliths did not contain at least 70 per cent of mineral type listed; no nucleus and shell detected.

§Uroliths containing an identifiable nucleus and one or more surrounding layers of different mineral type.

Summary

In summary, it appears that at least three different mechanisms may result in feline urinary struvite precipitates that are qualitatively similar but quantitatively and etiologically dissimilar. Formation of amorphous urethral plugs with a large quantity of matrix that is a result of unidentified mechanisms is one type. Formation of sterile struvite uroliths, perhaps as a result of certain dietary ingredients, is another type. Sterile struvite uroliths typically have less matrix than do urethral plugs. Formation of "infected" or "urease" struvite uroliths as a sequela to UTI with urease-producing bacteria is a third type. Infection-induced feline struvite uroliths appear to contain more matrix than sterile uroliths but typically contain less matrix than do urethral plugs. A combination of a sterile struvite nidus that predisposes to UTI with urease-producing bacteria and subsequent formation of infected struvite laminations around the sterile nidus may also occur. It is emphasized that not all feline uroliths are composed of struvite. Other mineral forms may also occur.

BIOLOGIC BEHAVIOR OF UROLITHS

The natural course of struvite urolithiasis has not been well documented in cats. Feline uroliths have been detected in cats ranging in age from 2 months to older than 16 years. We have observed spontaneous dissolution of naturally occurring bladder uroliths presumed to be struvite in two adult cats. In one, a 5-year-old female domestic shorthair, uroliths spontaneously dissolved 18 days after their radiographic detection. Radiographic evidence of uroliths was not detected during seven monthly follow-up examinations. However, on the eighth month, multiple urocystoliths were detected. They subsequently dissolved spontaneously during the next 3½ months.

In male and female cats, uroliths that form in the urinary bladder may pass into the urethra. Likewise, renoliths may pass into the ureters. Feline struvite uroliths have a tendency to recur. In one retrospective study of uroliths in cats, there were 25 known recurrences in 131 patients. Twenty-one cats had two recurrent episodes, whereas three cats had three recurrences and one cat had four recurrences.

It is generally accepted that feline urethral plugs are associated with a frequent but unpredictable tendency to recur. However, this appears to be an overstatement, since most investigators have considered urethral obstruction in male cats and struvite urethral plugs interchangeably. Recent clinical studies, however, indicate that urethral obstruction in male cats may be initiated and maintained at one or more sites by one or a combination of primary, secondary, or iatrogenic causes. Even in those instances in which recurrent obstruction is caused by urethral plugs, there have been no studies specifically designed to evaluate comparisons of the nature and composition of first-occurrence plugs and recurrent obstructing material.

DIAGNOSIS

Uroliths are usually suspected on the basis of typical findings obtained by history and physical examination. Urinalyses, urine culture, and radiography may be required to differentiate uroliths from other causes of clinical signs such as UTI, inflammatory polyps, and neoplasia. (Consult the article entitled Medical Dissolution and Prevention of Canine Struvite Uroliths for specific details.)

Formulation of therapy to reduce the composition of specific calculogenic crystalloids in urine is de-

***Table 4.** Checklist of Factors that May Aid in "Guesstimation" of Mineral Composition of Uroliths*

1. Radiodensity and physical characteristics of uroliths
2. Urine pH
   a. Sterile struvite—usually 6.5 or higher
   b. Infected struvite—usually 7.5 or higher
   c. Calcium phosphate—presumed to be alkaline
   d. Ammonium urate—presumed to be variable
   e. Uric acid—presumed to be acidic
   f. Calcium oxalate—presumed to be variable
   g. Cystine—not yet identified in cats
   h. Silica—not yet identified in cats
3. Identification of crystals in urine sediment
4. Type of bacteria, if any, isolated from urine
   a. Urease-producing bacteria, especially staphylococci, commonly associated with infected struvite uroliths
   b. Urinary tract infections often absent with sterile struvite uroliths and metabolic uroliths. When present they are associated with a variety of urease positive or urease negative bacteria
   c. Sterile struvite and metabolic uroliths may predispose cats to UTI. If infections are caused by urease-producing microbes, infected struvite may precipitate around them
5. Serum chemistry evaluation
   a. Hypercalcemia may be associated with calcium-containing uroliths (apparently uncommon in cats)
   b. Hyperuricemia may be associated with urate uroliths (apparently uncommon in cats)
   c. Hyperchloremia, hypokalemia, and acidemia may be associated with distal renal tubular acidosis and calcium phosphate uroliths (not yet documented in cats)
6. Urine chemistry evaluation
   a. Patient should be consuming a standardized diagnostic diet, or the diet consumed when uroliths were formed
   b. Although no controlled studies have been performed in cats, excessive quantities of one or more minerals contained in the urolith are expected.
7. Analysis of uroliths fortuitously passed during micturition (especially female cats)

pendent on knowledge of the composition of uroliths. For example, use of magnesium-restricted diets might enhance calcium oxalate urolith formation, since magnesium is an inhibitor of calcium oxalate crystal formation. On the other hand, use of magnesium-restricted diets might be beneficial in preventing recurrent formation of magnesium ammonium phosphate uroliths. In situations in which consideration is being given to medical therapy but uroliths are not available for analysis, one may be forced to make an educated guess about their composition (Table 4).

MEDICAL MANAGEMENT OF FELINE STRUVITE UROLITHS

Overview

Consult the article entitled Medical Management and Prevention of Canine Struvite Uroliths for specific details pertaining to indications for and objectives of medical dissolution of struvite uroliths.

Experimental and clinical studies of feline sterile struvite uroliths have confirmed the feasibility of inducing their dissolution by medical therapy. Key components in inducing dissolution of most struvite uroliths in cats appear to be (1) reduction of urine pH to 6.0 or less and (2) reduction of urine magnesium by feeding magnesium-restricted diets (Table 5). Although formation of dilute urine may enhance the rate of urolith dissolution, our preliminary results indicate that this factor is not an essential component of medical calculolytic protocols for treatment of sterile uroliths in cats.

Clinical Studies of Sterile Struvite Uroliths

In a pilot clinical study of three male and seven female cats with urocystoliths presumed to be composed of sterile struvite, patients were given a high-moisture magnesium restricted diet (Prescription diet c/d, Hill's Pet Products) supplemented with sufficient D,L-methionine (1000 to 1500 mg/day) or a mixture of ammonium chloride and D,L-methio-

***Table 5.** Summary of Recommendations for Medical Dissolution of Feline Struvite Uroliths*

1. Perform appropriate diagnostic studies including complete urinalyses, quantitative urine culture, and diagnostic radiography. Estimate urolith composition by evaluation of appropriate clinical data (Table 4).
2. Initiate dietary management designed to reduce the urine concentration of magnesium and create a pH of 6.0 or less. No other food should be fed to patients consuming calculolytic diets. Monitor urine pH 4 to 8 hours after eating. Urine that is acidic at this time is likely to be acidic throughout the day.
3. Although attempts may be made to stimulate thirst-induced diuresis by addition of sodium chloride to the diet, it is not essential. Thirst-induced diuresis may be of benefit to patients with slowly dissolving uroliths.
4. Attempt to eradicate or control secondary UTI with antimicrobial agents. Although control of secondary UTI is not essential to induce sterile struvite urolith dissolution, it is warranted to prevent damage of tissues of the urinary tract by bacteria and their metabolites.
5. Periodically (2- to 4-week intervals) monitor the size of uroliths by survey radiography. Survey radiography is preferable to retrograde contrast radiography to monitor urolith dissolution, since use of catheters during retrograde radiographic studies may result in iatrogenic UTI. Alternatively, intravenous urography may be considered.
6. Periodic evaluation of urine sediment for crystalluria may be considered. Struvite crystals should not form if therapy has been effective in promoting formation of urine that is undersaturated with magnesium ammonium phosphate.
7. Continue calculolytic diet therapy for at least 1 month after radiographic disappearance of uroliths.
8. If uroliths increase in size during dietary management or do not begin to decrease in size after approximately 4 to 8 weeks of appropriate medical management, alternative methods should be considered. Difficulty in inducing complete dissolution of uroliths by creating urine that is undersaturated with the suspected calculogenic crystalloid should prompt consideration that (1) the wrong mineral component was identified, (2) the nucleus of the urolith is of different mineral composition than other portions of the urolith, or (3) the owner of the patient is not complying with medical recommendations.

nine to induce urine pH values of 6.0 or less. All uroliths dissolved within a mean of 47 days (range = 29 to 100 days).

In a follow-up clinical study of eight male and seven female cats fed a high-moisture (canned) calculolytic diet (Prescription Diet Feline s/d, Hill's Pet Products), urocystoliths presumed to be composed of sterile struvite dissolved in a mean of 32 days (range = 14 to 82 days) (Figs. 2 and 3). The high-energy diet (720 calories/15 oz) containing 41.4 per cent dry weight protein was formulated to contain reduced quantities of magnesium (0.058 per cent dry weight) and to promote formation of acid urine (pH ± 6.0). The diet was also supplemented with sodium chloride (0.79 per cent of dry weight sodium) to stimulate thirst and promote diuresis.

Results of these clinical studies confirm that medical dissolution of sterile struvite uroliths in cats is a reasonable alternative to surgery.

Clinical Studies of Infected Struvite Uroliths

Infection-induced struvite uroliths occur in cats but are much less common than sterile struvite uroliths. The authors have induced dissolution of staphylococcus-associated cystoliths presumed to be composed of struvite in two cats by using a combination of antimicrobial agents and the calculolytic diet used for sterile struvite uroliths. We have not yet determined the relative benefit of restricting dietary protein (and thus urine urea concentration) in promoting dissolution of infection-induced struvite uroliths in such patients. This point is of considerable significance because of the relatively high protein requirement of cats. We emphasize that the calculolytic diet designed for use in dogs should not be given to cats because of the restricted quantity of protein that it contains.

Precautions

Since the calculolytic diet is supplemented with sodium chloride and since it has been formulated to produce aciduria, neither sodium chloride nor urine acidifiers should be given concomitantly with it. Likewise, the diet should not be given to cats that are acidemic (e.g., primary renal dysfunction, postrenal azotemia) or to cats with cardiac dysfunction or hypertension.

Monitoring Response to Therapy

The size of uroliths should be periodically monitored by survey radiography. We recommend that radiographs be taken at 2- to 4-week intervals.

Periodic evaluation of urine sediment for crystalluria also may be considered. Struvite crystals should not form if therapy has been effective in promoting urine that is undersaturated with magnesium ammonium phosphate.

Urine collected by cystocentesis from patients with concomitant UTI should be periodically cultured for microbes. If bacteriuria persists despite antimicrobic therapy, antimicrobial susceptibility tests should be re-evaluated to determine the antimicrobial agent of choice.

Since small uroliths may escape detection by survey radiography, we recommend that the calculolytic diet and (if necessary) antimicrobial agents be continued for at least 1 month after radiographic documentation of urolith dissolution.

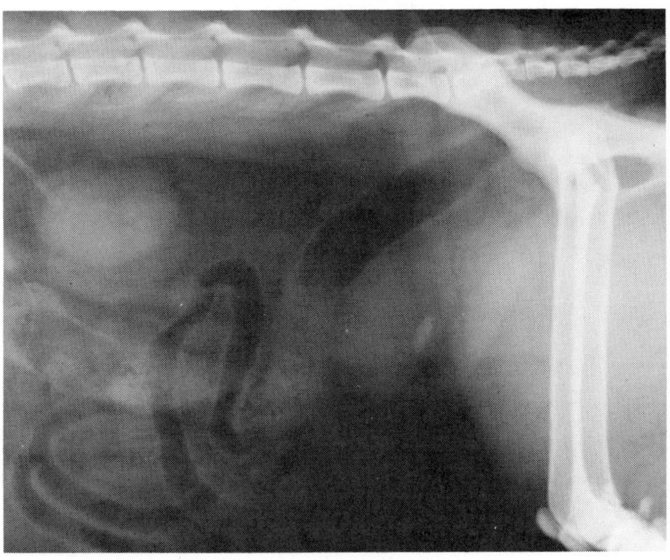

Figure 2. Survey radiograph of the lateral aspect of the abdomen of a 6-year-old spayed female domestic long-hair cat. Note the solitary radiodense urolith in the bladder lumen. Aerobic bacteria could not be cultured from a urine sample collected by cystocentesis.

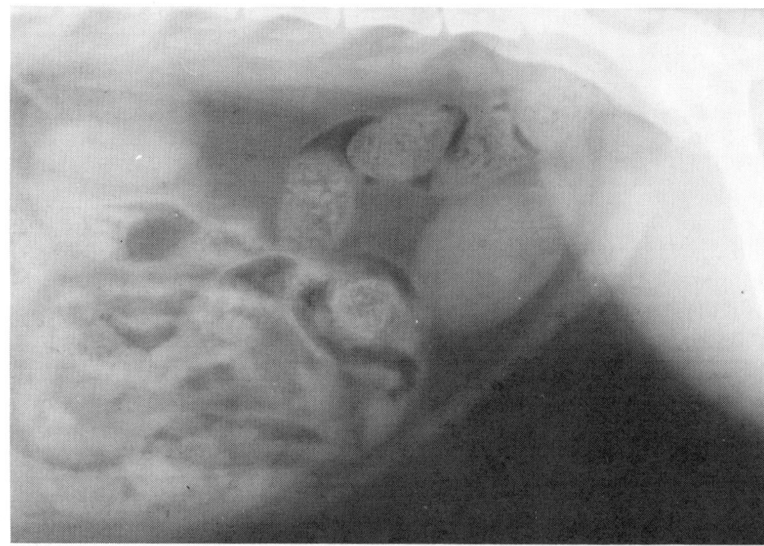

Figure 3. Survey radiograph of the lateral aspect of the cat described in Figure 2. They were obtained 5 weeks after initiation of a calculolytic diet. There are no radiodense uroliths in the urinary tract.

Difficulty in inducing complete dissolution of uroliths by creating urine that is undersaturated with struvite should prompt consideration that (1) the wrong mineral component was identified (Figs. 4 and 5), (2) the nucleus of the urolith is of different mineral composition than outer portions of the urolith, or (3) the owner or patient is not complying with therapeutic recommendations.

Prevention of Recurrence of Struvite Uroliths

Empirical clinical studies performed at the University of Minnesota Veterinary Teaching Hospital indicate that acidification of urine (pH less than 6.0) and consumption of low-magnesium diets are effective in preventing recurrence of sterile struvite cystoliths in male and female cats. No attempt was made to determine whether acidification of urine or the low-magnesium diet was the major factor responsible for the beneficial results.

Prevention of infection-induced struvite uroliths in cats should be based on the same principles as those described for dogs. The key to prevention of recurrence is eradication or control of infection.

MEDICAL MANAGEMENT OF FELINE URETHRAL PLUGS

The immediate need to remove urethral plugs within hours of their discovery precludes attempts

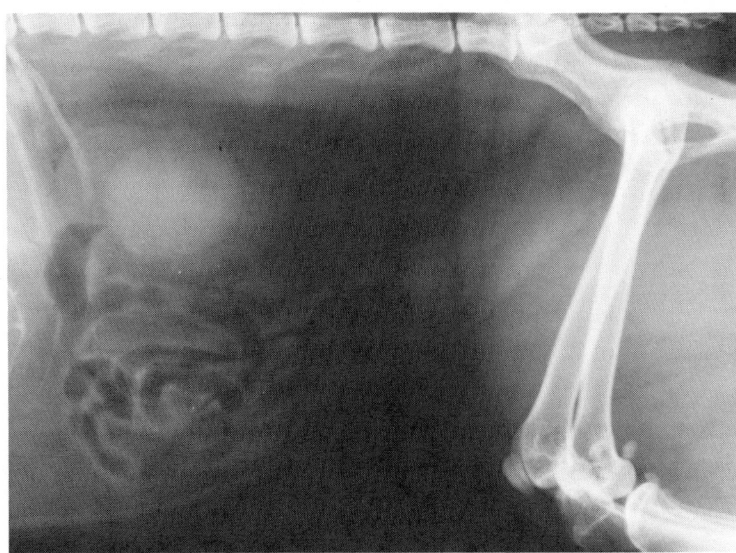

Figure 4. Survey radiograph of the lateral aspect of a cat, 12 weeks after initiation of therapy with a calculolytic diet. There has been no change in the size of the urolith from that seen in a pretreatment radiograph.

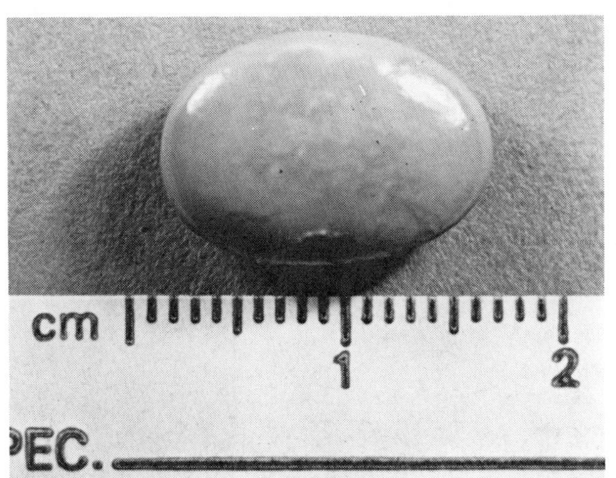

Figure 5. Urolith surgically removed from the urinary bladder of the cat shown in Figure 4. Quantitative analysis revealed that it was composed of 100 per cent ammonium acid urate.

to cause their dissolution over a period of days to weeks. However, it is often possible to repulse urethral plugs into the bladder lumen. Thus the question arises, "Can such plugs be dissolved by medical therapy?" As previously discussed, urethral plugs typically contain a substantially greater quantity of matrix than do classic uroliths. Although it is likely that medical protocols effective in inducing sterile struvite urolith dissolution would also be effective in dissolving the struvite crystalline component of urethral plugs located in the bladder lumen, it is difficult to comprehend how such therapy would dissolve plug matrix.

If formation of insoluble crystals were a primary event that stimulated production of matrix substances by tissues lining the urethral lumen, one could hypothesize that prevention of crystal formation would in turn prevent matrix formation. Currently, there are no data to prove or disprove this hypothesis. Investigative progress has been hindered by lack of a reproducible model of feline lower urinary tract disease characterized by urethral plug formation.

METABOLIC UROLITHS

Recommendations for consistently effective medical dissolution of naturally occurring calcium oxalate, calcium phosphate, uric acid, and ammonium acid urate uroliths in cats remain a goal for the future. With our present knowledge of nonstruvite feline uroliths, surgery remains the most reliable way to remove them from the urinary tract.

References and Supplemental Reading

Bohonowych, R. O., Parks, J. L., and Greene, R. W.: Features of cystic calculi in cats in a hospital population. J.A.V.M.A. 173:301, 1978.

Finco, D. R., and Barsanti, J. A.: Diet-induced feline urethral obstruction. Vet. Clin. North Am. 14:529, 1984.

Johnston, G. R., Feeney, D. A., and Osborne C. A.: Urethrography and cystography in cats. Part II. Abnormal radiographic anatomy and complications. Comp. Cont. Ed. Pract. Vet. 4:931, 1982.

Osborne, C. A., Clinton, C. W., Brunkow, H. C., et al.: Epidemiology of naturally occurring feline uroliths and urethral plugs. Vet. Clin.. North Am. 14:481, 1984.

Osborne, C. A., Kruger, J. M., Polzin, D. J., et al.: Medical dissolution of feline struvite uroliths. Minn. Vet. 24:22, 1984.

Taton, G. F., Hamar, D. W., and Lewis, L. D.: Urinary acidification in the prevention and treatment of feline struvite urolithiasis. J.A.V.M.A. 184:437, 1984.

MEDICAL MANAGEMENT OF FELINE UROLOGIC SYNDROME

CARL A. OSBORNE, D.V.M.,
DAVID J. POLZIN, D.V.M.,
GARY R. JOHNSTON, D.V.M.,
and JOHN M. KRUGER, D.V.M.
St. Paul, Minnesota

DEFINITION

Available experimental and clinical data suggest that the term *feline urologic syndrome* (FUS) is in reality a synonym for a lower urinary tract disease resulting from fundamentally different causes that may be single, multiple and interacting, or unrelated. More than one causal agent may act dependently or independently in an affected cat. A change in the perspective with which we view naturally occurring forms of FUS is of considerable clinical significance because it tends to eliminate the stereotyped approach to treatment and prevention of FUS that is currently in vogue. We suggest that the term *feline urologic syndrome* be abandoned and replaced with descriptive terms pertaining to the site (e.g., urethra, bladder), causes (e.g., bacteria, parasites, neoplasms, metabolic disturbances, idiopathic forms), morphologic changes (e.g., inflammation, neoplasia), and pathophysiologic mechanisms (e.g., obstructive urethropathy, reflex dyssynergia) whenever possible. The same terminology and approach to diagnosis and treatment of lower urinary tract disorders of other species (e.g., dogs, humans) should be used for cats.

ETIOPATHOGENESIS

Feline Urethral Plugs versus Uroliths

We hypothesize that at least three different mechanisms may result in feline urinary struvite precipitates that are qualitatively similar but quantitatively and etiologically dissimilar. Formation of amorphous urethral plugs with a large quantity of matrix due to as yet unidentified mechanisms is one type. Formation of sterile struvite uroliths, perhaps as a result of certain dietary ingredients, is another. Sterile struvite uroliths typically have less matrix than do urethral plugs. Formation of "infected" or "urease" struvite uroliths as a sequela to urinary tract infection (UTI) with urease-producing microbes is a third. A combination of a sterile struvite nidus that predisposes to UTI with urease-producing bacteria and subsequent formation of infected struvite laminations around the sterile nidus also may occur. (Consult the article entitled Medical Dissolution and Prevention of Feline Struvite Uroliths for specific details.)

Causes and Sites of Urethral Obstruction

CAUSES. Survey and contrast radiographic studies of male cats with naturally occurring urethral obstruction have revealed that urethral obstruction may be associated with urethral plugs, uroliths, strictures caused by connective tissue, lesions of the prostate gland, and extraluminal masses that have compressed the urethral lumen (Table 1; Fig. 1). In some patients, an anatomic cause of partial or total obstruction could not be identified. These observations prompt consideration of whether inflammatory swelling of the urethral wall or spasm of musculature associated with inflammation is primarily involved in some cases. Functional outflow obstruction caused by reflex dyssynergia is an additional possibility.

SITES. Radiographic studies of male cats with naturally occurring urethral obstruction have revealed that partial or total urethral obstruction may occur at sites other than, or in addition to, the penile urethra. These observations suggest that surgical procedures designed to minimize obstruction of the distal urethra of male cats by amputating the penis may be partially or totally ineffective in some cases. In addition, persistence of unrecognized concomitant abnormalities may contribute to what is perceived to be the recurrent nature of

Table 1. Possible Causes of Urethral Obstruction in Male Cats

Primary Causes	Perpetuating Causes	Iatrogenic Causes
Intraluminal	Intraluminal	Tissue damage
Plugs (matrix and crystals)	Sloughed tissue	Reverse flushing solutions
Uroliths	Inflammatory cells, fibrin and RBC (clots)	Catheter trauma
Sloughed tissue (uncommon)	Overproduction of mucoprotein	Catheter-induced foreign body reaction
Mural or extra-mural	Mural	Post-surgical dysfunction
Neoplasms	Inflammatory swelling	
Strictures	Muscular spasm	
Anomalies	Strictures	
Reflex dyssynergia		
Combinations	Combinations	
Other (?)	Other (?)	

lower urinary tract disease in male cats. Therefore, prior to irreversible amputation of the distal urethra, radiographic procedures are recommended to localize the sites of obstruction and, if possible, to determine the causes of obstruction (Fig. 2).

Infectious Agents

VIRUSES. Although published data about experimentally induced viral FUS are impressive, the inability of some investigators to reproduce this experimental model of FUS and the inability of others to isolate herpesvirus or calicivirus from naturally occurring cases of FUS have prompted questions about the relationship between this model and naturally occurring forms of the disease. Attempts to induce viral lower urinary tract disease experimentally in female cats have apparently not been performed.

The role of viruses as causative agents in naturally occurring FUS remains unresolved. In light of the fact that a substantial number of male and female cats develop hematuria, dysuria, and urethral obstruction without demonstrable cause, and in light of the difficulty in routinely isolating viruses from naturally occurring cases, the search for viral pathogens must continue.

BACTERIA. The initial episode of feline lower urinary tract disorders typically occurs in the absence of significant numbers of detectable bacteria in the urine. When significant bacteriuria has been confirmed, it frequently (but not invariably) occurred as a secondary or complicating rather than a primary etiologic factor. The infrequency with which bacteria have been isolated from urine of cats during the early phases of lower urinary tract disease may be related to highly effective local host defense mechanisms in this species.

Despite these obstructions, it is possible that primary bacterial infection has a role in at least an occasional case of feline lower urinary tract disease. Further studies are required to determine whether or not viable pathogens are present in tissues that line the lumen of the urinary system. Pending the outcome of these studies, routine screening by quantitative urine culture is recommended prior to the administration of diagnostic or therapeutic agents. It is emphasized that bacterial infection may also occur as a sequel to FUS, especially in patients with open indwelling urethral catheters.

Dietary Factors

Current data suggest that the composition of diets may have a primary role in formation of sterile struvite uroliths in cats with naturally occurring urolithiasis. The relationship of diets to formation of urethral matrix plugs is not clear. (Consult the article entitled Medical Dissolution and Prevention of Feline Struvite Uroliths for additional information.)

The role of diet in formation of infection-induced struvite uroliths occasionally encountered in cats has not been evaluated. As is the situation in dogs, we presume that formation of infection-induced feline struvite uroliths is dependent on urease-producing pathogens in the urinary tract and urinary excretion of sufficient urea to alkalinize urine, which in turn promotes supersaturation of urine with magnesium, ammonium, and phosphate.

Urachal Anomalies

Anomalies of the urachus, especially bladder diverticula associated with partial patency of the urachus, have frequently been identified in cats with lower urinary tract disease. Unlike the condition in dogs, the significance of vesicourachal diverticula in cats is more difficult to assess. In a study performed at the University of Minnesota, 60 per cent of male and female cats evaluated for signs of lower urinary tract disease had vesicourachal diverticula detected by contrast cystography. Surprisingly, only 40 per cent of these cats had bacterial UTI. This finding may be related to the inherent resistance of the cat's urinary tract to bacterial infection, or it may suggest that vesicourachal diverticula in cats are less likely to predispose the host to bacterial UTI than in dogs.

The prevalence of urachal diverticula in cats without signs of lower urinary tract disease must be determined in order to prevent overinterpretation of the significance of these anomalies. The fact that urachal diverticula do not commonly cause recognizable clinical signs in cats younger than 1 year

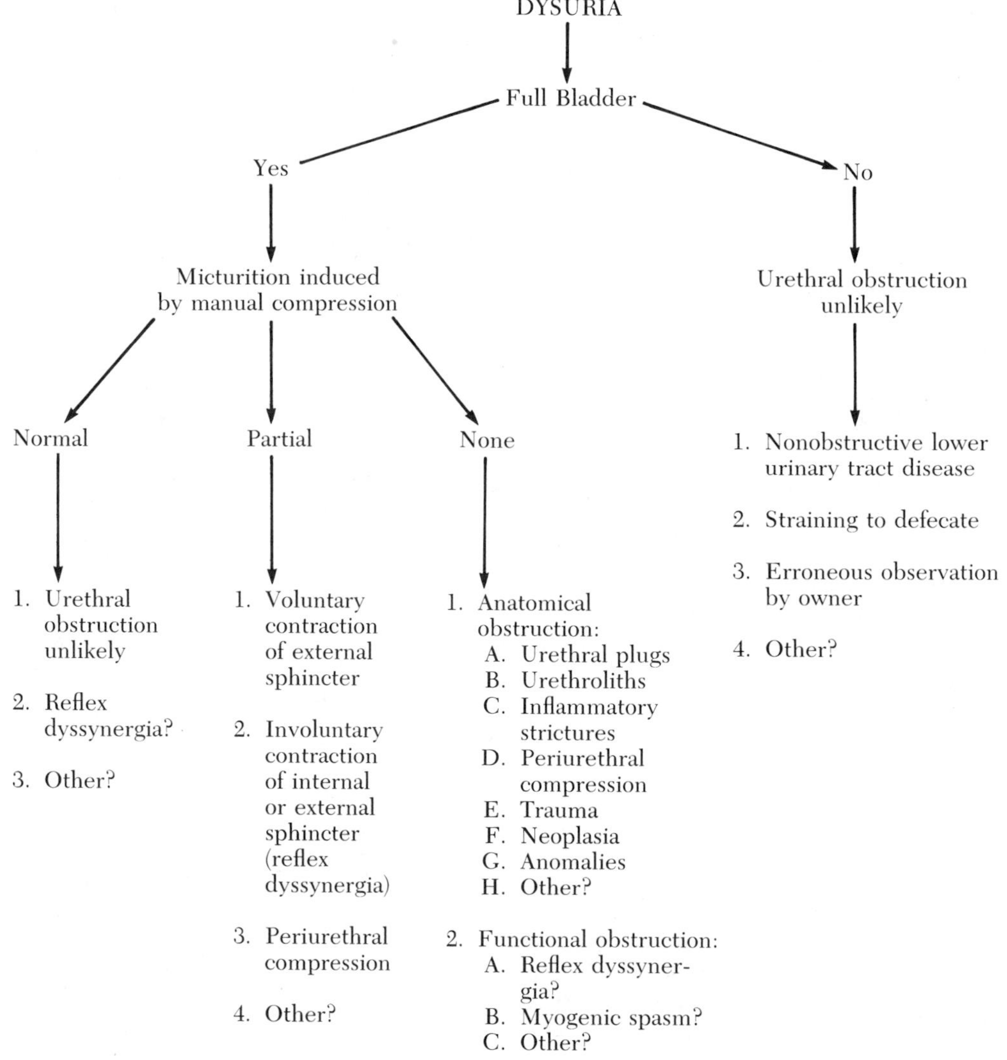

Figure 1. Clinical confirmation of suspected urethral obstruction.

also must be considered. Although it appears that they represent a predisposing cause to infectious disorders of the urinary tract of cats, the relationship, if any, of urachal diverticula to clinical signs of lower urinary tract disease in cats with sterile urine remains unexplained.

BIOLOGIC BEHAVIOR

Overview

The biologic behavior of naturally occurring forms of the feline lower urinary tract disorders has not been evaluated by prospective studies of a suitably large population of male and female cats. The difficulty in formulating generalities from studies reported in the literature is that the authors' definition of FUS is frequently not stated. In addition, the natural course of the disease in most reports cannot be followed because of therapeutic intervention or because the interval of the case study was too short.

Nonobstructed Cats without Uroliths

Preliminary clinical observations of untreated naturally occurring lower urinary tract disease in abacteriuric nonobstructed male and female cats admitted to the University of Minnesota Veterinary Technical Hospital revealed that the clinical signs often subsided in approximately 1 week. Our findings are comparable with those of investigators at the University of Georgia who reported amelioration of clinical signs of FUS in nonobstructed male and female cats treated with chloramphenicol or a placebo. Spontaneous resolution of clinical signs in this subset of cats with lower urinary tract disease may be the rule rather than the exception.

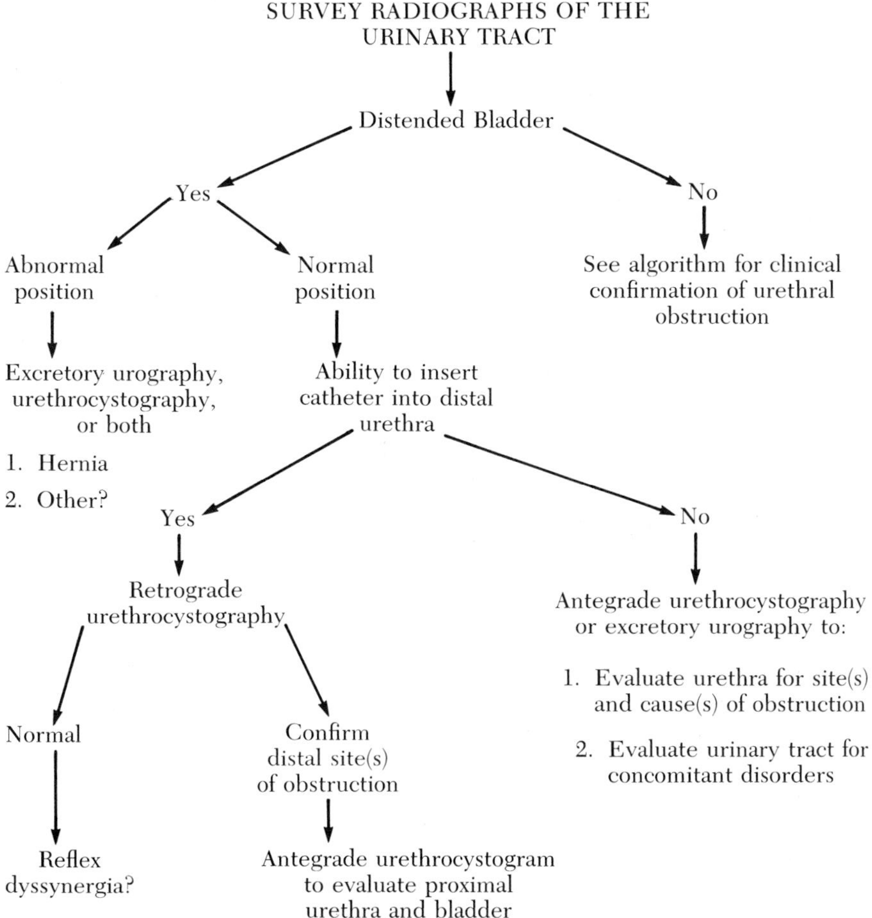

Figure 2. Algorithm for radiographic confirmation and localization of urethral obstruction.

Obstructed Cats

The biologic behavior of any disorder is influenced by its cause. Future studies of the biologic behavior of obstructive uropathy in male cats must encompass efforts to detect and specify the nature of the obstruction (Table 1).

Of the various manifestations of FUS, the consequence of urethral obstruction and postrenal azotemia have received the greatest emphasis. There is general agreement that obstruction of urine outflow produces predictable clinical and biochemical abnormalities that vary with the duration and degree of obstruction. However, systemic abnormalities in fluid, acid-base, and electrolyte balance caused by urethral obstruction probably occur irrespective of specific cause (e.g., uroliths, plugs, strictures).

RECURRENCE

The fact that signs of lower urinary tract disease may recur in male and female cats is common knowledge. Unfortunately, the causes of recurrence have not been carefully considered. Possibilities include (1) a recurrent episode of the original disease induced by the same mechanisms, (2) late occurring sequelae of the original disease (e.g., spontaneous or iatrogenic urethral stricture), (3) onset of a different disease associated with clinical manifestations similar or identical to the original disorder, and (4) various combinations of these factors. These factors must be considered when evaluating the etiopathogenesis of recurrence of different *forms* of feline lower urinary tract disease and when evaluating methods to treat and prevent them. The unpredictability with which signs of lower urinary tract disorders undergo remission and exacerbation mandates carefully designed and controlled double-blind clinical trials in patients known to have an identical disorder to prove efficacy of treatment and prevention.

DIAGNOSIS

Detection of FUS (e.g., hematuria, dysuria, or urethral obstruction) is a starting point of diagnostic evaluation. In addition to an appropriate history and physical examination, complete urinalyses and the screening of quantitative urine cultures performed on samples that have not been altered by reverse flushing solutions should be routinely obtained. Survey and contrast radiography may be required to aid in localization of problems in addition to identifying the underlying causes of persistent or recurrent clinical signs (Fig. 2). Localization of the site and cause of urethral obstruction is especially important if urethrostomy is being considered. A neurologic examination may be helpful in identifying abnormalities of micturition. Patients with postrenal azotemia caused by urethral obstruction should be evaluated with the aid of hemograms, blood chemistry profiles (especially potassium and bicarbonate concentrations), and perhaps electrocardiograms (for the cardiotoxic effect of hyperkalemia). Analysis of uroliths and urethral plugs should be routine. According to the principles of good surgical practice, any tissue removed surgically (including the penile urethra) should be routinely fixed in formalin and saved so that it is available for examination by light microscopy.

A problem-specific data base for feline lower urinary tract disorders (or FUS) has been developed (Table 2). Selected items in this problem-specific data base may be deleted, depending on the goal of the client and veterinarian. Likewise, additional items may be added to various components of this problem-specific data base. Note that some items have been preceded with the word "consider," indicating that they are optional.

Table 2. *Problem-Specific Data Base For Feline Lower Urinary Tract Disease*

History Checklist
1. Changes in frequency and location of voiding?
2. Apparent difficulty or pain on voiding?
3. Size and velocity of urine stream?
4. Quantity of urine passed during each attempt to void?
5. Changes in urine, odor, color, or clarity?
6. Presence of sand or larger uroliths in urine?
7. Changes in urine production and/or water consumption?
8. Ability to void normally?
9. Licking of vulva or prepuce?
10. Duration of problem?
11. Are problem(s) increasing in severity, decreasing in severity, or remaining the same?
12. Other signs not directly related to the urinary system?
13. Type of diet?
14. Medications given? Type? Dose? Response?

Physical Examination Checklist
1. Kidneys
   - Position? Number?
   - Size? Shape? Consistency? Surface contour? Pain?
2. Bladder
   - Position?
   - Size? Shape? Consistency?
   - Surface contour? Thickness of bladder wall?
   - Grating or nongrating masses within or adjacent to bladder lumen?
   - If present, constant or variable in location?
   - Pain?
3. Urethra
   - Position?
   - Size? Shape? Consistency?
   - Uroliths or masses palpable?
   - Discharge, urethral plugs, or uroliths visible at urethral orifice?
   - Size of urethral orifice?
   - Pain?
4. Genital system
   - Prostate: Position? Size? Shape? Consistency? Pain?
   - Penis and prepuce: Size? Shape? Consistency? Pain?
   - Vulva: Size? Shape? Consistency? Pain?
   - Testicules: Present or absent?

Laboratory and Specialty Examinations
1. Complete blood count
2. Urinalysis
3. Quantitative urine culture
4. Consider blood chemistry profile, especially if urethra is obstructed
5. Consider quantitative urolith or urethral plug analysis
6. Consider special urine culture techniques (e.g., mycotic, mycoplasmal, or viral isolations)
7. Consider neurologic examination
8. Consider cystometrogram and urethral pressure profile
9. Consider bladder biopsy if bladder surgery is performed for therapeutic reasons

Radiographic Studies
1. Survey abdominal radiographs
2. Consider contrast urethrocystogram
3. Consider double-contrast cystogram

MANAGEMENT

A detailed review of all aspects of management of feline lower urinary tract disorders is beyond the scope of this discussion. The following discussion is limited to recommendations for immediate relief of urethral obstruction and symptomatic and supportive therapy of nonobstructed cats with hematuria and dysuria. (Consult the article entitled Medical Dissolution and Prevention of Feline Struvite Uroliths for additional information.) Consult previous editions of *Current Veterinary Therapy* or reference material for information about management of the systemic consequences of obstructive uropathy.

Immediate Relief of Urethral Obstruction

Obstructive urethropathy may be caused by one or more intraluminal, mural, or extramural abnormalities located at one or more sites (Table 1; Fig. 1). It follows that reverse flushing solutions may be very effective in dissolving urethral plugs but would have no effect on obstructive lesions located in the urethral wall or periurethral tissue. Inability to restore patency by flushing the urethral lumen with a solution should arouse one's suspicion that the problem could be a mural or periurethral lesion in addition to, or instead of, a firmly lodged urethral plug or urethrolith.

RESTRAINT

Physical restraint alone or in combination with topical anesthesia may be sufficient for relief of urethral obstruction in patients that are particularly docile or severely depressed. Wrapping the cat in a bath towel may help to protect the patient and the assistant. If local anesthetics are used to anesthetize the urethral mucosa, they should be administered only in a quantity sufficient to accomplish this goal. We do not recommend use of local anesthetic agents as primary reverse flushing solutions since they may induce systemic toxicity if absorbed in sufficient quantity. Their absorption may be enhanced by damage to the urothelium, and their toxic potential may be enhanced by postrenal uremia.

Because of an increased risk of adverse drug reactions associated with obstructive uropathy, pharmacologic restraint should be avoided when feasible. However, the risk of adverse drug reactions must be weighed against the possibility of iatrogenic trauma to the urethra in an uncooperative patient. If the disposition of the patient is such that attempts to dislodge the urethral obstruction are likely to be associated with additional damage to the urethra, or if there is a high risk of iatrogenic UTI, some form of pharmacologic restraint should be considered. Short-acting barbiturates (thiamylal) that are metabolized by the liver or inhalant anesthetics may be considered if general anesthesia is required. Anesthetics must be given cautiously, since dosages less than those recommended for patients with normal renal function are required in patients with postrenal azotemia. If ketamine hydrochloride is used, similar caution must be exercised since it is excreted in active form by the kidneys. Low doses (1 to 2 mg/kg IV) have been successfully used by many clinicians. However, if difficulty is encountered in relieving outflow obstruction, it is generally inadvisable to administer additional quantities of ketamine.

PRIORITY OF PROCEDURES

We recommend the following priority of procedures when attempting to restore urethral patency of an obstructed male cat: (1) massage of the distal urethra; (2) attempt to induce voiding by gentle palpation of the urinary bladder; (3) cystocentesis; (4) retrograde urethral flushing; (5) combinations of (1) to (4); (5) muscle relaxants; (6) diagnostic radiology to determine if the cause of urethral obstruction is intraluminal, mural, or extramural; and (7) surgical procedures.

Urethral Massage. Gentle massage of the penis between the thumb and fingers may help to dislodge plugs located in the penile urethra. If necessary, the penis may be manipulated while it is retracted within the prepuce. Plugs located in the preprostatic (abdominal) or membranous (pelvic) urethra may occasionally be dislodged by massaging the urethra through the rectum. Although these methods are often ineffective, their simplicity and occasional success make them worth trying prior to consideration of cystocentesis or catheterization.

Palpation of the Urinary Bladder. Inability of a cat to void urine spontaneously indicates that increasing intraurethral pressure by digitally compressing the urinary bladder is unlikely to be effective. However, if this technique is used after urethral massage, sufficient intraluminal pressure may be generated to dislodge fragments of urethral precipitates. Appropriate caution should be used to prevent iatrogenic damage to the urinary bladder. If UTI is likely, the consequences of inducing vesicoureteral reflux during palpation should be considered, since microbes may be forced into the upper urinary tract.

Cystocentesis. Because solutions used to flush the urethral lumen may alter the composition of urine in the bladder lumen and therefore may alter results of diagnostic tests (e.g., urinalyses, urine culture), serious consideration should be given to collection of a urine sample by cystocentesis prior to attempts to restore urethral patency with reverse flushing solutions. This strategy has many advantages and some disadvantages. In addition to preserving the diagnostic value of a urine sample, simultaneous decompression of an overdistended urinary bladder by removing most (but not all) of the urine provides a mechanism to halt temporarily the continued adverse effects of obstructive uropathy irrespective of cause. This may provide additional time to remove or bypass the obstructive urethral lesion without further deterioration of renal function. It also may decrease intraluminal pressure at the proximal site of urethral obstruction, which in turn may facilitate repulsion of a urethral plug or urolith into the bladder lumen. In addition, the gross character of aspirated urine may provide valuable clues about the nature of the obstructive disorder (intraluminal precipitates of matrix and crystalline material versus extraluminal compression). The potential disadvantages of the procedure are that (1) it may result in extravasation of urine into the bladder wall or peritoneal cavity and (2) it may injure the bladder wall or surrounding structures. Although these complications could be severe in patients with a devitalized bladder wall, in our experience this has been the exception rather than the rule if most of the urine is removed from the bladder. Loss of a small quantity of urine into the peritoneal cavity is usually of little consequence, especially if it does not contain pathogens. The potential of trauma to the bladder and adjacent structures can be avoided by using good technique.

We are not advocating an "always or never" recommendation regarding diagnostic and therapeutic cystocentesis. Clinical judgment is required regarding its use in each patient. However, it is preferable to decompress the urinary bladder by cystocentesis (saving an aliquot for appropriate diagnostic tests) prior to use of reverse flushing procedures in the following patients: (1) those that are likely to have adequate integrity of the bladder wall and (2) those in which immediate overdistension of the bladder lumen is not allowed to recur (consult Osborne et al., 1980).The bladder should be emptied as completely as is consistent with atraumatic technique. It is undesirable to attempt complete evacuation of the bladder lumen, since this will allow the sharp point of the needle to damage the bladder wall.

The need for prophylactic antibacterial therapy after cystocentesis must be determined on the basis of the status of the patient and retrospective evaluation of technique. If subsequent restoration of urethral patency requires intermittent or indwelling catheterization, preventive antimicrobial therapy should be considered.

Reverse Flushing Techniques. Flushing the urethral lumen with sterilized solutions after urethral catheterization may dislodge urethral plugs and calculi. However, it is emphasized that urethral obstruction may be caused by a combination of intraluminal precipitates (uroliths or urethral plugs), swelling of the urethral wall, and spasm of urethral musculature (Table 1).

Reverse flushing solutions should be used cautiously, since accumulation and absorption of large quantities of acid or anesthetic solutions by way of an inflamed urinary bladder may cause systemic toxicity. The authors prefer lactated Ringer's solution because it is sterilized, nontoxic, nonirritating, economical, and readily available.

A variety of catheters may be used, including disposable flexible catheters (Open-end Tomcat catheters, Sherwood; Brunswick sterile disposable feeding tube and urethral catheter, Sherwood; Jackson cat catheter, Portex), synthetic tubing (Intramedicpolyethylene tubing, PE 60 or PE 90, Clay Adams), intravenous catheters, and silver abscess cannulas (Becton Dickinson). Hypodermic needles with blunted ends, metal lacrimal cannulas, and other instruments that can easily damage the urethral mucosa should be avoided. We have had favorable results with a recently developed semiflexible olive-tipped metal urethral catheter for retrograde flushing of the feline urethra (VetLab, Inc.) (Fig. 3). Every effort should be made to protect the patient from iatrogenic complications associated with catheterization, including UTI and trauma to the urinary tract. Since the urine of most affected cats is bacteriologically sterile and since inflammation of the urethra and bladder, together with stagnation of urine within the bladder, predispose the patient to bacterial UTI, appropriate precautions must be taken to prevent iatrogenic infection. Only sterile catheters should be used. In addition, the penis and prepuce should be washed with warm water prior to catheterization. Regardless of the method employed, meticulous aseptic and feather-touch technique should be used to prevent damage to delicate tissues of the urethra and urinary bladder.

After the penis is cleaned with warm water, a catheter coated with sterilized aqueous lubricant should be carefully advanced to the site of obstruction, which is indicated by the distance the catheter can be inserted. This information should be recorded since it may be of value when considering use of muscle relaxants and when considering urethral surgery to prevent recurrent obstruction. However, caution must be used not to mistake resistance induced by the natural curvature of the feline male urethra for a site of obstruction. A large quantity of lactated Ringer's solution (as much as several hundred milliliters) should then be flushed into the urethral lumen and allowed to reflux out of the external urethral orifice. When possible, the catheter should be advanced toward the bladder. As a result of this maneuver, the obstructing urethral plugs may be gradually dislodged and flushed around the catheter and out through the urethra. Application of steady but gentle digital pressure to the bladder wall after the urethra has been flushed with lactated Ringer's solution may result in expulsion of the urethral plug or urolith out of the urethra. Excessive pressure should not be used because it may result in (1) trauma to the bladder, (2) reflux of potentially infected urine into the ureters and renal pelves, and (3) rupture of the bladder wall.

If the aforementioned procedure is unsuccessful, it may be necessary to attempt repulsion of suspected urethral plugs or uroliths back into the bladder lumen by occluding the distal end of the urethra around the catheter before injecting fluid into the urethra. By preventing reflux of solution out of the external urethral orifice, this maneuver will tend to dilate the urethral lumen. If the obstruction persists, an attempt may be made to gently advance the suspected plug or urolith toward the bladder. Excessive force should not be used. Prior to advancement of the catheter, the extended penis

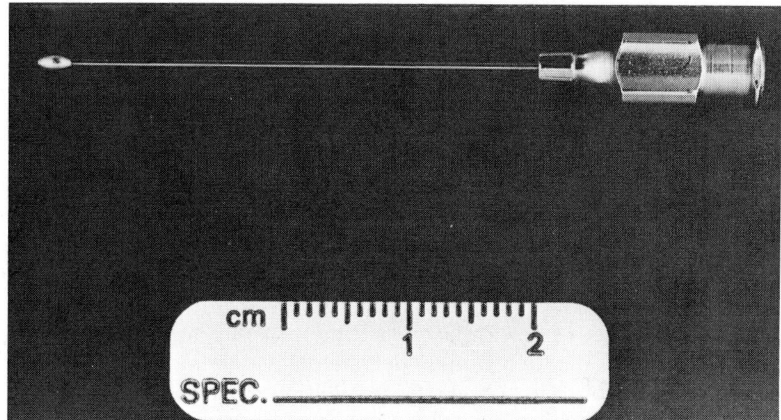

Figure 3. Photograph of a semiflexible, olive-tipped, feline urethral catheter (VetLab, Inc.).

should be displaced dorsally until the long axis of the urethra is approximately parallel to the vertebral column. This maneuver facilitates catheterization by reducing the natural curvature of the caudal urethra.

On occasion, it is advantageous to allow the reverse flushing solution to soften the obstructing urethral plugs (this technique is ineffective for most uroliths) before attempts are made to propel them back into the bladder. Allowing several hours to elapse between attempts to remove firmly lodged plugs by reverse flushing has been effective. Likewise, a probe made from monofilament stainless steel suture material may be used to attempt to gently disrupt plugs that have become firmly lodged in the urethra.

MUSCLE RELAXANTS. The bladder muscle of nonobstructed male and female cats with lower urinary tract disease is frequently in a state of contraction. Such cats frequently have urge incontinence; their bladders are small (presumably due to detrusor contraction or spasm) and painful. The possibility that inflammation of the urethra also may induce spasm of the smooth or skeletal muscle layers surrounding the urethra has also been hypothesized.

In the past, there has been no consensus about the value of smooth and skeletal muscle relaxants as adjunct therapy in cats with urethral obstruction. The value of propantheline in causing relaxation of the smooth muscle of the male or female feline urethra is unknown. Since propantheline exerts its effect primarily by interfering with impulse transmission of parasympathetic receptors (it has very little direct effect on smooth muscle) and since the highest density of postganglionic parasympathetic receptors are thought to be located in the urinary bladder of many species, this drug may exert greater effect on smooth muscle of the urinary bladder than on circular smooth muscle fibers of the urethra.

Conceptually, direct acting–antispasmodics (oxybutynin, dicyclomine, and flavoxate) should have greater action on the urethra. However, there have apparently been no studies to evaluate the efficacy (if any) and potential toxicity of these drugs in male or female cats with urethral obstruction. Further controlled experimental and clinical trials using contemporary diagnostic techniques are needed to evaluate the value of smooth muscle and skeletal muscle relaxants in cats with urethral obstruction. Studies designed to distinguish between nonspecific muscle spasm secondary to inflammation and detrusor-urethral reflex dyssynergia are also needed. Although α-adrenergic blocking agents such as phenoxybenzamine would be expected to be beneficial in the treatment of functional outflow obstruction caused by smooth muscle detrusor–urethral reflex dyssynergia, a direct smooth muscle or skeletal muscle relaxant might be required to counteract nonspecific spasm that persists during the storage and voiding phases of micturition.

DIAGNOSTIC RADIOLOGY AND SURGERY. Inability to establish adequate urethral patency by the use of catheters and reverse flushing should arouse a high index of suspicion that the underlying cause is not a urethral plug (Table 1; Fig. 1). Appropriate diagnostic procedures should be considered (Fig. 2). We do not recommend surgical intervention to correct obstructive urethropathy in uremic cats unless no reasonable alternative exists.

IMMEDIATE AFTERCARE

After urine flow has been re-established by nonsurgical techniques, most of the urine should be removed from the bladder lumen. It is unnecessary and inadvisable to remove all the urine from the bladder lumen, since trauma associated with such efforts may aggravate the severity of bladder lesions. Manual compression may be used provided it does not require substantial pressure to induce voiding. Manual compression of the bladder is not necessarily the procedure of choice if an overdistended bladder has been recently decompressed by cystocentesis, since it may result in extravasation of urine into the bladder wall or peritoneal cavity. Alternative methods include use of a catheter and syringe or cystocentesis. Each of these procedures has advantages and disadvantages that must be considered in light of the status of the urinary bladder and urethra of each patient. If the gross appearance of voided or aspirated urine suggests that reobstruction due to intraluminal debris is likely, removal of this material with saline or lactated Ringer's solution flushes of the bladder lumen may be of value in minimizing reobstruction. Local instillation of antimicrobial agents into the bladder lumen in an attempt to prevent or treat UTI is of unproven value. Unless the bladder wall is hypotonic or atonic, the antimicrobial agent is likely to be voided soon after instillation. If circumstances dictate the need for antimicrobial agents, oral or parenteral administration is recommended to maximize the effectiveness.

The urinary bladder should be periodically evaluated after restoration of adequate urethral patency to ensure that urethral obstruction has not recurred and that the detrusor muscle is not hypotonic. Micturition induced by gentle digital compression of the bladder may facilitate evaluation of urethral patency.

INDWELLING URINARY CATHETERS

We do not recommend routine use of indwelling urinary catheters in cats after relief of urethral obstruction because they may induce further damage to the urinary tract. Indwelling urinary catheters may be indicated after relief of urethral obstruction to (1) facilitate measurement of urine formation rate during intensive care of critically ill cats, (2) promote recovery of detrusor atony by maintaining an empty bladder, and (3) prevent recurrence of urethral obstruction in high-risk patients. The likelihood that a cat will voluntarily resume micturition may be assessed by evaluation of (1) the caliber of the urine stream during the voiding phase of micturition, (2) the amount of material in the urine that can potentially occlude the urethral lumen, and (3) the adequacy of detrusor tone immediately after relief of urethral obstruction. When indwelling urinary catheters are used, every effort should be made to minimize complications.

IDIOPATHIC HEMATURIA AND DYSURIA IN NONOBSTRUCTED MALE AND FEMALE CATS

Antibacterial Agents

The infrequency with which bacteria have been identified at the onset of clinical signs of lower urinary tract disorders has been well established. The uselessness of antimicrobial agents in the treatment of abacteriuric cats with lower urinary tract disease has also been documented. Indiscriminate use of antimicrobial agents has undoubtedly been responsible—at least in part—for the emergence of the resistant strains of microbes that populate veterinary hospitals.

Urinary Tract Antiseptics

Urinary tract antiseptics are sometimes used as adjunctive agents in the treatment, control, and prevention of UTI in humans. Although their use is frequently acknowledged in treatment of bacterial UTI in dogs and is occasionally mentioned for treatment of lower urinary tract disorders in cats, there have been no studies to substantiate their effectiveness in these species.

Methenamine (Mandelamine, Parke-Davis) is a cyclic hydrocarbon. In an acid environment (pH less than 6.0), methenamine hydrolyzes to form formaldehyde, an essential component of its antimicrobial activity. Because of the necessity of acid urine for formation of formaldehyde, methenamine is usually given in combination with acidifiers such as mandelic acid (methenamine mandelate) or hippuric acid (methenamine hippurate). It may be necessary to administer more potent acidifiers in addition to these combinations of drugs to acidify urine, especially if infection with urease-producing bacteria is present. Methenamine must remain in the urinary tract for a sufficient period to allow generation of effective concentrations of formaldehyde. However, once generated in sufficient concentration, formaldehyde is capable of killing microbes at any urine pH.

In light of the hypothesis that some forms of lower urinary tract disorders in cats are caused by viruses, the unproven suggestion that methenamine may have virucidal action in urine is of interest. However, definitive proof that viruses are a cause of naturally occurring lower urinary tract disorders in cats, and further studies of the efficacy of methenamine in such patients, are required before recommendations can be formulated.

Methylene blue (tetramethylthionine chloride) is a weak antiseptic agent that at one time was popularly used in combination products (Uritin, Burns-Biotic; Azo Gantrisin, Roche) designed to treat animals with signs of lower urinary tract infection. *Use of medications containing methylene blue is contraindicated in cats* because methylene blue has the potential to cause Heinz bodies and severe anemia.

Urinary Tract Analgesics

Phenazopyridine is an azo dye that is commonly used as a urinary tract analgesic in humans. Its use alone or in combination with sulfa drugs (Azo Gantrisin, Roche) *is contraindicated in cats* because it has the potential to cause methemoglobinemia and irreversible oxidative changes in hemoglobin resulting in formation of Heinz bodies and anemia. Cats have been very susceptible to dose-related toxicity of this agent.

Smooth Muscle Antispasmodics

Many cats with inflammation of the lower urinary tract develop urge incontinence, which is an uncontrollable desire to void that results in involuntary loss of urine. Incontinence occurs soon after the sensation of bladder fullness. It is characterized by inability to control micturition between the time of urge to micturate and the actual time of voiding. Micturition usually occurs at a low volume of bladder filling. Apparently there is no damage to the urethral sphincter mechanisms, because continuous loss of urine is not observed.

Because the exact mechanism of urge incontinence is unknown, details about specific therapy are unavailable. It is logical to consider smooth muscle antispasmodics as symptomatic treatment of urge incontinence. Combination preparations designed to treat signs of lower urinary tract disorders frequently contain atropine, hyoscyamine, and scopolamine (Urised, Conal). The efficacy, if any, of these agents in cats with dysuria has not been established by properly controlled clinical trials.

Propantheline (Pro-Banthine, Searle & Co.) minimizes the force and frequency of uncontrolled detrusor contractions but has negligible effect on urethral sphincter pressure. In a controlled clinical study of the efficacy of propantheline (7.5 mg given orally on one occasion) in the treatment of naturally occurring hematuria and dysuria in nonobstructed male and female cats, no difference in rate of recovery was observed between cats treated with propantheline and control groups. This is not an unexpected finding, because the administration of propantheline represents a symptomatic form of therapy.

Propantheline may be considered to reduce the severity and frequency of urge incontinence in nonobstructed male and female cats. It has a rapid onset of action. However, care must be used to prevent urinary retention resulting from using excessive quantities in cats. Because the smallest tablet is 7.5 mg, the suggested dose is 7.5 mg given orally approximately every 72 hours. Further studies using appropriate dosages and maintenance intervals are required to substantiate a beneficial symptomatic effect of propantheline in cats with urge incontinence.

Anti-Inflammatory Agents

OVERVIEW. It is reasonable to assume that most cats with hematuria and dysuria have an inflammatory lesion of the lower urinary tract. Hematuria is indicative of (but not pathognomonic of) inflammation; dysuria indicates involvement of the lower urinary tract. The cause of the inflammation in many cats is unknown. In many patients, however, it can be established what the cause is *not*.

Lack of specific therapy for abacteriuric, nonurolith-forming cats with hematuria and dysuria has stimulated many clinicians to question the value of anti-inflammatory agents to reduce the severity of clinical signs. Success in minimizing the frequency of voiding would not only be beneficial to affected cats, it would eliminate owner frustration associated with the socially unacceptable problem of frequent voiding on floors, carpets, and furniture. Unfortunately, there have been no controlled clinical trials to study the short- and long-term effectiveness of anti-inflammatory agents in the symptomatic treatment of dysuria and hematuria in cats. We emphasize that hematuria and dysuria in abacteriuric cats without uroliths are often self-limiting.

GLUCOCORTICOIDS. Consideration of glucocorticoids to minimize persistent signs associated with *inflammation in cats with idiopathic dysuria* and hematuria is logical. Consideration of glucocorticoids to symptomatically treat signs associated with microbe-induced inflammation, urolith-induced inflammation, urolith-induced inflammation, neoplasia-induced inflammation, and so on is illogical.

It is emphasized that hematuria and dysuria in many nonobstructed cats with idiopathic lower urinary tract disease will spontaneously undergo remission within a few to several days. Therefore, appropriate caution must be used in assessing the therapeutic value of glucocorticoids in these patients.

Because of their catabolic effect, glucocorticoids are generally contraindicated in cats with urethral obstruction and postrenal azotemia. They should not be considered in such patients until deficits and excesses in fluid, electrolyte, and acid-base balance have been corrected. Likewise, glucocorticoids are contraindicated in cats with bacterial UTI. Use of glucocorticoids in cats with indwelling catheters is especially apt to be hazardous.

DIMETHYL SULFOXIDE (DMSO). DMSO is an analgesic anti-inflammatory agent with weak antibacterial, antifungal, and antiviral activity. It has been reported to be effective in the treatment of a variety of genitourinary disorders of humans, including interstitial cystitis, radiation cystitis, chronic prostatitis, and female chronic trigonitis. Retrograde infusion of 50 per cent solutions of pyrogen-free DMSO into the bladder lumina of humans with interstitial cystitis has been reported to minimize associated clinical signs in more than 50 per cent of the patients.

DMSO has been used to treat FUS in cats, presumably because of its reported efficacy in humans with interstitial cystitis. However, it is not known whether any type of lower urinary tract disease in cats is morphologically similar to interstitial cystitis in humans.

Appropriately controlled clinical trials that are designed to evaluate the effectiveness of local instillation of DMSO into the urinary bladders of cats with signs of lower urinary tract disease have not been reported. Dosages and frequency of administration have been entirely empiric. Side effects of DMSO therapy reported in humans include (1) alteration of the refractive index of the ocular lens; (2) garliclike taste; (3) offensive breath odor; (4) nausea; (5) diarrhea; (6) headaches; and (7) skin irritation.

Local instillation of varying quantities (up to 25 ml) of solutions containing 25 to 50 per cent DMSO into the urinary bladders of dogs weighing 15 to 40 kg (33.6 to 88 lb) every other week for up to 6 months revealed no detectable side effects. Use of solutions containing 100 per cent DMSO caused mucosal edema and hemorrhage. Licensed products available to veterinarians contain 90 per cent DMSO and are not pyrogen-free (Domoso, Diamond); licensed products available to physicians contain 50 per cent DMSO and are pyrogen-free (Rimso-50, Research Industries). Side effects of DMSO in cats have apparently not been evaluated.

Diverticulectomy

Diverticulectomy and antimicrobial therapy are recommended for vesicourachal diverticula associated with bacterial UTI. Pending results of evaluation of the clinical significance of urachal diverticulae of the bladder in abacteriuric cats with signs of lower urinary tract disease (e.g., hematuria, dysuria), the value of diverticulectomy remains questionable. Rather than adopt an "always-or-never" recommendation, we recommend that diverticulectomy be considered as an option if clinical signs persist despite medical therapy. Owners should be forewarned that surgical excision of the diverticulum may not result in amelioration of clinical signs. Likewise, diverticulectomy may not prevent recurrence of signs of lower urinary tract disease.

If a urachal diverticulum is detected by contrast radiography in an abacteriuric male cat being evaluated for perineal urethrostomy, the client should be informed that removal of the penile urethra (and its contribution to local host defenses) may result in bacterial UTI and possibly development of infection induced struvite uroliths. Rather than recommend a combined perineal urethrostomy and diverticulectomy, re-evaluate the indications for urethral surgery. If a perineal urethrostomy is subsequently performed, the cat should be periodically monitored for bacterial UTI. If bacterial UTI occurs after perineal urethrostomy, diverticulectomy should then be considered.

References and Supplemental Reading

Barsanti, J. A., Finco, D. R., Shotts, E. B., et al.: Feline urologic syndrome: Further investigation into etiology. J. Am. Anim. Hosp. Assoc. 18:391, 1982.

Barsanti, J. A., Finco, D. R., Shotts, E. B., et al.: Feline urologic syndrome: Further investigation into therapy. J. Am. Anim. Hosp. Assoc. 18:387, 1982.

Burrows, C. F., and Bovee, K. C.: Characterization and treatment of acid-base and renal defects due to urethral obstruction in male cats. J.A.V.M.A. 1972:801, 1978.

Finco, D. R.: Induced feline urethral obstruction: Response of hyperkalemia to relief of obstruction and administration of parenteral electrolyte solution. J. Am. Anim. Hosp. Assoc. 12:198, 1976.

Finco, D. R., Barsanti, J. A., and Crowell, W. A.: The urinary system. *In* Pratt, P. W. (ed.): *Feline Medicine*, 1st ed. Santa Barbara, CA: American Veterinary Publications, 1983, pp. 363–410.

Johnston, G. R., Feeney, D. A., Osborne, C. A.: Urethrography and cystography in cats. Part II. Abnormal radiographic anatomy and complications. Comp. Cont. Ed. Pract. Vet. 4:931, 1982.

Klausner, J. S., Osborne, C. A., and Stevens, J. B.: Screening tests for the detection of significant bacteriuria. *In* Kirk, R. W. (ed.): *Current Veterinary Therapy, VII*. Philadelphia: W. B. Saunders, 1980, pp. 1154–1157.

Lees, G. E., and Osborne, C. A.: Use and misuse of intermittent and indwelling urinary catheters. *In* Kirk, R. W. (ed.): *Current Veterinary Therapy VIII*. Philadelphia: W. B. Saunders, 1983, pp. 1097–1100.

Lees, G. E., and Osborne, C. A.: Feline urinary tract infections. *In* Kirk, R. W. (ed.): *Current Veterinary Therapy VIII*. Philadelphia: W. B. Saunders, 1983, pp. 1058–1061.

Lees, G. E., Osborne, C. A., Stevens, J. B., et al.: Adverse effects of open indwelling urethral catheterization in clinically normal male cats. Am. J. Vet. Res. 42:825, 1981.

Osborne, C. A., Johnston, G. R., Polzin, D. J., et al.: Feline urologic syndrome: A heterogeneous phenomenon? J. Am. Anim. Hosp. Assoc. 20:17, 1984.

Osborne, C. A., Lees, G. E., and Johnston, G. R.: Cystocentesis. *In* Kirk, R. W. (ed.): *Current Veterinary Therapy VII*. Philadelphia: W. B. Saunders, 1980, pp. 1150–1153.

Schecter, R. D.: The significance of bacteria in feline cystitis and urolithiasis. J.A.V.M.A. 156:1567, 1970.

Symposium on feline lower urinary tract disorders. Vet. Clin. North Am. 14:407, 1984.

PHARMACOLOGIC MANIPULATION OF URINATION

DENNIS J. CHEW, D.V.M.,
STEPHEN P. DIBARTOLA, D.V.M.,
and WILLIAM R. FENNER, D.V.M.
Columbus, Ohio

REVIEW OF PHYSIOLOGY

Normal micturition requires that both storage of urine (filling phase) and voiding of urine (emptying phase) be normal. Urinary continence implies voluntary ability to control micturition, whereas incontinence is the loss of this voluntary control. In normal animals, pressure within the urethra exceeds pressure within the bladder during the filling phase, preventing leakage of urine. During the emptying phase, these pressures are reversed, and intraluminal pressure exceeds the pressure generated by the sphincter, thus allowing complete emptying of the bladder.

Micturition is a reflex centered in the sacral spinal cord (S1–S3 parasympathetic and somatic) and cranial lumbar (L1–L4 sympathetic) segments, but it is modified by impulses from the brain stem (pons and medulla), cerebral cortex, cerebellum, and thalamus. Normal micturition involves a complex interaction of all these levels of the nervous system, with resulting effects on the muscles of the bladder and urethra. Figures 1, 2, and 3 show the anatomy of the parasympathetic (emptying function), sympathetic (filling function), and somatic (filling function) innervation involved in micturition. Three functional muscle groups of the lower urinary system operate to maintain normal micturition. Smooth muscle of the bladder cranial to the ureteral openings is referred to as the body (fundus, dome). It has predominantly β-adrenergic (sympathetic) and cholinergic (parasympathetic) neuroreceptors. The smooth musculature of the urethra and of the bladder distal to the ureteral openings is referred to as the internal sphincter and is dominated by α-adrenergic neuroreceptors. Striated muscle of the urethra is referred to as the external sphincter and is largely under the control of somatic neurons of the pudendal nerve. The external sphincter is located in the midurethral region in females and in the membranous urethra in males.

Stimulation of sympathetic receptors in the bladder and urethra facilitates relaxation of the body of the bladder and contraction of the internal sphincter, both of which facilitate urine storage. This is because stimulation of α-receptors induces contraction of smooth muscle, whereas stimulation of β-receptors results in relaxation of smooth muscle. Inhibition of parasympathetic impulses along with normal or enhanced tone from somatic impulses to the external sphincter further facilitates urine storage. Stimulation of the parasympathetic receptors in the body of the bladder causes smooth muscle contraction that, when coordinated with relaxation of the internal and external sphincters, facilitates emptying.

DIFFERENTIAL DIAGNOSIS OF INCONTINENCE

Neurogenic

1. Upper motor neuron bladder or urethra (lesions cranial to sacral spinal cord)
   a. Cerebral disease (inappropriate micturition, but reflex urinations still occur)
   b. Cerebellar disease—detrusor hyperexcitability
   c. Brain stem disease—loss of normal reflex micturition
   d. Spinal cord disease—loss of normal reflex micturition (disk protrusion, tumor, trauma, fibrocartilaginous infarct, infections)
2. Lower motor neuron bladder or urethra—reduced or absent pelvic and pudendal nerve stimulation causes loss of reflex urinations; autonomous contractions of bladder smooth musculature can result in ineffective urination (partial emptying)
   a. Sacral spinal cord lesions
   b. Caudal equina lesions
   c. Bilateral pelvic nerve or pudendal nerve injury (trauma or surgery)
   d. Detrusor muscle lesions—muscle not capable

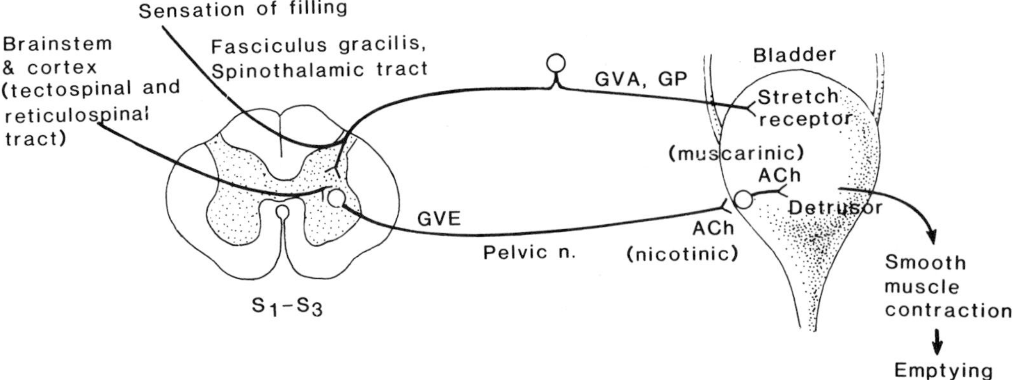

Figure 1. Stimulation of the pelvic nerve results in contraction of the detrusor muscle and emptying of the bladder. ACh = acetylcholine; GP = general proprioception; GVA = general visceral afferent; GVE = general visceral efferent.

of responding to normal neurologic stimulation, usually owing to overdistension

3. Reflex dyssynergia (detrusor urethral dyssynergia) partial spinal cord or cauda equina lesion results in failure of adequate urethral relaxation when bladder contraction occurs

Non-neurogenic

1. Hormone-responsive
   a. Estrogen-responsive (older spayed female dogs)
   b. Testosterone-responsive (older castrated male dogs)
2. Anatomic abnormalities—congenital
   a. Ectopic ureters (most common)
   b. Patent urachus
   c. Urethral fistula (rectal or vaginal)
   d. Female pseudohermaphroditism
   e. Exstrophy of urinary bladder
   f. Urethral diverticulum
   g. Vestibulovaginal stenosis
3. Anatomic or structural abnormalities—acquired
   a. Infiltrative disease of bladder or urethra—

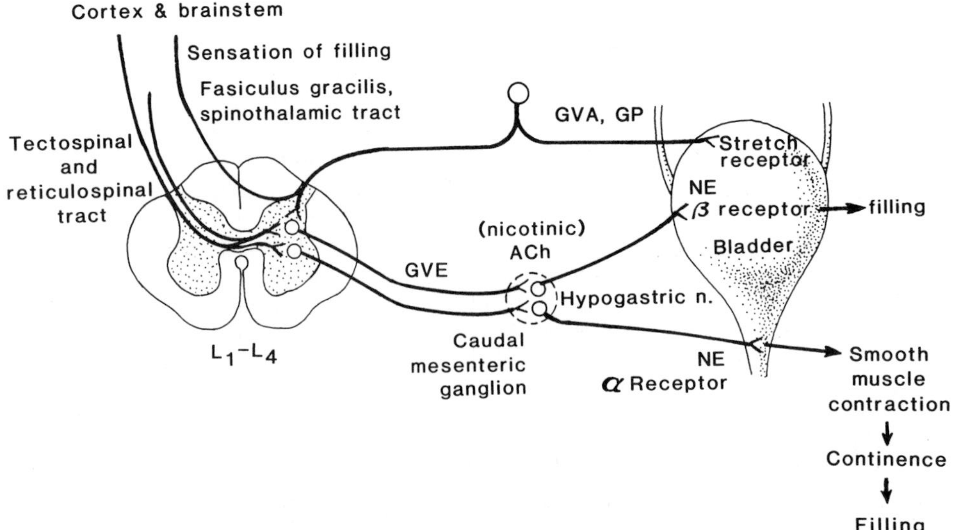

Figure 2. Stimulation of sympathetic nerves facilitates urine storage by increasing tone of the internal urethral sphincter and by decreasing tone to the detrusor muscle in the body of the bladder. ACh = acetylcholine; GP = general proprioception; GVA = general visceral afferent; GVE = general visceral efferent; NE = norepinephrine.

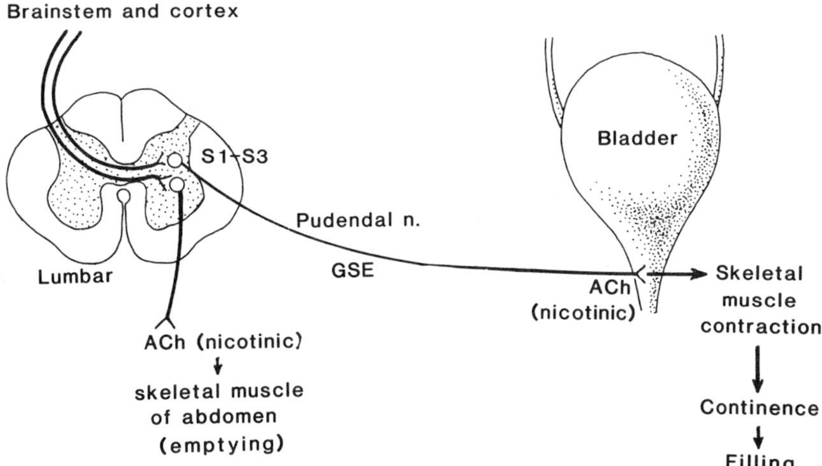

Figure 3. Stimulation of the pudendal nerve results in increased tone to the skeletal muscle of the external urethral sphincter; this favors urine storage. Stimulation of nerves supplying the abdominal wall of skeletal muscle favors voiding urine when the abdomen is pressed. ACh = acetylcholine; GSE = general somatic effect.

reduced filling capacity or reduced sphincter closure
1. Chronic cystitis
2. Chronic urethritis
3. Neoplasia
4. Urolithiasis

b. Infection or inflammation of uterine stump after ovariohysterectomy
c. Urethral fistula after trauma or surgery
d. Ureterovaginal fistula after surgery

4. Paradoxic (obstructive) incontinence—partial obstructive lesion of urethra that results in leakage of urine around the obstruction as pressure within the bladder increases
   a. Neoplasia
   b. Urolithiasis
   c. Stricture
   d. Granulomatous urethritis
   e. Prostatic disease
5. Urge incontinence—often associated with urinary infection or inflammation
6. Severe polyuria—volume overflow from a normal bladder, often presenting as nocturia or as urge incontinence if awake
7. Pelvic bladder
8. Infectious—feline leukemia virus
9. Idiopathic

GENERAL APPROACH TO WORKUP OF URINARY INCONTINENCE

The initial clinical goal should be to determine whether incontinence is neurologic or non-neurologic in origin. Subsequently, it should be determined whether the defect involves urine storage, urine emptying, or both. A combination of history, physical examination, neurologic examination, observation of voiding pattern (including palpation or catheterization of the bladder both before and after micturition to determine residual volume), urinalysis, urine culture, and plain and contrast uroradiographic studies may be needed to determine whether incontinence is neurogenic or non-neurogenic.

The signalment can suggest possible causes of incontinence. Young animals are more likely to have congenital disorders and older animals more frequently have acquired disorders such as hormone-responsive incontinence or neoplasia. The sex of the animal also can give insight into the probable cause of incontinence, such as the increased frequency of ectopic ureters in female dogs and hormone-responsive incontinence in older neutered male and female dogs. Siberian huskies, miniature poodles, Labrador retrievers, terriers, collies, and corgis are known to be at increased risk of ectopic ureters.

Ascertain from the history whether there is voluntary initiation and maintenance of urination. The ability to voluntarily initiate and maintain urination suggests that the detrusor muscle is capable of normal reflex activity. The absence of this ability suggests an interruption in reflex detrusor contraction (either upper or lower motor neuron bladder), obstruction, or failure of urine to enter the bladder. Stranguria, dysuria, and pollakiuria in the history suggest inflammatory or obstructive disease of the lower urinary tract as a cause of urge or paradoxic incontinence. A normal urine stream that rapidly diminishes to dribbling suggests reflex bladder dyssynergia. Constant dribbling of urine suggests ectopic ureters, severe failure of urethral resistance, or paradoxic obstructive incontinence. Dribbling of urine during periods of recumbency or sleeping is characteristic of the initial phases of hormone-responsive incontinence as well as early phases of severe polyuria. Intermittent dribbling of urine can also suggest expulsion of urine due to automatic or autonomous discharges of the detrusor muscle in animals with upper and lower motor neuron disease, respectively. A history of major abdominal trauma (resulting in damage to pelvic or pudendal nerves or spinal cord) or surgery in the area of the urogenital tract (prostate, uterus, bladder, or urethra) may provide insight into possible causes of incontinence.

Verification of incontinence due to any cause may be gained by observing for a wet perineum, staining of the perineal hair, or urine scalding. Abdominal and rectal palpation of the urinary tract during the physical examination may disclose an obvious non-neurogenic cause for incontinence (e.g., calculi, neoplasms, stricture, changes in thickness of the bladder or urethral wall). Vaginoscopy may disclose structural abnormalities, and rarely ectopic ureteral openings can be seen. Palpate the bladder and note whether it is normal, large and flaccid (suggesting bladder atony from an emptying disorder), or small and thickened (suggesting cystitis). Try to manually express urine from the bladder and note if resistance is offered by the urethra. Expelling urine easily during bladder palpation suggests decreased urethral resistance (lower motor neuron or primary urethral disease—urine storage disorders).

Palpation of the bladder before and after voiding can be helpful in determining residual urine volume. The volume of remaining urine can be verified by urethral catheterization (normal is approximately 0.2 to 0.4 ml/kg). A large residual volume may be encountered in disorders of emptying (upper and lower motor neuron bladders) and with functional or structural obstruction to outflow of urine. Obstruction may be ruled out if catheterization can be performed without difficulty.

A complete neurologic examination should be performed, and special emphasis given to sacral reflexes. Anal tone, the perineal reflex, and bulbocavernosus reflex all depend on an intact sacral reflex arc and pudendal nerve. If these functions are normal, then it is likely that the sacral reflex arc and pudendal nerve function to the urethra are intact.

Laboratory evaluation should always include a complete urinalysis. Persistently dilute urine should alert the clinician to suspect polyuria leading to or exacerbating incontinence. Urine sediment examination may reveal pyuria or bacteriuria caused by urinary infection. Urine culture should be performed on urine from animals suspected of urinary tract infection. Routine serum biochemistry evaluation can be helpful in disclosing causes of polyuria contributing to incontinence.

Contrast radiographic studies are often necessary to document anatomic abnormalities contributing to urinary incontinence. Excretory urography (IVP) can be helpful in documenting ectopic ureters or in evaluation of the lower urinary tract when it is difficult to perform retrograde contrast studies. Double-contrast cystography or positive contrast urethrography may be necessary to characterize structural abnormalities of the lower urinary tract.

Special urodynamic studies have recently become available at some referral centers. These studies include the cystometrogram, urethral pressure profile, and simultaneous cystometry and uroflowmetry. Use of these tests allows localization and functional characterization of a lesion causing abnormal urine storage or emptying. Clinical experience with these tests in veterinary patients has been limited.

USE OF PHARMACOLOGIC AGENTS

Pharmacologic agents are selected for management of incontinence after paradoxic obstructive incontinence, anatomic abnormalities of the urinary tract, and urinary tract infection have been ruled out as possible causes. Surgery may successfully correct anatomic abnormalities as well as provide relief of obstruction. Successful management with pharmacologic agents depends on an accurate diagnosis.

Failure to Store Urine Adequately

Urge incontinence:

1. Appropriate antimicrobial therapy if urinary tract infection is present
2. Propantheline (Pro-Banthine, Searle & Co.)
   Mechanism: provides anticholinergic effect, reducing contractions of the detrusor smooth muscle
   Dose: 5 to 30 mg PO t.i.d. in dogs; 5 to 7.5 mg PO t.i.d. in cats
   Side effects: dryness of mucous membranes; constipation
3. Aminopromazine (Jenotone, Jensen Salsbery Labs)
   Mechanism: direct rather than neurotropic smooth muscle relaxant
   Dose: 2 mg/kg b.i.d. for both dogs and cats; available in oral and injectable preparations

Side effects: potentiation of central nervous system depressants, organophosphates, and procaine hydrochloride

Estrogen-responsive incontinence (spayed female dogs):

1. Diethylstilbestrol
   Mechanism: unknown, but may increase internal sphincter sensitivity to catecholamines
   Dose: 0.1 to 1.0 mg PO for 3 to 5 days followed by 1.0 mg weekly or less often; occasionally animals will require greater than 1.0 mg weekly to maintain continence
   Side effects: signs of estrus and possibly bone marrow suppression (unlikely with this regimen)
2. Repositol estrogen such as estradiol cypionate (ECP) is not recommended because of the potential for bone marrow toxicity
3. Ephedrine sulfate—may be used alternatively in some animals
   Mechanism: α-adrenergic stimulation of internal sphincter
   Dose: 25 to 50 PO mg per dog b.i.d.
   Side effects: central nervous system stimulation and tachycardia

Testosterone-responsive incontinence (neutered male dogs):

1. Injectable testosterone
   Mechanism: unknown
   Dose: 2.2 mg/kg testosterone cypionate IM every 30 days or 2.2 mg/kg testosterone propionate IM as often as three times weekly (oral medication is not recommended because of the level of hepatic degradation after absorption)
   Side effects: possible recurrence or worsening of perianal adenoma, perineal hernia, and prostatic enlargement or disease

Idiopathic incontinence—for urinary incontinence that cannot be treated by definitive means:

1. Ephedrine sulfate
   Mechanism: stimulation of α-adrenergic receptors of internal sphincter
   Dose: 25 to 50 mg PO in dogs b.i.d. or t.i.d.; 2 to 4 mg/kg PO b.i.d. to t.i.d. in cats
   Side effects: minimal, but may include excessive central nervous system stimulation and tachycardia
2. Phenylpropanolamine (Propagest, *Carnick*; 12.5 mg/5 ml)
   Mechanism: α-adrenergic receptor stimulation of internal sphincter
   Dose: 12.5 to 50 mg PO t.i.d. in dogs
   Side effects: less central nervous system stimulation than with ephedrine
3. Imipramine (Tofranil, Geigy) is a drug with α-adrenergic activity that is effective experimentally in increasing pressure along the canine urethra, but clinical experience is lacking in dogs and cats

Failure to Empty Urine Adequately

Failure to empty urine adequately from the bladder can occur whenever there is excessive resistance to outflow of urine by the caudal bladder or urethra (increased internal or external sphincter tone—failure of relaxation) or when there is failure of adequate contraction of the detrusor muscle to expel urine (detrusor hyporeflexia). Abnormal micturition caused by neurologic disorders is often difficult to treat when definitive neurologic cure is not possible. Pharmacologic management of these disorders only partially improves micturition, and other supportive measures such as bladder expression and sterile intermittent urethral catheterization may have to be employed.

Upper motor neuron bladder—loss of detrusor reflex with increased tone to the urethra (uninhibited sympathetic and somatic input); dribbling is usually intermittent

1. Phenoxybenzamine (Dibenzyline, Smith Kline & French)
   Mechanism: α-adrenergic antagonist that reduces internal sphincter tone
   Dose: 5 to 15 mg PO once daily per dog; 2.5 to 7.5 mg PO once daily per cat (0.25 to 0.50 mg/kg t.i.d.)
   Side effects: hypotension
2. Bethanecol (Urecholine, Merck Sharp & Dohme)
   Mechanism: stimulation of cholinergic detrusor receptors results in contraction that would otherwise not occur until greater intravesical pressure was achieved
   Dose: 5 to 15 mg PO t.i.d. in dogs; 1.25 to 5.0 mg PO t.i.d. in cats; often used in conjunction with phenoxybenzamine
   Side effects: lacrimation and abdominal cramping
3. Diazepam or dantrolene to relax external sphincter (see below)

Lower motor neuron bladder/urethra—dribbling is often constant

1. Bethanecol (Urecholine) as discussed above to increase the tone of the flaccid detrusor
2. Phenoxybenzamine: α-adrenergic blockade as discussed above; this drug is not often necessary when somatic tone to the external sphincter is lost; possibly helpful when resistance to outflow is due to remaining sympathetic tone

Functional outlet obstruction (detrusor-urethral ataxia; detrusor-urethral dyssynergia)—no mechanical obstruction is detectable yet increased urethral resistance inhibits free flow of urine

1. Alpha-adrenergic blockers such as phenoxybenzamine (Dibenzyline) as discussed before to reduce internal sphincter tone
2. Diazepam (Valium, Roche)
   Mechanism: centrally acting skeletal muscle relaxant may reduce tone to the external sphincter

Dose: 2 to 10 mg PO t.i.d. in dogs; 2 to 5 mg PO t.i.d. in cats; 0.50 mg/kg IV in both dogs and cats
Side effects: sedation

3. Dantrolene (Dantrium, Eaton)—may have a veterinary role in the future, but clinical evidence is lacking
   Mechanism: direct-acting skeletal muscle relaxant may reduce tone to the external sphincter
   Dose: 1 mg/kg PO t.i.d. but can be increased to 5 mg/kg if necessary; dose only for dogs
   Side effects: may cause generalized weakness and is potentially hepatotoxic

References and Supplemental Reading

Awad, S. A., Downie, J. W., and Kiruluta, H. G.: Pharmacologic treatment of disorders of bladder and urethra: A review. Can. J. Surg. 22:515, 1979.

Barsanti, J. A., Edwards, P. D., and Losonsky, J.: Testosterone-responsive urinary incontinence in a castrated male dog. J. Am. Anim. Hosp. Assoc. 17:117, 1981.

de Lahunta, A.: *Veterinary Neuroanatomy and Clinical Neurology*. Philadelphia: W. B. Saunders, 1983, pp. 123–127.

Khanna, O. P.: Disorders of micturition, neuropharmacologic basis and results of drug therapy. Urology 8:316, 1976.

Moreau, P. M.: Neurogenic disorders of micturition in the dog and cat. Comp. Cont. Ed. Pract. Vet. 4:12, 1982.

Rosin, A. H., and Ross, L.: Diagnosis and pharmacological management of disorders of urinary continence in the dog. Comp. Cont. Ed. Pract. Vet. 3:601, 1981.

Section 14

REPRODUCTIVE DISORDERS

DONALD H. LEIN, D.V.M.
Consulting Editor

***Additional Pertinent Information Found in* Current Veterinary Therapy VIII:**

Concannon, P. W.: Fertility Regulation in the Bitch: Contraception, Sterilization, and Pregnancy Termination, p. 901.
Concannon, P. W.: Reproductive Physiology and Endocrine Patterns of the Bitch, p. 886.
Concannon, P. W., and Lein, D. H.: Feline Reproduction, p. 932.
Johnston, S. D.: Management of the Post-Partum Bitch and Queen, p. 959.
Johnston, S. D.: Management of Pregnancy Disorders in the Bitch and Queen, p. 952.
Larsen, R. E.: Breeding Soundness Examination of the Male Dog, p. 956.
Lein, D. H.: Examination of the Bitch for Breeding Soundness, p. 909.
Lein, D. H.: Pyometritis in the Bitch and Queen, p. 942.
Lein, D. H., and Concannon, P. W.: Infertility and Fertility Treatments and Management in the Queen and Tom Cat, p. 936.
Lindsay, F. E. F.: Endoscopy of the Reproductive Tract in the Bitch, p. 912.
Olson, P. N., et al.: Infertility in the Bitch, p. 925.
Reimers, T. J.: Endocrine Testing for Infertility in the Bitch, p. 922.
Rendano, V. T., Jr.: Radiographic Evaluation of Fetal Development in the Bitch and Fetal Death in the Bitch and Queen, p. 947.
Sonderberg, S. F., and Olson, P. N.: Abortifacients, p. 945.
Smith, F. O., and Larsen, R. E.: The Infertile Stud Dog, p. 962.

CLINICAL AND ENDOCRINE CORRELATES OF CANINE OVARIAN CYCLES AND PREGNANCY

P. W. CONCANNON, PH.D.
Ithaca, New York

The reproductive physiology of the domestic bitch has been reviewed extensively and in detail in recent years. The intention of the present article is therefore to provide only a brief review of major reproductive events in the bitch and introduce some recent published and unpublished observations of interest. The emphasis is on the considerable variation in clinical and endocrine measurements that must be considered in the course of reproductive evaluations of individual bitches. The major events and hormone changes of nonfertile and fertile cycles are summarized in Figures 1 and 2, respectively.

TIMING REPRODUCTIVE EVENTS

Preovulatory Surge of Luteinizing Hormone

The preovulatory surge of luteinizing hormone (LH) is the central event in both fertile and nonfertile cycles. It usually occurs over a 1- or 2-day period. With the exception of events best timed in relation to parturition or weaning, reproductive events in the bitch are best timed in relation to the preovulatory LH peak. In evaluating individual cycles it is often useful to estimate the time of the LH peak from changes in the more readily assessible clinical values, as outlined in Figure 3. The transition from proestrous to estrous behavior, when abrupt, often occurs within 1 day of the LH peak; however, first acceptance of a male may occur as early as 4 days before, or as late as 6 days after, the LH peak. A distinct softening of the swollen vulva, when observed, normally occurs 1 to 2 days after the LH peak. A distinct decrease in the abundance of cornified superficial cells in vaginal smears obtained in late estrus normally begins 7 to 9 days after the LH peak but in the extreme may occur as early as 6 days, or as late as 11 days, after the peak. Earlier changes in the epithelial cells of vaginal smears that might be predictive of the LH peak or ovulation are not consistent in either occurrence or timing. Maximum cornification may occur as early as 5 to 6 days before the LH peak or as late as 2 to 3 days after the LH peak. An abrupt decrease in either red blood cells or noncellular debris or both usually indicates the occurrence of the LH surge. Such changes, although useful, are inconsistent and therefore not reliable. A progressive wrinkling and loss of edema in the vaginal mucosa occurs during the period of the LH surge and ovulation. Monitoring of vaginal smears and the endoscopic appearance of the vaginal mucosa are considered in more detail at the end of this article.

Stages of the Cycle

The interval from one cycle to the next can range from 4 to 13 months. Signs of proestrus may last from 3 days to 3 weeks. Estrous behavior may also last 3 days to 3 weeks. The period of peak fertility lasts about 6 days, beginning with the start of the preovulatory LH surge, and it usually coincides with behavioral estrus. Metestrus, based on progesterone secretion profiles, usually lasts 2 to 3 months in the absence of pregnancy. Pregnancy terminates with parturition 64 to 66 days after the LH peak. Anestrus can range from 1 to 8 months.

Proestrus

The onset of proestrus, defined as the time when obvious vulval swelling or vaginal discharge of uterine blood begins, can occur as early as 3 weeks, or as late as 3 days, before the LH peak. Presumably, the associated follicular phases and rises in estrogen are correspondingly protracted or brief. Estradiol levels rise from 10 to 20 pg/ml at the start of proestrus to reach a peak of 50 to 100 pg/ml by 1 to 2 days before the LH peak; they then decline during and after the LH surge. Progesterone levels rise slowly from about 0.5 ng/ml to reach around 1

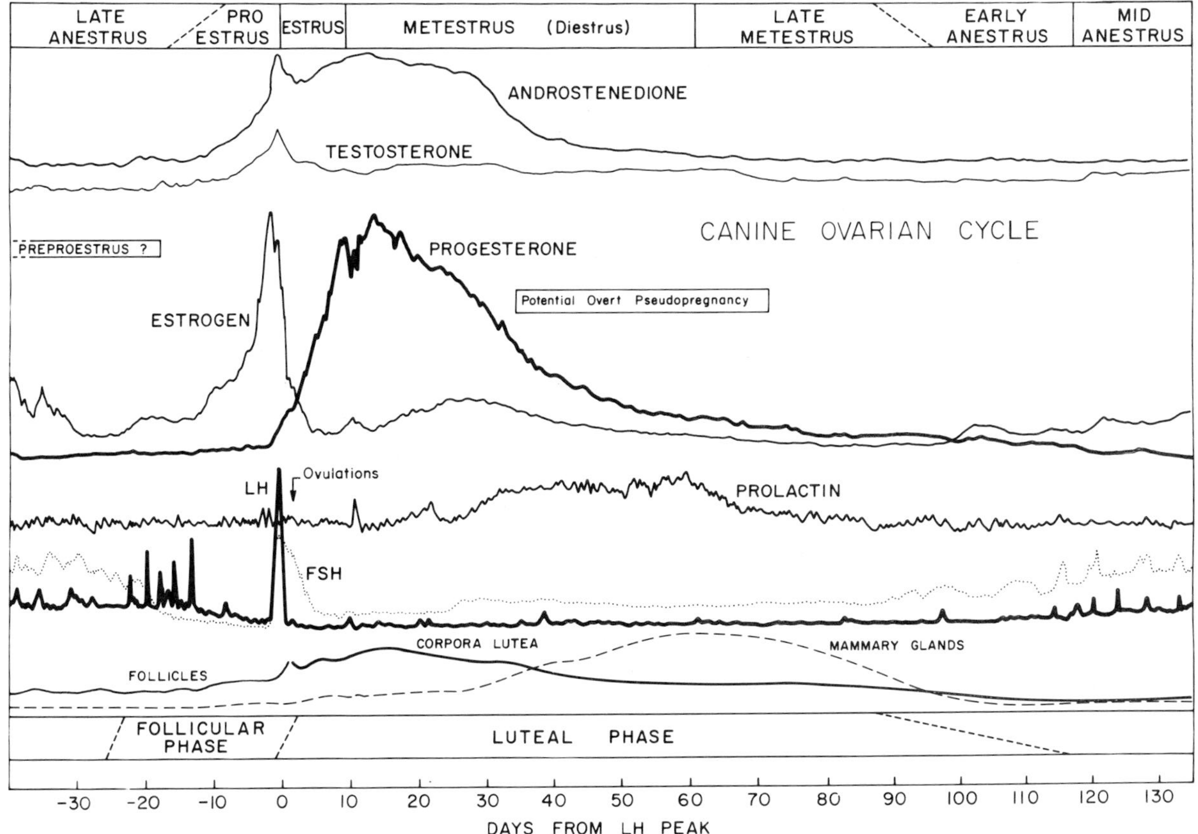

Figure 1. Schematic representation of typical changes in serum or plasma levels of estrogen, progesterone, LH, FSH, prolactin, testosterone, and androstenedione reported or presumed to occur during the canine ovarian cycle and their temporal relation to observable stages and functional phases of the estrous cycle. (From Concannon: Vet. Clin. North Am. [Small Anim. Pract.], in press, with permission.)

Basal and peak serum levels of steroids are, respectively, 5 to 10 and 50 to 100 pg/ml for estradiol, 0.2 to 0.5 and 15 to 90 ng/ml for progesterone, 0.1 and 1 ng/ml for testosterone, and 0.2 ng/ml and 2 ng/ml for androstenedione.

ng/ml at the start of the LH surge and then increase rapidly during and after the LH surge. This rapid rise in progesterone reflects the extensive preovulatory luteinization of follicles that occurs in the bitch.

Estrus

Behavioral estrus, characterized by the female's standing firmly for males and by reflex tail deviation, often begins within a day of the LH surge, but it may begin up to 4 days earlier or 6 days later. Therefore, ovulations, which occur 2 days after the LH surge, may occur early or late in behavioral estrus or may occur several days before acceptance of a male. This is the basis for recommendation of breeding during early, middle, and late estrus, to ensure that at least one mating occurs during the period of maximum fertility. Progesterone levels increase throughout the 1 to 2 weeks of estrus, approaching peak levels of 15 to 85 ng/ml, whereas estradiol levels decline. The duration of behavioral estrus is variable and at times unrelated to, and may be much longer than, the period of fertility, which is better reflected by the maintenance of vaginal cornification, assessed by vaginal cytologic or endoscopic examination.

Ovulation and Fertility

Ovulations usually occur synchronously 2 days after the LH peak. However, the dog, unlike most species, has oocytes that are ovulated as primary oocytes and do not mature and become capable of being fertilized until they reach the distal segments of the oviducts. The exact time course for the movement and maturation of oocytes has not been determined. Oocyte maturation may not occur until 2 or 3 days after ovulation and 4 or 5 days after the LH surge. The fertile life of mature oocytes may be another 2 or 3 days, since matings in late estrus (7 or 8 days after the LH peak) are often fertile. Pregnancies following matings delayed until 9 or 10 days after the LH peak are rare, produce litters of

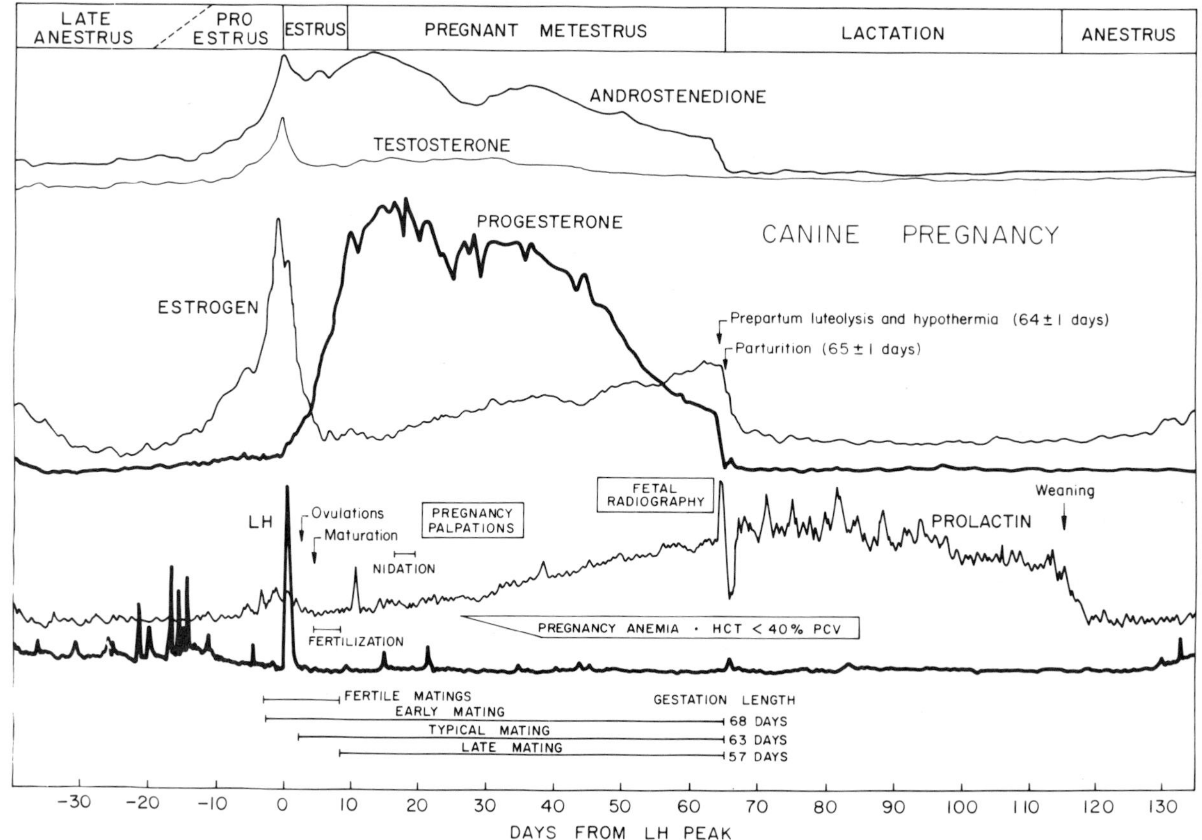

Figure 2. Schematic representation of typical changes in serum or plasma levels of estrogen, progesterone, LH, prolactin, testosterone, and androstenedione reported or presumed to occur during pregnancy and lactation in the bitch and their relation to indicated events considered important for breeding programs and clinical management of pregnancy. Actual ranges for basal and peak levels of steroids in serum or plasma are the same as in nonpregnant cycles (see Fig. 1). (From Concannon: Vet. Clin. North Am. [Small Anim. Pract.] in press, with permission.)

only one or two pups, and have an apparent gestation length of 55 to 57 days between mating and parturition. Fortuitous or forced matings more than 2 days before the LH peak are rarely fertile and result in mating-to-whelping intervals of 68 days or longer if they are fertile (or followed by other matings). The ability of canine sperm to remain fertile in the female tract (in some instances for 6 to 7 days) has been demonstrated (Concannon et al., 1983).

Events of Pregnancy

The timing of some of the physiologically important and clinically relevant events of canine pregnancy are outlined in Table 1. Practical aspects to note include the following: the variation in the timing of events based on time of breeding versus the time of the preovulatory LH peak; the potential to use vaginal cytologic or endoscopic examination to estimate the time of breeding in relation to the period of fertility; the limited period optimal for palpation of uterine implantation swellings; the ability to use ultrasonography to observe the amnion and embryo by day 22 after mating and to follow fetal well-being, heart beat, and position throughout pregnancy to parturition; the occurrence of an extensive anemia of pregnancy; the use of conventional radiography for pregnancy diagnosis limited to the last 3 weeks of pregnancy; and the consistency in gestation length in relation to periovulatory endocrine events but not in relation to the time of mating.

Postimplantation Pregnancy

Pregnancy-specific increases in progesterone and estrogen have been reported but appear to be only poorly reflected in blood levels owing to hemodilution associated with the normal anemia of pregnancy in the bitch. Body weight increases by 20 to 55 per cent. The maternal hematocrit declines, normally reaching 40 per cent (PCV) by 35 days and below 35 per cent at term. There is an associated decrease in hemoglobin and sedimentation rate. A moderate immunosuppression involving

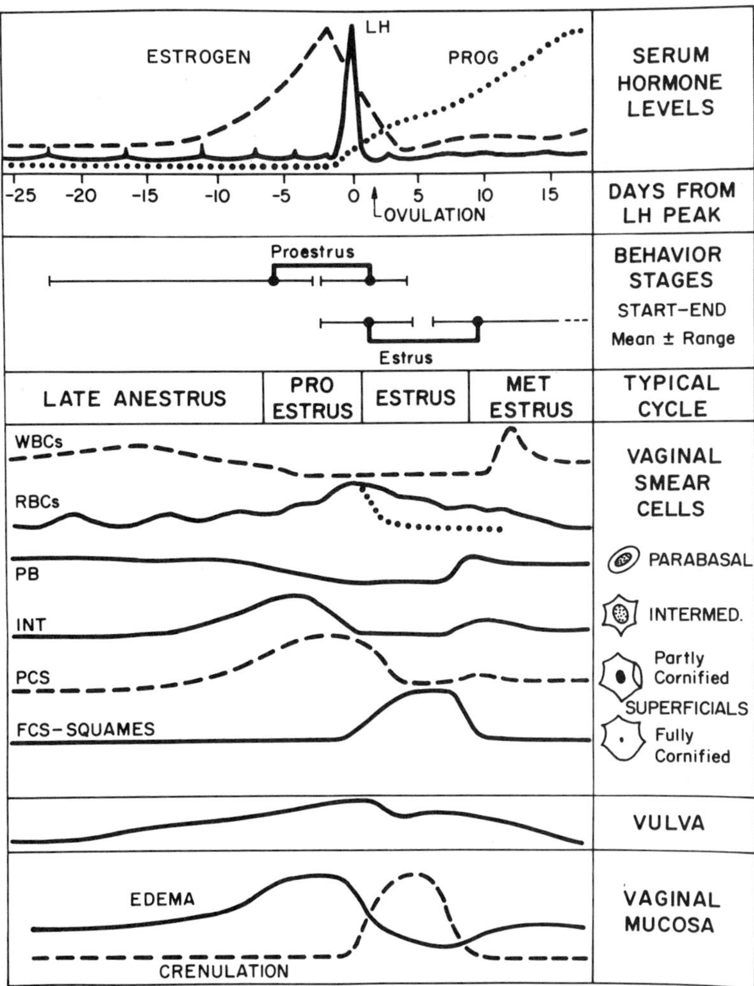

Figure 3. Schematic summary of the temporal relationships among the periovulatory endocrine events, behavioral and vulval changes, and changes in vaginal smears during proestrus, estrus, and early metestrus in the bitch. (From Concannon *in* Kirk (ed.): *Current Veterinary Therapy VIII*. Philadelphia, W. B. Saunders, 1983, pp. 886–901.)

Progressive increases in the superficial cell component of vaginal smears and in edema of the vaginal mucosa can be used to monitor the preovulatory rise in estrogen. Crenulation (wrinkling) of the vaginal mucosa is more reflective of the occurrence of the preovulatory LH peak and ovulation than any changes in the vaginal smear at that time, as the latter are inconsistent. The loss of vaginal crenulation and increase in nonsuperficial cells in the vaginal smear both occur rather abruptly 7 to 9 days after the LH peak and 5 to 7 days after ovulation, and they can be used to determine retrospectively the approximate times of those events. The latter relationship is the basis for considering the occurrence of a physiologically significant transition from "vaginal estrus" to "vaginal metestrus" independent of the termination of "behavioral estrus," which can be extremely variable (see text).

serum IgG levels below 500 ng/dl has been reported. The extent to which general metabolism and metabolic hormone activity are altered has not been fully determined. Thyroxine levels and post-ACTH cortisol levels may be elevated. A reduced sensitivity to insulin is common and pre-existing diabetic or prediabetic states are commonly aggravated. Fetal skeletons do not become radiopaque until after 44 days of gestation; i.e., 3 weeks prepartum (Concannon and Rendano, 1983).

Pseudopregnancy

Clinical pseudopregnancy refers to an overt pseudopregnancy or pseudocyesis of such an extent that aspects of mammary development, body conformation, and behavior are not clearly distinguishable from those of late pregnancy or lactation. It is usually, and appropriately, considered in contrast to the more modest mammary development that accompanies the extended luteal phase (or so-called physiologic or covert pseudopregnancy) of all nonfertile ovarian cycles in the bitch. Many of the symptoms of overt pseudopregnancy are apparently due to an excessive elevation in prolactin levels caused by an abrupt decline in progesterone (Smith and McDonald, 1974). Prolactin levels can be suppressed and pseudopregnancy terminated by administration of prolactin-lowering, dopamine-agonist compounds such as bromocriptine (Parlodel, Sandoz) and related ergot alkaloids, but none are marketed for veterinary use. Treatment with an androgen, such as mibolerone (Cheque, Upjohn), at a dose of 16 μg/kg for 5 days, is reported effective in terminating pseudopregnancy (Brown, 1984). Symptoms are suppressed by progestin, such as megesterol acetate (Ovaban, Schering), but often recur in response to progestin withdrawal.

Luteal Function and Pregnancy Maintenance

Maintenance of pregnancy is dependent on ovarian secretion of progesterone throughout gestation and will not tolerate abnormal elevations in estrogen (Concannon, et al., 1977). Luteal secretion of progesterone, in cycles of both pregnant and nonpreg-

Table 1. *Events of the Fertile Ovarian Cycle and Pregnancy of the Domestic Dog in Relation to the Preovulatory LH Peak and to Potential Times of Fertile Matings*

Selected Reproductive Events	Days After LH Peak*	Days After Fertile Mating†
Onset of proestrus	−25 to −3	
Full vaginal cornification reached	−4 to +3	
Onset of estrus	−4 to +5	
Estradiol peak	−3 to −1	
Decreased vaginal edema	−1 to 0	
LH surge and sharp rise in progesterone	−1 to 0	
LH peak	0	−9 to +3
First of multiple matings	−5 to +10	−12 to 0
First fertile mating	−3 to +9	0
Initial crenulation of vaginal mucosa begins	−2 to 0	
Peak vaginal crenulation	2 to 6	
Ovulation of primary oocyte	2	−7 to +5
Oviductal oocytes		
Resumption of meiosis	3	
Extrusion of first polar body	4	−4 to +7
Sperm penetration	3 to 9	0 to 7
Fertilization, formation of pronuculeus	4 to 9	0 to 7
Loss of unfertilized ova	6 to 9	
Two-cell embryo	6 to 10	1 to 12
Loss of vaginal crenulation	6 to 10	0 to 9
Reduced vaginal cornification	6 to 10	
Return of leukocytes to vaginal smear	5 to 12	
Morulae (8 to 16 cells) seen in oviduct	8 to 10	
Blastocyst (32 to 64 cells) entry into uterus	9 to 11	3 to 14
Intracornual migration (1-mm blastocysts)	10 to 13	
Transcornual migration (2-mm blastocysts)	12 to 15	
Attachment sites established, zonae pellucidae shed	16 to 18	9 to 21
Swelling of implantation sites, primitive streak formation	18 to 20	11 to 23
Palpable uterine swellings of 1-cm diameter	20 to 25	15 to 28
Ultrasound detection of amniotic cavities	21 to 26	12 to 29
Onset of pregnancy anemia	26 to 28	
Uterine swellings detectable by x-ray	30 to 32	
Reduced palpability of 3-cm swellings	32 to 34	27 to 38
Hematocrit below 40 per cent PCV	38 to 40	31 to 43
Hematocrit below 35 per cent PCV	48 to 50	41 to 53
Fetal skull and spine radiopaque	44 to 46	37 to 49
Radiographic diagnosis of pregnancy	45 to 48	39 to 50
Fetal pelvis becomes radiopaque	53 to 57	46 to 60
Fetal teeth radiopaque	58 to 61	50 to 64
Prepartum luteolysis and hypothermia	63 to 65	55 to 68
Parturition	64 to 66	58 to 70

*Conservative estimates based on published and unpublished observations.

†Based on fertile single matings from 3 days before to 9 days after the LH peak.

nant animals, is dependent on pituitary secretion of both LH and prolactin and can be depressed experimentally by administration of anti-LH serum or by ergocryptine treatment (Concannon, 1986). The uterus has little or no effect on canine luteal function, based on studies of the effects of hysterectomy (Olson et al., 1984a). Prostaglandin $F_{2\alpha}$ is luteolytic and abortifacient in dogs from midgestation to term, but repeated injections of doses of 50 to 250 μg/kg twice daily for several days are needed to effect a permanent luteolysis or abortion without excessive side effects (Concannon and Hansel, 1977; Paradis et al., 1983).

HORMONE LEVELS AND MANAGEMENT

Estrogen

Estradiol levels are at basal values of 5 to 10 pg/ml in very late anestrus, 10 to 20 pg/ml at the start of proestrus, at peak levels of 50 to 100 pg/ml in late proestrus and 1 or 2 days before the LH surge, reduced during estrus, and variable thereafter. Elevations to proestrous values with return to baseline have been reported during anestrus (Olson et al., 1982).

ESTROGEN ASSAYS. Diagnostic radioimmunoassays for estrogen and, more specifically, estradiol are available in many veterinary and human medical laboratories. However, except in cases of suspected estrogen-secreting tumors, their utility in canine reproduction cases is doubtful, for at least three reasons. Postprandial lipids in canine serum may interfere with the assays. Assays intended for human diagnostics may not be fully sensitive to the range appropriate for dogs. Interpretation of results is difficult. Near-peak estradiol levels of 40 to 100 pg/ml are expected in late proestrus and at reduced levels during estrus. However, estradiol levels are variable during metestrus in cycles of both pregnant and nonpregnant animals, and during anestrus levels of estradiol have been reported to be as high as those that occur during proestrus. Thus, the finding of either elevated or basal estradiol levels is unlikely to be as informative as a progesterone level in evaluating the reproductive status of a bitch. An ovarian response test involving measurement of increases in estradiol in response to administered gonadotropin might be considered in cases of chronic anestrus or suspected activity of accessory ovarian tissue in spayed bitches. However, increases in estradiol levels were inconsistent in bitches after administration of one or more injections of follicle-stimulating hormone (FSH) (Shille et al., 1984).

Progesterone

Progesterone levels are normally less than 1 ng/ml during anestrus and proestrus, 2 to 4 ng/ml during the LH surge, 4 to 10 ng/ml at ovulation, and at peak values of 15 to 80 ng/ml by day 15 to 30. In the absence of pregnancy progesterone levels progressively decline to fall below 1 ng/ml between days 50 and 130 of the cycle. In pregnancy, progesterone levels are always elevated above 3 to 15 ng/ml until 2 or 3 days before parturition, and they fall below 1 to 2 ng/ml during the 24 hours before parturition (Concannon, 1983).

PROGESTERONE ASSAYS. Assay of serum or plasma progesterone levels is particularly useful for confirming the occurrence or absence of prior ovulation and the subsequent luteal phase, and this procedure should be part of any evaluation in which the occurrence of ovarian cycles is in doubt. Progesterone assay can be used to evaluate the occurrence and normal duration of luteal function in a bitch that failed to conceive at an apparently normal estrus, or it can be used to detect a missed cycle in a bitch presented for persistent anestrus. Progesterone levels above 5 ng/ml would confirm the occurrence of ovulation within the previous 2 months; above 2 ng/ml, within the previous 3 to 4 months. Levels below 1 ng/ml confirm the absence of ovulation within the previous 2 months and the existence of a true anestrus state. Levels below 1 ng/ml are expected in anestrus. However, instances of progesterone levels of 1 to 3 ng/ml have been observed in some bitches as late as 80 days post partum or after 120 days of a nonpregnant cycle. The significance of this finding and whether the source of progesterone in such cases is follicular or luteal, or possibly adrenal, are not known.

When results of progesterone assays can be obtained nearby or with little delay, they can be used to time ovulation and schedule matings for bitches that are difficult to breed and those in which behavioral changes associated with normal periovulatory hormone changes are erratic, premature, or delayed. Levels below 1 ng/ml indicate that the LH peak has not yet occurred; levels of 6 to 10 ng/ml indicate that ovulation has occurred and that the fertile period is nearly or actually ended. Levels over 15 ng/ml occur near and after the end of the fertile period.

Androgens

Androgen levels have recently been determined for anestrus, proestrus, and estrus (Olson et al., 1984b) as well as during follicular and luteal phases in the cycles of pregnant and nonpregnant animals (Concannon and Castracane, 1985).

Serum testosterone levels are about 0.1 ng/ml during anestrus, and they increase slightly, along with those of estradiol, during proestrus to reach peak values of about 0.3 to 1.0 ng/ml shortly after the estradiol peak and coincident with the preovulatory LH peak. Testosterone levels then decline and remain below 0.2 ng/ml throughout the luteal phase. Serum androstenedione levels are less than 0.2 ng/ml during anestrus. They increase during proestrus and reach levels of 0.6 to 2.3 ng/ml at the time of the LH peak. During the luteal phase in cycles of pregnant and nonpregnant animals, androstenedione levels remain elevated and follow the pattern of luteal progesterone secretion; mean levels of 0.7 ng/ml at day 20 slowly decline to 0.5 ng/ml near day 40 and reach lower levels during the progession into anestrus. Elevated androgen levels during proestrus probably reflect excess production by follicles beyond that needed to provide androstenedione as the substrate for aromatase enzymes and synthesis of estrogens. The significance of luteal production of androstenedione in preference to testosterone during the luteal phase and pregnancy is unknown, but the levels produced are considerably lower than those in several noncarnivore species.

Gonadotropins

Different laboratories report gonadotropin levels in terms of standards of varying potency, and only relative changes can be reviewed. Levels of FSH rise along with those of LH during the preovulatory surge (Fig. 1). The surge represents a 20- to 40-fold increase in LH levels and a two- to fourfold increase in FSH levels. Mean levels of both LH and FSH are very low during most of proestrus, whereas they are moderately elevated during middle and late anestrus (Olson et al., 1982). Mean levels of FSH during anestrus may surpass levels seen during the preovulatory surge; those of LH during anestrus are only moderately elevated. LH release is episodic, and pulses of release occur at intervals of about 1 to 8 hours; reported elevations in mean levels presumably represent increased pulse amplitude or frequency. Preliminary results in the author's laboratory suggest that an increase in the LH pulse frequency often occurs in late anestrus just prior to the onset of proestrus. FSH levels appear to be increased slightly during late pregnancy (Reimers et al., 1978). Prolactin levels appear to be unaltered by endocrine events of proestrus and estrus. Prolactin levels are increased about three times normal in nonpregnant metestrus during the period when progesterone levels are declining. Declining progesterone has been suggested as a stimulus for prolactin release in the bitch (Concannon, 1986). Prolactin levels are elevated nine to ten times above basal values during late pregnancy, surge acutely to peak levels during the prepartum fall in progesterone, and remain elevated in response to suckling-induced reflex release during lactation (DeCoster et al., 1983; Concannon et al., 1979).

VAGINAL SMEARS AND VAGINOSCOPY

Vaginal Cytology

Recent reports and reviews have amply demonstrated that vaginal smears can be easily and routinely used to monitor the progression of proestrus and estrus (Olson et al., 1984d; Concannon and DiGregorio, 1985; Linde and Karlsson, 1984; Roszel, 1975). Any of several stains permit characterization of the various epithelial cell types based on size, shape, and nuclear conditions (Fig. 4).

Smears are best obtained from the cranial vagina by using a narrow spreading speculum and a lightly moistened cotton-tipped swab. Wiping of the mucosa should be deliberate, and the cells are transferred to the slide with a gentle, rolling motion. Fixation before drying, with an aerosol or liquid fixative, is preferred but not necessary. Among useful stains recently reviewed is a modified Wright's-Giesma staining set that is commercially available, rapid, and easy to use (Diff-Quik, Harleco). The normal progression of changes in relative incidences of different epithelial cell types in the smear is easy to follow (Figs. 5 and 6). Distinguishing between early proestrus and the period of very late estrus or early metestrus can be difficult if based on the study of only one smear of an unknown cycle.

Rounded nonsuperficial cells (parabasal and small intermediate cells) dominate the smear taken during early proestrus and virtually disappear from the smears 3 to 4 days before the LH peak or earlier. Maximum cornification may occur as early as 5 to 6 days before the LH peak, or may not occur until 2 to 3 days after the LH peak. Maximum cornification may be represented by nearly 100 per cent fully cornified anuclear superficials; by a high percentage of partly cornified cells containing distinct, condensed nuclei; or, in some cycles, by a retention of some large, well-nucleated intermediate cells along with the superficials (Concannon and DiGregorio, 1985). The variation in the extent of maximal cornification and in its timing preclude any reliable use of changes in epithelial cells to predict the times of the LH surge or ovulation with any immediacy. Because of the great variation in the relative incidence and progression of large intermediate cells among cycles, this cell type often poses the greatest problems in interpretation of the progression of changes in smears during proestrus and, for that reason, should be recognized and appreciated as a unique cell type. Large intermediate cells are unique in having large, healthy nuclei characteristic of nonsuperficial cells and the irregular, squamous, wrinkled shape characteristic of cornified superficial cells.

To repeat, there are no acute changes in epithelial cells routinely predictive of the LH peak or ovulation. In cases in which fully cornified cells completely replace partly cornified cells, the transition usually occurs around the time of ovulation. In cases of an abrupt decline in erythrocytes or in the amount of noncellular debris, the change often occurs between the LH peak and ovulation. More

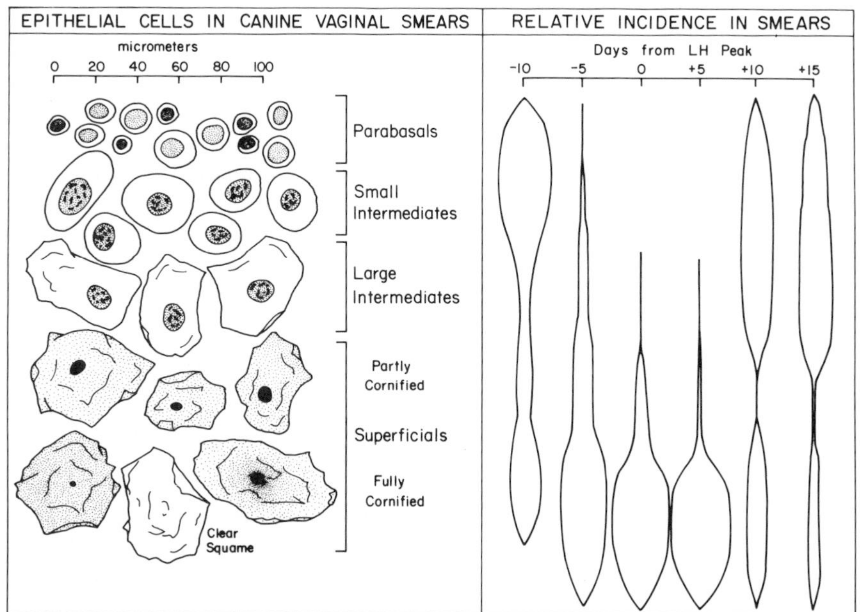

Figure 4. Types of epithelial cells commonly observed in canine vaginal smears, drawn to scale.

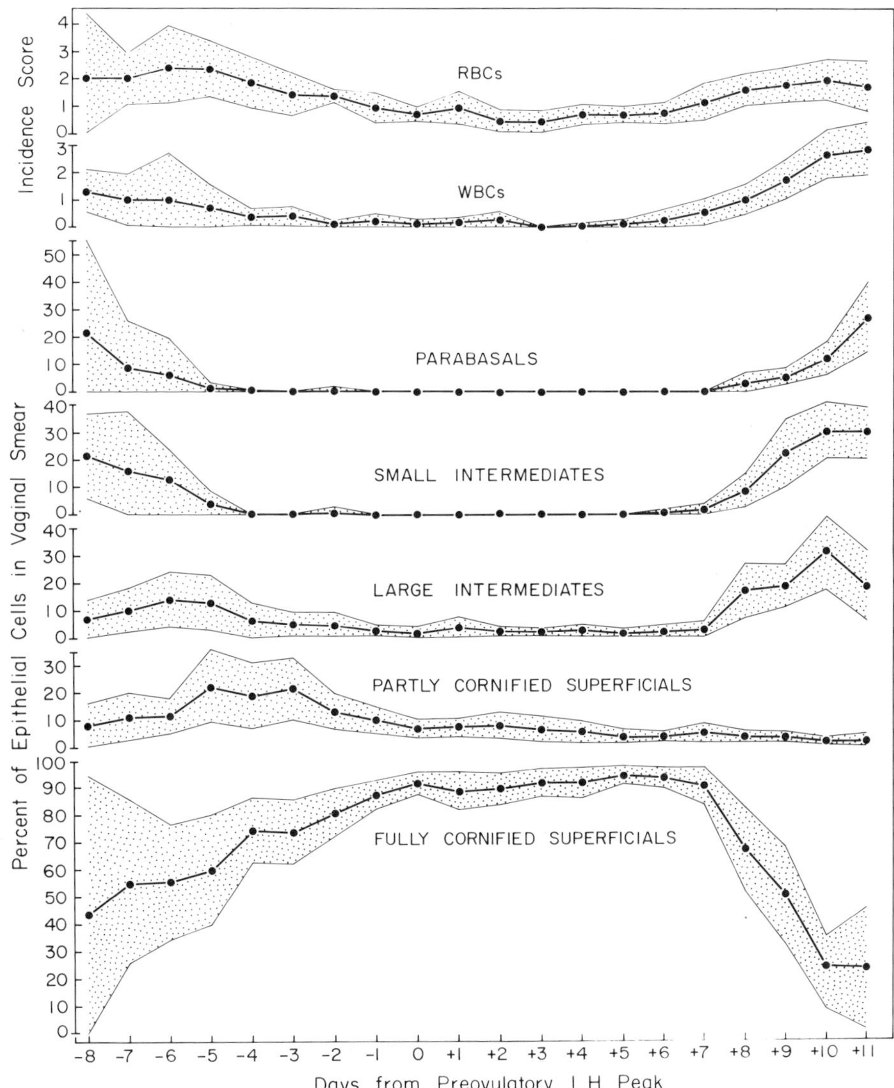

Figure 5. Mean incidence of blood cells (based on relative, subjective scoring) and of epithelial cell types (as actual percentages of epithelial cells present) observed in vaginal smears obtained at known times relative to the day of the preovulatory LH peak. Results are for 18 normal cycles in which the day of the LH peak was determined. (From Concannon and DiGregorio *in* Burke (ed.): *Canine and Feline Reproduction and Infertility.* Philadelphia: Lea & Febiger, 1986, pp. 92–107.)

often erythrocytes appear in the smear throughout and beyond estrus. When proestrus is unusually prolonged there may be a concern that behavioral estrus is overdue, and forced mating or artificial insemination warranted. No concern should exist, however, until 3 to 4 days after rounded nonsuperficial cells (parabasals and small intermediates) have been reduced to less than 1 per cent of epithelial cells present.

Smears continue to show near-maximum cornification throughout the fertile period of estrus, and continued collection of smears is useful for more accurate timing of reproductive events. The latter is based on the abrupt, initial reappearance of nonsuperficial cells that usually begins 7 to 8 days after the LH peak (Figs. 4 and 5). A range of 6 to 10 days after the LH peak has been observed for this metestrous shift. During this period oocyte fertility rapidly declines and subsequent matings are unlikely to be fertile if delayed more than 24 hours. Several studies suggest that the metrestrous or diestrous shift in vaginal cytologic characteristics can be used with considerable accuracy to time preceding and subsequent events of the fertility cycle (Table 2), since it occurs approximately 8 days after the LH peak in most cycles.

Individual smears obtained in early or mid-proestrus, without benefit of prior smears, vaginoscopy,

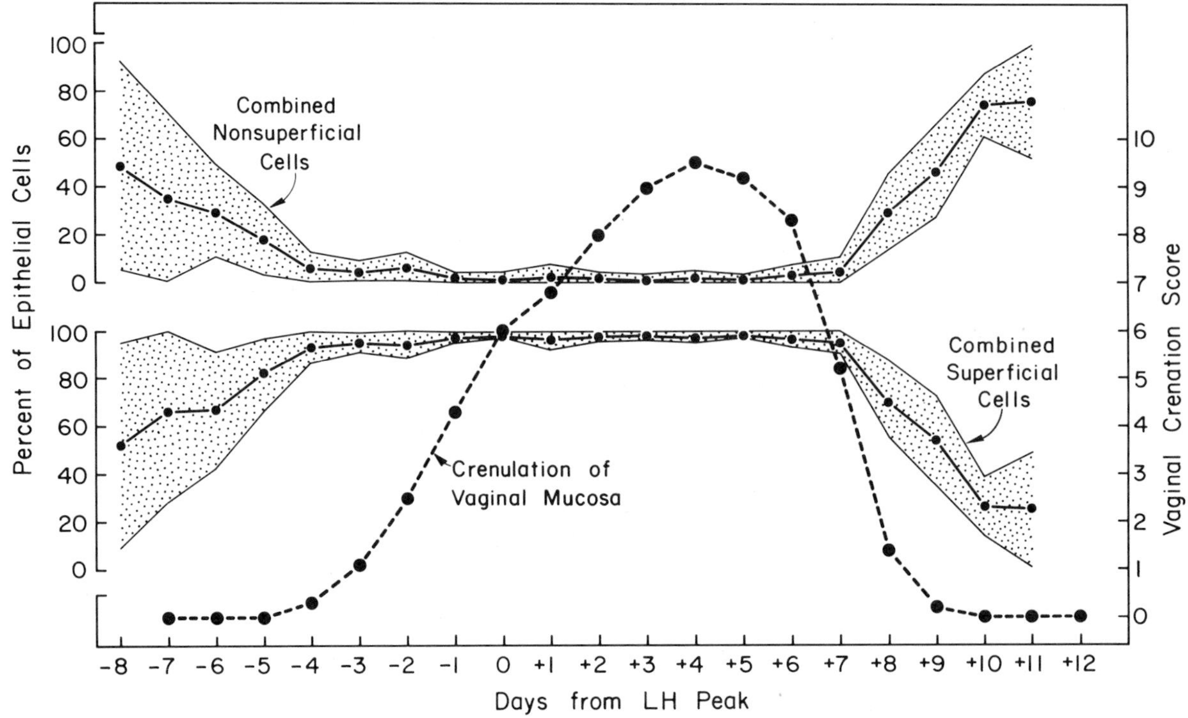

Figure 6. Summary of major changes in the incidence of epithelial cell types in canine vaginal smears; only the superficial and nonsuperficial cells in relation to the day of the LH peak are considered. Mean percentages and 95 per cent confidence intervals are shown for 18 dogs. Also shown are the mean scores for endoscopically viewed gross changes in the vaginal surface of the same dogs. The latter are based on a scoring system for extent of crenulation of mucosal folds, including the following in chronological order: 0—round and edematous; 4—obvious wrinkling and sacculation; 8—obvious, sharp angulation; 10—maximum angulation; 7—thinner, angulated mucosa; 3—very thin, but wrinkled, shedding epithelium; 0—flattened or small round folds with patchy coloration. (From Concannon and Lindsay *in* Burke (ed.): *Canine and Feline Reproduction and Infertility*. Philadelphia: Lea & Febiger, 1986, pp. 108–116.)

or genital exam, can often appear like a smear obtained during the above-mentioned transition from late estrus to early metestrus and thereby can cause confusion in interpretation. At both times, there can be a similar mixture of superficial and nonsuperficial cells and moderate numbers of both erythrocytes and leukocytes. Vaginoscopy and vulvar examination usually resolve the confusion.

***Table 2.** Timing of Reproductive Events in the Bitch in Relation to the Reappearance of Nonsuperficial Epithelial Cells in Vaginal Smears Observed During the Transition from Late Estrus to Early Metestrus*

Reproductive Event	Days From Smear Transition *Mean*	*Range*
Preovulatory LH peak	−8	−6 to −10
Onset of behavioral estrus	−7	−1 to −13
Ovulation	−6	−4 to −6
Oocyte maturation	−4	−2 to −4
End of peak fertile period	−2	−1 to −5
Metestrous shift in smear	0	
Latest possible fertilization	2	0 to 4
Early pregnancy palpation	12	9 to 15
Optimal pregnancy palpation	17	14 to 20
Questionable pregnancy palpations	26	22 to 30
Early fetal radiography	39	36 to 42
Prepartum hypothermia	56	53 to 59
Parturition	57	54 to 60

Vaginoscopy

As initially reported by Lindsay (1983), during proestrus and estrus obvious and dramatic changes occur in the gross appearance of vaginal mucosa. Recent observations demonstrate that the changes can be assessed by using either a small-diameter (5-mm) fiberoptic endoscope or an 11-mm diameter nonoptical pediatric or stricture proctoscope (Concannon and Lindsay, 1986). In contrast with vaginal cytologic events, the gross changes in the vaginal mucosa immediately before and after ovulation are sufficiently consistent in extent and timing to provide a reliable indicator of the onset of the period of fertility. In addition there is an abrupt change at the end of "vaginal" estrus that corresponds to the late-estrous shift seen in vaginal smears.

The changes observed in the surface of the vaginal mucosa begin with the enlargement and edema of mucosal folds during the rise in estrogen throughout

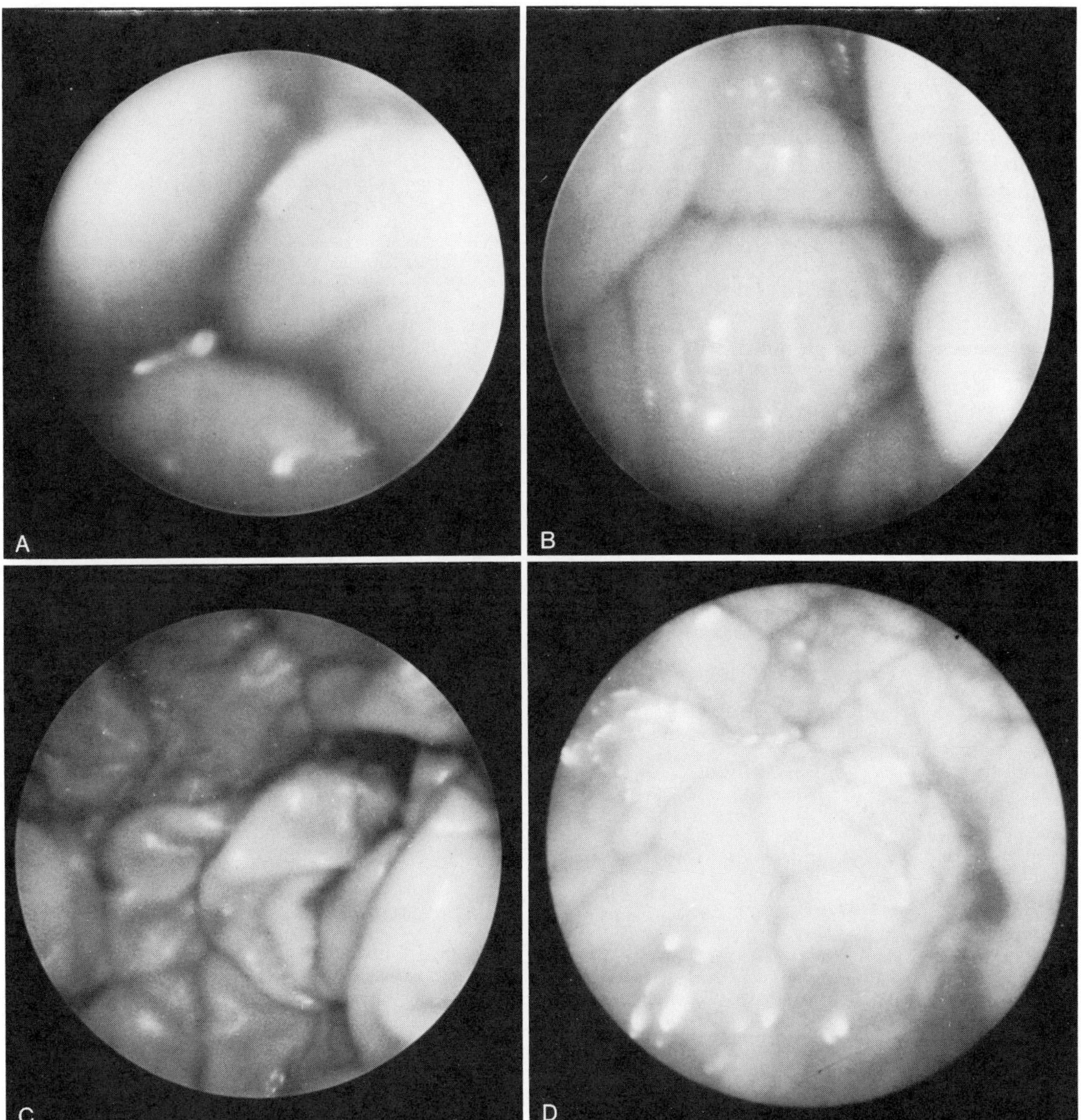

Figure 7. Endoscopic views of canine vaginal mucosal folds. *A*, Large, round, pink to white edematous folds normally seen during proestrus period of increasing estrogen levels; absence of wrinkles yields a crenulation score of 0. *B*, Initial wrinkling of surface of large round folds, normally seen shortly before and during the preovulatory LH surge and before ovulation, as estrogen levels decline; score of 2 to 4. *C*, Severe wrinkling, sacculation, and angulation of mucosa normally observed 2 days after the LH peak and during the peak of ovulation; crenation score of 6. Maximum angulation (score of 8 to 10) and sharpness of peaks normally occurs during oocyte maturation, about 4 days after the LH peak. *D*, Low, flat mucosa devoid of large wrinkles, with patchy red and white areas on the surface, normally seen at the end of vaginal estrus (7 to 10 days after the LH peak, during the termination of the period of fertility); crenulation score of 0. (Adapted from Concannon and Lindsay *in* Burke (ed.): *Canine and Feline Reproduction and Infertility*. Philadelphia: Lea & Febiger, 1986, pp. 108–116.)

most of proestrus. There then begins a progressive loss of edema and concomitant development of an increasingly wrinkled surface during the preovulatory fall in estrogen and rise in progesterone associated with the LH surge. Maximum wrinkling, or crenulation, and development of angulated folds that have sharp profiles are observed in the interval between ovulation and oocyte maturation. A few days later, around 7 to 8 days after the LH peak and toward the end of the period of fertility, there is an abrupt thinning and flattening of the mucosa over a 1- to 3-day period, resulting in a low, flaccid mucosa. It has a patchy or variegated appearance characteristic of metestrus; some of the surface is slightly thickened and white, and some is thinner and red. During anestrus the mucosa is extremely thin, red, and fragile and is unlike the thickened mucosa seen in the periovulatory period. A typical pattern of edema and wrinkling of vaginal mucosal folds is shown schematically in Figure 3 in relation to other periovulatory events. Shown in Figure 6 are the actual mean scores obtained for crenulation of the vaginal mucosa quantitated daily in a group of 18 bitches; results of vaginal smears and the relation of the crenulation to the day of the preovulatory LH peak are also included. Examples of the endoscopic appearance of the vaginal mucosa are shown in Figure 7.

References and Supplemental Reading

Brown, J.: Efficacy and dose titration study of mibolerone for treatment of pseudopregnancy in the bitch. J.A.V.M.A. 184:1467, 1984.

Concannon, P. W.: Effects of hypophysectomy and of LH administration on luteal phase plasma progesterone levels in the beagle bitch. J. Reprod. Fertil. 58:407, 1980.

Concannon, P. W.: Prolactin and LH: Two luteotrophic requirements in the dog. Program of the Annual Conference of the Society for the Study of Fertility, Edinburgh, 1981, p. 19.

Concannon, P. W.: Reproductive physiology and endocrine patterns of the bitch. *In* Kirk, R. W. (ed.): *Current Veterinary Therapy VII*. Philadelphia: W. B. Saunders, 1983, pp. 886–901.

Concannon, P. W.: Canine reproductive physiology. *In* Burke, T. (ed.): *Canine and Feline Reproduction and Infertility*. Philadelphia: Lea & Febiger, 1986, pp. 23–77.

Concannon, P. W.: Canine pregnancy and parturition. Vet. Clin. North Am. [Small Anim. Pract.], in press.

Concannon, P. W.: Physiology and endocrinology of canine pregnancy. *In* Morrow, D. (ed.): Current Therapy in Theriogenology, Vol. II. Philadelphia: W. B. Saunders, in press.

Concannon, P. W., Butler, W. R., Hansel, W., et al.: Parturition and lactation in the bitch: Serum progesterone, cortisol and prolactin. Biol. Reprod. 19:1113, 1978.

Concannon, P. W., and Castracane, V. D.: Serum androstenedione and testosterone concentrations during pregnancy and nonpregnant cycles in dogs. Biol. Reprod., in press.

Concannon, P. W., Cowan, R. G., and Hansel, W.: LH release in ovariectomized dogs in response to estrogen withdrawal and its facilitation by progesterone. Biol. Reprod. 20:523, 1979.

Concannon, P. W., and DiGregorio, G.: Canine vaginal smears. *In* Burke, T. (ed.): *Canine and Feline Reproduction and Infertility*. Philadelphia: Lea & Febiger, 1986, pp. 92–107.

Concannon, P. W., and Hansel, W.: Prostaglandin $F_{2\alpha}$-induced leutolysis, hypothermia and abortions in beagle bitches. Prostaglandins 13:533, 1977.

Concannon, P. W., Hansel, W., and McEntee, K.: Changes in LH, progesterone and sexual behavior associated with preovulatory luteinization in the bitch. Biol. Reprod. 17:604, 1972.

Concannon, P. W., Hansel, W., and Visek, W.: The ovarian cycle of the bitch: Plasma estrogen, LH and progesterone. Biol. Reprod. 12:112, 1975.

Concannon, P. W., and Lindsay, F.: Normal canine vaginoscopy. *In* Burke, T. (ed.): *Canine and Feline Reproduction and Infertility*. Philadelphia: Lea & Febiger, 1986, pp. 108–116.

Concannon, P. W., Powers, M. E., Holder, W., et al.: Pregnancy and parturition in the bitch. Biol. Reprod. 16:517, 1977.

Concannon, P. W., and Rendano, V.: Radiographic diagnosis of pregnancy: The onset of fetal skeletal radiopacity in relation to times of breeding, preovulatory LH release and parturition. Am. J. Vet. Res. 44:1506, 1983.

Concannon, P. W., Whaley, S., Lein, D., et al.: Canine gestation length: Variation related to time of mating and fertile life of sperm. Am. J. Vet. Res. 44:1819, 1983.

DeCoster, R., Beckers, J. F., Beerens, D., et al.: A homologous radioimmunoassay for canine prolactin: Plasma levels during the reproductive cycle. Acta Endocrinol. 109:473, 1983.

Holst, P. A., and Phemister, R. D.: Temporal sequence of events in the estrous cycle of the bitch. Am. J. Vet. Res. 36:705, 1975.

Linde, C., and Karlsson, I.: The correlation between the cytology of the vaginal smear and the time of ovulation in the bitch. J. Small Anim. Pract. 25:77, 1984.

Lindsay, F. E. F.: Endoscopy of the reproductive tract in the bitch. *In* Kirk, R. W. (ed.): *Current Veterinary Therapy VIII*. Philadelphia: W. B. Saunders, 1983, pp. 912–921.

Lindsay, F. E. F.: The normal endoscopic appearance of the caudal reproductive tract of the cyclic and non-cyclic bitch: Post-uterine endoscopy. J. Small Anim. Pract. 24:1, 1983.

Nett, T. M., and Olson, P. N.: Reproductive physiology of dogs and cats. *In* Ettinger, S. J. (ed.): Textbook of Veterinary Internal Medicine. 2nd ed. Philadelphia: W. B. Saunders, 1983, p. 1698.

Olson, P. N., Bowen, R. A., Behrendt, M. D., et al.: Concentrations of reproductive hormones in canine serum throughout late anestrus, proestrus and estrus. Biol. Reprod. 27:1196, 1982.

Olson, P. N., Bowen, R. A., Behrendt, M. D., et al.: Concentrations of progesterone and luteinizing hormone in the serum of diestrous bitches before and after hysterectomy. Am. J. Vet. Res. 45:149, 1984a.

Olson, P. N., Bowen, R. A., Behrendt, M. D., et al.: Concentrations of testosterone in canine serum during late anestrus, proestrus, estrus and early diestrus. Am. J. Vet. Res. 45:145, 1984b.

Olson, P. N., Bowen, R. A., Behrendt, M. D., et al.: Validation of radioimmunoassays to measure prostaglandins $F_{2\alpha}$ and E_2 in canine endometrium and plasma. Am. J. Vet. Res. 45:119, 1984c.

Olson, P. N., Thrall, M. A., Wykes, P. M., et al.: Vaginal cytology. Part 1. A useful tool for staging the canine estrous cycle. Comp. Cont. Ed. Pract. Vet. 6:288, 1984d.

Paradis, M., Post, K., and Mapletoft, R.; Effects of prostaglandin $F_{2\alpha}$ on corpora lutea formation and function in mated bitches. Can. Vet. J. 24:239, 1983.

Phemister, R. D., Holst, P. A., Spano, J. S., et al.: Time of ovulation in the beagle bitch. Biol. Reprod. 8:74, 1973.

Reimers, T., Phemister, R., and Niswender, G.: Radioimmunological measurement of follicle-stimulating hormone and prolactin in the dog. Biol. Reprod. 19:673, 1978.

Rendano, V., Lein, D., and Concannon, P. W.: Radiographic evaluation of prenatal development in the beagle: Correlation with times of breeding, LH release and parturition. Vet. Radiol. 25:132, 1978.

Richkind, M.: Possible use of early urine for detection of pregnancy in dogs. V.M./S.A.C. 78:1067, 1983.

Roszel, J. F.: Genital cytology of the bitch. Vet. Scope 19:3, 1975.

Shille, V. M., and Stabenfeldt, G. H.: Current concepts in reproduction in the dog and cat. Adv. Vet. Sci. Comp. Med. 24:211, 1980.

Shille, V. M., Thatcher, M., and Simmons, B.: Efforts to induce estrus in the bitch using pituitary gonadotropins. J.A.V.M.A. 184:1469, 1984.

Smith, M. S., and McDonald, L. E.: Serum levels of luteinizing hormone and progesterone during the estrous cycle, pseudopregnancy and pregnancy in the dog. Endocrinology 94:404, 1974.

Wildt, D., Seager, S., and Chakraborty, P.: Behavioral, ovarian and endocrine relationships in the pubertal bitch. J. Anim. Sci. 53:182, 1981.

MANAGEMENT OF REPRODUCTIVE DISORDERS IN THE BITCH AND QUEEN

VICTOR M. SHILLE, D.V.M.
Gainesville, Florida

DATA BASE

Define the present complaint as precisely as possible.

Summarize or tabulate the reproductive history of the patient so that information can be easily correlated. For each cycle the following information should be noted:

Onset of proestrus, estrus, diestrus; date of mating; occurrence of pseudopregnancy, unusual signs or behavior.

Results of vaginal cytologic and culture tests; results of *Brucella canis* test (not cats).

Was bitch (queen) diagnosed pregnant at 30 days?

Description of parturition and puerperium.

Number of live and dead neonates delivered.

Number of pups (kittens) weaned.

If similar problems are seen in related bitches or queens, construct pedigree chart.

Ask about environmental or iatrogenic factors such as:

Stress or emotional factors.

Amount of light (cats).

Use of nutritional supplements containing hormonal substances, anabolics.

Use of estrus-controlling drugs, dermatologic treatments.

Use of any drugs, supplements, or treatments during pregnancy.

Ask about fertility of the male.

Ask about the management of the breeding act—coitus or artificial insemination (AI).

Complete physical examination should include:

Palpation of mammae and uterus.

Digital examination of vestibule and posterior vagina.

Collection of vaginal smear from posterior vagina for cytologic exam.

Visual inspection of vagina with long, sterile speculum.

Collection of vaginal smear for culture through a guarded culture instrument from anterior vagina.

Laboratory tests include at least:

Hematocrit, leukocyte total count, and leukocyte differential.

Urinalysis.

Brucella rapid slide agglutination test.

Laboratory tests, as indicated, include:

Serial vaginal smears for cytologic tests and serial blood samples for estrogen and progesterone analysis. Vaginal smears should be done at least three times weekly starting as soon as possible after onset of vulval swelling and discharge (proestrus) to determine day when only anuclear cells and cells with pyknotic nuclei (superficial cells) are present (usually associated with start of estrus) and subsequently to determine the day when the noncornified cells again appear in the vaginal smear (day 1 of diestrus). Blood samples should be collected at the same time as the vaginal swabs.

Hormone analysis after appropriate stimulation by trophic hormones: TSH or ACTH stimulation tests, gonadotrophic hormone stimulation tests (cats only).

Exploratory laparotomy and culture or biopsy of uterus.

DEFINE THE PROBLEM

Conditions are grouped by primary presenting complaint.

A. Delayed onset of puberty
   1. Causes of delay
      a. Variability from the normal

In dogs, first estrus is associated with attainment of a specific body weight between the ages of 6 and 24 months. Crude rule of thumb: estrus occurs 2 months after reach-

Table 1. *Reproductive History Form*

Recorded Events	Cycle Number I	II	III	IV
Onset of proestrus	02–11–81	09–08–81	05–12–82	
Mating date	—	09–18–81	—	
Sire		Gator Joe		
B. canis titer	—	neg	—	
Pregnant at 30 days		yes		
Parturition		11–21–82		
Whelped live/dead		9/0		
Postpartum period		ok		
Weaned		7		

ing 70 per cent of breed-specific mature body weight. For example (using canine growth charts):

Pomeranian: mature weight is 10 lbs at 9 months
70 percent = 7 lbs (reached at 4 months)
puberty: 4 + 2 = 6 months

Great Dane: mature weight is 120 lbs at 24 months
70 per cent = 84 lbs (reached at 8 months)
puberty: 8 + 2 = 10 months

Full reproductive performance not reached until second (or third) estrus.

In cats, onset of puberty is influenced by time between birth and onset of breeding season. Kittens born in October may not become sexually mature until onset of new breeding season in January and may be 14 months of age at first estrus.

b. Unobserved estrus
c. Delayed maturity (genetic, nutritional)
d. Iatrogenic (androgens, progestins used in patient)
e. Intersex (chromosomal disorders; use of androgens, progestins in dam of patient)
f. Developmental anomalies (imperforate hymen, atresia of tubular genitalia)
g. Gonadal-pituitary-hypothalamic (or higher) factors, such as developmental anomalies, neoplasia, or traumatic insult
h. Miscellaneous endocrine defects, such as hypothyroidism, diabetes mellitus, or adrenal disorders

2. Diagnostic procedures
a. Detailed reproductive history of patient, littermates, dam
b. Physical examination (this may be sufficient information for a diagnosis)
c. Laparotomy and biopsy of appropriate internal genitalia
d. Karyotyping
e. Laboratory tests to rule out adrenocortical or thyroid disease
f. Serial stimulation of ovarian-pituitary-hypothalamic axis by trophic hormones has been recommended in humans as a means to monitor the ability of the ovary and of the pituitary to respond to hormonal signals. Since the response to trophic hormones in the bitch is quite variable, no recommendations can be given for this procedure.
In the queen, 2 mg follicle-stimulating hormone (FSH) daily until onset of estrus when functional ovaries are present.

3. Suggested treatment: Depends on primary condition, varies from untreatable to not requiring any treatment
4. Client education: Heroic diagnostic methods not needed in most cases; counsel client to be patient; above all, resist indiscriminate shotgun use of hormones

B. Prolonged Anestrus
1. Causes
a. Silent heat
b. Iatrogenic (administration of drugs containing androgen or progestogen)
c. Long interestrous interval
1) Genetic
2) Due to stress
3) Seasonal (cats only)
4) Effect of insufficient light period or intensity (cats only)
d. Diseases of gonads, pituitary, or hypothalamus
e. Diseases of thyroid, adrenals, or pancreas
f. Debilitating systemic diseases
2. Diagnostic procedures: Similar to those for delayed puberty.
3. Suggested treatment: Depends on primary condition.
a. For cats, ensure a period of twelve hours light provided by 100-watt incandescent or 40-watt fluorescent bulb 8 to 10 feet above the floor.
b. Several regimens have been devised for induction of estrus in the bitch; none can be unequivocally recommended
c. In cats, inject 2 mg of follicle-stimulating hormone (FSH) daily until estrus is shown (for no more than 5 days); then breed daily until estrus stops. Ovulation in the queen can be induced by coitus or by injection of 250 IU (single total dose) human chorionic gonadotropin (hCG), or 2 μg/kg gonadotropin hormone–releasing hormone (GnRH) given on the first and second days of estrous behavior.

C. Persistent proestrual bleeding (animal is attractive to males but refuses males)
1. Causes
a. Cystic follicle in ovary, no ovulation
b. Administration of exogenous estrogens for pregnancy prevention
c. Granulosa-cell tumor
2. Differential diagnostic procedures:
a. Normal, slightly prolonged proestrus; uninformed owner; vaginitis
b. Some wild canids have 2-month proestrus; cross-breeds have been reported to have long proestrous phases
3. Suggested treatment:
a. 250 to 500 units hCG intramuscularly; allow full estrous period for complete

recovery (2 to 3 weeks); induced ovulation probably does not produce fertile ova

b. Surgical puncture of cysts not recommended
c. Ovariohysterectomy
d. May use melengestrol acetate (Ovaban, Schering) 2 mg/kg for 8 days for negative feedback on the pituitary and to diminish clinical signs; MUST spay within 3 to 4 weeks to avoid possible pyometra

D. Short interestrous interval (less than 120 days)
  1. Cause: Unknown, may be associated with cystic ovarian follicles
  2. Suggested treatment: May postpone onset of next cycle with mibolerone (not proved)

E. Will not allow breeding during apparently normal estrous cycle
  1. Causes
     a. Agenesis, strictures, persistent hymen, persistent Mullerian duct structures
     b. Vaginal estrous hyperplasia in boxers and other large breeds occurs during proestrual period, often in first heat period (young bitches)
  2. Diagnostic procedures: Swelling and hyperplasia of the vaginal mucosa, which eventually prolapses through vulva; characteristically it is possible to enter vagina, usually over top of the mass, since it arises from the floor of vagina
  3. Differential diagnostic procedures: Neoplasia will persist after estrus; primary vaginal prolapse is usually postpartum; secondary prolapse may accompany hyperplasia
  4. Suggested treatment:
     a. Manual replacement, protection from injury with ointments, pads
     b. Surgical resection—condition will tend to recur if not done
     c. Hormonal treatment has been tried but is not effective (testosterone) or may predispose to pyometra (progestins, progesterone)
     d. Ovariohysterectomy
  5. Client education: Breeding can be done only by artificial insemination; mass will regress after estrus and will not interfere with parturition; if mass is not treated, severe ulceration or necrosis will result

F. Failure to conceive in presence of adequate estrous cycles
  1. Causes
     a. Male infertility
     b. Improper timing of breeding or AI
     c. Obstruction of semen flow in vagina, uterus, oviduct
     d. Disturbed endometrial integrity (short cycles, subclinical cystic endometrial hyperplasia)
     e. Inadequate luteal function
     f. Infectious causes (vaginitis, endometritis, brucellosis, leptospirosis, canine herpes)
  2. Diagnostic procedures: The approach to the problem should best combine diagnostic procedures, treatment, and client education; an educated cooperative client is required who is willing to spend time and money on solving the problem
     a. Accurate history is absolutely essential
     b. Conduct breeding soundness examination of the male or look for proof of fertility by litters conceived AFTER the bitch (queen) in question has been bred
     c. Evaluate breeding (AI) procedure
     d. Evaluate female for nonreproductive disorders
     e. Evaluate breeding behavior by daily teasing with a male; at the same time establish correct time for breeding either by teasing or by a series of vaginal smears taken three times weekly from the first day of noticeable proestrus (swelling, bleeding); breed (AI) every other day from the day of first acceptance or when there are fewer than 20 per cent noncornified vaginal epithelial cells on the vaginal smear; insist on local stud to avoid travel stress

        Establish time of ovulation and adequacy of luteal function by measurement of progesterone levels in plasma samples taken at the same time as the vaginal smears during proestrus and estrus; also take samples on days 1, 10, 30, and 40 of diestrus, as established by the vaginal smear; there should be a total of nine samples during proestrus and estrus and four during pregnancy
     f. Rule out infection of genitalia by culture of vagina at least twice during early proestrus; use guarded culture instrument and a long scope to sample from anterior vagina; be aware that normal vagina harbors bacteria particularly in late proestrus and in estrus; disagreement between serial culture results or finding more than one isolate suggests nonclinical condition
     g. Rule out brucellosis by two measurements for *B. canis* titer, taken 30 days apart
     h. Differentiate lack of conception from early embryonic death by examining bitch on days 25 to 32 of diestrus (par-

turition is on days 56 to 59 of diestrus); daily exams during critical period may be needed; a diagnosis of nonpregnant at this time may warrant a laparotomy and uterine biopsy or culture; ultrasonography is the recommended means of pregnancy diagnosis

i. Confirm pregnancy diagnosis by radiography on day 45 to 50 from the last breeding; evaluate viability of the fetuses; ultrasonography recommended

j. Within 24 hours postpartum, sample uterus for bacterial culture with a guarded swab and a long vaginoscope; enhance speed of uterine involution by ergonovine 0.1 to 0.2 mg once to three times daily

k. Perform necropsy on all dead fetuses and neonates:
   1) Refrigerate but do not freeze tissues to be used for histologic sections
   2) If within 4 hours of death, culture stomach contents and heart blood
   3) If after 4 hours postmortem, culture brain and interior of eye
   4) Examine and describe gross lesions
   5) Submit tissues from lungs, liver, kidneys, intestines, and spleen for histopathologic exam

G. Abortion Diseases
1. Unknown causes
2. Canine brucellosis
   a. History
      1) Failure to conceive in presence of normal estrus
      2) Abort on day 48 to 60, with minimal signs
      3) Interrupted whelping pattern
      4) Birth of weak pups that die quickly; pups are seropositive
   b. Diagnostic procedures: Serologic and culture tests of blood, fetal fluids, membranes
   c. Suggested treatment: Identify affected dogs, remove from breeding facility; test animals every 30 days until all negative for 90 days; to enter kennel, dogs must have two negative tests, taken 30 days apart

H. Cystic endometrial hyperplasia—pyometra
1. Causes
   a. In dogs, combined effects of estrogen and progesterone on endometrium result in cystic hyperplasia of endometrial glands; prolonged or repeated insult terminates in continuous hyperplastic state (and, therefore, infertility); invasion of bacteria brings on endometritis, acute or chronic; pseudopregnancy does not predispose animal to pyometra
   b. Probably the same in cat, but poorly investigated
2. Diagnostic procedures (see Hardy and Osborne, 1974)
3. Suggested treatment
   a. Ovariohysterectomy
   b. Select patient for alternative treatment that will preserve reproductive capacity: young bitches and queens with open (draining) pyometras and "good" presenting signs; drainage and flushing of uterus is essential; breeding on estrus immediately following is imperative; prognosis is guarded—recurrence rate is quite high
      1) Prior to treatment: Conduct complete blood count, blood chemistry tests (at least for blood urea nitrogen, creatine kinase, and electrolytes), and culture and sensitivity tests of the anterior vagina; stabilize, hydrate, give antibiotics; rule out pregnancy
      2) Treatment:
         a) Give prostaglandin $F_{2\alpha}$ (Lutalyse, Upjohn, *not FDA approved*); 0.1 or 0.25 mg/kg once daily until discharge stops but no more than 5 days; re-examine in 2 weeks and repeat treatment at 0.25 or 0.5 mg/kg if discharge has recurred; a third course of treatment should not be administered; if bitch has not responded, perform ovariohysterectomy; antibiotic therapy (ampicillin or a combination of sulfadiazine and trimethoprim [Tribrissen, Burroughs Wellcome]) is essential
         b) Alternately insert drainage catheters (one per horn) via an abdominal approach through an incision in body of uterus; catheter tips protrude through vagina and are used for flushing; flush twice daily with 50 ml sterile saline containing antibiotic (according to results of culture and sensitivity tests of material taken from uterus), mucolytics (detergents—Alevaire, Tergemist; acetylcysteine—Mucomist, Mead Johnson), and enzymes (trypsin, pancreatic dornase); also treat with systemic drugs—give an appropriate antibiotic for 14 days (Ergonovine 0.1–0.2 mg once to three times daily)

References and Supplemental Reading

Al-Bassam, M. A., Thomson, R. G., and O'Donnell, L.: Normal postpartum involution of the uterus in the dog. Can. J. Comp. Med. 45:217, 1981.

Chakraborty, P. K., Wildt, D. E., and Seager, S. W. J.: Induction of estrus and ovulation in the cat and dog. Vet. Clin. North Am. 12:85, 1982.

Hardy, R., and Osborne, C.: Canine pyometra: pathophysiology, diagnosis and treatment of uterine and extra-uterine lesions. J. Am. Anim. Hosp. Assoc. 10:245, 1974.

Hirsch, D. C., and Wiger, N.: The bacterial flora of the normal canine vagina compared to that of vaginal exudates. J. Small Anim. Pract. 18:25, 1977.

Johnston, S. D.: Diagnostic and therapeutic approach to infertility in the bitch. J.A.V.M.A. 176:1335, 1980.

Lein, D. H. (ed.): Reproductive disorders (Section 12). *In* Kirk, R. W. (ed.): *Current Veterinary Therapy VIII*. Philadelphia: W. B. Saunders, 1983, pp. 885–964.

Mara, J. L.: Pyometra. *In* Kirk, R. W. (ed): *Current Veterinary Therapy IV*. Philadelphia: W. B. Saunders, 1971, pp. 762–764.

Nelson, R. W., Feldman, E. C., and Stabenfeldt, G. H.: Treatment of canine pyometra and endometritis with prostaglandin $F_{2\alpha}$. J.A.V.M.A. 181:899, 1982.

Olson, P. N. S., and Mather, E. C.: Canine vaginal and uterine bacterial flora. J.A.V.M.A. 172:708, 1978.

Olson, P. N., Thrall, M. A., Wykes, P. M., et al.: Vaginal cytology. Part I. A useful tool for staging the canine estrous cycle. Comp. Cont. Ed. Pract. Vet. 6:288, 1984.

Olson, P. N., Thrall, M. A., Wykes, P. M., et al.: Vaginal cytology. Part II. Its use in diagnosing canine reproductive disorders. Comp. Cont. Ed. Pract. Vet. 6:385, 1984.

Pollock, R. V. H .: Canine brucellosis: Current status. Comp. Cont. Ed. Pract. Vet. 1:255, 1979.

Shille, V. M., Thatcher, M. J., and Simmons, K. J.: Efforts to induce estrus in the bitch using pituitary gonadotropins. J.A.V.M.A. 184:1469, 1984.

DIFFERENTIAL DIAGNOSIS OF VULVAR DISCHARGE IN THE BITCH

DONALD H. LEIN, D.V.M.
Ithaca, New York

Causes	Discharge Appearance	Diagnostic Aids
Normal Estrous Cycle		
Proestrus	Bloody mucus	Vaginal cytology, vaginoscopy, sex behavior, vulvar size
Estrus	Clear to bloody mucus (variable)	
Metestrus/Diestrus	Clear to bloody to brown mucus (variable)	
Postbreeding Vaginitis	Mucopurulent, possible bloody to brown	Vaginal cytology, vaginoscopy
Gestation and Parturition		
Late gestation	Mucus, tenacious and gray (scant)	Vaginoscopy, vaginal cytology
Parturition	Bloody mucus	
Postpartum (normal, 7 to 14 days)	Blood tinged, sanguinous to mucoid	
Subinvolution of placental sites (weeks, months)	Continuous to intermittent blood	
Dystocia	Green (uteroverdin) and/or tinged with blood	Vaginoscopy, radiography, ultrasonography
Abortion	Bloody and/or green to mucopurulent, possibly odorous	
Emphysematous dead pups	Fetid: bloody, serosanguinous, and/or green	
Retained pups or placenta	Bloody and/or green, possibly odorous	
Embryonal or fetal resorption	Mucus is not present or slightly tinged with blood	
Postpartum metritis	Serosanguinous to mucopurulent, usually odorous	Vaginal cytology, vaginal culture, vaginoscopy

Table continued on following page

Causes	Discharge Appearance	Diagnostic Aids
Congenital Deformities		
Intersexes	Mucus may be absent, seromucoid, or mucopurulent	Karyotype, vaginal exams, vaginoscopy, contrast radiology
Vulvar and vaginal strictures, stenosis, imperforate hymen, double vagina, segmental aplasia	Mucus may be absent, seromucoid, or mucopurulent	Vaginal exam, vaginoscopy, contrast radiology
Enlarged clitoris	Mucopurulent	Vulvar exam, animal may attract male dogs
Pathological Conditions		
Local Inflammation		
Perivulvar dermatitis	Bloody to mucopurulent, pyodermatitis	Vulvar exam, animal may attract male dogs
Vulvitis (may be granular)	Mucopurulent to bloody	Vulvar exam, animal may attract male dogs
Clitoritis	Mucopurulent	Clitoral exam, animal may attact male dogs
Foreign body	Mucopurulent to bloody, may be fetid	Vulvar exam, animal may attract male dogs
Deep Inflammation		
Juvenile vaginitis	Mucopurulent to seromucoid	Vaginal cytology, vaginal cultures, vaginoscopy
Vaginitis	Mucopurulent	
Endometrial hyperplasia or endometritis	Mucopurulent to bloody	
Cystic endometrial hyperplasia or endometritis	Mucopurulent to bloody	Vaginoscopy, ultrasonography
Pyometritis		
Open	Mucopurulent	Radiology, ultrasonography, vaginal culture, vaginoscopy
Closed	None to slightly mucopurulent	
Uterine stump abscess (spayed)	Mucopurulent to bloody, possibly odorous	Vaginoscopy, vaginal cytology, vaginal culture, radiography
Tumors		
Vulva		
Squamous cell carcinoma	Bloody, fetid, possibly mucopurulent	Vulvar exam, biopsy, vulvar cytology
Transmissible venereal tumor (TVT)	Bloody, fetid, possibly mucopurulent	
Vagina		
Leiomyoma, fibroid	Bloody	Vaginoscopy; vaginal cytology, biopsy
Transmissible venereal tumor (TVT)	Bloody, fetid, possibly mucopurulent	
Transitional cell tumor (Urethral extension)	Bloody	
Uterus		
Endometrial polyps	Mucus may be absent, bloody, or mucopurulent; may be fetid	Vaginoscopy, radiography
Leiomyoma, fibroid	If present, bloody	Abdominal exam, radiography, palpation, vaginal cytology
Adenocarcinoma	If present, bloody	
Ovary		
Granulosa cell tumor	Mucus may be absent, or mucopurulent	Animal may attract dogs; radiography, laparoscopy, vaginal cytology (estrus)
Cystic follicular degeneration	Mucus may be absent, or mucopurulent	
Papillary Cystadenocarcinoma	Mucus may be absent, or mucopurulent	Ascites, radiography, laparoscopy
Cystadenoma	None	
Dysgerminoma	If present, bloody	Radiography, laparoscopy
Parovarian cyst	None	
Infectious Diseases		
Canine herpes (genital)	Bloody to mucopurulent	Vaginal culture, serology, vulvar exam for vesicles, biopsy
Canine distemper	If present, bloody	Vaginal cytology, clinical exam

Table continued on opposite page

Causes	Discharge Appearance	Diagnostic Aids
***Infectious Diseases** (Continued)*		
Bacterial		
Brucella canis	Mucus may be absent, mucopurulent, or bloody	Serology, blood culture, vaginal culture, abortion
Escherichia coli, beta-hemolytic *Streptococcus, Klebsiella* spp., *Streptococcus* spp., *Haemophilus canis, Proteus* spp., or *Pseudomonas* spp.	If present, mucopurulent, occasionally bloody	Vaginal culture, vaginal cytology, vaginoscopy
Mycoplasma and *Ureaplasma* spp.	If present, mucopurulent	Vaginal culture, vaginal cytology, vaginoscopy
Mycotic and Fungal Organisms	If present, mucopurulent	Vaginal culture, vaginal cytology, vaginoscopy, check for diabetes mellitis
Associated Urinary Tract Disorders		
Ectopic ureters	Seromucoid to bloody	Vaginoscopy, contrast radiography
Cystitis	Bloody to mucopurulent	Urinalysis, vaginoscopy, urine culture, abdominal palpation
Nephritis	Bloody	Urinalysis, urine culture, vaginoscopy
Pyelonephritis	Bloody to mucopurulent	Urinalysis, urine culture
Uroliths	Bloody	Radiography, abdominal palpation, urinalysis
Systemic disease or toxicity with hemoglobinurea or hematuria	Bloody	Clinical exam, urinalysis, hemogram

SUBINVOLUTION OF PLACENTAL SITES

SHIRLEY D. JOHNSTON, D.V.M.
St. Paul, Minnesota

Subinvolution of placental sites (SIPS) is a canine disorder of unknown etiology associated with persistent postpartum sanguinous vulvar discharge. Presumptive diagnosis is based on persistence of this discharge in the absence of clinical signs of metritis. Definitive diagnosis is based on histologic examination of the postpartum uterus.

Postpartum uterine involution occurs over 12 weeks in the normal bitch. Involution is complete when both placental and interplacental regions of the endometrium have undergone proliferation of collagen fibers, sloughing of the collagen masses, and replacement of the endometrial lining by a single layer of small basophilic cells. Soon after parturition, trophoblast-like cells invade the canine endometrium and myometrium along the uterine arteries, where they degenerate and die. Failure of these cells to degenerate is associated with failure of the normal involution process. Hemorrhage occurs with SIPS because of failure of thrombosis and occlusion of the endometrial blood vessels, perhaps caused by damage to the vessels by persistence of these trophoblastlike cells.

Range in days of duration of lochial discharge in the normal bitch is not known. Dark brown mucus and blood clots covering the mucosal surface of the endometrium (placental and interplacental sites) have been reported to persist for 3 weeks postpartum in the bitch; by the fourth week postpartum the mucosal surface of the interplacental sites is covered with clear mucus, and only a few pinpoint hemorrhagic foci and blood clots are seen within small grayish nodules spread randomly over the placental sites. Mucus is not observed at the mucosal surface of uteri removed from normal bitches and examined between 5 and 12 weeks postpartum. This suggests that lochial discharge persists in the normal bitch until 3 to 4 weeks postpartum.

The high incidence of SIPS in first-litter bitches suggests that prior uterine disease is not a major predisposing factor. One, some, or all placental sites in a single uterus may be affected; this is evidence against a hormonal cause. Although luteal progesterone was once implicated in the pathogenesis of this disorder (because of observation of corpora lutea in affected bitches), it is now known that corpora lutea persist structurally beyond parturition in all bitches and that serum progesterone in both SIPS and normal postpartum bitches is low. No histologic changes associated with bacterial infection have been observed in SIPS. Glenn (1968) reported that 8 of 26 dogs with histologically confirmed SIPS did not have a persistent sanguinous vulvar discharge, suggesting that SIPS may be present in some clinically normal dogs; its influence on subsequent fertility and pregnancy is unknown.

INCIDENCE

SIPS has been reported in 54 cases in the veterinary literature. Twenty-nine cases were detected in routine pathologic examination of 450 ovariohysterectomy (OHE) specimens. Twenty were detected in 95 (21 per cent) tracts examined in a study of postpartum uterine involution. SIPS generally occurs in dogs less than 3 years of age (range = 1 to 7.5 years), and there is no breed predisposition. Twenty-four of 26 affected animals were reported to have delivered normal litters with uneventful whelping prior to clinical signs of this disorder.

CLINICAL SIGNS

The presenting complaint in clinical patients is that of sanguinous vulvar discharge that persists more than four weeks after whelping; in some patients the discharge persists for 12 to 16 weeks or until onset of the next proestrus. Quantity of the discharge is variable, and character may range from serosanguinous to frank hemorrhage with blood clots and flecks of necrotic debris. Affected bitches are usually bright and active and have normal appetite, temperature, and pulse and respiration rates. Uterine size at abdominal palpation may be normal, or spherical enlargements (one and one-half to three times the diameter of the uninvolved portions of uterine horn) may be palpated.

DIAGNOSIS

Differential diagnoses for a persistent hemorrhagic vulvar discharge in the postpartum bitch include SIPS, metritis, vaginal inflammation or trauma, endogenous or exogenous estrogen influence, and uterine or vaginal neoplasia. Diagnostic plans should include cytologic characterization of the discharge and determination of its site of origin by vaginoscopy. Uterine size should be determined by abdominal palpation, radiography, or both. Bacterial culture of the discharge should be performed if cytologic examination or the hemogram supports a diagnosis of metritis; in most SIPS patients, culture reveals the presence of a mixed population of normal vaginal flora (such as α- and β-hemolytic streptococci, staphylococci, *Escherichia coli*, enterococci, and *Proteus* spp.). A complete blood count is indicated to help rule out metritis (usually associated with neutrophilia) and to monitor the effect of chronic hemorrhage on the hematocrit. Serologic tests for *Brucella canis* are indicated for all bitches with persistent vaginal discharges.

Presumptive diagnosis is based on persistence for more than 4 weeks postpartum of a nonpurulent sanguinous discharge of uterine origin in the absence of vaginal epithelial cornification and systemic illness. Although uterine neoplasia cannot be ruled out by the initial diagnostic plan, neoplasia usually occurs in bitches older than the SIPS population, it is not generally associated with sanguinous vulvar discharge, and it has not been reported to occur in concert with pregnancy in the bitch.

Definitive diagnosis is based on histologic examination of the placental sites at excision or incision biopsy of the uterus. One, some, or all of the sites may be affected. On gross examination affected sites are elliptical, are larger than involuted sites, and contain nodular protrusions of the endometrium that may project into or even through the endometrium. In one case a fetus was expelled through an area of rupture at the placental site and was found mummified in the peritoneal cavity at OHE 6 weeks postpartum. Histologic examination reveals the presence of large lobulated masses of eosinophilic tissue extending toward the lumen from the underlying endometrium; necrosis and hemorrhage are present at the endometrial surface. Glenn (1968) reported the presence of ill-defined syncytial masses of closely packed trophoblastlike cells encroaching on the endometrium.

TREATMENT AND PROGNOSIS

Because the cause, natural course, and likelihood of recurrence of SIPS are unknown, treatment is supportive and prognosis is uncertain. Of the 54 cases in the veterinary literature in which definitive histologic diagnosis was made, 53 were from tracts taken at OHE; only one was from uterine biopsy. The biopsied bitch conceived at her next season and whelped nine normal puppies without clinical recurrence of SIPS. Pregnancy has been reported in four affected bitches after uterine curettage, but biopsy confirmation of the diagnosis was not presented. Many bitches with persistent sanguinous vulvar discharge postpartum reproduce normally at subsequent cycles, but they cannot be said definitively to have had SIPS without the results of a uterine biopsy. Effect of oxytocin, ergonovine, and prostaglandin $F_{2\alpha}$ on these patients is unknown.

At present, OHE is recommended for SIPS patients not intended for further breeding. Breeding bitches should be treated supportively if such is indicated by their laboratory data. (Blood transfusions can be given for severe anemia or specific antibiotics can be administered if the hemogram or serial cytologic examination of the discharge supports development of uterine infection during the course of SIPS.) Reports of serial uterine biopsy and of fertility at subsequent cycles are needed for SIPS patients.

References and Supplemental Reading

Al-Bassam, M. A., Thomson, R. G., and O'Donnell, L.: Involution abnormalities in the postpartum uterus of the bitch. Vet. Pathol. 18:208, 1981.

Al-Bassam, M. A., Thomson, R. G., and O'Donnell, L.: Normal postpartum involution of the uterus in the dog. Can. J. Comp. Med. 45:217, 1981.

Andersen, A. C., and Simpson, M. E.: The Ovary and Reproductive Cycle of the Dog (Beagle). Los Altos, CA: Geron-X, 1979, p. 290.

Beck, A. M., and McEntee, K.: Subinvolution of placental sites in a postpartum bitch. A case report. Cornell Vet. 56:269, 1966.

Buckner, R. G.: Placental subinvolution. *In* Catcott, E. J. (ed.): *Canine Medicine*, 4th ed. Santa Barbara: American Veterinary Publications, 1979, p. 507.

Glenn, B. L.: Subinvolution of placental sites in the bitch. 18th Gaines Veterinary Symposium. White Plains, NY: Gaines Dog Research Center, 1968, pp. 7–10.

Nye, S. S.: Even areas of uterine necrosis following parturition in the bitch. Vet. Rec. 62:118, 1950.

Schall, W. D., Duncan, J. R., Finco, D. R., et al.: Spontaneous recovery after subinvolution of placental sites in a bitch. J.A.V.M.A. 159:1780, 1971.

PROSTAGLANDIN THERAPY IN SMALL ANIMAL REPRODUCTION

DONALD H. LEIN, D.V.M.
Ithaca, New York

Prostaglandin $F_{2\alpha}$ ($PGF_{2\alpha}$) is used in the bitch and queen for luteolysis and smooth muscle contraction, which causes cervical dilatation and uterine contraction. Luteolysis and abortion occur in mid-pregnancy after a daily series of $PGF_{2\alpha}$ injections from approximately 30 and 40 days to parturition in the bitch and queen, respectively. It is also used clinically to treat pyometra and endometritis in the bitch and queen. Experimental prostaglandin analogues have been studied in the bitch and cause luteolysis and abortion.

TOXICITY AND REACTIONS

The median subcutaneous lethal dosage of $PGF_{2\alpha}$ in the bitch was determined to be 5.13 mg/kg. Clinical signs of reactions and toxicosis include excessive salivation, vomiting, diarrhea, hyperpnea, ataxia, urination, anxiety, and pupillary dilatation followed by constriction. Severity of side effects are dose dependent. At low dosages, defecation is more frequent, whereas at intermediate dosages, hyperpnea, anxiety, hypersalivation, vomiting, and defecation have been observed. Higher doses have caused ataxia and slight depression. The reported dose range has been from 0.02 to 1.0 mg/kg (20 to 1000 μg/kg) in the bitch and 0.220 to 1.0 mg/kg (220 to 1000 μg/kg) in the queen. It is usually administered intramuscularly or subcutaneously.

Side reactions are seen 20 to 120 minutes after injection, and death in animals given lethal doses occurs from 2 to 12 hours after the injection is given. Bitches appear to adapt to $PGF_{2\alpha}$ and side effects diminish by the fourth or fifth treatment. Cats appear to tolerate higher doses. Prostaglandin $F_{2\alpha}$ or its analogues should not be used in dogs or cats with asthma or liver, kidney, or heart problems. Prostaglandins have not been approved for use in small animal medicine and should be considered experimental by clinicians. Owners of pets should be warned that these are not approved drugs.

LUTEOLYSIS AND ABORTION

Early researchers thought that $PGF_{2\alpha}$ was not luteolytic in the dog. Concannon was the first to show that 20 μg/kg every 8 hours or 30 μg/kg every 12 hours for 3 days caused abortion in four of seven bitches when treatment started on days 33 to 53 of gestation; abortion occurred 56 to 80 hours after initial treatment. Hypothermia following the initial injection of $PGF_{2\alpha}$ was also found to be correlated to the drop of progesterone level. Progesterone plasma levels were 0.6 to 1.4 ng/ml when abortion occurred. The three bitches that did not abort had a mean low value of 2.1 ng/ml of plasma progesterone during $PGF_{2\alpha}$ treatment beginning on days 31 to 40 of gestation. Their plasma progesterones recovered to levels of 5 to 10 ng/ml and were maintained until the normal prepartum decline. In this study, eight nonpregnant bitches in middle or late luteal phase were also treated, but all eight had afterwards complete luteolysis with low anestrus baseline levels of plasma progesterone. Two nonpregnant bitches in early luteal phase (days 5 and 20) were also treated, and their plasma progesterone levels were not drastically altered.

In another study ten mated bitches were given 250 μg/kg of $PGF_{2\alpha}$ twice daily; five dogs received it between the first and fifth days of metestrus, and five were given $PGF_{2\alpha}$ between 31 and 35 days of metestrus. Bitches in early metestrus were not affected and appeared the same as the five nontreated controls, whereas all five in midgestation had complete luteolysis and hypothermia following the initial injection of $PGF_{2\alpha}$ and aborted after the fourth to eighth injections.

The above research indicates that early canine corpora lutea are quite resistant to exogenous $PGF_{2\alpha}$ until midgestation (the period from 25 to 30 days) to term. The author has treated six clinically confirmed pregnant mismated bitches of the following breeds: Laborador retriever, Chesapeake Bay retriever, Siberian husky, vizsla, cocker spaniel and coonhound. Their ages ranged from 8 months to 5 years; gestations ranged from 31 to 60 days. A range of 2 to 8.5 days of $PGF_{2\alpha}$ treatments was needed to cause abortion.

Treatment consisted of 25 to 50 μg/kg of $PGF_{2\alpha}$ (Lutalyse, Upjohn) intramuscularly, given twice a day. All bitches were hospitalized, secluded as much as possible in a quiet, comfortable area, and observed quietly for signs of abortion. The lower dose was given the first day or two to observe the severity of side effects and to relax the cervix. These bitches showed nesting signs 24 to 48 hours prior to abortion. Vaginoscopic examination of three of the six revealed daily changes in the anterior vagina and increasing edema of the vaginal and cervical folds, presence of fluid, and dilatation of the cervix 24 to 48 hours prior to abortion. The two late-gestation bitches, at 57 to 60 days of gestation, aborted after 2 and 4.5 days of treatment, respectively, and both had live pups. Live pups can be expected at 55 days to term. The bitch at 31 days of gestation aborted three pups 6 days after initial treatment and by palpation and behavior appeared to have completed the abortion. She was given 10 IU of oxytocin intramuscularly the following day to enhance uterine involution. Two weeks later, two retained viable fetuses were noted on palpation and radiographs. The bitch whelped two normal live pups at term and has had three normal litters since. All bitches returned to estrus at normal intervals. One bitch had prolonged postpartum hemorrhage for 6 weeks and was diagnosed as having subinvolution of placental sites. In the first 15 to 60 minutes after injection, all bitches showed varying individual minor side effects, including increased salivation, diarrhea, emesis, and panting.

This evidence shows that $PGF_{2\alpha}$ can be used to cause abortion in healthy bitches from midgestation to term. A dose range of 25 to 250 μg/kg, given intramuscularly twice daily, is effective. During this period hospitalization and close observation are necessary. The later the stage of gestation in which treatment is started, the quicker the effect. Vaginoscopy can be done on a daily basis to detect dilation of the cervix. Ultrasonography or radiography is performed every 3 to 5 days during the treatment period if it is difficult to tell by uterine palpation when the bitch has completed the abortion process. These procedures should also be followed when abortion is attempted in a pregnant queen.

Luteal function in the pseudopregnant and pregnant queen can also be altered by $PGF_{2\alpha}$. Pregnancy was terminated in 13 queens after day 40 of gestation with one or two injections of either 0.50 or 1.00 mg/kg of $PGF_{2\alpha}$. Two injections of 0.25 mg/kg caused abortion in three of six queens. Parturition or abortion occurred within 8 to 24 hours in nine cats and within 8 to 24 hours after the second injection in four queens. Queens treated at gestation times prior to 40 days were not affected. Minimal side effects were also seen in these queens. Longer daily dose schedules should be studied in queens earlier in the gestation period.

A luteolytic effect was seen in pseudopregnant queens administered either 220 or 440 μg/kg every 12 hours on days 21 to 25, but minimal depression of plasma progesterone levels was produced in queens treated on days 11 to 15. The concentration of plasma progesterone was significantly higher in the refractory queens treated early than it was in controls treated on days 33 and 36 after breeding.

PYOMETRA AND ENDOMETRITIS

Several investigators have reported the clinical treatment of bitches with pyometra or endometritis. Prostaglandin $F_{2\alpha}$ is effective in causing luteolysis, cervical dilatation, and myometrial contraction during late metestrus in bitches that have closed-cervix pyometra. It is also highly effective in stimulating uterine evacuation in bitches that have open pyometra or endometritis and varying degrees of abnormal discharge. Within 48 to 96 hours of treatment, there is usually a great reduction in uterine size, improved myometrial tone, and an abundant vulvar discharge.

Bitches are usually treated with $PGF_{2\alpha}$ to effect. It is approximately 3 to 5 days after treatment before vaginal discharge is scant or stops and the uterus is reduced to a firm small size. Parenteral antibiotic therapy should always be given during treatment and continued for at least 10 to 36 days. Deep vaginal or cervical swabs for bacterial, mycoplasmal, and ureaplasmal culture and sensitivity should be taken to determine the most beneficial antibiotic therapy. Therapeutic levels of parenteral chloramphenicol, ampicillin, or a combination of sulfadiazine and trimethoprim (Tribrissen, Burroughs Wellcome) are given initially until culture results are known. Chloramphenicol is the author's drug of choice, because it is a broad-spectrum agent that is usually highly effective against *E. coli*, mycoplasma, and ureaplasma infections. Daily anterior vaginal douches with 200 to 500 ml of warm 1 per cent tamed iodine solution (Betadine Solution, Purdue Frederick) are beneficial during the $PGF_{2\alpha}$ treatment.

Dosages of $PGF_{2\alpha}$, from 25 to 1000 μg/kg, have been used for bitches with pyometra. Success has been obtained with single doses of 250 to 1000 μg/kg or with multiple injections of 25 to 50 μg/kg every 12 hours. Daily single injections of 250 μg/kg have also been effective. Most of these dosage regimens were given to effect (usually 3 to 5 days). The lower the dosage, the fewer the side effects. Burke recommends a final dose be given 3 to 5 days after the last dose of the series to ensure that the uterus is not refilling with exudate. The author uses multiple dosages of 25 to 250 μg/kg every 12 hours to effect. Dosage depends on the clinical condition and side effects exhibited by individual bitches. The lower dosage is used first to evaluate the effect of the drug on each individual.

$PGF_{2\alpha}$ (Lutalyse, Upjohn) is commercially available for cattle use and comes in a preparation containing 5 mg per ml of $PGF_{2\alpha}$. For small dogs and cats, 1 ml of this product is diluted to 25 ml with sterile water for injection. Thus 5 mg or 5000 μg in 25 ml of water will give a concentration of 200 μg/ml, which is easier to deliver accurately.

Bitches that develop pyometra as a sequela of endometrial cystic hyperplasia or endometritis should be bred at the next estrus after treatment, since recurrence of pyometra after nonpregnant cycles is high. If further litters are not planned, ovariohysterectomy is recommended.

Prior to the next estrus, brood bitches should have a culture and cytologic study of the anterior vagina. This should be done in late anestrus or early proestrus. Treatment with appropriate parenteral or topical antibiotics is indicated prior to breeding. Bitches highly susceptible to postcoital infections should be bred by artificial insemination; semen should be mixed with antibiotic-treated extenders to reduce the number of potential infectious organisms. Discharge from these bitches should also be cultured after the animals are bred and they should be treated again if necessary.

Prognosis depends on the age of the bitch, the severity of degenerative lesions in the uterus, and the degree of care given prior to breeding. Older bitches with severe uterine degenerations or with renal, pulmonary, or cardiac disorders are poor risks. Pyometritis in some cases of cystic hyperplasia can be a positive factor, since the suppuration and necrosis acts to slough the uterine lining and results in destruction of the degenerative endometrium and regrowth of a new endometrium. Some bitches will conceive if bred the next estrus after treatment. Bitches with minimal degenerative endometrial conditions (such as the young bitch with pyometra after a mismating injection of estradiol) can be highly successful breeders following treatment with $PGF_{2\alpha}$.

Queens with pyometritis can be treated the same as bitches, with the same dosages of $PGF_{2\alpha}$ and antibiotics. The prognosis for these queens is similar to that for the bitches.

In addition to the use of prostaglandins for pyometra or endometritis and for abortion, future studies and research with new analogues may lead to their successful use early in metestrus as injections for mismating. They may also control the length of luteal function throughout the nonpregnant estrous cycle of the bitch and queen. Intravaginal administration of prostaglandin $F_{2\alpha}$ or its analogues also may lead to effective luteolysis with fewer side effects.

References and Supplemental Reading

Burke, T. J.: Prostaglandin $F_{2\alpha}$ in the treatment of pyometra-metritis. Vet. Clin. North Am. [Small Anim. Pract.] 12:107, 1982.

Concannon, P. W., and Hansel, W.: Prostaglandin $F_{2\alpha}$-induced luteolysis, hypothermia, and abortions in beagle bitches. Prostaglandins 13:533, 1977.

Jackson, P. S., Furr, B. J. A., and Hutchinson, F. G.: A preliminary study of pregnancy termination in the bitch with slow-release formulation of prostaglandin analogues. J. Small Anim. Pract. 23:287, 1982.

Johnson, S. D.: Use of prostaglandins in reproduction. D.V.M. 10:18, 1979.

Lein, D. H.: Pyometritis in the bitch and queen. *In* Kirk, R. W. (ed.): *Current Veterinary Therapy VIII*. Philadelphia: W. B. Saunders, 1983, pp. 942–944.

Nachreiner, R. F., and Marple, D. N.: Termination of pregnancy in cats with prostaglandin $F_{2\alpha}$. Prostaglandins 7:303, 1974.

Nelson, R. W., Feldman, E. C., and Stabenfeldt, G. H.: Treatment of canine pyometra and endometritis with prostaglandin $F_{2\alpha}$. J.A.V.M.A. 181:899, 1982.

Paradis, M., Post, K., and Mapletoft, R. J.: Effects of prostaglandin $F_{2\alpha}$ on corpora lutea formation and function in mated bitches. Can. Vet. J. 24:239, 1983.

Shille, V. M., and Stabenfeldt, G. H.: Luteal function in the domestic cat during pseudopregnancy and after treatment with prostaglandin $F_{2\alpha}$. Biol. Reprod. 21:1217, 1979.

Sokolowski, J. H.: Prostaglandin $F_{2\alpha}$-THAM for medical treatment of endometritis, metritis and pyometritis in the bitch. J. Am. Anim. Hosp. Assoc. 16:119, 1980.

Sokolowski, J. H., and Gent, S.: Effect of prostaglandin $F_{2\alpha}$-THAM in the bitch. J.A.V.M.A. 170:536, 1977.

Vickery, B., and McRae, G.: Effect of synthetic prostaglandin analogue on pregnancy in beagle bitches. Biol. Reprod. 22:438, 1980.

Vickery, B. H., McRae, G. L., Kent, J. S., et al.: Manipulation of duration of action of a synthetic prostaglandin analogue (TPT) assessed in the pregnant beagle bitch. Prostaglandins Med. 5:93, 1980.

TERMINATING CANINE AND FELINE PREGNANCIES

PATRICIA N. OLSON, D.V.M.,
RICHARD A. BOWEN, D.V.M.,
PAUL W. HUSTED, V.M.D.,
and TERRY M. NETT, PH.D.

Fort Collins, Colorado

Approximately 20 million pets in the United States are euthanized each year or die of exposure, starvation, or trauma. Most animals euthanized at humane shelters are healthy abandoned or unwanted dogs and cats (Hodge, 1984). It is estimated that 4 million pregnancies would have to be intercepted or terminated to prevent the births of the 20 million puppies and kittens destined to someday be surrendered or abandoned. Spaying, or performing an ovariohysterectomy on females, is a practical way to attenuate this problem. In fact, efforts by humane societies and veterinarians that encourage owners to have their pets neutered, along with comprehensive animal legislation and enhanced public awareness about the reasons that pets become unwanted and subseqently abandoned, have resulted in 31 per cent fewer dogs and 37 per cent fewer cats impounded in 1982 than in 1972 (Humane Society Newsletter, 1984). In spite of this improvement, there has been little change in the percentage of animals euthanized each year.

Although ovariohysterectomy prevents pregnancy in a bitch, many owners delay having their animals neutered for a variety of reasons. It has been speculated that most spay procedures are performed for esthetic reasons rather than for birth control (Burke, 1979). Some owners present proestrous bitches to be neutered only after the hemorrhagic discharge passes from the vulva onto carpets and floors. Estrous bitches attracting males from miles away become a nuisance. The queen may not be neutered until her constant yowling prevents owners from sleeping. Veterinarians are often reluctant to spay an animal in estrus since the uterus is very vascular at this time and can hemorrhage with minimal handling. Hence, owners may attempt to confine their estrous pets but often discover a few minutes of inattention affords a persistent suitor the opportunity to mate with the fertile bitch or queen. Confining an estrous bitch or queen can be particularly troublesome if the animal remains in estrus for several weeks.

If a bitch or queen is bred and the owners do not want the puppies or kittens, the female can be spayed or the pregnancy aborted. Spaying a pregnant bitch or queen during the first 3 weeks of pregnancy can be done easily and safely. Although animals can also be spayed during late gestation, the very vascular and enlarged uterus must be removed with care to prevent hemorrhage and shock. Fluids may be needed intravenously and animals may need close monitoring (e.g., continuous EKG, blood pressure, hematocrit, total serum proteins). These precautionary measures increase the cost of surgery, and owners may elect to let their pets deliver offspring. This soon poses additional problems, as owners are unwilling or reluctant to euthanize the newborn offspring. Owners frequently are unable to find suitable homes for newborn puppies or kittens allowed to grow to weaning age. In desperation, some of the puppies or kittens may be surrendered or abandoned.

Although owners should be encouraged to have their pets neutered and not to perpetuate the pet population problem, several methods of pregnancy termination may be necessary to alleviate the problem, since one method may not appeal to all owners or be the best method at all stages of gestation.

ESTROGENS

Regimens Previously Used to Terminate Pregnancy in the Bitch

Estrogens have been used by veterinarians for many years to terminate canine and feline pregnancies. This method has not proved to be consistently effective in terminating pregnancy, and serious side effects may occur. Evaluating efficacy and toxicity has been difficult, since various estrogens with varying dosage regimens have been utilized. Estrogens may be toxic to the bone marrow, resulting in an aplastic anemia that is frequently fatal (Mills and Slatter, 1981; Legendre, 1976; Lowenstine et al., 1972). Furthermore, estrogens apparently increase the incidence of pyometra (Dow, 1959), presumably through increasing concentrations of progesterone receptors in the endometrium (Lessey et al., 1981). Therefore, bitches receiving the abortifacient in an attempt to terminate pregnancy without surgical removal of the reproductive tract may still have to undergo ovariohysterectomy.

Although various regimens have been reported for terminating pregnancy with estradiol cypionate (Burke, 1977; Jackson and Johnston, 1980; Olson and Nett, 1983; Soderberg and Olson, 1983), most authors urge that the drug never be repeated during a single estrus nor given at a dose of greater than 10 μg/lb intramuscularly. Additionally, no bitch should receive a total dose of estradiol cypionate greater than 1.0 mg, regardless of the animal's size. Most reported cases of aplastic anemia have involved dogs receiving total doses of estradiol cypionate exceeding 1.0 mg or 10 μg/lb or dogs receiving more than one injection during a single estrus. However, aplastic anemia was diagnosed in a dog that was presented to the Colorado State University Veterinary Teaching Hospital and which was correctly dosed, suggesting extreme variability in sensitivity to the drug.

Unfortunately, some manufacturers still market estradiol cypionate for mismating and recommend that doses of 0.5 to 5.0 mg be administered to bitches to terminate pregnancy. Therefore, some veterinarians may unknowingly administer toxic doses of estradiol cypionate because directions with the product are incorrect.

Diethylstilbestrol (DES) has also been used by veterinarians for many years to terminate canine and feline pregnancies. After the parenteral formulation of DES was no longer marketed, a regimen utilizing the oral form of DES was reported (Soderberg and Olson, 1983). Unfortunately, little data exists on the efficacy of this treatment.

Recent Work on the Efficacy and Toxicity of Estrogens Used to Terminate Pregnancy in the Bitch

Recently, estradiol cypionate and DES have been evaluated at Colorado State University for efficacy in terminating canine pregnancies (Bowen et al., 1985). Bitches were either given DES (1 mg/30 lbs) orally for 7 days (n = 12), or a single intramuscular injection of estradiol cypionate (10 μg/lb, n = 12, or 20 μg/lb, n = 12). Treatments were given once (estradiol cypionate) or commenced to be given (DES) during late proestrus, 4 days after the onset of behavioral estrus, or on the second day of cytologic diestrus. Diethylstilbestrol was not effective in terminating pregnancy (Table 1). Estradiol cypionate was most efficacious in terminating pregnancy when administered during estrus or early diestrus. However, two of eight dogs (25 per cent) treated with estradiol cypionate during diestrus developed pyometra. None of the treatments was efficacious when administered during proestrus.

Although signs of toxicity to the bone marrow (e.g., leukocytosis, thrombocytopenia, or severe anemia) were not observed in treated animals up to day 25 of diestrus (when animals were spayed and evaluated for pregnancy), further work is necessary to determine the incidence of aplastic anemia when estradiol cypionate is administered at the different dose ranges. Although the numbers are small, it appears that the 20 μg/lb dose may be more efficacious in terminating pregnancy than the 10 μg/lb dose. The authors, however, still recommend that the total dose of estradiol cypionate not exceed 1.0 mg.

Recommendation to an Owner Presenting a Bitch for Pregnancy Termination

Since bitches receiving estrogens are at risk for developing aplastic anemia, pyometra, and possibly

Table 1. *Efficacy of Estrogens to Terminate Canine Pregnancies*

Times of Drug Administration	Drug Dose	Number of Dogs	Pregnancy Rate (%)
Proestrus	DES: 1 mg/30 lb	4	100
Estrus	orally for 7	4	100
Diestrus (day 2)	days	4	75
Proestrus	Estradiol cypio-	4	50
Estrus	nate: 10 μg/lb	4	50
Diestrus (day 2)	IM once	4	25*
Proestrus	Estradiol cypio-	4	100
Estrus	nate: 20 μg/lb	4	0
Diestrus (day 2)	IM once	4	0*

*One case of pyometra in each group.

Table reprinted with permission from Bowen et al.: J.A.V.M.A., 186:783, 1985.

cystic ovaries, *owners should be routinely discouraged from having their bitches undergo abortion with estrogens.*

Owners still requesting termination of pregnancy with estrogens after being informed about potential side effects should be made aware that a bitch receiving estrogens may remain in behavioral estrus for several days after treatment. If such a bitch is again mated, estrogens should *never* be administered a second time. Repeated administration of estradiol cypionate appears to increase the risk of aplastic anemia (Legendre, 1976; Lowenstine et al., 1972; Maddux and Shaw, 1983). Additionally, such a bitch is probably receptive to mating owing to the previous hormonal therapy, not because she is in her fertile period again. Therefore, there is little if any justification for a second administration of estrogens. Bitches that are receptive for longer than 21 days after therapy with estradiol cypionate should be evaluated for cystic ovaries. Two of 16 bitches with cystic ovaries presented to the Colorado State University Veterinary Teaching Hospital over a 2-year period had received estradiol cypionate during their previous "heat period" to terminate pregnancy.

Since bitches treated with estrogens are at increased risk for developing pyometra and aplastic anemia, owners should be watching for signs of these disorders for at least 4 to 8 weeks after treatment. Lethargy, anorexia, vomiting, diarrhea, abnormal discharge passing from the vulva, excessive water consumption, and excessive urination are signs that can occur in bitches with pyometra. Abnormal bleeding or bruising may occur in bitches with suppressed bone marrow function.

Clinical Approach for Determining Candidates for Abortifacients

In many cases in which bitches are presented for pregnancy termination, the use of an abortifacient will be of no value. Since estrogens potentially have very significant, adverse side effects, it is extremely important that veterinarians make every effort to determine if these drugs are indicated prior to administration. A complete history, thorough physical examination, and careful evaluation of vaginal smears serve as the basis for making this determination. (For a review on vaginal cytology, see Olson et al., 1984.)

Occasionally a bitch is presented to a veterinarian because the owner is afraid that a mismating occurred, even though an actual mating was not observed. Stud dogs can be attracted to bitches producing odors for a variety of reasons (e.g., hormonal stimulation of the vagina, vaginitis, cystitis, infections of the anal sacs). If the vaginal smear indicates genitourinary tract infection and not estrus, the infection should be treated and no abortifacient administered. If a bitch's vaginal smear suggests proestrus, terminating pregnancy is unnecessary because proestrous bitches attract males but are usually not receptive to mating. Additionally, estrogens administered during proestrus do not reliably terminate pregnancy in bitches subsequently bred during the fertile period (Table 1). If the vaginal smear suggests diestrus (which may be indistinguishable from proestrus) the bitch should not be aborted. Although a bitch entering diestrus (as based on vaginal smears) may be receptive to mating for a few days, conception rates and number of offspring produced are low. Also, bitches in diestrus have had elevated concentrations of progesterone in the serum for several days and are more likely to develop pyometra.

Therefore, only bitches with smears that indicate estrus at the time of presentation should be considered candidates for receiving estradiol cypionate. Since estrogens are believed to terminate pregnancy by interfering with transit of ova through the uterine tubes (oviducts), the ideal time to administer estrogens for maximal efficacy is when ova are in the uterine tubes (i.e., from the third day of estrus to the fourth day of diestrus). Treatment should not be given during diestrus since, as previously noted, diestrous bitches receiving estradiol cypionate are at increased risk for developing pyometra.

Spermatozoa are sometimes observed in vaginal smears from mated bitches, but the period during which they are present varies among dogs. The presence of spermatozoa therefore confirms a mating, but the absence of spermatozoa does not ensure that a bitch was not bred. In one preliminary study, sperm heads (rarely intact spermatozoa) were observed in approximately 65 per cent and 50 per cent of the vaginal smears obtained 24 and 48 hours after a natural mating, respectively (Bowen et al., 1985).

Terminating Pregnancy in the Queen

Early therapeutic abortion of queens can be induced by the administration of 250 μg estradiol cypionate 40 hours after copulation (Herron, 1977; Herron and Sis, 1974). As little as 125 μg has been reported effective in the queen (Lein and Concannon, 1983). Estrogens reportedly delay the transport of ova through the uterine tubes of queens. Therefore, the ova are no longer viable and able to implant when they reach the uterus. Unfortunately, little data exists describing efficacy and toxicity of estrogens in terminating feline pregnancies.

PROSTAGLANDINS

Maintenance of pregnancy in the bitch throughout gestation is dependent upon the continued production of progesterone from the ovaries (Sokolowski, 1971). In cats, however, ovariectomy during the last third of pregnancy does not interrupt gestation (Scott, 1970; Courrier and Gros, 1935), since the feline placenta is able to synthesize progesterone (Malassine and Ferre, 1979). Any drug that causes regression of corpora lutea could theoretically interrupt pregnancy if it were administered at a time when pregnancy depended on the production of progesterone by the ovaries. Prostaglandin $F_{2\alpha}$ is a drug that causes corpora lutea to regress and secretion of progesterone to cease in many species. Prostaglandin $F_{2\alpha}$ has been experimentally used to abort bitches and queens *but is not approved for clinical use in these species.*

Concannon and Hansel (1977) demonstrated that injections of 20 μg/kg prostaglandin $F_{2\alpha}$ every 8 hours or 30 μg/kg every 12 hours for 3 days caused abortion in four of seven bitches when treatment was initiated on days 33 to 53 of pregnancy. Abortion occurred 56 to 80 hours after the initial treatment. Serum concentration of progesterone fell to less than 2.0 ng/ml in the four bitches that aborted; thus, $PGF_{2\alpha}$ was luteolytic in some animals. Two nonpregnant bitches in early diestrus (day 5 or 20) were also treated with $PGF_{2\alpha}$, but serum concentrations of progesterone were not altered, suggesting that luteal tissue is more resistant to the effect of $PGF_{2\alpha}$ during the early luteal phase than during mid-pregnancy. In another study, five bitches treated with 250 μg/kg $PGF_{2\alpha}$ twice daily from days 31 to 35 of pregnancy aborted, whereas pregnancy was not terminated in five bitches treated similarly during days 1 to 5 of diestrus (Paradis et al., 1983).

Prostaglandin $F_{2\alpha}$ administered intramuscularly at a dose of 25 to 50 μg/kg twice daily terminated pregnancy in bitches within 2 to 8.5 days of initiation of therapy when treatment was begun after day 30 of gestation (Lein, in press). All bitches showed increased salivation, diarrhea, emesis, and panting the first 15 to 60 minutes after injection. Therefore, the lower dose (25 μg/kg) was given the first day or two so that the severity of side effects could be observed. The one bitch treated on day 31 aborted three pups 6 days after the initial treatment and appeared to have completed delivery. However, two viable fetuses were palpated abdominally two weeks later and were subsequently delivered at term.

Therefore, $PGF_{2\alpha}$ may or may not be luteolytic in the bitch, depending on when the drug is administered during diestrus. Unfortunately, late gestation is not an ideal time for abortion, since treatment either requires hospitalization or owners willing to observe well-formed fetuses expelled at home.

Newer prostaglandin analogues are being developed and may offer prolonged action and reduced side effects yet may safely terminate pregnancy in dogs and cats. Preliminary work indicates, however, that some analogues also may be less likely to cause luteolysis during early diestrus (Jackson et al., 1982) and that pregnancy termination may not always be induced (Vickery et al., 1980). It is crucial that veterinarians are aware of dosage differences when utilizing the parent compound ($PGF_{2\alpha}$) and its analogues. Dosages given in this text are for $PGF_{2\alpha}$ and not prostaglandin analogues. *Using similar doses for analogues could likely result in the death of the bitch.*

Nachreiner and Marple (1974) reported that pregnancy was terminated in 12 of 15 cats treated with $PGF_{2\alpha}$ after 40 days of gestation. All 11 queens treated prior to day 40 did not abort. Nine queens over 40 days of gestation aborted when given two subcutaneous injections of either 0.5 or 1.0 mg/kg (500 or 1000 μg/kg) $PGF_{2\alpha}$ 24 hours apart. Three of six queens receiving 0.25 mg/kg (250 μg/kg) $PGF_{2\alpha}$ at the same frequency aborted. Wycokoff and Ganjam (1979), however, failed to induce abortion with similar regimens. Only when adrenocorticotropin was administered prior to $PGF_{2\alpha}$ did serum concentrations of progesterone decrease. These authors speculated that increased levels of corticoids might be necessary to accelerate $PGF_{2\alpha}$-induced pregnancy termination in the cat.

SUMMARY

Reliable and safe methods of terminating pregnancy in pets with pharmacologic agents are unavailable. Canine pregnancy can be terminated with estrogens, but there are severe limitations with regard to both efficacy and safety. In view of the increased risk of pyometra, aplastic anemia, and possibly cystic ovaries in estrogen-treated dogs, it may be best to advise against using estrogens for pregnancy termination in the bitch. Although efficacious during late gestation, prostaglandins are not currently approved for use in the bitch or queen. Unfortunately, this leaves the owners with the options of having an ovariohysterectomy performed or allowing the animals to deliver offspring. It is hoped that new abortifacients that are safe and efficacious will be developed for use in pets.

References and Supplemental Reading

Bowen, R. A., Olson, P. N., Behrendt, M. D., et al.: The efficacy and toxicity of estrogens commonly used to terminate canine pregnancy. J.A.V.M.A. 186:783, 1985.

Burke, T. J.: Pregnancy prevention and termination. *In* Kirk, R. W. (ed.): *Current Veterinary Therapy VI.* Philadelphia: W. B. Saunders, 1977, pp. 1241–1242.

Burke, T. J.: Birth control for dogs. D.V.M. 10:6, 1979.

Concannon, P. W., and Hansel, W.: Prostaglandin $F_{2\alpha}$ induced luteolysis, hypothermia, and abortion in beagle bitches. Prostaglandins 13:533, 1977.

Courrier, R., and Gros, G.: Contributions a l'endocrinoligie de la grossesse chez la chatte. C. R. Soc. Biol. 102:5, 1935.

Dow, C.: Experimental reproduction of the cystic endometrial hyperplasia-pyometra complex in the bitch. J. Pathol. Bacteriol. 78:267, 1959.
Herron, M. A.: Feline reproduction. Vet. Clin. North Am. 7:715, 1977.
Herron, M. A., and Sis, R. F.: Ovum transport in the cat and the effect of estrogen administration. Am. J. Vet. Res. 35:1277, 1974.
Hodge, G. R.: Personal communication. Humane Society of the United States, Washington, DC, 1984.
Humane Society Newsletter 29:4, 1984.
Jackson, P. S., Furr, B. J. A., and Hutchinson, F. G.: A preliminary study of pregnancy termination in the bitch with slow-release formulations of prostaglandin analogues. J. Small Anim. Pract. 23:287, 1982.
Jackson, W. F., and Johnston, S. D.: Pregnancy prevention and termination. *In* Kirk, R. W. (ed.): *Current Veterinary Therapy VII*. Philadelphia: W. B. Saunders, 1980, p. 945.
Legendre, A. M.: Estrogen-induced bone marrow hypoplasia in a dog. J. Am. Anim. Hosp. Assoc. 12:525, 1976.
Lein, D. H .: Prostaglandins in small animal reproduction. *In* Morrow, D. A. (ed.): *Current Therapy in Theriogenology*, 2nd ed. Philadelphia: W. B. Saunders, in press.
Lein, D. H., and Concannon, P. W.: Infertility and fertility treatments and management in the queen and tom cat. *In* Kirk, R. W. (ed.): *Current Veterinary Therapy VIII*. Philadelphia: W. B. Saunders, 1983, p. 936.
Lessey, B. A., Wahawisan, R., and Gorell, T. A.: Hormonal regulation of cytoplasmic estrogen and progesterone receptors in the beagle uterus and oviduct. Mole. Cell. Endocrinol. 21:171, 1981.
Lowenstine, L. J., Ling, G. V., and Schalm, O. W.: Exogenous estrogen toxicity in the dog. Calif. Vet., August 1972, p. 14.
Maddux, J. M., and Shaw, S. E.: Possible beneficial effect of lithium therapy in a case of estrogen-induced bone marrow hypoplasia in a dog.: A case report. J. Am. Anim. Hosp. Assoc. 19:242, 1983.
Malassine, A., and Ferre, F.: 5,3-β-Hydroxysteroid dehydrogenase activity in cat placental labyrinth: Evolution during pregnancy, subcellular distribution. Biol. Reprod. 21:965, 1979.
Mills, J. N., and Slatter, D. H.: Stilbestrol toxicity in a dog. Aust. Vet. J. 57:39, 1981.
Nachreiner, R. F., and Marple, D. N.: Termination of pregnancy in cats. Prostaglandins 7:303, 1974.
Olson, P. N. S., and Nett, T. M.: Small animal contraceptives. *In* Ettinger, S. J. (ed.): *Textbook of Veterinary Internal Medicine*, 2nd ed. Vol. 2. Philadelphia: W. B. Saunders, 1983, p. 1725.
Olson, P. N., Thrall, M. A., Wykes, P. M., et al.: Vaginal cytology. Part I. A useful tool for staging in the canine estrous cycle. Comp. Cont. Ed. Pract. Vet. 6:288, 1984.
Olson, P. N., Thrall, M. A., Wykes, P. M., et al.: Vaginal cytology. Part II. Its use in diagnosing canine reproduction disorders. Comp. Cont. Ed. Pract. Vet. 6:385, 1984.
Paradis, M., Post, K., and Malpletoft, R. J.: Effects of prostaglandin $F_{2\alpha}$ on corpora lutea formation and function in mated bitches. Can. Vet. J. 24:239, 1983.
Scott, P. P.: Cats. *In* Hafez, E. S. E. (ed.): *Reproduction and Breeding Techniques for Laboratory Animals*. Philadelphia: Lea & Febiger, 1970, p. 192.
Soderberg, S. F., and Olson, P. N.: Abortifacients. *In* Kirk, R. W. (ed.): *Current Veterinary Therapy VIII*. Philadelphia: W. B. Saunders, 1983, p. 945.
Sokolowski, J. H.: Effects of ovariectomy on pregnancy maintenance in the bitch. J. Anim. Sci. 21:696, 1971.
Vickery, B. H., McRae, G. T., Kent, J. S., et al.: Manipulation of duration of action of a synthetic prostaglandin analogue (TPT) assessed in the pregnant bitch. Prostagland. Med. 5:93, 1980.
Wycokoff, J. T., and Ganjam, V. K.: Successful termination of pregnancy in cats by the administration of a combination of adrenocorticotropin hormone (ACTH) and prostaglandin $F_{2\alpha}$-THAM salt. Fed. Proc. 38:5071, 1979.

CANINE MYCOPLASMA, UREAPLASMA, AND BACTERIAL INFERTILITY

DONALD H. LEIN, D.V.M.
Ithaca, New York

Mycoplasmas and ureaplasmas are classified as the smallest free-living microorganisms. Ureaplasmas (formerly called T-strain mycoplasmas, "T" standing for "tiny") are part of the order called Mycoplasmatales, simply referred to as mycoplasmas. The family Mycoplasmataceae is divided into two genera, *Mycoplasma* and *Ureaplasma*. Both require sterol for growth. Ureaplasmas have the ability to hydrolyze urea. They are highly pleomorphic in shape because they lack a rigid cell wall. Like bacteria, these organisms can be grown on synthetic media enriched with sera. Mycoplasmas and ureaplasmas are frequently opportunistic and can be carried as normal flora on the mucosal membranes of the nasopharyngeal cavity or urogenital tract with no clinical expression until the right conditions or numbers of organisms are present.

Urogenital disease caused by mycoplasmas and ureaplasmas have been recognized for years in humans and cattle. The infertility caused by these microorganisms can result in male or female genital tract disease, poor conception, early embryonic death, abortion, postparturient septicemia, or weak and diseased newborns. Carrier states (with no clinical expression) and venereal spread are common and reported in both humans and cattle. Poor quality semen has been associated with these microorganisms in both species.

Eleven species of *Mycoplasma*—*M. canis*, *M. spumans*, *M. maculosum*, *M. opalescens*, *M. ed-*

wardii, M. cynos, M. molare, M. feliminutum, M. gateae, M. arginini, M. bovigenitalium—Acholeplasma laidlawii, and four serologic groups of *Ureaplasma* as well as an unclassified strain of *Mycoplasma* were reported as the mycoplasmal flora of the dog by Rosendal (1982). *Mycoplasma felis* was also reported from the canine genital tract by Doig and coworkers (1981). *Mycoplasma canis* was the most common isolate from the canine genital tract; it was followed in frequency by *M. cynos*. Ureaplasmas are frequently isolated with a concomitant species of *Mycoplasma* from the genital tract of the dog. Mycoplasmas tend to be species-specific, but in the above-mentioned reports, both bovine and feline strains are reported. *M. bovigenitalium* has been reported in other species, including humans. Mycoplasmas and ureaplasmas most often cause disease of the mucosal epithelium or serous membranes and often are associated with diseases of the lungs, joints, urogenital tract, mammary glands, and eyes of affected animals. In the dog, they have caused or been associated with diseases of the lungs, heart, urogenital tract, intestinal tract, eyes, and tonsils. Experimental chronic orchitis and epididymitis in the dog and endometritis in the bitch were induced by using a strain of *M. canis* isolated from the vagina of a bitch with an abnormal estrous cycle. Mycoplasmic agents have been isolated and reported by the author from three cases of unilateral epipididymo-orchitis. Canadian workers have found association between infertility and canine mycoplasmas or ureaplasmas in stud dogs and breeding bitches. They found a significantly higher incidence of ureaplasmas in the prepuces of infertile stud dogs than in those that were fertile; bitches that were infertile and had purulent vulvar discharge had a higher rate of isolation of these organisms than did those dogs that were clinically normal. In this study, ureaplasmas were always isolated in association with a concomitant *Mycoplasma* infection in the female. *Ureaplasma* was isolated in pure culture from the prepuce of one infertile male, whereas all other dogs also were infected with *Mycoplasma*.

Our laboratory and clinic have confirmed the findings of the Canadian workers. Clinical studies recognize a syndrome of infertility characterized by poor conception, early embryonic death, embryonal or fetal resorption, abortion, stillborn pups, weak newborns, and neonatal death. We have isolated mycoplasmas or ureaplasmas (or both) from animals in all phases of this syndrome. This syndrome is most frequently recognized in breeding kennels where close, intensive living conditions and the environment provide an opportunity for large numbers of these organisms to develop and affect the bitch and stud dog. The same is seen with bacterial opportunistic infections, such as the beta-hemolytic streptococci, *Haemophilus canis*, *Escherichia coli*, species of *Pseudomonas* and *Proteus*, and other bacteria. At times, bacterial and mycoplasmal or ureaplasmal infections are mixed. Historically, mycoplasmas and concomitant bacteria cause severe diseases as mixed infections, such as chronic respiratory disease of birds and kennel cough in dogs. Intensive husbandry with large numbers of animals grouped closely together are common denominators in ureaplasmal and mycoplasmal infertility of cattle. The single house pet or small, less intensively managed kennel is not likely to be affected. In some infected kennels, several bitches will be involved and fertility rates will drop drastically. Normal, reproductively sound dogs can also harbor these agents. Bitches and stud dogs that are infertile may show no clinical manifestation of overt urogenital tract infections, but embryos, fetuses, or newborn pups may become infected *in utero* after conception, during pregnancy, or at the time of whelping by organisms in the vaginal cavity. In others, mucopurulent vulvar discharges associated with vaginitis and probably upper tract infections can be seen. In the stud dog, balanoposthitis and possibly upper tract infections, including prostatitis and epidiymo-orchitis, can be diagnosed.

Infertility caused by mycoplasmas, ureaplasmas, or bacteria in the bitch and stud dog should be suspected when a history of infertility is given and characterized by reduced conception, early embryonal or fetal death, abortion, stillborns, fading pups, or neonatal deaths. Individual animals with mucopurulent urogenital discharges and upper tract infections are also suspect.

Diagnosis is made by isolation of the organisms. A deep vaginal swab for culture from the affected bitch is taken by passing a guarded culture swab (Guarded Culture Instrument, Kalayjian Industries, or Playtex Gentle Glide, Playtex, Inc.) to the anterior vagina during anestrus, early proestrus, or whenever a mucopurulent discharge is present. The aborted pups, any placenta, and postresorption discharges should all be fully examined. They can be either submitted whole or cultured by swabbing the affected tissues or discharges, placenta, and major organs of the aborted or recently dead pups. Swabs should be placed in Amies transport media (Difco Laboratories) without charcoal and sent in a Styrofoam shipping box containing ice. Entire tissues or pups should be shipped on ice instead of frozen.

To obtain a deep anterior vaginal culture, a sterile vaginal speculum without lubrication should be passed into the caudal vagina. Through the speculum, the sterile, guarded swab is passed to the anterior vagina and the culture swab is then exposed and rotated in the anterior vagina so that sufficient mucosa is contacted. The swab is then pulled back into the protective guard for removal. In small dogs the head of a sterile, small otoscope can be passed into the vagina and a nonguarded swab (4 mm in diameter) is passed through the otoscope and to the anterior vagina. Cleaning of the vulva, perineum, and surrounding hair (if needed) should be done 12 to 24 hours prior to obtaining the specimen, since a wet skin surface frequently causes contamination of the area, especially with species of *Pseudomonas* or *Proteus*. Long leg hair or feathers should be pinned to the side of the dog with a clip, and long tail hair can be covered with a tail wrap of 2- to 3-inch gauze roll bandage. Care should be taken not to contaminate the specimen as it passes through the vestibule or cranial vagina. The culture swab should either be processed for mycoplasmas, ureaplasmas, and bacteria within minutes or placed in Amies transport media without charcoal, refrigerated, and sent on ice in a Styrofoam mailing pack to a laboratory capable of culturing these microorganisms. Antimicrobiologic sensitivity tests should be done on significant bacterial isolations.

A vaginal smear for cytologic examination is obtained from the anterior vagina at the same time the culture specimen is taken. Evidence of no inflammatory response or active response with several degenerate polymorphonuclear leukocytes and bacteria is recorded for correlation with the eventual culture results. The stage of the estrous cycle and evidence of neoplastic disorders will also be determined from studying the vaginal cells. A vaginoscopic examination is then carried out to ascertain evidence of active inflammation, which is characterized by mucopurulent debris on the floor of the vagina, severe congestion, or ulceration and fibrin on the vaginal wall. Exudate may be seen coming from the cervical area; this indicates a uterine infection.

Cultures of bacteria, mycoplasmas, or ureaplasmas in high numbers, either pure or mixed, are significant if signs of active inflammation are present or if an infertility syndrome is present (even if no active inflammation is demonstrated). Isolation of these organisms from aborted or stillborn pups, dead neonates, or resorption discharge is highly significant. These bitches should be treated.

Preputial swabs, semen, or prostatic fluid from suspect or affected male dogs can be placed in Amies transport media and submitted for culture. Serologic diagnosis by blood test is not reliable, since many of the infections or carrier states are on mucosal epithelium and are not systemic, resulting in poor serologic response and a high canine population with low-level titers. Since the mycoplasmal and ureaplasmal organisms are very fastidious and need special media and different atmospheres for growth, laboratories should be consulted to see if they are able to isolate and identify these agents.

Kennels that are affected with this syndrome are difficult to treat, since there appears to be little immunity developed in the urogenital tract against these organisms and the carrier state. Therefore, the syndrome continues through repeated breeding periods if adequate numbers of organisms are available. The best control in kennels affected with this type of infertility is to alter the husbandry and management practices by isolating bitches and stud dogs that do or do not receive chemotherapy into smaller, less intense groups. This reduces contact between dogs and, therefore, the number of microorganisms and carrier states.

Treatment for mycoplasmal and ureaplasmal infections or carrier states consists of parenteral treatment of small isolated groups of animals with chloramphenicol or tetracycline, the drugs of choice for these microorganisms. Treatment should be given for 10 to 14 days. These drugs are contraindicated in pregnant bitches. Erythromycin and ampicillin, although not as effective against these agents, are safe to use in early pregnancy. Chloramphenicol is reported to be safe in the latter half of pregnancy. A mild 1 per cent povidone-iodine vaginal douche may be administered two or three times during the parenteral treatment. Parenteral treatment is preferred to local topical treatment, since both the urogenital tract and nasopharyngeal areas of affected animals can harbor these microorganisms. Bacterial infections should be treated with the antibiotic showing the best antimicrobial sensitivity. Records of pregnancy rate, litter size, and weaned numbers of pups are then studied for improvement. Routine periodic cultures of the deep vaginal cavity of breeding bitches and the prepuce or semen of stud dogs prior to mating are necessary to check for reinfection by bacteria, mycoplasmas, or ureaplasmas. Single affected dogs are quite easy to treat and remain free of infection if kept isolated.

Research is needed to establish the definite role of these agents in breeding dogs. Species differences and pathogenicity of different species and strains should be studied. Looking for infection with mycoplasmas, ureaplasmas, and bacteria should be a part of every diagnostic workup in cases of infectious canine infertility.

References and Supplemental Reading

Bruchim, A., and Lutsky, I.: Isolation of mycoplasmas from the canine genital tract: A survey of 108 healthy dogs. Res. Vet. Sci. 25:243, 1978.

Doig, P. A., Ruhunke, H. L., and Bosu, W. T. K.: The genital mycoplasma and ureaplasma flora of healthy and diseased dogs. Can. J. Comp. Med. 45:223, 1981.

Holzmann, A., and Laber, G.: Experimentally induced mycoplasmal infection in the genital tract of the male dog. I. Andrological-spermatological investigation before infection. Theriogenology 7:167, 1977.

Holzmann, A., and Laber, G.: Experimentally induced mycoplasmal infection in the genital tract of the male dog. II. Andrological and microbiological investigations after exposure to mycoplasmas. Theriogenology 7:177, 1977.

Holzmann, A., Laber, G., and Walzl, H.: Experimentally induced mycoplasmal infection in the genital tract of the female dog. Theriogenology 12:355, 1979.

Johnston, S. D.: Diagnostic and therapeutic approach to infertility in the bitch. J.A.V.M.A. 176:1335, 1980.

Lein, D. H.: Canine orchitis. *In* Kirk, R. W. (ed.): *Current Veterinary Therapy VI*. Philadelphia: W. B. Saunders, 1977, pp. 1255–1259.

Olson, P. N. S.: Canine vaginitis. *In* Kirk, R. W. (ed.): *Current Veterinary Therapy VII*. Philadelphia: W. B. Saunders, 1980, pp. 1219–1222.

Olson, P. N., Thrall, M. A., Wykes, P. M., et al.: Vaginal cytology. Part II. Use in diagnosing canine reproductive disorders. Comp. Cont. Ed. Pract. Vet. 6:385, 1984.

Rosendal, S.: Canine mycoplasmas: Their ecologic niche and role in disease. J.A.V.M.A. 180:1212, 1982.

UPDATE ON FREEZING CANINE SEMEN

FRANCES O. SMITH, D.V.M.
St. Paul, Minnesota

Despite the American Kennel Club's approval of registration of litters resulting from insemination with thawed frozen canine sperm in 1981 (Fig. 1), there is an impression among breeders and veterinarians alike that performance is poor. As of May 1, 1985, only 29 litters had been registered as a result of insemination with frozen semen. Canine sperm can be successfully frozen and, when inseminated, can result in pregnancy. In other species, thawed frozen semen must be inseminated into the uterus (i.e., not the vagina) in order for normal conception rates to occur. Work at the University of Minnesota College of Veterinary Medicine indicates this may also occur in dogs. Because one cannot cannulate the cervix of most bitches, surgical insemination (injection of thawed semen via needle and syringe through the uterine wall exteriorized at surgery) has been necessary at this institution to achieve normal conception rates. With surgical insemination into the uterus, conception rates have ranged from 66 to 83 per cent.

The reason for poor performance with vaginal insemination is not well defined but may be related to sperm transport through the cervix. Timing of insemination of frozen semen is also critical, since thawed sperm do not survive in the female tract as long as fresh sperm. The best insemination time in our laboratory has been on the third to fourth day

Table 1. *Litter Size and Sex Ratios in Litters Resulting from Various Insemination Methods*

Reference	Breed	Thawed Frozen Semen, Artificial Insemination			Fresh Semen, Artificial Insemination			Natural Mating		
		Mean Litter Size	*Number of Litters*	*Sex Ratio*	*Mean Litter Size*	*Number of Litters*	*Sex Ratio*	*Mean Litter Size*	*Number of Litters*	*Sex Ratio*
Seager, 1969		1	1	NR				6.9		
Gill, 1970	Beagle	0		0						
Van Gemert, 1970	Rhodesian ridge-back	9	1	NR						
Andersen, 1972	NR	3	1	NR						
Seager and Fletcher, 1973	Labrador	P 3.75 M —	4 —	0.88:1.00	P 7.07 M 6.79	42 39	P 1.03:1.00 M 1.25:1.00	P 7.10 M 9.63	72 51	P 1.16:1.00 M 1.22:1.00
	Crossbred	P 1.40 M 11.00	5 1	0.75:1.00 0.83:1.00	P 7.08 M 9.25	12 12	P 1.18:1.00 M 1.31:1.00	P 6.44 M 7.07	55 15	P 1.08:1.00 M 0.89:1.00
Seager et al., 1975	Labrador	N 3.7 M 4.0	10 5	1.81:1.00 1.50:1.00		NR			NR	
	Crossbred	N 2.0 M 8.5	2 4	1.00:1.00 1.26:1.00						
	Beagle	N 4.0 M 5.2	18 16	0.76:1.00 1.44:1.00						
Andersen, 1976	NR	3.7	15	NR	5.0	13	NR			
Takeishi et al., 1976		NR	3	NR						
Lees and Castleberry, 1977	German shepherd	4.25	8	1.33:1.00				7.8	8	
Platz and Seager, 1977	Beagle	6.7	12	1.14:1.00				6.2		

Key: M = multiparous; NR = not reported; N = nulliparous; P = primiparous.

AKA REGULATIONS APPLYING TO THE REGISTRATION OF LITTERS PRODUCED THROUGH ARTIFICIAL INSEMINATION USING FROZEN SEMEN

These Regulations shall supplement the "Regulations for Record Keeping and Identification of Dogs."

Each person* engaged in the collection, freezing, storage, shipping and insemination of frozen semen shall follow such practices and maintain such records as will preclude any possibility of error in identification of any individual dog or doubt as to the parentage of any dog or litter.

RECORDS:

To provide a source of reference for the registration of litters of pure-bred dogs produced by artificial insemination, using frozen semen, applications for which have been made, or may later be made, to the American Kennel Club, and to assure the accuracy of such applications, certain minimum records must be kept.

All required records shall be made immediately, when dog has been delivered for the purpose of semen collection, at time of shipment of frozen semen, and insemination of same; shall be kept on forms devoted to that exclusive purpose; and shall be consecutive, accurate and up-to-date. Such records shall be maintained for a period of no less than five years from the point in time when the last of the frozen semen from a given donor-dog is used.

NOTE: *At this time there are no provisions for registering litters that result from imported frozen canine semen.*

I RECORDS TO BE KEPT BY COLLECTOR:

A. *Dog Identification:*

Breed
AKC registered name and number of donor-dog
Sex, color, markings of donor-dog (include tattoo, if any)
Color photographs of donor-dog (full front and full side views)
Date of birth
AKC registered name and number of sire and dam
Name and address of owner of donor-dog
(AKC suggests that collector also keep a health work-up of donor-dog as part of donor-dog's identification)

B. *Collection of Semen:*

Date on which donor-dog was received
Owner's authorization of semen collection
Date semen collected, frozen and stored
Number of breeding units stored
Form of semen storage (Pellets, Ampules, Vials, Straws, etc.)
Container in which each breeding unit is stored shall be indelibly imprinted to show: Breed, AKC registration number of donor-dog; Date semen collected

C. *Disposition of Semen:*

Identification of shipped semen
Number of breeding units shipped
Name and Address of person to whom semen shipped
Authorization of semen owner for shipment
Date(s) semen shipped

D. *Collector shall also maintain records of all transfers of ownership of stored semen (See Section VI below re: Transfer of ownership of semen)*

II RECORDS TO BE KEPT BY OWNERS OF DONOR-DOGS:

In addition to the records required to be kept by owners and breeders, as provided in AKC pamphlet "Regulations for Record Keeping and Identification of Dogs," owners of dogs from which semen has been collected, frozen and stored, shall include the following:

AKC registered name and name of donor-dog
Date dog shipped to collector
Name and address of collector
Number of breeding units collected, frozen and in storage
Location of semen storage
Transfer of ownership of semen (see Section VI below)

III RECORDS TO BE KEPT BY OWNERS OF SEMEN OF DONOR-DOGS WHEN BREEDING HAS BEEN ARRANGED:

Identification of semen (Breed, AKC registered name and number of donor-dog, date semen collected)
Number of breeding units authorized for shipment and insemination
Date of shipment
To whom semen shipped
AKC registered name and number of bitch to be inseminated Name and address of owner of bitch

IV RECORDS TO BE KEPT BY BREEDERS:

In addition to the records required to be kept by owners and breeders, as provided in AKC's pamphlet "Regulations for Record Keeping and Identification of Dogs," owners (or lessees) of bitches inseminated shall include the following:

Name and address of veterinarian who handled insemination
AKC registered name and address of bitch inseminated
Date(s) of insemination
Identification of semen (Breed, AKC registered name and number of donor-dog, date semen collected)

V NOTIFICATION OF AKC BY COLLECTOR:

The AKC shall be immediately notified by collector of collection and freezing of canine semen. Such notification shall identify donor-dog by its breed; AKC registered name and number; the number of breeding units collected; date stored; address of storage facility; name and address of owner of donor-dog.

VI TRANSFER OF OWNERSHIP OF SEMEN:

Records required to be kept by owners of dogs from which semen has been collected and stored, and records required to be kept by collector (if semen is held in storage) must also note transfers of ownership of semen. Such records to include:

Authorization of transfer
Number of breeding units transferred
Date of transfer
Name and address of new owner

The AKC shall be immediately notified of such transfer of ownership of frozen semen.

VII LOCATION OF STORED SEMEN:

In the event semen is stored at a facility other than the facility at which it was collected, frozen and initially stored—or—in the event all or part of the collected frozen semen is transferred to a new owner (see Sections II and VI above), the owner or new owner shall immediately notify AKC. Such notification shall include:

Identification of semen (Breed, AKC registered name and number of donor-dog, date semen collected)
Number of breeding units relocated
Date transferred to new storage facility
Name and address of storage facility

VIII CERTIFICATION:

The AKC shall require such certifications from semen owner, owner (or lessee) of bitch, and veterinarian who inseminated bitch as shall be necessary to support an application for registration of a litter of dogs produced by the use of frozen semen.

IX INSPECTION:

The rules provide that the AKC or its duly authorized representatives shall have the right to inspect the records required to be kept and the practices required to be followed by these regulations and to examine any dog registered or to be registered with the AKC.

X PENALITIES:

The rules provide that the AKC may refuse to register any dog or litter or to record the transfer of any dog, for the sole reason that the application is not supported by the records required by these regulations.

The rules also provide that the Board of Directors of the AKC may suspend from all privileges of the AKC any person who fails to observe the above regulations.

**Chapter 3A Section 1 of Rules Applying to Registration and Dog Show defines "Person" as ". . . any individual, partnership, firm, corporation, association or organization of any kind."*

Figure 1. American Kennel Club regulations on artificial insemination using frozen semen.

Table 2. Characteristics of Canine Semen

Reference	Collection Technique	Number of Dogs (collections)	Volume (ml) Frxn 1	Frxn 2	Frxn 1+2	Frxn 3	Total	Percentage of Progressive Motility	Sperm Numbers × 10^6 (per ml)	(per ejaculate)	Percentage of Morphologic Abnormalities Normal	Primary	Secondary	pH
Amann, in press														
	10–34# AV	30			2.4 + 0.3				209+42	400				
	35–59# AV	53			3.9 + 0.5				359+72	1120				
	60–84# AV	32			5.4 + 1.3				228+58	1430				
Boucher et al., 1958														
	AV without teaser	5(14)					2.0–8.5	0–40	4.2–130.6	13–965	73–94			6.3–6.9
	Hand manipulation without teaser	9(37)					1.8–16.5	60–90	2.5–246.4	5.4–966	77–98			6.23–6.95
	Hand manipulation with teaser	15(74)					0.5–20.4	30–90	27.2–388.8	93.1–1427	34–97			6.49–7.10
	Initial trial	(65)	0.25–2.8	0.4–2.0			1.1–16.3							
Chatterjee et al., 1976														
	Normal masturbation 90						0.2–22	50–100	30–570	9–5940	74.5–96	0.2	NR	6.4–6.9
	Vasectomized, masturbation	39					0.2–10	0–40	10–95	9–300	29.5–88	14.0	65.75	6.6–6.9
Heywood and Sortwell, 1971	AV	6(41)					0.3–8.0	20–100	4–276	2.1–591	0–97			
James et al., 1979	AV	8					2.8–3.4	40–80	57–164	154–449	90–97			
Schutte and Bezuidenhout, 1965	AV	16			1.5–11.5									
Seager, 1972	AV	5	0.25–2.0	0.5–4.0	3.0–25.0	3.75–31.0		75–99	103–708					5.5–6.5
Taha et al., 1981	Masturbation	5					3.8–10.15	70–82	207–608	173–310	84–91			
Wildt et al., 1982	Outbred AV	14					3.2	66.0	69.6+34	366+98				
	Inbred AV	4					1.9	23.4	17.6+15	117+31				

Table 3. *Semen Cryopreservation Techniques and Performances of Frozen Semen in the Dog*

Reference	Extender	Glycerol (%)	Yolk (%)	Freeze Method	Motility Post-thaw (%)	Conception Rate	Volume (ml)	Total Number of Sperm Inseminated ($\times 10^6$)
Gutierrez Nales, 1957	3% sodium citrate in DW	5.5	37.5	DI	NR	R	NR	NR
Bahlau, 1958	3% sodium citrate in DW	6.5	20.0	NR	NR	NR	—	—
Harrop, 1961	Skim milk (heat treated)	NR	10	NR	50	—	—	—
Martin, 1963a	120 mM Krebs-Henseleit-Ringer solution (KHR),* 20 mM phosphate buffer	2, 4, 8§	25	A, F	4–30	—	—	—
	86 mM sodium citrate, 20 mM sodium phosphate buffer	2, 4, 8§	25	A, F	4–30	—	—	—
	90 mM KHR,* 20 mM sodium phosphate buffer, 46 mM fructose	8	0	A, F	4–30	—	—	—
Martin, 1963b	9% skim milk powder (w/v) in DW	7.5–10	0	A, F	36.7	—	—	—
	3 parts (v/v) 120 mM KHR,* 1 part (v/v) 0.1 M sodium phosphate buffer, 1 part (v/v) 0.308 M fructose	7.5–10	0	A, F	17.7	—	—	—
	3 parts (v/v), 0.3 M sodium citrate, 1 part (v/v) 0.1 M sodium phosphate buffer, 1 part (v/v) 0.308 M fructose	7.5–10	0	A, F	6.2	—	—	
Foote, 1964	0.2 M Tris,† 1.25% glucose	11	20	A, DI	41	—	—	—
	2.17% sodium citrate, 1.25% glucose	8	20	A, DI	27	—	—	—
Seager, 1969	11% lactose (w/v)	4	20	P	40–50	—	—	—
Van Gemert, 1970	11% lactose (w/v)	4	20	P	25	1/1	12	200
Gill et al., 1970	Tris-citric acid, fructose‡	8.8	20	NA	28	0	1.5	60–64
Andersen, 1972	11% lactose	4.7	20	S	40–60	0	1.5	200
	0.2 M Tris	7	20	S	40–60	1/4 (25%)	1.5	200
Seager and Fletcher, 1973	11% lactose	4	20	P	NR	15/32 (46%)	—	—
Andersen, 1974	0.2 M Trisfructose citrate	8	20	S	—	9/10	—	150
Andersen, 1976	0.2 M Trisfructose citrate	8	20	S	50–70	10/11	2.0–2.5	200
Andersen, 1976	0.2 M Trisfructose citric acid	8	20	S	50–70	16/20 (80%)	2.0	200–300
Takeishi et al., 1976	12% milk; 1.2% glucose, sodium citrate, phosphate	4	4	S	35–70	75%	NR	NR
Platz and Seager, 1977	11% lactose	4	20	P	48.7	12/13 (92%)	3.7	NR
Lees and Castleberry, 1977	11% lactose	4	20	P	50	8/14 (57%)	72.5	100–150
Christiansen, 1980	Tris-fructose-citrate	0–16	20	S	50–70	—	—	—
Bowen et al., 1984	Tris	—	20	S	40–60	15%	NR	300

Key: A = ampule; DI = dry ice; DW = distilled water; F = automated freeze; NR = not reported; P = pellet; R = pregnancies reported; S = straw.

*100 ml 0.9% NaCl, 4 ml 1.15% HCl, 1 ml 2.11% KH_2PO_4, 1 ml 3.82% $MgSO_4$, and 2 ml 1.3% $NaHCO_3$.

†3.028 gm Tris buffered with 1.692 gm citric acid monohydrate and 1.25 gm glucose in 100 ml DW.

‡2.4 gm Tris hydroxymethyl aminomethane, 1.3 gm citric acid monohydrate, and 1.0 gm fructose in 72.2 ml DW.

§One amount of each percentage was used in a separate portion of the same experiment.

***Table 4.** Facilities Approved for Freezing Canine Semen*

Canine Breeder Service, Inc. 432 North Homer Road Lansing, MI 48912 (517) 337-2892	Canine Cryobank 861 Via De La Paz #F Pacific Palisades, CA 90272 (213) 459-5068
Cryo-Genetic Laboratories Ludwig's Corner, Rt. 100 & Black Horse Road Box 256-A Chester Springs, PA 19425 (215) 458-5888	Herd's Merchant Semen RR 1, Box 151 Old Lake Street Elgin, IL 60120 (312) 289-2976
International Canine Semen Bank P.O. Box 5506 Kingwood, TX 77325 (713) 354-3800	Life Forces, Inc. Southwest Center P.O. Drawer EK College Station, TX 77841
Preservation, Inc. South Hill Veterinary Clinic 9702 11th Street Puyallup, WA 98371 (206) 848-1503	Carol Schubert 23415 Western Park Forest, IL 60466 (312) 748-0954
Spermco P.O. Box 4267 Burlingame, CA 94011 (415) 347-1284	University of Minnesota Department of Small Animal Clinical Sciences College of Veterinary Medicine 1988 Fitch Avenue St. Paul, MN 55108 (612) 373-0779

after onset of receptivity to mating (i.e., behavioral estrus). With traditional vaginal insemination techniques, conception rates are approximately 10 per cent in experimental studies and not known in field conditions, since only litters born are reported and there is no tally of unsuccessful inseminations.

Table 1 compares the reproductive performances of bitches bred with thawed frozen semen, those bred by artificial insemination with fresh semen, and those that were naturally bred. Generally, litter size is slightly smaller after insemination with thawed frozen semen.

Successful semen freezing requires good-quality semen. A semen evaluation, including assessment of color, volume, motility, total numbers, and morphology, is necessary in order to predict how well it will freeze. Table 2 summarizes characteristics of canine semen. Ejaculates with poor motility and poor morphology do not freeze well. Freezability may be affected by the composition of the buffer or extender used in the freezing process.

From carbon decay studies it appears that dog semen may be stored in liquid nitrogen for virtually thousands of years without loss of sperm viability after thawing. When semen is shipped in liquid nitrogen transport tanks, the sperm must be used before the liquid nitrogen evaporates (usually 14 days) unless additional liquid nitrogen is added.

In normal dogs studied at the University of Minnesota Veterinary College, the number of insemination doses (IDs) has ranged from one to 19; most dogs average five to seven IDs per ejaculate. Semen is mixed with a buffer and frozen in 0.5-ml French straws. The number of IDs per straw varies with the concentration of each dog's semen. An insemination dose at the University of Minnesota contains 100×10^6 sperm. The actual minimum insemination dose required to achieve pregnancy in the dog is unknown.

The buffer developed by the author may be formulated by making a 0.3 M solution of PIPES (Piperazine-*n,n bis* ethane sulfonic acid, mw = 342.4, Sigma) and 0.3 M potassium hydroxide (KOH). The two solutions are titrated to pH 7.0 ± 0.1 by adding 0.1-ml aliquots of the base to the acid. After titration, osmolality is adjusted to 300 ± 10 mOsm with double-distilled, deionized water (DDDW). The PIPES/KOH buffer is 50 per cent by volume of the extender, which also contains 25 per cent by volume 0.3 M dextrose and 25 per cent 0.3 M sodium citrate. After 20 per cent egg yolk by volume is added, the mixture is centrifuged and the supernatant is saved. Glycerol (9 per cent by volume) is added to the supernatant; this is then mixed and stored frozen in 10-ml aliquots.

A number of other different buffer and extender combinations have been used with varying degrees of success for cryopreservation of canine semen. Each of these buffers and cryopreservatives has been used effectively by the investigators listed. Table 3 summarizes the components of the buffers and extenders and the post-thaw motility resulting from their use.

There are currently ten AKC-approved facilities for freezing canine semen in the United States. Approval is based on record-keeping practices as outlined in the American Kennel Club Form R-198-1 (8-81). These facilities are listed in Table 4.

In summary, cryopreservation of semen is a practical reality. Performance to date is disappointing. However, the problem apparently is not with the fertilizing capacity of the thawed ejaculate, since fertility has resulted from its use. Instead, additional research is necessary to overcome the formidable cervical barrier to nonsurgical intrauterine insemination and to better identify best days for insemination. Clients should be encouraged to use semen cryopreservation to preserve genetic material of valued stud dogs. The insemination problems will be overcome in the future.

References and Supplemental Reading

Aamdal, J., Andersen, K., and Fougner, J. A.: Insemination with frozen semen in the blue fox. 7th Int. Cong. Anim. Repro. A. I., Munich, 1976, pp. 1713, 1716.

Adler, H. C.: The comparative efficiency of the intracervical and intrauterine insemination of cattle with streptomycin-treated and non-treated semen. Acta Vet. Scand. 1:105, 1960.

Amann, R. P.: Reproductive physiology and endocrinology. *In* Morrow, D. A. (ed.): *Current Therapy in Theriogenology*. 2nd ed. Philadelphia: W. B. Saunders, in press.

Andersen, K.: Fertility of frozen dog semen. Proc. 7th Int. Cong. Anim. Repro. A. I., Munich, 1972, pp. 1703–1706.

Andersen, K.: Intrauterine insemination with deep frozen semen in the dog. Proc. 12th Nordic Vet. Cong., Reykjavik, 1974, pp. 153–154.

Andersen, K.: Artificial uterine insemination in dogs. 7th Int. Cong. Anim. Repro. A. I., Krakow, 1976, p. 960.

Andersen, K.: Artificial insemination and storage of canine semen. *In* Morrow, D. A. (ed.): *Current Therapy in Theriogenology*, 1st ed. Philadelphia: W. B. Saunders, 1980, pp. 661–665.

Anderson, V. K., Amdahl, J., and Fougner, J. A.: Intrauterine and deep cervical insemination with frozen semen in sheep. Zuchthegiene 8:113, 1973.

Bahlau, E.: Untersuchen über die Konservierung von Hundesperma. V.M.D. thesis, University of Munich, 1958.

Boucher, J. H., Foote, R. M., and Kirk, R. W.: The evaluation of semen quality in the dog and the effects of frequency of ejaculation upon the semen quality, libido and depletion of sperm reserves. Cornell Vet. 48:67, 1958.

Bowen, R. A., Amann, R. P., Fromen, D. P., et al.: Artificial insemination with frozen semen in the dog. Dog World 69:66, 1984.

Chatterjee, S. N., Meenakshi, R. N. S., and Kar, A. B.: Semen characteristics of normal and vasectomized dogs. Indian J. Exp. Biol. 14:414, 1976.

Christiansen, I. J., and Schmidt, M.: Freezing of dog semen. Preliminary report. Institute for Sterilitetesforskning, Kongelige Veterinaer-og Landbohojskole, 23:67, 1980.

Foote, R. H.: The effects of electrolytes, sugars, glycerol and catalase on survival of dog sperm in buffered yolk mediums. Am. J. Vet. Res. 25:32, 1964.

Gill, H. P., Kaufman, C. F., Foote, R. W., et al.: Artificial insemination of beagle bitches with freshly collected liquid stored and frozen stored semen. Am. J. Vet. Res. 31:1807, 1970.

Graham, E. F., Crabo, B. G., and Brown, K. I.: Effect of some zwitter ion buffers on storage of spermatozoa. I. Bull. J. Dairy Sci. 55:1, 1972.

Graham, E. F., Schmehl, M. K. L., Evenson, B. K., et al.: Semen preservation in nondomestic mammals. Symp. Zool. Soc. Lond. 43:153, 1978.

Gutierrez Nales, N. N.: The dilution and storage of canine semen. Reo. Patron. Biol. Anim. (Madr.) 3:189, 1957.

Harrop, A. E.: Semen preservation and canine artificial insemination. IVth Int. Cong. An. Reprod., 4:898, 1961.

Heywood, R., and Sortwell, R. J.: Semen evaluation in the beagle dog. J. Small Anim. Pract. 12:343, 1971.

James, R. W., Heywood, R., and Street, A. F.: Biochemical observations of beagle dog semen. Vet. Rec. 104:480, 1979.

Lees, G. E., and Castleberry, M. W.: The use of frozen semen for artificial insemination of German Shepherd dogs. J. Am. Anim. Hosp. Assoc. 13:382, 1977.

Martin, I. C. A.: The freezing of dog spermatozoa to −79C. Res. Vet. Sci. 4:304, 1963a.

Martin, I. C. A.: The deep freezing of dog spermatozoa in dilutents containing skim milk. Res. Vet. Sci. 4:315, 1963b.

Platz, C. C., and Seager, S. W. J.: Successful pregnancies with concentrated frozen canine semen. Lab. Anim. Sci. 17:1013, 1977.

Schutte, A. P., and Bezuidenhout, J. P.: Practical aspects of A. I. in dogs. I: Collection of semen. J. S. Afr. Vet. Med. Assoc. 36:345, 1965.

Seager, S. W. J.: Successful pregnancies utilizing frozen dog semen. A. I. Digest 27:6, 1969.

Seager, S. W. J., and Fletcher, W. S.: Collection, storage and insemination of canine semen. Lab. Anim. Sci. 22:177, 1972.

Seager, S. W. J., and Fletcher, W. S.: Progress on the use of frozen semen in the dog. Vet. Rec. 92:6, 1973.

Seager, S. W. J., Platz, C. R., and Fletcher, W. S.: Conception rates and related data using frozen dog semen. J. Reprod. Fert. 45:189, 1975.

Smith, F. O.: Cryopreservation of canine semen: Technique and performance. Ph.D. thesis, University of Minnesota, 1984.

Taha, M. B., Noakes, D. E., and Allen, W. E.: The effect of season of the year on the characteristics and composition of dog semen. J. Small Anim. Pract. 22:177, 1981.

Takeishi, M., Mikami, T., Kodama, Y., et al.: Studies on reproduction in the dog. VIII. Artificial insemination using frozen semen. Jpn. J. Anim. Reprod. 22:28, 1976.

Van Gemert, W.: Deep-freeze pups. Tijdrschr. Diergeneesk. 95:697, 1970.

Wildt, D. E., Baas, E. J., Chakraborty, P. K., et al.: Influence of inbreeding on reproductive performance, ejaculate quality and testicular volume in the dog. Theriogenology 17:445, 1982.

NORMAL DEVELOPMENT AND CONGENITAL BIRTH DEFECTS IN THE CAT

DREW M. NODEN, PH.D.
Ithaca, New York

"What caused this?" and "Is it inherited?" are the questions most frequently asked by clients, especially breeders, when confronted with a stillborn or congenitally malformed kitten. During the 9 to 10 weeks it takes for a fertilized, single-cell egg measuring approximately 1/250 inch to develop into a newborn kitten, the embryonic organism undergoes tremendous growth and major transformations that bring about the formation of unique tissues and organs, each in its proper location and with appropriate functions. This article first outlines when and how some of these changes occur in the embryo and then uses this information to explain the bases for some of the common inherited, induced, and spontaneous congenital malformations in cats.

NORMAL DEVELOPMENT

Feline development can be divided into three phases: (1) preimplantation, days 0 to 12; (2) embryogenesis, days 12 to 24; and (3) fetal growth, days 24 to term. Unlike dogs, cats ovulate in response to mating. A queen may accept more than one male, which can result in a litter having multiple parentage. At the time of fertilization the female gamete is encased by an inert sheath, the zona pellucida, which is surrounded by several hundred ovarian follicular cells (the corona radiata). The sperm penetrates both of these layers by using lytic enzymes released by rupture of the acrosome, which is a membranous sac encasing the head of the sperm. After contact and fusion with the ovum, both the zona pellucida and the cell surface of the egg are biochemically altered to prevent penetration by additional sperm.

During the preimplantation stage, the organism undergoes cell division while traveling down the oviduct, and it enters the body of the uterus on about the sixth day of development (Table 1). It forms a *blastocyst*, which is a hollow sphere containing about 250 cells. Most of the cells establish a thin superficial epithelial layer; these are called trophoblast cells, and most will contribute to the placenta. Clustered at one pole are cells destined to form all tissues of the embryo as well as parts of the placenta; this aggregate is the embryonic disk. Studies on laboratory animals have shown that by this stage the genetic programming within embryonic disk cells is different from that of trophoblast cells. During the second week of development the blastocyst expands and breaks free of the zona pellucida.

Embryogenesis is the most critical phase of mammalian development. It is during this period that the embryonic disk becomes totally reorganized and forms the primordia of every organ system in the body. Apposition between maternal and embryonic tissues occurs at the beginning of this stage, around day 12 of gestation.

The first stage of embryogenesis is called *gastrulation* (*gaster* = belly). At this time the embryonic cells form three separate layers of tissues, which expand rapidly beneath the trophoblast layer. This results in the formation of three concentric epithelial layers. The middle layer, mesoderm, soon splits into separate deep (visceral) and superficial (somatic) layers with a cavity, the coelom, between.

Immediately thereafter the organism enters the *neurula* stage, during which time the primordia of the nervous system, the heart, and the vertebral column are established. This is accomplished by rearrangements of all three cell layers, a process called *morphogenesis* (*morphos* = form or shape; *genesis* = beginning). Also, blood vessels are formed both within the embryo and throughout the extraembryonic tissues that are forming the placenta. As indicated in Table 1, these two embryonic stages occur very rapidly in cats and dogs.

Neurulation is followed by a period of embryonic *organogenesis*, during which the primordia of most of the other organs, including the liver and digestive tract, respiratory system, limbs, sense organs, skull, and urogenital structures, are formed (Fig. 1). This stage is completed by about 3½ weeks of gestation in the cat (6 weeks in humans), by which time the embryo is slightly over ½ inch in length.

Fetal development is characterized by rapid growth of the organism (Fig. 2). The organ primordia established earlier assume their correct shapes and configurations, many nerves develop their projections, and the endocrine and secretory glands of the organism begin to function and control many physiologic processes. Cats are born in a very immature condition, and all these developmental processes continue after birth. For example, full development of the visual system is not accomplished until 5 to 6 weeks after birth, and a full complement of cortical neurons in the cerebellum is not present for several months postnatally in the cat (3 years in humans).

DEVELOPMENTAL MECHANISMS

Understanding how populations of embryonic cells become transformed from a homogeneous cluster in the embryonic disk to highly organized, patterned arrays of tissues, each with the correct biochemical characteristics and in the proper location, is a major frontier in biologic research today. This is not simply a matter of scientific curiosity. Rather, locked in the embryo are the secrets to mechanisms of tissue repair and organ regeneration, genetic programming, and the control of cell proliferation which, when unchecked in adult tissues, can result in tumor formation and metastasis.

Table 1. *Timetable of Early Developmental Stages*

Species	Gestation Length	Two Cells	Eight Cells	Blastocyst	Gastrula	Neurula	4-mm Embryo	9-mm Embryo	16-mm Embryo
Cat	62 days	3*	3.5*	5*	12	13	15	21	24
Dog	63 days	4	6	8	16	17	22	25	30
Cow†	280 days	1	3	7	14	19	23	28	35
Human	266 days	1.5	2.5	4	14	20	28	37	43

*Age in days after fertilization.

†Horses (340 days gestation) initially develop at a similar rate.

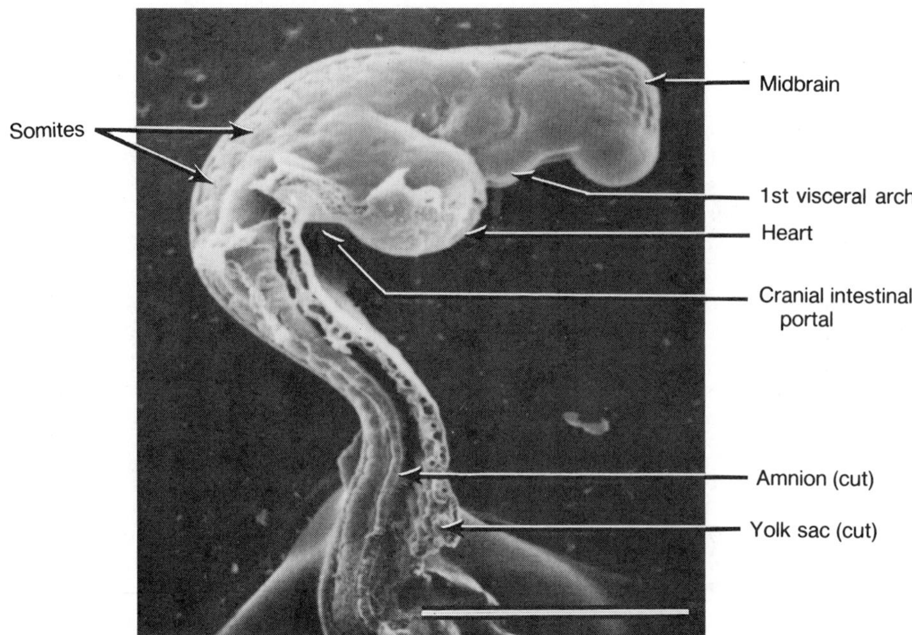

Figure 1. Scanning electron micrograph of the right side of a 22-somite cat embryo, approximately 15 to 16 days of gestation. The amnion was cut off close to the body of the embryo during preparation of this specimen. Note that future cephalic and cardiac tissues develop earlier than abdominal structures, and that the heart forms initially beneath the first visceral arch (future jaw). Bar: 1 mm. (From Noden and de Lahunta: *The Embryology of Domestic Animals*. Baltimore: Williams & Wilkins, 1985.)

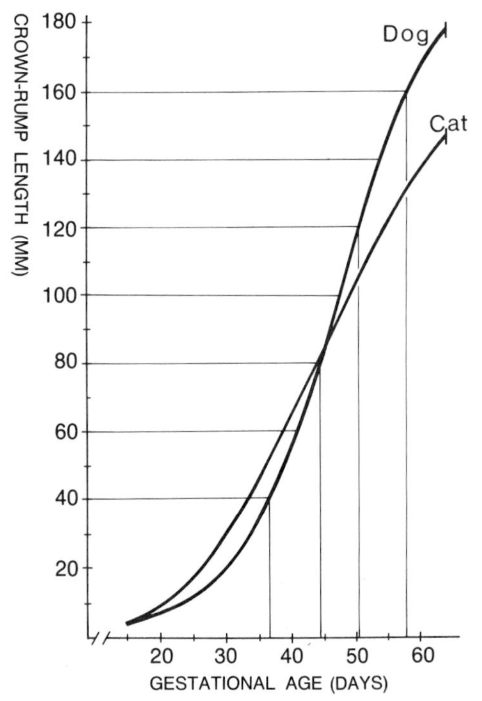

Figure 2. Comparative fetal growth rates in dogs and cats.

The problems confronting the whole embryo can readily be appreciated by focusing on a developing limb (Fig. 3). Here a few hundred embryonic cells localized at four discrete regions of the embryo must proliferate and form a structure with muscles, cartilages and bones, tendons and ligaments, blood vessels, nerves, claws, fur, and so forth. Moreover, each of these tissues must have a precise shape and relation to the others and collectively constitute a mirror image of the contralateral limb. Finally, both limbs must be the same length and must grow synchronously after birth. This example illustrates the four basic processes that operate during the development of every organ:

GROWTH
MORPHOGENESIS
CYTODIFFERENTIATION (the formation of unique cell types)
PATTERNING

Although none of these processes is fully understood, developmental biologists have learned several general features about them. It is known, for example, that all four are interdependent and inseparable. Thus, a genetic or teratogenic disruption of one will usually alter the others. Also, each of these processes requires that adjacent cells and tissues interact with one another. Sometimes this is by direct contact between them; more often the intercellular dialogue is facilitated by chemicals released by cells into the extracellular matrix. Later in development, circulatory growth factors and hormones play critical roles. Often the same molecules will have different effects, depending upon the type of receptors a target cell has or upon subtle differences in the particular combination of molecules present.

CRITICAL PERIODS AND MALFORMATIONS

The kinds of processes and interactions described above for limb development occur in every tissue and organ in the kitten embryo. These events are extremely sensitive to any kind of chemical or genetic disruption. Also, the complex spatial and temporal relationships that must be established for a structure to develop normally will on occasion spontaneously go awry, resulting in a congenital malformation.

The stage during which each developing tissue or organ is most sensitive to disruption is called the *critical period* in its development. As indicated in Figure 4, the critical period for most structures occurs in the embryonic stage of development, during the third and fourth weeks of gestation in the cat, the third through sixth weeks in the human. The end of the critical period does not mean that a particular developing structure is no longer susceptible to disruption. Rather, its sensitivity declines, and abnormalities are more likely to be very localized.

Errors in development that are expressed during the first 2 weeks of gestation are usually lethal, resulting either in the immediate death of the embryo or in failure to establish normal relations with the uterine wall. Statistically, the late blastocyst and gastrula stages, which include the time of initial contact between the embryo and the wall of the uterus, *are the times of greatest loss of embryos* in all mammals.

The final general point to be made about embryonic malformations is that in many cases a defect in one system will result in abnormal development of others. For example, some cardiovascular defects deprive peripheral tissues of a sufficient blood supply for their normal growth, and many vertebral

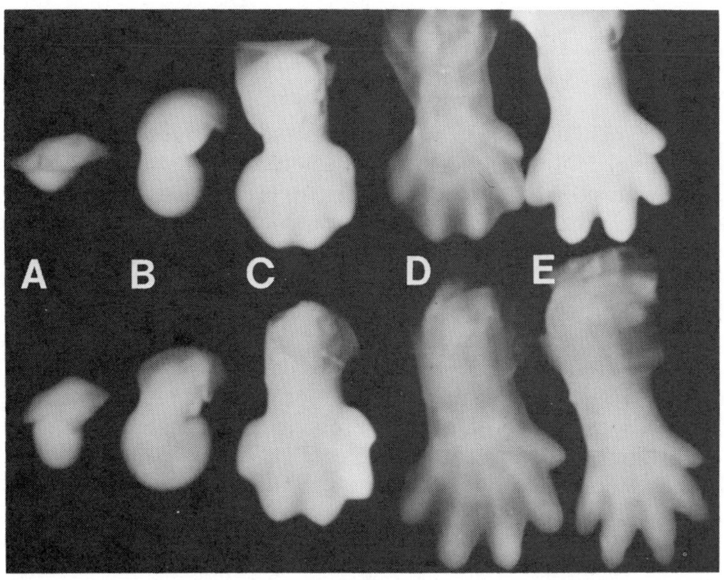

Figure 3. Early development of the limbs in a typical carnivore (ferret). Note that the forelimbs (lower row) are consistently more advanced than the hind limbs (upper row). Dog or cat limbs would have a similar appearance at stages *A*, 8- to 10-mm; *B*, 12- to 13-mm; *C*, 15- to 16-mm; *D*, 18- to 19-mm; and *E*, 21- to 23-mm. (From Noden and de Lahunta: *The Embryology of Domestic Animals*. Baltimore, Williams & Wilkins, 1985.)

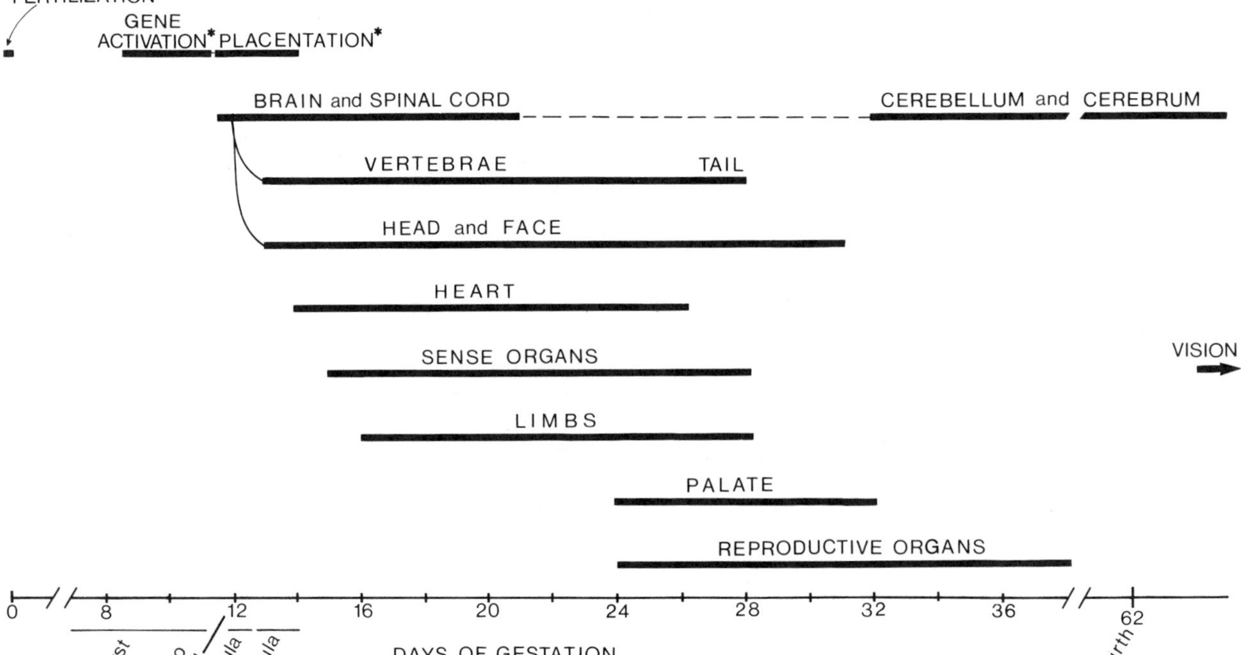

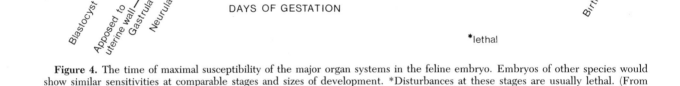

Figure 4. The time of maximal susceptibility of the major organ systems in the feline embryo. Embryos of other species would show similar sensitivities at comparable stages and sizes of development. *Disturbances at these stages are usually lethal. (From Noden and de Lahunta: *The Embryology of Domestic Animals*. Baltimore: Williams & Wilkins, 1985.)

malformations affect the spinal cord. A compromise of the nerve supply to any target tissue will result in secondary atrophy of the muscles and immobilization of the joints in that region. Thus, the clinician must often sort through several secondary defects to ascertain the primary lesion.

CAUSES OF CONGENITAL MALFORMATIONS

Many malformations, especially those associated with highly inbred breeds, have a heritable basis. This means that the frequency or severity of the anomaly is directly affected by the genome of the developing organism. Occasionally this may be due to a single gene alteration or mutation, as is the case for certain enzyme deficiencies (mucopolysaccharidosis, gangliosidosis).

More often the precise genetic basis is less obvious, because many genes regulate or are affected by the products of other genes. Problems associated with pigmentation (including defects in vision and hearing in Siamese and Persian cats), with the spinal cord and vertebral column (spina bifida in the Manx), with the limbs (polydactyly, ectrodactyly, and hemimelia), and with the head (hydrocephalus, anencephaly, and facial defects in Burmese cats) fall into this broad category. Finally, genetic heterogeneity may create a situation in which no single gene product is abnormal but the collective effects of many genes is inadequate to support the normal development of an organ.

The probability that interactions between families of genes will have a deleterious effect is directly correlated with the amount of inbreeding. Every breeder must recognize that *there is no amount of inbreeding that is without risk* of increasing the incidence of birth defects. Unless extensive breeding studies are done, it is usually impossible to define the genetic basis for most congenital malformations.

Induced congenital defects are no easier to deal with. An agent that disrupts a normal developmental process is called a *teratogen*. Any chemical that has toxic effects on the queen is likely to have severe effects on developing systems. Included in this category are dioxin (a component of Agent Orange), heavy metals (especially lead and mercury), most complex organic hydrocarbons (particularly pesticides), and most antimitotic agents, such as hydroxyurea. In addition, embryos are particularly sensitive to excess vitamin A or ethanol during the neurula stage, to some normal body products (e.g., most steroid hormones) delivered at the wrong time or in excess amounts, or to pathogens such as panleukopenia virus that cross or impair the placental barrier.

In many cases a chemical entering the mother is converted by her into other metabolites that cross the placenta. This feature makes comparative teratology a difficult scientific discipline, because each species and often every individual has its own unique metabolic processes and rates. The picture is further complicated by the varied structures and transport mechanisms present in the placentas of various mammals. With any suspected teratogen, the time of exposure and dose delivered to the queen are critical factors in the outcome.

Although a few chemicals and other factors (x-rays, hyperthermia) are known to be teratogenic, there is little direct proof linking most chemicals found around the home and yard to specific birth defects. *The absence of such proof does not mean they have been proved to be completely harmless.* Most chemicals have never been formally tested on companion animals, nor have the possible teratogenic effects of very low intake of many different combinations of normally safe chemicals been tested.

COMMON CONGENITAL MALFORMATIONS IN CATS (Table 2)

Axial Duplications

Conjoined twins are an anomaly in which two embryos or parts of embryos are attached to one another. In some cases both may be fully formed and attached only at the head, thorax, or abdomen (often called "Siamese" twins). In other situations only one part will be duplicated; for example, kittens with two faces (diprosopus), two heads (dicephalus), or two tails have been reported. These anomalies result from duplications that occur between the blastocyst and neurula stages, and those occurring earlier are more complete. There is no known genetic or teratogenic cause of these duplications in cats and dogs.

Table 2. *Incidence of Congenital Malformations**

System	Dog	Cat	Cow	Horse
Musculoskeletal	29.0	2.4	2.4	8.0
Urogenital	5.0	1.3	9.6	20.1
Cardiovascular	3.5	0.8	1.2	0.3
Gastrointestinal	2.2	0.4	1.8	1.5
Sensory	8.2	1.3	1.2	1.3
Neurologic	1.7	1.7	1.8	1.7
Other	9.7	4.3	13.7	10.7
TOTAL	59.3	12.2	31.7	43.6

*Data presented as incidence per 1000 births, based on a 5-year survey of 137,717 patients at ten North American veterinary clinics. From Priester et al.: Am. J. Vet. Res. 31:1871, 1970.

Axial Defects

Malformations of the brain and spinal cord or the skeletal tissues surrounding them (vertebral column and skull) are the most common congenital defects in all domestic animals and humans. Most early defects in neurogenesis will cause abnormalities in development of the surrounding skeletal structures, and vice versa. This is because there are several sequential, reciprocal interactions between the spinal cord, somites (vertebral precursors), notochord, and spinal ganglia that are necessary for the establishment of axial tissues and correct alignment of all parts of the vertebrae.

Spina bifida is a broad term that includes all failures of the vertebrae to close normally around the spinal cord. If, as usually occurs, the spinal cord is abnormal or secondarily compromised by incomplete or malformed vertebrae, there will be motor and sensory deficits in structures innervated by nerves whose roots emerge at or caudal to the site of the lesion. The Manx line is an example of inherited spina bifida. Here, it is caused by a dominant autosomal gene that shows incomplete penetrance (i.e., other genes modify the severity of expression). It is impossible to breed for "optimal" Manx features without being at risk of producing severe lumbosacral and urogenital malformations.

Failure of the roof of the skull to form (cranioschisis) is usually correlated with an increased, abnormal expansion of the brain (*encephalocele*, or more severely, *exencephaly*) or in severe cases with failure of the brain to form a closed tube (*anencephaly*). In the last situation, brain tissue secondarily degenerates before birth, leaving an empty crater open to the top of the head. These lethal conditions are frequently caused by teratogens but may occur spontaneously or as a result of genetic factors.

Hydrocephalus usually results from swelling of the fluid-filled lateral ventricles within the forebrain that secondarily causes an abnormal expansion of the roof of the skull. This condition can result from heritable factors (in Siamese cats), pathogenic organisms, or spontaneous developmental errors.

Malformations of the Face and Mouth

Cleft palate (Fig. 5) and *cleft lip* result from failure of embryonic facial tissues to grow and fuse together. According to the published literature, these defects are rare in all breeds of cats except the Siamese, in which there is evidence for an inherited predisposition. However, the impression

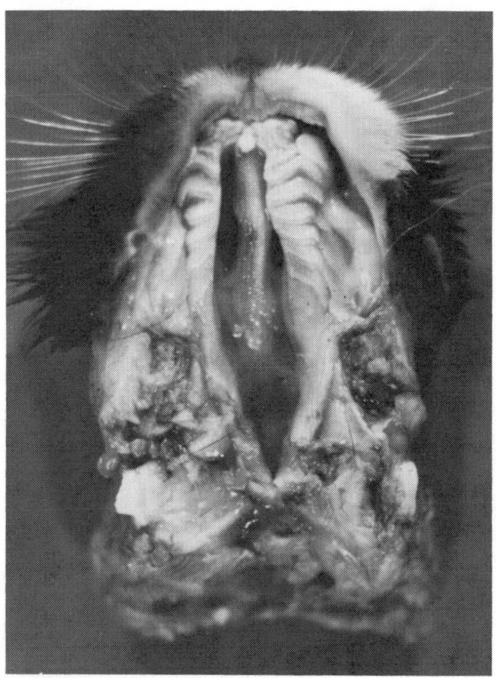

Figure 5. Ventral view of the roof of the oral cavity in a neonatal kitten that was born to a queen treated orally with 1000 mg/week of the antifungal agent griseofulvin, starting the day after breeding. Note the bilateral cleft palate that exposes the nasal cavity. (From Noden and de Lahunta: *The Embryology of Domestic Animals*. Baltimore: Williams & Wilkins, 1985.)

of many veterinarians and cat breeders is that the incidence of these malformations has been underestimated in other breeds.

The hard palate develops from a pair of lateral palatine processes that shift from being nearly vertical, extending on either side of the tongue, to being oriented horizontally above the tongue. This occurs on day 32 of development in the cat and is followed immediately by fusion of the two palatal processes to form the roof of the mouth. Ossification begins a few days after fusion. Any deviation in the timing of elevation, size of palatal processes, size or location of the tongue, or width of the oral cavity will increase the likelihood that fusion will not occur, resulting in a cleft.

These conditions reduce the ability of the neonate to suckle, and the animals often die of choking. In humans and some breeds of companion animals, cleft palate sometimes shows a familial pattern (as in the Siamese) and may be accompanied by malformations of other systems. Many teratogens can also cause cleft palate.

Dog and cat breeders frequently select for animals having extreme facial profiles, a potentially disastrous practice that is often encouraged by show judges and breed standards. However, *selecting for any extreme in facial proportions inevitably increases the incidence of craniofacial malformations.* For example, in collies the incidence of collie eye anomaly is directly related to the ratio of snout length to width. When this ratio is very high, the eyes develop too close together, compromising the formation of blood vessels to the retina and resulting in partial loss of vision. The opposite extreme, exemplified by bulldogs, pugs, and Persian cats, greatly increases the incidence of cleft palate and creates abnormalities of tooth eruption as well as chronic corneal and nasolacrimal disorders.

A tragic example of this has happened in the "new look" strain of Burmese cats. These animals are *brachycephalic* (abnormal shortening of the face); their snout area is reduced in length and they have a heavy crown. Unfortunately, the same genetic changes that brought about this shortening cause a lethal birth defect in nearly one out of four kittens born to "new-look" parents. The gross features of the malformation are exencephaly, involuted eyelids due to the degeneration of the eyes, the absence of all nasal tissues, and the presence of four whisker pads. Dissection of the heads of these neonates reveals that all the incisive, nasal, and ethmoidal skeletal components are absent, and that there are two complete sets of maxillary structures. This condition is inherited as an autosomal dominant but has variable expression. As in Manx cats, the malformation is inseparably linked to the phenotype favored by judges and many breeders, which presents a difficult moral choice to those fond of this breed.

Cardiovascular Malformations

The heart begins as a simple, straight tube formed on day 14 of development, and during the following 2 weeks it becomes transformed into a four-chambered organ with separate pulmonary and systemic channels (Fig. 6). Throughout this period of change,

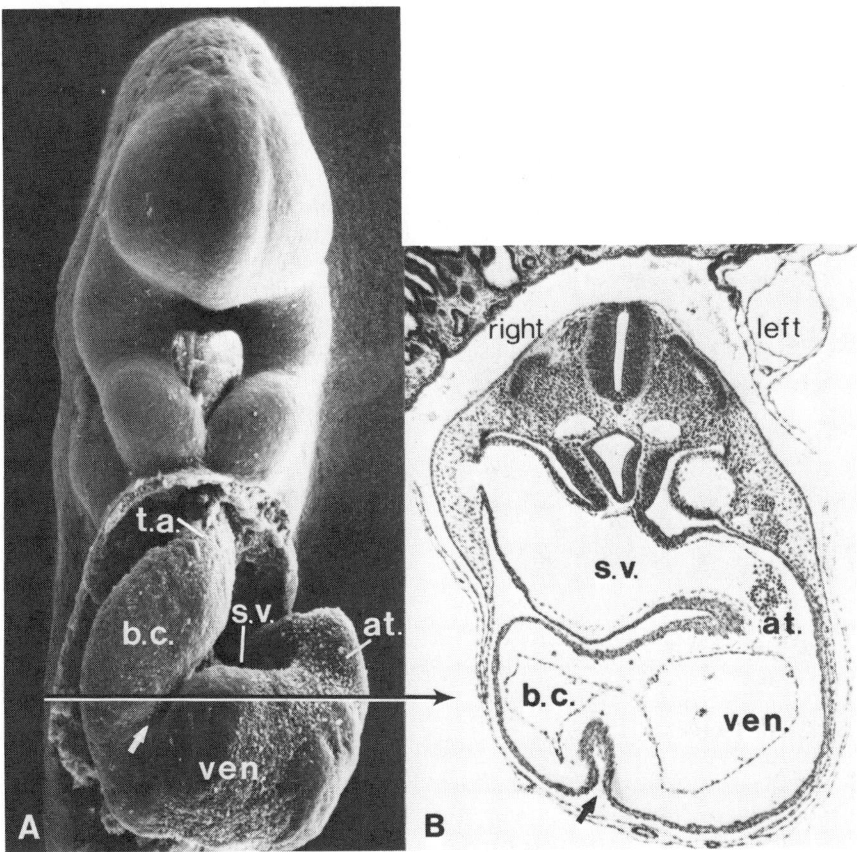

Figure 6. Early development of the heart. *A*, Ventral view of a 19-somite canine embryo in which the ventral pericardial and body wall tissues have been removed to reveal the heart loop. *B*, Transverse section through the heart loop of a 22-somite feline embryo at the level of the fourth somite, indicated by the bar/arrow in *A*. Blood flows from the sinus venosus (*s.v.*) to the atrium (*at.*), ventricle (*ven.*), and bulbus cordis (*b.c.*) and leaves the heart through the truncus arteriosus (*t.a.*). The small arrows point to the bulboventricular sulcus. (From Noden and de Lahunta: *The Embryology of Domestic Animals.* Baltimore: Williams & Wilkins, 1985.)

the heart is functional and supplies blood to all parts of the embryo and placenta without interruption—a remarkable feat of biological engineering.

Congenital heart defects are common in all animals and represent about 10 per cent of diagnosed cardiovascular problems in young animals. Included in this category are failures of the four chambers to become fully separated (*septal defects*), constrictions of a major blood vessel (*aortic* or *pulmonary stenosis*), histogenic changes such as endothelial fibroelastosis (which occurs in Siamese and Burmese breeds), and abnormal retention of an embryonic blood vessel. The latter includes *patent ductus arteriosus* (*PDA*), *vascular ring defects*, and *portosystemic shunts*.

PDA is the most common of these disorders. In the embryo and fetus the ductus arteriosus connects the left pulmonary artery directly to the aorta. This permits oxygen-rich blood entering the right side of the heart from the placenta to bypass the nonfunctional lungs and flow directly into the systemic circulation. Normally the ductus arteriosus closes a few days after birth. If it remains open, pulmonary and systemic blood streams mix, which causes the heart to work harder and can lead to many secondary complications. PDA appears with increased frequency in some lines of dogs; no data on heritability are available for cats.

Similarly, a portosystemic shunt usually is due to the persistence of an embryonic vein joining the major systemic venous channel of the trunk (the vena cava) with portal veins carrying blood from the intestines to the liver tissues, where it will be filtered and detoxified. If the shunt persists postnatally, this permits nonfiltered blood to enter the systemic venous channel and create serious metabolic imbalances in the animal. Occasionally these shunts may develop as a result of formation of new blood vessels, which is usually associated with chronic liver disease. Both PDA and portosystemic shunts are medically and surgically treatable if they are diagnosed early and are not severe.

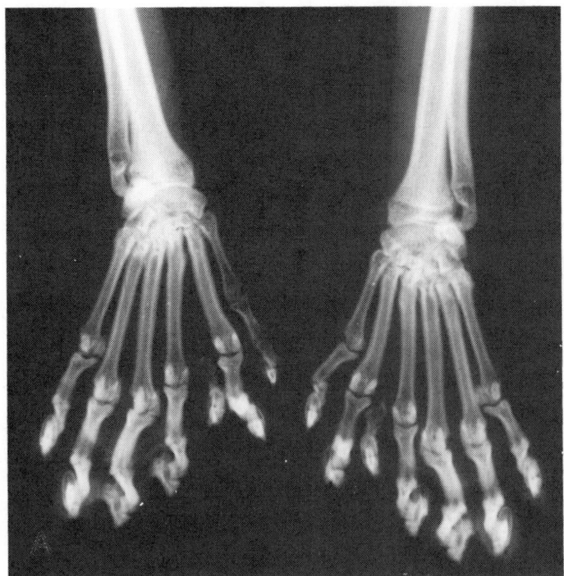

Figure 7. Radiograph showing polydactyly in a cat. (From Noden and de Lahunta: *The Embryology of Domestic Animals.* Baltimore: Williams & Wilkins, 1985.)

Limb Defects

Malformations involving the absence of some or all structures of the digits or limb are common. In cats, *radial hemimelia* (congenital absence of the radius) and *ectrodactyly* and *ectromelia* (absence of the digits and of an entire limb) are the most frequently seen reductions. *Syndactyly* is the condition in which only a single digit is present. This malformation is debilitating in dogs and humans, although it is normal in horses.

The cause of most limb reductions is not known, nor do we understand why forelimbs are usually more likely to be affected than hindlimbs. The drug thalidomide causes a reduction in proximal limb structures in humans such that the hands or feet develop close to the shoulder or hip, a condition known as *phocomelia* (seal-shaped limb). Despite many years of intensive study, the exact mechanisms underlying this disastrous teratogenic insult are not known.

Congenital limb duplication can include an entire limb (*dimelia*) or only the digits (*polydactyly*). There are cases in which each of these has been suspected of being inherited in cats; polydactyly (Fig. 7) due to an autosomal dominant is the most common and also the least detrimental malformation.

Other Common Feline Congenital Malformations

During the fourth week of development the gut tube elongates rapidly, so much so that much of the future intestinal tract herniates into the umbilical stalk (Fig. 8). At this time the intestinal loop rotates, bringing the end of the duodenum, the ascending colon, and the cecum into their definitive locations. Failure of the midgut to be fully withdrawn into the abdominal cavity results in an *omphalocele*.

Gastroschisis is a lethal condition in which the kitten is born with its intestines protruding outside of the ventral abdominal wall. This results from a failure of abdominal wall tissues to form a constriction around the base of the umbilical stalk.

A congenital *diaphragmatic hernia* is an opening in the diaphragm that permits abdominal organs to enter the pericardial or pleural cavities and impinge upon the normal development and functioning of thoracic organs. This condition arises during the early stages in the development of the liver and

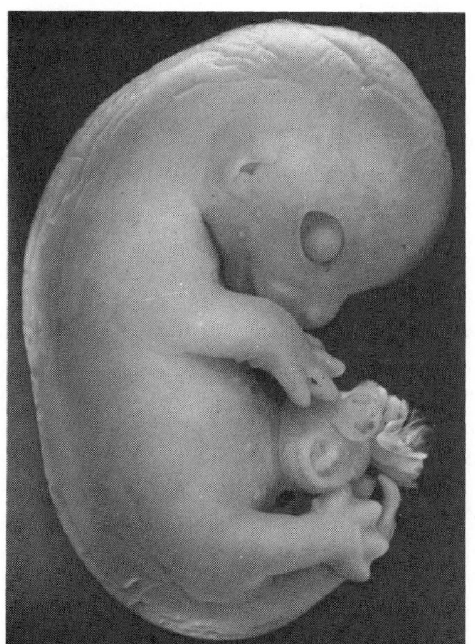

Figure 8. A 16-mm (25-day) feline embryo. Note the presence of the intestinal loop in the umbilical stalk. (From Noden and de Lahunta: *The Embryology of Domestic Animals.* Baltimore: Williams & Wilkins, 1985.)

heart and is common in cats. It has been estimated to occur once in every 1000 live births, and in some cases it is a result of an autosomal recessive gene.

Congenital anomalies of sense organs are reportedly less frequent in cats than in most other domestic animals. *Convergent strabismus* in the Siamese is correlated with abnormal optic nerve projections, and both conditions result from expression of the gene for albinism. *Heterochromia* occurs in Persians and Angoras. There is a high incidence of deafness on the blue-eyed side, which is due to the pleiotropic action of a dominant white gene.

PERSPECTIVES

In order to eliminate congenital malformations in the domesticated cat, there are several problems that must be resolved. First, we must continue research by using laboratory animals, tissues and cells grown in culture, and other model systems to understand better the normal mechanisms of embryonic development. Next, research on the physiology, pathology, and reproduction of cats must be increased to reflect more accurately the interest in and concern for this species in our society. These two tasks are the proper responsibility of the scientific and veterinary communities.

A third and equally important area in which data are needed concerns the results of current and past cat breedings. Except in the cases of a few popular breeds, there have been very few thorough, systematic studies of congenital problems in cats. Most of the available data represent isolated case reports. The type of study needed requires that the incidence and types of malformations present in a breeding line be accurately documented and that careful analysis of the pedigree and all relatives of affected kittens be made. Often it is necessary to perform test matings to establish the exact mode of genetic transmission. These critical analyses are possible only if cat breeders and fanciers familiarize themselves with the problems, keep accurate records of all litters, are especially watchful for the appearance of similar anomalies in more than one litter, and bring all specimens and data to their veterinarian for examination.

The final factor in our attempt to reduce the incidence of congenital malformations in cats falls again on the cat breeders and show judges. Each must decide what is acceptable and tolerable in order to obtain a champion. In the human population any situation in which a birth defect appears once per 1000 births is considered a major public health issue, and teams of researchers descend upon the area to discover the causes. Yet many dog and cat breeders will grimly accept an appalling 10 to 25 per cent mortality rate. *In nearly every case this tragedy is preventable.* The choice is between adherence to traditional breed descriptions written with no regard to basic principles of developmental genetics and the production of healthier cats.

References and Supplemental Reading

David, L. E.: Adverse effects of drugs on reproduction in dogs and cats. Modern Vet. Pract. 1:969, 1983.

Foley, C. W., Lasley, J. F., and Osweiler, G. D.: *Abnormalities of Companion Animals.* Ames, IA: Iowa State University Press, 1979.

Merton, D. A.: Selective breeding in the dog and cat, Part II: Known and suspected genetic diseases. Comp. Cont. Ed. Pract. Vet. 4:332, 1982.

Noden, D. M., and de Lahunta, A.: *The Embryology of Domestic Animals: Developmental Mechanisms and Malformations.* Baltimore: Williams & Wilkins, 1985.

Priester, W. A., Glass, G. G., and Waggoner, N. S.: Congenital defects in domesticated animals: General considerations. Am. J. Vet. Res. 31:1871, 1970.

Saperstein, G., Harris, S., and Leipold, H. W.: *Congenital Defects in Domestic Cats.* St. Louis, MO: Ralston Purina Co., 1978.

USE OF REAL-TIME ULTRASOUND SCANNING IN THE DIAGNOSIS OF SMALL ANIMAL REPRODUCTIVE CONDITIONS

AMY DIETZE, D.V.M.
Ithaca, New York

In the past several years, real-time ultrasound scanning has found its way into veterinary medicine as a diagnostic tool. Reasons for this are the current rapid advancements made in real-time ultrasound technology, the proven usefulness and acceptance of ultrasound as an imaging modality in the human medical field, the increasing variety and availability of scanning equipment, and the decreasing cost of this equipment. The ability to noninvasively reveal the soft tissue structures of the abdomen, and especially the ability to distinguish between fluid-filled and solid, soft tissues, justifies the use of ultrasound scanning in veterinary theriogenology. Detection of pregnancy and fetal viability in the small animal by real-time ultrasound scanning and ultrasonic evaluation of the canine prostate are described in the veterinary literature. Imaging of tumors, ovarian cysts, cystic endometrial hyperplasia, testicular tumors, mineralization and fibrosis, and some inflammatory conditions of the reproductive organs such as pyometra will be further uses of diagnostic ultrasound in the practice of small animal theriogenology.

EQUIPMENT

Real-time ultrasound scanners are available as portable and mobile units. Portable equipment is light enough to carry. It is electronically less sophisticated, has less image-recording apparatus, and is less expensive than the mobile units. Mobile ultrasound equipment can be rolled from room to room but is not readily transportable to distant locations. It is electronically more sophisticated than portable units and has more image processing and image display capabilities, often has built-in image recording apparatus, and is more expensive to purchase because of these additional features.

Ultrasound transducers house one or more piezoelectric crystals that emit and receive ultrasonic waves. Transducers can be categorized into two types, which differ in the geometric shape of the image they produce. Linear array transducers produce a rectangular image, and sector transducers create a pie-shaped image. Both types are applicable to ultrasonic scanning of the reproductive tracts of small animals, and selection of a transducer is a matter of personal preference.

Transducers are available in a range of sound-wave frequencies. Commonly manufactured frequencies that would be useful for imaging the abdomen of a small animal range from 3.0 to 7.5 megahertz (MHz). The sound waves from transducers of lower frequencies are more penetrating and are focused at a greater depth than are those at higher frequencies, resulting in images that depict soft tissue structures at a greater distance away from the skin surface. Transducers of higher frequencies create images of tissue at less depth but with resolution that is superior to that of transducers at lower frequencies. Ideally, one should have a range of transducers available and should tailor transducer selection for optimal ultrasound imaging to patient size and depth of the structure to be studied. A 5.0-MHz transducer would be the best single selection for scanning the reproductive tract of small animals.

PATIENT RESTRAINT AND PREPARATION

Minimal patient restraint is required for an ultrasonic examination of the small animal's abdomen. The procedure is neither painful nor unpleasant, it does not require elaborate or precise patient positioning, and it is not deterred by a small amount of patient motion, so tranquilization of the patient is rarely necessary.

The main intent of patient preparation for ultrasonic examination is the elimination of gas pockets between the ultrasound transducer and the soft tissue to be imaged. Gas is an "enemy" of ultrasound. When ultrasound waves strike a gas–soft tissue interface, a very strong echo is generated and essentially no ultrasound waves are left to create an image of the structures deep to the gas pocket. This phenomenon is termed "acoustical shadowing." The gastrointestinal tract and the animal's hair both contain gas. For this reason, it is preferred that the patient have an empty gastrointestinal tract when the abdominal viscera are scanned. When there is less gas in loops of gut, there will be fewer acoustical shadows to obscure visceral images. Fasting patients for 12 hours and administering laxatives are recommended prior to ultrasonic examination. In regard to the coat, the best ultrasonic image will be obtained if hair is clipped over the area to be scanned with a No. 40 blade. An ultrasonic coupling gel must then be applied to the skin surface to establish air-free contact between the transducer and the skin. If the coat cannot be clipped, copious amounts of coupling gel applied to the hair will allow imaging of the abdominal viscera; however, the image quality will be degraded.

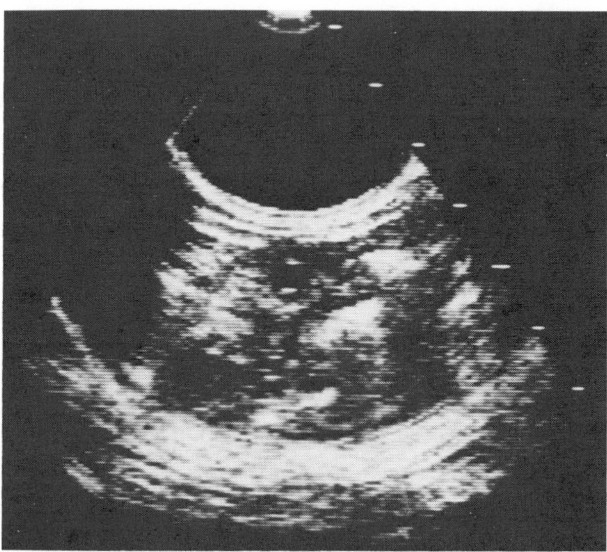

Figure 1. Ultrasound scan of a bitch, 19 days after breeding, was made with a 7.5 MHz mechanical sector transducer with a built-in stand-off. The scan shows the cross section of a 5-mm anechoic gestational sac surrounded by hypoechoic uterine wall. Several sections of small intestine containing hyperechoic gas are adjacent to the uterus.

DETECTION OF PREGNANCY AND FETAL VIABILITY IN THE BITCH

The uterus of a recumbent or standing pregnant animal can be scanned through the lateral or ventral abdominal body wall. Scanning in the first two weeks after breeding may demonstrate sequential enlargement of the part of the uterus located dorsal to the bladder, which is indicative of a possible pregnancy (Cartee and Rowles, 1984). A positive diagnosis of pregnancy can be made when a focal, spherical, anechoic structure (the gestational sac) is identified; this is surrounded by a hypoechoic wall (the uterus and placenta) and contains a hyperechoic area (the fetal tissue) (Figs. 1 and 2). These ultrasonic findings have been seen as early as 10 days after the last observed breeding in one bitch (Cartee and Rowles, 1984). However, positive detection of pregnancy by real-time ultrasonic scanning methods will occur with reliability at 24 to 28 days of gestation (Johnston et al., 1983). At 28 days of gestation the embryo is shaped like a question mark. Starting at this time, crown-rump length and biparietal diameter can be measured. Between 38 to 45 days of gestation, organ development becomes ultrasonographically detectable (Cartee and Rowles, 1984) (Fig. 3).

Real-time ultrasonic detection of pregnancy in the bitch was shown to be 99.3 per cent accurate when performed 28 days after the last breeding (Bondestam et al., 1984). Pregnancy detection by abdominal palpation performed between 26 to 35 days of gestation was shown to be 87 per cent accurate in those bitches that did whelp and 73 per cent accurate in those that were not pregnant (Allen and Meredith, 1981). Fetal viability can be assessed ultrasonographically. Because real-time ultrasonic images display motion, the fetal heart beat—a definitive sign of life—and fetal activity can be observed. When the fetal tissues inside the gestational sac are first observed at 24 to 28 days of gestation, the fetal heart beat is detectable (Johnston et al., 1983). If a pregnancy is followed by sequential

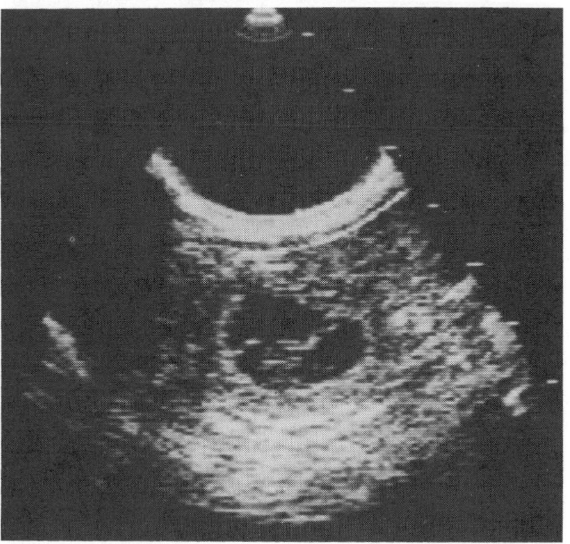

Figure 2. Ultrasound scan of the same bitch as in Figure 1 (23 days after breeding) demonstrates a 15-mm anechoic gestational sac that contains fetal tissue and is surrounded by uterine wall.

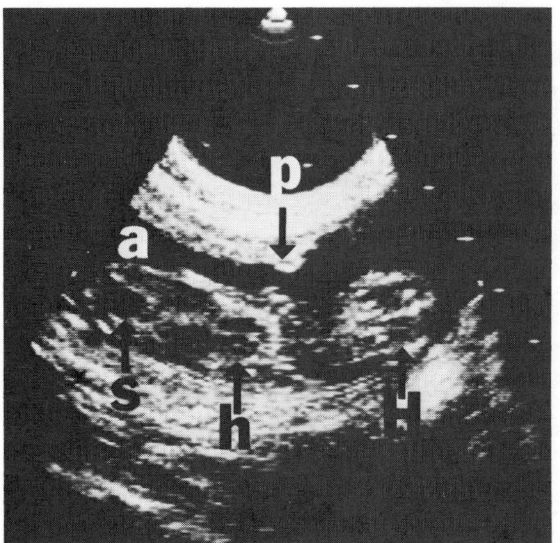

Figure 3. Ultrasound scan of a canine fetus on day 40. At this stage of gestation various organ structures can be distinguished: *p*, zonary placenta; *a*, amniotic fluid; *s*, anechoic stomach caudal to the hypoechoic liver; *h*, cardiac chambers surrounded by hyperechoic lung; *H*, head (note lateral ventricles).

imaging, fetal growth can be monitored. Failure of the fetus to grow indicates an abnormality. Near the time of parturition, if fetal distress is suspected, fetal heart rate can be counted from a real-time ultrasonic image. One normal heart rate value of the near-term canine fetus is given as 120 to 140 beats per minute (Johnston et al., 1983).

Determination of litter size by ultrasonic scanning gives a fairly reliable estimation when litter size is small. Fetuses are most easily counted at about 28 days of gestation, when they are small and not confluent (Bondestam et al., 1983). Usually litter size is overestimated in litters of five or fewer. When more than eight puppies are present, litter size is often greatly underestimated. Estimation of litter size by ultrasonic examination should not be off by more than two fetuses when litter size is smaller than five (Bondestam et al., 1984).

ULTRASONIC EVALUATION OF THE CANINE PROSTATE

The canine prostate is scanned through the ventral abdominal body wall as the dog is positioned in dorsal recumbency. The size and contour of the prostate can be seen. Thus, ultrasound can be used as a tool to detect and measure prostatomegaly and to differentiate the prostate from the bladder or other caudal abdominal masses.

Ultrasonic imaging of the prostate will help narrow the list of differential diagnoses when prostatomegaly is present (Johnston and Feeney, 1984; Cartee and Rowles, 1983). The prostatic parenchyma may appear as a solid, soft tissue structure (which may indicate hyperplasia or neoplasia), it may contain hyperechoic areas of calcification, or it may have fluid-filled cavities associated with it. These fluid cavities may be intraparenchymal and represent cystic hyperplasia or abscessation of the prostate (Fig. 4, *A* and *B*). The fluid cavities may be extraparenchymal and indicative of prostatic cysts (Fig. 5, *A* and B).

Since ultrasonic scanning is noninvasive and harmless, prostatic disease can be followed by serial ultrasonic examinations. Response to treatment or

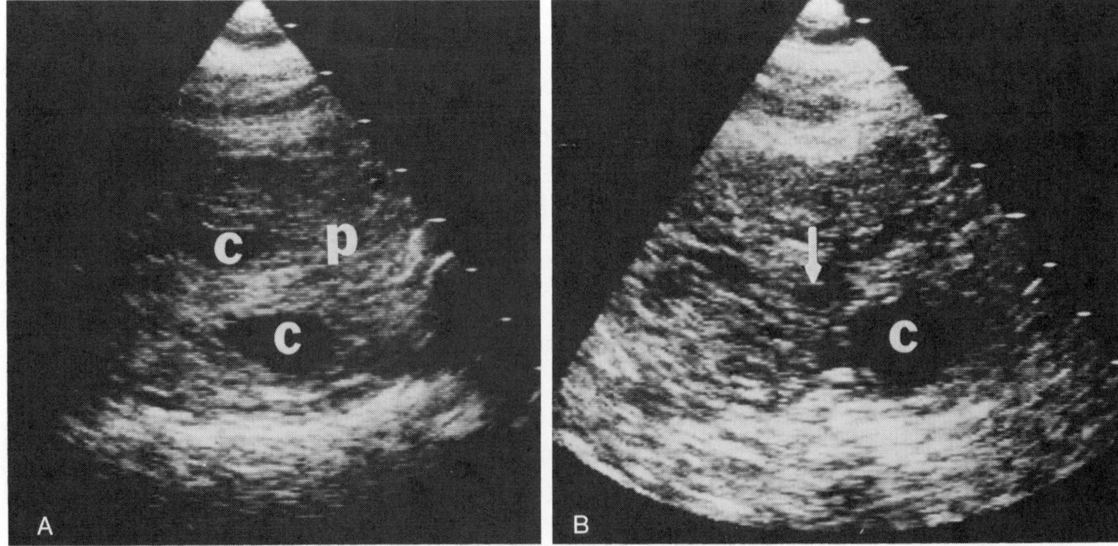

Figure 4. *A*, Longitudinal ultrasound scan of a canine prostate, made with a 5 MHz mechanical sector transducer, shows two fluid-filled cavities (*c*) contained within the hypoechoic prostate (*p*). *B*, This transverse ultrasound scan of the prostate depicted in A shows it to have a symmetrical, bilobed shape. There are multiple, small spaces containing fluid and one larger fluid-filled cavity (*c*) within the prostate. The neck of the bladder is seen at the arrow.

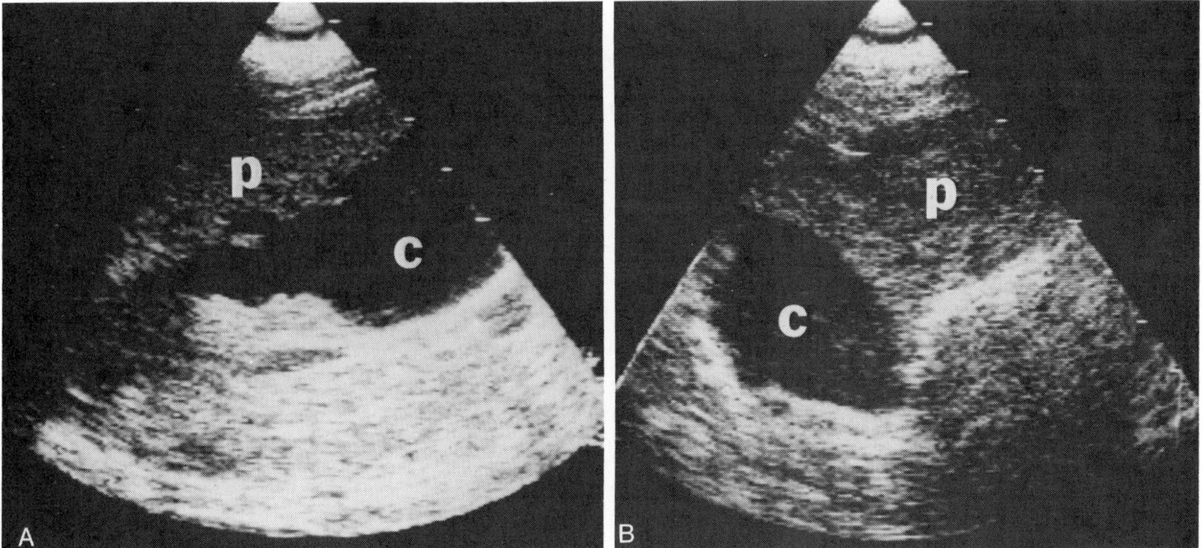

Figure 5. *A*, Longitudinal ultrasound scan of a canine prostate (*p*) with one large, extraparenchymal, fluid-filled cavity (*c*). *B*, The transverse plane reveals one large, fluid-filled cavity (*c*) that lies outside the left lobe of the prostate (*p*).

progression of disease can be ascertained. When focal prostatic lesions exist, ultrasound-guided needle biopsy or aspiration can be performed.

The future use of ultrasonography to detect and diagnose endometrial cystic hyperplasia, pyometritis, and cystic ovarian disease in both the bitch and queen has great potential. In the male, testicular neoplasia, fibrosis, and calcification should be definable and prognostic. Segmented aplasias of the reproductive tract, which become cystic with age and are seen frequently in intersexes and occasionally as congenital defects in dogs and cats, will be detectable by ultrasonic scanning. Ultrasonography has become an important procedure and valuable adjunct to the diagnosis of reproductive problems in small animals and holds a great possibility for future applications.

References and Supplemental Reading

Allen, W. E., and Meredith, M.: Detection of pregnancy in the bitch: A study of abdominal palpation, A-mode ultrasound, and Doppler ultrasound techniques. J. Small Anim. Pract. 22:609, 1981.

Bondestam, S., Alitalo, I., and Karkkainen, M.: Real-time ultrasound pregnancy diagnosis in the bitch. J. Small Anim. Pract. 24:145, 1983.

Bondestam, S., Karkkainen, M., Alitalo, I., et al.: Evaluating the accuracy of canine pregnancy diagnosis and litter size using real-time ultrasound. Acta Vet. Scand. 25:327, 1984.

Cartee, R., and Rowles, T.: Transabdominal sonographic evaluation of the canine prostate. Vet. Rad. 24:156, 1983.

Cartee, R., and Rowles, T.: Preliminary study of the ultrasonographic diagnosis of pregnancy and fetal development in the dog. Am. J. Vet. Res. 45:1259, 1984.

Johnston, O., and Feeney, D.: Comparative organ imaging: Lower urinary tract. Vet. Radiol. 25:146, 1984.

Johnston, S., Smith, F., Bailic, N., et al.: Prenatal indicators of puppy viability at term. Comp. Cont. Ed. Pract. Vet. 5:1013, 1983.

APPENDICES

ROBERT W. KIRK, D.V.M.
Consulting Editor

A ROSTER OF NORMAL VALUES FOR DOGS AND CATS

JOHN BENTINCK-SMITH, D.V.M.
Mississippi State, Mississippi

Age, sex, breed, diurnal periodicity, and emotional stress at the time of sampling can be expected to cause variation in normal values. The methodology will also affect the biologic measurements.

For these reasons practitioners are well advised to employ the normal values supplied by the laboratory that they patronize. However, this laboratory must have determined their normal ranges and means by a sufficient number of normal samples to provide statistical validity. The laboratory should run control serum samples and provide other means of quality control.

Since biochemical results are most frequently determined on Technicon SMA, equipment values for this method are provided (through the courtesy of Dr. A. I. Hurvitz and Dr. Robert J. Wilkins of the Animal Medical Center, New York). Other data are derived from the New York State College of Veterinary Medicine, the Ralston Purina Corp., Biozyme Veterinary Laboratory (a division of Biozyme Medical Laboratories, Inc.), standard texts, and the literature. References are cited as footnotes within the tables and appear in full at the end of this appendix. Values for reptiles and exotic animals can be found in *Current Veterinary Therapy VII*, pages 748 and 749, and in *Current Veterinary Therapy VI*, page 795.

In appropriate collection and preparation, prolonged storage, hemolysis, lipemia, and hyperbilirubinemia may invalidate the laboratory results.

Normal Blood Values*

Erythrocytes	Adult Dog	Average	Adult Cat	Average
Erythrocytes (millions/μl)	5.5–8.5	6.8	5.5–10.0	7.5
Hemoglobin (gm/dl)	12.0–18.0	14.9	8.0–14.0	12.0
Packed cell volume (vol. %)	37.0–55.0	45.5	24.0–45.0	37.0
Mean corpuscular volume (femtoliters)	66.0–77.0	69.8	40.0–55.0	45.0
Mean corpuscular hemoglobin (picograms)	19.9–24.5	22.8	13.0–17.0	15.0
Mean corpuscular hemoglobin concentration (gm/dl)				
Wintrobe	31.0–34.0	33.0	31.0–35.0	33.0
Michrohematocrit	32.0–36.0	34.0	30.0–36.0	33.2
Reticulocytes (%) (excludes punctate retics.)	0.0–1.5	0.8	0.2–1.6	0.6
Resistance to hypotonic saline (% saline solution producing)				
Minimum	0.40–0.50	0.46	0.66–0.72	0.69
Initial and complete hemolysis				
Maximum	0.32–0.42	0.33	0.46–0.54	0.50
Erythrocyte Sedimentation Rate	PCV 37	13	PCV 35–40	7–27
(mm at 60 min)	PCV 50	0		
RBC life span (days)	100–120		66–78	
RBC diameter (μm)	6.7–7.2	7.0	5.5–6.3	5.8
Leukocytes	**Adult Dog**	**Average**	**Adult Cat**	**Average**
Leukocytes (no/μl)	6,000–17,000	11,500	5,500–19,500	12,500
Neutrophils—Bands (%)	0–3	0.8	0–3	0.5
Neutrophils—Mature (%)	60–77	70.0	35–75	59.0
Lymphocyte (%)	12–30	20.0	20–55	32.0
Monocyte (%)	3–10	5.2	1–4	3.0
Eosinophil (%)	2–10	4.0	2–12	5.5
Basophil (%)	Rare	0.0	Rare	0.0
Neutrophils—Bands (no/μl)	0–300	70	0–300	100
Neutrophils—Mature (no/μl)	3,000–11,500	7,000	2,500–12,500	7,500
Lymphocytes (no/μl)	1,000–4,800	2,800	1,500–7,000	4,000
Monocytes (no/μl)	150–1,350	750	0–850	350
Eosinophils (no/μl)	100–1,250	550	0–1,500	650
Basophils	Rare	0	Rare	0

*From Schalm et al., 1975.

*Canine Blood Values at Different Ages—Average Values**

Age	RBC Millions/μl	Retic. %†	Nucl. RBC/ 100 WBC†	Hb gm/dl	PCV Vol. %	WBC/dl	Neut./dl	Bands/dl	Lymph./dl	Eos./dl
Birth	5.75	7.1	1.8	16.70	50	16,500	1,300	400	2,500	600
2 weeks	3.92	7.1	1.8	9.76	32	11,000	6,500	100	3,000	300
4 weeks	4.20	7.1	1.8	9.60	33	13,000	8,600	0	4,000	40
6 weeks	4.91	3.6	1.8	9.59	34	15,000	10,000	0	4,500	100
8 weeks	5.13	3.9	0.3	11.00	37	18,000	11,000	234	6,000	270
12 weeks	5.27	3.9	Rare	11.60	36	15,300	9,400	115	4,600	322

*From Andersen and Gee, 1958.
†See Ewing et al., 1972.

*Canine Blood Values at Different Ages**

	Sex	Birth to 12 Mo.	Average	1–7 Yr.	Average	7 Yr. and Older	Average
Erythrocytes (million/μl)	Male	2.99–8.52	5.09	5.26–6.57	5.92	3.33–7.76	5.28
	Female	2.76–8.42	5.06	5.13–8.6	6.47	3.34–9.19	5.17
Hemoglobin (gm/dl)	Male	6.9–16.5	10.7	12.7–16.3	15.5	14.7–21.2	17.9
	Female	6.4–18.9	11.2	11.5–17.9	14.7	11.0–22.5	16.1
Packed Cell Volume (vol. %)	Male	22.0–45.0	33.9	35.2–52.8	44.0	44.2–62.8	52.3
	Female	25.8–55.2	36.0	34.8–52.4	43.6	35.8–67.0	49.8
Leukocytes (thousands/μl)	Male	9.9–27.7	17.1	8.3–19.5	11.9	7.9–35.3	15.5
	Female	8.8–26.8	15.9	7.5–17.5	11.5	5.2–34.0	13.4
Neutrophils Mature (%)	Male	63–73	68	65–73	69	55–80	66
	Female	64–74	69	58–76	67	40–80	64
Lymphocytes (%)	Male	18–30	24	9–26	18	15–40	29
	Female	13–28	21	11–29	20	13–45	29
Monocytes (%)	Male	1–10	6	2–10	6	0–4	1
	Female	1–10	7	0–10	5	0–4	1
Eosinophils (%)	Male	2–11	3	1–8	4	1–11	4
	Female	1–9	5	1–10	6	0–19	6

*From *1975 Normal Blood Values for Dogs.*

*Feline Blood Values at Different Ages**

Age	RBC Millions/μl	Hb gm/dl	PCV Vol. %	WBC/dl	Neut./dl	Lymph./dl
Birth	4.95	12.2	44.7	7,500		
2 weeks	4.76	9.7	31.1	8,080		
5 weeks	5.84	8.4	29.9	8,550		
Average†	4.80	7.5	26.2	11,770	4,600	6,970
Range†	3.90–5.70	6.6–8.4	21.0–33.5	7,500–14,500		4,500–9,400
6 weeks	6.75	9.0	35.4	8,420		
8 weeks	7.10	9.4	35.6	8,420		4,900
Average†	5.90	7.5	26.2	12,400	7,500	1,925–10,100
Range†	3.30–7.30	7.6–15.0	22–38	6,900–23,100		

*From Schalm et al., 1975.
†See Anderson et al., 1971.

*Feline Blood Values at Different Ages**

	Sex	Birth to 12 Mo.	Average	1–5 Yr.	Average	6 Yr. and Older	Average
Erythrocytes (millions/μl)	Male	5.43–10.22	6.96	4.48–10.27	7.34	5.26–8.89	6.79
	Female	4.46–11.34	6.90	4.45–9.42	6.17	4.10–7.38	5.84
Hemoglobin (gm/dl)	Male	6.0–12.9	9.9	8.9–17.0	12.9	9.0–14.5	11.8
	Female	6.0–15.0	9.9	7.9–15.5	10.3	7.5–13.7	10.3
Packed Cell Volume (vol. %)	Male	24.0–37.5	31	26.9–48.2	37.6	28.0–43.8	34.6
	Female	23.0–46.8	31.5	25.3–37.5	31.4	22.5–40.5	30.8
Leukocytes (thousands/μl)	Male	7.8–25.0	15.8	9.1–28.2	15.1	6.4–30.4	17.6
	Female	11.0–26.9	17.7	13.7–23.7	19.9	5.2–30.1	14.8
Neutrophils	Male	16–75	60	37–92	65	33–75	61
Mature (%)	Female	51–83	69	42–93	69	25–89	71
Lymphocytes (%)	Male	10–81	30	7–48	23	16–54	30
	Female	8–37	23	12–58	30	9–63	22
Monocytes (%)	Male	1–5	2	1–5	2	0–2	1
	Female	0–7	2	0–5	2	0–4	1
Eosinophils (%)	Male	2–21	8	1–22	7	1–15	8
	Female	0–15	6	0–13	5	0–15	6

*From *1975 Normal Blood Values for Cats.*

*Effect of Pregnancy and Lactation on Blood Values of the Dog**

	Gestation				Term	Lactation		
	2 Weeks	*4 Weeks*	*6 Weeks*	*8 Weeks*	*0 Weeks*	*2 Weeks*	*4 Weeks*	*6 Weeks*
RBC (millions/dl)	8.85	7.48	6.73	6.26	4.53	5.13	5.65	6.15
PCV (Vol. %)	53	47	44	37	32	34	38	42
Hb (gm/dl)	19.6	16.4	14.7	13.8	11.0	11.7	12.8	13.4
Sedimentation Rate (mm at 60 min)	0.6	11.0	31.0	14.0	12.0	14.0	14.0	13.0
WBC (thousands/dl)	12.0	12.2	15.7	19.0	18.9	16.9	17.1	15.9

*From Andersen and Gee, 1958.

*Effect of Pregnancy and Lactation on Blood Values of the Cat**

	Gestation					Term	Lactation	
	1 Day Past Conception	*2 Weeks*	*4 Weeks*	*6 Weeks*	*8 Weeks*	*0 Weeks*	*2 Weeks*	*4 Weeks*
RBC (millions/dl)	8.0	7.9	7.1	6.7	6.2	6.2	7.4	7.4
PCV (Vol. %)	36.1	37.0	33.0	32.0	28.0	29.0	33.0	33.0
Hb (gm/100 ml)	12.5	12.0	11.0	10.8	9.5	10.0	11.5	11.2
Reticulocytes (%) (includes punctate retics.)	9	11	9	10	20.1	15	9	6

	Adult Dog	Average	Adult Cat	Average†
Thrombocytes × 10^5/μl	2–5	3–4	3–8	4.5
Icterus Index	2–5 units		2–5 units	
Plasma Fibrinogen (gm/L)	2.0–4.0		0.50–3.00	

*From Berman, 1974.
†From Schalm et al., 1975.

Normal Bone Marrow (Percentage)

Erythrocytic Cells	Dog*	Cat†
Rubriblasts	0.2	1.71
Prorubricytes	3.9	12.50
Rubricytes	27.0	
Metarubricytes	15.3	11.68
Total Erythrocytic Cells	46.4	25.89
Granulocytic Cells		
Myeloblasts	0.0	1.74
Progranulocytes	1.3	0.88
Neutrophilic Myelocytes	9.0	9.76
Eosinophilic Myelocytes	0.0	1.47
Neutrophilic Metamyelocytes	7.5	7.32
Eosinophilic Metamyelocytes	2.4	1.52
Band Neutrophils	13.6	25.80
Band Eosinophils	0.9	—
Neutrophils	18.4	9.24
Eosinophils	0.3	0.81
Basophils	0.0	0.002
Total Granulocytic Cells	53.4	58.542
M:E Ratio—Average	1.15:1.0	2.47:1.0
M:E Ratio—Range (Schalm)	0.75–2.50:1.0	0.60–3.90:1.0
Other Cells		
Lymphocytes	0.2	7.63
Plasma Cells	0	1.61
Reticulum Cells	0	0.13
Mitotic Cells	0	0.61
Unclassified	0	1.62
Disintegrated Cells	0	4.60

*From Schalm et al., 1975.
†From Penny et al., 1970.

Blood, Plasma, or Serum Chemical Constituents: Part I
(B) = Blood, (P) = Plasma, (S) = Serum

Chemical constituents are liable to show markedly different values, depending on the method employed.

Constituent	Adult Dog: *Coulter Chemistry**	Adult Dog: *Technicon SMA†*	Adult Cat: *Coulter Chemistry**	Adult Cat: *Technicon SMA†*
Urea N(s) (mg/dl)	8–23	10–22	18–32	5–30
Glucose (S) (mg/dl)	71–115	50–120	66–95	70–150
Total bilirubin (S) (mg/dl)	0.1–0.6	0–0.6	0.15–0.3	0–0.8
Total protein (S) (gm/dl)	5.2–7.0	5.4–7.8	5.9–7.3	5.5–7.5
Albumin (S) (gm/dl)	2.7–3.8	2.2–3.4	2.2–3.0	2.2–3.5
Alkaline phosphatase (S) (IU/L)	10–82	20–120	7–30	10–80
Calcium (S) (mg/dl)	9.8–11.4	9–11.6	8.9–10.6	7.6–11.0
Inorganic phosphorus (S) (mg/dl)	2.8–5.1	3.9–6.3	4.3–6.6	3.2–6.3
LDH (S) (IU/L)	8–89	40–200	33–99	10–200
AST or SGOT (S)	13–93‡	5–80§	32–58‡	10–60§
ALT or SGPT (S) (IU/L)	15–70	5–25	10–50	10–60
Total CO_2 (S) (mEq/L)	18–25	17–25‖	18–25	16–25‖
Creatinine (S) (mg/dl)	0.5–1.2	0.4–1.5‖	0.5–1.7	1.3–2.1‖
Uric acid (S) (mg/dl)		0.2–0.8‖		0.1–0.7‖
Total cholesterol (S) (mg/dl)	82–282	156–294‖	41–225	116–126‖
Triglycerides (S) (mg/dl)		10–42‖		6–58‖
CPK (S) (IU/L)	12–84	27–93‖	6–130	62–262‖
GGT (S) (IU/L) (Centrifugal Analysis**)	1.4–11.5		1.8–18.3	

Chemical Values Affected by Age	Dog < 6 Mo–SMA†	Cat < 6 Mo–SMA†
Inorganic phosphorus (S) (mg/dl)	3.9–9.0	3.9–8.1
Calcium (S) (mg/dl)	7.0–11.6	7.0–11.0
Alkaline phosphatase (S) (IU/L)	20–200	10–120
LDH (S) (IU/L)	40–400	10–300

	Sex	Dogs†† and Cats‡‡: *Birth to 12 mo.*	*Average*	*1–5 yr.*	*Average*	*6 yr. and Older*	*Average*
Total Protein (S) (gm/dl)	Male	3.90–5.90	5.15	4.90–9.60	6.33	5.5–7.3	6.4
(Dogs)	Female	4.00–6.40	5.58	5.50–7.80	6.34	4.7–7.5	6.2
Total Protein (S) (gm/dl)	Male	4.3–10.0	6.4	6.8–10.0	8.1	6.2–8.5	7.2
(Cats)	Female	4.8–9.1	6.4	6.6–8.9	7.4	6.0–9.0	7.3

Electrophoresis	Dog	Cat
Albumin (S) (gm/dl)	2.3–3.4	2.3–3.5
Globulin (S) (gm/dl)	3.0–4.7	2.6–5.0
Alpha 1 (S) (gm/dl)	0.3–0.8	0.3–0.5
Alpha 2 (S) (gm/dl)	0.5–1.3	0.4–1.0
Beta (S) (gm/dl)	0.7–1.8	0.6–1.9
Gamma (S) (gm/dl)	0.4–1.0	0.5–1.5
Albumin/globulin ratio, A/G (S)	0.7–1.1	0.5–1.0

*From Tasker, 1978.

†From Wilkins and Hurvitz, 1978.

‡Trans Act Units/liter (General Diagnostics). 1 Trans Act Unit of GOT activity is the amount of enzyme in 1 liter of sample that will form 1 mM of oxalic acid in 1 minute under specified conditions.

§U/liter.

‖See Biozyme Veterinary Laboratory, 1978.

**From Boyd, 1984.

††From *1975 Normal Blood Values for Dogs.*

‡‡From *1975 Normal Blood Values for Cats.*

Blood, Plasma or Serum Chemical Constituents: Part II
(B) = Blood, (P) = Plasma, (S) = Serum

Chemical constituents are liable to show markedly different values depending on the method employed.

Other Constituents	Adult Dog	Adult Cat
Lipase (S)		
(Sigma Tietz Units/ml)	0–1	0–1
Roe Byler Units (S)	0.8–12	0–5
IU (S)	13–200	0–83
Amylase (S)		
Harleco Units/dl	0–800	0–800
Harding Units/dl	1600–2400	0–2700**
Dy Amyl (General Diagnostics)	<3200**	0–2600**
Caraway Units/dl*	330–1530	170–1170
Lactic acid (S) (mg/dl)	3–15	
Pyruvate (B) (mEq/l)	0.1–0.2	
Cholesterol esters (S) (mg/dl)	84–168	45–120
Free cholesterol (S) (mg/dl)	28–84	15–60
Total lipid (P) (mg/dl)	47–725	145–607
Free glycerol (S) 24-hr fast (mg/dl)†	14.2–23.2	
Bromsulfalein retention test (P) (%)	<5	
Iron (S) (μg/dl)	94–122	68–215
Total iron-binding capacity (S) (μg/dl)	280–340	170–400
Lead (B) (μg/dl)	0–35	0–35

Electrolytes	Dogs		Cats	
	Coulter‡	*Technicon*§	*Coulter*‡	*Technicon*§
Sodium (S) (mEq/L)	143–151	144–154	150–162	147–161
Potassium (S) (mEq/L)	4.1–5.7	3.8–5.8	3.7–5.5	3.7–4.9
Magnesium (S) (mEq/L)	1.4–2.4	1.07–1.73	2.2	1.92–2.28
Chloride (S) (mEq/L)	103–115	93–121	114–124	80–158
Sulfate (S) (mEq/L)	2.0			
Osmolality (S) (mOsm/kg)	280–310		280–310	
pH (Corning)	7.31–7.42		7.24–7.40	

Blood Gases	Adult Dog	Adult Cat
P_{O_2} (B) mm Hg (arterial)‖	85–95	—
(B) mm Hg (venous)‖	40–60	—
P_{CO_2} (B) mm Hg (arterial)‖	29–36	—
(B) mm Hg (venous)‖	29–42	—
Base excess (B) (mEq/L)	±2.5	±2.5
Bicarbonate (P) (mEq/L)	17–24	17–24

*From *Chemassay Amylase.*
†From Rogers et al., 1975.
‡From Tasker, 1978.
§From Biozyme Veterinary Laboratory, 1978.
‖Standard temperature and pressure.
**From Benjamin, 1978.

Blood, Plasma or Serum Chemical Constituents: Part III
(B) = Blood, (P) = Plasma, (S) = Serum

Chemical constituents are liable to show markedly different values depending on the method employed.

	Adult Dog		Adult Cat	
Endocrine Secretions	*Resting Level*	*Post-ACTH**	*Resting Level*	*Post-ACTH**
Cortisol (S) (RIA) (mg/dl)†	1.8–4	3–4 × Pretreatment	1–3	3–4 × Pretreatment
Cortisol (S) (CPB) (mg/dl)‡	2–6	3–4 × Pretreatment§	2–5	3–4 × Pretreatment§
Cortisol (S) (fluorometric) (μg/dl)	5–10	10–20		
	Resting Level	*Post-TSH‖*	*Resting Level*	*Post-TSH*
T_4 (P) (RIA) (μg/dl)**	1.52–3.60	At least 3- to 4-fold	1.2–3.8	
T_3 (P) (RIA) (ng/dl)**	48–154	More than 10 ng increase		
Protein-bound iodine (μg/dl)††	1.6–3.0	Increase of 3 μg/dl (mean)		

T_4 Changes With Age	Dog	Cat
T_4 (S) (RIA)	Decrease of 0.07 μg/dl per year of age**	No values for cat
T_4 (S) (CPB) (μg/dl)		
10–12 wk‡‡	3.24 ± 0.51	2.82 ± 0.73
1 yr‡‡	2.25 ± 0.33	2.43 ± 0.55
	Adult Dog	**Adult Cat**
Thyroid uptake of radioiodine (^{131}I)(%)‡‡	17–30	
Insulin (S) (RIA) (μU/ml)§§	0–30	0–50

Plasma Proteins

Basenji Dogs‖‖		*Cats****	
Age	*Plasma Proteins (gm/dl)*	*Age*	*Plasma Proteins (gm/dl)*
6–8 weeks	5.33 ± 0.29	Adults (younger animals have lower values)	6–8
9–12 weeks	5.87 ± 0.46		
4–6 months	6.6 ± 0.25		
1–2 years	7.03 ± 0.33		

*Two μg ACTH gel IM 2 hours after injection.

†Data from Thomas J. Reimers, Assistant Professor and Director of the Endocrinology Laboratory, New York State College of Veterinary Medicine, Cornell University, Ithaca, New York.

‡Data from R. Wallace, Research Support Specialist, New York State College of Veterinary Medicine, Cornell University, Ithaca, New York.

§Data from D. W. Scott, Assistant Professor of Medicine, Department of Clinical Sciences, New York State College of Veterinary Medicine, Cornell University, Ithaca, New York.

‖Five μg TSH IV 4–6 hours after injection.

**From Belshaw and Rijnberk, 1979.

††From Benjamin, 1978.

‡‡From Kallfelz and Erali, 1973; personal communication from F. A. Kallfelz, Associate Professor of Clinical Nutrition, Department of Large Animal Medicine, Obstetrics, and Surgery, New York State College of Veterinary Medicine, Cornell University, Ithaca, New York.

§§Data from R. J. Wilkins, Animal Medical Center, New York, New York.

‖‖From Ewing et al., 1972.

***From Schalm et al., 1975.

*Hemostatic Values**

	Adult Dog	Adult Cat
Bleeding time	2–4	1–5†
Dorsum of nose (min)	85–110	
Lip (sec)	2.5–3	
Ear (min)	1–2	
Abdomen (min)		
Whole blood coagulation time		
Glass (Lee and White) (min)	6–7.5	8†
Silicone (Lee and White) (min)	12–15	
Capillary tube (min)‡	3–4	5.2 ± 0.2§
Activated coagulation time of whole blood		
Room temp. (sec)	60–125‖ 83–129**	A limited number of cats have shown a range similar to that of the dog.
37°C (sec)	64–95**	
Prothrombin time (sec)‡	6–10	8.6 ± 0.5§
Puppies 1–4 hours old (sec)††	42.2	
6–12 hours old (sec)	49.1	
16–48 hours old (sec)	36.8	
48 hours old (sec)	24.5	
Russell's viper venom time (sec)‡‡	11	9
Partial thromboplastin time (sec)	15–25	
Prothrombin consumption (sec)‡‡	20.5	20
Fibrin degradation products (μg/ml)	<10	

*No test should be interpreted without an accompanying normal control.
†From Seager and Fletcher, 1972.
‡From Coles, 1974.
§From Osbaldiston et al., 1970.
‖From Byars et al.,. 1976.
**From Middleton and Watson, 1978.
††From Benjamin, 1978.
‡‡From Rowsell, 1969.

Normal Renal Function and Urine Values

Urine*	Adult Dog	Adult Cat
Specific Gravity		
Minimum	1.001	1.001
Maximum	1.060	1.080
Usual Limits (normal water and food intake)	1.018–1.050	1.018–1.050
Volume (ml/kg body weight/day)	24–41	22–30
Osmolality Urine (mOsm/kg)		
Usual Range	500–1200	
Maximal Limits	2000–2400	
Osmolality Plasma	300	
Urine Constituents†	**Adult Dog**	**Adult Cat**
Creatinine (mg/dl)	100–300	110–280
Urea (gm/dl)	1.0–2.5	1.0–3.0
Protein (mg/dl)	0–30	0–20
Amylase (Somogyi units)	50–150	30–120
Sodium (mEq/L)	20–165	
Potassium (mEq/L)	20–120	
Calcium (mEq/L)	2–10	
Inorganic phosphorus (mEq/L)	50–180	
Urinalysis—Semiquantitative Values	**Adult Dog**	**Adult Cat**
Protein sulfosalicylic acid	0–trace	0–trace
Protein Multistix (Miles Laboratories)‡	0–1+	0–1+
Glucose	0	0
Ketones	0	0
Bilirubin	0	0
10–20% Dogs—high specific gravity	1+	
5% Cats—high specific gravity		1+
Urobilinogen (Ehrlich unit)	0–1	0–1
(Wallace and Diamond)	<1:32	<1:32

Table continued on opposite page

Normal Renal Function and Urine Values Continued

Urine Total Protein Excretion (24 hr) in the Dog (Trichloroacetic Acid Ponceau Method)			
N	*Range (mg)*	$\bar{X}$	*SD*
17‡	48–1040	333 mg	± 309 mg
10§	8–151	38 mg	

Renal Function—Dog*	
Effective renal plasma flow	266 ± 66 ml/min/m² body surface 13.5 ± 3.3 ml/min/kg body weight
Glomerular filtration rate	84.4 ± 19 ml/min/m² body surface 4 ml/min/kg body weight

Renal Function Tests—Dog	
Phenolsulfonphthalein	
Excretion in urine at 20 min, 6-mg dose‖	21–66%
Clearance (P) 1 mg/kg at 60 min**	<80 μ/ml
$T_{1/2}$ clearance 5 mg/kg††	19.6 min
Creatinine, endogenous clearance*	60 ± 22 ml/min/m² body surface 2.98 ± 0.96 ml/min/kg body weight

*From Osborne et al., 1972.
†Data from R. J. Wilkins, Animal Medical Center, New York, New York. Values are markedly affected by degree of concentration.
‡From DiBartola et al., 1980.
§From Barsanti and Finco, 1979.
‖From Coles, 1974.
**From Kaufman and Kirk, 1973.
††From Brobst et al., 1967.

Cerebrospinal Fluid and Synovial Fluid

Cerebrospinal Fluid*	Adult Dog	Adult Cat
Color	Clear, colorless	Clear, colorless
Pressure (mm H_2O)	<170	<100
Cells/μl	<5 lymphocytes	<5 lymphocytes
Protein (ml/dl)	<25	<20
Glucose (mg/dl)	61–116	85

Normal Synovial Fluid—Carpal, Elbow, Shoulder, Hip, Stifle, and Hock Joints†	Adult Dog	
	Range	*Mean*
Amount (ml)	0.01–1.00	0.24
pH	7–7.8	7.33
Leukocytes (× 10^3/μl)	0–2.9	0.43
Erythrocytes (× 10^3/μl)	0–320.0	12.15
Neutrophils/μl	0–32	3.63
Neutrophils(%)‡	10	
Monocytes/μl	0–838	230.77
Lymphocytes/μl	0–2436	245.6
Clasmatocytes/μl	0–166	14.69
Mononuclear cells(%)‡	90	
Mucin clot	Tight, ropy clump; clear supernatant	

*Data from A. de Lahunta, Professor of Anatomy, Department of Clinical Sciences, New York State College of Veterinary Medicine, Cornell University, Ithaca, New York.
†From Sawyer, 1963.
‡From Miller et al., 1974.

*Canine Semen**

Regular Collection by Hand Manipulation With a Teaser (125 Ejaculates From Small Dogs, Mostly Beagles)†	Mean	Standard Deviation	Range
Volume (ml)	-5	4.3	0.5–20.4
% Motile sperm	75	7.5	30–90
% Normal sperm	86	14.7	34–97
pH	6.72	0.19	6.49–7.10
Concentration/mm^3 (10^3)	148	84.6	27.2–388.8
Total sperm per ejaculate (10^6)	528	321.0	94–1428

Fractionated Ejaculates (Based on 65 Ejaculates)	Mean	Range	pH
First Fraction	0.8 ml.	0.25–2.00	6.37
Second Fraction	0.6 ml.	0.40–2.00	6.10
Third Fraction	0.4 ml.	1.0–16.3	7.20

Ejaculates From Purebred Labrador Retrievers, 18 to 48 Months Old‡	Mean	Range
Volume (ml)	2.2§	0.5–6.5
% Motile sperm	93	75–99
% Unstained sperm (eosin-nigrosin)	84	61–99
Concentration/mm^3 (10^3)	564	103–708

*Revisions and corrections courtesy of R. H. Foote, Professor of Animal Physiology, Department of Animal Science, New York State College of Life Sciences, Cornell University, Ithaca, New York.

†From Boucher, 1957.

‡From Seager and Fletcher, 1972.

§Only the first two fractions were collected, resulting in smaller volume and higher concentration of sperm/mm^3 than would result if all the prostatic fluid (third fraction) were obtained.

References and Supplemental Reading

Andersen, A. C., and Gee, W.: Normal values in the beagle. Vet. Med. 53:135, 156; 1958.

Anderson, L., Wilson, R., and Hay, D.: Haematological values in normal cats from four weeks to one year of age. Res. Vet. Sci. 12:579, 1971.

Baker, H. J.: Laboratory evaluation of thyroid function. *In* Kirk, R. W. (ed.): *Current Veterinary Therapy IV.* Philadelphia: W. B. Saunders, 1971.

Barsanti, J. A., and Finco, D. R.: Protein concentration in urine of normal dogs. Am. J. Vet. Res. 40:1583, 1979.

Belshaw, B. E., and Rijnberk, A.: Radioimmunoassay of plasma T_4 and T_3 in the diagnosis of primary hypothyroidism in dogs. J. Am. Anim. Hosp. Assoc. 15:17, 1979.

Benjamin, M.: *An Outline of Veterinary Clinical Pathology,* 3rd ed. Ames, IA: Iowa State University Press, 1978.

Berman, E.: Hemogram of the cat during pregnancy and lactation and after lactation. Am. J. Vet. Res. 35:457, 1974.

Biozyme Veterinary Laboratory (a division of Biozyme Medical Laboratories, Inc.): *Normal Ranges Chemistry.* Olean, NY: Biozyme Veterinary Laboratory, 1978.

Boucher, J. H.: Evaluation of semen quality in the dog and the effects of frequency of ejaculation upon semen quality, libido and restoration of sperm reserves. M.S. Thesis, Cornell University, Ithaca, N.Y., 1957.

Boyd, J. W.: The interpretation of serum biochemistry test results in domestic animals. Vet. Clin. Pathol. 13(2):7, 1984.

Brobst, D. F., Carter, J. M., and Horron, M.: Plasma phenolsulfonphthalein determination as a measure of renal function in the dog. 17th Gaines Veterinary Symposium, University of Minnesota, 1967, p. 15.

Byars, T. D., Ling, G. V., Ferris, N. A., and Keeton, K. S.: Activated coagulation time (ACT) of whole blood in normal dogs. Am. J. Vet. Res. 37:1359, 1976.

Chemassay Amylase. Pitman-Moore, Inc., Washington Crossing, N.J. 08560.

Coles, E. H.: *Veterinary Clinical Pathology,* 2nd ed. Philadelphia: WB Saunders, 1974.

DiBartola, S. P., Chew, D. J., and Jacobs, G.: Quantitative urinalysis including 24-hour protein excretion in the dog. J. Am. Anim. Hosp. Assoc. 16:537, 1980.

Ewing, G. O., Schalm, O. W., and Smith, R. S.: Hematologic values of normal Basenji dogs. J.A.V.M.A. 161:1661, 1972.

Kallfelz, F. A., and Erali, R. P.: Thyroid function tests on domesticated animals. Am. J. Vet. Res. 34:1449, 1973.

Kaufman, C. F., and Kirk, R. W.: The 60-minute plasma phenolsulfonphthalein concentration as a test of renal function in the dog. J. Am. Anim. Hosp. Assoc. 9:66, 1973.

Kraft, W.: Schielddrusenfunktionsstörunge. beim Hund. (Thyroid function disturbances in the dog). Thesis, Justus Liebig University, Giessen, West Germany, 1964. (Cited by Belshaw.)

Middleton, D. J., and Watson, A. D. J.: Activated coagulation times of whole blood in normal dogs and dogs with coagulopathies. J. Small Anim. Pract. 19:417, 1978.

Miller, J. B., Perman, V., Osborne, C. A., Hammer, R. F., and Gambardella, P. C.: Synovial fluid analysis in canine arthritis. J. Am. Anim. Hosp. Assoc. *10*:392, 1974.

1975 Normal Blood Values for Cats. Ralston Purina Co., Professional Marketing Services, Checkerboard Square, St. Louis, Missouri 63188.

1975 Normal Blood Values for Dogs. Ralston Purina Co., Professional Marketing Services, Checkerboard Square, St. Louis, Missouri 63188.

Osbaldiston, G. W., Stowe, E. C., and Griffith, P. R.: Blood coagulation: Comparative studies in dogs, cats, horses and cattle. Br. Vet. J. 126:512, 1970.

Osborne, C. A., Low, D. G., and Finco, D. R.: *Canine and Feline Urology.* Philadelphia: W. B. Saunders, 1972.

Penny, R. H. C., Carlisle, C. H., and Davidson, H. A.: The blood and marrow picture of the cat. Br. Vet. J. 126:459, 1970.

Rogers, U. A., Donovan, E. F., and Kociba, G. J.: Lipids and lipoproteins in normal dogs and dogs with secondary hyperlipoproteinemia. J.A.V.M.A. 166:1092, 1975.

Rowsell, H. C.: Blood coagulation and hemorrhage disorders. *In* Medway, W., Prier, J. E., and Wilkinson, J. S. (eds.): *Textbook of Veterinary Clinical Pathology.* Baltimore: Williams & Wilkins, 1969, p. 247.

Sawyer, D. C.: Synovial fluid analysis of canine joints. J.A.V.M.A. 143:609, 1963.

Schalm, O. W., Jain, N. C., and Carroll, E. J.: *Veterinary Hematology,* 3rd ed. Philadelphia: Lea & Febiger, 1975.

Seager, S. W. J., and Fletcher, W. S.: Collection, storage, and insemination of canine semen. Lab. Anim. Sci. 22:177, 1972.

Tasker, J. B.: Reference values for clinical chemistry using the Coulter Chemistry System. Cornell Vet. 68:460, 1978.

Wilkins, R. J., and Hurvitz, A. I.: *Profiling in Veterinary Clinical Pathology.* Tarrytown, NY: Technicon Instruments Corp., 1978, pp. 17, 19.

63-DAY PERPETUAL GESTATION CHART

Conception—Jan.	1 2 3 4 5 6 7 8 9 10 11 12 13 14 15 16 17 18 19 20 21 22 23 24 25 26 27		28 29 30 31
Due—March	5 6 7 8 9 10 11 12 13 14 15 16 17 18 19 20 21 22 23 24 25 26 27 28 29 30 31	April	1 2 3 4
Conception—Feb.	1 2 3 4 5 6 7 8 9 10 11 12 13 14 15 16 17 18 19 20 21 22 23 24 25 26		27 28
Due—April	5 6 7 8 9 10 11 12 13 14 15 16 17 18 19 20 21 22 23 24 25 26 27 28 29 30	May	1 2
Conception—Mar.	1 2 3 4 5 6 7 8 9 10 11 12 13 14 15 16 17 18 19 20 21 22 23 24 25 26 27 28 29		30 31
Due—May	3 4 5 6 7 8 9 10 11 12 13 14 15 16 17 18 19 20 21 22 23 24 25 26 27 28 29 30 31	June	1 2
Conception—Apr.	1 2 3 4 5 6 7 8 9 10 11 12 13 14 15 16 17 18 19 20 21 22 23 24 25 26 27 28		29 30
Due—June	3 4 5 6 7 8 9 10 11 12 13 14 15 16 17 18 19 20 21 22 23 24 25 26 27 28 29 30	July	1 2
Conception—May	1 2 3 4 5 6 7 8 9 10 11 12 13 14 15 16 17 18 19 20 21 22 23 24 25 26 27 28 29		30 31
Due—July	3 4 5 6 7 8 9 10 11 12 13 14 15 16 17 18 19 20 21 22 23 24 25 26 27 28 29 30 31	August	1 2
Conception—June	1 2 3 4 5 6 7 8 9 10 11 12 13 14 15 16 17 18 19 20 21 22 23 24 25 26 27 28 29		30
Due—August	3 4 5 6 7 8 9 10 11 12 13 14 15 16 17 18 19 20 21 22 23 24 25 26 27 28 29 30 31	Sept.	1
Conception—July	1 2 3 4 5 6 7 8 9 10 11 12 13 14 15 16 17 18 19 20 21 22 23 24 25 26 27 28 29		30 31
Due—September	2 3 4 5 6 7 8 9 10 11 12 13 14 15 16 17 18 19 20 21 22 23 24 25 26 27 28 29 30	Oct.	1 2
Conception—Aug.	1 2 3 4 5 6 7 8 9 10 11 12 13 14 15 16 17 18 19 20 21 22 23 24 25 26 27 28 29		30 31
Due—October	2 3 4 5 6 7 8 9 10 11 12 13 14 15 16 17 18 19 20 21 22 23 24 25 26 27 28 29 30	Nov.	1 2
Conception—Sept.	1 2 3 4 5 6 7 8 9 10 11 12 13 14 15 16 17 18 19 20 21 22 23 24 25 26 27 28		29 30
Due—November	3 4 5 6 7 8 9 10 11 12 13 14 15 16 17 18 19 20 21 22 23 24 25 26 27 28 29 30	Dec.	1 2
Conception—Oct.	1 2 3 4 5 6 7 8 9 10 11 12 13 14 15 16 17 18 19 20 21 22 23 24 25 26 27 28 29		30 31
Due—December	3 4 5 6 7 8 9 10 11 12 13 14 15 16 17 18 19 20 21 22 23 24 25 26 27 28 29 30 31	Jan.	1 2
Conception—Nov.	1 2 3 4 5 6 7 8 9 10 11 12 13 14 15 16 17 18 19 20 21 22 23 24 25 26 27 28 29		30
Due—January	3 4 5 6 7 8 9 10 11 12 13 14 15 16 17 18 19 20 21 22 23 24 25 26 27 28 29 30 31	Feb.	1
Conception—Dec.	1 2 3 4 5 6 7 8 9 10 11 12 13 14 15 16 17 18 19 20 21 22 23 24 25 26 27		28 29 30 31
Due—February	2 3 4 5 6 7 8 9 10 11 12 13 14 15 16 17 18 19 20 21 22 23 24 25 26 27 28	March	1 2 3 4

From Kirk, R. W., and Bistner, S. I.: *Handbook of Veterinary Procedures and Emergency Treatment*, 4th ed. Philadelphia: W. B. Saunders, 1985.

CONVERSION TABLE OF WEIGHT TO BODY SURFACE AREA (IN SQUARE METERS) FOR DOGS*

Kg	M^2	Kg	M^2
0.5	0.06	26.0	0.88
1.0	0.10	27.0	0.90
2.0	0.15	28.0	0.92
3.0	0.20	29.0	0.94
4.0	0.25	30.0	0.96
5.0	0.29	31.0	0.99
6.0	0.33	32.0	1.01
7.0	0.36	33.0	1.03
8.0	0.40	34.0	1.05
9.0	0.43	35.0	1.07
10.0	0.46	36.0	1.09
11.0	0.49	37.0	1.11
12.0	0.52	38.0	1.13
13.0	0.55	39.0	1.15
14.0	0.58	40.0	1.17
15.0	0.60	41.0	1.19
16.0	0.63	42.0	1.21
17.0	0.66	43.0	1.23
18.0	0.69	44.0	1.25
19.0	0.71	45.0	1.26
20.0	0.74	46.0	1.28
21.0	0.76	47.0	1.30
22.0	0.78	48.0	1.32
23.0	0.81	49.0	1.34
24.0	0.83	50.0	1.36
25.0	0.85		

*Although the above chart was compiled for dogs, it can also be used for cats. A formula for more precise values follows:

$$\text{BSA in } M^2 = \frac{K \times W^{2/3}}{10^4} \quad \textit{Given that} \quad \begin{array}{ll} \text{BSA} & = \text{body surface area} \\ M^2 & = \text{sq meters} \\ W & = \text{weight in gm} \\ K & = 10.1 \text{ (dogs), } 10.0 \text{ (cats)} \end{array}$$

From Ettinger, S. J.: *Textbook of Veterinary Internal Medicine.* Vol. I. Philadelphia, W. B. Saunders, 1975, p. 146.

TABLES OF NORMAL PHYSIOLOGIC DATA

Electrocardiography*

It is recognized that normal and abnormal electrocardiographic measurements overlap and that the criteria for the normal electrocardiogram serve only as a guide for the clinician. Deviations from normal in an individual electrocardiogram suggest but are not always diagnostic of heart disease. As additional statistical data become available for the electrocardiograms of dogs of each breed, body type, age, and sex, the data herein may require revision and "normal" may be more precisely defined. The *value of serial electrocardiograms* from an individual cannot be overemphasized, since serial changes best demonstrate electrocardiographic abnormalities.

Criteria for the Normal Canine Electrocardiogram†

Heart rate—60 to 160 beats per minute for adult dogs; up to 180 beats per minute in toy breeds, and 220 beats per minute for puppies.

Heart rhythm—Normal sinus rhythm; sinus arrhythmia; and wandering sinoatrial pacemaker.

P wave—Up to 0.4 millivolt in amplitude; up to 0.04 second in duration; always positive in leads II and aVF; positive or isoelectric in lead I.

P-R interval—0.06 to 0.14 second duration.

QRS complex—Mean electric axis, frontal plane, 40 to 100 degrees.

Amplitude—Maximum amplitude of R wave 2.5 to 3.0 millivolts in leads II, III, and aVF. Complex positive in leads II, III, and aVF; negative in lead V_{10}.

Duration—To 0.05 second (0.06 second in dogs over 40 lbs).

Q-T segment—0.15 to 0.22 seconds duration.

ST segment and T wave—ST segment free of marked coving (repolarization changes).

ST segment depression not greater than 0.2 millivolt.

ST segment elevation not greater than 0.15 millivolt.

T wave negative in lead V_{10}.

T wave amplitude not greater than 25 per cent of amplitude of R wave.

Criteria for the Normal Feline Electrocardiogram†

Heart rate—240 beats per minute maximum.

Heart rhythm—Normal sinus rhythm or, infrequently, sinus arrhythmia.

P wave—Positive in leads II and aVF: may be isoelectric or positive in lead I; should not exceed 0.03 second in duration.

P-R interval—0.04 to 0.08 second duration (inversely related to the heart rate).

QRS complex—More variable than in the canine; the mean electric axis in the frontal plane is often insignificant. Often the QRS complex is nearly isoelectric in all frontal plane limb leads (so-called horizontal heart).

Amplitude—The amplitude of the R wave is usually low; marked amplitude of R waves (over 0.8 millivolt) in the frontal plane leads may suggest ventricular hypertrophy.

Duration—Less than 0.04 second.

Q-T segment—0.16 to 0.18 second duration.

ST segment and T wave—ST segment and T wave should be small and free of repolarization changes as well as marked depression of elevation.

*From Ettinger, S. J., and Suter, P. F.: *Canine Cardiology.* Philadelphia: WB Saunders, 1970, pp. 102–169.
†From Ettinger, S. J.: *Textbook of Veterinary Internal Medicine*, 2nd ed. Vol. I. Philadelphia: WB Saunders, 1983, p. 984.

RECOMMENDED NUTRIENT ALLOWANCES FOR DOGS (PER LB OR KG OF BODY WEIGHT PER DAY)*

Nutrient	Per Lb	Per Kg	Nutrient	Per Lb	Per Kg
Protein (gm)	2.25	5.0	Vitamins		
Fat (gm)	0.70	1.5	Vitamin A (IU)	50	110
Linoleic acid (gm)	0.1	0.22	Vitamin D (IU)	5	11
Carbohydrate†	—	—	Vitamin E (μg)	0.55	1.2
			Thiamine (μg)	11.0	24
Minerals			Riboflavin (μg)	22.0	48
Calcium (mg)	120	265	Pyridoxine (μg)	11.0	24
Phosphorus (mg)	100	220	Pantothenic acid (μg)	100	220
Potassium (mg)	65	144	Niacin (μg)	114	250
Sodium chloride (mg)	91	200	Folic acid (μg)	1.8	4
Magnesium (mg)	6.4	14	Vitamin B_{12} (μg)	0.5	1.1
Iron (mg)	0.6	1.32	Biotin (μg)	1.0	2.2
Copper (mg)	0.07	0.16	Choline (mg)	11.8	26
Manganese (mg)	0.05	0.11			
Zinc (mg)	1.0	2.2			
Iodine (mg)	0.015	0.033			
Selenium (mg)	1.1	2.42			

*1977 modification by Cornell Research Laboratory for Diseases of Dogs; data taken from NAS-NRC Publication No. 8, Nutrient Requirements of Dogs, 1974.

†Carbohydrate as such has not been shown to be required. As a common ingredient of most dog foods, it serves as an excellent source of energy and may be required for reproduction.

From Sheffy, B. E.: Nutrition and nutritional disorders. Vet. Clin. North Am. 8:10, 1978.

CALORIC REQUIREMENTS FOR ADULT DOGS BASED ON PHYSICAL ACTIVITY AND BREED SIZE*

	Mature Weight Kg	Lb	House Dog† Calories	Active Dog‡ Calories	Working Dog§ Calories
Small Breeds	2.3	5	200	250	300
	4.5	10	400	500	600
	6.8	15	600	750	900
	9.1	20	800	1000	1200
Medium Breeds	9.1	20	560	700	840
	11.4	25	700	875	1050
	13.6	30	840	1050	1260
	15.9	35	930	1225	1470
	18.2	40	1120	1400	1680
	20.5	45	1260	1575	1890
	22.7	50	1400	1750	2100
	25.0	55	1540	1925	2310
	27.3	60	1680	2100	2520
	29.5	65	1820	2275	2730
	31.8	70	1980	2450	2940
	34.1	75	2100	2625	3150
Large Breeds	34.1	75	1800	2250	2700
	36.4	80	1980	2400	2880
	38.6	85	2040	2550	3060
	40.9	90	2160	2700	3240
	43.2	95	2280	2850	3420
	45.5	100	2400	3000	3600
	47.7	105	2520	3150	3780
	50.0	110	2640	3300	3960
	52.3	115	2760	3450	4140
	54.5	120	2880	3600	4320
	56.8	125	3000	3750	4500
	59.1	130	3120	3900	4680
	61.4	135	3240	4050	4860
	63.6	140	3360	4200	5040
	65.9	145	3480	4350	5220
	68.2	150	3600	4500	5400

*These are average daily requirements. Animal requirements may vary according to age, breed, body and environmental temperature, temperament, and degree of activity. Owing to temperament, there is some overlap between the largest animals of some breeds and the smallest of others.

†Caloric requirements of house dogs = adult dogs maintained in laboratory cages.

‡Active dogs = adult dogs allowed to free run in outside pens, 125 to 480 square feet in size.

§Working dogs = adult dogs running at 5 mph on a 6 per cent incline for 4 hours each day.

Data courtesy of Ralston Purina Company, St. Louis, Missouri.

From Kirk, R. W., and Bistner, S. I.: *Handbook of Veterinary Procedures and Emergency Treatment*, 4th ed. Philadelphia: W.B. Saunders, 1985.

RECOMMENDED DAILY CALORIC INTAKE DURING FIRST FOUR WEEKS OF LIFE

Dog			Cat (Estimated)	
Kcal/oz BW	*Kcal/gm BW*	*Week*	*Kcal/gm BW*	*Kcal/oz BW*
3.8	0.133	1	0.20	5.7
4.4	0.155	2	0.22	6.3
5.0–5.7	0.175–0.20	3	0.27	7.7
5.7+	0.20+	4	0.29	8.3

*Amount of formula per day (ml) = weight of young (in gm) times kcal factor (per gm BW) for age.

From Kirk, R. W., and Bistner, S. I.: *Handbook of Veterinary Procedures and Emergency Treatment,* 4th ed. Philadelphia: W. B. Saunders, 1985.

COMPOSITION OF MATERNAL MILK AND SUBSTITUTES

	Kcal Per ml	% Solids	Fat	Protein	Carbohydrate
Bitch milk	1.5	24.0	44.1	33.2	15.8
Esbilac powder*†	1.0	98.4	44.1	33.2	15.8
Esbilac liquid*	0.9	15.3	44.1	33.2	15.8
Cow milk	0.7	12.0	30.0	25.6	38.5
Evaporated milk‡	1.2	14.0	15.8	13.9	19.5
Cat milk	0.9	18.2	25.0	42.2	26.1
KMR*	0.9	18.2	25.0	42.2	26.1

*Manufactured by Pet-Vet Products, Borden Chemical Company, Borden, Inc., Norfolk, Virginia 23501.

†1 volume to 3 volumes water.

‡4 volumes to 1 volume water.

From Kirk, R. W., and Bistner, S. I.: *Handbook of Veterinary Procedures and Emergency Treatment,* 4th ed. Philadelphia: W. B. Saunders, 1985.

NUTRITIONAL REQUIREMENTS (AMOUNTS PER POUND OF BODY WEIGHT PER DAY) OF ADULT CATS AND 10-WEEK-OLD KITTENS*

Nutrients	Adult	Kittens
Protein (gm)†	2.9	8.6
Energy (kcal)	40.0	115.0
Fat (gm)‡	1.5	3.2
Minerals		
Calcium (mg)	90	290
Phosphorus (mg)	80	230
Magnesium (mg)	5	14
Potassium (mg)	30	90
Sodium chloride (mg)	50	140
Iron (μg)	10	30
Copper (μg)	0.5	1.4
Manganese (μg)	0.9	2.8
Zinc (μg)	3.2	8.6
Iodine (μg)	0.1	0.3
Sodium (μg)	0.01	0.03
Vitamins		
Vitamin A (IU)§	100	290
Vitamin D (IU)	10	29
Vitamin E (IU)	1	3
Thiamine (mg)	0.05	0.14
Riboflavin (mg)	0.05	0.14
Pantothenic acid (mg)	0.10	0.28
Niacin (mg)‖	0.50	1.0
Pyridoxine (μg)	45	140
Folic acid (μg)	9	30
Biotin (μg)	0.5	1
Vitamin B_{12} (μg)	0.2	0.6
Choline (mg)	20	57

*Modified by F. A. Kallfelz from Nutrient Requirements of Cats. Publication No. 13. Washington, D. C., National Academy of Sciences–National Research Council, 1978.

†In addition to the essential amino acids, the cat (particularly the growing kitten) has a requirement for the amino-sulfonic acid taurine, which is found in highest concentrations in certain seafoods. Cat foods should contain at least 0.02 per cent taurine on a dry basis.

‡Although this may represent basal fat requirements, fat enhances palatability and is found at high levels in many cat foods. The cat has an absolute requirement for arachidonic acid, which should compose 0.02–0.05 per cent of the diet on a dry basis.

§The cat cannot convert β-carotene to vitamin A and thus has an absolute requirement for this vitamin.

‖The cat cannot use tryptophan as an adequate source of niacin and must have niacin in the diet.

RECOMMENDED DAILY METABOLIZABLE ENERGY ALLOWANCES FOR CATS*

Kitten (wk of age)	Kcal/kg BW†	Adult‡	Kcal/kg BW
10	250	Inactive	70
20	130	Active	85
30	100	Gestation	100
40	80	Lactation	250

*Metabolizable energy allowances based on 4 kcal/gm of dietary protein and carbohydrate (nitrogen-free extract), and 9 kcal/gm of dietary fat. These allowances are presumed to apply in a thermoneutral environment (approximately 22°C).

†Body weight.

‡Fifty weeks of age and older.

From Nutrient Requirements of Cats. Publication No. 13. Washington, D.C., National Academy of Sciences–National Research Council, 1978.

A CATALOGUE OF CONGENITAL AND HEREDITARY DISORDERS OF DOGS (BY BREED)

Breed	Mode*	Disorders
Aberdeen terrier		Primary uterine inertia
Afghan hound	R	Cataract (bilateral)
		Elbow joint malformation
	R	Necrotizing myelopathy
Airedale terrier		Cerebellar hypoplasia
		Trembling of the hind quarters
		Umbilical hernia
Alaskan malamute		Anemia with chondrodysplasia
	R	Dwarfism
	R	Factor VII deficiency
	R	Hemeralopia
		Renal cortical hypoplasia
American foxhound		Deafness
		Microphthalmia
Antarctic husky	D	Entropion
	SLR	Hemophilia A
Australian shepherd	R	Microphthalmia and multiple colobomas
Basenji	R	Coliform enteritis
		Hemolytic anemia
		Inguinal hernia
	D	Persistent pupillary membrane
		Pyruvate kinase deficiency
		Umbilical hernia
Basset hound	D	Achondroplasia
	SLR	Anomaly of third cervical vertebra
		Inguinal hernia
	ID	Platelet disorder
		Primary glaucoma
Beagle		Atopic dermatitis
		Bladder cancer
		Bundle branch block
		Cataract (unilateral)
	D	Cataract with microphthalmia
	P	Cleft lip and palate
		Distemper
Beagle (*Continued*)	R, P	Epilepsy
	R	Factor VII deficiency
	SLR	Hemophilia A
		Hypercholesterolemia
		Intervertebral disc disease
		Lymphocytic thyroiditis
	R	Mononephrosis
		Multiple epiphyseal dysplasia
		Necrotizing panotitis
	P	Otocephalic syndrome
	R	Primary glaucoma
	P	Pulmonic stenosis
		Renal hypoplasia
	R	Retinal dysplasia
	R	Short tail
		Thyroiditis
		Unilateral kidney aplasia
Bedlington terrier		Renal cortical hypoplasia
	R	Retinal dysplasia
Bernese sennehund	P	Cleft lip and palate
Black and tan coonhound	SLR	Hemophilia B
Bloodhound		Distemper
Blue tick hound		Globoid cell leukodystrophy
Border collie		Central progressive retinal atrophy
Boston terrier		Aortic and carotid body tumors
	R	Cataract (bilateral)
		Craniomandibular osteopathy
		Hemivertebra
		Mastocytoma
		Oligodendroglioma
		Patellar luxation
		Pituitary tumor
Boxer		Abnormal dentition (extra incisor)
		Aortic and carotid body tumors
		Aortic stenosis
		Atrial septal defects

Table continued on following page

Breed	Mode*	Disorders
Boxer (*Continued*)	SLR	Cystinuria
		Dermoid cysts
		Endocardial fibroelastosis
		Fibrosarcoma
		Gingival hyperplasia
		Histiocytoma
		Intervertebral disk disease
		Mastocytoma
		Melanoma
		Oligodendroglioma
		Persistence of right venous valve
		Pulmonic stenosis
	P	Subaortic stenosis
		Superficial corneal ulcer
Brussels griffon		Short skull
Bull mastiff		Abnormal dentition (extra incisor)
Bull terrier	R	Deafness
		Inguinal hernia
		Umbilical hernia
Cairn terrier		Craniomandibular osteopathy
	SLR	Cystinuria
	R	Globoid cell leukodystrophy
	SLR	Hemophilia A
	SLR	Hemophilia B
		Inguinal hernia
Ceylon		Hairlessness
Chihuahua		Collapsed trachea
		Dislocation of the shoulder
	SLR	Hemophilia A
	R	Hydrocephalus
		Hypoplasia of dens
		Mitral valve defects
		Patellar luxation
		Pulmonic stenosis
Cocker spaniel	P	Behavioral abnormalities
	R	Cataract (bilateral)
		Cataract with microphthalmia
	P	Cleft lip and palate
	R	Cranioschisis
		Distichiasis
	D	Factor X deficiency
		Hip dysplasia
English bulldog		Abnormal dentition (extra incisor)
		Anasarca
		Arteriovenous fistula
	P	Cleft lip and palate
		Hemivertebra
	R	Hydrocephalus
		Hypoplasia of trachea
		Mitral valve defects
		Oligodendroglioma
		Predisposition to dystocia
		Pulmonic stenosis
		Short skull
	R	Short tail
		Spina bifida
English cocker spaniel	SLR	Hemophilia A
	R	Juvenile amaurotic idiocy
	R	Neuronal ceroid lipofuscinosis
English springer spaniel	D	Cutaneous asthenia
	ID	Factor XI deficiency
	R	Retinal dysplasia
Foxhound		Deafness
		Osteochondrosis of the spine
Fox terrier	R	Ataxia
		Atopic dermatitis
		Deafness
		Dislocation of the shoulder
		Esophageal achalasia
		Glaucoma
		Goiter
		Lens luxation
		Oligodontia
		Pulmonic stenosis
French bulldog		Hemivertebra
German shepherd		Atopic dermatitis
	P	Behavioral abnormalities
	D	Cataract (bilateral)
	P	Cleft lip and palate
	SLR	Cystinuria
		Dermoid cyst
		Ectasia syndrome
		Enostosis
	R, P	Epilepsy
		Esophageal achalasia
		Eversion of nictitating membrane

Breed	Inheritance	Disorder
	R	Hydrocephalus
		Inguinal hernia
		Intervertebral disk disease
		Over- and undershot jaw
	P	Patent ductus arteriosus
		Primary glaucoma
		Primary peripheral retinal dystrophy
		Renal cortical hypoplasia
		Skin neoplasms
	R	Tail abnormalities
		Umbilical hernia
	P	Ununited anconeal process
Collie		Bladder cancer
	R	Collie eye anomaly
	R	Cyclic neutropenia
		Deafness
	R, P	Epilepsy
	SLR	Hemophilia A
		Inguinal hernia
	ID	Iris heterochromia
		Microphthalmia
		Nasal solar dermatitis
		Optic nerve hypoplasia
	P	Patent ductus arteriosis
		Umbilical hernia
	D	Achondroplasia
Dachshund	P	Cleft lip and palate
	SLR	Cystinuria
		Deafness
		Diabetes mellitus
		Ectasia syndrome
		Intervertebral disk disease
	ID	Iris heterochromia
		Microphthalmia
		Osteopetrosis
		Over- and undershot jaw (long-haired Dachshund)
		Renal hypoplasia
Dalmatian		Atopic dermatitis
		Deafness
	R	Excess uric acid excretion
		Globoid cell leukodystrophy
Doberman pinscher		His bundle degeneration
		Polyostotic fibrous dysplasia
		Renal cortical hypoplasia
		Spondylolisthesis
		Liver copper storage disease
		Persistent primary hyperplastic vitreons
	SLR	Hemophilia A
	P	Hip dysplasia
	R	Pancreatic insufficiency
	P	Persistent right aortic arch
		Pituitary dwarfism
		Renal cortical hypoplasia
	P	Subaortic stenosis
	P	Ununited anconeal process
	D	Von Willebrand's disease
German short-haired pointer	R	Amaurotic idiocy
	R	Eversion of nictitating membrane
		Fibrosarcoma
	D	Lymphedema
		Melanoma
		Subaortic stenosis
Golden retriever	D	Cataract (bilateral)
		Cataract with microphthalmia
Gordon setter		Generalized progressive retinal atrophy
Great Dane	SLR	Cystinuria
		Deafness
		Eversion of nictitating membrane
	ID	Iris heterochromia
		Mitral valve defects
		Spondylolisthesis
	P	Stockard's paralysis
Great Dane × bloodhound		Paralysis of the hind limbs
Greyhound		Esophageal achalasia
	SLR	Hemophilia A
		Predisposition to dystocia
	R	Short spine
Griffon		Dislocation of the shoulder
Griffon bruxellois × dachshund		Susceptibility to rickets
Irish setter	SLR	Carpal subluxation
		Generalized myopathy
	R	Generalized progressive renal atrophy
	SLR	Hemophilia A
		Persistence of right aortic arch
	R	Quadriplegia with amblyopia
Irish terrier	SLR	Cystinuria
Jack Russell terrier		Ataxia
		Lens luxation
Keeshond	P	Conus septal defects
	R, P	Epilepsy
		Mitral valve defects
	P	Tetralogy of Fallot

Table continued on following page

Breed	Mode*	Disorders
Kerry blue		Hair follicle tumor
	P	Ununited anconeal process
King Charles spaniel		Diabetes mellitus
Labrador retriever		Carpal subluxation
	ID	Cataract (bilateral)
		Craniomandibular osteopathy
	SLR	Cystinuria
	SLR	Hemophilia A
	R	Retinal dysplasia
Labrador × American foxhound		Diaphragmatic hernia
Labrador × poodle	D	Lymphedema
Lhaso apso		Inguinal hernia
		Renal cortical hypoplasia
Mexican, Turkish, and Chinese breeds	D	Hairlessness
Miniature pinscher		Dislocation of the shoulder
Miniature poodle	R	Achondroplasia
		Cerebrospinal demyelination
	SLR	Cystinuria
		Dislocation of the shoulder
		Ectasia syndrome
		Ectodermal defect
	R	Generalized progressive retinal atrophy
		Globoid cell leukodystrophy
		Hypoplasia of dens
		Partial alopecia
		Patellar luxation
	P	Patent ductus ateriosus
Miniature schnauzer	R	Cataract (bilateral)
		Pulmonic stenosis
	D	Von Willebrand's disease
Mongrel		Black hair follicular dysplasia
	SLR	Cystinuria
		Multiple cartilaginous exostoses
Newfoundland		Eversion of nictitating membrane
	P	Subaortic stenosis
Norwegian dunkerhound		Deafness
		Microphthalmia
Norwegian elkhound	R	Generalized progressive retinal atrophy
		Keratoacanthoma
		Renal cortical hypoplasia

Breed	Mode*	Disorders
Scottish terrier		Bladder cancer
		Atopic dermatitis
		Achondroplasia
		Craniomandibular osteopathy
	SLR	Cystinuria
		Deafness
		Melanoma
		Primary uterine inertia
	R	Scottie cramp
	D	Von Willebrand's disease
Sealyham terrier		Atopic dermatitis
		Lens luxation
	R	Retinal dysplasia
Shetland sheepdog		Bladder cancer
	R	Collie eye anomaly
	SLR	Hemophilia A
		Hip dysplasia
	ID	Iris heterochromia
		Nasal solar dermatitis
	P	Patent ductus arteriosus
Shiba ina	R	Short spine
Shih tzu	P	Cleft lip and palate
		Renal cortical hypoplasia
Siberian husky	ID	Iris heterochromia
Silver grey collie		Cyclic neutropenia
	ID	Iris heterochromia
Skye terrier	R	Hypoplasia of the larynx
Springer spaniel	D	Ehlers-Danlos syndrome
	ID	Factor XI deficiency
	R	Retinal dysplasia
Staffordshire bull terrier	R	Cataract (bilateral)
	P	Cleft lip and palate
Standard poodle	R	Cataract (bilateral)
Swedish lapland	R	Neuronal abiotrophy
Swiss dogs		Generalized progressive retinal atrophy
Swiss sheepdog	P	Cleft lip and palate
Tervueren shepherd	R	Epilepsy
Toy poodle		Ectasia syndrome
		Fibrosis of the plantaris muscle
	R	Generalized progressive retinal atrophy
		Patellar luxation
	P	Patent ductus arteriosus
		Tracheal collapse

Breed	Mode*	Disorders
Old English sheepdog	R	Cataract, bilateral
Otterhound	ID	Platelet disorder
Pekingese		Distichiasis
		Hypoplasia of dens
		Inguinal hernia
		Intervertebral disk disease
		Short skull
		Trichiasis
		Umbilical hernia
Pointer		Bithoracic ectomelia
	R	Cataract (bilateral)
	R	Neuromuscular atrophy
	R	Neurotropic osteopathy
		Umbilical hernia
Pomeranian		Dislocation of the shoulder
		Hypoplasia of dens
		Patellar luxation
	P	Patent ductus arteriosus
		Tracheal collapse
Poodle (see also miniature, standard, and toy poodle)		Atopic dermatitis
	P	Behavioral abnormality
	SLR	Cystinuria
		Distichiasis
	R	Epilepsy
	P	Patent ductus arteriosus
Pug		Male pseudohermaphroditism
		Trichiasis
Rhodesian ridgeback		Dermoid sinus
Rottweiler		Diabetes mellitus
St. Bernard		Aphakia with multiple colobomas
		Dermoid cysts of cornea
		Eversion of nictitating membrane
	SLR	Hemophilia A
	SLR	Hemophilia B
	P	Stockard's paralysis
St. Bernard × Great Dane		Paralysis of the hind limbs
Samoyed		Atrial septal defects
		Diabetes mellitus
	SLR	Hemophilia A
		Pulmonic stenosis
Vizsla	SLR	Hemophilia A
Weimaraner		Eversion of nictitating membrane
		Fibrosarcoma
	SLR	Hemophilia A
		Melanoma
		Spinal dysraphism
		Umbilical hernia
Welsh corgi	SLR	Cystinuria
		Generalized progressive retinal atrophy
		Predisposition to dystocia
West Highland white terrier		Atopic dermatitis
		Craniomandibular osteopathy
	R	Globoid cell leukodystrophy
		Inguinal hernia
Whippet		Partial alopecia
Yorkshire terrier		Hypoplasia of dens
		Patellar luxation
	R	Retinal dysplasia
All breeds	D	Blood group incompatibility
Brachycephalic breeds		Pituitary cysts
		Stenotic nares and elongated soft palate
Giant breeds		Elbow dysplasia
		Hip dysplasia
		Osteogenic sarcoma
Many breeds	P	Behavioral abnormalities
	SLR	Cryptorchidism
		Demodectic mange
	D	Dewclaws
		Ectropion
		Elbow dysplasia (especially large and giant breeds)
		Entropion
		Esophageal dilation
		Hip dysplasia (especially large and giant breeds)
Many miniature breeds		Collapsed trachea
		Glycogen storage disease
		Legg-Calvé-Perthes syndrome
		Patellar luxation
		Predisposition to dystocia
		Tracheal collapse
Miscellaneous		White breed deafness

*Mode of inheritance: R = recessive; D = dominant; ID = incomplete dominance; SLR = sex-linked recessive; and P = polygenic.
Modified from Patterson, D. F.: A catalogue of genetic disorders of the dog. *In* Kirk, R. W. (ed.): *Current Veterinary Therapy VII*. Philadelphia: W. B. Saunders, 1980, with permission.

IMMUNIZATION PROCEDURES

IMMUNIZATION OF WILD ANIMAL SPECIES AGAINST COMMON DISEASES

As with domestic animals, there is no unanimous opinion as to the proper methods that should be used in immunizing wild animals. The following information represents current approaches to vaccination in managing wild species maintained in zoos or game parks. *Private ownership of wild animal species as pets is strongly discouraged! No rabies vaccine is approved for any wild species.*

FAMILY CANIDAE. Coyote, fox, jackal, wolf, dingo, cape hunting dog, and so on.

Canine distemper—infectious canine hepatitis (ICH). Administer modified live virus (MLV) vaccine as for domestic dogs. Revaccinate annually and prior to anticipated possible exposure if 6 months have elapsed since last vaccination.

Parvovirus. Canine parvovirus vaccines are being used on wild canids, but there are no data to support statements on efficacy or safety.

Rabies. No rabies vaccine is licensed for use. Limited testing indicates that wild animals have unpredictable responses to rabies vaccinations. If vaccination *must* be used in animals confined in zoos or game parks, administer only inactivated rabies vaccine.

FAMILY FELIDAE. Tiger, leopard, lion, cheetah, jaguar, lynx, ocelot, margay, bobcat, mountain lion, jungle cat, golden cat, and so on.

Feline panleukopenia. Wild felids appear to be exquisitely susceptible to the feline panleukopenia virus. Proper and adequate vaccination is a *must!*

Vaccinate with MLV vaccine containing rhinotracheitis and calicivirus vaccines. Begin vaccination when the animal is 6 to 8 weeks of age, and repeat two or three times at 4-week intervals. Revaccinate adults at 12-month intervals. Use manufacturers' recommendations.

Pneumonitis. The use of MLV pneumonitis vaccine is definitely an *elective procedure* and cannot be recommended as a routine procedure for the individual cat. Pneumonitis vaccine might best be administered to wild felids with anticipated exposure to other domestic or wild felids (such as at cat shows). In this situation, the vaccine should be administered 10 to 14 days prior to anticipated exposure.

Rabies. No rabies vaccine is licensed for use. Limited testing indicates that wild animals have unpredictable responses to rabies vaccinations. If vaccination *must* be used in animals confined in zoos or game parks, administer only inactivated rabies vaccine.

FAMILY PROCYONIDAE. Lesser panda, raccoon, coatimundi, and kinkajou.

Canine distemper. MLV vaccine may be administered according to the manufacturers' recommendations. Adults should be revaccinated annually.

Infectious canine hepatitis. Limited data available; inapparent infection may occur in raccoons. No recommendations.

Feline panleukopenia. Although proven cases have been reported only in the raccoon and the coatimundi, the current trend is to vaccinate all captive members of the family Procyonidae. MLV vaccine may be used according to the manufacturers' recommendations. Adults should be revaccinated every 12 months.

Pneumonitis. Elective procedure as per family Felidae.

Rabies. No rabies vaccine is licensed for use. Limited testing indicates that wild animals have unpredictable responses to rabies vaccinations. If vaccination *must* be used in animals confined in zoos or game parks, administer only inactivated rabies vaccine.

FAMILY VIVERRIDAE. Binturong, fossa, linsang, mongoose, and civet.

Canine distemper. Cases of proven canine distemper have been reported in the biturong and civet. It is suggested that all captive viverrids be vaccinated for canine distemper as per the family Canidae.

Infectious canine hepatitis. No data available.

Feline panleukopenia. Cases are poorly documented, but it has been recommended that at least the binturong if not all captive viverrids be vaccinated for feline panleukopenia as per the family Felidae.

Rabies. No rabies vaccine is licensed for use. Limited testing indicates that wild animals have unpredictable responses to rabies vaccinations. If vaccination *must* be used in animals confined in zoos or game parks, administer only inactivated rabies vaccine.

FAMILY URSIDAE. Bears.

Canine distemper. Although several species of

*See also compendia on rabies, canine, and feline vaccines, which follow.

From Kirk, R. W., and Bistner, S. I.: *Handbook of Veterinary Procedures and Emergency Treatment,* 4th ed. Philadelphia: W. B. Saunders, 1985.

bears are reported to be susceptible to canine distemper, bears are not routinely vaccinated at zoos. In some cases it may be advisable to use MLV vaccine as per family Canidae.

Infectious canine hepatitis. Infection of bears with ICH has been described but not confirmed. No recommendations.

Feline panleukopenia. Cases of panleukopenia (not verified by virus isolation) have been reported in young bear cubs. No recommendations can be given at this time as to the advisability of vaccinating bears for feline panleukopenia.

Rabies. No rabies vaccine is licensed for use. Limited testing indicates that wild animals have unpredictable responses to rabies vaccinations. If vaccination *must* be used in animals confined in zoos or game parks, administer only inactivated rabies vaccine.

FAMILY HYAENIDAE. Hyenas.

Canine distemper. All species of hyena are susceptible and should be vaccinated for canine distemper as per family Canidae.

Infectious canine hepatitis. No data available.

Rabies. No rabies vaccine is licensed for use. Limited testing indicates that wild animals have unpredictable responses to rabies vaccinations. If vaccination *must* be used in animals confined in zoos or game parks, administer only inactivated rabies vaccine.

FAMILY MUSTELIDAE. Ferret, mink, otter, skunk, wolverine, badger, marten, sable, grison, and fisher.

Canine distemper. The mink, ferret, and skunk are susceptible, and probably all captive mustelids should be vaccinated for canine distemper using an MLV vaccine as per family Canidae.

Infectious canine hepatitis. Limited data available. No recommendations.

Viral enteritis (may be variant of feline panleukopenia). Mink only. Administer autogenous or commercial mink enteritis formalized vaccine or killed feline panleukopenia virus vaccine. Kits, 6 to 8 weeks of age; adults should be revaccinated annually. Follow manufacturers' recommendations.

Feline panleukopenia. It has been suggested that all mustelids except the ferret are susceptible to feline panleukopenia and should receive vaccine as per the family Felidae. Mink should receive either killed panleukopenia vaccine or formalized mink enteritis vaccine. They need not receive both.

Botulism (mink and ferret). *Clostridium botulinum* type C toxoid. Kits can be vaccinated at 10 to 12 weeks of age; adults should be revaccinated yearly.

Rabies. No rabies vaccine is licensed for use. Limited testing indicates that wild animals have unpredictable responses to rabies vaccinations. If vaccination *must* be used in animals confined in zoos or game parks, administer only inactivated rabies vaccine.

ORDER MARSUPIALIA, FAMILY DIDELPHIDAE. Opossum.

The opossum is highly resistant to infection by canine distemper and rabies and probably does not need to be vaccinated for these diseases.

ORDER PRIMATES. Subhuman.

Poliomyelitis (apes only—gorilla, orangutan, chimpanzee, and gibbon). Live oral polio virus vaccine. Adults, one 12-month booster with trivalent vaccine. Initial dose, a child's dose of trivalent vaccine administered twice at 6- to 8-week intervals.

Rabies. No rabies vaccine is licensed for use. Limited testing indicates that wild animals have unpredictable responses to rabies vaccinations. If vaccination *must* be used in animals confined in zoos or game parks, administer only inactivated rabies vaccine.

Tuberculosis (immunization not recommended). Susceptible nonhuman primates should be subjected to periodic tuberculin tests and either eliminated or vigorously treated with appropriate medication if found to be positive. Test procedure (WHO recommendations): Koch's Old Tuberculin (full strength) 0.1 cc. *intradermally* in the upper eyelid. Read test at 24, 48, and 72 hours postinjection; positive test is characterized by swelling and erythema with closure of the eye. Should have three successive negative tests at 2-week intervals.

Measles, smallpox, and similar diseases. Vaccination of primates (especially apes) against the common childhood diseases is an elective procedure and depends on the degree of exposure to which the primate may be subjected. Consult with a pediatrician on the choice of immunizing agent(s).

Hepatitis. Where the possibility of disease exists or where there is known exposure to a hepatitis patient, gamma globulin IM may be administered prophylactically.

ORDER RODENTIA. Mouse, rat, hamster, gerbil, guinea pig, and squirrel.

Rabies. Vaccination is not recommended for these animals if they remain caged.

Ectromelia (mice and rats). Routine vaccination is not recommended, because this viral disease does not appear to be a problem in the United States.

ORDER LAGAMORPHA. Rabbit and hare.

See order *Rodentia.*

References and Supplemental Readings

Fowler, M. E.: Immunoprophylaxis in nondomestic carnivores. *In* Kirk, R. W. (ed.): *Current Veterinary Therapy VIII.* Philadelphia, W. B. Saunders Company, 1983, p. 1129.

Compendium of Animal Rabies Vaccines, 1986*

Prepared by The National Association of State Public Health Veterinarians, Inc.

Part I: Recommendations for Immunization Procedures

The purpose of these recommendations is to provide information on rabies vaccines to practicing veterinarians, public health officials, and others concerned with rabies control. This document will serve as the basis for animal rabies vaccination programs throughout the United States. Its adoption will result in standardization of procedures among jurisdictions, which is necessary for an effective national rabies control program. These recommendations are reviewed and revised as necessary prior to the beginning of each calendar year. All animal rabies vaccines licensed by the USDA and marketed in the United States are listed in Part II of the Compendium, and Part III describes the principles of rabies control.

A. **VACCINE ADMINISTRATION:** It is recommended that all animal rabies vaccines be restricted to use by or under the supervision of a veterinarian.

B. **VACCINE SELECTION:** The use of vaccines with three-year duration of immunity is recommended since their use constitutes the most effective method in increasing the proportion of immunized dogs and cats in comprehensive rabies control programs.

C. **ROUTE OF INOCULATION:** Unless otherwise specified by the product label or package insert, all vaccines must be administered intramuscularly at one site in the thigh.

D. **WILDLIFE VACCINATION:** Vaccination is not recommended since no rabies vaccine is licensed for use in wild animals and since there is no evidence that any vaccine will protect wild animals against rabies. It is recommended that neither wild nor exotic animals be kept as pets. Offspring born to wild animals bred with domestic dogs or cats will be considered as wild animals.

E. **ACCIDENTAL HUMAN EXPOSURE TO VACCINE:** Accidental inoculation may occur in individuals during administration of animal rabies vaccine. Such exposure to inactivated vaccines constitutes **no known** rabies hazard. There have been no cases of rabies resulting from needle or other exposure to a licensed modified-live-virus vaccine in the United States.

F. **IDENTIFICATION OF VACCINATED DOGS:** It is recommended that all agencies and veterinarians adopt the standard tag system. This will aid the administration of local, state, national and international procedures. Dog license tags should not conflict in shape and color with rabies tags. It is recommended that anodized aluminum rabies tags should not be less than 0.064″ in thickness.

1. *RABIES TAGS.*

CALENDAR YEAR	COLOR	SHAPE
1986	Orange	Fireplug
1987	Green	Bell
1988	Red	Heart
1989	Blue	Rosette

2. *RABIES CERTIFICATE:* All agencies and veterinarians should use the NASPHV form #50 Rabies Vaccination Certificate, which can be obtained from vaccine manufacturers.

THE NASPHV COMPENDIUM COMMITTEE
Melvin K. Abelseth, DVM, PhD, Chairman
Russell W. Currier, DVM, MPH
John I. Freeman, DVM, MPH
Russell J. Martin, DVM, MPH
Grayson B. Miller, Jr., MD
James M. Shuler, DVM, MPH
R. Keith Sikes, DVM, MPH

*Address all correspondence to:
Melvin K. Abelseth, DVM, PhD
Bureau of Communicable Disease Control
New York State Department of Health
Empire State Plaza, Corning Tower, Room 651
Albany, NY 12237

CONSULTANTS TO THE COMMITTEE
Leslie Paul Williams, Jr., DVM, Dr. PH AVMA Council on Public Health and Regulatory Veterinary Medicine
Kenneth L. Crawford, DVM, MPH
David A. Espeseth, DVM, Veterinary Biologics Staff, APHIS, USDA
Howard Koonse, Representative, Veterinary Biological Section, Animal Health Institute
Suzanne Jenkins, VMD, MPH, CDC, PHS, HHS

ENDORSED BY:
Conference of State and Territorial Epidemiologists
AVMA Council on Public Health and Regulatory Veterinary Medicine

Part II: Vaccines Marketed in the United States, and NASPHV Recommendations

PRODUCT NAME	PRODUCED BY	MARKETED BY	FOR USE IN[1]	DOSAGE[2]	AGE AT PRIMARY VACCINATION[3]	BOOSTER RECOMMENDED
A) MODIFIED LIVE VIRUS						
ENDURALL-R	NORDEN License No. 189	Norden	Dogs	1 ml	3 mos. & 1 yr. later	Triennially
			Cats	1 ml	3 months	Annually
NEUROGEN-TC	BOEHRINGER INGELHEIM License No. 124	Bio-Ceutic	Dogs	1 ml	3 mos. & 1 yr. later	Triennially
B) INACTIVATED						
TRIMUNE	FORT DODGE License No. 112	Ft. Dodge	Dogs Cats	1 ml 1 ml	3 mos. & 1 yr. later	Triennially Triennially
ANNUMUNE	FORT DODGE License No. 112	Ft. Dodge	Dogs Cats	1 ml 1 ml	3 months 3 months	Annually Annually
BIORAB-1	DOUGLAS License No. 165-B	Schering Veterinary and Tech/America	Dogs Cats	1 ml 1 ml	3 months 3 months	Annually Annually
BIORAB-3	DOUGLAS License No. 165-B	Schering Veterinary and Tech/America	Dogs	1 ml	3 mos. & 1 yr. later	Triennially
			Cats	1 ml	3 months	Annually
RABMUNE 3	DOUGLAS License No. 165-B	Beecham	Dogs	1 ml	3 mos. & 1 yr. later	Triennially
			Cats	1 ml	3 months	Annually
DURA-RAB 1	Wildlife Vaccines Inc. KUNZ-TEBBIT License No. 277	Wildlife Vaccines & Kunz-Tebbit	Dogs Cats	1 ml 1 ml	3 months 3 months	Annually Annually
RABCINE	BEECHAM License No. 225	Beecham	Dogs Cats	1 ml 1 ml	3 months 3 months	Annually Annually
ENDURALL-K	NORDEN License No. 189	Norden	Dogs Cats	1 ml 1 ml	3 months 3 months	Annually Annually
RABGUARD-TC	NORDEN License No. 189	Norden	Dogs Cats	1 ml 1 ml	3 mos. & 1 yr. later	Triennially Triennially
			Sheep Cattle Horses	1 ml 1 ml 1 ml	3 months 3 months 3 months	Annually Annually Annually
CYTORAB	COOPERS ANIMAL HEALTH INC. License No. 107	Coopers	Dogs Cats	1 ml 1 ml	3 months 3 months	Annually Annually
TRIRAB	COOPERS ANIMAL HEALTH INC. License No. 107	Coopers Durvet	Dogs	1 ml	3 mos. & 1 yr. later	Triennially
			Cats	1 ml	3 months	Annually
RABVAC 1	FROMM License No. 195-A	Fromm	Dogs Cats	1 ml 1 ml	3 months 3 months	Annually Annually
RABVAC 3	FROMM License No. 195-A	Fromm	Dogs Cats	1 ml 1 ml	3 mos. & 1 yr. later	Triennially Triennially
IMRAB	MERIEUX License No. 298	Pitman-Moore	Dogs Cats Sheep	1 ml 1 ml 1 ml	3 mos. & 1 yr. later	Triennially Triennially Triennially
			Cattle Horses	2 ml 2 ml	3 months 3 months	Annually Annually
IMRAB-1	MERIEUX License No. 298	Pitman-Moore	Dogs Cats	1 ml 1 ml	3 months 3 months	Annually Annually
C) COMBINATION						
ECLIPSE 3 KP-R	FROMM License No. 195-A	Fromm	Cats	1 ml	3 months	Annually
ECLIPSE 4 KP-R	FROMM License No. 195-A	Fromm	Cats	1 ml	3 months	Annually
CYTORAB RCP	COOPERS ANIMAL HEALTH INC. License No. 107	Coopers	Cats	1 ml	3 months	Annually
FEL-O-VAX PCT-R	FORT DODGE License No. 112	Ft. Dodge	Cats	1 ml	3 mos. & 1 yr. later	Triennially

1. Refers only to domestic species of this class of animals.
2. All vaccines must be administered intramuscularly at one site in the thigh unless otherwise specified by the label.
3. Three months of age (or older) and revaccinated one year later.

Part III: Principles of Rabies Control

These guidelines have been prepared by the National Association of State Public Health Veterinarians (NASPHV) for use by government officials, practicing veterinarians and others who may become involved in certain aspects of rabies control. It is intended that the NASPHV will annually review and revise these recommendations as necessary. Standardized control procedures are needed to deal effectively with the public health aspects of rabies.

A. PRINCIPLES OF RABIES CONTROL

1. *THE DISEASE IN HUMANS:* Rabies in humans can be prevented by eliminating exposure to rabid animals, and prompt local wound treatment and immunization when exposed. Current recommendations of the Immunization Practices Advisory Committee (Rabies) for pre-exposure and post-exposure prophylaxis are suggested for attending physicians. These recommendations, along with the current status of animal rabies in the region and information concerning the availability of rabies biologics, are available from state health departments.

2. *DOMESTIC ANIMALS:* Local governments should initiate and maintain effective programs to remove stray and unwanted animals and ensure vaccination of all dogs and cats. Since cat rabies cases now exceed the annually reported cases in dogs, immunization of cats should be required. Such procedures in the United States have reduced laboratory-confirmed rabies cases in dogs from 8,000 in 1947 to 97 in 1984. The recommended vaccination procedures and the licensed animal vaccines are specified in Parts I and II of the NASPHV's annually released Compendium.

3. *RABIES IN WILDLIFE:* The control of rabies in foxes, skunks, raccoons, and other terrestrial animals is very difficult. Selective reduction of these populations when indicated may be useful, but the utility of this procedure depends heavily upon the circumstances surrounding each rabies outbreak (See C. Control Methods in Wild Animals).

B. CONTROL METHODS IN DOMESTIC AND CONFINED ANIMALS

1. *PRE-EXPOSURE VACCINATION AND MANAGEMENT*
Animal rabies vaccines, because of species limitations, techniques and tolerances, should be administered only by or under the direct supervision of a veterinarian. Within one month after vaccination, a peak rabies antibody titer is reached and the animal can be considered to be immunized. (See Parts I and II of the Compendium for recommended vaccines and procedures.)

(a) DOGS AND CATS
All dogs and cats should be vaccinated against rabies commencing at three months of age and revaccinated in accordance with Part II of this Compendium.

(b) LIVESTOCK
It is not economically feasible, nor is it justified from a public health standpoint, to vaccinate all livestock against rabies. Owners of valuable animals, and veterinary clinicians, may consider immunizing certain livestock located in areas where wildlife rabies is epizootic.

(c) OTHER ANIMALS

(1) *Animals Maintained in Exhibits and in Zoological Parks*
Captive animals not completely excluded from all contact with local vectors of rabies can become infected with rabies. Moreover, such animals may be incubating rabies when captured. Exhibit animals, especially those carnivores and omnivores having contact with the viewing public, should be quarantined for a minimum of 180 days. Since there is no rabies vaccine licensed for use in wild animals, vaccination even with inactivated vaccine is not recommended. Pre-exposure rabies immunization of animal workers at such facilities is recommended to protect the workers and to reduce the need for euthanasia of valuable animals for rabies testing after they have bitten a handler.

(2) *Wild Animals*
Because of the existing risk of rabies in wild animals such as raccoons, skunks and foxes, the AVMA, the NASPHV and the Conference of State and Territorial Epidemiologists strongly recommend the enactment of state laws prohibiting the interstate and intrastate importation, distribution and relocation of wild animals and wild animals crossbred to domestic dogs and cats. Further, these same organizations continue to recommend the enactment of laws prohibiting the distribution or keeping of wild animals as pets.

2. *STRAY ANIMAL CONTROL*
Stray dogs or cats should be removed from the community, especially in rabies-epizootic areas. Local health department and animal control officials can enforce the pickup of strays more efficiently if owned animals are confined or kept on leash when not confined. Strays should be impounded for at least three days to give owners sufficient time to reclaim animals apprehended as strays and to determine if human exposure has occurred.

3. *QUARANTINE*

(a) INTERNATIONAL. Present regulations (CFR No. 71154) governing the importation of wild and domesticated felines, canines, and other potential vectors of rabies are minimal for preventing the introduction of rabid animals into the United States. All dogs and cats imported from countries with endemic rabies should be vaccinated against rabies at least 30 days prior to entry into the United States. The Centers for Disease Control (CDC) are responsible for these animals imported into the United States. Their requirements should be coordinated with interstate shipment requirements. The health authority of the state of destination should be notified within 72 hours of any animal conditionally admitted into its jurisdiction.

The conditional admission into the United States of such animals must be subject to state and local laws governing rabies. Failure to comply with these requirements should be promptly reported to the director of the CDC.

(b) INTERSTATE. Prior to interstate shipment, dogs and cats should be vaccinated against rabies according to the Compendium's recommendations and preferably shall be vaccinated at least 30 days prior to shipment. While in shipment, they should be accompanied by a currently valid NASPHV Form #50 Rabies Vaccination Certificate. One copy of the certificate should be mailed to the appropriate Public Health Veterinarian or State Veterinarian of the state of destination.

(c) HEALTH CERTIFICATES. If a certificate is required for dogs and cats in transit, it must not replace the NASPHV rabies vaccination certificate.

4. *ADJUNCT PROCEDURES*

Methods or procedures which enhance rabies control include:

(a) LICENSURE. Registration or licensure of all dogs and cats may be used as a means of rabies control by controlling the stray animal population. Frequently a fee is charged for such licensure and revenues collected are used to maintain a rabies or animal control program. Vaccination is usually recommended as a prerequisite to licensure.

(b) CANVASSING OF AREA.This includes house-to-house calls by members of the animal control program to enforce vaccination and licensure requirements.

(c) CITATIONS. These are legal summonses issued to owners for violations including the failure to vaccinate or license their animals.

(d) LEASH LAWS. All communities should adopt leash laws which can be incorporated in their animal control ordinances.

5. *POST-EXPOSURE MANAGEMENT*

ANY DOMESTIC ANIMAL THAT IS BITTEN OR SCRATCHED BY A BAT OR BY A WILD, CARNIVOROUS MAMMAL WHICH IS NOT AVAILABLE FOR TESTING SHOULD BE REGARDED AS HAVING BEEN EXPOSED TO A RABID ANIMAL.

(a) When bitten by a rabid animal, unvaccinated dogs and cats should be destroyed immediately. If the owner is unwilling to have this done, the unvaccinated animal should be placed in strict isolation for six months and vaccinated one month before being released. Dogs and cats that are currently vaccinated should be revaccinated immediately and observed by the owner for 90 days.

(b) *Livestock.* All species of livestock are susceptible to rabies infection; cattle appear to be among the most susceptible of all domestic animal species. Livestock known to have been bitten by rabid animals should be destroyed (slaughtered) immediately. If the owner is unwilling to have this done, the animal should be kept under very close observation for six months.

The following are recommendations for owners of livestock exposed to rabid animals:

(1) If slaughtered within seven days of being bitten, tissues may be eaten without risk of infection, providing liberal portions of the exposed area are discarded. Federal meat inspectors will reject for slaughter any animal that has been exposed to rabies within eight months.

(2) No tissues or secretions from a clinically rabid animal should be used for human or animal consumption. However, as pasteurization temperatures will inactivate rabies virus, the drinking of pasteurized milk or eating of completely cooked meat does not constitute a rabies exposure.

C. CONTROL METHODS IN WILD ANIMALS

Bats and wild carnivorous mammals, as well as wild animals crossbred with domestic dogs and cats, that bite people should be killed and appropriate tissues should be sent to the laboratory for examination for rabies. A person bitten by a bat or any wild animal should immediately report the incident to a physician who can evaluate the need for antirabies treatment (See current Rabies Prophylaxis Recommendations of the Immunization Practices Advisory Committee: Rabies.)

1. *TERRESTRIAL MAMMALS*

Continuous and persistent government-funded programs for trapping or poisoning wildlife as a means of rabies control are not cost-effective in reducing wildlife reservoirs or rabies incidence on a statewide basis. However, limited control in high-contact areas (picnic grounds, camps, suburban areas) may be indicated for the removal of selected high-risk species of wild animals. The public should be warned not to handle wild animals. The state wildlife agency should be consulted early to manage any elimination programs in coordination with the state health department.

2. *BATS*

(a) Rabid bats have been reported from every state except Hawaii, and have caused human rabies infections in the United States. It is neither feasible nor practical, however, to control rabies in bats by areawide bat population reduction programs.

(b) Bats should be eliminated from houses and surrounding structures to prevent direct association with people. Such structures should then be made bat-proof by sealing routes of entrance with screen or other means.

COMPENDIUM OF CANINE VACCINES, 1985

FREDRIC W. SCOTT, D.V.M.
Ithaca, New York

Vaccine Name	Manufacturer	Type	Vaccine Components									
			CDV	*CA1*	*CA2*	*CPI*	*Lep*	*Bor*	*Rab*	*MV*	*CPV*	*FPV*
Adenomune-7L	TechAmerica	A/I	x	x	x(i)	x	x(i)					x
Adenomune-7	TechAmerica	A/I	x	x	x(i)	x	x(i)					x(i)
Annumune	Fort Dodge	I							x			
Biorab-1	Schering	I							x			
Biorab-3	Schering	I (3)							x			
Bronchicine	TechAmerica	I						x				
Canine Distemper-Hepatitis	Colorado Serum	A	x	x								
Canine Distemper-Hepatitis-Leptospira	Colorado Serum	A/I	x	x			x(i)					
Cytorab	Coopers	I							x			
D-Vac-6	Bio-Ceutic	A/I	x	x		x	x(i)				x	
D-Vac-M	Bio-Ceutic	A								x		
Duramune DHLP + PV	Fort Dodge	A/I	x	x		x	x(i)				x	
Duramune-DA$_2$P + PV	Fort Dodge	A	x		x	x					x	
Duramune-PV	Fort Dodge	A									x	
Dura-Rab 1	TechAmerica	I							x			
Endurall-K	Norden	I							x			
Endurall-R	Norden	A (3)							x			
EPIvaxine DA$_2$P	Coopers	A	x		x	x						
EPIvaxine DA$_2$PPv	Coopers	A/I	x		x	x					x(i)	
EPIvaxine DA$_2$PL	Coopers	A/I	x		x	x	x(i)					
EPIvaxine DA$_2$PPvL	Coopers	A/I	x		x	x	x(i)				x(i)	
ERA Strain Rabies	Coopers	A							x			
Fromm D	Fromm	A	x									
Galaxy DA$_2$	Fromm	A	x		x							
Galaxy DA$_2$PL	Fromm	A/I	x		x	x	x(i)					
Galaxy VI	Fromm	A/I	x		x	x	x(i)					x(i)
Galaxy VI MHP	Fromm	A	x		x	x					x	
Galaxy VI MHP-L	Fromm	A/I	x		x	x	x(i)				x	
Galaxy VI MP	Fromm	A	x		x	x						x
Galaxy VI MP-L	Fromm	A/I	x		x	x	x(i)					x
Imrab	Pitman-Moore	I (3)							x			
Imrab 1	Pitman-Moore	I							x			
Intra-Trac-II	Schering	A (1)				x		x				
Leptobac	Fromm	I					x					
Leptoferm C-I	Norden	I					x					
Naramune 2	Bio-Ceutic	A				x		x				
Neurogen-TC	Bio-Ceutic	A (3)							x			
Paramune V	TechAmerica	A/I	x	x		x	x(i)					
Paramune VI	TechAmerica	A/I	x	x		x	x(i)					x(i)
Parvac	Fromm	I										x
Parvocine	TechAmerica	I										x
Parvocine-MLV	TechAmerica	A										x
Parvoid	Fromm	A										x

Vaccine Name	Manufacturer	Type	Vaccine Components									
			CDV	*CA1*	*CA2*	*CPI*	*Lep*	*Bor*	*Rab*	*MV*	*CPV*	*FPV*
Parvoid II	Fromm	A									x	
Quantum 4	Pitman-Moore	A	x	x		x					x	
Quantum 6	Pitman-Moore	A/I	x	x		x	x(i)				x	
Rabcine	Beecham	I							x			
Rabguard-TC	Norden	I (3)							x			
Rabies Vacc	Guardian	I							x			
Rabvac 1	Fromm	I							x			
Rabvac 3	Fromm	I (3)							x			
Sentrypar	Beecham	A									x	
Sentryvac-DHP	Beecham	A	x	x		x					x	
Sentryvac-DHP/L	Beecham	A/I	x	x		x	x(i)				x	
Tissuvax 5	Pitman-Moore	A/I	x	x		x	x(i)				x	
Tissuvax 6	Pitman-Moore	A/I	x	x		x	x(i)					x
Trimune	Fort Dodge	I							x			
Trirab	Coopers	I(3)							x			
Unirab	Bio-Ceutic	A							x			
Vanguard CVP (ML)	Norden	A									x	
Vanguard CPV (killed)	Norden	I									x	
Vanguard D-M	Norden	A	x							x		
Vanguard DA_2	Norden	A	x		x							
Vanguard DA_2L	Norden	A/I	x		x		x(i)					
Vanguard DA_2P	Norden	A	x		x	x						
Vanguard DA_2P+CPV	Norden	A	x		x	x					x	
Vanguard DA_2PL	Norden	A/I	x		x	x	x(i)					
Vanguard DA_2MP	Norden	A	x		x	x				x		
Vanguard DA_2PL + CPV	Norden	A/I	x		x	x	x(i)				x	
Vanguard DMP	Norden	A	x			x				x		
Vovax	Coopers	I									x	

A = Attenuated (modified live virus or MLV)
I = Inactivated (killed)
A/I = Combination of attenuated and inactivated
(i) = Inactivated components of mixed attenuated and inactivated vaccine
Bor = *Bordetella bronchiseptica*
CA1 = Canine adenovirus-1 (infectious canine hepatitis)
CA2 = Canine adenovirus-2
CDV = Canine distemper virus
CPI = Canine parainfluenza
CPV = Canine parvovirus
FPV = Feline parvovirus (feline panleukopenia)
Lep = Leptospirosis (usually *L. canicola* plus *L. icterohaemorrhagica*)
MV = Measles virus
Rab = Rabies virus

(1) = Intranasal administration
(3) = Administered triennially

Modified from *Veterinary Pharmaceuticals and Biologicals*, 4th ed. Edwardsville, KS: 1982–1983, Veterinary Medicine Publishing Co., 1985/1986; and *Compendium of Animal Rabies Vaccines*, 1985.

COMPENDIUM OF FELINE VACCINES, 1985

FREDRIC W. SCOTT, D.V.M.
Ithaca, New York

Vaccine Name	Manufacturer	Type	Vaccine Components					
			FPV	*FVR*	*FCV*	*FP_n*	*Rabies*	*FeLV*
Annumune	Fort Dodge	I					x	
Biorab-1	Schering	I					x	
Biorab-3	Schering	I					x	
Cytorab	Coopers	I					x	
Cytorab RCP	Coopers	A/I	x	x	x		x(i)	
Dura-Rab I	TechAmerica	I					x	
Eclipse I	Fromm	A	x					
Eclipse I-KP	Fromm	I	x					
Eclipse III	Fromm	A	x	x	x			
Eclipse III-KP	Fromm	A/I	x(i)	x	x			
Eclipse III-KP-R	Fromm	A/I	x(i)	x	x		x(i)	
Eclipse IV	Fromm	A	x	x	x	x		
Eclipse IV-KP	Fromm	A/I	x(i)	x	x	x		
Eclipse IV-KP-R	Fromm	A/I	x(i)	x	x	x	x(i)	
Endurall-K	Norden	I					x	
Endurall-R	Norden	A					x	
Epifel RCP	Coopers	A/I	x(i)	x	x			
Fel-O-Vax PCT	Fort Dodge	I	x	x	x			
Fel-O-Vax PCT-R	Fort Dodge	I (3)	x	x	x		x	
Felipan	Coopers	I	x					
Felocell CVR	Norden	A	x	x	x			
Felocine	Norden	I	x					
Felomune CVR	Norden	A (1)		x	x			
FVR C-P	Pitman-Moore	A/I	x(i)	x	x			
FVR C-P (MLV)	Pitman-Moore	A	x	x	x			
Imrab-1	Pitman-Moore	I					x	
Imrab	Pitman-Moore	I (3)					x	
Leukocell	Norden	I						x
Panacine	Beecham	A	x					
Panacine RC	Beecham	A	x	x	x			
Panagen	Pitman-Moore	I	x					
Panavac	Beecham	I	x					
Panavac RC	Beecham	A/I	x(i)	x	x			
Premune RC/KP	Coopers	A/I	x(i)	x	x			
Premune RCN/KP	Coopers	A/I	x(i)	x	x	x		
Premune RCP	Coopers	A	x	x	x			
Premune RCPN	Coopers	A	x	x	x	x		
Psittacoid	Fromm	A				x		

Table continued on opposite page

Vaccine Name	Manufacturer	Type	Vaccine Components					
			FPV	*FVR*	*FCV*	*FP_n*	*Rabies*	*FeLV*
Rabcine	Beecham	I					x	
Rabguard-TC	Norden	I (3)					x	
Rabvac 1	Fromm	I					x	
Rabvac 3	Fromm	I (3)					x	
Respomune CP	TechAmerica	A/I	x(i)	x	x			
Rhinolin-CP	Bio-Ceutic	A (1)	x	x	x			
Rhinopan KP	TechAmerica	I	x	x	x			
Rhinopan MLV	TechAmerica	A	x	x	x			
Trimune	Fort Dodge	I (3)					x	
Trirab	Coopers	I					x	

A = Attenuated (modified live virus or MLV)
I = Inactivated (killed)
A/I = Combination of attenuated and inactivated
(i) = Inactivated component of mixed attenuated and inactivated vaccine
FPV = Feline parvovirus (panleukopenia)
FVR = Feline viral rhinotracheitis
FCV = Feline calicivirus
FeLV = Feline leukemia virus
FP_n = Feline pneumonitis (chlamydia)

(1) = Intranasal administration
(3) = Triennial booster after primary vaccination at 3 months and 1 year later

Modified from *Veterinary Pharmaceuticals and Biologicals*, 4th ed. Edwardsville, KS: 1982/1983, Veterinary Medicine Publishing Co., 1985/1986; and *Compendium of Animal Rabies Vaccines*, 1985.

TABLE OF COMMON DRUGS: APPROXIMATE DOSES

Drug Name	Dog	Cat
Acetazolamide	10 mg/kg q6h PO	Same
Acetylcysteine (Mucomyst)	*Eye:* Dilute to 2% of soln with artificial tears and apply topically q2h to eye for maximum of 48 h *Respiratory:* 50 ml/h for 30–60 min q12h by nebulization	Same
Acetylpromazine (acepromazine)	0.055–0.11 mg/kg IV, IM, SC 0.55–2.2 mg/kg PO	0.055–0.11 mg/kg IM, SC 1.1–2.2 mg/kg PO
Acetylsalicylic acid (aspirin)	*Analgesia:* 10 mg/kg q12h PO *Antirheumatic:* 40 mg/kg q18h PO or 25 mg/kg q8h	*Analgesia:* 10 mg/kg q52h PO *Antirheumatic:* 40 mg/kg q72h
ACTH	2 units/kg/day IM (therapeutic) or 20 units/dog IM (response test; take post sample in 2 hr)	10 units/cat IM (response test)
Actinomycin D (Cosmegen)	0.015 mg/kg/once daily for 5 days	None
Aldactone (spironolactone)	1–2 mg/kg q12h	Same
Allopurinol (Zyloprim)	10 mg/kg q8h PO, then reduce to 10 mg/kg PO daily	None
Amatraz (Mitaban)	10.6 ml in 2 gallons water, dip q2wk for 3 treatments, let dry on	None
Amforol	2–6 tablets/9 kg initially *Maintenance:* 1–3 tabs/9 kg q8h	None
Amikacin	5 mg/kg q8H IM, IV	None
Aminophylline	10 mg/kg q8h PO, IM, IV	6.6 mg/kg q12h PO
Ammonium chloride	100 mg/kg q12h PO	¼ tsp powder/feeding
Amoxicillin	22 mg/kg q12h PO	Same
Amphetamine	4.4 mg/kg IV, IM	Same
Amphotericin B	0.15–1.0 mg/kg dissolved in 5–20 ml 5% dextrose and water given rapidly IV 3 times weekly for 2–4 mo; do not exceed 2.0 ml/kg; pretreat with antiemetics if needed; monitor BUN.	Same
Ampicillin (Polyflex, Princillin)	10–20 mg/kg q6h PO; 5–10 mg/kg q6h IV, IM, SC	Same
Amprolium	100–200 mg/kg/day in food or water for 7–10 days	None
Anterior pituitary gonadotropin	*Bitches:* 100–500 units once daily to effect	None
Apomorphine	0.02 mg/kg IV or 0.04 mg/kg SC; ¼–½ tablet in conjunctival sac, flush once emesis begins	None
Ascorbic acid (vitamin C)	100–500 mg/day (maintenance) or 100–500 mg q8h (urine acidifier)	100 mg/day (maintenance) or 100 mg q8h (urine acidifier)
L-Asparaginase	10,000–20,000 IU/M² weekly IP or 400 IU/kg weekly	Same
Atropine	0.05 mg/kg q6h IV, SC, IM or 1% soln in eye *Organophosphate poisoning:* 0.2–2.0 mg/kg IV, SC, IM. Give ¼ dose IV and remainder IM or SC as needed	Same
Aurothioglucose (Solganol)	First wk 5 mg IM; second wk 10 mg IM; then 1 mg/kg once/wk IM, decreasing to once/mo	First wk, 1 mg IM, second wk, 2 mg IM; then 1 mg/kg once/wk IM, decreasing to once/mo
Azathioprine	2 mg/kg q24h PO	None
BAL	4 mg/kg q4h IM until recovered	None
Betamethasone (Betasone)	0.028–0.055 ml/kg IM; give only once	None
Bethanechol (Urecholine)	5–25 mg q8h PO	2.5–5.0 mg q8h PO
Bismuth, milk of	10–30 ml q4h PO	Same
Bismuth (subnitrate, subgallate, or subcarbonate)	0.3–3.0 gm q4h PO	Same
Bleomycin (Blenoxane)	10 mg/m² daily IV or SC for 4 days, then 10 mg/m² weekly to a maximum total dose of 200 mg/m²	None
Blood	20 ml/kg IV or IP or to effect	Same
Brewer's yeast	0.2 gm/kg once daily PO	Same
Bromsulphalein (BSP) (5% solution)	*Test only:* 5 mg/kg IV; post sample in 30 min	None
Bunamidine (Scolaban)	25–50 mg/kg PO. Fast 3 hr before and after administration.	Same
Busulfan (Myleran)	4.0 mg/m² daily PO; 0.1 mg/kg daily	None
Butorphanol	0.055–0.11 mg/kg q6–12h SC up to 7 days; 0.55 mg/kg q6–12h PO	None
Caffeine	0.1–0.5 gm IM	None

Table continued on opposite page

Drug Name	Dog	Cat
Calcium carbonate	1–4 gm/day PO	Same
Calcium chloride (10% solution)	1–2 ml IV, IC	0.05–0.1 mg/kg IV, IC
Calcium EDTA	100 mg/kg diluted to 10 mg/ml in 5% dextrose and given SC in 4 divided doses; continue for 5 days	Same
Calcium gluconate (10% solution)	10–30 ml IV (slowly)	5–15 ml IV (slowly)
Calcium lactate	0.5–2.0 gm PO	0.2–0.5 gm PO
Canine DA_2P vaccine	1 vial SC at 8, 12, and 16 wk of age; annual booster	None
Canine parvovirus vaccine (MLV)	1 ml SC 8, 12, 16, and 20 wk; annual revaccination	None
Captan	0.2–0.25% soln topically, 2 to 3 times weekly	Same
Captopril	1–2 mg/kg q12h PO	None
Carbenicillin	15 mg/kg q8h IV	Same
Castor oil	8–30 ml PO	4–10 ml PO
Cefadroxil	22 mg/kg q12h PO	
Cefoxitin	22 mg/kg q8h IV, IM	
Cephalexin (Keflex)	30 mg/kg q12h PO	Same
Cephalothin sodium	35 mg/kg q8h IM, IV	Same
Cephapirin	10–20 mg/kg q6h IM, IV	Same
Charcoal, activated (Requa)	0.3–5 gm q8–12h PO *Poisoning:* 1–2 tsp/10–15 kg in 200 ml tap water; administer by stomach tube	Half the canine dose
Cheracol	5 ml q4h PO	3 ml q4h PO
Chlorambucil (Leukeran)	0.2 mg/kg PO once daily 1.5 mg/m² PO as single dose; decrease for repeated dosage	Same
Chloramphenicol	50 mg/kg q8h PO, IV, IM, SC	Same, except q12h
Chlordane	0.5% solution on dog or premises	None
Chlorethamine	0.2–1.0 gm q8h PO	100 mg q8h PO
Chlorpheniramine	4–8 mg q12h PO	2 mg q12h PO
Chlorpromazine (Thorazine)	3.3 mg/kg PO once to 4 times daily 1.1–6.6 mg/kg IM once to 4 times daily 0.55–4.4 mg/kg IV once to 4 times daily	Same
Chlortetracycline	20 mg/kg q8h PO	Same
Chlorthiazide (Diuril)	20–40 mg/kg q12h PO	Same
Cimetidine (Tagamet)	5–10 mg/kg q6–12h	None
Clavamox	13.75 mg/kg q12h PO	
Cloxacillin	10 mg/kg q6h PO, IV, IM	Same
Cod liver oil	1 tsp/10 kg once daily PO	Same
Codeine	*Pain:* 2 mg/kg q6h SC *Cough:* 5 mg/dose q6h PO	None
Colistimethate (Coly-Mycin)	1.1 mg/kg q6h IM	Same
Cyclophosphamide (Cytoxan)	6.6 mg/kg PO for 3 days, then 2.2 ml/kg PO once daily; 10 mg/kg q7–10 days IV; 50 mg/m² PO, IV, once daily for 3–4 days/wk; repeat as needed	Same
Cyclothiazide	0.5–1.0 mg/PO once daily	None
Cytarabine (Cytosar)	5–10 mg/kg once daily for 2 wk, or 30–50 mg/kg IV, IM, SC once/wk; 100 mg/m² once daily IV, IM for 4 days, then 150 mg/m²	Same
Dapsone	1.1 mg/kg q8h PO	None
Darbazine	0.14–0.2 ml/kg q12h SC; 2–7 kg: 1 #1 capsule q12h PO; 7–14 kg: 1–2 #1 capsules q12h PO; Over 14 kg: 1 #3 capsule q12h PO	0.14–0.22 ml/kg q12h SC
Delta Albaplex	3–7 kg: 1–2 tablets/day PO; 7–14 kg: 2–4 tablets/day PO; 14–27 kg: 4–6 tablets/day PO; Over 27 kg: 6–8 tablets/day PO	1 tablet q12h PO
Depo-penicillin	15,000–30,000 U/kg q48h IM, SC	Same
Desoxycorticosterone acetate (Doca)	1–5 mg q24h IM	0.5–1.0 mg q24h IM
Desoxycorticosterone pivalate	Each 25 mg releases 1 mg Doca/day for 1 mo IM dose: 5–10 mg once/mo to effect	Same
Dexamethasone (Azium)	0.25–1.0 mg IV, IM once daily; 0.25–1.25 mg PO once daily *Shock:* 5 mg/kg IV	0.125–0.5 mg once daily PO, IV, IM *Shock:* same
Dextran	20 ml/kg IV to effect	Same
Dextrose solutions (5% in water, saline, or Ringer's)	40–50 mg/kg q24h IV, SC, IP	Same
Diazepam (Valium)	2.5–20 mg IV, PO; 10-mg bolus IV (slowly) if in status epilepticus; repeat if no effect	2.5–5.0 mg IV, PO

Table continued on following page

Drug Name	Dog	Cat
Diazoxide	10–40 mg/kg/day divided PO	None
Dichlorphenamide	2–4 mg/kg q8h PO	10–25 mg q8h PO
Dichlorvos (Task)	26.4–33 mg/kg PO; in risk animals divided dose, give remaining half 8–24 h later	None
Dicloxacillin (Dicloxin)	11–55 mg/kg q8h PO	Same
Diethylcarbamazine (Caricide, Cypip, Filaribits)	*Treatment of ascarids:* 55–110 mg/kg PO *Prevention of ascarids:* (Cypip) 3.3 mg/kg PO once daily *Prevention of heartworms:* (Caricide, Filaribits) 6.6 mg/kg PO once daily	*Treatment of ascarids:* 55–110 mg/kg PO
Diethylstilbestrol (DES)	0.1–1.0 mg/day PO	0.05–0.10 mg/day PO (caution)
Di-Gel (liquid)	30–60 ml PO	Half the canine dose
Digitoxin (Foxalin-Vet)	0.033–0.11 mg/kg PO, divided twice daily	None
Digoxin (Lanoxin, Cardoxin)	*Digitalization:* 0.028–0.055 mg/kg q12h PO for 2 days *Maintenance:* 0.0055–0.011 mg/kg q12h PO; 0.01 mg/kg IM q6–12h to digitalize (maximum dose 0.04–0.06 mg/kg), then switch to ¼ total amount given q24h for maintenance; 0.044 mg/kg IV to digitalize, then switch to oral maintenance; or 0.01 mg/kg IV q1h to digitalize (maximum dose 0.04–0.06 mg/kg), then switch to ¼ total amount given q24h for maintenance	0.0055 mg/kg q12h (tablet only)
Dihydrocodeinone	5 mg q6h PO	None
Dihydrostreptomycin	10 mg/kg q8h IM, SC	Same
Dihydrotachysterol	0.01 mg/kg/day	1–2 drops q12–24 h PO
Dimenhydrinate (Dramamine)	25–50 mg q8h PO	12.5 mg q8h PO
Dioctyl sulfosuccinate (Surfak, Permeatrate)	10–15 ml of 5% soln with 100 ml water q12h PO, per rectum as needed; 1 or 2 50-mg capsules q12–24h PO	2 ml of 5% soln with 50 ml water q12h PO, per rectum as needed 1 50-mg capsule q12–24h PO
Diphenhydramine (Benadryl)	2–4 mg/kg q8h PO; 5–50 mg q12h IV	Same
Diphenylhydantoin (Dilantin) See *Phenytoin*		
Diphenylthiocarbazone	60 mg/kg q8h PO for 5 days beyond recovery	None
Dipyrone	25 mg/kg SC, IM, IV, may repeat q8h	Same
Disophenol (DNP)	10 mg/kg SC; may be repeated in 2–3 wk	None
Disopyramide	6–15 mg/kg q8h PO	None
Dithiazanine (Dizan)	6.6–11 mg/kg PO once daily for 7–10 days	None
Dobutamine HCl (Dobutrex)	250 mg in 1,000 ml 5% dextrose, IV at a rate of 2.5 μg/kg/min	None
Domeboro's solution	1–2 tablets/pint water; apply topically q8h; store soln no longer than 7 days	Same
Dopamine HCl (Intropin)	40 mg in 500 ml lactated Ringer's, IV at a rate of 2–8 μg/kg/min	Same
Doxapram (Dopram)	5–10 mg/kg IV *Neonate:* 1–5 mg SC, sublingual or umbilical vein	5–10 mg/kg IV *Neonate:* 1–2 mg SC, sublingual vein
Doxorubicin (Adriamycin)	30 mg/m² IV q 3 wk	None
Doxylamine succinate	1–2 mg/kg q8h IM	Same
Edrophonium	0.11–0.22 mg/kg IV	None
Emetrol	4–12 ml q15min PO until emesis ceases	Same
Enflurane (Ethrane)	*Induction:* 2–3% *Maintenance:* 1.5–3%	Same
Ephedrine	5–15 mg PO	2–5 mg PO
Epinephrine (1:1000 soln)	0.1–0.5 ml SC, IM, IV, or intracardiac	0.1–0.2 ml SC, IM, IV, or intracardiac
Erythromycin	10 mg/kg q8h PO	Same
Estradiol cyclopentyl propionate (ECP)	0.25–2.0 mg IM *once* *Abortifacient:* 22 μg/kg IM to maximum 1.0 mg at time of estrus; never repeat in same estrus	0.25–0.5 mg IM *once* *Abortifacient:* 250 μg IM 40 hr after copulation
Ether	0.5–4.0 ml (*Induction:* 8%; *Maintenance:* 4%; inhalant to effect)	Same
Ethoxzolamide (Cardrase)	4 mg/kg q12h PO	Same
Feline leukemia vaccine	—	1 ml IM at 9 wk or older; repeat in 2–3 wk; booster dose in 2–4 mo; annual revaccination
Feline panleukopenia vaccine	Used, but not FDA-approved	1 vial SC at 1, 12, and 16 wk of age; annual booster
Fenbendazole	50 mg/kg/day for 3 days	*Lungworms:* 50 mg/kg PO once
Fentanyl (Sublimaze)	0.02–0.04 mg/kg (preanesthetic) IM, IV, SC	Same, but use with tranquilizer to prevent excitation

Table continued on opposite page

Drug Name	Dog	Cat
Ferrous sulfate	100–300 mg q24h PO	50–100 mg q24h PO
Festal	1–2 tablets PO with or immediately after feeding	1 tablet PO with or immediately after feeding
Flucytosine (Ancobon)	100 mg/kg q12h PO	Same
Fludrocortisone (Florinef)	0.2–0.8 mg once daily PO	0.1–0.2 mg once daily PO
Flumethasone (Flucort)	0.06–0.25 mg once daily PO, IV, IM, SC	0.03–0.125 mg once daily PO, IV, IM, SC
Flunixin	0.3 mg/kg IM	None
5-Fluorouracil	5 mg/kg IV q5–7 days; 200 mg/m² IV once daily for 3 days, followed by 100 mg/m² IV on alternate days until signs of toxicity appear; then 200–400 mg/m² IV weekly	None
Folic acid	5 mg/day PO	2.5 mg/day PO
Furosemide (Laxis)	2.5–5.0 mg/kg once or twice daily at 6- to 8-h intervals PO, IM, IV	2.5 mg/kg once or twice daily at 6- to 8-h intervals PO, IM, IV
Gentamicin	2 mg/kg q8h IM, SC	Same
Glucagon	*Tolerance test:* 0.03 mg/kg IV	None
Glycerin	0.6 ml/kg q8h PO	Same
Glycopyrrolate	0.01 mg/kg IM or SC	None
Griseofulvin	50 mg/kg PO once daily with fat for 6 wk	Same
Halothane (Fluothane)	*Induction:* 3% *Maintenance:* 0.5–1.5%	Same
Heparin	Initial IV dose: 200 units/kg; continue by SC administration q8h	Same
Hetacillin (Hetacin)	10–20 mg/kg q8h PO	Same
Hydralazine	1 mg/kg q8h PO	None
Hydrochlorothiazide (Hydrodiuril)	2–4 mg/kg q12h PO	Same
Hydrocortisone (Solu-Cortef)	4.4 mg/kg q12h PO *Shock:* 50 mg/kg IV	Same
Hydrogen peroxide (3%)	5–10 ml q 15 min PO until emesis occurs	Same
Hydroxyurea (Hydrea)	80 mg/kg q 3 days PO; 40–50 mg/kg divided twice daily PO; 20–30 mg/kg PO as a single daily dose	Same
Imidazole (DTIC)	200 mg/m² for 5 days IV; repeat 5-day cycle q 3 wk	None
Innovar-Vet	0.1–0.14 ml/kg IM; 0.04–0.09 ml/kg IV; Administer with atropine to minimize bradycardia and salivation	CNS excitation—do not use.
Insulin (regular)	2 units/kg q2–6h IV (ketoacidosis), modified to effect *Hyperkalemia:* 0.5–1.0 units/kg with 2 gm dextrose per unit of insulin	3–5 units SC q6h, modified to effect
Insulin (intermediate)	0.5–1.0 units/kg q24h SC, modified as needed	3–5 units q24h SC, modified as needed
Isoproterenol (Isuprel)	0.1–0.2 mg q6h IM, SC; 15–30 mg q4h PO 1 mg in 250 ml 5% dextrose, IV at a rate of 0.01 μg/kg/min	Same 0.5 mg in 250 ml 5% dextrose, IV to effect
Isuprel	Elixir: 0.44 ml/kg q8h PO	
Ivermectin	*Microfilaricide:* 0.25 mg/kg PO 2 wk after adulticide therapy	
Jenotone	2 mg/kg q12h IM, SC	Same
Kanamycin (Kantrim)	10 mg/kg q6h PO; 7 mg/kg q6h IM, SC	Same
Kaopectate	1–2 ml/kg q2–6h	Same
Ketamine (Vetalar)	None	*Restraint:* 11 mg/kg IM *Anesthesia:* 22–33 mg/kg IM; 2.2–4.4 mg/kg IV
Ketoconazole	10 mg/kg/day PO	Same
Lactated Ringer's solution	40–50 ml/kg/day IV, SC, IP	Same
Lactulose	*Constipation:* 1 ml/4.5 kg q8h PO to start, then adjust *Hepatic encephalopathy:* 30–45 ml q8h PO	Same
Laxatone	*Laxative:* 2–4 ml PO 2–3 days/wk	*Laxative:* 1–2 ml PO 2–3 days/wk *Hairballs:* 2–4 ml/day PO for 2–3 days; then 1–2 ml 2–3 days/wk
Leucovorin	3 mg/m² within 3h of methotrexate administration	None
Levamisole (L-tetramisole)	*Microfilariae:* 10 mg/kg once daily PO for 6–10 days	*Lungworms:* 20–40 mg/kg PO every other day for 5 or 6 treatments
	Immunostimulant: 0.5–2 mg/kg 3 times weekly PO	None
Levarterenol (norepinephrine)	1–2 ml in 250 ml of drip, IV to effect	None
Levo-Thyroxin	22 μg/kg q12h PO	0.05–0.1 mg PO once daily

Table continued on following page

Drug Name	Dog	Cat
Lidocaine (without epinephrine) (Xylocaine)	1–2 mg/kg IV bolus, followed by IV drip, 0.1% soln at 30–50 μg/kg/min	Do *not* use as antiarrhythmic.
Lime sulfur	3% solution, dip once a week for 4–6 wk, let dry on	Same
Lincomycin	15 mg/kg q8h PO; 10 mg/kg q12h IV, IM	Same
Lindane	0.025–0.1% aqueous soln topically	None
Liothyronine	4 μg/kg q8h PO	None
Lomotil	2.5 mg q8h PO	None
Magnesium hydroxide (milk of magnesia)	*Antacid:* 5–30 ml PO *Cathartic:* 3–5 times the antacid dose	*Antacid:* 5–15 ml PO
Magnesium sulfate (Epsom salts)	8–25 gm PO	2–4 gm PO
Mannitol (20% soln)	1.0–2.0 gm/kg q6h IV	Same
Measles vaccine	1 vial SC to dogs between 6 and 8 wk of age	None
Mebendazole (Telmintic)	22 mg/kg with food q24h for 3 days	None
Meclizine (Bonnie)	25 mg once daily PO	12.5 mg once daily PO
Megestrol acetate (Ovaban)	*Skin:* 1 mg/kg/day PO	*Skin:* 5 mg/day PO for 1 wk, then twice weekly
	Behavior: 2–4 mg/kg once daily; reduce to half dose at 8 days for maintenance	*Behavior:* 2–4 mg/kg once daily; reduce to half dose at 8 days for maintenance
	To postpone estrus: In proestrus: 2 mg/kg PO daily for 8 days In anestrus: 0.5 mg/kg PO daily for 32 days False pregnancy: 2.0 mg/kg PO daily for 8 days	None
Melatonin	1–2 mg once daily SC for 3 days; repeat monthly as needed	None
Melphalan (Alkeran)	0.05–0.1 mg/kg PO once daily; 1.5 mg/m² PO once daily for 7–10 days, then no therapy for 2–3 wk	Same
Meperidine (Demerol)	10 mg/kg IM as needed	3 mg/kg IM as needed
6-Mercaptopurine (6-MP)	50 mg/m² daily PO or 2 mg/kg daily	None
Metamucil	2–10 gm q12–24h in wetted or liquid food	2–4 gm q12–24h in wetted or liquid food
Metaraminol (Aramine)	2–10 mg SC, IM; 10–50 mg/500 ml saline infused IV to effect	None
Methenamine mandelate (Mandelamine)	10 mg/kg q6h PO to effect	None
Methicillin	20 mg/kg q6h IV, IM	Same
DL-Methionine	0.2–1.0 gm q8h PO	0.2 gm q8h PO
Methischol	1 capsule/15 kg q8h PO	1 capsule q12h PO
Methocarbamol	44.4–222.2 mg/kg IV 44.4 mg/kg q8h PO first day, then 22.2–44.4 mg/kg q8h	Same
Methohexital (Brevital)	11 mg/kg IV (2.5% soln)	Same
Methotrexate	0.06 mg/kg once daily PO; 0.3–0.8 mg/kg IV weekly; 2.5 mg/m² once daily PO, IV, IM	Same
Methoxamine	0.2 mg/kg IV	Same
Methoxyflurane (Metofane)	*Induction:* 3% *Maintenance:* 0.5–1.5%	Same
Methylprednisolone (Medrol, Depomedrol)	See *Prednisolone* 1.0 mg/kg IM every 2 wk	Same 20 mg/cat IM once
Methyltestosterone	0.5 mg/kg q24h PO	Same
Metoclopramide	0.2–0.4 mg/kg q6–8h PO, SC 1.0–2.0 mg/kg/24 hr in IV continuous infusion	Same
Metronidazole	60 mg/kg q24h PO for 5 days	Same
Metropine	0.5–1.0 mg q8h PO	None
Mibolerone	30 mcg/0.45–11.3 kg, 60 mcg/11.8–22.7 kg, 120 mcg/23–45.3 kg, 180 mcg/45.8 kg and over daily PO German shepherd and German shepherd mix: 180 μg all weights daily PO	None
Milk of Magnesia. See *Magnesium hydroxide*		
Mineral oil	2–60 ml PO	2–10 ml PO
Mithramycin	2 μg/kg IV once daily for 2 days	Same
Morphine	1 mg/kg SC, IM as needed	0.1 mg/kg SC, IM as needed
Nafcillin	10 mg/kg q6h PO, IM	Same
Nalorphine	1.0 mg/kg IV, IM, SC	None
Naloxone (Narcan)	0.04 mg/kg IV, IM, SC	None
Nandrolone decanoate	1.0–1.5 mg/kg/wk IM	

Table continued on opposite page

Drug Name	Dog	Cat
Natamycin	*Nasal flush:* 0.1% soln infused over 15- to 25-min period twice weekly for 2–3 wk	
Neo-Darbazine	1 #1 capsule q12h PO (4.5–9 kg) 2 #1 capsules q12h PO (9–13.6 kg) 3 #1 capsules or 1 #3 capsule q12h PO (13.6–27.3 kg) 1 or 2 #3 capsules q12h PO (over 27.3 kg)	None
Neomycin (Biosol)	20 mg/kg q6h PO; 3.5 mg/kg q8h IV, IM, SC	Same
Neostigmine (Stiglyn)	1–2 mg IM as needed; 5–15 mg PO as needed	None
Niclosamide (Yomesan)	157 mg/kg PO; overnight fast; repeat in 2– 3 wk	Same
Nikethimide (Coramine)	7.8–31.2 mg/kg IV, IM, SC	Same
Nitrofurantoin	4 mg/kg q8h PO; 3 mg/kg q12h IM	Same
Novobiocin	10 mg/kg q8h PO	Same
Nystatin	100,000 units of q6h PO	Same
Octin	0.5–1.0 ml IM; 1 tablet q8–12h PO	0.25–0.5 ml IM; ½–1 tablet q12h PO
o,p-DDD(Lysodren)	50 mg/kg once daily PO to effect (approx. 5–10 days), then once every 2 wk	None
Orgotein	5 mg once weekly SC	None
Ouabain	0.02–0.04 mg/kg total dose IV, ¼–½ dose initially, then ¼ dose q30min *Maintenance dose:* ¼ of total dose q3h	None
Oxacillin	11–22 mg/kg q8h PO	Same
Oxymetholone	1 mg/kg q8–24h PO	Same
Oxymorphone (Numorphan)	0.1–0.2 mg/kg SC, IM, IV as needed	Same
Oxytetracycline	20 mg/kg q8h PO; 7 mg/ q12h IV, IM	Same
Oxytocin	5–10 units IM, IV; repeat q 15–30 min	0.5–3.0 units IM, IV
2-PAM	40 mg/kg IV over 2-min period, q12h as needed (may be given IM or SC)	20 mg/kg q12h
Pancreatin	2–10 tablets with food	1–2 tablets with food
Pancuronium	0.1 mg/kg IV	None
Papavatrol-10	None	¼–½ tablet q8–12h PO
Paregoric	3–5 ml q6h PO	None
D-Penicillamine (Cuprimine)	10–15 mg/kg q12h	None
Penicillin G, benzathine	40,000 U/kg q 5 days IM	Same
Penicillin G (Na or K)	40,000 U/kg q6h PO (not with food); 20,000 U/kg q4h IV, IM, SC	Same
Penicillin G, procaine	20,000 U/kg q12–24h IM, SC	Same
Penicillin V	10 mg/kg q8h PO	Same
Pentazocine (Talwin)	0.5–1.0 mg/kg IM maximum. **Never IV.**	None
Pentobarbital	*Sedation: 2–4 mg/kg IV* *Anesthesia:* 30 mg/kg IV to effect	Same
Pepto-Bismol	2.2 ml/kg PO	None
Phenethicillin	10 mg/kg q8h	Same
Phenobarbital	*Status epilepticus:* 6 mg/kg q6–12h IM, IV as needed *Less severe conditions:* 2 mg/kg PO twice daily	Same
Phenoxybenzamine	0.25–0.5 mg/kg q6–8h PO	Same
Phenylephrine (Neo-Synephrine)	0.15 mg/kg IV; 10% soln topically in eye	Same
Phenytoin (Dilantin)	*Antiepileptic:* 50–80 mg/kg q8h PO *Antiarrhythmic:* 50–100 mg IV over 5-min period, maximum total dose 24 mg/kg 8–15 mg/kg q8h PO	*Antiepileptic:* 2–3 mg/kg/day; 20 mg/kg/wk *Antiarrhythmic:* None
Phthalofyne (Whipcide)	180 mg/kg PO after 24-hr fast; repeat in 3 mo	None
Phthalylsulfathiazole (Sulfathaladine)	50 mg/kg q6h PO; 100 mg/kg q12h PO	Same
Phytonadione (vitamin K_1)	5–20 mg q12h IV, IM, SC Following IV therapy, 5 mg q12h PO for 7 days	1–5 mg q12h IV, IM, SC
Piperacetazine (Psymod)	*Tranquilization:* 0.11 mg/kg PO 2 to 4 times daily; IV, IM, SC *Sedation:* 0.44 mg/kg IV, IM, SC	Same
Piperazine	110 mg/kg PO, repeat in 21 days	Same

Table continued on following page

Drug Name	Dog	Cat
Pitressin (ADH)	10 U IV, IM (aqueous) or 0.5–1.0 ml IM every other day (oil)	Same
Polymyxin B	2 mg/kg q12h IM; Aerosol: Nebulize 300,000 units in 2.5 ml saline q8–12 h	Same
Potassium chloride	1–3 gm/day PO IV: maximum 10 mEq/hr and 40 mEq/day/dog	0.2 gm/day PO
Praziquantel (Droncit)	½ tablet/2.3 kg and under 1 tablet/2.7–4.5 kg 1½ tablets/5–6.8 kg 2 tablets/7.3–13.6 kg 3 tablets/14–20.5 kg 4 tablets/20.9–27.3 kg 5 tablets/maximum over 27.3 kg	½ tablet/1.8 kg and under 1 tablet/2.3–5.0 kg 1½ tablets/5 kg and over
Prazosin	1–2 mg 18–12h PO	None
Prednisolone (Solu-Delta-Cortel)	*Allergy:* 0.5 mg/kg twice daily PO or IM *Immune suppression:* 2.0 mg/kg twice daily PO or IM *Prolonged use:* 0.5–2.0 mg/kg every other morning *Shock:* 5.5–11 mg/kg IV, then q 1, 3, 6, or 10 h as needed	1.0 mg/kg twice daily PO or IM 3.0 mg/kg twice daily PO or IM 2.0–4.0 mg/kg every other evening PO Same
Primidone	55 mg/kg PO once daily	None
Procainamide (Pronestyl)	10–12 mg/kg q6h PO sustained-release (SR) 10–12 mg/kg q8h PO 11–22 mg/kg IM q3–6h; 100-mg bolus IV, followed by IV drip at 10–40 μg/kg/min	None
Promazine (Sparine)	2.2–4.4 mg/kg IV, IM	Same
Promethazine (Phenergan)	0.2–1.0 mg/kg q8–12h PO, SC	None
Propantheline (Pro-Banthine)	Small: 7.5 mg q8h PO Medium: 15 mg q8h PO Large: 30 mg q8h PO	7.5 mg q8h PO
Propiopromazine (Tranvet)	1.1–4.4 mg/kg PO once or twice daily	None
Propranolol (Inderal)	0.2–1.0 mg/kg q8h PO 0.04–0.06 mg/kg IV slowly	Same 0.25 mg diluted in 1 ml saline, 0.2 ml IV boluses to effect
Propylthiouracil	11 mg/kg q12h PO	Same
Prussian blue	0.1 gm/kg/day PO q8h	None
Pyrantel pamoate	5 mg/kg PO, repeat in 3 wk	10 mg/kg PO, repeat in 3 wk
Pyrimethamine	1 mg/kg q24h PO for 3 days, then 0.5 mg/kg q24h PO	Same
Quadrinal	¼ to ½ tablet q4–6h PO	¼ tablet q4–6h PO
Quibron	1–3 capsules q8h PO Elixir: 5 ml/15 kg q8h PO	½ capsule q8h PO Elixir: 2 ml q8h PO
Quinacrine (Atabrine)	50–100 mg q12h PO for 3 days, repeat in 3 days	None
Quinidine gluconate (Quinaglute)	8–20 mg/kg q8–12h PO 8–20 mg/kg IM or slow IV q8h	None
Quinidine polygalacturonate (Cardioquin)	8–20 mg/kg q8–12h PO	None
Quinidine sulfate	8–20 mg/kg q6–8h PO	None
Rabies vaccine (CEO)	1 vial IM (as per state regulations)	Same
Rabies vaccine (TCO)	1 vial IM (as per state regulations)	Same
Ranitidine	2.2–4.4 mg/kg q12h PO	None
Riboflavin	10–20 mg/day PO	5–10 mg/day PO
Ringer's solution	40–50 ml/kg/day IV, IP, SC	Same
Rompum. See *Xylazine*		
Septra	30 mg (combined)/kg q24h PO or 15 mg/kg q12h	None
Sodium bicarbonate	50 mg/kg q8–12h PO (1 tsp powder equals 2 gm) 1 mEq/kg IV immediately, add 3 mEq/kg to drip	Same Same
Sodium chloride (0.9% soln)	40–50 ml/kg/day IV, IP, SC	Same
Sodium dioctyl sulfosuccinate	100–300 mg q12h PO	100 mg q12–24h PO
Sodium iodine (20% soln)	1 ml/5 kg q8–12h PO, IV	Same
Sodium sulfate (Glauber's salt)	*Purgative:* 10–25 mg PO *Laxative:* 1/5 the purgative dose	*Purgative:* 2–4 gm PO
Spectinomycin	5.5–11 mg/kg q12h IM; 22 mg/kg q12h PO	None
Stanozolol (Winstrol-V)	½–2 tablets q12h PO 25–50 mg IM weekly	½ tablet q12h PO 25 mg IM weekly
Styrid-Caricide	1 ml/10 kg once daily PO for heartworm prevention	None
Sucralfate	½–1 tablet q6–8 PO	

Table continued on opposite page

Drug Name	Dog	Cat
Sulfonamides:		
Phthalylsulfathiazole	100 mg/kg q12h PO (not absorbed)	Same
Sulfadiazine	220 mg/kg initial dose, then 110 mg/kg q12H	Same
Sulfadimethoxine	25 mg/kg q24h PO, IV, IM	Same
Sulfamethazine, sulfamerazine, sulfadiazine (Triple sulfa)	50 mg/kg q12h PO, IV	Same
Sulfasalazine (Azulfidine)	10–15 mg/kg q6h PO	None
Sulfathalidine	100 mg/kg q12h PO (not absorbed)	Same
Sulfisoxazole, sulfamethizole	50 mg/kg q8h PO	Same
Tannic acid (Tannalbin)	1 tablet/5 kg q12h PO; decrease dose for several days after diarrhea is under control	Same
Tan-Sal (5% tannic acid, 5% salicylic acid, and 70% ethyl alcohol)	Topical, q8h; no more than 2 treatments	Same
Temaril-P	1 capsule PO q24h (up to 5 kg) 2 capsules PO q24h (5–10 kg) 4 capsules PO q24h (10–20 kg) 6 capsules PO q24h (over 20 kg)	Same
Terbutaline	1.25–5 mg q8–12h PO	1.25 mg q8–12h PO
Testosterone	2 mg/kg once daily q 2–3 days PO up to 30 mg total; 2 mg/kg (up to 30 mg total) IM (repositol) q 10 days	Same
Tetanus antitoxin	100–500 U/kg, maximum 20,000 U (initial test of 0.1–0.2 ml SC 15–30 min prior to IV dose)	Same
Tetracycline	20 mg/kg q8h PO; 7 mg/kg q12h IV, IM	Same
Thenium closylate	500 mg PO for dogs heavier than 4.55 kg; 250 mg twice daily for those 2.27–4.55 kg; repeat in 2–3 wk	None
Thiabendazole	50 mg/kg once daily PO for 3 days; repeat in 1 mo	None
Thiarcetamide (Caparsolate)	2.2 mg/kg IV twice daily for 2 days	None
Thiamine	10–100 mg/day PO	5–30 mg/day PO
Thiamylal (Surital, Bio-Tal)	17.5 mg/kg IV (4% soln)	Same, but use 2% soln
6-Thioguanine (6-TG)	1 mg/kg/day PO	Same
ThioTEPA	0.5 mg/kg once daily for 10 days IV or intralesionally; 9 mg/m^2 as single dose or in 2–4 divided doses on successive days IV or intracavitary	Same
Thyroid (desiccated)	10 mg/kg/day PO	Same
Timolol	1 drop in the eye q12–24h	
Toluene (methylbenzene)	200 mg/kg PO	Same
Tresaderm	Topically, q12h; maximum duration of treatment 7 days	Same
Triamcinolone (Vetalog)	0.25–2 mg once daily PO for 7 days; 0.11–0.22 mg/kg IM, SC	0.25–0.5 mg once daily PO for 7 days 0.11–0.22 mg/kg IM, SC
Trichlorfon (Neguvon)	3% solution to whole body q 3 days	None
Trifluomeprazine (Nortran)	0.55–2.2 mg/kg PO, q12–24h	Same
Trimethobenzamide (Tigan)	3 mg/kg q8h IM	None
Trimethoprim and sulfadiazine (Tribrissen)	15 mg (combined)/kg q12h, or 30 mg (combined)/kg q24h PO, SC	None
Tripelennamine	1.0 mg/kg q12h PO; 1 ml/20 kg IM	Same
Trisulfapyrimidine	50 mg/kg q12h PO	None
TSH (thyroid-stimulating hormone)	1 unit IV (response test); post sample in 4 h	1 unit IM or SC
Tylosin	10 mg/kg q8h PO; 5 mg/kg q12h IV, IM	Same
Verapamil	0.1–0.3 mg/kg IV slowly, not to exceed 5 mg total dose 1–3 mg/kg q6–8h PO	None
Vermiplex	*Single-dose method:* 1 #000 capsule/0.23 kg 1 #00 capsule/0.57 kg 1 #0 capsule/1.14 kg 1 #1 capsule/2.27 kg 1 #2 capsule/4.55 kg 1 #3 capsule/9.1 kg 1 #4 capsule/18.2 kg Can be repeated in 2–4 wk	Same
	Divided-dose method: Divide body weight by 5 and administer appropriate size capsule once daily for 5 days; can be repeated in 2–4 wk	Same

Table continued on following page

Drug Name	Dog	Cat
Vinblastine (Velban)	3.0 mg/m^2 weekly IV, or 0.1–0.5 mg/kg weekly	Same
Vincristine (Oncovin)	0.025–0.05 mg/kg q7–10 days; 0.5 mg/m^2 IV weekly or biweekly	Same
Viokase	Mix into food 20 min prior to feeding; 1–3 tsp/lb of food	Same
Vi-Sorbin	1–3 tsp/day PO	½ tsp/day PO
Vitamin A	400 units/kg/day PO for 10 days	Same
Vitamin B complex	0.5–2.0 ml q24h IV, IM, SC	0.5–1.0 ml q24h IV, IM, SC
Vitamin B_{12}	100–200 μg/day	50–100 μg/day
Vitamin D	30 units/kg/day PO for 10 days	Same
Vitamin E	500 mg/day PO	100 mg/day PO
Xylazine (Rompun)	1.1 mg/kg IV; 1.1–2.2 mg/kg IM. SC	Same

Compiled by Richard Johnson, Reg. Ph.

Modified from Kirk, R. W., and Bistner, S. I., *Handbook of Veterinary Procedures and Emergency Treatment,* 4th ed. Philadelphia: W. B. Saunders, 1985.

USE OF ANTIMICROBIAL AGENTS FOR TREATMENT OF INFECTIONS

Organism	Disease	Drugs of Choice	Alternative Drugs
Actinomyces	Actinomycosis	Penicillin G*	Tetracyclines
Anaerobic organisms *Peptococcus, Peptostreptococcus, Lactobacillus*	Soft tissue infections, granulomas, wound infections after GI surgery	Chloramphenicol, ampicillin, clindamycin/lincomycin	Penicillin, cephaloridine, erythromycin
Bacillus anthracis	Anthrax	Penicillin G	Erythromycin, cephalosporin, tetracyclines
Bacteroides	Wound infections	Chloramphenicol, clindamycin	Tetracycline, cephalosproin
Blastomyces, Candida, Coccidioides, Cryptococcus, Mucor, Aspergillus	Pneumonia, skin and soft-tissue lesions, bone lesions, disseminated disease	Amphotericin B	2 hydroxystilbamide† *(Blastomyces)*, flucytosine† (Candida, Cryptococcus)
Bordetella bronchiseptica	Respiratory infections	Tetracyclines	Chloramphenicol
Brucella canis	Abortions	Tetracyclines with streptomycin	Chloramphenicol with streptomycin
Chlamydia psittaci	Respiratory infections, conjunctivitis	Tetracyclines	Chloramphenicol
Clostridium tetani	Tetanus	Penicillin G*	Erythromycin
Clostridia (other)	Gas gangrene	Penicillin G*	Tetracyclines
Coccidia	Coccidiosis	Sulfonamides	Nitrofurazone
Escherichia coli	Urinary tract infections	Gentamicin, ampicillin	Cepahlosporins, nitrofurantoin, chloramphenicol, tetracyclines, sulfonamides, Tribrissen
	Other infections	Ampicillin, chloramphenicol, tetracyclines	Aminoglycosides, polymyxins
Fusobacterium	Ulcerative stomatitis	Penicillin G	Tetracyclines, metronidazole
Giardia	Enteritis	Penicillin G	Quinacrine, glycobiarsol
Haemobartonella	Infectious anemia	Tetracycline‡	Chloramphenicol‡
Klebsiella, Enterobacter	Respiratory, urinary tract infections	Kanamycin, gentamicin	Cephalosporins, chloramphenicol
Leptospira	Leptospirosis	Penicillin G with streptomycin	Tetracyclines
Microsporum, Trichophyton, Epidermophyton	Skin, hair, and nail bed infections	Griseofulvin	—
Mycobacterium	Tuberculosis	Isoniazid with streptomycin or *p*-aminosalicylic acid	—
Mycoplasma	Respiratory infection (?), conjunctivitis	Erythromycin Chloramphenicol, tetracycline	
Neorickettsia	Salmon disease	Tetracyclines	Chloramphenicol
Nocardia	Nocardiosis	Sulfonamides with ampicillin or Tribrissen	Ampicillin with erythromycin
Pasteurella multocida	Abscesses, respiratory infections	Penicillin G*	Tetracyclines, ampicillin
Pentatrichomonas	Trichomonal enteritis	Metronidazole	Glycobiarsol
Pityrosporum	Skin and ear infections	2% "tame" iodine or 25% glyceryl triacetate topically	—
Proteus mirabilis	Urinary tract and soft-tissue infections	Ampicillin, cephalosporin, nitrofurantoin§	Chloramphenicol, aminoglycosides
Pseudomonas	Urinary tract and soft-tissue infections, burns	Gentamicin, tobramycin	Carbenicillin with amikacin
Salmonella	Gastroenteritis	Chloramphenicol	Ampicillin, nitrofurantoin

Table continued on following page

Organism	Disease	Drugs of Choice	Alternative Drugs
Staphylococcus aureus	Pyoderma, endocarditis, osteomyelitis, soft-tissue infections	Penicillin G–sensitive: penicillin G Penicillin G–resistant: cloxacillin, erythromycin	Ampicillin, macrolides, lincomycin Cephalosporins, chloramphenicol, lincomycin
Streptococcus	Urinary tract infections, otitis, soft-tissue infections, upper respiratory infections	Penicillin G	Ampicillin, cephalosporins, erythromycin
Toxoplasma	Toxoplasmosis	Pyrimethamine with sulfonamide	—

*Large dosage.
†Used to treat these infections in humans; efficacy in dogs and cats uncertain.
‡Efficacy questionable.
§Urinary tract infections only.
Modified from Aronson, A. L., and Kirk, R. W.: Antimicrobial drugs. *In* Ettinger, S. J. (ed.): *Textbook of Veterinary Internal Medicine.* Philadelphia, W. B. Saunders Company, 1975, pp. 338–366.

MOST EFFECTIVE pH FOR OPTIMAL ANTIBACTERIAL ACTIVITY

Antimicrobial Drug	pH	5.5	6.0	6.5	7.0	7.5	8.0
[x]Ampicillin		+	+	+			
[x]Cephalothin*			+	+	+	+	+
[x]Chloramphenicol*						+	+
Colistin						+	+
Erythromycin†							+
[x]Gentamicin						+	+
Kanamycin						+	+
Lincomycin						+	
[x]Methenamine mandelate		+	+				
Neomycin†						+	+
[x]Nitrofurantoin			+				
Novobiocin		+	+				
Oxacillin			+				
[x]Penicillin G			+	+			
Polymyxin*							+ (best)
Streptomycin‡						+	+
[x]Sulfonamides* (pH not important except as it affects solubility)			+	+	+	+	+
[x]Tetracycline*			+	+	+		
Oxytetracycline*		+	+	+			
Chlortetracycline†			+				

*The pH is not important, since effectiveness of the drug is not highly dependent on pH, but (+) indicates optimal range.

†The pH is very important, since effectiveness of the drug is highly dependent on pH; (+) indicates optimal range.

[x]Especially useful in urinary infections.

From Kirk, R. W., and Bistner, S. I.: *Handbook of Veterinary Procedures and Emergency Treatment*, 4th ed. Philadelphia: W. B. Saunders, 1985.

DIGITALIZATION AND MAINTENANCE GUIDE FOR VETERINARY DIGOXIN ELIXIR (LANOXIN—0.05 MG/ML)

Digitalization (Guide to 48-Hour Loading-Dose Method)*			Maintenance (Guide to Maintenance Dosage)†		
Weight (lb)	*Dosage (ml)*	*Dosage (mg)*	*Weight (lb)*	*Dosage (ml)*	*Dosage (mg ± ml)*
5	1.2–2.4	0.06–0.12	5	0.45	0.022 ± 0.15
10	1.4–4.8	0.12–0.24	10	0.90	0.045 ± 0.24
15	3.6–7.2	0.18–0.36	15	1.50	0.075 ± 0.36
20	4.8–9.6	0.24–0.48	20	1.80	0.090 ± 0.45
30	7.8–9.9	0.40–0.50	30	3.00	0.15 ± 0.75
40	9.9–15.0	0.50–0.75	40	3.60	0.18 ± 0.90
50	15.0	0.75	50	4.50	0.225 ± 1.20
over 50	19.8	1.0	over 50	6.00	0.30 ± 1.50
over 100	30.0	1.5	over 100	9.00	0.45 ± 3.00

*Guide refers to the approximate amount of the glycoside usually required by dogs in each weight group. Individual variations will occur and must be considered. Digoxin is given every 12 hours for 48 hours. Dosage to be given for four full doses unless intoxication develops first. Signs of digitalis intoxication indicate that full digitalization has been reached, regardless of the dose administered.

†Guide refers to the approximate amount of the glycoside usually required by dogs in each weight category for daily maintenance therapy. Individual variations require individual titration of the actual dosage. Digoxin is given twice daily, preferably at 12-hour intervals.

Modified from Kirk, R. W., and Bistner, S. I.: *Handbook of Veterinary Procedures and Emergency Treatment*, 4th ed. Philadelphia: W. B. Saunders, 1985.

Data courtesy of Burroughs Wellcome Company.

DIGITALIZATION THERAPY

1. There is no specific dosage for digitalization.
2. Every cardiac glycoside dose must be adjusted to the individual animal at time of administration.
3. Accumulation of digitalis in the body is dependent on the maintenance dose. Rapid loading dose of digitalis should be used only in acute cardiac failure.
4. *Do not* give digitalizing dose to the point to toxicity.
5. Give digoxin on the basis of lean body weight, which is total body weight minus 15 per cent.

THERAPEUTIC BLOOD LEVELS OF DIGOXIN IN THE DOG

Determinations of digoxin serum concentration by radioimmunoassay can be obtained after constant maintenance dosages have been given for at least 3.5 half-lives (10 days) of the drug. Dogs with digoxin levels between 1 and 3.0 ng/ml are adequately digitalized. Dogs with digoxin levels less than 1 ng/ml are not adequately digitalized.

THERAPEUTIC BLOOD LEVELS OF DIGOXIN IN THE CAT

The toxic range of digoxin in the cat is 2.4 to 2.9 ng/ml. The mean therapeutic concentration is 1.4 ng/ml and biological half-life is 33 ± 9.5 hours.

DRUGS USED TO TREAT SOLID TUMORS IN DOGS AND CATS

Drug	Suggested Dosages
Plant Alkaloids	
Vincristine (Oncovin, Eli Lilly), 1- and 5-mg vials	0.5 mg/m² weekly or biweekly, IV 0.0125–0.025 mg/kg weekly, IV
Vinblastine (Velban, Eli Lilly), 10-mg vials	2 mg/m² weekly or biweekly, IV 0.05–0.1 mg/kg every 7–10 days, IV
Antimetabolites	
Methotrexate (Lederle Labs), 2.5-mg tablets, 5- and 10-mg vials	0.06 mg/kg daily, PO (may vomit) 2.5 mg/m² daily PO (may vomit) 5–10 mg/m² once per day × 4 days weekly, PO or IV 0.3–0.8 mg/kg weekly, IV 15 mg/m² for dogs ≤ 15 kg, or 20 mg/m² for dogs ≥ 16 kg, IV every 3 weeks in combination therapy
5-Fluorouracil (Roche Labs), 500-mg vials	DO NOT USE IN CATS 100–200 mg/ml² weekly, IV 2–5 mg/kg weekly, IV
Alkylating Agents	
Cyclophosphamide (Cytoxan, Mead Johnson), 25- and 50-mg tablets; 100-, 200- and 500-mg vials	50 mg/m² once per day for 3 to 4 days, weekly, IV or PO 10 mg/kg every 7–10 days, IV 200 mg/m² or 10 mg/kg, every 3 weeks, IV, in combiantion therapy
n, n′, n″ Triethylenethiophosphoramide (thio-TEPA, Lederle Labs), 15-mg vials	9 mg/m² as single dose or as 2–4 divided doses on successive days, IV or intracavitary 0.2–0.5 mg/m² as single dose repeated weekly, IV or intracavitary 0.2–0.5 mg/kg daily for 5 to 10 days, repeat every 3 weeks
Antibiotics	
Actinomycin D (Cosmegan, Merck, Sharp, and Dohme), 500-μg vials	0.015 mg/kg every 3–5 days, IV, wait 3 weeks for marrow recovery 1.5 mg/m² once weekly
Doxorubicin hydrochloride (Adriamycin, Adria Labs), 10- and 50-mg vials	30 mg/m² every 21 days, IV, maximum cumulative dose 300 mg/m², dose every 5 weeks in cats
Bleomycin (Blenoxane, Bristol Labs), 15 U/vials	10 mg/m³ once per day for 3 or 4 days, IV or SC, repeat weekly, maximum cumulative dosage 200 mg/m² 0.3–0.5 units/kg weekly, IM
Hormones	
Adrenal corticosteroids (prednisone)	0.5–1.0 mg/lb divided twice daily, PO 10–40 mg/m² daily, PO gradually change to 10–20 mg/m² every 2 days 30 mg/m² once per day, PO, decreasing weekly
Miscellaneous	
Dacarbazine (DTIC, Dome Labs), 100- and 200-mg vials	100 mg/m² IV, days 1–5 every 3 weeks in combination therapy 200 mg/m² for 5 days every 3 weeks, IV 300 mg/m² IV, every 3 weeks

From Brown, N.: Management of solid tumors. *In* Kirk, R. W. (ed.): *Current Veterinary Therapy VII.* Philadelphia, W. B. Saunders, 1983, p. 416.

INDEX

Note: Page numbers in *italics* refer to illustrations; page numbers followed by "t" refer to tables.